Disorders Quick Look Up

Page numbers followed by "f" denote figures, "t" denotes tables, "b" denotes boxes, and proceeded by "e" denotes online only.

A
Abdominal hernias, 650–653, 652f
Abdominal pain, 603–604, 604–606f, 606, 609
Abnormal uterine bleeding (AUB), 750–751
Aches, leg, 526
Acne vulgaris, 239–248, 241f
Acquired immunodeficiency syndrome (AIDS), 1164–1171
Actinic keratosis, 254–256
Acute coronary syndrome (ACS), 553–565, 556–558f, 561–562f
Acute kidney injury (AKI), 729–735
Acute musculoskeletal injury, 884–893
Acute pancreatitis, 681–685
Adhesive capsulitis, 945–946
Adrenal insufficiency, 152, 1011–1013
Allergic reactions, 1104–1113
Alopecia, 147–150
Alzheimer's disease (AD), 104–109, 108f
Amenorrhea, 809–811
Amyotrophic lateral sclerosis (ALS), 114–115
Anemia, 1066–1067
   macrocytic, 1079–1083
   microcytic, 1067–1074
   normocytic, 1074–1079
   sickle cell, 1083–1088
Ankle pain, 905
Ankle sprains, 886–887, 953
Anorexia nervosa (AN), 304, 776, 809, 1198, 1305, 1307–1308
Anxiety disorders, 1274–1275
Appendicitis, 637–639
Arrhythmias, 577–585, 578–580f
Arthropod bites and stings, 1346–1355
Asthma, 465–474, 470–471f
Atomic dermatitis, 215–222
Attention deficit-hyperactivity disorder (ADHD), 1188–1194, 1209
Autism spectrum disorder (ASD), 1194–1197
Avascular necrosis (AVN), 949–950

B
Back pain, 896–898, 915–922, 920f
Bell's palsy, 136–137
Benign prostatic hyperplasia (BPH), 752, 833–839
Binge-eating disorder (BED), 304, 1304–1305, 1308
Bipolar and related disorders (BD), 1198, 1209, 1250–1264
Bites and stings, arthropod, 1346–1355
Bladder tumors, 744–747
Blepharitis, 270–272
Body dysmorphic disorder (BDD), 1177, 1299–1300
Bowel obstruction, 659–661
Breast cancer, 798–808
Breast mass, 749–750, 800
Bronchitis, chronic, 475–486
Bruising, 1063–1064
Bulimia nervosa (BN), 304, 1305, 1308
Bursitis, 935–937

C
Calcific tendinitis, 947
Cancer, 1439–1447
   bladder tumors, 744–747
   breast, 798–808
   cervical, 750–751, 819–824
   colorectal, 672–677
   endometrial, 824–827
   ovarian, 827–830
   prostate, 842–846
   renal tumors, 742–744, 743f
   skin, nonmelanomatous, 261–264
   testicular, 860–865
Candidiasis, 172–180
Carbuncles and furuncles, 197–199
Carpal tunnel syndrome (CTS), 941–943
Cataracts, 288–290
Cauda equina syndrome (CES), 928–930
Celiac disease, 657–658
Cellulitis, 199–204, 1336
Cerebrovascular accident (CVA), 116–123, 124f
Cervical cancer, 750–751, 819–824
Cervical muscle sprain/strain, 910–913
Cervical spondylosis, 913–915
Chalazion and hordeolum, 272–273
Chest pain, 521–523, 522f
Cholecystitis, 678–681
Chronic bronchitis and emphysema, 475–486
Chronic fatigue syndrome (CFS), 1124–1128
Chronic kidney disease (CKD), 736–742
Chronic obstructive pulmonary disease (COPD), 475–485
Chronic pancreatitis, 685–688
Chronic pelvic pain syndrome
   in females, 753–754
   in males, 754–755
Chronic venous insufficiency, 597–600
Cirrhosis and liver failure, 690–698
Colorectal cancer, 672–677
Compassion fatigue and burnout, e1560–e1561
Confusion, 73–76, 74f
Conjunctivitis, 280–284
Constipation, 600–609, 608f
Contact dermatitis, 223–226
Coronary heart disease (CHD), 547–553
Cough, 417–419, e1496
Cushing's syndrome, 1006–1011, 1089

D
Deep vein thrombosis (DVT), 596–600
Depressed mood, 1178–1179
Depression, 1178–1179, 1209, 1239
   major depressive disorder, 1239–1250, 1296
De Quervain's tenosynovitis, 943–945
Dermatitis
   atopic, 215–222
   contact, 223–226
   seborrheic, 226–228
Dermatophytoses, 180–186
Diabetes mellitus (DM)
   type 1, 1014–1027, 1015f
   type 2, 1027–1039
   type 3, 1039–1041
Diabetic retinopathy, 295–296
Diarrhea, 607, 609–610, 610–611f, 1168
Diverticular disease, 661–664
Dizziness and vertigo, 76–77, 78f, 320–321, 321f
Dry eye, 267–268, 274–277
Dupuytren's contracture, 945
Dyslipidemia, 543–547, 741
Dysmenorrhea, 812–814
Dyspareunia, 751–752
Dyspepsia and heartburn, 611–612, 613f
Dysphagia, 615, 617–618
Dysphonia, 412–415
Dyspnea, 419–421, 524–526, 1409, e1495–e1496
Dysuria, 701

E
Ear pain (otalgia), 303
Eating disorders, 1304–1311
Edema, peripheral, 526–528, 527f
Elbow pain, 899–900
Emphysema, 475–486
Encephalitis, 129–131
Endometrial cancer, 824–827
Endometriosis, 814–818
Epididymitis, 854–856
Epistaxis, 306, 401–406, 403f
Erectile dysfunction (ED), 847–854, 848f
Excessive tearing (epiphora), 268, 277–280
Eye pain, 268

F
Family planning, 760–771, 762f
Fatigue, 1064
Fertility problems, 771–778
Fever, 1064–1065
Fibromyalgia syndrome (FMS), 1124–1128
Folliculitis, 194–197
Foot pain, 906–907
Fractures, 889–893
   vertebral, 931–933
Frostbite, 1388–1389
Furuncles and carbuncles, 197–199

G
Ganglion cyst, 944
Gastroenteritis, 614–615, 618–628
Gastroesophageal reflux disease (GERD), 640–645, 641f
Generalized anxiety disorder (GAD), 1275–1281, 1296
Glaucoma, 286t, 291–295
Gout, 1055–1062
Greater trochanteric pain syndrome (GTPS), 903, 949
Grief, 1179–1181
Guillain-Barré syndrome (GBS), 137–138
Gynecomastia (GM), 980–981

H
Hand, tendon injuries of the, 945, 945f
Hand and wrist pain, 900–901, 902
Headache, 77, 79–90, 80b, 82f, 84f
Hearing, impaired, 303–304, 310–316, 311f
Hearing loss, 303–304, 310–316, 311f, 1429–1430
Heartburn, 611–612, 613f
Heart failure (HF), 565–573
Heat-related illnesses, 1382–1386
Hematuria, 701–704
Hemoptysis, 421–422

Hemorrhoids, 648–650
Hepatitis, 628–636, 1345–1346, 1429
Hernias, abdominal, 650–653, 652f
Herniated lumbar disc (herniated nucleus pulposus), 922–926
Herpes simplex infections, 210–214, 1169
Herpes zoster, 90, 131–134, 1169
Hip pain, 901, 903
Hirsutism, 981–982
Hoarding disorder (HD), 1296, 1300–1302
Hoarseness, 305
Hordeolum and chalazion, 272–273
HIV infection, 1147–1163, 1156f, 1159f
Hydrocele, 857–859
Hypertension (HTN), 529–535, 739–740, 1026, 1038
Hyperthyroidism, 984–993
Hypocalcemia, 979–980
Hypoglycemia, 1023, 1037, 1041–1046
Hypothermia, 1386–1388
Hypothyroidism, 993–1002

I

Impaired hearing, 303–304, 310–316, 311f
Impaired vision, 288–300
Impetigo, 190–194
Increased neck size, 982–983
Infectious mononucleosis, 1139–1142
Inflammatory bowel disease (IBD), 664–672
Influenza, 432, 433, 435
Insomnia disorder, 1311–1317
Intellectual disability (ID), 1197–1201
Interstitial lung disease (ILD), 486–493
Intimate partner violence (IPV), 1182–1184
Irritable bowel syndrome (IBS), 653–657

J

Jaundice, 612

K

Keratosis
    actinic, 254–256
    seborrheic, 251–253
Knee pain, 903–905

L

Leg aches, 526
Leiomyomas (uterine fibroids), 817–819
Leukemia, 1092–1102
Liver failure, cirrhosis and, 690–698
Lou Gehrig's disease, 114–115
Low back pain (LBP), 915–922, 920f
Lower urinary tract infections (UTIs), 714–721
Lumbar spinal stenosis, 926–928
Lyme disease, 1142–1147
Lymphadenopathy, 1065–1066

M

Macrocytic anemia, 1079–1083
Macular degeneration, 296–300
Major depressive disorder (MDD), 1178, 1239–1250, 1296
Malignant melanoma, 256–264
Mastitis, 794–798
Melena, 612–613
Ménière's disease, 327–330
Meningitis, 126–129
Menopause, 782–792
Meralgia paresthetica, 949
Microcytic anemia, 1607–1704
Mood, depressed, 1058–1060
Mouth sores, 304–305
Multiple sclerosis (MS), 138–144
Muscle cramps, 893
Musculoskeletal injury, acute, 884–893
Myasthenia gravis (MG), 138
Myofascial pain, 894–895

N

Nausea and vomiting, 614–615
Neck pain, 895–896
Neck size, increased, 982–983
Nephrolithiasis, 724–728
Nocturia in males, 752, 837
Nonmelanomatous skin cancers, 261–264
Normocytic anemia, 1074–1079

O

Obesity, 1047–1054
Obsessive-compulsive disorder (OCD), 1293–1299
Obstruction, bowel, 659–661
Onychomycosis, 187–189
Osteoarthritis (OA), 958–967, 963f
Osteoporosis, 790–791, 967–975, 972f
Otalgia, 303
Otitis externa (swimmer's ear), 334–341
Otitis media (OM), 336, 337, 341–348
Ovarian cancer, 827–830

P

Pain, 1469–1488
    abdominal, 603–604, 604–606f
    ankle, 905
    back, 896–898
    chest, 521–523, 522f
    ear, 303
    elbow, 899–900
    eye, 268
    foot, 906–907
    greater trochanteric pain syndrome (GTPS), 949
    hip, 901, 903
    knee, 903–905
    low back, 915–922, 920f
    myofascial, 894–895
    neck, 895–896
    shoulder, 898–899
    testicular, 755–756
    wrist and hand, 900–901, 902
Palpitations, 523–524, 525f
Pancreatitis
    acute, 681–685
    chronic, 685–688
Panic disorder, 1177–1178, 1184, 1281–1284
Paresthesia and paresis, 92–93, 797
Parkinson's disease (PD), 109–114
Pediculosis, 167–171
Peptic ulcer disease (PUD), 645–648
Peripheral artery disease (PAD), 594–596, 927
Peripheral edema, 526–528, 527f
Pharyngitis, 305–306
    and tonsillitis, 392–398
Pigmentation changes, 150–153
Pneumonia, 438–448, 441f
Poisoning, 1375–1382
Polycythemia, 1088–1092
Polydipsia, 983–984, 983f
Polyphagia, 983–984, 983f
Polyuria, 983–984, 983f
Posttraumatic stress disorder (PTSD), 1173, 1177, 1184, 1188, 1285–1289, 1322, 1430
Precancerous lesions and cancer of the cervix, 819–824
Premenstrual syndrome (PMS) and premenstrual dysphoric disorder (PMDD), 778–782
Prostate cancer, 842–846
Prostatitis, 840–842
Proteinuria, 704–705
Proximal femoral (hip) fracture, 890–891
Pruritus, 153–156
Psoriasis, 228–238
Pyelonephritis, 721–723

R

Rash, 156–158
Red eye/conjunctivitis, 268–269, 280–284

Refractive errors, 285–288
Renal tumors, 742–744, 743f
Restless legs syndrome (RLS), 1317–1318
Rheumatoid arthritis (RA), 1113–1124
Rheumatoid disease, 936
Rhinitis, 350–365
Rhinosinusitis, 365–377
Rosacea, 242, 248–251
Rotator cuff syndrome, 899
Rotator cuff tear, 947–948

S

Scabies, 163–167
Schizophrenia spectrum disorders, 1226–1236
Seborrheic dermatitis, 226–228
Seborrheic keratosis, 251–253
Seizures, 98–102
Sexual assault, 1320–1326
Sexually transmitted infections (STIs), 866, 872–875
Shoulder pain, 898–899
Shoulder sprains, 886
Sickle cell anemia, 1083–1088
Sjögren's syndrome (SS), 1128–1131
Skin cancer, 152–153, 378
    nonmelanomatous, 261–264
Sleep apnea, 423–431, 426f
Sore throat, 305–306
Stroke, 81, 116–123, 124f
Substance use disorders (SUDs), 1181–1182, 1209–1222, 1296
Suicide, 1250, 1254, 1264–1269, 1431
Swimmer's ear, 334–341
Syncope, 524, 1410
Systemic lupus erythematosus (SLE), 1132–1138, 1136f

T

Tearing, excessive, 268, 277–280
Temporomandibular joint (TMJ) disease, 407
Tendinitis/tenosynovitis, 937–940
Tendon injuries, 1336
    of the hand, 945, 945f
Testicular cancer, 860–865
Testicular pain, 755–756
Testicular torsion, 856–857
Testosterone deficiency, 756
Thyroid cancer, 378, 985, 1003–1005
Tic disorders, 1201–1204, 1296
Tinnitus, 304, 316–320
Tremors, 90, 92–93, 92f
Trigeminal neuralgia, 134–135
Trigger finger, 944–945
Tuberculosis (TB), 452–464
Type 1 diabetes mellitus, 1014–1027, 1015f
Type 2 diabetes mellitus, 1027–1039
Type 3 diabetes mellitus, 1039–1041

U

Upper respiratory infections (URIs), 431–436
Urinary incontinence (UI), 706–714, 707f
Urinary tract infections (UTIs)
    lower, 714–721
    upper, 721–723
Urticaria, 158–161, 160f
Uterine fibroids, 732–734, 817–819

V

Varicocele, 859–860
Vertebral fracture, 931–933
Vision, impaired, 288–300
Visual disturbances, 269, 288–300
Vulvodynia, 830–832
Vulvovaginitis, 756–759

W

Warts, 205–209
Wrist and hand pain, 900–903

YOUR GUIDE TO

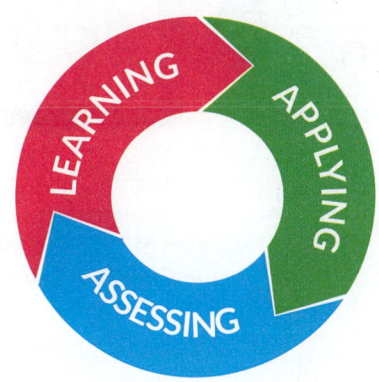

PRIMARY CARE

The Art and Science of Advanced Practice Nursing —An Interprofessional Approach

BUILDING CONFIDENCE & KNOWLEDGE for
- Class
- Exams
- Board Certification

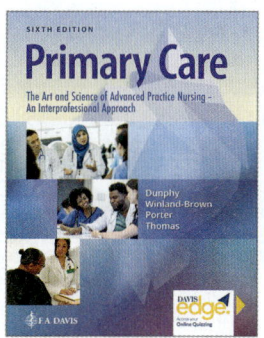
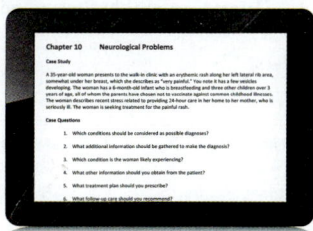
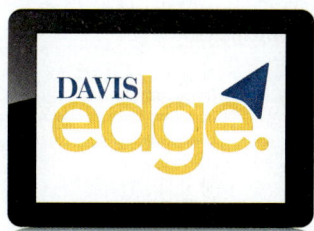

LEARNING
Your text provides the foundational knowledge you need to know.

APPLYING
Online Case Studies with Critical-Thinking Questions hone your clinical reasoning skills.

ASSESSING
Davis Edge's online Q&A review platform evaluates your understanding of key content.

Your journey to success begins here!

Your text works together with online Case Studies and Davis Edge to help prepare you for your role as an Advanced Practice Nurse in the primary care setting.

Don't miss everything that's waiting online to enrich your learning experience!

Follow the instructions on the inside front cover.
UNLOCK YOUR RESOURCES TODAY!

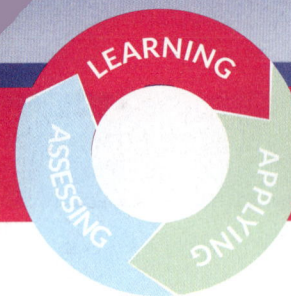

LEARNING

STEP #1 Build a solid foundation.

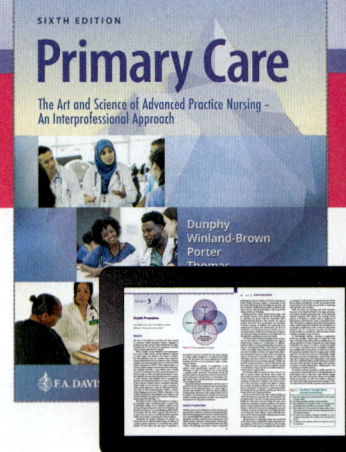

Color-coded icons categorize and emphasize three major areas for Advanced Practice Nurses.

An integrated eBook version of your text lets you study anytime, anywhere.

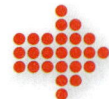

Nursing Assessment

Nursing Therapies

Nursing Perspectives

Differential Diagnosis 12.2: Pediculosis

Rash present
- Atopic dermatitis (eczema)
- Bullous pemphigoid
- Burrowing insects/larvae (scabies)
- Contact dermatitis
- Dandruff
- Dermatitis herpetiformis
- Dermatographism (Darier's disease)
- Drug eruptions
- Ecthyma
- Erythroderma
- Folliculitis
- Impetigo
- Insect bites
- Lichen planus
- Malignancy (cutaneous T-cell lymphoma)
- Miliaria (heat rash)
- Neurotic excoriation
- Pityriasis rosea
- Pregnancy induced
- Prurigo nodularis
- Pyoderma (impetigo)
- Psoriasis
- Scabies
- Seborrheic dermatitis
- Tinea (capitis, corporis, pedis, cruris)

No rash pre...

Drugs Commonly Prescribed 12.2: Pediculosis

DRUG	INDICATION	ADVERSE REACTIONS AND PRESCRIBING CONSIDERATIONS
Topical		
Permethrin 1% lotion or 5% cream OTC (Nix)	Presence of lice/nits; may use on children older than 2 months	May need to reapply in 7–14 days. Use nit-remover products before application of permethrin. Apply to towel-dried, affected area; leave on 10 minutes, then wash off.
Pyrethrin 0.3% with piperonyl butoxide shampoo or gel OTC (RID, R&C shampoo)	Presence of lice/nits	May need to reapply in 7–14 days. Use shampoo for head or pubic lice, gel for body lice. Contraindicated in persons sensitive to ragweed. Apply to dry hair until wet; leave on 10 minutes, then wash off.

Differential Diagnosis boxes help you reach the specific diagnosis to determine the best treatment.

Drugs Commonly Prescribed charts summarize the key drugs used to treat a particular condition.

The Patient's Voice 10.1: Postherpetic Neuralgia

My mother died of postherpetic neuralgia (PHN).

My mother was 80 years old and had recently won the golf championship at her club. She had been a widow for 25 years and decided that she wanted to move in with me, her daughter, and her only granddaughter (age 3). We lived 4 hours away. At first she was very independent, driving around by herself and going shopping while I worked. That only lasted a few months. Then the decline began. First, she broke a wrist, which incapacitated her, and then she got pneumonia, which weakened her. Then she got "shingles" (herpes zoster), which did her in. She was diagnosed at the earliest onset of pain, yet treatment wasn't started until the vesicles erupted. She had ophthalmic herpes, so her vision was affected. She developed PHN very early, and due to the persistent pain, she became reclusive. She stopped going out, retreating to her room, and eventually wouldn't get out of bed. Nothing helped the pain. I'm convinced it was because preventive treatment wasn't started early. As she became more depressed and stayed in bed, she got weaker and weaker and just gave up. She complained of shooting pain over half of her head that was worse at night, so she'd be awake all night, and sleep all day. Nobody could help—not her primary-care provider, neurologist, ophthalmologist, psychologist, or me. She died in her sleep, and I'm convinced it was the result of PHN.

I've learned three things from this experience. First, if older persons are optimally functioning, don't move them out of their familiar supportive environment. Second, treat all cases of herpes aggressively, as you don't know who is going to develop PHN. As my mom used to say, "An ounce of prevention is worth a pound of cure." This leads to the third, probably most important lesson: get every older adult vaccinated!

The Patient's Voice highlights the important role of the Advanced Practice Nurse as a holistic practitioner through stories that illustrate how a disorder can affect patients and their families.

Pediatric/Adolescent Considerations: Wilson's Disease

Wilson's disease should be ruled out in all young patients presenting with a movement disorder because it is easily treatable. Most people are diagnosed between the ages 5 and 35 years. This disease is inherited as an autosomal recessive trait and is present at birth, but the signs and symptoms do not appear until around adolescence when copper builds up in the brain, liver, or other organs. The most common sign is uncontrolled movements or muscle stiffness. Other signs and symptoms include fatigue, loss of appetite or abdominal pain, jaundice, fluid buildup in the legs or abdomen, golden-brown eye discoloration (Kayser-Fleischer rings), and problems with speech or swallowing. When untreated, the condition may be fatal. Complications included cirrhosis, liver failure, neurological problems, kidney stones, psychological problems, and hemolysis. Treatment includes chelating agents that bind the copper to release it into the bloodstream, and then the copper is filtered out by the kidneys. A liver transplant may be necessary.

Geriatric Considerations: Alzheimer's Disease

One in 10 people aged 65 and older have dementia from AD. Many people with Alzheimer's disease and other types of dementia along with their caregivers are unaware of their diagnosis, and therefore they are unlikely to get information about it and its treatment. The earlier the diagnosis of dementia, the better the health outcomes.

In 2019, costs were estimated to be $290 billion for services for people older than 65 years with dementia. Caregivers should consider some therapies mentioned below (e.g., pet therapy, music therapy, art therapy, reminiscence, and storytelling) that might help with memory skills, communication, and motor skills.

> **NEW! Pediatric/Adolescent Considerations** and **Geriatric Considerations** allow you to hone in on specific populations.

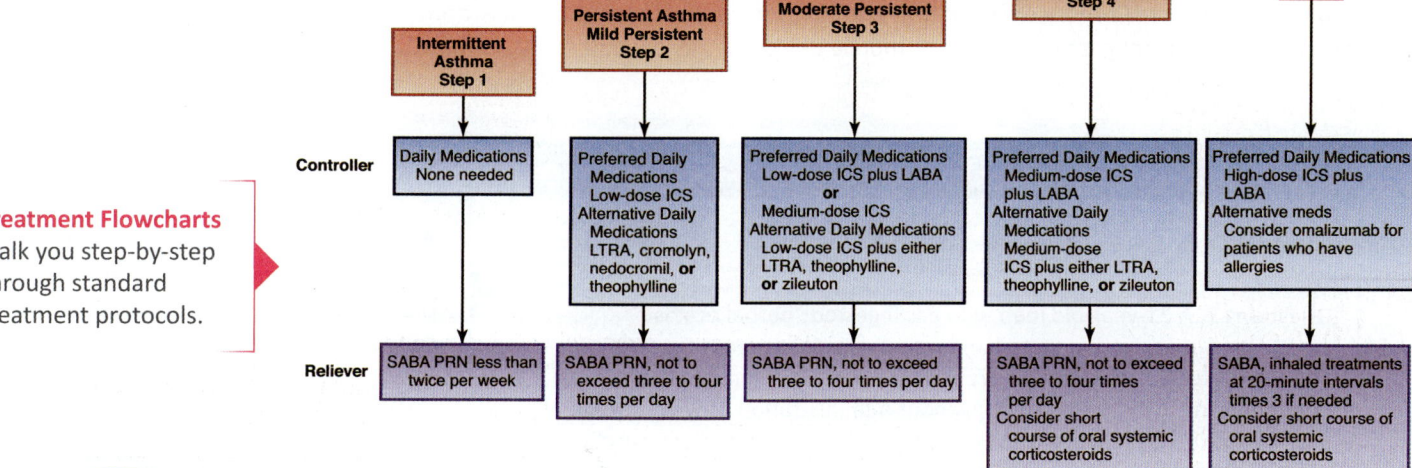

> **Treatment Flowcharts** walk you step-by-step through standard treatment protocols.

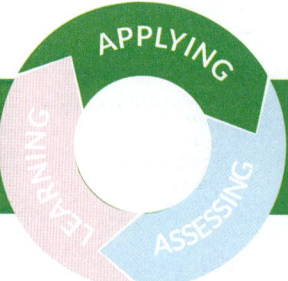

APPLYING

STEP #2 — Practice in a safe environment.

Online Case Studies with Critical-Thinking Questions hone your clinical decision-making skills with real-world scenarios that challenge you to diagnose and treat patients successfully.

Chapter 10 — Neurological Problems

Case Study

A 35-year-old woman presents to the walk-in clinic with an erythemic rash along her left lateral rib area, somewhat under her breast, which she describes as "very painful." You note it has a few vesicles developing. The woman has a 6-month-old infant who is breastfeeding and three other children over 3 years of age, all of whom the parents have chosen not to vaccinate against common childhood illnesses. The woman describes recent stress related to providing 24-hour care in her home to her mother, who is seriously ill. The woman is seeking treatment for the painful rash.

Case Questions

1. Which conditions should be considered as possible diagnoses?
2. What additional information should be gathered to make the diagnosis?
3. Which condition is the woman likely experiencing?
4. What other information should you obtain from the patient?

Topics include...

- Ears, Eyes, Nose & Throat Problems
- Cardiovascular Problems
- Neurological Problems
- Respiratory Problems
- Endocrine and Metabolic Problems
- Skin Problems
- Health Promotion
- Care of Older Adults
- Palliative/Chronic Pain
- Sports Physicals
- Human Trafficking
- Genetic and Genomic Assessments
- Suicide Risk Assessment
- Opioid Addiction

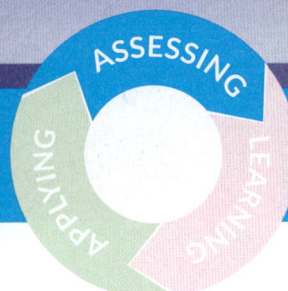

ASSESSING

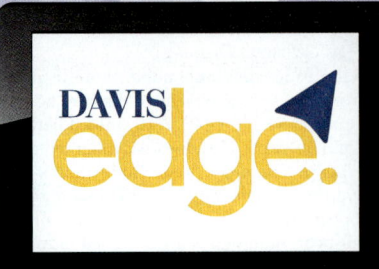

STEP #3

Study smarter, not harder.

Davis Edge is the interactive, online Q&A review platform that provides the practice you need to master *Primary Care* content and to improve your scores on classroom exams. Access it from a laptop, tablet, or mobile device for review and study on the go.

Quiz

Assignment 1

Questions 1. A 21-year-old man who has ingested "herbal ecstasy" containing ephedrine is agitated and tremulous. Blood pressure 230/128 mm Hg; pulse 152/min; and respirations 24/min. Sinus tachycardia is noted on cardiac monitoring. Intravenous administration of which of the following is the preferred initial therapy to reduce the blood pressure?

- Acetazolamide
- Adenosine
- ● Nifedipine
- Phentolamine

Assignments are made by your instructor. Or, create your own practice quizzes as a study tool to review before an exam.

Question 4. A 21-year-old man who has ingested "herbal ecstasy" containing ephedrine is agitated and tremulous. Blood pressure 230/128 mm Hg; pulse 152/min; and respirations 24/min. Sinus tachycardia is noted on cardiac monitoring. Intravenous administration of which of the following is the preferred initial therapy to reduce the blood pressure?

- 1. Acetazolamide
- 2. Adenosine
- ✗ 3. Nifedipine
- ✓ 4. Phentolamine

Rationales

Option 1:	Acetazolamide is a carbonic anhydrase inhibitor diuretic that is used to prevent and treat acute high mountain sickness. It has no sympatholytic effect.
Option 2:	Adenosine is administered to patients who have paroxysmal supraventricular tachycardia. However, this agent should not be given to patients who have asthma or chronic obstructive lung disease because adenosine can precipitate acute bronchospasm.
Option 3:	Nifedipine is a dihydropyridine calcium channel blocker. It has no anti-arrhythmic effect. It is a potent vasodilator that elicits a strong reflex beta adrenergic response resulting in tachycardia. This limits its efficacy in treatment of angina pectoris unless the patient is also taking a beta adrenergic blocker. Long-acting nifedipine is commonly used to treat the patient who has isolated systolic hypertension.
Option 4:	Ephedrine and cocaine cause stimulation of the sympathetic nervous system in the brain and peripherally. Patients have hypertension, tachycardia, agitation, psychosis, and seizures. Intravenous administration of phentolamine (an alpha-adrenergic blocker) is indicated to lower blood pressure.

Comprehensive rationales explain why your responses are correct or incorrect. Page-specific references direct you to the relevant content in your textbook.

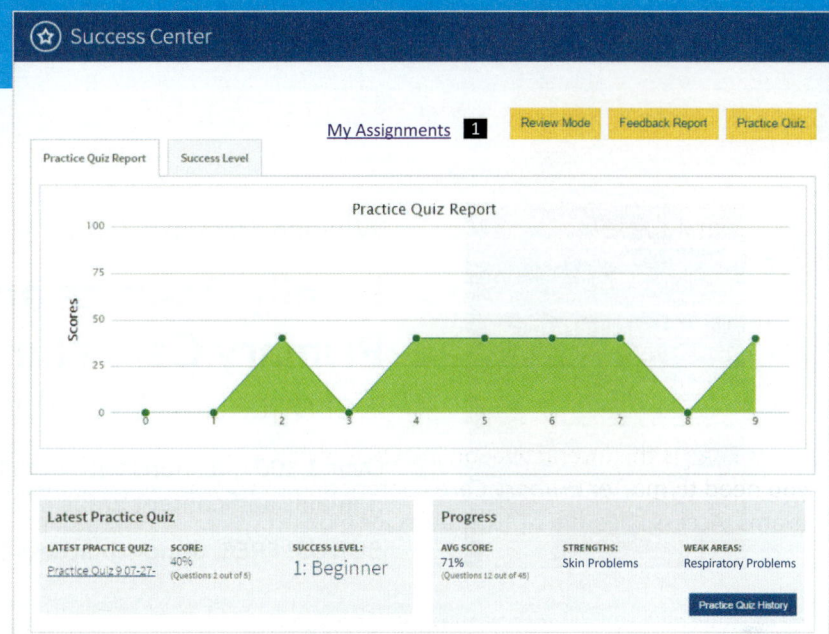

The Success Center is where you can access your quizzing assignments from your instructor and see a snapshot of your progress to identify your strengths and weaknesses.

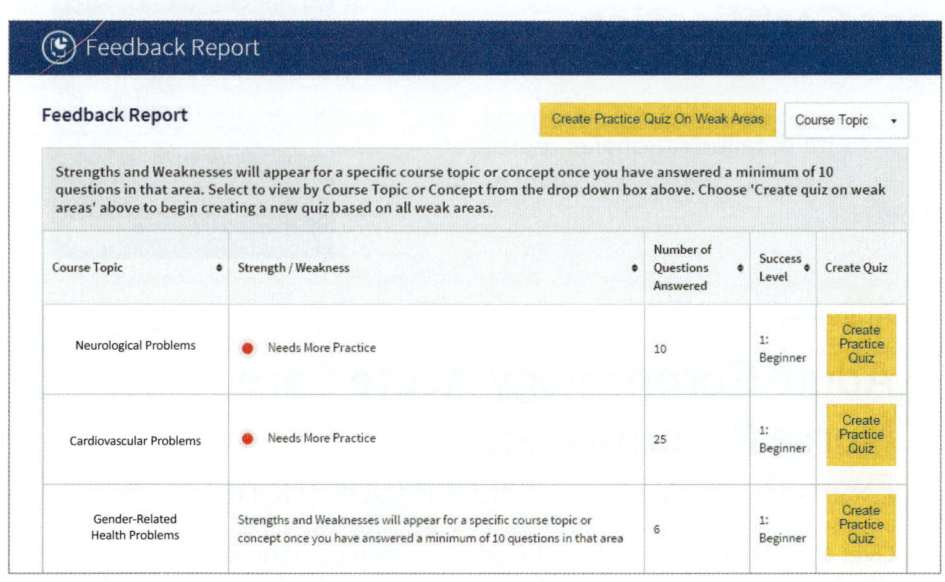

The Feedback Report drills down to show your performance in individual content areas. It's easy to create new practice quizzes that focus on your areas of weakness or to select the topics or areas of practice where you want to focus your studies.

"My experience with Davis Edge not only helped my scores, but my confidence as a test taker and a student. Without this powerful tool, I don't think I would be where I am today."

— Rachel O., Online Reviewer

95%

of students surveyed received a B or higher in their class using Davis Edge.

STRESSED ABOUT NP CERTIFICATION?

Here's what you need to pass your exams.

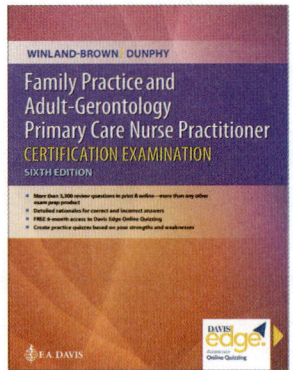

Winland-Brown | Dunphy

Family Practice and Adult-Gerontology Primary Care Nurse Practitioner
Certification Examination

Over 3,300 questions with detailed rationales parallel the domains and content areas of the FNP and AGNP exams.

BONUS! FREE, 6-month access to Davis Edge.

Fitzgerald

Nurse Practitioner Certification Exam Prep

Over 2,500 exam-prep questions with detailed rationales represent every major clinical condition. Plus, two comprehensive online exams mirror the FNP and AGPCNP board exams.

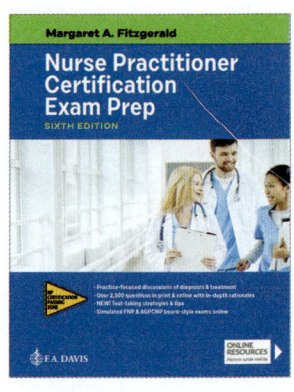

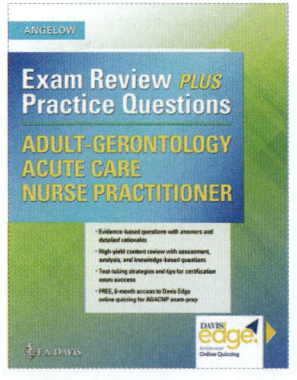

Angelow

Adult-Gerontology Acute Care Nurse Practitioner,
Exam Review Plus Practice Questions

Over 1,200 questions reflect the domains and content areas of the American Nurses Credentialing Center and the American Association of Critical Care exams.

BONUS! FREE, 1-year access to Davis Edge.

SAVE 20% + FREE SHIPPING
Use Promo Code: **DAVIS20**

ORDER TODAY!
Visit **FADavis.com**

Promotion subject to change without notice. Offer valid for individual purchases from FADavis.com in the US only.

PRIMARY CARE
The Art and Science of Advanced Practice Nursing —An Interprofessional Approach

SIXTH EDITION

Lynne M. Dunphy, PhD, APRN, FNP-BC, FAAN, FAANP
Professor Emerita
Christine E. Lynn College of Nursing
Florida Atlantic University
Boca Raton, Florida
Director, Nurse Practitioner Education
Visual Diagnosis (VDX)
Rochester, New York

Jill E. Winland-Brown, EdD, APRN, FNP-BC, FAANP
Professor Emeritus
Christine E. Lynn College of Nursing
Florida Atlantic University
Boca Raton, Florida
Family Nurse Practitioner
VIM/Hands Clinic
Ft. Pierce, Florida
Teaching Faculty I
Florida State University, College of Medicine

Brian Oscar Porter, MD, PhD, MPH, MBA
Clinical Drug Development Physician-Scientist
Biopharmaceutical Industry
and
Medical House Officer
Veterans Affairs New Jersey Health Care System–Lyons Campus
Lyons, New Jersey

Debera J. Thomas, PhD, RN, FNP/ANP
Dean and Professor, Emerita
Orvis School of Nursing
University of Nevada–Reno
Professor Emeritus
Northern Arizona University
Flagstaff, Arizona

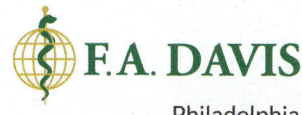

Philadelphia

F. A. Davis Company
1915 Arch Street
Philadelphia, PA 19103
www.fadavis.com

Copyright © 2023 by F. A. Davis Company

Copyright © 2023 by F. A. Davis Company. All rights reserved. This book is protected by copyright. No part of it may be reproduced, stored in a retrieval system, or transmitted in any form or by any means, electronic, mechanical, photocopying, recording, or otherwise, without written permission from the publisher.

Printed in the United States of America

Last digit indicates print number: 10 9 8 7 6 5 4 3 2 1

Publisher: Susan Rhyner
Manager of Project and eProject Management: Catherine Carroll
Content Project Manager: Amanda Minutola
Design & Illustration Manager: Carolyn O'Brien

As new scientific information becomes available through basic and clinical research, recommended treatments and drug therapies undergo changes. The author(s) and publisher have done everything possible to make this book accurate, up-to-date, and in accord with accepted standards at the time of publication. The author(s), editors, and publisher are not responsible for errors or omissions or for consequences from application of the book, and make no warranty, expressed or implied, in regard to the contents of the book. Any practice described in this book should be applied by the reader in accordance with professional standards of care used in regard to the unique circumstances that may apply in each situation. The reader is advised always to check product information (package inserts) for changes and new information regarding dose and contraindications before administering any drug. Caution is especially urged when using new or infrequently ordered drugs.

Library of Congress Cataloging-in-Publication Data

Names: Dunphy, Lynne M. Hektor, editor. | Winland-Brown, Jill E., editor. |
  Porter, Brian Oscar, editor. | Thomas, Debera J., editor.
Title: Primary care : the art and science of advanced practice nursing - an
  interprofessional approach / [edited by] Lynne M. Dunphy, Jill E.
  Winland-Brown, Brian Oscar Porter, Debera J. Thomas.
Other titles: Primary care (Dunphy)
Description: Sixth edition. | Philadelphia, PA : F.A. Davis Company, [2023]
  | Includes bibliographical references and index.
Identifiers: LCCN 2022008196 (print) | LCCN 2022008197 (ebook) | ISBN
  9781719644655 (hardcover) | ISBN 9781719644686 (ebook)
Subjects: MESH: Advanced Practice Nursing | Primary Care Nursing
Classification: LCC RT82.8 (print) | LCC RT82.8 (ebook) | NLM WY 128 |
  DDC 610.73--dc23/eng/20220412
LC record available at https://lccn.loc.gov/2022008196
LC ebook record available at https://lccn.loc.gov/2022008197

Authorization to photocopy items for internal or personal use, or the internal or personal use of specific clients, is granted by F. A. Davis Company for users registered with the Copyright Clearance Center (CCC) Transactional Reporting Service, provided that the fee of $.25 per copy is paid directly to CCC, 222 Rosewood Drive, Danvers, MA 01923. For those organizations that have been granted a photocopy license by CCC, a separate system of payment has been arranged. The fee code for users of the Transactional Reporting Service is: 978-0-7196-4465-5/22 0 + $.25.

The contents of this textbook and the independent contributions of Dr. Porter do not represent official views of Novartis, the VA, the FDA, the NIH, or any other U.S. federal government agency.

To Our Families:

*To my husband, Jim, for his patience, support, and affection, which have been ENDLESS . . .
To my parents, Joan and Arthur, for their immense love,
and to my brother, Jim, for his good humor,
steadfastness, and vacation planning!
I must add my nieces, Andrea and Autumn Hektor,
and my nephew, Bradley James Arthur Hektor,
for their love and support.*

Lynne M. Dunphy

*To my husband, Harvey, who is my soulmate.
To my parents, who instilled a sense of purpose in me and never let me give up on myself.
To my children: my sons, who have grown into wonderful friends—Ken, Nathan, Eddie,
and Mason—and my daughter, Cydney, for all that we've shared in the past
and look forward to in the future.
To my students, past, present, and future, who I have learned so much from.*

Jill E. Winland-Brown

*As with all my professional endeavors, this work is ultimately for my family—my beautiful
and endlessly supportive wife, Carolyn; our gifted and talented sons, Mitchel and MJ; our
creative and loving daughter, Cheyanne; and our brilliant yet goofy youngest son, Brennan.
I also dedicate this work to my mother and professional inspiration, Dr. Luz Sobong Porter,
the first Filipina nurse to earn a Ph.D. in nursing science, and my dear aunt, Dr. Loreto
Calibo Sobong, who earned a Ph.D. in education, both pioneers in their fields, as well as the
physician role models in my family—Uncle Boy, Auntie Espie, Uncle En, and Auntie Esther.*

Brian Oscar Porter

*To my husband, Bob Coan, who manages to do all the ranch
chores when I am too busy.
To my parents, who inspired me to believe that I could do anything.
To my cat, Neffer Kitty, for never failing to wake me up at 4:00 a.m. for breakfast
and start the day early! To my donkeys, Obie and Oscar, for always managing
to make me laugh, and the girls (chickens) for the endless supply of eggs!*

Debera J. Thomas

We, the co-editors, dedicate the sixth edition of Primary Care: The Art and Science of Advanced Practice Nursing: An Interprofessional Approach in honor of our esteemed and much beloved professor, mentor, mother, and dear friend:
Luz Sobong Porter, PhD, ARNP, FNP, FAANP, FAAN

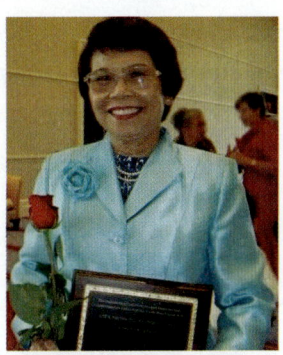

A brilliant, internationally renowned nursing researcher, author, professor, and compassionate nurse practitioner, Dr. Porter passed away on November 17, 2021, leaving behind a remarkable legacy of inspiration, kindness, excellence, and notable contributions to the profession of nursing and academia.

Born and raised in Oroquieta City, Philippines, Dr. Porter received her bachelor's degree in Nursing in 1958 as a scholar at Silliman University, where she would eventually return to begin her clinical nursing and teaching career as Distinguished and Visiting Professor and Assistant Dean in the College of Nursing. After emigrating to the U.S., she earned her master's degree in Nursing at the University of California-Los Angeles. In 1967, Dr. Porter became the first Filipina nurse ever to earn a Ph.D. in Nursing Science, awarded from New York University, with a focus on Parent-Child Nursing, which remained an ongoing passion of hers throughout her entire career.

Among her many distinguished honors, Dr. Porter was a Fellow of the American Academy of Nursing, the American Academy of Nurse Practitioners, the Robert Wood Johnson Foundation, Sigma Theta Tau, and the W.K. Kellogg Foundation, through which she completed her Family Nurse Practitioner Fellowship at the University of Tennessee-Memphis in 1997. She was also selected as a Senior Fulbright Scholar and served as a Visiting Fulbright Professor at Alexandria University in Egypt and was a member of the Congress of Minority Nurse Leaders. She served as a consultant and reviewer to numerous U.S. and global higher education institutions and organizations focused on graduate and doctoral nursing education and pediatric nursing, selflessly engaging in community service and membership with countless professional and advocacy organizations throughout her life, notably Sigma Theta Tau, the National Coalition of Ethnic Minority Nurse Associations, and the Philippine Nurses Association of South Florida.

Indeed, Luz led a truly multifaceted and full life, which included being a devoted sister to nine siblings, a mother to three children (the youngest being Dr. Brian Oscar Porter), and a grandmother to nine grandchildren and one great grandchild. She was a devoted mentor, friend and colleague to many, including Dr. Lynne Hektor Dunphy, serving as Matron of Honor at her wedding. An avid and adventurous traveler, Dr. Porter snorkeled Australia's Great Barrier Reef and visited New Zealand as recently as 2018, as well as her home country of the Philippines in 2019.

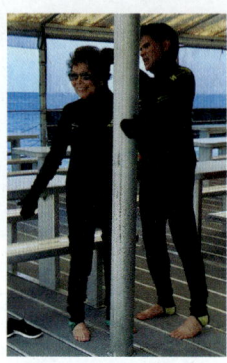

*We offer this as a reflection of a life well-lived, with much love, inspiration, joy, and [always.] laughter and music.
Luz remains in our hearts forever.*

Preface

We are enthused and proud to present this sixth edition of *Primary Care: The Art and Science of Advanced Practice Nursing – An Interprofessional Approach*. Continuing our commitment to a holistic, caring-based approach to primary care practice, the *Circle of Caring* model presented in Chapter 1 keeps persons and family - in the context of the community - at the center of care, surrounded by a team of care providers. Never has this been more important in this age of the COVID-19 pandemic.

There are many new and exciting changes to announce in the sixth edition of the textbook:

Additions to Our Editorial Team

The sixth edition welcomes new expertise and voices in Consulting Editor, Dr. Michael Zychowicz, as well as Section Editor, Dr. Karen Jennings Mathis. Dr. Zychowicz acted as Section Head and provided editorial guidance and oversight for Unit 2, Section 4: Ear, Nose and Throat Problems as well as Section 10: Musculoskeletal Problems, and Dr. Jennings Mathis assumed editorial responsibility for Unit 2, Section 13: Psychosocial Problems. We are delighted with the fresh energy and perspectives that Drs. Zychowicz and Jennings Mathis brought to this new edition and thank them for their important contributions, as well as their friendship and camaraderie along the way.

Sixth Edition Updates: New Section, New Chapters, and Expanded Content

The sixth edition afforded us the opportunity to add a significant amount of new information to the text, including an entirely new section in Unit 3 and six new chapters frequently requested by faculty, and students.

New Section: Unit 3, Caring for Vulnerable Populations

This new section of the text focuses on client populations that merit special attention and consideration in the practice of primary care. Four brand new chapters to the textbook are presented in this section:

- Primary Care of Adolescents
- Primary Care of Patients Who Are Transgender
- Primary Care of Veterans
- Primary Care of the Patient With Cancer

The special needs of these various populations are carefully discussed and detailed, in order to best prepare students for the wide variety of client needs that they will encounter in future practice. This section is also rounded out with thoroughly revised and updated chapters on Sports Physicals, Primary Care of the Older Adult, and Pain Management.

Additional New and Reorganized Chapters

Unit 2, and Unit 3 Section 2, of the text have also been revised to provide two new chapters and three substantially reorganized chapters:

- Common Reproductive System Issues
- Sexual Assault (new)
- Human Trafficking (new)
- Palliative and End-of-Life Care
- Pain Management

Expanded Content

In addition to six new chapters in the book, twelve chapters within Units 2 and 3 in the sixth edition have been significantly expanded:

- Common Ear, Nose, and Throat Complaints
- Hearing and Balance Disorders
- Inflammatory and Infectious Disorders of the Nose, Sinuses, Mouth, and Throat
- Infectious Respiratory Disorders
- Disorders of the Vascular System
- Infectious Gastrointestinal Disorders
- Common Musculoskeletal Complaints
- Spinal Disorders
- Soft Tissue Disorders
- Immunological Disorders
- Neurodevelopmental Disorders
- Mood Disorders

All of these changes – combined with thorough and detailed updating of all other chapters – was a daunting task, but one that we hope brings new insights and knowledge to your students and to the faculty that we serve.

How The Text Is Organized

Unit 1, *Caring-Based Nursing: The Art*, contains five chapters that continue to provide a caring-based interprofessional approach to primary care, conceptualized by the *Circle of Caring*, presented in Chapter 1, which is further operationalized in the remainder of the text. Chapter 2 lays out an ontological base for caring-in-practice and extends this across disciplines. We continue to expand our contributors to include physician and physician assistant colleagues, in addition to nurse practitioners, and are pleased to embrace a truly interprofessional approach to primary care, which leads to sound, team-based practice. We have never believed that caring is the domain of any one discipline; rather, we embrace caring as a mode of relating, accessible to all, and lived out between the care provider/s across the team and the person seeking care.

Chapter 3 grounds caring-based primary care in the context of community and health promotion, and Chapter 4 reviews the basis for a caring-based, interprofessional approach to diagnosis and treatment that includes precision medicine. Chapter 5 discusses evidence-based practice, critical to providing value-based care.

Unit 2, *Caring-based Nursing: The Science*, uses the traditional system-based approach to provide the essential information necessary to deliver safe and effective primary care to patients. Each body system section has chapters that begin with "Common Complaints," a symptom-based approach to clinical phenomena that lays out the associated differential diagnoses of each complaint with which a patient may present, as well as emphasizing the correct questions that a new practitioner needs to ask.

Following "Common Complaints," each section then provides chapters on the most frequently encountered of these differential diagnoses under "Common Problems." Each problem is defined, and the associated epidemiology and causes are outlined, as well as the pathophysiological processes. Dr. Brian Porter has again provided a thoughtful and in-depth update on the pathophysiology of the disorders developed within these chapters, as well as a thorough review of diagnostic processes and management plans. As noted, we have added Drs. Zychowicz and Jennings Mathis for content strength. Additionally, we added content as appropriate; under Dr. Jennings Mathis direction we added new chapters on Sexual Assault and Human Trafficking, as these are critically important issues for today's primary care providers. The addition of more medical and physician assistant colleagues as content experts and authors have also provided a true team-based interprofessional approach, new insights, and depth to the information presented, including cutting-edge content on current medical topics, such as primary care and preventive practices during the COVID-19 pandemic, as well as treatment.

Within each disorders-based chapter, the subjective and objective manifestations of each problem are elaborated, as well as the associated diagnostic testing that might typically be used in a comprehensive work-up. A review of potential differential diagnoses for the disorder is provided, including the underlying reasoning and critical thinking involved in reaching a specific diagnosis. This helps shape team-based treatment decisions, made in concert with patient and family preferences. Consistent with our caring model, a holistic database is established and built on the patient's voice and experience. Management strategies, including pharmacological therapy and surgical interventions, when indicated, are described, as well as complementary therapies and behavioral health interventions to provide a holistic plan of care. There is also a focus on community-based approaches, practices, and involvement. Follow-up and referral practices are included, along with patient education—the all-important teaching-learning component of caring-based primary care practice.

Unit 3, *Caring-based Nursing: The Practice,* is composed of critical content for advanced practice that does not fit into a structured body system approach. As mentioned previously, for this sixth edition, we have expanded this content to include two sections: Section 1: Care of Vulnerable Populations and Section 2: Special Topics in Advanced Practice. The brand new content in Section 1 we hope will serve the many populations that are deserving of special attention while under the care of primary care practitioners. Section 2: Special Topics in Advanced Practice consists of updated and cutting edge content on Palliative and End-of-Life Care, ethical and legal issues affecting advanced practice nursing, and a substantive chapter on the business of practice. We also include an update of a practical approach to psychotherapy for primary care. This is especially important in an age of rising behavioral health issues and the need for integrated mind-body approaches. Finally, we include an important message for all advanced practice nurses: a chapter on caring for self, *NEVER* more important than during the COVID-19 pandemic, which has taken such a toll on *all* health care providers. To provide caring-based care, care of self is critical.

Pedagogical Tools and Color-Coding

To aid students in making connections and retaining information, the pedagogy, key features, and boxes in the text are color-coded to one of three major categories:

- Nursing Assessments features - Red
- Advanced Practice Nursing Therapies features – Yellow
- Advanced Practice Nursing Perspectives features - Blue

As in past editions, tables, figures, and recurring displays are provided throughout the text, including drugs commonly prescribed, therapeutic procedures that a primary care clinician might be called on to perform, screening guidelines, diagnostic reasoning algorithms, treatment standards and guidelines, advanced assessment techniques, as well as sidebars for history-taking and risk factors. Also included are "Nursing Situations" (essential case studies), along with abstracts of current nursing-based research, and anecdotes from patients drawn directly from practice experience in "The Patient's Voice." This variety of information will assist any primary care provider, regardless of discipline or training background, in establishing and implementing a holistic, caring practice base.

FACULTY AND STUDENT RESOURCES

We provide an array of faculty and student resources to enhance student learning and provide faculty and preceptor support. These resources include:

Davis Edge Online Quizzing

Davis Edge is an adaptive platform that affords faculty and students access to more than 1,000 board-style questions, with complete and detailed rationales for all correct answers and incorrect distractors. Davis Edge provides faculty with a powerful assessment tool that seamlessly integrates with learning management systems and gradebooks. As students take quizzes in Davis Edge, the system provides data back to faculty as well, tracking student progress and reporting on areas of student strengths and weaknesses (as individuals and at the cohort level) to assist with remediation. **All questions in Davis Edge are completely different from those in the faculty test bank described below,** so that quizzing and exams are separate experiences.

For students, the Davis Edge platform offers nearly endless opportunities to ensure that they comprehend and retain the information presented in the disorders-based chapters. The platform also provides integrated access to the e-book version of the text, so students can quickly look up and refresh their knowledge base as a part of their quizzing experience. Most importantly, Davis Edge Online Quizzing is included at no additional fee whether the student purchases a print or an online version of the textbook, making it accessible to all.

Additional instructor resources include:

- **Faculty test bank** – over 800 questions for exams that are unique and different from those provided in Davis Edge online quizzing.
- **Online case studies** – 58 case studies, including 5 to 6 critical thinking questions per case with model answers for instructors, to help evaluate student responses. These cases are available online to students (without the answers), so instructors can easily assign them as homework or for classwork discussion.
- **PowerPoint presentations** – provide detailed content overviews to support faculty lectures and course packs.

Conclusion

As long-time nurse practitioner faculty and practicing clinicians, we remain committed to providing an in-depth book with a comprehensive and holistic approach that can be used across the nurse practitioner curriculum, as well as in a variety of other primary care curricula—and that includes participation and review by practitioners from other disciplines, such as medicine, pharmacy, and social work. This text provides a high-level pathophysiological foundation, evidence-based diagnostic and management strategies, and a holistic plan of care that is consistent with this advanced level of practice. Although we realize that health professional students will always need supplementary information to provide the currency and depth of information required for clinical practice, the reader will be able to find a large amount of information in this comprehensive and complete text, complemented by an ever-expanding collection of instructor and student resources to enhance teaching and learning. We hope that the sixth edition of *Primary Care: The Art and Science of Advanced Practice Nursing – An Interprofessional Approach* brings faculty and students the most up-to-date, comprehensive information and resources needed to teach and successfully bring forth a new generation of primary care practitioners.

Acknowledgments

There are numerous people to thank for helping this book become a reality: Susan Rhyner, Publisher—our wonderful, *patient*, always supportive, and ever optimistic editor, whom we have come to know well, and who is, most of all, our dear friend.

Amanda Minutola, our Content Project Manager, who has had to work *very* hard to keep us all in line—and always managed to do this with professionalism and humor.

The entire F. A. Davis production team—Bob Butler, Production Manager; Carolyn O'Brien, Design/Illustrations Manager; and Daniel Domzalski, Illustration Coordinator—*all* of whom were always patient, flexible, and terrific!

All of our students, past and present, who continue to teach us as much, if not more, than we teach them!

We also acknowledge and thank the many authors who collaborated with us and contributed to prior editions of the textbook over the past 21 years; without their generosity of time and expertise, this new edition would not have been possible.

Finally, but most of all, we acknowledge all our patients over the years, who taught us to "hear" their voices.

About the Authors

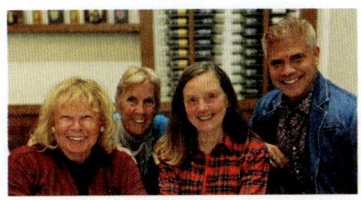

Lynne M. Dunphy, PhD, APRN, FNP-BC, FAAN, FAANP Dr. Lynne Dunphy is a Professor Emerita from the Christine E. Lynn College of Nursing, Florida Atlantic University, Boca Raton, Florida. She held the inaugural role of Associate Dean for Practice and Community Engagement from 2014-18, and Research Professor from 2018-22. Dr. Dunphy was the Inaugural Routhier Chair for Practice from 2006–2014 at the College of Nursing at the University of Rhode Island, Kingston, Rhode Island. She also served as Associate Dean for External Affairs during 2012–2014. She was a Robert Wood Johnson Executive Nurse Fellow (2009-12) and was the founding nursing lead of the Rhode Island Action Coalition (RIAC), dedicated to the implementation of the Institute of Medicine's recommendations for the Future of Nursing. Dr. Dunphy served for 4 years on the Board of the National Organization of Nurse Practitioner Faculties (NONPF) and as Co-Chair and Lead Co-chair of the American Academy of Nursing's Primary Care Expert Panel. She currently is the Director of Nurse Practitioner Education for Visual Dx, Rochester, New York.

Jill E. Winland-Brown, EdD, APRN, FNP-BC, FAANP Dr. Winland-Brown was born in Boston but raised in Pennsylvania. After high school, she went to Newport Hospital School of Nursing, Salve Regina College, Newport, Rhode Island, for her BSN; Boston College for her MS; and Florida Atlantic University for her EdD and post master's FNP. Her first teaching position was at the University of Rhode Island, after which she moved to Florida. She taught in the undergraduate and graduate programs at FAU and was Assistant Dean and then moved to the Northern Campus as Director. Children include his, mine, and ours, although after 41 years, all five are ours. In whatever little free time is left, her loves are the beach and tennis. Dr. Winland-Brown was also on the ANA Center for Ethics and Human Rights Advisory Board. She currently volunteers 8 hours per week as a nurse practitioner at a Volunteers in Medicine Clinic and precepts NP students as well as MD students.

Brian Oscar Porter, MD, PhD, MPH, MBA Dr. Porter is a triple board–certified and licensed immunologist/allergist, internist, and pediatrician. After completing both his MD and PhD in immunology and microbiology at the University of Miami School of Medicine (Miami, Florida), as well as his MPH at the Harvard School of Public Health (Boston, Massachusetts), Dr. Porter completed combined residency training in internal medicine and pediatrics at the Virginia Commonwealth University Medical Center (Richmond, Virginia), followed by fellowship training in allergy and immunology at the National Institutes of Health (Bethesda, Maryland), where he also served as an Adjunct Intramural Investigator in the Laboratory of Immunoregulation and Principal Investigator on two NIH–based clinical and translational research protocols in primary and acquired immunodeficiency in the National Institute of Allergy and Infectious Diseases. Dr. Porter then joined the U.S. Food and Drug Administration's Center for Drug Evaluation and Research (Silver Spring, Maryland) as a Primary Reviewer and Medical Officer, before transitioning into the private pharmaceutical industry as a clinical drug development physician-scientist, focusing on biologic immunotherapies and global product development strategy. To complement this work, Dr. Porter further earned an Executive MBA from the Northwestern University–Kellogg School of Management

(Miami, Florida). Dr. Porter has held leadership roles in several biopharmaceutical companies, including Human Genome Sciences, GlaxoSmithKline, and most recently Novartis Pharmaceuticals, where he currently serves as Vice-President and Clinical Development Head for Immunology* (East hanover, New Jersey), Hepatology, and Dermatology* (East Hanover, New Jersey). He also continues to work actively as a clinician in the Veterans Affairs New Jersey Health Care System as a Medical House Officer* (Lyons, New Jersey). Dr. Porter credits his multidisciplinary approach to human health largely to the influence and encouragement of his mother, Dr. Luz Sobong Porter, a nurse clinician, educator, and researcher, who always involved him in her work and was one of his primary research collaborators.

Debera J. Thomas, PhD, RN, FNP/ANP Dr. Thomas is Professor and Dean, Emerita of Nursing at the Orvis School of Nursing at the University of Nevada, Reno, and a Professor Emeritus at Northern Arizona University in Flagstaff, Arizona. Her teaching career began in 1978 at Augustana Hospital School of Nursing in Chicago, Illinois. She has held numerous faculty and administrative positions at institutions including Kent State University, Case Western Reserve University, Florida Atlantic University, University of Connecticut, Northern Arizona University, and the University of Nevada Reno. In her free time, Debera is a potter, hiker, winemaker, and skier. On most weekends, you can find her caring for her 10 acres of gardens, vineyard, and house outside of Reno, NV.

*The contents of this textbook and the independent contributions of Dr. Porter fall outside of his current employment and do not represent official views of Novartis Pharmaceuticals, the U.S. Department of Veterans Affairs, or any other U.S. federal government agency.

Contributors

Sherley Belizaire, DNP, PMHNP-BC, FNP-BC
Nurse Practitioner
Mental Health Services Director
Nurse Practitioner Residency Program
Mental Health VA Boston Healthcare System
Brockton, Massachusetts
  Chapter 80 Primary Care of Veterans

Kara Birch, DNP, PMHNP, FNP
HS Associate Clinical Professor
University of California San Francisco
San Francisco, California
  Chapter 68 Schizophrenia Spectrum and Other Psychotic Disorders; Chapter 70 Anxiety Disorders and Post-Traumatic Stress Disorder

Anne Boykin, PhD, RN
Founding Dean and Professor Emeritus
Florida Atlantic University
Christine E. Lynn College of Nursing
Boca Raton, Florida
  Chapter 2 Caring and the Advanced Practice Nurse

Katelyn Brady, MSN, PMHNP-BC
Psychiatric Nurse Practitioner
BOLD Health
San Diego, California
Assistant Professor
University of California San Francisco
San Francisco, California
  Chapter 70 Anxiety Disorders and Post-Traumatic Stress Disorder

Rebecca Carley, DNP, APRN-CNP
Associate Clinical Professor
University of Rhode Island
Kingston, Rhode Island
  Chapter 88 Putting Caring Into Practice: Caring for Self

Janet G. Campbell, DNP, ANP-BC, ACNS, COHN-S
Coach/Mentor Nurse Practitioner
Office of Academic Affiliations
Veterans Health Administration
Department of Veterans Affairs
Washington, DC
  Chapter 80 Primary Care of Veterans

Deirdre Carolan, PhD, ANP-BC, GNP-BC, FAANP
Assistant Professor
Conway School of Nursing, The Catholic University of America
Washington, District of Columbia
  Chapter 82 Primary Care of Older Adults

Katherine Chadwell, DNP, MBMSc, APRN, GNP-BC
Christine E. Lynn College of Nursing
Boca Raton, Florida
  Chapter 4 The Art of Diagnosis and Treatment

Maria Colandrea, DNP, NP-C, CORLN, CCRN, FAANP
Nurse Practitioner, Department of Otolaryngology Head and Neck Surgery
Adjunct Faculty
Durham Veterans Affairs Healthcare System
Duke School of Nursing
Durham, North Carolina
  Chapter 21 Common Ear, Nose, and Throat Complaints; Chapter 22 Hearing and Balance Disorders; Chapter 23 Inflammatory and Infectious Disorders of the Ear; Chapter 24 Inflammatory and Infectious Disorders of the Nose, Sinuses, Mouth, and Throat; Chapter 25 Epistaxis; Chapter 26 Temporomandibular Disorders; Chapter 27 Dysphonia

Debbie Conner, PhD, MSN, ANP/FNP-BC, FAANP
Professor and Chair Family Nurse Practitioner Program
Franklin University
Columbus, Ohio
  Chapter 43 Common Urinary Complaints; Chapter 44 Urinary Tract Disorders; Chapter 45 Kidney and Bladder Disorders; Chapter 50 Prostate Disorders; Chapter 51 Penile and Testicular Disorders

Sean Convoy, DNP, PMHNP-BC
Assistant Professor
Duke University. School of Nursing, Adult Health Systems
Durham, North Carolina
  Chapter 67 Substance-related and Addictive Disorders

Didier Demesmin, MD, MBA
University Pain Medicine Center
New Jersey
  Chapter 83 Pain Management

Cameron Duncan, PhD, DNP, MS, APRN, FNP-BC, PMHNP-BC
Interim Dean
Associate Professor
Orvis School of Nursing
University of Nevada Reno
Reno, Nevada
Chapter 79 Primary Care of Patients Who Are Transgender

Dorothy J. Dunn, PhD, APRN, FNP-BC, AHN-BC
Retired Professor
University of Massachusetts Dartmouth
Dartmouth, Massachusetts
Chapter 3 Health Promotion

Lynne M. Dunphy, PhD, APRN, FNP-BC, FAAN, FAANP
Professor Emerita
Christine E. Lynn College of Nursing
Florida Atlantic University
Boca Raton, Florida
Chapter 1 Primary Care in the Twenty-First Century: A Circle of Caring; Chapter 18 Common Eye Complaints; Chapter 19 Lid and Conjunctival Pathology; Chapter 20 Visual Disturbances and Impaired Vision; Chapter 82 Primary Care of Older Adults; Chapter 83 Pain Management; Chapter 84 Palliative and End-of-Life Care; Chapter 87 Primary Care Approaches to Behavioral Health

Terry Eggenberger, PhD, RN
Associate Professor/Director of Interprofessional Education and Practice
Florida Atlantic University
Boca Raton, Florida
Chapter 2 Caring and the Advanced Practice Nurse

Tiffany Ellis, MSN, ANP-C, CORLN
Nurse Practitioner
Department of Otolaryngology
Durham VA Health Care System
Durham, North Carolina
Chapter 24 Inflammatory and Infectious Disorders of the Nose, Sinuses, Mouth, and Throat

Kim Ferguson, DNP, APRN, FNP-BC, PMHNP-BC
Assistant Professor
East Tennessee State University
Johnson City, Tennessee
Chapter 71 Obsessive-Compulsive and Related Disorders

John Fraleigh, MSN, RN, CFRN
Faculty Clinical Instructor
University of Arizona College of Nursing
Tucson, Arizona
Chapter 74 Human Trafficking

Susan Garnett, MSN, APRN, FNP-BC
Chapter 11 Common Skin Complaints; Chapter 13 Mucocutaneous Fungal Infections; Chapter 14 Bacterial Skin Infections; Chapter 15 Viral Skin Infections

Michelle Gibson, MSN, PMHNP-BC, CARN-AP
Psychiatric Nurse Practitioner
North Ridgeville, Ohio
Chapter 80 Primary Care of Veterans

Teresa Gibson, DNP, APRN, FNP-BC
Family Nurse Practitioner
Jensen Beach, Florida
Chapter 4 The Art of Diagnosis and Treatment

Monica Giovannini, MD
Clinical Development Head-Oncology
Novartis Pharmaceuticals
East Hanover, New Jersey
Chapter 61 Common Hematological and Immunological Complaints; Chapter 62 Hematological Disorders

Margaret M. Harding, MSN, RN, AGPCNP-BC, RNFA, CPAN
Nurse Practitioner
Duke University Hospital and Duke University School of Nursing
Durham, North Carolina
Chapter 56 Osteoarthritis and Osteoporosis

Nancy Harris, DNP, APRN, FNP-BC
Assistant Professor
Christine E. Lynn College of Nursing, Florida Atlantic University
Boca Raton, Florida
Chapter 12 Parasitic Skin Infestations; Chapter 17 Skin Lesions

Michaela K. Hogan, DNP, APRN, PMHNP-BC
Clinical Assistant Professor
Track Coordinator: Psychiatric-Mental Health DNP Program
University of Florida
Gainesville, Florida
Chapter 69 Mood Disorders

Sarah Horn, MD
Neurologist
Philadelphia, Pennsylvania
Chapter 6 Common Neurological Complaints; Chapter 7 Seizure Disorders; Chapter 8 Degenerative Disorders; Chapter 9 Cerebrovascular Accident (Stroke); Chapter 10 Infectious and Inflammatory Neurological Disorders

Elizabeth Hutson, PhD, APRN-CNP, PMHNP-BC
Associate Professor
Psychiatric Mental Health Nurse Practitioner Program Director
Texas Tech University Health Sciences Center School of Nursing
Lubbock, Texas
Chapter 66 Neurodevelopmental Disorders; Chapter 87 Primary Care Approaches to Behavioral Health

Karen Jennings Mathis, PhD, APRN-CNP, PMHNP-BC, FAED
Assistant Professor
University of Rhode Island College of Nursing
Providence, Rhode Island
*Chapter 65 Common Psychological Complaints;
Chapter 66 Neurodevelopmental Disorders;
Chapter 67 Substance-related and Addictive Disorders;
Chapter 68 Schizophrenia Spectrum and Other Psychotic Disorders; Chapter 69 Mood Disorders; Chapter 70 Anxiety Disorders and Post-Traumatic Stress Disorder;
Chapter 71 Obsessive-Compulsive and Related Disorders;
Chapter 72 Other Psychiatric Disorders; Chapter 73 Sexual Assault; Chapter 74 Human Trafficking*

Kathryn B. Keller, PhD, RN, CNE
Professor
Christine E. Lynn College of Nursing
Boca Raton, Florida
*Chapter 34 Common Cardiovascular Complaints;
Chapter 35 Cardiac and Associated Risk Disorders;
Chapter 36 Dysrhythmias and Valvular Disorders;
Chapter 37 Disorders of the Vascular System*

Michael B. Keller, MD
Department of Medicine
Johns Hopkins Hospital and School of Medicine
Baltimore, Maryland
*Chapter 36 Dysrhythmias and Valvular Disorders;
Chapter 37 Disorders of the Vascular System*

Meredith Kells, PhD, RN, CPNP
Assistant Professor
University of Rochester School of Nursing
Rochester, New York
Chapter 72: Other Psychiatric Disorders

Amie M. Koch DNP, FNP-C, RN, ACHPN
Assistant Professor and Family Nurse Practitioner
Duke University School of Nursing
Durham, North Carolina
Chapter 84 Palliative and End-of-Life Care

Benjamin G. Kuhar, DO
Resident Physician
Ophthalmology Resident
Madigan Army Medical Center
Tacoma, Washington
Chapter 18 Common Eye Complaints; Chapter 19 Lid and Conjunctival Pathology; Chapter 20 Visual Disturbances and Impaired Vision

Mary Lavin, DNP, APRN-CNP
Associate Clinical Professor
University of Rhode Island
Kingston, Rhode Island
Chapter 88 Putting Caring Into Practice: Caring for Self

Amanda Ling, MS, RN, PMHNP
Assistant Clinical Professor
University of California San Francisco
San Francisco, California
Chapter 68 Schizophrenia Spectrum and Other Psychotic Disorders; Chapter 70 Anxiety Disorders and Post-Traumatic Stress Disorder

Rachele Lipsky, PhD, APRN, PMHNP
Fellow
Duke University
Durham, North Carolina
Chapter 65 Common Psychological Complaints

Janine Llamzon, DNP-C, MS, AGNP-C, RN, CEN, NEA-BC
Assistant Vice President of Emergency Services
Department of Emergency Medicine
Montefiore Medical Center
The University Hospital for Albert Einstein College of Medicine
Bronx, New York
Chapter 30 Infectious Respiratory Disorders

Bernadette M. Longo, PhD, RN, CNL, FAAN
Associate Professor Emerita
Orvis School of Nursing, University of Nevada Reno
Reno, Nevada
Chapter 5 Evidence-Based Practice

Jamison Lord, DNP, APRN, PMHNP-BC
Faculty
Duke University School of Nursing
Durham, North Carolina
*Chapter 65 Common Psychological Complaints;
Chapter 67 Substance-Related and Addictive Disorders*

Ashley Love, DNP, PMHNP-BC
Psychiatric Nurse Practitioner
Boulder Community Health
Boulder, Colorado
Chapter 69 Mood Disorders

Rene Love, PhD, DNP, PMHNP-BC, FNAP, FAANP
Associate Dean for Academic Affairs for Graduate Clinical Education
University of Florida
Gainesville, Florida
Chapter 69 Mood Disorders

Deborah Lowell Shindell, PhD, FNP-BC, CNE
Associate Professor
Orvis School of Nursing
University of Nevada Reno
Reno, Nevada
Chapter 52 Sexually Transmitted Infections

Donna Maheady, EdD, APRN, PNP-BC
Adjunct Faculty
Utica College
St. Petersburg, Florida
>Chapter 16 Dermatitis

Katerina Melino, MS, PMHNP
Assistant Clinical Professor and PMHNP Program Director
University of California San Francisco
San Francisco, California
>Chapter 65 Common Psychological Complaints;
>Chapter 73 Sexual Assault

Michael Anthony Moore, MSN, NP-C, RN, HIV-PCP
Harborview Medical Center
University of Washington
Seattle, Washington
>Chapter 80 Primary Care of Veterans

Erica Muniz, DNP, APRN, FNP-BC
>Chapter 4 The Art of Diagnosis and Treatment

Nilesh Patel, DO, FAAEM, FACOEP
Vice Chair, Emergency Medicine
St. Joseph's Health
Paterson, New Jersey
>Chapter 30 Infectious Respiratory Disorders

Brian Oscar Porter, MD, PhD, MPH, MBA
Clinical Drug Development Physician-Scientist
Private Biopharmaceutical Industry
and
Medical House Officer
Veterans Affairs New Jersey Health Care System–Lyons Campus
Lyons, New Jersey
>Chapter 1 Primary Care in the Twenty-First Century: A Circle of Caring; Chapter 11 Common Skin Complaints; Chapter 12 Parasitic Skin Infestations; Chapter 13 Mucocutaneous Fungal Infections; Chapter 14 Bacterial Skin Infections; Chapter 15 Viral Skin Infections; Chapter 16 Dermatitis; Chapter 17 Skin Lesions; Chapter 18 Common Eye Complaints; Chapter 19 Lid and Conjunctival Pathology; Chapter 20 Visual Disturbances and Impaired Vision; Chapter 21 Common Ear, Nose, and Throat Complaints; Chapter 22 Hearing and Balance Disorders; Chapter 23 Inflammatory and Infectious Disorders of the Ear; Chapter 24 Inflammatory and Infectious Disorders of the Nose, Sinuses, Mouth, and Throat; Chapter 25 Epistaxis; Chapter 26 Temporomandibular Disorders; Chapter 27 Dysphonia; Chapter 28 Common Respiratory Complaints; Chapter 30 Infectious Respiratory Disorders; Chapter 31 Inflammatory Respiratory Disorders; Chapter 32 Lung Cancer; Chapter 33 Smoking Addiction; Chapter 34 Common Cardiovascular Complaints; Chapter 35 Cardiac and Associated Risk Disorders; Chapter 36 Dysrhythmias and Valvular Disorders; Chapter 37 Disorders of the Vascular System; Chapter 43 Common Urinary Complaints; Chapter 44 Urinary Tract Disorders; Chapter 45 Kidney and Bladder Disorders; Chapter 46 Common Reproductive System Complaints; Chapter 47 Common Reproductive System Issues; Chapter 48 Breast Disorders; Chapter 49 Vaginal, Uterine, and Ovarian Disorders; Chapter 50 Prostate Disorders; Chapter 51 Penile and Testicular Disorders; Chapter 52 Sexually Transmitted Infections; Chapter 57 Common Endocrine and Metabolic Complaints; Chapter 58 Glandular Disorders; Chapter 59 Diabetes Mellitus; Chapter 60 Metabolic Disorders; Chapter 61 Common Hematological and Immunological Complaints; Chapter 62 Hematological Disorders; Chapter 63 Immunological Disorders; Chapter 64 Infectious Disorders; Chapter 75 Common Injuries; Chapter 76 Toxic and Environmental Exposures; Chapter 83 Pain Management

Megan R. Pratt, DNP, APRN, FNP-BC, GS-C
Associate Professor
Orvis School of Nursing
University of Nevada Reno
Reno, Nevada
>Chapter 47 Common Reproductive System Issues; Chapter 48 Breast Disorders; Chapter 49 Vaginal, Uterine, and Ovarian Disorders

Luminita Pricop, MD
Senior Global Program Clinical Head
Novartis Pharmaceuticals
East Hanover, New Jersey
>Chapter 63 Immunological Disorders

Angela Richard-Eaglin, DNP, MSN, FNP-BC, CNE, FAANP
Associate Dean for Equity
Associate Clinical Professor
Yale School of Nursing
Orange, Connecticut
>Chapter 80 Primary Care of Veterans

Marcella M. Rutherford, PhD, MSN, MBA, RN
Dean, College of Nursing
Nova Southeastern University
Ft. Lauderdale, Florida
>Chapter 86 Quality & Value-Based Payment: Making an Economic Impact on Health Care

Denese Sabatino, MSN, APRN, NP-C, CCRN
Lead ARNP Department Surgical Critical Care
Cleveland Clinic Florida
Weston, Florida
>Chapter 36 Dysrhythmias and Valvular Disorders

Carol Savrin, DNP, CPNP, FNP-BC, FAANP, RN
Associate Professor
Frances Payne Bolton School of Nursing
Case Western Reserve University
Cleveland, Ohio
>Chapter 77 Primary Care of Adolescents

Savina O. Schoenhofer, PhD, RN
Professor Emeritus
Alcorn State University
School of Nursing
Natchez, Mississippi
>Chapter 2 Caring and the Advanced Practice Nurse

Anna L. Schwartz, PhD, FNP-BC, FAAN
Professor
University of Nebraska
Lincoln, Nebraska
Chapter 81 Primary Care of the Patient With Cancer

Virginia Sheikh, MD, MHS
Medical Officer
U.S. Food and Drug Administration
Silver Spring, Maryland
Chapter 64 Infectious Disorders

John Suen, MD
Clinical Assistant Professor
College of Medicine
Florida State University
Vero Beach, Florida
Chapter 29 Sleep Apnea

Debera J. Thomas, PhD, RN, ANP/FNP
Family and Adult Nurse Practitioner
Dean and Professor, Emerita
Orvis School of Nursing
University of Nevada Reno
Reno, Nevada
and
Professor Emeritus
Northern Arizona University
Flagstaff, Arizona
Chapter 1 Primary Care in the Twenty-First Century: A Circle of Caring; Chapter 3 Health Promotion; Chapter 5 Evidence-Based Practice; Chapter 38 Common Abdominal Complaints; Chapter 39 Infectious Gastrointestinal Disorders; Chapter 40 Gastric and Intestinal Disorders; Chapter 41 Gallbladder and Pancreatic Disorders; Chapter 42 Cirrhosis and Liver Failure; Chapter 43 Common Urinary Complaints; Chapter 44 Urinary Tract Disorders; Chapter 45 Kidney and Bladder Disorders; Chapter 46 Common Reproductive System Complaints; Chapter 47 Common Reproductive System Issues; Chapter 48 Breast Disorders; Chapter 49 Vaginal, Uterine, and Ovarian Disorders; Chapter 50 Prostate Disorders; Chapter 51 Penile and Testicular Disorders; Chapter 52 Sexually Transmitted Infections; Chapter 57 Common Endocrine and Metabolic Complaints; Chapter 58 Glandular Disorders; Chapter 59 Diabetes Mellitus; Chapter 60 Metabolic Disorders; Chapter 77 Primary Care of Adolescents; Chapter 79 Primary Care of Patients Who Are Transgender

Josie Weiss, PhD, FNP-BC, PNP-BC, FAANP
Associate Professor
College of Nursing
University of Central Florida
Orlando, Florida
Chapter 85 Ethical and Legal Issues of a Caring-Based Practice

Susan Wilkinson, MSN, PMHNP-BC
Psychiatric Nurse Practitioner
Ally Integrated Health Care
Boston, Massachusetts
Chapter 80 Primary Care of Veterans

Jill E. Winland-Brown, EdD, APRN, FNP-BC, FAANP
Professor and Family Nurse Practitioner
Christine E. Lynn College of Nursing
Florida Atlantic University
Boca Raton, Florida
Chapter 1 Primary Care in the Twenty-First Century: A Circle of Caring; Chapter 4 The Art of Diagnosis and Treatment; Chapter 6 Common Neurological Complaints; Chapter 7 Seizure Disorders; Chapter 8 Degenerative Disorders; Chapter 9 Cerebrovascular Accident (Stroke); Chapter 10 Infectious and Inflammatory Neurological Disorders; Chapter 11 Common Skin Complaints; Chapter 12 Parasitic Skin Infestations; Chapter 13 Mucocutaneous Fungal Infections; Chapter 14 Bacterial Skin Infections; Chapter 15 Viral Skin Infections; Chapter 16 Dermatitis; Chapter 17 Skin Lesions; Chapter 28 Common Respiratory Complaints; Chapter 29 Sleep Apnea; Chapter 30 Infectious Respiratory Disorders; Chapter 31 Inflammatory Respiratory Disorders; Chapter 32 Lung Cancer; Chapter 33 Smoking Addiction; Chapter 34 Common Cardiovascular Complaints; Chapter 35 Cardiac and Associated Risk Disorders; Chapter 36 Dysrhythmias and Valvular Disorders; Chapter 37 Disorders of the Vascular System; Chapter 61 Common Hematological and Immunological Complaints; Chapter 62 Hematological Disorders; Chapter 63 Immunological Disorders; Chapter 64 Infectious Disorders; Chapter 75 Common Injuries; Chapter 76 Toxic and Environmental Exposures; Chapter 85 Ethical and Legal Issues of a Caring-Based Practice

Michael E. Zychowicz, DNP, ANP, ONP, FAAN, FAANP
Clinical Professor of Nursing
Co-Director, Durham VA-Duke Primary Care NP Residency
Lead Faculty, Orthopedic NP Specialty
Duke University School of Nursing
Durham, North Carolina
Chapter 21 Common Ear, Nose, and Throat Complaints; Chapter 22 Hearing and Balance Disorders; Chapter 23 Inflammatory and Infectious Disorders of the Ear; Chapter 24 Inflammatory and Infectious Disorders of the Nose, Sinuses, Mouth, and Throat; Chapter 25 Epistaxis; Chapter 26 Temporomandibular Disorders; Chapter 27 Dysphonia; Chapter 53 Common Musculoskeletal Complaints; Chapter 54 Spinal Disorders; Chapter 55 Soft Tissue Disorders; Chapter 56 Osteoarthritis and Osteoporosis; Chapter 78 Sports Physicals; Chapter 80 Primary Care of Veterans

Previous Edition Contributors

Rehan Aziz, MD

Ronke Babalola, MD, MPH

Barbara Beausejour, MSN, APRN, FNP-BC

Cesar Benarroche, MD

Susan J. Bulfin, DNP, APRN, FNP-BC

Margaret Colyar, DSN, APRN, FNP-BC, PNP-BC

Brandi Cotton-Parker, PhD, APRN, PMHNP-BC

Mae De La Calzada-Jeanlouie, DO, MS

Ilene Decker, PhD, RN

Sally Doshier, EdD, MS, RN

Dorothy J. Dunn, PhD, APRN, FNP-BC, AHN-BC

Jacinta D. Elder, MD, MSc

Angela K. Golden, DNP, APRN, FNP-C, FAANP

Kimberly Rae Gould, DNP, RN, FNP-BC

Kim S. Griswold, MD, MPH, AS, RN

Joseph Holbrook, MSN, APRN

Mary Hooshmand, MSN, PhD, RN

Bette K. Idemoto, PhD, RN, ACNS-BC, CCRN

Beth M. King, PhD, APRN, PMHCNS-BC, PMHNP-BC

Jason V. Lambrese, MD

Dianne M. Loomis, DNP, APRN, FNP-BC

Conor Luskin, PA-C

Lori Martin-Plank, PhD, APRN, FNP-BC, GNP-BC, FAANP

Ruth McCaffrey, DNP, APRN, FNP-BC, GNP, FAAN, FAANP

Eugenia Millender, PhD, RN, MS, PMHNP-BC, CDE

Patricia A. Pastore, MS, APRN, FNP-BC

Cathleen Provins, RN, MSN, PhD, CCRN-K, NE-BC, ACNP-BC

Humberto Reinoso, PhD, FNP-BC, ENP-BC

Edwin W. Schaefer, ND, APRN, FNP-BC

Martin T. Strassnig, MD

Michael E. Thase, MD

Denise Vanacore, PhD, APRN, ANP-BC, FNP, PMHNP-BC

Patricia Vanhook, PhD, MSN, APRN, FNP-BC, FAAN, FAANP

Timothy Wilson, DNP, APRN, FNP, PMHNP

Reviewers

Nadine M. Aktan, PhD, APN-BC
Professor of Nursing, Family Nurse Practitioner
William Paterson University
Wayne, New Jersey

Elizabeth Blunt, PhD, RN, CRNP
Clinical Professor & Director NP Programs
Villanova University
Villanova, Pennsylvania

Lynn Chilton, BSN, MSN, DSN, FNP-BC, GNP-BC
Professor of Nursing
University of South Alabama
Mobile, Alabama

Patsy E. Crihfield, DNP, APRN, FNP-BC, PMNHP-BC
Associate Dean of Graduate Programs
Union University
Jackson, Tennessee

Maura Farrell Miller, PhD, APRN, GNP-BC, PMHCNS-BC, ACHPN
Director of Hospice and Palliative Care Program
Director of Therapeutic Gardening Program
Adjunct Professor
Florida State University
College of Nursing
West Palm Beach, Florida

MaryAnn Troiano, DNP, APN-C
Associate Professor, Family APN
Monmouth University
West Long Branch, New Jersey

Margaret Whelan, EdD, APRN, FNP-BC
Professor
Molloy College
Rockville Centre, New York

Contents

Unit I Caring-Based Nursing: The Art 1

Chapter 1
Primary Care in the Twenty-First Century: A Circle of Caring 3

Jill E. Winland-Brown, EdD, APRN, FNP-BC, FAANP
Lynne M. Dunphy, PhD, APRN, FNP-BC, FAAN, FAANP
Debera J. Thomas, PhD, RN, ANP/FNP
Brian Oscar Porter, MD, PhD, MPH, MBA

- Where We Are and Where We Are Going 3
- The Tip of the Iceberg 7
- Prevention as Health Promotion 8
- Historical Perspectives on Advanced Practice Nursing 9
- Changing Models of Advanced Nursing Practice 10
- Changing Models of Medical Practice 12
- A Transformative Template: The Circle of Caring 13
- Interprofessional Care: From Patient to Population 15
- Further Understanding the Circle of Caring 15

Chapter 2
Caring and the Advanced Practice Nurse 19

Anne Boykin, PhD, RN
Savina O. Schoenhofer, PhD, RN
Terry Eggenberger, PhD, RN

- Caring 19
- Caring Processes 22

Chapter 3
Health Promotion 25

Dorothy J. Dunn, PhD, APRN, FNP-BC, AHN-BC
Debera J. Thomas, PhD, RN, ANP/FNP

- Health 25
- Health Promotion 25
- Risk Factors in Health Promotion 28
- Influences on Health Promotion 29
- Practical Epidemiology 34
- Conclusion 36

Chapter 4
The Art of Diagnosis and Treatment 38

Teresa Gibson, DNP, APRN, FNP-BC
Erica Muniz, DNP, APRN, FNP-BC
Jill E. Winland-Brown, EdD, APRN, FNP-BC, FAANP
Katherine Chadwell, DNP, MBMSc, APRN, GNP-BC

- Clinical Judgment in Primary Care 38
- The Clinical Process and Its Limitations 40
- Diagnostic Process Overview 41
- Elements of the Diagnostic Process 42
- Current Diagnostic Process Trends 49
- Documentation 50
- Reduction of Medical Errors 52
- The Digital Future and Telehealth 52
- Artificial Intelligence 53
- Precision Health Care 54
- Ethics 54

Chapter 5
Evidence-Based Practice 56

Bernadette M. Longo, PhD, RN, CNL, FAAN
Debera J. Thomas, PhD, RN, ANP/FNP

- The Aims of Nursing Research for Clinical Application 56
- A Brief History of Evidence-Based Practice 58
- Development of Best Practice Guidelines 58
- Application of Clinical Practice Guidelines 63
- Searching the Literature 64
- Developing a Point-of-Care Strategy 65
- EBP Clinical Decision Making 68

Unit II Caring-Based Nursing: The Science 71

Section 1 NEUROLOGICAL PROBLEMS 73
Section Editor: Jill E. Winland-Brown, EdD, APRN, FNP-BC, FAANP

Chapter 6
Common Neurological Complaints 73

Sarah Horn, MD
Jill E. Winland-Brown, EdD, APRN, FNP-BC, FAANP

- Confusion 73
- Dizziness and Vertigo 76
- Headache 77
- Paresthesia and Paresis 90
- Tremors 90

Chapter 7
Seizure Disorders 94
Sarah Horn, MD
Jill E. Winland-Brown, EdD, APRN, FNP-BC, FAANP
- Epidemiology and Causes 95
- Pathophysiology 96
- Clinical Presentation 96
- Diagnostic Reasoning 97
- Management 97
- Follow-Up and Referral 100

Chapter 8
Degenerative Disorders 102
Sarah Horn, MD
Jill E. Winland-Brown EdD, APRN, FNP-BC, FAANP
- Dementia 102
- Alzheimer's Disease 104
- Parkinson's Disease 109
- Amyotrophic Lateral Sclerosis (Lou Gehrig's Disease) 114

Chapter 9
Cerebrovascular Accident (Stroke) 116
Sarah Horn, MD
Jill E. Winland-Brown, EdD, APRN, FNP-BC, FAANP
- Epidemiology and Causes 117
- Pathophysiology 117
- Clinical Presentation 119
- Diagnostic Reasoning 120
- Management 122
- Follow-Up and Referral 123

Chapter 10
Infectious and Inflammatory Neurological Disorders 126
Sarah Horn, MD
Jill E. Winland-Brown, EdD, APRN, FNP-BC, FAANP
- Meningitis 126
- Encephalitis 129
- Herpes Zoster 131
- Trigeminal Neuralgia 134
- Bell's Palsy 136
- Guillain-Barré Syndrome 137
- Myasthenia Gravis 138
- Multiple Sclerosis 138

Section 2 SKIN PROBLEMS 147
Section Editor: Jill E. Winland-Brown, EdD, APRN, FNP-BC, FAANP

Chapter 11
Common Skin Complaints 147
Susan Garnett, MSN, APRN, FNP-BC
Jill E. Winland-Brown, EdD, APRN, FNP-BC, FAANP
Brian Oscar Porter, MD, PhD, MPH, MBA
- Alopecia 147
- Pigmentation Changes 150
- Pruritus 153
- Rash 156
- Urticaria 158

Chapter 12
Parasitic Skin Infestations 163
Jill E. Winland-Brown, EdD, APRN, FNP-BC, FAANP
Nancy Harris, DNP, APRN, FNP-BC
Brian Oscar Porter, MD, PhD, MPH, MBA
- Scabies 163
- Pediculosis 167

Chapter 13
Mucocutaneous Fungal Infections 172
Susan Garnett, MSN, APRN, FNP-BC
Jill E. Winland-Brown, EdD, APRN, FNP-BC, FAANP
Brian Oscar Porter, MD, PhD, MPH, MBA
- Candidiasis 172
- Dermatophytoses 180
- Onychomycosis 187

Chapter 14
Bacterial Skin Infections 190
Susan Garnett, MSN, APRN, FNP-BC
Jill E. Winland-Brown, EdD, APRN, FNP-BC, FAANP
Brian Oscar Porter, MD, PhD, MPH, MBA
- Impetigo 190
- Folliculitis 194
- Furuncles and Carbuncles 197
- Cellulitis 199

Chapter 15
Viral Skin Infections 205
Susan Garnett, MSN, APRN, FNP-BC
Jill E. Winland-Brown, EdD, APRN, FNP-BC, FAANP
Brian Oscar Porter, MD, PhD, MPH, MBA
- Warts 205
- Herpes Simplex Infections 210

Chapter 16
Dermatitis 215
Donna Maheady, EdD, APRN, PNP-BC
Jill E. Winland-Brown, EdD, APRN, FNP-BC, FAANP
Brian Oscar Porter, MD, PhD, MPH, MBA
- Atopic Dermatitis 215
- Contact Dermatitis 223
- Seborrheic Dermatitis 226
- Psoriasis 228

Chapter 17
Skin Lesions 239
Jill E. Winland-Brown, EdD, APRN, FNP-BC, FAANP
Nancy Harris, DNP, APRN, FNP-BC
Brian Oscar Porter, MD, PhD, MPH, MBA

- **Benign Lesions** 239
  - Acne Vulgaris 239
  - Rosacea 248
  - Seborrheic Keratosis 251
- **Premalignant Lesions** 254
  - Actinic Keratosis 254
- **Malignant Lesions** 256
  - Malignant Melanoma 256
  - Nonmelanomatous Skin Cancers 261

Section 3 EYE PROBLEMS 267
Section Editor: Lynne M. Dunphy, PhD, APRN, FNP-BC, FAAN, FAANP

Chapter 18
Common Eye Complaints 267
Benjamin G. Kuhar, DO
Lynne M. Dunphy, PhD, APRN, FNP-BC, FAAN, FAANP
Brian Oscar Porter, MD, PhD, MPH, MBA

- Dry Eye 267
- Excessive Tearing (Epiphora) 268
- Eye Pain 268
- Red Eye 268
- Visual Changes 269

Chapter 19
Lid and Conjunctival Pathology 270
Benjamin G. Kuhar, DO
Brian Oscar Porter, MD, PhD, MPH, MBA
Lynne M. Dunphy, PhD, APRN, FNP-BC, FAAN, FAANP

- Blepharitis 270
- Hordeolum and Chalazion 272
- Dry Eye 274
- Excessive Tearing (Epiphora) 277
- Red Eye/Conjunctivitis 280

Chapter 20
Visual Disturbances and Impaired Vision 285
Benjamin G. Kuhar, DO
Brian Oscar Porter, MD, PhD, MPH, MBA
Lynne M. Dunphy, PhD, APRN, FNP-BC, FAAN, FAANP

- Refractive Errors 285
- Cataracts 288
- Glaucoma 291
- Diabetic Retinopathy 295
- Macular Degeneration 296

Section 4 EAR, NOSE, AND THROAT PROBLEMS 303
Section Editor: Michael E. Zychowicz, DNP, ANP, ONP, FAAN, FAANP

Chapter 21
Common Ear, Nose, and Throat Complaints 303
Maria Colandrea, DNP, NP-C, CORLN, CCRN, FAANP
Michael E. Zychowicz, DNP, ANP, ONP, FAAN, FAANP
Brian Oscar Porter, MD, PhD, MPH, MBA

- Ear Pain (Otalgia) 303
- Impaired Hearing 303
- Tinnitus 304
- Mouth Sores 304
- Hoarseness 305
- Sore Throat 305
- Epistaxis 306
- Sinus Complaints 306
- Neck Masses 307

Chapter 22
Hearing and Balance Disorders 309
Maria Colandrea, DNP, NP-C, CORLN, CCRN, FAANP
Michael E. Zychowicz, DNP, ANP, ONP, FAAN, FAANP
Brian Oscar Porter, MD, PhD, MPH, MBA

- Hearing Loss 309
- Tinnitus 316
- Vestibular Disorders 320
- Benign Paroxysmal Positional Vertigo 321
- Ménière's Disease 327
- Vestibular Neuritis and Labyrinthitis 330

Chapter 23
Inflammatory and Infectious Disorders of the Ear 334
Maria Colandrea, DNP, NP-C, CORLN, CCRN, FAANP
Michael E. Zychowicz, DNP, ANP, ONP, FAAN, FAANP
Brian Oscar Porter, MD, PhD, MPH, MBA

- Otitis Externa (Swimmer's Ear) 334
- Otitis Media 341

Chapter 24
Inflammatory and Infectious Disorders of the Nose, Sinuses, Mouth, and Throat 350
Maria Colandrea, DNP, NP-C, CORLN, CCRN, FAANP
Tiffany Ellis, MSN, ANP-C, CORLN
Michael E. Zychowicz, DNP, ANP, ONP, FAAN, FAANP
Brian Oscar Porter, MD, PhD, MPH, MBA

- Rhinitis 350
- Rhinosinusitis 365
- Neck Masses 377
- Stomatitis and Glossitis 382
- Oral Cancer 389
- Pharyngitis and Tonsillitis 392

Chapter 25
Epistaxis 401
Maria Colandrea, DNP, NP-C, CORLN, CCRN, FAANP
Michael E. Zychowicz, DNP, ANP, ONP, FAAN, FAANP
Brian Oscar Porter, MD, PhD, MPH, MBA

    Epidemiology and Causes 401
    Pathophysiology 402
    Clinical Presentation 403
    Diagnostic Reasoning 404
    Management 404
    Follow-Up and Referral 405

Chapter 26
Temporomandibular Disorders 407
Maria Colandrea, DNP, NP-C, CORLN, CCRN, FAANP
Michael E. Zychowicz, DNP, ANP, ONP, FAAN, FAANP
Brian Oscar Porter, MD, PhD, MPH, MBA

    Epidemiology and Causes 407
    Pathophysiology 407
    Clinical Presentation 407
    Diagnostic Reasoning 408
    Management 408
    Follow-Up and Referral 411

Chapter 27
Dysphonia 412
Maria Colandrea, DNP, NP-C, CORLN, CCRN, FAANP
Michael E. Zychowicz, DNP, ANP, ONP, FAAN, FAANP
Brian Oscar Porter, MD, PhD, MPH, MBA

    Epidemiology and Causes 412
    Pathophysiology 412
    Clinical Presentation 412
    Diagnostic Reasoning 413
    Management 414
    Follow-Up and Referral 415

Section 5   RESPIRATORY PROBLEMS 417
Section Editor: Jill E. Winland-Brown, EdD, APRN, FNP-BC, FAANP

Chapter 28
Common Respiratory Complaints 417
Jill E. Winland-Brown, EdD, APRN, FNP-BC, FAANP
Brian Oscar Porter, MD, PhD, MPH, MBA

    Cough 417
    Dyspnea 419
    Hemoptysis 421

Chapter 29
Sleep Apnea 423
John Suen, MD
Jill E. Winland-Brown, EdD, APRN, FNP-BC, FAANP

    Epidemiology and Causes 424
    Pathophysiology 424
    Clinical Presentation 425
    Diagnostic Reasoning 427
    Management 428
    Follow-Up and Referral 430

Chapter 30
Infectious Respiratory Disorders 431
Jill E. Winland-Brown, EdD, APRN, FNP-BC, FAANP
Nilesh Patel, DO, FAAEM, FACOEP
Janine Duran Llamzon, DNP-C, MS, AGNP-C, RN, CEN, NEA-BC
Brian Oscar Porter, MD, PhD, MPH, MBA

    Upper Respiratory Infections 431
    Cystic Fibrosis 436
    Pneumonia 438
    Tuberculosis 452

Chapter 31
Inflammatory Respiratory Disorders 465
Jill E. Winland-Brown, EdD, APRN, FNP-BC, FAANP
Brian Oscar Porter, MD, PhD, MPH, MBA

    Asthma 465
    Chronic Bronchitis and Emphysema (Chronic Obstructive Pulmonary Disease [COPD]) 475
    Interstitial Lung Disease 486

Chapter 32
Lung Cancer 494
Jill E. Winland-Brown, EdD, APRN, FNP-BC, FAANP
Brian Oscar Porter, MD, PhD, MPH, MBA

    Epidemiology and Causes 494
    Pathophysiology 495
    Clinical Presentation 497
    Diagnostic Reasoning 500
    Management 504
    Follow-Up and Referral 506

Chapter 33
Smoking Addiction 508
Jill E. Winland-Brown, EdD, APRN, FNP-BC, FAANP
Brian Oscar Porter, MD, PhD, MPH, MBA

    Epidemiology and Causes 508
    Pathophysiology 511
    Clinical Presentation 512
    Diagnostic Reasoning 513
    Management 513
    Follow-Up and Referral 518

Section 6 CARDIOVASCULAR PROBLEMS 521

Section Editor: Jill E. Winland-Brown, EdD, APRN, FNP-BC, FAANP

Chapter 34
Common Cardiovascular Complaints 521

Kathryn B. Keller, PhD, RN, CNE
Jill E. Winland-Brown, EdD, APRN, FNP-BC, FAANP
Brian Oscar Porter, MD, PhD, MPH, MBA

- Chest Pain 521
- Palpitations 523
- Syncope 524
- Dyspnea 524
- Leg Aches 526
- Peripheral Edema 526

Chapter 35
Cardiac and Associated Risk Disorders 529

Kathryn B. Keller, PhD, RN, CNE
Jill E. Winland-Brown, EdD, APRN, FNP-BC, FAANP
Brian Oscar Porter, MD, PhD, MPH, MBA

- Hypertension 529
- Dyslipidemia 543
- Coronary Heart Disease 547
- Acute Coronary Syndrome 553
- Heart Failure 565

Chapter 36
Dysrhythmias and Valvular Disorders 575

Kathryn B. Keller, PhD, RN, CNE
Denese Sabatino, MSN, APRN, NP-C, CCRN
Jill E. Winland-Brown, EdD, APRN, FNP-BC, FAANP
Michael B. Keller, MD
Brian Oscar Porter, MD, PhD, MPH, MBA

- Arrhythmias 575
- Valvular Disorders and Murmurs 586

Chapter 37
Disorders of the Vascular System 594

Kathryn B. Keller, PhD, RN, CNE
Jill E. Winland-Brown, EdD, APRN, FNP-BC, FAANP
Brian Oscar Porter, MD, PhD, MPH, MBA
Michael B. Keller, MD

- Peripheral Artery Disease 594
- Deep Vein Thrombosis/Chronic Venous Insufficiency 596

Section 7 ABDOMINAL PROBLEMS 603

Section Editor: Debera J. Thomas, PhD, RN, ANP/FNP

Chapter 38
Common Abdominal Complaints 603

Debera J. Thomas, PhD, RN, ANP/FNP

- Abdominal Pain 603
- Constipation 604
- Diarrhea 607
- Dyspepsia and Heartburn 611
- Jaundice 612
- Melena 612
- Nausea and Vomiting 614
- Dysphagia 615

Chapter 39
Infectious Gastrointestinal Disorders 618

Debera J. Thomas, PhD, RN, ANP/FNP

- Gastroenteritis 618
- Hepatitis 628
- Appendicitis 635

Chapter 40
Gastric and Intestinal Disorders 640

Debera J. Thomas, PhD, RN, ANP/FNP

- Gastroesophageal Reflux Disease 640
- Peptic Ulcer Disease 645
- Hemorrhoids 648
- Abdominal Hernias 650
- Irritable Bowel Syndrome 653
- Celiac Disease 657
- Bowel Obstruction 659
- Diverticular Disease 661
- Inflammatory Bowel Disease 664
- Colorectal Cancer 672

Chapter 41
Gallbladder and Pancreatic Disorders 678

Debera J. Thomas, PhD, RN, ANP/FNP

- Cholecystitis 678
- Acute Pancreatitis 681
- Chronic Pancreatitis 685
- Pancreatic Cancer 688

Chapter 42
Cirrhosis and Liver Failure 690

Debera J. Thomas, PhD, RN, ANP/FNP

- Epidemiology and Causes 690
- Pathophysiology 691
- Clinical Presentation 692
- Diagnostic Reasoning 693
- Management 695
- Follow-Up and Referral 698

Section 8 RENAL PROBLEMS 701
Section Editor: Debera J. Thomas, PhD, RN, ANP/FNP

Chapter 43
Common Urinary Complaints 701
Debbie Conner, PhD, MSN, ANP/FNP-BC, FAANP
Debera J. Thomas, PhD, RN, ANP/FNP
Brian Oscar Porter, MD, PhD, MPH, MBA

- Dysuria 701
- Hematuria 701
- Proteinuria 704

Chapter 44
Urinary Tract Disorders 706
Debbie Conner, PhD, MSN, ANP/FNP-BC, FAANP
Debera J. Thomas, PhD, RN, FNP/ANP
Brian Oscar Porter, MD, PhD, MPH, MBA

- Urinary Incontinence 706
- Lower Urinary Tract Infections 714
- Upper Urinary Tract Infection: Pyelonephritis 721
- Nephrolithiasis 724

Chapter 45
Kidney and Bladder Disorders 729
Debbie Conner, PhD, MSN, ANP/FNP-BC, FAANP
Debera J. Thomas, PhD, RN, ANP/FNP
Brian Oscar Porter, MD, PhD, MPH, MBA

- Acute Kidney Injury 729
- Chronic Kidney Disease 736
- Renal Tumors 742
- Bladder Tumors 744

Section 9 GENDER-RELATED HEALTH PROBLEMS 749
Section Editor: Debera J. Thomas, PhD, RN, ANP/FNP

Chapter 46
Common Reproductive System Complaints 749
Debera J. Thomas, PhD, RN, ANP/FNP
Brian Oscar Porter, MD, PhD, MPH, MBA

- Breast Mass 749
- Abnormal Uterine Bleeding 750
- Dyspareunia 751
- Nocturia in Males 752
- Chronic Pelvic Pain Syndrome in Females 753
- Chronic Pelvic Pain Syndrome in Males 754
- Testicular Pain 755
- Testosterone Deficiency 756
- Vulvovaginitis 756

Chapter 47
Common Reproductive System Issues 760
Megan R. Pratt, DNP, APRN, FNP-BC, GS-C
Debera J. Thomas, PhD, RN, ANP/FNP
Brian Oscar Porter, MD, PhD, MPH, MBA

- Contraception and Family Planning 760
- Fertility Problems 771
- Premenstrual Syndrome and Premenstrual Dysphoric Disorder 778
- Menopause 782

Chapter 48
Breast Disorders 793
Megan Pratt, DNP, APRN, FNP-BC, GS-C
Debera J. Thomas, PhD, RN, ANP/FNP
Brian Oscar Porter, MD, PhD, MPH, MBA

- Mastitis 794
- Breast Cancer 798

Chapter 49
Vaginal, Uterine, and Ovarian Disorders 809
Megan Pratt, DNP, APRN, FNP-BC, GS-C
Debera J. Thomas, PhD, RN, ANP/FNP
Brian Oscar Porter, MD, PhD, MPH, MBA

- Amenorrhea 809
- Dysmenorrhea 812
- Endometriosis 814
- Leiomyomas (Uterine Fibroids) 817
- Precancerous Lesions and Cancer of the Cervix 819
- Endometrial Cancer 824
- Ovarian Cancer 827
- Vulvodynia 830

Chapter 50
Prostate Disorders 833
Debbie Conner, PhD, MSN, ANP/FNP-BC, FAANP
Debera J. Thomas, PhD, RN, ANP/FNP
Brian Oscar Porter, MD, PhD, MPH, MBA

- Benign Prostatic Hyperplasia 833
- Prostatitis 840
- Prostate Cancer 842

Chapter 51
Penile and Testicular Disorders 847
Debbie Conner, PhD, MSN, ANP/FNP-BC, FAANP
Debera J. Thomas, PhD, RN, ANP/FNP
Brian Oscar Porter, MD, PhD, MPH, MBA

- Erectile Dysfunction 847
- Epididymitis 854
- Testicular Torsion 856
- Hydrocele 857
- Varicocele 859
- Testicular Cancer 860

Chapter 52
Sexually Transmitted Infections 866
Deborah Lowell Shindell, PhD, FNP-BC, CNE
Debera J. Thomas, PhD, RN, ANP/FNP
Brian Oscar Porter, MD, PhD, MPH, MBA

Epidemiology and Causes 866
Pathophysiology 872
Clinical Presentation 872
Diagnostic Reasoning 873
Management 874
Follow-Up and Referral 874

Section 10 MUSCULOSKELETAL PROBLEMS 877
Section Editor: Michael E. Zychowicz, DNP, ANP, ONP, FAAN, FAANP

Chapter 53
Common Musculoskeletal Complaints 877
Michael E. Zychowicz, DNP, ANP, ONP, FAAN, FAANP

Acute Musculoskeletal Injury 884
Muscle Cramps 893
Paresthesias 894
Myofascial Pain 894
Regional Musculoskeletal Complaints 895
Neck Pain 895
Back Pain 896
Shoulder Pain 898
Elbow Pain 899
Wrist and Hand Pain 900
Hip Pain 901
Knee Pain 903
Ankle Pain 905
Foot Pain 906

Chapter 54
Spinal Disorders 910
Michael E. Zychowicz, DNP, ANP, ONP, FAAN, FAANP

Cervical Muscle Sprain and Strain 910
Cervical Spondylosis 913
Low Back Pain 915
Herniated Lumbar Disc (Herniated Nucleus Pulposus) 922
Lumbar Spinal Stenosis 926
Cauda Equina Syndrome 928
Vertebral Fracture 931

Chapter 55
Soft Tissue Disorders 935
Michael E. Zychowicz, DNP, ANP, ONP, FAAN, FAANP

Bursitis 935
Tendinitis/Tenosynovitis 937
Hand and Wrist Disorders 941
Carpal Tunnel Syndrome 941
De Quervain's Tenosynovitis 943
Ganglion Cyst 944
Trigger Finger 944
Tendon Injuries of the Hand 945
Dupuytren's Contracture 945
Shoulder Disorders 945
Adhesive Capsulitis 945
Impingement Syndrome 946
Calcific Tendinitis 947
Rotator Cuff Tear 947
Hip Disorders 949
Greater Trochanteric Pain Syndrome 949
Meralgia Paresthetica 949
Avascular Necrosis 949
Bone Tumors 950
Knee Disorders 951
Cruciate Ligament Injury 951
Medial Collateral Ligament Injury 951
Meniscus Tear 952
Foot and Ankle Disorders 952
Plantar Fasciitis 953
Interdigital Neuroma 953

Chapter 56
Osteoarthritis and Osteoporosis 956
Margaret M. Harding, MSN, RN, AGPCNP-BC, RNFA, CPAN
Michael E. Zychowicz, DNP, ANP, ONP, FAAN, FAANP

Osteoarthritis 956
Osteoporosis 967

Section 11 ENDOCRINE AND METABOLIC PROBLEMS 979
Section Editor: Debera J. Thomas, PhD, RN, ANP/FNP

Chapter 57
Common Endocrine and Metabolic Complaints 979
Debera J. Thomas, PhD, RN, ANP/FNP
Brian Oscar Porter, MD, PhD, MPH, MBA

Hypocalcemia 979
Gynecomastia 980
Hirsutism 981
Increased Neck Size 982
Polydipsia, Polyphagia, and Polyuria 983

Chapter 58
Glandular Disorders 984
Debera J. Thomas, PhD, RN, ANP/FNP
Brian Oscar Porter, MD, PhD, MPH, MBA

Hyperthyroidism 984
Hypothyroidism 993
Thyroid Cancer 1003
Cushing's Syndrome 1006
Adrenal Insufficiency 1011

Chapter 59
Diabetes Mellitus 1014

Debera J. Thomas, PhD, RN, ANP/FNP
Brian Oscar Porter, MD, PhD, MPH, MBA

- Diabetes Mellitus Type 1   1014
- Diabetes Mellitus Type 2   1027
- Diabetes Mellitus Type 3C   1039

Chapter 60
Metabolic Disorders 1047

Debera J. Thomas, PhD, RN, ANP/FNP
Brian Oscar Porter, MD, PhD, MPH, MBA

- Obesity   1047
- Gout   1055

Section 12 HEMATOLOGICAL AND IMMUNOLOGICAL PROBLEMS 1063

Section Editor: Brian Oscar Porter, MD, PhD, MPH, MBA

Chapter 61
Common Hematological and Immunological Complaints 1063

Monica Giovannini, MD
Jill E. Winland-Brown, EdD, APRN, FNP-BC, FAANP
Brian Oscar Porter, MD, PhD, MPH, MBA

- Bruising   1063
- Fatigue   1064
- Fever   1064
- Lymphadenopathy   1065

Chapter 62
Hematological Disorders 1066

Monica Giovannini, MD
Jill E. Winland-Brown, EdD, APRN, FNP-BC, FAANP
Brian Oscar Porter, MD, PhD, MPH, MBA

- Anemia   1066
- Microcytic Anemia   1067
- Normocytic Anemia   1074
- Macrocytic Anemia   1079
- Sickle Cell Anemia   1083
- Polycythemia   1088
- Leukemia   1092

Chapter 63
Immunological Disorders 1104

Brian Oscar Porter, MD, PhD, MPH, MBA
Jill E. Winland-Brown, EdD, APRN, FNP-BC, FAANP
Luminita Pricop, MD

- Allergic Reactions   1104
- Rheumatoid Arthritis   1113
- Chronic Fatigue Syndrome and Fibromyalgia Syndrome   1124
- Sjögren's Syndrome   1128
- Systemic Lupus Erythematosus   1132

Chapter 64
Infectious Disorders 1139

Virginia Sheikh, MD, MHS
Jill E. Winland-Brown, EdD, APRN, FNP-BC, FAANP
Brian Oscar Porter, MD, PhD, MPH, MBA

- Infectious Mononucleosis   1139
- Lyme Disease   1142
- HIV Infection   1147
- AIDS   1164

Section 13 PSYCHOSOCIAL PROBLEMS 1173

Section Editor: Karen Jennings Mathis, PhD, APRN-CNP, PMHNP-BC, FAED

Chapter 65
Common Psychological Complaints 1173

Jamison Lord, DNP, APRN, PMHNP-BC
Rachele Lipsky, PhD, APRN, PMHNP
Katerina Melino, MS, PMHNP
Lynne M. Dunphy, PhD, APRN-CNP, PMHNP-BC, FAED

- Anxiety Disorders   1176
- Depressed Mood   1178
- Grief   1179
- Substance Use Disorder   1181
- Intimate Partner Violence   1182

Chapter 66
Neurodevelopmental Disorders 1187

Elizabeth Hutson, PhD, APRN-CNP, PMHNP-BC
Karen Jennings Mathis, PhD, APRN-CNP, PMHNP-BC, FAED

- Attention Deficit-Hyperactivity Disorder   1188
- Autism Spectrum Disorder   1194
- Intellectual Disability   1197
- Tic Disorders   1201

Chapter 67
Substance-Related and Addictive Disorders 1209

Jamie Lord, DNP, APRN, PMHNP-BC
Sean Convoy, DNP, PMHNP-BC
Karen Jennings Mathis, PhD, APRN-CNP, PMHNP-BC, FAED

- Epidemiology and Causes   1210
- Pathophysiology   1212
- Clinical Presentation   1213
- Diagnostic Reasoning   1218
- Management   1218
- Follow-Up and Referral   1220

Chapter 68
Schizophrenia Spectrum and Other Psychotic Disorders 1226

Amanda Ling, MS, RN, PMHNP
Kara Birch, DNP, PMHNP, FNP
Karen Jennings Mathis, PhD, APRN-CNP, PMHNP-BC, FAED

　　Epidemiology and Causes   1227
　　Pathophysiology   1227
　　Clinical Presentation   1228
　　Diagnostic Reasoning   1228
　　Management   1230
　　Follow-Up and Referral   1235

Chapter 69
Mood Disorders 1239

Michaela K. Hogan, DNP, APRN, PMHNP-BC
Ashley Love, DNP, PMHNP-BC
Rene Love, PhD, DNP, PMHNP-BC, FNAP, FAANP
Karen Jennings Mathis, PhD, APRN-CNP, PMHNP-BC, FAED

　　Major Depressive Disorder   1239
　　Bipolar and Related Disorders   1250
　　Suicide   1264

Chapter 70
Anxiety Disorders and Post-Traumatic Stress Disorder 1274

Kara Birch, DNP, PMHNP, FNP
Katelyn Brady, MSN, PMHNP-BC
Amanda Ling, RN, PMHNP
Karen Jennings Mathis, PhD, APRN-CNP, PMHNP-BC, FAED

　　Generalized Anxiety Disorder   1275
　　Panic Disorder   1281
　　Phobias   1284
　　Post-Traumatic Stress Disorder   1285

Chapter 71
Obsessive-Compulsive and Related Disorders 1293

Kim Ferguson, DNP, APRN, FNP-BC, PMHNP-BC
Karen Jennings Mathis, PhD, APRN-CNP, PMHNP-BC, FAED

　　Obsessive-Compulsive Disorder   1293
　　Body Dysmorphic Disorder   1299
　　Hoarding Disorder   1300

Chapter 72
Other Psychiatric Disorders 1304

Karen Jennings Mathis, PhD, APRN-CNP, PMHNP-BC, FAED
Meredith Kells, PhD, RN, CPNP

　　Feeding and Eating Disorders   1304
　Sleep–Wake Disorders   1311
　　Insomnia Disorder   1311
　　Restless Legs Syndrome   1317

Chapter 73
Sexual Assault 1320

Katerina Melino, MS, PMHNP
Karen Jennings Mathis, PhD, APRN-CNP, PMHNP-BC, FAED

　　Epidemiology and Causes   1321
　　Pathophysiology   1321
　　Clinical Presentation   1322
　　Diagnostic Reasoning   1322
　　Management   1322
　　Follow-Up and Referral   1324

Chapter 74
Human Trafficking 1327

John Fraleigh, MSN, RN, CFRN
Karen Jennings Mathis, PhD, APRN-CNP, PMHNP-BC, FAED

　　Epidemiology and Causes   1327
　　Clinical Presentation   1329
　　Diagnostic Reasoning   1330
　　Management   1331
　　Follow-Up and Referral   1331

Section 14 URGENT CARE PROBLEMS 1333

Section Editor: Jill E. Winland-Brown, EdD, APRN, FNP-BC, FAANP

Chapter 75
Common Injuries 1333

Jill E. Winland-Brown, EdD, APRN, FNP-BC, FAANP
Brian Oscar Porter, MD, PhD, MPH, MBA

　　Wounds and Lacerations   1333
　　Animal and Human Bites   1342
　　Arthropod Bites and Stings   1346
　　Burns   1356
　　Head Trauma   1362
　　Pneumothorax and Hemothorax   1369
　　Foreign Body Obstruction   1371

Chapter 76
Toxic and Environmental Exposures 1375

Jill E. Winland-Brown, EdD, APRN, FNP-BC, FAANP
Brian Oscar Porter, MD, PhD, MPH, MBA

　　Poisoning   1375
　　Heat-Related Illnesses   1382
　Cold-Related Illnesses   1386
　　Hypothermia   1386
　　Frostbite   1388

Unit III Caring-Based Nursing: The Practice 1391

Section 1 CARE OF VULNERABLE POPULATIONS 1393

Chapter 77
Primary Care of Adolescents 1393
Carol Savrin, DNP, CPNP, FNP-BC, FAANP, RN
Debera J. Thomas, PhD, RN, ANP/FNP

Adolescence Overview 1393
Conclusion 1404

Chapter 78
Sports Physicals 1406
Michael E. Zychowicz, DNP, ANP, ONP, FAAN, FAANP

Introduction 1406
Examination Timing 1406
Examination Formats 1407
Components of Sports Physical: History, Physical Examination, and Clearance 1407

Chapter 79
Primary Care of Patients Who Are Transgender 1417
Cameron Duncan, PhD, DNP, MS, APRN, FNP-BC, PMHNP-BC
Debera J. Thomas, PhD, RN, ANP/FNP

Introduction 1417
Prevalence and Demographics of Transgender Patients 1418
Assessment 1418
Common Gender-Affirming Treatment – Trans Men 1419
Common Gender-Affirming Treatments – Trans Women 1420
Pharmacological Considerations 1420
Gender-Appropriate Care 1421
Conclusion 1422

Chapter 80
Primary Care of Veterans 1424
Michael E. Zychowicz, DNP, ANP, ONP, FAAN, FAANP
Sherley Belizaire, DNP, PMHNP-BC, FNP-BC
Janet G. Campbell, DNP, ANP-BC, ACNS, COHN-S
Angela Richard-Eaglin, DNP, MSN, FNP-BC, CNE, FAANP
Michelle Gibson, MSN, PMHNP-BC, CARN-AP
Michael Anthony Moore, MSN, NP-C, RN, HIV-PCP
Susan Wilkinson, MSN, PMHNP-BC

Introduction 1424
Non-VA Health-Care Providers 1424
Military Separation 1425
Military and Veteran Families 1425
Exposure to Risks for Illness and Injury 1427
Veteran Mental Health Needs 1430
Conclusion 1436

Chapter 81
Primary Care of the Patient With Cancer 1439
Anna L. Schwartz, PhD, FNP-BC, FAAN

Introduction 1439
Health Promotion 1445

Chapter 82
Primary Care of Older Adults 1448
Deirdre Carolan, PhD, ANP-BC, GNP-BC, FAANP
Lynne M. Dunphy, PhD, APRN, FNP-BC, FAAN, FAANP

Introduction 1448
Demographics and the Changing Face of Aging 1448
Processes of Aging 1449
A Focus on Healthy Aging 1450
Health Screening for Older Adults 1455
Immunizations 1460
Geriatric Syndromes 1460
Medications in the Older Adult 1462
Special Topics in Aging 1463
End-of-Life Decision Making 1465
Conclusion 1465

Chapter 83
Pain Management 1469
Didier Demesmin, MD, MBA
Lynne M. Dunphy, PhD, APRN, FNP-BC, FAAN, FAANP
Brian Oscar Porter, MD, PhD, MPH, MBA

Introduction 1469
Pain Mechanisms: Pathophysiology 1469
Classifications of Pain 1471
Assessment of Acute and Chronic Pain 1473
Pain Management 1474
Vulnerable and Special Populations 1482

Section 2 - eBook Only

Section 2 SPECIAL TOPICS IN ADVANCED PRACTICE 1489
Section Editor: Lynne M. Dunphy, PhD, APRN, FNP-BC, FAAN, FAANP

Chapter 84
Palliative and End-of-Life Care 1489
Amie M. Koch, DNP, FNP-C, RN, ACHPN
Lynne M. Dunphy, PhD, APRN, FNP-BC, FAAN, FAANP

History of Palliative Care and Hospice 1489
Differences Between Hospice and Palliative Care 1490

Hospice Care Utilization 1491
Death and Dying in the United States 1491
Utilization of Palliative Care 1492
Professional Educational Efforts to Improve the Practice of Palliative Care 1492
Suffering 1493
Advance Directives 1494
Specialty Populations 1495
The Role of the Primary Care Provider in Palliative Care 1497
Conclusion 1509

Chapter 85
Ethical and Legal Issues of a Caring-Based Practice 1513
Jill E. Winland-Brown, EdD, APRN, FNP-BC, FAANP
Josie Weiss, PhD, FNP-BC, PNP-BC, FAANP

Ethical Issues 1513
Legal Issues 1521

Chapter 86
Quality & Value-Based Payment: Making an Economic Impact on Health Care 1530
Marcella M. Rutherford, PhD, MSN, MBA, RN

Introduction 1530
Third-Party Payer Rules 1531
Affordable Care Act: Impact and Status 1536
Reimbursement Rules—Billing and Coding 1540
Value-Based Reimbursement and Performance-Based Care 1544
Conclusion 1547

Chapter 87
Primary Care Approaches to Behavioral Health 1551
Elizabeth Hutson, PhD, APRN-CNP, PMHNP-BC
Lynne M. Dunphy, PhD, APRN, FNP-BC, FAAN, FAANP

Stress 1551
Brain Changes in Response to Stress and Counseling 1552
Health Coaching Using Cognitive and Behavioral Techniques 1552
Motivational Interviewing 1554
Summary 1555

Chapter 88
Putting Caring Into Practice: Caring for Self 1558
Mary Lavin, DNP, APRN-CNP
Rebecca Carley, DNP, APRN-CNP

Background: Caring and Self-Care 1558
Challenges to Self-Care Inherent in Advanced Practice Nursing 1559
Compassion Fatigue and Burnout 1560
The Principles of Self-Care Management 1561
The Process of Self-Care Management 1561
Conclusion 1562

Index I-1

Special Features

Page numbers preceeded by "e" denotes online only.

ASSESSMENT FEATURES

Advanced Assessment

- 4.1 Functional Health Patterns: Questions to Elicit Data 45
- 8.1 Alzheimer's Disease: Signs and Symptoms for Further Assessment 106
- 8.2 Functional Activities Questionnaire 106
- 13.1 KOH Examination 174–175
- 16.1 Atopic Dermatitis 217
- 16.2 Contact Dermatitis 224
- 30.1 Sputum Staining 445
- 35.1 Hypertension 534
- 35.2 Assessing Axis Deviation 558
- 36.1 Cardiac Examination and Assessment of Heart Murmurs 589–590
- 39.1 Physical Examination Maneuvers for Diagnosing Appendicitis 638
- 43.1 Urinalysis 702
- 53.1 Physical Examination for Musculoskeletal Disorders 880
- 53.2 Synovial Fluid Analysis 883
- 53.3 Assessing Ankle Ligaments—Special Tests 887
- 53.4 Assessing Knee Ligaments—Special Tests 887
- 53.5 Ottawa Ankle and Foot Rules 889
- 53.6 Reading an Extremity X-Ray 892
- 53.7 Paresthesias and Affected Nerve Roots 894
- 53.8 Spurling's Maneuver 895
- 53.9 Straight-Leg-Raise Test 897
- 53.10 Tests for Wrist and Hand Problems 901
- 53.11 Assessing the Meniscus and the Patella—Special Tests 905
- 54.1 Assessing the Lower Back—Special Tests 919
- 54.2 Common Findings of Nerve Irritation From Disc Herniation 924
- 64.1 HIV-positive Individual 1164–1165
- 65.1 The *Diagnostic and Statistical Manual of Mental Disorders, Fifth Edition, Text Revision (DSM-5-TR)* 1176
- 75.1 Wounds and Lacerations 1335–1336
- 75.2 Rapid Neurological Examination 1366–1367

Differential Diagnosis

- 7.1 Seizures 98
- 11.1 Alopecia 148
- 11.2 Pruritus 153
- 12.1 Scabies 165
- 12.2 Pediculosis 169
- 13.1 Mucocutaneous Candidiasis 175
- 13.2 Tinea Infections 184
- 16.1 Atopic Dermatitis 218
- 16.2 Psoriasis 232–233
- 22.1 Tinnitus 319
- 24.1 Rhinitis 352–355
- 24.2 Rhinosinusitis 369–370
- 24.3 Neck Mass 382
- 24.4 Common Benign Oral Lesions 386–387
- 24.5 Common Premalignant and Malignant Oral Lesions 391
- 25.1 Epistaxis 405
- 26.1 Temporomandibular Disorder 408
- 27.1 Dysphonia 414
- 40.1 Irritable Bowel Syndrome 655
- 40.2 Bowel Obstruction 660
- 43.1 Hematuria 704
- 46.1 Pelvic Pain 753–754
- 46.2 Vulvovaginitis 757–758
- 50.1 Benign Prostatic Hyperplasia 836
- 53.1 Muscle Cramps 893
- 53.2 Shoulder Pain 899
- 53.3 Foot Pain 906
- 54.1 Low Back Pain 921
- 56.1 Osteoarthritis 959
- 65.1 Anxiety Disorders 1177
- 65.2 Types of Depression 1179
- 65.3 Substance Use Disorders 1182
- 66.1 Attention Deficit-Hyperactivity Disorder 1190
- 66.2 Autism Spectrum Disorder 1197
- 66.3 Intellectual Disability 1200
- 66.4 Tic Disorders 1203
- 71.1 Obsessive-Compulsive Disorder 1295–1296

Screening Recommendations/Guidelines

Screening for Tuberculosis 455
Colon Cancer Screening, American Cancer Society, (2020) 676
Breast Cancer 799

ADVANCED PRACTICE NURSING THERAPIES FEATURES

Therapeutic Procedures

- 16.1 The Skin "Punch" Biopsy 231
- 17.1 Removal of Seborrheic Keratoses 253
- 17.2 Cryosurgery for Actinic Keratoses 255
- 49.1 Smear and Liquid-Based Cervical Cell Collection (Pap Test) 823
- 53.1 Removing Rings 902
- 62.1 Bone Marrow Transplantation 1101
- 63.1 Seven-step Treatment for Anaphylaxis 1105
- 75.1 Abscess Drainage 1337
- 75.2 Suturing Techniques/Materials 1340–1341

Complementary Therapies

- 6.1 Headaches 89
- 16.1 Herbal Treatments for Eczema 222
- 35.1 Cardiac Conditions 551–552
- 38.1 Complementary Therapies for Gastrointestinal Problems 609
- 40.1 Irritable Bowel Syndrome (IBS) 656
- 47.1 Female Health 783
- 49.1 Women's Health Problems 817
- 50.1 Benign Prostatic Hyperplasia 838
- 56.1 Osteoarthritis and Musculoskeletal Problems 962
- 70.1 Relaxation Therapy Techniques 1281

Drugs Commonly Prescribed

- 6.1 Migraine Headache: Adults 87-88
- 7.1 Seizure Disorders (Monotherapy Only) 99–100
- 8.1 Alzheimer's Disease 109
- 8.2 Parkinson's Disease 113
- 10.1 Multiple Sclerosis 141–142
- 12.1 Scabies 166
- 12.2 Pediculosis 170
- 13.1 Candidal and Tinea Infections 176-179
- 14.1 Folliculitis 196
- 15.1 Herpes Simplex Infections 213
- 17.1 Acne and Rosacea 243–245
- 19.1 Conjunctivitis 279
- 20.1 Glaucoma 294
- 20.2 Wet Acute Macular Degeneration 299
- 23.1 Bacterial Otitis Externa 340
- 23.2 Acute Otitis Media (AOM) in Children and Adults 345–347
- 24.1 Rhinitis 356–362
- 24.2 Acute Viral Rhinosinusitis (AVRS) and Acute Bacterial Rhinosinusitis (ABRS) 372–376
- 26.1 Temporomandibular Disorder 409
- 30.1 *CFTR* Modulators 438
- 30.2 Tuberculosis 459
- 31.1 Asthma 471–473
- 33.1 Therapies for Smoking Cessation—Prescribing Considerations 517
- 35.1 Hypertension 538–541
- 35.2 Statin Therapy for Hyperlipidemia 546
- 36.1 Antithrombotic Treatment Options for Stroke Prevention in Nonvalvular Atrial Fibrillation 584
- 38.1 Constipation 609
- 38.2 Nausea and Vomiting 617
- 39.1 Symptomatic Treatment of Acute Diarrhea 627
- 39.2 Chronic Hepatitis B Infection 635
- 39.3 Treatment for HCV 636
- 40.1 Treatment for GERD 644
- 40.2 Peptic Ulcer Disease 648
- 40.3 Inflammatory Bowel Disease 670
- 44.1 Urinary Incontinence 711–712
- 44.2 Urinary Tract Infection (UTI) 717–719
- 46.1 Vulvovaginitis 758–759
- 47.1 Hormone Therapy for the Treatment of Menopausal Symptoms 789–790
- 51.1 Erectile Dysfunction 851-852
- 56.1 Osteoarthritis 965
- 56.2 Osteoporosis 974
- 58.1 Hyperthyroidism 991
- 58.2 Hypothyroidism—Lifelong Pharmaceutical Treatment 1000
- 58.3 Corticosteroid Replacement Therapy 1010
- 59.1 Diabetes Mellitus Type 1 Insulin Regimens 1021–1022
- 59.2 Noninsulin Agents for Diabetes Mellitus Type 2 1034–1035
- 63.1 Over-the-Counter (OTC) Drugs for Allergic Reactions 1109–1110
- 63.2 Disease-modifying Antirheumatic Drugs (DMARDs) 1122–1123
- 66.1 Attention Deficit-Hyperactivity Disorder (ADHD) Medications 1191–1192
- 66.2 Medications Used in the Treatment of Autism Spectrum Disorder 1198
- 66.3 Medications for Tic Disorders 1203–1204
- 68.1 Typical Antipsychotics 1231
- 68.2 Atypical Antipsychotics 1232–1233
- 69.1 Major Depressive Disorder 1245–1248
- 69.2 Bipolar Disorder 1257–1260
- 70.1 Antianxiety Agents 1278–1279
- 71.1 Obsessive-Compulsive Disorder (OCD) 1297–1298
- 72.1 Sedatives and Hypnotics 1314–1315
- 75.1 Burns 1361
- 79.1 Medications Used for Gender Affirmation 1420–1421
- 83.1 Dosage of Common NSAIDs 1476
- 83.2 Anticonvulsant Drugs 1477
- 83.3 Antidepressants 1477
- 84.1 Pharmacological Management of Nausea and Vomiting e1502
- 84.2 Delirium e1505

Treatment Standards/Guidelines

Empiric Antimicrobial Choices for Community-Acquired Pneumonia (CAP)   449
Maintenance Medications in COPD   481–482
Infective Endocarditis Prophylaxis   592
Initiation of ARV Therapy   1160

ADVANCED PRACTICE NURSING PERSPECTIVE FEATURES

The Patient's Voice

3.1   The Wellness Visit   35
4.1   Artificial Intelligence and Health Care   54
10.1   Postherpetic Neuralgia   133
20.1   Macular Degeneration   300
30.1   Cystic Fibrosis   439
33.1   Battleground   519
35.1   Myocardial Infarction   564
40.1   Crohn's Disease   664
48.1   A Breast Mass   800
49.1   Endometriosis   818
50.1   Nocturia   837
58.1   Hypothyroidism   1002
63.1   Chronic Fatigue Syndrome   1128
64.1   Occupational Exposure and HIV Infection   1154
68.1   Schizophrenia   1230
69.1   Suicide   1265
82.1   My Children Are Coming Today   1459
83.1   Pain Management   1481
84.1   End-of-Life Care   1490
84.2   Palliative Care   1490

Evidence-Based Nursing Practice

8.1   Alzheimer's Disease   110
10.1   Multiple Sclerosis   144
16.1   Atopic Dermatitis   219
31.1   COPD   486
33.1   Smoking Cessation   519
34.1   Chest Pain   521

35.1   Heart Failure   570
48.1   Breast Cancer   808
63.1   Chronic Fatigue Syndrome   1129
64.1   Human Immunodeficiency Virus (HIV)   1162
69.1   Depression   1239
75.1   Abscess Drainage   1337
85.1   Institutional Ethics Committees   e1521
85.2   Malpractice   e1525
85.3   Interprofessional Education   e1526

DIAGNOSTIC REASONING ALGORITHMS

6.1   Confusion   74
6.2   Dizziness and Vertigo   78
6.4   Headache   84
6.5   Paresthesia and Paresis   91
6.6   Tremor   92
8.1   Alzheimer's Disease   108
34.1   Chest Pain   522
34.2   Palpitations   525
34.3   Peripheral Edema   527
38.1a   Abdominal Pain—Sudden Onset   604
38.1b   Abdominal Pain–Burning   605
38.1c   Abdominal Pain–Cramping   605
38.1d   Abdominal Pain–Visceral   606
38.2   Constipation   608
38.3   Diarrhea   610–611
38.4   Heartburn and Dyspepsia   613
38.5   Nausea and Vomiting   616
53.1   Articular and Musculoskeletal Disorders   885
57.1   Polydipsia, Polyphagia, and Polyuria   983

TREATMENT FLOWCHARTS

31.1   Asthma   470
31.2   Self-management of asthma exacerbations   471
32.1   Non-small-cell lung cancer   504
33.1   Smoking cessation strategies   515
35.4   Unstable angina   562
64.1   Management of early HIV infection   1159

Nursing—The Seasons of My Life

Nursing is the spring of my life—
Each experience is fresh and new.
There's wonderment
Like flowers washed with morning dew.

Nursing is the summer of my life—
A time to perfect all I know.
There's confidence
A world where I can grow.

Nursing is the autumn of my life—
Ablaze with experience rich and glowing.
There's compassion
From richness of caring and knowing.

Nursing is the winter of my life—
A tapestry, a mosaic of all I am.
There's challenge
To find the spring again.

—Charlotte Dison, RN

Unit I

Caring-Based Nursing
The Art

High-quality primary care is the foundation of a robust healthcare system, and perhaps more importantly, it is the essential element for improving the health of the U.S. Population. High-quality primary care is a critical component to achieve the quadruple aim of a healthcare-enhancing patient experience, improving population health, reducing costs, and improving the healthcare team experience—and it can both make healthcare more personal and address the inequities that currently plague the U.S. healthcare system.

—National Academies of Sciences, Engineering, and Medicine, 2021, p 19

Chapter 1

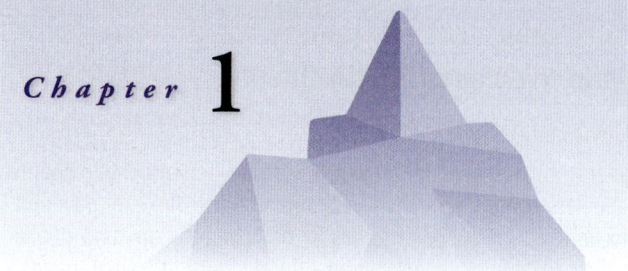

Primary Care in the Twenty-First Century:
A Circle of Caring

Jill E. Winland-Brown, EdD, APRN, FNP-BC, FAANP
Lynne M. Dunphy, PhD, APRN, FNP-BC, FAAN, FAANP
Debera J. Thomas, PhD, RN, ANP/FNP
Brian Oscar Porter, MD, PhD, MPH, MBA

Because advanced practice nurses comprise much of the primary health-care workforce, they are in an ideal situation to bring the caring "piece" into advanced practice primary care nursing. As this chapter will illustrate, the art of caring in practice is an essential element for improving the health of the nation.

WHERE WE ARE AND WHERE WE ARE GOING

Our health-care system is in flux, as issues of systemic racism and recovery from the COVID-19 pandemic dominate the national agenda and as political battles over health-care funding shift rapidly. Educational models are also in the process of being reformed; interprofessional education and team-based care are required norms, and clinical education is moving increasingly toward competency-based assessments and curricula. It "takes a village" to provide quality, cost-effective, population-based, and person-centered primary care. This book is dedicated to the notion that advanced practice registered nurses (APRNs), specifically primary care nurse practitioners (NPs), are ideal care providers to take a leadership role in our continually evolving health-care delivery system, especially in safety net settings, such as federally qualified health centers.

This chapter describes the disciplines of nursing and medicine, highlighting the different strengths that each disciplinary background brings to the care of patients. The Circle of Caring practice model on which this text is based is presented as a way of making primary care practice, which incorporates aspects of what has been traditionally defined as medical practice, richer by integrating nursing-based understanding of the lived experiences of patients and families in the context of community and caring relationships.

The Future of Nursing Reports

Heeding the recommendation of the initial Institute of Medicine's (IOM) report *The Future of Nursing: Leading Change, Advancing Health* (2011) that all nurses practice to their full scope of education, many states have implemented important changes in APRN scope of practice regulations. Nonetheless, the scope of practice for APRNs remains inconsistent across the United States, and APRN autonomy faces persistent threats, even though certain practice restrictions were lifted during the COVID-19 pandemic, starting in 2020.

The second IOM report in 2016, *Assessing Progress on the Future of Nursing,* found that there was much more to be done and suggested three themes necessary for future success: 1) the need for nurses to play a full role in practice, education, collaboration, and leadership; 2) the need for diversity in the nursing workforce; and 3) the need for better data to evaluate progress.

The third report, *The Future of Nursing 2020-2030: Charting a Path to Achieve Health Equity* (2021) (Box 1.1), continues to advocate for full practice authority for APRNs, as well as major changes to the structure of our health-care system to improve the culture of health for all. With nurses experiencing first-hand the inequitable impact of the COVID-19 pandemic's effects on the United States, they have stepped up to address these inequities. As this report highlights, the COVID-19 pandemic has taught us that the American health-care system continues to struggle with fiscal realities, as well as questions of quality, health-care disparities, structural racism, access to care, and potential burnout of the primary care workforce. Emerging pandemics (as illustrated by COVID-19), technological advances, an aging population, chronic illnesses, and alarming increases in behavioral health issues, such as those manifested by the U.S. opioid epidemic and ever-increasing gun violence, color the ongoing political debate over the American health-care system, as politicians and the public debate whether health care is a right or a privilege. For example, the Affordable Care Act of 2010, which was rejuvenated in 2021 under the Biden administration, has achieved major reforms, despite ongoing political, legal, and policy efforts to dismantle it. Within the context of legislative initiatives, payment reform has continued to evolve from a fee-for-service payment system to payment for quality, cost, and satisfaction with care (see Chapter 86). However, illnesses often continue to be treated episodically, outside the context of home, family, community, and people's day-to-day lives, in isolation from the trajectory of individuals' lives.

> **Box 1.1** The Future of Nursing 2020-2030: Charting a Path to Achieve Health Quality
>
> *Recommendation 1:*
> In 2021, all national nursing organizations should initiate work to develop a shared agenda for addressing social determinants of health and achieving health equity. This agenda should include explicit priorities across nursing practice, education, leadership, and health policy engagement. The Tri-Council for Nursing and the Council of Public Health Nursing Organizations, with their associated member organizations, should work collaboratively and leverage their respective expertise in leading this agenda-setting process. Relevant expertise should be identified and shared across national nursing organizations, including the Federal Nursing Service Council and the National Coalition of Ethnic Minority Nurse Associations. With support from the government, taxpayers, health and health-care organizations, and foundations, the implementation of this agenda should include associated timelines and metrics for measuring impact.
>
> *Recommendation 2:*
> By 2023, state and federal government agencies, health-care and public health organizations, taxpayers, and foundations should initiate substantive actions to enable the nursing workforce to address social determinants of health and health equity more comprehensively, regardless of practice setting.
>
> *Recommendation 3:*
> By 2021, nursing education programs, employers, nursing leaders, licensing boards, and nursing organizations should initiate the implementation of structures, systems, and evidence-based interventions to promote nurses' health and well-being, especially as they take on new roles to advance health equity.
>
> *Recommendation 4:*
> All organizations, including state and federal entities and employing organizations, should enable nurses to practice to the full extent of their education and training by removing barriers that prevent them from more fully addressing social needs and social determinants of health and by improving health-care access, quality, and value. These barriers include regulatory and public and private payment limitations; restrictive policies and practices; and other legal, professional, and commercial impediments. The term "commercial" refers to contractual agreements and customary practices that make antiquated or unjustifiable assumptions about nursing.
>
> *Recommendation 5:*
> Federal, tribal, state, local, and private payers and public health agencies should establish sustainable and flexible payment mechanisms to support nurses in both health care and public health, including school nurses, in addressing social needs, social determinants of health, and health equity.
>
> *Recommendation 6:*
> All public and private health-care systems should incorporate nursing expertise in designing, generating, analyzing, and applying data to support initiatives focused on social determinants of health and health equity, using diverse digital platforms, artificial intelligence, and other innovative technologies.
>
> *Recommendation 7:*
> Nursing education programs, including continuing education, and accreditors and the National Council of State Boards of Nursing should ensure that nurses are prepared to address social determinants of health and achieve health equity.
>
> *Recommendation 8:*
> To enable nurses to address inequities within communities, federal agencies and other key stakeholders within and outside the nursing profession should strengthen and protect the nursing workforce during the response to such public health emergencies as the COVID-19 pandemic and natural disasters, including those related to climate change.
>
> *Recommendation 9:*
> The National Institutes of Health, the Centers for Medicare & Medicaid Services, the Centers for Disease Control and Prevention, the Health Resources and Services Administration, the Agency for Healthcare Research and Quality, the Administration for Children and Families, the Administration for Community Living, and private associations and foundations should convene representatives from nursing, public health, and health care to develop and support a research agenda and evidence base describing the impact of nursing interventions, including multi-sector collaboration, on social determinants of health, environmental health, health equity, and nurses' health and well-being.
>
> Source: National Academies of Sciences, Engineering, and Medicine (2021). *The Future of Nursing 2020-2030: Charting a Path to Achieve Health Equity.* Washington, DC: The National Academies Press.

Healthy People 2030

Healthy People 2030 (U.S. Department of Health and Human Services, 2020), the fifth iteration of the Healthy People initiative, highlights the importance of addressing social determinants of health (SDOH) (Table 1.1). However, three of the major goals of *Healthy People 2030*—to attain healthy, thriving lives and well-being, free of preventable disease, disability, injury and premature death; to eliminate health disparities, achieve health equity, and attain health literacy to improve the health and well-being of all; and to create social, physical, and economic environments that promote attaining full potential for health and well-being for all—are far from being met. In fact, after decades of improvement, reversals are being seen in these areas, which are more apparent than ever under the relentless lens of the COVID-19 pandemic. In turn, there is resonance with the 2021 recommendations from *The Future of Nursing 2020-2030* report (Box 1.1).

TABLE 1.1 Social Determinants of Health
Addressing Social Determinants of Health (SDOH) to achieve health equity requires multisectoral and multilevel collaboration
BUILT ENVIRONMENT
Built environment is human-made surroundings that influence overall community health and individual behaviors that drive health.
COMMUNITY-CLINICAL LINKAGES
Community-clinical linkages are connections made among health-care systems and services, public health agencies, and community-based organizations to improve population health.
FOOD AND NUTRITION SECURITY
Food and nutrition security exists when all people, at all times, have physical, social, and economic access to food that is safe and consumed in sufficient quantity and quality to meet their dietary needs and food preferences, and it is supported by an environment of adequate sanitation, health services, and care, allowing for a healthy and active life.
SOCIAL CONNECTEDNESS
Social connectedness is the degree to which individuals or groups of individuals have and perceive a desired number, quality, and diversity of relationships that create a sense of belonging and being cared for, valued, and supported.
TOBACCO-FREE POLICY
Tobacco-free policies are population-based preventive measures to reduce tobacco use and tobacco-related morbidity and mortality.
By using this framework, we intend to achieve equity, which requires acknowledging and addressing unfair, avoidable, and solvable differences in opportunities for health that systematically disadvantage people.

Source: CDC (2021). National Center for Chronic Disease Prevention and Health Promotion (NCCDPHP). Social Determinants of Health. https://www.cdc.gov/chronicdisease/programs-impact/sdoh.htm

Implementing High-Quality Primary Care Report

This report defines quality primary care in the following way: "...[primary care] provides continuous, person-centered, relationship-based care that considers the needs and preferences of individuals, families, and communities. Without access to high-quality primary care, minor health problems can spiral into chronic disease, chronic disease management becomes difficult and uncoordinated, visits to emergency departments increase, preventive care lags, and health care spending soars to unsustainable levels." Using team-based, interprofessional approaches that integrate behavioral health, high-performing primary care practices should be able to seamlessly combine the strengths of various disciplines to provide quality primary care at affordable prices. The consensus group, charged with creating an implementation plan for the IOM's 1996 report, *Primary Care: America's Health in a New Era*, has provided an extensive and detailed report targeting primary care stakeholders. It is an effort to support local fit with national needs and priorities. See Box 1.2 for five identified objectives to make high-quality primary care available for all in the nation.

Challenges

Despite increasing evidence of the need for strengthening health promotion and disease prevention strategies, including principles of behavioral change and the need for caring and relationship-building interactions in the clinician-patient relationship, these shifts are not easily accomplished. Health-care disciplines are in the throes of change, and change is never easy. Disciplinary and professional turf battles abound as health-care reimbursement shrinks. For example, the American Nurses Association (ANA) recognizes that changes in U.S. federal Medicaid laws are still needed to "expand fee-for-service Medicaid to include direct payment for services provided by all nurse practitioners; recognize all NPs as primary care case managers; and require Medicaid managed care panels to include NPs" (ANA, 2021).

Increased access to quality primary care for more of the population, although morally imperative, continues to be difficult to achieve, yet the need is critical. It is well-documented that where people live and what educational level they have achieved influence life expectancy. One of the fundamental ways scientists measure the well-being of a nation is by tracking the rate at which its citizens die and how long they can be expected to live. Currently in the United States, Asian Americans live the longest (86.3 years), followed by European

---

Box 1.2 Implementation Plan to Make High-Quality Primary Care Available for All in the U.S.

1. Pay for primary care teams, not doctors, to care for people and deliver services.
2. Ensure that high-quality primary care is available to every individual and family in every community.
3. Train primary care teams where people live and work.
4. Design information technology that serves the patient, family, and interprofessional care team.
5. Ensure that high-quality primary care is implemented in the United States.

Source: National Academies of Sciences, Engineering, and Medicine (2021). *Implementing High-Quality Primary Care: Rebuilding the Foundation of Health Care.* Washington, DC: The National Academies Press. https://doi.org/10.17226/25983.

Americans (78.6 years), Native Americans (77.4 years), and African Americans (75.0 years). There are clear racial gaps in life expectancy in the United States. For all races, average life expectancy is 78.9 years.

For the first time in more than 100 years, life expectancy in the United States fell in 2015. Between 1960 and 2015, life expectancy for the total population in the United States increased by almost 10 years from 69.7 years in 1960 to 79.4 years in 2015. However, total life expectancy is projected to increase only 6.1 years between 2016 and 2060. This trend is concerning, especially as death rates are decreasing and life expectancy is increasing in most other industrialized countries. Negative economic factors, unresolved since the Great Recession of 2008, and the rise in opioid addictions and overdoses—called "deaths of despair"—have contributed to this decline in U.S. life expectancy. Job losses, unemployment, a weakening social structure, and a divisive political environment have all contributed to a declining quality of life. Rural areas have been especially hard hit. The wide availability of guns in the United States accounts in part for the rise in unintentional injuries and suicide. As of this writing, mass shootings continue to occur on almost a daily basis. The trend of decreasing life expectancy has continued, although it had plateaued for all races and ethnicities by 2019, before the start of the COVID-19 pandemic. However, by 2020, the age-adjusted death rate for Americans rose by 15.9%, as mortality from heart disease and stroke increased after having declined for years and the COVID-19 pandemic led to more than half a million deaths over just 12 months. Deaths were also up from Alzheimer's disease, respiratory disease, kidney disease, and diabetes mellitus, reflecting increases in mortality rates from eight of the top 10 leading causes of death in the United States.

Moreover, the COVID-19 pandemic has spotlighted long-simmering deficiencies in the U.S. health-care system that contribute to this disparity and the disproportionate burden carried by ethnic minorities. For example, throughout the COVID-19 pandemic, Latino and African Americans have died from COVID-19 at disproportionately higher rates than the general U.S. population. African Americans comprised 30% of hospitalized patients with COVID-19 but only 13% of the U.S. population.

As the population ages and the number of older Americans rises, so will the burden of chronic illness. Increasing numbers of older adults live with multiple chronic illnesses. Currently, 87% of Americans 65 to 79 years of age live with one chronic condition, and more than 45% have three or more chronic comorbidities. Cancer, cognitive disorders, and diabetes are projected to increase 50% by 2023. The number of individuals with disabilities is projected to grow from approximately 5.1 million in 1986 to 22.6 million by 2040, an increase of nearly 350%, even as the overall population of older adults grows by only 175%.

Whereas in the past, the burden of chronic illness care was shouldered by hospitals and specialty practices, today a substantial portion of that care must be provided in community-based primary care settings. In turn, there is a rising demand for primary care services and a decreasing supply of professionals providing these services. The empowerment of individuals, families, and communities is critical, and primary care practices and community-based services must join forces to ensure a seamless journey through a system of care across the life span.

Nursing Perspectives Needed

In this milieu, APRN care providers will be needed more than ever, specifically NPs who provide primary care. Nurses have *always* cared for community, since the time of Florence Nightingale, often focusing explicitly on health in a community context. Nurses excel in the coordination of community care services; their nursing background is situated in the empowerment of person, family, and community, and it builds on health promotion and disease prevention. Nurses know that good health starts in homes, schools, places of worship, workplaces, neighborhoods, and communities. Health means self-care, eating well, staying active, not smoking, getting recommended immunizations and health screening tests, and seeing a health-care provider when sick. Health is determined in large part by access to social and economic opportunities; the resources and supports available in homes, neighborhoods, and communities; the quality of schooling; the safety of workplaces; the cleanliness of water, food, and air; and the nature of social interactions and relationships. This is what the SDOH are all about (see Table 1.1). The conditions in which people live explain why some Americans are healthier than others and why Americans generally are not as healthy as they could be. In turn, differences in the SDOH contribute to health disparities, especially among ethnic minority populations.

The Agency for Healthcare Research and Quality (AHRQ) has developed a tool to help primary care clinicians screen and refer patients for SDOH, such as food or housing. It is one of the Tools for Change developed as part of AHRQ's EvidenceNOW: Advancing Heart Health Initiative, and it will be an additional resource on AHRQ's Social Determinants of Health site.

The tool helps primary care practices (AHRQ, 2021. New Tool Helps Primary Care Practices Screen Patients for Social Needs):

- Find resources and information to get started on patient screening and referral
- Consider what approaches work best for their practice
- Understand how to use collected information to address patients' social needs, tailor care to their circumstances, and maximize reimbursement.

In a keynote address at the Centennial Conference of the National League for Nursing in 1993, Donna

Shalala, secretary of the Department of Health and Human Services in the Clinton administration (1993 to 2001), stated that patients, families, groups, and communities are calling for the appearance of the "good fairy" in health care—someone who really hears them and their concerns, the details of their day-to-day experiences and struggles. She suggested that *nurses* are the "good fairies" that are needed. Shalala went on to chair the first IOM *Future of Nursing Report* (2011), and that report is firmly rooted in this view. This has only been accentuated during the COVID-19 pandemic.

We as primary care providers need to hear why patients and families did not take the medications that were prescribed because they could not tolerate them, could not afford them, could not get to the pharmacy to pick them up, could not remove the pill bottle cap, or could not understand or even read the directions for administration. Patients and their families need us to hear why they did not undergo the mammogram that was ordered, get the COVID-19 test and/or vaccine that was recommended, or immunize their baby because they were afraid, they had no transportation, or because putting food on the table was more important. APRNs are uniquely in tune with these day-to-day realities of patients and can work to overcome these barriers to care.

THE TIP OF THE ICEBERG

The health problems encountered in day-to-day practice are merely the tip of the iceberg on which our health-care system has traditionally focused. Reimbursement streams pay for the "tip" of this iceberg: a visit to a primary care provider to place a diagnostic label, for billing purposes, on the symptomatology of the patient and a "treatment"—typically a pharmaceutical product—aimed at treating that symptom or the underlying disease. Whether any type of health-care reform will be able to continue to effect meaningful change within a value-based system of reimbursement rooted in quality outcomes, cost-containment, and patient satisfaction remains to be seen.

The true causality of what brought the patient into the primary care setting is the much larger part of the iceberg; it lies under the surface and has often been invisible in health care. This hidden "understructure" is composed of the SDOH (see Table 1.1) built upon various lifestyle and health equity issues, such as environmental challenges, the overall health and safety of communities, food and nutrition security, social connectedness, and institution of tobacco-free policies. Socioeconomic status, spiritual issues, family concerns, psychological stressors, and biological–genetic factors that have an effect on health are challenges APRNs are well-suited to face, and the nursing perspective—Donna Shalala's "good fairy"—is even more critical in today's world than it was in 1993. Nurses understand the *whole* of the "patient's iceberg" (Fig. 1.1). They are educated to see both above *and* below

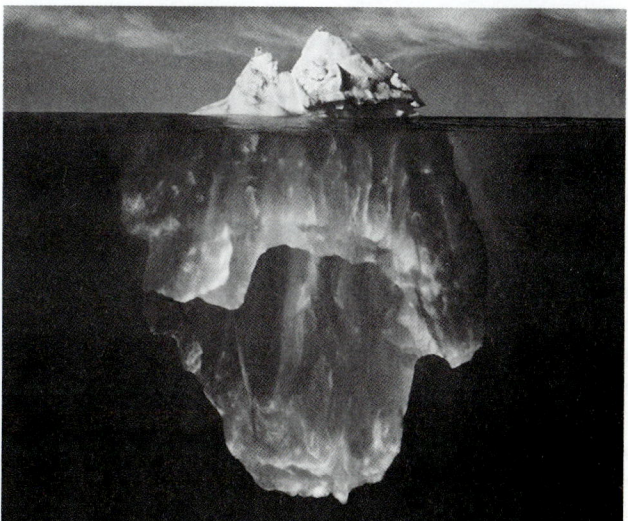

Figure 1.1 The Patient's Iceberg: Nurses understand the *whole* of the patient's "iceberg"; they are educated to see both above *and* below the water and to intervene accordingly.

the waterline and to intervene accordingly. In turn, the SDOH are inextricably bound to the lower part of the iceberg—often unseen, invisible, and unidentified. This point was made by Judge-Ellis and Wilson (2017) who issued a call to action for each NP to "...name a personal philosophy, claim the nursing identity and time needed to practice advanced practice nursing and explain the value of this practice to all" (p 588). In short, NPs need to "own" their individual practice.

The classic medical model, on the other hand, focuses on disease and abnormalities in the structure and function of genes, organs, or systems; it is concerned primarily with the malfunction or maladaptation of genetic, biological, and/or psychophysiological processes of the individual. In their textbook of family practice, Rakel and Rakel (2021) make a distinction between the terms *disease* and *illness*. *Illness* is "all the sensations of a patient and all the ramifications of a disorder." *Disease,* however, "is a theoretical and taxonomic concept, a useful tool that enables the health care provider to make inferences and predictions concerning phenomena." As such, the concepts of illness and disease belong to two different universes of discourse: *disease* in the world of theory and *illness* in the lived experience of the patient. Benner and Wrubel (1989) also distinguish between disease and the experience of disease, or illness. Illness is defined as the way sick people and their social networks perceive and respond to disease. Illness is inextricable from the context of the patient's life, including the intersections of social, political, economic, spiritual, and cultural factors—in other words, the whole of the iceberg, which includes all community-based, socially constructed determinants of health.

Historically, nursing has been concerned with the whole person and the promotion of health across the life span—what Florence Nightingale referred to as "the Laws of Health." Nurses also have traditionally focused on people's responses to the illness experience in the context of their day-to-day lives. Much of the challenge in the role of the APRN is the negotiation of seemingly disparate worlds: the reconciliation of an essentially holistic nursing model with a health-care system still focused predominantly on disease-oriented care. It is precisely this nexus between more discrete diagnostic categories of disease and a more holistic view of the continuum between health and illness—the whole iceberg—that gives nursing its identity, richness, diversity, and usefulness.

Today's primary care NPs must dwell in this nexus and bridge these two realities—the world of disease and the world of illness, including the context of the patient's life in all its complexity. The increasing and necessary placement of APRNs in primary care settings and teams across the health-care continuum provides nursing with the opportunity to effect change on both micro and macro levels—in the lives of individual patients and families, as well as on the well-being of the organizations in which they work and the communities in which they live. When APRNs fully actualize their role, the impact can ultimately extend to the larger global community, a phenomenon by which the COVID-19 pandemic has highlighted the interconnectedness of us all.

PREVENTION AS HEALTH PROMOTION

Clinicians agree that patients need to be encouraged to change their health behaviors. This is a skill that needs to be taught, but it is not included in many nursing and medical curricula, although for the health-care provider, healthful behavioral change is undergirded by the context of a caring provider–patient relationship. The challenge in making the prevention of illness through preventive care a meaningful part of health-care reform involves changing both behavior *and* reimbursement streams.

Changing health behaviors involves altering habits that have "complex developmental, psychological, cultural, and socioeconomic roots" (Blacksher, 2009). In addition, health promotion and disease prevention require comprehensive policy changes that support the often tedious, unglamorous work of behavioral change, as well as community-based services. The care of the sick, the real-life day-to-day health needs of people, their social and economic circumstances, and the health of their communities are all part of the traditional domain of nursing practice. Florence Nightingale understood these links and discussed them in her prophetic *Notes on Nursing* (1860). More recently, nurse theorist Margaret Newman and colleagues (Newman et al, 2008) asserted that the NP–patient relationship has become the central focus of the nursing discipline: "It is the nature of the nurse-patient relationship that unites the practice of nursing ... nursing actions occur within the context of a unified commitment. That commitment is to a caring relationship focused on understanding the meaning of the current situation for the people involved and appreciating the pattern of evolving forces shaping health, so that appropriate actions can be realized."

Nurse historian Ellen Baer noted that the services demanded today of primary care providers are broader in scope than those within the domain of medicine before the 1960s. Supportive functions, previously the domain of the clergy or multigenerational families, began falling within the purview of the primary care provider. Likewise, the conceptual shift to health promotion, coupled with increased knowledge about healthy lifestyles, requires that primary care providers be well-grounded in their patients' community context. In making her case for the role of the nurse in primary care, Baer (1993) concludes: "The best reason for nurses to provide primary care is because they are nurses. Nursing's focus on people; its blend of medical, behavioral, and social science expertise; and its commitment to caring, teaching, counseling, and supporting patients are the characteristics of nursing that make nurses so uniquely qualified to provide primary health care services."

This text provides a nursing-based approach to primary care and includes content on health promotion and disease prevention, as well as the diagnosis, management, and treatment of disease in the primary care setting. The essentials of disease pathology and management necessary for safe and satisfactory functioning in primary care practice are integrated into a view of the wholeness of people, an understanding of human responses, and a repertoire of therapeutic options. This perspective will enable the primary care provider, regardless of disciplinary background, to become an orchestrator of health and wellness, as well as a skilled negotiator and mediator in the space that exists between health and illness—in other words, between disease and the "lived experience of the patient" in the context of their community.

Self-actualization Through Advanced Practice

APRNs must understand the discipline of nursing to effectively fill the gap between health and illness with true nursing care. Nurses on teams and in interprofessional educational settings must be confident and secure about their knowledge base and its intrinsic value, as well as the critical nature of their contributions to the care of the patient and the subsequent outcomes of that care. To this end, the American Association of Colleges of Nursing (AACN) has called for all APRN preparation to take place in practice-based programs at the doctoral level—the Doctor of Nursing Practice (DNP)—by 2025. The DNP is a catalyst, allowing nursing to develop and expand nursing knowledge and practice through health promotion and disease prevention practices, essential for disciplinary distinction and growth.

The AACN, the "voice of academic nursing," approved and published a new document *The Essentials: Core Competencies for Professional Nursing Education* (AACN, April 2021). In it, the AACN lays out a category for specialty/role requirements/competencies beyond the DNP. A variety of postgraduate education and certifications have emerged, sometimes called *residencies* or *fellowships,* some housed in educational institutions and others in clinical settings.

This document affirms that all professional nursing education has the foundation of a liberal education, built on the knowledge of nursing as a discipline, and utilizes the principles of competency-based education (AACN, 2021, p 3). The *Essentials* documents a framework reflecting requirements across nursing educational levels that include nursing-based knowledge and applied experience. They have outlined the following 10 Domains with descriptors. The Domains are as follows:

- Domain 1: Knowledge for Nursing Practice
- Domain 2: Person-Centered Care
- Domain 3: Population Health
- Domain 4: Scholarship for Nursing Practice
- Domain 5: Quality and Safety
- Domain 6: Interprofessional Partnerships
- Domain 7: Systems-Based Practice
- Domain 8: Information and Healthcare Technologies
- Domain 9: Professionalism
- Domain 10: Personal, Professional, and Leadership Development

There is tremendous congruence between the recommendations in *Implementing High-Quality Primary Care* and the more broadly worded new AACN Domains. The remainder of this chapter will discuss the essential nursing knowledge that professional nursing education builds upon, as well as some of the history of the evolution of this knowledge, and contrasts this with the emergence of medical knowledge and concepts. Advanced practice nursing knowledge and its relation to care of people are further detailed.

HISTORICAL PERSPECTIVES ON ADVANCED PRACTICE NURSING

As far back as 1860, Nightingale proclaimed in *Notes on Nursing* that there were laws of sickness and laws of health. However, there was not enough known, she wrote, about the laws of health. Nursing the "room" (meaning the environment surrounding the patient) was as important as nursing the patient. Somewhat more controversially, she also wrote that nursing and medicine were like "cats and dogs" and should not be mixed.

The early public health nurses of Lillian Wald's Henry Street Settlement House at the turn of the 20th century created their own vision of health and illness, living and working in the community they served. Lavinia Dock, one of the first Henry Street nurses, evolved a model of nursing (Fig. 1.2) that still has important implications for the current health-care system. New and emerging primary care models are attempting to recapture population-based care, health promotion, and disease prevention in more meaningful and reimbursable ways, such as through team approaches, patient-centered medical homes (PCMHs), and affordable care organizations, in which health-care systems are integrated across the continuum of care.

As noted by Blacksher in an editorial in the *Hastings Center Report on Prevention,* "Health happens where people live, learn, pray, love, work, and play" (2009). These activities flow from the spirit, science, and art of nursing or the "heart, head, and hand" of nursing (a phrase popularized by Virginia Henderson [1966]). The first instances of standardized nursing care protocols, for example, evolved from the work of early school nurses and the New York City Public Health Department. These early public health nurses enjoyed an autonomy of practice similar to that exercised by today's primary care providers. Dock and Stewart (1920) likened the relationship between nursing and medicine to workers on a team who complement and supplement each other; the relationship is based on neither independence nor subordination but on interdependence and cooperation.

Henderson's 1966 book, *The Nature of Nursing,* was an attempt to provide nursing with its own explanatory model for practice. Building on her own experiences in nursing (Henderson also spent time as a public health nurse at the Henry Street Settlement) and on her understanding

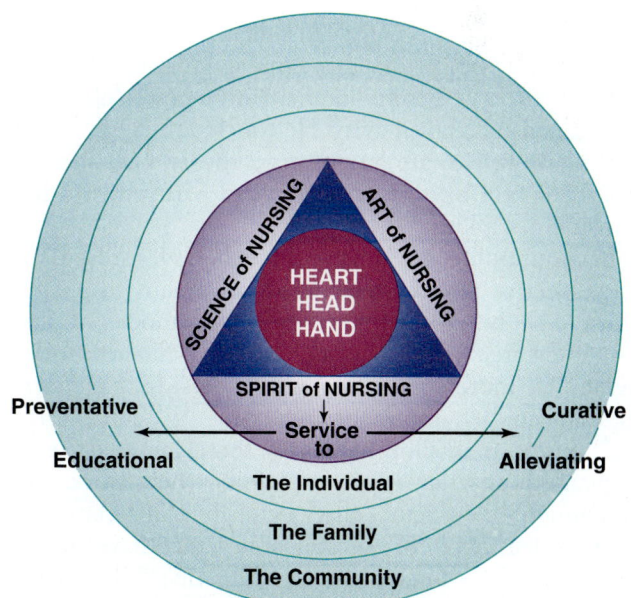

Figure 1.2 Dock Model of Nursing: The professional equipment of the modern nurse and the scope of responsibilities. Source: *Dock LL, Stewart IM.* A Short History of Nursing: From the earliest times to the present day. *3rd ed. New York, NY: G.P. Putnam's Sons; 1931: 337.*

of physiology, she tried to place nursing on a continuum with medical care. Henderson argued that nurses had to place themselves (figuratively) "inside" patients to become their "counterpart, alter ego, or helper."

Martha Rogers, another foundational nurse-theoretician, argued for the necessity of an independent basis of nursing science, out of which autonomous nursing practice grows. According to Rogers, "Primary care by nurses is as old as modern nursing," citing examples rooted in her early public health nursing experiences (as quoted by Hektor, 1989). Those patients who ended up in hospitals were, in her words, "our mistakes" (as quoted by Hektor, 1989). Overall, the early nurse practitioner "movement" evolved with little connection to academia and the flurry of nursing conceptual models and theories that proliferated throughout the 1970s and 1980s. These pioneering nurse practitioners, rooted in clinical practice, usually in a primary care setting, and often "trained" in certificate programs, had little patience with the abstractions of nursing theory that provided little meaning for their day-to-day practices. They needed and valued the medical model to care for their patients. Yet most remained nurses at heart, devoted to health promotion and disease prevention and providing holistic care to their patients.

Very few nursing models have addressed or attempted to make sense of the dichotomy of nurse practitioner practice and medical care. Some practitioners argue that no dichotomy exists, while others have identified the relationship between advanced nursing practice and medical practice as an issue requiring ongoing attention. Cody (1994) views medicine as still dominating nursing politically, and he states that many nurses "actually value having medical tasks delegated to them." On a more ominous note, he points out that nursing must realize what is merely delegated from another (more powerful) discipline can also be taken away. He concludes, "Only when nurses everywhere are guided by a theory base specific to nursing will nursing have achieved parity with other scholarly disciplines."

In an unpublished paper, Lynaugh (1989) discussed the respective roles of nurses and physicians in greater depth. She noted that the biomedical model of disease and cure, which swept across the Western world, seemed far more compelling and promising than nursing's holism, environmentalism, and "watchful waiting" approach to illness. Nurses, she elaborated, seem to be both inarticulate in explaining their work and "touchingly confident" that altruism will eventually be rewarded. Years of medical dominance have drawn a veil over the work of nursing. This invisibility has a broad impact because it compromises the public's access to good nursing care in an era in which reimbursement for care is restricted to payment based exclusively on the phenomena of interest to physicians. The power relationships among patient, nurse, and physician are complicated by economic issues, professional territoriality on all sides, and profound questions of disciplinary identity; therefore, adjustments in these relationships will come slowly, step by step, but inevitably. An essential component of this process is making the "invisible" work of nurses more visible. It is the part of the iceberg that is below the water that takes up so much of nursing's time and energy and is so unnamed and unseen. The demonstration of nursing's contribution to patient care is vital, and this is accomplished, in part, through the clear articulation of nursing's theoretical base.

In the day-to-day realities of practice and the needs of patients and families, these issues are often obscured. After all, the needs of patients unite APRNs and physicians. As clinicians, APRNs and MDs work well together and will engage in collaborative relationships most often when caring for patients. The real tension between nursing and medicine lies in the politicized agendas of each, as advanced by their respective professional organizations.

As nursing theory embraces the mode of midrange theory development and testing, with real-life clinical applications for practice, the applicability to advanced practice nursing and the utilization of theory-based practice should increase. This still begs the question, however, of an underlying theoretical basis for advanced practice nursing. It can be argued, as Burman et al (2009) do in an article titled "Reconceptualizing the Core of Nurse Practitioner Education and Practice," that "the heart and soul of nursing is health promotion both in healthy persons and those dealing with chronic illness." Nursing practice as a DNP should focus more explicitly on health promotion, changing health behaviors, and chronic disease management, thus advancing a unique nursing science. These are traditional nursing domains and strengths.

CHANGING MODELS OF ADVANCED NURSING PRACTICE

Advanced practice nursing is not filling the gap with medical care where it does not exist; it is filling the existing gap in healthcare with the core of nursing practice... The core of advanced practice nursing lies within nursing's disciplinary perspective on human–environment and caring relationships that facilitate health and healing. This core is delineated specifically in the theoretic foundations of nursing. True advanced nursing practice is theory-based [and] fully integrated into the nurse's way of being and practicing.

—Marlaine Smith. The core of advanced practice nursing. Nurs Sci Q. 1995;8(1):2–3.

In a study by Lewis and Brykczynski (1994), the authors elaborated on the *practical* knowledge as well as the *healing* role of nurse practitioners. In the discussion of their findings, the authors state that to bring about healing, nurse practitioners fight for patient's rights and access to care—going beyond the call of duty by visiting diverse care settings, such as schools, jails, prisons, homeless shelters, residential housing communities, federally qualified health centers (FQHCs), and community health centers; making phone calls; driving patients to appointments; and attending funerals. The practitioners in the study described both the professional and personal satisfaction derived from their caring practices, even when the rewards of such actions were limited. The authors situate the work of these practitioners within a caring paradigm, citing Sally Gadow, Jean Watson, and Madeline Leininger. They also cite the 1991 work of Benner, who, in studying the effectiveness of expert nurses, found that mere technique and knowledge were not enough and that caring, or a certain level of human involvement, was required for expert "human practice." Indeed, such expert "human practice" should be a goal of all primary care providers.

Johnson (1993) cites clear evidence of a nursing perspective in NP primary care practice. According to Johnson, nurse practitioner–patient dialogue incorporates the voice of medicine and the voice of the "lifeworld" (of the patient). A skilled practitioner "knows self" and how to share personal experience to either enhance the patient's progress or strengthen the provider–patient bond. An element of camaraderie was viewed as positive and not in opposition to maintaining a professional stance. *Coordination, continuity,* and *advocacy* were the major functions the NPs in this study believed that they contributed to this practice. All primary care practices need these functions, which constitute some of the foundational ideas of a PCMH.

Swanson (1995) proposed "A Spirit-Focused Conceptual Model of Nursing for the Advanced Practice Nurse" in which she identified the core of every person, both patient and nurse, as the spirit. She describes the act of nursing as a goal-directed interpersonal relationship between the patient and nurse, based on traditional nursing process components, including assessing, planning, intervening, and evaluating. These broad-based interventions range from play, music, and stories to utilization of counseling principles, such as active listening and anticipatory guidance. Indeed, the use of this approach in primary care nursing practice could be adapted by any primary care practitioner.

The Shuler Nurse Practitioner Practice Model (Shuler & Davis, 1993) is an ambitious attempt to describe the nurse practitioner's integrated role. Building on a holistic nursing assessment, the key step is a mutual identification of unmet patient health needs to identify health problems. The treatment plan must then be mutually agreeable and oriented toward self-care, with disease prevention and health promotion activities incorporated into the treatment plan. Nonpharmacological treatments, including alternative and complementary healing practices, are also integrated into the treatment plan. These approaches are framed within the concept of functioning within a multidisciplinary team and could be seen as particularly relevant in today's team-based clinical care settings.

In addition, Shuler's model is seen as enhancing both the patient's and the nurse practitioner's personal movement toward wellness. Patients are encouraged to examine their lives honestly and to identify areas that are not "balanced." The patient's physical and psychological ability to participate in wellness activities is assessed, and creative, uninhibited problem-solving and identification of appropriate wellness activities are pursued. The model emphasizes that the primary care practitioner's personal commitment to health and wellness can have a direct effect on the ability to influence positive patient outcomes.

Snyder (1996) conceptualizes advanced practice within a nursing paradigm built around human responses as a focus for nursing interventions. They identify the following focuses for advanced practice nursing:

1. Self-care limitations
2. Impaired functioning in the areas of rest, sleep, ventilation, circulation, nutrition, and the like
3. Pain and discomfort
4. Emotional problems related to illness and treatment, life-threatening events, or daily experiences, such as anxiety, loss, or loneliness
5. Distortion of symbolic functions reflected in interpersonal and intellectual processes, such as hallucinations
6. Deficiencies in decision-making ability to determine personal choices
7. Self-image changes required by health status
8. Dysfunctional perceptual orientations to health
9. Strains related to life processes, such as birth, development, and death
10. Problematic affiliative relationships

Patient problems, conceptualized in this manner, are amenable to uniquely nursing-based interventions, as well as medical approaches. Attention to human responses, as such, provides the missing link to much that is absent within today's health-care system. Many of these responses are tied to SDOH—such as where one lives and works. Our current health-care system, however, is not structured in such a way to make many of these practices sustainable, because such interventions are not typically coded for reimbursement.

Another promising direction is Nurse Coaching, which promotes integrative approaches for health and well-being and can be used by APRNs to promote behavioral change. It supports the need for clinicians to help their patients develop a plan for healthy living and to support them in making the stepwise journey to health. This builds on the theoretical model of health and health promotion that embraces the integration of body, mind, and spirit. Utilizing motivational interviewing, nonjudgmental acceptance of the patient, the transtheoretical model of behavioral change, appreciative inquiry, cultural perspectives, and "rituals of healing," this largely nursing-based model extends nursing practice.

CHANGING MODELS OF MEDICAL PRACTICE

Advances in therapeutics over the course of the 20th century, which are often taken for granted today, were far more effective than therapeutic advances before this period. Medicine was able to intervene—specifically, powerfully, and radically—in the course of previously fatal diseases. Today, no disorder, however complex, seems beyond the possibility of understanding and cure, provided the health-care system is willing to invest in research and development. As a result, the effects of medicine is felt far beyond the immediacies of the patient–provider encounter. Alcoholism, for example, viewed as a moral disorder in earlier times, is now a phenomenon conceptualized as a disease, with an array of psychological and pharmacological interventions available to practitioners.

A review of the progress of medicine in combating disease is a journey from an integrated view of illness and therapeutics to one of discrete diseases with distinct causes and an armamentarium of ever-expanding and specific therapeutics. From the time of the ancient Greeks and Romans until well into the 19th century, illness was seen as an imbalance in the economy of the entire body, which could be expressed in the relationships between input or output of food, sweat, secretions, urine, phlegm, and the like. Treatment was focused on restoring harmony and balance between body and environment (a view promulgated by Nightingale, 1860/1969). Specific symptoms were not treated; instead, a systemic physiological effect was sought through such methods as inducing or facilitating sweating, fever, diuresis, and/or vomiting. These interventions, it was theorized, would assist the body to recover its balance.

Throughout the course of the 19th century, however, this integrated view of disease and therapeutics was increasingly challenged by notions of discrete disease states with specific causes. Illnesses seemed less amenable to purges, bleeding, and diuretics (the so-called *holistic approaches*) than was previously thought. Late in the modern era, the first active principles of some of the oldest and most useful botanicals were isolated, and later some were even synthesized. A new dimension was added to the emerging concept of specificity of therapeutics by the discovery of sulfonamides in the late 1930s and penicillin in the early 1940s. Not only could therapy be directed at particular symptoms, but for the first time, therapeutics also could become "radical," matching the power of the surgeon's knife—that is, they could eradicate the primary cause of an illness, in this case, specific microorganisms.

Increasingly tailored therapies, such as disease-specific antisera, highly fractionated blood components, polypeptide hormones, biological immunotherapeutics, and individualized gene therapies, comprise the modern pharmaceutical treatment armamentarium. Advances in laboratory analysis and diagnostic techniques confer the potential for these therapies to effect cures at the molecular level, related, for example, to genetic abnormalities in the patient or at the loci of infection or other eternal insult. The era of specific and radical therapeutics has only just begun, as the continued trend toward even greater specificity in the diagnosis and management of disease, extending to the genetic level, is the hallmark of this era of precision medicine. This will continue to have profound effects on the medical profession, society, and the inherent power imbalances among patients, nurses, and physicians. Newly developed diagnostic and therapeutic technologies will require increasingly sophisticated and specialized health-care providers, whose training must cover precision medicine treatment strategies. In turn, the costliness of these interventions and the practitioners who provide them will surely raise questions of access to care and equitable distribution among all patients, as there is overwhelming evidence that technological innovations are some of the most important drivers of health-care costs. For this reason, primary care practice is likely to remain at the vanguard of disease prevention and health promotion, which are key elements for countering increasing health-care costs.

Against the backdrop of this historical context, medicine's successes led to a generation of physician-specialists with an increasingly narrow focus on human disease and technologically advanced medical interventions that are often far removed from the day-to-day lives of patients. Although this has been a useful stance for the creation of highly effective medical interventions, when universalized to all realms of medical practice, this approach may be antithetical to the fulfillment of the core moral and social responsibilities of medicine. Care—when defined as helping the patient and family to cope, offering reassurance, educating, and relieving worry—does not require a high level of scientific sophistication or technological advancement; however, it does require human understanding and empathy.

In the past, when physician remuneration was less driven by technological advances and physicians were highly integrated members of the community, issues of care could be negotiated more successfully between doctor and patient, with more dedicated time for two-way physician-patient interaction. Today, however, physicians are increasingly at risk of being seen as unfamiliar interventionists, with multiple competing priorities and limited time for direct patient interaction. This raises a fearful dilemma for patients who must trust physicians because of their specialized knowledge and power to heal, as that trust may be undermined by suspicion of the physician's self-interest. Additionally, social responsibilities in a broader public health sense have become neglected, as population-based health indicators in the United States continue to lag behind those of other developed nations.

Despite the emphasis on medical advancements purported by many sectors of the health-care industry—including for-profit pharmaceutical and medical device companies, as well as large health-care delivery systems—there is nonetheless recognition of the limits of medical progress and technological innovation on community-based and population health. Beginning with the AIDS epidemic in the early 1980s through today's struggle with multidrug-resistant organisms and pandemic-level infectious disease, it has become increasingly clear that not all aspects of human health and wellness can be controlled solely through medical technology and the development of newer therapeutics. In numerous studies over time, 60% of the improvement in population-based health status is tied to improved socioeconomic factors, particularly education and income. With the notable exception of health care for the older adult population, only approximately 40% of improvements in health status result from medical care.

For example, the unprecedented speed with which highly effective COVID-19 vaccines were developed—thanks to cutting-edge, mRNA-based technology—was critical to address the COVID-19 pandemic. However, without the infrastructure and coordinated plans to manufacture, distribute, and administer these vaccines globally, their impact would be minimal. Likewise, the unwillingness of large numbers of people to receive these vaccines due to fear, suspicion, or a misunderstanding of their safety and efficacy profile has the potential to render this technological advancement largely moot. However, primary care practice is well-positioned to address these barriers at the patient level through supportive, understanding, and caring provider-patient relationships.

In turn, there has been an increasing call for a better balance between cure-oriented and care-oriented medicine. Chronic disease continues to be the most difficult and expensive type of health problem to manage. People are living longer with chronic conditions and significant morbidity, and much of primary care is focused on long-term management of chronic disease. To address this, care-oriented medicine reflects the well-coordinated assistance from all relevant providers to enable patients to manage disease, combined with the marshaling of critical family-based and social supports.

A TRANSFORMATIVE TEMPLATE: THE CIRCLE OF CARING

Both the traditional medical and nursing models are predicated on a subjective and objective clinical database, a labeling of the patient's problems and responses, a therapeutic plan, and an evaluation of patient outcomes. The Circle of Caring model builds on these features and expands them to include the following:

- A broadened and contextualized database, more typical of a holistic nursing assessment, that gives the health-care provider a more in-depth understanding of the patient's situation, life, strengths, and weaknesses, including SDOH.
- A labeling of the patient's concern that more actively incorporates the patient's responses to the meaning of illness in day-to-day life, as well as standard medical diagnostic language.
- A holistic and creative approach to an individualized therapeutic plan that utilizes nursing interventions based on evidence, including complementary therapies as appropriate, incorporated with standardized pharmacological, surgical, and other nonpharmacological interventions.
- A view of outcomes based on the patient, family, social group, and community perceptions of improvement, as well as the more traditional quantified outcome measures, such as mortality and morbidity, with emerging primary care quality indicators and costs of care also built into these outcomes. This integrates the health of populations into the outcomes of care.

The Circle of Caring model is a synthesized view of the problem-solving methodology that may be used in a variety of settings—primary care, acute care, and community-based settings. The model is diagrammed in Figure 1.3. The basic problem-solving process used by nurses is represented by the boxes in the middle of the diagram. This process is encircled by a visual representation of caring—the interpersonal process that occurs between the caregiver and the patient and reflects the patient's family, social group, and community.

The ability to provide effective and meaningful care for the patient is based on the qualities of authentic presence, patience, courage, advocacy, commitment, and knowing. These qualities of caring enable the nurse to hear the patient's "call" and to fashion creative nursing responses. It is this authenticity in the nurse–patient encounter that allows the nurse to enter the lifeworld of that person and be truly compassionate in providing care.

A Broadened, Contextualized Database

A contextualized approach—the lived experience of the patient in the context of community—is central to this model and is one that most nurses have learned in their undergraduate nursing programs. Although the patient's subjective perception of this experience is captured in the history portion of the assessment database, the Circle of Caring is based on hearing the patient's story in all its complexity, as well as eliciting the patient's own unique meaning of *health*. In addition, increased attention is focused on the interplay among perceptual, psychodynamic, socioeconomic, cultural, and environmental factors that have an effect on the patient's health status—in other words, increased awareness and attention to the SDOH.

The Nature of Patient Responses

The ANA's Social Policy Statement has many essential features of professional nursing. Among the definitions of nursing are "provision of a caring relationship that

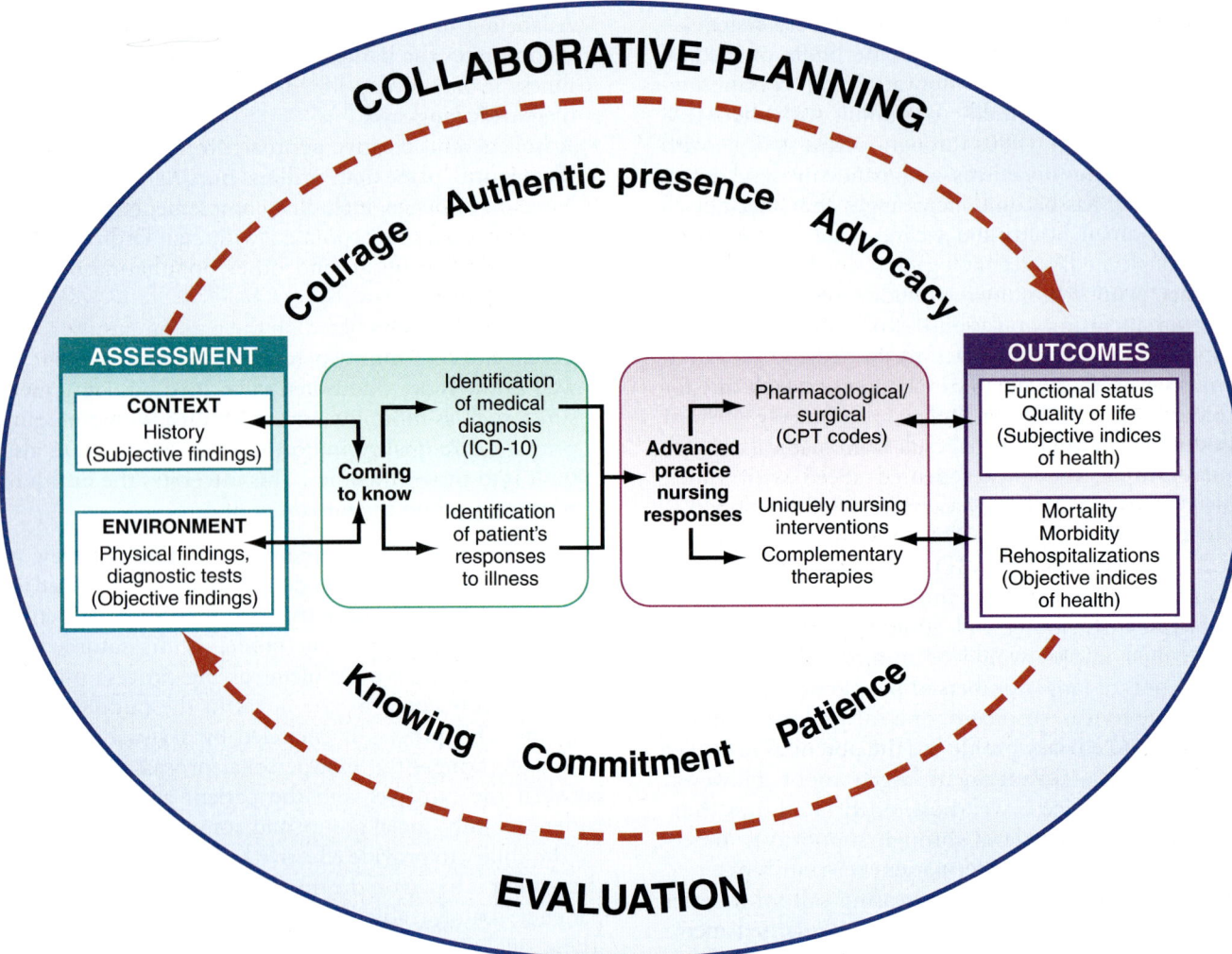

Figure 1.3 The Circle of Caring model.

facilitates health and healing and attention to the range of human experiences and responses to health and illness within the physical and social environments." Given this context, the Circle of Caring model may be used effectively with the traditional tools of nursing diagnosis. Boykin and Schoenhofer (2001) conceptualized the phenomenon of human responses as "calls for nursing." As such, these calls remain unique, interactional, and contextualized, and thus unamenable to any form of generic labeling. By coming to know people as caring persons, the nurse is able to fully hear each patient's call.

Labeling the patient's problem (i.e., the "call for nursing"), be it in medical or nursing diagnostic terminology or in a more generic format, helps to address patient responses more effectively. Thus, labeling involves acknowledgment and knowledge of the complex interplay of perceptual, psychodynamic, socioeconomic, cultural, and environmental factors that contribute to health. APRNs are especially skilled at eliciting and understanding this complexity and fashioning nursing-based responses that are uniquely suited to the individual.

A Creative Approach to Therapeutics and Interventions

Another hallmark of the Circle of Caring model is its broadened approach to therapeutics and interventions. This approach should be actualized in day-to-day practice by APRNs, yet it remains a particularly invisible piece of nursing work. This flexible nursing-based approach entails working with the individual patient to tailor evidence-based interventions geared toward the meaning of *health* as defined by that patient. Building on today's standards of medical and nursing practice, interventions are fine-tuned for each patient, in the context of their community. Although a focus of this text is to provide today's evidence-based standards of care, this approach often requires care providers to make decisions through narrowly prescribed filters. As noted by Payne, "There is an art to clinical practice that extends beyond hard science and numbers and often requires swift, sound decision making in an environment of incomplete evidence. Sometimes no formula or calculation based on quantified evidence and data can determine the appropriate action" (2009).

Alternative and complementary therapies are considered within their evidentiary basis and meaningfulness for the patient. This requires a creative approach to therapeutics that includes a holistic approach to healing, as well as a sophisticated understanding of evidence-based practice. Patients increasingly call for alternative and complementary approaches to their treatment in the face of rapid growth of this multibillion-dollar industry and largely unregulated direct-to-consumer marketing.

In the practice of nursing as caring (see Chapter 2), the nurse is described as "an artist who responds creatively to calls for nursing with unique nursing responses." Any taxonomy of nursing must, by necessity, have universal applicability. What distinguishes so many of nursing's interventions, however, is precisely their uniqueness and the tailoring of an individual response to each patient. A broadened approach to therapeutics and interventions based on a contextualized database implies attention to the context of a patient's life, including the SDOH for the patient, as well as the patient's family and community.

INTERPROFESSIONAL CARE: FROM PATIENT TO POPULATION

Current outcomes-based research demonstrates the need to incorporate patients' perceptions as measured both objectively (by functional assessments and similar methods) and subjectively. Quality-of-life measures and, most important, the various and individualistic meanings of health and illness must be taken more fully into consideration. The patient experience is a frequently used measure of quality care in both acute and primary care settings. Treatment plans must be assessed according to their potential to assist patients, families, social groups, and communities to meet their goals in ways that are meaningful to them, not just as standard items on a checklist of preventive measures. The voice of an increasingly informed, information-savvy health-care consumer demands no less.

The PCMH as a model of health care puts patients at the center of care. Multiple social and environmental factors affecting health are recognized as additional pieces of the health-care puzzle—the traditional realm of public health. SDOH are becoming increasingly recognized as key components of the enormous understructure of the primary care iceberg discussed earlier—the all-too-often "unseen" and invisible aspects beneath the water (Fig. 1.1). Sometimes labeled community-oriented primary care or *primary health care* (according to the World Health Organization, 2008), approaches to care that incorporate these social and environmental factors are now understood to be essential elements of a truly reformed health-care system.

Although this holistic perspective was largely abandoned by allopathic medicine in the earlier part of the 20th century in favor of technology-based interventions and medical specialization, modern medicine recognizes the need for multidisciplinary interventions to provide more effective care with lasting effects. An interprofessional approach to patient care is also needed to deal with health-care realities that highlight the interplay among human health and environmental and social influences (e.g., the health effects of community violence, gun violence, teen pregnancy, sexual and physical abuse, and HIV infection). As with medicine, nursing has renewed its emphasis on population-based approaches, reaffirming its historic roots. There is now a shared understanding of the importance of these approaches. In turn, today's health-care climate is ideal to build an interprofessional educational base, consisting of shared core understandings of care, but with variations to implement or practice these understandings.

FURTHER UNDERSTANDING THE CIRCLE OF CARING

The Circle of Caring model has grown out of, and is rooted in, the assumption that caring is the central concept of nursing. Boykin and Schoenhofer (2001) contend that the special contributions of nursing are to nurture the wholeness of people and their environment through caring. Additionally, they affirm all nursing care takes place within nursing situations, as "shared lived experiences in which caring between the persons of nurse and nursed enhances the process of living and growing in caring" (see Chapter 2 of this text). Watson (1988) viewed caring as an intersubjective human process based on the belief that "persons learn from one another how to be human by identifying ourselves with others or finding their dilemmas in ourselves." Boykin and Schoenhofer (2001) extended this concept and defined caring in nursing as "the intentional and authentic presence of the nurse with another who is recognized as a person living caring and growing in caring."

Mayeroff (1971) discussed the primacy of caring as a process in contrast to caring as a product, with caring viewed as an end in and of itself. Mayeroff also identified "ingredients" of caring: knowing, alternating rhythms, patience, honesty, courage, humility, trust, and hope. Boykin and Schoenhofer (2001) viewed caring in nursing "as a mutual human process in which the nurse responds with authentic presence to a call from another." The caring attributes of the Circle of Caring are based on these—knowing, patience, authentic presence, commitment, courage, and advocacy—and are elaborated by Boykin and Schoenhofer in Chapter 2 of this text. These caring attributes characterize the nurse-patient relationship, enabling healing. In this context, healing is meant in the broadest sense of the word, as it may even imply a peaceful and comforted death.

While this chapter has focused on the complementary professions of nursing and medicine, the Circle of Caring is grounded in interprofessional practice that may include many other disciplines, such as dentistry, social work, pharmacy, and physical and occupational therapy. Seemingly disparate partners may also play a role in health care, such as lawyers and advocates working for social equity, local and global businesses creating healthier communities, and local, state, and federal governments developing healthier housing and safer community environments.

No single discipline, perspective, or role can heal the problems ailing the U.S. health-care system. All are needed more than ever to shape a healthful future, and all must rethink their roles, functions, and professional cultures. Moving away from the hierarchical role structures of the traditional hospital setting creates an opportunity to redefine the content and processes of clinical practice and negotiate a new and as yet undefined space. The boundaries of practice continue to expand or contract for various health-care stakeholders during this transformative period, and the larger questions for all health-care professions include the following:

- How will all health-care professionals be accountable to their patients?
- Are physicians and APRNs willing to share accountability in a responsible manner?
- How can disciplines work together in a meaningful way to achieve the goals and objectives of *Healthy People 2030*?
- How can medicine and nursing, as well as other disciplines, work together to achieve the triple aim of health-care reform: improving the patient experience of care (including quality and satisfaction), improving the health of populations, and reducing the per capita cost of health care?

Lynaugh, in an unpublished paper from 1989 specifically discussing medicine and nursing, suggests that both disciplines can occupy the same territory to the benefit of patient care; however, she notes that tension is created by proximity, stating that "physicians and nurses quarrel occasionally when they jostle each other in the narrow passageway of patient care." This can be further extrapolated to other health-care professions. However, Lynaugh makes the case that tension is preferable to the distrust and ignorance that stem from silence and distance between disciplines. She advocates a "productive tension" and social parity between health-care professions that will benefit the care of all people. Health-care professionals are *all* natural allies, with the best interests of the patient at their core. In turn, all perspectives are needed, working together, for effective change to occur in the health-care system. This provides a useful way to view true interprofessional practice. All disciplines have a unique view—working together provides a richness and depth that no one single discipline can provide.

In daily practice, primary care providers hear the frustration of patients and their families in dealing with today's health-care system. Although the technology of medical care continues to advance—telehealth, digital health apps, and precision medicine being prime examples—the interactional and collaborative aspects of care are often underdeveloped. Gradually, these technologies move toward providing more meaningful person engagement and experiences, which are examples of Circles of Caring. As a model for patients, families, social groups, and communities, the Circle of Caring model is also a way to document and describe the practice of primary care providers, who respond to calls from patients and who imaginatively, creatively, and powerfully foster meaningful responses in a situational context. These responses may be fashioned on the micro level in the one-to-one clinician-patient relationship in primary or acute care or on the macro level, as nursing-based knowledge unites with traditional public health approaches and is applied to the care of communities and populations (see Chapter 3).

In turn, this transformative model incorporates the strengths of nursing, public health, and medicine, and reformulates them in a new model of care. Primary care practitioners, now educated in interprofessional models, are the appropriate providers to demonstrate the efficacy of an integrated model of caregiving, rooted in the lived experience of the patient, as experienced in the context of the larger community. This text offers the necessary tools to provide care in ways that will be meaningful for patients, their families, their social groups, and the larger communities in which they live.

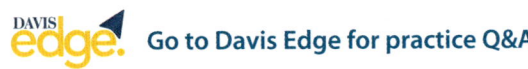 Go to Davis Edge for practice Q&A

REFERENCES

Ahmad FB, Cisewski JA, Minifio A, et al. Provisional Mortality Data—United States, 2020. Morbidity and Mortality Weekly Report (MMWR). *Weekly* / April 9, 2021 / 70(14);519–522. Centers for Disease Control and Prevention.

AHRQ, 2021. New Tool Helps Primary Care Practices Screen Patients for Social Needs. 6/22/2021.

American Association of Colleges of Nursing—The Voice of Academic Nursing (2021) The Essentials: Core competencies for professional nursing education. April 6, 2021.

American Association of Nurse Practitioners. All about NPs. (2021). https://www.aanp.org/about/all-about-nps/whats-a-nurse-practitioner. Accessed 6/6/2021.

American Nurses Association (ANA). *Nursing: A social policy statement.* Kansas City, MO: ANA; 2010.

American Nurses Association (2021). Medicaid Coverage of Advanced Practice Nursing. https://www.nursingworld.org/practice-policy/aprn/medicaid-coverage-of-advanced-practice-nursing/. Accessed 5/29/2021.

Arias E, Tejada-Vera B, Ahmad F. Provisional life expectancy estimates for January through June, 2020. Vital Statistics Rapid Release; no 10. Hyattsville, MD: National Center for Health Statistics. February 2021. doi: https://dx.doi.org/10.15620/cdc:100392.

Baer E. Philosophical and historical bases of primary care nursing. In: Mezey MD, McGivern DO, eds. *Nurses, nurse practitioners: Evolution to advanced practice.* 2nd ed. New York, NY: Springer; 1993:114.

Benner P. *From novice to expert.* Menlo Park, CA: Addison-Wesley; 1984.

Benner P, Wrubel J. *The primacy of caring.* Menlo Park, CA: Addison-Wesley; 1989.

Bodenheimer T, Chen E, Bennett HD. Confronting the growing burden of chronic disease: Can the U.S. healthcare workforce do the job? *Health Aff.* 2009;28:64–74.

Bodenheimer T, Grumbach K. *Understanding health policy: A clinical approach.* 7th ed. New York, NY: Appleton & Lange; 2016.

Boykin A, et al. Aesthetic knowing grounded in an explicit conception of nursing. *Nurs Sci Q.* 1994;7(4):158–161.

Boykin A, Schoenhofer S. *Nursing as caring: A model for transforming practice.* Sudbury, MA: Jones and Bartlett and National League for Nursing Press; 2001.

Brandt AM. Just say no: Risk, behavior, and disease in twentieth-century America. In: Walters R, ed. *Scientific authority and twentieth century America.* Baltimore, MD: Johns Hopkins University Press; 1997:82–98.

Burman ME, et al. Reconceptualizing the core of nurse practitioner education and practice. *Am Acad Nurse Pract.* 2009;21:11–17.

Callahan D. Medical progress: Unintended consequences. In: Callahan D, ed. *Connecting American values with health reform.* Garrison, NY: Hastings Center; 2009:12–14.

Carlson R. The racial life expectancy gap in the U.S. *U.S. & World Economies,* May 27, 2021.

Cody WK. Nursing theory-guided practice: What it is and what it is not. *Nurs Sci Q.* 1994;7(4):144–145.

Cooke M, et al. American medical education 100 years after the Flexner Report. *N Engl J Med.* 2006;355(13):1339–1344.

Dacher E. Reinventing primary care. *J Altern Ther Health Med.* 1995;1(5):29–34.

Decker J, et al. Use of medical care for chronic conditions. *Health Aff.* 2009;28(1):26–35.

Dock LL, Stewart IB. *A short history of nursing.* New York, NY: G.P. Putnam's Sons; 1920.

Doctor of Nursing Practice—DNP. Will the DNP make it over the top as the new standard for advanced practice nursing by 2025? https://www.doctorofnursingpracticednp.org/2020/01/will-the-dnp-make-it-over-the-top-as-the-new-standard-for-advanced-practice-nursing-by-2025/. Accessed 6/6/2021.

Dols J, Hernández C, Miles H. The DNP project: Quandaries for nursing scholars. *Nurs Outlook.* 2017;65(1):84–93.

Dunphy LM. Doing what had to be done. In: Joel L, ed. *Advanced practice nursing: Essentials for role development.* 4th ed. Philadelphia, PA: F.A. Davis; 2017:2–15.

Eisenberg L. Disease and illness: Distinctions between professional and popular ideas of sickness. *Cult Med Psychiatry.* 1977;1:9.

Fairman J, D'Antonio P. Reimagining nursing's place in the history of clinical practice. *J Hist Med Allied Sci.* 2008;63(4):435–446.

Gordon M. *Nursing diagnosis: Process and application.* 2nd ed. New York, NY: McGraw-Hill; 1987.

Harris KM, Woolf S, Gaskin DJ. High and Rising Working-Age Mortality in the US—A Report From the National Academies of Sciences, Engineering, and Medicine. *JAMA* May 25,2021;325(20):2045-2046.

Hektor (Dunphy) LM. Martha E. Rogers: A life history. *Nurs Sci Q.* 1989;2:63–73.

Henderson V. *The nature of nursing.* New York, NY: Macmillan; 1966.

Hooker SA, Punjabi A, Justesen K, et al. Encouraging health behavior change: Eight evidence-based strategies. http://www.aafp.org/fpm Mar/Apr. 2018. https://www.aafp.org/fpm/2018/0300/fpm20180300p31.pdf. Accessed 5/29/2021.

Institute of Medicine. *Health professions education: A bridge to quality.* Washington, DC: National Academy Press; 2003.

Institute of Medicine. *The future of nursing: Leading change, advancing health.* Washington, DC: National Academy Press; 2011.

Johnson R. Nurse practitioner–patient discourse: Uncovering the voice of nursing in primary care practice. *Schol Inq Nurs Pract Int J.* 1993;7(3):143.

Judge-Ellis T, Wilson TR. Time and NP practice: Naming, claiming, and explaining the role of nurse practitioners. *Nurse Pract.* 2017;13(9):583–589.

Kochanek KD, Anderson RN, Arias E. Changes in life expectancy at birth, 2010–2018. NCHS Health E-Stat. 2020.

Kochanek KD, Murphy SL, Xu JQ, Arias E. Mortality in the United States, 2016. NCHS Data Brief, no 293. Hyattsville, MD: National Center for Health Statistics. 2017.

Kolata G. Death rates rising for middle-aged white Americans, study finds. *New York Times.* November 2, 2015. https://nyti.ms/1KUrGdg. Accessed 11/24/17.

Kolata G, Cohen S. Drug overdoses propel rise in mortality rates for young whites. *New York Times.* January 16, 2016. https://www.nytimes.com/2016/01/17/scence/drug-overdoses-propel-rise-in-mortality-rates-of-young-whites.html. Accessed 11/24/17.

Lewis PH, Brykczynski KA. Practical knowledge and competencies of the healing role of the nurse practitioner. *J Am Acad Nurse Pract.* 1994;6(5):207–213.

Livanos N. Physicians look to disrupt longtime regulatory tradition for APRNs. *J Nurs Regul.* 2017;9(3):59–62.

Lynaugh J, Bates B. The two languages of nursing and medicine. *Am J Nurs.* 1973;73(1):66.

Lynaugh, J. Personal communication shared with L. Hektor-Dunphy, 1988.

Mayeroff M. *On caring.* New York, NY: Harper & Row; 1971.

Mishler EG. *The discourse of medicine: Dialectics of medical interviews.* Norwood, NJ: Ablex; 1984.

Mitchell G. Nursing diagnosis: An obstacle to caring ways. In: Boykin A, ed. *Power, politics, and public policy.* New York, NY: National League for Nursing Press; 1995.

National Academies of Sciences, Engineering, and Medicine. 2021. Implementing high-quality primary care: Rebuilding the foundation of healthcare. Washington, DC: The National Academies Press. https://doi.org/10.17226/25983.

National Academies of Sciences, Engineering, and Medicine. 2021. The Future of Nursing 2020–2030: Charting a Path to Achieve Health Equity. Washington, DC: The National Academies Press. https://doi.org/10.17226/25982.

Newman MA, Smith MC, Pharris MD, et al. The focus of the discipline revisited. *Adv Nurs Sci.* 2008;31(1):16–27.

Nightingale F. *Notes on nursing: What it is and what it is not.* Dover, New York; 1860/1969.

Parker M. Exploring the aesthetic meaning of presence in nursing practice. In: Gaut D, ed. *The presence of caring in nursing.* New York, NY: National League for Nursing Press; 1992.

Pew Research Center (2018). *What Unites and Divides Urban, Suburban and Rural Communities.*

Philips RL, McCauley LA, Koller CF. Implementing High-Quality Primary Care—A Report from the National Academies of Sciences, Engineering, and Medicine. *JAMA.* 2021;325(24):

2437–2438. https://jamanetwork.com/journals/jama/fullarticle/2779749. Accessed 6/24/2021.

Rakel RE & Rakel DP ed. (2021). *Textbook of family practice*. 9th ed. Philadelphia, PA: Elsevier WB Saunders; 2021.

Reed PG. A treatise on nursing knowledge development for the 21st century: Beyond postmodernism. *Adv Nurs Sci*. 1995;17(3):70.

Rogers ME. Nursing: To be or not to be? *Nurs Outlook*. 1972;20: 42–46.

Rogers ME. The nurse practitioner movement: Pro and con. *Am J Nurs*. 1975;75(10):1834–1843.

Scoville R, Little K. Comparing lean and quality improvement. IHI white paper. Cambridge, MA: Institute for Healthcare Improvement; 2014.

Shalala DE. Nursing and society: The unfinished agenda for the 21st century. *Nurs Healthcare*. 1993;14(6):4–7.

Shuler PA, Davis JE. The Shuler Nurse Practitioner Practice Model. *J Am Acad Nurse Pract*. 1993;5(1):11–17.

Snyder M. Defining nursing interventions. *Image J Nurs Sch*. 1996;28(2):137.

Social Determinants of Health. Healthy People 2030. U.S. Department of Health and Human Services. https://health.gov/healthypeople/objectives-and-data/social-determinants-health. Accessed 6/6/2021.

Stewart M, et al. *Patient-centered medicine: Transforming the clinical method*. Thousand Oaks, CA: Sage; 1995.

Swanson C. A spirit-focused conceptual model of nursing for the advanced practice nurse. *Issues Comp Pediatr Nurs*. 1995;18:267–275.

Thurman W, Pfitzinger-Lippe M. Returning to the profession's roots: Social justice in nursing education for the 21st century. *Adv Nurs Sci*. 2017;40(2):184–193.

Vakil K. "Those numbers take your breath away': Why Black Americans are dying from COVID-19 at alarming rates. *Courier* May 11, 2020. https://couriernewsroom.com/2020/04/20/why-black-americans-are-dying-from-covid-19-at-alarming-rates/. Accessed 5/29/2021.

Watson J. *Nursing: Human science and human care*. Norwalk, CT: Appleton-Century-Crofts; 1988.

World Health Organization, Commission on Social Determinants of Health. Closing the gap in a generation: Health equity through action on the social determinants of health. https://www.who.int/social_determinants/final_report/csdh_finalreport_2008.pdf Accessed 8/18.

Xu J, Murphy SL, Kochanek KD, et al. *Mortality in the United States, 2018* (National Center for Health Statistics, 2020).

Xu J, Murphy SL, Kochanek KD, et al. *Mortality in the United States, 2015* (National Center for Health Statistics, 2016).

RESOURCES

American Association of Colleges of Nursing—The Voice of Academic Nursing. (April 6, 2021). The Essentials: Core Competencies for Professional Nursing Education.

Future of Nursing Toolkit
https://www.nap.edu/resource/25982/interactive/. Accessed 6/24/2021.

U.S. Dept. of Health and Human Services. Office of Disease Prevention and Health Promotion. Healthy People 2030.
https://health.gov/healthypeople. Accessed 6/24/2021.

U.S. Department of Health and Human Services Office of Minority Health. HHS.gov.
https://www.minorityhealth.hhs.gov/. Accessed 6/6/2021.

Chapter 2

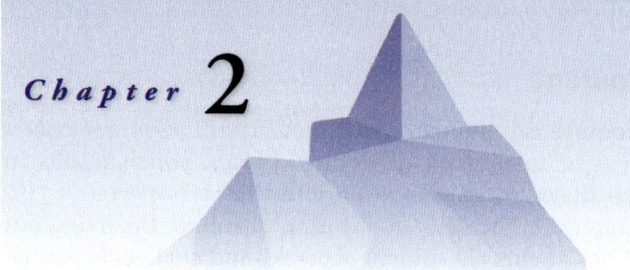

Caring and the Advanced Practice Nurse

Anne Boykin, PhD, RN
Savina O. Schoenhofer, PhD, RN
Terry Eggenberger, PhD, RN

Advanced practice registered nursing (APRN) is a special way of nursing. Although the APRN role blends elements of medical practice and generic primary care, it is based on the traditional nursing approach of caring as a way of being, knowing, and doing. The emphasis on learning medical and scientific knowledge and acquiring skills in advanced nursing science programs sometimes obscures the fact that these programs are aimed at the development of advanced practice nurses, not physicians. This is further confounded by the need for competency in collaborative practice for all health-care professionals (Interprofessional Education Collaborative, 2016). These competencies must include the ability of all health-care providers to integrate knowledge of caring with interprofessional competencies.

The importance of relationships in care of patients should be viewed through an interprofessional lens. The Dance of Caring Persons, a value-based model grounded in the theoretical framework of Nursing as Caring, offers a perspective that celebrates and appreciates the unique gifts that each health-care professional brings to practice. The image of dancers in a circle conveys a way of being in relationship where each person is valued and respected. A fundamental belief of the theory of Nursing as Caring is that all people are caring by virtue of their humanness. The model calls for one to grow in an understanding of what it means to be caring. Mayeroff (1971) in his book, *On Caring*, describes eight expressions of caring that provide a core language for all health professionals. These expressions include knowing, alternating rhythms, patience, honesty, trust, humility, courage, and hope. The focus of each dancer in the circle is to come to know the person as caring and respond to a particular form of care. The 2017 Summer Academy of the Anne Boykin Institute (ABI) for the Advancement of Caring in Nursing focused on "Interprofessional Relationships Grounded in Caring Science." Colleagues from various disciplines engaged in dialogue on how caring is lived uniquely in their roles. The ABI Web site features a video depicting how the integration of caring with interprofessional competencies enriches practice; the Web site also has a Tool Kit.

The advanced practice of nursing must be firmly grounded in the knowledge and skills of caring. The framework presented in this text is intended to help students, faculty, and providers retain a caring-based nursing focus while addressing advanced practice nursing within an interprofessional collaborative practice (IPCP) environment. The World Health Organization (2010) defines IPCP as different professionals working together with patients, families, and communities to "deliver the highest quality of care."

Dunphy's advanced practice nursing model, the Circle of Caring (see Chapter 1), introduces the term "caring process" as a pivotal element. In familiar usage, the term "process" (e.g., "nursing process" or "problem-solving process") means a series of cognitive or psychomotor steps or things to do. In the Circle of Caring model, "process" means "unfolding." Caring processes express a way of being and living as a caring person in the profession of advanced nursing. There is no defined set or list of caring processes; rather, there are as many caring processes as there are persons and situations.

CARING

Caring is the essence of being human, and nursing is a deeply human relationship; thus, caring is the essence of nursing. The meaning of caring as the essential nature of humanness cannot be condensed within a single limiting definition; however, caring can be understood, recognized, and developed both philosophically and practically. Caring expressed in nursing is the intentional and authentic presence of the nurse with another person who is living, caring, and growing in caring (Boykin & Schoenhofer, 2001).

All human service disciplines are based on caring. Nursing is unique in that caring directly characterizes a nurse's knowledge base and service. In contrast, in the discipline of medicine, the fundamental commitment to caring is directly reflected in the diagnosis and treatment of human structural and functional problems manifested primarily in physical terms. The nature of the APRN role permits a direct focus on care and caring that also incorporates the focus of medicine. An APRN does not practice medicine but instead draws on and transforms characteristic medical methods of practice for nursing purposes, just as the practice of holistic medicine draws on and transforms characteristic nursing ways of practice for medical purposes.

Caring is the matrix, the medium, the "stuff" within which APRN–patient relationships come to life. In these relationships, APRNs live the commitment to caring by facilitating a personal connection that communicates "I acknowledge you as a caring person, one who is worthwhile and deserving of my respect, my attention, my commitment, my care." That effort to create a personal connection also communicates practitioners' acceptance of the trust placed in them as caring people who are available and able to participate effectively in the lives of others. Within a caring relationship, each participant has the opportunity to enhance personhood, that is, for living life grounded in caring and for growing in one's capacity to express caring in meaningful and satisfying ways.

Knowing another as a caring person requires a commitment to entering the world of the nursed with the explicit intention of knowing the person individually and uniquely. Entering the world of another with caring intention requires practitioners to know themselves as caring and be open to growing in such relationships. A truly collaborative relationship (in contrast to one in which the collaboration is taken at face value or is in some way limited) emerges in the context of this caring intention.

All APRNs, including nurse practitioners (NPs) in primary care, practice a specialized form of nursing. In APRN practice, specialized opportunities for creating situations of care call forth unique patterns of caring. Although a person seeking care may present with an issue that is characterized as typically medical, the APRN is cocreating a relationship with the person in which care is experienced and possibilities for personally meaningful ways of living unfold.

Specialized patterns of caring in the role of APRN blend knowledgeable perspectives of the health situation and recommendations for characteristically medical ways of ameliorating presenting issues (treatment) with generalized patterns of nursing care. Generalized patterns of nursing care are represented in the Circle of Caring model as follows:

- Courage
- Authentic presence
- Advocacy
- Knowing
- Commitment
- Patience

Specialized patterns of care are incorporated in the uniqueness of caring processes. Knowledge of general patterns of care is important; however, that knowledge must be creatively used in actual, unfolding processes of care if the situation is to be considered nursing. Documentation of these situations is highlighted in this text as Nursing Situation features, which are used throughout the text to illustrate the lived experience of caring between nurse and those "nursed." These themes of caring can serve as a conceptual structure or framework to assist the practitioner in examining, recognizing, and understanding the fullness of caring in advanced nursing practice. Though interconnected, each individual theme is addressed theoretically and then in action in a practice situation to illustrate caring processes.

Courage

Courage is a human act (Tillich, 1952). Courage comes to light in making deliberate choices, which results in acts that express who we are and what is important to us. Courage is the daily application of values, the living out of one's beliefs in spite of obstacles and challenging situations. Expressions of courage affirm our being.

This understanding of courage offers an ethical grounding for the practice of advanced nursing. It requires that in each nursing situation, the nurse live the values held dear. The nurse risks entering each situation with the fullness of being, willing to be rejected or not understood, or, perhaps equally risky, being accepted and known.

As part of courage, the nurse also understands and acts on the obligation to come to know what matters to those seeking care. What shapes the moments the nurse has with people is the intention to know them as caring, hear their stories, and create nurturing responses reflective of the uniqueness of the situation. Courage manifests because of the nurse's deliberate choices to carry out, in a particular time and place, the beliefs that serve as the core of advanced nursing practice. Courage manifests in making one's nursing vocation a commitment to these values and beliefs that undergird caring.

Authentic Presence

Nursing is communicated through authentic presence. Authentic presence is a unique way of being with others, in that it is a way of ordering and balancing self so as to grow in one's beauty and spirit. Such presence with self requires trust, courage, and the desire to know. One who is authentic with self and others is able to see things from the inside that others see only from the outside. There is an inner genuine awareness that is congruent with feelings, attitudes, and actions lived moment to moment. The commitment to truly know oneself frees one to be with others in authentic presence.

Authentic presence may be understood as intentionally being with another in the fullness of one's personhood. The caring that is communicated through authentic presence is the initiating and sustaining medium of nursing within the nursing situation. Nurses are called to be authentically present in nursing situations. Stories of nursing practice portray the depth of such experiences. The degree to which one knows oneself influences one's presence with others and thus the degree of commitment possible in the situation.

Advocacy

Advocacy is a way in which nurses have traditionally expressed caring. There are many opportunities for advocacy, that is, many situations in which "speaking up for" another is an important aspect of the role. From a depth of knowledge and understanding, the practitioner speaks up for the person as unique and worthwhile, as having personal hopes, dreams, intentions, and preferences that are honorable. Gadow's (1990) formulation of existential advocacy calls for the nurse to advocate for alternative interpretations of the situations that arise from experience and specialized knowledge. Existential advocacy is contrasted with advocacy that is either paternalistic or consumer oriented. Paternalistic advocacy is characterized by a sense of "as the expert, I know what is best for you and your life." Consumer-oriented advocacy takes the approach that "I'll just give you the facts and options; you sort them out by yourself."

In existential advocacy, self is brought into the situation as a full partner, sharing alternative perspectives for consideration, although not insisting on them or imposing them. The patient enters the relationship, seeking to connect with the practitioner as a whole person, not just as a set of facts. When the practitioner takes the paternalistic stance (dismissive and overbearing, offering an all-or-none option) or the consumer-oriented stance (withdrawn to an objective distance, offering an essentially value-free set of options), the patient experiences loss of an opportunity to connect with another assumed to be truly concerned, knowledgeable, and giving. When the nurse offers existential advocacy, the nursed feels truly known, respected, and connected in a way that affirms humanity and being.

Knowing

Knowing as an aspect of caring encompasses "knowing that," "knowing about," "knowing directly," and "unknowing." "Knowing that" and "knowing about" refer to descriptions and analyses of the patient's situation in the context of facts and information. Caring competence requires knowledge of facts and data points that are empirically and objectively derived. "Knowing directly" involves being deeply attuned to the person-as-person, and this comes through as an intentionality and authentic presence. "Unknowing" refers to an openness toward unfolding, a humble sense that all is not yet known. The practitioner who truly embraces unknowing recognizes that what might be right or timely in general terms may be neither right nor timely for the particular person seeking care in a particular moment.

Carper (1978) described patterns of knowing fundamental to nursing: personal, empiric, ethical, and aesthetic knowing. The practitioner draws on the personal way of knowing as essential intuitive knowing. Empiric knowing is an avenue for drawing on science and skilled observation. Ethical knowing prompts the practitioner to ask, "What are the personal and professional values that enter into this situation?" And thus, "What is right for this situation?" Aesthetic knowing develops as the practitioner incorporates knowing gained from the other patterns in the context of fully living the situation while cocreating with the nursed an integrated understanding of the unfolding whole picture.

The Circle of Caring is developed and strengthened as the practitioner and patient communicate their unfolding knowing of self, of each other, and of the situation. Knowing, as described briefly here, contributes to enhanced personhood, to the affirmation and growth of self and other as caring persons.

Commitment

Is there any greater act of courage than the commitment to another? Commitment is a sign of that which we value. Choosing to be a member of the discipline and profession of nursing speaks to the deep valuing and lifelong commitment of service to humankind. Commitment directs obligations or what "ought to be" in particular situations. Because these commitments are so internalized as values, however, one's obligation is not experienced as a burden but as a response that is right, deliberate, conscious, and caring (Roach, 2002).

Nurses in advanced practice roles frequently face challenges to commitment. Choices made in practice reflect one's devotion to particular commitments. Often, the values of an economically based health-care system, of which nursing is such an integral part, do not support or seem to be in line with the substantive nature of caring and its essential relation to practice. A struggle to preserve nursing's values often results. The APRN has the unique opportunity to demonstrate how a commitment to the values of nursing influences the outcomes of care.

The practice of advanced nursing must be firmly rooted in the values of the nurse. In addition to many essential types of knowledge and skills, a nurse must be able to draw on the knowledge of nursing, especially knowledge of caring, to create environments for care that honor person-as-person and that humanize care.

Nursing always occurs in a relational context. As a human science, nursing calls for the continued commitment to understand better the lived experience of the nursed, to truly hear their stories, and to respond in ways that matter, ways that nurture and sustain persons as they live and grow in caring. Central to advanced practice is the commitment to know self and others as caring.

Patience

Patience as a key theme in caring refers to trusting people to grow in their own time and in their own way (Mayeroff, 1971). Patience is not passive, but rather an active openness to "the moment alive with possibilities." Humility and courage are intimately connected to patience. The ability to remain actively engaged with the person while honoring individual circumstances and freedom of choice is an act of courage leading to the kind of patience that communicates caring.

CARING PROCESSES

The following two Nursing Situations illustrate ways in which advanced nursing practice is truly an expression of caring processes. The first story was shared by a family nurse practitioner (FNP) in practice in a family clinic in a small rural southern town.

Nursing Situation: Like a Pebble in a Pond—The Circle of Caring

The incident that I am describing involved an 18-year-old female college student—I'll call her Lucy—and her mother, Mrs. K. Lucy presented at my clinic with a history of shortness of breath and flu-like symptoms for several months. She and her mother had been to multiple health-care providers, seeking a diagnosis and resolution of Lucy's problem. I had never seen this patient, so I went through the usual process of taking a history of the present illness, past medical history, social history, and a thorough physical examination. I then ordered what I determined to be the necessary tests. The outcome was a referral to a pulmonologist in a nearby city with the eventual successful resolution of her illness.

The interesting part of this story is what happened years later regarding this clinical incident. My husband and I went into a newly opened used bookstore in our community. On entering, there was no one but the owner and the two of us in the store. When the owner saw me, she came over and hugged me like a long-lost friend—it was Mrs. K! I did not even remotely recognize her and was sure she had mistaken me for someone else. She looked at my husband and stated, "She saved my daughter's life." She then began to cry as she related her feelings about the event and what had transpired. Mrs. K was embarrassed by her emotions (so was I), but she was determined to tell her story.

Mrs. K said that she had taken her daughter to multiple health-care providers, seeking help for her child. She felt they did not take the case seriously and "blew her off" even as her daughter worsened. When Mrs. K and Lucy came to me, Mrs. K was desperate for help for her daughter. Mrs. K described her feelings regarding the clinical visit, grateful that I had listened and believed what she was saying. She then quoted something I had said to her that she said had given her hope and comfort. I told her, "I will do everything possible to find out what is wrong in order to help Lucy get better. We will not give up until we know what is going on with Lucy." Mrs. K said a burden was lifted from her because at last she felt that "someone cared." Mrs. K told us that with the referral, the problem was diagnosed and resolved. It was her profound belief that I had literally saved her daughter's life. I do not remember Lucy's final diagnosis now, and I don't know how much actual assistance I gave in the final resolution of her illness, but I will always remember Mrs. K's gratitude for a caring response to her feelings of helplessness while dealing with the health-care system. Mrs. K's belated description of her heartfelt feelings regarding her daughter's illness and my interventional actions made a profound impression on me as a provider. The need for a caring response to each of our patients is evident, yet we may never know how much such caring can impact a life.

As shared by Carolyn B. Dollar, PhD, APRN-BC, FNP

In this story, the most prominent caring processes are authentic presence and commitment, as the FNP offered self in a way that truly communicated caring to this beleaguered family. The FNP's commitment to caring for the family and her courage and patience in tackling an issue that obviously had been given a "pass" by previous health-care providers illustrate the importance of opportunities to hear and respond effectively to calls for caring in advanced nursing practice. Referral is an act of advocacy that is frequently an element of NP practice, and when it is recognized as an opportunity for caring through advocacy, it becomes an even more integral expression of advanced nursing. Referral also is recognition of the value of interprofessional practice. The fact that the FNP offered this particular story as an exemplar of caring in advanced nursing practice makes evident the merging of knowing in past–present–future: the FNP continues to be open to knowing self and others through appreciation of the mother's report of the impact of an act of caring initiated in the rather distant past.

A second story from an APRN practicing in a specialty clinic in an urban health sciences center showcases the centrality of the nurse–patient caring relationship in the midst of treatment situations involving complicated biomedical technology.

Nursing Situation: Spirited Caring

My APRN role has been a rewarding challenge. The story that I am going to share was pivotal to my development as an APRN. The story focuses on a pleasant, jolly, gem of a patient, with a warm smile—I'll call her Mrs. J. Her energy lit up the room. This independent free spirit also worked as a volunteer at the clinic. She served cookies and other baked goods to the patients undergoing chemotherapy. Her strong faith and compassion for others impressed me as a busy provider. To the nursing staff, she stood out as a patient and volunteer. Her faith helped her in aiding the sicker patients to maintain hope. Her genuine concern for others encouraged nursing staff and family members to have compassion for others. Mrs. J was always the first to ask, "How are you doing?" This unique patient was a beacon of light in a dark, sobering environment.

My favorite patient and I developed a good rapport as I saw her weekly in the Coumadin clinic. She was my first patient on my very first day. When she stepped into my office and noted my frazzled appearance, she grabbed my hands and prayed with me. Because we are in the Bible belt, I considered that to be normal. She later apologized because she did not know my religious beliefs. I assured her that her actions had calmed me and made my day go a little better. Mrs. J had been doing exceptionally well although she had been diagnosed with cancer. She had a history of stage II breast cancer but had been in complete remission for 2 years.

One Friday, she presented to the clinic at 4 o'clock in the afternoon. She had been complaining of vision changes and had her son bring her to the clinic. I knew something was wrong because this independent woman always presented to visits alone. Mrs. J's primary care provider was not available by phone and her oncologist was out of town. She reported a headache with vision changes, which seemed strange for a woman who had undergone chemotherapy with adjuvant radiation therapy without difficulties. She explained that 4 days before this clinic visit, she experienced the worst headache she had ever had. Her clinical presentation led me to order a computed tomography (CT) scan of the head with contrast. After reading her CT, the radiologist called me immediately. He had identified a large mass that was pressing against her sulcus. At this point, I had to find her hematologist, start her on high-dose steroids, find the neurosurgeon on call, and prepare her for everything that was about to take place. I was so consumed by my actions that I nearly forgot to care for the patient.

Mrs. J demonstrated sincere compassion when I had to give her the hard news. She grabbed my hands and prayed for me and the other health-care providers. She prayed that we would make the right decisions regarding her health care. Just as we had started our relationship, we were ending it. Her demonstration of faith was a unique testament to her life. Her strength in a time of weakness showed the vigor of her faith. Though she was a devout Catholic and I am a Methodist, we had to rely on our genuine concern for each other and our beliefs in a higher being to get us through this difficult time. Compassion and faith were integral components in our provider–patient relationship.

The experience taught us that compassion and faith coupled with therapeutic communication can get you through the toughest situation. In revisiting this story, I am reminded of the need to foster a sense of caring and respect for patients' beliefs as I mature and develop as a nurse. The patient's actions were surprising. I had been taught about putting my compassion and faith into action; however, I had never seen it done. It was affirming as an APRN to recall how we cried and laughed and came to the sobering realization that this disease might beat her. However, we had given it our best effort. This experience was beneficial to me because it was my first time being the bearer of bad news to a patient. Consumed as we are with time management, compassion and faith are not always exhibited, shared, or utilized in my daily practice. However, by revisiting this story, I am challenged to treat others as I treated my special patient. The core values that guided my practice in the past have been rekindled while reflecting on my nursing experience. Nursing is a rewarding challenge if you allow it to be.

As shared by C'Sara Strong, MSN, CFNP

This story needs no interpretation; it can be easily recognized as an exquisite example of creating a holistic fabric of caring integrating a multitude of harmonious patterns: interpersonal, interprofessional, clinical, and technological.

These stories illustrate the use of caring processes. As these Nursing Situations are studied and relived, students, faculty, and providers discover the limitless ways caring is expressed. As nurses, we live out our personhood—our living grounded in caring—in unique and special ways. We bring to our practice our humanness, our expertise in caring, and our intention to participate fully in the life experiences of those we are privileged to nurse and, thus, to bring the benefits of nursing to those seeking care.

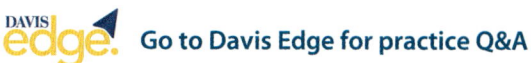

Go to Davis Edge for practice Q&A

REFERENCES

Boykin A, Schoenhofer SO. *Nursing as caring: A model for transforming practice.* Sudbury, MA: Jones & Bartlett; 2001.

Carper B. Fundamental patterns of knowing in nursing. *Adv Nurs Sci.* 1978;1(1):13–23.

Gadow S. A model for ethical decision making. In: Pence T, et al, eds. *Ethics in nursing: An anthology.* New York, NY: National League for Nursing; 1990:52–55.

Interprofessional Education Collaborative. (2016). Core competencies for interprofessional collaborative practice: 2016 update. Washington, DC: Interprofessional Education Collaborative.

Johns C. *Becoming a reflective practitioner.* 4th ed. Hoboken, NJ: Wiley-Blackwell; 2013.

Leininger M, McFarlane MR. *Transcultural nursing: Concepts, theories, research, and practice.* New York, NY: McGraw-Hill, Medical Publishing Division; 2002.

Locsin RC. *Technological competency as caring in nursing: A model for practice.* Indianapolis, IN: Sigma Theta Tau International Honor Society of Nursing; 2005.

Mayeroff M. *On caring.* New York, NY: Harper Perennial; 1971.

Paterson J, Zderad LT. *Humanistic nursing.* New York, NY: National League for Nursing; 1988.

Roach MS. *The human act of caring: A blueprint for the health professions.* Ottawa, ON: Canadian Hospital Association; 1987.

Roach S. *Caring: The human mode of being. A blueprint for the health professions.* Ottawa, ON: CHA Press; 2002.

Smith MC, Turkel MC, Wolf ZR. *Caring in nursing classics: An essential resource.* New York, NY: Springer Publishing Co; 2012.

Tillich P. *The courage to be.* New Haven, CT: Yale University Press; 1952.

Watson J. *The philosophy and science of caring.* Revised edition. Boulder, CO: University Press of Colorado; 2008.

Watson J. *Assessing and measuring caring in nursing and health sciences.* New York, NY: Springer Publishing Co; 2009.

Wolf Z, King B, France N. Antecedent context and structure of communication during a caring moment: Scoping review and analysis. *Int J Hum Caring.* 2015;19(2):7–21.

RESOURCES

Anne Boykin Institute (ABI) for Advancement of Caring in Nursing
http://nursing.fau.edu/outreach/anne-boykin-institute/resources.php

Archives of Caring of the Christine E. Lynn College of Nursing
    http://nursing.fau.edu/archives/
Institute for Healthcare Improvement. (2020). *What Matters.*
    http://www.ihi.org/Topics/WhatMatters/Pages/default.aspx
International Association for Human Caring (IAHC)
    http://www.humancaring.org/
International Journal for Human Caring (IJHC)
    http://www.humancaring.org

Journal of Art and Aesthetics in Nursing and Health Sciences
    http://www.JAANHS.org
Watson Caring Science Institute
    http://watsoncaringscience.org/
World Health Organization. (2010). Framework for action on interprofessional education and collaborative practice (No. WHO/HRH/HPN/10.3). Geneva: World Health Organization.

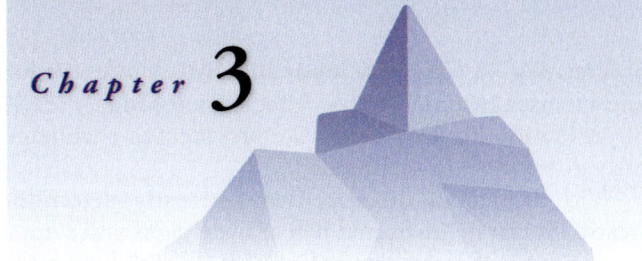

Chapter 3

Health Promotion

Dorothy J. Dunn, PhD, APRN, FNP-BC, AHN-BC
Debera J. Thomas, PhD, RN, ANP/FNP

HEALTH

The goal of all health-care providers and their patients is to promote health and prevent disease. Engaging in health-promoting activities helps individuals live longer, healthier lives. To put this goal in perspective, the basic tenets of health must first be explored.

What is health? Several disciplines and organizations have tried to define health, and the definition continues to evolve. Some view health as the absence of disease, but this definition does not consider other important human characteristics that have physical, social, spiritual, cultural, and emotional dimensions. In 1948, the World Health Organization (WHO, 1948) defined health as a "state of complete physical, mental and social well-being"; this definition provides a more holistic view of health because it incorporates the social and mental aspects of a human being, as well as the physical dimension. In fact, this definition has not been amended since its inception in 1948. However, this definition fails to recognize the spiritual and cultural dimensions of a person. According to the American Holistic Nurses' Association (Mariano, 2016), health can be described as a state or process in which people experience a sense of well-being, harmony, and unity of their body-mind-spirit within a continuously changing environment. Health is, therefore, a state in which the physical, psychological, social, spiritual, and cultural attributes of a person are in balance, creating harmony within the body (Fig. 3.1).

The balance of each of these dimensions is an important parameter when considering health. A patient may be physically healthy, but the spiritual, cultural, social, and psychological dimensions may not be balanced, and therefore the patient is not experiencing optimal health. If we believe that the whole is greater than the sum of its parts, then we cannot accurately determine someone's health status without evaluating all of these attributes.

Historically, the medical evaluation of a patient was based only on the clinical manifestations of a disease. If a patient lacked symptoms, we considered that patient healthy. We now know that this type of assessment is incomplete; it does not consider how the other attributes of a person either contribute to or subtract from health status. We also know that many patients have medical problems that have not yet presented as signs or symptoms of a disease.

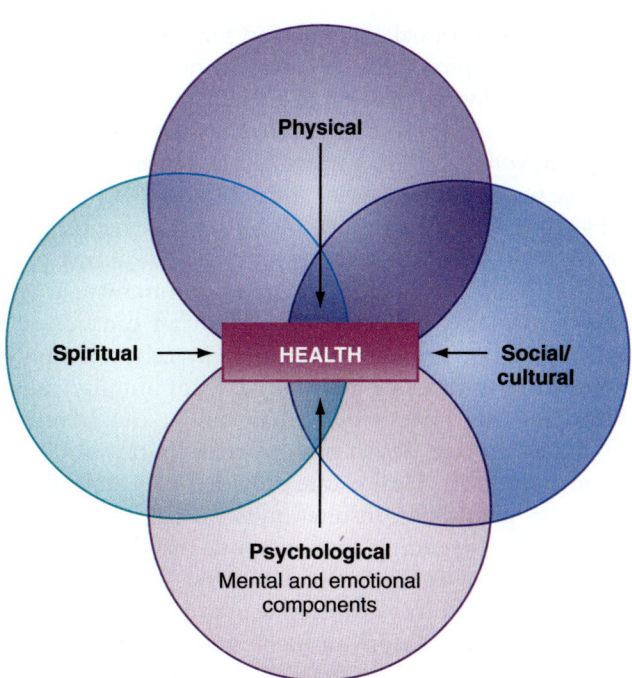

Figure 3.1 The components of health.

When assessing a patient, it is imperative to also evaluate social, psychological, spiritual, and cultural well-being, as well as the physical state. In performing a complete health assessment, the provider should ask questions related to the person's social and dietary habits; current living and work situation or environment; feelings, beliefs, values, and life satisfaction; and philosophical and spiritual beliefs.

Along with physical manifestations, all these parts of a patient's history inform diagnosis and treatment plans. The focus on all component parts of a person helps to provide a more holistic view, which can assist in making a comprehensive assessment of the current health status of the patient. The determination of health is based on the synthesis of all the parameters of health, and it should be incorporated into all patient assessments.

HEALTH PROMOTION

Health promotion can be defined as activities and preventive measures that contribute to a person's state of optimal health. Such activities and preventive measures include immunizations, fitness/EXERCISE programs, breast self-awareness, appropriate nutrition, relaxation, stress management, social support, prayer, meditation, healing rituals, cultural practices, and promotion of environmental health and safety. Health and well-being stem from a balance of physical, psychological, spiritual, cultural, and social components of health. Health promotion requires a commitment on the part of the individual patient, the health-care provider, and the community. Health-promotion efforts are effective only when everyone works in partnership to achieve goals that enhance health and well-being.

Health-promotion efforts should always begin with the clinician because of the pivotal role clinicians play in educating the patient and the community about health-promoting behaviors. The clinician can educate patients about how their environment can contribute to health or disease. In addition, the community must understand the impact that environment can have on individuals so that health-promotion activities can be a community effort. Health-care providers play an important role by providing consultation to the community and the legislature regarding environmental health.

Consultation with influential members of the community can assist efforts to develop legislation that supports healthy living conditions in a community. In addition, legislative efforts can help provide funding to maintain or improve environmental health. When patients commit to their own health, living conditions in the community must also be healthy to sustain and support their efforts. Basic community resources, such as water and sanitation, must be monitored for potential threats to health and well-being, and these resources are the responsibility of community and local government agencies. Health-care providers and patients need to work in collaboration with these agencies to ensure that resources essential to health are maintained or improved. To be successful, health promotion must be a group effort.

Historically, health promotion has been viewed as an effort to prevent disease and illness. Most sources cite three levels of prevention: primary prevention is the prevention of disease; secondary prevention consists of early screening and detection of disease; and tertiary prevention is the restoration of health after illness or disease has occurred. Focusing health-care efforts on all three levels of prevention is important to promoting health, but during the last two decades, primary prevention has become the focus of health promotion.

During the first half of the 20th century, health-care efforts were directed at patients who were already ill. The prevailing belief at the time was that patients should seek health care when they were ill. During this time, most health-care practitioners cared for patients at the tertiary level by (1) preventing further insult or injury after the disease or illness had occurred by stabilizing the patient's condition to prevent deterioration; (2) helping patients recover from the current illness or disease through treatment; and (3) whenever possible, helping restore patients to their previous state of health.

Advancements in technology during the second half of the 20th century contributed to better diagnostic testing, helping to shift the focus of health care to secondary prevention. Providers began to emphasize the importance of screening "at risk" patients at appropriate intervals for known diseases and illnesses. A focus on secondary levels of prevention has led health-care providers to encourage early detection and treatment.

With the focus on screening and early detection, treatment can be instituted before overt signs and symptoms appear, thereby preventing some of the long-term sequelae associated with disease. For example, blood pressure is checked in a patient with no symptoms of hypertension, and if elevated, a plan of treatment is initiated. The goal is to maintain the patient's blood pressure within normal limits and minimize the development of catastrophic complications such as stroke or myocardial infarction. Box 3.1 summarizes questions the clinician should consider in consultation with the patient before routinely screening for any condition.

In determining whether screening is appropriate, health-care providers should keep in mind that early signs of chronic disease often surface in midlife; that is, in persons aged 40 to 65 years. In general, the earlier disease is identified, the easier it is to treat, and the more likely it is to have a successful outcome. In addition, individuals in midlife tend to focus more on behaviors to extend life and prevent disability than do younger people. Adults aged 20 to 40 years focus more on relationships, family, self-image, and career development, whereas those older than age 65 spend more time responding to and coping with overt, established illness. As life expectancy increases and older adults anticipate living longer, more attention is focused on health enhancement, adding quality years to the life span of older persons.

Focusing on primary prevention enables providers to assess patients' potential risk factors, including lifestyle and family history, and to help them make lifestyle changes that will foster health and prevent disease and disability. Health-care providers are aware that health or wellness is best achieved through primary prevention strategies. However, when this is not possible, secondary and tertiary levels

---

Box 3.1 Questions to Consider Before Ordering Screening Tests

1. Does the condition have a significant effect on the quality and span of life?
2. Are there acceptable treatment options available?
3. Does detection of the condition while it is asymptomatic significantly reduce morbidity and mortality if treated?
4. Does treatment in the asymptomatic phase yield a therapeutic result superior to that obtained by delaying treatment until symptoms appear?
5. Are there tests available acceptable to patients at a reasonable cost that detect the condition in the asymptomatic period?
6. Is evidence of the condition sufficient to justify the cost of the screening?

of prevention are employed. Each health-care interaction between a patient and clinician is an opportunity to promote health at the primary, secondary, and tertiary levels. Optimal wellness or health for all patients is the goal.

Health-care providers can use the levels of prevention in several ways: on an individual level, with small groups (families), and with larger groups such as a community. Individual encounters provide an opportunity to educate patients about their individual risk factors and changes they can make to prevent, or at least delay, the onset of disease(s) and the potential sequelae of disease (implementing primary and secondary prevention strategies). Incorporating family members into the educational process of health promotion can provide support and reinforcement for patients during the early phase of risk reduction. This incorporation of family may also serve individual family members by educating them regarding their own risk for disease. Family members can also serve as advocates for patients by helping to synthesize the information given and providing the patient with a support system to make healthy lifestyle changes.

Health-care providers can be instrumental in developing health-promotion strategies in a community. This can be accomplished by developing interventions that include identifying community groups at risk for certain diseases and developing community-wide programs to educate these groups about their potential risks. Community-based educational programs reach a broad audience with the potential to have a significant impact on the health status of a community (Fig. 3.2).

Expanding knowledge has increased our awareness that today many diseases, including hypertension, cardiovascular disease, and diabetes, can be minimized or potentially avoided with early assessment and management. For example, most patients diagnosed with diabetes have had the disease for at least 5 years. Diabetes has serious consequences in many organ systems if it is not diagnosed early and treated aggressively. The development of a community-wide diabetes education and screening program can help identify patients who are at high risk for the disease. With early diagnosis and treatment, long-term complications associated with diabetes,

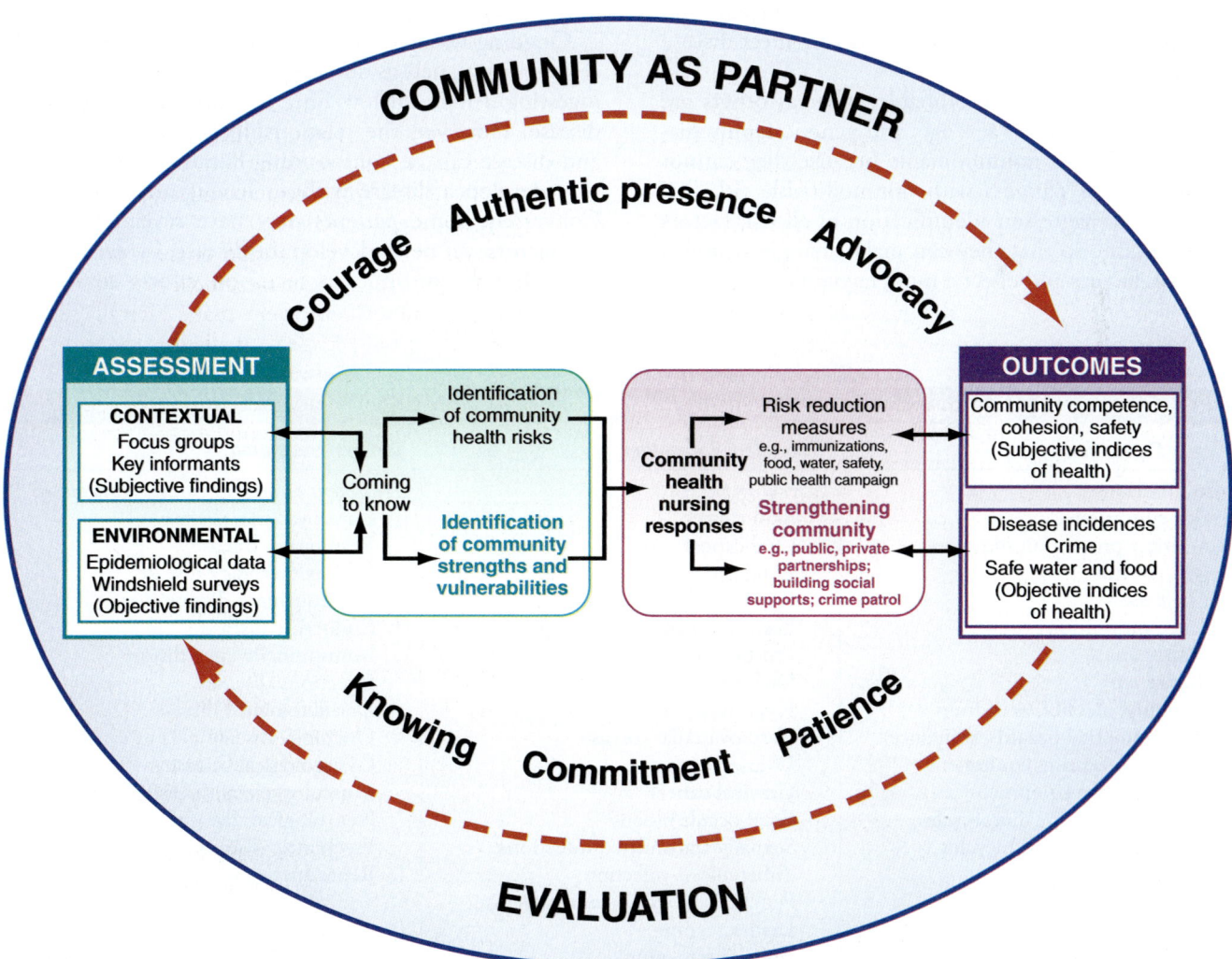

Figure 3.2 The community-based *Circle of Caring*.

such as peripheral neuropathy, cardiovascular complications, and retinopathies, can be minimized.

Clinicians can take a leadership position within a community by developing targeted programs for early identification and treatment. This type of wide-scale intervention can reduce morbidity and mortality rates. Early diagnosis, before signs/symptoms of a disease are present, can have a significant effect on the outcomes of disease. If patients are identified early, educated about the importance of healthy nutrition and lifestyle, and treated aggressively, the outcome may be a long, healthy life. Table 3.1 provides examples of primary, secondary, and tertiary prevention.

RISK FACTORS IN HEALTH PROMOTION

The identification of risk factors is an essential component of health promotion. Some patients have no known risk factors, whereas others have many. The key component of effective health promotion is to screen patients for potential known risk factors and to intervene. Not all diseases can be prevented, and not every person with an unhealthy lifestyle will get a disease, but the elimination or alteration of certain risk factors can affect disease outcomes.

Some risk factors are modifiable, whereas others are not. Such risk factors as sex, age, and genetic/family history are considered nonmodifiable because they cannot be changed. For patients with nonmodifiable risk factors, early and aggressive identification of all risk factors should be done so that they can make changes in modifiable risk factors and effect a more favorable outcome.

Modifiable risk factors include weight, diet, exercise, social habits, lifestyle choices, and stress. For example, 38-year-old Mr. Hart is being seen for a physical examination. He has not had a physical in 20 years. His past medical history is negative for any diseases, surgeries, or illnesses. His social history includes the use of alcohol and cigarettes; he works an average of 60 hours per week as an emergency medical technician and does not exercise. His family history reveals that his father, paternal uncle, and grandfather all had a myocardial infarction before age 50. Mr. Hart's physical examination reveals the following: height, 69 inches; weight, 230 pounds; and a body mass index (BMI) of 34. Mr. Hart's laboratory results include a cholesterol level of 250 mg/dL, a high-density lipoprotein (HDL) of 30 mg/dL, and a low-density lipoprotein (LDL) of 160 mg/dL. Box 3.2 reviews the risk factors for heart disease for Mr. Hart.

Although Mr. Hart cannot change his age, sex, or family history, there are several factors that he can change. With improvements in his diet, regular exercise, stress reduction, moderation of alcohol intake, and smoking cessation, Mr. Hart can reduce his risk for heart disease. This case illustrates the importance of early identification of risk factors for intervention.

Ongoing research has shown the relationship between certain risks, such as smoking, consuming alcohol, and ingesting a high-fat/low-fiber diet, and the presence of disease. However, the relationship between risk factors and disease can be confounding because often a person may develop a disease without having any risk factors. Conversely, some patients may have several identified risk factors, yet never develop the disease. Evidence-based research will continue to focus on efforts to identify

TABLE 3.1 Examples of Primary, Secondary, and Tertiary Prevention

Primary Prevention	Secondary Prevention	Tertiary Prevention
Immunizations	*Screening for:*	*Treatment to prevent further sequelae of:*
Health education	Skin cancer	Cardiovascular disease
Skin cancer prevention measures	Oral cancer	Respiratory disease
Weight control	Lung cancer	Gastroenterology disease
Seat belt use	Breast cancer	Genitourinary disease
Violence prevention	Testicular cancer	Endocrine diseases
Substance abuse	Prostate cancer	Immunodeficiency disease
Education on:	Diabetes	Infectious disease
Smoking, alcohol, and drugs	Hypertension	Dermatological disease
Environmental hazards avoidance	Cardiovascular disease	Oncology disease
Protective hearing equipment	Ovarian cancer	Gynecological disease
Protective eye equipment	Cervical cancer	Musculoskeletal disease
Safety helmets for motorcycles, skateboards, and bicycles	Fecal occult blood	Neurological disease
	Sexually transmitted infections	Psychiatric disease
Nutrition counseling	Tuberculosis infection	Reproductive disease
Exercise	Pediatric developmental screening	
Stress reduction	Lead screening	
Eliminating allergen exposure	Anemia screening	
	Height, weight, and BMI screening	

> **Box 3.2 Risk Factors for Mr. Hart**
>
> **Nonmodifiable Risk Factors**
> - Male sex
> - Age
> - Family history
>
> **Modifiable Risk Factors**
> - Weight
> - Sedentary lifestyle
> - Elevated cholesterol
> - Elevated LDL and suboptimal HDL
> - Alcohol consumption
> - Smoking
> - Stress level

unknown risk factors or health-promoting determinants that could influence the outcomes for disease.

INFLUENCES ON HEALTH PROMOTION

Many factors influence health-promotion activities today. Government initiatives, community health programs, and the media all focus attention on the importance of health literacy, health promotion, and disease prevention.

Health Literacy

Most people encounter health information when they seek health care, and most people encounter health information that they cannot understand. More than a measurement of reading skills, health literacy also includes conceptual knowledge and writing, listening, speaking, and mathematical skills. *Health literacy* is commonly defined as the degree to which individuals have the capacity to obtain, process, and understand basic information and services needed to make appropriate decisions regarding their health (Affordable Care Act [ACA], 2010).

Health literacy is required when acute illness, injury, or chronic-disease management necessitates that a person seek health care. Consider that nurses are charged with "the protection, promotion, and optimization of health and abilities, prevention of illness and injury, alleviation of suffering through diagnosis and treatment of human response, and advocacy in the care of individuals, families, communities, and populations" (American Nurses Association, 2010, p 10). Therefore, nurses must accept the challenge to screen and assess for health literacy levels at each health-care encounter. Many instruments are available to assess a person's level of health literacy. For example, the Newest Vital Scale (NVS) instrument can be used to assess health literacy within 3 minutes. The NVS can provide results comparable to more time-consuming literacy tests such as the Test of Functional Health Literacy in Adults or Rapid Estimate of Adult Literacy in Medicine—Short Form. Other instruments have been developed for other languages (AHRQ, 2016).

By identifying those at risk for misunderstanding instructions and failing to adhere to recommendations in all aspects of care, health-care providers have a positive effect on health promotion, prevention strategies, and successful treatment adherence for individuals who seek health care.

Government Initiatives

Three major government initiatives that have had great impact on health promotion in the United States are the National Prevention Strategy (NPS), *Healthy People 2030*, and the U.S. Preventive Services Task Force (USPSTF).

National Prevention Strategy

The ACA of 2010 created the National Prevention Council, which in turn developed the NPS. In 2011, the National Prevention Council released *National Prevention Strategy: America's Plan for Better Health and Wellness*, a comprehensive plan that describes evidence-based and achievable means for improving health and well-being for all Americans at every stage of life. These efforts were designed to stop disease before it starts and to create strategies for a healthy, fit nation, recognizing that prevention must be part of daily life. The goal of the NPS is to transform us from a system of sick care to one based on wellness and prevention. In addition, an Advisory Group on Prevention, Health Promotion, and Integrative and Public Health made final recommendations to the U.S. surgeon general and National Prevention Council that reaffirm the value of and the group's commitment to the following four strategic directions of the NPS (Surgeon General, 2014):

- Health and safe community environments
- Clinical and community preventive services
- Empowered people
- Elimination of health disparities

Within this framework, seven priorities were identified to reduce the burden of the leading causes of preventable death and major illness:

- Tobacco-free living
- Preventing drug abuse and excessive alcohol use
- Healthy eating
- Active living
- Injury and violence-free living
- Reproductive and sexual health
- Mental and emotional well-being

Healthy People 2030

Healthy People 2030: Building a healthier future for all, launched August 18, 2020, is a foundational resource for the NPS's four strategic directions and seven priorities. It is based on the accomplishments of five previous *Healthy People* initiatives: (1) the 1979 *Healthy People: The Surgeon General's Report on Health Promotion and Disease Prevention*; (2) *Healthy People 1990: Promoting Health/Preventing Disease: Objectives for the Nation*; (3) *Healthy People 2000: National Health Promotion and Disease Prevention Objectives*; (4) *Healthy People 2010: Objectives for Improving Health*; and (5) *Healthy People 2020: Objectives for Improving Health*.

The stated purpose of *Healthy People 2030* is to guide the United States in achieving the population's full potential for health and well-being across the lifespan. The mission is to promote, strengthen, and evaluate the nation's efforts toward this goal and to set national goals and measurable objectives guiding evidence-based policies, programs, and other actions (U.S. Department of Health & Human Services, Office of Disease Prevention and Health Promotion, 2020).

Healthy People 2030's seven foundational principles were developed over the course of the decade (2010-2020), and they appear in Box 3.3. The five overarching goals are:

- Attain healthy, thriving lives and well-being, free of preventable disease, disability, injury, and premature death.
- Eliminate health disparities, achieve health equity, and attain health literacy to improve the health and well-being of all.
- Create social, physical, and economic environments that promote attaining full potential for health and well-being for all.
- Promote healthy development, healthy behaviors, and well-being across all life stages.
- Engage leadership, key constituents, and the public across multiple sectors to take action and design policies that improve the health and well-being of all.

Healthy People 2030 objectives are organized into related topic areas. They are Health Conditions, Health Behaviors, Populations, Settings and Systems, and Social Determinants of Health. Experts from numerous federal agencies developed the topic areas. These agencies include the Administration on Aging, Agency for Healthcare Research and Quality, Centers for Disease Control and Prevention (CDC), and the U.S. Food and Drug Administration. The topic areas for *Healthy People 2030* are listed in Box 3.4. For further data, information, and relevant objectives, go to https://health.gov/healthypeople/objectives-and-data/browse-objectives.

Each of the *Healthy People 2030* topic areas includes related evidence-based interventions and resources from the USPSTF Clinical Preventive Services, *Guide to Community Preventive Services*, and Healthfinder.gov's *Quick Guide to Healthy Living Information for Consumers*. *Healthy People 2030* also hosts an online community, using Twitter, LinkedIn, and webinars. Leading health indicators reflect high-priority health issues and communicate actions that can be taken to address them. These indicators will be used to assess the health of the nation from 2020 to 2030; facilitate collaboration across sectors; and motivate action at the national, state, and community levels to improve the health of the U.S. population.

According to the *Healthy People* initiative, *health promotion* is defined as any strategy helping individuals make personal choices in a social context about lifestyle that will have a positive influence on the individual's health prospects. *Health protection* is defined as interventions related to the environment made by regulatory bodies to protect a large population group. *Preventive services* include screening for disease, counseling, medication to prevent disease, and immunization interventions for individuals in the clinical setting. The last priority—surveillance and data systems—is essential to track all of the changes that occur with programs focusing on meeting the goals of *Healthy People 2030*.

The *Healthy People* initiatives continue to have a significant impact on primary health care in the United States. The incorporation of health-promoting and disease prevention strategies has become the foundation for primary care. It is believed that all of the goals of *Healthy People 2030* are achievable with support from individual healthcare providers, local and national government agencies, and most importantly, the active participation of individual patients.

Box 3.3 *Healthy People 2030* Foundational Principles

- Foundational principles explain the thinking that guides decisions about *Healthy People 2030.*
- Health and well-being of all people and communities are essential to a thriving, equitable society.
- Promoting health and well-being and preventing disease are linked efforts that encompass physical, mental, and social health dimensions.
- Investing to achieve the full potential for health and well-being for all provides valuable benefits to society.
- Achieving health and well-being requires eliminating health disparities, achieving health equity, and attaining health literacy.
- Healthy physical, social, and economic environments strengthen the potential to achieve health and well-being.
- Promoting and achieving the nation's health and well-being is a shared responsibility that is distributed across the national, state, tribal, and community levels, including the public, private, and not-for-profit sectors.
- Working to attain the full potential for health and well-being of the population is a component of decision making and policy formulation across all sectors.

Source: U.S. Department of Health & Human Services, Office of Disease Prevention and Health Promotion (ODPHP). Healthy People 2030. https://health.gov/healthypeople.

Box 3.4 Topic Areas for *Healthy People 2030*

- Access to Health Services
- Adolescent Health
- Arthritis, Osteoporosis, and Chronic Back Conditions
- Blood Disorders and Blood Safety
- Cancer
- Chronic Kidney Disease
- Dementias, Including Alzheimer's Disease
- Diabetes
- Disability and Health
- Early and Middle Childhood
- Educational and Community-Based Programs
- Environmental Health
- Family Planning
- Food Safety
- Genomics
- Global Health
- Health Communication and Health Information Technology
- Health-Care–Associated Infections
- Health-Related Quality of Life and Well-being
- Hearing and Other Sensory or Communication Disorders
- Heart Disease and Stroke
- HIV
- Immunization and Infectious Diseases
- Injury and Violence Prevention
- Lesbian, Gay, Bisexual, and Transgender Health
- Maternal, Infant, and Child Health
- Medical Product Safety
- Mental Health and Mental Disorders
- Nutrition and Weight Status
- Occupational Safety and Health
- Older Adults
- Oral Health
- Physical Activity
- Preparedness
- Public Health Infrastructure
- Respiratory Diseases
- Sexually Transmitted Diseases
- Sleep Health
- Social Determinants of Health
- Substance Abuse
- Tobacco Use
- Vision

Source: U.S. Department of Health & Human Services, Office of Disease Prevention and Health Promotion (ODPHP). Healthy People 2030. https://health.gov/healthypeople.

The action plan for *Healthy People 2030* includes:

- Setting national goals and measurable objectives to guide evidence-based policies, programs, and other actions to improve health and well-being
- Providing data that are accurate, timely, accessible, and can drive targeted actions to address regions and populations with poor health or at high risk for poor health in the future
- Fostering impact through public and private efforts to improve health and well-being for people of all ages and the communities in which they live
- Providing tools for the public, programs, policymakers, and others to evaluate progress toward improving health and well-being
- Sharing and supporting the implementation of evidence-based programs and policies that are replicable, scalable, and sustainable
- Reporting biennially on progress throughout the decade from 2020 to 2030
- Stimulating research and innovation toward meeting *Healthy People 2030* goals and highlight critical research, data, and evaluation needs
- Facilitating the development and availability of affordable means of health promotion, disease prevention, and treatment.

(U.S. Department of Health & Human Services, Office of Disease Prevention and Health Promotion, 2020)

U.S. Preventive Services Task Force

The USPSTF is composed of private-sector experts who make recommendations to the health-care community regarding clinical prevention strategies. This group was first convened by the U.S. Public Health Service in 1984, but since 1998, it has come under the umbrella of the Agency for Healthcare Research and Quality. The USPSTF's mission, as mandated by Public Law Section 915, is to conduct scientific evidence reviews of a broad array of clinical preventive services; develop recommendations for the health-care community; and provide ongoing administrative, research, and technical support to disseminate the findings.

The USPSTF meets and systematically reviews scientific evidence for each of the current health-care screening guidelines, as well as preventive medications, immunizations, and counseling, and makes recommendations based on these reviews. Through consensus, the task force assigns a grade to each recommendation based on net benefits for patients and the strength of evidence for each of the current recommendations.

The result of the task force's efforts is an online *Procedure Manual* that can be used by clinicians who provide preventive services. The *Procedure Manual* provides recommendations for screening, including the following: cancer screening and chemoprevention strategies; screening for heart and valvular disease, infectious disease, injury and violence, mental health issues, and substance abuse; metabolic, nutritional, and endocrine screening; and pediatric screening guidelines. Nurse practitioners can use its evidence-based recommendations for clinical preventive services. The USPSTF *Procedure Manual* (2017) is available for distribution from several sources and has its own Web site: https://www.uspreventiveservicestaskforce.org/uspstf/procedure-manual. An evidence-based prevention resource for nurse practitioners is available through the USPSTF Web site: https://www.uspreventiveservicestaskforce.org/uspstf/evidence-based-prevention-resource-nurse-practitioners.

The USPSTF not only makes recommendations for screening select populations (https://www.uspreventiveservicestaskforce.org/uspstf/recommendation-topics/uspstf-and-b-recommendations#:~:text=The%20USPSTF%20recommends%201-time%20screening%20for%20abdominal%20aortic,to%2070%20years%20who%20are%20overweight%20or%20obese), but it also prioritizes services. All of the recommendations issued by the USPSTF are optional; providers and patients may decide not to implement certain recommendations based on shared decision making. For example, a patient who has a significant family history for a particular type of cancer may need to be screened earlier than recommended for the general population but only after careful discussion allowing the patient to weigh the pros and cons and the possibility of false-positive results.

The work of this task force continues. Some of the current recommendations such as lead poisoning and iron-deficiency anemia screenings have been included for many years as part of well-child visits in pediatrics. It is important that screening programs be continued or eliminated based on the strength of scientific evidence available and not just on tradition (see Box 3.1).

With the rapid evolution of technology in health care, it is important to be knowledgeable about current health-care information. Such resources as the NPS, *Healthy People 2030*, and the USPSTF recommendations are essential tools to help clinicians keep up to date with current best practices. These initiatives have Web sites that provide updates to the current printed reports. The NPS encourages partnerships among federal, state, tribal, local, and territorial governments; business, industry, and other private sector partners; philanthropic organizations; community- and faith-based organizations; and everyday Americans to improve health through prevention. Initiatives such as *Healthy People 2030* and the USPSTF recommendations are excellent examples of well-researched tools that can enhance health promotion and disease prevention. The result will be comprehensive care of patients with the goal of optimal health for all.

Immunization Practices

Immunization administration is one of the best examples of primary health promotion. Immunizations provide the patient's body with the ability to build up antibodies to a potential life-threatening illness before exposure to the offending agent. The guidelines for immunization continue to evolve over time; the most current information can be obtained from the CDC's Web site, which offers current immunization guidelines for children and adults (https://www.cdc.gov/vaccines/schedules/). For more information on immunizations, please see Chapter 77.

Immunizations are an effective form of primary health promotion, but they are not without controversy. Over the past several years, some consumers have argued that immunizations are not safe and, in fact, cause diseases such as autism and attention deficit-hyperactivity disorder. There is no evidence to support that theory, however.

Each clinician must provide patients and their families with accurate information regarding immunization administration, including potential side effects and known contraindications to immunization, and keep a copy of a written consent for each immunization on file. This consent must be obtained for each immunization before it is administered. If, after administration of a vaccine, a patient develops a significant reaction (such as a very high fever, uncontrollable crying for more than 2 hours, lethargy, a coma, etc.), the patient should be evaluated in a timely manner, and the potential adverse reaction to the vaccine should be reported. In 1986, the National Childhood Vaccine Injury Act required that all health-care providers report any severe adverse reactions to the Vaccine Adverse Event Reporting System and the CDC. The length of time from administration to the appearance of a reportable adverse reaction is between 7 and 30 days and is dependent on whether the vaccine contains a live virus. When in doubt, it is best to report the event.

Information regarding potential reactions for each vaccine is available in the *Red Book* developed by the American Academy of Pediatrics or on the CDC Web site's Morbidity and Mortality Weekly Report *(MMWR)*, at https://www.cdc.gov/mmwr/index.html. Immunization is still one of the best methods for preventing illness and disease or the serious sequelae that can develop from specific diseases such as polio, diphtheria, *Haemophilus influenzae*, and others.

Individual Influences

The key to successful health promotion is the motivation and commitment of the patient. To obtain a successful outcome, the patient must be willing to make lifestyle changes. The clinician should provide patients with health education that informs them of their current risk factors, the possibility of reducing or eliminating risk factors by lifestyle changes, and the potential benefits of implementing these changes. Once the clinician has provided the information to the patient, the decision to act rests with the patient. An ideal scenario for health promotion would involve both patient and clinician working in partnership toward mutually agreed-upon health goals. However, the choice to engage in this partnership is the patient's decision. For example, 36-year-old K.J. is being seen for a routine physical examination and reveals a smoking history of a pack a day of cigarettes for 20 years. The provider counsels her about her smoking habit and the associated risk for cardiac, respiratory, and peripheral vascular disease. She states that she understands that smoking is not good for her health but currently is not willing to quit. This scenario illustrates that despite the best efforts of the clinician, the patient still has the right to not engage in health-promoting behaviors.

Many factors can influence a patient's motivation to engage in health-promotion activities, such as willingness to alter lifestyle practices, belief that making the changes will affect health, and belief that promoting health can prevent disease. These factors influence whether a patient decides to make lifestyle changes. Several health models have been developed to identify factors that influence a patient's willingness to act and make changes. Nola Pender's Health Promotion Model provides a framework for health-care providers to use in assessing patients' readiness to make lifestyle changes to promote their own health (2017). Pender's model has four assumptions: (1) People seek active participation to regulate their own behavior; (2) people interact with the environment and are transformed as they transform their environment; (3) health professionals, including nurses, are part of the interpersonal environment that has influence on people throughout their life span; and (4) people reconfigure the person-environment interactive patterns, and this is essential to change behavior. There are several factors that affect a patient's decision to act. Pender divides these factors into two types: cognitive-perceptual factors and modifying factors. Cognitive-perceptual factors include items such as importance of health, perceived control of health, and perceived barriers to health-promoting behaviors. Modifying factors include biological characteristics, situational factors, and demographic characteristics.

Pender states that these factors will affect a patient's willingness to act (which she terms "cues to take action"). For example, 17-year-old Jonathan had not been consistently wearing a seat belt while riding in or driving a car until 2 months ago. His friend Kyle was involved in a motor vehicle collision (MVC) in which Kyle was seriously injured. Kyle's parents informed Jonathan that Kyle's injury could have been prevented if Kyle had been wearing a seat belt. In this situation, Jonathan has changed his perception (cognitive-perceptual factors) about the importance of wearing a seat belt (health-promoting behavior) based on interpersonal influences (his friend's involvement in an MVC). His "cue to action" was hearing that the injuries incurred by Kyle could have been avoided had Kyle been wearing his seat belt.

This scenario illustrates that although various factors can influence positive health changes, the "cues to action" for patients may vary. In this scenario, it would be interesting to find out if the MVC caused Kyle to change his behavior regarding seat belt use. It is important that clinicians strive to offer patients a variety of scenarios to promote health.

Today's focus on primary disease prevention is empowering for patients, in contrast to the situation 20 years ago, when most patients were not given the option of actively participating in their health care. Health care today provides many opportunities for patients and clinicians to optimize health through health promotion and disease prevention.

Community Influences

Community efforts can also substantially enhance health-promotion efforts. As described previously, the burden of responsibility regarding sanitation, hygiene, and clean water supplies rests with the local community government. A person who lives in a community that lacks appropriate waste disposal, air pollution controls, or law enforcement is exposed to greater health risks than is an individual who lives in a community in which each of these environmental issues has been effectively addressed.

Health-care providers need to work in partnership with local government agencies to ensure that healthy living conditions are a right for each citizen and not dependent on an individual's race or ethnicity, geography, or socioeconomic status. Clinicians can provide education and expertise to local government agencies for understanding the connection between effective sanitation measures and health. Each health-care provider can also alert the local community to possible outbreaks of illness and disease that can affect the greater community at large.

One of the major transitions that occurred from the earlier initiatives of *Healthy People* to *Healthy People 2000/2010/2020/2030* was the shift from a largely federal government initiative to more involvement from local and community agencies. It was believed that this shift in responsibility would result in a significant improvement in meeting the goals of the initiative.

Community programs aimed at providing health information are one way that local communities can assist with this initiative. Offering forums for dialogue between health-care providers and local citizens is an excellent way to educate a broader audience. If community leaders support these types of efforts, there will be a larger impact on the community. The development of health-promoting legislation is another way that local communities can help affect change. For example, the passage of smoking restrictions in public areas is an excellent example of how local efforts can improve the health of the communities they serve. Legislative policies and interventions that affect the health of individuals and communities, such as housing, labor, energy, transportation, education, justice, and so forth, can be initiated by local and regional agencies. *Healthy People 2030* encourages the active participation of all civic and community agencies to help meet the goals for 2030.

Communities can also respond to the "call for action" from *Healthy People 2030* by ensuring that their citizens have equal access to health care, which is a priority for the *Healthy People* initiatives. For example, it is often difficult for Indigenous populations to access health-care services because of the rural nature of their communities. The Navajo Nation, for instance, covers 27,000 square miles and includes parts of Utah, Arizona, and New Mexico. The nearest health-care facility can be a 3-hour drive away.

In addition, many communities do not have systems in place to support the efforts of patients who have language or financial barriers to seek care in their communities. Often, patients from underserved populations only have access to care through a hospital emergency department. At that time, tertiary measures of prevention are employed, and they are very costly. Community hospitals can work together with local government agencies to develop health programs/settings that will provide access to health care for all citizens.

The long-range goals of establishing these types of health programs are a reduction in direct hospital costs and an improvement in the quality of life for all citizens. Saving money is a major concern for hospitals and local communities; improving access to nonemergent health care can provide significant savings to both. Ensuring access to health-care services for underserved populations will do much to improve the health disparities affecting our nation.

The ACA was signed into law on March 23, 2010, and the U.S. Supreme Court rendered a decision on June 28, 2012, to uphold the heath-care law. The ACA puts consumers in charge of their health care, allowing for improved access to care, stability and flexibility of care, and access to information that helps them make informed choices about their health. Although there have been efforts to eliminate the ACA, none have been successful as of this writing.

Other Influences

Health-promotion strategies can be effective only when we have adequate knowledge of diseases affecting any given population. With this knowledge, individuals, families, health-care providers, community partners, and governmental agencies can work together to alleviate or minimize the impact of disease on patients. The evaluation of current health indicators is important to change the course of illness and disease. Evaluating the current leading causes of death in the United States is one way to evaluate past trends. Once this evaluation is made, it can be determined whether these diseases can be prevented or reversed with lifestyle changes.

A list of the leading causes of death in this country is published by the National Center for Health Statistics. The top 10 causes of death in the United States for 2017 and February 1, 2020, to June 27, 2020, are listed in Table 3.2. Our knowledge regarding these diseases indicates that healthy lifestyles can indeed positively affect their outcomes. For example, heart disease has been the leading cause of death in the United States for many years. A healthy lifestyle can prevent or at least ameliorate heart disease in most individuals. The previously discussed health scenario of Mr. Hart is an excellent example of risk factors for heart disease. Mr. Hart had several lifestyle factors that put him at risk for heart disease: smoking, alcohol consumption, being overweight, and elevated cholesterol and LDL levels. Making different lifestyle choices could potentially help Mr. Hart to control his heart disease to live a long and healthy life, without the devastation of a myocardial infarction or possibly even death from heart disease.

Most of the top 10 causes of death could be avoided or delayed with healthy lifestyle choices, providing hope for the future health status of patients. With early health assessment and screenings, clinicians can intervene by helping patients make healthier life choices and lowering their risks for devastating health consequences.

PRACTICAL EPIDEMIOLOGY

It is essential for clinicians to monitor trends in health and disease that may affect patients' health. In the role of health promoters for both their patients and the larger

TABLE 3.2 Top 10 Causes of Death (National Vital Statistics Report for 2017 and for USAFacts.org for February 1 to June 27, 2020)

Cause of Death	Statistics	Cause of Death	February 1 to June 27, 2020 (USAFacts.org)
Heart disease	647,457	Heart disease	353,727
Cancer	599,108	Cancer	311,008
Accidents (unintentional injuries)	169,936	COVID-19	156,975
Chronic lower respiratory disease	160.201	Stroke	81,254
Stroke (cerebrovascular disease)	146,383	Chronic lower respiratory disease	81,153
Alzheimer's disease (AD)	121,404	AD	68,786
Diabetes mellitus (DM)	83,564	DM	51,070
Influenza & pneumonia	55,672	Influenza & pneumonia	31,006
Nephritis, nephrotic syndrome, & nephrosis	50,633	Septicemia	20,520
Intentional self-harm (suicide)	47,173		

Sources: Heron, M. (2019). Deaths: leading causes for 2017. *National Vital Statistics Report, 68*(6); USAFacts.org. Top causes of death in the United States: Heart disease, cancer and COVID-19. https://usafacts.org/articles/top-causes-death-united-states-heart-disease-cancer-and-covid-19/.

community, clinicians gather and contribute raw epidemiological data to various health organizations. Clinicians then consume the analyses of these data in the research reports and journals produced by these organizations.

Epidemiology is the evaluation of distribution patterns and determinants of health and disease in populations. The focus of epidemiology is to study the trends of disease occurrences in groups rather than in individuals. The goal of epidemiological studies is to discover and evaluate the trends of illness or disease in groups of people to determine cause and effect and thereby to prevent further disease. For example, a single case of swine flu (H1N1) is a concern, but it is not the focus of epidemiology. Instead, increasing numbers of cases of the H1N1 virus become an epidemiological issue when they occur at the same time and in the same place. When susceptible populations are studied for the presence of a particular infection or disease, distribution patterns and symptoms may begin to emerge.

When disease statistics are given, reports often refer to the prevalence and incidence rates of a certain disease. The terms prevalence and incidence are commonly used to describe disease trends (Table 3.3). The *prevalence* rate refers to the number of cases of a particular disease at a particular point in time divided by the percentage of the population at a point in time. Prevalence does not distinguish between *new* and *old* cases. For example, if the current prevalence rate for a disease is 1 million, it indicates the number of new and old cases of the disease in the current population. The *incidence rate* is the number of *new* cases of a disease diagnosed at a point in time (e.g., 1 year).

Additional common terms used to study trends include *morbidity, mortality, sporadic, endemic, pandemic,* and *epidemic*. Morbidity and mortality rates are often described together. *Morbidity* is the number of people who have been diagnosed with a disease divided by the number of total population at risk. The number of people who have died from a particular disease divided by the total population is the *mortality* (Table 3.4).

To understand the difference between morbidity and mortality, consider HIV. During 2003, the estimate for the number of people living with HIV/AIDS in the United States was 1,185,000 (morbidity rate). During the same year, the total number of deaths from AIDS was 17,934 (mortality rate). The most updated rates for HIV infection (2018) indicate that significant strides have been made in prevention of HIV, which has in turn influenced the incidence, prevalence, morbidity, and mortality associated with the disease. As of 2018, there were 1,040,352 people living with HIV, and deaths fell to 15,820. More people are living longer with HIV as a result of significant advances in treatment and management.

Certain illnesses affect the population during annual predictable cycles. Terminology regarding these cycles includes *epidemic, endemic, sporadic,* and *pandemic* (Table 3.5). For example, the influenza (flu) virus is known to be prevalent during the winter season, and it can cause significant morbidity and mortality. The ability to predict the active cycle of this virus helps health-care practitioners educate and immunize patients before predicted outbreaks. These health-promotion efforts are effective means of decreasing the prevalence and incidence of the influenza virus. Each year, predictions are made regarding the number of patients who without health-promotion efforts will experience the flu. In the past, there have been years in which the number of patients experiencing the flu was significantly higher than expected, which is called an *epidemic*.

Although there is some seasonal variation in the incidence of the common cold, it is known to be present throughout the year. *Endemic* is the term used when the presence of an event is constant at or about the same frequency as expected based on past history. A *sporadic* outbreak occurs when

TABLE 3.3 Prevalence and Incidence Rates

Prevalence Rate	Incidence Rate
New and old cases of "B" disease at a specific point in time	New cases of "C" disease at a specific point in time
Number of cases divided by total population at a specific point in time	Number of cases divided by total population at a specific point in time

TABLE 3.4 Morbidity and Mortality Formulas

Morbidity Formula	Mortality Formula
Number of new cases of "D" disease divided by total population at risk	Number of deaths from "E" disease divided by total population at risk

The Patient's Voice 3.1

THE WELLNESS VISIT

Delia, a 41-year-old woman, comes in for a complete physical examination and fills out a primary health-promotion questionnaire. "This is the first time any primary care provider has asked me so many in-depth questions about my own health and well-being. After doing this, I realize that there are many things in my life that impact my health. It made me take a personal inventory of everything from emotional, social, cultural, and psychological aspects of my life." She indicates that she is willing to work with her primary care provider to begin to change some of her current health and lifestyle patterns to enhance her own health and well-being. "This has been a very enlightening exercise for me, and I can't wait to begin the journey to balance my life to be healthier."

TABLE 3.5 Epidemiological Terms

Term	Definition
Sporadic	Outbreaks of an illness/disease that occur occasionally and are unrelated in space and time
Epidemic	Presence of an event (illness or disease) at a much higher rate than expected based on past history
Endemic	Presence of an illness/disease constantly present or present at a rate that is expected based on history
Pandemic	Presence of an event in epidemic proportions affecting many communities and countries in a short period of time

there are occasional cases of an event unrelated in space or time. For example, a gastrointestinal virus may be present in three patients this month, 20 patients 2 months from now, and 100 patients in 6 months. The virus is present but is not causing illness at a specific time and place. It is rare to hear of a patient having the flu during the summer season. A *pandemic* is defined as the presence of an event in epidemic proportions affecting many communities and countries in a short period of time.

In 1918, the great influenza pandemic was known as the deadliest one in history. Today, we are in the midst of a global pandemic. The WHO declared the outbreak a pandemic in March 2020, and it has spread to more than 200 countries, with severe public health and economic consequences (https://covid19.who.int). The pandemic is a result of a novel (new) coronavirus (SARS-CoV-2), which causes severe acute respiratory syndrome, among other manifestations. The disease was first identified in Wuhan, Hubei, China, in December 2019. In March 2020, the WHO declared the COVID-19 outbreak a pandemic. Public health groups, including the CDC and WHO, are monitoring the pandemic.

At the time of this writing 8 months after the virus was first identified, there continues to be a rise in illness and deaths, continued quarantines, development of COVID testing, research on medication for treatment, and the hope of a vaccine. COVID-19 vaccines (2 doses—Pfiser and Moderna) were approved by the FDA for emergency use in December 2020 with full approval in August 2021. The single dose Janssen vaccine was approved for emergency use in February 2020 with full approval in November 2021. The impact on day-to-day life and front-line health-care workers caring for affected people has been globally significant. Around the world, there have been mass closings of schools, factories, and businesses and orders for everyone to stay at home. These measures were initially effective in reducing the number of cases. As more and more businesses and schools opened and stay-at-home restrictions were eased, the number of cases in the United States began to rise. Some states and/or localities instituted mandatory face coverings when in public, which has shown to be effective. Currently, face coverings, keeping at least 6 feet of physical distance from others, and practicing handwashing and disinfection are the methods used worldwide to combat the spread of the virus.

The CDC generally monitors and reports the incidence, prevalence, morbidity, and mortality rates of diseases and specifically monitors the rates of infectious diseases. This information is distributed in the weekly *MMWR Report*. The report contains useful information about current infectious diseases that are a threat to local and global communities and provides the latest guidelines for treatment of infectious diseases. It is a helpful tool to investigate current infectious disease trends and potential health-promotion practices that may minimize or eliminate the threat of infectious disease.

CONCLUSION

Health promotion is one of the most powerful tools available today to prevent disease and disability. Clinicians should use health-promotion strategies at the primary, secondary, and tertiary levels of prevention. Each level of prevention is important, but the ultimate goal is primary prevention because it has the most significant impact on disease. Actively engaging in primary prevention strategies, such as health promotion, creates a wonderful opportunity for patients and health-care providers to work together as a team with the common goal of wellness and the prevention of disease. When primary prevention strategies are not feasible, *Healthy People 2030* and the USPSTF provide clinicians with guidelines to initiate secondary prevention strategies, such as early screening and detection of illness and disease. The utilization of these guidelines and health-focused initiatives will help to improve the health of the nation. With all health-promotion strategies in place and a focus on disease prevention, it may be possible to eliminate or minimize the most expensive level of health promotion: tertiary prevention. As we embrace the third decade of the 21st century, we continue to build momentum for primary health-promotion strategies with the goal of ensuring optimal health and wellness for all citizens.

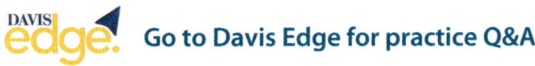
Go to Davis Edge for practice Q&A

REFERENCES

Advisory Committee on Immunization Practices (ACIP). Vaccine Recommendations and Guidelines of the ACIP. https://www.cdc.gov/vaccines/hcp/acip-recs/index.html. Accessed 8/25/2020.

The Affordable Care Act. U.S. Department of Health & Human Services. https://www.hhs.gov/healthcare/about-the-aca/index.html. Accessed 10/19/2020.

Agency for Healthcare Research and Quality (AHRQ). *Health literacy*, https://dev.ahrq.gov/topics/health-literacy.html. Accessed 8/25/2020.

Agency for Healthcare Research and Quality (AHRQ). Ten Attributes of Health Literate Health Care Organizations. Content last reviewed August 2019. Agency for Healthcare Research and Quality, Rockville, MD. Created June 2019 and last reviewed August 2019 https://www.ahrq.gov/professionals/quality-patient-safety/quality-resources/tools/literacy/ten-attributes.html

American Nurses Association. *Nursing's social policy statement: The essence of the profession.* 3rd ed. Silver Spring, MD: American Nurses Association; 2010.

Dossey B, Keegan L. *Holistic nursing: A handbook for practice.* 7th ed. Burlington, MA: Jones & Bartlett Learning; 2016.

Heron M. Deaths: Leading causes. *National Vital Statistics report,* 2019:68(6) https://www.cdc.gov/nchs/data/nvsr/nvsr68/nvsr68_06-508.pdf

Mariano C. *Holistic nursing: scope and standards of practice.* In: Dossey B, Keegan L, eds. *Holistic nursing: A handbook for practice.* 7th ed. Burlington, MA: Jones & Bartlett Learning; 2016.

Murdaugh CL, Parsons MA, & Pender N. *Health promotion in nursing practice.* 8th ed. Upper Saddle River, NJ: Prentice-Hall; 2018.

National Center for Health Statistics. https://www.cdc.gov/nchs/index.htm. Accessed 8/25/2020.

Surgeon General. The national prevention strategy: prioritizing prevention to improve the nation's health. U.S. Department of Health and Human Services; 2014. https://prevention.nih.gov/education-training/methods-mind-gap/national-prevention-strategy-prioritizing-prevention-improve-nations-health#:~:text=About%20the%20National%20Prevention%20Strategy&text=The%20Strategy%20provides%20evidence%2Dbased,health%20in%20their%20own%20communities.

U.S. Department of Health & Human Services. Office of the Surgeon General's Priorities. https://www.hhs.gov/surgeongeneral/priorities/index.html. Accessed 10/16/2020.

U.S. Department of Health and Human Services. *Healthy people 2000.* Washington, DC: U.S. Government Printing Office; 1996.

U.S. Department of Health and Human Services. *Healthy people 2010.* Washington, DC: U.S. Government Printing Office; 2000.

U.S. Department of Health and Human Services. *Healthy people 2020.* www.healthypeople.gov/2020/topicsobjectives2020/default.aspx. Accessed 8/18.

U.S. Department of Health & Human Services, Office of Disease Prevention and Health Promotion (ODPHP). *Healthy People 2030 Framework,* https://www.healthypeople.gov/2020/About-Healthy-People/Development-Healthy-People-2030-Framework. Updated 8/14/2020.

U.S. Department of Health, Education, and Welfare, Public Health Service. The Surgeon General's report on health promotion and disease prevention. Washington, DC: U.S. Department of Health and Human Services; U.S. Government Printing Office; 1979.

U.S. Preventive Services Task Force. Procedure Manual. https://www.uspreventiveservicestaskforce.org/uspstf/procedure-manual. Accessed 8/25/2020.

U.S. Preventive Services Task Force. An Evidence-Based Prevention Resource for Nurse Practitioner. https://www.uspreventiveservicestaskforce.org/uspstf/about-uspstf/methods-and-processes/evidence-based-prevention-resource-nurse-practitioners. Accessed 8/25/2020.

U.S. Preventive Services Task Force. Screening Recommendations. https://www.uspreventiveservicestaskforce.org/uspstf/recommendation-topics/uspstf-and-b-recommendations#:~:text=The%20USPSTF%20recommends%201-time%20screening%20for%20abdominal%20aortic,to%2070%20years%20who%20are%20overweight%20or%20obese. Accessed 8/25/2020.

World Health Organization. Constitution of the World Health Organization, 45th edition, October 2006. https://www.who.int/publications/m/item/constitution-of-the-world-health-organization. Accessed 10/16/2020.

RESOURCES

Agency for Healthcare Research and Quality
http://www.ahrq.gov

American Academy of Family Physicians
http:// www.aafp.org

American Academy of Nurse Practitioners
http:// www.aanp.org

American College of Nurse Practitioners
http:// www.nurse.org/acnp

American College of Sports Medicine
http:// www.acsm.org

Centers for Disease Control and Prevention
http:// www.cdc.gov/cdc.html

National Institute of Nursing Research
https://www.ninr.nih.gov/

National Institutes of Health
http:// www.nih.gov

National Library of Medicine
http:// www.nlm.nih.gov

Occupational Safety and Health Administration
http:// www.osha.gov

U.S. Department of Health and Human Services
http:// www.hhs.gov

U.S. Food and Drug Administration
http:// www.fda.gov

U.S. Preventive Services Task Force
https://www.uspreventiveservicestaskforce.org/Page/Name/home

Chapter 4

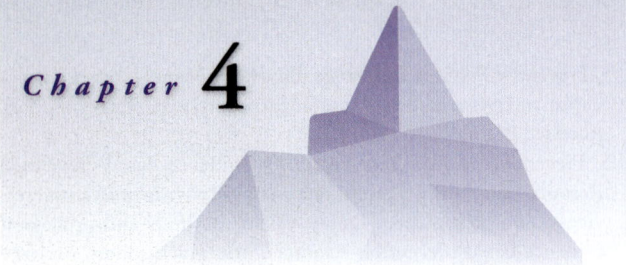

The Art of Diagnosis and Treatment

Teresa Gibson, DNP, APRN, FNP-BC
Erica Muniz, DNP, APRN, FNP-BC
Jill E. Winland-Brown, EdD, APRN, FNP-BC, FAANP
Katherine Chadwell, DNP, MBMSc, APRN, GNP-BC

Health-care policy reform continues to drive critical changes in the health-care system. Regardless of how the system evolves, nurse practitioners (NPs) will be central in delivering much of primary care. NPs are able to offer unique services in primary care for several reasons. All NPs provide care by making treatment and screening choices, based on current research findings. Evidence-based care works best when systems of care are established so that local protocols and tracking systems support the diagnosis and treatment decisions of providers and adhere to a standard of care.

NPs are able to provide evidence-based care particularly well because they bring a nursing perspective of whole-person care to patient encounters in settings that in some cases have been traditionally more disease centered than person centered. Instead of focusing solely on diagnoses, clinicians can work with patients to improve overall health by considering each person's life situation. A care plan may include medications as well as recommendations for diet, activity, rest, stress management, and health promotion. Evidence-based practice requires more than a "diagnose-and-treat" mentality. There is more to do in a primary care visit than set up a treatment plan. Treatment decisions are made based on patient values, preference, and resources while also considering guidelines and research-based recommendations. Learning to practice primary care is an art, and it requires a certain kind of thinking.

CLINICAL JUDGMENT IN PRIMARY CARE

Clinical Judgment and the Circle of Caring

The Circle of Caring model introduced in Chapter 1 provides a framework for advanced practice nursing. It includes aspects of the more traditional medical model approach within a model that has nursing as its origin. The Circle of Caring incorporates elements of the patient's experience, including the context of that experience in the patient's life and the environment in which care is delivered. It includes traditional modes of assessment, such as history taking, that are similar to those of the medical model but also are grounded in the nursing perspective, functional health patterns, and other holistic measures. Objective findings include physical assessment data, laboratory test data, and functional measures. The Circle of Caring demonstrates that the clinician uses these data as part of a data collection process that leads to the identification of both medical diagnoses as listed in the International Classification of Diseases, 10th revision and to human responses to those specific diagnoses. A full understanding of the patient's situation provides a basis for planning interventions based on the best available evidence. Patient preferences are considered as the patient and clinician together design a treatment plan that may include pharmacological measures in addition to lifestyle choices and complementary modalities to approach healing and wellness. The Circle of Caring reflects that outcomes of NP practice include improved mortality and morbidity statistics for aggregates of patients; optimized use of the health-care system that provides early, relatively inexpensive treatments to prevent more expensive problems later; and improved functional status and quality of life, as judged by the patient. All of this occurs in an environment consistent with the Institute of Medicine's recommendations that all patients have access to care based on best available evidence, as well as care that takes into account the patient's preferences and values.

Not only is the Circle of Caring an expanded way of thinking about the nursing and medical clinical process, but it also denotes the way in which the NP and patient relate to each other within this model. The NP is able to make appropriate diagnoses and intervention selections on the basis of knowing the patient, being committed to using appropriate clinical guidelines, and having patience when working with the patient, who may be required to make substantial lifestyle changes as a result of illness or risk factors. In addition, both patient and nurse exhibit courage, in that they engage in this most human of endeavors, that of caring. Throughout assessment, diagnosis, and treatment, the NP brings an authentic presence, which is in itself humanizing and healing, and is willing to be an advocate for the patient in personal or professional realms. The Circle of Caring requires a balance. The nurse and patient working together need to create meaningful plans for treatment and follow-up support. The Circle of Caring depicts a complex yet rewarding practice that enriches both patient and nurse.

Essential to high-quality clinical judgment is the ability of the nurse to form a link between the patient's experience of health concerns and the range of diagnostic and therapeutic choices available to achieve a range of possible outcome states. The clinician must be expert at eliciting the true story of the patient ("entering their world") and recognizing patterns that are presented in the data to arrive at an appropriate diagnosis and therapeutic plan. This chapter focuses on merging the results of research with diagnostic reasoning and clinical judgment to facilitate their application by the clinician.

Purpose and Goal of Diagnostic Reasoning

From the patient's point of view, the purpose of a visit to a clinician may be to solve a physical problem. Beyond problem-solving, the practitioner must always keep in mind that every visit is an opportunity for disease prevention, screening for high-risk problems, and health promotion based on appropriate guidelines. The patient must know that initial concerns are taken seriously and are not ignored. The clinician can establish a tone that attends to body, mind, and spirit in every visit. Diagnostic reasoning to solve problems, promote health, and screen for disease or illness all require sensitivity to complex stories, contextual factors, and a sense of probability and uncertainty. At times, the patient will schedule a visit, stating one concern, but during the visit, other issues arise that become more important. Headache might be caused by a stressful job or family situation, or the patient might not want to tell the scheduler that domestic violence or a sexual concern is really what is bothering them. Clinicians learn to pay attention to the "By the way, I was wondering about..." lead-ins to real concerns. Chapter 87 deals with mental health coaching in primary care; it provides strategies for getting to the heart of the patient's true concerns and introduces motivational interviewing and coaching techniques to assist the patient and family in making needed behavioral changes.

The mental tasks of eliciting and sorting through large amounts of data, clustering data elements into meaningful patterns, connecting patterns to reasonable diagnostic statements, considering risk factors, and selecting appropriate interventions require the highest order of cognitive processes. These analytical functions distinguish advanced practice nursing, and patients seek our services because of them. The human element of caring helps elicit rich data and establish the trust necessary to encourage patients to adjust their living patterns in the short or long term.

Unique Aspects of Primary Care

Many students come to advanced practice programs with extensive experience in acute- or critical-care nursing. They are committed to learning an expanded mode of practice but may be overwhelmed by the amount of new material that must be mastered. Even students with community health experience find that issues faced in primary care differ from those encountered in previous practices and require new knowledge and skills. Primary care is a new world with a different set of problems to be solved, different kinds of constraints on choices, and a different culture of care. Entering this world with sensitivity to its differences can help reduce anxiety for new NP students and can explain other reactions to this new nursing setting that might arise.

The types of problems addressed in primary care are different from those encountered in acute- or critical-care settings. Upper respiratory infections, common abdominal complaints, skin rashes, and vaginal discharges are problems not often encountered in acute-care settings. Even chronic conditions present differently in primary care. Hypertension, heart failure, arthritis, and diabetes present day-to-day management problems that are different from the crises to which acute-care nurses must respond. Patients with psychosocial problems, such as anxiety and depression, frequently present with vague, nonspecific somatic complaints.

The pace of care is different in primary care. Nurses who are seeking refuge from busy acute-care duties will be surprised by the mental fatigue that comes from diagnosing and treating up to 30 different patients or families in a day. The sheer variety of possible problems faced in a day's time is exciting and interesting, but it is also challenging. Primary care includes more than problem-solving and symptom management. It involves screening for problems as yet undetected and supporting health promotion and disease and injury prevention at every opportunity. It also involves dealing with patients who have chronic diseases and need to make behavioral changes, which can present challenges. Teaching patients of all ages about how their bodies work, risk reduction, and treatment options helps patients assume more responsibility for their own wellness. These activities support patients in increasing their health literacy so that they can be active participants in their own care. Establishing trust and believing that the NP cares about the whole person promote true person-centered care.

Uncertainty

Primary care and the increased autonomy that NPs enjoy also bring increased uncertainty. Patient problems are not always labeled when the NP sees the patient. Many different conditions present in similar ways. Even the "hard numbers" of laboratory tests must be evaluated for their reliability. Once a diagnosis is made, multiple treatment approaches are available even for simple problems. Furthermore, patients do not always carry out recommended treatment plans. Many problems require lifelong lifestyle adjustment. At the end of the day, the clinician may have nagging doubts about the decisions that were made on many levels. New practitioners especially need support to develop confidence in their diagnostic and treatment-planning capabilities, but even experienced practitioners describe learning to live with the uncertainties involved in primary care. Intellectual honesty and humility are important aspects of thoughtful practice; they can be cultivated, but they must be balanced with confidence based on experience.

Nursing and the Medical Model

NPs perform in both nursing and medical domains. The nursing domain considers individual and family responses to actual or potential threats to health. It involves helping patients cope with disease processes that may be occurring, and it anticipates human distress and works on the level of what an illness experience means to the patient. By becoming an NP, nurses do not leave their nursing model of practice. As NPs gain skill in the medical domain of practice, they learn new diagnostic reasoning possibilities and new treatment options for specific medical problems. These new skills are built on the nursing framework, but they do not replace the nursing basis for practice. NPs have been proven to be effective and efficient care providers for patients with acute and chronic health problems. The process of clinical judgment is unique in primary care because patients and their families are actively involved, and the clinician must take that into account in designing a treatment or health-promotion plan. Although much of this textbook is designed to provide a background for managing medical problems, all that the nurse has learned in caring for patients still applies. An NP's approach to patient problems is invariably very individualized and, therefore, not as easy to summarize in a textbook. Nevertheless, the nursing model supports and nurtures the NP's practice. It provides the basis for the Circle of Caring.

Communication

A model for how clinicians comanage patients elicits three attributes to effectively provide care. These involve communication, mutual respect and trust, and clinical alignment. Communication is essential so that all clinicians caring for the patient are on the same "wavelength" and provide effective feedback to improve the quality of care for the patient. Reciprocal trust and respect are necessary to prevent looking over one's shoulder and help reduce redundancy of documentation and diagnostic testing. *Clinical alignment* refers to having a shared philosophy with respect to approaches to care management (Norful, de Jacq, Carlino, et al, 2018).

Effective communication is an intentional process that involves providing authentic presence and finding out from patients what matters most so that they will listen to their clinicians. Gaining feedback is essential to validate that the clinician and the patient both understand what's being communicated. The Agency for Healthcare Research and Quality cites the SHARE approach as a model for shared decision making. SHARE stands for **S**eek your patient's participation, **H**elp your patient explore and compare treatment options, **A**ssess your patient's values and preferences, **R**each a decision with your patient, and **E**valuate your patient's decision. The quality of communication and agreement about what the encounter is meant to accomplish will improve both effectiveness and satisfaction with the patient encounter for both parties.

THE CLINICAL PROCESS AND ITS LIMITATIONS

Human Memory Limitations

One of the most useful models for understanding diagnostic reasoning is the information-processing model. This model is built on the premise that the human brain has both short- and long-term memory and that these forms of memory are different from each other. Short-term memory is the processing space that can hold new pieces of information and elements of the patient history and physical data. It has the limitation of being able to hold only approximately seven "bits" of information. Much of the mental activity used in diagnostic reasoning is done to maximize the active processing space and to cluster or "chunk" cues into collections of data that can be managed together, which helps to maximize processing capacity.

In contrast, long-term memory is practically unlimited. It can hold vast quantities of facts, sensations, and experiences. To bring these facts or experiences to bear on a given situation, long-term memories must be accessible. Research has shown that the ability to retrieve a fact depends on the frequency with which the fact is brought forward for use. This is why in some cases repetitive exercises assist in cementing long-term memory. Another factor that affects retrievability of facts from long-term memory is the organizational structure with which the fact is associated. Body systems and functional health patterns are systems of data organization that help busy clinicians retrieve relevant bits of information as needed.

Although the information-processing model is a useful starting point, it leaves out many of the complexities of the human experience. The human brain is able to sense patterns of data and include emotional responses to interactions with human beings. The ability to empathize with a patient, to be authentically present, and to be invested with the patient in maximizing health make the human decision maker much more valuable than any computer or protocol system could ever be. Patients come to a clinician for more than a diagnosis; they come for a human connection. The human aspect of the nurse–patient relationship adds to, rather than detracts from, diagnostic accuracy. Research suggests NPs create equalitarian relationships by being present, listening to, and communicating effectively with patients, leading to improved patient satisfaction and outcomes in the primary care setting (Rickards & Hamilton, 2020).

Critical Thinking

Diagnostic reasoning can be seen as a kind of critical thinking. *Critical thinking* has been defined as reflective thinking because the process involves questioning one's thinking to determine whether all possible avenues have been explored and whether the conclusions that are being drawn are based on evidence. This kind of thinking supports clinical judgment in several ways. First, it becomes a habit of mind to have humility about one's thought processes and to know that even the most experienced thinker can be mistaken. Second, it becomes a systematic way of generating creative ways of thinking about problems. Third, critical thinking returns one to an examination of the strength of evidence for a given conclusion. "Evidence" in this context means more than "hard" data such as laboratory values. Even laboratory values must be examined critically when they are used to assist diagnostic reasoning. The type of evidence that is useful includes subjective impressions of the ways patients present themselves. The patient's initial complaint may be fatigue, but any patient who describes a bone-chilling inability to generate energy for daily living (compared with a fulfilled fatigue that comes after a challenging situation is completed) is providing data the clinician can use to investigate potentially serious health problems.

Critical thinking can include creative thinking—in this sense, the clinician is creative in developing potential problem lists. A patient may complain of abdominal pain. The pattern is unclear, or it may indicate irritable bowel syndrome. The creative clinician will explore stress management issues as a way of generating diagnostic and therapeutic choices that could include a diet and symptom log, increased fiber in the diet, a walking program, or a quick follow-up visit to check on symptoms. Creativity may also be required in developing goals with patients for their short- or long-term problems. In addition to creative processing, critical thinking includes systematic thinking that evaluates each new piece of data as it either supports some diagnostic hypotheses or reduces the likelihood of others.

Intuition

Another kind of thinking that develops with experience is that of intuition. Research on intuition shows that it develops after long experience in a particular setting and that it is based on unconscious thought that is probably exquisite pattern matching. The experienced clinician is reminded of a situation that occurred in the past when presented with a certain new situation. Experience provides a picture of what will likely happen. The experienced clinician often could not list the specific data points that led to the conclusion. In fact, in some studies of artificial intelligence, experienced clinicians were asked to "think aloud" as a research device aimed at identifying the steps involved in reaching a diagnosis. Experienced clinicians reported that being asked to do that kind of thinking changed their thought processes and slowed them down. Although intuition characterizes expert practice, it is not a goal in itself. Being able to reflect on one's thinking processes opens the process to analysis, sharing, and improvement.

Developing Expertise

Benner et al (1996) have done extensive work describing differences in clinical judgment based on experience. Benner first published her work in 1982. NP students, even those who are experts in hospital or specialty care, find it disconcerting to enter a world where they feel like novices again. Even skills that were part of their old practices feel awkward. Their minds often do not generate ideas smoothly, and they focus on execution of skills more than on patients' situations. With the experience of the clinical practicum, however, the student gains skill and by graduation is probably functioning at the advanced beginner level. Features of diagnostic reasoning used in the various stages of expertise are summarized in Table 4.1.

DIAGNOSTIC PROCESS OVERVIEW

In general, the diagnostic process involves collecting data from a variety of sources (e.g., the history, physical examination, and diagnostic test results) and then generating a working hypothesis about the cause of the patient's signs and symptoms. In collecting data and generating a hypothesis, the clinician uses probabilistic reasoning, pattern matching, planning, problem-solving, and critical reflection. These processes are commonly summarized by describing the steps in the nursing process or the clinical reasoning process. Research has shown that many clinicians, physicians, nurses, occupational and physical therapists, dentists, and others use a similar method. Although research that uses simulated case studies to examine methods of clinician reasoning tends to oversimplify what happens in real life, it is helpful to review a simplified description of the diagnostic process.

TABLE 4.1 Skill Acquisition in Advanced Practice Nursing

Skill Level	Features of Clinical Judgment
Novice	Rule-based actions, unaware of context
Advanced beginner	Sensitive to aspects of the situation, able to formulate principles, needs help setting priorities
Competent	Goal-directed actions, feeling of mastery based on experience, deliberate planning
Proficient	Sees situation as a whole, immediate grasp of meaning, recognizes patterns of normalcy or aberrance, uses maxims to guide action
Expert	Transcends rules, intuitive grasp of the wholeness of situation, creative response to particularities of situation, flexible response to situations

Research indicates that expert clinicians generate a list of possible diagnoses or diagnostic hypotheses early in the clinical encounter. The likelihood that the diagnostic choice will be correct is higher if the correct diagnosis is included in the initial hypothesis list. In generating hypotheses, the clinician considers a number of labels that could be associated with the initial complaint and considers potential problems for each patient, based on the patient's age and demographics and the setting of the practice.

For experienced clinicians, data acquisition during history-taking and physical examination is most effective if it is hypothesis driven—that is, when the information selected and gathered is related to the list of possible diagnoses. For common problems, the data collection approach becomes routine and, therefore, takes less active processing space in short-term memory. In contrast, novices tend to use a "shotgun" approach and ask a little bit about everything that might be possible, not considering which diagnoses are most likely. Hypothesis-driven data collection means that data that would confirm or disprove a specific hypothesis are specifically sought and recorded. It is not enough to note only those data that fit with one possible problem. Competing hypotheses must be ruled out by seeking nonconfirmatory data. In doing this, the clinician must be open to changing the priority list of hypotheses based on new information. For example, rhinitis may present similar to a viral infection; however, when asked whether the symptoms have occurred before, the patient says, "Yes, I had the same thing 2 weeks ago." This response decreases the likelihood of viral illness and increases the likelihood of allergy.

An approach to data collection that is completely symptom driven, however, can result in leaving out important concepts. The agenda for the visit includes not only the patient's agenda but also expands the visit to provide health promotion.

Data are clustered together into meaningful "chunks" of information that explain and account for different elements of the history. Clinicians are alert to any data bits that do not fit the pattern of what is expected. They are alert to the feeling in themselves that "something is just not right here." This feeling can indicate that the problem is more serious than it initially appeared or that there are data bits that are not yet accounted for. Diagnosticians are persistent in trying to fit the pieces of data into a coherent picture. One must be on guard not to ignore discrepant data. Research has shown that "we see what we expect to see" in many cases, so openness to the patient situation must be maintained to continue "seeing" all the data present.

A maxim of practice is that "common things occur commonly." Students are frequently excited to make a diagnosis for the rare or exotic condition. This can be the result of a rich experience in acute- or critical-care settings where the most serious cases are seen. In primary care, common problems predominate. The adage "When you hear hoofbeats, think horses, not zebras" applies. In real life, "zebra" diagnoses are rare. Rare conditions can be considered with the differential list, but their lower probability must be taken into consideration.

Experienced clinicians keep their antennae raised for the most serious conditions. Abdominal pain could be from gas, but if it is from a ruptured ectopic pregnancy, a dissecting abdominal aortic aneurysm, or a ruptured appendix, immediate surgical consultation is necessary. The clinician must make it a point to collect and document data that rule out any potentially life-threatening condition.

Diagnoses are frequently interrelated. Obesity, hypertension, hyperlipidemia, and type 2 diabetes mellitus (DM) frequently occur together. When evaluating competing hypotheses, the clinician can cluster related problems together. The lifestyle recommendations for all these conditions are the same. The medication approach might differ. Clinicians should try to approach the core diagnosis, which, if managed appropriately, will ameliorate all the others. By dealing with the underlying problem, the other problems might not need direct intervention. If the clinician focuses only on the superficial problem level, the problems may still remain.

Clustering history data into a likely problem list helps to focus the physical examination, laboratory test evaluation, and initial management plan. Physical examination for a problem-focused visit serves to rule in or rule out competing diagnostic hypotheses. A new hypothesis rarely emerges during a physical examination, but it might emerge for a problem that the patient cannot see or that causes no symptoms, such as a skin lesion. Laboratory tests also provide information that is not available any other way.

Finally, a working diagnosis is reached, even though there might still be some uncertainty. A management plan is discussed with the patient in light of mutually shared goals and guidelines for practice based on published research. Honest conversation about the patient's ability and willingness to follow treatment recommendations will result in more realistic plans. Written instructions often help patients implement complicated treatment directions. Part of the treatment plan always includes a plan for follow-up. Patients need to know when to return for a visit and under what circumstances they should telephone. Documenting these plans in the patient record reduces the possibility of misunderstanding and places appropriate responsibility with the patient. Some patients need support in learning how to engage the health-care system in an effective way. This is one aspect of health literacy that the clinician can support.

ELEMENTS OF THE DIAGNOSTIC PROCESS

A more detailed examination of each step in the diagnostic reasoning process is presented in the following sections.

History

History of Present Illness

Taking a history is the first step in the diagnostic reasoning process. Problems cannot be found, strengths identified, or appropriate direction known without a real grounding in the lived experience of the individual patient. If the patient's visit is for "episodic" care or if it is for addressing a new complaint, the history begins with a history of present illness (HPI). Mnemonics can help the clinician remember the essential data elements; the "OLD CART" mnemonic is presented in Box 4.1.

Immediately on hearing the chief complaint, the clinician begins to sort out diagnostic possibilities. The list of possibilities helps to generate questions to follow up on the HPI and in other areas of the history. Specific questions are asked that help distinguish between competing diagnostic hypotheses. For example, the question, "Do you feel the pain more often on an empty stomach or several hours after eating?" helps distinguish between an ulcer and gallbladder disease. In general, asking open-ended questions helps patients give their perspectives and provides richer databases. An open-ended question is one that cannot be answered by a "yes" or "no" response. Eliciting the patient's story will assist the clinician in understanding the illness experience from the patient's point of view. Frequently interrupting the patient's story distracts and places the story in the context of the examiner and not in the context of the patient's own life.

The clinician continues to clarify the patient's story until a clear picture of the illness appears. This can require patience because patients do not know which facts "fit together" to support diagnostic hypotheses. Patients may get the chronological order confused or not recall the exact onset of their problems. They may also have more than one problem and may not be able to distinguish which symptoms cluster together. The picture may not be completely clear at this point of history-taking, but other areas of history can fill in some gaps. Periodically, the clinician can restate the emerging understanding of the story to clarify and summarize it. This summary allows the patient to clarify any misunderstandings. One important issue to address as part of the HPI is what the *patient* thinks may be wrong. Patients know their own bodies, and parents know their own children better than anyone. They may have important insights to share. On the other hand, if patients share their fears of serious diagnoses, the clinician can also explain reasons why many of those fears may be unfounded. A recurring headache does not necessarily indicate a brain tumor.

Visits to get periodic health screening, to establish a new patient–provider relationship, or to follow up on an existing problem do not use the HPI in the same sense unless a new problem is also identified. The clinician can ask, "What do you want to accomplish today?" or "What matters most to you today?" Such questions are particularly useful for the patient with a long list of problems or complaints. A plan for follow-up for other problems may need to be addressed.

Past Medical History

Past medical history (PMH) helps refine the hypothesis list by offering new explanations for symptoms or by ruling out others. The PMH also gives suggestions of risk factors for other problems that are being considered. If a patient reports that the gallbladder was removed 10 years ago, cholecystitis is now off the hypothesis list, but abdominal adhesions might go onto the list. PMH is frequently divided into childhood and other illnesses, surgical history, other hospital admissions, history of trauma, pregnancies, and psychiatric diagnoses. Travel outside the United States and any possible exposure to infectious or toxic agents can be explored. Treatment for cancer in the distant past is important in that the treatments may have increased the risk for other conditions. For example, use of some chemotherapy agents can lead to heart failure in later years.

The PMH includes information regarding all medications that the patient takes, including prescription and over-the-counter medications, such as vitamins and herbal remedies. Patients also need to be asked whether they take any medications that have been prescribed for other members of the family. Even for patients who are well known to the practice and whose medications are

Box 4.1 OLD CART Mnemonic

Onset	When did this problem start? How did it start? Has it changed over time? For an injury, exactly how did the injury occur (the mechanism of injury)?	**Duration**	Are the symptoms constant, fluctuating, getting better or worse?
		Characteristics	How are the symptoms experienced? Dull ache, sharp pain, heat, or electrical?
Location	Where exactly are the symptoms experienced? Can a specific location be identified, or is the problem more generalized? Has the symptom moved?	**Aggravating factors**	What makes the symptoms worse?
		Relieving factors	What makes the symptoms better?
		Treatment	What have you done so far to try to help the problem?

listed on the chart, asking a patient what medications he or she is currently taking allows the clinician to learn what the patient remembers about the medication regimen. For patients with multiple prescriptions, it sometimes helps to use the "brown bag" method: Ask the patient to bring in all the medications they are taking, then go over them one by one. This helps determine whether the medications that have been ordered are really being taken. This review of medications also gives the clinician information about the patient's understanding of the medications and helps determine any difficulties the patient is having with the prescribed regimen. Immunization status is part of the PMH. Many parents bring their child's immunization cards with them to office visits. This allows any additional immunization series to be documented. Adults often forget that they need immunizations for things such as tetanus, influenza, or pneumonia. Verification of the COVID-19 vaccine is also essential.

Allergies can be discussed at this time and reviewed. The kind of reaction the medications or food caused can help to distinguish an adverse effect from a true allergy. By noting the adverse effect, one can avoid confusing it with an allergy, which is characterized by rash, hives, wheezing, or other hypersensitivity reactions.

Health maintenance practices can be questioned, as well as risk reduction techniques such as seat-belt use and exercise habits. This may lead to a teaching moment, stressing the need for helmets when riding a bike or knee pads when skateboarding.

Family History

Family history provides information for a part of the risk factor pattern for this patient. The most efficient way to represent the family history is to draw a genogram (Fig. 4.1). This method of representation can be used to record family patterns of births, ages at death, and causes of death. The genogram can also record family members with whom the patient currently lives. Try to include information for at least two generations back, as well as for any children and their health status. The genogram can be used to map difficulties, such as alcohol use disorder or the quality of relationships in the family, by drawing slashes across the relationship lines that are troubled or by using thick lines to represent relationships that are strongly supportive. Judgment is required to determine whether this level of information is useful. If there is no room in the patient's record for a genogram, list the major diseases that have familiar patterns, such as diabetes, heart disease, arthritis, psychiatric problems, alcohol use disorder, and cancer.

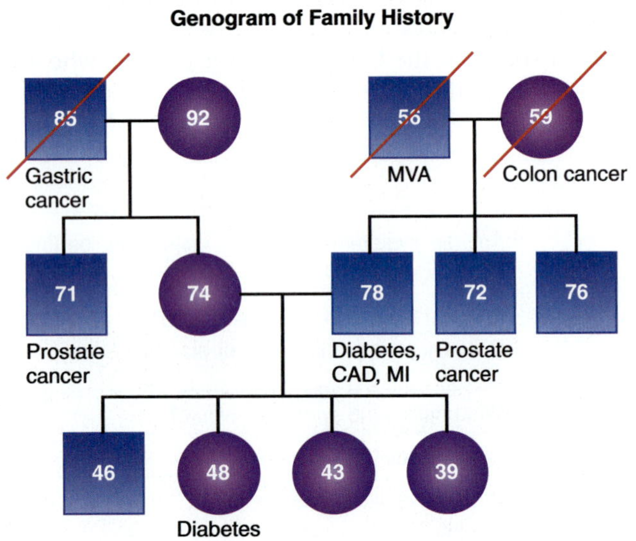

Social History

Social history in a medical model interview includes such things as work patterns. Even if the patient is retired, the type of work in which the patient had engaged is important because worksite exposures can be risk factors for many potential problems. Work background also gives the clinician a sense of how the person might handle new information and what kind of resources are available. Medical model histories also include the use of alcohol, tobacco, and street drugs. Nursing histories are more expanded in this area. Include such information as leisure time activities, risk factors and exposures, and the patient's resources and activity level. If a full functional health pattern is collected, much of this information can be recorded there. If the documentation system in use in a particular setting does not accommodate functional health patterns, expand the social history section to reflect nursing issues.

Review of Systems

This section of the history is often completed by the patient immediately before the physical examination. It is organized by body systems. Whenever the review is completed, it can include problems and symptoms that are current or related to PMH and prompt the patient to report any past difficulties. This also helps remind patients of conditions they may have forgotten and can help to refine the hypothesis list further or to screen out potential new problems. When introducing a body system, start questions in general terms and then proceed to more specific items. When documenting this section, students frequently forget that these data are appropriately recorded as subjective data because they are reported from the patient's point of view.

Functional Health Patterns

Functional health patterns, developed by Marjory Gordon in 1987, serve as a database for determining nursing diagnoses. NPs engage in some activities that require making medical diagnoses, but their practice base

Figure 4.1 Genogram of family history.

is always nursing. The value that NPs bring to a practice is an enhanced ability to assist patients with lifestyle changes and an ability to support patients as they cope with illness. The openness and thoroughness that patients report when cared for by an NP are dependent on the NP practicing from a database that is broader and more personal than that of the traditional medical model. Even in practice settings using a medically dominated model, the nurse has an obligation to represent nursing's contribution to care. The type of data recorded in the functional health pattern in the medical record can reflect a nursing approach.

For episodic visits, some patterns are more important than others, and the list can be prioritized accordingly. For example, for a patient with a sore throat, important data cover nutrition (Are they able to eat and drink sufficiently?), sleep and rest (Is sleep interrupted?), activity and exercise (Do they feel fatigued?), and role relationship (Are they able to work? Are there children in the home?). Inability of the patient to carry out normal day-to-day functions is often a "red flag"—an indicator for the NP that a potentially serious disease process may be developing.

The purpose of the functional health pattern is to determine the extent to which illness is affecting the person's ability to live a "normal" life. What accommodations must be made, even for a self-limiting condition? This is nursing's central question. What is the human response to the health problem? Advanced Assessment 4.1 presents the 11 functional health patterns and sample questions that can be used to elicit data for each functional pattern area.

At this phase of history-taking, the hypothesis list is taking shape. The initial diagnostic possibilities generated are weighed as each new piece of information is

Advanced Assessment 4.1: Functional Health Patterns: Questions to Elicit Data

Pattern	Sample Questions	Pattern	Sample Questions
Health perception	Do you have a regular health-care provider?	Cognitive/perceptual concept	Any hearing or vision problems? Any memory changes? How do you like to learn new things? Any pain or discomfort?
Health management	How often do you go to your health-care provider? What do you do to stay healthy?	Self-perception/self-concept	How would you describe yourself? Do you feel good about yourself? Any changes in how you feel about your body? Do you get angry or down at times?
Nutrition/metabolic	What did you eat yesterday or on a typical day? What do you drink? How is your appetite? Any skin problems?	Role relationship self-perception/self-concept	Who lives with you? Do you have friends? What kind of work do you do? Do you have other responsibilities?
Elimination	What are your bowel and bladder elimination patterns? Do you have unexpected loss of control?	Sexuality/reproductive Role relationship	Any problems with your sexuality? Any changes? If sexually active, do you practice safe sex? Do you use birth control? What mode of birth control do you use?
Activity/exercise	How far can you walk before feeling tired? Do you have energy to do the things you want? Do you need any assistance with feeding, bathing, toileting, dressing, getting around (activities of daily living)? Do you need any help with cooking, shopping, or cleaning (instrumental activities of daily living)?	Coping/stress tolerance	How do you cope with stress? Any use of alcohol, drugs? Do you have someone to talk things over with?
Sleep/rest	How many hours do you sleep? Any trouble falling asleep or with early wakening? Do you feel rested?	Value/belief	What is most important to you in your life? Are you religious? Any values about life that health-care providers should know? Do you have a health-care proxy (medical power of attorney) or living will (advance directive)?

Karaca, Turkan, Functional Health Patterns Model – A Case Study (2016). Case Studies Journal ISSN (2305-509X) Volume 5, Issue 7, July 2016.

gathered. Some data serve to support one hypothesis in favor of another; some data are noncontributory. Some data serve to rule out specific hypotheses. The problem list may contain physical disorders with signs or symptoms that are visible, along with other physical disorders that are presumed to be present based on the patient's story, emotional distress related to specific disorders, general emotional disorders, family or social disorders, or even spiritual distress. The patient's problem list may contain more than one diagnosis from any of the biological, psychosocial, or spiritual realms. It may also include health risks. Further data are available to help refine the hypothesis list by performing the physical examination and ordering diagnostic tests.

Physical Examination

The physical examination serves to clarify diagnostic hypotheses and to detect unanticipated problems of which the patient is unaware. In primary care, there is a wide range of ways of performing the physical examination. Textbooks of physical assessment outline a general head-to-toe model that is useful for an initial visit with a full physical examination or a periodic reassessment. In most practices, an initial patient visit is scheduled for more time, and in coding schemes the visit may be reimbursed at a higher level because of its comprehensiveness. Students in nursing or medical school learn to perform the head-to-toe examination in an organized way. In actual practice, however, clinicians must learn to focus their physical assessment skills and make the physical examination appropriate to the patient's complaint and history. If the patient complains of headache, a review of head, eyes, ears, nose, and throat and a neurological examination are indicated. For joint pain, a review of musculoskeletal tenderness, range of motion, and strength might be indicated. The body systems that are examined depend on the working hypothesis list that the clinician has generated. Examination skills need to be organized at a general screening level, with subroutines of examination techniques that can be adapted to specific findings and complaints. Positive or negative findings that serve to refine the hypothesis list must be noted and recorded in the documentation system that is in use. At times, a condition is in evolution, and the symptoms may not be clear when the patient comes for a visit. Nonetheless, the rich data reporting from that visit—even though the diagnosis is not clear—can serve to make the diagnosis more accurate later, when the condition evolves further. Full documentation serves to protect both patient and provider. The physical examination can also be a time to provide feedback and teaching about findings and about self-care. There is some evidence that thorough physical examinations are becoming rarer in medicine. An overreliance on blood work, radiology, and other tests to confirm diagnoses increases costs of care and reduces contact with the patient. The ritual of the physical examination is evidence of person-to-person attention and may be perceived as the kind of professional caring expected in a health-care visit.

Diagnostic Tests

Diagnostic tests can be used to confirm or to rule out diagnostic hypotheses or as screening devices for conditions with subtle presentations that need to be picked up early, such as lead poisoning in children. Diagnostic tests vary in their usefulness, based on their sensitivity, specificity, and predictive value. When considering or evaluating a test, consider that there are patient, test, and disease factors that affect interpretation of the tests. The prevalence of a condition is the number of cases present in a given population at a particular point in time. The incidence of a condition reflects the total number of cases during a specified time period. For example, the number of cases of flu in a year (incidence) is greater than the number of people who have the flu on a given day (prevalence). Both incidence and prevalence rates are important considerations in making accurate diagnoses. Laboratory tests and radiographic or other imaging can assist in screening for conditions and in making diagnoses. For chronic conditions, tests are used to monitor progress in managing the condition.

No test is perfect, and test results can be inaccurate. When a patient who does not have a condition has a positive test result, it is called a "false-positive result." When a patient does have a condition but has a negative test result, it is called a "false-negative result." The sensitivity of a test is greater when it has few false negatives. Sensitivity equals the number of true positives for a test divided by the number of tested individuals who truly have the disease. The specificity of a test is greater when it has few false positives. The specificity of a test is equal to the number of true negatives divided by the number of all tested individuals who do not have the disease. Table 4.2 represents the relationship between test results and actual conditions.

TABLE 4.2	Tests: Characteristics and Diseases		
Test Reading	*Disease Present*	*Disease Absent*	**Total**
Positive	True positive (TP) A	False-positive (FP) B	All positives A + B
Negative	False-negative (FN) C	True negative (TN) D	All negatives C + D
Totals	All diseased A + C	All healthy B + D	Grand Total

Source: Brown, S. (2020). Medical False Positives and False Negatives (Conditional Probability). https://brownmath.com/stat/falsepos.htm; Paulos, John Allen (1995). *A Mathematician Reads the Newspaper*. Basic Books.

In clinical practice, the predictive value of a test is the important consideration. Given a positive test result, what is the likelihood that the patient actually has the condition? Positive predictive value is equal to true positives divided by all positives. Negative predictive value is equal to true negatives divided by all negatives. Predictive value is in part dependent on the prevalence of the condition. If a condition is highly likely, a positive test result is more likely to be accurate. If a condition is very unlikely, a positive test result needs to be questioned, perhaps with different tests.

When deciding whether to order a test, cost, convenience, sensitivity and specificity, and risk of missing a condition are considered. One can ask whether the test result would affect the potential treatment plan. If not, the test might not be necessary. It is not appropriate to order a test merely to increase the clinician's confidence and comfort. Appropriate screening for life-threatening or life-altering conditions must be considered. Clinicians can use the U.S. Preventive Services Task Force guidelines or other research-based guidelines for deciding on screening tests for specific patients. It is important to always consider the individual patient's situation. For example, age for the first mammogram has changed over the years, based on research data, and is dependent, in part, on a strong family history or other risk factors for breast cancer.

Genetic Influences

"Genomic discoveries and technology are improving our ability to predict disease susceptibility, provide individualized preventive screening and risk reduction interventions, and target disease treatment" (Greco, Tinley, & Seibert, 2011). Depending on the patient's history, it may be appropriate to order genetic/genomic tests and/or studies to assist in a diagnosis. In a family practice, patients who are planning on getting pregnant may need genetic/genomic education and counseling. Clinicians should have knowledge of prescribing pharmacogenomic-based drugs and use of the information in symptom management. A genetic specialist may need to be consulted to help develop a comprehensive plan to manage these patients.

Differential Diagnosis

A differential diagnosis list is the list of possible diagnoses, usually in priority order. When clinicians discuss a case, the list of differential diagnoses is usually considered. Supports for developing a rich differential diagnosis list include several guides. One approach suggests considering the problem from the "skin in." This means that if the patient complains of chest pain, the clinician can consider all possible causes of chest pain, beginning at the skin, and visualize all structures in the area that could possibly be affected. For example, chest pain at skin level could indicate early herpes zoster sensitivity and pain.

Below the skin, the musculoskeletal system (including the rib cage) could be causing pain from costochondritis or from muscle strain. The clinician can consider pain below the rib cage as a source of pain. Could the patient have pneumonia, pneumothorax, or pulmonary embolus? Next is the esophagus. Could the pain be from esophagitis, gastroesophageal reflux, or hiatal hernia? Next consider the pericardium as a possible source of pain, as with pericarditis. Finally, consider cardiac pain. This "skin in" approach keeps the student from jumping to early conclusions without considering a wide range of problems. Thus, it avoids the common diagnostic error of premature closure.

An evolving problem list can become quite long, even on an initial visit. The following Nursing Situation describes one approach to differential diagnosis.

Nursing Situation: A Nurse Practitioner's Approach to Differential Diagnosis

An NP describes her approach to a new patient.

My initial diagnosis at that time, just by speaking with him, without any laboratory test results and examining him physically, was this: his diabetes was in poor control. His hypertension was in poor control. He had some rhinitis, probably allergic, but he was not having a problem. He has known unequal pupils since he had surgery and had damage to the pupillary musculature, but it does not affect his vision; if you did not happen to know that, you might be very concerned about it, you know? It is real important to put that in the problem list. He had a transurethral resection for benign prostatic hyperplasia. He had a real bad pes planus with secondary hip pain, and he kept going to people with back pain, and nobody ever stood him up and looked at his feet. He also had seborrheic dermatitis. The guy is an Irishman with pale skin and washed-out blue eyes, and he never used sunscreen. He had lots of skin cancers. The doctor kept calling him back to cut out the skin cancers but never told him to use sunscreen.

For this patient, the NP goes on to describe her approach to ordering diagnostic tests. Note that the hypotheses precede the test consideration. She describes her initial treatment plan:

OK, first thing you need is your laboratory parameters to check the problems that you have just defined. I would do blood counts, chemistries, thyroid function, glycohemoglobin, urines, prostate-specific antigen. The first time I see a patient, I always do the whole gamut. This guy also had had a bilateral total hip replacement, so I reviewed the subacute bacterial endocarditis prophylaxis because he had never been told about it. I started him on Prinivil, an angiotensin-converting enzyme inhibitor, because he has diabetes and had previously been on Hytrin, but it was not doing the trick, and it was not protecting his kidneys. I started him on Glucotrol. He had not been on anything other than Micronase, which he quit using because he really did not know how to use the stuff. I also talked to him about his seborrhea and sunscreen.

The NP sees the wholeness of the patient's situation. This is a different approach than treating discrete problems as they come up. The NP's description of her approach to this patient continues:

> He had had previous health care, and he thought he was doing fine. He just had never had it all put together. As far as he was concerned, he happened to have some elevated blood pressure and some elevated blood glucose, but nobody had ever put it all together in terms of the effects on the whole body. He went to someone for his glucose, and he went to somebody for his blood pressure. The guy was not a train wreck, but he had a number of problems that had been overlooked until he saw me and somebody (me) made a list. For example, he had not had a recent eye examination. For any patients with diabetes, I make sure they get an eye examination every single year. And that is how I started. His wife is also a patient of mine—a great cook, which is a tragedy for a diabetic—and he, like most husbands, will eat what he is given. So she needed some education as to what is the proper thing to eat and when and how they could cheat.

The NP is able to pull all of this patient's concerns and problems together in a way that honors his wholeness and his family dynamics. Her concern is for preventing future problems that are likely to develop, given his pattern of risk factors. Her method of collecting data and clustering it together to form a comprehensive picture of his life results in an effective, personal plan.

The differential diagnosis list should always include any conditions that are life-, organ-, or function-threatening. An NP describing a different patient situation stated:

> I always think in terms of the most dangerous or the most serious thing first—not necessarily the most catastrophic, but the most serious problem. If I know somebody has an abdominal aortic aneurysm (AAA) and he comes in with abdominal pain and it's sensitive, well, he probably has diverticulitis, but if I blow the diagnosis and go that way and it turns out that his aneurysm is dissecting, then he is dead. So I will treat his diverticulitis, but I will get the abdominal ultrasound right away. I consider the most urgent, deadly thing first. Cancer can be deadly, but it usually is not an emergency. It will kill you, but it is not going to kill you tomorrow. But an AAA can blow at any time. I had someone with an aneurysm blow in here once while I had the surgeon and the OR team waiting for him in the ER. We knew we had an aneurysm that was about to blow because I put my hand on his belly, and it was throbbing, and the patient was hypotensive, and he was sweating. He had come into the hospital because he was ready to go on vacation and just wanted to check this out before he left. So, you think of the most life-threatening situation first.

The following Nursing Situation illustrates how the diagnosis often involves more than medical problems.

Nursing Situation: An Advanced Practice Nurse's View of Nursing Versus Medical Problems

One pediatric NP described her interaction with an immigrant father who brought in a 3-year-old girl with a runny nose. The father was not disciplining the child, even though she was being difficult, because he had been reported to child protective services for hitting this child previously at 8 months of age.

> I see myself making a dual diagnosis—a nursing diagnosis as well as a medical diagnosis. If the father does not discipline his child at the appropriate time in an appropriate way, that is a knowledge deficit. So I made a nursing decision there, and I intervened on the basis of that nursing decision, but I also made a medical decision, in that the child had an upper respiratory infection, and I prescribed what I thought to be the appropriate medication for that. So, I see myself making nursing diagnoses as well as medical diagnoses and trying to somehow mesh these two to care for the family holistically because there is no way you can care for a child without caring for the family. That is my belief.

When asked if her full response was documented in the treatment plan, she responded:

> Yeah, well, it sure does not fall under "upper respiratory infection." In this case, I did not know when the family was going to apply for insurance, so I certainly did not want to put "behavior disorder" down. Instead, I put down under my diagnosis "knowledge deficit, re: discipline." In my treatment plan, I noted that I discussed discipline and that I gave the father "time out" guidelines and how to reward good behavior. I also noted that the father is coming back to me in 2 weeks to report differences in his approach to discipline and how it worked out. Nobody ever leaves my office without knowing when he or she needs to come back, and I document when I tell them to come back in my treatment plan.

Developing a Management Plan

Once the problem list has been clarified, the clinician needs to use clinical judgment about how to best manage those problems. Although NPs bill for services in the medical realm, meaning selecting an International Classification of Diseases (ICD) code for billing that designates a medical diagnosis and Current Procedural Terminology (CPT) code for treatment (see Chapter 86), they also operate in the nursing domain. NP students learn by "presenting the patient" to their preceptors. This skill involves presenting the data collected in history and physical assessment; organizing the content, along with major findings, in a coherent way to the preceptor; and then reviewing treatment options. The preceptor then confirms and clarifies the data collection with the patient and proceeds to treatment planning. Initially, students may need to use a template to ensure that they are organized as they begin this process. With experience, the organization of patient data will become more obvious. This same skill of organizing patient data is useful when communicating with consulting providers. They need a clear summary of the case for efficient consultation.

Clinicians should consider a broad range of interventions for patients in addition to prescription medications.

Different levels of interventions are useful when addressing patient problems. At the most basic level, interventions deal with symptom relief such as ice for acute muscle pain, followed by heat application for strained muscles or a prescription for muscle spasms. At a higher level of complexity, interventions address functional patterns such as stress and coping. The clinician could schedule a follow-up visit to determine whether a stressful condition is being managed more successfully after a brief teaching or counseling session. An intervention could be concerned with life patterns such as recommending a course of rehabilitation to help a patient regain confidence in exercising after a cardiac event. Finally, interventions such as spiritual support could be chosen to help patients and their families cope with life processes, such as a terminal condition. If, for example, a patient has been unable to lose weight using simple diet instruction, a more personal intervention such as counseling may be required to address the source of the problem at a deeper level.

The Diagnostic Process in Action

A simple encounter for a self-limiting acute illness might proceed as follows:

A patient requests an appointment for a "sore throat." The patient is known by the clinician as a resourceful, independent young adult. Before even entering the room, the clinician draws from experience with other patients who have complained of sore throat and begins to generate a list of hypotheses. Contextual factors enter into the reasoning: It may be allergy season in that particular area, or the clinician may have seen a large number of other patients with similar complaints who have tested positive for *Streptococcus* infection. The clinician enters the room and notes the general appearance of the patient. Does the patient appear ill, flushed, fatigued, or mildly irritated? These observations may serve to adjust the hypothesis list. The patient's story is elicited, beginning with HPI, along with a review of data already present in the record regarding PMH and medications. Further questions regarding current life stresses and exposures may also serve to adjust the hypothesis list. The history narrows the hypothesis list to a short one, although experienced clinicians have ways of preventing the common diagnostic error of premature closure and work to consider alternative conditions that could also be represented by the same cluster of symptoms.

The physical examination serves to verify hypotheses and to screen out unlikely, though troubling, alternative diagnoses. The hypothesis list is narrowed further as data are weighed to see whether they fit the pattern of the highest-favored hypothesis; disconfirming data are also elicited to avoid leaping to conclusions too early. Finally, diagnostic tests may be chosen to firm up the diagnosis if the findings of the tests will have a bearing on how the patient's care is to be managed.

Once findings of relevant tests have been obtained, treatment decisions are considered, including patient factors such as resources, reliability, and the risk of the patient's not following through on instructions. For example, insufficiently treated strep throat could result in rheumatic heart disease. In addition to prescribing medication, the clinician should consider comfort measures that are likely to assist the patient and judge the appropriateness of health promotion and educational opportunities. For example, is this a good time to give the patient smoking cessation materials? Finally, a plan to evaluate the treatment plan is made. Is a follow-up appointment necessary? Would a telephone call be useful? For which date should the next "well" visit be scheduled? The list of decisions made in this rather simple example is long. Given few data or situational changes, the management of the patient's care could be quite different, and a new-patient visit would require even deeper background data collection. Patients who present with more complex, long-term problems require even more complex decision making by the clinician. In observing the experienced clinician, many of these mental processes may not be apparent. Many of these processes occur as a kind of internal dialogue, but they occur nonetheless.

CURRENT DIAGNOSTIC PROCESS TRENDS

Evidence-Based Practice

There is an emphasis in health care today to promote evidence-based practice (EBP) (see Chapter 5). In a just society, patients have equal access to the most up-to-date treatment approaches and are able to make informed choices about their treatment. To justify a treatment approach, proponents of EBP argue that there must be evidence, either from clinical trials or from case studies, that the approach is likely to benefit the patient. Obviously, it is easier to demonstrate the benefit of a certain drug that has been tested on a large number of individuals than it is to demonstrate the effectiveness of individual counseling. However, it is important for clinicians not to limit their practices to medicine based on clinical trials alone. This may require clinical research to demonstrate case studies of creative nursing intervention success. Guidelines for practice are available from government agencies or from specialty or disease-related groups, such as the American Heart Association, the American Academy of Pediatrics, or any of the specialty organizations.

Shared Decision Making

With the increased availability of health-care choices and treatment options, providers as well as families are faced with multiple treatments and care options, including choice of medications, laboratory tests, procedures, surgeries, and home versus inpatient care, to name a few. In the past, these choices were driven primarily by provider preferences, affiliations, and insurance plans. As clinicians strive to incorporate evidence into practice, providers must balance choices with the needs and desires of the individual patient and family.

Shared decision making is a person-centered care model that encourages the patient and family to be involved, fully informed, and engaged in all decisions related to care with the premise that they can ask questions and express personal values and opinions about care. The process includes the use of evidence-based decision aids that provide patients and families with updated clinical information and decision tools based on current standards. Additionally, this process presumes the clinician will respect the patient's preferences, values, and opinions, and incorporate them into the recommendations and treatments. This type of shared decision making by engaging patients assists them in making informed individualized health decisions, resulting in improved patient satisfaction, improved health outcomes, and reduced costs by complying with suggested treatment regimens as agreed to by both the patient and clinician. With NPs historically at the forefront of person-centered care, they are in a pivotal position to promote shared decision making for all recipients of health care.

Outcome Considerations

In many instances, the patient's and clinician's chosen outcomes for an encounter are clear. The simple, acute health problem is to be resolved. The screening measures recommended for the person's age group are ordered to rule out the presence of nascent disease. When dealing with more chronic problems or problems that cause the patient what may be reduced quality of life, the clinician must be more sensitive to outcome determination.

DOCUMENTATION

Preparing concise, comprehensive, and meaningful documentation of one's thoughts and activities as a provider of primary care is a skill that takes time to develop. The purposes of documentation are to record the patient's report of symptoms, PMH, lifestyle and family factors, positive and negative findings on physical examination, and the clinician's decisions and actions. An accurate record is essential to remind the clinician of findings and actions for the next follow-up visit. In a large practice, other providers will be seeing the patient and will need the benefit of the clinician's observations and actions during previous visits. The effectiveness of a treatment plan can be judged only if the plan has been adequately described. For example, if teaching about diet was provided at one visit but not recorded, the same teaching might be repeated at the next visit to the frustration of the patient who was looking for new information. This frustration might be misunderstood by the next provider as a lack of cooperation with the treatment plan. Finally, documentation can serve as protection for the provider or the practice in the rare case in which litigation is brought by the patient or family. In addition, third-party payers may be auditing the patient's record to determine whether the level of the visit that was billed was justified and whether the interventions billed were actually delivered. Additional details on billing and coding are provided in Chapter 86. In the student situation, the depth and comprehensiveness of documentation can assist the preceptor or faculty in determining the student's progress in learning judgment.

SOAP Format

General principles for documentation are commonly applied, using the subjective, objective, assessment, and plan (SOAP) format of charting. If other systems of charting are used, the principles still apply.

Subjective

The subjective portion of the record includes all data from the patient's report: the HPI, PMH, family history, social history, functional health patterns data, and review of systems. The clinician can include here, in an easily visible way, current medications, immunization status, allergies to foods or medications, past hospitalizations (if appropriate), and, for females, the last menstrual period and menstrual cycle information. Even when a female patient is being treated for simple problems, pregnancy status must be known before certain medications are prescribed. It is an error to confuse physical findings noticed during the examination with subjective data from the patient. If the patient's particular way of describing a problem seems important, use the patient's exact words and include quotes. This is not necessary if the description is simple and without nuance.

It is helpful to develop an outline form for documentation that includes all essential data elements in a way that is retrievable. Writing in full sentences and paragraphs does not allow for easy retrieval of data by other providers. An outline template also serves as a memory tool for the new clinician. This template is useful in organizing patient presentation for the preceptor.

Objective

The objective section of the record includes all data obtained through objective means. This is not limited to numerical data. The objective portion of the record should begin with a brief description of the overall impression of the patient. Such phrases as "tired looking," "energetic," or "worried" can convey much of the patient impression that is useful in diagnostic reasoning. Vital signs and pertinent findings from the physical examination, as well as laboratory data, should also be included. Diagnostic judgments should not be included in this section; this part of the record should consist of "just the facts."

At first, students may not be able to focus on which pieces of data are significant to a problem; they tend to include every piece of data available. All data need not be recorded, but "pertinent negatives" need to be recorded. These include data that by being normal tend to rule out a possible diagnosis. Recording pertinent negatives helps to show that a diagnosis was considered and why it was ruled out. It does not take long, however, for both the subjective and objective sections to be recorded with reasonable skill, even for advanced beginner students. When following patients over time, flow sheets can be useful for tracking data. For example, a flow sheet can show the effect of a change in medication management of hyperlipidemia or blood pressure or track a patient's weight over months or years.

Assessment

The assessment portion is an area of documentation in which much variability can be found. The assessment must include active problems that are being managed during the current visit. It can also include chronic problems that may have an impact on the treatment plan. Often, practices include a health-promotion line on the problem list to remind each clinician that the visit should reflect the preventive focus of that practice. For the list to serve both patient and practitioner well, a simple diagnostic label may not be enough. For example, if the patient has hypertension that is being managed by lifestyle changes and medication, the effectiveness of control of the problem can be recorded in the assessment section. Assessment is ongoing in the management of health problems. For example, a patient's problem list might read as follows: (1) hypertension (HTN) stage 1, well controlled; (2) type 2 DM, poorly controlled; (3) obesity, unchanged. This documentation directs evaluation and intervention adjustment much more clearly than a simple list of "HTN, DM, obesity." It is helpful for practices to maintain an active problem list near the front of the patient record or in a part of the electronic record; this is particularly useful when dealing with chronic conditions and is recommended. The clinician can initiate such a tool in any practice, even if a blank progress note sheet is filed at the beginning of that section of the patient's record.

When reviewing the assessment part of the record, students can evaluate their own thinking by asking themselves if all data that were used to justify the naming of a problem are included in the subjective and objective section of the note. Further, one can ask whether all data were accounted for in the assessment section. In some cases, a clear problem cannot be identified. Abdominal pain that does not fit a clear diagnostic pattern can be reported in the problem list by simply naming the complaint. The clinician can reflect diagnostic hypotheses by writing "abdominal pain, rule out (R/O) irritable bowel syndrome." Or "cough, viral bronchitis versus allergy." Students are often reluctant to admit that they cannot name the problem. It is a mistake, however, to name a problem in error, simply to have a problem on the list. The patient will not be well served if the record fails to reveal competing diagnostic hypotheses. In primary care, uncertainty is reasonable and expected. Even if the problem is not completely specified, the problem list is the basis for the intervention schedule in the treatment plan.

Plan

The plan for treatment is most effective if it is described in detail, including specific directions for each intervention. Three general sections are included in planning. First, any diagnostic testing that is to be conducted should be listed. The results of these diagnostic tests will help to clarify the assessment, but, of course, they are not yet available to the provider. Second, educational approaches are to be laid out. Every visit is a teaching opportunity. Patient education might include specifics of the problems being managed, such as symptom control for upper respiratory infections; medication teaching; diet and activity recommendations; and risk reduction, such as smoking cessation information or a discussion of seat-belt usage. The documentation of the plan includes details regarding any therapeutic plan that is to be carried out—including prescriptions, various therapies, counseling, activity promotion or restriction, dietary changes, or any of the therapeutics discussed earlier. When recording prescriptions, be sure to include all the data that were written on the prescription list including the number or volume of doses to be dispensed and the number of refills allowed. This is important because patients may call for refills before they are due, and if a different provider takes the call, that provider may have an unclear idea of how the patient's condition has been managed. This is especially important when prescribing drugs that are prone to abuse.

Finally, the treatment plan is not complete without clear plans for follow-up. When will the patient be seen again, and under what circumstances is the patient instructed to call back? For example, when treating a viral infection, remind the patient to call back if not better in 2 days or if a fever develops. By documenting your instructions for follow-up, you allow other providers to better manage the patient's care if the patient calls when you are not available.

Plans are most effective when they include a sense of the goal of treatment. If the condition is simple and self-limiting, the goal of treatment may be obvious and need not be stated. For chronic or complex problems, however, the short- and long-term goals of therapy need to be discussed and recorded. By engaging the patient in this discussion, the choices that the patient makes in altering lifestyle and following a treatment plan may be clearer. For example, the patient with hypertension, diabetes, and obesity might have a goal to lose 4 pounds in a month. The plan to help the patient achieve this goal might include walking three times a week and eating one fewer restaurant meal a week. The feedback on the short-term goal at the next visit can help keep the patient motivated to sustain lifelong change.

Finally, when reviewing the documentation for personal or peer evaluation, the clinician must consider whether the note conveys the scope and tone of the visit. Does it reflect the type of visit that occurred? If the patient were to ask to see the record, would the information be clear? The NP should write the note in such a way that the patient could agree with what has been stated. Discussions of sensitive issues such as family problems can be left in general terms. This is a useful approach when one considers that others, such as third-party payers or lawyers, might have access to the record in the future. If the provider and the patient disagree on a treatment plan—for example, on the use of medications—the record can reflect the disagreement in nonjudgmental terms, such as "Patient requested prescription for muscle relaxants, which was discussed as being unlikely to benefit the shoulder pain described." This kind of note can assist in determining patterns of behavior or documenting difficulties over time.

Documentation is an opportunity for clinicians at all levels to review the level of their thoughts. In general, NPs document visits more completely and have their charts refused less frequently for payment by third-party payers than other clinicians do. It is best to develop a system for maintaining current, accurate records. Saving quick scratches of notes and writing all formal patient notes at the end of a busy day do not correspond with the recommended approach. Dictation and computer systems allow for complete record-keeping and help manage time spent on the task.

Documentation Systems

Documentation systems vary greatly from practice to practice. There are hundreds of electronic medical record (EMR) software programs available. Different software programs are geared toward different settings. Most software designed for primary care settings includes EMR features such as tracking and storage of patients' demographics, histories, systems reviewed, assessments, tests ordered, results, medications, SOAP notes, diagnoses, and treatments. In addition to the EMR features, primary care documentation systems software also has features for managing the business. Management features can include automatic billing, claim tracking, referrals, reports, and scheduling. Many documentation systems include patient features, so patients may look up their scheduled visits, tests ordered, and any test results through online patient portals. Many large practices and hospital systems have robust documentation software, which can be integrated with smaller software programs for continuity of patient care. Becoming familiar with any new documentation system takes time and practice; however, it is crucial to use the system in favor of improved patient outcomes. For example, Tapp et al (2020) reported a significant increase in hepatitis C and HIV screening after implementing an EMR alert in the primary care setting.

Many documentation systems have alerts for providers, identifying which patients are due for their preventive screenings, such as a mammogram, depression questionnaire, or colorectal examination. Ultimately, EMRs have the potential to help providers optimize their time spent documenting, as well as standardize preventive care and allow more time for hands-on patient care.

REDUCTION OF MEDICAL ERRORS

The reduction of medical errors and the support of patient safety are important in the health-care arena. The Institute of Medicine has called for attention to processes and systems of care to reduce error and enhance safety. Most medical errors in primary care are considered administrative; such errors include information filed in the wrong place or at the wrong time, computers being "down," and lack of documentation. Errors also occur in obtaining or processing a laboratory specimen. Some errors are due to lack of clinical knowledge or skills; these include a wrong or missed diagnosis or wrong treatment choices. Attention to decision making and follow-through is important to all primary care providers. NPs can contribute to shaping the practice in their setting by, for example, developing systems to ensure that important laboratory results are addressed in a timely manner. All of these efforts are part of quality-oriented guidelines developed for the patient-centered medical homes (PCMHs) discussed in Chapter 1. These are the health-care systems of the future, and they are still emerging. NPs have an opportunity and an obligation to participate in and influence that emergence with their own unique knowledge base, to translate their knowledge into systems that support patient engagement.

The importance of accurate diagnostic reasoning to prevent errors and thus patient harm cannot be stressed. See Evidence-Based Nursing Practice 4.1 for an abstract of a research study that integrates strategies for improving diagnostic reasoning and reducing errors.

THE DIGITAL FUTURE AND TELEHEALTH

The American Recovery and Reinvestment Act was designed to create a means to electronically capture and store patient medical records and to make "meaningful use" of these data. This legislation mandated adoption of EMRs by 2014. EMRs are now required for all health-care providers; those who are not in compliance are subject to penalties. The Medicare Access and CHIP Reauthorization Act (MACRA) further impacts the reporting of all providers, requiring each to declare their track—the Alternative Payment Model (APM) or the Merit-based Incentive Payment System (MIPS)—which will centralize the reporting of quality outcome measures for each provider and direct reimbursement.

Evidence-Based Nursing Practice 4.1

Nordick, CL. (2021). Integrating strategies for improving diagnostic reasoning and error reduction. Journal of the American Association of Nurse Practitioners: May 2021 - Volume 33 - Issue 5 - p 366-372.

Errors of diagnostic reasoning contribute significantly to patient harm. Students, novice diagnosticians, and even experienced clinicians often have difficulty understanding or describing the processes of diagnostic reasoning. Inappropriate use of cognitive heuristics and poor logical reasoning by novice or experienced diagnosticians may result in missed or delayed diagnoses. Reduction of diagnostic errors through knowledge acquisition, self-reflection, and checklists has individually demonstrated some improvements in diagnostic reasoning. Implementing the diagnostic and reasoning tool (DaRT), a method of reasoning that integrates the evidence-based strategies of knowledge acquisition, metacognition, and logical reasoning skills throughout the patient encounter, results in improvement in diagnostic reasoning in advanced practice nurses. Use of the DaRT in one university setting resulted in significant improvement in advanced health assessment skills and diagnostic reasoning abilities as demonstrated by improvements of 28% to 55% end-of-program Health Education Systems Incorporated scores. Translation into practice settings may further support the use of this multiple-modality tool.

Box 4.2 Additional Benefits of EMRs

1. Provides a longitudinal account of patient care
2. Allows tracking of care from the acute-care setting to nursing homes, retirement homes, or patients' private residences
3. Focuses on measurement of care quality across all settings rather than on episodes of care
4. Facilitates patient identification that allows providers to track the patient throughout the care delivery system and across the continuum of providers, offering information in a need-to-know environment
5. Provides practitioner alerts and reminders, communicates up-to-date resources, and links evidence-based bodies of knowledge used for clinical decision support
6. Presents real-time cost-effective options and enhances timely reimbursement through interconnectivity to payers, offering patient eligibility and authorization requirements
7. Matches patients to medications
8. Facilitates electronic transmission of payment to providers

The importance of all providers using EMRs is based on the principles of securing patient information and reducing administrative health-care costs. Standardizing EMRs and billing data will also improve provider cash flow, allowing carriers to process claims more efficiently and reduce health-care costs. Box 4.2 lists additional benefits.

Telehealth is not a new concept in health care, but it has become more prominent over the last few years, especially in the midst of the COVID-19 pandemic. Using telehealth in primary care has played an integral role in promoting health and wellness, managing chronic illnesses in the home setting, and reducing hospital visits. These advantages are crucial to note as many primary care practices have begun to adopt this service. Telehealth can be performed between clinician and patient over the telephone without video or via live-video conferencing, remote patient monitoring, and asynchronous video. Advantages of telehealth include reduction in transportation concerns and costs, the ability to receive care from any setting patients choose, and health promotion through education. Disadvantages include inadequate assessments based on patient complaints, technical glitches, inability to physically examine or observe the patient (if by phone), and physician or clinician resistance. As the art of telehealth becomes more incorporated into primary care, clinicians have the opportunity to stay connected to patients and provide holistic care when they need us most.

ARTIFICIAL INTELLIGENCE

Over the past several decades, person-centered care has become the standard when assessing, diagnosing, and treating patients. Because empathy and compassion are part of the fundamental values in the clinician–patient relationship, it is important not to lose these aspects when applying artificial intelligence (AI) to a treatment plan. AI encompasses machine-learning algorithms and software to simulate human intelligence in the analysis, presentation, and comprehension of complex medical and health-care data (Kerasidou, 2020). With this in mind, AI could help improve diagnosis and treatment accuracy. The development and assessment of an AI-based tool for skin condition diagnosis by primary care physicians and nurse practitioners in teledermatology practices provide one example of how AI can help improve diagnoses, thus improving the quality of patient care (Jain, Way, Gupta, et al, 2021). Several forms of AI allow patients to help manage their own chronic conditions and promote a healthier lifestyle. These include:

- Smartphone technology with health apps to track calories and manage weight
- Smartwatches that can detect one's heart rate, heart rhythm, and oxygen saturation
- Continuous glucose monitors, such as Dexcom and Freestyle Libre
- Insulin pumps, including Medtronic and Omnipod
- Software programs in the clinician's EMR, such as AdvancedMD, CareCloud, and Athenahealth, which collect patient data to help identify different diagnoses or areas of concern

As more patients become willing to participate in their own care, the use of AI in diagnosing and monitoring health conditions may be a true asset to clinicians. See The Patient's Voice 4.1 for a personal experience with AI.

PRECISION HEALTH CARE

Personalized, predictive, and precision are similar terms referring to health care that considers individual genetic variations, lifestyle, and environmental factors in the treatment and prevention of disease. Many developments have the potential to transform health care, including the completion of the Human Genome Project; advances in molecular biology, particularly those related to "-ome" science (e.g., genome, epigenome, metabolome, proteome, and transcriptome); considerable advances in biotechnology; and improved ability to analyze large data sets. These scientific and technological advances have given rise to the exciting field of precision health care, which refers to a prevention-and-treatment approach targeting groups or individuals based on genes, environment, and lifestyle. For example, various forms of cancers such as breast cancer may be treated differently, based on a person's genetics, with specific, targeted medications. Consumers and providers alike are seeking patient-specific solutions to address health-care concerns. People are interested in precision health care and want to know more about their health in this way. As precision health care progresses, the goal will be to advance treatments targeted specifically to the individual, which will truly create a paradigm shift in health-care delivery. NPs in primary care settings can anticipate rapid growth of precision health care and increased consumer knowledge. It is anticipated that precision health care will open the door for more targeted and effective treatment plans for multiple disease conditions to further improve patient outcomes. NPs will be challenged to translate this evidence as it evolves into practice solutions, and ultimately, individual patient treatment plans.

Health care approached from a personalized medicine perspective creates a different model of care that calls for a more holistic approach and requires personal engagement to be successful. Nursing theories on caring are well suited to addressing precision health concerns and challenges as we come to know the wholeness of a person in the moment. Caring in nursing is relational, steeped in deep moral and ethical foundations, examined through deliberation, and expressed through moral actions. This is an important nursing perspective in the personalized health-care initiative as many concerns with its implementation are related to ethical, legal, and social issues. Nursing has a unique view, and the very act of nursing engagement in precision health is creating a caring environment. The successful navigation of precision health challenges through the lens of caring offers an opportunity to illuminate patients and create an enduring spirit of what matters most.

ETHICS

Every clinical judgment is an ethical judgment. Clinical judgment begins with respect for people and supports each individual's autonomy. Some decisions call for balancing such principles as beneficence against autonomy, for example, when a patient chooses not to follow a treatment plan. Truth-telling by the clinician can do much to establish trust and develop a plan the patient can accept. Ethical judgments are involved as well in the allocation of scarce resources, the most prominent for clinicians being their own time. If one patient constantly requires more time than is allotted, other patients are made to wait or are given less time for their visits. Being a patient advocate means ascertaining that the health-care system provides for each patient everything that is reasonable to which the patient is entitled. Such advocacy is a role of the NP. Fidelity to the patient until the problem has been solved or resolved is another aspect of NP practice that is based on ethical principles. One could make the case that NPs have an ethical and professional responsibility to help design and implement systems to collaborate in the establishment of PCMHs that truly reflect the intent of the model that "hears" the voice of the patient.

Additionally, as technology advances, the NP is in a prime position to ensure that ethical considerations are integrated into the decision-making, planning, and integration phases, ensuring balance between technology and ethical principles: autonomy, beneficence, nonmaleficence,

---

 The Patient's Voice 4.1: Artificial Intelligence and Health Care

At the age of 20, I was diagnosed with type 1 diabetes. While going to college, managing my mealtime insulin and blood glucose checks in between classes was difficult, to say the least. At times, I would have approximately half an hour to get food and then race back to class, making the process very stressful. Fast-forward 12 years, and I no longer have to prick my fingers six or seven times a day. I currently use a Dexcom G6 continuous glucose monitor (CGM). This device has completely changed my life and has improved the way I manage my diabetes care. I'm able to view my blood sugar every minute of every day instead of trying to capture my blood glucose level for one moment at a time but several times throughout the day. All the guesswork has been removed from the situation, and I can adjust my insulin therapy at any moment in time, depending on what my blood glucose reading is. My system is a hybrid, with my Dexcom G6 linked via Bluetooth to an insulin pump. These two devices communicate with each other to effectively maintain my blood glucose levels. The system alerts me to the changes being made in my insulin delivery, so I can also make the necessary adjustments to help the device maintain normal glucose ranges and reduce the highs and lows that come along with this disease.

Erica Muniz

other groups may develop both practice standards and guidelines.

Practice standards are intended to be used under all circumstances and define correct overall practice. They are generally considered to be inflexible and should not be interpreted as adaptable to fit different contexts. The American Nurses Association (ANA) has issued practice standards for nurses, which include broad requirements for nursing practice in any setting and at any level of practice. Practice standards are designed to provide direction to nurses to guide and evaluate their practices (Spring, 2015).

Two types of standards are delineated by the ANA: standards of care for clinical practice and standards of professional performance. Standard 13 (2015) describes the nurse's obligation to utilize research findings in practice. This expectation indirectly refers to the use of clinical guidelines and other resources. The American Association of Nurse Practitioners (AANP) establishes the standards of practice for nurse practitioners. The standards encompass many aspects of practice, including qualifications, processes of care, care priorities, and research as a basis for practice (AANP, 2019).

Practice guidelines are not cookbooks that take the decision making away from providers; instead, they allow flexibility when making individual patient-care decisions. Guidelines are intended to provide a reference point and general direction for decision making and are not meant to be interpreted as rigid criteria that must be followed regardless of the context. Nonetheless, guidelines should be followed in the majority of cases unless there is a clear rationale for deviating from them to serve the particular needs of individuals. Tailoring care to the needs of a particular patient is a cornerstone of EBP. The usefulness of applying guidelines in clinical decision making has become increasingly recognized over the past decade and is now an expectation in the delivery of health care. A current definition from the Institute of Medicine states "Clinical Practice Guidelines are statements that include recommendations intended to optimize patient care that are informed by a systematic review of evidence and an assessment of the benefits and harms of alternative care options" (2011, p 4).

Developing the Guidelines

The essential components of guideline development are as follows: (1) identification/clarification of the topic, (2) establishment of an expert panel, (3) a systematic review of the literature, (4) development of an evidence-based table, (5) writing draft recommendations based on the evidence, (6) external review of the recommendations, and (7) final acceptance of the revised recommendations by the panel. Panel members are chosen according to the focus and intent of the guidelines, and they may include expert researchers on the topic, physicians, APRNs, clinical nurse specialists, ethicists, pharmacists, therapists, and health-care consumers. Ultimately, the expert panel seeks consensus on the guideline that will inform practitioners about the current best practice.

Grading the Evidence

One of the most important aspects of developing guidelines is appraising the quality of the evidence used to make each recommendation and then grading the recommendation based on the level of evidence. Various grading systems are currently in use. For example, the U.S. Preventive Services Task Force (USPSTF) uses a three-tiered system to rate evidence and a five-point rating scale (A through E ratings) to grade recommendations. Another system, known as GRADE, is a relatively new methodology that is becoming more popular among medical organizations (Grade Working Group, 2004-2022). It is important to keep in mind the lack of standardization for defining the level of evidence. This must be considered when selecting criteria and the appropriate rating scale based on the clinical question.

Table 5.1 describes various databases and scales that are used to rate evidence.

The following discussion explains a common hierarchy used to evaluate evidence based on research design. This hierarchy was modified by Melnyk and Fineout-Overholt (2015) from Guyatt and Rennie (2002). It rates evidence on a scale of I to VII based on the type of research design.

Level I Evidence—Systematic Review or Meta-Analysis of RCTs

Systematic reviews and meta-analyses are considered among the highest levels of evidence on which to base a change in practice. The systematic review includes all RCT studies and quantitative studies with similar methods that address a clinical question. A meta-analysis is a specific type of statistical analysis that pools the results of a group of similar RCTs conducted on an intervention or treatment. The result is an overall *effect size* that estimates the average size of the relationship between the intervention and the desired outcome. A review of the literature allows for a compilation of all the studies to give strength to outcomes. This review is a rigorous approach, and it provides a high level of evidence due to the minimization of bias. Thus, you can see how systematic reviews and meta-analyses are especially suitable for determining if there is significant evidence on the effectiveness of an intervention or practice. This level of evidence is generally used in the development of clinical practice guidelines. The Cochrane Library has an extensive compilation of systematic reviews.

Level II Evidence—Single Well-Designed RCTs

RCTs are increasingly considered the most respected method for establishing the cause of disease or the efficacy of a treatment/intervention. For example, the U.S. Food and Drug Administration requires evidence of a

TABLE 5.1 Sources of Evidence and Level of Evidence

Sources of Evidence	Different Types of Evidence	Specific Use	Examples of Types/Levels of Evidence
Cochrane Library[1] SR and meta-analyses attempt to identify, appraise, and synthesize empirical evidence to inform decision making.	Five types: • Intervention reviews • Diagnostic test accuracy reviews • Methodology reviews • Qualitative reviews • Prognosis reviews	Findings are based on results that meet certain criteria; reliable studies provide the best evidence, reducing impact of bias. • Identification of relevant studies from different sources • Selection for inclusion and evaluation of strengths and limitations based on predefined criteria • Systematic collection of data • Appropriate synthesis of data	• Database of SRs • DARE: Database of Abstracts of Reviews of Effects • Cochrane Central Register of Controlled (Clinical) Trials • National Health Service Economic Evaluation Database • Gold standard for developing SRs. Flow chart created from preappraised studies and clinical trials
Preferred Reporting Items for Systematic Reviews and Meta-Analyses (PRISMA)[2] Starting point for developing clinical practice guidelines. Addresses several conceptual and practical advances in the science of SRs.	Reporting reviews of evaluating randomized trials, reviews of interventions (meta-analyses).	Adopts the definitions of SR and meta-analysis used by Cochrane Collaboration.	• Identification: Records identified through database searching, then records duplicates removed • Screening: Records screened, records excluded • Eligibility: Full-text articles assessed for eligibility; full-text articles excluded with reasons • Included: Studies included in qualitative synthesis, studies included in quantitative syntheses
Johns Hopkins Nursing[3] Evidence Levels and Quality Guide	Level I: experimental, RCT, SR of RCTs Level II: quasi-experimental Level III: nonexperimental, qualitative Level IV: opinion of expert(s), consensus panels Level V: literature reviews, quality improvement, case reports, experiential opinions of experts	PET framework P: practice question E: evidence T: translation Problem-solving approach to clinical decision making within a health-care organization	Levels I–III A: High quality—consistent, generalizable results; thorough reference to scientific evidence B: Good quality—reasonable, consistent results; some reference to scientific evidence C: Low quality/major flaws—inconsistent results, insufficient sample size, conclusions cannot be drawn Levels IV–V A: High quality—consistent results; sponsored by professional, public, private, or government agencies; developed or revised within 5 years B: Good quality—reasonably consistent results C: Low quality/major flaws—not sponsored by an official organization, limited literature search, not revised in 5 years

TABLE 5.1 Sources of Evidence and Level of Evidence—cont'd			
Sources of Evidence	**Different Types of Evidence**	**Specific Use**	**Examples of Types/Levels of Evidence**
Melnyk & Fineout-Overholt (2018)[4] Rating system for the hierarchy of evidence for intervention/treatment questions	Level I: SR or meta-analysis of RCTs Level II: at least one RCT Level III: controlled trial without randomization Level IV: case–control or cohort studies Level V: SR of descriptive and qualitative studies (meta-synthesis) Level VI: single descriptive or qualitative study Level VII: opinion of authorities or reports of expert committees	PICOT question format to determine key search parameters in databases Quick critical appraisal guides for evaluating specific evidence depending on level	

Abbreviations: PICOT, patient or population/intervention/comparison/outcome/time; RCT, randomized clinical trial; SR, systematic review.
1. Cochrane Review-Cochrane Library. About Cochrane reviews. http://www.cochranelibrary.com/about/about-cochrane-systematic-reviews.html. Published 1999–2017.
2. Moher D, Liberati A, Tetzlaff J, et al. Preferred Reporting Items for Systematic Reviews and Meta-Analyses: The PRISMA statement. *PLoS Med.* 2009;6(7):e1000097.
3. *Johns Hopkins Nursing evidence-based practice: Model and guidelines.* 3rd ed. Indianapolis, IN: Sigma Theta Tau International; 2017.
4. Melnyk BM, Fineout-Overholt E. *Evidence-based practice in nursing & healthcare: A guide to best practice.* 4th ed. Philadelphia, PA: Wolters Kluwer; 2018.

drug's efficacy from two independently conducted RCTs before approving the drug's use in the United States. The National Institutes of Health is increasingly funding RCTs, and agencies or organizations developing clinical guidelines now consider the evidence from RCTs to supersede findings from case–control or cohort studies.

The strength of RCTs to establish cause or efficacy lies in the ability of this design to maintain a high degree of control within experimental conditions. If there are different effects between the groups (e.g., blood pressure, the development of pressure ulcers, the prevention of pregnancy), the differences can generally be attributed to the intervention, exposure, or treatment rather than "extraneous" factors. Moreover, the random assignment of subjects to the treatment or control group allows for a high degree of confidence in making causal inferences about the effects of an exposure, intervention, or treatment.

RCTs also frequently employ the use of double-blinding to further strengthen support for identifying a cause-and-effect relationship. When RCTs are double-blind, neither the principal investigators nor the participants know who is in the control or experimental group until either significant differences are noted in a (blind) analysis of the data or the study is complete. The purpose of double-blinding is to eliminate the potential for participants in the experimental or control group to treat themselves differently or to be treated differently by investigators.

Level III Evidence—Well-Designed Controlled Trials Without Randomization

Quasi-experimental research designs evaluate the effectiveness of an intervention/treatment, but subjects are not randomly assigned to either the treatment or control group. In these designs, many of the same methods to ascertain the internal validity of a study instituted in RCTs, such as control of extraneous variables and standardization of treatment, are implemented. For example, de Cunto Taets and de Figueiredo (2016) conducted a study to verify whether comatose patients experience pain during bed baths. They collected saliva from patients before and during bed baths and measured substance P levels in the saliva samples. This study evaluated the effects of a common nursing intervention but did not randomize the patients to a treatment or control group.

Level IV Evidence—Well-Designed Case–Control or Cohort Studies

These types of studies are especially useful in answering clinical questions that address prognosis or causation. With this design, the study is generally initiated after the disease has developed. A group of individuals who have the disease (cases) and a group of individuals who do not (controls) are selected and compared in terms of prior exposures thought to be associated with the development of a particular type of disease. Case–control studies are also considered observational studies because they do not manipulate the exposure (what may also be referred to as the intervention). The course of the disease is observed without interference. The lack of control over the exposure in case–control studies (along with other observational studies) risks introducing selection bias into the study, which may confound the results. These potential shortcomings have some researchers arguing that case–control studies are essentially worthless because of the inherent potential for bias.

Despite the arguments against the value of the case–control design, it is the most commonly used epidemiological design in the medical literature today. For example, the association between unopposed estrogen use in postmenopausal women and the development of endometrial cancer was established through several case–control studies.

The Nurses' Health Study is an example of a well-known prospective cohort study. It is a large, ongoing cohort study that enrolled more than 120,000 married female nurses who were aged 30 to 55 years in 1976. The nurses completed a baseline questionnaire about a number of demographic and health characteristics. Follow-up questionnaires at 2-year intervals asked about the development of disease and any new exposures. By comparing the exposed and unexposed groups on a number of variables (e.g., those who took hormone replacement and those who did not; those who ate high-fat foods and those who did not) and the onset of disease within each group, the study has provided important information about the relationships of these variables with the development of cancer and cardiovascular disease in women.

Another example of a prospective cohort study is the Framingham Heart Study. In this study, investigators identified and examined 5,127 men and women from Framingham, Massachusetts, who were 30 to 59 years old in the 1950s. When the study was initiated, all 5,127 participants were determined to be free from coronary heart disease. Participants in the study provided ongoing lifestyle and health status information and had been re-examined at regular intervals since 1952 for the development of coronary events. Prospective data from this study have been pivotal in identifying several major risk factors associated with coronary artery disease (CAD) and have been one of the sources of evidence for recommending lifestyle modifications to prevent CAD.

Level V Evidence—Systematic Reviews of Descriptive and Qualitative Studies

The purpose of descriptive research is to accurately portray the characteristics of a population or a clinical situation. Descriptive research can be quantitative or qualitative in design. In quantitative designs, the findings address the incidence, prevalence, or measurable characteristics of the population, using descriptive statistics (frequencies, means, mode, etc.). These studies seek to answer research questions and lay the groundwork for future studies that will test hypotheses. The design of quantitative descriptive studies can identify *associations* between variables but cannot provide evidence of *causation*.

In qualitative designs, the population or clinical situation is displayed in a narrative format for the purpose of increasing the understanding of the various dimensions of the phenomena of interest. Common qualitative designs used in nursing research include phenomenology, ethnography, grounded theory, and historical analysis.

Level VI Evidence—Single Descriptive or Qualitative Studies

Along with the single quantitative descriptive or qualitative study, the case study design falls into this category. Case studies are ranked lower because of their likelihood of decreased objectivity. These studies describe the history of one individual or a small group of patients. Case studies are generally told in story form with rich descriptions of the signs, symptoms, and events. The value of this study type is to alert a provider to an adverse event or a rare disease or to add to a provider's knowledge base. It is important to recognize that no inferences can be made from a case study to the general population.

A thought-provoking example of a case study is the NASA Twins Study (Garrett-Bakelman et al, 2019). Long-duration space missions over 300 days are rare; however, public and private entities plan on taking humans into Earth orbit and plan for space travel to the moon and Mars in the near future. Comprehensive studies are needed to assess the impact of long-duration space flight on the human body, brain, and overall physiology. Hence, genetically identical twin brothers Mark and Scott Kelly were the astronaut cases for this study that measured and compared various attributes at baseline and during and after long-duration space flight.

Level VII Evidence—Opinion of Authorities and/or Reports of Expert Committees

This level of evidence is just as it states: it is someone's opinion. This type of evidence follows the traditional approach for "correct" or "common" practice and may or may not be based on strong evidence. This level of evidence should not be a sole determination of changing practice or determining the proper course of treatment. However, there are times when this is the only evidence, and it is utilized to begin treatment in rare situations that do not have higher levels of evidence.

It is important to note that there is an increasing trend toward regarding evidence from RCTs as the only valid type of evidence appropriate for use in the practice setting. The danger in this perspective is disregarding what we have learned and can continue to learn from observational studies such as case–control and cohort studies.

The most sobering outcome of reliance on RCTs is the failure to teach providers to think and critically evaluate information. There are many circumstances in which randomization is impossible and where observational methods have provided invaluable information. For example, how did we come to understand the relationship between alcohol use in pregnancy and fetal alcohol syndrome; smoking and cardiopulmonary disease; birth defects and thalidomide; the transmission of HIV and viral hepatitis; and the development of endocarditis with intravenous drug use? Knowledge of these associations came from observational studies. Randomizing pregnant women into experimental or control group to either drink alcoholic beverages or not or designing an experimental trial to determine how the transmission of HIV in humans occurs is not ethically possible (or desirable). How we know what we know in practice must be determined through a critical appraisal of the information available.

Sources of Clinical Practice Guidelines

There is ongoing development of clinical practice guidelines as new research contributes to the body of knowledge on a topic. Existing guidelines are often reviewed and updated, requiring the APRN to be engaged in a continual process of reviewing sources to practice from an evidence base.

The Agency for Health Care Policy and Research was instrumental in leading the way toward EBP, improving outcomes, and publishing national guidelines on a variety of health-care problems, such as smoking cessation, early detection and treatment of Alzheimer's disease, and caring for patients with HIV. The Healthcare Research and Quality Act of 1999 reauthorized this agency and renamed it the Agency for Healthcare Research and Quality (AHRQ). The mission of the AHRQ has been to improve the quality, safety, efficiency, and effectiveness of health care for all Americans. An extremely important source for evidence-based guidelines was the National Guideline Clearinghouse (NGC). The NGC was an initiative of AHRQ, created in 1997 in partnership with the American Medical Association and the American Association of Health Plans. The Web site was made available to the public in 1999, and it was maintained for nearly 20 years, closing in 2018 due to a lack of funding. However, a study by AHRQ was still underway in 2020 with an aim to help identify new models for disseminating and accessing evidence-based clinical practice guidelines.

An excellent source for EBP guidelines is the Cochrane Collaboration and Library. Many national and professional health-care organizations offer guidelines (Box 5.2). Large health-care systems also offer publicly available guidelines such as the Veterans Health Administration in collaboration with the Department of Defense. In addition, searches using the databases PubMed and the Cumulative Index to Nursing and Allied Health Literature (CINAHL) can locate published clinical practice guidelines.

APPLICATION OF CLINICAL PRACTICE GUIDELINES

Providers who use clinical guidelines must learn techniques and skills that focus on finding and evaluating relevant practice guidelines. They must also develop a systematic method with which to evaluate EBP guidelines at the point of patient care.

> **Box 5.2 Examples of Clinical Practice Guidelines and Evidence-Based Guidelines Developed/Published by Organizations and Agencies**
>
> Alzheimer's Association
> Guideline for Alzheimer's disease management
> www.alz.org
> American Academy of Allergy, Asthma & Immunology
> Allergen immunotherapy: a practice parameter second update
> www.aaaai.org
> American College of Physicians
> Guidelines follow a rigorous development process and are based on the highest-quality scientific evidence
> www.acponline.org/clinical_information/guidelines
> Faculty of Sexual and Reproductive Healthcare
> Contraception for women aged over 40 years
> www.fsrh.org
> Society for Acupuncture Research
> Acupuncture evidence-based treatment guidelines
> www.acupunctureresearch.org
> Global Initiative for Asthma
> Global strategy for asthma management and prevention
> http://ginasthma.org
> National Association of Pediatric Nurse Practitioners
> Identifying and preventing overweight in childhood (clinical practice guideline)
> www.napnap.org
> National Health Care for the Homeless Council, Inc.
> Adapting your practice: general recommendations for the care of homeless patients.
> www.nhchc.org
> World Health Organization (WHO)
> WHO recommendations for the prevention of postpartum hemorrhage
> www.who.int/reproductivehealth/publications/maternal_perinatal_health/9789241548502/en

Evaluation of Clinical Practice Guidelines

Clinicians who use clinical guidelines should evaluate their usefulness by examining the following major characteristics:

- **Who created the guideline, and what is the date of revision or origination?** Authorship and funding of the guideline may be important if there is the potential for bias. In addition, the best guideline will be created by using multidisciplinary groups and following a systematic approach as recommended by AHRQ. The guideline must be current, meaning it was created or revised in the past 2 to 3 years and it used the most current evidence.
- **Are the guidelines clinically important?** To establish clinical importance, guidelines should convince you that following them will provide more benefits for your patients than their potential associated harms or costs.

- **How strong are the recommendations?** As discussed previously, the strength of a recommendation is largely determined by the strength of available evidence used to make the recommendations (see Table 5.1).
- **Are the guideline recommendations applicable to your patients?** Guidelines are developed for a variety of settings and for different practitioners. First, it is necessary to determine the group for whom the guidelines were written (e.g., primary care providers, specialists, or quality assurance reviewers) and whether they suit the intended purpose. Second, a determination is made on whether the individual patient has the characteristics of patients for whom the guidelines were intended. For example, if the patients you care for have a higher or lower prevalence of a disease or a different set of risk factors for disease than those in the guidelines, the recommendations may not apply. The patient population for whom the guidelines are intended will likely be dictated by the sample characteristics of the studies used to develop them as evidence. Before applying recommendations to any one patient, first determine whether this patient's characteristics are consistent with those for whom the guideline was intended and modify the guidelines when required (remember, they are meant to be flexible and adapted to individual needs when necessary). Third, a determination is made whether the guideline is appropriate for the setting and environmental conditions of the patient (e.g., inpatient, long-term care, outpatient care settings, or homebound).

Examples of Applying Clinical Guidelines

APRNs are challenged with decisions on using guidelines to change practice. The following example serves as a brief case study in applying clinical guidelines: a 52-year-old male patient with hypertension is in the office. The patient is on a diuretic and a beta blocker with well-controlled blood pressure. The provider is trying to determine whether the patient should be tested for causes of secondary hypertension. According to the Eighth Report of the Joint National Committee on Prevention, Detection, Evaluation, and Treatment of High Blood Pressure (JNC 8), the evidence demonstrates that the improved clinical outcomes associated with treating underlying causes of secondary hypertension are based on several well-designed studies; however, the costs and risks of adverse outcomes associated with diagnostic tests to rule out a cause such as renal artery stenosis may be greater than the benefits when applied to the entire population. Thus, guidelines do not recommend that every person who develops hypertension undergo extensive testing. Rather, specific characteristics of patients presenting with hypertension assist us in narrowing the population to those individuals who would reap the benefits of screening beyond any potential harm of the tests. A second patient presents with new-onset elevated blood pressure. He is 28 years old with no family history of hypertension. This patient would meet the criteria in the JNC 8 for investigation of possible renal stenosis.

Distinguishing between intermediate and clinical outcomes is also critical before applying research findings to practice. In outcomes research, as described earlier in the chapter, an outcome is generally considered the dependent variable of the study. Intermediate outcomes include measurements such as bone mineral density, hemoglobin levels, and eosinophil level. Clinical outcomes include measurements such as the number of hip fractures, a person's functional status, peak flow values, and the number of acute asthma exacerbations experienced.

Improvement in intermediate outcomes does not necessarily lead to improvements in clinical outcomes. For example, in early studies of using fluoride to treat osteoporosis, bone mineral density values improved greatly when fluoride was given to osteoporotic women, but the number of fractures over time did not differ from those in women who were given placebos. Thus, intermediate outcomes, although important to study to gain an understanding of disease processes and treatment, should not be substituted for clinical outcome data.

Another example of evaluating evidence to change practice is the use of angiotensin-converting enzyme (ACE) inhibitors in patients with congestive heart failure (CHF). In the early 1990s, several clinical trials demonstrated that the use of ACE inhibitors improved clinical outcomes in patients with CHF, not only with regard to mortality but also in exercise tolerance, symptom severity, progression to left ventricular dysfunction, and lower hospitalization rates. The consistency of the findings and the fact that they came from well-designed RCTs provided unequivocal evidence that ACE inhibitor use was beneficial for the majority of patients with CHF. As a result, the American College of Cardiology, the American Heart Association, and the AHRQ developed clinical guidelines for the treatment of CHF that strongly encourage ACE inhibitors as standard therapy. The use of ACE inhibitors is now considered a standard of care, and it should be incorporated into the care of people with CHF. For the provider at the point of care, the clinical guideline produced by these organizations provides point-of-care evidence to utilize with a patient.

SEARCHING THE LITERATURE

There are numerous examples of nursing research that have contributed to the knowledge base of nursing. Critically appraising studies regarding the appropriate use of results is one of the most important skills APRNs will need in practice. Using a framework for guidance can assist clinicians in taking the appropriate steps toward meeting this obligation. Some of the steps in applying the framework presented here are similar to those used for evaluating clinical practice guidelines. Two of the many sources to find literature are PubMed and CINAHL. A framework for evaluating journal articles in the health science literature is presented in Box 5.3. This framework provides an organized approach to interpreting the information found in a variety of articles, be it a review of the current knowledge in an area or original research findings.

Many methods of knowing contribute to our knowledge or understanding of the world, and a combination of methods (or various ways of triangulating) will provide a clearer, more encompassing answer to questions asked within the discipline to provide the best individualized care for patients. The example (Box 5.4) of using multiple types of research to care for a family with a child diagnosed with diabetes demonstrates the value of multiple methods of using evidence.

DEVELOPING A POINT-OF-CARE STRATEGY

One aspect of providing evidence-based care is the ability to access summaries of large amounts of information using mobile technologies. During a busy clinical day, it is unlikely that providers will implement the full EBP process. For example, it is not practical for a busy clinician to collect the most relevant, best evidence from a review of the literature including published literature reviews, meta-analyses, and clinical practice guidelines and to critically evaluate the evidence. Providers need key answers to their questions at the point of care.

Ely et al (1999) reported that providers generally have 2 minutes or less to spend searching for answers to clinical questions. Therefore, it is more feasible for clinicians to use preappraised summaries of evidence to assist them in making clinical decisions.

Box 5.3 A Framework for Evaluating Health Science Literature

Learning to evaluate health science literature is critical. It can be a time-consuming process, but it is necessary for reading an article for use in practice.

1. Look at the title to determine whether it reflects your specific interest.
2. Validate that the content is relevant to your original interest by reading the abstract.
3. Evaluate and determine what is being studied:
   - What are the study questions or hypotheses?
     - Often called "aims," these are found at the end of the Introduction section.
   - What are the specific variables under study?
     - These are the data and outcomes.
   - How are the variables defined and measured?
     - Operational definition, reputable survey, or tools used.
4. Evaluate and determine who is being studied:
   - What are the characteristics of the study sample or subjects?
   - How were subjects selected for the study?
     - *Most important* for generalizing the findings. Probability-based sampling (e.g., random) or purposive (e.g., convenience).
   - Is there an adequate sample size?
     - Look for a power analysis in the Methods section. There is risk of Type II error.
5. Evaluate and determine the type of study design and assess its validity:
   - Is the design used appropriate to answer the research question?
   - Does the design test for associations, correlations, or causation?
     - Strength of evidence; look up the design on evidence pyramid or grade of evidence.
   - Have other studies in similar (or different) samples found consistent results?
     - Found in the Discussion or Introduction section.
     - Important for building the body of knowledge/evidence on the topic.
6. Evaluate and determine how data have been analyzed:
   - What are the descriptive statistics used to describe the sample characteristics?
   - Could the degree or pattern of missing data influence the results?
   - Were the inferential statistics used on the variables appropriate for the study question and design?
   - Remember that statistical tests of significance (p-values, risk estimates with confidence intervals, effect measures) do not determine causation or clinical significance; they estimate the risk of Type I error (shows a difference, but there is actually no difference).
7. Evaluate what you have determined thus far:
   - Have you been skeptical? Do you see limitations or problems with the study?
   - Have you judged the quality of the literature based on the journal in which it was published?
   - Do you realize that there is no such thing as a "perfect" study?
   - How have you judged the author's treatment of contradictory results?
   - Remember that validity and reliability are crucial aspects of the study.
8. Discuss your evaluation with colleagues and seek other opinions (such as in a journal club):
   - Do your colleagues agree with your evaluation?
   - Do the results or recommendations suggest a change in your clinical practice? If so, what change is suggested, and how will it be implemented?

Box 5.4 Example: Integration of Evidence-Based Practice and Nursing Research–Based Practice

The management of an 8-year-old child with type 1 diabetes requires a multidisciplinary approach of which the family is an integral part. Following are two resources available to the APRN to assist in the management of the child with diabetes.

Evidence-Based Practice Guidelines

The American Diabetes Association (ADA) Professional Association supports the development of clinical guidelines for the management of diabetes. The ADA uses an evidence-grading system for standards of medical care in diabetes (levels of evidence are graded A to E). The foundation of the guideline for the management of diabetes is the recommendations made regarding glycemic control. These include the following:

1. Lowering A1C has been associated with a reduction of microvascular and neuropathic complications of diabetes (A).
2. Developing or adjusting the management plan to achieve normal or near-normal glycemia with an A1C goal of less than 7% is reasonable if it can be achieved without excessive hypoglycemia (B).
3. A lower A1C is associated with a lower risk of myocardial infarction and cardiovascular death (B).
4. Aggressive glycemic management with insulin may reduce morbidity in patients with severe acute illness, preoperatively, after myocardial infarction, or in pregnancy (B).
5. Less stringent treatment goals may be appropriate for patients with a history of severe hypoglycemia, patients with limited life expectancies, very young children or older adults, and individuals with comorbid conditions (E).

The panel rated the strength of the evidence supporting the first recommendation as "A." An "A" indicated that there was clear evidence from well-conducted, generalizable, randomized clinical trials that were adequately powered, or at the least, supportive evidence from well-conducted, randomized controlled trials that were adequately powered, including evidence from a well-conducted trial at one or more institutions. Evidence supporting the second through fourth recommendations was rated as "B." An evidence rating of "B" indicated that there was supportive evidence from well-conducted cohort studies. The final recommendation was given an evidence rating of "E." Evidence rated as E indicated that support for the recommendation was from expert consensus or clinical experience.

The guidelines also addressed nutrition and psychosocial assessment and care. The recommendations listed under psychosocial assessment and care are as follows:

1. Preliminary assessment of psychological and social status should be included as part of the medical management of diabetes (E).
2. Psychosocial screening should include but is not limited to attitudes about the illness; expectations for medical management and outcomes; affect/mood; general and diabetes-related quality of life; resources (financial, social, and emotional); and psychiatric history (E).
3. It is preferable to incorporate psychological treatment into routine care rather than to wait for identification of a specific problem or deterioration in psychological status (E).

Nursing Research

Sullivan-Bolyai and colleagues (2004) conducted a study to describe the experiences of parents managing their child's type 1 diabetes with the use of continuous subcutaneous insulin infusions (CSII), commonly referred to as the insulin pump. In this qualitative study, 14 mothers and seven fathers were interviewed and asked to describe the day-to-day experience of managing their child's diabetes. The children ranged in age from 2 to 11 years, and their mean age was 7.2 years of age. Parents in this study agreed that the pump was very effective in managing their child's diabetes and believed that their child's glucose was under much better control with the pump compared with using multiple daily injections (MDIs). The results of Sullivan-Bolyai et al's research indicated that some parents are reluctant to change to an alternative method of achieving glycemic control for their child. But all of the parents in their study, once familiar with the device, were very satisfied with the results and reported a better quality of life after they changed methods. Another important finding was that parents reported more freedom and flexibility in their lives once their child was switched from MDIs to the insulin pump. Some parents reported that once the child was placed on the insulin pump, they often were tempted to impose stricter controls on their child's glucose levels.

Impact on Advanced Practice Nursing

The ADA guidelines indicate that there is strong, reliable evidence to support interventions that assist the child with diabetes to maintain normal to near-normal glycemic levels, with less convincing evidence given to support less stringent control in very young children. Two methods currently used to achieve control are MDI and CSII, commonly called the insulin pump.

These guidelines also include a mandate for the primary care provider to provide psychosocial assessment and care. One assessment needed is the parents' comfort with technology and resources. Technology once limited to secondary and tertiary health-care settings is now available in the community and is often managed by laypersons and caregivers.

The method used to achieve glycemic control of the child is ultimately the parents' decision. However, APRNs who care for these children and families will be influential in the education and support of these families as they make complex health-care decisions for their child. Using the guidelines as the goals for management, APRNs can provide parents with evidence-based rationales for glycemic management of their child and assist them in their choices.

Relaying information to parents based on nursing research, such as the research conducted by Sullivan-Bolyai et al, may

Box 5.4 Example: Integration of Evidence-Based Practice and Nursing Research–Based Practice—cont'd

relieve some initial hesitancy in parents about switching from MDI to SCII to manage their child's diabetes. One important consideration in using this research in practice is that the sample for the above research was described as Caucasian and well educated. Will these same experiences be similar in other samples? However, perceptions of parents that their child's diabetes is under better control with the insulin pump and that this method has improved their quality of life can be useful to APRNs in their care of families managing this complex health condition.

This brings the evidence to the point of care, and using the providers' confidence in the evidence, their own experience with MDI or CSII, and the parents' comfort with technology demonstrates the essence of evidence-based practice.

Sources: American Diabetes Association Professional Association. *Standards of medical care in diabetes. Diabetes Care* 2017;40:S4–S5; Sullivan-Bolyai S, et al. Parents' reflections on managing their children's diabetes with insulin pumps. *J Nurs Scholarsh.* 2004;36:316–323.

A point-of-care strategy involves the following tasks: (1) asking a clinical question, (2) having evidence resources readily available, (3) completing the search using those resources, (4) examining the results of the search, and finally (5) applying the findings to the individual patient. Box 5.5 describes a framework for point-of-care search strategy for EBP. Education of practitioners in developing point-of-care use of EBP should become an essential part of nursing degree programs.

The first step in the process of sorting through information relevant to any given clinical situation is to formulate the clinical issue into a searchable, answerable question. To do this, the clinician asks two types of questions. The first is a clinical question such as "What is the best method for X?" The second is a question essential to find evidence to answer the clinical question. For example, "Between the two best methods for X, which one will work the best in my clinical situation and population?"

Box 5.5 A Framework for Point-of-Care Search Strategy

1. Ask the clinical question.
2. Select the evidence resource. The following lists suggested resources:
   - Cochrane Collaboration: www.cochrane.org
   - Essential Evidence Plus: www.essentialevidenceplus.com
   - UpToDate: www.uptodate.com/home/index.html
   - DynaMed: https://dynamed.ebscohost.com
   - Smartphone or tablet options:
     - PubMed4Hh from the National Library of Medicine offers "PICO search" box https://pubmedhh.nlm.nih.gov/nlmd/pico/piconew.php
     - Skyscape Clinical Constellation: www.skyscape.com/estore/ProductDetail.aspx?ProductId=1180
     - PEPID Primary Care Plus Ambulatory Care: www.pepid.com
3. Search.
4. Examine the evidence found in the search. Consider the level of evidence the search provided (meta-analysis, systematic reviews).
5. Apply the evidence to your patient.

Case scenario 1: A 72-year-old man is in the office for recent onset and worsening difficulty breathing. Pulse oximetry reading is 88 (sea level), and he is complaining of difficulty in completing activities of daily living due to the shortness of breath even while at rest. His wife states that he is more lethargic, and this is confirmed on examination.

1. The question: What are the treatment options for a patient with an acute exacerbation of chronic obstructive pulmonary disease (COPD)?
2. Selected resource: AHRQ—Guidelines and Measures https://www.ahrq.gov/gam/index.html
3. Search term: "COPD acute exacerbation"
4. Examine the evidence: This 2019 guideline ("Pharmacologic and Nonpharmacologic Therapies in Adult Patients with Exacerbation of COPD") lists key messages such as "antibiotic therapy increases the clinical cure rate and reduces the clinical failure rate;…corticosteroids improve dyspnea and reduce the clinical failure rate;…titrated oxygen reduces mortality compared with high flow oxygen;" and many more.
5. Explain the guideline recommendations to the patient and discuss the options.

Case scenario 2: A 3-year-old child is diagnosed in the clinic with acute otitis media (AOM). He appears mildly ill and has an axillary temperature of 100.6°F. Child has no known allergy to medication and is otherwise a healthy 3-year-old. Child is in day care during the day at a camp; parents are migrant workers.

1. The question: What is the recommended antibiotic for AOM in a 3-year-old child?
2. Selected search places: AAFP Clinical Practice guidelines (https://www.aafp.org/family-physician/patient-care/clinical-recommendations/clinical-practice-guidelines.html
3. Search term: "AOM children"
4. Examine the evidence:
   - Pain should be assessed in children with AOM and treated.
   - In children 6 months and older with severe symptoms (otalgia for at least 48 hours or fever of 39°C [102.2°F] or higher), antibiotics should be prescribed.

Continued

| Box 5.5 | A Framework for Point-of-Care Search Strategy—cont'd |

- In children 6 months to 24 months of age without severe signs or symptoms, antibiotics should be prescribed for bilateral AOM.
- For children 6 months to 23 months of age with nonsevere unilateral AOM or in children 24 months of age or older with nonsevere AOM (either unilateral or bilateral), observation offered with close follow-up, or antibiotics should be prescribed. There must be a mechanism in place to ensure proper follow-up and initiation of antibiotic therapy if the child's condition worsens or does not improve within 48 to 72 hours of onset of symptoms.
- Amoxicillin is the drug of choice for AOM unless the child has received amoxicillin in the past 30 days, has concurrent purulent conjunctivitis, is allergic to penicillin, or has a history of recurrent AOM unresponsive to amoxicillin.

5. Explain to the patient (family) the results found and discuss the options.

Sources: Agency for Healthcare Research and Quality (AHRQ). Guidelines and Measures; AAFP. Clinical Practice Guideline: Otitis Media. https://www.aafp.org/family-physician/patient-care/practice-guidelines.html. Endorsed, July 2013 and Reaffirmed 2019.

Evidence for clinical questions is best found when the question is posed in a searchable format. In the foregoing example, the clinical question asks, "In X population, how does X compare with Y affect Z?"

There is an abundance of readily available resources that provide access to summaries of the best evidence on specific clinical issues. These resources facilitate the retrieval and use of preappraised information for use at the point of care. Campbell et al (2015), building on the work of Banzi et al (2010), identify available EBP point-of-care resources as "web-based medical compendia specifically designed to deliver predigested, rapidly accessible, comprehensive, periodically updated, and evidence-based information (and possibly also guidance) to clinicians" (p 313). The authors present a comprehensive evaluation of 20 point-of-care resources. These resources were evaluated for general characteristics, content presentation, and editorial quality. The top resources identified were UpToDate, Nursing Reference Center, Mosby's Nursing Consult, British Medical Journal (BMJ) Best Practice, and Joanna Briggs Institute (JBI) COnNECT+. Many point-of-care resources are downloadable databases for smartphones and tablets that are periodically updated. Decisions about which resources to use depend on the provider's specific needs.

Applying evidence to care can be a complicated process. Research is establishing a number of moderating factors for applying evidence in practice. Often, it is difficult for providers to trust the information and balance the findings with their personal clinical knowledge and expertise. In addition, patient preference may conflict with EBP recommendations and preclude their implementation.

EBP CLINICAL DECISION MAKING

The decisions APRNs make in practice are fundamental to the quality of care given. Although collecting and evaluating evidence are critical to providing safe care, the importance of taking into consideration the patient's beliefs and desired outcomes is basic to making any health-care decision. There are two main steps of decision making in clinical practice: (1) collecting and analyzing evidence (or data) on the benefits, potential harms, and costs of various options, and (2) making a judgment about how to use the available evidence to achieve the health outcome desired. This last step includes the provider's experience with the population of patients served and knowledge of available resources in the community.

The components of EBP for clinical decisions are depicted in Figure 5.2. Using the *Circle of Caring* as an underlying practice model, the APRN considers the best evidence, their own clinical expertise and attitude, the patient's preferences and values, and the environmental and sociocultural influences on health.

EBP: The Patient

Applying analytical procedures for determining the credibility or reliability of data to be employed as evidence is only one aspect of the decision-making process. An equal challenge in making practice decisions involves making a judgment about how to use the evidence. This second step is not a question of facts but of patient values or

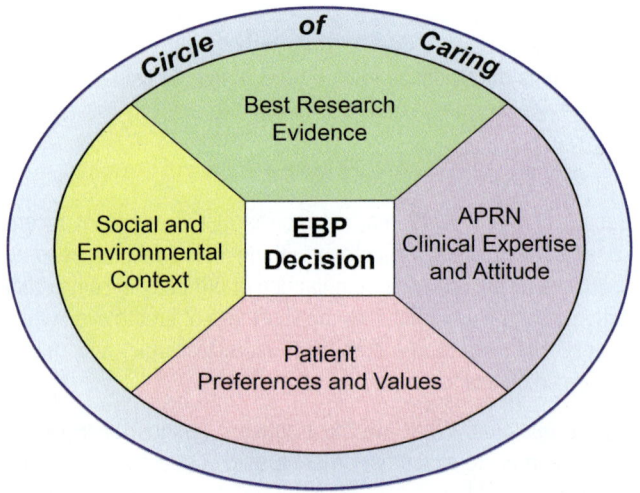

Figure 5.2 EBP Decision Making for the APRN

preferences. Ultimately, the issue is one of the patient's receptiveness to the mutual decisions about their clinical care. One of the most substantial qualities of advanced practice nursing is establishing a relationship with patients, providing them with the most current information, and allowing them to make health-care decisions they determine are best for them.

There will be times, however, that what the patient desires is not appropriate. Ms. Smith, who is 22 years old, comes to the office, asking for Synthroid. The patient explains that she has tried everything to lose weight and has a friend who was started on Synthroid and lost 30 pounds. The APRN performs a review of systems and a physical examination and orders the appropriate diagnostics. When the patient's laboratory results do not confirm a need for thyroid hormone replacement, the APRN educates the patient about the results and explains the reasons for not prescribing the medication simply because the patient is asking for it. Clearly, this case identifies consideration of a patient's preference when the evidence will support a change in the "best" option while not prescribing based solely on patient preference.

EBP: Environmental and Sociocultural Influences

The APRN further considers the patient's current environmental circumstances such as type of living situation (e.g., built environment, residence, household members), sources of transportation, access to quality food sources, and exposure to environmental contaminants in the home or community. It cannot be emphasized enough the importance of knowing your patient's economic circumstances and their ability to follow through on the clinical decisions. The APRN is also sensitive to the patient's cultural factors and seeks to integrate culture care into the decision-making process. Moreover, it is important to consider the patient's ability to understand and use health information to make the best-informed decision. In the recent *Healthy People 2030*, personal health literacy is defined as the degree to which individuals have the ability to find, understand, and use information and services to inform health-related decisions and actions for themselves and others (HHS, 2020). Using effective communication techniques to hear the patient's story as described in the *Circle of Caring* model leads the APRN to the best EBP clinical decisions.

EBP: The APRN

Clinical expertise is essential, yet it is caring that is central to making EBP clinical decisions. Considering the *Circle of Caring* model, the APRN is courageous when being open to change their practice based on new clinical evidence-based guidelines. Just as changes over the years have occurred in first-responder care for cardiac arrest, the sense of comfort in knowing is disrupted. Barriers to EBP have persisted over time due to a lack of education and skill to use EBP, the perception that it takes too much time, and the lack of a supportive environment (Melnyk & Fineout-Overholt, 2018). Many times, clinical practice changes require acquisition of new skills or routines in care delivery, thereby requiring the APRN to be committed to learning and being patient with themselves as they seek mastery of the new practice. Change is constant in health care, and open-mindedness can augment the APRN's attitude toward engaging in EBP. An ongoing spirit of inquiry and a coalition of practitioners in the practice environment support evidence-based clinical decision making as a standard approach to patient care (Melnyk & Raderstorf, 2021).

APRNs have the opportunity to engage in a career-long process of learning and leading EBP. It is fulfilling to learn and share the skills involved in searching and critiquing research findings that ultimately lead to improvements in patient care. As the APRN grows in EBP and sees the results of practice changes in their patients' health, there will be improved satisfaction with daily work and renewed commitment to this important health-care role.

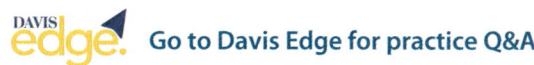
Go to Davis Edge for practice Q&A

REFERENCES

Ackley BJ, Swan BA, Ladwig G, et al. *Evidence-based nursing care guidelines: Medical-surgical interventions.* St. Louis, MO: Mosby Elsevier; 2008.

Agency for Healthcare Research and Quality. (1999). Reauthorization fact sheet. http://archive.ahrq.gov/about/ahrqfact.htm.

Agency for Healthcare Research and Quality. Guidelines and Measures. https://www.ahrq.gov/gam/index.html.

Amend R, Golden A. Practice at the point of care. *J Nurse Pract.* 2011; 7(4): 303–308.

American Association of Nurse Practitioners. (Revised 2019). Standards of practice for nurse practitioners. https://www.aanp.org/advocacy/advocacy-resource/position-statements/standards-of-practice-for-nurse-practitioners.

American Diabetes Association. *Standards of medical care in diabetes. Diabetes Care.* 2017;40:S4–S5. https://professional.diabetes.org/sites/professional.diabetes.org/files/media/dc_40_s1_final.pdf

American Nurses Association (ANA). *Nursing: scope and standards of practice.* 3rd ed. Silver Spring, Maryland: 2015. https://www.nursebooks.org

Banzi R, Liberati A, Moschetti I, et al. A review of online evidence-based practice point-of-care information summary providers. *J Med Internet Res.* 2010;12(3):e26.

Branham S, DelloSritto R, Hilliard T. Lost in translation: The acute care nurse practitioners' use of evidence based practice. A qualitative study. *J Nurs Educ Pract.* 2014;4(6):53–59.

Burns PB, Rohrich RJ, Chung KC. The levels of evidence and their role in evidence-based medicine. *Plastic Reconstr Surg.* 2011;128(1):305–310.

Campbell JM, Umapathysivam K, Xue Y, et al. Evidence-based practice point of care resources: A quantitative evaluation of quality, rigor, and content. *Worldviews Evid Based Nurs.* 2015;12(6): 313–327.

Cochrane AL. Effectiveness and efficiency: Random reflections on health services. Nuffield Provincial Hospitals Trust, London, 1972.

de Cunto Taets GG, de Figueiredo NMA. A quasi-experimental nursing study on pain in comatose patients. *Rev Bras Enferm.* 2016;69(5). https://www.scielo.br/scielo.php?pid=S0034-71672016000500927&script=sci_arttext&tlng=en.

Donabedian A. *Explorations in quality assessment and monitoring. Volume I. The definition of quality and approaches to its assessment.* Ann Arbor, MI: Health Administration Press; 1980.

Ely JW, et al. Analysis of questions asked by family doctors regarding patient care. *BMJ.* 1999; 319(7206):358-361. https://doi.org/10.1136/bmj.319.7206.358)

Garrett-Bakelman FE, Darshi M, Green SJ, et al. The NASA Twins Study: A multidimensional analysis of a year-long human spaceflight. *Science.* 2019;364(6436):eaau8650. doi:10.1126/science.aau8650

Grade Working Group. What is GRADE? http://www.gradeworkinggroup.org/#. Accessed 4/12/2022.

Grey JR, Grove SK. *Burns and Grove's the practice of nursing research: Appraisal, synthesis, and generation of evidence.* 9th ed. St. Louis, MO: Elsevier; 2021

Guyatt G, Rennie D, eds. *Users' guides to the medical literature: A manual for evidence-based clinical practice.* Chicago, IL: American Medical Association; 2002.

Institute of Medicine. (2011). *Clinical Practice Guidelines We Can Trust.* Washington, DC: The National Academies Press. https://doi.org/10.17226/13058.

Mackey A, Bassendowski S. The history of evidence-based practice in nursing education and practice. *J Prof Nurs.* 2017;33(1): 51–55.

Melnyk BM, Fineout-Overholt E. *Evidence-based practice in nursing & healthcare: A guide to best practice.* 3rd ed. Philadelphia, PA: Wolters Kluwer; 2015.

Melnyk BM, Fineout-Overholt E. *Evidence-based practice in nursing & healthcare: A guide to best practice.* 4th ed. Philadelphia, PA: Wolters Kluwer; 2019.

Melnyk BM, Raderstorf T. *Evidence-based leadership, innovation, and entrepreneurship in nursing and healthcare.* New York, NY: Springer Publishing Company, LLC; 2021.

Sackett DL. Rules of evidence and clinical recommendations on the use of antithrombotic agents. *Chest.* 1989;95:2S–4S.

Sackett DL, Rosenberg W, McGray JA, et al. Evidence-based medicine: What it is and what it isn't. *BMJ.* 1996;312:71–72.

Spring S. *Scope and standards of practice.* 3rd ed. American Nurses Association; 2015.

Stetler CB. Updating the Stetler Model of research utilization to facilitate evidence-based practice. *Nurs Outlook.* 2001;49(6):272–279.

Stevens KR. Critically appraising knowledge for clinical decision making. In: Melnyk BM, Fineout E, eds. *Evidence-based practice in nursing & healthcare: A guide to best practice.* 3rd ed. Philadelphia, PA: Wolters Kluwer; 2015.

Sullivan-Bolyai S, Knafl K, Tamborlane, W, et al. Parents' reflections on managing their children's diabetes with insulin pumps. *J Nurs Scholarsh.* 2004;36(4):316–323.

Teeling Smith G, Wells N, eds. *Medicines for the year 2000.* A symposium held at the Royal College of Physicians, September 1978, by the Office of Health Economics. London: Office of Health Economics. https://www.ohe.org/publications/medicines-year-2000.

United States Department of Health and Human Services. *Health Literacy in Healthy People.* Healthy People 2030. Updated August 18, 2020. Available at: https://health.gov/our-work/healthy-people-2030/about-healthy-people-2030/health-literacy-healthy-people

U.S. Preventive Services Task Force. Methods and processes. https://www.uspreventiveservicestaskforce.org/uspstf/about-uspstf/methods-and-processes. Accessed 12/9/2020.

RESOURCES

Agency for Healthcare Research and Quality
https://www.ahrq.gov/

Cochrane Library
https://www.cochranelibrary.com/

U.S. Preventive Services Task Force
https://www.uspreventiveservicestaskforce.org/uspstf/

Unit II

Caring-Based Nursing
The Science

The march of professionally educated nurses onto the panoramic scene in the nation's health services re-defines the boundaries of nursing practice.... Inter-professional collaboration is imbued with the essence of conjoined learning to provide a higher degree of service than could be offered by one profession.

–Martha E. Rogers: *Reveille in Nursing.* Philadelphia, PA: F.A. Davis: 1964: 77.

Section 1 NEUROLOGICAL PROBLEMS

SECTION EDITOR
Jill E. Winland-Brown, EdD, APRN, FNP-BC, FAANP

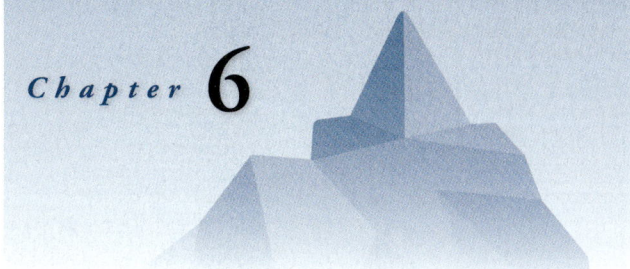

Chapter 6

Common Neurological Complaints

Sarah Horn, MD
Jill E. Winland-Brown, EdD, APRN, FNP-BC, FAANP

CONFUSION

Confusion is not a disease process or disease state but rather a symptom. Confusion is an inability to think quickly or coherently. A confused patient may be disoriented to time, place, or person, and usually demonstrates impairment of global cognitive functioning. The impairment is usually demonstrated by inappropriate reactions to environmental stimuli; it may arise suddenly or gradually, and it may be either temporary or irreversible. Medical illness, stressful events, lack of sleep or food, or sensory deprivation may precipitate confusion. Age is not a reliable predictor; however, older adults are most at risk because of polypharmacy (multiple prescription drugs), the aging process, preexisting cognitive impairment, and the presence of chronic disease (see Geriatric Considerations).

DIFFERENTIAL DIAGNOSIS

Confusion is a key sign of neurological disorders. The clinician must be diligent in determining its cause. The physical examination will provide clues. One major difficulty lies in differentiating symptoms of delirium from dementia. The clinician must establish whether the patient has delirium; a delirium superimposed on another condition such as Alzheimer's disease (AD); or another neurocognitive disorder apart from delirium, such as dementia. Once the disease has been identified and treatment started, the symptom of confusion may disappear. Differential diagnoses for confusion involve almost all body systems (Fig. 6.1).

Dementia

Dementia is a decline in mental functioning affecting memory, cognition, language, and personality. An acute transient disturbance in thought process is a result of delirium, whereas persistent or more severe confusion, with or without psychomotor hyperactivity characterized by a significant time span between symptom appearance and death, defines dementia. Clinically significant confusion in older patients may lead the practitioner to suspect a neurodegenerative dementia such as AD; vascular dementia; depression, which can cause pseudodementia; or excessive consumption of alcohol or drugs, which can also cause dementia. (More information about dementia is discussed in Chapter 8, and vascular disease is discussed in Chapter 9.)

Delirium

Delirium is sometimes called an acute confusional state. The clinician must distinguish between delirium and dementia when evaluating confusion in the older adult patient. Patients with a history of dementia have a higher incidence of delirium, whereas delirium may also exist as a state by itself without any evidence of dementia. See Table 6.1 for the differences between delirium and dementia. The two, however, do share common characteristics. Once the cause of the delirium is corrected, the patient should return to their previous state of cognitive functioning.

There are many screening tools with varying degrees of sensitivity and specificity to detect cognitive changes that may be used to aid the clinician in the first step toward an accurate diagnosis (see Table 6.1). It is helpful to use the same tool at each visit for consistency in monitoring the patient's mental function.

Metabolic Disturbances

Fluid, electrolyte, and acid–base imbalances such as hyponatremia, hypercalcemia, and lactic acidosis may be the result of metabolic problems, which can alter a patient's level of consciousness, producing confusion. The extent of the imbalance determines the severity of the patient's confusion. Often, the patient is dehydrated and

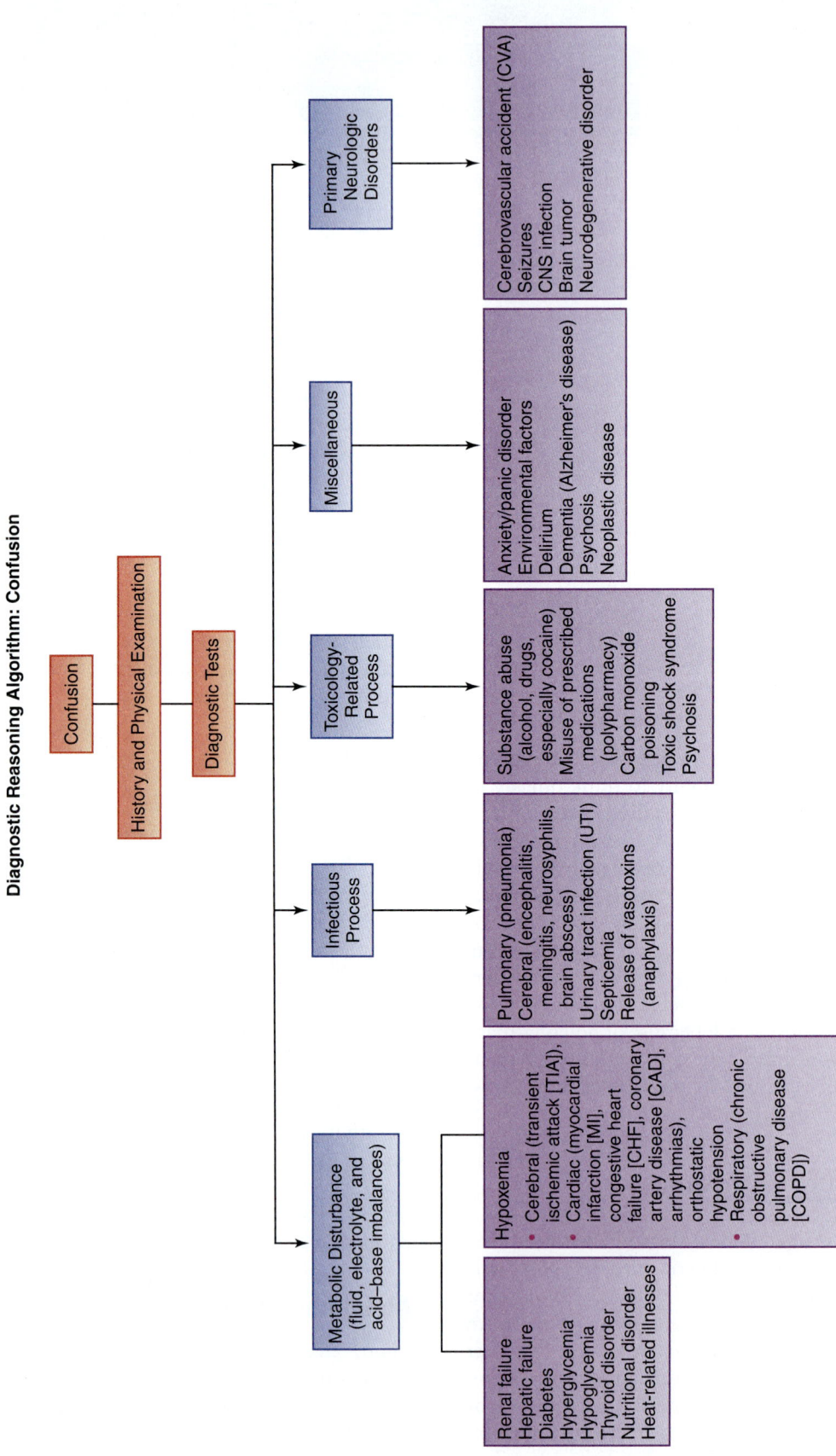

Figure 6.1 Diagnostic reasoning algorithm: confusion.

TABLE 6.1 Delirium Versus Dementia

	Delirium (Acute Confusional State)	**Dementia (Chronic)**
Onset	Abrupt onset over a short period of time—days to weeks	Gradual onset over months or years
Timing	Confusion fluctuates throughout the day	Slow progressive decline
Duration	Hours to weeks	Months to years
Causes	Cerebral event Organic brain syndrome Distended bladder, constipation Sensory deprivation (poor eyesight/poor hearing) Fever, infection—sepsis, glomerulonephritis, chronic kidney disease Actively dying Polypharmacy Adverse reaction to/abrupt withdrawal of a medication, serotonin syndrome Alcohol withdrawal delirium Hypoxemia Metabolic (thyroid function or organ failure) Stroke	*Neurodegenerative diseases:* Alzheimer's disease Dementia with Lewy bodies Parkinson's disease dementia Frontotemporal dementia Huntington disease Chronic traumatic encephalopathy *Nonneurodegenerative causes:* Alcohol-related dementia Vascular dementia Normal pressure hydrocephalus Chronic subdural hematoma CNS infections (syphilis, HIV, prion disease, etc.)
Symptoms	Hallmark—inattention (73%) Sleep–wake cycle disturbance (73%) Memory problems Psychomotor retardation (37%) Agitation (27%) Perceptual disturbances and hallucinations (26%) Language disturbance (25%)	*Mild/moderate:* Multidomain cognitive deficits—aphasia, apraxia, agnosia, impairment of occupational and social functioning A failing sense of direction Being repetitive Struggling to adapt to change Requiring help with activities of daily living *Severe:* Incontinence, inability to perform ADLs, inability to speak more than six intelligible words in a day, progressive weight loss of 10% of body weight in the past 6 months

Screening tools	MMSE
	MOTYB screening tool
	CAM
		SLUMS
		MoCA
		AD8 informant interview
		MC-FAQ
		MMSE:
		    24 early dementia
		    12–24 intermediate dementia
		    Less than 12 severe dementia
		    FAST: score of 7—admit to hospice
		    Clock-drawing test

Treatment	Stabilize the environment; glasses or hearing aids if sensory deprivation; antipsychotics (haloperidol, olanzapine) if sedation is required for acute agitation	*Nonpharmacological interventions:* Behavior management Caregiver intervention programs Cognitive stimulation Reality orientation therapy Recreational activities *Pharmacological interventions:* Cholinesterase inhibitors Antidepressants Antipsychotics

Continued

TABLE 6.1 Delirium Versus Dementia—cont'd

	Delirium (Acute Confusional State)	Dementia (Chronic)
Prevention/help	Avoid illness—health-promotion efforts Avoid alcohol Decrease number of medications Normalize environment Check eyeglass prescription Use hearing aids if needed	Regular exercise, healthy diet No sure way to prevent dementia; support families in ways to assist the patient's brain to stay healthy longer (e.g., being physically and socially active, mind exercises) Reduce blood pressure; reduce homocysteine and cholesterol levels; control diabetes mellitus; healthy diet; cease smoking; being current on vaccines

Abbreviations: ADLs, activities of daily living; CAM, confusion assessment method; FAST, Functional Assessment Staging Tool; MC-FAQ, Mini-Cog with Functional Assessment Questionnaire; MMSE, Mini-Mental State Examination; MoCA, Montreal Cognitive Assessment; MOTYB, months of the year backward; SLUMS, St. Louis University Mental Status Examination.

has poor skin turgor and dry skin. Infectious symptoms, such as fever and tachycardia, may be present. Additional signs and symptoms along with an extensive history and physical examination will usually lead the clinician to a diagnosis. Routine laboratory tests, including electrolyte panel, urinalysis, chest x-ray (CXR) examination, and electrocardiogram (ECG), may be performed. Treatment should be focused on restoration of appropriate fluid and electrolyte balance by specific correction of the primary metabolic disorder.

Infectious Process

Confusion from toxic metabolic encephalopathy may also be the result of an infectious process, particularly in the setting of preexisting neurological disease. Severe generalized infections, such as septicemia or bacteremia (e.g., from a urinary tract infection), can cause delirium and coma. If the infectious process continues to worsen, hypotension, multiorgan failure, and death may ensue. Infections that directly affect the nervous system (such as viral meningoencephalitis and bacterial meningitis) cause confusion, headache, and nuchal rigidity. Specific signs and symptoms of infections include fever, tachycardia, tachypnea, and decreased blood pressure. Diagnostic studies should include routine tests and those associated with the suspected infectious agent. Treatment should focus on managing the primary cause of the infection.

Tissue Hypoxia and Ischemia

Cardiovascular disorders can cause confusion as a result of tissue hypoxia and ischemia. Confusion may be insidious and may come and go. The patient typically appears ill and has significant changes in vital signs (decreased blood pressure, elevated and/or irregular pulse, and tachypnea); edema; cyanosis; and hypoxia. Diagnostic examinations should include routine laboratory testing, analysis of arterial blood gases, CXR, and ECG. Treatment depends on the problem or disease identified.

Neoplasm

Neoplastic diseases that cause confusion include cancers causing organ dysfunction leading to metabolic derangement, intracranial lesions to the brain, and paraneoplastic neurological syndromes causing autoimmune encephalopathy. Signs and symptoms depend on the areas of the body where the cancer is located. Large brain tumors can cause extensive cerebral edema with increased intracranial pressure resulting in confusion, headaches, seizures, gait disturbances, changes in levels of consciousness, vomiting, and sensory and motor deficits. If left untreated, brain herniation and death may ensue. Diagnostic studies should include basic routine tests. Additional studies and treatment measures will vary, depending on the type of cancer.

DIZZINESS AND VERTIGO

Dizziness and vertigo are often used synonymously, but they do not have the same meaning. *Dizziness* is a nonspecific term describing a sensation of unsteadiness or feeling off-balance, light-headedness, or spinning/movement. Underlying etiologies include orthostatic hypotension, a medication side effect, and balance disorders. If severe, orthostatic hypotension can lead to loss of consciousness, but the feeling of faintness encourages the patient to lie down, which may cause the dizziness to disappear. *Vertigo* describes the false sensation of rotation or movement of the patient or the patient's surroundings. Vertigo may result from an inner ear disease or a disturbance of the vestibular center or pathways in the central nervous system (CNS).

It is important to distinguish vertigo from other causes of dizziness. Episodes of dizziness may be brief or prolonged, mild or severe, with an abrupt or gradual onset. Both dizziness and vertigo may be accompanied by unsteady gait. Vertigo is often accompanied by nausea, vomiting, and nystagmus. If other neurological symptoms occur, such as ataxia, cranial nerve dysfunction, numbness, or weakness, a CNS etiology affecting the cerebellum or brainstem must be investigated.

DIFFERENTIAL DIAGNOSIS

Differential diagnoses of dizziness are classified into four categories: peripheral vestibular disease, systemic disorders (causing global cerebral hypoperfusion), CNS disorders, and balance disorders causing dysequilibrium. The history and physical examination are essential to pinpoint a diagnosis (Fig. 6.2). Key questions to ask a patient with vertigo cover duration of attacks, severity, triggers (such as positional changes), and any associated symptoms such as hearing loss and weakness. Key points to assess include physical examination of the ear to rule out otitis media or shingles infection; hearing tests, including whisper, Weber, and Rinne; and a thorough neurological assessment. For episodic vertigo, the Dix-Hallpike maneuver can distinguish benign paroxysmal positional vertigo (BPPV) from other causes of episodic vertigo. The Dix-Hallpike maneuver is performed by rotating the patient's head to one side and then lowering it slowly to 30 degrees below the body-line. The patient should be observed for nystagmus during head rotation and vertical positioning. In patients with BPPV, rotational or horizontal unidirectional nystagmus begins after a short latency, with recurrence of vertigo. This is transient and is less pronounced with repeating the maneuver. The clinician should suspect a central lesion when the nystagmus is direction changing or vertical, or other neurological abnormalities are seen on examination such as cranial nerve palsies, hemiparesis, sensory loss, or dysmetria. If the vertigo is sustained and no other neurological signs are present on examination, a Head Impulse test, Nystagmus, and Test of Skew (HINTS) examination can differentiate between a peripheral inner-ear issue and a central lesion.

Peripheral Vestibular Disease

Peripheral vestibular disease accounts for up to 44% of all cases of vertigo. Many patients who experience dizziness may have a diseased vestibular nerve. Examination of patients with peripheral vestibular disease is notable for unidirectional horizontal nystagmus, a positive head impulse test, and absence of other neurological abnormalities. Vestibular neuritis is a viral or postviral inflammatory disorder of the cranial nerve (CN) VIII, causing severe sustained vertigo accompanied by nausea, vomiting, and gait instability. When accompanied by unilateral hearing loss, it is called labyrinthitis. Ménière disease causes a triad of symptoms: episodic vertigo, tinnitus, and hearing loss. It is likely caused by endolymphatic hydrops of the labyrinthine system of the inner ear. BPPV is caused by dislodged otoliths in the semicircular canal, and it can be cured with the Epley maneuver (demonstrated on several YouTube videos listed in the resource section). This may need to be repeated, and patients with BPPV are prone to recurrent attacks of vertigo.

Diagnostic studies may include audiological evaluation, electronystagmography, magnetic resonance imaging (MRI), magnetic resonance angiography, brainstem-evoked responses, and basic laboratory screening as guided by history and physical examination. Antihistamine/anticholinergic medications, such as meclizine (Antivert) or promethazine, are the most commonly prescribed medications for acute vertigo. Patients are instructed to take the medication as needed on a short-term basis. Antiemetics should be considered when nausea and vomiting are severe. Prochlorperazine (Compazine) orally (PO) or by suppository or trimethobenzamide (Tigan) PO or by suppository will usually bring relief to the patient. Vestibular rehabilitation and exercises can help the patient with the symptoms of vertigo.

Systemic Disorders

Systemic disorders that cause cerebral hypoperfusion may cause dizziness described as light-headedness. Patients typically complain of light-headedness or feeling that they are about to faint or pass out. Dizziness may be aggravated by postural changes (especially standing up) or exertion. Pallor, dyspnea, tachycardia, palpitations, fatigue, hypotension, blurred vision, and diaphoresis suggest systemic problems. These symptoms should prompt the practitioner to look for signs of anemia, cardiovascular disease, hyperventilation, drug reactions, endocrine disorders, fluid and electrolyte imbalances, and orthostatic hypotension. Systemic diseases require diagnostic examination and treatment that is specific for the cause of the dizziness.

Central Nervous System Disorders

CNS disorders that disrupt the pathway between the vestibular apparatus and the brain, such as lesions in the cerebellum or brainstem, may cause vertigo of central etiology. Accompanying neurological abnormalities on examination may include numbness, hemiparesis, diplopia, dysmetria, and dysarthria. The nystagmus in CNS disorders is often direction changing or vertical; there may be a vertical misalignment of the eyes (skew deviation); and the head impulse test should be negative. Diagnostic examination and treatment depend on the underlying disorder.

HEADACHE

One of the most common of all human ailments is thought to be the headache. A headache is a pain or ache in the head that sometimes restricts activity, reduces the

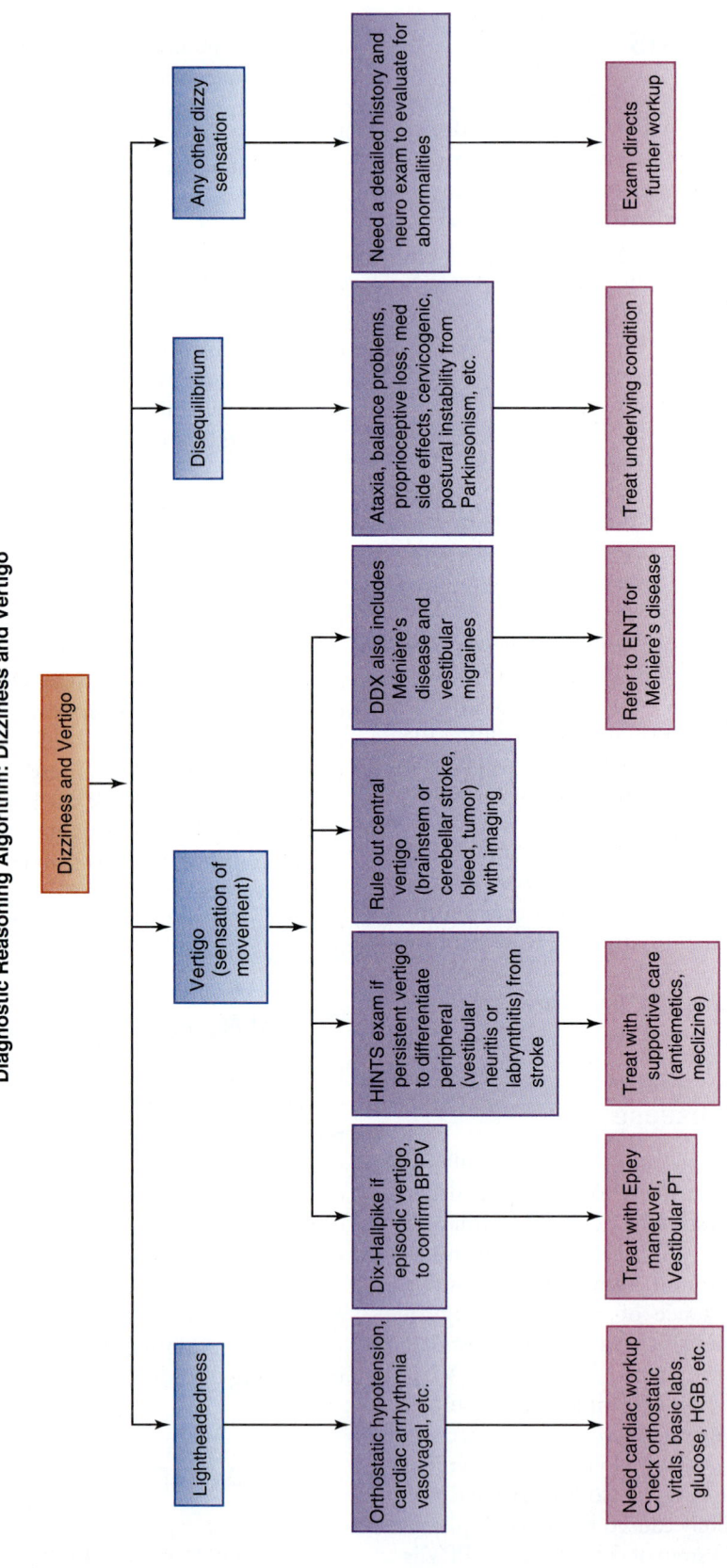

Figure 6.2 Diagnostic reasoning algorithm: dizziness and vertigo.

level of functioning, and decreases work performance. The prevalence of headaches has a great impact on society because of lost or reduced effectiveness at home, work, or school. Individual burdens result from pain and the disabling effects of various headache syndromes. About 90% of all headaches are primary headache disorders without pathological causes. However, practitioners need to avoid underestimating the significance of headache as an early manifestation of serious neurological disease.

Headaches may be classified into two general categories: primary and secondary headaches. Primary headaches include tension-type headaches, migraines, and cluster headaches. Table 6.2 presents a comparison of these three categories of headaches. Secondary headaches are a symptom of an injury or an underlying illness.

The Headache Classification Committee of the International Headache Society has a headache classification system and operational diagnostic criteria for the different headache syndromes. This system was designed to describe and identify headaches to allow for more accurate diagnosis and research.

Migraine has two major subtypes: migraine with aura and migraine without aura. The diagnosis of migraine with aura must include the presence of one or more of the following fully reversible neurological symptoms: visual, motor, sensory, speech, brainstem, or retinal. The symptoms of an aura typically develop gradually during or preceding a headache. Auras are fully reversible and last 5 to 60 minutes. For migraine without aura, two of the following characteristics are required for diagnosis: unilateral location, pulsating quality, moderate to severe intensity, and exacerbation by physical activity. In addition, at least one of the following must be present: nausea or vomiting, photophobia, or phonophobia. Chronic migraines are classified as those that occur on at least 15 days of the month for more than 3 months.

EPIDEMIOLOGY AND CAUSES

More individuals complain about headaches than any other condition experienced, and they affect anyone of any age. Each year, approximately 45 million individuals complain of headaches, and more than 8 million individuals of all ages visit a health-care provider with this complaint annually, with the incidence decreasing with age. In the United States, some researchers estimate the annual cost of headaches, including costs of direct medical care and lost productivity, to exceed $17 billion. Women are two to three times more likely to be affected than men across all age groups, with the incidence in women increasing during adolescence and peaking at menopause.

Tension-Type Headaches

Tension-type headache is a highly prevalent condition that can be disabling. It is the most common type of headache, with an estimated 80% to 90% of the population experiencing tension headaches at some period in their lives. It occurs more often in women (86%) than

TABLE 6.2 Primary Headaches: A Comparison of the Different Types

Assessment/Plan	Tension-Type Headache	Migraine	Cluster
Signs and symptoms	Bilateral pressure or bandlike pain	Unilateral pulsating episodic pain Nausea and vomiting Photophobia and phonophobia	Periorbital nighttime unilateral, nonpulsatile pain Photophobia Tearing Nasal stuffiness
History and physical examination findings	Sleep cycle disturbances Social stressors Neck arthritis Neck muscle spasm	May be similar	May be similar
Diagnostic tests	MRI: rule out lesions, hemorrhage, cerebral venous sinus thrombosis, etc. CT: rule out hemorrhage LP: measure opening pressure, rule out meningitis	Same	Same
Treatment	Support Biofeedback Stress management Massage Drugs: aspirin, acetaminophen (Tylenol), NSAIDs, muscle relaxants Preventive treatment	Avoidance education Drugs: Abortive: triptans, NSAIDs, antiemetics Prophylactic: propranolol, nortriptyline, topiramate, CGRP inhibitors, Botox	100% oxygen by mask, sumatriptan, indomethacin

Abbreviations: CGRP, calcitonin gene-related peptide; CT, computed tomography; LP, lumbar puncture; MRI, magnetic resonance imaging.

in men (65%). Its prevalence peaks at about age 30 to 38. Tension headache occurs more frequently in whites (40%), especially with increasing educational levels (48%). Although few people with tension-type headaches lose time from work, more than 40% of people affected reported decreased effectiveness at work, home, or school because of this type of headache. These muscle contraction headaches may either be primary (without underlying pathology) or secondary (the result of pathology such as trauma, infection, arthritis, or tumor).

Migraine Headaches

Migraine headaches are the second most common type of headache with high prevalence and socioeconomic impacts. Migraines are the third most prevalent disorder with the seventh highest specific cause of disability in the world. Racial differences in migraine prevalence are striking: black people and nonwhite people of Hispanic or other nonspecified ethnic origin are at least twice as likely as White or Asian people to be migraine sufferers. An inverse relationship exists between migraine and age. Prevalence of migraine is highest in adults younger than age 40 and lowest in those older than age 60. Migraine headaches occur in 4% to 5% of school-age children. It is not unusual for migraine headaches to begin during childhood. Migraine syndromes are painful and often disabling, accounting for a loss of more than 157 million workdays to headache pain each year. About 5 million people in the United States have at least one migraine attack per month. More than 11 million people with migraines claim moderate to severe disability. In one study of patients who met the International Headache Society's criteria for migraine, fewer than half had actually received a diagnosis of migraine.

Migraine headaches are often hereditary. In familial hemiplegic migraine, the cause is associated with mutations in calcium, sodium, or potassium channel genes. In women, menstrual migraines are triggered by hormonal fluctuations typically occurring around the time of menstruation. Decreasing estrogen levels can trigger a migraine that is either endogenously or exogenously induced (e.g., by a week-off [21-day] oral contraceptive pill or by hormone replacement therapy).

There are multiple, varied precipitating factors of migraine headaches, which differ from person to person. A migraine headache may occur with sleep deprivation, skipped meals, odors, neck pain, or emotional stress. Certain foods, such as chocolate, alcohol, and caffeine (consumption or withdrawal), are common triggers. Box 6.1 presents common triggers of migraine headaches.

Cluster Headaches

Cluster headaches fall under the category of trigeminal autonomic cephalalgias, which are a group of primary headache disorders associated with severe, unilateral head pain accompanied by ipsilateral autonomic symptoms. Cluster headaches are named for their pattern of occurrence: they usually come in groups (clusters) over the span of several weeks or months and then disappear for months or even years. Cluster headaches are one of the most painful types of headaches. They typically occur in middle-aged men, with the first onset between ages 20 and 30, and typically cluster on a seasonal basis, with anywhere from 3 to 18 months between headaches. Approximately 69 out of 100,000 individuals have cluster headaches. A dysfunction of the hypothalamus may account for the periodicity and clocklike regularity of cluster headaches.

Other Types of Headaches

Older adults have fewer headaches overall. However, when an older adult presents with a new-onset headache, suspicion should be high for an underlying systemic disease such as temporal arteritis or intracranial lesion

---

Box 6.1 Common Triggers of Migraine Headaches

Hormonal
- Low estrogen level, increased prostaglandin level

Environmental
- High-pitched noises, excessive sun, bright lights, weather changes, strong odors, video display terminals

Diet
- Alcohol, sodium nitrate, caffeine, chicken livers, yogurt, avocado, sour cream, artificial sweeteners
- Tyramine (bananas, ripe cheese, nuts, pods of broad beans [Italian pole, lima, or butter beans])
- Phenylethylamine (some cheeses, red wine, chocolate)
- Monosodium glutamate (some fast foods, canned soups, frozen dinners)

Lifestyle
- Stress, sports, swimming, cycling, hockey, weight lifting, running, inadequate warm-ups

Physical activity at high altitudes
- Cycling, climbing, skiing

Fatigue

Changes in sleep schedule
- Excessive sleep, too little sleep

Cigarette smoking

Dehydration

(see Geriatric Considerations). These headaches require immediate medical evaluation.

Temporal arteritis or giant cell arteritis (GCA) affects men and women equally and occurs predominantly in adults older than age 60. Its incidence increases with age, and it is rare in younger people. Associated symptoms include scalp allodynia, jaw claudication, and concurrent polymyalgia rheumatica. Other symptoms are local swelling; tenderness and pulselessness of the temporal artery; and systemic symptoms of fever, anorexia, weight loss, and chills. Systemic markers of inflammation also are present. Prompt diagnosis is important because temporal arteritis can cause permanent vision loss if left untreated.

A "thunderclap headache" is an abrupt and severe, sudden onset headache that reaches maximal intensity in under 1 minute. This type of headache requires emergent evaluation because it is often caused by a subarachnoid hemorrhage. The headache from subarachnoid hemorrhage commonly occurs from a ruptured intracranial aneurysm, such as a "berry" aneurysm or dissecting arterial aneurysm of the carotid or vertebral vessels. A berry aneurysm, named for its shape, results from a congenital abnormality of intracranial vessels, primarily at the circle of Willis. Ruptured intracranial aneurysms are the primary cause of subarachnoid hemorrhage. Less often, a subarachnoid hemorrhage is caused by an atrioventricular malformation (AVM) or bleeding disorder. An AVM is a congenital disorder that results in the formation of a tangled collection of dilated arteries and veins. Symptoms are usually seen in people aged 20 to 40 years. Two-thirds of people affected by a subarachnoid hemorrhage are aged 40 to 60 years; women are affected slightly more frequently. In the United States, 10 to 15 cases occur per 100,000 people per year. Activities such as lifting, straining, sexual intercourse, and emotional excitement can precipitate a hemorrhage.

The headache from a subdural hematoma is of venous origin, typically resulting from a head injury that is usually mild and easily forgotten by the patient. It occurs predominantly in people older than age 50 and is more common in men. Alcohol abuse and use of anticoagulants contribute to its occurrence. It rarely is associated with a fractured skull.

Arterial dissection, although occurring infrequently in young adults, is characterized by cephalic pain or headache of sudden onset, often preceding transient ischemic attack (TIA) or stroke symptoms. Carotid or vertebral artery dissection causes acute unilateral neck pain that is sudden and often radiates to the ipsilateral face or eye. The headache is related to cervical manipulation, sustained exertion, or trauma. Recognition and proper treatment are important since arterial dissections can lead to stroke.

Increased intracranial pressure causes headaches that worsen with lying flat, bending over, or doing the Valsalva maneuver. There may be an associated CN VI palsy, pulsatile tinnitus, or transient visual obscuration, which is a graying-out of vision, typically with position changes. Funduscopic examination reveals papilledema. Idiopathic intracranial hypertension (pseudotumor cerebri) is a common cause, although it is a diagnosis of exclusion after mass lesion, cerebral venous sinus thrombosis, and meningitis are ruled out. Proper diagnosis of cerebral venous sinus thrombosis is important since it can lead to life-threatening infarcts and brain hemorrhage. Common causes associated with this type of thrombosis are pregnancy and oral contraceptive use. In meningeal irritation, headache is often the most prominent feature, along with photophobia, pain with eye movement, neck stiffness, and positive Brudzinski's and Kernig's signs. Encephalitis is associated with a new-onset generalized headache, accompanied by confusion, altered level of consciousness, focal neurological signs, or seizures. Signs of infection and meningismus may be present. Changes associated with these conditions can be detected with lumbar puncture (LP) and brain imaging.

PATHOPHYSIOLOGY

Inside the skull, only certain structures are sensitive to pain; these include the meninges, arteries, and skull. The brain parenchyma itself is not sensitive to pain. Increased pressure on and inflammation of the meninges, as well as distention of or traction on the arteries, will cause pain. Head trauma usually causes headaches through all these pain-inducing mechanisms.

Beside head trauma, many other medical problems can initiate a headache secondarily—strokes (ischemic and hemorrhagic); intracranial infections; tumors; metabolic disorders (hypercapnia, hypoglycemia, and hypoxia); sudden hypertension; changes in intracranial pressure; drugs and drug withdrawal syndrome; cranial nerve pain; and eye, ear, nose, sinus, teeth, and jaw disorders. The primary headache syndromes—chronic tension-type headaches, migraine headaches, and cluster headaches—are those in which the headache is the primary problem.

Pain signals are transmitted from most structures in the head by branches of the trigeminal nerve (Fig. 6.3), although pain from the back of the head and the posterior fossa of the skull are transmitted by branches of the first three cervical spinal nerves. First-order pain fibers from these nerves synapse in the brainstem and upper spinal cord, and from there, the second-order pain fibers project to sensory nuclei in the thalamus. Regardless of its cause, headache pain is the result of activating these trigeminothalamic and cervicothalamic pain circuits.

Primary headache syndromes, however, are not caused only by the normal activation of trigeminal or cervical pain receptors inside the skull. In addition, primary headache syndromes require hypersensitization of the trigeminothalamic or cervicothalamic circuitry at one or more points along their route from the primary afferent axons to the thalamic sensory nuclei.

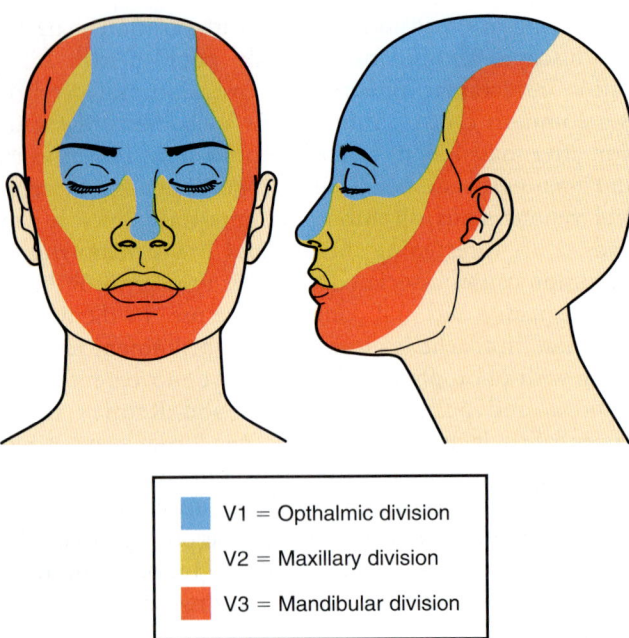

Figure 6.3 The three branches of the trigeminal nerve.

V1 = Opthalmic division
V2 = Maxillary division
V3 = Mandibular division

One part of this circuitry on which many headache studies have focused is the thalamus. When pain stimuli pass through the thalamus, the signals are modulated by serotonergic axons coming from the dorsal raphe nuclei in the midbrain. It is thought that an abnormal reduction in serotonergic activity in the thalamus is a part of the hypersensitization in primary headache syndromes. Among the observations consistent with this idea are the following:

- Serotonin agonists (ergotamine, dihydroergotamine, and triptans) can reduce the pain and frequency of migraines and can reduce the duration and frequency of cluster headaches.
- Increasing the effectiveness of serotonergic synapses with a selective serotonin reuptake inhibitor can reduce the frequency of tension-type headaches.
- Reserpine, a drug that depletes CNS synapses of serotonin, can precipitate migraine headaches.

Chronic Tension-Type Headaches

Chronic tension-type headaches produce mild to moderate pain that feels like a constant, bilateral head tightness and lasts from a half hour to a week. These headaches do not pulsate, do not cause nausea, and usually are not made worse by physical activity. Chronic tension-type headaches occur repeatedly (typically many times a month), have a gradual onset during the day, and are more common in people with depression.

Although patients with chronic tension-type headaches have muscle tenderness, their headaches do not appear to be caused by unusual muscle tension or contraction. Instead, in patients with this type of primary headache, the head and neck pain circuitry is hypersensitized so that normal stimuli and typical muscle strains lead to headaches. The basic cause of the hypersensitization is not known, although it is thought that chronic tension-type headaches result from abnormalities in the serotonin, norepinephrine, or dopamine pathways that originate in the brainstem and that modulate the trigeminothalamic or cervicothalamic pain circuits.

Migraine Headaches

Migraine headaches produce moderate to severe unilateral head pain lasting from 4 hours to 3 days. These headaches throb, cause nausea, and are made worse by activity. Migraine headaches happen repeatedly (typically one to three times per month) and can be triggered by certain stimuli, most commonly alcohol, stress, menstruation, or diet.

Migraine headaches occur as a set of events that unfold in a predictable pattern. First, there is a prodrome, which begins hours or days before the headache. The prodrome is often a psychological change—it can be drowsiness; depression; euphoria; hyperactivity; difficulty concentrating; irritability; or increased sensitivity to noises, lights, or smells. The prodrome is thought to reflect disturbances in the hypothalamic-limbic system.

After the prodrome, patients with migraine experience a unilateral throbbing headache, which is accompanied by anorexia and nausea (with vomiting in one-third of cases) and by a heightened sensitivity to noises, lights, and smells. The basis for the pain is a hypersensitized trigeminothalamic circuit, which makes the normally innocuous pulsing of cerebral blood flow feel painful. The hypersensitivity can affect all trigeminal nerve stimuli on the same side of the head so that normal pressures (caused by, e.g., combing, shaving, taking a shower, or wearing glasses or earrings) on the skin of the face or scalp also feel painful.

In an experimental model, migraine-like headaches can be initiated by electrical stimulation of areas in the midbrain. In this region, focal stimuli set off a cascade of specific reactions including an increase in local blood flow and a hypersensitization of the trigeminothalamic pain circuits.

In the less common type of migraine (migraine with aura), the headache is preceded by sensory phenomena called an aura. An aura is usually a visual phenomenon, often with a geometric pattern spreading across a visual field; less commonly, the aura may cause tingling or weakness to slowly spread across one side of the body over a period of minutes. The aura coincides with a spreading wave of chemical and metabolic changes that moves across the cerebral cortex from an initial focus in the occipital lobe (in visual aura). As the wave reaches a region, it briefly activates the local neurons and increases the local blood flow. After the wave passes, the neurons are refractory and the local blood flow decreased. It is thought that this wave contributes to the hypersensitization tension-type headache. Drug therapy for acute headache should generally not exceed more than 3 days per week on a regular basis. More frequent treatment may result in medication-overuse chronic daily headaches.

Migraine treatment can be divided into abortive, prophylactic, and nonpharmacological treatment. Nonpharmacological measures are useful for minor migraines or as an adjunct to pharmacological treatment to prevent or decrease the severity of a headache. These methods include identifying and eliminating known triggers. Maintaining a regular schedule for sleep and meals can prevent a headache related to fatigue and hunger. If exercise precipitates an attack, an adequate warm-up before working out is recommended. Biofeedback, relaxation techniques, and regular aerobic exercise are encouraged. Deep breathing, massage, and hot or cold therapy sometimes ease the pain, but use of excessive cold (e.g., ice packs) or caffeine can backfire.

Most migraine attacks vary in their effects on the patient's ability to function. In mild attacks, the effect is minimal. In moderate attacks, visual activities are moderately impaired. In severe attacks, however, the patient is unable to continue normal activities or can continue them only with severe discomfort. In some severe attacks, the patient is incapacitated, requiring treatment in the provider's office, urgent care setting, or emergency department.

Drug therapy should be added when these measures are not completely effective. Early abortive treatment of migraines with effective medications improves a variety of outcomes, including duration, severity, and associated disability. It is appropriate for the clinician to take a trial-and-error approach to identify medications most successful in the relief of headaches and associated symptoms with the fewest adverse effects, minimal costs, and a return to normal functioning for each patient. Some patients may require a combination of medications, such as a triptan as an abortive medication and a daily preventive medication. NSAIDs are a common first-line abortive treatment for patients with migraine. Triptans are also a commonly prescribed abortive migraine treatment. Drugs Commonly Prescribed 6.1 and Complementary Therapies 6.1 present a list of medications commonly used to treat migraines and complementary therapies that may help treat headaches.

Recommended first-line treatment for the relief of acute attacks of cluster headaches includes subcutaneous injection of sumatriptan or intranasal use of zolmitriptan orally or intranasally. Oxygen inhalation is highly effective for cluster headaches when administered at the beginning of an attack with a nonrebreathing facial mask at 7 to 15 L/min. Most patients will obtain relief within 15 minutes.

FOLLOW-UP AND REFERRAL

Referral to a neurologist should be considered for any patient with episodes of transient neurological deficits; increasing frequency and severity of unilateral headaches; atypical auras; changes in personality; excessive sleepiness; and new onset of progressive deficits suggesting a mass lesion, hemorrhage, or structural disorder. GCA must be carefully considered in a middle-aged or older

Drugs Commonly Prescribed 6.1: Migraine Headache: Adults

DRUG	ADVERSE REACTIONS AND PRESCRIBING CONSIDERATIONS
Abortive	
Triptans (serotonin receptor agonists)	
Almotriptan (Axert) Eletriptan (Relpax) Frovatriptan (Frova) Naratriptan (Amerge) Rizatriptan (Maxalt) Sumatriptan (Imitrex, Alsuma) Naratriptan (Amerge) Zolmitriptan (Zomig)	Side effects: paresthesia, asthenia, nausea, dizziness, chest or neck tightness, heaviness, somnolence Contraindicated in ischemic heart disease or other significant cardiovascular disease or cerebrovascular disease There is a risk of rebound headache if triptans are used more than twice a week. Imitrex is also available as an injection and nasal spray.
Ergot derivatives	
Ergotamine 1 mg/caffeine 100 mg (Cafergot) Ergotamine 2 mg/caffeine 100 mg (Cafergot supp) Dihydroergotamine (DHE 45, Migranal)	Contraindicated in peripheral vascular disease, coronary heart disease, hypertension, and hepatic or renal disease Intravenous route preferred when rapid relief is desired Migranal is a nasal spray.

Continued

Drugs Commonly Prescribed 6.1: Migraine Headache: Adults—cont'd

DRUG	ADVERSE REACTIONS AND PRESCRIBING CONSIDERATIONS
Antiemetics Metoclopramide Prochlorperazine	Adverse effects: extrapyramidal side effects, fatigue, restlessness, sedation, dizziness
NSAIDs Ibuprofen (Advil, Motrin) Acetylsalicylic acid (ASA—aspirin) Naproxen sodium (Aleve, Naprosyn)	For mild to moderate pain. Increased risk of gastrointestinal (GI) bleed with alcohol Adverse reactions: GI upset, GI bleed
Combination analgesics Butalbital 50 mg/acetaminophen 325 mg/caffeine 40 mg (Fioricet) Butalbital 50 mg/ASA 325 mg/caffeine 40 mg (Fiorinal)	Potentiation with alcohol Adverse effects: drowsiness, dizziness, GI disturbances Use of butalbital-containing medications is not recommended as first-line treatment for migraine headaches; avoid if possible.
Opiates Morphine Oxycodone	Adverse effects: sedation, respiratory failure, constipation, addiction Use of opiates is not recommended as first-line treatment for migraine headaches; avoid if possible.
Steroids Medrol Dose Pack (methylprednisolone) Dexamethasone intramuscular (IM)/IV	Can use as adjunct therapy for severe, refractory migraine headaches
Prophylactic Medications	
Beta blockers Propranolol (Inderal) Timolol (Blocadren) Metoprolol (Lopressor, Toprol) Atenolol (Tenormin) Nadolol (Corgard)	Preferred if patient is hypertensive or has angina Contraindicated in asthma, sinus bradycardia, second or third atrioventricular block Potentiated by alcohol May cause weight loss, asthenia, mental fuzziness
Antidepressants Venlafaxine (Effexor XR) Nortriptyline Amitriptyline	May cause sedation (especially amitriptyline) so recommend nighttime dosing
Calcium channel blockers Verapamil (Calan)	May take several months to be effective Contraindicated in pregnancy Adverse effects: bradycardia, fatigue, weight gain, constipation, nausea, edema, muscle pain
Anticonvulsant agents Topiramate (Topamax) Gabapentin (Neurontin) Valproic acid (Depakote)	Adverse effects: dizziness, somnolence, tremor, weight gain, teratogenic effects, paresthesia, kidney stones Adverse effects: somnolence, dizziness, asthenia Preferred for patients with seizure disorders or diabetic peripheral neuropathy
CGRP antagonists Erenumab (Aimovig) Fremanezumab (Ajovy) Galcanezumab (Emgality) Eptinezumab (Vyepti)	Newer medications approved for migraine prevention Monoclonal antibodies that block calcitonin gene-related peptide (CGRP) activity. Injectable medications given every 1 to 3 months
Botulinum toxin injections onabotulinumtoxinA (Botox)	For chronic migraine. Injected into the muscles of the face and neck every 3 months

Complementary Therapies 6.1: Headaches

Acupuncture/acupressure
Aroma and herbal therapy

- Apply lavender oil to the temples (women).
- Apply peppermint oil to the temples (men).
- Use eucalyptus for sinus headaches.
- Drink rosemary tea or mix the essential oil in hot water and inhale.
- Take evening primrose oil 500 mg.
- Apply cold black tea bags to the eyes for 15 minutes.
- Take *Ginkgo biloba* 120 to 240 mg of dried extract in two to three doses daily.
- Take valerian *(Valeriana officinalis)* 2 to 3 g one to three times per day.

Biofeedback
Diet therapy

- At the first sign of a migraine, drink one to two cups of strong coffee (effective for some individuals) or a glass of carrot or celery juice.
- To reduce throbbing and contractions, eat foods high in magnesium such as dark, leafy greens; fresh seafood; sea vegetables; nuts; whole grains; and molasses.
- Eat vitamin C–rich foods such as broccoli, hot and bell peppers, sprouts, cherries, citrus.
- Drink green tea.
- Avoid foods known to trigger headache: additive and chemical-based foods (monosodium glutamate, sulfites [red wine]; condiments; nitrates [aged and smoked meats]; pickled fish and shellfish; caffeine-containing foods, including chocolate; cultured foods [e.g., yogurt]; refined sweeteners); red meats; dairy products (cheese); soft drinks (the phosphorus binds magnesium); alcohol; salty, sugary, and wheat-based foods.

Exercise
Massage

- Massage the temples for 5 minutes.
- Do 10 neck rolls.
- Pull ear lobes for 5 seconds.
- Rub back of ear and all around ear shell.
- Apply an ice pack to the back of the neck or put feet in a cold water bath.

Poultices

- Rub capsaicin (Zostrix) cream on the forehead.
- Apply onion or horseradish poultices to the nape of the neck or soles of the feet.

Reflexology

- Apply pressure to the inside base of the foot and big toe three times for 10 seconds each.

Relaxation therapy

- Perform deep breathing.

Vitamins

- Take magnesium citrate 800 mg daily.
- Take niacin 100 to 500 mg daily.

Other

- Avoid smoking and secondhand smoke.

Transcutaneous supraorbital nerve stimulation (Cefaly headband)

---

patient who presents with a new and unexplained headache. Surgical referral may be necessary for a temporal artery biopsy and definitive diagnosis or possible use of chronic steroid therapy.

Patient Education: Migraine Headache

The management of migraine is a team effort in which the patient plays an equal role. Patients must be convinced of the practitioner's interest in their complaints and commitment to their treatment. Realistic outcomes should be discussed because treatment is often ineffective or can be used for only a short period of time. Patients should be educated about the nature of migraine and given additional literature. Patients should keep a diary of any events that may be associated with an attack. This helps identify and avoid triggers associated with a single episode and distinguish them from triggers that lead to an increase in the frequency and severity of attacks. Although clinicians may not help patients deal with endogenous triggers (e.g., genetic tendencies), they may help the patient identify other triggers. Exogenous triggers include foods—for example, red wine and other alcoholic beverages, aged cheese, monosodium glutamate, aspartame (dietary sweetener), and chocolate—the frequency and pattern of light; and oral contraceptives. Environmental triggers include stress and stressful family events, air travel, weather changes, odors (bad and good), and meteorological depression. Having an awareness of the triggers may help the patient avoid them, which should diminish the frequency and intensity of the attacks. The clinician should explain the importance of warming up before exercise and avoiding tight-fitting goggles, sunglasses, helmets, or other headgear and suggest that regular exercise may prevent or decrease the headaches. If exercise is found to trigger an attack, discuss the importance of adequate nutrition and fluids before and after such activities.

Women who have migraines with aura have a higher risk of stroke with the use of estrogen-containing contraceptives compared with those without migraines. Alternative forms of birth control should be used. When discussing migraine therapy with women of childbearing age, the clinician should ask what method of birth control the individual is using.

Stress-management strategies and relaxation techniques are commonly taught to patients to manage frequent, unavoidable family- or work-related stress and emotional problems. When pharmacological treatment is necessary, the family should fully understand the treatment. Impaired judgment may occur with severe attacks, and the patient may not remember what drugs or dosages were used. The patient should understand each medication type; its proper use; adverse effects of the medications, including interactions with other medications; and any contraindications, such as pregnancy. The patient should be asked to record in a headache diary the medications used (including any OTC or other medications); dosages; response to medication; and evaluation of treatment, including adverse effects. Clinicians should advise patients not to take headache medications other than those prescribed. Excessive use of other analgesics may reduce their effectiveness. Using triptans and analgesics frequently can lead to rebound headaches or chronic daily headaches. Adverse effects are common, and the patient must keep the practitioner informed in case changes in medicine are needed. Patients should discuss with the practitioner if they desire to become or are pregnant.

PARESTHESIA AND PARESIS

Paresthesia is an abnormal sensation described as numbness or tingling, cramping, or pain without a known stimulus, felt along peripheral nerve pathways. Paresis is weakness that may be local to a single extremity or the face, or it may involve more than one extremity. Paresis may develop suddenly or gradually and may be permanent or transient. Feelings associated with paresthesia are annoying "pins and needles" sensations that often cause the patient to touch or rub the affected area. Paresthesia is a common complaint, especially in patients with certain systemic diseases or those taking certain medications.

DIFFERENTIAL DIAGNOSIS

Paresthesia is usually due to damage or irritation anywhere along the sensory pathway in the nervous system, from the cerebral cortex in the parietal lobe to the thalamus, brainstem, spinal cord, and peripheral nerves. It is important to explore the symptom of paresthesia by asking the patient to describe when it first began; the character, duration, and distribution of the paresthesia; and any other associated signs and symptoms such as sensory or motor loss. A medical history may reveal neurological, cardiac, vascular, endocrine, renal, or inflammatory diseases the patient may have had or still has. Recent trauma, surgery, or invasive procedures may reveal possible causes of peripheral nerve injury. The physical examination should focus on the neurological system, assessing level of consciousness; cranial nerve function; reflexes; motor strength; and touch, pain, and temperature sensations. Skin color and the quality of all pulses should also be noted. If the patient has diabetes, symptoms of diabetic neuropathy such as a bilateral loss of pain sensation and diminished touch, temperature sensation, and proprioception may be present. They may present in a stocking-glove distribution.

The most common diagnoses associated with paresthesia symptoms are arterial occlusion (stroke or TIA), nerve entrapment syndrome, neuropathy, peripheral vascular disease, and herpes zoster (Fig. 6.5).

A stroke is a sudden loss of neurological function caused by impaired blood flow to the brain, often due to arterial occlusion. The loss of function can last from a few minutes to 24 hours; after a TIA, normal function returns. If some residual weakness remains, the patient has had a stroke. Arterial occlusion is an emergency. An acute occlusion may be either an arterial embolism or a thrombosis. Immediate thrombolysis followed by embolectomy is the treatment of choice but must be performed early, preferably within 6 hours of the embolic event.

Arteriosclerosis obliterans is a disorder that involves the pathological process of atherosclerosis, which causes progressive narrowing of the arteries with subsequent obstruction of blood flow, resulting in diminished or decreased flow of blood to the legs and feet.

Nerve entrapment syndrome results from compression of a nerve pathway along the root of the nerve, which results in paresthesia or weakness. Trauma, repetitive use, edema, infection, prolonged standing or sitting, and tight clothing can all cause entrapment of the nerve.

Neuropathy is usually the result of underlying diseases such as diabetes, renal failure, cancer treatments, autoimmune disease, vasculitis, thyroid disease, ingestion of toxins, or nutritional deficiency. Glucose intolerance is the most common cause of peripheral neuropathy. This typically causes diminished sensation in a stocking-glove distribution. The neuropathy is painful in a minority of patients.

Herpes zoster is caused by the varicella-zoster virus, which causes an acute vesicular eruption in adults, especially in immunocompromised patients. An early symptom of herpes zoster is paresthesia, which occurs as a result of infection, inflammation, and compression along the dermatomal distribution of a spinal nerve.

TREMORS

Tremors are rhythmic, involuntary, oscillating muscle movements across a joint. A resting tremor occurs in a relaxed extremity and stops when the extremity is lifted or moved. Conversely, an action tremor occurs with posture

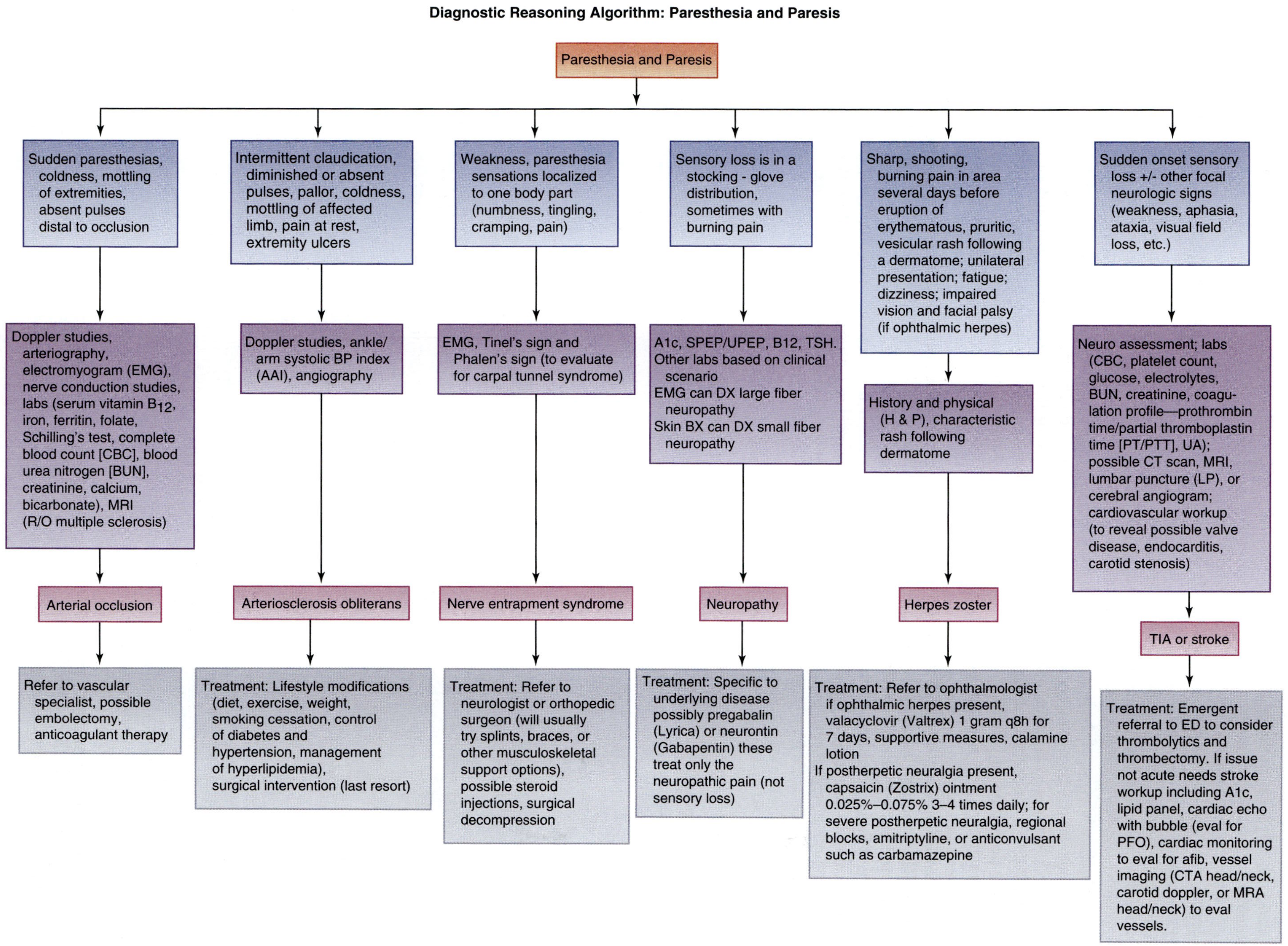

Chapter 6 Common Neurological Complaints

Diagnostic Reasoning Algorithm: Paresthesia and Paresis

Paresthesia and Paresis

- Sudden paresthesias, coldness, mottling of extremities, absent pulses distal to occlusion
  - Doppler studies, arteriography, electromyogram (EMG), nerve conduction studies, labs (serum vitamin B₁₂, iron, ferritin, folate, Schilling's test, complete blood count [CBC], blood urea nitrogen [BUN], creatinine, calcium, bicarbonate), MRI (R/O multiple sclerosis)
    - **Arterial occlusion**
      - Refer to vascular specialist, possible embolectomy, anticoagulant therapy

- Intermittent claudication, diminished or absent pulses, pallor, coldness, mottling of affected limb, pain at rest, extremity ulcers
  - Doppler studies, ankle/arm systolic BP index (AAI), angiography
    - **Arteriosclerosis obliterans**
      - Treatment: Lifestyle modifications (diet, exercise, weight, smoking cessation, control of diabetes and hypertension, management of hyperlipidemia), surgical intervention (last resort)

- Weakness, paresthesia sensations localized to one body part (numbness, tingling, cramping, pain)
  - EMG, Tinel's sign and Phalen's sign (to evaluate for carpal tunnel syndrome)
    - **Nerve entrapment syndrome**
      - Treatment: Refer to neurologist or orthopedic surgeon (will usually try splints, braces, or other musculoskeletal support options), possible steroid injections, surgical decompression

- Sensory loss is in a stocking - glove distribution, sometimes with burning pain
  - A1c, SPEP/UPEP, B12, TSH. Other labs based on clinical scenario. EMG can DX large fiber neuropathy. Skin BX can DX small fiber neuropathy
    - **Neuropathy**
      - Treatment: Specific to underlying disease possibly pregabalin (Lyrica) or neurontin (Gabapentin) these treat only the neuropathic pain (not sensory loss)

- Sharp, shooting, burning pain in area several days before eruption of erythematous, pruritic, vesicular rash following a dermatome; unilateral presentation; fatigue; dizziness; impaired vision and facial palsy (if ophthalmic herpes)
  - History and physical (H & P), characteristic rash following dermatome
    - **Herpes zoster**
      - Treatment: Refer to ophthalmologist if ophthalmic herpes present, valacyclovir (Valtrex) 1 gram q8h for 7 days, supportive measures, calamine lotion. If postherpetic neuralgia present, capsaicin (Zostrix) ointment 0.025%–0.075% 3–4 times daily; for severe postherpetic neuralgia, regional blocks, amitriptyline, or anticonvulsant such as carbamazepine

- Sudden onset sensory loss +/- other focal neurologic signs (weakness, aphasia, ataxia, visual field loss, etc.)
  - Neuro assessment; labs (CBC, platelet count, glucose, electrolytes, BUN, creatinine, coagulation profile—prothrombin time/partial thromboplastin time [PT/PTT], UA); possible CT scan, MRI, lumbar puncture (LP), or cerebral angiogram; cardiovascular workup (to reveal possible valve disease, endocarditis, carotid stenosis)
    - **TIA or stroke**
      - Treatment: Emergent referral to ED to consider thrombolytics and thrombectomy. If issue not acute needs stroke workup including A1c, lipid panel, cardiac echo with bubble (eval for PFO), cardiac monitoring to eval for afib, vessel imaging (CTA head/neck, carotid doppler, or MRA head/neck) to eval vessels.

Figure 6.5 Diagnostic reasoning algorithm: paresthesia and paresis.

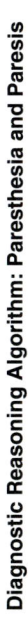

1. NEUROLOGICAL PROBLEMS

or movement and disappears at rest. An intention tremor is seen with cerebellar pathology and worsens when an extremity approaches a target.

A complete history and physical examination are necessary to obtain important subjective data on the tremor's characteristics, including duration, onset of action, progression, alleviating factors, and associated symptoms (e.g., memory loss, agitation, and nausea). It is important to note when the tremor is present (e.g., with rest or action), what part of the body is affected, whether it is bilateral, and the type of movement produced by the tremor (e.g., flexion or extension, pronation, supination, or pill-rolling). The patient's muscle tone should also be assessed to determine whether it is normal or increased (cogwheel rigidity). The patient's speech, gait, and posture all must be assessed. A thorough drug history is essential, including a list of any OTC drugs the patient is taking. The clinician should note whether the tremors affect the patient's activities of daily living and if there is any history of family members' having tremors. A review of systems may disclose a history of endocrine, metabolic, or neurological disorders. A complete musculoskeletal and neurological examination must be done to assess range of motion, mental status, strength and sensitivity, cranial nerve function, deep tendon reflexes, and gait.

DIFFERENTIAL DIAGNOSIS

Common causes of tremor include essential tremor, Parkinson's disease, and enhanced physiological tremor. Figure 6.6 presents common differential diagnoses of tremor.

Essential tremor is an isolated tremor disorder that causes an action tremor of the arms and possibly the head, voice, and/or face. It is estimated that at least 10 million people in the United States have essential tremor. As the most common movement disorder, it is apparent in one in 20 Americans older than age 40 and one in five older than age 65 (see Geriatric Considerations). It often runs in families, may improve with alcohol intake, and is slowly progressive over years. First-line treatment options include propranolol and primidone. When the tremor is refractory and severe enough to affect daily function, these patients should be referred to a neurologist. Surgical management options can be very effective for severe tremor and include deep brain stimulation and focused ultrasound thalamotomy.

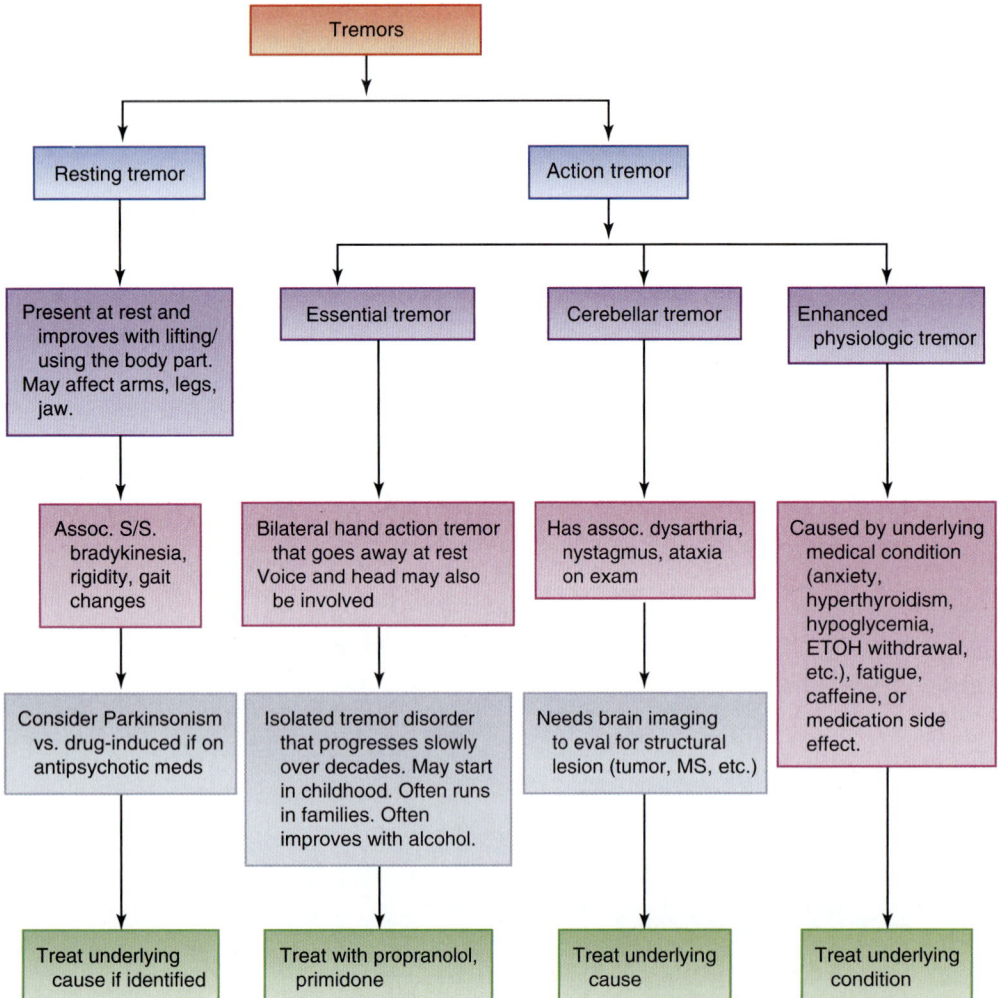

Figure 6.6 Diagnostic reasoning algorithm: tremor.

> **Geriatric Considerations: Common Neurological Complaints**
>
> There are three neurological conditions that affect older adults more than other age groups.
>
> 1. Older patients are more prone to confusion due to polypharmacy. Clinicians should be familiar with the Beers Criteria, which list medications that should be used with caution in older adults.
> 2. Temporal arteritis is more common in older adults, typically occurring with new-onset headache. Other symptoms are cited in this chapter.
> 3. The most common movement disorder is an essential tremor, which is more common in older patients.

Parkinson's disease is a neurodegenerative disease that causes a resting tremor in most but not all patients, in addition to bradykinesia (slowness of movement) and rigidity. Parkinson's disease is further discussed in Chapter 8.

An enhanced physiological tremor is a fine, fast postural tremor that is typically mild and triggered by an underlying cause, such as hyperthyroidism, hypoglycemia, or other metabolic derangement; anxiety or stress; caffeine; or medications. Treatment is aimed at identifying and treating the underlying cause.

REFERENCES

General

American Geriatrics Society. For older people, medications are common; updated AGS Beers Criteria aims to make sure they're appropriate, too. https://www.americangeriatrics.org/media-center/news/older-people-medications-are-common-updated-ags-beers-criteriar-aims-make-sure. Accessed 1/11/2021.

Delirium and Dementia

Alzheimer's Association. Delirium or dementia—do you know the difference? http://www.alz.org/norcal/in_my_community_17590.asp. Accessed 10/30/20.

American Psychiatric Association. *Diagnostic and statistical manual of mental disorders, 5th edition, Text Revision*. DSM-5-*TR* Washington, DC: American Psychiatric Association; 2013.

Hendry K, Quinn TJ, Evans J, et al. Evaluation of delirium screening tools in geriatric medical inpatients: a diagnostic test accuracy study. *Age Ageing*. 2016;45(6):832–837.

Montreal Cognitive Assessment. https://www.parkinsons.va.gov/consortium/moca.asp. Accessed 10/30/2020.

St. Louis University Mental Status (SLUMS) Examination. https://globalrph.com/medcalcs/slums-screening-for-cognitive-impairment-in-older-adults/. Accessed 10/30/2020.

Tombaugh TN, McIntyre NJ. The mini-mental state examination: a comprehensive review. *J Am Geriatr Soc*. 1992;40(9):922–935.

University College London (UCL) Institute of Neurology. Queen Square Brain Bank. https://www.ucl.ac.uk/ion/research/departments/clinical-and-movement-neurosciences/centres-and-projects/queen-square-brain-0. Accessed 10/30/2020.

Dizziness and Vertigo

Kaylie DM. (2019). Dizziness and vertigo. Merck manual—professional version. http://www.merckmanuals.com/professional/ear,-nose,-and-throat-disorders/approach-to-the-patient-with-ear-problems/dizziness-and-vertigo#v943820. Accessed 10/30/2020.

Headaches

Curtis KM, Tepper NK, Jatlaoui TC, et al. U.S. medical eligibility criteria for contraceptive use, 2016. *MMWR Recomm Rep*. 2016;65(3):1–103.

Hain TC. (2016). Migraine headache in women. http://www.dizziness-and-balance.com/disorders/central/migraine/migraine%20in%20women.html. Accessed 7/25/2017.

Hammond A, Holcomb M. Exploring treatment options for migraine headache. *Clin Advisor*. 2015;18(8):35–43.

McCarthy M. Practical evaluation and treatment of headaches. Lecture presented at Pri-Med. Ft. Lauderdale, FL. February 5, 2017.

Olesen J. International Headache Society classification of headache disorders. 3rd ed. Updated 2016. https://www.ichd-3.org/. Accessed 10/30/2020.

Tremor

Bhatia KP, et al. "Consensus statement on the classification of tremors. From the task force on tremor of the International Parkinson and Movement Disorder Society." Movement Disorders 33.1 (2018): 75–87.

RESOURCES

Eply Maneuver

American Academy of Neurology
https://www.youtube.com/watch?v=hq-IQWSrAtM

Dementia

Alzheimer's Association
http://www.alz.org

Headache

National Headache Foundation
1-888-NHF-5552
http://www.headaches.org

Chapter 7

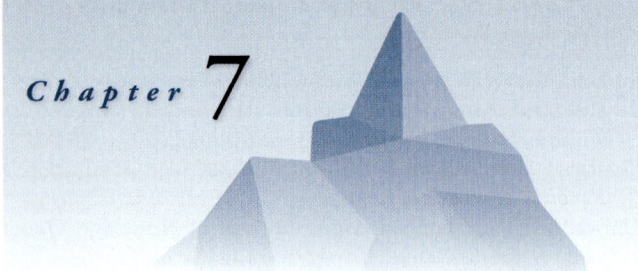

Seizure Disorders

Sarah Horn, MD
Jill E. Winland-Brown, EdD, APRN, FNP-BC, FAANP

The term "seizure" refers to sudden, transient symptoms and/or changes in behavior caused by abnormal, synonymous electrical activity within the brain. Seizures can be provoked by an underlying medical condition or unprovoked. A provoked seizure may never recur nor require treatment beyond treating the underlying medical condition. Causes of provoked seizures include febrile-related seizure in infancy, trauma, hypoglycemia, hyponatremia, hypocalcemia, substance use disorder, and withdrawal from alcohol. Provoked seizures are most often generalized tonic-clonic seizures. Epilepsy, by definition, is a condition in which an individual is predisposed to seizures and has had two or more unprovoked seizures during their lifetime. Seizure disorders referred to in this chapter include the diagnosis of epilepsy. Status epilepticus is defined as a seizure lasting longer than 30 minutes or multiple seizures without return to baseline in a 30-minute period. This is a medical emergency; discussion of management of status epilepticus is beyond the scope of this chapter.

A seizure occurs when an abnormal electrical discharge in the brain causes a sudden, involuntary, typically time-limited alteration in behavior. The manifestations of a seizure can be quite varied and relate to the area of the brain affected by the seizure. Seizures can cause changes in the following functions:

- Motor activity—jerking or stiffening of a limb
- Autonomic function—tachycardia or sweating
- Vision—seeing colored shapes
- Olfaction—smelling strange odors
- Language—aphasia
- Psychological feeling—déjà vu
- Sensation—paresthesias in one area of the body
- Consciousness—loss or impairment

Seizures can be focal (affecting just one part of the brain) or generalized (affecting the entire brain). Individuals with epilepsy, however, tend to have stereotypical seizures; they look the same every time. Figure 7.1 presents the different types of common seizures.

Focal onset seizures are those in which the first clinical and electroencephalographic (EEG) changes of the seizure are limited to one part of the cerebral hemisphere. Focal onset seizures are typically caused by an underlying focal lesion or abnormality in the brain that acts as an epileptogenic seizure focus. A seizure focus can lie in any area of the cerebral cortex; thus, different patients' seizures can vary quite dramatically, depending on the area of brain affected. A focal onset seizure is further classified on the basis of whether consciousness is impaired during the attack and whether there is motor involvement at onset, such as repetitive and rhythmic jerking of one limb. Focal impaired awareness seizures, previously called complex partial seizures, are the most common type of seizure in adults with epilepsy. Typically, patients appear awake, although they are not aware of their surroundings and do

ILAE 2017 Classification of Seizure Types Expanded Version

Focal Onset
Aware or Impaired awareness

Motor Onset
Automatisms
Atonic
Clonic
Epileptic spasms
Hyperkinetic
Myoclonic
Tonic

Nonmotor Onset
Autonomic
Behavior arrest
Cognitive
Emotional
Sensory

May progress to focal to bilateral tonic-clonic

Generalized Onset

Motor
Tonic-clonic
Clonic
Tonic
Myoclonic
Myoclonic-tonic-clonic
Myoclonic-atonic
Atonic
Epileptic spasms

Nonmotor (absence)
Typical
Atypical
Myoclonic
Eyelid myoclonia

Unknown Onset

Motor
Tonic-clonic
Epileptic spasms

Nonmotor
Behavior arrest

Unclassified

Figure 7.1 International League Against Epilepsy (ILAE) classification of seizure types. *Source:* Fisher RS, Cross JH, D'Souza C, et al. Instruction manual for the ILAE 2017 operational classification of seizure types. Epilepsia. 2017;58(4):531–542.

not respond appropriately to others. These seizures may be associated with repetitive behaviors called automatisms, such as chewing, lip-smacking, repeating words, or gestures. During focal aware seizures, previously referred to as seizure auras or simple partial seizures, awareness is preserved, such as with olfactory hallucinations in temporal lobe epilepsy. Focal onset seizures may progress to a generalized seizure, called a focal to bilateral tonic-clonic seizure.

Generalized onset seizures are those that begin with generalized abnormal electrical activity in the brain. Examples include generalized tonic-clonic, absence, myoclonic, tonic, and atonic seizures. Generalized onset seizures are often associated with childhood onset generalized epilepsy syndromes. Since both hemispheres are involved, consciousness is typically transiently impaired (except in myoclonus). Motor manifestations are bilateral. The EEG shows bilateral and widespread seizure activity in both hemispheres.

An absence seizure is a nonmotor seizure that causes a sudden interruption of ongoing activities, typically with a blank stare. If the patient is speaking, speech will be slowed or interrupted; if the patient is walking, they will stand transfixed; if eating, the food will be stopped on the way to the mouth. The attack typically lasts a few seconds.

Tonic-clonic seizures, which used to be referred to as grand mal seizures, are the most frequently encountered generalized seizures. There is a sudden tonic stiffening of muscles, often associated with stridor or an ictal cry, and the patient falls to the ground in the tonic state. The patient lies rigid; during this state, tonic contraction inhibits respiration, and cyanosis may occur. The tongue may be bitten, and urine may be voided involuntarily. The tonic stage then leads to clonic convulsive movements lasting a variable period of time. At the end of this stage, deep respiration will occur, and all muscles will relax. In the postictal period (the stage following a tonic-clonic seizure), the patient will have a depressed level of consciousness. The individual frequently goes into a deep sleep and may have a significant headache when awakened. Tonic-clonic seizures may be generalized onset, meaning that the seizure begins as a tonic-clonic seizure or focal onset that then progresses to a bilateral tonic-clonic seizure.

Myoclonic jerks are sudden, brief, shock-like contractions, which may be generalized or confined to the face and trunk or to one or more extremities. They occur predominantly during sleep and are associated with certain generalized epilepsy syndromes.

Atonic seizures cause a sudden loss of muscle control. Tonic seizures cause sudden muscle stiffening. Both are also associated with generalized epilepsy syndromes and cause "drop attacks" (sudden falls without warning). These types of seizures typically begin in childhood and can lead to injuries.

Psychogenic nonepileptic seizures (PNES) are paroxysmal seizure-like events that arise from psychological disturbances rather than abnormal electrical brain activity. The previously used term "pseudo-seizures" has fallen out of favor in the neurology community. Because these may mimic true seizures, confirming the diagnosis is key. PNES often can be distinguished from epileptic seizures by history and examination during an event, but EEG monitoring sometimes is required for accurate diagnosis. History may reveal that the events are triggered by stressful events. Features of the seizure-like events may be atypical for epileptic seizures and may include preserved consciousness despite having bilateral motor involvement; lack of response to antiepileptic medications; variation of events over time; nonrhythmic movements; and lack of typical associated features such as incontinence, tongue biting, and postictal period. During a nonepileptic seizure, the EEG will be normal. PNES are often comorbid with epilepsy and can be considered to be a type of conversion disorder. It can cause significant morbidity including repeated hospitalizations and intensive care unit admissions. Typically, psychotherapy and psychiatric medications are used to treat this condition.

EPIDEMIOLOGY AND CAUSES

Seizures are common and affect 8% to 10% of people during their lifetimes. Each year, approximately 300,000 individuals in the United States seek medical attention because of a first-time seizure, representing an incidence of 120 per 100,000. The majority of patients are younger than age 5 and present with a febrile seizure.

Epilepsy is among the most common neurological conditions, affecting more than 2.5 million people in the United States, with a cumulative lifetime incidence of approximately 3%. Each year, 50 per 100,000 individuals in the United States are diagnosed with epilepsy, which is approximately 125,000 new cases each year. Although epilepsy may start at any age, the incidence is bimodal with the highest frequency in young children and people older than age 65.

In most newly diagnosed cases, no specific cause is identified. Many factors have been implicated in the etiology of seizure disorders, such as severe head trauma, central nervous system (CNS) infections, mesial temporal sclerosis, and stroke. Children with brain injury present from birth, such as those with cerebral palsy, have an increased risk of seizures. Children who are intellectually challenged and who may or may not have genetic disorders may have an increased risk for a seizure disorder. When the conditions coexist, 50% or more of patients affected can be expected to develop a seizure disorder by age 20. Although most children with a history of febrile seizures do not develop epilepsy, there is a slightly increased risk for developing a seizure disorder during their lives.

Seizure disorders frequently occur in families. The parents, siblings, and offspring of a patient with a seizure disorder are more likely (3% to 5%) than the general population to have a seizure as a result of both genetic and environmental causes.

PATHOPHYSIOLOGY

A seizure is an uncontrollable paroxysm caused by abnormal, synchronous, repetitive firing of neurons in the brain. The motor cortex, the hippocampal formation, and the amygdaloid complex are regions that are especially susceptible to seizures.

Many disorders can initiate seizures, including drug overdose (e.g., from antihistamines, cholinesterase inhibitors, methylxanthines, muscarinic agonists, and tricyclic antidepressants), drug withdrawal (e.g., from alcohol, benzodiazepines, and barbiturates), head trauma, strokes, degenerative brain diseases, mesial temporal sclerosis, infections, tumors, and developmental brain defects (e.g., cortical dysgenesis and vascular malformations). The common epileptogenic feature of all these disorders is that they can cause populations of brain neurons to become hyperexcitable.

One category of disorders that cause hyperexcitable neurons includes systemic problems—fever, infection, sleep deprivation, and metabolic imbalances (hypocalcemia, hypoglycemia, hyponatremia, and hypoxia). These problems cause ionic changes throughout the body. For example, hyponatremia causes a relative increase in extracellular potassium concentrations systemically. In the CNS, increased extracellular K+ at the neuron cell membrane lowers the threshold for triggering axon potentials, and for this reason, acute hyponatremia (typically at levels less than 120 mEq/L) leads to seizures.

The excitability of neuron cell membranes is regulated by intramembrane molecular complexes that either actively move molecules from one side to the other (i.e., ion pumps) or control gated ion channels. Genetic defects in the structure of ion pumps or ion channels can cause seizures. Some of the uncommon heritable epilepsies (e.g., generalized epilepsy with febrile seizures and benign familial neonatal convulsions) are known to be caused by genetic defects in ion channels. It is believed that other heritable seizure disorders are caused by as-yet unidentified genetic defects in ion pumps or ion channels.

The antiepileptic drugs phenytoin (Dilantin), carbamazepine (Tegretol), and lamotrigine (Lamictal) reduce the hyperexcitability of neuron cell membranes by slowing the activation of sodium channels; ethosuximide (Zarontin) decreases the activity of certain calcium channels.

Much of the excitatory activity throughout the brain occurs via glutamatergic synapses, and increasing the amount or the effect of glutamate in the brain predisposes a person to seizures. Normally, the amount of extracellular glutamate in the brain is minimized by astrocytes, which selectively take up glutamate. Experimental studies have shown that seizures will occur if astrocytes cannot efficiently clear extracellular glutamate from the vicinity of synapses.

Glutamate depolarizes neurons by activating specific receptors that open channels for small cations, such as Na+ and K+. These are called ionotropic receptors, and the CNS contains at least three different ionotropic glutamate receptors. High brain concentrations of agonists, such as the street drugs cocaine and phencyclidine (angel dust), may induce seizures. These agonists (chemicals) bind to a receptor and activate it to produce a biological response (the seizure).

Much of the inhibitory transmission throughout the brain is via gamma-aminobutyric acid (GABA)ergic synapses. In general, neurons use the neurotransmitter GABA to prevent the spread of abnormal bursts of neuronal discharges. Reducing the availability of GABA predisposes a person to seizures. Drugs that interfere with the synthesis of GABA, such as 3-mercaptopropionic acid, cause seizures. Vitamin B_6 (pyridoxine) is required for the biosynthesis of GABA, and genetic forms of vitamin B_6 deficiency can cause epilepsy. Drugs that interfere with GABA receptors or with GABA binding to receptors can also cause seizures; such drugs include bicuculline, penicillin, and picrotoxin.

GABA agonists have the opposite effect: they counteract a person's tendency to have seizures. Benzodiazepines (e.g., diazepam [Valium] and lorazepam [Ativan]) are GABA agonists and are used to treat seizure disorders. Gabapentin (Neurontin) and pregabalin (Lyrica) are drugs that increase GABA. Barbiturates, which potentiate the actions of both GABA and benzodiazepines, are antiepileptic drugs. Likewise, the antiepileptic drugs tiagabine and vigabatrin both work by enhancing GABA-mediated inhibition of the circuitry. Besides the GABAergic pathways, noradrenergic circuits (originating mainly in the reticular formation of the brainstem) also appear to play an antiseizure role, because damage to noradrenergic pathways can predispose a person to seizures.

During a seizure, brain metabolism accelerates in the affected areas. Oxygen consumption, glucose use, and lactate levels increase; free fatty acids are released into the blood; extracellular concentrations of neurotransmitters rise; and cerebral blood flow increases. Between seizures, metabolism in the affected areas drops below normal. Prolonged seizures increase the local transcription of certain genes and the synthesis of certain proteins (although the synthesis of most proteins declines). The abnormal metabolic activities associated with repeated seizures produce long-term changes in brain circuitry that make further seizures more likely, a phenomenon referred to as kindling. One reason for controlling epilepsy is to prevent these lasting increases in neural sensitivity.

CLINICAL PRESENTATION

Subjective

The patient may or may not be aware of a seizure. They may wake up slightly confused, on the floor, or in a different position. The patient may have been incontinent. If an aura was present at the start of a seizure, the patient may know that a seizure took place.

Objective

In evaluating a presumed seizure, it is important to determine whether the event in question was a seizure or another type of condition that mimics seizure (such as syncope, PNES, or a panic attack). Not all events associated with abnormal body movements are seizures. Some events may be mistaken for seizures on initial presentation, but accurate diagnosis is essential for successful treatment. Careful and detailed history taking remains the cornerstone of accurate diagnosis of a seizure. Epilepsy is primarily a historical diagnosis; the initial assessment and approach to management are based on the patient's clinical history, especially on an accurate description of the event in question. It is important to ask the patient for a description of the event in chronological order, for example: What circumstances surrounded the seizure? Did any factors bring it on? What did you feel before, during, and after the seizure? These chronological questions may reveal the presence of an aura at the start. The patient also should be asked about the last attack witnessed, the first seizure, presence of risk factors, and provoking factors. The setting in which the attacks occurred may be significant for differential diagnoses. A careful review of the events occurring days before the seizure is important. Points of particular interest include relation of events to the sleep–wake cycle, concurrent infections, recent medication changes, or other factors that lower the seizure threshold. It is important to determine if the seizure was provoked by an underlying medical condition, such as withdrawal from alcohol. Questions need to be asked to determine whether the patient experienced an aura or other focal feature at onset, which indicates the seizure is probably focal onset. Obtaining a history of the patient's social, behavioral, and cognitive functioning, as well as a previous health history, including prior CNS insults (such as trauma, infections, stroke); history of febrile seizures; and family history of seizure disorders or neurological disorders, is crucial because this may reveal risk factors for the development of epilepsy. History of postictal behaviors should also be elicited; for example, how long did it take to return to normal function?

The physical examination should take into account the interval since the patient's most recent seizure. If the examination is performed within minutes or hours of an attack, the practitioner should look for postictal signs, including confusion, depressed level of consciousness, or Todd's paralysis, which is a transient hemiparesis following some seizures. When the examination is performed after some time has elapsed since the last seizure, the practitioner's main objective is to determine whether there are signs of baseline neurological dysfunction indicating evidence of a focal brain lesion, favoring a diagnosis of symptomatic epilepsy due to an underlying brain lesion. A full neurological examination should be performed to evaluate for focal neurological signs. The examination may also reveal papilledema, indicating elevated intracranial pressure or evidence of drug toxicity. A general medical examination should also be performed to detect the presence of a heart arrhythmia or murmur or other abnormalities, which may suggest an alternate diagnosis such as syncope.

DIAGNOSTIC REASONING

Diagnostic Tests

Initial tests should be done to assess for provoking factors and seizure mimics. Tests may include electrocardiogram; complete blood count (CBC) with differential; blood glucose level; serum electrolytes; liver function tests; serum calcium; urinalysis; a drug screen or blood alcohol level, if appropriate; and blood levels to assess target levels if the patient is on antiseizure medications. Serum prolactin, white blood cell count, creatine kinase, and lactate levels assessed soon after a seizure may be elevated, although these findings are nonspecific and are not recommended for the routine evaluation of seizure.

All patients who present with a first-time seizure should have brain imaging, either with a computed tomography (CT) or magnetic resonance imaging (MRI) scan, to evaluate for a structural lesion, such as a hemorrhage or tumor, as the cause of the seizure. A brain MRI provides a more detailed view of the brain than CT scan and may reveal more subtle seizure focuses, such as mesial temporal sclerosis, that can be missed on CT scan. EEG is helpful in the evaluation of patients with seizures. Between seizures, an EEG can support a diagnosis of epilepsy if epileptiform discharges are present. An EEG also can help differentiate between focal onset and generalized onset epilepsy. A lumbar puncture should be done if CNS infection is suspected.

Differential Diagnosis

Two of the most common seizure mimics are syncope and PNES. Benign sleep myoclonus, breath-holding spells in children, movement disorders, migraine aura, transient ischemic attacks, parasomnias, hemifacial spasm, and tic disorders can also be mistaken for seizures. Additional differential diagnoses are included in Differential Diagnosis 7.1.

MANAGEMENT

The main principle of epilepsy management is to prevent the recurrence of seizures with anticonvulsant medications while avoiding adverse effects from the drugs. The clinician should refer the patient to a neurologist, who should make the decision to start treatment after a complete review of the risk of further seizures is discussed with the patient. Before initiating treatment, the type of

Differential Diagnosis 7.1: Seizures

Type of Disorder	Specific Conditions Associated With Seizure
Cerebrovascular disorders	Transient ischemic attack (carotid artery, vertebrobasilar); ischemic stroke; intracerebral hemorrhage; vascular malformations
Diencephalic and brainstem disorders	Decorticate and decerebrate posturing, diencephalic attacks, nonepileptic paroxysmal laughter, peduncular hallucinosis, Kleine-Levin syndrome
Headaches	Classic migraine (with aura), basilar artery migraine, cluster headache, chronic paroxysmal hemicrania, ice pick headache, trigeminal neuralgia
Infant and pediatric disorders	Jitteriness, shuddering, esophageal reflux (Sandifer's syndrome), breath-holding attacks, alternating hemiplegia
Miscellaneous	Transient global amnesia, toxic metabolic encephalopathy
Movement disorders	Hemifacial spasm, tic, paroxysmal kinesigenic dyskinesia, dystonia, paroxysmal ataxia, tremor, chorea
Nonepileptic myoclonus	Hypnic jerks; myoclonus or other etiologies (spinal, reticular, palatal, essential); myoclonus and asterixis in toxic metabolic encephalopathy
Psychiatric disorders	Psychogenic nonepileptic seizures, depersonalization, psychogenic amnesia, psychogenic fugue, panic attacks, hyperventilation anxiety attacks, intermittent explosive disorder (episodic dyscontrol), schizophrenia
Sleep disorders	Pavor nocturnus, jactatio capitis nocturna, confusional arousals, somnambulism, periodic limb movements of sleep, nocturnal myoclonus, sleep apnea syndrome, narcolepsy, rapid eye movement behavior disorder
Startle disorders	Startle reaction, startle disease (hyperekplexia), jumping Frenchman, Malay latah, etc.
Syncope disorders	Vasovagal syncope; convulsive syncope; cardiac syncope (Stokes-Adams attack, tachyarrhythmias, prolonged QT syndrome aortic stenosis, hypertrophic cardiomyopathy); orthostatic syncope (idiopathic orthostatic hypotension, Shy-Drager syndrome, autonomic neuropathy); deliberate syncope ("fainting lark"); syncope in specific situations (micturition syncope, tussive syncope, carotid sinus hypersensitivity, glossopharyngeal neuralgia)
Toxic metabolic or infectious disorders	Alcoholic blackouts, hallucinogen ingestion (Lysergic acid diethylamide [LSD], mescaline), strychnine and camphor poisoning, tetanus, rabies, hypoglycemia, porphyria, pheochromocytoma, carcinoid syndrome, mastocytosis

seizure the patient experiences should be identified and classified accordingly. In adults presenting with a first-time unprovoked seizure, the risk of recurrent seizure is greatest in the first 2 years after the seizure (21% to 45%). Typically, after a single, isolated seizure, a work-up is done to identify the cause of the seizure, but antiepileptic therapy is usually not required unless the patient experiences recurrent seizure activity or an underlying disorder with a high predisposition to future seizures is revealed. Some structural lesions are clearly associated with recurrent seizures. These include brain tumor and arteriovenous malformation (AVM). When these conditions are diagnosed after a single seizure, patients usually begin pharmacological treatment; however, a more common situation is one in which the initial evaluation fails to reveal a specific causative factor for the seizure. Then the neurologist must carefully evaluate the risk of subsequent seizures. The choice of antiepileptic therapy must be individualized for each patient. Choice of therapy is contingent on comorbid conditions, medication interactions, adverse side effects, patient age, and type of seizure.

If the decision to treat is made, accurate identification of the seizure type is helpful in choosing the drug for the best outcome. Drugs Commonly Prescribed 7.1 presents suggested medications based on the different types of seizures. Although it is not a complete list, it includes the more commonly prescribed antiepileptic medications. These can be used as monotherapy or in combination. If a patient has uncontrolled epilepsy requiring multiple antiepileptic drugs, consultation with a neurologist should be considered. It is worth noting that in 2008, the U.S. Food and Drug Administration issued a warning about a possible increased risk of suicidality linked to antiepileptic drugs. Thus, patients who are taking an antiepileptic drug should be monitored for notable

Drugs Commonly Prescribed 7.1: Seizure Disorders (Monotherapy Only)

DRUG	INDICATION	ADVERSE REACTIONS AND PRESCRIBING CONSIDERATIONS
Benzodiazepines: Clonazepam (Klonopin), clobazam (Onfi), lorazepam (Ativan), diazepam (Valium)	Focal and generalized onset seizures • Lorazepam and diazepam generally used in the acute setting to abort seizures • Clonazepam and clobazam can be used for chronic epilepsy treatment (although typically not used in monotherapy)	Formulations: PO and IV (lorazepam and diazepam) May cause sedation, fatigue, ataxia, nystagmus, depression, dependence, withdrawal seizures with abrupt discontinuation Potentiates CNS depression with alcohol
Carbamazepine (Tegretol)	Focal onset seizures May worsen generalized onset seizures	Recommended therapeutic range is 4 to 12 mg/L. Formulation: PO Adverse reactions: hyponatremia, nausea, headache, dizziness, sedation, cognitive impairment, leukopenia, weight gain, decreased bone density, rare aplastic anemia, teratogenicity, rash, hepatotoxicity. With elevated levels: blurry vision, double vision, nystagmus, gait unsteadiness, incoordination, tremor Inducer of liver enzymes
Ethosuximide (Zarontin)	Absence seizures	Formulation: PO Adverse reactions: nausea, anorexia, vomiting, diarrhea, dizziness, insomnia, fatigue, behavioral changes, rash, Stevens-Johnson syndrome, headaches, psychosis, depression, hallucinations, thrombocytopenia, rare aplastic anemia
Gabapentin (Neurontin)	Focal onset seizures • May worsen absence and myoclonic seizures	Formulation: PO Adverse events: weight gain, peripheral edema, behavioral changes, dizziness, ataxia
Lacosamide (Vimpat)	Focal onset seizures	Formulations: PO and IV Adverse reactions: PR interval prolongation (obtain baseline and steady-state ECG), dizziness, nausea, vomiting, headache, diplopia, fatigue
Lamotrigine (Lamictal)	Focal and generalized onset seizures	Formulation: PO Adverse reactions: Stevens-Johnson syndrome, rash (requires slow titration to avoid), hepatic and renal failure, disseminated intravascular coagulation, tics, insomnia, dizziness, blurry vision, unsteadiness, diplopia, headache, tremor Note: Interaction with valproic acid necessitates lower doses when used in combination.
Levetiracetam (Keppra)	Focal and generalized onset seizures	Formulations: PO and IV Adverse reactions: irritability and behavior change, depression, dizziness, somnolence
Oxcarbazepine (Trileptal)	Focal onset seizures • May worsen generalized onset seizures	Formulation: PO Adverse reactions: hyponatremia, rash, drowsiness, headache; high doses can cause dizziness, blurry vision, diplopia, nausea, vomiting, and ataxia

Continued

Drugs Commonly Prescribed 7.1: Seizure Disorders (Monotherapy Only)—cont'd

DRUG	INDICATION	ADVERSE REACTIONS AND PRESCRIBING CONSIDERATIONS
Phenobarbital	Focal or generalized onset seizures • May worsen absence seizures	Formulations: PO and IV Recommended therapeutic range is 15 to 40 mg/L. Adverse reactions: respiratory depression, irritability, folate deficiency, sedation, nystagmus, cognitive function, long-term connective tissue effects, teratogenicity Formulations: IV and PO Inducer of liver enzymes
Phenytoin/fosphenytoin (Dilantin)	Focal onset seizures • May worsen absence and myoclonic seizures	Recommended therapeutic range is 10 to 20 mg/mL. Formulations: PO and IV Adverse reactions: ataxia, cognitive effects, dysarthria, nystagmus, diplopia, rash, rare Stevens-Johnson syndrome. Long-term use can cause gingival hyperplasia, acne, hirsutism, cerebellar atrophy, decreased bone density, anemia, and peripheral neuropathy; hypotension, local reactions, and arrhythmias using IV formulation. Inducer of liver enzymes
Topiramate (Topamax, Trokendi XR)	Focal and generalized onset seizures	Formulation: PO Adverse reactions: weight loss, cognitive slowing and language dysfunction, paresthesias, kidney stones, glaucoma, hypohidrosis, metabolic acidosis, fatigue, ataxia, depression, birth defects
Valproic acid (Depakene, Depakote)	Focal and generalized onset seizures	Recommended therapeutic range is 50 to 100 mcg/mL. Formulations: PO and IV May cause depression, hair loss, weight gain, peripheral edema, pancreatitis, thrombocytopenia, coagulopathy, upset stomach, tremor, elevated ammonia, rare severe hepatotoxicity. Has highest risk of birth defects among anticonvulsants. Inhibitor of liver enzymes; interacts with lamotrigine
Zonisamide (Zonegran)	Focal and generalized onset seizures	Recommended therapeutic range is 10 to 40 mg/L. Formulation: PO Adverse reactions: kidney stones, hypohidrosis, irritability, weight loss, photosensitivity, rash, dizziness, nausea, cognitive slowing, rare Stevens-Johnson syndrome, metabolic acidosis. Avoid if history of sulfonamide allergy

Abbreviations: CNS, central nervous system; ECG, electrocardiogram; IV, intravenous; PO, by mouth.

changes in behavior that could indicate new or worsening depression or suicidal thoughts.

Once the appropriate drug has been chosen based on the seizure type, baseline CBC, electrolytes, and liver function tests may be done. Depending on the agent chosen, monitoring of serum drug levels and trending of the laboratory test results also may be done.

Surgery may be performed to treat partial epilepsy. The portion of the brain that triggers the seizure is removed. This is the only potential cure for epilepsy.

FOLLOW-UP AND REFERRAL

If the seizures are controlled, the clinician can monitor the patient routinely for side effects and seizure control. Drug levels are routinely available for some antiepileptics and can be helpful to assess for compliance and toxicity. If the seizures are not controlled with adequate doses and levels of the medication, the clinician should refer the patient to a neurologist for a second opinion and possible combination therapy. Patients may be taken off medications after a few years in some types of epilepsy, while other types may require lifelong therapy. If attempting to discontinue antiepileptics, medications should be weaned gradually.

Patient Education: Seizure Disorders

Education about seizure disorders can provide the patient with understanding and a sense of control over the illness. It is necessary to recognize that to the affected individual, this condition is more than seizures. The patient and family may be overwhelmed by thoughts of disability and impaired quality of life. Such factors as age at onset, duration of seizure activity, frequency, seizure type, associated neurological abnormalities, and associated environmental factors contribute to the degree of disability in each patient. Education is ongoing and should be constantly reinforced. Patients and their families should be referred to seizure literature available through the Epilepsy Foundation of America as soon as they are diagnosed, because the well-informed patient is the best advocate for their own care. Using the Circle of Caring model and coming to know the patient and what matters most to them will assist in helping the patient reach their highest potential.

Other treatments for refractory epilepsy include the ketogenic diet and vagal nerve stimulator implantation. A diet high in fat and low in carbohydrates has helped reduce the burden of seizures in the pediatric population. Several studies have shown this diet reduces or prevents seizures in some children who could not be controlled by medications alone. A vagal nerve stimulator is an implanted device used in the treatment of patients with refractory epilepsy. These treatments should typically be done in consultation with a neurologist.

A patient with a seizure disorder lives with the fear that a seizure may strike at any moment. People with a seizure disorder fear dying during a seizure. They also fear personal injury. This fear is justified; therefore, health-care providers need to counsel patients regarding safety issues. People with a seizure disorder should take showers instead of baths to reduce their risk of drowning. If they take a bath, they should only do it with the door unlocked and when someone else is home. Automatic safety devices that adjust water temperature and shut off water when the shower drain is blocked can be installed. They should swim only with a partner who is aware of their diagnosis and knows what to do if a seizure occurs (Box 7.1). When cooking, patients should be instructed to use the microwave or back burners on the stove and keep pot handles turned inward. They should be encouraged not to smoke, but if they decline to quit, they should never smoke when alone. Their home should be evaluated to identify any safety hazards, and they should develop a risk-reduction plan. Families, friends, and coworkers need to be taught what to do in case of a seizure. They should avoid climbing ladders or doing other activities that could be dangerous if a seizure occurs.

Patients with a seizure disorder and their caregivers should be apprised of the risks of harm. Compared with the general population, children and adolescents with seizure disorders have a 1,000-fold greater risk of drowning during bathing and a 70-fold greater risk of drowning while swimming. Burns tend to occur in the home and are most commonly associated with cooking, showering, and use of space heaters. Driving needs to be discussed at length. The loss of driving privileges is serious because it restricts a patient's mobility, and therefore, their independence. Each state has different laws governing the granting of driver's licenses for individuals with a seizure disorder that will dictate a period of time patients must refrain from driving after having a seizure. At the federal level, the U.S. Department of Transportation has regulations that bar anyone with a history of seizures from being licensed to drive in interstate trucking. The purpose of the driving restrictions is obvious: to protect the public. Although only six states require health-care providers to report patients who have been diagnosed with seizure disorder, all practitioners have the responsibility to advise their patients of the medical risks, legal requirements, and recommendations regarding driving. Educational and support materials are available through the Epilepsy Foundation of America.

Box 7.1 Emergent Care for Seizures

Partial Seizures

The patient may resemble an intoxicated or drugged person. They may stare without focusing or speaking, appear to be fidgeting, make chewing movements, or smack the lips.

During the seizure:

- Do not attempt to restrain the patient.
- Gently move the patient away from dangerous objects.

After the seizure:

- Stay with the patient until the patient is fully alert.
- Reassure others that the behavior was medically caused.

Generalized Seizures

The patient may issue a warning sign, cry out or scream, and then fall down and rhythmically jerk arms and legs in a strong movement that cannot be stopped.

Before or during the seizure:

- Remove the patient's glasses (if wearing) and help the patient lie down on their side, but do not restrain them.
- Clear the area of dangerous objects.
- Loosen tight clothing around the patient's neck.
- Do not put any object into the patient's mouth.

After the seizure:

- Stay with the patient until they are fully awake.
- If the patient has a known seizure disorder, it may not be necessary to call for medical help, depending on the preference of the patient and family unless an injury has occurred, the seizure lasts longer than 3 minutes, a second seizure occurs, or the patient requests help.

> **Pediatric/Adolescent Considerations:**
> **Seizure Disorder**
>
> Adolescents with a seizure disorder have an increased risk of:
>
> - Drowning while swimming
> - Suffering burns while cooking
> - Having an accident while driving

REFERENCES

Abou-Khalil BW. Antiepileptic drugs. *Continuum (Minneap Minn)*. 2016;22(1 Epilepsy):132–156.

Fisher RS, Cross JH, D'Souza C, et al. Instruction manual for the ILAE 2017 operational classification of seizure types. *Epilepsia*. 2017;58(4):531–542.

Mula M, Kanner AM, Schmitz B, et al (2012). Antiepileptic drugs and suicidality: An expert consensus statement from the Task Force on Therapeutic Strategies of the ILAE Commission on Neuropsychobiology. *Epilepsia*. https://onlinelibrary.wiley.com/doi/full/10.1111/j.1528-1167.2012.03688.x. Accessed 1/7/2021.

RESOURCE

Epilepsy Foundation
1-800-EFA-1000
　https://www.epilepsyfoundation.org

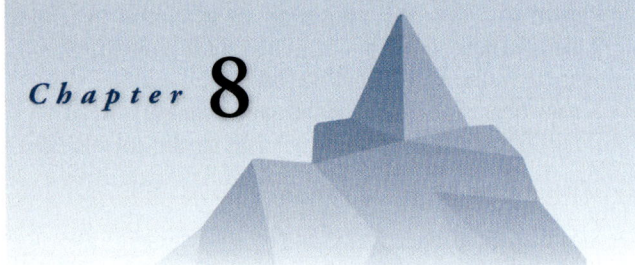

Chapter 8

Degenerative Disorders

Sarah Horn, MD

Jill E. Winland-Brown, EdD, APRN, FNP-BC, FAANP

DEMENTIA

Dementia is a decline in mental functioning, affecting memory, cognition, language, and/or personality. *The Diagnostic and Statistical Manual of Mental Disorders, 5th edition, Text Revision* (*DSM-5-TR*; American Psychiatric Association, 2013) defines *dementia* as significant cognitive impairment that represents a significant decline from a previous level of functioning. *Cognitive impairment* refers to a decline in at least one of the following cognitive domains: language, executive function, complex attention, perceptual-motor function, social cognition, learning, and memory. The disturbance must interfere with independence in everyday activities and not be better explained by another neurocognitive disorder.

EPIDEMIOLOGY AND CAUSES

Dementia may be reversible or irreversible. Reversible causes include delirium, normal pressure hydrocephalus (NPH), chronic long-term dementia (only partially reversible), vitamin B_{12} deficiency, subdural hematomas, and thyroid disease, among others. The irreversible dementias include Alzheimer's disease (AD), vascular dementia, Parkinson's disease (PD), and others listed in Table 8.1. The most common type of dementia in adults is from AD, comprising 60% to 80% of cases.

TABLE 8.1 Causes of Dementia

Neurodegenerative Diseases	Nonneurodegenerative Diseases
Alzheimer's disease (AD)	Vascular dementia
Dementia with Lewy bodies (DLB)	Alcohol-related dementia
Parkinson's disease dementia (PDD)	Normal pressure hydrocephalus (NPH)
Frontotemporal dementia (FTD)	Chronic subdural hematoma
Huntington's disease (HD)	Neurosyphilis
Chronic traumatic encephalopathy (CTE)	HIV-associated dementia (HAD)
Corticobasal degeneration (CBD)	Creutzfeldt–Jakob disease (CJD)
Progressive supranuclear palsy (PSP)	

PATHOPHYSIOLOGY

Dementing illnesses are caused by widespread degeneration of the brain and have a variety of causes. Most dementias are considered neurodegenerative diseases, caused by progressive neuron loss over time due to the accumulation of abnormal proteins, namely beta-amyloid, tau, and/or alpha-synuclein (depending on the type of dementia). These conditions invariably progress over time, with no currently available treatments to slow or halt the progression. Dementia with Lewy bodies (DLB) involves small, circular deposits of proteins that interfere with the functioning of dopamine and acetylcholine. There typically is no family history of DLB.

Nonneurodegenerative dementias may be reversible, or their progression slowed, if the underlying cause is identified. The most common nonneurodegenerative dementia is vascular dementia, caused by stroke and/or cerebral small vessel disease. Vascular dementia is also caused by atherosclerosis, which restricts blood flow to the brain, resulting in anoxic tissue.

Other examples of dementia include alcohol-related dementia, normal pressure hydrocephalus, chronic subdural hematoma, and chronic central nervous system (CNS) infections (such as HIV and syphilis).

CLINICAL PRESENTATION

Subjective

Patients with dementia often do not report cognitive decline themselves; rather, a spouse or other informant typically brings it to the clinician's attention. The cognitive impairment in dementia must be a change from previous baseline, insidious in onset, progressive, not due to an alternate medical problem, and severe enough to impact independence in daily functioning. History taking should include questions about sedating medications, sleep disorders, and screening for depression, all of which cause or contribute to cognitive impairment.

Objective

A complete physical examination, including a detailed neurological examination, should be performed to both exclude alternate medical diagnoses, as well as confirm the presence of cognitive impairment. A thorough examination can also elucidate the underlying etiology of the dementing illness (such as resting tremor and cogwheel rigidity in DLB).

Brief bedside screening tools such as the Mini-Mental State Examination (MMSE) and Montreal Cognitive Assessment (MoCA) can be administered during routine appointments. These tools are limited in breadth, and more detailed mental status testing is often warranted, including referral to a neuropsychologist for psychometric testing.

DIAGNOSTIC REASONING

Diagnostic Tests

Laboratory tests should be obtained to screen for hypothyroidism and vitamin B_{12} deficiency. Other tests can be considered on a case-by-case basis, including electrolytes, calcium level, liver function tests, and tests for syphilis and HIV. Brain imaging with head computed tomography (CT) or magnetic resonance imaging (MRI) should also be done to rule out mimics or reversible causes of dementia and to assist in diagnosing the underlying etiology of the dementia.

The diagnosis of major neurocognitive disorder (previously referred to as *dementia*), based on *DSM-5-TR* diagnostic criteria, requires:

1. Evidence of significant cognitive decline from a previous level of performance in one or more cognitive domains: learning and memory, language, executive function, complex attention, perceptual-motor, and social cognition.
2. The cognitive deficits must be severe enough to interfere with the ability to perform everyday activities, such as paying bills or managing medications.
3. The cognitive deficits do not occur exclusively in the context of a delirium (see Chapter 6).
4. The cognitive deficits are not better explained by another mental disorder (such as depression, substance use disorder, etc.).

Differential Diagnosis

The normal cognitive changes associated with aging include mild memory and processing issues that generally do not progress over time nor interfere with daily functioning. Mild cognitive impairment (MCI) is an intermediary diagnosis between normal cognition and dementia, in which a patient has demonstrable cognitive decline on examination, though not severe enough to affect independence in daily functioning. Delirium is an acute and reversible confusional state due to an underlying medical condition (further discussed in Chapter 6). So-called "pseudo-dementia" is a phenomenon in which depression mimics the symptoms of dementia.

MANAGEMENT

Treatment for dementia consists of both pharmacological and nonpharmacological measures. All treatment options are symptomatic in nature. There are currently no disease-modifying agents to slow down or reverse the progression of neurodegenerative diseases.

Nonpharmacological Treatment

The mainstay of management in dementia is symptomatic, including treatment of behavioral issues, optimizing the environment to support daily functioning, and counseling regarding safety issues.

Traditional nonpharmacological measures include cognitive rehabilitation, exercise, and occupational therapy. Additionally, modifying the environment to reduce clutter and noise to help focus attention can reduce agitation and aggressive behaviors that often accompany late-stage dementia. Vitamin E and omega-3 fatty acids show some evidence of improved attention in dementia patients.

Some nontraditional therapies can help with some dementia symptoms such as memory loss, agitation, and depression. Pet therapy, providing the patient with an animal companion to interact with and pet, has been shown to decrease depression and anxiety and encourage communication. Music therapy has also been found to be a powerful memory stimulator, and listening to familiar music can be comforting (Gomez & Gomez, 2017). Art therapy, such as walking through a gallery or museum or painting and drawing, can improve motor skills and help the patient with dementia to express feelings (Chancellor, Duncan, & Chatterjee, 2014). Reminiscence and storytelling are methods for exercising long-term memory, especially in the early stages of this disease (Kapucu & Asiret, 2017).

Certain preventive measures have been shown to reduce the risk of dementia. There is evidence that regular physical exercise reduces the risk of dementia. A diet rich in grains, fruits and vegetables, fish, nuts, and healthy fats has also been shown to decrease the risk for dementia.

Pharmacological Treatment

Pharmacological therapy for cognitive impairment consists primarily of cholinesterase inhibitors (such as donepezil and rivastigmine) and *N*-methyl-D-aspartate (NMDA) receptor antagonists (memantine). Memantine regulates glutamate, a chemical messenger, while cholinesterase inhibitors reduce the breakdown of acetylcholine, which sustains the level of this neurotransmitter in the brain longer to promote brain function. For patients with newly diagnosed dementia—including Alzheimer disease, DLB, vascular dementia, and Parkinson disease dementia—initiation of a cholinesterase inhibitor is recommended. Memantine should be considered in moderate to advanced dementia, typically in combination with a cholinesterase inhibitor. The benefit of these medications is typically modest at best.

Antipsychotic drugs such as haloperidol (Haldol), quetiapine (Seroquel), risperidone (Risperdal), olanzapine (Zyprexa), and aripiprazole (Abilify) continue to be used to treat severe agitation, aggression, and associated psychosis. However, they can be sedating, worsen confusion, and increase the risk of mortality and so should be used with caution. In patients with Parkinson's disease dementia and DLB, only antipsychotics with lower dopamine blockade should be used (i.e., quetiapine, clozapine, or pimavanserin).

Patients with panic disorders may respond to benzodiazepines such as lorazepam (Ativan) or diazepam (Valium), although these medications should be used judiciously due to risks of side effects including sedation, confusion, falls, and long-term dependence. Referral to a specialist may help in treatment of agitation and confusion. Management goals for the family and caregivers should be supportive, specific, and consistent.

FOLLOW-UP AND REFERRAL

Dementia not only affects the patient but also the entire family and/or support person(s). For this reason, it is often called a family disease. For a health-care provider, it is important to assess not only the patient but the support persons as well. Providing resources for support persons to obtain the assistance they need is an important part of providing health care to patients and their significant others dealing with dementia. Patients should be followed up every few months to make sure they are not regressing too fast and to support the family and/or support persons. Tests listed in Chapter 6, such as the clock test, months of the year backward (MOTYB) test, and others, can be used to follow up on any declining function. Patients and families/support persons can do word search puzzles together and play card games to maintain brain function as much as possible.

The care of patients is often multidisciplinary, and referrals to neuropsychology for cognitive testing, neurology for diagnosis of the underlying etiology, and to psychiatry for management of neuropsychiatric symptoms, social work, occupational therapy, and palliative care can be considered.

ALZHEIMER'S DISEASE

Alzheimer's disease (AD) is a progressive neurodegenerative condition and the most common form of dementia (60% to 80%) in the older population. One in three older individuals dies with AD or another form of dementia. AD accounts for about $100 billion per year in medical and custodial expenses, with approximately $27,000 per year for each patient for medical and nursing care.

AD is characterized by an insidious onset; slow, progressive cognitive decline; and an array of emotional and behavioral problems that result from cognitive decline. The cognitive impairment in AD manifests as a decline in memory and learning, with at least one additional cognitive domain: language (aphasia), executive function, learned motor function (apraxia), visuospatial, and complex attention. Recent advances in understanding AD have modified both diagnostic and treatment choices. Most cases are sporadic, although there are rare familial forms of the disease.

AD was named after Dr. Alois Alzheimer, who in 1906 noticed changes in the brain tissue of a woman who had died of an unusual mental illness. She had symptoms of memory loss, language problems, and inappropriate behavior. On autopsy, he found microscopic clumps of abnormal proteins in her brain: amyloid plaques and neurofibrillary tangles (comprised of the protein tau).

EPIDEMIOLOGY AND CAUSES

The incidence of the sporadic form of AD in the general population increases rapidly with age. It affects an estimated one in 10 people older than 65 years. AD is the sixth leading cause of death in the United States and the fifth leading cause of death among people older than 65 years. An estimated 5.8 million Americans have dementia from AD. By 2050, this figure is estimated to rise to 18.8 million. The increase in people with dementia from AD in the United States increases with age—16% or 0.9 million people aged 65 to 74; 45% or 2.6 million people aged 75 to 84; and 36% or 2.1 million people aged 85 and older.

The prevalence of AD dementia is higher in people of color than in whites. Additional risk factors that have been identified include lower educational and occupational levels, family history, head injury, Down syndrome, and vascular disease. Because onset is insidious, it is difficult to accurately predict duration or survival time with the disease. For 60- to 70-year-old individuals with AD, the average life expectancy is 7 to 10 years after diagnosis. AD is the sixth leading cause of death overall and the fifth leading cause of death for individuals older than 65 years. More than 60% of patients with AD are expected to die before age 80 years compared with 30% of people without AD. However, it is not just a disease of old age. Early-onset AD affects approximately 200,000 individuals younger than age 65.

The rare familial form of AD typically has an earlier onset. Inheritance is autosomal dominant; if a parent has the familial form of AD, offspring have a 50% chance of developing the disease.

PATHOPHYSIOLOGY

AD is a progressive and irreversible neurodegenerative syndrome. The disease depletes the cerebral cortex of neurons, causing generalized cortical atrophy. Neurons that use the neurotransmitter acetylcholine are especially susceptible to the disease. Cortical areas that are preferentially affected include the hippocampus, the amygdala, the temporal cortex, the olfactory system, and intercortical connections.

Pathological changes seen in brains of patients with AD include neuritic plaques and neurofibrillary tangles. Neuritic plaques are microscopic spherical lesions found throughout the cortex (although they are relatively sparse in the primary motor and sensory areas), hippocampus, and amygdala. Each plaque has a core of beta-amyloid, an insoluble peptide. The core is surrounded by swollen and degenerating neurites, which are encased in a layer of microglia and astrocytes. Excess beta-amyloid is also found diffusely throughout the cerebral cortex, cerebellar cortex, and basal ganglia, especially in and around blood vessels.

Neurofibrillary tangles are microscopic collections of intertwined cytoskeletal fibers that form inside neurons. The tangles are best seen in silver-stained tissue, and their density correlates with the degree of the patient's dementia. One major protein in these tangles is an aberrant form of *tau* protein (which, in its normal form, stabilizes microtubules), and patients with AD have elevated concentrations of *tau* proteins in their cerebrospinal fluid. The formation of neurofibrillary tangles immobilizes or otherwise deactivates the neuron's normally dynamic cytoskeleton and leads to the cell's death. The tangles are insoluble and remain after the neurons have degenerated.

The central biochemical problem in AD appears to be a defect in the metabolism of beta-amyloid precursor protein, leading to accumulation of beta-amyloid. Normally, many types of cells, including neurons, make beta-amyloid precursor protein, the function of which is not yet fully understood. When this protein is broken down, the by-products include beta-amyloid peptides. One current theory proposes that beta-amyloid deposition is the primary problem in AD and that intracellular neurofibrillary tangles are the consequence of the toxic effects of beta-amyloid on neurons.

CLINICAL PRESENTATION

Subjective

The patient usually presents with complaints of memory problems. Often, it is a family member who mentions this because patients with AD do not typically have insight into their memory difficulties. Recognition of cognitive difficulty on the part of the patient or family is often related to a change in pattern: getting lost in familiar places, inability to accomplish a demanding task at work, or increasingly slow response to any cognitive challenge. Difficulties with balancing the checkbook, preparing dinner, traveling alone, or maintaining employment are frequent problems reported by family members when the disease has progressed to the point where it is noticeable to others. In the later stages, the person needs help dressing and bathing and becomes incontinent. Eventually, the person loses the capacity to converse, walk, sit, or hold up the head. Eighty percent of patients in nursing homes with AD have behavioral problems. These may include hostility, aggression, suspiciousness and paranoia, delusions, agitation, sundowning, and inappropriate or impulsive sexual behavior (see Advanced Assessment 8.1).

Advanced Assessment 8.1: Alzheimer's Disease: Signs and Symptoms for Further Assessment

LEARNING AND MEMORY

The patient becomes repetitive; has trouble remembering recent conversations, events, appointments; or frequently misplaces objects. These problems disrupt daily life.

HANDLING COMPLEX TASKS

The patient has trouble following a complex set of tasks that require many steps, such as organizing bills or following a recipe.

REASONING ABILITY

The patient is unable to respond with a reasonable plan to challenges at work or home, such as knowing what to do if the kitchen sink is plugged; shows poor judgment.

SPATIAL RELATIONSHIPS

The patient has trouble remembering directions or driving to what once was a familiar place, organizing objects around the house, unfamiliarity with familiar objects and places.

SPEECH

The patient has increasing difficulty with finding the words to express themselves and following along with conversations.

CHANGES IN BEHAVIOR

The patient appears less social and responsive; is more irritable, depressed, anxious, and suspicious than usual.

Geriatric Considerations: Alzheimer's Disease

One in 10 people aged 65 and older have dementia from AD. Many people with Alzheimer's disease and other types of dementia along with their caregivers are unaware of their diagnosis, and therefore they are unlikely to get information about it and its treatment. The earlier the diagnosis of dementia, the better the health outcomes.

In 2019, costs were estimated to be $290 billion for services for people older than 65 years with dementia. Caregivers should consider some therapies such as pet therapy, music therapy, art therapy, reminiscence, and storytelling that might help with memory skill, communication, and motor skills.

Objective

Concern about cognitive decline expressed by the patient or family or changes in behavior or cognition should trigger an initial assessment for dementia. Cognitive assessment is central to diagnosis and management of dementias, and it should be performed for all patients. Routine social conversation and questions that can be answered automatically will not elicit symptoms of early AD. Instead, the clinician should probe the patient's memory further with such questions as "Do you remember what you did last Sunday?" or "What did you have for breakfast this morning?" The importance of maintaining the patient's dignity by examining the patient alone before interviewing others cannot be overemphasized. The patient should be informed if others are to be interviewed. It is also important to be alert to the possibility that family members at times may minimize or exaggerate their report of symptoms, depending on their motives. Family members can report on the patient's ability to perform independent activities of daily living (ADLs), using the Functional Activities Questionnaire (FAQ) (see Advanced Assessment 8.2).

The clinician should take a focused history documenting signs and symptoms related to the dementia; chronology of the problem (including onset, duration, and stepwise vs. continuous progression); and family history. Other causes of cognitive impairment, such as medication side effects, thyroid disease, low levels of B_{12}, depression, anxiety, and sleep issues, should be evaluated and addressed. The physical examination should include a neurological evaluation and evaluation of any factors contributing to delirium (see Chapter 6). Formal neuropsychological testing can pinpoint the types

Advanced Assessment 8.2: Functional Activities Questionnaire

The Functional Activities Questionnaire (FAQ) is an informant-based measure of functional abilities. The caregiver or informant provides a score of dependent (3); requires assistance (2); has difficulty but does by self (1); or normal (0) on 10 functional items. Other responses include the following: never did the activity but couldn't do it now (0) and never did the activity but would have difficulty now (1).

The 10 activities are as follows:

1. Maintains financial records.
2. Collects information for IRS purposes.
3. Shops alone for necessities.
4. Does an intellectual activity.
5. Heats water and turns off the stove.
6. Cooks a healthy meal.
7. Has knowledge of what is going on in the world.
8. Carries on a conversation about something in the media.
9. Remembers medications and significant dates.
10. Arranges own travel for activities.

The sum of scores for the 10 items ranges from 0 to 30. The higher the score, the poorer the function.

For a complete discussion and instructions for administering this test, see Pfeffer RI, Kurosaki TT, Harrah CH, et al. Measurement of functional activities of older adults in the community. *J Gerontol.* 1982;37(3):323–329.

and severity of impairments in language, reasoning, visuospatial, and memory deficits.

An easily administered bedside test for cognition is the Montreal Cognitive Assessment (MoCA; https://www.parkinsons.va.gov/resources/MOCA-Test-English.pdf). Asking the patient to name the months of the year backward (MOTYB) or spell the word "world" backward are two easy tests to evaluate attention. Functional assessment tests are also very basic screening tools. These may include the timed "get up and go," a gait assessment, or the FAQ (see Advanced Assessment 8.2), which may be performed by the clinician. The FAQ is also a useful measure that is reported to discriminate well at higher functional levels. One of the easiest tests to administer and informative of various areas of cognition is the clock-drawing test. The patient is asked to draw a clockface with all the numbers in place, set to a specific time. The drawing can be placed in the patient's record, and the test can be repeated periodically. Asking the patient to name items, follow commands, repeat a phrase, and write a sentence tests language function. These tests are appropriate for initial assessment. The results also provide a baseline from which any further decline can be quantitatively compared. The clinician should refer the patient to a memory disorder center or a specialist in dementing diseases if the initial assessment is suggestive of AD, particularly when atypical presentation, severe impairment, or complex comorbidities are present. Other assessment tests are listed in Chapter 6.

DIAGNOSTIC REASONING

Diagnostic Tests

Laboratory tests (complete blood count, electrolytes, blood glucose, serum calcium, thyroid-stimulating hormone level, and vitamin B_{12}) may be used to rule out other conditions that impair brain function. Structural magnetic resonance imaging (MRI) of the brain can rule out alternate diagnoses, as well as evaluate for radiological biomarkers of AD such as generalized cortical atrophy and focal hippocampal atrophy. Functional brain imaging with 18-F fluorodeoxyglucose positron emission tomography (FDG-PET) or single-photon emission computed tomography (SPECT) can look for regions of hypometabolism (PET) and hypoperfusion (SPECT) seen in AD. Positron emission tomography (PET) imaging using amyloid tracers may be used to detect amyloid deposits. Studies show that this test is 86% accurate in predicting which individuals will develop AD within 2 years and 92% accurate in ruling out the likelihood of developing AD.

Cerebrospinal biomarkers including beta-amyloid and *tau* can be helpful in the evaluation for AD. Genetic testing is available for patients with a family history, although less than 1% of AD cases are caused by the three known genetic mutations (Amyloid precursor protein [APP] on chromosome 21; Presenilin 1 [PSEN1] on chromosome 14; and Presenilin 2 [PSEN2] on chromosome 1). AD-related brain changes may occur 20 years before symptoms begin. An individual with early brain changes has preclinical AD or MCI due to AD.

Differential Diagnosis

To some extent, the diagnosis of AD is still a process of excluding other causes of cognitive impairment (Fig. 8.1). Medical conditions and drug-related adverse effects need to be ruled out in patients suspected of AD. Infection, structural CNS lesion, traumatic conditions, metabolic derangements, and vitamin B_{12} deficiency need to be considered. In addition, depression, drug and alcohol use disorder, delirium, and psychosis need to be ruled out. Other common causes of dementia to consider include vascular dementia, frontotemporal dementia, and DLB.

Patients may present with a combination of issues. Delirium or depression may be superimposed on AD; vascular dementia (or other dementia) can also coexist with AD, causing a mixed dementia.

Depression can mimic AD and is frequently mistaken for AD in older adults. Information from multiple sources—patient self-report, family members/support persons, health-care provider observations, and patient history—should be considered when making a diagnosis.

The following signs are highly suggestive of the diagnosis of AD:

- Absence of a precipitating medical illness
- Absence of a drug-related phenomenon
- Presence of objective, well-documented, progressive, and worsening deficits in new learning and memory
- Signs of functional impairment

MANAGEMENT

The principles of management of AD are directed toward slowing progression of the disease pharmacologically, protecting physical health, providing emotional support, and maintaining optimal function through prevention or reduction of excess disability. Maintaining as much normalcy as possible in relationships and everyday activities may be the most effective way to prevent the development of excess disability, defined as the difference between the observed function and the actual underlying impairment.

Family members/significant others have reported that sensitivity to their distress, acknowledgment of their contributions, and information about the disease and its management have not always been dealt with adequately in encounters with primary care providers. Both patient and family/support persons need assistance in understanding and coping with a diagnosis of AD. Most patients are eager to try approved and research-stage drugs. Support group attendance can be helpful but should be relevant to the stage of the disease. Anxiety and depression should be recognized and treated vigorously. Legal and financial

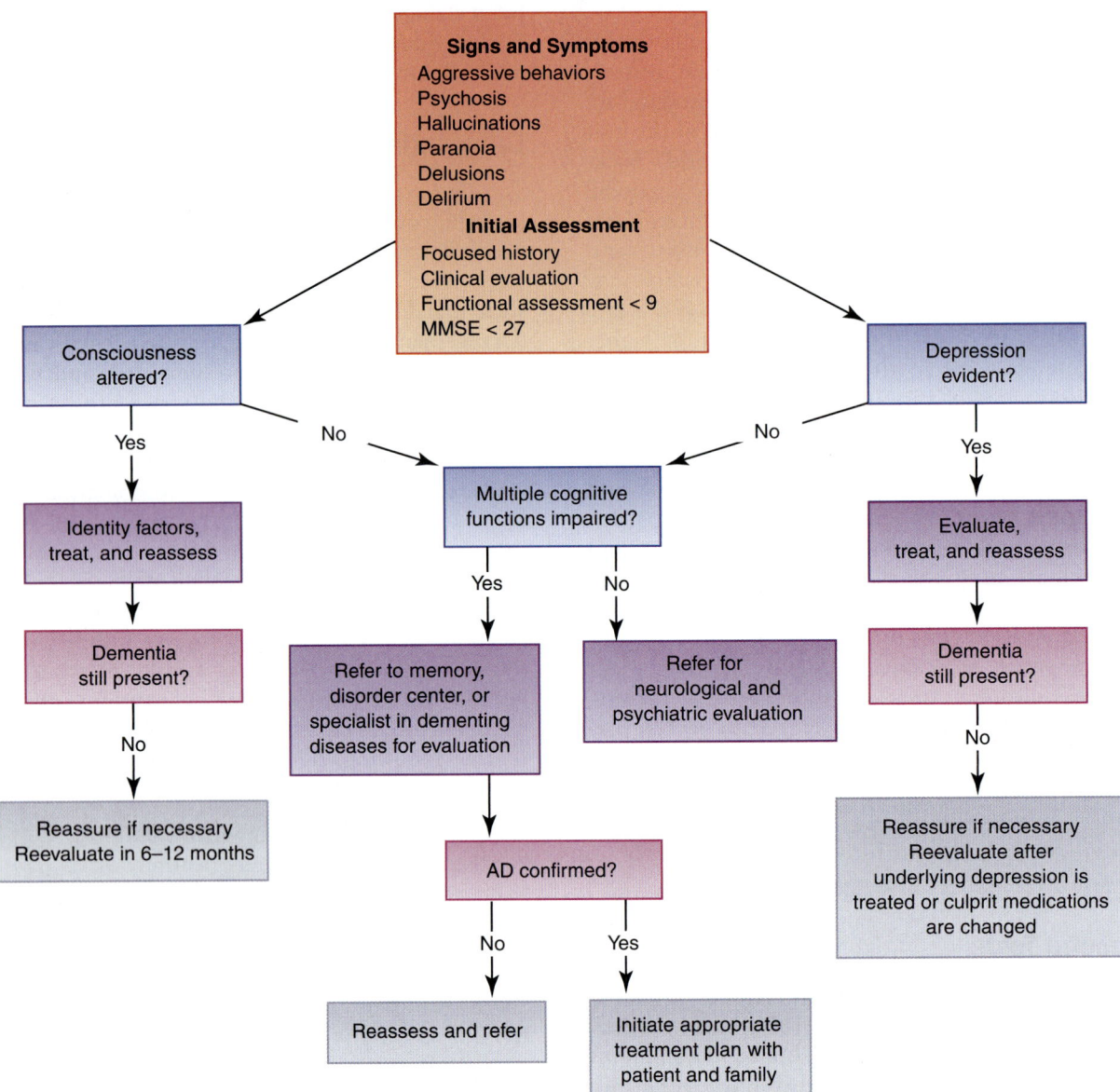

Figure 8.1 Diagnostic reasoning algorithm: Alzheimer's disease.

planning and discussion of future care options should take place early in the disease course.

Medications may improve cognitive function in mild to moderate AD. Treatment with cholinesterase inhibitors should be considered at the time of diagnosis, taking into account expected therapeutic benefits and potential safety issues (see Drugs Commonly Prescribed 8.1). The dosages for the following drugs are adjusted gradually as tolerated: donepezil (Aricept), galantamine (Razadyne), and rivastigmine (Exelon). An *N*-methyl-D-aspartate receptor antagonist, memantine (Namenda), has been effective in moderate to severe AD by improving cognitive function and has additive effects to cholinesterase inhibitors.

Donepezil does not prevent progression of AD, but it seems to slow the rate of decline. Patients who stop and restart donepezil may not reach the level of function that they had before stopping the drug. Antidepressant drugs have shown to be effective in patients with depressive symptoms. Anxious and agitated behavior may respond to anxiolytic drugs; however, use of pharmacological agents for noncognitive symptoms such as anxiety, depression, and insomnia should be reserved for instances where behavioral intervention is ineffective.

Because of their side effects, antipsychotics should be used with caution and reserved for patients who exhibit persistent disruptive or dangerous behavior. Precautions include avoidance of drugs that have even a moderate anticholinergic effect and drugs that sedate, affect balance, or are known to cause confusion in older individuals. Atypical antipsychotic medications—risperidone (Risperdal), olanzapine (Zyprexa), and quetiapine (Seroquel)—are usually well tolerated. Federal regulations require that

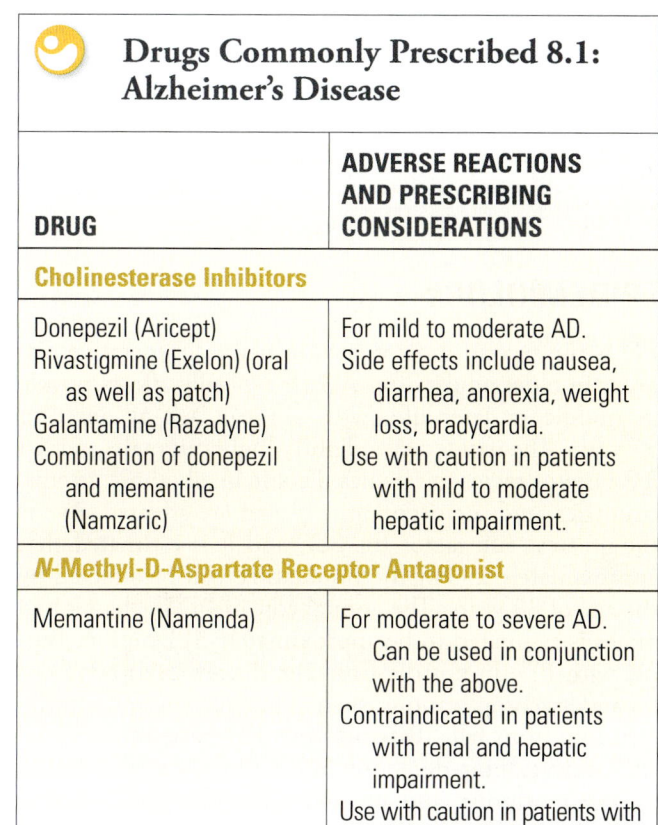

Drugs Commonly Prescribed 8.1: Alzheimer's Disease

DRUG	ADVERSE REACTIONS AND PRESCRIBING CONSIDERATIONS
Cholinesterase Inhibitors	
Donepezil (Aricept) Rivastigmine (Exelon) (oral as well as patch) Galantamine (Razadyne) Combination of donepezil and memantine (Namzaric)	For mild to moderate AD. Side effects include nausea, diarrhea, anorexia, weight loss, bradycardia. Use with caution in patients with mild to moderate hepatic impairment.
***N*-Methyl-D-Aspartate Receptor Antagonist**	
Memantine (Namenda)	For moderate to severe AD. Can be used in conjunction with the above. Contraindicated in patients with renal and hepatic impairment. Use with caution in patients with cardiac conduction abnormalities and peptic ulcer.

Abbreviation: AD, Alzheimer's disease.

if antipsychotic agents are used in nursing homes, an effort should be made to reduce the dosage at least every 6 months. Alpha-tocopherol (vitamin E) may help to slow progression of AD in some patients.

The failure to institute timely pharmacological management in patients with AD may result in a more rapid need for institutionalization, an increase in aggression, further difficulty with ADLs, and further cognitive decline.

Given the advanced age, compromised brain function, and frequent presence of other chronic medical conditions in most patients with AD, close monitoring of response to any drug regimen is advisable. In addition, as the patient becomes less able to communicate physical or emotional distress, more careful observation of general health and well-being is needed.

Attention to good nutrition, exercise, and preventive care (immunizations and dental, vision, and hearing care) should not be reduced. Patients and their families/significant others also need continued support and assistance related to changes that occur as the disease progresses. Recognition of and respect for the patient's humanity can be difficult to maintain in the face of declining cognition, leading to the unfortunate temptation to care for family members/significant others while ignoring the patient.

FOLLOW-UP AND REFERRAL

Referral to a memory disorder center is usually warranted. These centers offer multidisciplinary services ranging from diagnosis and access to experimental medications to counseling and support groups. They are excellent sources of accurate information about AD. Most cities also have local chapters of national organizations for patients with AD and their caregivers that usually offer referrals and support groups as well. Respite care, both at home and overnight in participating health-care facilities, and adult day care centers provide social outlets for people with AD and a break in the constant care demands for family members and support persons. Family members/significant others must be cared for as well; if the clinician is unable to support them, it is essential to find social service agencies that will be able to help.

Patient Education: Alzheimer's Disease

Both the patient and family members/significant others need to understand the disease, its ramifications, its future course, and treatment options. Memory aids and environmental modifications can prolong independent function. Specialized communication techniques, memory training, exercise, training in independent and basic ADLs, and therapeutic recreational activities can all contribute to improve function and quality of life as the disease progresses. Patients need information on legal and financial issues related to the capacity to make decisions, including end-of-life decisions. Driving and living alone are safety issues that arise in the earlier stages; wandering and falls become issues in the later stages. Both patient and support persons must deal with changes in ability, lifestyle, and relationships with others. Finally, family members/significant others need to learn how to help the patient while taking care of themselves as well. There are negative consequences of caregiving such as depression, anxiety, and failure to care for self.

Many patients with advanced disease are taking as many as eight to 10 medications daily, and many of these medications have side effects that affect cognition and result in falls. Fall precautions need to be taken at home, as well as in long-term care facilities, and clinicians should educate families and support persons regarding these at every visit (see Evidence-Based Nursing Practice 8.1).

PARKINSON'S DISEASE

Parkinson's disease is a chronic, progressive, degenerative disorder of the basal ganglia in the CNS. The disease usually begins insidiously and eventually leads to disability. Parkinsonian syndrome is any disorder that manifests symptoms of parkinsonism, which include rest tremor, rigidity, bradykinesia, and postural instability. Idiopathic PD is the most common cause of parkinsonism, but other causes include

> **Evidence-Based Nursing Practice 8.1**
>
> **ALZHEIMER'S DISEASE**
>
> Yueh-Feng Y, Ellis J, Yang Z, et al. Satisfaction with a family-focused intervention for mild cognitive impairment dyads. *J Nurs Scholarsh*. 2016;48(4);334–344.
>
> This study describes the satisfaction that people with mild cognitive impairment and their caregivers had with the Daily Enhancement of Meaningful Activity (DEMA) intervention. The dyads work together to meet goals and remain engaged in meaningful activities. A randomized study compared satisfaction with DEMA to an information support group (both patients and caregivers) as well as to a control group. Six biweekly sessions were given. Data analysis included descriptive statistics, independent-sample *t* tests, and content analysis. Results documented patients' satisfaction with their caregivers and intervention of DEMA. The study findings provide preliminary support of DEMA as a means to improve quality of life by helping to support patient and caregiver engagement in meaningful activities and problem-solving.

atypical parkinsonian syndromes, secondary parkinsonism, and certain genetic disorders. Patients with idiopathic PD make up the largest subgroup, which represents 78% of the affected population. Atypical parkinsonian syndromes cause more widespread neurodegeneration and are characterized by neurological signs and symptoms in addition to parkinsonism. Examples in this category include progressive supranuclear palsy, multiple systems atrophy, DLB, and corticobasal degeneration. Secondary parkinsonism is symptomatic of an underlying cause of the disorder, such as cerebrovascular disease, drugs, infections, trauma, or exposure to toxins. Common causes of secondary parkinsonism include exposure to dopamine-blocking medications, such as antipsychotics or certain antiemetics. There are some rare hereditary causes of parkinsonism. Only 15% of patients have a family history of PD.

One of the more common causes of parkinsonism is Wilson's disease, which causes an abnormal accumulation of copper.

EPIDEMIOLOGY

PD is the second most common neurodegenerative disorder in older adults after AD. It typically affects people in middle to later life, with a mean age at onset of 57 years. The incidence is slightly higher in males, with a 3:2 ratio of males to females. People in all ethnic groups, countries, and socioeconomic classes are affected. Age is the greatest risk factor for PD, and it is estimated that approximately 2% of the population will be affected by the age of 80 years. The annual cost of PD in the United States is estimated to be approximately $11 billion. People with PD do not die from the disease itself but from secondary complications, such as pneumonia and injuries resulting from falls. Patients with PD have an increased risk of developing dementia in their lifetime (Fig. 8.2).

The morbidity and mortality rate for PD is higher than the general population. An estimated 9% of patients become disabled or die within 1 to 5 years of diagnosis, 21% in 6 to 10 years, and almost 38% in 11 to 15 years.

> **Pediatric/Adolescent Considerations: Wilson's Disease**
>
> Wilson's disease should be ruled out in all young patients presenting with a movement disorder because it is easily treatable. Most people are diagnosed between the ages of 5 and 35 years. This disease is inherited as an autosomal-recessive trait and is present at birth, but the signs and symptoms do not appear until around adolescence when copper builds up in the brain, liver, or other organs. The most common sign is uncontrolled movements or muscle stiffness. Other signs and symptoms include fatigue, lack of appetite or abdominal pain, jaundice, fluid buildup in the legs or abdomen, golden-brown eye discoloration (Kayser-Fleischer rings), and problems with speech or swallowing. When untreated, the condition may be fatal. Complications included cirrhosis, liver failure, neurological problems, kidney stones, psychological problems, and hemolysis. Treatment includes chelating agents that bind the copper to release it into the bloodstream, and then the copper is filtered out by the kidneys. A liver transplant may be necessary.

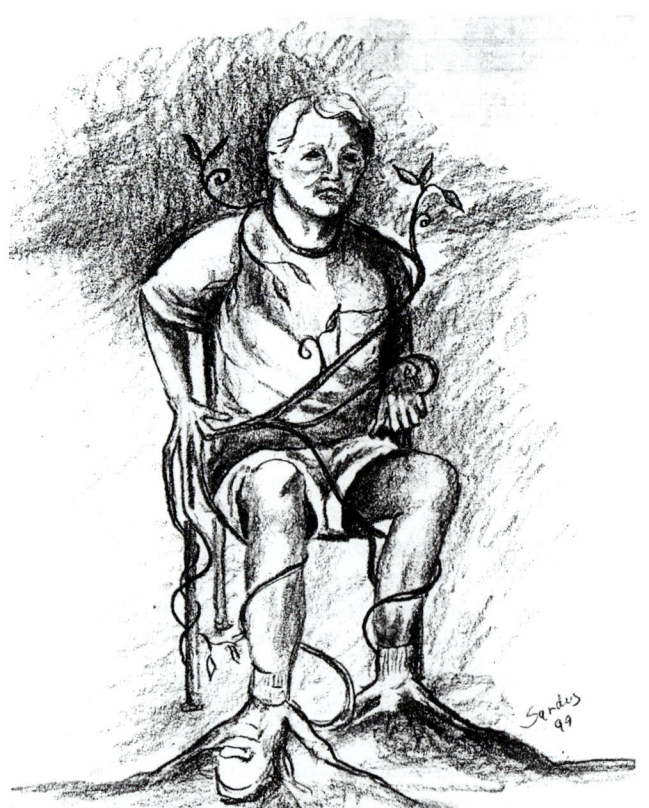

Figure 8.2 One man's depiction of having Parkinson's disease. *(Illustration by Christine Sanders.)*

Michael J. Fox, the actor, was first diagnosed with young-onset PD at age 30 and has raised public awareness for the disease. His foundation for PD research has funded more than $1 billion to find a cure for PD (see Resources).

PATHOPHYSIOLOGY AND CAUSES

Pathologically, PD causes abnormal accumulation of Lewy bodies and degeneration of the pigmented dopaminergic cells of the substantia nigra (located in the brainstem). Lewy bodies are spherical, eosinophilic inclusions in the cytoplasm consisting primarily of alpha-synuclein.

The substantia nigra is part of the basal ganglia, a group of subcortical nuclei with strong connections to the cortex, thalamus, and brainstem. The main components of the basal ganglia include the caudate, putamen, globus pallidus, subthalamic nucleus, and substantia nigra. It is a critical part of the motor system, through its interactions with the motor pathways of the thalamus and cortex.

The main input to the basal ganglia is from the cerebral cortex, and these inputs are mostly excitatory, using the neurotransmitter glutamate. The main output of the basal ganglia is to the thalamus; these outputs are mostly inhibitory and use the neurotransmitter GABA (gamma-aminobutyric acid). Within the basal ganglia lie intrinsic excitatory and inhibitory connections named the direct pathway and indirect pathway, respectively. Aberrations in these pathways lead to hyperkinetic and hypokinetic movement disorders. PD depletes the dopaminergic neurons of the substantia nigra. Dopamine has both excitatory effects in the direct pathway and inhibitory effects in the indirect pathway. Thus, loss of dopaminergic neurons in PD causes a blanket inhibition of the motor activity passing through the thalamus. Clinically, this leads to the rigidity and bradykinesia seen in PD.

In addition to cell loss in the substantia nigra, PD also causes Lewy body accumulation and destruction of cells in other areas of the nervous system, leading to other associated signs and symptoms seen in PD. Cortical Lewy bodies can lead to dementia, either in DLB or PD dementia. Differentiation between these conditions depends on the timing of dementia onset as it relates to the development of parkinsonism and can be somewhat arbitrary, given they are variations of the same pathological disorder.

The cause of sporadic idiopathic PD is unknown. The pathogenesis is thought to be multifactorial, resulting from a combination of genetic predisposition, exposure to possible environmental toxins, and endogenous factors. Research indicates that oxidative stress, mitochondrial dysfunction, and accumulation of toxic proteins play a role. A positive family history increases the lifetime risk of developing PD from 2% to 4%. Numerous genes have been found that cause a hereditary form of PD, although this type is rare.

CLINICAL PRESENTATION

Subjective

Presentation of the disease is variable. The major manifestations of **T**remor at rest, **R**igidity, **A**kinesia (or bradykinesia), and **P**ostural disturbances form the mnemonic "TRAP."

A tremor may be the reason the patient or family first seeks care, and it is recognized as the first symptom of PD in 70% of patients at initial diagnosis. The classic rest tremor of PD is a low-frequency tremor that appears distally in the extremities when the extremity is motionless and at rest. It can mimic the motion of rolling an object between the thumb and forefingers; because of this, it is also called a "pill-rolling tremor." This resting tremor disappears with action but often reemerges as the limb maintains a posture. A resting tremor is most common in the hands but can also be present in the jaw and feet. The resting tremor of the hands tends to increase when the patient is walking and may be an early sign of PD before other signs are visible. Stress tends to worsen the tremor, and it is absent during sleep.

In addition to the motor symptoms of tremor, slowness, and stiffness, a variety of nonmotor symptoms are common in PD, including cognitive decline, anxiety, depression, apathy, orthostatic hypotension, overactive bladder, fatigue, drooling, constipation, loss of sense of smell, and REM sleep behavior disorder (an abnormal acting out of dreams during REM sleep). Constipation, REM sleep behavior disorder, and anosmia frequently predate symptoms of PD by several years. Progressive bradykinesia may contribute to slowness and difficulty in the performance of ADLs. Swallowing problems may be prominent in advanced disease, causing aspiration and choking. Both the motor and nonmotor symptoms can have a major impact on the quality of life of patients with PD.

Objective

The three cardinal manifestations of PD are bradykinesia, rigidity, and rest tremor. Parkinsonism is defined as bradykinesia (slowness of movement) in combination with rest tremor and/or rigidity. A standardized approach to examination of parkinsonism is presented in the Unified Parkinson's Disease Rating Scale and allows for objective quantification of parkinsonism.

Bradykinesia is defined as slowness of movement and decreased amplitude or speed of movement. This can be evaluated by assessing finger and toe tapping. Rigidity is a state of increased muscle tone felt when the clinician passively moves a patient's neck and limbs when they are completely relaxed. This resistance is independent of velocity (as opposed to spasticity, which increases with increased velocity). Rigidity is equal in all directions. "Cogwheeling," a ratchet-like quality to the rigidity, is also commonly found on examination in patients with PD and is caused by an underlying tremor, even in the absence of a visible tremor. When another limb is engaged in voluntary movement, rigidity of the passive limb increases. Rest tremor is a low-frequency tremor in a fully resting limb that is suppressed by active movement. Of note, although postural instability is a feature of parkinsonism, it is not part of the diagnostic criteria for PD because it is typically a later manifestation, and its presence early in the disease process suggests a parkinsonism-plus disorder. The clinician can assess postural reflexes with the pull test, in which the examiner stands behind the patient, gives a sudden and firm pull on the patient's shoulders, and checks for retropulsion.

Patients with PD typically have a stooped posture. The head is bowed, the trunk is bent forward, and the back posture is kyphotic. Extreme truncal flexion is called *camptocormia*; this trunk flexion resolves when in the supine position. There may be a "striatal hand" deformity including ulnar deviation, fingers flexed at the metacarpophalangeal joints, and extension of interphalangeal joints. Walking is slow, with a shortened stride length and tendency to shuffle. Freezing, also called "motor block," is the transient inability to perform active movements. Most often, the legs are affected and become stuck to the floor when trying to walk, but it may also involve eyelid opening, speaking, and writing. Freezing is transient and occurs suddenly. It typically occurs when the patient begins to walk, attempts to turn while walking, or approaches a destination. The patient may be fearful about the inability to handle perceived barriers such as elevator doors and heavily trafficked streets.

Other common manifestations of PD include drooling as a result of decreased frequency of swallowing, dysphagia secondary to the neuromuscular incoordination of the pharyngeal musculature, excessive perspiration as a result of a disorder of the hypothalamic heat-regulating mechanism and impairment of perspiration controls, constipation secondary to hypomotility of the gastrointestinal tract, orthostatic hypotension as a result of deterioration of the peripheral autonomic nervous system, and urinary urgency secondary to autonomic dysfunction. The patient may also demonstrate a "masklike" face (hypomimia); soft speech (hypophonia); and small, slow handwriting (micrographia).

Many patients with PD exhibit behavioral changes. Apathy, anxiety, and depression are common. More than 50% of patients with PD experience depression, and this may precede motor symptoms. There may also be confusion, agitation, and hallucinations, often in combination with cognitive decline and/or as side effects of dopaminergic PD medications as well.

Patients with PD commonly experience cognitive decline. The patient may be slow to answer questions and may be unable to change mental set rapidly.

Autonomic dysfunction such as constipation, bladder dysfunction, sexual dysfunction, and orthostatic hypotension is common.

DIAGNOSTIC REASONING

Diagnostic Tests

Usually, the history and physical examination lead the clinician to the diagnosis of PD. Diagnosis requires the presence of parkinsonism (bradykinesia plus rigidity and/or rest tremor) and absence of exclusion criteria, which include cerebellar abnormalities, vertical supranuclear gaze palsy, treatment with antidopaminergic medication and time course consistent with drug-induced parkinsonism, absence of response to high-dose levodopa, signs of cortical dysfunction on examination, and normal functional neuroimaging of the presynaptic dopaminergic system. Red flags that indicate an alternative diagnosis include rapid progression of gait impairment, absence of progression over years, severe early bulbar dysfunction, severe early autonomic failure, recurrent early falls, and symmetric signs.

Genetic testing may be used in the diagnosis of PD along with other specific features such as family history and early age of onset. An MRI of the brain may be performed to exclude structural brain lesions but not to demonstrate pathological changes indicative of PD. A SPECT scan and a PET scan may show a pattern of reduced dopaminergic activity in the basal ganglia and may help in diagnostic accuracy. Levodopa may be given on a trial, as the patient's response to levodopa is helpful diagnostically. Patients with PD usually have improvement in rigidity, bradykinesia, and tremor with levodopa, whereas patients with other forms of parkinsonism are less likely to respond.

Differential Diagnosis

PD may be mistaken for essential tremor, although the latter is characterized by postural and action tremor, not resting tremor. Idiopathic PD needs to be differentiated from atypical parkinsonian syndromes. In progressive supranuclear palsy, parkinsonism is accompanied by a supranuclear disorder of eye movements, pseudobulbar palsy, and axial dystonia. Multiple system atrophy (previously known as *Shy-Drager syndrome, striatonigral degeneration,* or *olivopontocerebellar atrophy*) causes a combination of parkinsonism, cerebellar signs, and autonomic symptoms. Corticobasal degeneration causes highly asymmetric parkinsonism in addition to dystonia, myoclonus, and cortical signs (such as neglect and apraxia). Buildup of Lewy bodies causes early dementia in addition to parkinsonism. Reversible parkinsonism may be caused by dopamine-blocking or dopamine-depleting medications such as antipsychotics and antiemetics. Vascular disease, other causes of dementia, Wilson's disease, and Huntington's disease can have features of parkinsonism.

It is important to recognize Wilson's disease because it is treatable. Onset of symptoms usually occurs in childhood or early adulthood. It also causes psychiatric and liver disease. Signs include Kayser-Fleischer rings in the cornea, chronic hepatitis, and increased concentrations of copper.

Patients with Huntington's disease can also present with rigidity and bradykinesia, but the cardinal clinical manifestation is chorea (dance-like movements), which will be absent in untreated PD.

MANAGEMENT

The principle of management is to control the symptoms of PD because no drug or surgical approach has been found to definitively prevent the progression of the disease. Each patient has a unique set of signs, symptoms, and responses to medications, so treatment must be individualized. Patients also have social, occupational, and emotional needs to be considered. Treatment is lifelong; the goal is to keep patients functioning independently for as long as possible.

The decision of when to initiate symptomatic treatment for PD should be individualized. In early PD when symptoms are mild and not disrupting daily activity, treatment may be deferred. When PD symptoms begin to interfere with activities, treatment should be initiated. Numerous medications are available. Levodopa is the most efficacious drug for PD; characteristically, the motor problems of PD improve when a patient is treated with levodopa. However, over time, patients can develop motor complications including wearing off and dyskinesia, which can affect quality of life. Often, other medications are used before and in combination with levodopa to delay and treat these complications. Some experts prefer using dopamine agonists first if the patient is younger with milder deficits, although these agents can have cognitive side effects and lead to compulsive behaviors. Medications prescribed for the management of PD are presented in Drugs Commonly Prescribed 8.2.

Drugs Commonly Prescribed 8.2: Parkinson's Disease

DRUG	ADVERSE REACTIONS AND PRESCRIBING CONSIDERATIONS
Monoamine Oxidase (MAO)-B Inhibitors	
Selegiline (Eldepryl) Rasagiline (Azilect) Safinamide (Xadago)	Adverse effects include nausea, headache, confusion, hallucinations, insomnia. When given with levodopa, can increase dopaminergic effects
Dopaminergic Medications	
Carbidopa/levodopa (Sinemet, Sinemet CR, Rytary) Duopa (gel form for use with gastrostomy tube) Parcopa (oral disintegrating table) Inbrija (inhaled)	Gradually titrate to relief of symptoms. Consider Parcopa if swallowing dysfunction is present though it must be swallowed to be absorbed. Duopa requires placement of gastrostomy tube. Adverse effects include nausea, headache, orthostatic hypotension, somnolence, hallucinations, psychosis. Inbrija can be used as a rescue medication.
Dopamine Agonists	
Pramipexole (Mirapex) Ropinirole (Requip) Apomorphine (injectable, sublingual)	Apomorphine can be used as rescue therapy because of its quick onset of action. Adverse effects include nausea, sleepiness, orthostatic hypotension, confusion, hallucinations, peripheral edema, compulsive behavior.
COMT (Catechol-O-Methyl Transferase) Inhibitors	
Entacapone (Comtan) Opicapone (Ongentys)	Only beneficial in combination with carbidopa/levodopa. Helpful in patients with motor fluctuations and with wearing off Adverse effects include diarrhea and orange urine, and it can worsen adverse effects of levodopa.
Anticholinergics	
Trihexyphenidyl (Artane) (Trihex) Benztropine mesylate (Cogentin)	Adverse effects include confusion, hallucinations, dry mouth, urinary retention.
Antiviral Medications	
Amantadine (Symmetrel) Amantadine ER (Gocovri, Osmolex)	Unknown mechanism of action in PD Can treat dyskinesia Adverse effects include ankle edema, confusion, hallucinations.

Once levodopa therapy is started, the rule of thumb is to administer the lowest dosage that controls symptoms. An adequate trial with a reasonably high dose should be tried before deciding a patient does not respond to levodopa. With more advanced disease, patients may also experience the "on–off" phenomenon. After 2 to 5 years of treatment, more than 50% of patients experience fluctuations in their response to levodopa with dyskinesia (extra hyperkinetic choreiform movements) at peak doses and recurrence of parkinsonism as the medication wears off. Rasagiline is a monoamine oxidase (MAO)-B inhibitor that is often used as an adjunct to levodopa. It has fewer side effects than levodopa, but the benefit tends to be only mild to moderate. Dopamine agonists presumably act directly on striatal dopamine receptors and do not require metabolic conversion to an active product to exert effects. They are slightly less effective than levodopa but are alternative first-line agents for PD. Anticholinergic agents are centrally acting drugs and are often used to treat PD. These drugs are typically prescribed for patients aged 70 years or younger in whom tremor is the dominant clinical feature and whose cognitive function is preserved. These agents are useful for treating resting tremors; however, adverse effects, including memory impairment, hallucinations, and confusion, are common with these drugs. Adverse CNS effects of drugs used to treat PD include dysphagia, sedation, and dyskinesia. These drugs should always be tapered gradually.

Peripheral catechol-O-methyl transferase (COMT) inhibitors such as entacapone (Comtan) and opicapone (Ongentys) can be used as adjunctive therapies to levodopa. These drugs increase the bioavailability of levodopa, thereby extending the duration of levodopa's effect. COMT inhibitors have been shown to be effective in both nonfluctuating and fluctuating patients.

Patients with severe symptoms, such as tremor, that are refractory to medications may require referral to a movement disorder neurologist or neurosurgeon to discuss deep brain stimulation. This therapy can be helpful in patients with refractory tremor or significant motor fluctuations with levodopa. In deep brain stimulation, electrodes are placed in subthalamic nuclei or globus pallidus.

For PD dementia, cholinesterase inhibitors such as rivastigmine or donepezil can be helpful. Hallucinations can be exacerbated by medications used to treat PD, particularly dopamine agonists and anticholinergics. If an antipsychotic needs to be used to treat psychosis in PD patients, the drugs of choice include quetiapine, clozapine, or pimavanserin because they are less likely to worsen parkinsonism.

FOLLOW-UP AND REFERRAL

The frequency of follow-up visits is based on the patient's response to treatment, adverse effects of medications, and disease progression. Follow-up should be early and repeated initially, especially during the introduction of a new medication or dose change. The decision for referral to a specialist should be made based on the practitioner's knowledge level and comfort treating PD and on the severity of symptoms. As the disease progresses, especially in the area of tremor, it may become necessary to refer the patient to a movement disorder neurologist or to a stereotactic neurosurgeon to consider surgical treatment options, such as deep brain stimulation.

Rating scales are frequently used to evaluate and monitor a patient's response to medications. The Unified Parkinson's Disease Rating Scale (UPDRS) is a comprehensive evaluation tool that assesses mental, historical, and motor features and the complications of dopaminergic therapy. A subscale of the UPDRS is the Activities of Daily Living Scale, which assesses speech, salivation, swallowing, handwriting, cutting food, handling utensils, hygiene, turning in bed, falling, freezing, walking, tremor, and sensory symptoms.

Patient Education: Parkinson's Disease

Patients should be educated on all issues of the disease, medications, adverse effects, complications, and progression. Patients with PD should be encouraged to exercise regularly, and a referral to physical therapy may be indicated. Nutrition in patients with advanced PD is an important component of care, particularly if the patient develops swallowing difficulties. The patient should also be assessed for physical and psychological problems, which may interfere with eating and nutrition. Functional capacity may be limited, hindering the patient's ability to prepare meals.

Speech therapy can be helpful in treating hypophonia from PD. Swallowing assessments and therapies may be needed to assist with problems of dysphagia.

Patients must also be instructed to continue routine health maintenance and screenings. In addition, both patient and caregiver must be educated about the risk for falls in patients with decreased mobility, as well as other home safety issues. There is an increase in mortality from influenza and pneumonia among patients with PD, so guidance for immunizations must be given. The patient and support persons may benefit from referral to a support group.

AMYOTROPHIC LATERAL SCLEROSIS (LOU GEHRIG'S DISEASE)

Amyotrophic lateral sclerosis (ALS) is a progressive neurological disorder that involves destruction of motor neurons. Both upper motor neurons (located in the motor cortex) and lower motor neurons (located in the anterior horn of the spinal cord and the motor nuclei of cranial nerves in the brainstem) are affected, distinguishing ALS from other motor neuron diseases. On examination, upper motor neuron signs localize to the CNS, including spasticity, hyperreflexia, and positive Babinski sign. Lower motor neuron signs localize to the peripheral nervous system, including muscle atrophy, fasciculations, and hyporeflexia. The etiology of ALS is not known, although approximately 10% of cases are genetic. Researchers are studying possible causes, which may include abnormal ribonucleic acid (RNA) processing, mitochondrial dysfunction, viral infection, disorganized immune response, toxicity, and others (Peters et al, 2015). Slightly more men than women have ALS. Age, family history, and possibly tobacco use are the only known risk factors. It is universally fatal with a median survival of 3 to 5 years.

Symptoms typically start in one limb or region in the spinal cord ("limb onset"), although in 20% of patients, the symptoms begin in the cranial nerve nuclei ("bulbar onset"). Bulbar onset portends a poorer prognosis because swallowing and breathing functions are affected sooner. Presentations may vary considerably between patients, as motor functions of any area of the body may be affected.

Over time, weakness will spread to other areas of the body. Signs of both upper and lower motor neuron dysfunction affecting multiple regions of the body occur, which is the hallmark of ALS. Gold standard diagnostic criteria are defined by the El Escorial World Federation of Neurology criteria. Given the complexity of these criteria, a consensual recommendation in 2019 proposed the Gold Coast criteria for diagnosing ALS, which include:

- Either progressive upper and lower motor neuron symptoms and signs in one limb or body segment or progressive lower motor neuron symptoms and signs in at least two limbs or body segments
- Absence of an alternative diagnosis to explain the neurological dysfunction

Bowel and bladder control is usually not affected. There is comorbid development of frontotemporal dementia in approximately 15% of patients. The diagnosis is clinical, although it can be confirmed with electromyography and nerve conduction studies. There is no treatment to reverse ALS; however, treatment may slow the progression of symptoms. Riluzole is an oral medication that has been shown to improve survival in ALS. The mechanism of action is unknown, but it may be related to a reduction in excitotoxicity caused by glutamate, a chemical messenger in the brain. Edaravone is an IV medication that was FDA approved in 2017 to treat ALS. It works as a free radical scavenger and has been shown to slow functional decline in patients with ALS, particularly those early in the disease process. Other treatments are aimed at managing the symptoms of the disease.

REFERENCES

Alzheimer's Disease

Alzheimer's Association. 2019 Alzheimer's disease facts and figures. https://www.alz.org/media/Documents/alzheimers-facts-and-figures-2019-r.pdf. Accessed 3/27/2021.

Corbett A, Burns A, Ballard C. Don't use antipsychotics routinely to treat agitation and aggression in people with dementia. *BMJ*. 2014;349:g6420.

Filippi M et al. European Federation of the Neurologic Societies. EFNS task force: The use of neuroimaging in the diagnosis of dementia. *Eur J Neurol*. 2012;19(12):1487–1501.

Langman N. Caregivers of dementia patients: Mental health screening & support. *Clin Rev*. 2016;26(6):42–49.

Shanley A. Is it Alzheimer disease? Guidelines for evaluating patients with mild memory loss. *Consultant*. 2016;56(12): 1074–1078.

Yueh-Feng Y, Ellis J, Yang Z, et al. Satisfaction with a family-focused intervention for mild cognitive impairment dyads. *J Nurs Scholarsh*. 2016;48(4);334–344.

Amyotrophic Lateral Sclerosis

Abe K et al. Safety and efficacy of edaravone in well defined patients with amyotrophic lateral sclerosis: a randomised, double-blind, placebo-controlled trial. The Lancet. 2017;16(7):505-512.

Amyotrophic lateral sclerosis (ALS). http://www.mayoclinic.org/diseases-conditions/amyotrophic-lateral-sclerosis/diagnosis-treatment/treatment/txc-20247219. Accessed 3/27/2021.

Hannaford A, Pavey N, van den Bos M, et al (2021). Diagnostic utility of Gold Coast criteria in Amyotrophic Lateral Sclerosis. *Ann Neurol*. 2021; Feb 9. https://pubmed.ncbi.nlm.nih.gov/33565111/. Accessed 4/1/2021.

Miller RG, Mitchell JD, Moore DH. Riluzole for amyotrophic lateral sclerosis (ALS)/motor neuron disease (MND). *Cochrane Database Syst Rev*. 2012;(3):CD001447.

Peters OM, Ghasemi M, Brown RH Jr. Emerging mechanisms of molecular pathology in ALS. *J Clin Invest*. 2015;125(5): 1767–1779.

Sanofi-Aventis, U.S. LLC. Survival rates of patients with ALS treated with Rilutek (riluzole). [Drug insert study.] http://products.sanofi.us/rilutek/rilutek.pdf.

Shefner JM et al. A proposal for new diagnostic criteria for ALS. *Clin Neurophysiol*. 2020;131(8):1975-1978.

Dementia

Causes of Dementia. https://www.dementia.org/causes. Accessed 4/1/2021.

Chancellor B, Duncan AC, Cjatterjee A. Art therapy for Alzheimer's disease and other dementias. *J Alzheimers Dis*. 2014;39(1):1–11.

Gomez GM, Gomez GJ. Music therapy and Alzheimer's disease: Cognitive, psychological, and behavioural effects. *Neurologia*. 2017;32(5):300–308.

Kapucu S, Asiret GD. The Use of Reminiscence Therapy in Alzheimer Patients. *J Neurol Stroke*. 2017;6(2):00198. doi: 10.15406/jnsk.2017.06.00198

Knopman DS et al. Practice parameter: diagnosis of dementia (an evidence-based review): report of the Quality Standards Subcommittee of the American Academy of Neurology. *Neurology*. 2001;56(9):1143–1153.

Parkinson's Disease

American Sleep Association. REM Behavior Disorder. https://www.sleepassociation.org/sleep-disorders/more-sleep-disorders/rem-behavior-disorder/. Accessed 4/1/2021.

Dancis A, Cotter VT. Diagnosis and management of cognitive impairment in Parkinson's disease. *J Nurse Pract.* 2015;11(3):307–313.

Fahn S, Jankovic J, Hallett M. *Principles and practice of movement disorders.* 2nd ed. Philadelphia, PA: Elsevier Health Sciences; 2011.

Kochanek KD, Murphy SL, Xu J, et al. Deaths: Final data for 2014. *Natl Vital Stat Rep.* 2016;65(4):1–122.

Medifocus Guidebook on Parkinson's Disease. A comprehensive patient guide to symptoms, treatment, research, and support. http://www.medifocus.com/parkinsons/?assoc=Bing&keyword=parkinsons. Updated January 6, 2021. Accessed 3/27/2021.

Movement Disorder Society Task Force on Rating Scales for Parkinson's Disease. The Unified Parkinson's Disease Rating Scale (UPDRS): Status and recommendations. *Mov Disord.* 2003;18(7):738–750. https://pubmed.ncbi.nlm.nih.gov/12815652/. Accessed 3/27/2021.

MoCa. Montreal Cognitive Assessment. https://www.mocatest.org/. Accessed 3/27/2021.

Postuma RB et al. MDS clinical diagnostic criteria for Parkinson's disease. *Mov Disord.* 2015;30(12):1591–1601.

Postuma RB, Aarsland D, Barone P, et al. Identifying prodromal Parkinson's disease: Pre-motor disorders in Parkinson's disease. *Mov Disord.* 2012;27(5):617–626.

Unified Parkinson's Disease Rating Scale. In: Fahn S, Elton R, Members of the UPDRS Development Committee. In: Fahn S, Marsden CD, Calne DB, et al, eds. *Recent developments in Parkinson's disease*; vol 2 Florham Park, NJ: Macmillan Health Care Information; 1987, 153–163, 293–304. http://img.medscape.com/fullsize/701/816/58977_UPDRS.pdf. Accessed 3/27/2021.

RESOURCES

Alzheimer's Disease

Alzheimer's Association
1-800-272-3900
  https://www.alz.org
Alzheimer's Foundation of America
1-866-232-8484
  http://alzfdn.org

Amyotrophic Lateral Sclerosis

Amyotrophic Lateral Sclerosis (ALS) Association
Washington, DC
  https://www.alsa.org

Parkinson's Disease

The Michael J. Fox Foundation for Parkinson's Research
  https://michaeljfox.org
Parkinson Foundation
1-800-327-4545
  https://www.parkinson.org

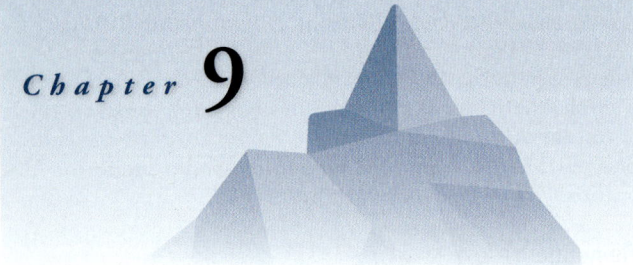

Chapter 9

Cerebrovascular Accident (Stroke)

Sarah Horn, MD

Jill E. Winland-Brown, EdD, APRN, FNP-BC, FAANP

Stroke, also referred to as a *cerebrovascular accident (CVA),* causes acute onset of neurological deficits caused by decreased blood flow or bleeding in a localized area of brain tissue. Although the incidence of stroke has decreased in the past 25 years because of risk-factor management and improved treatment, it has continued to be a significant public health problem in terms of both mortality and permanent disability. Stroke is a leading cause of disability in adults, incurring major economic burdens on the patient, family, and public as a result of direct medical costs and lost employment. The impact of cerebrovascular disease as a major health problem with demands on health care and other support systems will continue to grow as the number of stroke survivors living with disabilities increases and the population continues to live longer. The need for continued improvement in stroke prevention, the control of risk factors, and acute management of stroke is critical.

There are two kinds of strokes: hemorrhagic and ischemic. Approximately 80% of strokes are ischemic and 20% hemorrhagic. Ischemic stroke, also called an *ischemic cerebral infarct,* is caused by decreased blood flow to and subsequent tissue necrosis of a localized part of the brain supplied. Etiologies include embolism, thrombosis, and hypoperfusion. A transient ischemic attack (TIA) is a temporary episode of focal cerebral ischemia that resolves spontaneously and does not leave permanent damage. People who have had a TIA are at higher risk for future stroke.

EPIDEMIOLOGY AND CAUSES

Stroke is the fifth leading cause of death in the United States after heart disease, cancer, accidents, and chronic lower respiratory diseases. The rate of stroke is highest in the southeastern United States. There are approximately 150,000 deaths from stroke annually in the United States (one in every 20 deaths), and an estimated 795,000 people have a stroke each year. About 610,000 are first-time strokes. Every 40 seconds, someone has a stroke. Someone dies from a stroke every 3.7 minutes. More females than males (about 3:2) die from a stroke. In reviewing long-term survival, 25% of people who have an initial stroke die within 1 year, and two-thirds die within 12 years.

Health costs associated with stroke are significant. The average health-care costs per person (inpatient and outpatient) for strokes have been estimated to be between $8,000 and $16,500. These numbers do not include the additional costs of morbidity-related expenses (lost time from work, additional nursing care, etc.). The total direct and indirect costs to the nation are projected to reach $140 billion by 2030. This will be a 238% change in direct costs when compared to 2010 and a 73% change in indirect costs.

Age, sex, race, ethnic origin, and heredity have been identified as nonmodifiable risk factors for stroke, helping to identify those at greatest risk. Compared with European Americans, young African Americans are at two to three times greater risk of stroke, and they are two and a half times more likely to die from one. A higher incidence of stroke is also noted in Hispanic and Asian Americans, particularly people of Chinese and Japanese descent, than in European Americans. For people older than 55 years, the incidence of stroke more than doubles in each successive decade. Thirty-four percent of people who suffer a stroke are younger than age 65 years. An increased incidence of stroke in some families has been noted, probably because of a genetic tendency and familial exposure to similar environmental or lifestyle risks. Pregnant women are at higher risk of stroke compared with the general population.

Important modifiable risk factors for stroke include hypertension, cardiac disease, diabetes, hypercholesterolemia, smoking, illicit drug use, and lifestyle factors. There is a fourfold increase of stroke when a patient is hypertensive with a blood pressure (BP) greater than 160/95 mm Hg. Studies show that with treatment for hypertension, there is a 38% reduction in strokes and a 40% reduction in mortality from strokes. Atrial fibrillation is associated with a threefold to fivefold increased risk for stroke. Other cardiac diseases related to increased risk for stroke include artificial cardiac valves, cardiac structural abnormalities such as patent foramen ovale (PFO), and heart failure with low ejection fraction. People with diabetes are more prone to develop atherosclerosis, thus increasing the risk of stroke.

PATHOPHYSIOLOGY

Cerebral Ischemia

Cerebral ischemia is caused by a reduction in blood flow to the brain. Neurons stop functioning after less than 10 seconds of insufficient blood flow, but they can recover fully if circulation is restored promptly. After a few minutes without oxygen and glucose, however, neurons begin to die. The specific neurological deficits caused by cerebral ischemia reflect the functions of the brain region affected by the ischemia. Ischemia can be subdivided into three subtypes: thrombosis, embolism, and hypoperfusion.

Thrombosis

Thrombosis refers to local obstruction of an artery. Common causes include atherothromboses, dissection of an artery, and other disease of the arterial wall. Atherosclerosis produces atheromatous plaques—gummy bulges that protrude from the inner walls of arteries. Atheromatous plaques are masses of lipids, cell debris, collagen, fibrin, platelets, and blood cells covered by smooth muscle cells, macrophages, and lymphocytes. Plaques that erode can also initiate local blood clotting. When the clot sticks to the plaque, it often grows, occludes the arterial lumen, and leads to ischemia in the areas of the brain supplied by that occluded artery.

Embolism

Embolism refers to fragments of debris that travel downstream and occlude smaller arteries and arterioles, producing areas of ischemia. Occlusive emboli can be generated upstream some distance from the cerebral arteries. The two most common emboli are cardioembolic and artery to artery. Atrial fibrillation, prosthetic heart valves, valve vegetations, and myocardial infarcts can generate cardioembolic emboli. Artery-to-artery emboli are caused by clots and fragments of atherosclerotic plaque that form in the aorta, internal carotid arteries, or the vertebral arteries, dislodge, and are carried into more distal brain arteries, which then become occluded. Paradoxical embolism occurs when a venous thromboembolism passes through a PFO to enter the arterial system. Embolism of clots and clumps of platelets formed during conventional angiography procedures and cardiac surgery can become occlusive emboli. Hypercoagulability syndromes, elevated levels of blood platelets, calcified fragments of plaque and tissue, air, fat, cholesterol crystals, tumor fragments, bacterial vegetations, and foreign material (such as talc and cornstarch injected with illicit drugs) can all clog brain arteries either via embolism or thrombosis.

Decreased Brain Perfusion

Transient global low cerebral blood flow causes syncope (fainting). If brain perfusion remains low, for example, during shock or cardiac arrest, neurons begin to die, starting in the watershed areas—that is, at the borders between regions supplied by the major cerebral arteries. Watershed areas are located at the border between the areas supplied by the anterior cerebral artery and medial cerebral artery (MCA), as well as between the MCA and posterior cerebral artery (PCA) territories. Watershed infarcts are often bilateral and affect the brain more diffusely. In addition, certain hippocampal neurons are especially sensitive to loss of cerebral perfusion, and this may explain the memory deficits that occur after the hypoperfusion caused by even a brief cardiac arrest.

Cerebral Hemorrhage

The neurological symptoms of a cerebral hemorrhage result from the pressure of a hematoma. In some cases, this pressure causes infarcts in the compressed tissue. In others, there is less cell death so that when the hematoma is resorbed, the neurological deficits resolve to some degree. As a rule, the larger the hematoma, the greater and more permanent the damage.

Epidural Hematomas

Epidural bleeding is caused by severe head injuries. Epidural hematomas are most common along the temporal cranial wall and result from tears in the middle meningeal artery. The leaking arterial blood rapidly creates a hematoma between the dura and bone. This increases the overall intracranial pressure, which in turn reduces the cerebral blood perfusion. As the hematoma enlarges, it presses on adjacent brain tissue, causing contralateral hemiparesis. Next, the increasing pressure affects the diencephalon, and the patient becomes lethargic and drowsy. When the mid-brain becomes compressed against the dural rim of the tentorium, patients develop ipsilateral oculomotor nerve palsy and an enlarged pupil. Continued expansion of the hematoma compresses the contralateral cerebral peduncle, leading to hemiplegia. Eventually, the diencephalon and ipsilateral temporal lobe can be pushed down through the tentorial notch; such herniations compress the PCAs and press on the brainstem; they can be fatal.

Subdural Hematomas

Subdural bleeding is usually caused by blunt trauma that knocks the brain against the skull. Movement of the brain relative to the skull tears the thin superior cerebral veins (the bridging veins), which drain the external cerebral veins into the superior sagittal sinus. Minor repeated injuries can cause chronic venous leakage. Venous subdural hematomas expand more slowly than the higher-pressure arterial epidural hematomas. Small, self-limited subdural hematomas are often absorbed spontaneously, but subdural hematomas can also continue to enlarge slowly without severe or clear-cut neurological symptoms, especially in older adults. An untreated subdural hematoma can lead to permanent severe neurological deficits or death.

Intracerebral Hemorrhage

Also known as *intraparenchymal hemorrhage* (IPH), intracerebral hemorrhage refers to bleeding within the brain parenchyma. One of the most common causes of IPH is hypertension. Sudden increases in cerebral BP or cerebral blood flow can rupture intraparenchymal arteries, especially when the arteries have been weakened by chronic hypertension, aneurysms, or vascular malformations. Hypertensive IPHs most often develop from ruptures of arteries to the basal ganglia and thalamus, although hematomas can also form elsewhere in the cerebral lobes, cerebellum, and pons. Other etiologies include trauma, amyloid angiopathy, underlying tumor, clotting disorders, low platelet counts, anticoagulant drugs, vasoconstrictors (including amphetamine or cocaine use), and eclampsia during pregnancy. Hemorrhages from amyloid angiopathy tend to be in lobar locations (i.e., located more peripherally toward the cortex of the brain) as opposed to hypertensive hemorrhages, which tend to be located within deep structures in the brain.

The neurological symptoms of an IPH reflect the specific location of the hematoma—for example, a basal ganglia hematoma pressing on the internal capsule will cause contralateral motor weakness.

Subarachnoid Hemorrhage

Subarachnoid hemorrhages (SAHs) are caused by tears in the arteries running along the subarachnoid space at the surface of the brain. Ruptured arterial aneurysms are the most common source of subarachnoid bleeds. In the brain, these aneurysms usually occur at branch points of the large arteries, especially in the circle of Willis. Other causes include congenital vascular malformations, trauma, amyloid angiopathy, and bleeding diathesis.

Cerebrospinal fluid (CSF) circulates through the subarachnoid space, and blood from a subarachnoid hemorrhage will spread quickly throughout the CSF coating the brain and spinal cord. In SAH, a lumbar puncture (LP) produces CSF mixed with red blood cells. In this case, the CSF often assumes a yellowish tinge referred to as *xanthochromia*. Xanthochromia occurs as a result of the breakdown of hemoglobin in the CSF by enzymes producing yellow-pigmented bilirubin. Ruptures of arteries in the subarachnoid space cause a sudden increase in intracranial pressure and produce severe headache, vomiting, and drowsiness.

CLINICAL PRESENTATION

Subjective

A stroke should be suspected when a patient presents with sudden onset of focal neurological signs and symptoms. Particularly with ischemic strokes, maximum neurological deficits tend to occur at the onset and then improve over time as a patient recovers. Patients may complain of weakness or numbness on one side of the body, depending on the location of the stroke. Impairment may be seen in cognitive abilities, level of consciousness, vision, sensation, extraocular muscle functioning, coordination, and gait. Patients may or may not complain of a headache.

Unilateral weakness or numbness from a stroke is caused by damage to the opposite side of the brain that controls those functions. Patients may exhibit a variety of cognitive changes, depending on the location of the area of the brain affected by the stroke. A common cognitive change seen in a stroke affecting the right brain hemisphere, particularly in the territory of the right middle cerebral artery, is left-sided neglect. With this, patients lose awareness of the left side of their body and surroundings. They may not realize they have weakness or numbness on the left side of their body. In severe cases, they may not be able to recognize their own left hand. Lesions in the left middle cerebral artery territory commonly cause aphasia (language difficulty) in addition to right-sided weakness. Other possible cognitive changes include impairment of memory, decreased ability to concentrate on and attend to tasks, alexia (reading problems), and agraphia (difficulties writing). Strokes in the brainstem tend to cause cranial nerve (CN) abnormalities (such as double vision from extraocular movement abnormalities) in addition to weakness and/or numbness on one side of the body. Strokes in the PCA territory, which supplies the occipital lobes, can cause an isolated visual field deficit.

The primary care practitioner should ask about a history of cardiovascular risk factors, such as hypertension, hyperlipidemia, smoking history, diabetes, coronary artery disease (CAD), cardiac valvular disorders, atrial fibrillation, and recent myocardial infarction (MI). A list of current medications should be obtained, including prescribed, over-the-counter, recreational, and illicit drugs. The provider should be especially attentive to the use of anticoagulant, antiplatelet, and illegal drugs, which may provide clues to the cause of the stroke or affect treatment.

In brain hemorrhage, a severe headache of abrupt onset ("thunderclap headache"), possibly with a decreased level of consciousness, raises concern for subarachnoid hemorrhage. In subdural hematoma, headache is the single most common symptom and is more common in older adults. A subdural hematoma is often accompanied by focal neurological symptoms. IPH presents with focal neurological signs and symptoms similar to those seen in ischemic stroke.

Objective

Information obtained during the history and physical examination assists in identifying the area of the brain involved and the etiology of the stroke and in determining whether the stroke is hemorrhagic or ischemic. Relevant aspects of the history include the nature of the onset, the timing and duration of the neurological deficit, and whether the deficit is static, improving, or worsening. It is important to inquire specifically about the last time the patient was known to be well; the patient's activity when the symptoms began; how the symptoms progressed; the severity of the symptoms; and whether they have worsened, improved, or remained the same.

The hallmark of stroke is the sudden onset of symptoms, regardless of etiology. Headache is more common in hemorrhagic strokes, but it is also seen in ischemic strokes. The only definite way to differentiate between ischemic and hemorrhagic strokes is with brain imaging, typically computed tomography (CT) of the head. It is important to determine whether the symptoms are transient, which could indicate a TIA. To differentiate TIA from a stroke, the patient should undergo brain magnetic resonance imaging (MRI), which will indicate whether permanent damage to the brain has occurred. The causes of TIAs are the same as the causes of stroke. Expedited work-up and treatment of TIAs is important because the risk of stroke is elevated after a TIA. Table 9.1 presents the different etiologies of TIA and ischemic stroke.

Neurological examination aids in localization of the stroke. Signs and symptoms exhibited by the patient typically localize to a specific area of the brain (Table 9.2). Hemiparesis (i.e., weakness on one side of the body) indicates involvement of the motor pathway on the opposite side of the brain. Weakness may be evident in the lower face (a flattened nasolabial fold and asymmetrical smile), arm, and/or leg on one side of the body. This is often accompanied by sensory deficits as well. Aphasia typically localizes to the left middle cerebral artery territory. Left-sided neglect typically localizes to the right middle cerebral artery territory. Assessment of visual fields may identify deficits such as homonymous hemianopsia (complete loss of vision in the left or right visual field), blindness in one or both eyes, bitemporal hemianopsia, or homonymous quadrant defect. A visual field deficit helps localize the stroke along the visual pathways. CN abnormalities occur in brainstem strokes. A review of the CNs may indicate difficulties with eye movements (CNs III, IV, VI); facial sensation and chewing (CN V); facial weakness involving both the upper and lower face (CN VII); vertigo or impaired hearing (CN VIII); dysphagia and absent gag reflex (CNs IX and X); or impaired tongue movement (CN XII). Vertigo and unilateral ataxia typically indicate involvement of the cerebellum or brainstem. Alteration of consciousness indicates involvement of the reticular activating system and is typically caused by strokes in the upper brainstem or bilateral

TABLE 9.1 Pathologies of Ischemic Stroke and TIA

Etiology of Stroke and TIA	Signs and Symptoms	Physical Examination	Diagnostic Tests
Carotid artery pathology	Paresthesia Weakness of hand, arm, face Aphasia Dysarthria Unilateral neglect Transient blindness or blurred vision in one eye Cognitive/behavioral changes (rare)	Neurological examination Assess for carotid bruits Assess for retinal emboli (refer for complete ophthalmological examination) Cardiac auscultation	Laboratory tests: glucose, CBC, platelets, electrolytes, lipid panel, diabetes screen. Consider syphilis serology, toxicology screen, coagulation studies, hypercoagulability screen (antiphospholipid antibodies, PT/PTT, Russell's viper venom time for lupus anticoagulant), anticardiolipin antibodies, beta 2 glycoprotein, ESR, ANA Imaging studies: CT scan of the head and MRI brain (more sensitive than CT) Vessel imaging: Doppler studies of carotid vessels, magnetic resonance angiography, or CT angiography Echocardiography and Holter monitoring to evaluate for cardiac sources of emboli
Small cerebral vessel pathology	Pure motor hemiparesis Pure sensory stroke Ataxic hemiparesis Dysarthria—clumsy hand syndrome Sensorimotor stroke	As above	As above
Vertebrobasilar system pathology	Ataxia Dizziness, vertigo Dysarthria Alteration in consciousness, Diplopia, hemianopsia, or bilateral vision loss Unilateral or bilateral sensory or motor systems	As above	As above
Cardioembolic pathology	May cause any of the above symptoms. May also cause multiple areas of infarct	As above	As above

Abbreviations: ANA, antinuclear antibodies; CBC, complete blood count; CT, computed tomography; ESR, erythrocyte sedimentation rate; MRI, magnetic resonance imaging; PT/PTT, prothrombin time/partial thromboplastin time; TIA, transient ischemic attack.

thalami. The degree of infarction following a stroke varies, depending on the arteries involved, the duration of ischemia, and the adequacy of cerebral collateral circulation. The National Institutes of Health Stroke Scale (NIHSS; see Resources) is a standardized neurological examination designed to quickly identify the examination abnormalities caused by a stroke.

The physical examination can help discern the etiology of the stroke. An irregular heartbeat points toward atrial fibrillation. Severe hypertension often accompanies a hypertensive intracerebral hemorrhage. Patients with carotid atherosclerotic disease may have a carotid bruit. Detecting the presence of a bruit is significant. Not only does it indicate atherosclerosis and ischemic heart disease, but it may also increase the risk for a stroke. In caring for a patient with asymptomatic carotid bruit, the provider should begin with a thorough history for the presence of coronary and peripheral vascular occlusive disease. It is important to identify and manage stroke risk factors.

DIAGNOSTIC REASONING

Diagnostic Tests

Patients who present within the first few hours of stroke symptom onset may be eligible for acute stroke treatment with IV thrombolysis with tissue plasminogen activator (tPA) and/or mechanical thrombectomy and require

TABLE 9.2 Signs and Symptoms of Occlusion of Specific Areas of the Brain

Common Stroke Syndrome	Area of Brain	Signs and Symptoms of Occlusion
Right ICA, MCA, ACA	Right anterior hemisphere	Left-sided weakness Left-sided numbness Left-sided neglect Left visual field deficit Difficulty with leftward gaze
Left ICA, MCA, ACA	Left anterior hemisphere	Right-sided weakness Right-sided numbness Right visual field deficit Aphasia Difficulty with rightward gaze Difficulty with reading, writing, and calculations
PCA	Occipital lobe, thalamus, medial temporal lobes	Contralateral homonymous hemianopsia Left PCA lesion: alexia without agraphia, impaired color naming
Vertebrobasilar system	Cerebellum and brainstem	Contralateral hemiplegia Bilateral motor, sensory, and visual complaints Vertigo Diplopia Dysphagia Ataxia Dysconjugate gaze Crossed signs Horner's syndrome (ptosis of upper eyelid, slight elevation of lower lid, constriction of pupil, anhidrosis)
Pure motor stroke Ataxic hemiparesis	Small vessel occlusion ("lacunar infarct") Internal capsule Base of the pons	Weakness in the face, arm, and leg on one side of the body May be accompanied by ataxia on the side of the weakness Absence of other abnormalities on neurological examination
Pure sensory stroke	Thalamus	Numbness in the face, arm, and leg on one side of the body Absence of other abnormalities on neurological examination

Abbreviations: ACA, anterior cerebral artery; ICA, internal carotid artery; MCA, middle cerebral artery; PCA, posterior cerebral artery.

emergent evaluation in an emergency department. Evaluation should include vital signs, NIHSS, blood glucose level, head CT, CT-angiography of the head and neck vessels, and assessment of contraindications. Ideally, a neurological consultation should also be available within 30 minutes of the patient's arrival. In the clinician's physical and neurological examination and management of the stroke, the time at onset of symptoms is particularly important to determine the proper use of tPA and mechanical thrombectomy treatments.

It is strongly recommended that emergency CT be the initial brain imaging study for the emergency evaluation of a suspected ischemic stroke. Practice guidelines of the American Heart Association Stroke Council recommend the use of noncontrast CT of the head in patients with suspected acute stroke to exclude a nonvascular lesion as the cause of the signs and symptoms and to assess for an intracranial hemorrhage. If the patient is a candidate for mechanical thrombectomy, then CT-angiography should be performed as well to assess for a large vessel occlusion. Signs of an ischemic stroke are not initially apparent on a head CT. Detection of an ischemic stroke by CT depends on the location, extent, and duration of the infarct. Even large infarcts may not be apparent for several hours after onset. Some early infarct signs on head CT include hyperdensity in a segment of a blood vessel (representing clot at that location), loss of the "insular ribbon," loss of gray-white matter differentiation, hypoattenuation of the deep nuclei, and cortical edema. Eventually, an infarcted area appears hypodense on head CT. A CT during the first hours of symptoms can differentiate between a hemorrhagic and ischemic stroke and facilitate the decision to use early tPA and mechanical thrombectomy. Acute blood appears hyperdense on head CT. Other imaging techniques can help with diagnosis but should not delay treatment.

MRI is generally recommended for patients with stroke because it is more sensitive than CT for identifying small ischemic lesions, particularly in the acute period. It also can help identify the etiology of ischemic and hemorrhagic strokes. Abnormalities in MRI diffusion and perfusion sequences occur within minutes of ischemic stroke onset.

Pregnancy is not an absolute contraindication to emergent CT imaging in the setting of acute stroke nor treatment of stroke with IV tPA or mechanical thrombectomy. As with any patient, the risks and benefits of these interventions must be considered in pregnant patients with stroke.

After a stroke is diagnosed, it is important to discern the cause of the stroke because this will affect management. In ischemic stroke, large artery atherosclerosis, cardioembolic infarcts, and small-vessel occlusion are common etiologies. A basic stroke work-up for patients with ischemic stroke includes obtaining laboratory test results, electrocardiogram (ECG) and cardiac monitoring, brain MRI, vessel imaging, and echocardiogram. Patients with ischemic stroke should be screened for diabetes and hyperlipidemia. An ECG will detect the presence of risk factors increasing the probability of stroke, including a recent MI, atrial fibrillation, or left ventricular hypertrophy. Cardiomegaly may be seen on a chest x-ray. All patients with ischemic stroke should undergo cardiac monitor for underlying paroxysmal atrial fibrillation, a common cause of embolism. Vessel imaging is important to identify sources of artery-to-artery embolism and demonstrate large vessel occlusions amenable to mechanical thrombectomy in the acute setting. Magnetic resonance angiography, CT angiogram, color duplex ultrasound, and transcranial Doppler are acceptable noninvasive techniques to screen patients for vascular abnormalities in the setting of stroke. A cardiac echocardiogram should be obtained, preferably with a bubble study (which helps evaluate for a PFO), in patients with ischemic stroke to assess for cardioembolic source. A hypercoagulability screen may be warranted in cases of unexplained stroke. This can include laboratory testing and screening for underlying malignancy.

Patients with hemorrhagic stroke should also be evaluated to determine the etiology. BP must be closely monitored and severe hypertension treated. Angiography can assess for vascular abnormalities. Laboratory data may reveal a decreased platelet count or prolonged prothrombin time or partial thromboplastin time, which may indicate a bleeding disorder or use of anticoagulants, respectively. If the etiology is unclear, brain MRI can evaluate for evidence of underlying amyloid angiopathy, tumor, or hemorrhagic transformation of an ischemic infarct. The brain MRI may need to be repeated in several weeks after the blood resorbs if vascular malformation or tumor is suspected but not evident on initial imaging. An LP may be an additional test used to diagnose subarachnoid hemorrhage if the head CT is negative. Contraindications to this procedure include mass effect on head imaging, thrombocytopenia, and coagulation disorders.

Differential Diagnosis

Common conditions with similar signs and symptoms of stroke and TIA include focal seizure and complex migraine aura, both of which can cause focal neurological signs and symptoms. However, in seizure and migraine, these symptoms are transient, and the timing is different. In a stroke or TIA, the onset of symptoms is very sudden; in seizure, the symptoms can progress over seconds, and in migraine aura, the symptoms tend to progress over minutes.

Brain tumors can mimic stroke and cause focal neurological signs. Headache is often present, and patients may also develop seizures. Vomiting and papilledema may be present. Brain abscess, encephalitis, and meningitis can also cause focal neurological signs, although these are typically accompanied by headache and fever.

MANAGEMENT

The main principles in the management of stroke are prevention and early recognition and treatment. Patients with symptoms of a possible stroke require immediate referral to an emergency department for evaluation, CT scan of the brain, and possible use of IV thrombolysis and mechanical thrombectomy. Since the first positive studies demonstrating the safety and efficacy of mechanical thrombectomy were published in 2015, the landscape of acute stroke care has been constantly evolving (Mathews and De Jesus, 2021).

Initial management of a stroke is focused on addressing the patient's airway, breathing, and circulation to maintain adequate tissue oxygenation. Anaerobic metabolism with depletion of energy stores can increase the extent of brain injury and worsen the outcome. In the prehospital setting, special attention is given to monitoring the patient's oxygen status through pulse oximetry and the use of supplemental oxygen as needed to maintain oxygen saturation at greater than 94%. Maintaining an adequate airway is crucial, and intubation with mechanical ventilation is initiated when there is decreased level of consciousness or evidence of apparent hypoventilation. Hypotension is treated to maximize cerebral blood flow and minimize complications. Aggressive treatment of hypertension in the prehospital setting is not done in patients with known ischemic disease, because lowering the BP may precipitate hypoperfusion and injury. There is a permissive level of hypertension allowed in the days after the stroke as well. Prehospital evaluation and transport time can account for significant delays in initiation of thrombolytic therapy for patients with acute ischemic stroke who require it. Aggressive stroke protocols and educational programs keyed to emergency medical services can markedly reduce the time from stroke onset to initiation of treatment.

Once the clinical presentation, laboratory data, and results of the CT scan are completed and diagnosis of acute ischemic stroke is suspected, thrombolytic agents must be considered. The patient and/or family should understand that thrombolytic therapy carries a 6.4% risk of intracerebral hemorrhage. Intravenous thrombolytic therapy is effective in reducing the neurological deficits in some patients without CT evidence of intracranial hemorrhage within 3 to 4.5 hours after symptom onset. Although the 3-hour "rule" has been accepted, several studies extend this time frame for thrombolytic therapy and advanced imaging techniques, even allowing use beyond 4.5 hours in select patients. Contraindications to thrombolytic therapy include recent head trauma or stroke in the last 3 months, previous intracranial hemorrhage, recent intracranial or intraspinal surgery, untreated hypertension with blood pressure exceeding 185/110 mm Hg, active internal bleeding, known brain tumor, evidence of intracranial bleed on CT scan, international normalized ratio greater than 1.7, partial thromboplastin time greater than 40, platelet count of less than 100,000/mm³, infective endocarditis, and use of anticoagulants (unless on warfarin with International Normalized Ratio (INR) of 1.7 or less).

Edema in large-territory infarcts can lead to herniation and be life-threatening. This is often referred to as a "malignant" stroke. Large strokes in the cerebellum are particularly dangerous because swelling can compress the brainstem. Treatment options include hyperosmolar therapy and decompressive surgery. The use of corticosteroids is not indicated in the management of cerebral edema and increased intracranial pressure due to stroke.

Early ambulation and preventive measures against aspiration, malnutrition, pneumonia, deep vein thrombosis, pulmonary embolism, pressure injuries, contracture, and joint abnormalities are important goals in managing the patient with a stroke. It is important for the clinician to maintain normothermia and normoglycemia in patients with acute stroke.

It is important to investigate the etiology of the stroke because this affects management. Typically, either an antiplatelet or anticoagulant will be used for secondary stroke prevention, in addition to aggressive vascular risk factor management. In patients with a cardioembolic source of stroke, such as atrial fibrillation, anticoagulation is typically recommended. If a PFO is discovered on echocardiogram, it should prompt investigation for deep vein thrombosis. Sometimes PFOs are surgically closed. Patients with high-grade carotid artery stenosis ipsilateral to the side of a TIA or stroke may be referred for surgical management, in addition to aggressive medical management of vascular risk factors. Carotid endarterectomy is established as effective for symptomatic patients with 70% to 99% internal carotid artery stenosis. Carotid endarterectomy should not be considered for symptomatic patients with less than 50% stenosis.

A significant number of patients with carotid artery disease have concomitant CAD, and serum cholesterol in patients with CAD should be evaluated and treated. The hydroxymethylglutaryl–coenzyme A reductase inhibitors, or statins, reduce the risk of both nonfatal and fatal strokes, demonstrating a significant protective effect similar to that conferred by antiplatelet agents. Medical management is preferred to carotid endarterectomy for symptomatic patients with less than 50% stenosis.

One of the most significant changes in the approach to the medical management of patients with CAD with respect to stroke risk reduction has been the use of antiplatelet drugs, principally daily aspirin therapy (acetylsalicylic acid [ASA]) and clopidogrel (Plavix). Clinicians disagree as to whether high or low doses of aspirin are more efficacious; recommended dosages range from 81 to 325 mg per day. The recommended dosage of clopidogrel for stroke prevention is 75 mg daily.

In brain hemorrhage, severe hypertension must be treated. If the patient is taking anticoagulants, reversal agents must be given, if available.

FOLLOW-UP AND REFERRAL

Follow-up and rehabilitation focus on the return of the patient's optimal level of functioning. Following treatment and stabilization, the patient should be assessed for the potential for rehabilitation and transferred to a rehabilitation unit. The rehabilitation process involves six major areas of focus:

1. Preventing, recognizing, and managing comorbid illness and medical complications
2. Training for maximum independence
3. Facilitating psychosocial coping and adaptation by the patient and family/support person(s)
4. Preventing secondary disability by promoting community reintegration, including resumption of home, family/social, and vocational activities
5. Enhancing quality of life in view of residual disability
6. Preventing recurrent stroke and other vascular conditions, such as MI, that occur with increased frequency in patients with stroke

Patient Education: Stroke

Adjustments may need to be made in the home environment before discharge, such as building a ramp or removing a door to accommodate a wheelchair. Specific areas of teaching involve exercise and ambulation techniques, dietary requirements, recognition of symptoms of another stroke, and an understanding of the emotional lability and depression that commonly accompany strokes. Also important are knowledge of appropriate use of medications and the time, place, and frequency of occupational and physical therapy activities. To help prevent caregivers at home from becoming overburdened, clinicians should teach caregivers to plan for respite or time away from caregiving activities on a regular basis. Information regarding community, state, and national resources can be a welcome source of support to patients and their families. The American Stroke Association has resource information, including referral services and a quarterly newsletter. The American Heart Association provides a large variety of information regarding risk factors and referrals for assistive devices. Easter Seals also may provide assistance with wheelchairs or other assistive devices. Some communities have organizations to help with meals or transportation, along with self-help groups.

Education regarding the modification and reduction of risk factors plays a significant role in the reduction in the incidence of stroke and TIA. Risk factor reduction measures include control of hypertension, the use of ASA for prophylaxis in patients with a moderate to high risk of stroke or TIA, and the use of anticoagulants in patients with atrial fibrillation. In a summary of 17 treatment trials of hypertension throughout the world with nearly 50,000 patients, there was a 38% decrease in all strokes and a 40% decrease in fatal strokes after treatment of hypertension. In the Framingham Heart

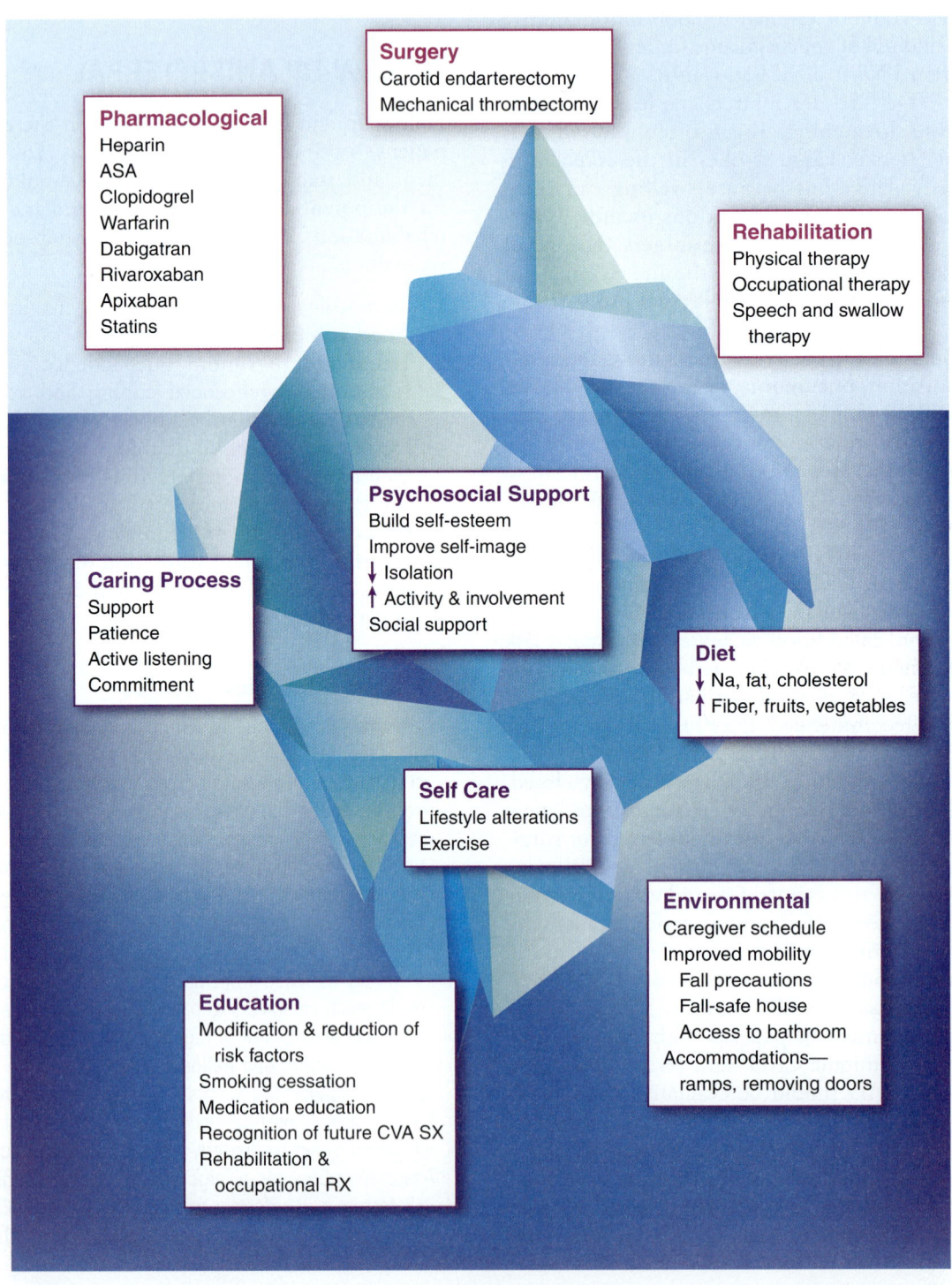

Study, smoking cessation promptly reduced the risk of stroke, with the major risk reduced within 2 to 4 years. Heavy use of alcohol also should be avoided. Moderate and intense levels of physical activity have been associated with a decrease in chronic incidence of stroke. Physical activity is believed to exert a beneficial influence on the risk factors for atherosclerotic disease by decreasing blood pressure, weight, and pulse rate; raising high-density lipoprotein cholesterol and lowering low-density lipoprotein cholesterol; decreasing platelet aggregability; increasing insulin sensitivity and improving glucose tolerance; and promoting a lifestyle conducive to changing diet and cessation of cigarette smoking. A diet low in fat, sodium, and cholesterol and high in fiber, fruits, and vegetables should be encouraged. Patients should also be encouraged to exercise moderately, avoid weight gain, and use stress-reduction techniques. If the patient has atrial fibrillation, anticoagulant therapy should be considered to prevent pooling of the blood in the atria that could promote potential emboli.

Because early treatment of a stroke is critical, successful treatment depends on educating the patient and the family/support person(s) to recognize stroke symptoms and access medical care by calling 911. Delay in treatment has been known to occur for patients who call their primary care provider instead of 911, live alone, have onset of stroke while asleep, have onset at home rather than work, and experience milder stroke symptoms. Studies have documented that 38% of patients and their families did not know a single warning sign of a stroke and that 28% could identify only one sign of seizures. They may attribute tingling or numbness of the fingers or mild gait clumsiness to a problem with the arm or leg. Patients may also feel they have dust in their eyes, when in fact they are experiencing amaurosis fugax. Patients may think such symptoms are trivial and may not seek attention, or if they do, they may not mention these symptoms to their provider. Older adults may simply forget that any symptoms occurred.

Education of the patient and family/support person(s) should include the importance of reporting any new neurological symptoms. Thorough education of high-risk patients and their families/support person(s) about the warning signs of a stroke, along with frequent evaluation and a careful review of symptoms by the primary care provider, will assist in detecting a problem and initiating treatment as soon as possible.

REFERENCES

Centers for Disease Control and Prevention. Pregnancy and Stroke: Are You at Risk? https://www.cdc.gov/stroke/pregnancy.htm. Reviewed 2021. Accessed 5/27/2021.

Centers for Disease Control and Prevention. Stroke facts. https://www.cdc.gov/stroke/facts.htm. Updated March 2021. Accessed 4/29/2021.

Centers for Disease Control and Prevention/National Center for Health Statistics. Leading causes of death. https://www.cdc.gov/nchs/fastats/leading-causes-of-death.htm. Updated March 2021. Accessed 4/29/2021.

Mathews S, De Jesus O. Thrombectomy. https://www.ncbi.nlm.nih.gov/books/NBK562154/. Updated August 2022. Accessed 4/9/2022.

Powers WJ et al. "Guidelines for the early management of patients with acute ischemic stroke: 2019 update to the 2018 guidelines for the early management of acute ischemic stroke: a guideline for healthcare professionals from the American Heart Association/American Stroke Association." *Stroke*. 2019;50(12): e344–e418.

Wolf PA, D'Agostino RB, Kannel WB, et al. Cigarette smoking as a risk factor for stroke. The Framingham Study. *JAMA*. 1988;259:1025–1029.

RESOURCES

Easter Seals
   https://www.easterseals.com/explore-resources/facts-about-disability/understanding-stroke.html
National Institutes of Health Stroke Scale
   https://en.wikipedia.org/wiki/National_Institutes_of_Health_Stroke_Scale
American Stroke Association
1-888-4STROKE
   https://www.stroke.org

Chapter 10

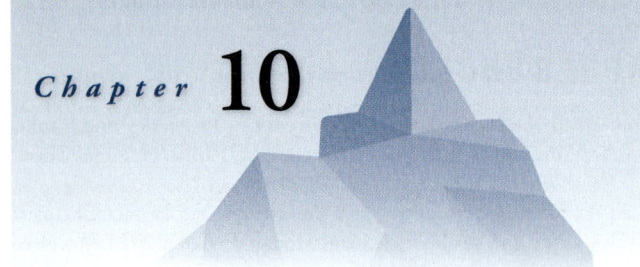

Infectious and Inflammatory Neurological Disorders

Sarah Horn, MD

Jill E. Winland-Brown, EdD, APRN, FNP-BC, FAANP

MENINGITIS

Meningitis is an inflammation of the meninges (pia, arachnoid, and dura) surrounding the structures of the central nervous system (CNS). It can be acute, subacute, or chronic, depending on the etiology. Causes include infection, neoplasm, autoimmunity, and drug-induction. The common factor shared by all types of meningitis is an increase in the number of white blood cells (WBCs) in the cerebrospinal fluid (CSF), typically with symptoms and signs of meningeal irritation.

Although most cases of infectious meningitis are caused by viral infections, bacterial and fungal infections also occur. Acute bacterial meningitis is a life-threatening infection. The most common organisms are *Streptococcus pneumoniae*, *Neisseria meningitidis*, and *Haemophilus influenzae* type B. When routine bacterial cultures are negative, meningitis is called *aseptic meningitis*, which has a very broad differential diagnosis. Viral infection is the most common cause of aseptic meningitis. Table 10.1 reviews the types of meningitis.

EPIDEMIOLOGY AND CAUSES

The incidence of meningitis is 15 per 100,000, with a prevalence of five cases per 100,000. Since the initiation of the widespread use of antibiotics in the 1950s, the mortality figures have remained steady at 10% to

TABLE 10.1 Types of Meningitis

Major Type	Description	Organism	Diagnostic Tests	Treatment
Bacterial	Rapid onset: hours or days after exposure	Age 3 months–18 years: *Haemophilus influenzae* *Neisseria meningitidis* *Streptococcus pneumoniae* Age 18–50: *S pneumoniae* *N meningitidis* Age 50 or older: *S pneumoniae* *N meningitidis* *Listeria monocytogenes* Gram-negative bacilli	CSF Gram stain analysis CSF culture (positive in 70%–85%) CSF PCR (putative transmembrane protein) for specific pathogenesis	Age 3 months–18 years: cefotaxime or ceftriaxone Age 18 or older: cefotaxime or ceftriaxone plus vancomycin; ampicillin if Listeria is suspected
Chronic/subacute	Symptoms develop over weeks to months; less acutely ill	*M tuberculosis* Fungi Spirochetes Virus Neoplastic Sarcoid Systemic lupus erythematosus Behçet's disease Vasculitis Drug-induced (NSAIDs, IV IgG)	CSF analysis (cell count, differential, glucose, protein) Culture PCR for specific pathogens	Tuberculosis: isoniazid, rifampin, pyrazinamide, and a fluoroquinolone Fungi: amphotericin flucytosine Spirochetes: penicillin G for syphilis Ceftriaxone for Lyme disease
Viral	More benign type; self-limited syndrome	Herpes simplex virus Enterovirus Varicella-zoster HIV EBV	CSF analysis (cell count, differential, glucose, protein) Culture PCR for specific pathogens	Supportive care in most cases Acyclovir can be used for HSV, VZV

Abbreviations: CSF, cerebrospinal fluid; EBV, Epstein-Barr virus; HSV, herpes simplex virus; PCR, polymerase chain reaction; VZV, varicella-zoster virus.

> **Pediatric/Adolescent Considerations:**
> **Meningitis**
>
> Meningitis may affect adolescents in crowded settings such as jails, prisons, college dormitories, and barracks. Adolescents should have received the meningococcal vaccine at age 11 to 18 years or older if going to college or into military service. It is crucial to diagnose and manage the disease early. Management includes antimicrobial therapy if meningitis is bacterial in origin. Fever, headache, and other symptoms should be treated, and the person should rest. It is also important for these people to avoid close contact with others.

15%. About one in five of those who do survive experience chronic, long-term problems, such as brain damage, kidney disease, hearing loss, or limb amputations. Susceptibility differs with the causative organism, but generally young people, older adults, and immunocompromised patients are at greatest risk. Bacterial meningitis affects more than 4,000 persons in the United States annually; 500 of those affected die from the disease. Fifteen percent of all cases involve adolescents and young adults. In adolescents, one in seven cases results in death.

The majority of cases of infectious meningitis are attributed to bacteria and viruses, with a much smaller occurrence caused by fungi or parasites. Among the viral causative agents, enteroviruses are the most common. Meningitis has a seasonal occurrence, with a higher incidence in the spring and fall. Infants and young children are particularly susceptible because of a lack of immunity and the higher rate of fecal-to-oral transmission that takes place in this age group. Arboviral infection is another common source during warm months when insect vectors are in abundance. The mumps virus can also be a causative factor in unimmunized populations. Various herpes viruses cause meningitis, and recurrent genital herpes can be associated with recurrent aseptic meningitis called *Mollaret's meningitis*.

Although anyone can get meningitis at any age, those most susceptible include the following groups:

- Infants younger than 1 year of age
- Adolescents and young adults (especially those living in crowded settings, such as dormitories or barracks)
- Travelers outside the United States (such as the meningitis belt in Africa)
- Laboratory personnel who may have been exposed to meningococcal disease during an outbreak

PATHOPHYSIOLOGY

Meningitis is an inflammation of the brain's meningeal membranes, most often caused by infection. Acute bacterial meningitis is a purulent infection that develops within the subarachnoid space. Signs and symptoms include fever, headache, and stiff neck, usually accompanied by vomiting, lethargy, confusion, seizures, or coma.

Bacteria enter the host via the nasopharynx, where they can enter the underlying blood vessels. *S pneumoniae* and *N meningitidis* are both encapsulated bacteria, and their capsules protect them from phagocytosis in the bloodstream.

From the circulation system, bacteria enter the CSF through the choroid plexuses in the ventricles and through injured or leaky areas of the blood–brain barrier. Bacteria can multiply rapidly in the subarachnoid space because normal CSF has few WBCs, no immunoglobulin M antibodies, and low concentrations of the complement components C3 and C4. Local monocytes, macrophages, astrocytes, and microglia react to components in the bacterial cell walls by releasing inflammatory molecules, which increase the permeability of the blood–brain barrier and attract polymorphonuclear leukocytes from the systemic circulation. Large numbers of WBCs enter the CSF and form a purulent exudate in the subarachnoid space. Meningeal irritation from the exudate causes nuchal rigidity (the neck resists passive flexion), and lumbar puncture (LP) in bacterial meningitis produces CSF with a high WBC count. The pus can reduce the flow of CSF and lead to increased intracranial pressure. LPs of patients with bacterial meningitis yield high CSF pressures.

CLINICAL PRESENTATION

Subjective

Subjective symptoms of meningitis include headache, photophobia, and neck pain and stiffness (nuchal rigidity).

Objective

Objective signs include fever, tachycardia, and tachypnea. Signs of meningeal irritation include photophobia, pain with eye movement, Brudzinski's sign (hip and knee flexion when the neck is flexed), and Kernig's sign (inability to fully extend the legs). Occasionally, opisthotonos (severe back spasm, causing arching) is observed. Bacterial meningitis can cause hydrocephalus, altered level of consciousness, and seizures. Cranial nerve dysfunction can occur, resulting in possible diplopia, deafness, facial weakness, and pupillary abnormalities.

History taking may yield clues to possible causative agents or risk factors for meningitis. Major areas to emphasize in taking the history include pertinent exposures, recent infectious symptoms, evidence of immunocompromise, underlying systemic disorders, and travel history.

DIAGNOSTIC REASONING

Diagnostic Tests

Initially, routine blood studies may show marked elevation of WBCs (neutrophils) in bacterial meningitis or mild elevation in viral meningitis. Electrolytes should be monitored. Hyponatremia may occur from a common complication of meningitis, the syndrome of inappropriate antidiuretic hormone secretion (SIADH).

If the clinical signs and symptoms indicate the possibility of meningitis, antibiotics should be started, and an LP should be done to obtain CSF studies. Treatment of bacterial meningitis with antibiotics should not be delayed while awaiting LP. CSF in bacterial meningitis is typically cloudy with elevated WBCs, elevated pressure, greater than 80% polymorphonuclear neutrophils, low glucose, and elevated protein. Gram stain and culture of CSF may assist in detecting causative organisms. A computed tomography (CT) examination of the head should be performed before LP in cases of an abnormal neurological examination (alteration of consciousness, focal findings, papilledema) to assess risk for herniation with LP.

Imaging studies such as a CT or magnetic resonance imaging (MRI) may reveal meningeal enhancement, basilar exudate, hydrocephalus, and associated focal lesions. Any other contributing abnormalities such as skin, lung, or sinus lesions should be investigated.

Differential Diagnosis

Many infectious and noninfectious conditions may mimic meningitis. Headache and alteration of consciousness are both nonspecific with many possible diagnoses (see Chapter 6, Common Neurological Complaints, and Fig. 6.4, Diagnostic reasoning algorithm: headache). Subarachnoid hemorrhage can cause meningeal irritation and headache. Meningitis should be differentiated from encephalitis, which affects the brain parenchyma but not the meninges. It is also important to establish the etiology of meningitis because this affects management.

MANAGEMENT

Meningitis can be life-threatening. If meningitis is suspected, the primary care practitioner should refer the patient to the collaborating physician for immediate hospitalization and extensive diagnostic examination and treatment. The principal goals for managing meningitis include eliminating infection, symptomatic care, and prevention or treatment of complications.

The first goal—and the priority—is to eliminate infection. This is achieved through the judicial use of specific antimicrobial therapy if the meningitis is bacterial in origin. If the diagnosis of bacterial meningitis is suspected, blood cultures and an LP should be performed immediately, and empiric antibiotic therapy should be initiated without delay. Antibiotic therapy should not be withheld if there is a delay in the performance of the LP. The choice of empiric therapy is based on the demographics of the patient (age, immunocompromised state, medical comorbidities). The patient's antibiotic regimen can be narrowed, based on the results of cultures of the CSF. The usual course of IV antimicrobials is 10 to 14 days. Some treatment regimens are included in Table 10.1. Adjunctive corticosteroids have been used in adolescents and adults with bacterial meningitis and have been shown to reduce hearing loss and mortality.

Chronic meningitis treatment is based on the underlying etiology. Symptomatic treatment includes reduction of fever with acetaminophen, headache management with analgesics, and treatment of nausea and vomiting with an antiemetic such as Zofran. Oversedation should be avoided because it may mask increasing intracranial pressure. Other supportive treatment includes rest in a quiet, darkened room; adequate liquids; and a nutritious diet as tolerated.

Several vaccines are available for the more common forms of meningitis. In some cases, prophylaxis is advised for documented exposure.

Of major concern as a complication of meningitis is increasing intracranial pressure caused by cerebral edema or hydrocephalus. Early signs include drowsiness, headache, double vision (from cranial nerve VI palsy), and confusion. Later signs include decreasing levels of consciousness; hemiparesis; pupillary changes; and Cushing's triad of hypertension, bradycardia, and respiratory changes. This serious complication requires emergent neurosurgical consult and intensive care unit admission, often with ventilatory support. Techniques to reduce intracranial pressure include hyperventilation, hyperosmolar therapy, and neurosurgical procedures such as drain placement.

FOLLOW-UP AND REFERRAL

All patients who are suspected of having any form of meningitis should be referred to the emergency department for urgent work-up and treatment. When the patient's condition is stable, the patient may be released to the care of the primary health-care practitioner to continue follow-up care, which consists of completion of the antibiotic regimen and monitoring of blood work. Any indication of a complicated course warrants close follow-up and neurological referral. Cases of uncomplicated acute meningitis such as aseptic meningitis may require only supportive care or home IV antibiotic therapy after discharge. Patients with chronic meningitis or with neurological deficits require rehabilitation and continuous follow-up. Choice of facility depends on the nature of the patient's needs and family resources.

Patient Education: Meningitis

Education regarding prevention of meningitis through available immunization or chemoprophylaxis, as well as observance for clues to impending complications, should be provided. The meningococcal vaccine is routinely recommended for all children and adolescents aged 11 to 18 years. If not administered in childhood, adults should also be vaccinated if they are college students leaving home to live in dormitories, military personnel living in barracks, laboratory workers exposed to specimens containing meningococcus isolates, travelers going to high-risk areas, or immunocompromised people.

Home management after hospital discharge includes assessing the need for assistance with routine activities while recovering. The patient should be encouraged to have frequent rest periods and gradually increase activities while looking for signs (e.g., shortness of breath, increased pulse) that the activity is too strenuous. The diet should be well-balanced and nutritious. Soft foods may be better tolerated. Plenty of fluids should be encouraged unless other conditions are present, such as congestive heart failure or kidney disease. Acetaminophen (Tylenol) may be taken as needed for pain or headache. The patient may feel more comfortable initially in a darkened, quiet room, which will prevent discomfort related to photophobia. The importance of completing the full course of antibiotic or antiviral medications exactly as prescribed must be stressed to the patient and family/caregiver(s). The patient initially needs to avoid close contact with others to whom the infection may be transmitted. The patient should be taught about potential complications and when it is necessary to call the health-care provider, for example, if there are any signs of an upper respiratory infection, any change in alertness or wakefulness, any recurrent fever, or any other sign of a worsening illness.

ENCEPHALITIS

In contrast to meningitis, which is inflammation of the meninges surrounding the brain, encephalitis is an inflammation of the parenchymal brain tissue. Symptoms and signs include fever and other systemic signs of infection, depressed level of consciousness, seizures, and focal neurological signs. Often, there are also associated signs of meningeal irritation such as headache and neck stiffness. Both conditions frequently occur together, which is referred to as *meningoencephalitis*. Whereas bacterial meningitis can cause signs of brain parenchyma involvement (new-onset seizures, focal neurological signs, and depressed level of consciousness), aseptic meningitis does not.

EPIDEMIOLOGY AND CAUSES

There are more than 100 infectious, postinfectious, and immune-mediated conditions known to cause encephalitis. Encephalitis remains a public health concern, with approximately 20,000 cases occurring annually in the United States. Worldwide, the cause of encephalitis is unknown for 37% to 85% of encephalitis cases. Viral pathogens are the most common with herpes simplex virus (HSV) being the most common cause of sporadic encephalitis. With overall mortality due to encephalitis averaging between 5% and 20% and with residual neurological deficits occurring in an additional 20% of cases, treatment and supportive care become important. Although most cases of encephalitis are viral, there are many nonviral infectious agents responsible for encephalitis including syphilis, *Rickettsia rickettsii* (responsible for Rocky Mountain spotted fever), mycoplasma, *Cryptococcus neoformans*, Lyme disease (*Borrelia burgdorferi*), and *Mycobacterium tuberculosis*.

Autoimmune encephalitis has a wide range of clinical presentations, and many causative autoantibodies have been discovered. Some antibodies are associated with underlying malignancies, known as *paraneoplastic encephalitis*. Common autoimmune encephalitides are outlined in Table 10.2.

Encephalitis may occur at any age, but very young children and older adults are at the highest risk. The incidence of encephalitis has been reduced, especially in children, by the elimination of smallpox and by vaccines against mumps, measles, and rubella. There is no significant ethnic predisposition, and encephalitis occurs equally among males and females. Arboviruses (carried by arthropods, such as mosquitoes) can cause seasonal epidemic encephalitis. These agents include Zika, West Nile virus, and the Eastern and Western equine encephalitis viruses.

PATHOPHYSIOLOGY

Patients typically present with encephalopathy, infectious symptoms, and diffuse or focal neurological symptoms. Encephalitis is often accompanied by inflammation of the meninges; therefore, headache and nuchal rigidity are also frequent symptoms. Encephalitis can produce a range of focal neurological problems, including seizures, muscle weakness or paralysis, and isolated cranial nerve palsies. Sometimes the inflammation disrupts the hypothalamic-pituitary axis, which can lead to diabetes insipidus, SIADH, or the inability to maintain a normal body temperature. When the infective agent is the HSV, the encephalitis has a predilection for the temporal lobes, and therefore it can cause memory problems, hallucinations, aphasia, and seizures.

Encephalitis is usually caused by a virus (in the United States, the most common cause is HSV), and the neurological signs and symptoms of encephalitis are usually preceded by other signs of viral infection, such as fever, malaise, muscle aches, rashes, gastrointestinal disturbances, or respiratory symptoms. Encephalitis viruses enter the body through a number of routes: HSV is transmitted through

TABLE 10.2 Common Autoimmune and Paraneoplastic Encephalitis Syndromes

Antibody	Typical Clinical Presentation	Common Tumor Association
NMDAR	Seizures, psychosis, limbic encephalitis, autonomic dysfunction	Ovarian teratoma
LGI1	Limbic encephalitis, faciobrachial dystonic seizures (pathognomonic), hyponatremia	Thymoma
Anti-Hu (ANNA-1)	Encephalomyelitis, cerebellar degeneration, sensory neuronopathy, and/or autonomic dysfunction	SCLC
Anti-Yo (PCA-1)	Cerebellar degeneration	Gynecological, breast
Anti-Ri (ANNA-2)	Cerebellar degeneration, brainstem encephalitis, opsoclonus-myoclonus	Breast, gynecological, SCLC
Anti-Ma (Ma1, Ma2)	Limbic and brainstem encephalitis	Testicular, lung, other solid tumors

Abbreviations: NMDAR: *NN*-methyl-D-aspartate receptor; LGI1: leucine-rich glioma inactivated 1; SCLC: small cell lung cancer.

person-to-person contact, enteroviruses are swallowed and invade through the gut, arboviruses are introduced by bites of insects, rabies enters through bites of mammals, and varicella-zoster virus is inhaled. In most cases, the viruses replicate, a viremia develops, and virus particles enter the CNS from the bloodstream. Some viruses (rabies, HSV, and varicella-zoster), however, are carried into the CNS in a retrograde fashion via axons.

The brain areas that sustain the most damage vary, and different causative agents have specific predilection for certain areas of the brain. Signs and symptoms also vary, depending on the affected areas of the brain. Seizures are common. When the brainstem becomes infected, coma or respiratory failure can result.

CLINICAL PRESENTATION

Subjective

Patients commonly present with confusion, alteration in level of consciousness, symptoms of meningeal irritation (headache, neck stiffness, photophobia), lethargy, behavioral or personality changes, amnesia, and/or lethargy.

Herpes simplex encephalitis caused by HSV may be heralded by bizarre behavior, aphasia, or hallucinations because the temporal and frontal lobes are selectively attacked by the virus. Other types of infectious agents (other herpes viruses, Lyme disease, varicella-zoster virus, *R rickettsii*) may produce a cutaneous rash in addition to neurological signs such as headache, seizures, or nuchal rigidity. The rash is a typical feature of many viral diseases.

Objective

Physical examination may reveal a fever, nuchal rigidity, hemiparesis, cranial nerve palsy, ataxia, movement disorders, focal seizures, encephalopathy, systemic signs of infection, and rash.

DIAGNOSTIC REASONING

Diagnostic Tests

Epidemiological clues and assessment of risk factors to identify potential etiological agents should be sought in all patients with encephalitis. When encephalitis is suspected, the patient should be referred to the collaborating physician and to a neurologist. Hospitalization is often required for work-up and treatment. Cultures of body fluid specimens (e.g., from blood, stool, nasopharynx, or sputum), if clinical and epidemiological clues are suggestive, should be performed to identify various viral, bacterial, and fungal etiologies of encephalitis. CSF testing reveals increased WBCs and an increased protein level. A Gram stain of CSF is useful to assess for bacterial meningitis as the cause of the symptoms. Polymerase chain reaction (PCR) tests of numerous common viral pathogens are commercially available and may identify the viral type. Serum antibody testing performed early in the infectious course and compared with a specimen drawn 1 to 3 weeks after onset of illness can reveal a significant increase in the antibody titer. Brain imaging is helpful to assess parenchymal involvement and rule out other causes of focal neurological signs (such as stroke and hemorrhage). Imaging can also provide clues to etiology; for example, HSV encephalitis commonly causes hemorrhagic necrosis in the frontal and temporal lobes. However, normal brain imaging does not rule out encephalitis.

Because changes in the CSF may not be apparent at the beginning of the infection, a repeat LP may be indicated if the first is negative and suspicion remains high. Electroencephalogram is nonspecific in establishing an etiology but has a role in identifying seizures, including nonconvulsive seizure activity, in patients who are confused, obtunded, or comatose.

Differential Diagnoses

There is significant overlap between organisms that cause aseptic meningitis and encephalitis. Therefore, patients often present with meningoencephalitis, with features of both meningeal irritation and brain parenchymal involvement. To differentiate meningitis from encephalitis (or meningoencephalitis), one must assess for signs of brain involvement such as confusion, seizures, or focal signs on examination. Encephalitis can also be postinfectious or autoimmune in etiology. Postinfectious encephalitis is part of acute demyelinating encephalomyelitis, which causes areas of demyelination in the brain and spinal cord after an infection. Autoimmune encephalitis is often, but not always, part of a paraneoplastic process. Identification and treatment of the underlying tumor is important for diagnosis and treatment. Anti-*N*-methyl-D-aspartate receptor encephalitis is one of the most common of the autoimmune encephalopathies and is typically associated with ovarian teratomas. Psychiatric manifestations are common early in the course of the disease. Seizures are also common in this population.

MANAGEMENT

A suspicion of encephalitis requires referral and patient hospitalization for definitive neurological diagnosis and treatment. Treatment includes antimicrobials, supportive care, and efforts to prevent complications.

If viral encephalitis is suspected, patients should be promptly started on treatment with IV acyclovir while awaiting further work-up because empirical treatment reduces both morbidity and mortality in HSV encephalitis.

Seizures should be treated with anticonvulsants like phenytoin (Dilantin), levetiracetam (Keppra), or other antiseizure medications. Safety must also be a consideration with these patients. Padding should be used to prevent seizure injury. Acetaminophen (Tylenol) is used to reduce hyperthermia and may be given as a rectal suppository if needed. Cerebral edema resulting in increased intracranial pressure is an ominous complication of encephalitis and can be treated with hyperosmolar therapy, hyperventilation, or neurosurgical intervention.

FOLLOW-UP AND REFERRAL

Patients suspected of having encephalitis are referred to the emergency department for urgent work-up and treatment and to a neurologist for definitive care and follow-up. When the patient is stabilized, the neurologist will release the patient's care to the primary care provider. The relative degree of neurological deficit determines the nature of follow-up care.

Patient Education: Encephalitis

Prevention of infection vectors through mosquito control and insect repellents should be one important focus of patient and community education. Early detection and proper removal of ticks are other important aspects. For convalescence, the importance of rest, fluids, rehabilitation, and nutrition is emphasized, as well as clues to impending complications. The patient should be encouraged to take frequent rest periods and to increase activities gradually while looking for signs that the activity is too strenuous, for example, shortness of breath and increased pulse. The patient should be instructed to eat a balanced diet to ensure the inclusion of nutrients such as protein and vitamin C. Fluids should be encouraged unless contraindicated. Acetaminophen may be used for pain or a headache. The patient may feel more comfortable in a darkened, quiet room if photophobia is present. The importance of taking the antibiotics or antiviral medications exactly as prescribed should be stressed to the patient. Patients should be instructed to avoid close contact with others who may be harboring germs. If they notice any signs of an upper respiratory infection, they should seek help from their health-care provider immediately. In the case of tick-borne infections, patients and families should be instructed to inspect the skin for ticks and to remove them intact. They should wear protective clothing to prevent tick bites. Last, patients should be instructed when to call the health-care provider, for example, if there are any changes in level of consciousness, recurrent fever, or any other signs of a worsening illness.

HERPES ZOSTER

Herpes zoster, commonly known as *shingles*, is an infection by the varicella-zoster virus occurring along dermatomal pathways and resulting in a vesicular skin rash.

EPIDEMIOLOGY AND CAUSES

Varicella-zoster virus becomes latent in the neurons of sensory ganglia after a primary infection of chickenpox; it then reactivates later in life in a dermatomal area as herpes zoster (shingles). One in three individuals in the United States will develop shingles. An estimated 1 million cases occur each year. Children may get shingles; however, the risk of disease increases with age; approximately one half of all cases occur in people aged 60 and over. Four percent of patients with herpes zoster experience a second episode but rarely a third. Immunocompromised patients are at a significantly increased risk for developing shingles, and they also have a higher incidence of complications.

PATHOPHYSIOLOGY

Varicella-zoster virus, which causes chickenpox, is also responsible for a number of neurological disorders, including encephalitis, meningitis, polyneuritis, multiple cranial neuropathies, and myelitis. Varicella-zoster virus initially infects people through the mucosa of the upper respiratory tract or the conjunctivae of the eyes. Within a week, the virus spreads throughout the body via the bloodstream, and approximately 1 week later, infections of the capillaries of the skin produce the vesicular lesions of chickenpox.

Once the lesions appear, virus particles are retrogradely transported inside sensory axons to dorsal root ganglia, where the viruses remain latent for the life of the patient. Varicella-zoster virus is most often found in the sensory ganglia of the ophthalmic division of the trigeminal nerve and in the dorsal root ganglia of the mid to lower spinal cord (ganglia T3 to L2). If viruses in a ganglion are reactivated, they replicate, destroy ganglion nerve cells, and migrate through the nerves to the innervated dermatomes, where they again produce vesicular skin lesions.

The destruction of sensory neurons in a ganglion produces pain in the innervated dermatome. This pain usually precedes the skin lesions by a few days, although sometimes pain is the only symptom. Typically, viruses are reactivated in only a single ganglion at a time; therefore, the symptoms are unilateral and affect a single dermatome. When the pain does not resolve within a few weeks, the syndrome is called *postherpetic neuralgia* (PHN). The pain of PHN can be either constant or intermittent, and it worsens at night and during temperature changes. Varicella-zoster virus that has been reactivated in the ophthalmic division of the trigeminal nerve can cause eye problems, including lesions of the cornea.

It is not known what triggers the reactivation of latent varicella-zoster viruses. The likelihood of developing this reactivation syndrome (called "herpes zoster" or "shingles") increases as a person ages and when a person's immune system becomes compromised. Herpes zoster is a frequent complication of HIV infection.

CLINICAL PRESENTATION

Subjective

Initially, the patient with herpes zoster may present with unexplained pain. The pain is described as constant or intermittent and may have a tingling or stabbing quality. The pain occurs along the involved dermatome, usually 48 to 72 hours before eruption of the classic vesicular skin rash. Pain acuity differs among individuals, but many patients say the pain becomes progressively worse at night or with changes in temperature. Herpes zoster ophthalmicus is a common complication of shingles in the V_1 distribution of the trigeminal nerve. This condition can cause blindness and requires immediate referral to an ophthalmologist for evaluation and treatment. Ocular involvement is more common in patients who have concurrent lesions at the tip of the nose, referred to as *Hutchinson sign*. Lesions located inside the mouth and in the external ear opening are often associated with unilateral facial weakness, vertigo, and hearing loss due to involvement of cranial nerves VII and VIII; this is referred to as *Ramsay Hunt syndrome*.

Another major characteristic of the disease is the occurrence of acute neuritis along the path of the rash dermatome. PHN occurs in approximately 25% to 50% of patients older than 60 years.

Objective

Herpes zoster is characterized by a unilateral vesicular rash along a dermatome, most commonly a thoracic or lumbar dermatome. The rash begins as erythema and then changes to papular lesions that rapidly form vesicles. The vesicles rupture, releasing infectious fluid, and then form scabs. Occasionally, the vesicles coalesce to form bullae. The skin lesions usually continue to develop for 3 to 5 days, and the entire disease course usually lasts 10 to 15 days. In some individuals, the skin lesions can persist for 30 days or longer. The pain caused by PHN may last much longer and at times may be permanent.

DIAGNOSTIC REASONING

Diagnostic Tests

Diagnosis is made after careful review of data obtained from the history and physical examination. The characteristic appearance and distribution of the lesions along with a history of preceding neuropathic pain help establish the diagnosis of herpes zoster. Usually the history and physical examination are all that are needed to make a definitive diagnosis.

If the diagnosis is questionable, a PCR assay, which detects the DNA sequence of the virus, may be done, along with an antibody titer (which requires more than one test for comparison). CSF analysis may be needed when CNS involvement is suspected.

Differential Diagnosis

Other conditions that cause similar rashes need to be ruled out. Impetigo may present as vesicles around an area of broken skin. The scrapings of these lesions can be sent for a Gram stain, which will reveal gram-positive cocci if Staphylococcus or Streptococcus bacteria are present. Viral cultures may be done to rule out HSV or Coxsackievirus infections that can appear in a dermatomal region. Cellulitis, bites and stings, candidiasis, and drug eruptions should all be ruled out.

MANAGEMENT

The principal goals are to manage the healed vesicles, obtain pain relief, and prevent secondary infection and other complications. Initial management of herpes zoster involves the use of antiviral agents. They reduce the impact of herpes zoster by diminishing neuritis and speeding the healing of the skin lesions. Early intervention in the treatment of herpes zoster produces the best results, and antiviral therapy should be started within the first 72 hours of symptom onset. Famciclovir (Famvir), acyclovir (Zovirax), or valacyclovir (Valtrex) may be used. Systemic corticosteroids such as prednisone were previously used in conjunction with antiviral therapy to prevent PHN. However, further research with a meta-analysis concluded that corticosteroids are ineffective at preventing PHN, and thus they are not recommended for the treatment of uncomplicated herpes zoster.

Skin lesions should be kept clean, dry, and covered to prevent secondary bacterial skin infection and spread of the varicella virus to others. Patients with ophthalmic herpes affecting the first branch of the trigeminal nerve must be referred to an ophthalmologist because this condition may result in blindness.

PHN is a persistent pain resulting from shingles that lasts more than 3 months after the disease has run its course. PHN rarely occurs in individuals younger than age 40, is more severe in individuals older than age 50, and may occur in up to one-half of untreated people over age 60. Even with treatment, PHN may occur. Analgesics (from nonnarcotic to narcotic agents in doses individualized for the patient) can reduce acute pain from neuritis and PHN. If PHN is present, the use of tricyclic antidepressants such as nortriptyline or amitriptyline taken each night may help if simple analgesics are ineffective and can be used long-term. For additional pain relief, gabapentin (Neurontin) may help. Topical capsaicin cream is approved by the U.S. Food and Drug Administration (FDA) for relief of PHN. Topical lidocaine patches may be helpful. If pain is persistent, chronic PHN may respond to a regional block with or without corticosteroids. Ideally, the patient should be referred to a pain center because PHN can have devastating effects (see The Patient's Voice 10.1.)

Geriatric Considerations:
Herpes Zoster

About half of all cases of shingles affect people older than 60 years. It is crucial to diagnose shingles early. The classic symptom is unexplained pain in the area 2 to 3 days prior to the vesicular skin rash. If not diagnosed at this early stage, it is easy to diagnose shingles because the rash only occurs on half of the body following the dermatomes and stops at midline on the body. The worst scenario is herpes zoster ophthalmicus, which may present as a lesion on the tip of the nose and may lead to blindness. It is essential to refer to an ophthalmologist as soon as this is seen.

Because PHN occurs in about 25% to 50% of older patients, treatment consisting of antiviral agents should be started early. See The Patient's Voice 10.1 for a devastating story of one woman's experience with PHN.

FOLLOW-UP AND REFERRAL

It is essential that any patient with ophthalmic herpetic lesions be referred to an ophthalmologist. Additional follow-up includes a return visit if skin lesions become infected or if PHN is present. Referral to a dermatologist may be required at any time if the patient does not respond to primary treatment plans. If neurological complications such as weakness occur, the patient should be referred to a neurologist and may require inpatient hospitalization. Patients should be referred to a pain center if PHN results in chronic persistent pain.

Patient Education: Herpes Zoster

Because herpes zoster is usually treated on an outpatient basis, patient and family/caregiver education is important. The clinician should encourage patients to complete the course of the antiviral agent, even if they feel the disease has abated or they feel the

---

The Patient's Voice 10.1: Postherpetic Neuralgia

My mother died of postherpetic neuralgia (PHN).

My mother was 80 years old and had recently won the golf championship at her club. She had been a widow for 25 years and decided that she wanted to move in with me, her daughter, and her only granddaughter (age 3). We lived 4 hours away. At first, she was very independent, driving around by herself and going shopping while I worked. That only lasted a few months. Then the decline began. First, she broke a wrist, which incapacitated her, and then she got pneumonia, which weakened her. Then she got "shingles" (herpes zoster), which did her in. She was diagnosed at the earliest onset of pain, yet treatment wasn't started until the vesicles erupted. She had ophthalmic herpes, so her vision was affected. She developed PHN very early, and due to the persistent pain, she became reclusive. She stopped going out, retreating to her room, and eventually wouldn't get out of bed. Nothing helped the pain. I'm convinced it was because preventive treatment wasn't started early. As she became more depressed and stayed in bed, she got weaker and weaker and just gave up. She complained of shooting pain over half of her head that was worse at night, so she'd be awake all night, and sleep all day. Nobody could help—not her primary care provider, neurologist, ophthalmologist, psychologist, or me. She died in her sleep, and I'm convinced it was the result of PHN.

I've learned three things from this experience. First, if older persons are optimally functioning, don't move them out of their familiar supportive environment. Second, treat all cases of herpes aggressively, as you don't know who is going to develop PHN. As my mom used to say, "An ounce of prevention is worth a pound of cure." This leads to the third, probably most important lesson: get every older adult vaccinated!

treatment is not as effective as they had hoped it would be. Patients should be informed that elimination of the disease could take longer than anticipated, and careful medication administration and follow-up care could mean fewer complications in the long run. Patients should be instructed that the medication may be better tolerated if taken with food. If adverse effects from the treatment plan occur, patients need to keep the practitioner informed so adjustments can be made. Education on the potential for spread of the herpes zoster virus via fluid from ruptured vesicles is important. Patients should be instructed that before the rash crusts, it can release fluid that will cause an infection in others. Patients must be careful in handling dressings, linens, towels, and clothes that they have used. They should not be around children who have not been vaccinated for chickenpox or those who have not had chickenpox yet; contact with pregnant females should also be avoided. Patients need to know that scratching the rash can lead to a bacterial skin infection. Patients should be instructed about the nature of the rash so that when they see it in varying stages of progression, they will not think that it is not healing. Again, the importance of completing all prescribed medications needs to be stressed. Patients need to know the reason they are taking other medications (for example, antidepressants that can treat PHN) so that they will continue taking them.

Research has shown that the shingles vaccine Zostavax has reduced the occurrence of shingles in people aged 60 and older and offers more than 50% protection. In addition, it reduces the incidence of PHN by almost 70%. The Advisory Committee on Immunization Practices recommends a single dose of Zostavax for adults aged 60 and older, even if they have already had shingles. The FDA has approved the vaccine for people older than age 50 years. Immunocompromised individuals should not receive the vaccine. Shingrix (Zoster Vaccine Recombinant, Adjuvanted) has proven to be more effective (at 97%) than Zostavax. It is recommended for those over age 50 years for the prevention of herpes zoster. It is given intramuscularly once, followed by another injection in 2 to 6 months. It may also be given to patients who have already received Zostavax.

TRIGEMINAL NEURALGIA

Trigeminal neuralgia is a distressing, painful idiopathic disorder of the trigeminal nerve (cranial nerve V). It is also known as *tic douloureux*. This excruciating facial pain is paroxysmal and usually lasts less than 3 seconds. For many individuals, the severity of the pain is disabling, and patients will do almost anything to prevent triggering an episode.

The lancinating, sharply cutting pain occurs along one or more of the three branches of the trigeminal nerve. Characteristically, the painful episodes occur when specific trigger zones are stimulated by touch, chewing, talking, shaving, or environmental temperature changes. Patients often describe the pain as "electric" or "stabbing" and penetrating. The pain of trigeminal neuralgia is chronic. Although patients may experience periods of spontaneous pain remission that may last weeks or months, the pain usually returns.

EPIDEMIOLOGY AND CAUSES

Trigeminal neuralgia occurs more frequently in females than in males and more often in individuals older than age 50. The incidence is 12 per 100,000 of the general population per year. A higher incidence of risk occurs in individuals with hypertension and multiple sclerosis (MS). These at-risk individuals are much younger than the characteristic age of patients with trigeminal neuralgia.

PATHOPHYSIOLOGY

Trigeminal neuralgia is sometimes caused by compression by a nearby artery and secondary demyelination of axons in the fifth cranial nerve, the trigeminal nerve. It is also associated with demyelination caused by MS. The trigeminal nerve has three main branches: V_1, the ophthalmic branch, which transmits sensation from the eye region and forehead; V_2, the maxillary branch, which transmits sensation from the midface and upper jaw; and V_3; the mandibular branch, which transmits sensation from the lower jaw. The neuron cell bodies for the sensory axons in these nerves are located in the trigeminal ganglion, which is inside the skull along the floor of the middle cranial fossa.

Trigeminal neuralgia most often affects the mandibular or maxillary branch of the trigeminal nerve. The problem tends to occur in middle-aged and older people. Patients with MS, another demyelinating syndrome, are affected by trigeminal neuralgia with a higher frequency than the rest of the population.

CLINICAL PRESENTATION

Subjective

The patient with trigeminal neuralgia presents with complaints of severe paroxysms of pain on one side of the face. The pain lasts for a few seconds, with no ache or pain between occurrences, and follows the trigeminal nerve distribution. The patient's history includes triggers of the pain including chewing, talking, brushing teeth, touching the face, or, in some cases, after physical activity, lowering of the head, and wind touching the face. The patient's history may include periods of remission with or without medical treatment.

During periods of exacerbation, the patient may be totally disabled by the severity of the pain. Patients may report refraining from eating, sleep deprivation, depression, and even suicidal thoughts, which reflect their willingness to go to great extremes to escape the severe paroxysmal pain.

Objective

On physical examination, the cranial nerves, specifically the trigeminal nerve, have normal motor and sensory function; facial muscle strength and reflexes are normal. Clinically, the cardinal signs of idiopathic trigeminal neuralgia are elicited when a facial trigger point is stimulated; the patient experiences a sharp, electric-type pain that follows the distribution of the trigeminal nerve and lasts for only a few seconds, and the patient's face grimaces. After the painful attack, there is usually no residual pain; however, patients with longstanding trigeminal neuralgia may have a constant dull pain present between spasms. Because of the many pathological and etiological theories regarding trigeminal neuralgia, the clinician must be alert to the characteristic symptoms of typical (idiopathic) trigeminal neuralgia. These are short periods of paroxysmal pain associated with triggers, pain limited to the distribution of the trigeminal nerve branches, and a normal neurological examination.

DIAGNOSTIC REASONING

Diagnostic Tests

Idiopathic trigeminal neuralgia can often be diagnosed based on clinical history that describes paroxysmal pain episodes triggered by specific activities in patients characteristically older than age 50.

Most patients undergo brain MRI as part of their work-up of trigeminal neuralgia to evaluate for underlying tumor or multiple sclerosis. This may or may not show vascular compression of the trigeminal nerve.

Differential Diagnosis

There are many causes for the general presentation of orofacial pain. These conditions can usually be categorized as inflammatory (e.g., dental pathology, sinusitis, parotitis, sialolithiasis, temporal arteritis, HSV), neurological (e.g., trigeminal, glossopharyngeal, or paratrigeminal neuralgia; cluster or migraine headaches; meningiomas; posterior fossa tumors), or musculoskeletal (e.g., temporomandibular joint pain, myofascial pain dysfunction syndrome). It is important, therefore, to identify whether the clinical presentation is either typical trigeminal neuralgia or some other orofacial pain.

MANAGEMENT

The major principles in the management of trigeminal neuralgia are to (1) elicit a remission by drug therapy, (2) prevent adverse effects in patients resulting from prescribed medications, and (3) help the patient avoid triggering painful episodes. Trigeminal neuralgia is a chronic condition that results in the need for the patient's chronic pain to be managed. In addition to interventions related to establishing remission and avoidance of painful episodes, the patient's psychological needs—related to depression, isolation, and possible suicidal thoughts—are significant areas in the plan of care.

Initially, pharmacological management is to initiate remission of the pain. Carbamazepine or oxcarbazepine are recommended as first-line agents for trigeminal neuralgia. If ineffective, alternative medications such as gabapentin, lamotrigine, or baclofen can be used. If the patient experiences good pain relief from the medication, it should continue while the patient is pain free for at least 6 weeks before attempting to slowly taper off.

Follow-up for complications of drug therapy with anticonvulsants is essential in the pharmacological management of typical trigeminal neuralgia. Carbamazepine has many potential adverse effects, including nausea, vomiting, dizziness, diplopia, skin rash, blood dyscrasias (aplastic anemia, agranulocytosis, thrombocytopenia, and leukopenia), fever, and chills.

In refractory cases, surgical management can be considered. The unrelenting paroxysmal pain of idiopathic trigeminal neuralgia is caused by vascular compression of the trigeminal nerve root. Microvascular decompression is performed to relieve the compression, although recurrence in 1 to 2 years is common after surgery, regardless of the surgical method chosen.

FOLLOW-UP AND REFERRAL

Because of the intense and chronic pain associated with trigeminal neuralgia, the patient may experience depression, social isolation, and suicidal ideation. The clinician must recognize these effects of the disease and reinforce coping mechanisms the patient may use during periods of exacerbation. Referral for counseling may be required if the patient is not able to cope with the chronicity and severity of the pain.

Patient Education: Trigeminal Neuralgia

The goals of patient instruction are the avoidance of triggering painful events, pharmacological management, and coping with chronic, severe pain. Nutritional counseling should encourage intake of soft or puréed, high-caloric foods, along with increased fluids. For hygiene, the use of soft washcloths and mouthwashes should be encouraged. Patients should be educated about adverse reactions (e.g., dizziness, sleepiness, ataxia, nausea, and vomiting) to their medications and about the necessity for follow-up blood studies to detect any blood dyscrasias. Intense counseling and supportive education are a continuous process in caring for the patient with trigeminal neuralgia. Recognition of the patient's educational needs based on their coping mechanisms, search for pain treatment, and the status of the neuralgia will direct the clinician in establishing an individualized plan.

BELL'S PALSY

Bell's palsy is an idiopathic cranial nerve VII palsy causing lower motor neuron facial paralysis, typically occurring on one side of the face. The peripheral facial palsy is self-limiting, and complete recovery usually occurs in a few weeks or months in 80% to 86% of patients. Initially, the facial paralysis may be incomplete and then worsen within 48 hours after onset. The sudden experience of facial paralysis can be frightening to the patient, who usually seeks medical care immediately.

EPIDEMIOLOGY AND CAUSES

The cause of Bell's palsy is most likely viral, typically from HSV infection. Approximately 40,000 individuals each year in the United States are affected by Bell's palsy. Males and females are affected equally, but it is less common in people younger than 15 years or older than 45 years. A higher incidence is seen in individuals with diabetes, hypertension, trauma, toxin exposure, Lyme disease, HIV, pregnancy, and those with upper respiratory ailments.

Recovery from facial paralysis usually occurs over 3 to 6 months. People at risk for incomplete recovery are those older than 55 or who have hypertension, experience pain other than ear pain, have complete facial paralysis, or have changes in lacrimation.

PATHOPHYSIOLOGY

Cranial nerve VII—the facial nerve—is mainly a motor nerve innervating the muscles of facial expression. It also has a small sensory component providing taste to the anterior two-thirds of the tongue and sensation to part of the external auditory canal. Its preganglionic, parasympathetic axons innervate the lacrimal and nasopalatine glands and all the salivary glands except the parotid.

The various classes of axons in the facial nerve peel off group by group as the nerve makes its way through the bony canals of the skull; therefore, pressure on or lesions of the nerve at different locations will produce different deficits. Inside the skull, the facial nerve runs with cranial nerve VIII, and lesions here may cause hearing loss and vestibular problems in addition to deficits in all the motor and sensory components of the facial nerve. Within the skull wall, the facial and vestibulocochlear nerves separate. After this, the first components to leave the facial nerve are the lacrimal and nasopalatine axons; therefore, damage to the facial nerve distal to this juncture will not affect a patient's ability to produce tears. The chorda tympani branch, which includes taste axons and the axons to the salivary glands, branches off next; therefore, damage to the facial nerve distal to this juncture will cause unilateral paralysis of all the muscles of facial expression but will not affect taste or the production of saliva. Most cases are thought to be caused by a reactivated herpes simplex infection of the geniculate ganglion, which leads to inflammation and swelling of the nerve inside its restrictive bony canal. Reactivated varicella-zoster virus can also cause Bell's palsy; this type also causes a rash in the external auditory canal or palate and can involve cranial nerve VIII, leading to hearing loss and vertigo.

CLINICAL PRESENTATION

Subjective

Patients with Bell's palsy present with an acute onset of partial or total paralysis on one side of the face that may worsen over a couple days. The patient has normal ocular movements. They may experience loss of taste (dysgeusia) on their ipsilateral tongue, postauricular pain, abnormal sensitivity to sound (hyperacusis), and a heavy feeling in the face.

Objective

On physical examination, the motor and sensory functions along the entire facial nerve should be assessed. Hallmarks of Bell's palsy are its acute onset and the fact that no other CNS symptoms exist. The physical assessment characteristically reveals the absence of forehead wrinkles on the affected side, wider palpebral fissure of the eye with weakness of eye closure, decreased corneal reflex, Bell's phenomenon (the eyeball turns upward when the patient tries to close the eyelid), flattening of the nasolabial fold, and loss of taste on the anterior two-thirds of the tongue. Lacrimation may or may not be affected. During the history, it is important to ask about pregnancy, diabetes, any recent infection, and rash.

A patient with Bell's palsy typically is unable to make the following movements on the affected side on request: raise the eyebrow, wrinkle the forehead, close the eyelid, whistle, or smile. When talking, the patient's cheek puffs out, and there is an inability to clearly pronounce words that require pursing of the lips. There appears to be a deviation of the tongue because of mouth paralysis on the affected side (although tongue deviation is not present when comparing tongue protrusion relative to the teeth). The patient is unable to suck or hold fluids in the mouth but is able to swallow.

Close inspection of the patient's ears and palate is done to assess for herpes zoster lesions that would indicate Ramsay Hunt syndrome, which is herpes zoster affecting the facial and auditory nerves, causing facial palsy and cutaneous herpes zoster lesions of the external ear, palate, and/or tympanic membrane. Associated symptoms include tinnitus, vertigo, and deafness.

DIAGNOSTIC REASONING

Diagnostic Tests

Diagnosis is based primarily on patient history and clinical examination. If the history and physical examination are inconclusive for Bell's palsy, the patient should be referred for further diagnostic work-up. A CT scan or MRI with contrast can rule out a tumor, stroke, MS, or other structural lesions.

Documentation of the extent of facial function at the time of initial diagnosis and at subsequent assessments is important to evaluate the course of the disease. The progression or lack of progression of the symptoms is important to differentiate Bell's palsy from other pathology.

Differential Diagnosis

Tumors, infections (HIV, infectious mononucleosis, Lyme disease), Guillain-Barré syndrome (GBS), trauma, stroke, sarcoidosis, and other inflammatory conditions can cause unilateral facial weakness that may appear similar to Bell's palsy. The history and physical examination are important to exclude other causes of facial weakness.

Damage to the facial nerve inside the skull wall can be caused by skull fractures, hemangiomas, tumors, and inflammation. When the facial nerve is damaged and no structural problems are found, the condition is called Bell's palsy. Bell's palsy always produces unilateral facial paralysis, and depending on the location of the nerve lesion, it may also include deficits in functions of the other components of the facial nerve.

In addition, a Bell's palsy–like facial paralysis is the most common neurological problem caused by Lyme disease, although this is often bilateral.

MANAGEMENT

The majority of patients with Bell's palsy will recover without treatment, although treatment with steroids starting within the first few days of symptom onset improves recovery and is recommended. Treatment with antiviral medications is controversial. Some practitioners prescribe antiviral medications in cases of particularly severe Bell's palsy and in cases of Ramsay Hunt syndrome.

Because Bell's palsy causes weakness of eye closure, it is important to protect the eye from injury, particularly during sleep. Loss of the ability to blink and close the eyelid subjects the cornea to drying and ulceration. The patient is instructed to keep the eye moist by topical application of artificial tears frequently during the day and use of an ocular lubricant ointment and eye patch at night. An ophthalmologist should be consulted if the patient experiences any signs of corneal irritation or injury.

Ear pain can be treated with acetaminophen (Tylenol) and ibuprofen (Advil, Motrin). Rest, earplugs, and decreased auditory stimulation may lessen the effects of hyperacusis.

FOLLOW-UP AND REFERRAL

The patient should be examined at regular intervals to assess for resolution or deterioration of Bell's palsy symptoms and adverse effects of medication, if prescribed. Special attention should be given to effectiveness of eye care by the patient. If the patient's symptoms do not improve, worsen beyond the acute setting, or if other neurological signs are evident, the patient should be referred to a neurologist.

Patient Education: Bell's Palsy

The clinician should provide essential teaching that supports the recovery process. Reassurance that Bell's palsy is usually a short-term and benign condition will allay some anxiety.

In addition to meticulous eye care, the patient should be taught to perform oral hygiene vigorously because food becomes trapped, and there can be a reduced amount of saliva. Foods may also need to be spicier than normal to compensate for loss of taste. The clinician should encourage the patient to eat soft foods of high nutritional value because patients often avoid eating because of difficulty holding food in the mouth. Drinking from a plastic, spouted bottle may be easier than drinking from a cup or glass because liquid can be squeezed into the back of the mouth.

GUILLAIN-BARRÉ SYNDROME

EPIDEMIOLOGY AND CAUSES

Guillain-Barré Syndrome (GBS) is an acute monophasic immune-mediated polyradiculoneuropathy. It is usually an ascending paralysis most often beginning in the legs and then progressing in an ascending fashion. Sensation can be involved, and patients usually report tingling in the extremities. Back pain and autonomic dysfunction are also common. It affects only about one to two people per 100,000 individuals. Incidence increases with age and in winter. There are many variations of GBS. The Miller Fisher variant causes brainstem symptoms such as ataxia and eye-movement abnormalities, in addition to loss of reflexes. GBS is often postinfectious, and there is a strong association with gastric *Campylobacter* infection. It is caused by the production of antibodies that attack nerves because of molecular mimicry. GBS can be mild or severe, causing respiratory failure. Most individuals reach the stage of greatest weakness within the first 2 to 3 weeks after the symptoms appear, and 90% will reach this point by the third week. Almost 30% of patients will experience residual weakness even after 3 to 5 years.

DIAGNOSISTIC REASONING

The diagnosis is made by history and physical examination. Spinal fluid analysis can be helpful to exclude alternate diagnoses, and it typically reveals elevated protein with little or no pleocytosis. Spot urine test for porphobilinogen can rule out porphyria. Nerve conduction studies and electromyography can also help aid in the diagnosis, although they may be normal initially. MRI with contrast of the spine may show enhancement of the nerve roots.

MANAGEMENT

The treatment involves IV gamma globulin or plasmapheresis. All patients suspected of having GBS, even if the case is mild, must be referred to the emergency department because respiratory failure can develop quickly and become life-threatening.

MYASTHENIA GRAVIS

EPIDEMIOLOGY AND CAUSES

Myasthenia gravis (MG) is a disorder of the neuromuscular junction. It is an autoimmune disease in which an antibody targets the receptor for acetylcholine at the neuromuscular junction. More women are affected than men, and it occurs in approximately five to 15 individuals per 100,000. Younger females, with peak onset at age 31 to 40, and males older than 60 years are most commonly affected.

MG causes muscle fatigue and weakness that worsens with use. Eye movements and speech are commonly affected. Weakness is usually worse later in the day, and the symptoms will usually ameliorate with rest.

DIAGNOSTIC REASONING

The diagnosis is made be demonstrating fatigable weakness on examination (weakness that develops or worsens with muscle activation). Diagnosis can be supported with the Tensilon test, in which use of edrophonium chloride results in resolution of the weakness. However, given the risk for systemic side effects, this test is less commonly used in practice. The presence of autoantibodies against the acetylcholine receptor supports the diagnosis, and electromyography can confirm the diagnosis.

MANAGEMENT

Symptomatic treatment is with anticholinesterase agents, which afford temporary relief. The major side effect is gastrointestinal irritability. Immunosuppressant drugs, IV immunoglobulins, and plasmapheresis are also used to reduce antibody levels. Because MG is associated with thymoma, all patients should be screened for this condition; in some patients, thymectomy can be curative.

MULTIPLE SCLEROSIS

Multiple sclerosis (MS) is a chronic and potentially disabling demyelinating disease of the CNS that begins most commonly in young adulthood. Common symptoms include visual changes (unilateral vision loss, double vision), weakness and numbness, and loss of balance.

MS is the most common cause of disability in young adults. It causes demyelination of the brain and spinal cord, which can be seen on MRI. MS is thought to be a disorder of the T and B lymphocytes in which the body's immune system attacks the myelin coating of the nerves in the CNS.

There are three classifications of MS that differ with patterns of progression:

- *Relapsing–remitting* MS is characterized by acute attacks, with recovery (either partial or full between episodes).
- *Primary progressive* MS has a steady disease progression from onset, with possibly some plateaus and remissions.
- *Secondary progressive* MS is a combination of the first two types, beginning as a relapsing–remitting disease but then transitioning to a progressive course.

MS phenotypes can be further described by disease activity. MS is active if there are clinical relapses or if contrast enhancement (which demonstrates active inflammation) is seen on MRI.

The clinical course of MS varies between patients. Prognosis is a common concern. Although there are no definitive prognostic indicators, the following are general guidelines. Good prognostic indicators include minimal disability after 5 years of onset, complete and rapid remission of initial symptoms, onset at age 35 or younger, only one symptom during the first year, acute onset of the first symptoms, brief duration of most recent exacerbation, long first remission, optic neuritis, or sensory symptoms. Poor prognostic indicators include late onset, chronic progressive course, motor symptoms, polysymptomatic onset, and vertigo. After 15 years, 50% to 60% of patients with MS remain ambulatory, 10% to 20% need assistance devices to ambulate, and 15% to 30% are bedridden.

EPIDEMIOLOGY AND CAUSES

MS occurs worldwide, but there are differences in both incidence and prevalence on the basis of race, sex, genetics, geographical location, and age at the time of probable exposure to a virus or other infectious agent. MS is most commonly diagnosed between ages 20 and 50 years, with a median onset at age 30. The first symptoms of the disease usually occur between ages 20 and 40. If the disease is diagnosed after age 50, it tends to have a more progressive course. The disease affects two to three times more women than men. It is more common among whites and people of northern or central European descent. People of Asian and African descent are at lower risk. About 450,000 people have MS in the United States.

Although the exact cause of MS is unknown, it is likely to be multifactorial. Some epidemiological findings suggest a relationship between MS and an unknown environmental factor, possibly a viral exposure during childhood. This exposure may lead to the entry of immune cells into the CNS, where a population of T cells becomes sensitized to a CNS antigen. After years of latency, an environmental agent may lead to an upregulation of circulating mediators or T-cell activation that may trigger an episode of demyelination and clinical disease. Other possible causes include genetic susceptibility, autoimmune mechanisms, and viral infections. One leading hypothesis is that of a cell-mediated immunopathological response directed against myelin in genetically predisposed people.

The possibility that susceptibility to MS is inherited is supported by its higher incidence in twins and in certain families. The major histocompatibility complex (MHC) on chromosome 6 has been identified as one genetic determinant for MS. Although genetic factors may contribute to an individual's susceptibility, they are neither sufficient nor necessary for development of MS. Clinical expression of the disease is likely to require additional exposure to one or more environmental factors, which are as of-yet undefined.

There is evidence of autoimmune mechanisms in the pathogenesis of MS. In a normal immune response, foreign antibodies are processed and presented to helper T cells by antigen-presenting cells and macrophages. These T-helper cells recognize foreign peptides bound to MHC molecules, become activated, and release various cytokines, tumor necrosis factor, and interleukins that augment the immune response to a particular antigen. These particular class II MHC molecules are usually found only on cells involved in an immune response. In MS, class II MHC induction has been shown to occur in CNS tissue. In peripheral blood of patients with MS, several nonspecific changes are seen that are similar to those in other autoimmune diseases. Suppressor T lymphocytes are decreased in both function and number. Excessive immunoglobulin is present, especially high levels of immunoglobulin G (IgG). Suppressor cell inducers are decreased in many patients with progressive disease.

PATHOPHYSIOLOGY

MS is a disease of the CNS stemming from progressive, patchy demyelination of axons. In MS, local immune reactions destroy CNS myelin and cause the death of oligodendrocytes, the cells that make myelin. Astrocytes react to these injuries by proliferating. At the same time, many of the axons remain intact.

MS is most commonly characterized by neurologic problems that periodically flare up and then abate. The symptoms reflect repeated episodes of demyelination in new parts of the white matter throughout the CNS. The specific neurological deficits of an MS patient depend on the regions of the CNS that have been affected. For example, lesions in the optic nerve produce unilateral vision loss, lesions in the corticospinal tracts produce weakness, lesions in the posterior column of the spinal cord produce unusual sensations or numbness, lesions in the medial longitudinal fasciculus produce double vision, and lesions in the vestibular pathways produce vertigo.

Areas of MS damage form sharply defined plaques, which are typically found around venules. MS plaques tend to be large (greater than 6 mm in diameter) and oval shaped; over time, the plaques become more widely distributed. Newly forming plaques, in which demyelination is not yet complete, are filled with lymphocytes, plasma cells, and macrophages. Older plaques have no myelin in their centers and contain only fibrous astrocytes and unmyelinated axons. Axon damage inevitably follows, but this appears to be a secondary phenomenon and occurs slowly. Between the plaques, myelin is also affected, although here the damage is not as dramatic.

MS plaques are the result of immune reactions, and the state of the disease is reflected in the immune indicators in the CSF. When the disease flares up, the CSF may have an increased number of lymphocytes (although usually less than 50/mcL). The CSF will also contain elevated levels of immunoglobulins, the majority of which are IgG. Oligoclonal bands are found in the CSF, regardless of the current state of the disease symptoms.

CLINICAL PRESENTATION

Subjective

The most common presenting symptoms in MS include weakness of the legs, bladder and bowel dysfunction, ataxic gait, paresthesias in the extremities, and optic neuritis. Seventy-five percent to 95% of patients with MS experience MS-related fatigue. Exacerbations and remissions occur, and signs and symptoms may localize to more than one lesion. The clinical course is variable. The subjective complaint at any one presentation depends on the location of the active lesion. Optic neuritis causes unilateral blurred vision, dulling of colors, or sometimes even blindness in one eye. Transverse myelitis (spinal cord inflammation) causes bilateral weakness, numbness, spasticity, and bladder dysfunction. Brainstem lesions can cause double vision, tremor, ataxia, and dizziness. When a patient presents with symptoms that may be from MS, it is important to ask about previous transient neurological symptoms. The diagnosis of MS requires demonstrating multiple lesions over time affecting different areas of the CNS.

Objective

Symptoms may begin to manifest over a period of hours to days. The clinician should assess the patient for common visual symptoms, including diplopia, blurred vision, diminution or loss of visual acuity unilaterally or bilaterally, and visual field defects. A patient with unilateral optic neuritis will have a relative afferent pupillary defect on examination. They may also have red desaturation, decreased visual acuity in one eye, and pain with eye movements. Demyelination in the brainstem of the fifth cranial nerve can cause trigeminal neuralgia. Limb weakness is a common sign of

MS, presenting as monoparesis, hemiparesis, or tetraparesis, and is typically caused by spinal cord lesions (myelitis). Over time, myelitis leads to hyperreflexia and spasticity. In patients with severe spasticity, there may be extensor or flexor spasms either spontaneously or on attempted movement. Spasticity may cause pain, interfere with sleep, or prevent movement. Cerebellar or brainstem involvement causes dysarthria, scanning speech, tremor, gait ataxia, and incoordination of limbs and trunk.

Bladder symptoms are common due to spinal cord involvement, and include incontinence, frequency, and urgency. Patients may have a small-capacity, spastic bladder or a large, flaccid bladder with overflow incontinence. Bladder dysfunction from myelitis may become chronic, requiring self-catheterization. Loss of libido and erectile dysfunction are common in men with MS; in women with MS, sexual dysfunction most commonly involves lack of lubrication and failure to reach orgasm. Although bowel incontinence is less common, constipation may occur.

Sensory impairment and paresthesias are common. Patients may complain of tingling or numbness in the face, limbs, or trunk. A sensation of "electricity" down the back after passive or active neck flexion, called *Lhermitte's sign*, is indicative of a lesion in the posterior column in the cervical spinal cord. Pain is common in MS. Pain may be associated with trigeminal neuralgia, flexor–extensor spasms, tonic spasms of the limbs, and local pain syndromes such as constricting pain around a limb, burning pain, pseudoradicular pain, foreign body sensation, headache, neuralgic pain, and pain caused by pressure injuries.

Patients may experience depression, euphoria, and cognitive changes. Patients may have difficulty with tasks that require processing new information rapidly, recalling newly acquired knowledge, and problem-solving. Attention deficits may be present early in MS, even before the onset of physical symptoms. In general, the longer the history of MS, the greater the attention impairment. Memory and abstract reasoning may be affected, as well as the capacity to direct attention.

DIAGNOSTIC REASONING

Diagnostic Tests

The diagnosis of relapsing-remitting MS requires the demonstration of multiple demyelinating CNS lesions that develop over time and in different locations. Diagnosis is based on patient history, neurological examination, and diagnostic tests. The key principles used for the diagnosis of MS include the presence of typical MS symptoms attributable to demyelination, objective evidence of CNS involvement, dissemination in space, dissemination in time, and lack of a better alternative explanation. With these principles, the McDonald criteria were created as standardized diagnostic criteria for MS. Although MS can cause a wide range of symptoms, the typical MS syndromes necessary for accurate MS diagnosis using the McDonald criteria are listed in Box 10.1.

Objective evidence of CNS involvement can come from a neurological exam, imaging, and/or neurophysiological tests with abnormalities corresponding to the abnormal presenting symptom. Dissemination in time can be demonstrated by having separate MS attacks at different points in time or having both gadolinium-enhancing and nonenhancing lesions simultaneously on MRI. Per the McDonald diagnostic criteria, the presence of oligoclonal bands in the CSF can act as a surrogate for dissemination in time. To demonstrate dissemination in space, MS lesions must be multifocal on brain MRI or exam, involving at least two of the characteristic MS regions, including periventricular, cortical or juxtacortical, infratentorial, and spinal cord.

An LP with an evaluation of CSF for the presence of lymphocytes and oligoclonal IgG bands may provide supportive data for a diagnosis of MS and help exclude other disorders with similar signs and symptoms.

Cortical-evoked responses or evoked potentials are of value in demonstrating clinically unsuspected lesions. Visual responses are abnormal in 75% to 97% of patients with MS. Somatosensory responses are abnormal in 72% to 87%, and brainstem responses are abnormal in 50% to 70% of patients with MS.

MRI is a sensitive, objective measure of plaques and is used to diagnose MS and measure the outcomes of treatment. Periodic recording of the volume and number of lesions detected in the brain by MRI can assist the clinician in monitoring the extent of the disease. Areas of contrast enhancement observed by MRI correlate with active inflammatory damage. In addition, the MRI should be

---

Box 10.1   McDonald's Criteria for Diagnosing MS

- Transverse myelitis: usually partial, causing sensory impairment, weakness, and bladder dysfunction
  - Examination abnormalities: quadriparesis, sensory level, position sense loss, spasticity, ankle clonus, positive Babinski sign
- Optic neuritis: usually unilateral, causing painful vision loss
  - Examination abnormalities: relative afferent pupillary defect (RAPD), decreased color vision (especially red desaturation), decreased visual acuity
- Brainstem syndrome: such as internuclear ophthalmoplegia ([INO] painless diplopia with nystagmus), trigeminal neuralgia
  - Examination abnormalities for INO: weakness of adduction in affected eye, with abduction nystagmus in the contralateral eye
- Cerebellar syndrome: causing balance and coordination issues with slurred speech
  - Examination findings: wide-based gait, dysmetria, nystagmus, scanning speech

obtained as soon as possible in all patients presenting with an isolated demyelinating syndrome involving the CNS to exclude other possible neurological conditions.

If only one clinical event can be demonstrated, the patient cannot be diagnosed with MS, but may have clinically isolated syndrome. Patients with clinically isolated syndrome are at risk for developing MS in the future if they develop another attack. Patients with evidence of demyelinating plaques consistent with MS on MRI but no clinical symptoms are described as having radiologically isolated syndrome. Patients who present with progressive disability at disease onset (as opposed to a relapsing-remitting course) have primary progressive MS.

Differential Diagnosis

Other CNS diseases may resemble MS clinically or radiologically, including cerebral small vessel disease; tumors such as lymphoma or glioma; infections such as Lyme, HIV, and other causes of encephalitis and/or myelitis; collagen vascular disease such as systemic lupus erythematosus, Behçet's disease, and sarcoidosis; other leukoencephalopathies; and other autoimmune demyelinating diseases of the CNS such as neuromyelitis optica spectrum disorders and acute disseminated encephalomyelitis.

MANAGEMENT

The principles of management include three major goals: to delay the progression of the disease, manage chronic symptoms, and treat acute exacerbations. There is no known cure for MS. Disease-modifying therapies are available; treatment decisions should be individualized, balancing the risks of the medications and the potential benefits. Disease-modifying medications include oral, injectable, and infusion methods. See Drugs Commonly Prescribed 10.1. Follow-up should be based on progression of disease and the treatment of symptoms and exacerbations.

Glucocorticoids are the mainstay of treatment for acute exacerbations. Glucocorticoids have both immunomodulatory and anti-inflammatory effects, which restore the blood–brain barrier, decrease edema, and may improve axonal conduction. The decision to treat an acute exacerbation depends on the functional limitations of the patient, the level of patient discomfort, and objective evidence of neurological dysfunction on examination. If symptoms of an exacerbation are severe enough to require treatment, high dose steroids, such as 1,000 mg daily of IV methylprednisolone (Depo-Medrol) for 3 to 5 days is administered, typically without an oral prednisone taper.

Drugs Commonly Prescribed 10.1: Multiple Sclerosis

DRUG	INDICATION	ADVERSE REACTIONS AND PRESCRIBING CONSIDERATIONS
Injectables		
Methylprednisolone (Depo-Medrol)	Acute exacerbation	• Side effects: glaucoma, cataracts, secondary infections, hypokalemia, hypocalcemia, hypernatremia, hypertension, psychotic disorders, myopathy, osteoporosis, peptic ulcer, dermal atrophy, increased intracranial pressure, glucose intolerance • Caution as some patients experience depression or suicidal ideation
Interferon therapies (Avonex, Rebif, Plegridy, Betaseron, Extavia)	Relapsing–remitting multiple sclerosis (RRMS), active secondary progressive (SPMS)	• May cause injection site reactions and flu-like symptoms • Monitor complete blood count (CBC) and liver function tests
Glatiramer acetate (Copaxone)	RRMS and active SPMS	• Side effects: reaction at injection site, flushing, sweating, shortness of breath, palpitations, chest tightness, anxiety • No routine monitoring required • Pregnancy class B
Ofatumumab (Kesimpta)	RRMS and active SPMS	• Monoclonal antibody • May cause injection site reactions and flu-like symptoms
Infusions		
Ocrelizumab (Ocrevus)	RRMS, active SPMS, primary progressive MS	• Monoclonal antibody • Contraindicated in patients with active hepatitis B virus infection • Infusions: two IV infusions 14 days apart, which are administered every 6 months • Side effects include infusion reactions and infection.

Continued

Drugs Commonly Prescribed 10.1: Multiple Sclerosis—cont'd

DRUG	INDICATION	ADVERSE REACTIONS AND PRESCRIBING CONSIDERATIONS
Natalizumab (Tysabri)	RRMS and active SPMS	• Monoclonal antibody • Infusion every 28 days • Monitor for progressive multifocal leukoencephalopathy (PML) • May cause infusion-related symptoms, hypersensitivity reactions • Only available through restricted distribution program, given safety profile
Alemtuzumab (Lemtrada)	RRMS and active SPMS	• Monoclonal antibody • Initial infusion for 5 consecutive days; repeat in 12 months for 3 days • Common side effects include infusion-related reactions • Secondary autoimmune diseases and development of cancer seen in trials • May cause immune thrombocytopenia and kidney damage • Only available through restricted distribution program, given safety profile
Oral Medications		
Cladribine (Mavenclad)	RRMS and active SPMS	• Causes lymphocyte depletion • Generally not a first-line treatment due to safety profile
Teriflunomide (Aubagio)	RRMS and active SPMS	• Avoid using in patients with any infection or PML • Use with caution in patients with liver disease, hypertension, immunosuppression, peripheral neuropathy, and respiratory problems • Contraindicated in pregnancy
Fumarates (dimethyl fumarate, diroximel fumarate, monomethyl fumarate)	RRMS and active SPMS	• Modulates immune system • PML risk • Monitor CBC, Liver Function Tests (LFTs) • Monitor for gastrointestinal (GI) side effects (especially dimethyl fumarate [Tecfidera])
Sphingosine 1P receptor modulators (fingolimod, siponimod, ozanimod, ponesimod)	RRMS and active SPMS	• Sequesters lymphocytes in lymph nodes • Monitor for bradycardia, macular edema • Risk of PML • Avoid foods with high tyramine content (ozanimod) • Monitor CBC and liver function tests • Fingolimod is U.S. Food and Drug Administration–approved for pediatric-onset MS
Symptomatic Medications		
Baclofen (Lioresal)	Symptomatic treatment for spasticity	• May cause drowsiness and confusion
Tizanidine (Zanaflex)	Spasticity	• May cause drowsiness • Do not use with clonidine (Catapres)
Diazepam (Valium)	Spasticity	• Contraindicated with acute narrow-angle glaucoma; potential for abuse

Patients with relapsing–remitting MS may benefit from early treatment with disease-modifying agents. Disease-modifying agents can reduce the frequency of MS exacerbations, new lesions noted on an MRI, and long-term disability. Efficacy and side effects vary, and choice of therapy must be individualized. Medications with higher efficacy in preventing MS relapses may increase the risk of opportunistic infections, which can be deadly. Progressive multifocal leukoencephalopathy is a CNS infection caused by the John Cunningham (JC) virus that can cause significant morbidity and mortality. JC antibody titers must be monitored when patients are taking certain disease-modifying medications.

Patients with MS should be referred to a neurologist for treatment with disease-modifying medications.

Physicians who prescribe these medications must be thoroughly familiar with dosage, possible adverse effects, and management of those adverse effects. Patients must be educated about side effects, injection techniques, storage, and care of the medications. Once appropriate drug therapy has been stabilized, the clinician may monitor the patient as described under Follow-up and Referral.

Symptomatic management and therapy are important in MS. Spasticity is a major cause of disability in 55% of patients with MS. Antispasmodics may be effective. If other noninvasive therapeutic measures for spasticity have failed, the patient may be referred to a neurosurgeon for evaluation of an implantable drug infusion pump to administer baclofen (Lioresal) intrathecally. This is highly effective because the drug can cross the blood–brain barrier. Adverse effects are minimal, and a test dose is administered intrathecally before implantation as part of the screening process for candidates.

Selective chemodenervation may be beneficial for localized spasticity in a single muscle or limb. This may be accomplished through administration of botulinum (*Clostridium botulinum*) toxin type A (Botox). Only a specialist familiar with the use, adverse effects, and injection sites for botulinum toxin should administer this medication.

The tremors associated with MS are usually cerebellar outflow tremors. Medications such as propranolol (Inderal), clonazepam (Klonopin), and primidone (Mysoline) may be effective.

Fatigue is a common problem in patients with MS. The existence of sleep apnea, pain, spasms, restless leg syndrome, and sleep quality and patterns should all be assessed. Other medical problems that may cause fatigue should be excluded. Patients should be instructed to take a daytime nap and remain in a cool environment and should be educated in energy conservation techniques. A referral for occupational therapy may be beneficial.

Neuropathic pain may be treated with antiepileptics such as gabapentin and/or antidepressants such as duloxetine and nortriptyline.

Providers should be aware of issues related to complementary therapies that may be raised by patients with MS. Complementary and alternative medicine (CAM) is used by up to 70% of persons affected with MS due to the progressive and debilitating nature of the disease. The following are frequently used complementary therapies for patients with MS: acupuncture, hypnotherapy and imagery, massage, biofeedback, tai chi, therapeutic touch, Reiki, bioelectromagnetic therapy, and chiropractic therapy. If referring a patient with MS to complementary therapy providers, it is important to suggest those who are experienced in treating people with MS. Relaxation and meditation, as well as yoga and spiritual practices, may all benefit people living with MS. Other CAM therapies need to be further researched.

FOLLOW-UP AND REFERRAL

Follow-up and referral should occur soon after diagnosis, and repeated initially at monthly intervals or more often as symptoms appear. During follow-up visits, the patient's level of functioning and the effectiveness of medications should be assessed, and dosage adjustments made if needed. The patient should be instructed to contact the clinician immediately if symptoms appear that may signal an exacerbation. Periodic MRIs are typically obtained to trend disease progression.

Patient Education: Multiple Sclerosis

Patients should be educated about all aspects of the disease, including medications and adverse effects, complications, progression, fatigue management, pain management, diet, and exercise. The weakness that results from MS may be amenable to strengthening exercises. Range-of-motion exercise is important to prevent contractures and joint restriction. Referral to a physical therapist experienced in the treatment of patients with MS may be beneficial. Regular exercise may change the course of the patient's response to illness by minimizing the deconditioning process and maintaining optimal levels of physical activity and functioning. The beneficial effects of prolonged activity are well-documented; it can help prevent muscular atrophy and weakness, fatigue, loss of flexibility, cardiovascular deficits, depression, and sleep disturbances. It is important to balance activity and exercise to prevent fatigue. There is no conclusive scientific evidence that any diet or nutritional therapy affects the course of MS. Many of the diets available are not harmful but may be tiring because of the attention to detail required, while offering no benefit. A generally well-balanced diet is recommended. Patients who have been diagnosed with MS may experience a wide range of emotions, from euphoria to depression, including helplessness, lack of hope, mental confusion, stress, and anxiety. These emotions can affect marital relationships and increase child-rearing stress. The chronic nature of MS and the inability to predict level of dysfunction contribute to difficulty coping with chronic illness and symptoms disruptive to daily living. Patients may also experience job loss, embarrassment, exhaustion, and the feeling of loss of contribution to society. It is important to teach patients health-promotion behaviors to emphasize emotional and social well-being.

Patients and families should also be educated in coping with possible behavior changes and mood swings. Patients with MS have reported feelings of hopelessness, loss of control, conflict, fear, loss, and uncertainty. Education in the management of problems related to sexual dysfunction may also need to be addressed. Caregivers should be educated not to neglect their own health because coping with a chronic illness may change and stress the dynamics both within a family and within other individual relationships. The complexity of issues surrounding caring for a person with MS is highlighted in Evidence-Based Nursing Practice 10.1.

> **Evidence-Based Nursing Practice 10.1**
>
> ### MULTIPLE SCLEROSIS ABSTRACT
>
> **Purpose:** The aim of the study was to explore the experience of male caregivers with a partner with MS.
>
> **Design and Methods:** A qualitative study was conducted with a grounded theory approach. Twenty-four partners of a man or woman diagnosed with MS were interviewed in depth. A thematic analysis of the narratives was done.
>
> **Findings:** Five major themes emerged: caregiving as a full-time job, changes in the couple, the importance of social support and social life, gender specificities, and fear of the future.
>
> **Conclusions:** Results highlight the complexity of issues surrounding this specific form of caregiving. Social expectations referring to the marital relationship and to gender norms play a central role.
>
> **Clinical Relevance:** Findings may help in developing ad hoc interventions to support male spousal caregivers to care for their partners.

Rollero C. The experience of men caring for a partner with multiple sclerosis. *J Nurs Scholarsh.* 2016;48(5);482–489.

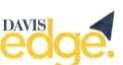 **Go to Davis Edge for practice Q&A**

REFERENCES

Bell's Palsy

Bell's Palsy Fact Sheet. (2018). National Institute of Neurological Disorders and Stroke. NIH Pub. No. 18-NS-5114. https://www.ninds.nih.gov/Disorders/Patient-Caregiver-Education/Fact-Sheets/Bells-Palsy-Fact-Sheet. Accessed 6/1/2021.

Encephalitis

Lancaster, E. Paraneoplastic disorders. *CONTINUUM: Lifelong Learning in Neurology* 2017;23(6): 1653–1679.

Parpia A, Li Y, Chen C, et al. Encephalitis, Ontario, Canada, 2002–2013. *Emerg Infect Dis.* 2016;22(3):426.

Schmidt A, Buhler R, Muhlemann K, et al. Long-term outcome of acute encephalitis of unknown aetiology in adults. *Microbiol Infect.* 2011;17:621–626.

Guillain Barré Syndrome

Grave C, Boucheron P, Rudant J. (2020). Seasonal influenza vaccine and Guillain-Barre syndrome—A self-controlled case series study. *Neurology:* 2020 May 19;94(20). https://n.neurology.org/content/94/20/e2168. Accessed 6/1/2021.

Willison HJ, Jacobs BC, van Doorn PA. Guillain-barre syndrome. *The Lancet,* 2016;388(10045):717–727.

Herpes Zoster

Centers for Disease Control and Prevention. (2018). What everyone should know about the shingles vaccine (Shingrix). Vaccines and preventable diseases. https://www.cdc.gov/vaccines/vpd/shingles/public/index.html. Accessed 5/31/2021.

Dooling KL, Guo A, Patel M. (2018). Recommendations of the Advisory Committee on Immunization Practices for Use of Herpes Zoster Vaccines. *CDC- Weekly* / 2018 Jan 26;67(3);103–108. https://www.cdc.gov/mmwr/volumes/67/wr/mm6703a5.htm. Accessed 6/1/2021.

Gross GE, Eisert L, Doerr HW, et al. (2020). S2k guidelines for the diagnosis and treatment of herpes zoster and postherpetic neuralgia. *J Dtsch Dermatol Ges.* 2020 Jan;18(1):55–78.

Han Y, Zhang J, Chen N, et al. (2013). Corticosteroids for preventing postherpetic neuralgia. Cochrane Database of Systematic Reviews (3).

Westmead Institute for Medical Research (2018, March 7). Why the latest shingles vaccine is more than 90 percent effective. https://www.sciencedaily.com/releases/2018/03/180307095243.htm. Accessed September 2018.

Meningitis

CDC. (2020). Meningitis. https://www.cdc.gov/meningitis/index.html. Accessed 6/1/2021.

National Meningitis Association. Statistics and disease facts. http://www.nmaus.org/disease-prevention-information/statistics-and-disease-facts/. Accessed May 31, 2021.

U.S. Department of Health and Human Services. (2016). Meningococcal vaccine. https://www.vaccines.gov/diseases/meningitis/index.html. Accessed May 24, 2021.

Multiple Sclerosis

Gross RH, Corboy JR. Monitoring, switching, and stopping multiple sclerosis disease-modifying therapies. *CONTINUUM: Lifelong Learning in Neurology.* 2019;25(3): pp.715–735.

Repovic P. Management of multiple sclerosis relapses. *CONTINUUM: Lifelong Learning in Neurology.* 2019;25(3):655–669.

Rollero C. The experience of men caring for a partner with multiple sclerosis. *J Nurs Scholarsh.* 2016;48(5):482–489.

Sierra Morales F, Koralnik IJ, Gautam S. Risk factors for lymphopenia in patients with relapsing–remitting multiple sclerosis treated with dimethyl fumarate. *J Neurol* 2020;267:132. https://doi.org/10.1007/s00415-019-09626-0

Solomon AJ. Diagnosis, differential diagnosis, and misdiagnosis of multiple sclerosis. *CONTINUUM: Lifelong Learning in Neurology* 2019;25(3):611–635.

Thompson AJ, Banwell BL, Barkhof F, et al. Diagnosis of multiple sclerosis: 2017 revisions of the McDonald criteria. *The Lancet Neurology* 2018;17(2):162–173.

Myasthenia Gravis

Myasthenia gravis foundation. (2015). Clinical overview of MG. https://myasthenia.org/Professionals/Clinical-Overview-of-MG. Accessed 6/1/2021.

Trigeminal Neuralgia

National Institute of Neurological Disorders and Stroke. Trigeminal neuralgia fact sheet. https://www.ninds.nih.gov/Disorders/

Patient-Caregiver-Education/Fact-Sheets/Trigeminal-Neuralgia-Fact-Sheet. Accessed 5/24/2021.

Gronseth G, Cruccu G, Alksne J, et al. Practice parameter: the diagnostic evaluation and treatment of trigeminal neuralgia (an evidence-based review): report of the Quality Standards Subcommittee of the American Academy of Neurology and the European Federation of Neurological Societies. *Neurology* 2008;71(15):1183–1190. Current practice guideline. Reaffirmed May 22, 2021.

RESOURCES

Bell's Palsy

National Organization for Rare Disorders (NORD)
   https://rarediseases.org/

Encephalitis

Nemours Foundation—Encephalitis (for children and teenagers)
   https://kidshealth.org/en/teens/encephalitis.html

Herpes Zoster

Centers for Disease Control and Prevention—Shingles (Herpes Zoster) https://www.cdc.gov/shingles/index.html

Meningitis

Centers for Disease Control and Prevention—Meningitis https://www.cdc.gov/meningitis/clinical-resources.html

National Institute of Neurological Disorders and Stroke—Meningitis and Encephalitis https://www.ninds.nih.gov/Disorders/All-Disorders/Meningitis-and-Encephalitis-Information-Page

Multiple Sclerosis

National MS Society
   https://www.nationalmssociety.org/

Myasthenia Gravis

Myasthenia Gravis Foundation of America
   Myasthenia.org
National Institute of Neurological Disorders and Stroke
   https://www.ninds.nih.gov

Section 2: SKIN PROBLEMS

SECTION EDITOR
Jill E. Winland-Brown, EdD, APRN, FNP-BC, FAANP

Chapter 11

Common Skin Complaints

Susan Garnett, MSN, APRN, FNP-BC
Jill E. Winland-Brown, EdD, APRN, FNP-BC, FAANP
Brian Oscar Porter, MD, PhD, MPH, MBA

ALOPECIA

Alopecia (baldness) is considered an autoimmune disease, which may be genetic in etiology with an environmental trigger. It can occur anywhere on the body where hair is present, although it is commonly associated with absence of hair in the scalp area. Scalp hair loss can occur in patches (patchy alopecia or alopecia areata [AA]) or over the entire scalp and face (alopecia totalis). Hair loss can also occur over the entire body (alopecia universalis) and can be either a temporary or permanent condition.

Hair loss is a gradual process; it is estimated that up to 50% of scalp hair can be lost before the loss becomes clinically apparent. Alopecia may be accompanied by psychological distress, even if the hair loss is temporary, as in AA. The most common cause of permanent hair loss is androgenic alopecia (AGA) or male-pattern baldness (common baldness). AGA has a polygenic inheritance pattern; thus, it is inherited from both parents, not only through maternal genes, which is a common myth. Another common misconception is that AGA is more common in men; in reality, it occurs in both sexes and all ethnicities.

There are four cycles of scalp hair growth. The growth phase (anagen) of scalp hair is the longest cycle, lasting from 2 to 6 years. The majority of hair on the scalp (90% to 95%) is in the anagen phase. The latent or involution phase (catagen) is the shortest cycle, which lasts only 2 to 3 weeks. The resting phase (telogen) lasts from 2 to 3 months, and hair is shed during the fourth phase (exogen). An average person loses 50 to 150 hairs daily, and the cycle is repeated. Both topical and systemic medications for hair loss affect some or all of the phases of hair growth.

Factors that influence normal hair development and cycling include estrogens, growth hormone, glucocorticoids, thyroid hormone, retinoid, prolactin, and androgens; these factors can be adversely affected by certain medications. The most important hair growth factors are the androgens testosterone and its active metabolite, dihydrotestosterone. During puberty, when androgen secretion starts, hair follicles become enlarged in certain areas of the body such as the beard area, chest, and extremities. Androgens have the opposite effect on the hair follicles of the scalp region; they cause a decrease in the size of the hair follicles (miniaturization) and can alter the hairline over the bitemporal region and the vertex area.

Alopecia affects an estimated 6.8 million people in the United States and 147 million people globally (National Alopecia Areata Foundation [NAAF], 2020) with an overall prevalence of 2%. The prevalence of AA has increased over time and varies significantly in its distribution around the world, thought to be due to regional variability in environmental factors such as nutrition and psychological stressors (Lee et al, 2020). Both men and women are affected equally. AA occurs more frequently than other kinds of alopecia in pediatric populations. Previously thought to occur equally among different ethnic groups, a recent meta-analysis suggests AA occurs more frequently in African Americans than European Americans, and less often in Asian Americans (Lee et al, 2019).

In reversible cases of nonscarring alopecia, regrowth of hair usually takes several months. Patients who are reassured of this important fact will have less anxiety about their condition. Two important factors that the clinician should address in the evaluation of alopecia are (1) whether it is scarring or nonscarring alopecia and (2) whether hair loss is in a small, well-circumscribed area (AA or compulsive hair pulling [trichotillomania]) or generalized (AGA). On the basis of these two general categories, the differential diagnosis is made easier for the clinician. Scarring alopecia (cicatricial alopecia) causes permanent hair loss and is not reversible. Hair loss from nonscarring alopecia (noncicatricial alopecia) can be either temporary or permanent.

DIFFERENTIAL DIAGNOSIS

A thorough history is important in the evaluation of alopecia. Information regarding family members—both male and female—with hair loss should be elicited. Because some medications affect hair growth, the patient's medication history should be reviewed. Drugs that cause hair loss include hormones, anticonvulsants, anticoagulants, oral contraceptives, beta blockers, antimetabolites, antithyroid drugs, and excessive amounts of vitamin A or topical Retin-A (see Differential Diagnosis 11.1).

A potassium hydroxide and Wood's light examination is helpful in the diagnosis of tinea capitis in cases of patchy hair loss. Although most cases of tinea capitis do not fluoresce, a fungal culture can provide definitive proof of fungal infection and should be performed if suspicion is high.

Some dermatologists use the telogen count, in which 100 hairs (only 50 hairs are needed for accuracy) are removed from different areas of the scalp and the number of hairs in telogen is counted. Telogen hairs are recognized because of the large white club on the end of each hair. The appearance of the skin on the scalp will give the clinician clues about the type of alopecia involved. In nonscarring alopecia, the scalp will have normal texture and color. In contrast, the scalp of a patient with scarring alopecia has no visible hair follicles (or no follicular openings) and is atrophied and smooth. The affected area of the scalp (or the entire scalp) is sometimes hypopigmented or hyperpigmented. Obvious scarring is seen in some patients, and some have erythema and scaling (in these cases, it is important to rule out fungal infection). Look for fine pitting of the dorsal nail plate (with the appearance of "hammered brass") on the physical examination.

Nonscarring Alopecia

Nonscarring alopecia has both systemic and nonsystemic causes. Nonsystemic causes of alopecia include trichotillomania, excessive traction of the frontal and temporal areas of the scalp (from tight cornrows or tight ponytails), trauma (both physical and chemical), radiation therapy to the head, local bacterial infection, and local fungal infection. Trichotillomania is more commonly seen in children and teens. It is usually on the same side as the dominant hand and may involve areas other than just scalp hair (e.g., eyelashes, eyebrows, and beard).

Systemic causes of nonscarring alopecia include AA, telogen effluvium (TE; discussed in the following section), androgenic baldness (common baldness), vitiligo, Hashimoto's thyroiditis, Addison's disease, systemic lupus erythematosus (SLE), hypothyroidism or hyperthyroidism, secondary syphilis, severe herpes zoster of the scalp, drug-induced alopecia (common in patients on cyclophosphamide therapy), iron-deficiency anemia, and pituitary insufficiency.

TE, excessive shedding of scalp hair that results from an increased number of hair follicles entering the resting stage (telogen), can be caused by fever and certain drugs; therefore, a search for these possible causes should be included in the history-taking. TE may also be caused by stress, pregnancy and/or childbirth, extreme weight loss, and general anesthesia. TE is almost nonexistent in men. In contrast, the classic signs of androgenic baldness are thinning hairs of various diameters and lengths ("miniaturized" hairs) located in typical areas of the scalp, which differ in men and women. In men, hair loss usually starts on the hairline and around the temples (bitemporal area) and at the vertex or crown (top of the head). In women, hair loss is much more diffuse and occurs mostly on top of the head. Hair loss is sometimes harder to recognize in women because of hairstyles that are used to camouflage the problem.

AA is a common condition in primary care practice. It is associated with autoimmune endocrinopathies such as Hashimoto's thyroiditis, Addison's disease, and pernicious anemia. The typical patient will present with well-circumscribed patches of hair loss on the scalp or sometimes on the face, in areas such as the eyebrows or beard area. Occasionally, only one patch is seen, although multiple patches of hair loss may be apparent. Because gray hair is spared, patients may complain of going gray overnight. When the scalp is examined closely with a magnifying lens, short, stubby hairs with tapered ends

Differential Diagnosis 11.1: Alopecia

Type of Alopecia	Differential Diagnosis
Scarring alopecia (cicatricial alopecia)	Trauma (chemical, physical, heat) Kerion formation in tinea capitis Chronic discoid lupus erythematosus Scleroderma Excessive radiation to scalp Lichen planopilaris Bacterial infection of scalp
Nonscarring alopecia (noncicatricial alopecia)	Alopecia areata Drug-induced hair loss Trichotillomania (hair pulling) Traction alopecia (from tight braids, cornrows, or ponytails) Telogen effluvium (after pregnancy, major surgery, major emotional stress) Androgenic baldness Tinea capitis (with no kerion formation) Hypothyroidism (Hashimoto's thyroiditis) Systemic lupus erythematosus Addison's disease

("exclamation point hairs") are seen on the periphery of the bald patch (or patches).

AA can occur once in a lifetime or it can be recurrent. There is no cure for AA, but in most patients, hair usually regrows spontaneously after several months, with new hairs that look thinner and finer than the original hair. The prognosis for AA is good if it occurs after puberty, as studies have found that up to 80% of these patients will regrow hair. Occasionally, a case of persistent AA that is unresponsive to treatment is seen; these cases are best referred to dermatologists for management.

Scarring Alopecia

Etiology of scarring (cicatricial) alopecia can include trauma (physical or chemical), severe bacterial or fungal infections of the scalp, scleroderma, discoid lupus, SLE, lichen planopilaris, and excessive radiation. Early recognition and treatment of bacterial or fungal infections can help prevent or minimize the incidence of scarring. Severe local infection with either bacteria or fungi can permanently damage hair follicles and cause a patchy (and scarring) alopecia that is permanent.

When an autoimmune disease is suspected, laboratory tests include antinuclear antibodies to rule out SLE or other autoimmune disorders, rheumatoid factor, and erythrocyte sedimentation rate (ESR), a nonspecific marker for inflammation. The rheumatology autoantibody profile or "arthritis panel" may help in the diagnosis of autoimmune disorders that can cause alopecia, such as SLE and scleroderma. Scleroderma (progressive systemic sclerosis) is a systemic and multisystem inflammatory disorder associated with sclerotic changes in the body that effect multiple organ systems, including the skin. The skin becomes diffusely thickened with frequent telangiectasias (small dilated blood vessels) visible at the skin surface.

In addition, serum testosterone, dehydroepiandrosterone, serum iron, total iron-binding capacity, and thyroid function tests, along with a complete blood count (CBC), will identify most other causes of hair thinning in premenopausal women. A scalp biopsy is usually reserved for difficult-to-treat and recalcitrant cases of scarring alopecia. Specimens must be obtained from the active border, rather than from the scarred central zone.

MANAGEMENT

Medical treatment is available but is not a permanent solution for alopecia. Patients should be educated that a total return to previous levels of hair growth rarely occurs, but cosmetically acceptable hair coverage is possible. Medical treatments must be used daily to maintain regrown hair. Stopping treatment will result in shedding of hair and a return to the previous levels of alopecia. Hair shedding is seen rapidly in a matter of days after stopping minoxidil (Rogaine), but is more gradual over several months with finasteride (Propecia).

Treatment options for alopecia are determined by the patient's age and severity of hair loss. For patients younger than 10 years of age, topical corticosteroids and/or topical 5% minoxidil are recommended, as children may not tolerate scalp injections. For patients older than 10 years of age with hair loss of less than 50%, treatment options include intralesional corticosteroid injections, topical 5% minoxidil solution or foam, and topical corticosteroid creams. Recalcitrant cases may require topical immunomodulator therapy.

Intralesional corticosteroid injection is considered first-line treatment for limited areas of involvement. After the application of a topical anesthetic 1.5 to 2 hours prior, small amounts (0.1 mL) of triamcinolone acetonide (Kenalog) 2.5 to 5 mg/mL may be injected intralesionally into the mid-dermal layer, spaced approximately 1 cm apart on bald patches and given every 4 to 6 weeks. New hair growth is usually seen in 6 to 8 weeks. Treatment is discontinued when hair growth is restored. Potential side effects of corticosteroid use are skin atrophy, telangiectasias, and hypopigmentation.

Treatments for more extensive (50% or greater) hair loss include topical and intralesional corticosteroids, oral corticosteroids, topical immunomodulator therapy, methotrexate, and oral immunomodulators. Oral corticosteroid therapy is known to have significant side effects with long-term use; therefore, a 6-week treatment course is recommended. In topical immunomodulator therapy, chemicals such as diphenylcyclopropenone (DPCP) and squaric acid dibutylester (SADBE) cause contact dermatitis when applied to the scalp, which modulates the autoreactive immune reaction driving hair loss. Oral immunomodulators such as Janus kinase (JAK) inhibitors have been effective in clinical trials. Existing medications such as statins and oral and topical phosphodiesterase-4 inhibitors are also being evaluated for the treatment of AA. The gut microbiome is also being evaluated as a causative factor in AA, with fecal microbiota transplants being studied as a potential treatment for the inflammatory autoimmune response underlying AA.

Nonmedical treatment options to address cosmetic concerns include hair weaves, and toupees and wigs, which are worn on top of the head. As the existing hair to which the weave is anchored grows, the weave must be readjusted periodically, which may impart increased stress on hair follicles, paradoxically resulting in traction alopecia. Surgical approaches to the treatment of extensive alopecia include hair transplantation and scalp restoration techniques.

Finasteride

Finasteride (Propecia, Proscar) is approved by the U.S. Food and Drug Administration (FDA) for use by men only. Systemic treatment for alopecia with finasteride should not be used in women of reproductive age because this drug can cause abnormalities of the external genitalia of male fetuses. In women of non-childbearing age, finasteride does not appear to be effective in treating AGA. Therefore, finasteride once daily is approved for the treatment of androgenic baldness in men only, whereas any use in women for female pattern baldness (with or without elevated androgen levels) is considered off-label and is not approved by the FDA.

Finasteride blocks the effects of 5-alpha reductase, an enzyme that converts dihydrotestosterone to testosterone and reduces the total amount of testosterone in the body. Because it is metabolized in the liver, finasteride should be used with caution in patients with liver disease. In men aged 60 years or older, finasteride may be less effective than in younger men because of decreased 5-alpha-reductase activity that occurs with age. Adverse effects include decreased libido (1.8%), erectile dysfunction (1.3%), and ejaculatory dysfunction (1.2%). In most men, these sexual side effects gradually resolve with prolonged treatment.

Minoxidil

Topical treatments for men and women containing minoxidil are available over the counter (OTC). Treatments for men include minoxidil 5% extra strength solution (Rogaine) and minoxidil 5% unscented foam, applied twice daily. Topical treatments available for women include minoxidil 5% foam applied once daily and 5% solution applied twice daily. At higher doses, oral minoxidil is a vasodilator and is used to treat hypertension. Topical minoxidil has not been found to cause lowering of systolic or diastolic blood pressure or pulse rate.

The best candidates for treatment with topical minoxidil are patients with recent onset of alopecia (less than 5 years), those younger than 50 years of age, and patients with smaller areas of hair loss. Up to 40% of patients who use topical minoxidil for a period of 1 year or more will experience moderate to dense hair regrowth. Minoxidil 2% solution has been consistently shown to reduce hair loss and induce new hair growth in females with female pattern hair loss. Because the 2% solution is used twice per day, the once daily 5% minoxidil foam for use in women is more effective because of improved compliance and patient-reported satisfaction, as well as milder side effects. Adverse effects include irritation, itching, dryness, scaling, and redness of the scalp, as minoxidil can sometimes cause contact dermatitis. An adverse effect that is more common in women is hypertrichosis (excessive hair growth on the body).

PIGMENTATION CHANGES

The skin is the largest and most visible organ of the body. Because of the skin's visibility, conditions affecting the skin cause not only physical discomfort but also have emotional overtones. Pigmentation disorders seen in primary care include both hyperpigmentation and hypopigmentation. Either condition can be a sign of disease or it can be considered a normal finding, depending on the clinical picture.

Melanin is a skin pigment produced by melanocytes that determines skin color. Although there is no difference in the average number of melanocytes among different ethnic groups, the ability of the melanocytes of darker-skinned people to produce and retain melanin (from melanosomes) is much greater than in people with lighter skin. Research has found that melanosome size is directly related to skin color: the larger the size of the melanosomes, the darker the skin color. Patients with light skin have fewer and smaller melanosomes compared with individuals with darker skin, especially people of African descent who can have melanosomes that are much larger and more numerous. Darker skin gives protection from ultraviolet (UV) radiation. Studies have shown that dark skin has a sun protection factor (SPF) between 5 and 13. Because of the protective aspect of darker skin, the incidence of nonmelanoma skin cancer in black people or people of African origin is much less than in white people or those with lighter skin. Studies have shown that basal cell carcinomas are extremely rare in individuals with darker skin.

Skin bleaching (or lightening) creams and ointments may be used by some patients wanting to lighten their overall skin tone. These creams, typically not prescribed, are sold OTC and may be prone to misuse or overuse. Their active ingredients are largely unregulated, and some preparations have been known to contain potential toxins, such as heavy metals. Patients should, therefore, be cautioned against the use of such nonprescription bleaching creams. The clinician should be sensitive to the fact that such discussions may also extend to the larger societal implications of skin color as perceived on a personal level by the patient.

Normal Variations of Pigmentation

Pigmentation disorders presenting in the primary care setting may include misclassifications of normal variations in skin color related to ethnic differences (e.g., oral hyperpigmentation in people with darker skin). Normal variations in pigmentation are commonly seen in patients with darker skin. In patients with dark skin or those of African descent, oral hyperpigmentation is considered a normal variant, but underlying pathology should be ruled out. One exception is newborn infants, in whom oral pigmentation should not be present at this early stage. The most common site of normal oral hyperpigmentation is the gingivae (the gums), but other sites such as the inside of the cheeks (buccal mucosa) and the tongue can be involved as well. The hyperpigmented areas can range from bluish black to deep brown in color. Another pigmentation change that is considered a normal variant of darker skin is hypopigmentation of the midsternal area. This type of hypopigmentation is seen in up to 70% of black children and in up to one-third of black adults and is more common in males.

Voigt or Futcher lines are seen in up to one-fourth of people with dark skin and less frequently in patients of Asian descent. These distinct lines appear down the length of each arm symmetrically, dividing lighter colored skin anteromedially from darker colored skin, with the lighter shade of skin touching the trunk. The nails of people with darker skin can also be pigmented, with involvement of the entire nail plate or in longitudinal bands or streaks of darker color. Normal nail pigmentation should be bilateral and symmetrical. Any asymmetry or new onset of pigmentation should arouse the clinician's suspicion for underlying disease, including acral melanoma. Pigmentation changes in people with darker skin do not necessarily point to pathology, but the clinician should not neglect the possibility of a disease process.

DIFFERENTIAL DIAGNOSIS

Pigmentation disorders can be clinical manifestations of diseases including endocrine, genetic, metabolic, or nutritional disorders or malignancy. Differential diagnoses to consider with oral hyperpigmentation include Peutz-Jeghers syndrome, pigmented tumors such as melanoma, Addison's disease (adrenal insufficiency), heavy metal exposure, and side effects of antimalarial medications. Peutz-Jeghers syndrome is an inherited disorder that presents with pigmented (dark brown–colored) macules on the lips and inside of the mouth on the mucous membranes. It is associated with multiple hamartomatous polyps in the stomach, the small intestine, and large bowel, causing abdominal pain and other gastrointestinal symptoms. Patients who are suspected of having this disease need to be referred to a gastroenterologist for further evaluation.

Vitiligo

Vitiligo, or the total loss of skin color in patchy areas of the body (rarely over the entire body), is recognized clinically as white macules or patches that are usually located on sun-exposed areas, such as the face, lips, arms, hands, and feet. Mucous membranes and the retina may also be affected, and premature graying of the hair may occur. Uveitis may be an associated finding. Vitiligo most often occurs in the 20s and 30s, although it may present at any age. Seventy percent to 80% of adults with vitiligo develop it before 30 years of age. Children represent nearly 30% of those affected. It occurs equally in both sexes and in all races. It is relatively common and affects 0.1% to 2% of the population.

Vitiligo is thought to be an autoimmune disorder in which the body produces antibodies against its own melanocytes. In support of an autoimmune etiology, vitiligo occurs more often in individuals with other autoimmune diseases such as Hashimoto's thyroiditis, Graves' disease, type 1 diabetes mellitus, AA, pernicious anemia, rheumatoid arthritis, psoriasis, inflammatory bowel disease, linear morphea, myasthenia gravis, discoid lupus, SLE, Sjögren syndrome, and autoimmune polyglandular syndrome. There is also some evidence that vitiligo may be inherited.

Another theory of causation is related to trigger events, such as emotional stress, a skin rash, sunburn, or other skin trauma, as well as to imiquimod exposure. Exposure to phenols in the environment (e.g., adhesives, paint, hair dye) may also contribute to depigmentation in people who are genetically predisposed.

The diagnosis of vitiligo is based on family history, a history of skin trauma, rash, or sunburn to the affected area, a personal or family history of other autoimmune disease, and physical examination. Biopsy may be done to confirm the absence of melanocytes in affected skin. A positive Wood's lamp examination of the affected area will show well-demarcated borders with a blue-white florescence. Laboratory studies include a CBC and peripheral smear (to detect pernicious anemia; i.e., megaloblastic anemia related to vitamin B_{12} deficiency), thyroid function studies, and an antinuclear antibody test. An eye examination to rule out uveitis may also be considered.

Current treatments for vitiligo include topical corticosteroids, topical tacrolimus (an immunosuppressive agent), narrowband ultraviolet B (NB-UVB) light therapy, psoralen (oral or topical) with UVA (PUVA) or UVB light therapy, depigmentation with topical creams, and surgical approaches, including skin grafting. No treatments are approved by the FDA for repigmenting skin affected by vitiligo; thus, all current therapies are used off-label. Topical corticosteroids should be cycled 1 week on and 1 week off to avoid adverse effects, such as skin thinning and striae. Light therapy, including excimer laser treatments, may require repeated sessions and may not have permanent results.

The side effects of oral psoralen include predisposition to sunburn, nausea, vomiting, hyperpigmentation, pruritus, and abnormal hair growth; oral PUVA may also cause skin cancer. Topical tacrolimus has a boxed warning in its drug label regarding cancer risk with long-term use. Depigmentation may be a viable choice for those with greater than 50% skin involvement; however, side effects of depigmentation creams may include redness, swelling, pruritus, or xerosis (dry skin). Surgical therapies are reserved for those who have vitiligo that is stable but unresponsive to other treatments. Camouflage techniques may also be used, such as self-tanning agents, pigmented cover creams, and tattooing. Multiple new approaches are under study in the treatment of vitiligo, including afamelanotide, a melanocyte-stimulating hormone (MSH; melanocortin 1 receptor agonist) used with NB-UVB, and targeted immunotherapy blocking the interferon-(-CXCL10 chemokine axis.

Melasma and Chloasma

Melasma is a common acquired condition of hyperpigmentation that develops in sun-exposed areas. Chloasma is a synonymous term for melasma when it occurs during pregnancy ("the mask of pregnancy"). Genetics, sun exposure, hormonal influences, and stress may all be components in the development of melasma. There is often a family history of hyperpigmentation. It is most common in females and in people with light-brown skin tones, i.e., Fitzpatrick skin color categories III to V. It may have a hormonal basis due to increased levels of estrogen, progesterone, and MSH during pregnancy, as well as oral contraceptive use.

Areas most commonly affected include the cheeks, forehead, upper lip, and chin, in a symmetrical pattern. The hyperpigmentation is worsened by exposure to sunlight, and patients should strictly avoid sun exposure, use sunblock such as iron oxide, and wear wide-brimmed hats and sun-protective clothing. Diagnosis of melasma/chloasma and the extent of epidermal/dermal involvement are determined by performing a Wood's lamp examination to visualize excess melanin in the epidermis.

Treatment of melasma/chloasma may include hydroquinone cream alone or in combination with a topical retinoid (tretinoin) and corticosteroids ("triple combination cream" or TCC). Other topicals include azelaic acid or kojic acid creams, glycolic and salicylic acid peels, and various laser and intense pulsed light photorejuvenation treatments. Oral tranexamic acid (TXA) has recently been shown to be effective for melasma that is unresponsive to topical therapy alone, but further study is needed. Laser treatments may be appealing to patients desiring faster results than bleaching agents provide; however, they are considered second-line therapy due to cost and limited access issues.

The current recommended first-line treatment for melasma is hydroquinone cream or TCC with a sunscreen with an SPF of greater than 30 and an iron oxide sunblock. TCC can be applied daily for up to 12 months. A 24-hour skin patch test to rule out allergy to any bleaching agent should be done before use. The patient should be advised to avoid the eye area and to use the cream cautiously in sensitive areas, such as the nose and lips. Safety of these treatments in pregnancy and lactation has not been established; pregnant or breastfeeding patients should be referred to an obstetrician for management. Due to the risk of postinflammatory hyperpigmentation, melasma can be difficult to treat in darker skin types, i.e., Fitzpatrick skin color categories IV to VI.

Drug-Induced Hyperpigmentation

Many classes of drugs have been implicated in hyperpigmentation, including antimalarials, chemotherapeutics, anticoagulants, antimicrobials, anticonvulsants, antipsychotics, antiretrovirals, NSAIDs, and heavy metals. Specific drugs that are known to cause diffuse hyperpigmentation (melanosis) include amiodarone, zidovudine, minocycline, clofazimine, psoralens, and cyclophosphamide. Photosensitivity reactions resulting in hyperpigmentation after sun exposure can also be caused by citrus oils present in fruits or certain perfumes and in commonly used essential oils. Thus, citrus oils should be not be applied to the skin before sun exposure.

Addison's Disease

Addison's disease is an adrenal insufficiency commonly caused by autoimmune destruction of the adrenal cortex, which results in the loss of the feedback loop to the hypothalamus and anterior pituitary. Continuous secretion of corticotropin and MSH occurs, resulting in the characteristic dermatological manifestations of Addison's disease, particularly hyperpigmentation of the skin and oral mucous membranes. (See Chapter 57 for a full discussion of adrenal insufficiency diagnosis and management.)

Addison's disease causes diffuse generalized hyperpigmentation, especially on skin creases. Classic areas where hyperpigmentation may be seen include the skinfolds; palmar creases; pressure points such as the elbows, knees, and knuckles; the oral mucosa; the vaginal and perianal mucosa; and on scars. However, lack of hyperpigmentation does not rule out Addison's disease as a potential diagnosis. Other symptoms of Addison's disease include generalized weakness, fatigue, poor appetite, weight loss, amenorrhea, and loss of axillary hair in women. Gastrointestinal symptoms may include nausea, vomiting, and diarrhea.

Skin Cancer

Skin cancer is the most common type of cancer and the incidence is increasing. The most common skin cancers are basal cell carcinoma, squamous cell carcinoma, and melanoma. In patients with pigmented nevi (moles), the presence of certain uncommon colors on a nevus, such as blue, gray, pink, white, or black (or a variegation of color), should raise suspicion for potential malignancy. Benign nevi are usually less than 6 mm (smaller than a pencil eraser) and have a well-defined border. Benign nevi should be only a single shade of color, usually brown, beige, or pink. The American Cancer Society mnemonic to help detect skin cancer is ABCDE: A, asymmetry; B, border (irregularity); C, color (variegation); D, diameter (greater than 6 mm); and E, evolving (changing in color, shape or size).

When evaluating nail pigmentation changes, symmetry and bilateral involvement of the nails and a history of stable pigmentation with no changes in color is reassuring. A variegated color or very dark color on one solitary nail should arouse suspicion for acral melanoma. Melanomas in people with darker skin are more likely to present on the extremities (acral areas) rather than on the trunk. The nailbeds, the palms, and the soles are sites where acral melanoma is more likely to be seen in darker skinned people. The differential diagnoses of nail pigmentation change include acral melanoma, Peutz-Jeghers syndrome, a subungual nevus, gold therapy, Addison's disease, hemochromatosis, and a history of taking antimalarial medications. If acral melanoma is suspected, referral to a dermatologist for a nail biopsy and definitive diagnosis is imperative.

Malignant melanoma, the deadliest of all skin cancers, requires a high index of suspicion. Risk factors for melanoma include sun exposure, especially to UVB light, having light hair and skin that burns easily, and having freckles or numerous (100 or more) benign nevi. Having a personal history of prior melanoma poses an increased risk of developing another, as well as having a family history of melanoma in a first-degree relative. Any mole presenting with asymmetry and changes in pigmentation, size, or surface features requires referral to a dermatologist for definitive diagnosis and treatment.

PRURITUS

Pruritus, the sensation of itching accompanied by the urge to scratch, is perceived as unpleasant; therefore, people often seek help in the primary care setting for this problematic symptom. Pruritus is a frequent symptom of dermatological disease; it can be acute or chronic and is sometimes so severe it interferes with sleep and daily life activities.

Pruritus generally has either a local (e.g., insect bite, contact dermatitis) or systemic (e.g., chronic renal failure, hyperbilirubinemia with skin deposition of bile salts) etiology. Rashes or other skin lesions generally accompany the sensation of itching on the skin, although in some cases of systemic etiology, no external findings on the skin are ever identified. Therefore, the finding of skin lesions or rashes is most useful in classification of the differential diagnosis of pruritus (see Differential Diagnosis 11.2).

DIFFERENTIAL DIAGNOSIS

A thorough and careful history is an important step in the evaluation of pruritus. If skin findings suggest an external causation (such as the linear striations characteristic of contact dermatitis), the history should be directed toward eliciting an external etiology. If the patient complains of generalized itching with no skin lesions, an internal or systemic etiology is more likely. The presence of a generalized rash should also arouse the clinician's suspicion of a drug reaction. Some systemic causes of pruritus include conditions such as allergies, drug reactions, malignancy (lymphomas and leukemias), chronic renal disease (especially with hemodialysis), pruritus from obstructive biliary disease due to elevated blood levels of unconjugated bilirubin, endocrine-related pruritus (hyperthyroidism and hypothyroidism, possibly diabetes mellitus), and hematological pruritus (polycythemia vera, possibly iron deficiency) (see Focus on History: Pruritus).

Differential Diagnosis 11.2: Pruritus

Condition	Differential Diagnosis
Pruritus—rash present	Atopic dermatitis (eczema) Bullous pemphigoid Burrowing insects/larvae (scabies) Contact dermatitis Dermatitis herpetiformis Dermatographism (Darier's disease) Drug eruptions Ecthyma Erythroderma Folliculitis Impetigo Insect bites/pediculosis Lichen planus Malignancy (cutaneous T-cell lymphoma) Miliaria (heat rash) Neurotic excoriation Pityriasis rosea Pregnancy-induced Prurigo nodularis Psoriasis Seborrheic dermatitis Tinea (capitis, corporis, pedis, cruris) Transient acantholytic dermatosis (Grover's disease) Urticaria (hives)
Pruritus—no rash present	Chronic renal disease, especially with hemodialysis Cholestatic liver disease Delusions of parasitosis Diabetes mellitus Hyperparathyroidism Hyperthyroidism/hypothyroidism Hodgkin's lymphoma Leukemia Polycythemia vera Iron deficiency

Focus on History: Pruritus

A thorough history of present illness for pruritus should include the seven variables of onset: location, duration, character, aggravating and relieving factors, timing, and severity. An in-depth investigation includes multiple areas of questioning.

History of contact with insects:

- Have you had any exposure to mosquitoes, fleas, sand flies, ticks, or spiders? (Brown recluse and black widow bites have necrotic centers.)

History of contact with the outdoors:

- Have you been to the beach, at a picnic, gone camping or swimming, or attended a sporting event (especially outdoors)?

History of contact with plants:

- Have you been in contact with plants or done any gardening?

History of contact with jewelry/metals:

- Any new watches, belts/belt buckles, earrings, or necklaces? Any contact with metals?

History of occupation:

- What is your occupation? (Gardeners and employees of prisons, day-care centers, and schools have the potential for scabies, pediculosis, or impetigo exposure.)

History of hobbies and sport participation:

- Any exposure to hobby paints and glues (agents of contact dermatitis)?
- Do you participate in any sports? (Weight lifters and athletes are prone to fungal skin infections.)

History of chemical exposure:

- Any use or exposure to pesticides, herbicides, fertilizers, or household cleaners?

History of medications:

- Any use of topical medications such as Neosporin ointment, Benadryl topical lotion, or anti-itch lotion or spray? If so, did it reduce the itching? (This would be consistent with contact dermatitis.)
- Any prescription or OTC medications, herbals, or vitamins?

Family history:

- Any family members or intimate friends with the same symptoms? (This raises suspicion for scabies, pediculosis, or tinea infections.)

Social history:

- Any history or current alcohol or drug abuse, emotional distress, or psychiatric illness?

Pruritus is a symptom and should elicit an investigation of its potential cause. External causes of pruritus include insect bites, insect infestations (scabies, pediculosis), pinworms (more common in children with perianal pruritus), larva migrans, contact dermatitis, fiberglass dermatitis, sea bather's eruption, and bacterial folliculitis. It is not uncommon for patients to deny the knowledge of insect bites (especially if the event occurred during sleep) because some insects do not have painful bites. The patient should be asked about any history of medication use, including prescription drugs, hormones, vitamin supplements, and the use of nutritional or protein supplements. The history should include a review of all detergents, soaps, creams, moisturizers, cosmetics, and perfumes. A history of alternative medicines should also be included, such as herbs, homeopathic remedies, and oils for aromatherapy. The use of recreational substances, including chewing tobacco, marijuana, and illicit drugs, should be considered as a potential cause of pruritus. Psychiatric illness as a cause of pruritus is a diagnosis of exclusion. With a psychogenic etiology, skin markings are seen more often on the extremities, and the urge to scratch even in the absence of itch is sometimes reported. The clinician should search for symptoms of depression or mood disorder. There is frequently a history of increased stress because of personal, financial, or familial problems.

The most predominant and disturbing symptom of scabies is pruritus, especially at night. On examination, the clinician may see the mites' burrows, which may be obliterated by scratching. Frequently, the rash has secondary changes, including excoriation, scaling, lichenification, and occasionally nodules (nodular scabies) due to the intense inflammatory response to the mites. The clinician should consider the diagnosis if the location of the rash is on the axilla, under the breast, on the waistline, on the penis, or between the fingers. Scabies is more common in group homes and nursing homes. For a full discussion of the diagnosis and management of scabies, see Chapter 12.

If a pruritic rash does not respond to symptomatic treatment, a work-up for systemic diseases is in order. Laboratory tests that should be ordered if systemic disease is suspected include a CBC with differential, ESR, fasting blood sugar, liver and renal function tests, a thyroid profile including thyroid-stimulating hormone (TSH) level, and a viral hepatitis profile. If the pruritic area is in the anus, an examination for external hemorrhoids should be done. In children or in adults with small children, a stool sample to check for ova and parasites or a Scotch tape test is recommended when pinworm infestation is suspected.

Dry skin, or *xerosis,* is a common finding in older adults. It is also seen in young adults who are overly meticulous with personal hygiene. Use of strong deodorant soaps or daily hot baths can precipitate dry skin and worsen pruritus.

Systemic causes of pruritus to consider include atopic dermatitis (eczema); psoriasis; drug reactions; urticaria (from exposure to any substance, including airborne allergens); urticarial eruptions of pregnancy; lichen planus; lichen simplex chronicus; prurigo nodularis; and malignancies such as Hodgkin's lymphoma (with pruritus seen in approximately 35% of cases), cutaneous

T-cell lymphoma (mycosis fungoides), and leukemia. A history of similar pruritic lesions in the past (especially if at the same location) should suggest an atopic history or urticaria. Atopic skin diseases that present predominantly with pruritus include atopic dermatitis (eczema) and psoriasis. The presence of hives or a history of hives to a known trigger is sufficient to diagnose urticaria. It is often seen with dermatographism, which can be elicited by rubbing a blunt object or finger on the skin firmly. An immediate response is seen, with formation of whealing that resolves within a few hours.

Lichen planus can mimic psoriasis and its cause is unknown. The lesions appear with shiny flat tops that are a red to violaceous color (red-violet tinged). Other presentations include small, flat-topped papules and a netlike lesion on the buccal mucosa (reticular lichen planus), penis, and external female genitalia. Malignant oral lesions occasionally occur, although oral carcinoma is rare. Lichen planus may have several presentations and locations. Lesions may be generalized, or they may be located on the arms, trunk, mouth, and genitalia. This disease may last for months to years; it does not have a cure and is best managed by a dermatologist.

MANAGEMENT

The treatment of pruritus depends on the correct diagnosis. The goal of treatment of pruritus is to relieve the itch, break the itch–scratch cycle, and maintain the barrier protection of the skin. Patients should be educated to avoid scratching, use cool compresses and apply pressure to itchy areas, and keep hands clean and fingernails trimmed. Wearing cotton gloves while sleeping may be advised to avoid the skin trauma from nighttime scratching.

Symptomatic treatment of pruritus includes systemic and topical treatments, or combinations of both. Systemic medications include classic oral H_1 antihistamines such as hydroxyzine (Vistaril), one of the most effective treatments for pruritus, given three to four times per day. Cyproheptadine is used two to three times per day. OTC antihistamines include loratadine, desloratadine, cetirizine, and fexofenadine, which can all be taken once daily. In addition, older generation agents such diphenhydramine, brompheniramine maleate, and chlorpheniramine maleate can be taken every 4 to 6 hours as needed. Newer generation agents such as cetirizine, levocetirizine, fexofenadine, and desloratadine cause less (or no) sedation when taken at their approved doses.

Any patient who is on antihistamines should be warned of possible drowsiness and should be cautioned against driving or operating dangerous machinery until the effects of the antihistamine on the individual patient are known. Alcohol and other central nervous system depressants worsen this effect. The sedating effects of first-generation antihistamines may be desirable when itching is interfering with sleep. First-generation antihistamines with anticholinergic properties such as diphenhydramine, cyproheptadine, brompheniramine maleate, and chlorpheniramine maleate should be avoided in older patients.

Topical treatments for pruritus include anesthetics such as lidocaine 2.5% and prilocaine 2.5% cream (EMLA) and pramoxine (ProctoFoam, Sarna Sensitive, Gold Bond Anti-Itch, Pramox). Topical antihistamines and capsaicin may provide relief from itching, and topical immunomodulators (pimecrolimus [Elidel], tacrolimus [Prograf]) may be used for atopic dermatitis. For anogenital pruritus, treatment includes the use of hydrocortisone and pramoxine cream 1% or 2.5% (Pramosone) on the anogenital area. Pramoxine preparations are effective and have a low incidence of sensitivity reactions compared with topical antihistamines and benzocaine. They are effective not only for anogenital pruritus but also for short-term relief of urticaria, insect bites, pruritus vulvae, and nummular eczema. Use of fluorinated and potent topical steroids on the anogenital area is not recommended because it can lead to atrophy and striae.

Symptomatic treatment for dry skin and resulting pruritus consists of avoidance of strong soaps; taking shorter, tepid showers (10 to 20 minutes) instead of hot baths; and the use of effective emollients. Mild, bland soaps (e.g., Dove, Basis, Purpose, Cetaphil, Neutrogena) are recommended. The patient should be educated to gently towel-dry after showering by patting the skin surface because rubbing the skin stimulates pruritus. To seal moisture into the skin, applying a bland emollient such as petroleum jelly, Eucerin, Lubriderm, or Alpha-Keri immediately after dabbing the skin with a towel to partially pat dry is helpful. Waiting too long (more than 5 minutes) after finishing a bath or shower allows moisture to evaporate from the skin. The strongest emollients are ointments that are petrolatum-based, followed by creams (oil in water), and then lotions (powder in water). Gels are alcohol-based; they should not be used for pruritus associated with dry skin because of alcohol's drying effect. Severe cases of dry skin may be treated using the "soak and smear" technique by wetting the skin for 20 minutes and then applying ointment directly to wet skin.

Pruritus of the scalp caused by seborrheic dermatitis (with dandruff and fine scales at the hairline, around the nares, and at the ears) should be treated with ketoconazole 2% shampoo (Nizoral shampoo). The rash of seborrheic dermatitis is best treated with hydrocortisone 1% (OTC) used two to three times a day. Fluorinated topical steroids should not be used on the face because of the risk of skin atrophy. If the etiology is an irritating external agent (such as fiberglass insulation), elimination of the agent may provide clinical relief of pruritus.

Lichen planus and its associated pruritus are treated with antihistamines, topical and systemic corticosteroids, retinoids, cyclosporine, PUVA, and tacrolimus or pimecrolimus topical preparations. The treatment of lichen planus is best managed by a dermatologist.

Other systemic treatments for persistent pruritus may include antidepressants such as the tricyclic doxepin or mirtazapine, as well as anticonvulsant/nerve pain agents such as gabapentin (Neurontin). The antinausea/antiemetic aprepitant (Emend) has also been shown to be effective in treating the itch of atopic dermatitis and prurigo nodularis.

If Hodgkin's lymphoma is suspected, the clinician should perform a thorough physical examination, looking especially for painless, enlarged lymph nodes and constitutional symptoms such as generalized pruritus, weight loss, night sweats, and fever. Cutaneous T-cell lymphoma (mycosis fungoides) is a malignancy of the helper T cells of the immune system. The onset of lesions may take many years, and intractable pruritus may sometimes be the only presenting symptom. Characteristic lesions may be misdiagnosed as psoriasis or as nummular dermatitis (eczema) because of their similar appearance. These lesions go through several stages and can present as red, scaly plaques that mimic the appearance of psoriasis; nodules and tumors can also be present, sometimes with ulceration. Diagnostic laboratory testing for suspected malignancy can include a CBC with differential, a peripheral smear, liver and renal function tests, ESR, a chest x-ray film, and directed computed tomography (CT) scanning. Patients with suspected malignancy should be referred to cancer specialists.

Pruritus associated with systemic disease requires treatment directed at the specific causation.

- Chronic renal failure: Pruritus of chronic renal failure responds well to NB-UVB therapy and activated charcoal. Topical treatments including capsaicin 0.025% cream (preceded by an application of EMLA cream to reduce the burning sensation), tacrolimus 0.03% ointment, topical γ-linolenic acid, and gabapentin cream have provided relief in some studies.
- Cholestasis: First-line treatment for pruritus associated with cholestasis is cholestyramine. Other therapies that have been effective include rifampin and opioid antagonists such as naloxone.
- Endocrine: Pruritus associated with hypothyroidism responds well to topical emollients and thyroid hormone replacement. Pruritus in this case is largely caused by dry skin typically associated with hypothyroidism, thus, itching usually improves with treatment of the underlying thyroid hormone deficiency.
- Hematological: Iron deficiency–associated pruritus is treated with iron supplementation, whereas the itch associated with polycythemia vera responds well to aspirin therapy.

RASH

The word *rash* refers to any pink- or red-colored skin eruption, although rash colors may differ depending on underlying skin color. Words that are synonymous with rash include *exanthem* and *eruption*. Rashes are clinical manifestations of skin irritation or inflammation and have multiple etiologies.

Skin cells (keratinocytes) originate in the basal layer of the epidermis. These cells take approximately 28 days to mature and migrate to the skin surface (stratum corneum). The epidermis has no blood supply of its own and is dependent on the dermis for its circulation. It is stratified into two main layers: the inner viable layer (stratum germinativum) and the outer layer of dead cells (stratum corneum or the horny layer). The stratum corneum consists of up to 25 layers of flat, tightly packed anucleate cells filled with keratin, a durable protein that limits the passage of molecules into and out of the skin. This tough outer layer is relatively impermeable to many external substances and prevents the evaporation of bodily fluids. It is also a protective barrier against numerous microorganisms.

When the stratum corneum is damaged by inflammation (i.e., a rash develops), it becomes more permeable to external substances, including microorganisms and chemicals. Not only do these substances and microorganisms have a greater chance of gaining entrance to the body, but therapeutic topical creams and ointments applied to inflamed skin also are more likely to be absorbed and thus have an increased risk of toxicity.

The dermis, which gives the skin its elasticity and strength, consists primarily of a complex network of collagen and elastic fibers interspersed with blood vessels, cutaneous nerves, apocrine glands, eccrine glands, lymphatics, and pilosebaceous units of the skin. The dermo-epidermal junction (the topmost section of the dermis) is the interface between the epidermis and the dermis. A defect in the dermoepidermal junction results in separation of these layers and the formation of bullae. Inherited autoimmune diseases of the skin resulting from abnormalities of the dermis include bullous pemphigoid and epidermolysis bullosa.

Gram-positive bacterial infections such as *Staphylococcus aureus* (the causative agent of toxic shock syndrome [TSS]) present with systemic symptoms such as fever, malaise, and an erythematous rash. Drug reactions can also present with a rash (e.g., erythema multiforme, urticaria). Many autoimmune disorders can cause characteristic rashes, including SLE (malar butterfly rash), erythema nodosum (painful red bumps under the skin of the extremities), Still's disease (evanescent salmon-colored rash), and Kawasaki disease (seen in children).

Viruses are responsible for many cases of rash and are usually self-limited in patients with intact immune systems. Viral infections that manifest with rash and systemic symptoms such as fever and malaise include measles, rubella (German measles), hand-foot-mouth disease (most commonly caused by coxsackievirus), erythema infectiosum (caused by parvovirus B19), herpes simplex infection, herpes zoster, varicella zoster (chickenpox), and roseola (also known as exanthema subitum) in children.

Rashes are more difficult to see in patients with darker skin because the typical red to dark pink color that is associated with rash becomes less visible. Instead of the pink to red color, a rash in a person with darker skin might appear as a dark-brown color. Thus, rashes on patients with darker skin can sometimes go unnoticed unless the patient complains of the problem to the clinician. The clinician must learn to use other dermatological clues besides skin color to differentiate rashes in this population. These include the history of the rash and associated symptoms, the type of lesions present (macule, papule, pustule), the texture of the lesions (flat, raised, rough), and the pattern of distribution (central vs. on the extremities) (see Focus on History: Rash).

Focus on History: Rash

Onset of skin lesions:
- When did the skin lesions first appear?
- How did the skin lesion appear at onset?
- Where did the skin lesion first appear?

Spread of skin lesions:
- Have the skin lesions spread? Where?

Change in skin lesions:
- Has the appearance of the skin lesions changed over time?
- Have the skin lesions gotten better or worse?

Symptoms associated with the skin lesion:
- Are there any associated symptoms, such as itching, burning, or pain?

History of skin treatment:
- What type of self-treatment have you attempted?
- Have you seen another health-care provider for the skin lesions? What type of treatment was given? Was it effective?
- Have you recently used any new skin care products, cosmetics, topical creams or lotions, shampoos, soaps, or clothing detergents?

History of food reactions:
- Do you have any food allergies or sensitivities, such as to dairy, seafood, peanuts, tree nuts, strawberries, tomatoes, or alcoholic drinks (such as red or white wine, beer, or mixed drinks)?

History of medications:
- Are you taking any prescription medications (e.g., antibiotics such as penicillin or sulfa drugs or pain medications such as codeine) and/or OTC medications such as aspirin, NSAIDs, cold medicines, or vitamins?
- Do any of these medications contain artificial colors or preservatives?

Alternative medicine:
- Are you taking any herbal medicines or teas, homeopathic remedies, aromatherapy, juices, or other alternative medicines?

Atopic history:
- Do you have a history of the same rash developing before? What was the diagnosis? How was it treated?
- Do you have a family history of skin conditions or rashes?
- Have you or a family member ever been diagnosed with eczema (atopic dermatitis), psoriasis, skin allergies, asthma, or other allergies?

Infectious disease exposure (any exposure up to 2 weeks before the onset of rash):
- Were you exposed to other people with the same symptoms?
- Were you exposed to small children, day-care, or school environments?
- Have you had sexual activity with a new partner (known to you for less than 3 months)?

Systemic symptoms (infectious, autoimmune, malignancies, metabolic):
- Do you have any systemic symptoms, such as sore throat or rhinitis (viral etiology), fever, fatigue, myalgia, joint pain, nausea, night sweats, weight loss (malignancy), or weight gain (diabetes mellitus)?

DIFFERENTIAL DIAGNOSIS

Because the differential diagnosis of rash is so broad, this section presents a framework to elicit information designed to determine the etiology of rash. Key considerations are discussed regarding rashes that are associated with serious health consequences. Clinicians should become familiar with these rashes, given their potential for serious sequelae, including death, if the diagnosis is missed.

Paget's Disease

Mammary Paget's disease is an uncommon form of breast cancer that presents with a rash that looks like eczematous dermatitis of the nipple and areola. The clinician should be careful not to overlook this rare intraepithelial adenocarcinoma. Its onset is gradual, ranging from several months to years. Early in its course, the disease is asymptomatic except for the rash. During the later stages, however, it may be accompanied by pruritus, discharge, bleeding, and ulceration. The size of lesions can range from less than 1 cm to several centimeters in diameter. Sometimes an underlying breast mass is palpable during the later stages of the disease; a worse prognosis is associated with this ominous finding. Patients with suspected mammary Paget's disease should be referred to a breast specialist.

The usual location of the classic rash of mammary Paget's disease is on one nipple (or areola); rarely, it is seen on both breasts. The skin lesion appears as an oval-shaped, erythematous scaling plaque with sharp margins. Because of its similar appearance, this lesion can be misdiagnosed as eczema, psoriasis, contact dermatitis, or impetigo. However, the lesions of eczematous dermatitis typically involve both breasts, last from 2 to 3 weeks, and respond to treatment with topical corticosteroids. Contact dermatitis usually involves only one breast (although sometimes both, depending on the extent of exposure to the triggering agent), resolves in 2 weeks, and responds to topical corticosteroids. If a rash on the nipple or areolar region lasts longer than 2 weeks and does not resolve with topical corticosteroids, a high index of suspicion for Paget's disease is imperative, and the patient should be referred to a breast specialist for further evaluation.

Toxic Shock Syndrome

TSS is an acute illness caused by toxin-producing *S. aureus*. In the United States, TSS occurs in both male and female patients, with an overall incidence of 0.8 to 3.4 per 100,000; among menstruating women its incidence is 1 per 100,000. However, 50% of TSS cases are nonmenstrual in etiology and males comprise 25% of these patients. Men can acquire TSS when the bacterium *S. aureus* gets into the bloodstream and produces toxins. Risk factors for menstrual TSS include tampon use in general, using tampons regularly during the menstrual cycle, and leaving tampons inserted for extended periods of time. Cases of menstrual TSS have progressively declined over the past 20 years after superabsorbent tampons were taken off the market. In these cases, symptoms begin within 5 days of the onset of menstruation in women who have used tampons. Nonmenstrual TSS can occur after childbirth or an abortion or as a result of surgical wounds, nasal packs, burns, catheters, or intravaginal occlusive birth control devices such as the sponge, diaphragm, or cervical cap. The amount of time a diaphragm or cervical cap remains in the vagina, particularly if greater than 30 hours, seems to be a factor in the development of TSS, as well as if pieces of a contraceptive sponge are retained in the genital tract. Women younger than 19 years of age account for one-third of TSS cases, and these women are prone to recurrence. The mortality rate for TSS is less than 5%. Severe group A beta-hemolytic *Streptococcus* (GABHS) infection can mimic TSS, except that GABHS is also associated with necrotizing fasciitis and has a higher mortality rate (30% to 70%).

TSS presents with a sudden onset of high fever (higher than 102°F [38.8°C]) and vomiting. It is associated with a tingling sensation of the hands and feet, myalgia, weakness, headache, and diarrhea, and in severe cases, it is associated with confusion, hypotension, and shock. It is accompanied by a bright-red, fine maculopapular (scarlatiniform) rash and is sometimes accompanied by petechiae and bullae. The skin on the palms of the hands and the soles of the feet is very erythematous, and in 1 to 2 weeks, the palms and soles start to desquamate. Abnormal laboratory results include leukocytosis, thrombocytopenia, abnormal liver function tests, elevated creatinine levels, and abnormally low levels of platelets (thrombocytopenia).

Complications of TSS include multisystem organ failure (e.g., acute respiratory distress syndrome, acute kidney failure), metabolic acidosis, disseminated intravascular coagulation, septic shock, and death. Thus, patients with suspected TSS should be referred immediately to a physician or an emergency department. Menstruating women who are using a tampon should be advised to remove the tampon immediately. Treatment consists of hospitalization in the intensive care unit for aggressive systemic antibiotic treatment and supportive therapy.

URTICARIA

Urticaria (hives or wheals) is a common problem seen in primary care. It affects 15% to 20% of the population at least once and occurs more frequently in females. Urticaria is a sudden generalized eruption of pale, evanescent wheals or papules associated with severe itching. Angioedema is urticaria that involves not only edema of the dermis, as in uncomplicated urticaria, but the subcutaneous tissues as well, which results in prominent and more extensive swelling. Angioedema and urticaria can be part of a life-threatening immunoglobulin E (IgE)–dependent anaphylactic reaction, which involves bronchospasm, laryngeal edema, and shock due to peripheral vasodilation. If anaphylaxis is not treated and reversed immediately with subcutaneous epinephrine, it can be fatal. However, angioedema associated with chronic urticaria is rarely life-threatening. In these cases, the patient will report a history of angioedema but without significant compromise of the throat or airway.

Urticarial wheals (hives) and angioedema are produced by the degranulation of mast cells when an offending allergen to which the patient has been sensitized is encountered. Degranulated mast cells release inflammatory factors, including histamines, that increase vascular permeability and cause pruritus. On microscopic examination, edema within the dermis is manifested by the wide separation of dermal fibers in cells from urticarial lesions, along with dilation of venules and lymphatics. Angioedema may also result from non–IgE-dependent immune reactions involving bradykinin and the complement cascade. Notably, chronic urticaria may be a symptom of an underlying autoimmune condition.

DIFFERENTIAL DIAGNOSIS

There are multiple diseases and syndromes that present with urticarial wheals and angioedema, which underscore the necessity of a thorough history and physical examination to differentiate etiology, particularly with regard to systemic disease. The typical patient with urticaria will present with a complaint of numerous, intensely pruritic hives or wheals that appear regularly at certain times of the day, then spontaneously resolve within a few hours (and typically within no more than 24 hours), only to reappear again the next day. The wheals typically enlarge and coalesce, forming round or irregular shapes.

Urticaria is classified as either acute or chronic. Eighty percent of cases of acute urticaria resolve in 6 weeks or less; however, 20% to 45% of patients with acute urticaria will develop chronic urticaria. As a result, some authorities recommend waiting at least 2 weeks before initiating an extensive (and expensive) laboratory workup for urticaria, as laboratory results are usually normal when testing is done.

Urticaria that lasts longer than 6 weeks is classified as chronic urticaria. Studies of patients with chronic urticaria have found clinically relevant changes in quality of life, including sleep deprivation, social isolation, negative body image, and mood changes.

Chronic urticaria is subclassified into chronic spontaneous urticaria and chronic inducible urticaria. Chronic spontaneous urticaria is characterized by the sudden onset of wheals and/or angioedema lasting longer than 6 weeks. It can be precipitated by infections (commonly upper respiratory infection [URI]), food allergies, drugs (especially angiotensin-converting enzyme [ACE] inhibitors and NSAIDs), emotional stress, and a chronic autoimmune response.

Chronic inducible urticaria includes physical urticaria and other inducible urticarias that are precipitated by an exogenous stimulus and can be provoked/reproduced. Chronic inducible urticaria accounts for 20% to 30% of all cases of urticaria. It occurs immediately or shortly after exposure to a physical stimulus such as pressure (dermatographism), cold, heat, sunlight (solar urticaria), or vibrations. Urticarial episodes resulting from exposure to these stimuli are usually of short duration; most last only 2 hours. Other inducible urticarias include cholinergic, contact, and aquagenic urticaria. Cholinergic urticaria is triggered by exercise, anxiety, elevated body temperature (e.g., fever, exercise, sweating), hot or spicy foods, and hot baths or showers. The lesions usually resolve within 30 minutes after the offending activity is stopped. The hives are small (2 to 4 mm), highly pruritic, surrounded by erythema, and commonly appear on the upper trunk and arms. Contact urticaria is an immediate response to skin contact with external substances such as latex, cosmetics, and sorbic acid (used as a food preservative), whereas aquagenic urticaria is a rare condition triggered by skin contact with water, regardless of the temperature.

Some pregnant women develop an extremely pruritic eruption known as pruritic urticarial papules and plaques of pregnancy (PUPPP) or polymorphic eruption of pregnancy. It occurs in 1 in 160 pregnancies. These lesions appear as erythematous urticarial papules and plaques (striae distensae) that usually start on the striae of the abdomen and spread to the thighs, buttocks, and occasionally, the arms. The lesions can start at any time during the third trimester, but they are frequently seen during the last 2 to 3 weeks of pregnancy. The cause is unknown. PUPPP is not associated with increased maternal or fetal morbidity and usually resolves after delivery of the fetus. Risk factors for the development of PUPPP include pregnancy with a male fetus (accounting for 70% of pregnancies that develop PUPPP), primigravid (first) pregnancy, multiple pregnancy, and pregnancy in women with hypertension (Pierson, 2020).

Treatment of PUPPP during the last trimester of pregnancy involves the use of a moderate to high-potency topical corticosteroid, such as fluticasone or fluocinonide. With topical treatment, improvement of the lesions should be seen in a few days. Topical corticosteroids should not be applied to rashes that are suspected to be of viral etiology (such as herpes simplex or varicella zoster) because corticosteroids can worsen them. Those cases that are unresponsive to topical corticosteroids are best referred to an obstetrician for possible treatment with antihistamines or systemic corticosteroids. There are no antihistamines that are considered completely safe in pregnancy. However, the first-generation antihistamine diphenhydramine is considered by many sources to be the safest antihistamine to recommend in pregnancy due to its long history of availability and use during pregnancy. It is recommended that second-generation antihistamines be utilized at the lowest possible dose for the shortest duration of time in pregnant or lactating women.

MANAGEMENT

The goal of treatment for urticaria is to identify the cause of the skin rash and stop exposure to the sensitizing allergen. Certain drugs such as aspirin, ACE inhibitors, and NSAIDs should be avoided in patients with urticaria. Tight clothing should be avoided because wheals tend to occur in areas with increased pressure or friction. Showering or bathing with hot water should be avoided because this worsens itching. Cool environmental temperatures in the home are helpful and aid in sleep.

The trigger for acute urticaria is identified in less than 50% of patients; URI is the most common etiology, followed by drug reactions and intolerance to foods. Viral infections that have been implicated in causing urticaria include herpes, hepatitis, acute mononucleosis, and rubella. Bacterial infections such as sinusitis and fungal infections have also been implicated. Allergens that can cause both acute and chronic urticaria include drugs; foods; food preservatives; insect bites; and bacterial, fungal, viral, or parasitic infections. If the patient is taking vitamins, herbs, or supplements that are not critical, they should all be stopped; "natural" vitamins and herbal preparations should not be exempted. The patient can start a trial of eliminating certain highly allergenic foods such as eggs, strawberries, tomatoes, chocolate, citrus fruits, peanuts, tree nuts, all vinegars and wines (due to allergenic sulfites), other alcoholic beverages, and shellfish, although this is cumbersome and bothersome for most patients. In addition, broad food elimination in children by concerned parents or overzealous health-care providers increases the risk of malnutrition and social isolation. Food allergens can be occasionally confirmed by antigen-specific serum IgE testing or by skin-prick tests performed by allergists, although interpretation of these test results is complicated by high false-positive rates, which may be overinterpreted by the patient and primary care provider.

The clinical evaluation of chronic urticaria should look for a contributory underlying disease, although the trigger of most cases of chronic urticaria is never found, with etiologies being even more elusive than in acute urticaria. A detailed history of present illness should include timing of onset and the patient's situation at onset (including prior travel), location and duration of lesions, character of rash (itchy or painful), history of similar episodes, known triggers of past reactions, past treatment and response to treatment, and any associated systemic symptoms. A thorough medication list and family history should be included, as well as a standardized urticaria score or scale for comparison over time, which is available on https://www.MDcalc.com/urticaria-activity-score-uas (see Resources).

A thorough physical examination should assess the distribution and characteristics of the lesions, as well as look for signs of localized or systemic disease such as chronic sinusitis, tooth abscess, low-grade fungal infection (candidiasis), intestinal parasites, or chronic hepatitis. Although guidelines do not recommend extensive laboratory testing for urticaria, some studies that may be helpful, depending on the history, include CBC with differential, ESR, C-reactive protein, liver and renal profiles, TSH, and cryoglobulins. Diagnosis of the subtype of chronic inducible urticaria may be made by provocation testing, by reproducing the suspected stimuli, such as rubbing the skin with a tongue depressor to confirm dermatographism, applying wet compresses for possible aquagenic urticaria, or engaging in moderate exercise for suspected cholinergic urticaria. Skin biopsy is not routinely recommended but may be used for recalcitrant cases of chronic urticaria or when another diagnosis is suspected.

Current practice guidelines recommend a stepwise approach to the treatment of urticaria (see Figure 11.1). First-line therapy (Step 1) for urticaria includes second-generation (nonsedating) H_1 antihistamines and avoidance of triggers if they have been identified. Fexofenadine, loratadine, desloratadine, cetirizine, levocetirizine, and azelastine are available OTC; once-daily dosing is recommended.

If the urticaria is not relieved with Step 1 therapy, guidelines suggest progressing to Step 2, which includes increasing the dose of the second-generation H_1 antihistamine two

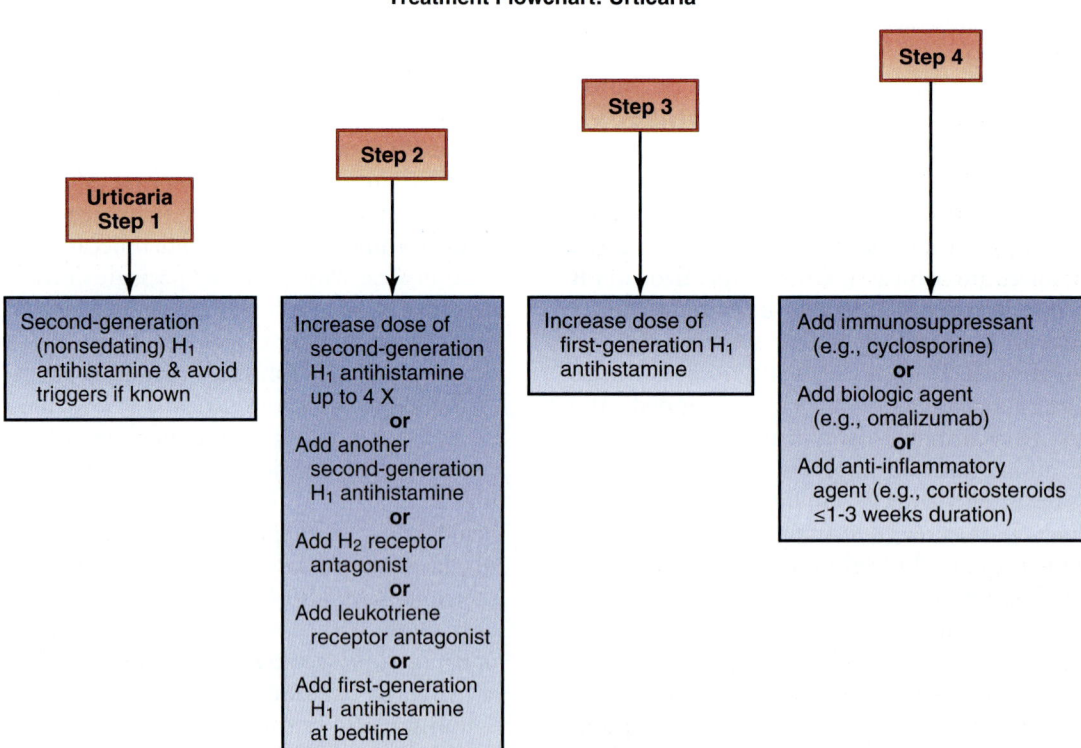

Figure 11.1 Treatment Flowchart: Urticaria. Data from Antia C, Baquerizo K, Korman A, et al. Urticaria: A comprehensive review: Treatment of chronic urticaria, special populations, and disease outcomes. *J Am Acad Dermatol*. 2018;79(4):617–633.

to four times the recommended dosage, adding another second-generation H_1 antihistamine, adding an H_2 blocker such as cimetidine, adding a leukotriene receptor antagonist such as montelukast, or adding a first-generation (sedating) H_1 antihistamine at bedtime. A combination of H_1 and H_2 antihistamines (e.g., cimetidine, famotidine) may be used by some clinicians in refractory cases, but the evidence does not support using these combinations versus H_1 antihistamines alone. Leukotriene receptor antagonists, such as zafirlukast, montelukast, and the 5-lipoxygenase-inhibitor zileuton, are commonly used in asthma and may be useful in patients who are unresponsive to antihistamine therapy.

First-generation H_1 antihistamines, such as hydroxyzine, diphenhydramine, and cyproheptadine, are faster-acting than second-generation agents but have greater sedative effects (which may nonetheless be desirable at bedtime) and shorter half-lives (requiring more frequent dosing for a prolonged effect). The timing of administration of antihistamines should be tailored so that bloodstream levels of the drug will peak during the time of day when urticarial lesions are most likely to occur, which will differ among individuals. All antihistamines, even the so-called nonsedating antihistamines, have the potential for sedation, particularly at high doses and in children and older patients. Patients should be warned against driving or operating heavy machinery while using these medications, particularly if the effects of the medication on the patient are unknown. The combination of antihistamines with other central nervous system depressants, such as alcohol, tranquilizers, and certain antidepressants, will increase this risk of sedation, and many states have restrictions against driving while taking antihistamines.

Due to their anticholinergic effects, first-generation H_1 antagonists such as diphenhydramine and certain H_2 antagonists such as cimetidine should be avoided in older adults, as they may cause arrhythmias, urinary retention, and dizziness, with an increased risk for falls. They may also precipitate confusion, with concerns for potentially increasing the risk of delirium or dementia.

If adequate relief is not achieved with these first- and second-line therapies, Step 3 calls for increasing the dosage of the first-generation H_1 antihistamine at bedtime, given the known sedating effects of these agents. Of note, despite being taken at bedtime, the sedative effects of these agents may carry over to waking hours and impair school or work performance, despite their shorter half-lives and more frequent dosing recommendations.

Patients with severe or refractory urticaria unresponsive to these therapies should be referred to a specialist (allergist or dermatologist), including for urticaria associated with angioedema of the tongue or throat, peanut allergy, latex allergy, or urticaria that persists beyond 6 weeks (chronic urticaria). Alternative treatment options for these difficult cases (Step 4) include immunosuppressants such as cyclosporine, the biological agent omalizumab (an anti-IgE monoclonal antibody also approved for moderate to severe persistent asthma), and anti-inflammatory agents such as corticosteroids. Corticosteroid therapy should be limited to the lowest dose for the shortest duration due to its known adverse effects; less than 3 weeks is recommended.

REFERENCES

Addison's Disease

Liotta E. Dermatologic aspects of Addison Disease. Accessed August 8, 2020. https://emedicine.medscape.com/article/1096911-overview#a5. Updated: Jul 18, 2017.

Alopecia

Borde A, Åstrand A. Alopecia areata and the gut-the link opens up for novel therapeutic interventions. *Expert Opin Ther Targets*. 2018;22(6):503–511.

Choe SJ, Lee S, Pi LQ, et al. Subclinical sensitization with diphenylcyclopropenone is sufficient for the treatment of alopecia areata: Retrospective analysis of 159 cases. *J Am Acad Dermatol*. 2018;78:515.

Lee H, Gwillim E, Patel KR, et al. Epidemiology of alopecia areata, ophiasis, totalis, and universalis: A systematic review and meta-analysis. *J Am Acad Dermatol*. 2020;82(3):675–682.

Lee H, Jung SJ, Patel AB, et al. Racial characteristics in alopecia areata in the United States. *J AM Acad Dermatol*. 2019;83(4):1064–1070.

Lee S, Kim BJ, Lee YB, et al. Hair regrowth outcomes of contact immunotherapy for patients with alopecia areata: A systematic review and meta-analysis. *JAMA Dermatol*. 2018;154:1145.

Lee S, Lee WS. Home-based contact immunotherapy with diphenylcyclopropenone for alopecia areata is as effective and safe as clinic-based treatment in patients with stable disease: A retrospective study of 40 patients. *J Am Acad Dermatol*. 2018;78:599.

National Alopecia Areata Foundation. In this together. https://www.naaf.org. Accessed 12/10/2020.

Phan K, Ramachandran V, Sebaratnam DF. Methotrexate for alopecia areata: A systematic review and meta-analysis. *J Am Acad Dermatol*. 2019;80:120.

Pourang A, Mesinkovska NA. New and emerging therapies for alopecia areata. *Drugs*. 2020;80(7):635–646. doi:10.1007/s40265-020-01293-0 https://pubmed.ncbi.nlm.nih.gov/32323220/.

Strazzulla LC, Wang EHC, Avila L, et al. Alopecia areata: Alopecia areata. An appraisal of new treatment approaches and overview of current therapies. *J Am Acad Dermatol*. 2018;78(1):1–12.

Strazzulla LC, Wang EHC, Avila L, et al. Alopecia areata: Disease characteristics, clinical evaluation, and new perspectives on pathogenesis. *J Am Acad Dermatol*. 2018;78(1):1–12.

Wu SZ, Wang S, Ratnaparkhi R, Bergfeld WF. Treatment of pediatric alopecia areata with anthralin: A retrospective study of 37 patients. *Pediatr Dermatol*. 2018;35:817.

Xie WR, Yang XY, Xia HH, et al. Hair regrowth following fecal microbiota transplantation in an elderly patient with alopecia areata: A case report and review of the literature. *World J Clin Cases*. 2019;7(19):3074–3081. https://pubmed.ncbi.nlm.nih.gov/31624757/.

Drug-Induced Hyperpigmentation

Elston DM. Drug-induced pigmentation (Updated 2018 Apr 30). https://emedicine.medscape.com/article/1069686-overview#a1. Accessed 8/8/2020.

Hassan S, Zhou, X. Drug induced pigmentation. (Updated 2019 Jun 30). In: StatPearls (Internet). Treasure Island (FL). StatPearls Publishing; 2020 Jan. https://www.ncbi.nlm.nih.gov/books/NBK542253/.

Melasma and Chloasma

Hardy CL. Laser treatment of benign pigmented lesions. (Updated 2019 Dec 13). https://emedicine.medscape.com/article/1120359-overview#a1. Accessed 8/4/2020.

Lyford WH. Melasma. (Updated 2020 Apr 27). https://emedicine.medscape.com/article/1068640-overview. Accessed 8/3/2020.

McKesey J, Tovar-Garcia A, Pandya AG. Melasma treatment: An evidence-based review. *Am J Clin Dermatol*. 2020;21(2):173–225.

Sarkar R, Bansal S, Garg VK. Chemical peels for melasma in dark-skinned patients. *J Cutan Aesthet Surg*. 2012 Oct–Dec;5(4):247–253.

Pruritus

Butler DF. Pruritus and systemic disease. https://emedicine.medscape.com/article/1098029-overview.

Rash

Ross A, Shoff H. Toxic shock syndrome. (Updated 2020 Aug 10). In: StatPearls (Internet). Treasure Island (FL): StatPearls Publishing 2020 Jan. https://www.ncbi.nlm.nih.gov/books/NBK459345/. Accessed 8/18/2020.

Schwartz RA. Mammary Paget disease. (Updated 2020 Apr 28). https://emedicine.medscape.com/article/1101235-overview. Accessed 8/12/2020.

Venkataraman R. Toxic shock syndrome. (Updated 2018 May 7). https://emedicine.medscape.com/article/169177-overview. Accessed 8/12/2020.

Skin Cancer

Holtel MR. Skin cancer-melanoma (Updated 2018 June 21). https://emedicine.medscape.com/article/846566-overview#a2. Accessed 8/10/2020.

Urticaria

Antia C, Baquerizo K, Korman A, et al. Urticaria: A comprehensive review: Epidemiology, diagnosis, and work-up. *J Am Acad Dermatol*. 2018;79(4):599–614.

Antia C, Baquerizo K, Korman A, et al. Urticaria: A comprehensive review: Treatment of chronic urticaria, special populations, and disease outcomes. *J Am Acad Dermatol*. 2018;79(4):617–633.

Bernstein JA, Lang DM, Khan DA. The diagnosis and management of acute and chronic urticaria: 2014 update. *J Allergy Clin Immunol* 2014;133(5).1270–1277. https://www.aaaai.org/Aaaai/media/MediaLibrary/PDF%20Documents/Practice%20and%20Parameters/Urticaria-2014.pdf. Accessed 9/7/2020.

Pierson JC. Polymorphic eruption of pregnancy. (Updated 2020 Feb 21). http://emedicine.medscape.com/article/1123725-overview#a5. Accessed 8/19/2020.

Wong HK. Urticaria. (Updated 2018 Jun 13). http://emedicine.medscape.com/article/762917-overview#a1. Accessed 8/19/2020.

Vitiligo

National Institutes of Health. Vitiligo. https://www.niams.nih.gov/health-topics/vitiligo. Accessed 12/10/2020.

Rodrigues M, Ezzedine K, Hamzavi I, et al. Current and emerging treatments for vitiligo. *J Am Acad Dermatol*. 2017;77(1):17–29.

Rodrigues, M, Ezzedine, K, Hamzavi, I, et al. New discoveries in the pathogenesis and classification of vitiligo. *J Am Acad Dermatol*. 2017;77(1):1–13.

RESOURCES

General

American Academy of Dermatology
https://www.aad.org
American Society of Dermatology
https://www.asd.org

Alopecia

National Alopecia Areata Foundation
https://www.naaf.org
National Institute of Allergy and Infectious Disease
https://www.niaid.nih.gov

Skin Cancer

The Skin Cancer Foundation
https://https://www.skincancer.org

Urticaria

Urticaria Activity Score (UAS).
https://www.mdcalc.com/urticaria-activity-score-uas

Chapter 12

Parasitic Skin Infestations

Jill E. Winland-Brown, EdD, APRN, FNP-BC, FAANP
Nancy Harris, DNP, APRN, FNP-BC
Brian Oscar Porter, MD, PhD, MPH, MBA

SCABIES

Scabies is a highly contagious mite infestation that occurs mainly in children, young adults, health-care workers, and institutionalized persons of all ages. It is characterized by generalized intractable pruritus, often with minimal cutaneous manifestations. The diagnosis of scabies infection is easily missed and should be considered in patients of any age with persistent and severe pruritus. Scabies can develop into a chronic condition.

EPIDEMIOLOGY AND CAUSES

Human scabies is caused by the itch mite *Sarcoptes scabiei* var. *hominis,* which infects human skin. The adult female measures 0.3 to 0.5 mm long and has a rounded body with four pairs of short legs. Scabies infestations occur worldwide, are endemic in most parts of the world, and affect people of all races and social classes. Epidemics are historically associated with war, conditions of poverty, overcrowding, poor hygiene, malnutrition, and sexual promiscuity. The World Health Organization estimates that there are about 300 million cases of scabies worldwide. Some studies suggest 6% to 27% of the general population has scabies, but other surveys find a lower prevalence. Close personal contact is the major mode of transmission for scabies, although casual contact such as nursing care may be sufficient for transmission to occur. Institutional epidemics have been reported in which caregivers were infested. Live mites have been discovered in dust samples from the homes of infested persons, suggesting fomite (shared objects, such as furniture or linens) transmission as a possibility. Although mites typically survive for only 24 to 36 hours off of the skin, they survive longer in cold weather.

PATHOPHYSIOLOGY

The scabies itch mite is an aerobic organism and thus requires exposure to surface air to survive. The male mite dies shortly after mating, but the female mite may live 4 to 6 weeks. As an obligate parasite, the scabies mite burrows into the skin shortly after contact. It both resides and reproduces in human skin. The female mite can lay two to three eggs per day (up to 10 to 25 total) in burrows created at the base of the stratum corneum of the epidermis, traveling up to 2 to 3 mm per day. Burrows average 5 mm in length, allowing for continued exposure to surface air, but soon after egg laying is completed, the female mite dies. Eggs hatch, and larvae emerge in 72 to 84 hours, molting at least three times before reaching adulthood. Mating of these new mites thus occurs after approximately 17 days.

Interestingly, sensitivity to *S. scabiei* must take place for pruritus to occur. Initial sensitivity takes several weeks to develop after primary infection and is caused by a foreign body inflammatory reaction to either the mite itself or its feces. In persons with reinfestation, pruritus may occur within 24 hours because the immune system has been previously sensitized. Individuals who are immunocompromised or have a neurological disorder, such as Down's syndrome, stroke, dementia, neuropathy, or spinal cord injury, may be predisposed to a variant of scabies known as crusted scabies (*scabies crustosa;* previously known as "Norwegian scabies"). Scabies crustosa is characterized by scaly lesions at the sites of invasion that soon become warty and encrusted, creating a protective barrier for the mites. The number of mites infesting a patient with scabies crustosa can exceed more than a million, whereas infestation with classic scabies is usually limited to 10 or fewer mites. One-half of patients with crusted scabies do not experience pruritus, reflecting the absence of key inflammatory mediators seen in classic scabies. A nodular form of scabies also exists in which firm, erythematous, dome-shaped lesions roughly 0.5 cm in size develop over the groin, buttock, and axillary areas. Nodular scabies represents the body's reaction to the infestation and is not itself a different type of scabies infestation. Histamine-mediated urticarial lesions may accompany this rash, which is intensely pruritic. In all forms of scabies, if rashes go untreated, bacterial superinfection by *Staphylococcus* species may result, worsening acute inflammation.

CLINICAL PRESENTATION

Subjective

The typical patient usually presents with a complaint of intense itching that is usually described as being more severe at night. Mothers may report changes in feeding patterns of children and that they are more tired and irritable than usual. Itching may be widespread but is commonly located in the interdigital web spaces, wrists, anterior axillary folds, periumbilical skin, pelvic girdle, penis, and ankles. The palms, soles, face, neck, and scalp are more frequently involved in small children. The pruritus is usually described as not responding to treatment. Many patients will complain of a rash, whereas others experience itching for months with no apparent rash. Patients are often aware of similar symptoms in family members and/or in sexual contacts. Patients presenting with the described symptoms should be screened for possible scabies infestation.

Focus on History: Scabies

If scabies is suspected:

- Do you live or work in a nursing home or group home, in a school, or in a prison?
- Do you have any family members or sexual partners who have similar symptoms?
- Are young children displaying increased signs of fatigue or irritability?
- Have the eating patterns of children changed?

If the patient complains of pruritus:

- Where is the itching worse?
- What part of your body is itching?
- Is the itching worse at night?
- Does itching interfere with your ability to sleep?
- How long have you been itching?
- Is the itching relieved by anything? If so, what?
- Are any family members who live with you also complaining of itching?

Objective

The earliest physical signs of scabies are small, red, 1- to 2-mm papules located in areas of the body that are most attractive to mites. Because of the intense itching, excoriations from repeated scratching with crusting and scaling may also be present. It may be difficult to visualize scabies mites on the skin and the patient may complain only of incessant itchiness. Skin lesions occur at the sites of mite infestation or result from a hypersensitivity reaction to the scabies mite. Secondary skin lesions including lichenification and excoriations are the result of chronic rubbing or scratching of lesions. Secondary bacterial infections present with increased symptoms, pruritus, and crusting of lesions (secondary impetigo).

The classic scabies skin lesion is the intraepidermal burrow. Each female mite produces one burrow. In light-skinned people, burrows have a whitish color with black specks caused by fecal particles. In darker-skinned people, the burrows may be thin gray, brown, or red lines that branch out from the bumps. The female mite resides at the blind end of the tunnel and can burrow 2 to 3 mm per day. Burrows are usually distributed in areas where there are few or no hair follicles and where the stratum corneum is thin and soft.

Burrows are sometimes seen on the top of early scabetic nodules that occur in 7% to 10% of patients with scabies. Nodules vary in color from pink to brown and are 5 to 20 cm in diameter. They may become more visible after treatment.

DIAGNOSTIC REASONING

Clinical diagnosis of scabies is almost never made until hypersensitivity has occurred. The diagnosis is based on epidemiological history, the occurrence of intractable itching, and an assessment of the distribution of lesions and pruritus.

Diagnostic Tests

The clinician should search for the presence of mites. The highest yield of mites is in burrows located on the finger webs, penis, female genitalia, or wrists. The burrow ink test is performed by rubbing a felt-tip pen over the suspected burrow (blue and green markers work best because they do not interfere with microscopic results). Excess ink is removed with an alcohol wipe, while the remaining ink concentrates in the tunnel, indicating the location of the burrow.

Once a burrow has been located, the clinician should place a drop of mineral oil over it, then scrape off the burrow using a number 15 scalpel blade. The scrapings should be placed on a slide with a drop of oil and then sealed with a cover slip. The identification of the *S. scabiei* mite, its eggs, or fecal pellets is diagnostic of scabies. There are no serological tests currently available for scabies.

Failure to identify mites, their eggs, or burrows does not rule out scabies infestation. If scabies infestation is suspected because of clinical symptoms, empirical treatment should be tried. Resolution of symptoms within a few days is indicative of previous scabies infection.

Differential Diagnosis

The diagnosis of scabies can be easily missed. Although there are common skin findings (e.g., burrows), the clinical picture of scabies can be extremely variable, depending on the duration of the infection and the severity of the sensitivity reaction. Variants of scabies in immunocompromised persons and persons with neurological disorders further cloud the diagnosis. An accurate diagnosis is essential for effective treatment. It should be noted that it is possible for patients to have preexisting skin problems in addition to scabies. A thorough history can help minimize diagnostic pitfalls (see Differential Diagnosis 12.1).

Differential Diagnosis 12.1: Scabies

Scabies	Atopic dermatitis (eczema) Bullous pemphigoid Chronic renal disease, especially with hemodialysis (pruritus) Cholestatic liver disease (pruritus) Delusions of parasitosis Contact dermatitis Dermatitis herpetiformis Dermatographism (Darier's disease) Drug eruptions Ecthyma Erythroderma Folliculitis Hyperparathyroidism Hodgkin's lymphoma Impetigo Insect bites/pediculosis Lichen planus Malignancy (cutaneous T-cell lymphoma) Miliaria (heat rash) Neurotic excoriation Pityriasis rosea Polycythemia vera Pregnancy induced Prurigo nodularis Psoriasis Pyoderma Seborrheic dermatitis Tinea (capitis, corporis, pedis, cruris) Transient acantholytic dermatosis (Grover's disease) Urticaria (hives)
Nodular scabies	Darier's disease Insect bites Prurigo nodularis Secondary syphilis Urticaria pigmentosa (in young child)
Crusted scabies	Eczematous dermatitis Erythroderma Psoriasis Seborrheic dermatitis

MANAGEMENT

With proper adherence to treatment regimens, cure rates for scabies approach 100%. However, application of medicated creams or lotions is insufficient for an affected person if the entire household is not treated and if all environmental reservoirs of the scabies mite (such as bedding, clothing, and towels) are not sufficiently cleaned with hot water and detergents. Therefore, effective care of patients with scabies involves treating the patient, their close personal contacts, and the surrounding environment. Treating the source of the infestation and any secondary complications, such as bacterial infection (e.g., secondary impetigo) or dermatitis, should also be included in the management plan.

Initial management of the patient diagnosed with scabies is directed at killing all live mites (see Drugs Commonly Prescribed 12.1). Lotions containing scabicides (such as permethrin, lindane, crotamiton, or sulfur) are commonly used. Permethrin is the first-line treatment. Antihistamines and topical steroids are helpful for pruritus. Of the products containing scabicides, lindane is the most toxic. It is rapidly absorbed through the skin and has been associated with central nervous system (CNS) symptoms such as irritability, seizures, and, in cases of ingestion or overdose, death. Older patients, young children, and pregnant and lactating women have the greatest risk of toxicity. Therefore, the choice of scabicide should be based on the age of the patient, pregnancy status, resistance patterns, degree of toxicity, and severity of infestation. High mite populations, the presence of crusts, and decreased immune status of the host make treating crusted scabies more difficult. It may be necessary to remove crusts that protect mites from scabicides before treating.

The majority of patients require only medical treatment with a topical scabicide. However, some patients experience hypersensitivity to the mite and scabicide products and may require systemic corticosteroids for the relief of severe pruritus. Ivermectin 200 mcg/kg is administered as a single dose, followed by another dose 1 to 2 weeks later. This should be used in conjunction with a topical cream or lotion. Some patients may delay treatment until a secondary bacterial infection has occurred, necessitating the additional use of an anti-staphylococcal antibiotic. Cephalexin or dicloxacillin for 7 to 10 days may be prescribed.

In addition, patients with extensive dermatitis lesions may obtain relief with topical corticosteroids, such as triamcinolone 0.1% cream twice daily for 7 days. Fluorinated steroids must not be used on the face or on skinfolds (e.g., intertriginous areas) because of the increased risk of skin atrophy. Management must include a strict isolation protocol for scabies crustosa.

FOLLOW-UP AND REFERRAL

Uncomplicated scabies infestations should be followed up 1 week after the initial treatment. If generalized itching persists, hypersensitivity to the remaining dead mites and scabicide products should be considered. It may be necessary to repeat the scabicide treatment, however. Patients who experience persistent scabetic nodules or scabies crustosa may require advanced management and should be referred to a dermatologist.

Drugs Commonly Prescribed 12.1: Scabies

DRUG	INDICATION	ADVERSE REACTIONS AND PRESCRIBING CONSIDERATIONS
Topical		
Permethrin cream 5% (Elimite) A 30-g tube is sufficient for an average adult for 1 dose.	Presence of live mites (scabicide)	Safe in pregnant and lactating women. Mite resistance has been reported. Safe for use in children 2 months and older. Apply to all areas of body from the neck down. (In young children, may also need to treat head and neck.) Leave on for 8 to 14 hours. Repeat application in 1 week. May repeat a third time 1 week later.
Lindane 19% (gamma-benzene hexachloride)	Presence of live mites (scabicide)	Potential CNS toxicity (only use as alternative therapy). Rapidly absorbed through skin. Do not use on infants or young children, pregnant or lactating women, or if history of seizures. Mite resistance has been reported. May also need to treat head and neck. *Adults:* apply thinly to all areas of the body from the neck down. Wash off thoroughly after 8 hours. Do not retreat.
Crotamiton cream 10% (Eurax)	Presence of live mites (scabicide)	Reported failure rates of up to 50%; may need to be repeated. Shake well before using. Apply to all areas of the body from the chin down for 2 consecutive nights. Change clothing and bed linen the morning after each application; wash these articles in hot water with a strong detergent to avoid reinfection.
Sulfur ointment 8% to 10%	Presence of live mites (scabicide)	Extensive use suggests it is safe to use on pregnant and lactating women and infants. Malodorous and stains clothing. *Adults:* apply to all parts of the body from the neck down for 3 consecutive days. *Children:* may also need to treat head and neck.
Systemic		
Ivermectin (Stromectol)	Presence of live mites (scabicide)	Reported to be effective for common scabies refractory to topical treatment and crusted scabies in conjunction with topical cream/lotion. 200 mcg/kg dose given twice over a 7- to 10-day period. Can pass into breast milk.
Others		
Antihistamines	Eczematous dermatitis	Helps patient sleep at night. Hydroxyzine, diphenhydramine: 25 to 50 mg at bedtime.
Topical corticosteroid ointments	Extensive dermatitis	For mild to moderate pruritus. Apply to areas of extensive dermatitis.
Systemic corticosteroids	Severe hypersensitivity reaction	For severe pruritus. Prednisone: tapered course for 1 to 2 weeks.
Systemic and topical antibiotics	Secondary bacterial infection	*Staphylococcus* and *Streptococcus* species are common pathogens. Risk of acute poststreptococcal glomerulonephritis in severe cases Systemic: 7- to 10-day course.

> **Patient Education: Scabies**
>
> Patient education is an integral part of successfully treating scabies. Patients should be instructed to trim their fingernails to reduce the possibility of harboring mites and reinfesting themselves or passing the infestation to others. Safety information regarding the use of scabicides should be stressed, such as not exceeding recommended exposure times, reporting characteristic toxicity symptoms, and the secure storage of treatment products to prevent accidental ingestion by children. Patients should be informed that itching may continue for up to a week after successful treatment due to local irritation.
>
> Patients should also receive instruction about treating their home environment to avoid reinfestation. They should be reminded that the scabies mite lives on humans, so environmental spraying of pesticides is ineffective and not recommended. Bedclothes and clothing should be washed in hot, soapy water. Except in cases of crusted scabies, extensive decontamination of the environment is not necessary. Children in day care or school can return after treatment.

PEDICULOSIS

Pediculosis (infestation by lice) in humans has been documented for thousands of years. It is difficult to document the number of lice cases occurring annually in the United States because reporting is not required in most states. It is estimated that 6 to 12 million American children are infested with head lice (pediculosis capitis) each year.

EPIDEMIOLOGY AND CAUSES

Pediculosis infestations occur worldwide and are endemic in most parts of the world. Only three species of lice are known to infest humans: *Phthirus pubis* (the crab louse), *Pediculus humanus capitis* (the head louse), and *Pediculus humanus corporis* (the body or clothing louse). Lice infestations occur in people of all ages. Head lice are commonly seen in school-age children, whereas pubic (crab) lice are most often seen in sexually active young adults. Children aged 3 to 12 years are most commonly affected by head lice, with more frequent occurrences in girls. Black children are affected much less frequently than children of other races.

Lice are blood-obligate parasites that obtain all their nutritional requirements from the host. Both *P. capitis* and *P. pubis* lice reside and reproduce on the human host. The *P. humanus corporis* louse feeds on the human host but resides and lays its eggs in clothing fibers. Body lice are increasingly rare in the United States, but they can be seen in communities of persons who are homeless or among persons who live in crowded conditions without the ability to wash and change clothing. Body lice are the only lice associated with disease transmission. Infected feces of the body louse can transmit typhus, trench fever, and relapsing fever. However, lice-borne outbreaks of these diseases have not been seen for many decades in the United States.

Although epidemics of pediculosis in the United States are relatively rare, outbreaks of head lice are common in elementary school settings. Outbreaks usually occur at the start of the school year and after winter and spring breaks. One explanation for the timing of these outbreaks is that they occur after children have spent extended time in the community. Close personal contact is the major mode of transmission for all types of pediculosis.

The cost of treatments, lost wages, and school expenses related to lice outbreaks total an estimated $1 billion annually, making pediculosis a major public health concern and an economic burden on families.

PATHOPHYSIOLOGY

Pediculosis infestation may be asymptomatic or cause few symptoms in the first 2 weeks after exposure. Sensitivity to lice must take place before pruritus occurs. Therefore, in individuals who have never before been exposed to a lice infestation, it can take several weeks before clinical symptoms (e.g., pruritus) develop during the initial infestation. A foreign body inflammatory reaction is caused by lice saliva injected into the skin during the insect's bite. In individuals with a reinfestation, pruritus occurs rapidly within 24 to 48 hours, due to key inflammatory mediators including histamine.

Head lice infestation averages about 10 lice per patient. However, in severe cases, they can number in the hundreds. Head lice are transmitted through close contact rather than by fomites; they survive for approximately 2 days away from a human host, after which time they die of dehydration. Both males and females are equipped with specialized mouth parts adapted for sucking blood, as well as legs capable of adhering to human hair. Each female head louse may lay from 7 to 10 eggs per day for a month. Pubic lice ("crab lice") lay relatively fewer eggs (up to three per day) that incubate for 1 week before hatching. Severe lice infestations may be complicated by bacterial superinfection from *Staphylococcus* species that normally colonize the skin.

CLINICAL PRESENTATION

Subjective

Patients may present with complaints of intense itching in areas of the body preferred by the particular type of infesting louse. The itching is usually described as being more severe at night. Mothers may report changes in feeding patterns and that their children are tired and irritable. School-age children may become inattentive and restless in class, with frequent scratching of the scalp.

Some cases of pediculosis are asymptomatic or present with few symptoms.

Objective

The earliest physical signs of lice infestation are small (2 to 3 mm), red, erythematous macules or papules that may be pruritic. Skin lesions may appear within minutes or several days after initial infestation. Some patients develop an allergic urticarial reaction, with typical wheal-and-flare formation after lice infestation.

Pruritus is the hallmark of all types of pediculosis. Because of the intense itching, excoriations on the scalp, body, or pubic area (depending on the type of lice) with crusting and scaling may also be present. Fresh nits (lice eggs) on hair shafts are thought to be deposited closer to the scalp. As the hair grows (0.5 mm daily on the scalp), the nit moves further away from the scalp. Therefore, if nits are found at varying distances on the hair shafts, the infestation has been present for several weeks to months. Individual lice are difficult to see on the scalp and hair strands. They appear as six-legged, wingless insects from 1 to 4 mm in length that move extremely fast. When engorged with blood, the insect's abdomen appears dark red.

Nits (eggs) are much easier to see than live lice; the teardrop-shaped eggs are attached securely to the hair shaft by the female louse. Newly laid eggs may be tan to coffee-colored and are difficult to see. Hatched lice eggs are whitish in color and appear shiny. The cap (operculum) of the egg faces away from the scalp. The distribution of lice, itching, and lesions provide clues to the type of louse present on the host. Head lice (*P. humanus capitis*) prefer the scalp, and crab lice (*P. pubis*) infest the pubic and perianal region. However, head lice can be found in facial hair such as eyebrows, beards, and mustaches. Crab lice and their nits can also be found in such areas as the eyelids, mustache area, axillae, or on the scalp. Combing the hair to visualize the lice or nits is almost four times more effective than simple visual inspection. Visual inspection may actually miss up to half of infestations. Using a magnifying glass may be helpful.

DIAGNOSTIC REASONING

Clinical diagnosis of pediculosis, body lice, or pubic lice is based on both the history of pruritus (because of a hypersensitivity reaction to the lice) and the finding of white nits or lice on the hair shaft. Sometimes, a lice infestation may be picked up during a routine physical examination or a pre-camp screening inspection for children.

Diagnostic Tests

The clinician should search for lice and nits on the area of the body where the patient is complaining of pruritus. Lice and their nits can be seen with the naked eye or with a handheld magnifying lens. Gloves should be worn during this procedure. Microscopic examination is generally not required. A Wood's light examination can be done for mass screening (or individual screening), but it requires a darkened room and protective eyewear for both the clinician and the child. When the light is directed at the scalp, live nits appear with a pearl-like fluorescence, whereas empty (hatched) nits do not fluoresce. The Wood's light examination is impractical in school settings and not recommended for use with young children who might be afraid of the dark. If secondary bacterial infection (impetigo) is suspected, bacterial cultures should be done with a standard culturette swab.

Failure to identify the presence of lice or nits does not rule out lice infestation. When suspicion is strong based on history and clinical presentation, the patient should be treated empirically; the relief of signs and symptoms is indicative of lice infestation. Treatment for head lice should be limited to persons who are experiencing an active infestation, which is defined as the presence of live lice. Because pubic lice are considered a sexually transmitted disease (STD), patients with this type of infestation should be screened for other STDs, including syphilis, gonorrhea, chlamydia, and HIV infection.

Differential Diagnosis

The diagnosis of pediculosis may be easily confirmed. However, "pseudonits" (e.g., hair casts, dandruff, or sebaceous plugs) can be mistaken for nits, resulting in inappropriate treatment. A hallmark of nits is that they are firmly cemented in place; therefore, they do not slide easily on the hair shaft, compared with dandruff scales. Sebaceous plugs result from plugged oil glands on the scalp, and unlike nits, do not originate on the hair shaft. Secondary bacterial infection can also complicate the diagnosis. Secondarily infected skin lesions resemble impetigo lesions, with crusting and erythema (see Differential Diagnosis 12.2).

MANAGEMENT

Effective care of patients with pediculosis involves treating not only the patient but also their close personal contacts who have been diagnosed with an active infestation. Treatment involves both medication and environmental control measures. It is important to screen all close contacts for head lice, keeping in mind that the contacts may be asymptomatic and have a small number of live lice. Treating the source of the infestation (if identified) and any secondary complications, such as secondary bacterial infection (impetigo) or dermatitis, should also be included in the management plan. Patients need to be reevaluated after 1 week. If live lice are present or if fresh nits are seen close to the scalp, retreatment is necessary.

Differential Diagnosis 12.2: Pediculosis

Rash present	Atopic dermatitis (eczema)
	Bullous pemphigoid
	Burrowing insects/larvae (scabies)
	Contact dermatitis
	Dandruff
	Dermatitis herpetiformis
	Dermatographism (Darier's disease)
	Drug eruptions
	Ecthyma
	Erythroderma
	Folliculitis
	Impetigo
	Insect bites
	Lichen planus
	Malignancy (cutaneous T-cell lymphoma)
	Miliaria (heat rash)
	Neurotic excoriation
	Pityriasis rosea
	Pregnancy induced
	Prurigo nodularis
	Pyoderma (impetigo)
	Psoriasis
	Scabies
	Seborrheic dermatitis
	Tinea (capitis, corporis, pedis, cruris)
	Transient acantholytic dermatosis (Grover's disease)
	Urticaria (hives)
No rash present	Chronic renal disease, especially with hemodialysis (pruritus)
	Cholestatic liver disease (pruritus)
	Delusions of parasitosis
	Hyperparathyroidism
	Hodgkin's lymphoma
	Polycythemia vera

Initial management of patients who are diagnosed with pediculosis is directed at killing and/or removing lice and their nits. Shampoos, cream rinses, and lotions containing benzyl alcohol, ivermectin, permethrin, spinosad, pyrethrin, and malathion are commonly used to kill lice. Lindane is a second-line treatment due to possible CNS toxicity (see Drugs Commonly Prescribed 12.2). Treatment history should be explored with the patient or caregiver. It is common for persons with head lice to delay seeking professional help until three to five self-treatment failures have occurred. Products resulting in treatment failure should not be tried again.

Of these products, lindane is the most toxic. Lindane is rapidly absorbed through the skin and has been associated with CNS symptoms such as irritability, seizures, and, in cases of ingestion or overdose, death. Because lindane is an organochloride, lindane shampoo 1% is approved by the U.S. Food and Drug Administration (FDA) for a second-line treatment of head lice but it is no longer recommended by the American Academy of Pediatrics for use as a pediculicide.

Manual delousing and nit removal using a fine-toothed comb are gaining popularity in light of increasing reports of resistance to available pediculicides. Electronic combs are available that electrocute the lice. They are safe for children and should be used on clean, dry hair. The coated lice comb tips protect the scalp. Many of these products are battery-operated.

In children with respiratory allergies, asthma, or compromised immune status, manual delousing methods should be considered as an initial form of treatment. Petroleum jelly, mayonnaise, tea tree oil, or olive oil may be used as topical agents to suffocate the lice, as the product is massaged into the scalp and left on overnight with a shower cap in place.

Numerous nonpesticidal treatment options have recently become available. There is limited empirical evidence, however, to support their efficacy and safety. Clinicians should caution patients against the use of home remedies that include kerosene and agricultural-grade or veterinary pesticides as such remedies are unsafe and potentially fatal. The majority of patients with pediculosis require only pediculicide treatment or manual delousing. Some patients may delay treatment until secondary bacterial infection has occurred, necessitating the use of topical or systemic antibiotics. Complicating staphylococcal bacterial superinfection may be treated with cephalexin or dicloxacillin for 7 to 10 days.

Children who present with pediculosis pubis (infestation by *P. pubis*) in their eyelashes or hair should alert the clinician to the possibility of sexual abuse, although intimate (genital to face) contact is not the only mode of transmission. Eyelash infestation can be treated by applying petroleum jelly to the eyelid margins twice daily for 10 days. *Pediculosis ciliaris* (eyelash infestation) may also be treated with physostigmine ophthalmic ointment 0.25% to 1% twice daily for 8 to 10 days, but this treatment may cause eye spasms in younger adults. Lice and nits should be manually removed from the eyelashes by gently sliding them off the hairs.

FOLLOW-UP AND REFERRAL

Uncomplicated pediculosis infestations do not require follow-up. In some areas, however, the American head louse has demonstrated resistance to pyrethrin and permethrin, as well as to lindane, resulting in increased treatment failures. Follow-up in 1 week is recommended if symptoms persist; the patient or the parent of an affected child can call the clinic to report any further symptoms. The National Pediculosis Association recommends manual delousing methods at the first sign of medical treatment failure. Because of toxicity concerns and known resistance

Drugs Commonly Prescribed 12.2: Pediculosis

DRUG	INDICATION	ADVERSE REACTIONS AND PRESCRIBING CONSIDERATIONS
Topical		
Permethrin 1% lotion or 5% cream OTC (Nix)	Presence of lice/nits; may use on children older than 2 months	Use nit-remover products before application of permethrin. Apply to towel-dried affected area; leave on 10 minutes, then wash off. Reapply on day 9.
Pyrethrin 0.3% with piperonyl butoxide shampoo or gel OTC (RID, R&C shampoo)	Presence of lice/nits	Use shampoo for head or pubic lice, gel for body lice. Contraindicated in persons sensitive to ragweed. Apply to dry hair until wet; leave on 10 minutes, then wash off. Reapply on day 9.
Malathion 0.5% lotion or gel (Ovide)	Presence of live head lice (not approved for other lice species) Lotion for use on children older than 6 years; gel safe to use on children older than 2 years	No reported resistance. Product contains 78% isopropyl alcohol and is flammable. Apply to dry hair; use sufficient amount to thoroughly wet hair and scalp (cover all lice on the hair and scalp). Although some recommend leaving on for 20 minutes, others recommend 8 to 12 hours. Rinse off, then shampoo. Repeat in 1 week.
Benzyl alcohol 5% (Ulesfia) lotion	Use in patients older than 6 months	Leave on hair and scalp for 10 minutes. May repeat in 7 days if live lice are still present.
Ivermectin 0.5% lotion	May use on children 6 years of age and older	Apply to dry hair for 10 minutes. May repeat after 7 days.
Spinosad (Natroba) 0.9% topical suspension	May use on patients 4 years of age and older	Apply to dry hair for 10 minutes; rinse, then shampoo. May repeat after 7 days.
Systemic		
Ivermectin (Stromectol)	Resistant pediculosis Not FDA approved but some recommend "at your own risk"	For cases resistant to permethrin and malathion, 200 to 400 mcg/kg by mouth as a single dose, followed by another dose in 1 to 2 weeks.
Trimethoprim-sulfamethoxazole (Bactrim)	Not FDA approved but some recommend "at your own risk"	10 mg/kg/day in two divided doses. Potential to cause Stevens-Johnson syndrome reaction.

Abbreviation: FDA, U.S. Food and Drug Administration.

patterns, lindane should be used only as a last resort, and prescriptions should not be written with refills. Referrals for pediculosis infestations are usually not required.

Patient Education: Pediculosis

Patient education is an integral part of successfully treating pediculosis. Patients and parents should continue to be instructed not to share hats, combs, scarves, headsets, towels, and bedding; however, there is some controversy about the contribution of fomites in the spread of head lice. After removal of hair and debris, combs and brushes should be washed in hot, soapy water, rinsed in hot water, and allowed to air dry.

Safety information regarding the proper use of pediculicides should be stressed, including information about not exceeding recommended exposure times, possible toxicity symptoms that should be reported, and the safe storage of treatment products to prevent accidental ingestion by young children. When using head lice products, patients should be instructed to cover the eyes and rinse products over a sink (not in the shower or bathtub) to reduce unnecessary pesticide exposure. Patients should be informed that itching may continue after successful treatment for up to 1 week because of the slow resolution of the inflammatory reaction caused by the lice infestation.

Patients should also receive instruction on cleaning the environment. With the exception of the body louse, lice live only on humans; therefore, treatment of pets is not necessary. Excessive decontamination of the environment is also not necessary. Environmental spraying of pesticides is ineffective and may be dangerous, and is therefore not recommended. Bedclothes and clothing should be washed in hot, soapy water and dried in a hot dryer. Normal vacuuming of carpets, rugs, upholstery, mattresses, cars, and car seats should be sufficient.

Parents should devote their energy to removing lice and nits. Children in day care or school can return after treatment. Some schools have a "no-nit" policy that requires parents to remove all lice and nits before a child may reenter the classroom, but these policies are changing as they have not been demonstrated to reduce the spread of lice at school. Parents should be instructed to screen children once a week for head lice as part of their regular hygiene routine. Early detection of lice infestation results in fewer transmissions and more successful treatment regimens.

REFERENCES

General
Kimberlin DW, Brady MT, Jackson MA, Long S. *Red Book, 30th Edition. 2015 Report of the Committee on Infectious Diseases.* American Academy of Pediatrics; 2015.

Pediculosis
Brody JE. Parents, relax. Don't keep them from school. It's just lice. *The New York Times.* September 20, 2010. http://www.nytimes.com/2010/09/21/health/21brody.html. Accessed 6/27/2017.

Centers for Disease Control and Prevention. (2016). Pediculosis. DPDx—laboratory identification of parasitic diseases of public health concern. https://www.cdc.gov/dpdx/pediculosis/index.html. Accessed 7/7/2020.

Head Lice Treatment. Parasites–Diagnosis. https://www.cdc.gov/parasites/lice/head/diagnosis.html. Accessed 9/17/2020.

Lapeere H, Brochez L, Verhaeghe E, et al. Efficacy of products to remove eggs of Pediculus humanus capitis (Phthiraptera: Pediculidae) from the human hair. *J Med Entomol.* 2014;51:400.

Pediculosis capitis. BMJ Best Practice—pediculosis capitis. https://bestpractice.bmj.com/topics/en-us/677. Accessed 12/5/2020.

Scabies
Ahmad HM, Abdel-Azim ES, Abdel-Aziz RT. Clinical efficacy and safety of topical versus oral ivermectin in treatment of uncomplicated scabies. *Dermatol Ther.* 2016;29:58.

Centers for Disease Control and Prevention. (2010). Parasites—scabies. https://www.cdc.gov/parasites/scabies/index.html. Accessed 7/7/2020.

Executive Committee of Guideline for the Diagnosis and Treatment of Scabies. Guideline for the diagnosis and treatment of scabies in Japan (third edition): Executive Committee of Guideline for the Diagnosis and Treatment of Scabies. *J Dermatol.* 2017;44:991.

Salavastru CM, Chosidow O, Boffa MJ, et al. European guideline for the management of scabies. *J Eur Acad Dermatol Venereol.* 2017;31:1248.

Simon MW. Update on the diagnosis and treatment of head lice. *Clin Advisor.* 2016;19(9):43–51.

World Health Organization. Lymphatic filariasis: scabies. https://www.who.int/health-topics/lymphatic-filariasis#tab=tab_1. Accessed 7/7/2020.

RESOURCES

American Academy of Dermatology
https://www.aad.org

American Society of Dermatology
https://www.asd.org

Centers for Disease Control and Prevention
https://www.cdc.gov

National Institute of Allergy and Infectious Disease
https://www.niaid.nih.gov

National Institutes of Health
https://www.nih.gov

National Pediculosis Association
https://www.headlice.org

Chapter 13

Mucocutaneous Fungal Infections

Susan Garnett, MSN, APRN, FNP-BC
Jill E. Winland-Brown, EdD, APRN, FNP-BC, FAANP
Brian Oscar Porter, MD, PhD, MPH, MBA

CANDIDIASIS

Candidiasis (also known as moniliasis and candidosis) is defined as an infection with the fungal organism *Candida*. *Candida* is an opportunistic pathogen that causes not only superficial mucocutaneous infections but also systemic disease that can be fatal, especially in immunocompromised patients. *Candida* belongs to the yeast family of fungi. There are more than 20 species of *Candida* that can cause infections in humans, the most common of which is *Candida albicans*. *Candida* is part of the normal flora of both the oropharynx and gastrointestinal (GI) tract. In addition, up to 20% of women who are asymptomatic test positive for vaginal *Candida*.

Favorable environmental factors and a weakened immune system are the two most important factors contributing to candidal infections. Certain areas of the body are also more prone to fungal infection, such as those that tend to trap heat and moisture.

Risk factors for serious disease include conditions that alter cellular immunity, such as AIDS, diabetes mellitus, corticosteroid treatment, bone marrow transplant, chemotherapy, invasive parenteral catheterization (parenteral feeding catheters are considered high risk), and invasive monitoring devices in intensive care units. Broad-spectrum antibiotic therapy, including antibiotics after major surgery in normal hosts, can increase the risk of *Candida* infection. Superficial cutaneous infections are the focus of this chapter.

Cutaneous infections caused by *Candida* include the following:

- Infections of infancy: thrush, diaper dermatitis
- Oral infections: oral candidiasis (thrush), angular cheilitis
- Genital infections: vulvovaginitis, balanitis
- Intertriginous (skinfold) infections: cutaneous candidiasis of the inframammary area, groin, axillae, web spaces of the fingers and toes, perianal area
- Other infections: folliculitis, candidal paronychia, subungual candidiasis (beneath the nail)

EPIDEMIOLOGY AND CAUSES

Although *C. albicans* was once the most common of all yeast isolates found in specimens, there has been an increase in other types of *Candida* species identified, such as *C. tropicalis, C. glabrata, C. krusei, C. parapsilosis, C. dubliniensis,* and the emerging *C. auris.* This is thought to be a result of the widespread use of azole antifungals. Unfortunately, some of these candidal species (*C. krusei, C. glabrata*) have developed resistance to the common antifungal agent fluconazole. *Candida* infection can occur at any age and in either gender. A higher incidence of thrush is seen among patients with AIDS and in infants. A higher prevalence of vulvovaginal candidiasis occurs in women of reproductive age. Areas of the body where there is skin-to-skin contact are more prone to candidal infection. These include areas under the breast (inframammary candidiasis), between the fingers (interdigital candidiasis), between the toes, the groin, the axillae, and the genital area. Infections in these areas are collectively called intertrigo or intertriginous infections.

Cellular immunodeficiency states increase the risk of mucocutaneous disease. Conditions such as AIDS, diabetes mellitus, corticosteroid therapy, and immunosuppressive therapy increase an individual's susceptibility to infection with *C. albicans*. Infants, given their immature immune systems, can easily become infected with *Candida* through the birth canal or through oral contact with an infected caregiver. In infants, oral candidiasis (thrush) and diaper candidiasis are considered benign findings. In adults, however, mucocutaneous candidiasis is the most common AIDS-defining condition seen. In women with AIDS, one of the earliest and most frequent opportunistic infections is vaginal candidiasis. Frequent episodes of vaginal candidiasis that are not accompanied by an underlying predisposing condition (e.g., diabetes mellitus, antibiotic use, pregnancy, or oral contraceptive use) should prompt the clinician to consider HIV infection in the differential diagnosis, although most cases of candidal vaginal infections occur in HIV-negative hosts.

Vaginal infection with *C. albicans* is common; it occurs in up to 75% of women at some point in their lifetime (pregnant women and patients with diabetes mellitus are at increased risk). If left untreated, vaginal candidiasis (also called candidal vaginitis) will either resolve spontaneously or become a chronic low-grade infection. Men with diabetes mellitus, especially if uncircumcised, are at higher risk for candidal infections of the glans penis (balanitis). The uncircumcised foreskin holds heat and moisture and increases the risk of candidal overgrowth. Males may become infected with *Candida* organisms from female or male sexual partners through either vaginal, anal, or oral intercourse. In candidal paronychia, the patient will report a history of hangnail or minor trauma in the cuticle area before the infection. Dishwashing or frequent water exposure may be a predisposing factor.

PATHOPHYSIOLOGY

Candida organisms cause a strong inflammatory response on the skin, which accounts for the intense erythema and pruritus commonly seen with this infection. Microscopic examination of *Candida* lesions reveals a pseudomembrane composed of masses of yeast organisms that invade the superficial layer of the epithelium. Satellite lesions are small colonies of *Candida* that have spread beyond the main lesion, which eventually enlarge and become confluent, resulting in large erythematous patches. Normal commensal flora and intact cellular immunity, mediated primarily by cytotoxic T cells, are the body's primary defense against fungal overgrowth and invasive candidal infection. The use of systemic antibiotics has the potential for clearing normal microbial skin flora, which removes natural competition to candidal overgrowth. In addition, oral and inhaled corticosteroids, HIV infection and AIDS, malignancy, chemotherapy and other immunosuppressant drugs, diabetes mellitus, and senescence all contribute to decreased helper and cytotoxic T-cell function, thereby increasing the likelihood of candidal skin and mucosal infections.

CLINICAL PRESENTATION

Subjective

Cardinal symptoms of mucocutaneous candidal infection include pruritus and sometimes a burning sensation.

Oral Candidiasis (Thrush)

The patient will complain of a severe sore throat. Pain or difficulty is noted during swallowing (dysphagia), especially with acidic foods such as citrus fruits or juices (see Chapter 21 for more information). The patient may complain of seeing white, creamy patches in the mouth and the tongue may be tender to touch and bleed with minor trauma.

Vaginal Candidiasis

The patient, usually ranging in age from adolescence to middle age, typically complains of burning, itching, and irritation, either on the vulva or both the vulva and vagina (vulvovaginitis). Burning may be noted during intercourse (dyspareunia) or urination (dysuria). The patient may report the vaginal discharge as white in color, with a "cottage-cheese" or thick texture (see Chapter 49 for more information).

Balanitis

The typical patient is a sexually active adult man who complains of a reddish rash and itching on the glans penis. It is sometimes accompanied by penile burning after intercourse, although no burning is usually felt with urination. Some patients will report having a female sexual partner who is being treated for a yeast infection or who has irritative vaginal symptoms or a male sexual partner with anogenital or perianal candidiasis (see Chapter 51 for more information).

Intertriginous Candidiasis

The typical patient is an obese adult who complains of a red, itchy rash that is occasionally "weepy" (draining tissue fluid) and moist, and is sometimes accompanied by a burning sensation. The location of the rash may be in the inframammary area, the groin, the perianal area, or the interdigital spaces of the hands and/or feet.

Candidal Paronychia

The typical patient is an adult who complains of an extremely painful and inflamed fingertip. A history of frequent water immersion of the hands is common.

Subungual Candida

The typical patient is an adult who reports one or several discolored, yellow fingernails on the hands and/or feet for several weeks to months. A history of excessive contact with water from dishwashing, bartending, or other occupations is frequently present. No pain, itching, or nail tenderness is associated with this infection in contrast to candidal paronychia.

Objective

A cardinal sign of cutaneous candidal infections is a bright-red rash with macules or satellite lesions seen on the borders. Mucosal infections may present with different types of enanthema, depending on the location.

Oral Candidiasis (Thrush)

The anterior and posterior pharynx (including the tongue) are frequently involved. White, creamy patches are seen and can be easily scraped off with a tongue blade, leaving behind erythematous patches. In adults, the buccal mucosa, tongue, and lips may also be involved and the patches may extend to the angles of the mouth (angular cheilitis or perleche).

Vaginal Candidiasis

The vulva and surrounding area (in some patients) appear erythematous and irritated. During speculum examination, the vaginal tissue appears erythematous, with white, curd-like patches on the vaginal walls. The posterior fornix of the vagina may be full of thick white discharge.

Balanitis

The glans penis typically has small, erythematous, eroded patches that are tender to the touch. An alternative presentation may be small, white, round lesions with a red base on the glans penis.

Intertriginous Candidiasis

Any area of skin on the body where there is maceration (i.e., skin rubbing against skin) or increased heat and moisture can easily become colonized by *Candida*. These areas include the inframammary area, axilla, groin, perianal area, and interdigital areas between the fingers and toes. In some extremely obese patients, macerated skin may occur in other areas as well. The lesions appear as bright-red patches with satellite lesions. The skin will appear eroded and moist and is tender to the touch.

Candidal Paronychia

The area around the nail (the paronychium) is bright red, swollen, and extremely tender. A purulent pocket of discharge is sometimes present; when fluctuant, this abscess will usually rupture and drain pus.

Subungual Candida

Affected nails are typically discolored (yellowish) and thickened. The nail may be deformed and partially or totally separated from the nailbed.

DIAGNOSTIC REASONING

Diagnostic Tests

Skin infections caused by *Candida* are generally diagnosed by their classic appearance. *Candida* yeasts are normally present in the mouth, vagina, sputum, or stool. Candidal cultures can be obtained from the skin or mucous membranes by sampling with a culture swab (culturette). Because *Candida* is part of the normal flora, a positive culture from the mouth or vagina is of limited value unless confirmatory signs and symptoms accompany it. For vaginal candidal infections, a saline wet mount, pH test with litmus paper, and a potassium hydroxide (KOH) test to assess for fungal forms in vaginal discharge are helpful in the diagnosis (see Advanced Assessment 13.1). The whiff test will be negative and the vaginal pH is normal (acidic) at 4.5 or less.

Differential Diagnosis

The location of the skin lesions determines the differential diagnoses to be considered. Contact dermatitis lesions can appear similar to candidal skin lesions. Fungal infections caused by dermatophytes can be confused with candidiasis, as they may affect a variety of sites, including the nails (tinea unguium causing onychomycosis), groin (tinea cruris), scalp (tinea capitis), and foot (tinea pedis), or the body in general (tinea corporis or "ringworm") (see Differential Diagnosis 13.1).

Advanced Assessment 13.1: KOH Examination

When assessing for candidiasis, a saline wet mount of vaginal discharge or a potassium hydroxide (KOH) examination of vaginal discharge or superficial scrapings from a suspected focus of infection may be performed. The KOH slide examination is necessary to visualize *Candida* or tinea fungus; however, a KOH examination is not necessary to see yeast forms in vaginal infections. The saline wet mount works well for vaginal candidiasis and is faster to prepare than a KOH examination.

The KOH examination is used to determine the presence of mycelial fragments or budding yeast cells in a skin lesion or other focus of infection. The test involves adding KOH solution to a small amount of vaginal discharge or superficial skin scrapings on a glass slide, covering the slide, and applying gentle heat. This enhances the natural effect of the alkaline KOH in dissolving thick keratin in the scrapings, which otherwise obscure visualization of fungal forms. The slide is then examined microscopically for fungal hyphae, which become more visible once the KOH dissolves keratin elements.

PERFORMING A SALINE WET MOUNT MICROSCOPIC EXAMINATION

1. Take a small amount of vaginal discharge from the posterior fornix of the vagina with either a long, cotton-tipped applicator or from the end of a speculum.
2. Place a small amount of the vaginal discharge in the middle of a clean, dry glass slide.
3. Add one to two drops of normal saline solution to the vaginal discharge and stir/mix to produce a thin, milky mixture.
4. Add a cover slip.
5. View the specimen first under low power and then at 40x magnification. Look for pseudohyphae, spores, and leukocytes.

PERFORMING A POTASSIUM HYDROXIDE (KOH) MICROSCOPIC EXAMINATION

1. Scrape a portion of the suspected area (e.g., skin rash) with the edge of a clean glass slide or a no. 15 sterile scalpel blade moistened with tap water to obtain scales. Transfer the scraped tissue onto a slide and add a small droplet of plain water. A slide may also be prepared with a small amount of vaginal discharge.
2. Add one or two drops of KOH 10% solution onto the specimen slide, place a cover slip, and warm the slide carefully for 15 to 30 seconds using a match, small candle, or Bunsen burner (do not place the slide directly into the flame to avoid burning the sample and carbon buildup).
3. Examine the specimen under low power with minimal illumination.
4. Look for pseudohyphae and/or spores. Identify hyphae (thin tubular structures, often seen as branching strands of uniform diameter).
5. Switch to high dry (40x to 43x) magnification to confirm findings.

NOTE: Although a positive examination establishes the diagnosis, a negative test does not rule out the disease, given sampling variability.

MICROSCOPY TIPS: SALINE WET MOUNT AND KOH EXAMINATIONS

- Do not confuse a piece of hair or thread on the slide with pseudohyphae. Hair or threads will appear as black opaque lines, whereas hyphae are translucent and colorless.
- Pseudohyphae or hyphae (the stems) have thin translucent walls that have complete (hyphae) or partial (pseudohyphae) septa dividing each segment (appearing like a bamboo stem).
- Spores are small and oval to round in shape, seen either alone or in clusters.
- Leukocytes are round to oval and are the size of nuclei in epithelial cells.
- A large number of leukocytes are seen in vaginal discharge with candidal and trichomonal infections because of the inflammatory response.
- Few leukocytes are seen in bacterial vaginosis (which does not cause significant inflammation) unless there is concurrent infection with *Candida* or *Trichomonas*.
- Epithelial cells are the largest cells found on the slide. Superficial epithelial cells are the most numerous (about 90%) and appear as squares with rounded corners and edges.
- The presence of immature epithelial cells (from the basal and parabasal layer) indicates severe inflammation. The immature cells are smaller and have larger nuclei than superficial (mature) epithelial cells.
- Bacteria are too small to be visualized clearly with a regular light microscope. They will appear as extremely small dark "specks" on the slide, under both low- and high-power magnification.

Differential Diagnosis 13.1: Mucocutaneous Candidiasis

Type of Candidiasis	Differential Diagnosis
Thrush (oral candidiasis)	Milk curd (infants) Pharyngeal exudate (bacteria/viral)
Intertrigo (skinfolds)	Contact dermatitis Bacterial intertrigo (erythrasma)
Vaginal candidiasis	Trichomoniasis Bacterial vaginosis Contact dermatitis (on vulva and surrounding structures)
Balanitis (glans of penis)	Flat genital warts Erythroplasia of Queyrat (Bowen's disease of the penis) Contact dermatitis Balanitis plasmacellularis (Zoon's balanitis)
Candidal paronychia (tissue surrounding the nail)	Bacterial paronychia (*Pseudomonas, Proteus*) Herpetic whitlow
Subungual *Candida* (under nail)	Tinea unguium (onychomycosis)

MANAGEMENT

Most cases of mucocutaneous and vaginal candidal infections (and tinea infections) respond well to topical treatment with antifungal creams that are available over the counter (OTC) or by prescription. The formulation of the topical antifungal used will depend on the site of the infection and whether the rash is moist or dry. Powders work well with moist, macerated lesions. Creams work well on drier lesions. Solutions and sprays are alcohol-based and cause burning on inflamed or macerated skin; therefore, they should be avoided on those areas. Preparations in ointment form are more adherent than liquid, lotion, or cream formulations and tend to work best for intertriginous areas. Oral formulations include suspensions and troches.

Pharmacological Therapy

Many antifungal medications are available to treat candidal infections (see Drugs Commonly Prescribed 13.1). Topical antifungals such as nystatin (Nyamyc, Pedi-Dri, Nystop; effective for *Candida* only), clotrimazole (Lotrimin), miconazole (Monistat-Derm), naftifine (Naftin), terbinafine (Lamisil), and ciclopirox (Loprox) are typically effective. Most topical antifungal creams are applied twice per day for at least 2 weeks (and up to 4 weeks). The patient should be instructed to apply creams sparingly because too much cream may lead to skin maceration, especially in intertriginous areas. The cream is massaged gently into the rash and the surrounding area. The patient is advised that mild improvement in the rash may be seen in a week, but it frequently takes 2 to 4 weeks until the rash is cleared. Adverse reactions are usually mild and may include erythema, local irritation, itching, burning, and dryness. In some patients, sensitization occurs, and a contact dermatitis results. If this occurs, the medication should be discontinued.

First-line treatment of vulvovaginitis is a topical or oral azole. Topical creams and suppositories are available OTC and by prescription; oral therapy is by prescription only. For treatment of severe cases of candidal vulvovaginitis, a 7- to 14-day course of topical azole or two doses of oral fluconazole 72 hours apart are recommended. Cream formulations often yield better results than vaginal suppositories. Women should be cautioned

Drugs Commonly Prescribed 13.1: Candidal and Tinea Infections

DRUG	INDICATION	DOSAGE	COMMENTS
Topical Agents			
Miconazole 2% cream (Lotrimin AF, Micatin, Monistat-Derm)	Tinea: pedis, cruris, and corporis Cutaneous candidiasis Vaginal candidiasis Tinea versicolor	Twice daily for 2 weeks Vaginal candidiasis: once at bedtime for 3 to 7 days	Tinea pedis needs longer treatment, for 4 weeks
Clotrimazole 1% cream and solution (Lotrimin)	Tinea: pedis, cruris, corporis, versicolor	Twice daily for 2 to 8 weeks	Tinea pedis should be treated for at least 4 weeks
Betamethasone 0.05% and clotrimazole 1% cream and lotion (Lotrisone)	Fungal skin infections	Apply sparingly twice daily for 1 week and reevaluate Maximum: 2 weeks	Contraindications: varicella, herpes, vaccinia, other viral infections Do not use on face Can cause atrophic skin changes with prolonged use Do not use for diaper dermatitis
Terbinafine 1% cream (Lamisil AT)	Tinea: cruris, corporis, pedis Moccasin-type tinea pedis (plantar tinea pedis)	Tinea cruris/corporis: once daily for 1 week Tinea pedis between the toes: twice daily for 1 week Plantar tinea pedis: twice daily for 2 weeks	Improvement may continue to be seen for up to 2 to 6 weeks after therapy
Terbinafine 1% solution (Lamisil solution)	Tinea: versicolor (pityriasis), pedis, cruris, corporis	Tinea versicolor/pedis: twice daily for 1 week Tinea cruris/corporis: once daily for 1 week	Alcohol-based solution Use only for 1 week Apply on dry skin Do not use on face or mucous membranes; avoid broken or irritated skin
Ciclopirox 0.77% cream, lotion (Loprox)	Cutaneous candidiasis and fungal skin infections (tinea pedis, corporis, cruris, versicolor)	Twice daily for 2 to 4 weeks	Do not use in children younger than 10 years Avoid occlusion
Ciclopirox 1% shampoo	Seborrheic scalp dermatitis	Shampoo and leave on for 3 minutes, then rinse; repeat twice weekly, at least 3 days apart	Not recommended for children younger than 16 years Avoid eyes and mucous membranes
Ciclopirox 8% topical solution (Penlac nail lacquer)	Onychomycosis of fingernails and toenails	Apply thin coat once daily at bedtime	Remove with alcohol once per week; repeat for up to 1 year Do not use nail polish
Efinaconazole 10% topical solution (Jublia)	Onychomycosis	Apply once daily	Use for 48 weeks

Drugs Commonly Prescribed 13.1: Candidal and Tinea Infections—cont'd

DRUG	INDICATION	DOSAGE	COMMENTS
Tavaborole 0.5% topical solution (Kerydin)	Onychomycosis	Apply once daily	Use for 48 weeks
Ketoconazole 2% cream, shampoo (Nizoral)	Tinea: pedis, cruris, corporis, versicolor Cutaneous candidiasis Seborrheic dermatitis	One to two times daily for 2 to 4 weeks or until clinical clearing	Contains sulfites Treat tinea pedis for 6 weeks Seborrheic dermatitis: use cream twice daily for 4 weeks or until clear Tinea versicolor: use shampoo (1 application); apply to damp skin, leave on for 5 minutes, then rinse; use for 2 weeks
Econazole 1% cream, foam (Spectazole, Ecoza)	Tinea: pedis, cruris, corporis, versicolor Cutaneous candidiasis	Tinea: once daily Cutaneous candidiasis: twice daily	Treat tinea pedis for 4 weeks and other types for 2 weeks
Sulconazole 1% cream, solution (Exelderm)	Tinea: cruris, corporis, versicolor Tinea pedis: cream only	Tinea pedis: twice daily for 4 weeks Other tinea: once or twice daily for 3 weeks	Reevaluate if no improvement within 4 to 6 weeks
Sertaconazole 2% topical cream, tablet (Ertaczo)	Tinea pedis Vaginal candidiasis	Apply twice daily for 4 weeks Single-dose tablet	Reevaluate if no improvement
Oxiconazole cream, lotion (Oxistat)	Tinea: pedis, corporis, cruris, versicolor	Tinea pedis: apply once or twice daily for 4 weeks Tinea versicolor: apply once daily for 2 weeks Other tinea: once or twice daily for 2 weeks	Reevaluate if no improvement
Naftifine 1% cream, gel (Naftin)	Tinea: pedis, cruris, corporis	Cream: once per day Gel: twice daily for up to 4 weeks	Reevaluate if no improvement within 4 weeks Wash hands after application Not recommended for children
Luliconazole 1% cream (Luzu)	Tinea pedis Tinea corporis and cruris	Tinea pedis: once daily for 2 weeks Other tinea: once daily for 1 week	Wash hands after application
Nystatin cream (Mycostatin)	Cutaneous candidiasis (intertrigo)	Twice daily for 2 to 4 weeks	Apply liberally to affected area
Nystatin powder (Bio-Statin)	Candidiasis, especially moist lesions (under breast, groin, shoes, feet, body folds)	Two to three times a day for 2 to 4 weeks	Good for weeping lesions under breast, in groin, and bodily folds Irritation is rare
Nystatin suspension (Mycostatin)	Thrush (oral candidiasis)	Place ½ dose of dropper on each side of mouth four times daily for at least 2 weeks	Swish and retain in mouth as long as possible before swallowing or spitting out

Continued

Drugs Commonly Prescribed 13.1: Candidal and Tinea Infections—cont'd

DRUG	INDICATION	DOSAGE	COMMENTS
Systemic Agents			
Itraconazole (Sporanox, Sporanox PulsePak)	Onychomycosis of toenail or fingernail Tinea: capitis, corporis Recalcitrant tinea pedis Oral candidiasis	Toenail: 200 mg daily (tablet) for 12 consecutive weeks Fingernail: total of two "pulses"; 200 mg twice daily for 1 week, then 3 weeks off; repeat pulse of 200 mg twice daily for 1 week Recalcitrant tinea pedis: 200 mg daily for 2 weeks or 400 mg daily for 1 week Tinea corporis/severe cruris: 200 mg once daily for 1 to 2 weeks Oral candidiasis: 10 mL suspension, swish and swallow	Take capsules and tablets with food; use suspension form on an empty stomach Numerous drug interactions; check before prescribing Hypoglycemia may result from drug interactions with oral antihyperglycemic agents Check liver function tests before, during, and after treatment *FDA boxed warning: heart failure, cardiac effects, drug interactions* Avoid taking antacids 2 hours before and 2 hours after using itraconazole
Terbinafine (Lamisil)	Onychomycosis of toenail or fingernail due to tinea unguium Tinea: capitis, corporis, cruris, pedis	Toenail: 250 mg once daily for 12 weeks Fingernail: 250 mg once daily for 6 weeks Tinea capitis: 250 mg once daily for 6 weeks Tinea corporis, cruris: 250 mg once daily for 2 to 4 weeks Tinea pedis: 250 mg once daily for 2 to 6 weeks	Check liver function before starting; repeat with CBC, if treatment lasts longer than 6 weeks Use with caution in patients with liver/renal disease Clinical cure of onychomycosis may not be apparent for months
Fluconazole (Diflucan)	Oropharyngeal (thrush), esophageal, vaginal, systemic candidiasis Tinea versicolor	All candidiasis doses once daily, unless otherwise specified Thrush: 200 mg on day 1, then 100 mg/day for at least 2 weeks Esophageal: 200 mg on day 1, then 100 mg/day for at least 3 weeks, then for 2 weeks more after symptoms resolve Vaginal: 150 mg single dose or every 72 hours for 3 doses Recurrent vaginal: 150 mg by mouth daily for 10 to 14 days followed by 150 mg once weekly for 6 months Tinea versicolor: 150 to 300 mg single weekly dose for 2 to 4 weeks, or 300 mg weekly for 2 weeks	Check liver function tests Contraindicated in patients with liver disease Numerous drug interactions; check before prescribing
Posaconazole (Noxafil) oral suspension, delayed-release tablets	Oropharyngeal candidiasis primary treatment or refractory to itraconazole and/or fluconazole	Loading dose: 100 mg (2.5 mL suspension) twice daily on first day, then maintenance dose of 100 mg (2.5 mL suspension) once daily for 13 days Refractory: 400 mg (10 mL suspension) twice daily	Take tablets and oral suspension with food Check liver function tests before starting and during treatment Numerous drug interactions; check before prescribing

Drugs Commonly Prescribed 13.1: Candidal and Tinea Infections—cont'd

DRUG	INDICATION	DOSAGE	COMMENTS
Griseofulvin (Grifulvin V): microsize and ultramicrosize	Tinea capitis, onychomycosis, severe recalcitrant tinea cruris, pedis, and corporis	Tinea capitis: 250 to 500 mg twice daily in adults and once daily in children 50 lb or more for 2 to 4 months Tinea corporis, cruris: Microsize, 500 mg once daily for 2 to 4 weeks Ultramicrosize, 375 mg daily for 2 to 4 weeks Tinea pedis or unguium: Microsize, 1000 mg daily in single or divided doses every 12 hours for 1 to 2 weeks Ultramicrosize, 250 mg every 8 hours for 4 to 8 weeks (unguium 4 to 6 months) Onychomycosis, fingernail or toenail: Microsize, 1000 mg once daily or in two divided doses every 12 hours for 6 months Ultramicrosize, 250 mg every 8 hours for 4 to 6 months	Best absorbed when taken with fatty meals; ultramicrosize formulation better absorbed High rate of resistant strains of tinea capitis Use with caution in patients with liver and renal disease; monitor renal, hepatic, and hematopoietic indices Severe skin reactions; avoid sunlight due to phototoxicity Numerous drug interactions; check before prescribing; decreases effectiveness of oral contraceptives, oral anticoagulants, and barbiturates

that topical treatments may weaken latex condoms and diaphragms. Vaginal suppositories can become dislodged from the vagina when the patient is voiding or during defecation. For mild to moderate cases, suppositories work well and are available as 1- to 3-day treatment regimens. Current data do not support the treatment of sexual partners of women with vulvovaginal candidiasis. It is recommended that pregnant women with vulvovaginal candidiasis should be treated only with topical azole therapy for 7 days. Although a single, low-dose (150 mg) administration of oral fluconazole to treat vulvovaginal candidiasis has not been shown to be unsafe in pregnant women, a referral to the patient's obstetrician is indicated in recalcitrant cases.

Although women often prefer oral treatment for its convenience, some experts discourage the use of systemic therapies for mucosal or cutaneous candidiasis because of the potential for adverse effects and an increase in fungal resistance. Studies have found that the increased use of imidazoles for systemic therapy has been associated with an increase in the strains of *Candida* species resistant to the systemic antifungal fluconazole (Diflucan). Less common candidal species such as *C. glabrata* and *C. tropicalis* are also more likely to be resistant to treatment with topical imidazoles. If the patient is immunocompromised, has severe vaginal or perianal candidiasis, or is unresponsive to topical medications, systemic antifungal therapy may be justified.

Drug interactions may occur with many oral systemic antifungals that are available by prescription when given with warfarin (Coumadin), phenytoin (Dilantin), or rifampin. Although there is limited evidence that topical miconazole may potentiate warfarin, monitoring is advised. Serious adverse events that may occur with oral systemic antifungals include hepatotoxicity, angioedema, and anaphylaxis. For significant skin infections resistant to extended topical therapy, systemic antifungal treatment options include fluconazole for 10 to 14 days or itraconazole (Sporanox) for 2 to 3 weeks. Patients with skin infections resistant to these treatments should be referred to a dermatologist or infectious disease expert for further evaluation and treatment.

First-line treatment for mild oral candidiasis is clotrimazole troches 10 mg five times a day or miconazole 50 mg buccal tablet once a day for 7 to 14 days, applied to the upper gum over the incisor. Oral candidiasis (thrush) may also be treated with nystatin, which is available in suspension, pastilles, or troches. Nystatin is available in a 100,000 units/mL suspension, and 4 to 6 mL (or one teaspoon) is given (one-half dose on each side of the mouth) four times daily. The patient should be advised to retain the suspension inside the mouth as long as possible before swallowing. Nystatin is available in pastille form (200,000 units); the patient should allow one or two pastilles to dissolve slowly inside the mouth four times a day for 14 days. Of note, relapse frequently occurs after treatment of thrush in immunocompromised patients.

Oral fluconazole 100 to 200 mg daily for 7 to 14 days is recommended for the treatment of moderate to severe oropharyngeal candidiasis. A 28-day course of itraconazole solution 200 mg once daily or posaconazole suspension 400 mg twice daily for 3 days and then once daily is indicated for oral candidiasis that is unresponsive to fluconazole. Additional alternatives include voriconazole or amphotericin B deoxycholate suspension. Most oral antifungal medications have not been confirmed to be safe in pregnancy; thus, pregnant patients with recalcitrant fungal infections should be referred to their obstetrician.

In candidal paronychia, a warm compress on the affected fingertip will enhance drainage of purulent discharge and help relieve the pain. Incision and drainage of purulent material may speed resolution and provide relief. Candidal infections of the nailbed (subungual *Candida*) are best treated with systemic antifungals. Terbinafine (Lamisil) is the most effective antifungal but has a cure rate of much less than 100%.

FOLLOW-UP AND REFERRAL

The patient should be seen in 2 weeks to monitor response to treatment. If there is no response to treatment, the initial diagnosis should be reconsidered, or the patient should be referred to a dermatologist or infectious disease specialist. If a partial response is seen, treatment can be continued for another 1 to 2 weeks, after which the patient should be reevaluated. If there is poor response at that time, referral is then indicated.

> ### Patient Education: Candidiasis
>
> Patients must be taught to decrease favorable environmental conditions for *Candida* such as moisture, warmth, and poor air circulation of affected areas (e.g., tight clothing). To prevent diaper rash, infants should be kept as dry as possible, and the use of rubber or plastic pants and undergarments should be discouraged. Baby powder with cornstarch should not be used because it will worsen the infection (*Candida* can utilize the cornstarch as a nutrient).
>
> Patients using inhaled corticosteroids should be advised to rinse their mouth with water or brush their teeth after use.
>
> For obese patients, one method of keeping deep folds of skin apart is by using clean, dry, white tissues between the folds of skin. Educate the patient on the importance of keeping the affected area dry to assist in healing and to prevent future candidal infections. Patients may be instructed to use a hair dryer to dry moist areas but stress that it must be kept on the "low" heat setting to avoid burns.
>
> Patients with candidal paronychia should be advised to minimize exposure of hands to water and the prolonged use of rubber gloves. If a fluctuant abscess is present, the patient should apply a warm compress to the involved finger two to three times per day to assist in drainage.

DERMATOPHYTOSES

Dermatophytoses, or tinea, are superficial skin infections caused predominantly by three fungal species: *Trichophyton, Epidermophyton,* and *Microsporum.* Transmission occurs primarily through direct contact with an infected person or animal (e.g., dogs, cats). Other modes of transmission include contact with asymptomatic carriers who can infect family members and close contacts, or contact with soil (which contains a large number of fungal spores). Although this route of transmission is controversial, fomites (shared objects, such as combs or hats) have been implicated in spreading tinea infections. It is not uncommon to find two (or more) tinea infections in one patient. Tinea manuum often occurs in the "one hand, two feet" distribution. Tinea pedis ("athlete's foot") can occur simultaneously with both tinea unguium (onychomycosis) and tinea corporis ("ringworm"), as well as with other combinations. Multiple tinea infections are caused by spreading infection from one area of the body to another through scratching.

Environmental and host factors play an important role in the development of tinea infections. Favorable environmental factors that increase the risk of tinea infection include heat, moisture, and poor air circulation. Host factors include age (e.g., prepubertal children, young adults), broken skin, broken hair shafts, and excessive moisture on the skin or nails. Tinea infections are classified by their location on the body; different types include the following:

- Tinea capitis or "ringworm" of the scalp
- Tinea corporis or "ringworm" of the body, also known as tinea circinata
- Tinea cruris or "ringworm" of the groin, also known as "jock itch"
- Tinea pedis or "athlete's foot"
- Tinea manuum or tinea of the hands
- Tinea versicolor, also known as pityriasis versicolor
- Tinea unguium (onychomycosis; covered in a separate section)

Although tinea versicolor is caused by *Pityrosporum orbiculare* (the yeast form of *Malassezia furfur*) and is not considered a classic dermatophytosis, it is also discussed in this section.

EPIDEMIOLOGY AND CAUSES

The estimated lifetime incidence of tinea infections is between 10% and 20%. Tinea infections are more common in humid climates. Individuals with diabetes mellitus are at higher risk for tinea and yeast infections. Tinea pedis, or athlete's foot, is the most common fungal infection in the United States. Acute tinea pedis is caused by *Trichophyton mentagrophytes* var. *interdigitale,* and chronic tinea pedis, which is more common, is caused by

Trichophyton rubrum. Other less common causes of tinea pedis include *C. albicans* and *Epidermophyton floccosum.* Tinea cruris (jock itch) is more common in men, and *T. rubrum* is the typical agent. Tinea capitis (ringworm of the scalp) is most often caused by *Trichophyton tonsurans* and is more common in children until puberty when, for unknown reasons, the incidence markedly decreases. Tinea unguium (onychomycosis) occurs more frequently in adults and older patients.

The most contagious of all dermatophytoses is tinea capitis (scalp ringworm). It has been known to cause epidemics in crowded conditions, such as schools and group homes, and outbreaks among family members. Tinea capitis infections are more common in toddlers and school-age children from urban areas. Tinea capitis is easily transmitted because *Trichophyton tonsurans* tends to produce large numbers of infectious spores called arthroconidia. *T. tonsurans* causes up to 90% of all cases of tinea capitis in the United States and Western Europe. A minor cause of tinea capitis in the United States is *Microsporum canis,* a zoophilic fungus from dogs. Less common causes are *Microsporum audouinii* and *T. rubrum.*

Tinea barbae, an infection of the beard area, is more common in men who work with animals. Tinea manuum (tinea manus), or tinea of the hand(s), is relatively rare compared with other tinea infections. Tinea manuum infection frequently occurs with tinea pedis infection. The patient infects the hand by touching or scratching an infected foot. Unlike tinea pedis, in which both feet usually become infected, in tinea manuum infection, only one hand is usually involved. Tinea versicolor (pityriasis versicolor) infection is caused by the yeast *P. orbiculare* (which causes round lesions) or *Pityrosporum ovale* (which produces oval lesions). It is more common in the summertime and becomes more obvious with sun exposure, which exposes hypopigmented macules that do not tan.

PATHOPHYSIOLOGY

Three types of parasitic fungi are implicated in causing dermatophytic or tinea infections. *Microsporum* and *Epidermophyton* species both cause infections of the skin and nails. *Trichophyton* species cause infections not only of skin and nails but also of the hair. These fungal infections are superficial because all three types metabolize keratin, the protein that comprises the topmost layer of body surface epithelium, which normally serves as a protective barrier against microbial infection. The clinical presentation of tinea infections depends on their anatomical location and the species of fungi. Asymptomatic carriers do not show symptoms of disease but infect susceptible hosts through direct contact or by possibly depositing spores onto fomites such as combs, brushes, or hats.

Microscopic examination of tinea lesions reveals either acute or chronic inflammation and a spongelike texture in the infected tissue, aptly termed *spongiosis.* Fungal hyphae are seen on the superficial keratin layer of the epidermis. In tinea capitis, infection occurs either inside (endothrix) or outside (ectothrix) the hair shaft. In ectothrix infections, fungal hyphae and spores invade the hair shaft, leading to destruction of the hair cuticle. Ectothrix infections are caused by *Microsporum* species (*M. canis* and *M. audouinii*). In contrast, endothrix infections are caused by *Trichophyton* species (*T. tonsurans* in North America) and occur inside the hair shaft, leaving the hair cuticle intact. Spores are found inside the hair shaft, rather than on skin scrapings of surface scale. This type of infection is most common in African American children; coiling of the hair shaft may play a role in susceptibility to infection.

Kerion formation sometimes results from an endothrix infection and is associated with severe inflammatory changes of the scalp, consisting of nodules and boggy, exudative tissue. Secondary staphylococcal infection may complicate kerion, causing purulent drainage, with infection possibly spreading to draining lymph nodes and causing painful lymphadenitis. When it heals, it typically results in scarring and alopecia. A variant of endothrix infection that is uncommon in North America but more common in South Africa and the Middle East is favus infection, a severe form of tinea capitis caused most often by *Trichophyton schoenleinii* that results in extensive hair loss and scarring.

CLINICAL PRESENTATION

Subjective

Tinea Capitis

The typical patient with tinea capitis is a toddler or school-age child. The parent often reports a painless bald spot. If kerion formation accompanies the infection, the child will show signs of discomfort or will complain of pain. Systemic symptoms such as fever or malaise are not associated with kerion formation.

Tinea Corporis

The typical patient will report a history of an erythematous, round, elevated pruritic lesion that grows in size and starts to clear in the center (the classic shape of ringworm). Sometimes there is a history of another family member with the same infection, and patients may report a history of prior infection. The clinician should inquire about possible exposure through close contact with domesticated animals, such as cats or dogs.

Tinea Cruris

The typical patient is an obese adult man who complains of a pruritic rash on the groin that spreads to the medial inner aspect of the upper thigh. Sometimes the rash is not associated with pruritus.

Tinea Pedis

The typical patient is usually a male teenage athlete or an adult who comes to the clinic complaining of athlete's foot and strong foot odor. Most patients do not have pain with this infection unless it becomes secondarily infected with bacteria, causing cellulitis. The patient reports areas of macerated, soft, whitened skin between the toes. Some patients will complain of concurrent infections on the hand (tinea manuum), on the body (tinea corporis), or under the toenails (tinea unguium).

Tinea Versicolor

Most cases of tinea versicolor are recognized in the summer months because the hypopigmented spots become more visible at that time of year, as they do not tan. Tinea versicolor is asymptomatic and has a gradual onset. Rarely, a patient will complain of mild pruritus. The typical patient is a teen or young adult, although tinea can occur at any age. Darker skinned people with tinea will complain of either light-colored (hypopigmented) or dark-colored (hyperpigmented) spots. In adults, the usual sites are on the back, upper chest, arms, and sometimes the neck and face. In children, the rash is more likely to be on the face or forehead.

Objective

Tinea Capitis

Three clinical presentations are seen with tinea capitis infections. One presentation is "black dot" tinea capitis caused by *T. tonsurans*. The child with black dot tinea capitis presents with painless patchy alopecia (either in single or multiple patches). The skin on the scalp does not have erythema, and the black dot appearance results from broken hair stubble that remains on the scalp.

Another presentation is called "gray patch" tinea capitis. A child with this condition also presents with patchy alopecia, but the bald patches are covered with fine gray-white scales. The patch is made up of thick, keratinized skin that is grayish-white in color. Broken hair shafts of different lengths are present on the surface. Because the inflammatory response is minimal in both gray patch and black dot tinea capitis, pain, erythema, nodules, and kerion are not present.

An extremely painful and inflammatory presentation of tinea capitis is known as a kerion. A kerion appears as a large, bright-red, boggy "bump" on the scalp with alopecia. Purulent drainage can be expressed out of the kerion by gentle pressure, and pus can be seen oozing out of its tiny follicular openings. Kerion formation can result in scarring alopecia. The affected hair follicles atrophy and become permanently damaged; hair does not grow back, even when the scalp is healed. A permanent bald patch can result from this tinea infection if it is not treated aggressively or if the patient does not present early enough during the course of the disease.

Tinea Corporis

This infection presents as the classic ringworm infection and it is easy to recognize in the clinical setting. The patient will present with ringlike lesions with a bright-red elevated border (collarette) that is covered with scales. Tinea corporis can occur in any age group from child to adult, and the size of the lesions can range from small to large. The patient or parent will typically report that the lesion is getting bigger. Some patients have only one lesion, whereas others have numerous lesions. The lesions are usually very pruritic, but sometimes they may be asymptomatic.

Tinea Cruris

Tinea cruris (jock itch) is more common in men in the summer or during warm weather. It is usually extremely pruritic, and most lesions will show some lichenification from chronic scratching. The typical lesion is round to a half-circle and will spread to the inner medial upper thigh but spare the scrotum. In contrast, candidal intertrigo can affect not only the groin and thigh but also the penis and scrotum. The color of the lesion, depending on whether it is chronic or acute, can vary from bright red to a dull discoloration. The lesions can become macerated from infection and scratching; they may become secondarily infected with bacteria or *C. albicans*.

Tinea Pedis

Tinea pedis is usually asymptomatic, although the patient will sometimes complain of pain from a secondary bacterial infection. The infection usually starts in the third or fourth interdigital web space and sometimes spreads to all toe webs and the soles of the feet.

There are several distinctive clinical presentations of tinea pedis. The most common presentation of tinea pedis is macerated white skin between the web spaces of the toes; the infection can occasionally cause painful fissures and can be accompanied by an unpleasant foot odor. If it becomes infected with bacteria (usually *Staphylococcus aureus*), a tender cellulitis with redness and ulceration can develop in the web space between the toes. This condition is called ulcerative tinea pedis. Moccasin-type tinea pedis (plantar tinea pedis) is seen more often with *T. rubrum* infection, in which scaling and thickening of the skin is seen in a moccasin distribution on both feet.

Another presentation of tinea pedis is a dermatophytid or "id" eruption. Acute id eruptions are caused by a hypersensitivity reaction to the fungus. The id eruption presents as vesicles on the sides of the fingers and/or the palms of the hands. The vesicles do not contain fungus and are sterile. The patient may or may not be aware of a concurrent tinea pedis infection.

Another vesicular type of tinea pedis caused by *Trichophyton mentagrophytes* is associated with burning pruritus and sometimes pain. It is more likely to flare up during warm weather, forming multiple vesicles and bullae. It can become secondarily infected with bacteria, resulting in cellulitis or even lymphangitis.

Tinea Versicolor

Tinea versicolor is usually asymptomatic; it is not associated with pruritus. The patient will commonly present with oval or round pink macules. Lesions may also be hypopigmented or hyperpigmented and are located mainly on the back, chest, arms, and sometimes the neck and face. Tinea versicolor in children is more likely to present on the face, especially on the forehead. Sometimes very fine scales are visible, especially if the patient has not showered or bathed for several days; otherwise, daily bathing usually eradicates the scales.

DIAGNOSTIC REASONING

Diagnostic Tests

Tinea infections are usually diagnosed by their clinical presentation. The classic ringworm lesions are easy to recognize. The diagnosis can be confirmed via microscopy in the clinic or a specimen (skin scraping) can be sent to the laboratory in a sterile plastic cup. Fungal culture is usually not necessary except in cases where the diagnosis is in doubt, in resistant cases, or before treatment of onychomycosis (tinea unguium) or tinea capitis is initiated. Because of the length of treatment and the potential for adverse reactions from systemic antifungals, confirmatory evidence by fungal culture is necessary to justify systemic therapy. Standard fungal cultures can take up to 2 weeks for results to become available, although if done on Sabouraud's agar or with dermatophyte test medium, results may be obtained in 3 days. Polymerase chain reaction (PCR) assays may also be used to identify fungus in nails.

A fungal culture is recommended for onychomycosis (tinea unguium) and for tinea capitis. Because these two tinea infections require long-term therapy with systemic antifungals (with a high potential for serious side effects), physician consultation is recommended. Proof of the causative agent must be provided by a positive fungal culture. Fungal cultures are also useful if the clinician is unsure of the diagnosis or if the infection does not respond to treatment. For tinea capitis, hair bulbs and broken hair, along with scales from the active lesion, should be cultured. Specimens from the affected site should include scales and hair roots. It is important to look for spores and hyphae on the hair shaft, inside the hair shaft (endothrix), and outside the hair shaft (ectothrix) using microscopy. To obtain a fungal culture for suspected tinea capitis, the clinician may use a dry toothbrush to brush the areas of alopecia and then impregnate the culture medium with the bristles. Another method is to use a wet cotton swab, wipe it over the areas of alopecia, and then implant it on the medium. Growth is usually seen in 10 to 14 days of culture. If a secondary bacterial infection is suspected, a sample of the exudate must be taken for culture and sensitivity using a sterile culture tube.

Microscopy is the most useful diagnostic tool for tinea in the primary care setting (see Advanced Assessment 13.1).

A Wood's light examination should be used on any area of alopecia and hypopigmentation. Some fungi fluoresce when examined under a Wood's light, which emits ultraviolet light (black light). The examining room should be darkened for this examination. A characteristic color that is associated with two minor causes of tinea capitis is a blue-green or bright green color from *M. canis* or *M. audouinii*. However, in contrast, *T. tonsurans*, the most common cause of tinea capitis, does not fluoresce under a Wood's light examination.

Differential Diagnosis

Tinea infections have a wide differential diagnosis, which is largely dependent on location (see Differential Diagnosis 13.2). Almost all tinea infections tend to have a gradual onset, characterized by low levels of inflammation, which do not typically produce bothersome symptoms such as pruritus or pain. In turn, some tinea infections, such as tinea manuum and tinea unguium (onychomycosis), may be present for months to years before the patient reports them to a health-care provider. Sometimes tinea infections may only be recognized as an incidental finding during a routine physical examination. Tinea infections such as tinea cruris and tinea corporis tend to be more symptomatic, and the severe pruritus associated with these infections usually drives the patient to seek medical care. Onychomycosis is discussed separately in a subsequent section.

MANAGEMENT

Most cases of tinea infection (except tinea infections of the scalp and nails) respond well to a 2- to 4-week course of topical treatment with azole-class drugs, such as those listed in Drugs Commonly Prescribed 13.1. These agents should be continued for at least 1 week after the lesions have cleared. They should be applied a few centimeters beyond the edges of the skin lesions. Other drugs, including systemic formulations, are also included in this table.

As noted previously, for all patients who are on systemic antifungals, physician consultation is recommended because systemically absorbed antifungal drugs can cause hepatotoxicity. A baseline liver function profile should be done initially and repeated again in 4 weeks and periodically thereafter during the course of treatment. The patient should be told to report symptoms such as anorexia, nausea, vomiting, malaise, dark urine, jaundice, and rash to the clinician. If the clinician suspects hepatotoxicity, the offending drug should be stopped and consultation with the supervising physician is recommended. Griseofulvin can also cause leukopenia and granulocytopenia. A baseline

Differential Diagnosis 13.2: Tinea Infections

Location	Differential Diagnoses
Scalp (tinea capitis, tinea of the scalp)	Psoriasis Seborrheic dermatitis Alopecia areata
Body (tinea corporis, "ringworm")	Atopic or contact dermatitis Psoriasis Subacute cutaneous lupus erythematosus Granuloma annulare Erythema annulare centrifugum Nummular eczema Pityriasis rosea Disciform erythrasma
Hands (tinea manuum)	Atopic dermatitis Dyshidrotic eczema
Groin (tinea cruris, "jock itch")	Erythrasma Inverse psoriasis Seborrheic dermatitis Contact dermatitis Candidal intertrigo
Feet (tinea pedis, "athlete's foot")	Bacterial intertrigo Candidal intertrigo Psoriasis Contact dermatitis Dyshidrotic eczema Impetigo Erythrasma Atopic dermatitis Pitted keratolysis Juvenile plantar dermatosis Keratolysis exfoliative Keratodermas Palmoplantar pustulosis Scabies
Nails (tinea unguium, onychomycosis)	Psoriasis of the nail Trauma Onychogryphosis
Tinea versicolor (pityriasis versicolor)	Vitiligo Pityriasis alba Pityriasis rosea Seborrheic dermatitis Erythrasma Secondary syphilis Confluent and reticulated papillomatosis of Gougerot-Carteaud Mycosis fungoides Terra firma-forme dermatosis

complete blood count (CBC) and another repeated in 4 weeks are recommended. Thereafter, a follow-up CBC can be done at 4- to 6-week intervals.

Of note, interval laboratory testing of liver function and CBCs during systemic treatment with griseofulvin and terbinafine has become somewhat controversial. A 2018 study challenged the use of interval monitoring during therapy with griseofulvin and terbinafine, due to the low rate of abnormalities and associated unnecessary health-care costs. To date, however, the American Academy of Dermatology has not changed its guidelines for interval monitoring with these medications.

Oral systemic antifungals are generally contraindicated in pregnant women due to multiple reports of birth defects and miscarriage. Women who may become pregnant while undergoing systemic antifungal treatment should use two effective forms of contraception and begin therapy on day 2 or 3 after the onset of menses; such contraception should be continued for 1 to 2 months after the last dose of the antifungal.

Tinea Capitis

In tinea capitis, a kerion that looks like a honeycomb may be observed. It is an inflammatory boggy mass containing broken hairs and oozing purulent material from follicular orifices. This rare, delayed hypersensitivity reaction to fungal antigens may result in permanent hair loss. Kerion rarely needs to be treated with concurrent antibiotics, as a noninfected kerion may appear exudative. It should be treated with antibiotics only if a secondary staphylococcal infection is apparent. Tinea infections of the hair and nails do not respond to topical treatment, unlike other tinea infections. Tinea capitis should be treated with oral systemic antifungals, along with a topical antifungal for localized scalp lesions. A Wood's light examination should be done in all cases of scalp alopecia. Although some infections will fluoresce (*M. canis, M. audouinii*), others do not (*T. tonsurans, T. violaceum*). A fungal culture is necessary not only to help in the diagnosis but also to classify the species of fungi. It is important to examine the patient's close contacts, including family members (especially other children) and schoolmates. Fungal cultures of close contacts are recommended, if possible. Asymptomatic cases of tinea capitis can be treated with selenium sulfide shampoo (e.g., Selsun Blue). There is no need to wait for results of the fungal culture (which take 2 weeks) before initiating treatment, especially if there is kerion formation (see Drugs Commonly Prescribed 13.1).

The first-line treatment for symptomatic tinea capitis is griseofulvin or oral terbinafine. Griseofulvin (Grifulvin V) is given 250 to 500 mg by mouth twice per day for severe cases in adults or once per day for children weighing more than 50 pounds. For children who weigh 30 to 50 pounds, 125 to 250 mg daily is recommended. Treatment duration is from 2 to 4 months or at least 2 weeks after negative cultures are obtained. Some authorities recommend against griseofulvin as a first-line drug because of its potential adverse effects. Female patients must be cautioned that oral contraceptives may be less effective with griseofulvin and to use additional birth control, such as barrier protection, during treatment and for 1 month after treatment. Male patients on griseofulvin should be advised that this drug affects sperm and is teratogenic; thus, males should avoid fathering a child during treatment and for at least 6 months after stopping the drug.

The adult dosage of terbinafine for tinea capitis is 250 mg daily for 6 weeks. Terbinafine is prescribed to children older than 4 years based on weight: 10 to 20 kg, 62.5 mg daily; 20 to 40 kg, 125 mg daily; more than 40 kg, 250 mg daily. The recommended duration of therapy in pediatric patients is 4 to 6 weeks. Other effective alternatives used to treat tinea capitis include oral fluconazole and itraconazole. Concurrent treatment with selenium sulfide shampoo three times per week is used as adjunctive therapy to systemic antifungals.

Tinea Corporis

Topical antifungal therapy generally works well for tinea corporis. The patient must be reminded to continue to use the topical agent for at least 1 week after resolution of the lesions and to apply the cream a few centimeters beyond the edges of the affected area. Concomitant short-term treatment with a mild corticosteroid such as hydrocortisone 1% (available OTC) is effective in helping relieve itch and inflammation. In cases that do not respond to topical treatment, systemic antifungals such as itraconazole or terbinafine taken daily are effective.

Tinea Cruris

Topical antifungal therapy is effective for the treatment of jock itch. Concomitant short-term treatment with a mild corticosteroid such as hydrocortisone 1% (OTC) is effective in helping relieve itch and inflammation. If weeping areas are present, compresses made from Burow's solution are helpful to dry the affected area. Use of OTC antifungal powders helps prevent future recurrences. For cases unresponsive to topical therapy, a short course of a systemic antifungal treatment such as itraconazole or terbinafine is effective.

Tinea Pedis and Tinea Manuum

Tinea pedis and tinea manuum are both treated with topical antifungals. Treatment of tinea pedis should emphasize moisture control; drying foot powders (e.g., miconazole, tolnaftate) are very helpful. If weeping areas are present, compresses made from Burow's solution are beneficial to dry the affected area. The feet should be exposed to air as much as possible; during warm weather, the use of airy sandals or going barefoot is helpful. If socks are worn, cotton or a synthetic "wicking" blend is the best material. Socks should be changed once daily, and changing socks twice daily is indicated if the patient's feet become wet. An antiperspirant spray on the soles of the feet (to be applied on normal skin only) can help patients with excessively sweaty feet. Severe tinea pedis can be treated with oral agents such as itraconazole or terbinafine daily. After a short course of systemic therapy, the patient should be placed on maintenance topical therapy with an antifungal powder or a spray (e.g., miconazole, tolnaftate) to prevent recurrences.

Tinea Versicolor

Tinea versicolor is treated with topical selenium sulfide lotion (Selsun) applied daily for 7 days from neck to waist, "lathered" on with a small amount of water, and left on for 10 minutes before rinsing thoroughly. Treatment is repeated once a week for 1 month and then once a month for maintenance. Ketoconazole (Nizoral) shampoo can also be used weekly for maintenance. The clinician should advise the patient that treatment will eradicate the infection but will not remove the hypopigmented spots from the skin, which will take longer to resolve. Patients should also be warned of the high rate of recurrence, because *P. orbiculare* (*M. furfur*) is a normal inhabitant of the skin. Exposing the hypopigmented lesions to sunlight can speed up the process of resolution in some patients, although their appearance may also be enhanced, given that they will not tan in sunlight relative to the surrounding skin.

For patients who desire more aggressive treatment, fluconazole and itraconazole are the drugs of choice. Fluconazole 150 to 300 mg weekly for 2 to 4 weeks is considered the safest choice for systemic treatment. Fluconazole may also be given once monthly for 6 months. As an alternate treatment, itraconazole may be prescribed at 200 mg daily for 7 days. However, the patient should be advised that there is a risk of hepatotoxicity with systemic antifungals and that treatment does not prevent recurrence. Because tinea versicolor is a superficial benign disease, this fact should be given serious consideration. Some success has also been reported with the use of photodynamic therapy for tinea versicolor.

FOLLOW-UP AND REFERRAL

The patient should be seen for initial follow-up 2 weeks after the start of therapy. For resistant cases, the clinician should confirm the diagnosis with a fungal culture or the diagnosis should be reevaluated. Resistant cases should be referred to a dermatologist for reevaluation or for more aggressive treatment with systemic antifungals. If the patient was initially placed on topical therapy only, systemic therapy can be considered, as severe tinea corporis and tinea pedis respond well to oral terbinafine or itraconazole.

Some tinea infections have higher recurrence rates than others. Tinea versicolor (pityriasis versicolor), although not a true tinea (because it is caused by a yeast, rather than a dermatophyte), has a high recurrence rate because *P. orbiculare* and *P. ovale* are normal colonizers of the skin. Tinea pedis also tends to recur, so meticulous attention should be given by the patient to eradicating favorable environmental conditions for fungal growth (see previous discussion of tinea pedis for preventive measures). Maintenance therapy for tinea pedis with topical OTC agents in powder or spray form (e.g., miconazole, tolnaftate) is effective in helping prevent recurrences.

If the clinician suspects that a secondary bacterial skin infection (cellulitis) is complicating the tinea infection, a culture should be done on any purulent drainage. Empiric therapy for mild cellulitis, which is usually caused by gram-positive bacteria such as *Staphylococcus* or group A beta-hemolytic *Streptococcus*, includes oral antibiotics such as cephalexin or dicloxacillin for 7 to 14 days. For patients with penicillin allergy, either erythromycin or clarithromycin is an appropriate alternative. Toe web infection (ulcerative type) can be due to gram-negative bacterial infection (e.g., *Pseudomonas aeruginosa, Escherichia coli, Proteus*) and must be treated with systemic fluoroquinolones (e.g., ciprofloxacin). Patients with moderate or severe cellulitis should be referred to a physician for more aggressive treatment, including IV antibiotics.

Patient Education: Antifungal Therapy

Patients who are taking systemic antifungal therapy must be informed of the risk of hepatotoxicity and educated on the signs and symptoms of acute hepatitis, such as anorexia, nausea, vomiting, malaise, dark urine, jaundice, and rash. For all patients on systemic antifungals, consultation with a physician is recommended. A baseline liver function profile and CBC should be obtained before treatment is initiated and repeated in 4 weeks and periodically thereafter. Patients should also be made aware of other adverse reactions to oral antifungals, including GI upset, abdominal pain, dizziness, headache, rash, and taste disturbances (associated with terbinafine). Blood dyscrasias including granulocytopenia and leukopenia, a lupus-like syndrome, and proteinuria are also possible adverse effects of griseofulvin.

Patients should also understand the risk of drug interactions with systemic antifungals. Griseofulvin decreases the effectiveness of certain drugs, such as oral anticoagulants and barbiturates. Any woman of reproductive age who is on oral contraceptives and is prescribed griseofulvin should be warned that the contraceptive will become less effective, and therefore her risk of pregnancy will increase. The patient should be advised to see her gynecologist about using another effective method of birth control. If a patient who is on a barbiturate or an oral anticoagulant feels strongly about starting antifungal treatment, the patient should consult the physician who prescribed the original medication before starting treatment with systemic antifungals. Terbinafine (Lamisil) is potentiated by cimetidine and is antagonized by rifampin. Itraconazole (Sporanox) is contraindicated if the patient is taking any drug that is metabolized in the liver by the cytochrome p450 CYP3A enzyme system. Itraconazole increases the blood levels of triazolam (Halcion), diazepam (Valium), digoxin, dihydropyridine calcium channel blockers (e.g., amlodipine, nifedipine), and several other drugs.

For patients interested in complementary therapies, they may try *Melaleuca alternifolia* (tea tree oil) applied twice daily to the affected areas. Although sufficient research has not been done on this commonly used alternative treatment to confirm its efficacy, no adverse side effects are known.

The following measures should be recommended to help prevent spread or recurrence of tinea infections:

- Tinea capitis: Family members and pets should be assessed for signs of tinea capitis. Family members should be advised not to share combs, hats, or any headgear with affected individuals and to use an antifungal shampoo for 2 to 4 weeks.
- Tinea corporis: The patient should be advised to control excessive sweat and body moisture by wearing loose-fitting clothing and to change clothing when it becomes wet or damp. After bathing, a hair dryer on the low-heat setting may be used to dry intertriginous skinfolds.
- Tinea corporis: Given its colloquial name, some patients (especially children) may incorrectly think that an actual worm is the cause of ringworm infections. Reassuring these patients that the infection is actually caused by a fungus can significantly allay anxiety.
- Tinea cruris: Cotton boxer shorts are better at preventing infections than tight briefs. The patient should avoid wearing tight jeans, pantyhose, or tight shorts made of close-fitting material such as Spandex (e.g., bike shorts).
- Tinea pedis: The patient should be advised to avoid scratching the feet because the infection can spread to the hands (tinea manuum) and the body (tinea corporis). The patient should avoid tight shoes and moist socks, especially socks made out of synthetic material, unless they are designed to wick away moisture. Patients who are prone to athlete's foot should change socks two or three times a day and expose their feet to air; they should use sandals if possible in warm weather. Absorbent nonsynthetic socks are preferred. Feet should be washed daily and dried thoroughly (a hair dryer on a low-heat setting is helpful). Use of antiperspirant spray on the soles of the feet may decrease sweating. Patients should also be advised to clean their shower stalls with bleach and to wash all white sheets with bleach. When showering away from home, shower shoes should be worn.
- Tinea versicolor: Advise the patient that exposure to sunlight will help in repigmentation of hypopigmented areas in the long term, although without proper treatment, tanning tends to enhance the appearance of affected hypopigmented skin patches.

ONYCHOMYCOSIS

Onychomycosis (tinea unguium) is a benign superficial infection of the toenails and fingernails, which negatively affects their appearance and may lead to dystrophic changes. Most patients tolerate mild to moderate forms of tinea nail infections for many years. Patients who seek treatment are usually younger adults who are disturbed by the cosmetic effects of the infection. The most common etiology for onychomycosis is infection with dermatophytic fungi, but molds, yeast, and nondermatophytic fungi may be causative agents as well. Factors that increase the risk of onychomycosis include wearing occlusive shoes, diabetes mellitus, participation in sports, increasing age, and poor circulation of the lower extremities.

EPIDEMIOLOGY AND CAUSES

Onychomycosis is more common in adults and older patients than in children. The combination of poor circulation in the lower extremities as a result of peripheral vascular disease and the immunocompromising effects of advanced age makes this a common problem in older adults. Toenails are more likely to become infected than fingernails. Onychomycosis is a common infection worldwide; the incidence of disease is variable and is dependent on many factors. In the United States, 20% of all adults have onychomycosis. Onychomycosis is sometimes caused by the yeast *C. albicans*. Dermatophytic species of fungi commonly implicated in this tinea infection are *Trichophyton* species: *T. rubrum, T. mentagrophytes, T. schoenleinii*, and several others. A zoophilic fungus that is normally found in animal species that can cause onychomycosis is *T. verrucosum*.

Like many infections, onychomycosis frequently has a multifactorial etiology, including both fungal exposure and decreased immunity. The development of onychomycosis cannot be attributed solely to the presence of the offending organism because most causative yeasts and fungi are ubiquitous in the environment. Molds, for example, are plentiful in soil, and the soil mold *Scopulariopsis brevicaulis* is the most common nondermatophytic cause of onychomycosis. Other molds implicated in onychomycosis include *Aspergillus* and *Alternaria* species. In addition, *C. albicans* can be part of the normal flora of the mouth, GI tract, or vagina.

PATHOPHYSIOLOGY

Onychomycosis is classified as either a primary or secondary infection. Primary onychomycosis involves invasion of the healthy nail plate. In secondary onychomycosis, diseased nails (e.g., from psoriasis or trauma) are predisposed to develop infection. Factors that increase the risk of onychomycosis include a decrease in circulation, resulting from either a chronic process such as peripheral vascular disease or an acute traumatic process such as fracture of the lower extremity. Abnormal enervation due to spinal trauma has also been implicated. Tinea unguium can result from an extension of an infection with tinea pedis, tinea manuum, or tinea corporis.

Nail invasion can proceed in several ways. In proximal subungual onychomycosis, the pathogen enters the nailbed through the posterior nail and cuticle area, then migrates to the proximal nailbed. This form of onychomycosis is most commonly seen in immunocompromised individuals who exhibit suboptimal T-cell function. In distal and lateral subungual onychomycosis, infection starts at the distal or lateral margins of the nail. The infection then moves toward the center of the nail until the entire nail is affected. Distal subungual onychomycosis is almost always caused by *T. rubrum*. Superficial white onychomycosis involves infection of the nail surface only and is caused mainly by *T. mentagrophytes*. Total dystrophic onychomycosis is associated mostly with chronic candidiasis, which is seen in severely immunodeficient states such as AIDS.

CLINICAL PRESENTATION

Subjective

The typical patient who seeks treatment for onychomycosis is either a young or middle-aged adult who is bothered greatly by the negative cosmetic effects of the infection. The duration of the infection can range from a few weeks to many years. Onychomycosis is an asymptomatic infection, and there should be no pain involved. Some patients report having tried several OTC remedies with no result. The patient may complain of thickened dystrophic nails or nails with cloudy, white-colored patches. Some report nail discoloration ranging from yellow to green or brown to black. In more severe forms, some patients complain of nails that are partially detached from the nailbed (onycholysis).

Objective

Onychomycosis has several presentations, and in some patients, multiple types can occur simultaneously. Superficial white onychomycosis involves only the nail surface, but may occur with either distal or lateral subungual onychomycosis. Subungual onychomycosis may involve distal, lateral, and proximal sites of infection. The first or fifth toenail is more likely to become infected than the other toes. The infected nail typically appears dry and has an opaque white patch with sharp borders that start on the distal, lateral, or proximal subungual portion, or is limited to the nail surface (superficial white onychomycosis). As the infection persists, the nail becomes brittle and thickened. The area underneath the nail accumulates chalky material made up of hyperkeratotic debris that can be scraped off easily for fungal cultures. In some patients, the white opaque areas become discolored—either yellow or brown. A green-black color suggests complication with a bacterial *Pseudomonas* infection.

DIAGNOSTIC REASONING

Diagnostic Tests

All cases of presumed onychomycosis must be confirmed by laboratory findings. A positive result on fungal culture, which includes proper identification of the fungal species involved, is necessary to start treatment with systemic antifungals. Findings of the KOH examination on light microscopy typical of fungal infection are hyphae and spores with a classic "spaghetti and meatballs" appearance. Under the microscope, hyphae appear as long translucent tubes with septa denoting separate sections, whereas spores are small, round to ovoid shapes.

Fungal Culture

Fungal cultures done on Sabouraud's agar or with dermatophyte test medium produce results in up to 3 days. The area where the samples are to be taken should be cleansed with 70% alcohol and allowed to dry before specimen collection. Skin should be taken from the active border of the lesion. Nail samples should be taken from the subsurface of the infected nail. To obtain samples from underneath the nail, a scalpel can be used to scrape the underside of the infected nail. In proximal subungual onychomycosis, the affected part of the nail is at the proximal fold and cannot be sampled without nail removal. Nail removal is done with a bilateral digital nerve block and is contraindicated if the patient has a bleeding disorder. The patient should be referred to a podiatrist for nail removal and treatment.

KOH Examination

A laboratory examination using KOH is necessary for diagnosis, because only 50% of dystrophic nails are due to dermatophytosis (see Advanced Assessment 13.1).

Differential Diagnosis

The differential diagnosis of onychomycosis includes psoriasis of the nail, trauma to the nail, and congenital nail abnormalities. Onychomycosis accounts for only 50% to 60% of abnormally appearing or dystrophic nails. Lichen planus, eczematous conditions, and senile nailbed ischemia may all result in similarly appearing nails; however, fungal infection does not underlie such conditions, and antifungal medications would be inappropriate in such cases.

MANAGEMENT

In the past, onychomycosis of the toenail required long-term treatment with systemic antifungals and had a high recurrence rate. With the advent of newer antifungals (e.g., itraconazole, terbinafine), the cure rates for onychomycosis have greatly improved. Fluconazole (Diflucan) has consistently been shown to be less effective than either itraconazole or terbinafine, however, and is not typically recommended. Superficial infections are more responsive to treatment with prescription topical antifungals (e.g., naftifine gel) than subungual types, in which infection occurs beneath the nail. Alternative therapies include laser treatment (which is a temporary aesthetic treatment, but not a cure) and chemical or surgical nail removal, followed by treatment with antifungals. Photodynamic therapy and plasma therapy are being studied for treatment of onychomycosis, although further clinical trials are needed.

Fingernail infection is easier to cure and has a lower rate of recurrence than toenail infection. The decision to treat onychomycosis aggressively must be considered carefully because it is predominantly a benign cosmetic infection. The patient's desires for treatment and their health history are probably the strongest determinants in deciding whether to treat with systemic antifungals. Other important factors include the presence of any preexisting medical problems and the patient's past medical history. Patients who have liver disease should avoid systemic antifungal drugs because of the high risk of hepatotoxicity and liver failure. A history of infection with viral hepatitis can result in chronic infection with hepatitis B or C, and a history of excessive alcohol use can result in cirrhosis of the liver or elevations in liver function tests—both of which are considered high-risk conditions for starting systemic antifungal therapy.

Medication interactions with antifungal therapies are also problematic. Drugs metabolized by the cytochrome p450 3A enzyme system interact with systemic antifungals. Itraconazole potentiates the effects of many common prescription drugs, including diazepam (Valium), digoxin (Lanoxin), triazolam (Halcion), anticoagulants (Coumadin), HIV protease inhibitors (e.g., indinavir, ritonavir), methylprednisone, and verapamil. Patients who are taking vinca alkaloids (used in cancer chemotherapy) should not take itraconazole. In addition, itraconazole requires a low gastric pH (acidic) to be absorbed; therefore, H_2 blockers and antacids must be avoided within 2 hours of taking the drug.

Topical Therapy

Topical treatment of onychomycosis is generally not very effective (cure rates of 10% or less), but it is worth an attempt because topical therapy is not typically associated with any serious side effects. Good candidates for topical treatment are motivated patients with only mild involvement (i.e., one-half or less of distal nail plate infected) or with surface involvement only (superficial white onychomycosis). Also, patients unable to take systemic antifungals may benefit from topical formulations. A topical solution such as ciclopirox nail lacquer 8% (Penlac) applied twice daily for 6 to 18 months or either efinaconazole 10% topical or tavaborole 0.5% solution applied once daily for 48 weeks may be effective when applied consistently to toenails. Efinaconazole and tavaborole should be applied once daily over the entire nail surface and under the nail. Ciclopirox 8% (Penlac) is indicated for mild to moderate onychomycosis of the fingernails and toenails (without lunula involvement). Initial improvement may take up to 6 months, and treatment can continue up to 48 weeks. Ciclopirox should be applied evenly on the affected nail and surrounding 5 mm of skin once daily, preferably at bedtime. It should be applied over previous coats, then removed with alcohol once a week. Nail polish should not be used during this treatment period.

Systemic Therapy

For patients who desire treatment for onychomycosis, most authorities recommend systemic therapy. If concurrent tinea pedis, tinea manuum, or tinea corporis is present, it should be treated with topical antifungals, so that the source of infection is eradicated. Fingernails are easier to treat than toenails and have a higher cure rate from 50% to 70%. See Drugs Commonly Prescribed 13.1 for recommended systemic medications.

Itraconazole and terbinafine are considered first-line therapy for toenail infections, which are more difficult to treat; terbinafine is preferred due to superior cure rates and fewer drug interactions than itraconazole. Patients who are on H_2 blockers can also take these drugs. There is no role for griseofulvin in the treatment of toenail onychomycosis because up to 80% to 90% of patients will relapse with this drug; in addition, treatment with fluconazole is not approved by the FDA and is, therefore, off-label.

FOLLOW-UP AND REFERRAL

After the initiation of therapy, liver function tests should be rechecked every 4 weeks. The first follow-up visit is scheduled during the fourth week to monitor for symptoms of hepatotoxicity, adverse reactions, compliance with treatment, and to obtain a liver function panel. Thereafter, the patient should be seen for follow-up every 4 to 6 weeks, with follow-up liver function tests and monitoring of nail growth until the nails become clinically normal. Resistant cases of onychomycosis should be referred to a dermatologist or infectious disease specialist.

Patient Education: Onychomycosis

Strategies to prevent the recurrence of onychomycosis include observing the feet for signs of tinea pedis, refraining from trimming cuticles and sharing unsterilized nail grooming tools, keeping feet cool and dry, and wearing foot coverings such as flip flops in public showers and gyms. Prophylactic application of topical antifungals to the feet, especially in the web spaces between the toes, may be considered. Patients on itraconazole and terbinafine treatment should be advised that treatment should continue until full nail regrowth occurs, which is approximately 6 to 9 months for fingernails and 12 to 18 months for toenails.

Naturopathic approaches may also be considered in treating nail fungus. Some patients have had success with *Melaleuca alternifolia* (tea tree oil) when applied to the affected nail twice daily, although there is insufficient evidence from controlled clinical trials to confirm its efficacy. Additional home remedies for toenail fungus include topical treatments with castor oil, antiseptic mouthwash (e.g., Listerine), mentholated petrolatum (Vicks VapoRub), feminine hygiene wash (e.g., Vagisil), vitamin E oil, and white vinegar. Most reports of success with these topical treatments are anecdotal, although small studies with mentholated petrolatum and acetic acid (vinegar) have shown somewhat positive results. However, additional studies are needed to confirm the efficacy of such treatments. Moreover, the safety profiles of these treatments are not yet fully defined and they may have unrecognized adverse effects; for example, vitamin E oil has been associated with dermatitis in some patients. An OTC preparation of ethanoic acid (Nonyx nail gel) has been cosmetically successful in some patients, as it removes keratin debris and thus improves the appearance of brittle, lifted, and thickened nails.

REFERENCES

Candidiasis

Centers for Disease Control and Prevention. 2015 Sexually transmitted disease treatment guidelines: vulvovaginal candidiasis. https://www.cdc.gov/std/treatment-guidelines/candidiasis.htm. Accessed 9/4/2020.

Centers for Disease Control and Prevention. Candidiasis. https://www.cdc.gov/fungal/diseases/candidiasis/. Accessed 9/4/21.

Jeanmonod R, Jeanmonod D. (2020). Vaginal candidiasis. StatPearls[Internet]. https://www.ncbi.nlm.nih.gov/books/NBK459317/. Accessed 12/15/2020.

Pappas PG, Kauffman CA, Andes DR, et al. Clinical practice guideline for the management of candidiasis: 2016 update by the Infectious Diseases Society of America. *Clin Infect Dis.* 2016;62(4):409–417.

Onychomycosis

Lipner SR, Scher RK. Onychomycosis: treatment and prevention of recurrence. *J Am Acad Dermatol.* 2019;80(4):853–867.

The People's Pharmacy. (2019 Jan 17). Graeden's guide to hair and nail care: toenail fungus. Accessed 9/8/2020.

Tinea

American Academy of Dermatology Association. Tinea versicolor: diagnosis and treatment. https://www.aad.org/public/diseases/a-z/tinea-versicolor-treatment. Accessed 12/15/2020.

CDC Centers for Disease Control and Prevention. Fungal diseases. https://www.cdc.gov/fungal/index.html. Accessed 12/15/2020.

Heymann WR. Breaking the terbinafine laboratory habit. *Skinmed*. 2020;1(11):115–116. Accessed 9/10/2020.

Stolmeier DA, Stratman HB, McIntee TJ, et al. Utility of laboratory test result monitoring in patients taking oral terbinafine or griseofulvin for dermatophyte infections. *JAMA Dermatol*. 2018;154(12):1409–1416.

RESOURCES

American Academy of Dermatology
https://www.aad.org

Infectious Disease Society of America
https://www.idsociety.org

MedlinePlus. Dermatological drugs, herbs, and supplements
https://medlineplus.gov/druginformation.html

National Institute of Allergy and Infectious Disease
https://www.niaid.nih.gov/diseases-conditions/fungal-diseases

---

Chapter 14

Bacterial Skin Infections

Susan Garnett, MSN, APRN, FNP-BC
Jill E. Winland-Brown, EdD, APRN, FNP-BC, FAANP
Brian Oscar Porter, MD, PhD, MPH, MBA

IMPETIGO

Impetigo is a highly contagious, superficial vesiculopustular infection of the skin that is commonly seen in infants and children. Impetigo spreads readily through direct contact among family members, children in classrooms or play groups, participants of contact sports, and the general population via fomites (shared objects such as clothing or furniture). Impetigo infection in adults is not as contagious as impetigo infection in infants and younger children. Impetigo infection typically demonstrates a mixed flora of gram-positive bacteria that includes *Staphylococcus aureus* and group A or group B beta-hemolytic *Streptococcus*. Two forms of impetigo are commonly seen in clinics: bullous and nonbullous (vesiculopustular). Bullous impetigo occurs primarily in newborns and infants. Nonbullous impetigo is the more common form, constituting approximately 80% of impetigo cases; it is caused solely by *S. aureus*.

EPIDEMIOLOGY AND CAUSES

Impetigo primarily affects infants in hospital nurseries and young children aged 2 to 5 years, especially those with inadequate hygiene and who are in day-care groups; however, patients of all ages are susceptible. Impetigo makes up nearly 10% of skin complaints in pediatric practices. It is the most prevalent bacterial skin infection and the third most common skin condition that occurs in children. Impetigo is more common in hot, humid weather, when biting insects and mosquitoes are most pervasive. The trauma caused by these insect bites favors bacterial growth on moist skin. There is an increased incidence of impetigo in disadvantaged socioeconomic groups due to several factors, including overcrowding, inadequate personal hygiene, and a higher incidence of anemia, diabetes mellitus, and malnutrition. In addition, any preexisting skin disease that goes untreated (e.g., atopic dermatitis) may also predispose individuals to secondary infection. Staphylococcal impetigo may also be associated with immunodeficiency.

PATHOPHYSIOLOGY

The infectious process in impetigo is limited to the stratum corneum. The presence of numerous neutrophils within a subcorneal blister and the presence of gram-positive cocci are characteristic of impetigo infections. Etiological agents may be found alone or in combination.

In cases of impetigo caused by a combination of gram-positive bacteria, symbiosis promotes the growth of both types of bacteria and produces more rapid spread. *Staphylococcus* bacteria are usually noted during the early stages of the lesions, whereas *Streptococcus* bacteria tend to predominate in the later stages. In recent years, epidemiologists have noted an etiological shift in which *S. aureus*, either alone or in combination with group A *Streptococcus*, has replaced the latter as the most common causative organism. Thus, chronic skin colonization with either *S. aureus* or group A *Streptococcus* predisposes an individual to impetigo. Infected lesions typically result from sites of previous injury, such as insect bites. Blister formation is caused by the action of epidermolytic (exfoliative) exotoxins produced by the bacteria; blisters are the result of local separation (acantholysis) of keratinocytes in the underlying epidermal layer that form the floor of the blister. Group A *Streptococcus* is the primary etiological agent for a rare, severe ulcerative form of impetigo known as ecthyma. Ulcer formation is also aided by coagulase-positive *Staphylococcus*.

Bullous impetigo is caused by *S. aureus* infection in newborns and young children. In this condition, exfoliative toxin A causes loss of cellular adhesion in the superficial epidermis normally mediated by the protein desmoglein. This results in large, blistering lesions known as bullae, which eventually drain, leaving thin, nonpurulent crusts over the affected skin area.

Methicillin-resistant *S. aureus* (MRSA) has increasingly been identified as a causative agent in primarily nonbullous impetigo. In recent years, impetigo has more frequently been caused by strains of community-acquired MRSA and gentamicin-resistant *S. aureus*.

CLINICAL PRESENTATION

Subjective

The most common symptom of both types of impetigo is pruritus from the lesions. The parent of a young or school-aged child may report a red, crusty rash that is spreading or getting larger in size. The rash is usually located on the face or on the extremities. Parents or the child may report that a close friend or classmate of the patient has the same rash.

The provider should ask about the location, onset, and duration of the lesions and any associated symptoms. The clinician should also inquire if any other family member has been affected and if treatment has been effective. Fever is unusual in impetigo, but if present, it should prompt investigation for a deeper infection.

Objective

The plaques of impetigo begin as vesicles. The roofs of these vesicles break down, leaving shallow erosions with yellowish crusts. The lesions may be discrete or confluent in their distribution and are usually seen on the face. Early impetigo may resemble many vesicular skin conditions, such as herpes simplex.

The bullous form of impetigo may present with bullae that begin as small (1 to 2 mm) superficial vesicles with fragile roofs that rupture easily. The parent or patient may deny seeing bullae because the vesicles rupture so quickly that they are not recalled by the patient or the parent. The serous fluid inside the ruptured vesicles develops into a thin, transparent, and varnish-like crust. Hence, the vesicles become pustular in a matter of hours. The bullous type of impetigo is usually caused by *Staphylococcus* bacteria; it commonly occurs on the face, elbows, and knees.

In the nonbullous or vesiculopustular form, the lesions are characterized by thick, adherent, dark yellow–colored crusts that have erythematous margins. This type of impetigo occurs more often in older children. Both bullous and nonbullous types produce symptoms such as burning and pruritus. In addition, regional lymphadenopathy is seen. When the face is involved, the cervical lymph nodes (and sometimes the preauricular and submandibular nodes) are enlarged; when the lesions are present on the upper extremities, the axillary nodes become enlarged.

A variant of bullous impetigo that is caused exclusively by *S. aureus* is known as "Staphylococcal scalded skin syndrome." Exotoxins produced by the bacteria lead to bullous, sheetlike necrosis of the epidermis and cause the epithelial layer of the skin to peel off in large pieces. The "scalded skin" thus mimics a thermal burn. This serious infection is more commonly seen in children and usually begins in the intertriginous areas.

The less common, ulcerative form of impetigo known as ecthyma occurs predominantly on the feet, ankles, legs, and thighs. It affects mostly people who are homeless, sewage and garbage workers, people who have alcohol use disorder, and older individuals without access to proper care. It is a deeper form of impetigo and often results from an untreated or poorly treated superficial abrasion or from infected insect bites. Itching is common, and autoinoculation from scratching may cause satellite lesions that are annular in form. Ecthyma presents as pruritic, tender, red vesicles or pustules that are surrounded by erythema that eventually ulcerate. Because this process is superficial, healing often occurs spontaneously in the center of the lesion and results in scarring. The inflammatory process involves both dermal and epidermal layers. See Table 14.1 for the clinical presentation of the different types of impetigo.

During physical assessment, a thorough examination of the skin should search for erosions that are covered with moist, honey-colored crusts. The physical assessment should include an examination of the head, ears, pharynx, and neck, and the regional lymph nodes should be noted for lymphadenopathy. Firm and dry or dark crusts with surrounding erythema are characteristic of ecthyma.

DIAGNOSTIC REASONING

Diagnostic Tests

Diagnosis may be based solely on medical history and clinical presentation. Initial testing for impetigo may also

TABLE 14.1 Types of Impetigo

Types of Impetigo	Causative Agent	Clinical Presentation
Bullous impetigo	*Staphylococcus aureus*	Lesion starts as a 1- to 2-mm superficial vesicle with a fragile roof that is easily ruptured; ruptured vesicle forms a thin, transparent, varnish-like or classic "honey-colored" crust. Becomes pustular in a matter of hours; pruritic; burning sensation
Staphylococcal scalded skin syndrome (SSSS)	*S. aureus*	Variant of bullous impetigo: epidermal necrosis caused by bacterial exotoxins, resulting in the epithelial layer's peeling off in large, sheetlike pieces; mimics scalded skin thermal burn
Nonbullous impetigo	*Streptococcus, S. aureus*	Lesions are thick, adherent; recurrent with dark yellow–colored crusts and erythematous margins; pruritic; burning sensation
Ecthyma	*S. aureus, Streptococcus;* other infective organisms may be observed	Pruritic, tender, red vesicles or pustules surrounded by erythema; rash eventually ulcerates. Deeper impetigo resulting from inadequately treated or neglected skin infections; also seen in infected insect bites or abrasions

include a bacterial culture and sensitivity analysis from the moist crusts of the lesions. The results of the culture and sensitivity testing help to assess for antibiotic resistance of the responsible pathogen. Resistance patterns can vary from community to community. In addition, a Gram stain can be obtained; if the lesions are caused by impetigo, the stain will reveal gram-positive cocci. If herpes simplex is suspected, a viral culture can be obtained. If the patient is febrile or has systemic symptoms, a complete blood count (CBC) with differential should be obtained.

Differential Diagnosis

The typical honey-colored crust is almost pathognomonic of bullous impetigo, so much so that cultures are not necessary before treatment is started. Bullous impetigo should be differentiated from other vesicular and pustular skin conditions. Many skin diseases with weepy lesions may resemble impetigo, such as varicella-zoster virus, herpes simplex virus, eczematous dermatitis (atopic dermatitis), bullous pemphigus/pemphigoid, and contact dermatitis. The history, distribution, and morphological features of the primary skin lesions provide the best information to help in the differential diagnosis of other skin conditions.

Varicella-zoster infection (herpes zoster or chickenpox) produces a rash with widely distributed papules and vesicular lesions. The onset of the rash typically starts on the head and neck area. The lesions of herpes zoster follow a dermatomal pattern that consists of a group of uniform 2- to 3-mm vesicles on an erythematous base.

A localized group of vesicles located on a single anatomical site, with clear to cloudy fluid on an erythematous and edematous base, helps characterize herpes simplex lesions. These lesions are usually preceded by a prodrome of burning and tingling before the lesions erupt.

Bullous pemphigus and bullous pemphigoid are autoimmune diseases affecting the skin and causing bullae that can become eroded and infected. They should be included in the differential diagnosis for any vesicular or bullous skin disease.

Acute nummular eczema manifests as pruritic, coin-shaped plaques or patches on an erythematous base; the lesions may become exudative and crusted. Candidiasis lesions are bright red, and this rash forms satellite lesions along with macerated moist patches. Candidiasis is often accompanied by pruritus and burning in the macerated areas.

MANAGEMENT

There are two principles of therapy in the management of impetigo: (1) nonpharmacological measures are used to enhance resolution and reduce bacterial colonization on the skin surface, and (2) antibiotics are prescribed to help eradicate the responsible pathogen and prevent recolonization and complications. Even without treatment, impetigo usually heals within 2 to 3 weeks. With appropriate treatment, lesions usually resolve after 7 to 10 days. The key to treating and preventing impetigo is practicing good personal hygiene and maintaining a clean environment.

Nonpharmacological Management

Nonpharmacological management of impetigo involves the use of solutions or substances to débride the impetiginized lesions and expose the skin surfaces where the bacteria are present. Exudative impetigo lesions may benefit from drying compresses to remove thick crusts and desiccate (dry out) the lesions. Normal saline, plain tap water, or Burow's solution may be applied for 10 to 20 minutes, three to four times daily. Although the dehydrating effect of the compresses may help improve the appearance of the skin lesions, disinfectant solutions are not particularly effective in treating the underlying condition.

Pharmacological Management

Pharmacological treatment of impetigo includes the use of both topical and oral antibiotics. Mild cases of bullous and nonbullous impetigo can be treated effectively with a topical antibiotic, combined with cleansing and débridement. First-line topical treatments for impetigo include mupirocin 2% cream or ointment (Bactroban), as well as retapamulin 1% ointment (Altabax). Mupirocin is applied three times daily for 5 days in children 12 years and older. This is equivalent in efficacy to oral cephalexin. However, *S. aureus* and MRSA have developed resistance to mupirocin. Washing with chlorhexidine (Hibiclens) is a valuable adjunct because of its bactericidal properties. The patient should be instructed to wash the affected skin area with the bactericidal soap two to three times a day before the mupirocin cream is applied. Dilute bleach baths (i.e., one-fourth cup of bleach added to a half-filled bathtub) may also be considered. In recurrent cases of impetigo, mupirocin (Bactroban Nasal) may be utilized to treat nasal carriage.

Retapamulin (Altabax) is effective against mupirocin-resistant strains. Retapamulin is applied twice daily for 5 days in children 9 months of age and older. However, it is not intended for mucosal use and is not U.S. (FDA) approved for the treatment of MRSA or the prevention of nasal carriage. Ozenoxacin 1% cream, a quinolone antibiotic, was approved by the FDA in 2017 for the treatment of impetigo in children 2 months of age and older. Another topical therapy that is in clinical trials for the treatment of impetigo is minocycline foam.

Systemic antibiotics are indicated for all cases of bullous impetigo. They should also be prescribed for nonbullous impetigo when there are systemic symptoms such as fever, toxicity, or lymphadenopathy; when a large area of the skin is involved; and when there are deep lesions and oral mucosal lesions. They may also be considered within the context of athletic team, child-care, or family-based clusters. Antibiotic therapy should cover *S. aureus* and group A beta-hemolytic *Streptococcus*. The prevalence of MRSA and macrolide-resistant *Streptococcus* is a recent challenge. MRSA has been cited as the causative agent for nearly 80% of all community-acquired Staphylococcal skin and soft tissue infections.

Penicillin therapy is recommended for Streptococcal impetigo. Antibiotics effective against *S. aureus* such as amoxicillin-clavulanate, dicloxacillin, or cephalexin are given for 7 days. If MRSA is suspected, the choice of antibiotic should be doxycycline, clindamycin, or trimethoprim-sulfamethoxazole (TMP-SMX). TMP-SMX (Bactrim) should only be prescribed if group A *Streptococcus* is not the causative organism. Newer antibiotics prescribed for MRSA include dalbavancin (Dalvance) and tedizolid phosphate (Sivextro); however, these are not indicated for use in children.

Empirical treatment depends on the prevalence and sensitivities of MRSA in the patient's geographical area. Patients with penicillin hypersensitivity should take doxycycline or clindamycin. Because oral antibiotics have far more gastrointestinal and systemic side effects than topical therapy, topical treatment is preferred for mild to moderate infections.

In addition to topical and systemic antibiotic therapy, antihistamines may be prescribed if pruritus is problematic to prevent skin trauma from excoriation and decrease the potential for spreading the infection. Second-generation antihistamines (e.g., fexofenadine [Allegra], loratadine [Claritin], and cetirizine [Zyrtec]) are preferable, given once daily at bedtime to minimize associated sedation.

FOLLOW-UP AND REFERRAL

Follow-up for the patient with an uncomplicated case of impetigo should occur in 10 to 14 days after initiation of therapy. Patients who have a fever should be followed closely; consultation with or referral to a physician is recommended. Development of acute glomerulonephritis (acute nephritic syndrome), typically as a result of Streptococcal infection, requires referral to a nephrologist; symptoms include the abrupt onset of proteinuria, hypertension, edema, azotemia, and red blood cells in the urine.

The majority of cases of both types of impetigo (bullous and nonbullous) resolve uneventfully after 10 days of treatment. Patients with recurrent impetigo should be tested for nasal carriage of *S. aureus* with a culture of the anterior nares. If the culture is positive, treatment of the nares with topical mupirocin (Bactroban Nasal) is effective. Repeat culture should be done to confirm the patient's status. Chronic carriers may be treated with nasal mupirocin three times a day for 5 days of each month, and an antimicrobial skin cleanser (e.g., Hibiclens) or bleach baths may be indicated for body decolonization. In the event of treatment failure, consultation with an infectious disease specialist should be considered. Bullous impetigo typically resolves even without antibiotic treatment. Nonbullous impetigo generally has a good prognosis, although poststreptococcal glomerulonephritis is a possible complication of this infection.

Patient Education: Impetigo

The clinician plays a pivotal role in the treatment and prevention of impetigo, a highly contagious skin infection, through patient education and counseling. Good hand washing and personal hygiene are strongly recommended to reduce the likelihood of bacterial spread. The fingernails should be kept short so that there is less likelihood of spread to other areas of the body through self-inoculation.

Children and family members should be educated about the contagious nature of impetigo. Frequent hand washing is imperative. Affected individuals should be told to refrain from participation in any contact sport or activity that might spread the infection. Children should not attend day care or school for

24 hours after antibiotic therapy is started. Family members should not share clothing or personal hygiene items such as towels, robes, razors, or shavers. Towels and bed linens should be washed with soap and hot water and dried on high heat.

The patient should be instructed to gently clean the crusts from the lesions with antibacterial soap before applying mupirocin 2% cream or retapamulin. Nighttime application is also advised. Cover dressings should be used to prevent contact with the exudate; they should be discarded carefully to prevent the spread of infection. If the patient is taking oral antibiotics, the side effects and potential adverse reactions of the drug should be explained, as well as the importance of completing the course of antibiotic therapy to prevent the complication of poststreptococcal glomerulonephritis. Patients should be informed that good personal hygiene and cleanliness, along with prompt attention to skin trauma, may help prevent future breakouts of impetigo. Patients should not visit hospitals or nursing homes until the infection has resolved. If MRSA is involved, patients should stay at home and not handle food until they have been on antibiotics for 24 hours.

FOLLICULITIS

Folliculitis is a superficial-to-deep skin infection of the hair follicles. Lesions can range from minute white-topped pustules in newborns to large, tender, yellow-white pustules in adults. Bacteria infect the hair follicle at a superficial level, leading to erythematous papules and pustules. Although the main pathogens are gram-positive bacteria, occasional cases are caused by a fungus or by gram-negative bacilli. Folliculitis represents the start of a continuum of skin infections. Deeper infections (as complications of folliculitis) can include a furuncle (boil) or carbuncle (multiple boils), which are covered in depth later in this chapter.

EPIDEMIOLOGY AND CAUSES

Folliculitis is a common skin infection that occurs in all age groups and races and affects both males and females. It is often caused by coagulase-negative *Staphylococcus*. Predisposing factors include diabetes mellitus, obesity, a chronic carrier state of *Staphylococcus* (present in the nares, axillae, or perineum), inadequate hygiene, hyperimmunoglobulin E (Job's syndrome, a primary immunodeficiency disorder), exposure to chemicals and solvents (cutting oils), and chronic skin friction. However, folliculitis may have other etiologies as well. Gram-positive resident flora of the nasal mucosa and adjacent facial skin become suppressed by long-term oral antibiotic therapy and are replaced by gram-negative rods, namely *Klebsiella* and *Escherichia coli*. Thus, gram-negative folliculitis may develop in patients who are on long-term tetracycline therapy for acne or rosacea, as well as in older men with seborrhea. Patients whose sebaceous follicles of the perioral and perinasal areas have become colonized by gram-negative bacteria can become infected due to trauma (e.g., from shaving), resulting in a suppurative process within the hair follicle. This type of folliculitis is usually seen on the upper lip in men. In addition, antibiotic use also increases the risk of *Candida* folliculitis, due to clearance of the normal bacterial skin flora. Exposure to wet environments, such as hot tubs or inadequately chlorinated pools, which contributes to *Pseudomonas aeruginosa* infection, also predisposes to folliculitis. In addition, chronic corticosteroid use that compromises T-cell immunity contributes to folliculitis by *Candida albicans*.

Folliculitis may occur anywhere on the skin as a result of trauma or damage to the hair follicle from chronic irritation due to friction from clothing or blockage of the hair follicle. Occlusion of the skin with tight-fitting clothing made of synthetic fabric promotes infection, and symptoms may occur abruptly within 1 to 3 days of wearing such garments. Occlusive therapy (plastic wrap) used for other diseases such as severe psoriasis or eczema allows for significant bacterial multiplication in a moist environment, which can also lead to folliculitis. Spread of bacterial infection to the surrounding skin may develop from exudative or transudative discharge from wounds, abscesses, or any type of draining lesion.

Eosinophilic folliculitis (EF) is a form of noninfectious sterile folliculitis. On histological examination, the hair follicle in EF is invaded by eosinophils and lymphocytes. Three types of EF have been identified. Eosinophilic pustular folliculitis (Ofuji disease) generally occurs in men of Japanese descent in their 30s. Another form of pustular EF is associated with immunosuppression and presents in patients with HIV/AIDS with low CD4 T-cell counts. A third type of EF, eosinophilic pustular folliculitis in infants (EPFI), occurs most commonly in males.

Acne is another noninfectious form of folliculitis. Currently, acne is theorized to be a primary inflammatory condition. Acne is discussed in depth in Chapter 16.

PATHOPHYSIOLOGY

Infection of the hair follicle with *Staphylococcus* or *Streptococcus* is marked by suppuration and liquefaction necrosis of the follicular base, thus termed a *pyodermal* infection. It is usually localized and results in abscess formation. Liquefaction necrosis develops when lytic enzymes released by polymorphonuclear leukocytes (PMNs) digest bacteria and cellular material. Thus, a competent immune system is required for such a response, as large numbers of PMNs are found in the central area of the abscess, along with necrotic debris. Because this inflammatory response is localized, however, folliculitis rarely causes systemic manifestations in the immunocompetent individual. Interestingly, HIV-positive patients do not display this neutrophilic response because they typically experience an eosinophilic perifollicular pustular folliculitis.

CLINICAL PRESENTATION

Subjective

Generally, the patient will present with a "bumpy rash," which can appear on any area of the body. The rash can be located on the hair follicles of the face, forehead, back of the earlobes, neck, shoulders, buttocks, torso, or extremities. Usually, the rash is not accompanied by itching. Often there is no history of previous skin eruptions or of pertinent medical history such as diabetes. The patient is usually concerned about the cosmetic effect of the lesions. The patient may report a history of hot tub use or of borrowing a shaver or razor from a friend. The clinician should inquire about the onset, duration, and location(s) of the rash, its appearance, and whether purulent drainage was present. The patient should also be asked about any associated systemic symptoms of fever and chills.

Objective

The primary lesions in folliculitis are small pustules surrounded by 1 to 2 mm of erythema located over the pilosebaceous orifice or the ostium of the hair follicle. There is no involvement of the surrounding skin. The eyelids, face, scalp, and extremities are the most typical sites. A hair in the center of the pustule sometimes perforates the lesion. This presentation is a hallmark for diagnosis. The pustules resolve into red macules, which fade to leave postinflammatory hyperpigmented scars in susceptible people. Folliculitis is usually asymptomatic, but it can be very pruritic and is sometimes accompanied by burning. During the physical examination, checking vital signs, including temperature, is important to help rule out systemic involvement. The practitioner should inspect the lesion for signs of inflammation and suppuration (erythema, swelling, pustules) and palpate the surface of the pustule for fluctuance. It is also important to palpate the adjacent lymph nodes for evidence of spreading lymphadenitis

Folliculitis is divided into two main types—superficial folliculitis and deep folliculitis. Follicular impetigo (Bockhart's impetigo) is a superficial form of folliculitis that presents as small, dome-shaped pustules that occur over the opening of the hair follicle. It is more common on the scalps of children. When follicular impetigo becomes chronic, it may lead to follicular destruction and consequent permanent patchy alopecia.

The distinctive forms of deep folliculitis include barber's itch (sycosis barbae), pseudofolliculitis barbae, and *Pseudomonas* folliculitis. In addition, newer diagnoses have been established, based on the histological characteristics of the skin eruption, such as EF (e.g., HIV-EF) and nosocomial folliculitis.

Barber's itch is a chronic, recurrent staphylococcal infection of the hair follicles on the bearded area of the face in men (usually the upper lip). It is aggravated by shaving and is most commonly seen in men with curly hair. It is usually propagated by the autoinoculation of bacteria caused by shaving. Tinea barbae is similar to barber's itch, but the infection is caused by a fungus. Pseudofolliculitis barbae, another differential diagnosis for sycosis barbae, is caused by hair in the beard area and posterior scalp and neck that curls toward the skin, causing an inflammatory reaction that can mimic folliculitis. This can become a chronic problem, and the hair follicles involved can become infected with any variety of bacteria.

Pseudomonas folliculitis presents as follicular erythematous papules, pustules, or vesicles over the back, buttocks, and upper arms. Associated features include pruritus, malaise, low-grade fever, sore throat and eyes, and axillary lymphadenopathy. This type of folliculitis usually resolves spontaneously within 10 days.

Folliculitis decalvans is a rare disease that tends to occur in individuals who have coarse, bristly hair. The predisposing factors of this disease are still unknown. The infection begins as a localized area of follicular pustules or papules. Exudation or suppuration soon follows; as the crust accumulates, the hairs are shed. New follicles become involved at the periphery, while at the center, the process eventually subsides, with scarring and permanent hair loss.

Hot tub folliculitis is caused by *Pseudomonas aeruginosa*, which withstands temperatures of up to 107°F (41.6°C) and chlorine levels of up to 3 mg/L. The lesions of this variant of folliculitis are found on the trunk and lower extremities of patients who have a recent history of hot tub use. Superhydration of the stratum corneum softens this protective layer and allows the bacteria to cause infection.

There are documented cases of superficial actinic folliculitis characterized by recurrent skin eruptions occurring within 6 to 24 hours after sun exposure. Histologically, there is perivascular lymphocytic infiltration and intrafollicular accumulation of neutrophils in the upper infundibulum of the follicle; these findings indicate the presence of an inflammatory response and suppurative process.

DIAGNOSTIC REASONING

Diagnostic Tests

A Gram stain and culture of purulent discharge are obtained by rupturing a pustule and taking samples of the exudate. The culture is useful to distinguish Staphylococcal infections from other bacterial or fungal infections, as well as from epidermal and pilar cysts that are sterile lesions. The Gram stain is usually positive for clusters of gram-positive cocci (*S. aureus*) along with large numbers of PMNs. With deeper forms of folliculitis, the presence of systemic symptoms or positive blood cultures requires referral to a physician for hospitalization and IV antibiotics.

If fungal infection is suspected, a fungal culture or potassium hydroxide (KOH) microscopic examination is helpful; if results are positive, treatment should change to an antifungal agent.

Differential Diagnosis

Superficial folliculitis is differentiated from tinea barbae by performing a KOH examination (see Advanced Assessment 13.1) of the affected hair or by a fungal culture. Acne vulgaris and bullous impetigo may occasionally mimic folliculitis, but the patient's age (i.e., nonadolescent) and the absence of comedones (blackheads or whiteheads) suggest a diagnosis of folliculitis. The lesions of bullous impetigo are usually larger and rupture easily, and the exudate is serous, not purulent. Approximately 50% of people with HIV with scabies have coexistent *S. aureus* folliculitis.

Occasionally, follicular lesions extend more deeply, forming abscesses. Rarely, follicles covering an area several centimeters across become infected, forming large violaceous plaques. The plaque may be studded with pustules and have deep sinus tracts connecting infected follicles. Rarely, an abscess of the muscles (pyomyositis) may occur due to extension of the infectious process.

MANAGEMENT

Patients rarely consult a health-care provider for minor cases of folliculitis, except for infections that become recurrent and persistent. The goal of treatment of superficial and deep folliculitis is to make the skin inhospitable to pathogens. This includes both nonpharmacological and pharmacological approaches (see Drugs Commonly Prescribed 14.1).

Gentle cleansing by washing the skin twice a day with over-the-counter (OTC) antibacterial liquid or bar soap (e.g., Hibiclens, Safeguard, Dial) is as important as prescription antibacterial medicines. Large pustular lesions with necrotic areas should first be cleansed with a weak soap solution, followed by soaking or the application of compresses to affected skin, using saline or Burow's solution (aluminum subacetate) twice daily. When the skin is softened, the clinician can gently open large pustules and trim away necrotic tissue.

Clearance of nasal colonization of *S. aureus* by mupirocin treatment twice daily for 5 days and daily chlorhexidine baths has been shown to significantly reduce the incidence of recurrent folliculitis. Bleach baths (i.e., one-fourth cup of chlorine bleach added to a half-filled tub of water) or

Drugs Commonly Prescribed 14.1: Folliculitis

DRUG	TYPE	ADVERSE REACTIONS AND PRESCRIBING CONSIDERATIONS
Topical Antibiotics		
Mupirocin (Bactroban)	2% ointment or cream Three times a day for 5 to 14 days	Consider for secondarily infected skin lesions
Retapamulin (Altabax)	Twice daily for 5 days	Lotion less irritating May cause diarrhea Avoid in patients with colitis
Clindamycin	1% solution, lotion, gel, pledget—twice daily until lesions clear	
Erythromycin	2% solution, lotion or gel, twice daily until lesions clear	
Other		
Ketoconazole (Nizoral) Fluconazole (Diflucan) Itraconazole (Sporanox)	Topical—cream, shampoo, foam, gel Oral tablets	Prescribed for fungal forms of folliculitis Topical formulations are safer than systemic formulations. Fluconazole has fewer side effects and drug interactions than itraconazole. Multiple FDA precautions with azoles; use only when other antifungal treatment is ineffective; monitor hepatic function before and during therapy; check for numerous drug interaction warnings.

bleach compresses (i.e., soaked in 1 teaspoon of chlorine bleach per gallon of water) may also be used to reduce skin colonization. Frequent washing of towels, bed linens, and clothing may also be helpful in reducing recurrences. Systemic anti-Staphylococcal antibiotics may be ordered if the infection is resistant to local treatment or if the scalp is involved. Usually, however, systemic antibiotics are not helpful or advantageous over topical treatments.

For EPFI, the treatment is not with antibiotics. EPFI is treated with anti-inflammatory agents. First-line therapy is systemic indomethacin, in addition to topical corticosteroids.

FOLLOW-UP AND REFERRAL

A patient who does not respond to therapy should be evaluated for possible diabetes mellitus or for chronic carriage of S. aureus (in the nares, axillae, or perineum). Cultures of the anterior nares, axillae, and perineum are recommended. Topical mupirocin 2% (Bactroban) should be applied twice daily for 5 to 7 days to the sites that yielded a positive culture. Because most strains of MRSA are resistant to topical mupirocin, in cases of MRSA colonization, retapamulin (Altabax) should be applied twice daily for 2 weeks.

More severe forms of folliculitis and rare skin eruptions such as HIV-EF should be referred to a physician. Systemic IV antibiotics may be necessary. Referral for patients with recurrent or persistent infections that do not respond to a standard treatment regimen is recommended.

> ### Patient Education: Folliculitis
>
> The clinician should emphasize to the patient that good hygiene is essential in treating this condition. Effective hand-washing technique is the best approach in preventing the spread of folliculitis. Patients who are prone to folliculitis should be advised to use an antibacterial soap to wash affected areas twice a day before applying topical agents. Patients should also be informed that any source of friction can predispose to a recurrence of folliculitis.
>
> Men who are prone to recurrent sycosis barbae should be advised to avoid shaving during treatment to allow complete healing. A preventive approach is the best treatment for this condition. When shaving is resumed, an electric shaver may cause fewer breaks in the skin than a razor. Patients should be cautioned to avoid borrowing or using old razor blades when shaving infected areas.

FURUNCLES AND CARBUNCLES

A *furuncle* (boil) is a deep bacterial infection of a hair follicle with abscess formation. Furuncles are caused almost exclusively by gram-positive S. aureus. Furuncles are extremely tender to the touch and bright red in color. The most common locations for furuncles are the scalp, neck, axillae, buttocks, groin, and thighs. Furuncles frequently become fluctuant. With the application of warm compresses, most furuncles drain pus and resolve spontaneously.

A *carbuncle* is a large, multiloculated abscess comprising multiple furuncles in a contiguous area. Carbuncles, which are less common than furuncles, appear as large, red, painful lumps on the skin, with multiple follicular openings. Some carbuncles can be quite large—up to 10 cm in size. Eventually, a carbuncle spontaneously drains pus.

EPIDEMIOLOGY AND CAUSES

Furuncles and carbuncles are usually caused by S. aureus and rarely by other pathogens. In some patients, especially those who are immunocompromised, infection can be due to MRSA. Conditions predisposing patients to the formation of furuncles and carbuncles include diabetes mellitus, inadequate hygiene, incarceration, obesity, and immune system defects. Chronic Staphylococcal carriage in the anterior nares, axilla, or perineum also increases the risk of infection and should be explored in cases of recurrent infections. Favorable environmental conditions that predispose the individual to furuncle and carbuncle formation include areas of moisture, friction, or occluded skin. Any area of skin that is subject to friction, such as the axillae, buttocks, groin, or thighs, is at increased risk of infection.

PATHOPHYSIOLOGY

Both furuncles and carbuncles evolve from superficially infected hair follicles (folliculitis), mediated primarily by S. aureus. Thus, all factors that contribute to folliculitis also predispose to furunculosis and carbuncle formation. As this superficial infection extends along the hair shaft, a small, painful inflammatory nodule is formed at the follicular base that is termed a *furuncle*. Eventually, a series of abscesses form along the hair shaft involving dermal and subcutaneous layers, ultimately coalescing into a fluctuant, subcutaneous mass that develops a soft, pointed necrotic center. When the furuncle ruptures, it results in the extrusion of pus and a necrotic plug at the entrance to the follicle. A small opening or cavitation remains that eventually heals with scarring. Thus, the affected hair follicle is destroyed and does not regenerate, resulting in destruction of the hair itself.

Carbuncles ("boils") undergo a similar process, except on a larger scale. Carbuncles are comprised of several furuncles that form into a large, multiloculated abscess with multiple follicular openings that eventually drain pus. Carbuncles are significantly larger than furuncles, typically involving deeper skin layers. Both carbuncles and furuncles are considered boils. They are more likely to occur on thicker skin, in areas such as the nape of the neck and upper back. A systemic response including fever resulting from the production of pyogenic cytokines is more common with carbuncle formation than furunculosis.

Certain risk factors are associated with furunculosis and carbuncle formation. Obesity results in thick skinfolds that are closely approximated. This creates a moist environment in which bacteria are prone to reproduce. Impaired immune function from chronic corticosteroid use, underlying systemic disease such as HIV or diabetes mellitus, or impaired neutrophil function also predispose to this condition. The presence of a bacterial virulence factor known as Panton-Valentine leukocidin in certain strains of *S. aureus* has been associated with particularly aggressive skin infections.

CLINICAL PRESENTATION

Subjective

The typical patient will complain of a hot, tender, bright-red bump or "boil" of several days' duration that becomes progressively larger. Some furuncles will "come to a head" or become fluctuant and will drain spontaneously on their own. Some patients will report a history of manipulation of the furuncle or carbuncle, either by squeezing it or by puncturing it with a needle. Some patients may report a past history of boils and other skin infections.

Objective

Both furuncles and carbuncles are extremely tender to the touch and are bright-red in color. A furuncle initially appears as a small (0.5 to 1.0 cm), red, indurated nodule. As the nodule grows in size, it starts to develop a yellow-colored central plug and begins to appear conical, with a central "nipple" covered by thinning skin. The pus, which is yellow to green in color, gives the "nipple" its characteristic color. Most furuncles eventually spontaneously rupture and drain pus, which hastens their resolution. As the necrotic material and pus are discharged, a small cavitation is left that heals with minimal scarring. Carbuncles initially appear as multiple furuncles that develop into a large, erythematous lump that eventually starts to drain pus from multiple follicular openings. Patients with darker skin can have permanent hyperpigmentation changes as a result of severe inflammation.

DIAGNOSTIC REASONING

Diagnostic Tests

Although most cases of furuncles and carbuncles are caused by *S. aureus,* a Gram stain and culture of the fluctuant lesion are still recommended, because MRSA strains may be identified. A CBC with differential is not necessary unless the patient has a severe case with an underlying immunocompromising disease, such as diabetes mellitus, or shows systemic symptoms such as fever.

No subsequent testing is necessary unless a patient is a Staphylococcal carrier. The nares and anogenital region should be recultured after treatment with topical mupirocin (Bactroban) is finished. In resistant cases where no response is seen after 1 week of therapy, a repeat culture should be done.

Differential Diagnosis

Some skin conditions to consider in the differential diagnosis of furuncles include an epidermal inclusion cyst that is acutely inflamed. Epidermal inclusion cysts are usually located in areas of the body where there is thicker skin and a large number of sebaceous glands, such as on the back and upper shoulders. The patient with an epidermal inclusion cyst will report a history of the cyst on the same site for months to years. In contrast, furuncles are an acute process, taking only several days to form. Another characteristic of an epidermal inclusion cyst is a cheesy white discharge with a strong odor when it is expressed. A furuncle or carbuncle will have a purulent yellow to green-colored discharge when it ruptures.

Another differential diagnosis for a furuncle is a deep fungal infection of the soft tissue called *sporotrichosis*. It is more common in gardeners and other agricultural workers and is usually seen on the hands or arms. It is caused by injury from a thorn or wood splinter that has been contaminated with the common soil fungus *Sporothrix schenckii*. Because it is usually asymptomatic, patients tend to ignore it.

If the furuncle or carbuncle is located in the axilla, a differential diagnosis to consider is hidradenitis suppurativa. The lesions of hidradenitis suppurativa are also extremely tender and inflamed. Patients with this condition report a chronic history of recurrent infection in the axilla, groin, or anal region. It is a chronic disease of the apocrine glands of the axilla and groin and is associated with severe hypertrophic scarring and sinus tracts, which are not seen in furuncles or carbuncles. The classic finding in hidradenitis suppurativa that differentiates it from a furuncle or carbuncle consists of numerous hypertrophic scars and sinus tracts that are found on the affected skin.

MANAGEMENT

Carbuncles usually must drain before healing will take place, and this typically occurs spontaneously within 2 weeks. The application of warm compresses will promote the localization, spontaneous rupture, and drainage of a furuncle. If a furuncle has not come to a head by the time the patient is seen, the patient should be instructed to apply warm compresses two to three times per day until it becomes fluctuant. Randomized controlled trials have failed to consistently show the benefit of such treatment, although some clinicians continue to treat with topical antibiotics with sufficient gram-positive coverage (e.g., mupirocin [Bactroban] or retapamulin [Altabax]), which may be applied twice per day until resolution.

Treatment with systemic antibiotics is not necessary in a healthy patient if no surrounding cellulitis is present. Antibiotic therapy should be considered for immunocompromised patients, the very young or older adults, those with systemic symptoms such as fever, and patients with more than one lesion; it also should be considered when incision and drainage do not lead to improvement. For furuncles or carbuncles in an immunocompromised patient (or one who is at risk for bacteremia because of a preexisting condition), systemic antibiotics are always mandatory, and physician referral is recommended. In addition, incision and drainage will hasten the resolution of infection. Preexisting immunocompromising conditions such as diabetes mellitus or chronic corticosteroid use predispose a patient to more complications. These patients should be monitored closely or referred to a physician. An occasional patient with furuncles or carbuncles will have bacteremia as a complication, with possible hematogenous spread to the heart valves (endocarditis), kidneys (perinephric abscess), joints, spine, or long bones (osteomyelitis).

A furuncle (especially if it is located on the upper lip or the central area of the face) or a carbuncle located on the neck, face, or scalp should be treated with physician consultation or referred to a physician for management. A furuncle located on the central face can spread via venous drainage to the cavernous sinus and result in cavernous sinus thrombosis or meningitis.

Fluctuant furuncles are ideally treated with incision and drainage, followed by covering the lesion with a sterile dry dressing. After a furuncle has been incised, the patient should be instructed to use warm compresses twice daily to encourage the drainage of pus.

Systemic antibiotics and physician referral are always indicated for the treatment of carbuncles. Purulent carbuncles require incision and drainage to aid in recovery. Empiric treatment for moderate infections or for methicillin-sensitive *S. aureus* (MSSA) includes dicloxacillin, cephalexin, TMP-SMX, or doxycycline. Severe MSSA infections may be treated with nafcillin, cefazolin, or clindamycin. Moderate infections of community-acquired MRSA are susceptible to TMP-SMX. However, severe infections with MRSA or Panton-Valentine leukocidin–expressing strains of *Staphylococcus* may require inpatient IV antibiotic therapy; thus, physician consultation or emergency department referral is recommended.

If a patient has a history of frequent infections, a search for Staphylococcal carriage is recommended. Cultures should be taken from the patient's nares, perineum, and anogenital region. If a patient is found to be a *S. aureus* carrier, a daily shower with chlorhexidine wash is recommended. Mupirocin ointment (Bactroban) or retapamulin (Altabax) should be applied twice a day to the anatomical sites from which *S. aureus* was cultured (nares, body folds, perineum, anogenital region) for 5 days; however, retapamulin is not FDA approved for mucosal treatment. A repeat culture should be done to document clearance of the bacteria. This program will eliminate the Staphylococcal carrier state and reduce the incidence of recurrence. There is some evidence that vitamin C supplementation (1 g/day for 4 to 6 weeks) may also help prevent recurrent skin infection in people with impaired neutrophil function.

FOLLOW-UP AND REFERRAL

The patient should be seen for initial follow-up within a few days to 1 week to monitor response to therapy, compliance with treatment, and any adverse reactions. A subsequent visit can be scheduled in 7 to 10 days to monitor for continuing progress and resolution of the lesions. For carbuncles or multiple furuncles in immunocompromised patients (or patients at risk for bacteremia because of preexisting disease), a physician referral is recommended.

In addition, if a patient has systemic signs such as fever or appears toxic, physician consultation or referral is recommended. These patients frequently need multiple laboratory tests, including blood cultures, which can be done in a hospital setting, in addition to treatment with parenteral antibiotics.

> **Patient Education: Furuncles and Carbuncles**
>
> The patient should be cautioned not to pop, squeeze, or manipulate furuncles in any way, especially those that are located on the mid to upper lip or near the border of the nasolabial folds, given the risk of cavernous sinus thrombosis, which may be fatal.

CELLULITIS

Cellulitis is a bacterial infection of the skin involving both the dermis and subcutaneous tissue, which in certain cases may result in death. Most cases of cellulitis are caused by group A beta-hemolytic *Streptococcus* or by *S. aureus,* both being gram-positive bacteria. Less common bacteria that can cause cellulitis include *Haemophilus influenzae* (more common in children), *Eikenella corrodens* (human bites), *Pasteurella multocida* (cat bites), *Capnocytophaga canimorsus* (dog bites), and *Vibrio* species (seawater-exposed injuries).

The typical lesion of cellulitis is a wide, diffuse area of erythematous skin that is warm and tender to palpation. Infection is occasionally accompanied by severe edema. Systemic symptoms such as fever, chills, and malaise may accompany some cases as well. A cellulitic infection can occasionally result in the loss of a limb.

Cellulitis may become a life-threatening event that is heralded by systemic inflammatory response syndrome: fever, tachypnea, tachycardia, white blood cell count greater than 12,000 cells/mcL, and hypotension. Toxic shock syndrome (TSS) and multiple organ failure resulting from both Streptococcal and Staphylococcal infections have been reported. The clinician must learn to differentiate between a severe case of cellulitis that is potentially life-threatening and an uncomplicated case that can be treated on an outpatient basis. Special types of cellulitis that have potentially serious consequences discussed in this chapter include erysipelas, necrotizing fasciitis, and periorbital cellulitis (Box 14.1). Severe cases of cellulitis, such as necrotizing fasciitis, must be treated with surgical débridement in addition to parenteral antibiotics to stop the spread of rapid tissue destruction; such patients require hospitalization. Periorbital cellulitis, an emergent condition, should also be treated aggressively with parenteral antibiotics and hospitalization to prevent permanent vision loss and extension of infection into deep cranial structures.

EPIDEMIOLOGY AND CAUSES

There is usually an obvious portal of entry into the skin or mucous membranes, such as an insect bite or a wound, although in some cases there is no obvious point of entry (this is more common with recurrent cellulitis). Cellulitis may occur at any age, but some organisms are more common in certain age groups. *Haemophilus influenzae* type B infections are more common in children. In adults

Box 14.1	Types of Cellulitis
Erysipelas	Erysipelas is a Streptococcal infection of the superficial layers of skin that does not involve the subcutaneous layers, unlike more typical cellulitis. An older name for erysipelas is "St. Anthony's fire." Despite the superficial nature of this infection, erysipelas should not be taken lightly, because it can be fatal if it is not treated promptly—especially in the very young and older adults. Before the advent of antibiotics, this infection was associated with a high mortality rate. Most cases of erysipelas are caused by group A beta-hemolytic *Streptococcus pyogenes* and sometimes develop after an episode of Streptococcal pharyngitis (strep throat). The most common sites of involvement are the face (especially the cheeks) and lower legs. Patients usually have systemic symptoms such as high fever, chills, and malaise. Erysipelas on the face first appears as a bright-red lesion by the nares that can spread rapidly within a few hours to days. An enlarging shiny, bright-red, indurated plaque develops that is warm to the touch and has sharp, distinct borders, as opposed to cellulitis, which has more diffuse, flat borders. The affected skin appears shiny and taut because of the edema from the infection. Skin streaking and regional enlarged nodes indicate lymphatic involvement.
Necrotizing fasciitis	The hallmark of this infection is its rapid progression with tissue destruction and severe symptoms. The progress of the infection is measured in terms of hours instead of days, as the border of the affected area can be seen literally spreading over just a few hours. This infection is caused by "flesh-eating bacteria," and loss of life or limb is a potential complication. Most cases of necrotizing fasciitis are caused by group A *Streptococcus pyogenes*, although several kinds of bacteria have been implicated in these rapidly progressive infections, including *Staphylococcus aureus, Clostridium perfringens, Bacteroides fragilis,* and *Aeromonas hydrophila*. During the early phase of the infection, the lesion appears bright red with edema that progresses to purpuric (indicated by a purple color change), including gangrene (indicated by a black color change). The symptom that differentiates necrotizing fasciitis from cellulitis is severe pain at the affected site, which may be out of proportion to the appearance of the skin lesion. This pain is due to involvement of the fascia around the muscle and sometimes of the muscle itself (myositis). Pressure on the skin may reveal crepitus due to gas production by the anaerobic bacteria *Clostridium perfringens*. Gangrene can present in just a few hours, with hypotension and mental status changes regarded as particularly ominous signs. Other indications of severe infection include violaceous bullae, hemorrhage, sloughing of the skin, and localized sensory loss.
Periorbital cellulitis	Periorbital cellulitis is a potentially life-threatening form of cellulitis that should be treated as an emergent condition. The typical patient is a young child with erythema and edema over the affected periorbital area. The edema can be so severe that the entire affected side of the face may become puffy. Symptoms include pain with certain eye movements due to inflamed extraocular muscles. Other symptoms include high fever, tachycardia, lethargy or mental status changes, and other systemic symptoms. On physical examination, the involved eye will lose the ability to move into certain quadrants (e.g., lateral or downward gaze), and the examination of cranial nerves III, IV, and VI that control extraocular movements will be abnormal.

and older patients, *S. aureus* and *Streptococcus pyogenes* are more common. In patients with diabetes mellitus or who are immunocompromised, unusual bacterial pathogens may include *Escherichia coli* and other enteric species (e.g., *Enterobacter*), as well as *Proteus mirabilis, Pseudomonas aeruginosa, Acinetobacter, Mycobacterium fortuitum,* and *Cryptococcus neoformans.*

Any break of the skin or mucous membranes is a potential portal of entry for bacterial pathogens. Skin breaks can be caused by surgical incisions, skin tears and wounds, trauma, insect bites or stings, and animal or human bites. Preexisting skin conditions such as stasis ulcers, dermatitides (eczema, psoriasis, contact dermatitis), viral skin infections (herpes simplex, herpes zoster, or varicella zoster), superficial bacterial infections (acne, folliculitis), and bullous diseases (bullous pemphigoid, pemphigus vulgaris, burns) all have the potential for secondary bacterial infection. The likelihood and severity of cellulitis are affected by three important factors: (1) virulence of the pathogen, (2) host immune status, and (3) depth of infection.

Risk factors that predispose an individual to cellulitis include the following conditions that affect cellular immunity and lymphatic drainage:

- Diabetes mellitus
- Lymphatic blockage
- History of recurrent cellulitis
- Postmastectomy
- Postsaphenous vein grafting
- HIV infection and AIDS
- Chronic corticosteroid use
- Cancer chemotherapy
- Drug or alcohol abuse
- Peripheral vascular disease

PATHOPHYSIOLOGY

The skin and subcutaneous tissue respond to bacterial invasion with an acute inflammatory process. An increase in vascular permeability of the microcirculation of the skin allows protein-rich fluids to leak into the interstitial tissue. This results in tissue edema, which may become chronic in recurrent cellulitis. Agents that are released into the tissue and increase vascular permeability include histamine, cytokines, platelet-activating factor, bradykinin, complement proteins, and arachidonic acid metabolites, including leukotrienes and prostaglandins. Vasodilation also occurs, giving cellulitis its characteristic bright-red color and indistinct borders. In addition, during the cellular phase of inflammation, leukocytes accumulate at the site of injury and engulf particulate material such as bacteria, cellular debris, and antigen–antibody complexes. Engulfed bacteria and other cellular debris are digested inside phagolysosomes by potent hydrolytic enzymes. Interestingly, the bacterial burden in cellulitis may be low, except in cases where abscesses or skin ulcers are present.

The most predominant leukocyte during the cellular inflammatory phase is the PMN (or neutrophil) and, to a lesser extent, basophils, mast cells, and platelets. PMNs express at least three types of granules containing proteolytic enzymes. Necrosis of normal tissue may occur during the inflammatory process due to these proteolytic enzymes and reactive oxygen metabolites. Some aggressive cases of cellulitis may progress to TSS in which certain strains of *Staphylococcus* and *Streptococcus* produce toxins that stimulate a massive release of inflammatory cytokines. This in turn can result in shock, multiorgan failure, and ultimately death if untreated. In addition, bacterial exotoxins have been shown to potentiate hypersensitivity responses to fungal antigens such as *Trichophyton,* the primary agent involved in tinea pedis or "athlete's foot" infection. Such responses have been shown to contribute to the pathogenesis of cellulitis in certain individuals.

CLINICAL PRESENTATION

Subjective

The typical adult patient with cellulitis will complain of a tender, warm, and erythematous area of skin that is usually located on the face, neck, or extremities. The patient will usually report a precipitating condition such as an insect bite or small cut that "got infected." The patient might already have a preexisting skin condition such as acne, tinea pedis, or chronic eczema with breaks in the skin that serve as the portal of entry for bacteria, although this may not be apparent to the patient. In cases of recurrent cellulitis of the lower leg, the patient will frequently deny any trauma or injury but will report a history of repeated infections on the same leg. The size of involvement can vary from a few centimeters to a larger area, including the entire limb. The patient will report a history of the lesion or plaque getting progressively larger over several days, but in the case of necrotizing fasciitis, the border will literally spread in just a matter of hours. Some cellulitis patients will complain of tender and enlarged lymph nodes near the affected area. Patients with more severe cases of cellulitis or with specific types such as necrotizing fasciitis, erysipelas, and periorbital cellulitis are more likely to complain of systemic symptoms such as fever and chills, lethargy, and malaise.

Objective

In adults, the lower leg is usually the most common site of infection. In cases of lower extremity cellulitis, the clinician should search for signs of tinea pedis and areas of macerated or peeling skin in the interdigital areas of the toes. A chronic tinea pedis ("athlete's foot") infection can become a point of entry for bacteria. In children, and occasionally in adults, the cheeks and the periorbital area are common sites of involvement. In lighter-skinned patients, the area of infected skin will have a bright-red color that is warm and tender to the touch. In darker-skinned patients, the color of the affected skin area will be a darker red. Sometimes extensive edema will be present, especially if the arm or leg is involved.

The red borders seen in cellulitis are flat and diffuse, compared with the distinct raised border seen with an erysipelas infection. Serious signs of systemic toxicity to look for include high fever, hypotension, tachycardia, marked leukocytosis, and associated lymphangitis. If these signs are present, the patient must be treated aggressively with hospitalization and parenteral antibiotics. Referral to a physician is recommended for severe or certain highly morbid cases of cellulitis, as described earlier.

DIAGNOSTIC REASONING

Diagnostic Tests

Most cases of mild to moderate cellulitis are diagnosed by clinical presentation and history. In most cases of acute cellulitis, there is usually no discharge or obvious wound present; therefore, obtaining cultures is difficult. If an open wound or purulent discharge is present, a culture and Gram stain should be obtained. For patients who appear ill or have systemic symptoms such as fever, a CBC and consultation with a physician are necessary. If periorbital cellulitis is suspected due to swelling and redness of the eyelids, limited spontaneous extraocular movements (EOMs), or fever, formal testing for the full range of EOMs should be done, along with other tests of cranial nerve function. Leukocytosis is seen in periorbital cellulitis, as well as in necrotizing fasciitis and erysipelas.

Differential Diagnosis

The site of the infection helps guide the clinician in searching for a differential diagnosis. If a lower limb is affected, deep vein thrombosis (DVT) should be considered. It may be difficult to make the distinction between DVT and cellulitis. DVT presents as a swollen, warm limb with erythema that is tender to the touch and can be similar in presentation to acute cellulitis. A history of recent surgery, bedrest, or prolonged immobility points more toward DVT; however, DVT can also occur after cellulitis, although rarely. There are usually no systemic symptoms such as fever associated with DVT. If fever is present, it points more toward a diagnosis of cellulitis. If crepitus is noted on palpation or if violaceous bullae and intense pain are present, the clinician should rule out necrotizing fasciitis. Serious systemic symptoms that point to severe infection include hypotension, lethargy (or any change in mental status), nausea and vomiting, severe pain (which points to possible fascial involvement), and a toxic appearance. If these signs are present, immediate consultation with a physician or referral to the emergency department is necessary.

MANAGEMENT

Treatment of cellulitis should take into consideration several factors: severity of the infection, site of the infection, presence of underlying disease, and virulence of the pathogen. Patients with diabetes mellitus are known to have a higher incidence of complications from skin infections because of chronic hyperglycemia that adversely affects the immune system and the microcirculation. Patients who are under long-term treatment with corticosteroids or chemotherapy are also at increased risk because of immune system depression. Previous surgical procedures, such as a mastectomy or saphenous vein graft, predispose the affected limb to cellulitis because of defective lymphatic drainage. Some sites of the body, such as the hands, feet, and the face, must be treated more aggressively to prevent any potential loss of future function. Particular care must be taken with soft tissue infections of the hand because a compartment-like syndrome can ensue, in addition to destruction of complex structures.

Human bite wounds are known to have a higher rate of infection because of the large amounts of anaerobic bacteria present in the mouth. Because of increased vascularity, the face and neck areas are less likely to become infected than the hands and feet. Closed-fist injuries of the hand are more likely to become infected, probably because exposed tendons and tissue that become contaminated with oral flora (during a punch to the mouth) retract back into the skin under anaerobic conditions and allow bacteria to proliferate. Cat bites are more likely (30% to 50%) to become infected (with *Pasteurella multocida*) than human bites. To a lesser extent, some dog bites (only 5%) become infected with *P. multocida* or *Capnocytophaga canimorsus*. In addition, any injury that occurs in salty or brackish water has the potential for infection with *Vibrio* species of bacteria. Periorbital cellulitis is potentially life-threatening and should be regarded as an emergent condition. It is seen more commonly in children than in adults.

Although *Streptococcus* and *Staphylococcus* cause most cases of skin infections, it is still important to establish the specific etiology of any infection. If purulent discharge or an open wound is present, a culture and Gram stain should be obtained. Because it is difficult to culture most cases of cellulitis, diagnosis is based mostly on clinical presentation. Empirical treatment for cellulitis must provide good coverage for both *Staphylococcus* and *Streptococcus*. Good choices for uncomplicated cases of cellulitis that are not associated with human or animal bites include penicillin, dicloxacillin, clindamycin, or cephalexin for 5 days or longer if insufficient improvement is seen over the first several days of therapy.

Patients with penicillin allergy may be prescribed clindamycin, azithromycin, or clarithromycin. Infected human and animal (cat or dog) bites are best treated with amoxicillin–clavulanic acid (Augmentin) for at least 2 weeks. Physician consultation or referral is recommended in complicated cases of cellulitis. Prophylaxis (not treatment) for fresh, uncomplicated human and animal bites (less than 6 hours old) to prevent infection is amoxicillin–clavulanic acid for 3 to 5 days.

Management of cellulitis infection of the lower extremities requires bedrest (with bathroom privileges) and elevation of the infected leg. Patients who are at increased risk of thrombus formation should be referred to a physician for possible anticoagulation therapy. In a small study of patients with chronic edema of the leg and cellulitis, compression therapy was effective in reducing recurrence over patients not using compression therapy (Webb et al, 2020).

Erysipelas is treated in the hospital with parenteral antibiotics. Necrotizing fasciitis is a medical emergency and must be treated aggressively in the hospital with parenteral antibiotics, surgical débridement, and fluid replacement.

Patients with underlying conditions such as AIDS, diabetes mellitus, alcohol use disorder, injection drug use, neuropathy, arterial insufficiency, lymphatic drainage abnormalities, intermittent claudication, a history of recent trauma to the affected body part, those with a history of recent trauma to the affected body part, and those who are receiving chemotherapy or chronic corticosteroids are more prone to complications of cellulitis and infection with unusual bacterial pathogens (e.g., gram-negative bacteria, anaerobes) and require more aggressive treatment. These cases frequently require referral and consideration for hospitalization. Unusual pathogens that may cause cellulitis include *E. coli, Klebsiella, Enterobacter,* and *Pseudomonas,* which are more common in patients with impaired immune systems. Cellulitis of vital structures such as the hand, foot, or face also requires close follow-up as part of the overall treatment plan.

Patients suspected of having a complicated case of cellulitis, including, for example, bacteremia (with fever and chills), periorbital cellulitis, necrotizing fasciitis, or erysipelas, require immediate consultation with a physician or referral to an emergency department. The clinician should not rely solely on laboratory results (such as leukocytosis) to diagnose a serious cellulitis infection because clinical presentation and symptoms are more helpful in guiding the management of cellulitis than any laboratory test result.

For oral therapy, cefuroxime (Ceftin) can be used when *Haemophilus influenzae* is suspected. Azithromycin or clarithromycin is preferred as a macrolide over erythromycin for penicillin-allergic patients with suspected *H. influenzae.* If gram-negative microorganisms are suspected, fluoroquinolones such as levofloxacin are typically chosen for complicated skin infections in adult patients. Clindamycin may be added to extend the spectrum of gram-positive coverage. Importantly, however, *Clostridium difficile* colitis is associated with clindamycin usage. *Vibrio* infections from seawater-associated injuries are best treated with doxycycline plus ceftazidime, whereas cellulitis related to freshwater injuries must cover *Aeromonas* infection and include a fluoroquinolone such as ciprofloxacin combined with doxycycline. Diabetics are typically treated with amoxicillin-clavulanic acid (Augmentin), although this may produce significant gastrointestinal effects such as loose stools, due to alterations in gut flora. Table 14.2 lists medications used for pharmacological management of skin and soft tissue infections in primary care.

If tinea pedis infection is concurrent with cellulitis, treatment for this must be initiated using terbinafine or itraconazole (covered in Chapter 13). For information on community-acquired MRSA infection, refer to the earlier discussion in this chapter about furuncles and carbuncles regarding selected oral agents, such as TMP-SMX (Bactrim). For more serious MRSA infections, physician consultation or emergency department referral is recommended.

TABLE 14.2 Pharmacological Management of Skin and Soft Tissue Infections in Primary Care

Purulent (Furuncle/Carbuncle/Abscess)	Nonpurulent (Cellulitis/Erysipelas/Necrotizing Infection)
Mild* Incision and drainage	*Mild** Oral treatment: Penicillin *or* Cephalosporin *or* Dicloxacillin *or* Clindamycin
Moderate** Incision and drainage Culture and sensitivities Empirical treatment: TMP-SMX *or* doxycycline Defined treatment: MRSA: TMP-SMX MSSA: dicloxacillin *or* cephalexin	*Moderate*** Emergency department referral for IV antibiotic treatment
Severe*** Requires immediate physician consultation/emergency department referral for hospitalization and IV antibiotic treatment	*Severe**** Emergency department/immediate surgical referral for evaluation/débridement

Abbreviations: MRSA, methicillin-resistant *Staphylococcus aureus;* MSSA, methicillin-sensitive *Staphylococcus aureus;* TMP-SMX, trimethoprim-sulfamethoxazole.
Purulent: *Mild infection—no systemic signs of infection; **Moderate infection—systemic signs of infection (temperature greater than 38°C, tachycardia, tachypnea, white blood cell count greater than 12,000 cells/mcL), immunocompromised; ***Severe infection—systemic signs of infection; no improvement with incision and drainage and oral antibiotic treatment.
Nonpurulent: *Mild infection—cellulitis, erysipelas with no purulence; **Moderate infection: systemic signs of infection; ***Severe infection: systemic signs of infection; no improvement with oral antibiotic treatment; immunocompromised; signs of deep infection (e.g., bullae, sloughing of skin), increased blood pressure, organ failure.
Source: Stevens DL, Bisno AL, Chambers HF, et al. Practice guidelines for the diagnosis and management of skin and soft tissue infections: 2014 update by the Infectious Diseases Society of America. *Clin Infect Dis.* 2014;59(2):e10–e52.

FOLLOW-UP AND REFERRAL

Most cases of uncomplicated cellulitis resolve with adequate antibiotic treatment. Improvement is usually obvious within 48 hours, although some cases might take 72 hours before improvement is seen. If the patient is responding to treatment, follow-up can be done on an outpatient basis. Recurrent infections of cellulitis on a lower extremity can result in chronic nonpitting edema, and the patient should be advised of this potential complication. Patients with diabetes mellitus should be advised to adhere to dietary and lifestyle changes (in addition to diabetic medications) to control their blood glucose levels. Consistent diabetic control is associated with fewer and less serious complications of infection, including potential vascular, kidney, or eye damage.

Initial follow-up for cellulitis should be done within 48 hours or sooner for sicker patients. Improvement in signs and symptoms should be seen, including a decrease in swelling, erythema, and pain of the affected area. The borders of erythema should be receding and getting smaller at follow-up. The clinician should use a surgical skin marking pen (with the patient's permission) to delineate the borders during the initial visit; this will make any changes in size easier to notice at subsequent follow-up visits. If the patient's response is satisfactory, the next follow-up visit is usually done in 1 week (or sooner, if closer follow-up is necessary). Thereafter, the patient can be seen on a weekly basis until the cellulitis is largely resolved.

If the patient does not respond to treatment with oral antibiotics after 48 to 72 hours or starts to appear toxic, a CBC and consultation with a physician (or referral to an emergency department) are necessary.

Patient Education: Cellulitis

The clinician should instruct the patient to call their health-care provider if the infection worsens or if fever persists despite antibiotic treatment for at least 48 hours. The patient should also call the clinic in 3 days to report the progress of uncomplicated cellulitis. The patient should be advised to elevate the affected limb as much as possible to decrease swelling. If the patient has chronic tinea pedis ("athlete's foot"), an OTC antifungal powder or spray should be used daily to prevent a recurrence of secondary infection with bacteria.

REFERENCES

Cellulitis

Bowen AC, Carapetis JR, Currie BJ, et al. (2017). Sulfamethoxazole-Trimethoprim (Cotrimoxazole) for skin and soft tissue infections including impetigo, cellulitis, and abscess. *Open Forum Infect Dis* 2017;4:ofx232.

Gottlieb M, DeMott JM, Hallock M, et al. Systemic antibiotics for the treatment of skin and soft tissue abscesses: a systematic review and meta-analysis. *Ann Emerg Med* 2019;73:8.

Moran GJ, Krishnadasan A, Mower WR, et al. Effect of Cephalexin Plus Trimethoprim-Sulfamethoxazole vs Cephalexin alone on clinical cure of uncomplicated cellulitis: a randomized clinical trial. *JAMA* 2017;317:2088.

Raff AB, Kroshinsky D. (2016). Cellulitis: A review. *JAMA* 2016; 316:325.

Stevens DL, Bisno AL, Chambers HF, et al. Practice guidelines for the diagnosis and management of skin and soft tissue infections: 2014 update by the Infectious Diseases Society of America. *Clin Infect Dis* 2014;59(2):e10–e52.

Talan DA, Moran GJ, Krishnadasan A, et al. (2018). Subgroup analysis of antibiotic treatment for skin abscesses. *Ann Emerg Med* 2018;71:21.

Wang W, Chen W, Liu Y, et al. Antibiotics for uncomplicated skin abscesses: systematic review and network meta-analysis. *BMJ Open* 2018;8:e020991.

Webb E, Neeman T, Bowden FJ, et al. Compression therapy to prevent recurrent cellulitis of the leg. *N Engl J Med* 2020;383(7):630.

Folliculitis

Bohaty BR, Choi S, Cai C, et al. Clinical and bacteriological efficacy of twice daily topical retapamulin ointment 1% in the management of impetigo and other uncomplicated superficial skin infections. *Int J Women's Dermatol* 2015;1:13.

Durdu M, Güran M, Kandemir H, et al. Clinical and laboratory features of six cases of candida and dermatophyte folliculitis and a review of published studies. *Mycopathologia* 2016;181:97.

Wang X, Yang Y, Li R, et al. Two cases of dermatophytic granuloma successfully treated with terbinafine. *Mycopathologia* 2018; 183:611.

Furuncles and Carbuncles

Souli M, Ruffin F, Park L, et al. (2017). Twenty-one years of Staphylococcus aureus Bacteremia (SAB): Variations in bacterial genotype and clinical phenotype in the S. aureus Bacteremia Group Prospective Cohort Study (SABG-PCS) from 1995 to 2015. *Open Forum Infect Dis* 2017;4:S545.

Impetigo

Bowen AC, Mahé A, Hay RJ, et al. The global epidemiology of impetigo: a systematic review of the population prevalence of impetigo and pyoderma. *PLoS One* 2015;10:e0136789.

Liu C, Bayer A, Cosgrove SE, et al. Clinical Practice Guidelines by the Infectious Diseases Society of America for the treatment of methicillin-resistant staphylococcus aureus infections in adults and children. *Clinical Infectious Diseases* 2011 Feb 1;52(3): e18–e55.

Nardi NM, Schaefer TJ. Impetigo. (Updated 2020 Aug 8). In: StatPearls [Internet]. Treasure Island (FL): StatPearls Publishing; 2020 Jan-. Available from: https://www.ncbi.nlm.nih.gov/books/NBK430974/. Accessed 9/22/2020.

Romani L, Steer AC, Whitfeld MJ, et al. Prevalence of scabies and impetigo worldwide: a systematic review. *Lancet Infect Dis* 2015; 15:960.

Rosen T, Albareda N, Rosenberg N, et al. Efficacy and safety of ozenoxacin cream for treatment of adult and pediatric patients with impetigo: A randomized clinical trial. *JAMA Dermatol*. 2018;154(7):806–813.

Sahu JK, Mishra AK. Ozenoxacin: A novel drug discovery for the treatment of impetigo. *Curr Drug Discov Technol* 2019;16(3): 259–264.

Schachner L, Andriessen A, Bhatia N, et al. Topical Ozenoxacin Cream 1% for Impetigo: A Review. *J Drugs Dermatol.* 2019;18(7):655–661.

RESOURCES

National Institute of Allergy and Infectious Disease
https://www.niaid.nih.gov

American Society of Dermatology
https://www.asd.org

Infectious Diseases Society of America
https://www.idsociety.org

Information on dermatological drugs
https://www.nsc.com.sg/Patient-Guide/Health-Library/List-of-Dermatological-Drugs/Pages/List-of-Dermatological-Drugs.aspx

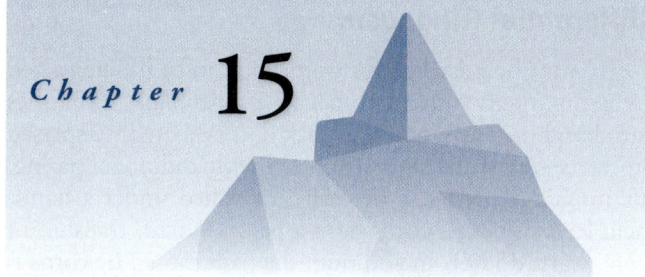

Chapter 15

Viral Skin Infections

Susan Garnett, MSN, APRN, FNP-BC
Jill E. Winland-Brown, EdD, APRN, FNP-BC, FAANP
Brian Oscar Porter, MD, PhD, MPH, MBA

WARTS

Warts (verruca vulgaris, plantar warts, and flat warts) are contagious skin lesions formed by infected keratinocytes caused by human papillomavirus (HPV). Warts are identified based on their morphology (flat, mosaic, digitate, or filiform) or anatomical location (e.g., plantar, anogenital, or palmar areas). See Chapter 52 for a full discussion of HPV-related anogenital warts.

EPIDEMIOLOGY AND CAUSES

Warts are a common skin disease throughout the world. Infection is more prevalent in children, with the highest incidence between the ages of 12 and 16 years. Individuals who walk barefoot, handle raw meat as an occupation, and/or bite their nails are at increased risk of acquiring warts. In addition, children and teens who use public showers and pools have a greater risk of developing warts, as do those with family members or schoolmates who have warts. Immunosuppression is an additional risk factor, as is having a preexisting atopic condition such as eczema (atopic dermatitis). Warts occur equally in males and females and in all ethnicities; however, common warts (verruca vulgaris) occur with twice the frequency among white people compared with all other ethnicities.

HPV is a small, double-stranded DNA virus that infects epithelial cells and causes hyperproliferation of these cells. HPV is species-specific and infects only humans, with a particular tropism for epithelial cells (such as keratinocytes) and the mucous membranes. There are more than 200 genomically distinct strains of HPV. Common warts are primarily caused by HPV serotypes 2 and 4, followed by 1, 3, 27, 29, and 57, whereas HPV serotypes 3, 10, and 28 cause flat warts. HPV serotypes 1 to 4, 27, and 57 typically cause plantar warts, whereas HPV serotypes 6 and 11 cause 90% of anogenital warts. It is estimated that high-risk HPV serotypes 16 and 18 are associated with more than 90% of anal and cervical cancers, 70% of vulvar and vaginal cancers, and 60% of penile malignancies.

In general, HPV and resultant warts can be transmitted by touch, by trauma to skin tissue such as from nail biting or shaving, and by fomites. HPV enters through breaks in the skin or mucosa. Viral particles contained within skin cells serve as the vehicle for person-to-person transmission. Plantar warts occur at points of maximum pressure (e.g., at the heads of metatarsal bones and heels); a thick, painful callus forms in response to the pressure. Anogenital warts are usually transmitted by genital-to-genital contact; penetrative intercourse is not necessary for transmission.

PATHOPHYSIOLOGY

Warts consist of infected keratinocytes, which form a mass in the epidermis that does not extend into the dermis or subcutaneous layers. It is a common misconception that warts have roots, as the underside of a wart is usually smooth and round. Several types of warts form tightly fused cylindrical projections resulting in a uniform mosaic pattern that is unique to warts. This pattern is a useful diagnostic sign. The black dots seen on the surface of common warts are thrombosed capillaries that became trapped in the cylindrical, fingerlike projections.

CLINICAL PRESENTATION

Subjective

Patients typically complain of a wart or small "bump" (or group of bumps) that has been present for several weeks to many months and sometimes for years. Some patients report the same wart being treated before and then recurring in the same area. Many adult patients with common warts attempt self-treatment with over-the-counter (OTC) wart remedies with limited to no success. Warts are usually asymptomatic but may be cosmetically undesirable. Plantar warts may cause discomfort when wearing shoes and weight-bearing.

Objective

Warts are small or large, fleshy or firm growths or lumps, which can be raised, flat, single, or multiple, isolated or clustered together to form a cauliflower-like shape. There are no skin lines crossing the surface, and examination with a hand lens reveals centrally located capillaries (black dots) that bleed with paring.

Varieties of warts include common warts (verruca vulgaris), filiform warts, flat warts (verruca plana), periungual warts, plantar warts, and deep palmoplantar warts. Common warts initially begin as smooth, flesh-colored papules. As they grow, they become dome-shaped, gray-brown hyperkeratotic masses with black dots on the surface. Although common warts can be found on any part of the body, the hands and knees are the most frequent sites of involvement. Filiform and digitate warts are fingerlike, flesh-colored projections that protrude from a narrow or broad base, usually on the face. Flat warts are small (0.1 to 0.3 cm), slightly elevated, flat-topped papules. They are usually numerous and involve the forehead, mouth, chin, eyes, dorsal surface of the hands, shins, and shaved areas. Scratching may produce a line of flat warts on shaved surfaces. Flat warts range in color from pink or light brown to light yellow.

Deep palmoplantar warts occur on the plantar surfaces of the hands and around or under the fingernails. They extend deeper than other warts and are, therefore, more painful. Mosaic warts are a group of plantar warts that form a plaque. Plantar warts occur on skin covering the heads of metatarsal bones and the heels (i.e., points of maximal pressure), appearing as thick, painful calluses. This may lead to repositioning of the foot while walking, causing a distortion in posture, as well as producing pain in other parts of the foot, leg, or back.

Cutaneous HPV infections (caused by serotypes 1, 2, 4, and 7) are more likely to be seen in children and young adults, with an incubation period of 2 to 6 months. As an individual reaches adulthood, the prevalence of cutaneous warts decreases, probably because of improved host immunity. Because these infections are usually benign, they are rarely brought to the attention of health-care providers. HPV serotypes 5, 8, 20, and 47 are closely linked with a rare form of hereditary skin cancer called epidermodysplasia verruciformis.

DIAGNOSTIC REASONING

Diagnostic Tests

If the clinician is unable to distinguish the lesion as a wart, a small skin biopsy specimen can be sent to the laboratory for identification.

Differential Diagnosis

Corns may be mistaken for warts and can be differentiated by paring them with a number 15 scalpel blade. Skin lines are absent on warts, and the black dots that are interspersed in the center of the wart will bleed with additional paring. Its mosaic pattern can be easily identified under a hand-held lens. Whereas corns have a painful, hard, translucent core, warts do not. In addition, the pain caused by corns is relieved when the hard central kernel is freed from the corn.

It is important to differentiate between the surface of the foot that is healing from recent trauma and warts that are undergoing spontaneous resolution (black warts). The black dots (thrombosed capillaries) seen on the plantar surface of a foot that has sustained a shearing injury may be confused with the black color of warts that are healing. It is hypothesized that the black color of warts that are spontaneously healing may be part of the process of regression and may represent a specific cell-mediated immune response to HPV-infected keratinocytes.

MANAGEMENT

There is no known cure for HPV infection. Studies suggest that one-half of warts resolve without treatment within 1 year, and two-thirds resolve within 2 years. Therefore, watchful waiting is recommended unless the warts are uncomfortable or cosmetically undesirable to the patient. Interestingly, multiple reports of cutaneous wart remission after the off-label administration of quadrivalent HPV vaccine have been noted. Thus, prospective, randomized, controlled clinical trials are recommended to establish whether HPV vaccine may provide prophylactic or therapeutic solutions for cutaneous warts.

Initial management for established warts should be geared toward relieving pain and pressure and minimizing skin trauma and scarring caused by available therapies. Although filiform and digitate warts are relatively easy to treat, flat warts present a unique therapeutic challenge. Their duration is prolonged, and they may be resistant to treatment. Because flat warts may be located in areas that are cosmetically important, treatment modalities that produce scarring should be avoided. It is important to note that several treatments for warts are contraindicated in pregnant women; however, salicylic acid applied to a small area of the skin for a short duration and liquid nitrogen cryotherapy are considered safe during pregnancy.

The treatment plan must be individualized because available therapies may produce unwanted effects such as pain, hyperpigmentation, scarring, damage to normal tissue, sun sensitivity, chemical sensitization, toxicity, and potential harm to pregnant women. In addition, it is important to identify previous treatment failures and successes, as well as the patient's risk factors (such as immunosuppression or lapses in therapy compliance) that may account for the failure of first-line therapy. Treatment intervals usually range from 1 to 2 weeks, but other patients may require prolonged therapy to eradicate more resistant lesions.

Treating cutaneous warts with a duct tape regimen was previously considered effective; however, recent studies have demonstrated little or no effectiveness with duct tape therapy alone. Duct tape occlusion is still used in combination with salicylic acid and 5-fluorouracil (Efudex 5%) in some treatment regimens. First-line treatments for warts include 17% salicylic acid and cryotherapy with liquid nitrogen.

Pharmacological Treatments

Keratolytic therapy in the form of salicylic acid plasters (Mediplast) or solution (Duoplant, Occlusal) is a safe, nonscarring, moderately effective, and low-cost OTC treatment of common warts, which patients can apply at home. First, the wart is pared with a number 15 scalpel blade, pumice stone, or emery board, and then the area is soaked in warm water to soften the surface and to facilitate penetration of the solution. In the case of salicylic acid solution, one drop or more is applied with an applicator to cover the surface of the wart. The surface is allowed to dry and covered with a piece of adhesive tape, duct tape, or bandage. This will enhance the penetration of the solution.

Tape occlusion may precipitate inflammation and soreness and may necessitate periodic interruption of treatment. The patient may prefer to apply the solution at bedtime. Within a few days, a soft white keratin layer will form; this layer should be pared or abraded until pink skin is exposed. This procedure may be better accomplished by an occasional office visit. When applying keratolytic plasters (40% salicylic acid), the patient may use the same procedure. The plaster is more useful when treating mosaic warts (i.e., a large cluster of warts). Once the plaster is cut to the size of the wart, the backing is removed, and the adhesive surface is attached to the wart and secured with adhesive tape. The plaster should be removed in 24 to 48 hours, and the surface should be pared as outlined earlier; a new plaster should then be applied to the area. Although this treatment may take several weeks to fully treat the wart, it is less irritating than salicylic acid solution.

Chemicals such as bichloracetic acid (BCA) or trichloroacetic acid (TCA) are caustic agents that destroy warts by chemical coagulation of the proteins. These chemicals are frequently used for recurrent warts or sometimes as initial therapy. The clinician should pare the excess calloused skin and apply petrolatum to the surrounding area before applying the acid with a cotton-tipped applicator. BCA or TCA should be applied sparingly because both are caustic agents that can damage adjacent normal tissue. These acids are self-neutralizing, although any excess amount can be wiped away with gauze. Repeat applications may be necessary every 7 to 10 days. A change of therapy should be considered if the patient has not improved substantially after three provider visits or if the warts have not cleared after six treatments.

Verruca plana (flat warts) are especially difficult to treat. While many formulations of tretinoin cream are available, the most effective for clearing warts in 80% of cases is 0.05% tretinoin cream applied nightly for 12 weeks. The frequency of application should be adjusted to elicit a fine scaling and mild erythema. If other treatment options fail, 5-fluorouracil (Efudex 5%) can be applied with tape occlusion one or two times a day for 3 to 5 weeks. Hyperpigmentation and recurrent warts at the site of inflammation are limitations of this therapy.

Podophyllin resin 10% to 25% in a compound tincture of benzoin can be used for external warts. Because of the potential complications associated with systemic absorption and toxicity, it is recommended that the treatment area be limited to 10 cm^2 per session, using 0.5 mL or less of solution. To minimize irritation, the area should be allowed to dry and then washed off 1 to 4 hours after application. Podophyllin is not used for cervical warts or dysplasia and is primarily reserved for exophytic lesions. It is contraindicated for use by pregnant or lactating women.

Surgical Treatments

Although cryosurgery with liquid nitrogen is effective for common warts and anogenital warts, it may produce severe pain around the palms, feet, and nail areas. Thermal injury to nerve tissue, epithelial cells, and melanocytes can occur and cause changes in pigmentation. Therefore, light applications of liquid nitrogen are preferable. More aggressive applications have been shown to be more effective; however, they may also cause more pain and blistering. Liquid nitrogen can be stored in 1- to 2-gallon tanks for approximately 10 days. Applications can be repeated every 1 to 2 weeks. OTC home-based cryotherapy kits are now available without a prescription for use on small, isolated warts in easily accessible areas, such as the hands and fingers. Directions for these kits must be followed closely to avoid damage to surrounding normal skin and tissue. These kits should not be used for warts located in highly sensitive areas, such as the face or genitalia; consultation with a health-care provider is warranted in such cases.

A recent meta-analysis suggests that intralesional injections of mycobacterial purified protein derivative (PPD) or the measles, mumps, and rubella vaccine (MMR) to elicit a local immune response are more effective than cryotherapy in the treatment of warts, with lower recurrence rates. Thus, these treatments may be considered first-line therapy administered by a qualified health-care provider, although as a live attenuated vaccine, MMR is contraindicated in pregnancy.

Surgical techniques such as blunt dissection or electrosurgery usually render patients wart free with a single visit; however, scarring may result, and recurrence has been reported. Additional clinical training, equipment, and longer patient visits are necessary for these procedures. Blunt dissection is relatively painless if performed on areas other than the plantar or palmar surface. After preparation with local anesthesia, a plane of dissection is established by inserting the tip of a pair of blunt-tipped scissors between the wart and normal skin. The wart is cut circumferentially, and the lesion is separated from the normal tissue with short, firm strokes. After the lesion is removed, the blunt dissector is moved firmly back and forth over the area of excision, to ensure that no tissue fragments remain. Liquid nitrogen should be applied to the base using a cotton-tipped applicator, which will destroy any remaining virus. Table 15.1 summarizes various treatment strategies for warts.

FOLLOW-UP AND REFERRAL

For the majority of common wart cases, a satisfactory response occurs after several treatments. For warts that are unresponsive or recalcitrant to treatment, more aggressive treatment options are available, which are recommended to be administered by a dermatologist.

Intralesional administration of interferon-alpha or interferon-beta in natural or recombinant forms is more effective than systemic treatment. The Centers for Disease Control and Prevention (CDC) does not recommend this treatment as first-line therapy, however, given the need for

TABLE 15.1 Treatment of Warts

Type of Wart	Description	Treatment Considerations
Common warts (verruca vulgaris)	Small, hardened growths of keratinized tissue. Warts usually grow around nails, on fingers, and on the backs of hands but can appear anywhere on the body.	• Salicylic acid solution/plasters • Cryotherapy with liquid nitrogen • Surgical excision
Flat warts (verruca plana)	Pink, light brown, or yellow; slightly elevated papules: 0.1 to 0.3 cm. Numerous sites: mouth, forehead, backs of hands, shaved areas (e.g., legs or beard area); may recur despite treatment. Frequently undergo spontaneous remission.	• May resolve without treatment • Avoid potentially scarring therapies • Tretinoin cream 0.025%, 0.05%, or 0.1%. Apply to involved areas at bedtime once or twice daily; adjust treatment to produce fine scaling and mild erythema; may require weeks to months of treatment • Cryotherapy with liquid nitrogen • 5-fluorouracil (Efudex 5%) once or twice daily for 3 to 5 weeks produces dramatic results, but may cause persistent hyperpigmentation (use ointment to minimize this adverse effect)
Filiform/digitate warts	Fingerlike, flesh-colored projections emanating from a narrow or broad base; common sites include the mouth, eyes, and ala nasi.	• Easiest to treat, but recur • Shaving spreads the lesions • Retract skin and use curette drawn across base to remove wart • May use light electrocautery • Cryotherapy with liquid nitrogen
Plantar warts	Lesions appear at maximum point of pressure (e.g., heads of metatarsal bones or heels) or anywhere on plantar surface; a thick, painful callus forms around lesion; pain is elicited on indirect pressure.	• More refractory to treatment • Remove surrounding callus with pumice stone or paring, after soaking feet in warm water to soften skin • Daily application of salicylic acid liquid, film, or plaster after soaking
Black warts	Warts become black when spontaneously healing	• Confirm spontaneous healing • Differential diagnosis includes black heel (calcaneal petechiae) caused by sheared capillaries due to trauma: normal skin lines present; when area is pared with no. 15 blade, skin underneath is soft and bleeds
Oral warts	Can be located on hard or soft palate or oral mucosa. Usually transmitted through oral–genital contact.	• Cryotherapy with liquid nitrogen • Surgical excision

frequent office visits and the high frequency of systemic side effects. In addition, the cure rate is similar to that of other available therapies.

When other treatments fail, intralesional bleomycin sulfate may be considered. Bleomycin is mixed with 5 mL of sterile water and 10 mL of lidocaine to form a solution, and then this solution is reconstituted with normal saline. With a 30-gauge needle, the solution is injected into the lesion to achieve blanching. The size of the wart will determine the amount of solution injected. Larger warts may require repeat injections. Leakage of the solution is unavoidable during the procedure. The cure rate has been reported at 48% for plantar warts and 71% for periungual warts. A multiple-puncture method can result in a 92% cure rate. Responsive warts produce hemorrhagic eschars that heal without scarring.

Another treatment modality that has been reported to be effective for refractory warts is photodynamic therapy with aminolevulinic acid, a photosensitizer. This treatment is costly and administered only by dermatologists.

The need for referral to a dermatologist is determined by several factors, including a lack of response to standard treatments, possible cosmetic consequences (especially with warts on the face and eyelids), and the clinician's knowledge, experience, and comfort in identifying and treating specific types of warts. If the clinician is unsure of the diagnosis or if the wart is resistant to multiple treatments, the patient should be referred to a dermatologist.

Patient Education: Warts

The clinician should educate the patient on the prevention of self-inoculation and the routes of transmission for common warts. These measures include limiting shaving of the affected area until warts are eradicated, strategies to control nail biting, and avoidance of scratching and rubbing warts. Wearing protective foot coverings in wet public areas such as showers, locker rooms, and pools and keeping warts dry are additional approaches to prevent infection (see Box 15.1).

Box 15.1 Basic Patient Information About Warts

About the Disease

- Warts are small growths or tumors produced by infection of normal skin tissue by human papillomavirus (HPV). The most common areas where warts are found include the plantar and palmar surfaces, nailbeds, hands, face, mouth, penis, vulva, cervix, and anus.
- One in four people are infected with HPV. Despite treatment, most warts will recur. Broken or abraded skin may facilitate transport of the virus. Lesions can be spread by skin-to-skin contact, including touch, vigorous rubbing, shaving, nail biting, and sexual intercourse.
- Contrary to popular belief, warts do not have roots. The underside of a wart is smooth and round. The black dots found in the center of a wart represent broken small blood vessels (capillaries).
- Strategies to prevent spreading warts:
  Avoid touching warts.
  Avoid nail biting.
  Wear waterproof foot coverings in public showers and locker rooms and around pools.
  Keep warts dry, as wetness facilitates spreading.
- Immunosuppression caused by diseases such as HIV or cancer, organ transplantation with antirejection therapy, and certain medications may reduce the efficacy of treatment. Cigarette smoking weakens the immune system and enhances the expression of HPV; therefore, smoking should be discontinued.

About Treatments

- For self-management of warts at home, refer to the American Academy of Dermatology for video instructions: https://www.aad.org/public/diseases/a-z/warts-self-care.
- Treatment often involves more than one session at 1- to 2-week intervals, and therapy may be prolonged.
- To minimize inflammation, do not apply medicated solutions, ointments, gels, creams, or plasters beyond the recommended duration.
- Cryotherapy may be available in a doctor's office or as an over-the-counter (OTC) wart freezing and removal kit for home use. Directions must be followed closely with home-based kits to avoid excessive damage to normal surrounding tissue.
- To improve efficacy, plasters should be cut to the size of the wart and kept in place with an adhesive for 24 to 48 hours. Pare or use a pumice stone to abrade the area and then reapply the plaster. The process may take several weeks to produce results.
- Podophyllin is applied only to external warts, and the area of application should be limited to 10 cm^2 per session. To minimize irritation, the area should be allowed to dry and washed off after 1 to 4 hours of therapy.
- Caustic acids, such as bichloracetic acid or trichloracetic acid, are very effective but may damage normal tissue if not allowed to dry properly. Repeat applications may be necessary every 7 to 10 days.
- With any topical treatment, wash the treated area after the recommended waiting period, and always check for signs and symptoms of bacterial superinfection, such as pus, severe pain, heat, redness, and swelling.
- For mild to moderate pain, take OTC analgesics.
- Pursue stress-reduction activities, such as exercise, imagery, biofeedback, meditation, and yoga, and maintain a healthy diet. Decreasing stress will boost the immune system and improve healing, as well as reduce the desire to smoke, overeat, and bite nails.

HERPES SIMPLEX INFECTIONS

Herpes simplex viruses (HSVs) are part of the Herpesviridae family and the Alphaherpesvirinae subfamily. HSV infections are caused by two types of viruses, HSV-1 and HSV-2, and can result in a wide range of clinical manifestations across age groups, depending on location (see Table 15.2). HSV-1 is associated primarily with oral infections, whereas HSV-2 is associated mainly with genital infections. HSV-1 genital infections are becoming more common, however, as are HSV-2 oral infections, likely due to oral–genital sexual contact. Herpes viral infections are lifelong; although there are effective antiviral medications for outbreaks, to date there is no known cure. Clinical studies on the development of herpes virus vaccines and topical microbicides are ongoing.

EPIDEMIOLOGY AND CAUSES

Both types of HSV produce identical patterns of infection. The World Health Organization (WHO) estimates that 3.7 billion people worldwide are infected with HSV-1 and 417 million people worldwide have HSV-2. The WHO further estimates that 67% of people younger than age 50 years are infected with HSV-1. According to the CDC, about 50 million people in the United States are thought to be infected with HSV-2, and there are 776,000 new cases of HSV-2 each year. It is estimated that 12% of people in the United States between the ages of 14 and 49 years have genital herpes caused by HSV-2. Including genital herpes caused by HSV-1, the prevalence for both types of HSV approaches 25% for women and 10% for men. *Healthy People 2030* has set a goal of maintaining the current baseline of 2.9% of people aged 15 to 24 years who have serological evidence of HSV-2. The prevalence of HSV-2 in women is nearly double that of men, with a 48% prevalence in black women in particular. People with HSV-2 are also three times more likely to acquire HIV.

PATHOPHYSIOLOGY

HSV infection has two phases: primary infection and secondary or recurrent infection. During the primary infection, the virus enters keratinocytes in the epidermis, eventually migrating to nerve endings. The virus then ascends via peripheral nerves to dorsal root ganglia, where it enters a latent stage without active viral replication, which can last for days to years. The trigeminal ganglia are the targets of oral herpes strains, whereas the sacral ganglia are the targets of genital herpes strains. Infection of the ganglia may occur within 24 hours of initial viral exposure and is essentially lifelong.

The majority of primary infections with HSV-1 and HSV-2 are subclinical and asymptomatic, and most HSV transmission occurs during periods of asymptomatic viral shedding. The severity of the viral infection increases with age, and oral–labial HSV infection may markedly compromise nutritional intake in older adults. HSV is spread by direct contact with active lesions, saliva, semen, or cervical secretions. Viral replication in the gingival epithelia facilitates oral shedding of the virus.

Symptoms may occur from 2 to 21 days after exposure. Tenderness, pain, mild paresthesias, or burning can

TABLE 15.2 Herpes Simplex Infections

Infection	Location	Commonly Affected Age Group
Oral–labial herpes simplex	Lips, oral cavity	Children aged 2 to 5 years, adults
Herpetic keratoconjunctivitis	Eyelids, periorbital area, cornea	Newborns, adults
Herpetic tracheobronchitis	Pharynx, trachea, bronchi	Older adults
Herpes simplex encephalitis	Temporal lobe of the brain	Any age, primarily immunocompromised adults
Herpes gladiatorum	Shoulder, neck, knuckles, areas of contact	Aged 14 years and older (commonly seen in wrestlers)
Herpetic whitlow	Fingertip	Aged 1 year and older
Lumbosacral herpes	Trunk or back	Adult
Herpes simplex of the buttocks	Buttocks	Adult
Genital herpes	Labia minora, labia majora, vagina, cervix, urethra, penis, rectal area	Young and older adults, 1% of pregnant women
Eczema herpeticum	Face or any area of active or recently healed atopic dermatitis	Infants, children, and adults, commonly with a history of atopic dermatitis
Erythema multiforme	Extremities, palms, soles of feet	Aged 20 to 30 years; more commonly seen in men than women

occur before the onset of lesions at the site of inoculation. Headache, fever, muscle aches, localized pain, and tender lymphadenopathy may occur as part of the prodrome, although some patients have no prodromal symptoms. Herpes infections may occur anywhere on the skin. After several days, grouped vesicles on an erythematous base appear, followed by ulcers or erosions that crust over with a characteristic honey color. Eventually, there is a loss of crusts, and reepithelialization occurs. In the moist genital region, crusts may not form; however, exudate may accumulate. Lesions typically heal in 7 to 10 days without scarring but may last up to 6 weeks or longer if they become secondarily infected with bacteria. Vesicles in primary HSV infection are more numerous and scattered than in recurrent infection.

Tissue destruction in HSV infection is mediated directly by viral replication within keratinocytes and other epithelial cells. A mononuclear and lymphocytic cellular infiltrate occurs at sites of infection, consisting primarily of CD4+ T cells early on, but eventually involving equal numbers of CD8+ T cells, as well as macrophages and cytotoxic natural killer cells that attempt to clear infected host cells. The cytokines interferon-γ and interleukin-6 are primary mediators of cytotoxic killing mechanisms. Interestingly, in animal models, nonclassical T cells endogenous to the skin and mucosal surfaces that express γ-δ rather than α-β antigen receptors have been shown to protect against severe mucocutaneous and encephalitic HSV infection.

Recurrent disease typically occurs at or near the site of primary infection. Physical and emotional stress, fever, exposure to ultraviolet light, chapping or abrasion of the skin, immune suppression, menses, or fatigue may cause reactivation of the virus, which descends spontaneously along sensory nerve axons to the skin surface. The anatomical site of infection and virus type affect the frequency of recurrence. Genital herpes recurs six times more frequently than oral–labial herpes. Genital HSV-2 infections recur more frequently than genital HSV-1 infections; however, oral–labial HSV-1 infections recur more often than oral–labial HSV-2 infections.

CLINICAL PRESENTATION

Subjective

HSV infections are usually oral or genital; however, any area of the body can be infected. The most common manifestation of HSV infection is oral–labial herpes (cold sores). Primary infection with HSV may present as herpetic gingivostomatitis in children and young adults, although most commonly, children aged 6 months to 5 years are affected. The patient may present with fever, sore throat, hypersalivation, and painful vesicles and ulcers on the tongue, palate, gingivae, buccal mucosa, and lips. In genital herpes, early symptoms may include pain in the legs, buttocks, or genital area, genital burning or itching, vaginal discharge, and lower abdominal pressure. Within a few days, lesions appear at the site of infection. With the first episode of genital herpes, fever, headache, muscle aches, painful or difficult urination, and inguinal lymphadenopathy may occur.

In older patients, primary infection or reactivation of oral HSV-1 can be extensive. Painful oral lesions make eating difficult and can compromise nutritional status. Superinfection with bacteria or *Candida* may further complicate HSV infection in older adults. Of major concern in older adults is autoinoculation of the eye, resulting in keratoconjunctivitis, which is the most frequent cause of corneal blindness. Signs and symptoms include unilateral excessive lacrimation, edema, chemosis, photophobia, and purulent exudate. Decreased visual acuity is a poor prognostic sign.

Herpetic whitlow is an HSV infection of the fingertip. This disorder was common among health-care practitioners before the use of gloves in universal precautions. Now, herpetic whitlow is commonly found in children with a recent history of gingivostomatitis and in women with genital herpes. Transmission apparently results from autoinoculation. Vesicles with a red halo may erupt on the finger, and lymphangitis may accompany generalized symptoms of chills, fever, and feeling ill.

A patient with a history of atopic dermatitis who presents with vesicles on the face or areas that have recently healed is likely to have eczema herpeticum. A patient who recently had an HSV infection but now presents with iris-shaped lesions on the palms and soles of the feet most likely has erythema multiforme. HSV lesions on the back are often misdiagnosed as varicella-zoster virus (VZV), and the correct diagnosis is often not made until there is a recurrence. The primary difference on clinical evaluation is that HSV vesicles are uniform in size, whereas varicella-zoster lesions vary in size.

Both HSV-1 and HSV-2 infection can cause encephalitis, in which patients present with an altered level of consciousness, personality changes, fever, and seizures. Patients may also experience olfactory and gustatory (taste) hallucinations and aphasia. Herpetic encephalitis is a medical emergency that requires immediate hospitalization and treatment with IV acyclovir (Zovirax). Herpes infections in immunocompromised patients are more severe, as frequent HSV recurrences often result in chronic and nearly continuous ulcerations. Focus on History lists key questions for eliciting information on HSV infection.

Focus on History: Herpes Simplex Virus Infections

General Questions

- When did the sores first appear?
- Have you ever had sores on the same area before?

- Before the appearance of the sores, did you experience burning, tingling, pain, or numbness?
- Do you have muscle aches, fever, and/or weakness?
- Are you able to swallow?
- Have you ever had this happen to you before? If so, when and how was it treated?
- Have you been around any person who may have had these same symptoms?
- Do you have a history of any skin problem?

Specific Questions for Genital Herpes

- How old were you at first sexual intercourse?
- How many total sexual partners have you had?
- How long have you been with your present sexual partner (if applicable)?
- Have you ever had a sexually transmitted infection (STI)?
- Do you use latex condoms? If so, do you use them correctly and consistently?
- Do you engage in oral sex? Vaginal sex? Anal sex? (For male patients) Do you have sex with other men?
- (For female patients) Have you ever had an abnormal Pap smear?

Objective

Lesions must be examined for their characteristic location, appearance, and distribution. Depending on the site of lesions, the anterior and posterior cervical, submental, or inguinal lymph node chains should be evaluated for lymphadenopathy. Grouped vesicles on an erythematous base occurring in the mouth or on the face or genitals are most likely the result of HSV infection. Vesicles on the eyelid, chemosis, or the presence of corneal dendrites requires prompt referral to an ophthalmologist.

DIAGNOSTIC REASONING

Diagnostic Tests

Viral culture and DNA studies such as polymerase chain reaction (PCR) testing are the standard methods of diagnosis. HSV can be cultured from vesicle fluid or from scrapings at the base of an erosion. Sampling must be done early (during the first 72 hours) in the course of an outbreak. The initial viral culture may be negative, but clinical evaluation and subsequent recurrence with early culture can verify HSV infection. Viral culture differentiates between HSV-1 and HSV-2 with high sensitivity. The Tzanck smear is rapid, easily performed, and can be used to identify multinucleated giant cells in vesicular fluid before the results of viral cultures become available. The Tzanck smear does not, however, differentiate among HSV-1, HSV-2, or VZV and is not considered reliable for this purpose. HSV antibodies can be detected in blood using type-specific serological tests based on the HSV glycoproteins G1 and G2, and PCR is useful in the diagnosis of central nervous system and systemic infections. However, viral culture remains the gold standard for the diagnosis of HSV infection when there is a lesion to sample.

Because persons with HSV-2 are three times more susceptible to infection with HIV, additional testing for HIV and other STIs is advisable in all patients infected with HSV. The U.S. Preventive Services Task Force does not recommend routine screening for HSV infection.

Differential Diagnosis

History and clinical presentation are the best guides to diagnosis, as several other conditions, both infectious and noninfectious, can mimic HSV infection. Aphthous stomatitis differs from HSV infection in that ulcerations of nonkeratinized mucosa occur. Therefore, lesions rarely appear on the gingivae or hard palate, as do herpetic ulcers. Also, no fever or lymphadenopathy occurs. In addition, an aphthous stomatitis ulcer is usually solitary and larger than a herpetic ulcer. Herpangina can also mimic HSV infection. Herpangina is seen predominantly in children and infrequently in adults; treatment is symptomatic. Hand-foot-and-mouth disease (caused by coxsackievirus) presents with red macules that progress to vesicles on an erythematous base. However, in this infection, the extremities—in particular, the hands and feet and the mouth—develop lesions. The characteristic target lesions of erythema multiforme can result from a hypersensitivity reaction to HSV or *Mycoplasma* infection or from a drug reaction. Treatment is based on the underlying cause, which may be directed to the infection, or by removing exposure to the offending agent. Pemphigus vulgaris is an autoimmune disorder that usually occurs in middle-aged patients (aged 40 to 60 years) in which erosions of the oral mucosa may mimic HSV infection. However, these are followed by distinctive bullae (large blisters) all over the body, due to the formation of autoantibodies against desmoglein, a protein that mediates attachments between adjacent epidermal cells.

MANAGEMENT

No cure for herpes exists; however, recurrences tend to be milder and of shorter duration than the primary infection. Therapy is primarily symptomatic and supportive, although oral antiviral medications are also used, especially in immunocompromised patients. Nutritional intake is important, especially in older patients, who may also benefit from using anesthetic mouth rinses for symptomatic relief. The goals for management include the reduction or elimination of pain, decreased viral shedding, and healing of ulcerated tissue. In cases of frequent recurrence of herpetic lesions, suppressive therapy may be needed. The social and psychological impact of a genital herpes diagnosis must also be addressed. Supportive counseling should include strategies for helping patients cope with the infection, informing sexual partners, and preventing transmission. Multiple patient resources are available through the CDC and the American Sexual Health Association.

Initial therapy for oral herpes is palliative and promotes healing. The primary care practitioner can initiate management with pharmacotherapy and self-help techniques, based on the location and extent of HSV infection. Acetaminophen can be used to control fever and pain. Lesions on the lip (if small) may require nothing more than applications of ice and analgesic lip ointments (e.g., Blistex). OTC docosanol 10% cream (Abreva) applied five times daily may also improve lesions. If lesions are more extensive, penciclovir 1% cream (Denavir) applied to the affected area every 2 hours while awake for 4 days promotes healing, shortens the course of the illness by several days, and substantially decreases viral shedding. Extensive oral lesions may require the use of oral anesthetics such as viscous lidocaine 2% (Xylocaine) or dyclonine hydrochloride 0.5% to 1% to control pain. In addition, acyclovir suspension 200 mg/5 mL can be used to treat oral lesions directly by rinsing the mouth with 1 teaspoon and swallowing (i.e., swish and swallow) five times a day for 7 days.

Initial treatment of genital herpes requires the use of oral antiviral drugs. Valacyclovir and famciclovir have greater bioavailability and require less frequent daily dosing than acyclovir, which makes them preferable. Comfort measures such as warm compresses or an oatmeal sitz bath several times a day can relieve pain and promote healing. A patient with genital or urethral herpes may find it easier to urinate into warm bath water. All patients with HSV infection benefit from increased fluid intake and rest.

The need for subsequent management is based on the recurrence of symptoms. A patient with a negative initial viral culture should be told to return to their primary care practitioner for another viral culture within the first 72 hours if symptoms recur. After the initial occurrence, a patient with genital herpes can be given a prescription for an antiviral drug and instructed to take the medication should they experience the beginning of symptoms in the future, such as tingling or burning at the site of previous lesions. A patient with genital herpes who experiences six or more recurrent episodes per year should be offered suppressive therapy (see Drugs Commonly Prescribed 15.1). Suppressive therapy will reduce recurrences by 70% to 80%,

Drugs Commonly Prescribed 15.1: Herpes Simplex Infections

DRUG	INDICATION	ADVERSE REACTIONS AND PRESCRIBING CONSIDERATIONS
Topical		
Acyclovir 5% cream Acyclovir 5% ointment Docosanol 10% cream (Abreva) (OTC)	Recurrent herpes labialis Initial genital herpes Herpes labialis	Apply five times daily for 4 days Apply six times daily for 7 days Begin at earliest sign or symptom, five times daily
Penciclovir 1% cream (Denavir) (OTC)	Recurrent herpes labialis on the lips and face	Every 2 hours while awake for 4 days
Systemic Therapy		
Famciclovir 125, 250, 500 mg tablet (Famvir)	Acute herpes zoster, treatment or suppression of recurrent genital herpes, treatment of recurrent herpes labialis in immunocompetent patients	No evidence of fetal harm when used during pregnancy Check prescribing reference or CDC guidelines for dosage regimens for initial outbreaks, recurrent episodes, and suppressive therapy
Valacyclovir (Valtrex)	Treatment of herpes zoster, herpes labialis, and varicella (chickenpox) Treatment or suppression of genital herpes in immunocompetent patients	As above
Acyclovir (Zovirax)	Genital herpes, herpes zoster, varicella, herpes labialis, herpetic whitlow	As above

> **Box 15.2 Basic Patient Information About Herpes Simplex Infection**
>
> - Fever, stress, sunlight, and menses can trigger recurrence of lesions.
> - Burning and tingling at the site may signal recurrence of the infection. If antiviral therapy is prescribed, begin it at the first sign of infection. If symptoms persist beyond 10 days, see your primary care practitioner.
>
> **Treatment**
>
> General:
> - Frequent hand washing, rest, and increased fluid intake are needed during a herpetic outbreak.
>
> Lip lesions:
> - Apply gel ice pack to lip lesions for 10 to 15 minutes as needed to relieve pain and decrease swelling.
> - Analgesic lip balm (e.g., Blistex) may be used on the lips to prevent drying of sores and to reduce pain.
> - Apply lip balm sunscreen (e.g., Chapstick) with an SPF of 15 or higher to lips before sun exposure.
>
> Oral lesions:
> - Apply a dental protective paste (e.g., Orabase) four times a day to prevent irritation of lesions by the teeth.
> - An equal mixture of diphenhydramine (Benadryl) syrup (12.5 mg/5 mL) and unflavored Maalox can be used as an oral rinse every 2 hours and then expectorated. Viscous lidocaine 2% (Xylocaine) 5 mL can be added to the mixture or used alone as an oral rinse before meals to decrease pain and facilitate eating.
> - For those with orolabial lesions, there should be no sharing of towels, silverware, or glasses; avoid oral contact until lesions are healed.
>
> Genital, anal, and/or buttocks lesions:
> - To soothe lesions, apply warm compresses or take a warm oatmeal sitz bath for 20 to 30 minutes as needed.
> - A blow-dryer placed on the cool setting can be used to thoroughly dry genital lesions.
> - Avoid sexual activity until lesions are healed. A latex condom must be used correctly and consistently during sexual intercourse to decrease viral spread, and not just during herpetic outbreaks.

with approximately a 50% reduced risk of transmission. Long-term suppressive therapy is safe, and after a period of 5 to 7 years, many patients discontinue such therapy with no relapses. In addition to suppressive therapy, correct and consistent condom use and abstaining from sexual activity during outbreaks are important to reduce the incidence of HSV transmission.

Pregnant women with preexisting HSV infection or infection acquired during pregnancy may be prescribed suppressive therapy to prevent transmission to the neonate during delivery, avoiding the need for a caesarean delivery. No evidence of fetal harm has been demonstrated with the use of antivirals for maternal herpes infection during pregnancy, whereas neonatal herpes may result in severe neurological disability or death.

Herpetic keratoconjunctivitis (herpes simplex keratitis) is an intraocular HSV infection that requires immediate referral to an ophthalmologist to prevent blindness. Treatment may include topical optic antiviral preparations and gentle epithelial débridement of the eye to remove infectious organisms and viral antigens that induce an ocular inflammatory response, as well as oral antiviral drugs, such as acyclovir.

FOLLOW-UP AND REFERRAL

Follow-up should be early and repeated, depending on the extent of disease. Lesions confined to the lip area may not need to be seen in follow-up unless they do not resolve. However, extensive oral or genital lesions should be seen on a weekly basis until resolution. As previously mentioned, herpetic lesions of the eye must be referred to an ophthalmologist immediately. A patient with genital herpes may benefit from referral to a local herpes health advocacy organization for continued counseling and emotional support.

Patient Education: Herpes Simplex Infections

Patient education is an integral component of the management of HSV infection. Most patients achieve relief of symptoms within 4 to 7 days of beginning therapy. Self-care techniques and instructions on the proper use of pharmacotherapy are vital. Box 15.2 provides basic information and guidelines about herpes infection.

REFERENCES

Herpes Simplex Infections

American Academy of Dermatology. Herpes Simplex. https://www.aad.org/public/diseases/a-z/herpes-simplex-overview. Accessed 10/10/2020.

Centers for Disease Control and Prevention. 2015 sexually transmitted diseases treatment guidelines. Genital HSV infections. https://www.cdc.gov/std/treatment-guidelines/herpes.htm. Accessed 9/21/2020.

Ferri FF. Herpes Simplex. *Ferri's Clinical Advisor 2021*. Philadelphia: Elsevier; 2021:681–682.e2.

James C, Harfouche M, Welton NJ, et al. Herpes simplex virus: Global infection prevalence and incidence estimates, 2016. *Bull World Health Organ.* 2020;98:315–329. doi: http://dx.doi.org/10.2471/BLT.19.237149

U.S. Preventive Services Task Force; Bibbins-Domingo K, Grossman DC, Curry SJ, et al. Serologic screening for genital herpes infection: US Preventive Services Task Force Recommendation Statement. *JAMA* 2016;316(23):2525–2530.

World Health Organization. WHO guidelines for the treatment of genital herpes simplex virus. http://www.who.int/reproductivehealth/publications/rtis/genital-HSV-treatment-guidelines/en. Accessed 9/21/2020.

Human Papillomavirus/Warts

Al Aboud AM, Nigam PK. Wart (Plantar, Verruca Vulgaris, Verrucae). 2020 Aug 11. In: StatPearls [Internet]. Treasure Island (FL): StatPearls Publishing; 2020 Jan–. PMID:28613701.

American Academy of Dermatology. Warts. https://www.aad.org/public/diseases/contagious-skin-diseases/warts. Accessed 9/22/2020.

Centers for Disease Control and Prevention. Anogenital warts. 2015 Sexually transmitted diseases treatment guidelines. https://www.cdc.gov/std/treatment-guidelines/anogenital-warts.htm

Pham, CT, Juhasz M, Sung CT, et al. The human papillomavirus vaccine as treatment for human papillomavirus-related dysplastic and neoplastic conditions: A literature review. *J Am Acad Dermatol* 2019;82(1):202–212.

Salman S, Ahmed, MS, Ibrahim AM, et al. Intralesional immunotherapy for the treatment of warts: A network meta-analysis. *J Am Acad Dermatol* 2019;80(4):922–930.e4.

Waldman A, Whiting D, Rani M, et al. HPV vaccine for treatment of recalcitrant cutaneous warts in adults: A retrospective cohort study. *Dermatol Surg* 2019;45(12):1739–1741.

RESOURCES

Centers for Disease Control and Prevention
   https://www.cdc.gov
Healthy People 2030.
   https://health.gov/healthypeople
Online Resource for Herpes and HPV
   https://www.herpes.org
American Sexual Health Association
   https://www.ashasexualhealth.org
National Institute of Allergy and Infectious Disease
   https://www.niaid.nih.gov
World Health Organization
   https://www.who.int

Chapter 16

Dermatitis

Donna Maheady, EdD, APRN, PNP-BC
Jill E. Winland-Brown, EdD, APRN, FNP-BC, FAANP
Brian Oscar Porter, MD, PhD, MPH, MBA

ATOPIC DERMATITIS

Atopic dermatitis is not considered a distinct disease entity but is a descriptive term for a group of skin disorders characterized by pruritus and inflammation whose exact cause is unknown. *Eczema* is a more general term that is often used collectively to describe skin of an erythematous and inflamed appearance, reflective of a superficial pathological process. Currently, the terms *eczema* and *dermatitis* are often used synonymously in the clinical arena in a nonspecific sense. The use of the term *eczematous rash*, although also indistinct, may be helpful both diagnostically and therapeutically because eczematous dermatitis may be classified into two major etiological categories—atopic dermatitis and contact dermatitis. Early in its presentation, atopic dermatitis is erythematous in appearance, with papulovesicular lesions that may ooze and crust. In its later stages, the rash becomes a red-purple color, dries, and develops scaling and lichenification, which is exacerbated by scratching resulting from its highly pruritic nature.

EPIDEMIOLOGY AND CAUSES

Atopic dermatitis is an inherited skin reaction that usually begins in infancy. Interestingly, children born to older women are more likely to develop eczema than children born to younger women. For unknown reasons, the prevalence of atopic disease has risen steadily over the past 30 years. Statistics vary, but overall the prevalence is estimated at one in 18 or 5.5%, which amounts to 17 million people in the United States. About 10% of the U.S. population will have atopic dermatitis at some point in their lifetime. It occurs across all ethnic groups and equally in both sexes.

Atopic dermatitis presents more severely in childhood. Onset during the first year of life occurs in up to 50% of patients, and in 85%, onset occurs before the age of 5 years. Up to 5% of all children are affected by atopic dermatitis, although many cases (40%) resolve by adulthood. The remainder of patients with atopic dermatitis are affected with a chronic disease course that is characterized by acute exacerbations (often during times of stress) and intermittent remissions.

The cause of atopic dermatitis is unknown, although family history is positive for atopy (allergic reaction) in two-thirds of all cases. A genetic predisposition toward allergic reactivity may be the most important etiological factor in all atopic conditions. A personal or family history of all or part of the "atopic triad"—asthma, allergic rhinitis, and eczema—is often present. It has been proposed that individuals with any of these three conditions have a preferential production of allergen-specific immunoglobulin E (IgE) and that the presence of such antibodies should be a mandatory criterion for the diagnosis of atopic dermatitis. Such a diagnostic test, however, only establishes the diagnosis of *atopic syndrome* and not atopic dermatitis. Any patient with a history of hives (urticaria), hay fever, or rashes should be considered to have an atopic history.

All atopic individuals seem to have itchier skin, yet what seems to be unique about the atopic patient's skin is its hypersensitivity. Many factors that do not make nonatopic individuals itch will make the atopic person feel itchy. Atopic patients are known to develop itch seconds after experiencing a stressful event. This type of reaction is thought to be caused by neuropeptide-induced vasodilation, which produces increased skin temperature and erythema. Symptoms are triggered or exacerbated through the interaction between genetic predisposition and environmental factors that trigger atopic dermatitis such as dust mites, animal dander, pollen, microbes, pollutants, climate, and emotional stress.

Excessively hot or cold climates or excessively dry or moist environments are particularly suitable for setting the stage for the atopic process. Anything that dries the skin can aggravate symptoms. Common triggers include excessive bathing, hand washing, lip licking, sweating, or swimming. Contact with irritants such as solvents, detergents, deodorants, tobacco, cosmetics, soap, and both wool and synthetic fabrics can precipitate an exacerbation of atopic dermatitis. Improperly fitting clothes can create friction and irritate the skin, thereby precipitating a flare-up. Other skin conditions or infections can also lead to an exacerbation of atopic dermatitis. Heat and sweat may also be aggravating factors for atopic dermatitis, including practices that generate an increase in body temperature, such as hot showers or baths, overdressing, use of heating pads, and electric blankets. Patients with atopy often are intolerant of heat, have difficulty with thermal sweating, and are more likely to develop heat exhaustion. Dysfunction of normal sweating may be a complicating factor in atopic patients. For example, excessive humidity may be a factor because it interferes with normal evaporation of sweat from the body.

PATHOPHYSIOLOGY

The inflammatory process in eczema causes erythema of the skin as a result of dilated blood vessels that are surrounded by inflammatory cells that migrate into the epidermis, resulting in edema both inside and between the epidermal cells (spongiosis). The epidermal cells malfunction as a consequence, resulting in thickening of the epidermis (acanthosis), excess production of keratin, and scaling. The outer epidermal layer of the skin, the stratum corneum, normally forms an impermeable barrier that protects the living cells beneath from environmental irritants and toxins. In atopic dermatitis, this outer barrier is impaired. There is an increase in water loss and a decrease in water binding, a process attributed to decreased functionality of filaggrin proteins in the skin, which leads to a brittle outer barrier. This condition is made worse by environmental factors such as physical trauma from scratching, cycles of wetting and drying, and the chemical erosion that is caused by detergents and solvents.

In addition, superinfection of eczematous skin by bacterial (e.g., *Staphylococcus aureus*) or fungal (e.g., *Malassezia furfur*) species and irritation from dust mites and their excrement are important factors that worsen atopic dermatitis by potentiating the immune response. Superinfection is also much more likely in atopic dermatitis than in other forms of dermatitis, such as psoriasis. Thus, infection may be thought of as both a trigger and a complication of atopic dermatitis.

Immunological abnormalities are key to the pathophysiology of the atopic response. These abnormalities can include elevated serum IgE levels (seen in 85% of affected individuals), hypereosinophilia, reduced cell-mediated immunity and antibody-dependent cellular cytotoxicity, slowed chemotaxis of neutrophils and monocytes, a relative increase in the number of CD4-positive (CD4+) Th2 helper T cells that secrete interleukin (IL)-4, and a decrease in CD4+ T helper cells that secrete interleukin-2 (IL-2). Interestingly, however, in later stages of the immune reaction, Th1 helper T-cell activity, which enhances cell-mediated immunity, appears to play an increasing role. In addition, the impairment of essential fatty acid metabolism has been identified as a causative factor of atopy.

Recently, Th17 cells and their associated cytokines (e.g., IL-17A) have also been implicated in this disease process, including in the protection against infection/colonization with superficial skin fungi (e.g., *Candida*) and bacteria (e.g., *Staphylococcus*) containing superantigens that are thought to trigger dysregulated immune responses, thereby resulting in eczematous lesions. However, reports in the literature are conflicting and have implicated Th17 cells in both proinflammatory and anti-inflammatory roles.

CLINICAL PRESENTATION

Subjective

Atopic dermatitis is characterized by an extremely low threshold for pruritus and has been referred to as "the itch that rashes." Usually, the itch occurs before the rash appears, and scratching the rash worsens it clinically. In fact, the cardinal sign of atopic dermatitis is severe pruritus, which is often extremely distressing in both the acute and chronic stages. In turn, the diagnosis of atopic dermatitis cannot be made without a history of pruritus, and if pruritus is absent, alternate diagnoses should be sought.

The patient may report a personal or family history of other atopic conditions (e.g., asthma, allergic rhinitis). In addition, the patient usually reports a history of episodic exacerbation of similar symptoms or a childhood rash or eczema. Often, the rash is reported as better in the warmer months and worse in the fall and winter. The clinician should inquire about any exposure to known or unknown common antigens and irritants, regardless of the history. Individuals with atopic dermatitis may also develop contact dermatitis; in fact, they are more susceptible to irritant reactions because of the impaired barrier function of their epidermal skin layer.

Objective

Atopic dermatitis usually begins as infantile eczema, with lesions affecting the cheeks, face, and upper extremities. Erythema is often seen before pruritus, and the acute lesions are excoriated, maculopapular, and inflamed. In infancy and early childhood, oozing and crusting usually characterize the erythema. As the child becomes older, the disease can go into remission or change to a flexural distribution (i.e., occurring in the antecubital fossae and neck area). Flexural eczema usually lasts until about age 4 to 10 years but may continue into adulthood.

In adults, eczema presents with symmetrical lesions that are crusting and excoriated. In its early stages, lesions may be erythematous, papulovesicular, edematous, and weeping. Later, the rash becomes crusted, scaly, thickened, and lichenified. The classic locations for lesions are noted to correspond to areas that are most accessible to rubbing and scratching. In addition, the typical flexural sites are more susceptible because they are in areas that are more likely to be hot and moist (see Advanced Assessment 16.1). Intergluteal involvement is uncommon and should raise suspicion of another diagnosis.

DIAGNOSTIC REASONING

Diagnostic Tests

Laboratory tests are usually not useful in the diagnosis of atopic dermatitis, but they can be helpful in ruling out other disorders or confirming that a patient is prone to atopy, as the etiology of the rash. Alterations in cell-mediated immune responses contribute to an increased susceptibility of atopic patients to cutaneous viral infections, such as herpes simplex virus, vaccinia, and molluscum contagiosum. Thus, if a viral etiology of the rash is suspected, a viral culture should be done on the exudate and moist parts of the rash. If atopy is suspected, skin prick testing, a serum radioallergosorbent test (RAST),

---

> **Advanced Assessment 16.1: Atopic Dermatitis**
>
> **DISTRIBUTION**
>
> Infants: trunk, face, extensor surfaces, scalp
> Children: antecubital fossae, popliteal fossae
> Adults: face, neck, upper chest, genital area, hands
>
> **STAGES**
>
> *Acute*
> Erosions with serous exudate
> Intense pruritus
> Papules and vesicles on an erythematous base
> Pain, heat, tenderness
>
> *Subacute*
> Scaly, excoriated
> Pruritus (may be intense)
> Papules or plaques over an erythematous base
> Secondary infection possible
>
> *Chronic*
> Lichenification, pigmentary changes (increased or decreased)
> Pruritus
> Excoriated papules and nodules
> Dryness, fissuring
>
> **OTHER CLINICAL MANIFESTATIONS**
>
> Keratosis pilaris ("chicken skin"): asymptomatic follicular papules, particularly on the posterolateral aspects of the upper arms and lateral thighs
> Lichenification of the skin, with a predilection for flexural creases
> Ichthyosis vulgaris: hyperlinearity of the palms and soles and fishlike scales, especially on the lower legs
> Dennie-Morgan lines (infraorbital folds) caused by edema
> Excessive fissuring of the earlobes, palms, soles, and fingers
> Pityriasis alba: hypopigmented asymptomatic areas on the face and shoulders
> Allergic "shiners": facial pallor and infraorbital darkening
> Anterior capsular cataracts
> Keratoconus: a cone-shaped cornea may develop in the second or third decade of life (in severe cases)
> Facial erythema, dry skin, history of wool intolerance, nonspecific hand dermatitis, and a tendency for skin infection (commonly impetiginization of excoriated skin)

or a second generation enzyme-linked immunosorbent assay test (ELISA) may be done. These tests are covered in Chapter 62, Hematological Disorders. An ELISA or fluorescent antibody staining technique (FAST) may be done to identify antigen-specific mast cell activation or to quantify levels of allergen-specific IgE, respectively.

The RAST or ELISA allergic (IgE) antibody test is usually available to primary care practitioners, whereas skin prick (scratch) testing is typically done only by board-certified allergists. Interpretation of RAST results requires specialized knowledge of the specificity and sensitivity of the assay because false-positive results are not uncommon. Thus, RAST should not be ordered arbitrarily or as a general atopic screening tool; instead, antigen-specific serum IgE testing should be directed by a detailed patient history. Commonly available RAST panels often include not only antigen-specific IgE levels but also antigen-specific IgG and IgM levels, which are not helpful in the diagnosis of atopic disease (hypersensitivity) and are therefore prone to misinterpretation.

A RAST panel may include testing for antigen-specific IgE to dust mites, mold, ragweed, animal dander, tree pollen, and many other allergens. RAST panels also exist for food allergens, which are often highly relevant in pediatric patients; however, true IgE-mediated food allergies are far less common in adults. Thus, RAST testing is useful for patients suspected of having an atopic history if directed by the patients' presenting signs, symptoms, and environmental exposures. An atopic or allergic tendency manifests as chronic or recurrent symptoms (in addition to dermatitis), which might include a history of allergic rhinitis (e.g., nasal congestion, chronic postnasal drip, sneezing, itchy nose) and asthma during childhood. Some patients will deny any allergic tendency but will report a history of frequent "sinus problems." A RAST is usually positive in patients with a history of symptoms of atopic dermatitis, but it often does not correlate well with clinical symptoms. Results appear to vary with the type of allergen being tested. Another potentially helpful marker for atopy is the total serum IgE level. Serum IgE levels are usually elevated during acute periods of dermatitis but may decrease during periods of remission. Higher levels of total serum IgE, however, also increase the tendency toward false-positive allergen-specific RAST results.

Allergen skin prick testing is considered useful because it is a direct functional test of a patient's allergic response, as it is based on antigen-specific IgE in the skin binding to mast cells and triggering an immediate hypersensitivity response. Patients should be advised to stop all antihistamines for at least 2 weeks before undergoing allergen skin testing, because these medications will interfere with skin prick test outcomes and may lead to false-negative results. In addition, delayed-type hypersensitivity responses to epicutaneously applied antigens (as used in scratch and skin-prick tests) may be blunted in atopic skin during periods of disease activity, so scratch tests should be avoided during flare periods to avoid uninterpretable results.

If the diagnosis proves elusive or if serious pathology (e.g., mycosis fungoides) is suspected, a skin biopsy can provide important information. The skin biopsy of atopic skin will reveal a thickened and hyperkeratoid epidermis, along with perivascular inflammation of the dermis. Patients with pustular superinfection should have their lesions cultured for antibiotic sensitivities if they do not heal in response to empiric therapy.

Differential Diagnosis

Both common and rare skin disorders can mimic atopic dermatitis. Common disorders include contact dermatitis, tinea infections (dermatophytosis), seborrheic dermatitis, and the early stages of mycosis fungoides (cutaneous T-cell lymphoma [CTCL]). In contact dermatitis, the characteristic linear or asymmetrical distribution of skin lesions helps to distinguish this condition from atopic dermatitis. The location and characteristic ring-like erythematous lesions with central clearing distinguish tinea corporis infections (ringworm) from atopic dermatitis. Mycosis fungoides skin lesions do not respond to topical corticosteroids; therefore, suspicious lesions in adults that do not respond to topical corticosteroids after a minimum of 2 weeks of treatment should be considered for skin biopsy.

If none of the common skin disorders apply, rare systemic diseases and skin disorders that can produce rashes that mimic atopic dermatitis should be considered (see Differential Diagnosis 16.1).

Differential Diagnosis 16.1: Atopic Dermatitis

Scabies
Seborrheic dermatitis
Allergic contact dermatitis
Tinea infections
Psoriasis
Ichthyosis
Dermatitis herpetiformis
Mycosis fungoides (cutaneous T-cell lymphoma)
Netherton's syndrome
Wiskott-Aldrich syndrome
Acrodermatitis enteropathica
Neurodermatitis
HIV infection (especially in children)
Phenylketonuria (if symptoms appear during the first year of life)
Hyper-immunoglobulin E syndrome
Dermatomyositis
Gluten-sensitive enteropathy
X-linked agammaglobulinemia
Selective IgA deficiency
Letterer-Siwe disease

MANAGEMENT

The primary aim in the management of atopic dermatitis is to control signs and symptoms, as no cure exists at present. The initial management of dermatitis embodies the fundamental principles of dermatology: precipitating factors should be eliminated, wet lesions should be dried, dried lesions should be hydrated, and inflammation should be treated with corticosteroids. Crucial to management is a careful and systematic assessment of trigger factors. The goals of management are to decrease pruritus, prevent secondary infection, and educate patients so that they can control the disease themselves. For example, atopic patients should be warned of their increased susceptibility to viral infections and encouraged to avoid exposure to infected individuals.

The critical importance of skin hydration cannot be overstated, as the chronic use and overuse of corticosteroids while neglecting sufficient skin hydration carry significant iatrogenic risks, including both local adverse effects (e.g., skin atrophy, local irritation, telangiectasias) and the potential adverse effects of systemic absorption (e.g., cataract formation, growth impairment, bone demineralization, adrenal suppression).

The benefits of primary prevention of atopic dermatitis, limitations of current research, and conflicting evidence are highlighted in Evidence-Based Nursing Practice 16.1.

Nonpharmacological Management

To avoid excessive irritation and skin dryness, patients with atopic dermatitis should use mild emollients (e.g., Cetaphil) as a substitute for soap. Controversy surrounds best bathing practices. Despite the chronic dryness of eczematous skin, showering has paradoxically been implicated in worsening the lesions of atopic dermatitis, possibly due to the physical trauma of strong water streams on the skin. Thus, soak baths are preferred, provided they are followed by the liberal application of moisturizers after partially patting dry the skin. This approach is referred to as "soak and smear." Soaps containing perfumes, coloring agents, or strong scents can be particularly irritating. If patients insist on the use of soap for cleanliness, glycerin soaps have been well tolerated and should be limited to the axilla, groin, and feet.

Excessive bathing can be detrimental in eczematous patients because bathing effectively removes the skin's protective oils. Older patients should take short, lukewarm showers with a mild water stream and avoid long, hot baths, which are extremely desiccating. The use of bubble baths and fragrance-containing oils should be discouraged. Bath oils are of minimal benefit because whatever oil remains on the skin after bathing is generally wiped off with toweling. Colloidal oatmeal baths (Aveeno) are soothing and may be helpful with more generalized lesions.

Evidence-Based Nursing Practice 16.1

ATOPIC DERMATITIS

Bawany F, Beck L, Järvinen K. Halting the March: Primary Prevention of Atopic Dermatitis and Food Allergies. *J Allergy Clin Immunol Pract*. 2020 Mar;8(3):860–875. doi:10.1016/j.jaip.2019.12.005.

Atopic dermatitis (AD) is one of the most common inflammatory skin conditions, affecting 15% to 30% of children and 2% to 10% of adults. Population-based studies suggest that having AD is associated with subsequent development of other atopic diseases, in what is known as the "atopic march." An overview of studies that investigate primary prevention strategies for the first two diseases in the atopic march, namely, AD and food allergies (FA), is presented. These strategies include emollients, breastfeeding, microbial exposures, probiotics, vitamin D and UV light, modifying water hardness, and immunotherapy. Some studies, including randomized controlled trials of emollients and microbial supplementation, have found encouraging results; however, the evidence remains limited and contradictory. With regard to breastfeeding, microbial and lifestyle exposures, vitamin D and UV light, water hardness, and immunotherapy, the lack of randomized controlled trials makes it difficult to draw definitive conclusions. Current American Academy of Pediatrics guidelines support the idea that breastfeeding for 3 to 4 months can decrease AD incidence in children younger than 2 years old. Recommendations regarding a direct relationship between breastfeeding and AD, however, cannot be made because of insufficient data. Regarding microbial supplementation, most guidelines do not recommend probiotics or prebiotics for the purpose of preventing allergic diseases because of limited evidence. Before definitive conclusions can be made regarding these interventions, more well-designed, longitudinal, and randomized controlled trials are required, particularly in at-risk populations.

Minimizing contact with cosmetics, deodorants, detergents, and solvents should be stressed. Moisturizers are useful in helping to prevent water loss and are most effective when applied immediately after patting the skin partially dry after a short shower or soak bath. Atopic dermatitis patients should be cautioned against using lotions and gels that contain alcohol, preservatives, and fragrances. Patients with atopic dermatitis should not use agents that contain lactic acid or other alpha-hydroxy/glycolic acids that can aggravate the condition.

Ointments that contain petroleum jelly form an occlusive layer and are more effective in preventing water loss than lotions, solutions, or creams. For less severe conditions or in hot, humid areas, creams that do not contain fragrance and have few preservatives are acceptable (e.g., Cetaphil cream, Eucerin, Dermabase, Unibase, and Vaseline Clinical Care Eczema Calming Lotion) and can be applied not only to dry eczematous lesions but also to all noninflamed areas of the skin to maintain hydration. Humidifiers are most helpful in maintaining skin hydration in cold and dry climates, but they can inadvertently contribute to an environment that is conducive to increased dust mite and mold growth. Acaricides are insecticides effective against dust mites; they may be used on all fomites (e.g., pillows, beds, sofas). After application, thorough vacuuming, preferably with a high-efficiency, particulate air–filtered apparatus, must be done to remove the insecticide. Antifungal cleaners for wet and damp areas are recommended for patients who are sensitive to mold. However, acaricides and other pesticides/chemical treatments have not been shown to be consistently helpful and are not first-line preventive treatments.

Pharmacological Management

If the skin lesions are wet, inflamed, or have an exudate, wet soaks or compresses with cool tap water, Burow's (aluminum acetate) solution (1:40 dilution), saline (1 teaspoon per pint of water), or silver nitrate solution (1% to 10%) can be used to dry the lesions and provide comfort. Burow's solution can be applied as a compress for 20 to 30 minutes four to six times throughout the day. Over-the-counter (OTC) topical corticosteroids should be immediately applied to inflamed areas after the soak. A prescription corticosteroid cream may be needed for more severe cases.

Although antihistamines are often used to relieve pruritus, they are usually ineffective in atopic dermatitis because histamine is not the only factor responsible for the mediation of pruritus in atopic dermatitis. The sedative effect of antihistamines may be more beneficial than their antipruritic properties if used at night. Individuals with atopic dermatitis have a tendency to scratch in their sleep, so sedation at bedtime may decrease the amount of scratching during sleep. First-generation H_1 blockers, such as ethanolamines (diphenhydramine) and phenothiazines (promethazine), are very sedating. Of note, sedating antihistamines are generally not recommended in children because they have been shown to lead to daytime drowsiness and impair school performance, as well as have a paradoxical effect of inducing hyperactivity in some children. Thus, sedating patients at night for severe atopic dermatitis, urticaria, or other forms of pruritus only applies to adults.

Some tricyclic antidepressants, such as doxepin (Sinequan), have potent antihistaminic activity as well and are useful in urticaria, atopic dermatitis, and other forms of pruritus. An added benefit to using an antidepressant agent is the relief of depression that may accompany severe atopic dermatitis.

Montelukast sodium (Singulair) 5 to 10 mg daily may contribute to the relief of atopic dermatitis in a patient with other forms of concurrent atopy. Montelukast is a leukotriene-receptor antagonist that inhibits eosinophilic infiltration in the skin, a major histological characteristic of atopic dermatitis. Of note, however, montelukast is not approved by the U.S. Food and Drug Administration (FDA) for the treatment of atopic dermatitis. In addition, the FDA issued a boxed warning for montelukast in 2020 regarding serious neuropsychiatric events, including behavioral and mood changes.

Corticosteroids are effective anti-inflammatory agents and are usually considered first-line pharmacotherapy for atopic dermatitis, although their use must always be preceded by optimal moisturization, because restoring skin hydration is the most important step in breaking the itch–scratch cycle of atopic dermatitis. In addition, the use of emollients (e.g., petroleum jelly, Eucerin, Lubriderm) will enhance the absorption and effectiveness of topical corticosteroids. Applying topical corticosteroids after hydrating the skin (after a brief shower or bath) may increase their absorption up to 10-fold. A weak coal tar preparation applied over a corticosteroid ointment can also reduce itching at night.

Crisaborole (Eucrisa) is a low molecular weight benzoxaborole, nonsteroidal, full-body topical ointment indicated for the treatment of mild to moderate atopic dermatitis in patients 3 months of age and older. Crisaborole's mode of action is not fully defined, although it appears to block overactive Phosphodiesterase-4 (PDE_4) enzymes within skin cells. Blocking PDE_4 is believed to reduce inflammation related to eczema.

Acute exacerbations of atopic dermatitis can be treated with a potent to mid-strength topical corticosteroid for a few days to quickly control acutely inflamed skin lesions, but the patient should switch to a weaker-strength agent once the lesion is under control. Medium- to high-potency topical corticosteroids (see Box 16.1) should not be used on the face or neck area because of potential adverse effects such as local irritation, atrophy of the skin, and formation of telangiectasias. Skin atrophy is more likely to occur when potent topical corticosteroids are applied repeatedly to thin and highly absorptive inflamed skin. In some instances, hypopigmentation has been associated with the use of topical corticosteroids, especially in darker-skinned individuals. Most cases of pigmentation changes are related to the underlying dermatitis, however, not the use of topical corticosteroids. Topical corticosteroids may also complicate treatment by masking underlying bacterial or fungal infections or impairing healing processes. Topical corticosteroids should never be used on ulcerated skin due to the risk of increased direct absorption and impaired skin healing.

Systemic corticosteroids are rarely necessary for the treatment of chronic atopic dermatitis, but they may be useful for an incapacitating acute exacerbation or when large numbers of weeping lesions are present. In these rare instances, the patient may benefit from a short course of oral prednisone (40 to 60 mg/day for adults and 1 mg/kg/day for children). Short-term therapy with prednisone does not require tapering if it is limited to 5 to 7 days and the patient does not have a history of recent oral prednisone use. As the lesions dry, topical

> **Box 16.1 Potency of Topical Corticosteroids**
>
> **Extremely High Potency**
> Betamethasone dipropionate, augmented 0.05%
> Clobetasol propionate 0.05%
> Fluocinonide 0.1%
> Flurandrenolide 4 mcg/cm^2 (tape)
> Halobetasol propionate 0.05%
>
> **High Potency**
> Amcinonide 0.1%
> Betamethasone dipropionate 0.05%
> Desoximetasone 0.05%, 0.25%
> Diflorasone diacetate 0.05%
> Fluocinonide 0.05%
> Halcinonide 0.1%
> Triamcinolone acetonide 0.5%
>
> **Intermediate Potency**
> Betamethasone valerate 0.05%, 0.12%
> Clocortolone pivalate 0.1%
> Desonide 0.05%
> Desoximetasone 0.05%
> Fluocinolone acetonide 0.025%
> Flurandrenolide 0.025%, 0.05%
> Fluticasone propionate 0.005%, 0.05%
> Hydrocortisone probutate 0.1%
> Hydrocortisone butyrate 0.1%
> Hydrocortisone valerate 0.2%
> Mometasone furoate 0.1%
> Prednicarbate 0.1%
> Triamcinolone acetonide 0.05%, 0.1%, 0.2%
>
> **Low Potency**
> Alclometasone dipropionate 0.05%
> Fluocinolone acetonide 0.01%
> Hydrocortisone base or acetate 1%, 1.85%, 2%, 2.5%
> Triamcinolone acetonide 0.025%

corticosteroids may be started. Of note, given the significant adverse effects associated with systemic corticosteroid use, such regimens should be considered a last resort and not used regularly. In some instances, the decision to use systemic corticosteroids to treat atopic dermatitis may signify the need for inpatient care to gain control of a debilitating exacerbation, particularly in pediatric patients.

When the acute inflammation subsides after 2 to 3 weeks, the patient should decrease the frequency of the topical corticosteroids and focus primarily on emollients such as petroleum jelly or Eucerin cream. The chronic use of topical corticosteroids (mid- to low-strength) should be limited to twice-weekly applications to any given area and should not be continued indefinitely.

Topical tacrolimus (Protopic) and the related agent pimecrolimus (Elidel), applied twice per day, have been shown to be effective and safe for use as second-line agents in atopic dermatitis. These are immunomodulating calcineurin inhibitors. Most patients experience a dramatic reduction of pruritus within 3 days of initiating treatment and have significant improvement in quality of life. When used as long-term maintenance therapy, topical preparations reduce the number of flares of atopic dermatitis and the requirement for corticosteroid treatment. Of note, given limitations in long-term safety data for these agents, including rare reports of malignancy, the FDA has issued a boxed warning for tacrolimus and pimecrolimus, warning clinicians against continuous long-term use of these agents in any age-group and highlighting the lack of approval of these agents in children younger than 2 years.

Aggressive treatment of refractory atopic dermatitis may also include cyclosporine A, an immunomodulatory drug, which may be as effective as corticosteroids with fewer adverse effects. It may be used in patients who have failed to respond to at least one systemic therapy or in patients for whom other systemic therapies are contraindicated or are intolerable. Its use can be highly beneficial in severe cases, but kidney function must be closely monitored, given the potential for renal vasoconstriction, and treatment courses must be restricted to 8 to 12 weeks. Azathioprine (Imuran) may also be used for maintenance therapy, but hematological parameters and hepatic function must be monitored, given its known toxicity risks. As with systemic corticosteroids, the use of a systemic immunosuppressant such as cyclosporine A or azathioprine for atopic dermatitis would strongly suggest the need for inpatient care to adequately control such an exacerbation.

Omalizumab (Xolair), an anti-IgE antibody that has been developed as an immunotherapeutic biological agent, has shown benefit in reducing atopy in highly allergic individuals, although it is not FDA approved to treat atopic dermatitis. In severe cases of atopic dermatitis, phototherapy with ultraviolet B radiation or PUVA (psoralen with ultraviolet A radiation) photochemotherapy may be used as an adjunct therapy. Lesions of patients with pustular superinfection should be cultured for antibiotic sensitivities if they do not heal in response to empiric antibiotic treatment, as bacterial or fungal superinfections must be treated appropriately.

Dupilumab (Dupixent), a subcutaneously injected cytokine-specific monoclonal antibody, has been approved by the FDA to treat adults with moderate to severe atopic dermatitis. By binding to the IL-4 receptor alpha (IL-4Rα), dupilumab inhibits inflammatory responses mediated by IL-4 and IL-13, which both utilize this shared cytokine receptor protein. Intended for patients whose atopic dermatitis is uncontrolled with topical therapies, dupilumab may cause side effects including conjunctivitis, corneal inflammation, and oral cold sores.

Complementary Therapies

There is limited evidence that mind–body relaxation techniques (e.g., yoga, meditation) may help improve symptoms of atopic dermatitis, particularly in the pediatric population. However, clinical studies of these therapies have not been methodologically rigorous.

Studies indicate that certain plants and herbs may be of value in the treatment of dermatological conditions. These include chamomile, arnica, calendula (marigold), hamamelis (witch hazel), aloe vera, cardiospermum, *Mahonia aquifolium*, oak bark, bittersweet stalk, and capsicum. Use of these herbs should be reserved for experienced practitioners in alternative health medicine because of the potential for allergic reactions. Complementary Therapies 16.1 lists herbs that are used in the treatment of eczema.

FOLLOW-UP AND REFERRAL

If basic management of atopic dermatitis fails, specialty referral to an allergist or dermatologist should be prompt. More aggressive treatment by a specialist is necessary for patients who have severe and extensive lesions or who do not respond to usual treatment with topical or systemic corticosteroids. Atopic skin is very susceptible to bacterial and viral infections. These patients may develop a widespread herpetic skin infection known as eczema herpeticum, which may be severe and life-threatening in children. Thus, patients with atopic dermatitis should avoid contact with people with active herpetic lesions. During an exacerbation, patients may contract secondary bacterial infections, and empiric therapy with erythromycin or penicillinase-resistant penicillin may be necessary.

Because *S. aureus* colonizes the skin of more than 90% of patients with atopic dermatitis (compared with only 5% of people without the disease), fingernails should be kept short, smooth, and clean to minimize trauma from scratching that exacerbates skin inflammation and allows microbes to be introduced into the skin. Bleach baths may be used one to two times per week as a means of decreasing the severity of atopic dermatitis by reducing bacterial skin colonization (i.e., one-half cup of unscented laundry bleach is added to a full bathtub of lukewarm water for a 20-minute soak). However, bleach baths may not be any more effective than water baths alone.

Patients should be informed that a change in seasons may cause an exacerbation of their disease, especially during the fall. Patients can be reminded to take extra care of their skin at this time by upgrading to stronger moisturizers (e.g., from lotions or creams to petroleum jelly). Refills of medications should be ordered before the recurrence of symptoms to allow for prompt treatment of acutely inflamed lesions. The primary care provider can assist the patient in developing a simple regimen of topical corticosteroid therapy for acute exacerbations. Patients with frequent exacerbations of skin lesions on their hands should avoid occupations that require repeated hand washing, immersion in water, or other wet conditions.

Food allergies are a common aggravating factor in up to 20% of patients with atopic dermatitis and are more common in children. Food sensitivities may be assessed through the judicious use of skin prick testing or RAST (food antigen–specific IgE) panels, provided interpretation of the results is done by an adequately trained clinician with the specialized knowledge to execute and interpret these tests. A dietitian should then be consulted when patients are eliminating foods from their diet because unsupervised food restriction may lead to malnutrition.

Complementary Therapies 16.1: Herbal Treatments for Eczema

HERB	COMMENTS
Chamomile (*Matricaria recutita*)	Topical application Anti-inflammatory properties Contraindicated in patients with ragweed allergy
Evening primrose (*Oenothera biennis*)	Should not be taken with phenothiazines
Marigold (*Calendula officinalis*)	Topical application—ointment or cream Anti-inflammatory properties
Goldenseal (*Hydrastis canadensis*)	Topical application Powdered root mixed with water to make a paste and applied to rash
Licorice (*Glycyrrhiza glabra*)	Topical application Anti-inflammatory properties
Turmeric (*Curcuma longa*)	Topical application Anti-inflammatory properties

> **Patient Education: Atopic Dermatitis**
>
> Patients with atopic dermatitis should be educated to be vigilant in watching for the signs of secondary bacterial infection and to report them immediately so that an oral antibiotic can be prescribed. Education about the importance of environmental measures in the prevention of disease exacerbations should be emphasized. House dust mites, animal dander, and pollen may all be identified as potential triggers based on antigen-specific IgE antibodies in the bloodstream and a consistent exposure-response history. In turn, avoidance of these triggers should be addressed when educating patients. Patients can also be counseled to reduce sweating, which may exacerbate wet lesions, by limiting the amount of bedclothes at night, avoiding hot occlusive garments, and keeping living areas cool. Patients should be encouraged to recognize their stress "triggers" and find measures to reduce their stress level, such as exercise.

CONTACT DERMATITIS

Contact dermatitis is a common condition categorized as either *irritant dermatitis* or *allergic dermatitis*. Although both of these conditions can have similar presentations, the etiology of each disease is what differentiates the two dermatitides. *Allergic contact dermatitis* is immunologically mediated, whereas *irritant contact dermatitis* is the result of repeated "insults" to atopic skin from caustic, irritant, or detergent-type substances.

EPIDEMIOLOGY AND CAUSES

Almost any substance may induce a cutaneous reaction depending on its concentration, the duration of contact, and the condition of the exposed skin. The etiology of allergic contact dermatitis may be from antimicrobials such as neomycin, antihistamines, anesthetics such as benzocaine, hair dyes, preservatives, latex, nickel, or adhesive tape. Hair-care practices of patients with tightly curled hair may also be contributing factors. The etiology of irritant contact dermatitis may be from soaps; detergents; organic solvents; or prolonged contact with masks, goggles, and protective gloves. Irritant contact dermatitis accounts for about 80% of all cases of contact dermatitis.

Delayed-type hypersensitivity reactions are immunological responses to contact allergens that occur in sensitized individuals. One of the most frequent causes of allergic contact dermatitis is from plants in the *Rhus* genus, which includes poison ivy, poison oak, and poison sumac. Other common topical sensitizers include ragweed pollen, dust mites, ethylenediamine (a stabilizer in many topical creams), potassium dichromate, paraphenylenediamine (dyes), nickel (10% of females are allergic to nickel often found in inexpensive jewelry, belt buckles, and metal fasteners on clothing), rubber compounds, and benzocaine (an OTC topical anesthetic for itching or pain). It is estimated that there are more than 6 million chemicals in the environment and that approximately 3,000 of them are potential sensitizers.

Contact dermatitis accounts for 4% to 7% of all dermatology consults. Hand dermatitis affects 2% of the population at any given time, and 20% of females will be affected at least once in their lifetime. Contact dermatitis is more common in adults than in children, and effects are more extreme in older patients. Women are twice as likely as men to develop dermatitis and are at highest risk after childbirth. White Americans are affected more frequently, and fair-skinned redheads are the most vulnerable population.

PATHOPHYSIOLOGY

Contact dermatitis is considered either allergic or irritant induced. A delayed-type hypersensitivity response (type IV immune reaction) elicits a non–IgE-mediated allergic response to specific antigens when applied to the skin, producing a local reaction characterized histologically by epidermal changes, including intracellular edema, spongiosis, and vesiculation. On initial contact with the offending agent, the antigen is taken up and processed by epidermal antigen-presenting cells known as Langerhans cells. These cells present antigens to naïve, antigen-specific CD4+ and CD8+ T lymphocytes, located in regional lymph nodes that drain the affected areas of skin. Over approximately 10 to 14 days, sensitized T cells migrate from the lymph nodes to sites of antigenic exposure, where subsequent reexposure to the same antigen results in an allergic reaction mediated by cytokine release. This response with notable skin surface changes typically occurs within 12 to 48 hours of reexposure to the antigen.

Irritant contact dermatitis is the result of a direct cytotoxic effect of an irritant on the cells of the epidermis, with a subsequent inflammatory response in the dermis. The main pathological feature of contact dermatitis is intracellular edema of the epidermis, which may result in intraepidermal vesicles and bullae formation in the acute phase. In chronic cases, papules, scaling, and lichenification occur. Irritants penetrate and disrupt the stratum corneum and injure the underlying epidermis and dermis as various immune cells congregate around dilated capillaries, contributing to the inflammatory process.

Rubber-glove dermatitis demonstrates the spectrum of pathophysiological mechanisms involved in contact dermatitis. Chemical irritants used in the glove manufacturing process (e.g., thiram, mercapto derivatives) may cause an allergic dermatitis via a delayed-type, T-cell–mediated hypersensitivity reaction. In addition, rubber glove components may result in a direct irritant effect on the moist skin of glove wearers. Finally, the natural rubber protein *latex,* once widely used in medical products, may elicit a profound, IgE-mediated, immediate hypersensitivity response, leading to systemic anaphylaxis and even death.

Interestingly, people with venous stasis (i.e., impaired venous return with pooling of blood in distended veins, particularly in the lower extremities) are more susceptible to irritant contact dermatitis, particularly from wood alcohols such as lanolin, fragrances, topical antibiotics such as neomycin, and methylparaben preservatives. Correctly diagnosing this condition is often difficult in these patients because contact dermatitis may be confused with stasis dermatitis.

CLINICAL PRESENTATION

Subjective

The cardinal symptom of contact dermatitis is a pruritic erythematous rash. Often, the patient is not aware of a previous history, but there may have been periodic episodes of a pruritic rash that resolved spontaneously. The patient may or may not be able to describe the conditions or substances contributing to the dermatitis, but the clinician should seek the patient's exposure history to known or unknown common antigens and irritants. In allergic contact dermatitis (in contrast to atopic dermatitis), the inflammatory reaction on the skin occurs much faster, typically within 6 to 12 hours of reexposure. In contrast to allergic contact dermatitis, irritant reactions do not always occur immediately after contact with the offending substance. The response time between the initial contact with the irritant and symptom development varies, and the severity of the reaction depends on the concentration, amount, and length of exposure to the irritating substance. The stages of clinical presentation of contact dermatitis are listed in Advanced Assessment 16.2.

Objective

Contact dermatitis presents with inflammation of the epidermis and is manifested by erythema (as in all types of dermatitis), but it does not present with the smooth, intact epidermal surface that characterizes hives (urticaria). The epidermal inflammation seen in acute contact dermatitis results in rough, reddened patches, but without the skin thickening and discrete demarcation of psoriasis. The acute presentation of contact dermatitis is characterized by weeping lesions with numerous tiny vesicles on an erythematous base that is pruritic or has a burning or stinging sensation. The surrounding area in severe cases is also erythematous, with edema and increased heat in the area, making it difficult to rule out secondary bacterial infection in some cases.

Lesions in nonallergic and delayed-type hypersensitivity contact dermatitis present in similar fashion, but the typical

>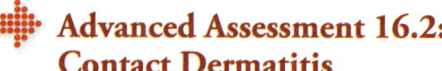
> ### Advanced Assessment 16.2: Contact Dermatitis
>
> **STAGES**
>
> ***Acute***
> Erythema and edema
> Clear, fluid-filled vesicles or bullae
> Exudate, clear fluid
> Distinct margins
> ***Subacute***
> Lessening edema
> Formation of papules
> Less distinct margins
> ***Chronic***
> Minimal edema
> Scaling skin
> Lichenification
> Minimal erythema

distribution and the lack of an atopic history are the most helpful factors in the diagnosis. Often, the location of the rash gives the clinician the best clue as to the possible etiological agent (see Advanced Assessment 16.1). Usually, the area of skin that has been the most heavily contaminated will break out first, followed by areas of lesser exposure.

For example, a patient with a rash on the scalp and the back of the neck might report a history of using a new shampoo, hair dye, or other scalp or hair treatment. A clothing- or detergent-related cause should be suspected if the lesions are generalized and primarily affect the borders of the axillae, waist, and upper thighs. Lesions in an area where jewelry has been worn recently (e.g., neck, wrist, earlobes) or where metal fasteners contact the skin (e.g., the infraumbilical area for belt buckles or snaps on denim pants) may indicate hypersensitivity to nickel. Reactions to toxic plants (e.g., *Rhus* or *Toxicodendron* species) are common on the extremities and follow a history of exposure. The characteristic rash is vesicular and linear (often asymmetrical) and is frequently found on the hands and ankles. *Rhus* dermatitis lesions may also be found on the facial area if the patient has inadvertently scratched the face with contaminated fingers.

DIAGNOSTIC REASONING

Diagnostic Tests

The diagnosis of contact dermatitis is based on the history of exposure to an irritant or allergen and the subsequent appearance of a rash on the exposed skin, either rapidly or one or more days after exposure (delayed hypersensitivity). If scabies is suspected, skin scrapings can be examined under a microscope to rule out that infestation. If tinea (corporis, cruris, pedis, capitis, manuum) infection is suspected, skin scrapings should be treated with potassium hydroxide (KOH) and gently heated on a glass slide; subsequent microscopic examination for tinea infection should search for septate hyphae and spores. If bacterial infection (impetigo) is suspected, cultures should be taken from the moist areas of the rash or from the discharge. Viral cultures can be done to rule out suspected viral etiology (e.g., herpes simplex, herpes zoster).

Laboratory tests that are done by specialists (e.g., allergists, dermatologists) include the scratch (skin prick), patch, and intradermal tests. These tests should not be done during an acute episode of contact dermatitis, however, because of an increased rate of false-positive reactions. The patch test is useful in identifying specific irritants in patients with histories that are suggestive of acute contact dermatitis. Allergens that are commonly responsible for such reactions are fixed in dehydrated gel layers or mixed in a small amount of petroleum jelly and taped against the skin of the patient's back for 48 hours and then removed. A negative control patch with only the vehicle without antigen should also be applied to rule out nonspecific reactions. A final reading done at 72 to 96 hours after initial application will usually reveal any evidence of contact dermatitis. In some patients, a complete blood count (CBC) with differential will show eosinophilia, but this blood test is neither sensitive nor necessary for the diagnosis. Skin biopsy is rarely necessary for diagnosis, particularly with a convincing contact exposure history.

Differential Diagnosis

The differential diagnosis of contact dermatitis is similar to that of atopic dermatitis and includes both common and rare disorders. Common disorders that have a similar presentation to contact dermatitis include seborrheic dermatitis, impetigo, and herpes zoster. Seborrheic dermatitis rashes, although erythematous, have a greasy and scaly appearance and appear only in certain areas of the body, such as the hairline, ears, scalp, and face. Impetigo, which is caused by gram-positive *Staphylococcus* or *Streptococcus* bacteria, is more common in children. A honey-colored crust is seen on top of erythematous lesions; impetigo also does not have a linear appearance like the rash of contact dermatitis. Herpes zoster is more common in older patients, and the lesions appear as multiple small vesicles on an erythematous base. Although herpes zoster has a linear distribution, it is more likely to occur on the trunk area (contact dermatitis occurs more often on the hands or face) and will follow the path of a dermatome.

MANAGEMENT

The clinical challenge in the treatment of contact dermatitis is to provide symptomatic relief to the patient while attempting to identify the underlying allergic precipitant. Identifying the antigen or irritant in contact dermatitis is critical, both to eliminate or minimize the current contact and to avoid future exposure. The responsible irritant should be identified and eliminated to prevent the cycle of itching, scratching, and skin disruption, which can lead to chronic changes in the skin. A careful history of exposures is key, in addition to a thorough skin examination. The effects of *Rhus* dermatitis (from poison ivy, poison oak, or poison sumac) may be lessened if the exposed skin is thoroughly rinsed in soap and water or with isopropyl alcohol as soon as possible after exposure. Exposed clothing should be discarded.

For localized contact dermatitis with weeping lesions, treatment with moist compresses and simple drying agents or antipruritic lotions (e.g., Burow's aluminum acetate solution, calamine lotion) applied several times a day is usually effective. For more extensive and severe cases, potent topical corticosteroids in cream form (avoiding the use of ointments on wet lesions because they can cause skin maceration) can be applied twice daily for the first few days to help decrease pruritus and inflammation. If treatment is necessary beyond 2 weeks, a less potent (mild or moderate) topical corticosteroid may be used twice daily until the rash resolves. High-potency corticosteroids (see Box 16.1) should not be used on the face or in body folds (intertriginous areas) because of their ability to thin the skin and cause hypopigmentation.

Oral systemic corticosteroids may be indicated in acute and particularly severe cases of contact dermatitis, offering relief within 12 to 24 hours. For example, relatively high doses of oral prednisone can be given for 10 to 14 days (or up to 21 days in the most severe cases). However, abrupt cessation of high-dose systemic corticosteroids given for more than 1 week should be avoided, with tapering used for regimens lasting longer than this to decrease the risk of adrenal suppression. Potential adverse effects of oral corticosteroid therapy are more likely with long-term use and may include any of the following: suppression of the hypothalamic-pituitary-adrenal (HPA) axis; hypokalemia; hypocalcemia; masking or worsening of infection; increased likelihood of secondary infection; carbohydrate intolerance and worsening of diabetes mellitus; glaucoma; cataracts; osteoporosis; dermal atrophy; skin hypopigmentation; and psychiatric disorders including depression, euphoria, or acute psychosis. It should also be noted that even systemic corticosteroids will likely prove ineffective if exposure to the offending allergen or irritant is not limited.

FOLLOW-UP AND REFERRAL

Follow-up and referral are determined by the patient's condition and response to therapy. Although most cases of contact dermatitis are effectively managed by the primary care practitioner, with at least one follow-up visit after a week to assess therapeutic response (thereby confirming the diagnosis), severe cases should be referred to a dermatologist or an allergist.

Patient Education: Contact Dermatitis

The provider should teach the patient and family about the disease course, how to recognize triggers (i.e., exposure to allergen or irritant 24 to 72 hours before the onset of rash) and prevent future contact, the appropriate use of medications, and signs of an exacerbation that should prompt the patient to seek care. The mainstay of prevention is helping patients to identify the agents causing the dermatitis and teaching them to avoid exposure; use protective clothing and gloves; and prevent the spread of contact allergens by avoiding scratching, trimming the fingernails, and thorough hand washing. Protective facial masks, which have become increasingly common in the avoidance of communicable diseases such as COVID-19, should be washed frequently if reusable (i.e., cloth masks).

SEBORRHEIC DERMATITIS

Seborrheic dermatitis is one of the most common skin conditions seen in primary care among adults and older patients. It is a chronic condition that is characterized by remissions and exacerbations and may be a sign of more serious underlying pathology, such as immune suppression. The rash of seborrheic dermatitis manifests on skin that is rich in sebaceous glands, such as the scalp, forehead, eyebrows, and areas surrounding the nose and ears.

EPIDEMIOLOGY AND CAUSES

Seborrheic dermatitis affects approximately 3% to 5% of the adult population. It runs in families and has a known genetic component. It may be an inflammatory reaction to *Malassezia furfur* yeasts. The occurrence of seborrheic dermatitis is most common during early infancy on the scalp ("cradle cap"), after the second decade of life, and in older adults or immunocompromised patients. A strong association with HIV infection and AIDS is well established, and severe or resistant cases of seborrheic dermatitis should prompt investigation for the risk factors of HIV infection. Emotional stress has also been associated with acute flares.

PATHOPHYSIOLOGY

This type of dermatitis was originally defined by excess oil secretion from the sebaceous glands and is thus found on areas of the body where such glands are most concentrated. In decreasing order, these include the scalp, face, chest, upper back, pubic area, and axillae. Interestingly, however, overproduction of sebum is not seen in all cases of seborrheic dermatitis. The condition is not thought to be a classic allergic reaction nor the result of poor hygiene. Skin biopsies typically reveal parakeratotic scale heaped around hair follicles and an inflammatory lymphocytic infiltrate. Thus, mild epidermal hyperproliferation has been cited as a contributing factor.

M. furfur commonly colonizes affected individuals. However, it is not known whether seborrheic dermatitis occurs in response to infection by saprophytic skin fungi or if the disease process creates conditions that may predispose affected skin to superficial fungal infection. Of note, the recurrence of symptoms has been linked to an increase in the number of *M. furfur* organisms found on the skin surface, and fungal-specific stains of affected skin reveal large numbers of fungal spores within the stratum corneum, the uppermost skin layer.

CLINICAL PRESENTATION

Subjective

The typical patient is an adult man who complains of a pink, scaling rash located on the face and scalp. Darker-skinned individuals may present with scaly, hypopigmented macules and patches. Infants of color often do not experience the "cradle cap" appearance that white infants do, and instead have erythema, flaking, and hypopigmentation of the scalp.

Seborrheic dermatitis can also be an incidental finding, as some patients are not bothered by the cosmetic effect of the rashes. The lesions are usually asymptomatic in most patients, but pruritus may be present and is aggravated by perspiration, especially with scalp lesions.

Objective

Seborrheic dermatitis presents as scaly patches that may be slightly papular; each patch is surrounded by erythema. The affected skin is pink, edematous, and covered with yellow to brown scales and crusts. The lesion borders are poorly defined, and the scales may appear greasy. The most frequently involved area is the scalp, and the condition is differentiated from common dandruff (pityriasis sicca) by the appearance of erythema, which may be minimal or moderate. Commonly affected areas include the forehead at the hairline, eyebrows, nasal folds, and the retroauricular and presternal areas. In more severe cases, intertriginous areas, the external ear canal, or the umbilicus may be involved. These rashes may be more difficult to recognize in fastidious patients because daily bathing removes some of the scale.

DIAGNOSTIC REASONING

Diagnostic Tests

The diagnosis of seborrheic dermatitis is based on clinical findings and the medical history. Dermatologists and allergists can test for *M. furfur*, using antigen-specific skin prick or serum RAST testing. Fifteen percent to 65% of patients with seborrheic dermatitis have positive responses to skin prick tests with *Malassezia* extracts. *Malassezia* antibodies have also been found in young adults with head and neck dermatitis. Fungal-specific periodic acid-Schiff and Gomori methenamine silver stains identify hyphae and spores in skin scrapings or biopsy samples; however, these specialized stains typically require specialist referral and are not commonly used in the primary care setting. Rather, the diagnosis of seborrheic dermatitis is most frequently based on the characteristic appearance and distribution of the rash, as well as its response to empiric therapy.

Differential Diagnosis

Skin conditions that mimic seborrheic dermatitis include impetigo, atopic dermatitis, psoriasis, scabies, tinea capitis, and Langerhans cell histiocytosis. A history of the same rash recurring at characteristic locations on the body (e.g., the scalp and hairline, sides of the nose and upper lip, eyebrows and eyelashes, cheeks, or ears) will give the clinician the best clues to identify seborrheic dermatitis accurately.

Impetigo, a bacterial infection of the skin caused by *Staphylococcus* or *Streptococcus* bacteria, has an acute onset and tends to occur on the extremities such as the sides of fingers (a location not seen in seborrheic dermatitis) or on the face under the nose (due to repeated wiping of nasal secretions with the hands). The most useful distinguishing feature between atopic dermatitis and seborrheic dermatitis is the increased number of lesions on the forearms in the former, compared with the increased number of lesions in the axillae in the latter. The erythema of seborrheic dermatitis typically has a pinkish hue, rather than the bright-red appearance of psoriasis.

Seborrheic dermatitis is also associated with several chronic conditions including Parkinson's disease, HIV infection and AIDS, phenylketonuria, cardiac failure, zinc deficiency, and epilepsy. This association is not specific, however, as other dermatological disorders such as acne vulgaris, rosacea, and psoriasis may also be associated with these diseases. Importantly, florid manifestations of seborrheic dermatitis may be an early cutaneous indicator of HIV infection, and these patients may demonstrate extensive symptoms that are often resistant to therapy.

MANAGEMENT

The high incidence and chronic benign nature of seborrheic dermatitis present a therapeutic challenge. Mild to moderate cases do not seem to bother some patients, especially those who frequently refuse treatment or are noncompliant. In contrast, younger patients who are bothered by the cosmetic effects of rashes on the face frequently request treatment. The therapeutic approach is aimed at managing symptoms and reducing the yeast count on the skin.

The regular use of an OTC antidandruff shampoo is sufficient to control most scalp lesions. The preparation must remain on the scalp for at least 5 to 7 minutes to be effective. Commonly used ingredients in these products include selenium sulfide, zinc pyrithione, coal tar, salicylic acid, sulfur, or ketoconazole. Zinc pyrithione and selenium sulfide are classified as keratolytic agents. They appear to be both fungicidal and cytostatic. The combination of sulfur and salicylic acid has keratolytic, antifungal, and antiseptic actions. Patients of color may require a modified treatment plan that takes into consideration differences in hair texture and frequency of hair washing. Coal tar shampoo should be used with caution in people with light-colored or dyed hair because changes in hair color may occur while the product is being used.

Resistant seborrheic dermatitis may require a prescription shampoo. Selenium sulfide 2.5% shampoo (Selsun 2.5%) and ketoconazole 2% shampoo (Nizoral 2%) are both available. Ketoconazole shampoo and similar antifungal products are recommended to be used every other day for resistant cases. When there is facial or chest involvement, ketoconazole 2% cream may be applied to the affected areas twice daily. Topical ketoconazole (Nizoral 1%) is available OTC. Keratolytic or oil-based lotions are recommended to soften heavy crusts.

A topical corticosteroid may be necessary when significant erythema is present. Selenium sulfide 2.5% shampoo (Selsun 2.5%)) for the face or betamethasone valerate 0.1% for the scalp should be applied after cleansing. Facial application and long-term use of topical corticosteroids should be avoided because of the risk of telangiectasias and dermal atrophy. These risks are not present with the topical use of ketoconazole (Nizoral 1%). Exudative lesions may require compresses of Burow's solution applied for 30 minutes three times daily for a drying effect.

Calcineurin inhibitors that decrease the activity of the immune system may be effective for recalcitrant cases, although these drugs are not FDA approved for seborrheic dermatitis. Such agents include tacrolimus (Protopic) and pimecrolimus (Elidel), which are available in topical formulations. As indicated for second-line therapy in atopic dermatitis, the FDA cautions against the chronic use of these medications in any age-group, given concerns over their long-term safety, including rare reports of malignancies.

Once symptoms resolve, maintenance therapy may be required with a once- to twice-a-week application of a topical product for prophylaxis, such as ketoconazole (Nizoral) shampoo or an OTC antidandruff shampoo (Head and Shoulders, Selsun Blue). For a superinfection of gram-positive skin bacteria, an appropriate antibiotic course is indicated, as guided by the patient's allergy history (e.g., cephalexin given for 7 to 10 days in patients without penicillin allergy). Similarly, given the strong association of severe seborrheic dermatitis with HIV infection and AIDS, treating a patient's underlying HIV infection with effective antiretroviral therapy is often the key to resolution of the patient's skin findings.

FOLLOW-UP AND REFERRAL

Although uncomplicated forms of seborrheic dermatitis are readily managed by the primary care practitioner, repeated secondary infections or resistance to standard management requires a prompt referral to a dermatologist. In addition, underlying exacerbating factors, such as immune suppression or neurodegenerative disorders that have an impact on self-care, also require appropriate referrals.

> **Patient Education: Seborrheic Dermatitis**
>
> Patients should be reassured that seborrheic dermatitis in and of itself is neither contagious nor progressive. They must understand the chronic nature of the condition and the need for continued management, as well as the potential for this condition to be associated with more serious underlying disorders, such as immunosuppression, poor self-care, or superinfection. The role of emotional stress in acute flare-ups should also be noted and addressed with self-relaxation techniques. If topical corticosteroids are used, the patient needs to be instructed in their proper application and the potential adverse effects of indiscriminate use. A list of effective OTC preparations should be provided, so each patient can select one that meets their personal preferences. Daily shampooing of oily hair is recommended for the first week, and then decreasing to two or three times a week as maintenance therapy.

PSORIASIS

Psoriasis is a chronic relapsing disorder of keratin synthesis that is characterized by well-circumscribed, raised, erythematous papules and plaques covered with silvery-white scales, usually involving extensor areas in adults such as the elbows and knees, the scalp, and, in some forms, the flexural surfaces of the body. The phrase "heartbreak of psoriasis" was coined because of the physically and emotionally disabling effects of the disease.

The more commonly seen variants of psoriasis are plaque, guttate, inverse, pustular, and erythrodermic psoriasis. Plaque psoriasis is the most common form in young adults; it presents as erythematous lesions with well-demarcated margins, topped with a thick, silvery scale. Plaque psoriasis accounts for approximately 80% of all cases of psoriasis. Guttate psoriasis is more common in children, presenting as an acute eruption of multiple smaller plaques (less than 1 cm). Inverse psoriasis is characterized by localization of psoriatic plaques to flexural (intertriginous) surfaces. Pustular psoriasis is the most serious form of the disease and is characterized by widespread scaling with a sheet of superficial pustules. Erythrodermic psoriasis may be considered a separate entity or the most severe form of pustular psoriasis; it may be life-threatening and is associated with chronic immunosuppression (e.g., HIV infection). Bright-red erythema affecting a large portion of the skin surface is the most prominent feature of erythrodermic psoriasis, which may present with variable keratotic scale and the presence of pustules.

EPIDEMIOLOGY AND CAUSES

Psoriasis is universal in occurrence, but the prevalence varies according to geography, race, and ethnicity. Approximately 7.5 million people in the United States have psoriasis, as well as 2% to 4% of the population worldwide. Geographic variations in prevalence (e.g., almost no cases in South Americans living in the Andes to nearly 3% of the population in Denmark) reflect the influence of both genetic and environmental factors. Psoriasis is less frequent among people of Asian descent and among North and South American native peoples, compared with people of European ancestry. It is also less frequent among West Africans. Prevalence among African Americans is lower than in European Americans, but African Americans were found to be less likely to report psoriasis than European Americans, which may explain the low reported incidence among this group. Prevalence is highest among Scandinavians, with rates slightly higher in northern rather than southern Sweden, further supporting the role of climate and sunlight exposure in the expression of the disease.

Adult men and women are affected with equal frequency. The two peak ages of onset are during the late teens to early 20s and in the late 50s to early 60s. Females tend to have an earlier onset than males, and earlier onset is associated with more severe disease. There is little to no epidemiological evidence that psoriasis is mediated by infectious agents.

Psoriasis has a strong genetic influence, with one-third of patients with psoriasis reporting having a relative with the disease. In family studies, when one parent is affected, 8% of offspring develop psoriasis and tend to have an earlier onset. When both parents have psoriasis, the percentage increases to approximately 40%. However, the mode of genetic transmission is not fully defined.

Environmental factors are known to precipitate the disease among genetically predisposed patients and include trauma to normal skin that results in psoriasis in areas of repeated friction (Köbner phenomenon), infections (e.g., upper respiratory infections, *Streptococcus pyogenes*, HIV), stress, fatigue, a warm and humid climate, sunlight, and certain drugs (e.g., systemic corticosteroids, lithium, beta-adrenergic blockers,

NSAIDs, and antimalarials). Risk factors for psoriasis are listed in the following box.

Risk Factors: Psoriasis

Trauma to normal skin (in patients with preexisting psoriasis) that develops into new psoriatic lesions (Köbner phenomenon)
    Physical, chemical, electrical, surgical, infective, or inflammatory insults
Infections
    Upper respiratory infections, HIV, *Streptococcus*
Endocrine and metabolic factors
    Postpartum period
    Hypocalcemia (e.g., after dialysis and parathyroidectomy)
Weather-related factors
    Extreme cold weather
    Prolonged exposure to sunlight* or hot, humid weather (more exacerbations occur in summer)
Medications
    Systemic corticosteroids
    Lithium
    Beta-adrenergic blockers
    Antimalarial drugs
    NSAIDs
Psychogenic factors
    Stress
    Mood disorders, e.g., depression
Other factors
    Fatigue
    Alcoholism
    Smoking

*Controlled exposure to sun/ultraviolet light can be therapeutic—see discussion in text.

Despite intensive investigation, the cause of psoriasis remains unknown, although it is thought to be a multifactorial disease, with genetic, environmental, biochemical, and immunological origins. Formerly theorized as an idiopathic skin disease, psoriasis is now known to be a genetically influenced, immune-mediated chronic disease.

Because the cutaneous lesions of psoriasis were originally thought to result from unregulated hyperproliferative activity in the epidermis, past treatment for psoriasis has been primarily directed toward normalizing hyperkeratinocytic activity. Currently, the speculation is that genetically predisposed people may experience clonal T-cell activation in response to antigenic stimulation. Proponents of this theory advance this view based on evidence that affected people have an increase of various human leukocyte antigens (HLAs), particularly certain class I HLAs such as HLA-B27, which is also seen in patients with psoriatic arthritis, a form of inflammatory arthritis with redness and painful swelling of peripheral joints that may co-occur with psoriasis. Although not all patients with psoriatic arthritis will have active skin manifestations, a personal or family history of psoriasis is required for diagnosis. In addition, psoriatic plaques have high numbers of activated T lymphocytes that are capable of both cellular proliferation and inflammation.

Current research is focused on the role of T cells and the ability of cytokines to influence the dermal immune response to an as-yet unidentified antigen. This focus is based on the finding that the immunomodulatory agent cyclosporine is capable of improving psoriatic symptoms, which led to a rethinking of disease pathogenesis. The genetic component of this disease has been the subject of extensive research, and a primary goal of psoriasis research is to elucidate the interplay of genetic and environmental influences on the errant cellular effects seen in the disease. A genetic region linking susceptibility to psoriasis in some individuals has been isolated on chromosome 6, and the first non–chromosome 6 genetic marker was identified on chromosome 17q. Subsequent research identified possible DNA loci on chromosomes 4, 8, and 16.

PATHOPHYSIOLOGY

Microscopic examination of psoriatic plaques typically reveals a thickened stratum corneum with hyperplasia of the epidermis and little inflammation. The basic histopathology of psoriasis is the uncontrolled hyperkeratinization of the stratum corneum layer of the skin. Hyperproliferation of keratins 6 and 16 (common to reactive and healing skin) predominates, whereas expression of keratins 1 and 10 (typically found in normal skin) is reduced. The psoriatic pathophysiological process occurs in varying degrees and results in a wide range of clinical symptoms. If increased mitosis or hyperkeratinization predominates, the result is a thick, silvery scale because of the separation of corneocytes with the presence of air in between. Despite this epidermal hyperplasia and parakeratosis, however, the granular layer of the epidermis is significantly thinned or absent. In contrast, if vasodilation predominates, the result is a presentation of diffusely reddened, hot, and slightly scaling skin. Of note, these two processes may coexist.

There are three stages to the psoriatic process: (1) an increased mitotic rate that results in rapid cellular turnover and shortened transit time from the basal layer to the stratum corneum or epidermis (3 to 4 days versus the normal 28 days); (2) dilation of upper dermal capillaries with intermittent extravasation of T cells and polymorphonuclear neutrophils into both the dermis and epidermis, leading to (3) faulty keratinization and accumulation of the stratum corneum, which clinically presents as raised papules and plaques covered with white, silvery scales.

Multiple growth factors (e.g., epidermal growth factor, transforming growth factor-α, tumor necrosis factor-α) and cytokines (e.g., interferon-γ, IL-2, IL-6, IL-8, and IL-17A) are overexpressed in psoriatic skin. Moreover, in plaque-type psoriasis, the T cells localized to the epidermis appear to express specific clonalities with regard to their antigenic receptors, implicating unrestrained T-cell replication in the pathogenesis of the disease. Interestingly, however, psoriasis is also associated with many causes of chronic immunosuppression and may be the presenting finding in newly diagnosed HIV infection—particularly the severe erythrodermic form.

Most recently, the importance of a novel subset of CD4 T helper T cells, known as Th17 cells, has been highlighted in the autoimmune pathogenesis of psoriasis, as they have also been isolated from psoriatic skin plaques. Activated Th17 cells produce multiple cytokines, including IL-17, IL-21, and IL-22, and proliferate in response to IL-23. Several studies have demonstrated the importance of Th17 cells in fighting infection by extracellular bacteria and fungi. Thus, one theory is that dysregulated Th17 function leads to an exuberant immune response to skin flora and ultimately the characteristic hyperkeratinization of psoriasis.

Drug-induced exacerbations of psoriasis can be unpredictable and severe. They are often delayed and may occur months after the start of drug use. Associations with specific drugs have offered some insights into the pathogenic mechanisms of psoriasis. Lithium is believed to act by enhancing the release of inflammatory mediators from neutrophils. Beta blockers lead to psoriasis by decreasing cyclic adenosine monophosphate-dependent protein kinase—an inhibitor of cellular proliferation. NSAIDs cause a buildup of the proinflammatory mediator arachidonic acid by inhibiting the enzyme cyclooxygenase. Antimalarials, the antifungal terbinafine (Lamisil), and angiotensin-converting enzyme (ACE) inhibitors are also associated with exacerbations of psoriasis, although these mechanisms are unclear.

CLINICAL PRESENTATION

Subjective

Patients with psoriasis usually present to the practitioner with concerns about itchy, red, dry, inflamed, and scaly plaques that have recently worsened. However, statements about the onset and course of the disease are highly variable among patients. Symptoms usually begin gradually and are confined to only a few areas (e.g., one or both elbows, the knees, buttocks, or scalp), but psoriasis can also be explosive in onset.

One cause of rapid-onset, explosive psoriasis is a preceding streptococcal throat infection, which can lead 2 to 3 weeks later to multiple, small, guttate lesions developing in a generalized distribution. Once the disease appears, it follows an irregular, chronic, and unpredictable course, as it may remain localized to a few areas or cause intermittent or persistent generalized lesions.

Itching is usually not a problem in most cases of psoriasis, but it may be severe in some patients. These patients often notice bloodstains on their bed sheets from traumatic, inadvertent scratching of the plaques during sleep. Lesions often occur at sites of trauma (Köbner phenomenon). A family history of psoriasis is elicited in one-third of patients, and 50% of these patients have an affected parent.

Three tools commonly used to assess the severity of psoriasis are as follows:

1. The Psoriasis Area and Severity Index combines the assessment of plaque severity (erythema, induration/thickness, and scaling) and the extent of skin surface area affected; it is the most widely used assessment tool for psoriasis in clinical research and practice settings.
2. The Dermatology Life Quality Index has the patient self-rate the impact of the condition on important aspects of their life.
3. Affected body surface area is an assessment of the overall skin area involved by percentage.

A Web site for accessing and automatically calculating disease severity scores using these tools is listed in the Resources section at the end of the chapter.

Psoriasis patients are known to be at greater risk for depressive symptoms, which may progress to suicidal ideation or behavior. The impact of psoriasis on one's quality of life and emotional state cannot be generalized, however, because this is largely dependent on the individual patient's coping skills. Thus, all psoriasis patients should undergo a screening mental health assessment for depression and suicidal ideation, regardless of the severity of disease.

Objective

Physical examination reveals erythematous plaques surrounded by a thick, silvery scale (which is not easily removed), resembling mica. When these micaceous scales are traumatically removed, multiple small sites of bleeding appear (Auspitz's sign). In intertriginous areas, maceration and moisture prevent dry scales from accumulating, but the lesions remain red and sharply defined.

Lesions usually are distributed symmetrically over areas of bony prominences such as the elbows and knees. Scaly plaques also occur frequently on the trunk, scalp, intergluteal cleft, and umbilicus. The latter three areas are frequently overlooked by the patient and clinician but are important in making the diagnosis, especially in patients with associated psoriatic arthritis and limited skin lesions. In fact, the nature of such inflammatory arthritis may only become apparent after typical psoriatic skin lesions are recognized.

A thorough examination of the entire skin surface is therefore crucial to the diagnosis and treatment of a patient with suspected psoriasis. Another helpful diagnostic feature is the Köbner phenomenon, in which physical trauma (e.g., at flexural surfaces) induces the formation of new skin lesions. Such isomorphic lesions can also be induced on the palms of patients whose hands are exposed to friction.

Nail involvement may include stippling or pitting of the nail plate or a yellow to red-brown coloring ("oil-staining") of the nails (nail psoriasis). An accumulation of yellow debris under the nails, simulating a tinea nail infection (tinea unguium), is seen in some patients. Swelling, redness, and scaling of the paronychial margins occur often and are associated with arthritis of the distal interphalangeal joints. The clinical course of this disease is characterized by chronicity and seasonal fluctuations, with improvement in the summer (due to sun exposure) and worsening in the winter as dry skin leads to epidermal injury.

Estimates of patients with psoriasis who also have inflammatory arthritis known as psoriatic arthritis range from 4% to 30%, although the most common form of arthritis seen in psoriasis patients, as in the general population, is osteoarthritis. The inflammatory joint manifestations of psoriatic arthritis may occur when psoriatic skin lesions are present, or they may precede initial skin manifestations, with psoriatic arthritis being suspected in a patient with inflammatory joint disease but no skin manifestations due to a family history of psoriasis. Associated inflammatory arthritis seen in psoriasis patients typically involves the distal interphalangeal joints of the hands and feet but may also involve the vertebrae of the spine, as seen with another form of seronegative (i.e., rheumatoid factor–negative) arthritis known as ankylosing spondylitis (see Chapter 56, Osteoarthritis and Osteoporosis for a more extensive discussion of the seronegative inflammatory arthritides).

DIAGNOSTIC REASONING

Diagnostic Tests

Initial laboratory studies include routine testing with a CBC with differential to assess for infection and a serum chemistry profile with a serum uric acid level. Laboratory tests are generally within normal limits in psoriasis, except for the serum uric acid level, which may be elevated (hyperuricemia). In more severe variants of psoriasis, other specific tests may be ordered. Throat culture is appropriate if *Streptococcus pyogenes* infection is suspected as the precipitating factor (as in guttate psoriasis). Immunoglobulins are generally normal, but selective IgA and IgG deficiencies are observed in some patients. In pustular psoriasis, leukocytosis and hypocalcemia are seen. An elevated erythrocyte sedimentation rate and decreased albumin levels, along with anemia, can be observed in chronic disease.

X-ray studies of the hands are sometimes helpful to search for associated psoriatic arthritis in patients who complain of joint pains in their hands. X-rays of patients with psoriatic arthritis will show extensive erosion and luxation of distal interphalangeal or metatarsophalangeal joints bilaterally, with characteristic "pencil-in-cup" erosive abnormalities of the interphalangeal joints. In these abnormalities, the distal head of a bone becomes pointed like a sharp pencil, while the adjacent articular surface becomes rounded, like a cup.

Biopsy is seldom necessary because the clinical features of psoriasis are so distinctive. Only in unusual circumstances (severe or unusual forms of the disease) are histological studies necessary to diagnose psoriasis. Biopsies should be planned to yield maximal information. When performing a biopsy, nonexcoriated intact lesions should be sampled. If there are lesions at different stages of eruption, more than one sample is necessary. Biopsies can include partial dermal thickness procedures, such as shave or curettage biopsy, or full-thickness sampling with punch or excisional biopsy.

A skin biopsy is done with the use of a local anesthetic to obtain sufficient tissue for an accurate diagnosis. Skin biopsy is a "clean" procedure and should be done simply and quickly. A standard 4-mm punch biopsy is often used and recommended because minimal scarring is the desired end result. It may be useful to take two or more samples at the first examination of complex cases. However, a biopsy should not be performed on infected skin, on any patient with a bleeding disorder, or on any individual who is allergic to local anesthetics. The key to an informative biopsy is careful selection of the sample based on experience. Clinicians who are not experienced in this procedure should refer the patient to a dermatologist (see Therapeutic Procedure 16.1).

Of note, the sudden onset of psoriasis, in particular erythrodermic forms, may be associated with HIV; thus, the presence of underlying HIV infection should be ruled out in such patients.

> **Therapeutic Procedure 16.1: The Skin "Punch" Biopsy**
>
> - Prep the area around the lesion that has been carefully selected.
> - Inject 1% lidocaine slowly and superficially at several sites around the lesion, for rapid effect and minimal injury. Epinephrine may be used to control bleeding except at certain distal sites, given the risk of tip necrosis (nose, ears, fingertips, toes, penis).
> - Punch into the skin with the punch biopsy tool around the lesion at a 90-degree angle to the plane of the skin, with a quick back-and-forth twisting motion, reaching in fast.
> - Carefully lift out the plug and snip it at the base with sharp tissue scissors.
> - Place the tissue plug in a formalin solution.
> - Apply pressure with sterile gauze for hemostasis.
> - Close with two sutures (4.0 or 5.0 size). (Suture removal will be determined according to the location—sutures on the face should be removed sooner than those on the extremities.)
>
> NOTE: Nerve damage can occur in areas where nerves are located superficially, such as the lateral aspects of fingers and the ulnar groove of the elbows. Any lesions in these areas (including the face for cosmetic reasons) should be referred to a dermatologist for biopsy, if needed.

Differential Diagnosis

It is not uncommon to see a patient with more than one variant of psoriasis at the same time, and the pattern may change over time. Often, psoriasis is mistaken for other dermatological conditions. Thus, other skin diseases should be ruled out by evaluating for characteristic clinical presentations, especially in atypical cases that are complicated by systemic manifestations. The differential diagnosis for psoriasis includes the following: atopic dermatitis, nummular eczema, CTCL (mycosis fungoides), tinea corporis, lichen planus, seborrheic dermatitis, drug eruptions, and secondary syphilis. The clinical characteristics of common variants of psoriasis (plaque, pustular, guttate, inverse, and erythrodermic) in comparison to these other similarly presenting diagnoses are detailed in Differential Diagnosis 16.2.

Differential Diagnosis 16.2: Psoriasis

Type of Psoriasis	Clinical Presentation	Differential Diagnosis	Distinguishing Differential from Psoriasis
Plaque psoriasis	• Plaques with silvery-white scales. In some cases, scales may be absent. • Seen on knees, extensor elbows, neck, scalp, between buttocks, or on back. May be erythematous with sharply defined margins • Usually bilateral involvement • Intertriginous areas may be involved. • Positive Auspitz sign and Köbner phenomenon • Gradual onset, chronic course	Seborrheic dermatitis	Sharply marginated yellowish-red to brown patches with sharp borders and greasy scales. Seen on the scalp (especially the hairline), central face, eyebrows, eyelids, nasolabial folds, and external ear. Can be pruritic
		Nummular eczema	Pruritic, coin-shaped plaques or papulovesicles on an erythematous base with uniform scaling; may become exudative and crusted. Typically seen on legs, upper extremities, and trunk.
		Lichen planus	Pruritic, flat, irregular purple papules with fine white lines and scales. Commonly seen on flexor surfaces, nails, and scalp
		Pityriasis rubra pilaris	Generalized erythematous, red-orange lesions with diffuse thickening, interspersed with areas of normal skin. The palms and soles are usually affected.
		Atopic dermatitis	Severe pruritus, palmar markings, increased creasing of infraorbital folds. The sides of the neck, hands, and flexural surfaces are most commonly affected after age 12 years.
		Cutaneous T-cell lymphoma (mycosis fungoides)	Sharply demarcated, scaly, raised plaques to violaceous nodules that may ulcerate
Pustular psoriasis	• Lesions may be localized, appearing on the hands and feet (Barber's disease) or involving the entire skin surface (Von Zumbusch's disease). • Onset is sudden. • Pustules appear on the edges of existing psoriatic plaques and on the palms. • Pruritus and intense burning sensation are present. • Patient may have a fever and systemic symptoms; systemic complications include pneumonia, congestive heart failure, and hepatitis.	Pustular dermatitis	Persistent or recurrent, dry, red, and scaly rash; first appearance in infancy, with history of dry skin since birth

Differential Diagnosis 16.2: Psoriasis—cont'd

Type of Psoriasis	Clinical Presentation	Differential Diagnosis	Distinguishing Differential from Psoriasis
Guttate psoriasis	• Characterized by small, red papules (less than 1 cm in diameter) • Discrete lesions, seen in a raindrop- or shower-like distribution, usually on the trunk and extremities • Triggered by streptococcal infection • May see Köbner phenomenon	Secondary syphilis	Base of lesion (ulcer) is clean and smooth; edges are raised and well circumscribed. Usually occurs in genital region or on lips
		Pityriasis rosea	Well-demarcated, salmon-colored herald patch, forming a collarette of fine scaling, followed by other lesions on trunk and proximal extremities. Christmas-tree distribution on exposed areas
Inverse psoriasis	• Involves the flexural areas (e.g., armpits, groin)	Candidiasis	Erythematous, macerated patches with sharp, scaling border. Satellite lesions (papules and pustules that are tender and pruritic) are common.
Erythrodermic psoriasis	• Severe form of pustular psoriasis • Generalized distribution • Erythema with variable scale • Fluid and electrolyte loss • May experience chills	Drug eruption	Massive superficial dermal edema that lifts off the epidermis, developing necrosis that appears as violaceous plaques or bullae, later healing with postinflammatory hyperpigmentation (e.g., Stevens-Johnson syndrome, toxic epidermal necrolysis).
		Pityriasis rubra pilaris	Fine to thick scales on the palms or soles; orange-red lesions with diffuse thickening.
		Eczematous dermatitis	See preceding descriptions for nummular eczema and atopic dermatitis.
		Mycosis fungoides	See description earlier in this Differential Diagnosis for cutaneous T-cell lymphoma.

Eczematous rashes may be mistaken for psoriasis, but several distinguishing characteristics may be noted. Hyperkeratotic eczema of the palms is a common cause of misdiagnosis, as psoriasis may also present in a palmoplantar distribution, but eczematous rashes tend to be more pruritic than psoriasis. Atopic dermatitis frequently has its first presentation in infancy or childhood, and the patient may report a persistent or recurrent dry, red, scaly, pruritic rash and a history of dry skin since birth. Atopic dermatitis at times develops a psoriasiform appearance, especially on the legs. Nummular eczema has a characteristic morphology that helps to distinguish it from other eczematous eruptions. Initially, nummular eczema presents with tiny papules and vesicles and then assumes its characteristic clinical appearance of coin-shaped plaques. It is typically seen on the legs, but it can also appear on the upper extremities and trunk; the lesions are pruritic, erythematous, and surrounded with uniform scaling.

CTCL can be difficult to diagnose in its early stages. Early on, the rash may appear as a single macule or as multiple erythematous, scaly macules. In its subsequent stage, which may occur anywhere from 6 months to 6 years later, sharply demarcated, scaly, elevated, red to violaceous indurated plaques develop, which typically begin on the thighs, buttocks, and trunk, known as mycosis fungoides. These plaques may coalesce to form larger plaques with annular, circinate, or serpiginous borders, or they may completely regress. The disease may further progress to brown or purplish-red dermal nodules (tumors). The nodules often occur on the face, the body folds, and the inframammary area in women. Mycosis fungoides lesions progress to violaceous, indurated plaques and nodules, which typically begin on the thighs, buttocks, and trunk. The tumors can progress further to exfoliative erythroderma. Through much of this process, CTCL may resemble atopic dermatitis with diffuse erythema and scaling; a definitive diagnosis can be made by skin biopsy.

Tinea corporis (ringworm) presents as erythematous patches and plaques with central clearing and peripheral scales, crusts, vesicles, and pustules; this fungal infection may spontaneously resolve or worsen with topical corticosteroid treatment. In seborrheic dermatitis, the lesions are lighter in color, less well-defined, and covered with a dull yellow scale. Lesions commonly occur in a similar psoriatic distribution, including face, scalp, and central chest. Lichen planus presents a diagnostic challenge if it presents as hypertrophic lesions on the legs, as penile lesions, or on the hands, which result from excessive scratching. In pityriasis rosea, a single herald patch occurs first, and subsequent smaller eruptions follow skin lines in a Christmas-tree pattern. Pityriasis rubra pilaris presents as generalized erythematous lesions with areas of normal skin; the palms and soles are usually affected. Drug eruptions resulting from beta blockers, methyldopa, and gold preparations can produce psoriatic-type lesions. Intertriginous psoriasis may appear similar to candidiasis but in most cases would be distinguishable through Wood's lamp examination and KOH wet mount testing, which will reveal fungal forms.

MANAGEMENT

The goal of therapy for psoriasis is to control the disease so that the patient no longer feels physically or psychologically hindered by the skin lesions. For sparse or mild lesions that do not bother the patient, no treatment may be needed. When treatment is indicated, however, the disease is controlled by decreasing epidermal proliferation and underlying dermal inflammation through the use of topical corticosteroids and other immunomodulatory agents, along with phototherapy in some patients. Systemic agents are reserved for moderate to severe or recalcitrant cases.

The chronic course of psoriasis and the lack of cure can be both discouraging and challenging for the patient and the clinician. Patients should be reassured that the therapeutic options today are much broader than in the past, and several new therapeutic approaches and medications, including highly effective biological therapies, are now available, as well as improvements in phototherapy and photochemotherapy.

Some patients find the presence of even a few small plaques highly objectionable because the location of the plaques in visible areas of the body is disfiguring or may hinder physical activity. Other patients are willing to accept the condition as bothersome but not debilitating, particularly when they realize there is no cure. A long-term individualized plan of disease management is therefore helpful for patients with psoriasis to deal with exacerbations, which cause frustration and discouragement.

Psoriasis is not simply localized skin disease. Its pathophysiology is characterized by systemic inflammation, in which other bodily systems, such as the cardiovascular network, may be affected by inflammation and subsequent high-risk events. In turn, the National Psoriasis Foundation (NPF) has established recommendations for comorbidity screening of adults with psoriasis. These include guidance on cardiovascular disease and metabolic syndrome, obesity, depression, infections, malignancy, and other immune-mediated inflammatory diseases such as Crohn's disease and psoriatic arthritis. Similarly, the Pediatric Dermatology Research Alliance and the NPF have also collaborated to develop evidence-based guidelines for comorbidity screening for patients with pediatric psoriasis. Appropriate therapy must be directed toward comorbidities identified through such screening.

Topical Therapy

Topical agents are first-line pharmacotherapeutics for psoriasis that are usually effective. If less than 20% of the body (e.g., no more than the elbows, knees, ears, and scalp) is involved, topical agents are usually sufficient. However, if more than 20% of the body is affected and manifestations are moderate to severe, systemic therapy may be warranted, and referral to a dermatologist is recommended. For stubborn, persistent, and widespread lesions, ultraviolet (UV) light treatment should be strongly considered. Systemic therapy in psoriasis is usually used as a last resort because the significant effectiveness of biological agents must be weighed against their high cost and side effect profile.

Widely used topical agents are available both as OTC and prescription formulations. OTC emollient creams or ointments applied to the skin at least twice daily are helpful in preventing cracking and fissuring of lesions, especially those on the palms and soles. Keratolytic agents, such as 1% to 5% salicylic acid preparations, may be combined with emollients to enhance the absorption of other drugs, such as topical corticosteroids, through thick psoriatic lesions. Keratolytic agents may be applied twice daily.

Topical corticosteroids are widely used because they are relatively easy to apply. Those with intermediate and strong potency (see Box 16.1) should be applied no more than once or twice daily. Topical corticosteroids are an appropriate treatment in cases involving 10% or less of the body surface (e.g., the face, neck, flexural surfaces, and genitalia). Psoriatic plaques usually blanch and thin in response to the treatment. More potent corticosteroids may be applied to achieve complete clearing of psoriasis and are helpful in treating exposed areas of the body. However, caution is needed regarding corticosteroid usage, because these drugs can cause skin atrophy and suppression of the HPA axis, resulting in Cushing's syndrome.

An effective treatment approach for exacerbations of psoriasis is to initially use "superpotent" topical corticosteroid preparations (e.g., Diprolene, Psorcon, Temovate, Ultravate) for not more than 2 weeks and then decrease to a less potent agent for maintenance therapy. Once symptoms are under control, other topical agents or a weaker corticosteroid may be substituted after gradually tapering the dose.

The penetration and absorption of topical corticosteroids will increase with occlusive dressing, but superpotent corticosteroids should not be applied with occlusion because of increased risk of HPA suppression from systemic absorption. Ointment preparations are preferred over creams or lotions if the psoriatic scale is thick. When heavy scaling is present, gentle brushing of the psoriatic scales after warm soaks or during warm baths before applying the topical agents will increase absorption. Hard scrubbing should be avoided, however, because skin trauma can exacerbate psoriasis.

Topical corticosteroid therapy has several drawbacks. Remission periods are often relatively short. Prolonged use produces striae and thinning of the skin (atrophy), and the rebound effect can worsen existing symptoms, possibly converting "stable" disease to an "unstable" state, if the dose of corticosteroid is suddenly discontinued. Prolonged use of corticosteroids has been associated with suppression of the HPA axis and Cushingoid syndrome, as noted earlier, due to suppression of endogenous glucocorticoid production.

Topical tar and anthralin are agents that can be used once daily in combination with topical corticosteroids. Scalp involvement may benefit from use of a tar shampoo (e.g., Zetar, Sebutone, Pentrax, Doak Tar) before the application of a topical corticosteroid. The tar shampoo is gently massaged on the scalp, left on for a few hours, and then rinsed off. Softened scales are gently removed. The scalp should be gently dried before application of the corticosteroid lotion. Wearing a shower cap after corticosteroid application enhances absorption and improves results. Excessive combing after washing the hair should be avoided to prevent trauma.

Anthralin (0.1% or 3.0% ointment) belongs to the class of trihydroxyanthracene compounds and is used topically for psoriasis. Anthralin is an antimitotic agent capable of inhibiting DNA synthesis. It is applied once or twice daily and should be washed off after 10 to 30 minutes. It produces quick remission of plaques after several weeks of use but has a tendency to irritate and stain adjacent skin and clothing, making it less preferable than other treatment options. Paradoxically, if topical corticosteroids are added to an anthralin regimen, there may be an increased risk of early relapse.

Another topical treatment includes calcipotriene (Dovonex), a vitamin D ointment derivative. Calcipotriene produces keratinocyte differentiation and controls proliferation. It is superior to a superpotent corticosteroid and is ideal for mild to moderate disease as a key alternative to topical corticosteroid therapy for plaque-type psoriasis. Studies have found it to be effective in nearly three-quarters of patients with plaque psoriasis, with relatively minor side effects. Calcipotriene foam 0.005% (Sorilux) is approved for the treatment of psoriasis of the scalp and body for patients aged 4 years and older. Calcipotriene-betamethasone dipropionate foam 0.005%/0.064% (Enstilar) is approved for the topical treatment of plaque psoriasis in patients aged 12 years and older. Calcipotriene-betamethasone dipropionate topical suspension 0.005%/0.064% (Taclonex) is approved for the treatment of 12- to 17-year-olds with plaque psoriasis of the scalp and for plaque psoriasis of the body in patients aged 18 years and older.

A topical agent with similar action to calcipotriene, tazarotene (Tazorac) interferes with excessive differentiation and proliferation of epidermal cells and also limits the migration of inflammatory mediators to areas of hyperkeratinization. It is available as an ointment, cream, or lotion preparation. Like other receptor-selective retinoids, tazarotene is considered teratogenic and should not be used by pregnant women. Halobetasol propionate/tazarotene lotion (Duobrii) is the first lotion indicated for adults with plaque psoriasis. It combines the corticosteroid halobetasol propionate with the vitamin A derivative tazarotene to clear psoriatic plaques while limiting the overgrowth of cells that cause plaque formation.

The topical calcineurin inhibitors tacrolimus (Protopic) and pimecrolimus (Elidel), applied twice per day, may be effective. These treatments have been particularly helpful for psoriasis in the facial and intertriginous areas where topical corticosteroid treatments (other than low-potency agents) should be avoided, given the risk of dermal atrophy.

Exposure to natural sunlight improves psoriasis and permits a more enduring remission than the use of topical corticosteroids. In some patients, topical corticosteroids may even be suspended during the summer. Although sun exposure to the point of mild erythema is helpful, sunburn exacerbates psoriasis and should be avoided. In 1925, W. H. Goeckerman, a physician at the Mayo Clinic, achieved encouraging results with experimental use of midrange ultraviolet B (UVB) light and coal tar ointment for patients whose psoriasis did not respond to topical therapy. With some modifications of the sunbeam spectrum and combined with topical agents, the traditional Goeckerman program is still being used. Crude coal tar of 1% to 2% in gel or ointment form is applied at night to the psoriatic plaques and is followed by UVB treatments, which are continued for 4 to 6 weeks, leading to remission (for up to 4 months) in 60% to 90% of patients, without evidence of increased skin cancer risk. Guttate psoriasis, in particular, responds well to UVB therapy.

A more aggressive treatment approach is photochemotherapy or PUVA, which has been reported to achieve an 80% to 90% rate of remission on otherwise recalcitrant and severe forms of psoriasis, such as the pustular type. The treatment inhibits mitosis by stopping DNA replication and is administered two to three times per week. PUVA involves ingestion of an oral psoralen compound (methoxsalen) before light exposure. Psoralen may be taken orally, or it can be added to a bath, but "bath PUVA therapy" is not widely used in the United States. Psoralen is inactive in the body, but on the skin it is activated by UVA (long-wavelength UVA light). The eyes must be protected during exposure to UVA light because of the potential for cataract formation. Because of the significant occurrence of nausea, body malaise, phototoxic erythema, premature aging of the skin, and pruritus following the administration of psoralen, the attrition rate of this treatment is high.

Although it can clear chronic plaque psoriasis in 6 to 8 weeks, overexposure to UVA light can cause acute sunburn in the short term, and in the long term, it can cause nonmelanoma skin cancer. Since the mid-1980s, the use of phototherapy has been shown to be associated with squamous cell carcinoma, and in 1991, some cases of melanoma began to surface among patients who had received more than 250 courses of treatment. Therefore, careful follow-up of patients who have had PUVA therapy is crucial. Patients considered at increased risk for skin cancer (those with fair skin who are easily sunburned or individuals who have had previous x-ray therapy to the skin) should not receive PUVA.

Systemic Therapy

Systemic therapy is reserved for patients with incapacitating psoriasis, such as severe or extensive plaque psoriasis, psoriatic arthritis, or pustular and guttate forms. Systemic therapy is administered by expert specialists such as rheumatologists or dermatologists who regularly use systemic antimitotic agents, including methotrexate, etretinate, and cyclosporine, as well as biological therapies.

Methotrexate (Rheumatrex) is a folic acid antagonist and a cytotoxic agent that inhibits cellular proliferation. It is used as chemotherapy for cancer, but it is also useful in patients with moderate to severe psoriatic arthritis. Oral regimens include every other day and once-weekly dosing. If nausea is significant, intramuscular administration can be used. A therapeutic response is usually seen within 2 to 3 weeks, at which time the dosage or dosing interval should be reduced. With prolonged use, cumulative doses of methotrexate could result in hepatotoxicity, nephrotoxicity, and bone marrow depression. Coadministration of folic acid 1 mg by mouth daily effectively protects against many of the side effects associated with this treatment, such as stomatitis. Methotrexate is contraindicated in patients with cirrhosis of the liver, immunodeficiency syndromes, or a history of alcoholism.

Monitoring of blood counts, including platelets, should be done weekly in patients taking methotrexate, followed by monthly testing if stable. Renal and liver function tests (baseline and follow-up studies) should be done. Intermittent liver biopsies may be needed with chronic dosing because hepatic fibrosis may occur with prolonged use. Methotrexate is teratogenic and should not be given to those who are pregnant or who want to become pregnant.

Apremilast (Otezla) may be used to treat moderate to severe plaque psoriasis and active psoriatic arthritis in adults. This oral drug inhibits the enzyme phosphodiesterase-4, which plays a role in the inflammation of psoriasis. Taken once daily, apremilast has no requirement for ongoing laboratory monitoring or initial laboratory testing. Of note, this drug contains a labeled warning for an association with an increase in depression and suicidal ideation.

Cyclosporine (Gengraf, Neoral) is an immunosuppressant that was originally used for the prevention of organ rejection in organ transplant recipients. Its efficacy in severe erythrodermic psoriasis and psoriatic arthritis was discovered serendipitously while the drug was being tested for rheumatoid arthritis. Significant improvement and even total clearing of psoriasis may become evident within days of administration in some patients, whereas withdrawal of cyclosporine is associated with relapse within weeks. Hypertension and nephrotoxicity can develop during cyclosporine treatment due to the development of interstitial fibrosis and tubular atrophy. Thus, serum creatinine levels should be monitored throughout the duration of treatment, although in the majority of patients, renal function subsequently normalizes after stopping the drug. Treatment with cyclosporine for more than 1 year is not recommended because it may cause prolonged immunosuppression and myalgias. Other systemic immunosuppressants such as hydroxyurea (Hydrea), azathioprine (Imuran), and tacrolimus have also been used for psoriasis. However, as with cyclosporine, these systemic agents all carry significant safety risks, and their use is reserved only for cases of sufficient severity.

An oral systemic agent, acitretin (Soriatane), is a retinoid that can be beneficial for patients with resistant and severe pustular and erythrodermic variants of psoriasis. About 50% of patients who are refractory to PUVA alone improve when a retinoid is added. Female patients who are treated with acitretin should be advised not to become pregnant for 3 years after ceasing treatment, because retinoids are teratogenic. Patients treated with this drug must also not donate blood for at least 3 years after taking it. Careful monitoring of blood counts, plasma triglycerides, and liver function tests is required.

The most significant development in the psoriasis treatment armamentarium in recent years has been the array of immunomodulatory injectable biological agents used for moderate to severe plaque psoriasis, psoriatic arthritis, and refractory disease. These initially included alefacept (Amevive), a recombinant CD2 antagonist fusion protein that inhibits T-cell activation, and efalizumab (Raptiva), a humanized monoclonal antibody against CD11a. However, efalizumab was withdrawn from the market by the FDA in 2009 due to its association with fatal cases of progressive multifocal leukoencephalopathy, and alefacept was voluntarily withdrawn from the market by its manufacturer in 2011.

Currently, the most widely used class of biological agents for psoriasis are the tumor necrosis factor–α (TNF-α) antagonists, which include the TNF receptor fusion protein etanercept (Enbrel), the human monoclonal antibodies adalimumab (Humira) and golimumab (Simponi), the human-murine chimeric monoclonal antibody infliximab (Remicade), and the monoclonal TNF-α-specific Fab fragment formulation certolizumab (Cimzia). These biological agents have been revolutionary in the treatment of moderate to severe and refractory psoriasis, and many are also approved for use in children. However, they require laboratory monitoring and carry the risk of significant side effects, including a boxed warning for serious infections and certain malignancies such as lymphoma. In addition, given their significant cost, these and other biological agents are typically considered second-line therapeutics when UV light therapy or other systemic agents fail. Given that the patents on many of these agents have expired, biosimilar versions (analogous to generic medications) are now becoming increasingly available for clinical use.

Alternative classes of biological agents have been developed to treat moderate to severe psoriasis. The human monoclonal antibody ustekinumab (Stelara) blocks the inflammatory activity of both IL-12 and IL-23 by binding their shared cytokine subunit p40, which has proven highly effective. Ustekinumab is also approved for use in children. The newer biologics risankizumab (Skyrizi), tildrakizumab (Ilumya), and guselkumab (Tremfya) work by blocking the action of IL-23 only, by binding to its specific p90 cytokine subunit.

Given the key role of Th17 cells in psoriasis, biological agents blocking the IL-17 pathway have also been developed to treat moderate to severe psoriasis in adults. These include the IL-17A-specific human monoclonal antibody secukinumab (Cosentyx), the IL-17A-specific humanized monoclonal antibody ixekizumab (Taltz), and the human monoclonal antibody brodalumab (Siliq), which blocks a specific type of IL-17 receptor and, therefore, the activity of multiple isoforms of IL-17 (IL-17A, IL-17F, IL-17C, IL-17A/F, IL-25). Ixekizumab is also approved for use in children. Because of their effects on the immune system, patients using these treatments may be at increased risk for infections. Suicidal ideation and behavior were also noted to have occurred in clinical trials of brodalumab; therefore, labeling for Siliq includes a boxed warning, and the drug is available only through a restricted program under an FDA-mandated Risk Evaluation and Mitigation Strategy.

Complementary Therapies

Utilization of complementary therapies for psoriasis is growing. Therapies include dietary modifications, herbs and supplements, mind–body therapies (e.g., aromatherapy, yoga, meditation), physical therapy, exercise, acupuncture, and tai chi. Much of the evidence supporting the use of complementary therapies for psoriasis and psoriatic arthritis is anecdotal, however, and certain practices such as dietary restrictions may actually be harmful, if key nutrients are removed from the diet.

FOLLOW-UP AND REFERRAL

Newly diagnosed patients and patients who have moderate to extensive skin involvement or severe disease (e.g., pustular psoriasis) should be referred to a dermatologist or psoriasis specialty treatment center. Patients with recalcitrant or frequent flare-ups should be referred to a dermatologist for UV light therapy and/or systemic treatment. An ophthalmology consultation is necessary before UV therapy to rule out the presence of cataracts. Patients with inflammatory arthritis should be referred to a rheumatologist for specialty care.

Patients with severe psoriasis are usually followed every 2 months by a specialist or more often as required by their particular treatment regimen. Patients who exhibit symptoms of depression or poor coping skills will benefit from referral to a psychiatrist, psychologist, or other mental health professional for psychological evaluation and therapy. Patient support groups that offer social support within the context of a shared patient experience may also be of great psychological help, regardless of the type of treatment initiated. In addition, because psoriasis and psoriatic arthritis patients have higher overweight and obesity rates than the general population, patients with these problems may benefit from dietary counseling and/or referral to a nutritionist.

Patient Education: Psoriasis

Psoriasis presents many challenges to both the patient and the health-care provider. For patients with disfiguring and difficult-to-control psoriasis, education and support are central to the treatment process. The patient should be informed of available community resources and support groups. Explanation of the disease process and treatment, including potential adverse effects of medications, is helpful. A newly diagnosed patient and their family should be reassured that the disease is not contagious or infectious. Patients need to understand that psoriasis may be an added risk for health problems in the future, such as cardiovascular and psychological comorbidities. Overweight and obese patients should also undergo dietary counseling.

Although the genetic aspects of psoriasis are complex and incompletely characterized, it may be explained to family members of a patient that if neither of the patient's parents has psoriasis, the chances are less than 10% that another child will develop the disease. If one parent is affected, the chance of a child developing psoriasis increases to 15%. If both parents are affected, the chance increases to approximately 60% that one or more children will have the disease.

The clinician should educate the patient that there are several ways to remain in remission, once treatments have taken effect. Patients with psoriasis should avoid skin trauma and should keep the skin relatively dry to decrease pruritus, scratching, and scaling. They should avoid photosensitizing medications such as tetracyclines, sulfa drugs, or phenothiazines. If drugs of these types are necessary, patients should be advised to inform the prescribing physician of their psoriasis and to ask for a possible alternative. Although photosensitizing drugs should be avoided, controlled sun exposure during the summer is beneficial; patients should be advised to use a high-SPF sunscreen to prevent sunburns. Patients should also be informed that they need to seek treatment immediately for streptococcal infections (e.g., skin infections, sore throats) and that other aggravating factors for psoriasis include increased stress and alcohol.

The clinician should explain to the patient that dietary manipulations do not appear to play a role in treating psoriasis. However, healthy eating habits support a strong immune system, and nutritionists recommend a low-fat, high-fiber diet for patients. Naturopaths recommend many herbal medicines to improve psoriasis and control or provide relief from the disturbing effects of these flare-ups (e.g., capsaicin, tea tree oil, turmeric, aloe vera, Oregon grape). Although many people subscribe to these therapies, there is a lack of data from randomized and controlled clinical trials to confirm their effectiveness.

REFERENCES

General

Errichetti E, Stinco G. Dermoscopy in general dermatology: a practical overview. *Dermatol Ther* 2016:6(4):471–507.

Utah Valley Dermatology. How to perform a punch biopsy of the skin by Jason Evans, PA-C.{Video file}(2016, January 19). https://www.youtube.com/watch?v=gCEvlzkmuyQ. Accessed 8/27/2020.

Atopic Dermatitis

Cardona ID, Stillman L, Jain N. Does bathing frequency matter in pediatric atopic dermatitis? *Ann Allergy Asthma Immunol.* 2016;117(1):9.

Drucker AM, Ellis AG, Bohdanowicz M, et.al. Systemic immunomodulatory treatments for patients with atopic dermatitis: a systematic review and network meta-analysis. *JAMA Dermatol* 2020:156(6), 659–659.

Frazier W, Bhardwaj N. Atopic dermatitis: diagnosis and treatment. *Am Fam Physician*, 2020:101(10):590–598.

Kumar R, Seibold MA, Burchard EG. Atopic dermatitis, race, and genetics. *J Allergy Clin Immunol* 2020:145(1):108–110.

Langan SM, Irvine AD, Weidinger S. Atopic dermatitis. *Lancet (London, England)* 2020;396(10247):345–360.

Perrett KP, Peters RL. Emollients for prevention of atopic dermatitis in infancy. *Lancet (London, England)* 2020;395(10228):923–924.

Sawada Y, Tong Y, Barangi M, et al. Dilute bleach baths used for treatment of atopic dermatitis are not antimicrobial in vitro. *J Allergy Clin Immunol* 2019;143(5):1946–1948

Sidbury R, Kodama S. Atopic dermatitis guidelines: diagnosis, systemic therapy, and adjunctive care. *Cl Dermatol* 2018;36(5): 648–652.

Contact Dermatitis

Fonacier L, Bernstein DI, Pacheco K. Contact dermatitis: a practice parameter—update 2015. *J Allergy Clin Immunol Pract.* 2015;3(suppl 3):S1–39.

Johnston GA, Exton LS, Mohd Mustapa MF. British Association of Dermatologists' guidelines for the management of contact dermatitis. *Br J Dermatol.* 2017;176(2):317–329.

Masood S, Tabassum S, Naveed S, et al. Covid-19 pandemic & skin care guidelines for health care professionals. *Pak J Med Sci* 2020; 36(Covid19-s4):117.

Psoriasis

Armstrong A, Aldredge L, Yamauchi P. Managing patients with psoriasis in the busy clinic. *J Cutan Med Surg.* 2016;20(3):196–206.

Armstrong A, Siegel M, Bagel J, et al. From the Medical Board of the National Psoriasis Foundation: Treatment targets for plaque psoriasis. *J Am Acad Dermatol.* 2017;76(2):290–298.

Elmets CA, Lim HW, Stoff B, et al. Joint American Academy of Dermatology–National Psoriasis Foundation guidelines of care for the management and treatment of psoriasis with phototherapy [published correction appears in *J Am Acad Dermatol.* 2020 Mar;82(3):780]. *J Am Acad Dermatol.* 2019;81(3):775–804.

Hjalte F, Carlsson K, Schmitt-Egenolf M. Sustained PASI, DLQI and EQ-5D response of biological treatment in psoriasis: 10 years of real-world data in the Swedish National Psoriasis Register. *Br J Dermatol.* 2018;178(1):245–252.

Menter A, Cordoro KM, Davis DMR, et al. (2020). Joint American Academy of Dermatology-National Psoriasis Foundation guidelines of care for the management and treatment of psoriasis in pediatric patients [published correction appears in *J Am Acad Dermatol.* 2020 Mar;82(3):574]. *J Am Acad Dermatol.* 2020;82(1):161–201.

Menter A, Gelfand JM, Connor C, et al. (2020). Joint AAD-NPF guidelines of care for the management of psoriasis with systemic non-biological therapies [published online February 28, 2020]. *J Am Acad Dermatol.* https://www.jaad.org/article/S0190-9622(20)30284-X/fulltext. Accessed 8/28/2020.

Menter A, Strober BE, Kaplan DH, et al. (2019). Joint AAD-NPF guidelines of care for the management and treatment of psoriasis with biologics. *J Am Acad Dermatol.* 2019;80(4):1029–1072.

Osier E, Tollefson MM, Wang AS, et al. Pediatric psoriasis comorbidity screening guidelines. *JAMA Dermatol.* 2017;153(7):698–704.

Talbott W, Duffy N. Complementary and alternative medicine for psoriasis: what the dermatologist needs to know. *Am J Clin Dermtol* 2015;16(3):147–165.

Vaughn A, Branum A, Sivamani RK. Effects of turmeric (*Curcuma longa*) on skin health: A systematic review of the clinical evidence. *Phytother Res.* 2016;30:1243–1264.

Yamauchi P, Bissonnette R, Texeira HD, et al. Systematic review of efficacy of anti–tumor necrosis factor (TNF) therapy in patients with psoriasis previously treated with a different anti-TNF agent. *J Am Acad Dermatol.* 2016;75(3):612–618.

Young M, Aldredge L, Parker P. Psoriasis for the primary care practitioner. *J Am Assoc Nurse Pract.* 2017;29(3):157–178.

Seborrheic Dermatitis

Borda LJ, Wikramanayake TC. Seborrheic dermatitis and dandruff: A comprehensive review. *J Clin Investig Dermatol.* 2015;3(2):10.

Elgash M, Dlova N, Ogunleye T, et al. Seborrheic dermatitis in skin of color: clinical considerations. *J Drugs Dermatol* 2019;18(1):24–27.

Gupta AK, Versteeg SG. Topical treatment of facial seborrheic dermatitis: A systematic review. *Am J Clin Dermatol.* 2017;18(2): 193–213.

RESOURCES

American Academy of Dermatology
https://www.aad.org
American Society of Dermatology
https://www.asd.org

Complementary and Alternative Treatments
   https://nationaleczema.org/eczema/treatment/complementary-and-alternative/
   https://www.psoriasis.org/treating-psoriasis/complementary-and-alternative/alternative-therapies
Dermatological drugs
   https://www.nsc.com.sg/Patient-Guide/Health-Library/List-of-Dermatological-Drugs/Pages/List-of-Dermatological-Drugs.aspx
National Eczema Association (USA)
   https://nationaleczema.org/about-nea/
Dermatology Life Quality Index (DLQI)
   www.dermatology.org.uk/quality/dlqi/quality-dlqi-questionnaire.html
National Eczema Society (UK)
   www.eczema.org
National Psoriasis Foundation (USA)
   www.psoriasis.org
Psoriasis Association (UK)
   https://www.psoriasis-association.org.uk

Psoriasis assessment

Corti M, Corti M. Psoriasis Area Severity Index (PASI) Calculator (2019) http://pasi.corti.li. Accessed 8/28/2020.
Psoriasis Area Severity Index (PASI) Calculator. pasi.corti.li

Dermoscopy education and training

Case presentations to educate practitioners—International Dermoscopy Society (IDS)
   www.dermoscopy-ids.org
   www.dermlite.com/cms/en/learn/for-professionals/video-course.html
   http://dermoscopic.blogspot.com
   http://dermnetnz.org/procedures/dermoscopy.html
Usatine & Erickson Media LLC. (Updated 2019 Aug 11). Dermoscopy Two Step Algorithm, Apple App Store. https://apps.apple.com/us/app/dermoscopy-two-step-algorithm/id731753300. Accessed 8/27/2020.

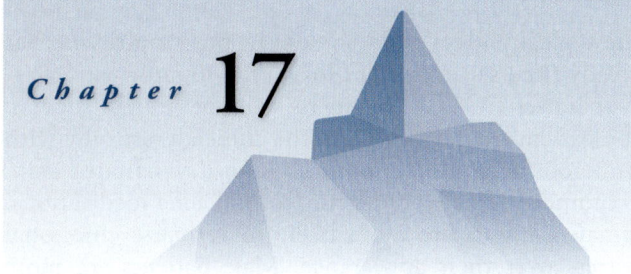

Chapter 17

Skin Lesions

Jill E. Winland-Brown, EdD, APRN, FNP-BC, FAANP
Nancy Harris, DNP, APRN, FNP-BC
Brian Oscar Porter, MD, PhD, MPH, MBA

BENIGN LESIONS

ACNE VULGARIS

Acne vulgaris (commonly called "acne") is the most common skin condition in the United States and one of the most common skin conditions that a clinician will see in the primary care setting. Sixty million Americans have active acne, and Americans spend an average of more than $3 billion annually on acne treatment.

EPIDEMIOLOGY AND CAUSES

Acne is derived from the Greek word *acme* meaning "prime of life" because it is a disease primarily of adolescence, although it may continue into adulthood. Acne vulgaris has the highest incidence among individuals 12 to 25 years of age, with an incidence peaking at 15 years of age. Twenty percent of all adults have active acne and 85% will experience acne at some point in their lives. Even after resolving in adolescence, acne can recur during adulthood, which is called *adult-onset acne*. Adult-onset acne is more commonly seen in females in their mid-20s to 40s in age, although an increasing number of females have acne in their third to fifth decades of life and beyond. Overall, however, the incidence of acne markedly decreases with age.

Although 80% of cases occur in females, acne is often more severe in males. Fifty percent of adult females have premenstrual flares of acne and many have their first flare, or worsening of existing acne, during pregnancy.

The etiology of acne is interdependent on several factors, including the following:

- An increase in production of sex hormones (androgens) in puberty and adolescence
- An increase in sebum production resulting from activation of the sebaceous glands (during puberty and adolescence) and genetic factors

- A disorder of epithelial cell "stickiness" (keratinization) and shedding (desquamation), leading to keratin plug formation
- Proliferation of *Propionibacterium acnes* bacteria inside the hair follicles
- The host inflammatory response

With the advent of the COVID-19 pandemic, a condition called *maskne*, the term coined for acne that results from wearing a mask, has become more prominent. This may also occur from wearing a sleep mask at night. The acne occurs under the mask and is due to rewearing of an unclean mask. The treatment of maskne is the same as for the more common types of acne, although the best approach is prevention. Washing the face twice daily is a must, and disposable masks should be used as recommended and not reworn. Cloth masks should be washed frequently, either in a mesh bag in the washing machine or by hand with dish soap.

PATHOPHYSIOLOGY

Acne is an inflammatory disorder of the sebaceous gland and accompanying hair follicle (known collectively as a *pilosebaceous unit*). Approximately 5,000 pilosebaceous units are present in the human body. Most of them are located on the face, back, chest, and upper arms, which are the most common sites for acne. Acne lesions include comedones, papules, nodules, and cysts. Painful nodules and cysts are found in severe forms of acne.

Comedones are the primary lesions of acne and are caused by a defect in desquamation at the opening of the pilosebaceous follicle. Instead of regular cellular shedding, desquamation is reduced, and shed epithelial cells become "sticky," forming plugs that block follicular openings in a process known as *retention hyperkeratosis*. It takes about 2 months for the accumulated shed epithelial cells, sebum, and keratin to produce a comedone. Comedones are noninflammatory lesions and are classified into two types: *closed* ("whiteheads") and *open* ("blackheads"). The black color of open comedones is caused by the oxidation of tyrosine (a substance normally present in the plug material) to melanin. Tyrosine is an amino acid precursor of melanin.

Enlargement of the sebaceous glands and increased sebum production triggered by adrenarche during adolescence provides a rich growth medium for the overgrowth of *P. acnes* bacteria within the pilosebaceous follicles. *P. acnes* is an anaerobic diphtheroid that is part of the normal skin flora in humans and is responsible in large part for triggering the inflammatory response observed in acne vulgaris. *P. acnes* bacteria utilize triglycerides as their primary source of nutrients by breaking down the sebum inside the affected hair follicle into its basic units, such as fatty acids and glycerol. Free fatty acids act as irritants and produce a sterile inflammatory response inside the sebaceous follicles. *P. acnes* also causes a direct inflammatory response by releasing proteolytic enzymes such as hyaluronidase, as well as chemotactic factors that attract neutrophils to the site of infection.

These neutrophils extrude lysozyme, which further degrades surface epithelia, leading to rupture of the previously closed comedone. When a comedone ruptures, its contents, which include sebum, bacteria, keratin, and free fatty acids, enter the dermis and elicit a severe inflammatory response. This results in the formation of deep abscesses, which present on the skin surface as nodules and cysts. Although androgen excess may lead to acne formation, most individuals with acne do not overproduce androgens. However, their pilosebaceous glands are likely hypersensitive to these hormones and are more prone to retention hyperkeratosis. Some studies have shown that the production of sebum is increased in patients with acne compared with control subjects of similar age, thus suggesting a possible genetic predisposition for acne vulgaris.

CLINICAL PRESENTATION

Subjective

The typical patient is an adolescent boy or girl who has already tried self-treatment for several months with over-the-counter (OTC) products without much success. The patient might present to the clinician not only with numerous acne lesions but also with dry, irritated skin, a common side effect of many topical acne medications. Female patients are more likely to verbalize emotional distress over their appearance. Male patients are more likely to wait until their acne is severe before they seek treatment from a clinician. Some patients with severe acne complain of pain and tenderness from multiple deep pustules, nodules, and cysts. Mild to moderate acne normally does not cause pain.

Objective

Mild Acne

In mild acne, lesions are primarily noninflammatory comedones with occasional small papules. Commonly, there is a mixture of both types of comedones. The location of the comedones and papules may vary, from predominantly facial involvement to other locations, such as the chest, back, and the upper outer arms. Closed comedones are small papules 1 to 3 mm in size that are the same color as the surrounding skin, sometimes with a visible white plug. Occasionally, a closed comedone can get irritated from trauma (e.g., scratching, scrubbing) and become inflamed. Open comedones have a black-colored central plug. The hard plug on some comedones can be removed easily by putting firm pressure on the sides of the lesion. See the Iceberg of Acne to appreciate all the issues involved.

The Iceberg of Acne

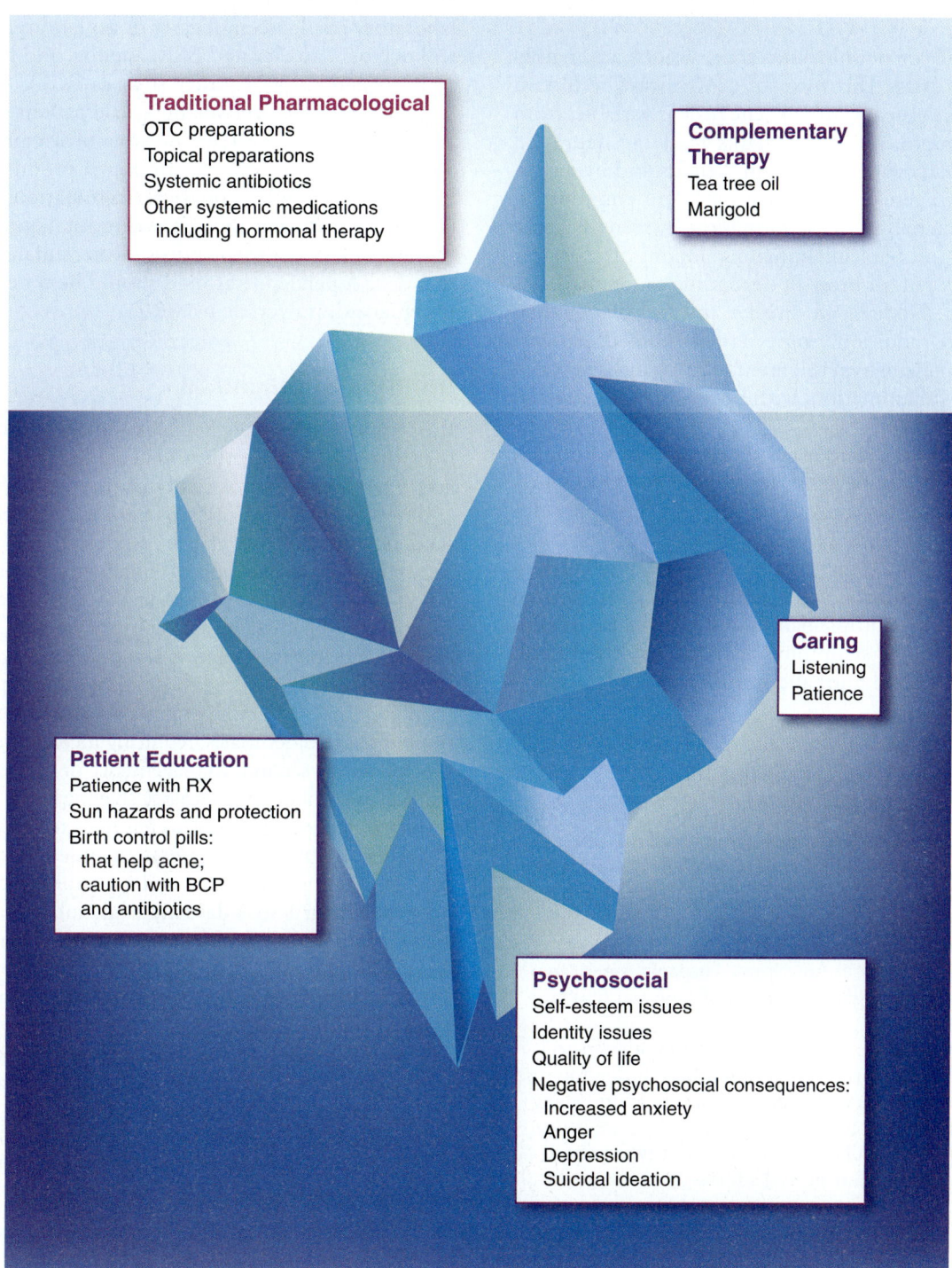

Traditional Pharmacological
OTC preparations
Topical preparations
Systemic antibiotics
Other systemic medications
  including hormonal therapy

Complementary Therapy
Tea tree oil
Marigold

Caring
Listening
Patience

Patient Education
Patience with RX
Sun hazards and protection
Birth control pills:
  that help acne;
  caution with BCP
  and antibiotics

Psychosocial
Self-esteem issues
Identity issues
Quality of life
Negative psychosocial consequences:
  Increased anxiety
  Anger
  Depression
  Suicidal ideation

Moderate Acne

In moderate acne, lesions are mainly inflammatory lesions such as papules and pustules. The papules range in size from a few millimeters to one-half centimeter. The color of the acne papules in light-skinned patients ranges from light pink to bright red. Papules in darker-skinned patients can be red to shades of brown. Pustules are easier to recognize; they appear like pointed papules, with yellow to green-colored tops. When pustules become fluctuant, they rupture spontaneously, providing relief from pain. Resolution of a pustule is usually rapid after rupture. Scarring is more likely with larger, deeper pustules. Postinflammatory hyperpigmentation can be problematic, especially in patients with darker skin; patients with olive-toned complexions and darker skin tones are more likely to have this problem. Patients who are prone to hyperpigmentation should be advised to avoid sun exposure to the face and to use oil-free sunblock on the face.

Severe (Nodulocystic) Acne

In severe acne, or nodulocystic acne, lesions are mainly nodules and cysts. This form of acne always results in scar formation. The severity of acne scars is variable, from numerous atrophic pits ("pockmarks") to large, depressed scars. In patients with darker skin, keloids and hypertrophic scars can result. Severe acne is more common in males. Occasionally, fistula formation is seen in some patients. Nodules are inflammatory lesions that appear bright to dark red (or brown), depending on the patient's shade of skin. Nodules are smaller and feel harder than acne cysts. In addition, some darker-skinned patients develop permanent hyperpigmentation changes secondary to severe inflammation, with brown to black-colored macules on the skin.

Acne conglobata is severe cystic acne in which nodules, cysts, and abscesses develop; lesions are predominantly located on the trunk instead of the face. Females with acne conglobata should be evaluated for polycystic ovary syndrome (PCOS). Acne fulminans is rare and is seen in young adolescent males. This condition is characterized by acute onset of multiple painful, ulcerated acne lesions, along with systemic symptoms such as fever, chills, malaise, and generalized joint and muscle aches.

Pediatric/Adolescent Considerations:
Acne Vulgaris

Although acne vulgaris has the highest incidence among individuals aged 12 to 25 years, the incidence peaks at 15 years of age. Racial and ethnic differences have also been noted. The average age of onset of acne is 16 years for Hispanic Americans, 19 years for Asian Americans, and 20 years for African Americans. Hispanic American teenagers have the highest incidence of acne and resultant scarring.

Treatment options should be offered to both affected teens and their parents or significant others during routine wellness visits, as well as during episodic visits. Many adolescents are reluctant to discuss this health-care issue, and the clinician should be proactive about treatment to prevent disfiguring scarring and address any associated mental health issues.

DIAGNOSTIC REASONING

Diagnostic Tests

Acne is diagnosed by its classic location and characteristic lesions. A complete history is crucial to the diagnosis and supplants the importance of most diagnostic tests, which are only needed when an underlying predisposing condition is suspected or for cases refractory to standard treatments. For acne fulminans, a complete blood count (CBC), blood chemistry panel, urinalysis, and erythrocyte sedimentation rate (ESR) can be helpful. Abnormal laboratory results seen in cases of acne fulminans include leukocytosis, an elevated ESR, anemia, and hematuria.

If an endocrine disorder such as PCOS is suspected (e.g., in a hirsute, overweight female patient with moderate to severe acne and amenorrhea or irregular menses), an evaluation for excessive androgen production should be done. A complete physical examination, along with laboratory tests that include serum total and free testosterone and dehydroepiandrosterone sulfate, is recommended. A pelvic ultrasound should be ordered to assess for enlarged, polycystic ovaries.

Differential Diagnosis

Rosacea, previously termed *acne rosacea*, should be ruled out. Rosacea is more common in adults and older patients and is located more centrally on the face, cheeks, chin, and nose. Comedones are not found in rosacea. There is a tendency for easy flushing in response to alcohol or heat. Telangiectasias (dilations of small groups of superficial blood vessels) may be present at the skin surface. Rosacea can be accompanied by eye complaints such as excessive dryness and irritation, and it is more common in patients of Irish, Scottish, or English descent. Chronic rosacea can result in rhinophyma (hyperplasia of nasal tissue) and is seen more often in older males, requiring medical treatment (see the following section Management) or more commonly surgical treatment (e.g., scalpel shaving, laser resurfacing, cryosurgery, dermabrasion) to remove excess tissue.

Other differential diagnoses include "hot tub folliculitis" (folliculitis lesions caused by staphylococci), which appears within 1 to 4 days after hot tub use, due to high water temperature and inadequate chlorination of the water. Patients will complain of small red pustules that are occasionally pruritic. Folliculitis is located on the areas of the body that were immersed in the water, such as the lower torso, buttocks, and legs. Perioral dermatitis is another similar presentation that appears as small, erythematous papules occurring around the mouth area and nasolabial folds, which is the main diagnostic clue. It is more common in adult females (usually 20 to 30 years old); treatment is similar to that for rosacea except that topical corticosteroids are not indicated.

MANAGEMENT

In the United States, of the 60 million individuals who have acne, 20 million will have lesions severe enough to cause scarring. However, only 10% of individuals with acne seek advice or treatment from a health professional. Although acne is not a life-threatening illness, it has the potential to cause physical scars and emotional trauma. The primary goal of acne treatment is to prevent and/or minimize scarring and permanent pigmentation changes, and most cases of acne can be treated safely in the primary care setting. However, the clinician should not ignore the effect of acne on self-esteem and identity, which are closely tied to physical appearance during the adolescent period. Research suggests that more than 90% of persons with acne have felt depressed, and 14% have considered suicide.

Patient education is important in acne management and should not be neglected. Mild acne is treated with topical medications only, whereas systemic antibiotics may be used in moderate cases that are unresponsive to topical agents and in severe cases (see Drugs Commonly Prescribed 17.1). Of note, numerous misconceptions regarding acne treatment abound in the community. Many patients and their family/significant others think that antibiotic treatment can result in a "quick cure." However, the response rate from acne treatment tends to be slow compared with most infections treated with antibiotics and can take up to 4 to 6 weeks before visible results are detected. More recently, clascoterone cream 1% (Winlevi), an androgen receptor inhibitor, received U.S. Food and Drug Administration (FDA) approval in 2020 for the topical treatment of acne vulgaris in patients older than 12 years.

Drugs Commonly Prescribed 17.1: Acne and Rosacea

DRUG	INDICATION	ADVERSE REACTIONS AND PRESCRIBING CONSIDERATIONS
Topical Anti-Inflammatory and Antibiotic Formulations		
Azelaic acid (Azelex) cream 20%	Acne vulgaris and inflammatory rosacea	Both bacteriostatic and bactericidal Avoid mouth, eyes, and mucous membranes Watch for hypopigmentation on darker-skinned patients Wash hands after use Adverse effects may include burning, dryness, stinging, erythema, and pruritus May use during pregnancy
Sulfacetamide (Rosula) gel, wash, and cream	Acne vulgaris, rosacea, and seborrheic dermatitis	Avoid mucous membranes
Benzoyl peroxide (Benzac) gel, wash, lotion, and foam	First-line therapy for acne	2.5% strength has similar efficacy as 10% strength but is less irritating; use water-based rather than alcohol-based formulation Adverse effects may include burning, dryness, stinging, erythema, and peeling May use during pregnancy
Metronidazole (Metrogel) 1% gel	Rosacea	Will not cure rosacea but reduces inflammatory lesions
Clascoterone (Winlevi) 1% cream	Acne vulgaris	Apply thin layer to affected area twice daily after washing Adverse effects may include erythema/reddening, pruritus, and scaling/dryness Research is still being done to assess safety in pregnancy
Clindamycin (Cleocin, Evoclin) 1% solution, lotion, gel, and pledget	Acne vulgaris and rosacea	Do not use alone, due to antibiotic resistance Lotion is less irritating May cause diarrhea; avoid in patients with colitis Other adverse effects may include pruritus, erythema, dryness, and peeling May use during pregnancy
Combination Topical Anti-inflammatory + Antibacterial Therapy		
Clindamycin + benzoyl peroxide (BenzaClin)	Acne vulgaris	Safety and efficacy in patients younger than 12 years have not been established Risk of severe pseudomembranous colitis; discontinue use if significant diarrhea occurs May bleach fabrics Avoid eyes and mucous membranes Caution in pregnant or breastfeeding patients

Continued

Drugs Commonly Prescribed 17.1: Acne and Rosacea—cont'd

DRUG	INDICATION	ADVERSE REACTIONS AND PRESCRIBING CONSIDERATIONS
Erythromycin + benzoyl peroxide (Benzamycin)	Acne vulgaris	Safety and efficacy in patients younger than 12 years have not been established Risk of severe pseudomembranous colitis; discontinue use if significant diarrhea occurs May bleach fabrics Avoid eyes and mucous membranes Transient skin discoloration Caution in pregnant or breastfeeding patients
Topical Retinoids: Not recommended for use in pregnancy unless otherwise stated		
Tretinoin (Renova) 0.05% cream	Acne vulgaris and rosacea	Not recommended for children younger than 10 years Do not use on sunburned skin
Tretinoin (Retin-A) cream, gel, and liquid	Acne vulgaris	Allow effects of other topical agents to subside before using
Tazarotene (Tazorac) 0.1%	First-line therapy for all acne variants	Female patients of childbearing potential should have a negative pregnancy test 2 weeks before starting and must use effective birth control Do not breastfeed while using
Adapalene (Differin)	First-line therapy for all acne variants	Less sun sensitivity than tretinoin Adverse effects may include burning, peeling, stinging, pruritus, erythema, and dryness May use during pregnancy
Isotretinoin (Amnesteem)	Severe recalcitrant nodular acne or rosacea unresponsive to conventional therapy (including antibiotics)	Teratogenic, must register patients in iPLEDGE program to avoid pregnancy Avoid sun exposure Monitor lipids, glucose, complete blood count, and liver enzymes Take with meals
Combination Topical Retinoid + Antibacterial Therapy		
Adapalene plus benzoyl peroxide (Epiduo gel)	Acne vulgaris	Ideal for teenage boys because they may be more likely to use just one topical product Apply a thin film once daily after washing
Systemic Therapies: Antibiotics		
Minocycline (Minocin)	Severe acne and rosacea	Take on an empty stomach with fluids
Doxycycline (Vibramycin, Oracea)	Severe acne and rosacea	Monitor blood, renal, and hepatic function with long-term use Adverse effects may include nausea, diarrhea, headache, photosensitivity, and tooth discoloration
Hormonal Therapy		
Norgestimate and ethinyl estradiol (Ortho Tri-Cyclen and others)	Oral contraceptive pills (OCPs) for moderate acne vulgaris in female patients older than 15 years	See Chapter 47 for precautions accompanying OCP use

Drugs Commonly Prescribed 17.1: Acne and Rosacea—cont'd

DRUG	INDICATION	ADVERSE REACTIONS AND PRESCRIBING CONSIDERATIONS
Norethindrone acetate and ethinyl estradiol (Estrostep FE, Loestrin, Loestrin FE)	Moderate acne vulgaris in female patients older than 15 years	See Chapter 47 for precautions accompanying OCP use
Drospirenone and ethinyl estradiol (Gianvi, Loryna, Nikki, Ocella, Syeda, Vestura, Yasmin, Yaz, Zarah)	Moderate acne vulgaris in female patients older than 15 years	See Chapter 47 for precautions accompanying OCP use

A combination of several types of acne lesions in a single patient is not uncommon, but the predominant lesions present will help in determining treatment choices. Other factors that help guide the choice of treatment include a higher risk of pigmentation changes (more common in patients with darker skin), a patient's refusal of systemic antibiotic treatment, and the severity of the acne. A parent's or guardian's permission is necessary to treat patients younger than 18 years.

Topical Treatment of Comedonal Acne

Comedones respond well to topical retinoids, which are derivatives of vitamin A and are available in multiple vehicles in a wide variety of concentrations. Synthetic retinoids such as tretinoin (Retin-A) and adapalene gel (Differin) decrease comedone formation by increasing cell turnover and decreasing epithelial cell cohesiveness. Mild adverse effects of tretinoin include dryness, erythema, scaling, and burning. Adapalene gel seems better tolerated on sensitive skin than tretinoin, but patients with extremely sensitive skin can still develop skin irritation. Adapalene 0.1% is an FDA-approved prescription-strength retinoid that is available OTC.

Tretinoin has been shown to cause thinning of the top layer of epidermis during the first 4 weeks of treatment and can result in dryness and irritation. During this period, patients may notice more skin sensitivity to the elements (e.g., cold air, wind, sun) and an increase in skin photosensitivity. Sunscreen or sunblock should be used during the entire treatment period, especially at this time. The thickness of the epidermis returns to normal after 4 to 6 weeks. It is important to warn patients and parents that tretinoin and, to a lesser extent, adapalene gel will cause a worsening of acne lesions during the first 4 to 6 weeks of treatment, as preexisting comedones will continue to surface during this time. Improvement should become visible by 6 to 8 weeks; however, a trial period of 2 months is generally recommended for topical retinoids, unless the patient develops contact dermatitis or other problems with the medicine.

To avoid excessive skin irritation, the patient should wait for at least 10 to 15 minutes after washing and should allow the skin time to dry before applying topical acne agents. Patients with a history of eczema or with sunburned skin should not use this medicine. The patient should avoid the eyes, mouth, angles of the nose, and mucous membranes when applying this medicine. Adverse reactions include excessive skin irritation, an apparent exacerbation of symptoms, transient pigmentation changes, stinging on application to the skin, and dry skin. The effects of other topical acne agents, such as benzoyl peroxide, sulfur, resorcinol, and salicylic acid, should be allowed to subside before the application of topical retinoids, such as tretinoin (Box 17.1). Given their teratogenic effects, retinoids should not be used by pregnant

Box 17.1 Initiating Tretinoin Therapy

Start with tretinoin 0.025% (Retin-A) cream (the least irritating formulation). Apply three to four times per week at bedtime on clean dry skin for the first 2 weeks until the patient can tolerate a daily dose. Wait 20 to 30 minutes after cleansing the face and ensure the face is completely dry before applying the cream. Give this dose a trial of 6–8 weeks.

- Gradually increase to a 0.05% cream or 0.025% gel if patient can tolerate the previous initial regimen and needs a stronger dose (i.e., if no reduction in acne lesions is seen after 8 weeks).
- If there is still no improvement of acne lesions, escalate to the 0.1% cream.

NOTE: The most potent and irritating dose of tretinoin is the 0.05% liquid formulation. Tretinoin 0.05% (Renova) has been shown to decrease the effects of solar damage and is approved by the U.S. Food and Drug Administration for the treatment of fine wrinkles, mottled hyperpigmentation, and tactile roughness of the skin. Remind the patient that acne breakouts may occur with up to 4–6 weeks of treatment, after which the skin will begin to clear.

or nursing females or children. The popular media have suggested that tretinoin has been associated with psychotic or suicidal behavior in teens, but this has not been substantiated by rigorous epidemiological data.

Topical Treatment of Inflammatory Acne

Patients with predominantly inflammatory lesions may respond well to topical antibiotics such as erythromycin or clindamycin, benzoyl peroxide, or a combination of benzoyl peroxide and erythromycin. Other good candidates for nonretinoid topical acne therapy include patients who cannot tolerate tretinoin or adapalene gel or patients who have concurrent eczema (atopic dermatitis). All topical antibiotics are applied once or twice daily and must be refrigerated when stored. The most common side effects include mild erythema or burning. Because topical antibiotic solutions use an alcohol base, they can cause excessive skin dryness. To avoid this problem, the clinician should tell patients to start their use gradually on a once-daily basis for 2 weeks.

Monotherapy with topical antibiotics may lead to bacterial resistance with a resultant slower therapeutic effect. Switching the patient to a combination of antibiotics and benzoyl peroxide has shown increased efficacy and a reduction of antibiotic resistance in *P. acnes*. The combination products are particularly effective in treating patients with postinflammatory hyperpigmentation or concomitant melasma.

Systemic Antibiotic and Hormonal Treatment of Moderate to Severe Acne

Topical acne medicines are a safer alternative than oral antibiotics, as they have less potential for adverse effects. Topical therapy has its limitations, however. Oral antibiotic treatment should generally be continued for 4 to 6 months, and maximal clinical results are typically not evident before 3 to 4 months.

Good candidates for oral antibiotic treatment include patients who:

- Have not responded to topical medications after a trial of at least 2 to 3 months,
- Are unable to tolerate topical acne treatment,
- Have large numbers of inflammatory lesions after several months on topical treatment,
- Have severe nodulocystic acne,
- Have large numbers of inflammatory lesions located on the back or upper outer arms (hard-to-reach areas),
- Want quick relief from inflammatory acne, and
- Are at increased risk of pigmentation changes or scarring.

Oral antibiotics are the standard of care in the management of moderate to severe acne and treatment-resistant forms of inflammatory acne. *P. acnes* is a biofilm-forming organism, and topical treatment is recommended along with oral antibiotics. Examples of oral antibiotics used in the treatment of inflammatory acne include doxycycline and minocycline, which are more effective than tetracycline. There is evidence that minocycline is superior to doxycycline in exerting not only an antibacterial effect against *P. acnes* but a direct anti-inflammatory effect as well. Trimethoprim-sulfamethoxazole and trimethoprim alone are also effective in instances where other antibiotics cannot be used.

The starting dose of minocycline (for tetracycline-resistant acne) is 50 mg at bedtime for 1 week; the dose is then gradually increased to 100 mg at bedtime. Once improvement is seen at 4 to 6 weeks, the dose can be decreased gradually every 6 to 8 weeks. The maintenance dose of minocycline is 50 mg once daily. The safety of minocycline has not been established for longer than 12 weeks. Adverse effects of minocycline include vertigo, dizziness, and ataxia (due to its effects on the vestibular apparatus of the inner ear). This effect can be avoided or decreased by starting the patient on a lower dose. Rare cases of blue-gray discoloration of the skin are sometimes seen in minocycline use. Other adverse effects associated with tetracycline antibiotics include serum sickness, hepatitis, and a lupus-like syndrome.

Doxycycline and minocycline are lipophilic and can be taken with food without affecting most of the drug's activity. Doxycycline should be taken with a full glass of water (if the pill becomes lodged in the esophagus, it can cause ulceration). Adverse reactions to doxycycline include photosensitivity, gastrointestinal upset, enterocolitis, rash, blood dyscrasias, and hepatotoxicity. If the patient's occupation or hobbies include plenty of sun exposure, another drug besides doxycycline should be considered. The patient must use strong sunscreen or sunblock while on this drug, in addition to avoiding excessive sun exposure.

Adverse reactions to tetracyclines in general include nausea, dizziness, rash, blood dyscrasias, pseudotumor cerebri, photosensitivity, and hepatotoxicity. Antacids, dairy products, and iron or magnesium-containing vitamins will inactivate tetracyclines due to binding of the drug with those substances. Tetracyclines should not be used in pregnant patients or those younger than 9 years because of the risk of tooth discoloration (during the second half of pregnancy when teeth are developed) and inhibited skeletal growth. In addition, tetracyclines reduce the effectiveness of oral contraceptives. Thus, patients on oral contraceptives should use a reliable second method of birth control, such as condoms.

Erythromycin is a macrolide antibiotic that prevents the production of bacterial proteins. Although erythromycin is effective, its use should be limited to patients who cannot use tetracyclines (e.g., pregnant patients or children younger than 9 years, due to the potential for damage to the skeleton and teeth). Adverse reactions to erythromycin include nausea, gastrointestinal upset, abdominal pain, anorexia, candidal vaginitis, hepatic dysfunction, rash, superinfection (overgrowth of non-susceptible bacteria or fungi), and pseudomembranous colitis (rare). The development of bacterial resistance by *P. acnes* is also more common with erythromycin treatment. Thus, erythromycin is usually considered a second-line agent, with doxycycline as an effective treatment for patients who develop erythromycin-resistant *P. acnes* infection.

In addition to antibiotic treatment, certain combination progestin plus estrogen hormonal therapies used for birth control are also approved for moderate acne in female patients 15 years of age or older and who have acne that is unresponsive to topical medications. The patient should have no known contraindications to hormonal therapy, such as a history of thrombophlebitis or thromboembolic disorders, cerebrovascular or cardiovascular disease, breast or other estrogen-dependent neoplasms, hepatic tumors, or undiagnosed genital bleeding. Norgestimate/ethinyl estradiol (Ortho Tri-Cyclen) is available with different doses of the progestin component (norgestimate), and Estrostep Fe is available with different doses of the estrogen component (ethinyl estradiol). Drospirenone/ethinyl estradiol (Beyaz) combines the estrogen component with an artificial form of progestin. Although thromboembolism is an established risk for all forms of hormonal birth control, birth control pills containing the synthetic progestin drospirenone may have an increased risk for thrombus formation compared with combination pills containing other types of progestins.

Severe Acne

Individuals with severe acne should be referred to a dermatologist for aggressive treatment with isotretinoin, a vitamin A derivative indicated for severe recalcitrant nodular acne that has not responded to conventional therapy (including oral antibiotics). Tretinoin and isotretinoin are confused by some patients as the same medication. Tretinoin is the active ingredient in Retin-A and is a topical medication. Isotretinoin is an oral acne medication that is the only treatment that works on all causes and types of acne. The most familiar brand name of this drug was Accutane, which has not been marketed in the United States since 2009 due to lawsuits related to inflammatory bowel disease claims. However, isotretinoin is now available generically under many brand names worldwide, include Sotret, Amnesteem, Claravis, and Roaccutane.

Isotretinoin induces sebaceous gland atrophy, normalizes follicular keratinocytes, reduces *P. acnes* colonization, and has direct anti-inflammatory effects. It is a highly potent teratogen and carries significant medicolegal implications for the clinician when prescribed to female patients of reproductive age. The manufacturers of isotretinoin require all prescribers to join the iPLEDGE program to minimize fetal exposure to the drug. The primary care practitioner should refer any female patient of reproductive age who is a candidate for isotretinoin therapy to a dermatologist for management, as specialty physician consultation is highly recommended. The risk and the benefits of therapy should be discussed with the female patient, including the possibility of pregnancy and contingency plans if they become pregnant (including a discussion regarding pregnancy termination, if this is an option). Two negative pregnancy tests must be obtained within 1 week of prescribing the isotretinoin, and two reliable forms of contraception must be used (unless abstinence is the chosen method). Monthly pregnancy tests must be ordered thereafter. The patient must have maintained effective contraception for at least 1 month before, during, and after therapy.

The dose usually starts at 0.5 mg/kg daily in two divided doses and may be increased gradually, depending on effect, to 1 mg/kg daily in two divided doses. Isotretinoin should generally be taken with food, although some formulations do not carry this recommendation. Only a 1-month supply of the drug should be prescribed at each visit, and it can be discontinued early if the patient's acne nodule count decreases by 70% or more. Isotretinoin will induce long-term remissions of acne in up to 40% of patients. After a period of 2 months or more off therapy, if persistent or recurrent severe nodular acne recurs, referral to a dermatologist is recommended.

The most frequent adverse effect of isotretinoin is cheilitis, which occurs in up to 90% of patients. Other common adverse effects include dry skin, dry nose, dry mouth, pruritus, epistaxis, and an increase in skin fragility. Patients who complain of headache should be evaluated for pseudotumor cerebri or benign intracranial hypertension. If the patient complains of moderate to severe myalgia, the medication should be discontinued immediately and creatine phosphokinase should be evaluated as a sign of muscle breakdown. Corneal opacities and decreased night vision have also been reported in patients taking isotretinoin. The link between isotretinoin and depression, psychosis, and suicide remains controversial, and some clinicians prefer not to prescribe this medication in patients with this type of psychiatric history.

The incidence of hypertriglyceridemia is high (25%) in patients taking isotretinoin, and some patients develop elevated liver transaminases. Elevated blood sugar levels have also been seen in some patients, as well as new-onset diabetes mellitus, although a causal association is unclear. Baseline laboratory testing, such as a fasting lipid panel and liver function tests, should therefore be done before starting treatment and weekly or biweekly thereafter until the patient's response to therapy is determined, after which laboratory monitoring can be done monthly.

Patients with acne fulminans present a particularly challenging situation because of the severity of the condition and the high potential for scarring. Patients should be referred as soon as possible to a dermatologist and treated with prednisone for its anti-inflammatory effects in combination with isotretinoin, which is the treatment regimen of choice for this condition, although other anti-inflammatory and immunosuppressant compounds (e.g., dapsone, cyclosporine A) have also been used.

Other Medical Therapies

Nonpharmacological therapies may be used in place of or in conjunction with medications to assist in the overall treatment of patients with acne. The surgical procedure of comedone extraction is common for the treatment of comedonal acne and may be used along with topical retinoids. Beta-hydroxy acid peels may also be effective against comedonal acne. To reduce acne scarring, Fraxel laser resurfacing, dermabrasion, and subcision (subcuticular cutting of fibrous scar tissue under the skin surface using a tri-beveled hypodermic needle inserted via a small puncture in the skin) or punch grafting (replacement of small plugs of scar tissue with punch grafts of healthy skin removed from an inconspicuous area, such as behind the ear) may be effective. In addition, dermal augmentation (soft tissue fillers) with autologous or nonautologous tissue may improve the appearance of atrophic scars. Photodynamic therapy with the use of a blue light or intense pulsed light and aminolaevulinic acid may be given every other week. Results are usually apparent after the second treatment.

FOLLOW-UP AND REFERRAL

Patients should be reevaluated in 4 to 6 weeks to monitor for response and any potential adverse effects of acne medication. Noncompliance issues should be addressed. In particular, female patients on oral antibiotics or isotretinoin should be monitored for their continued use of reliable methods of birth control. By the third month of treatment, clinical improvement of acne lesions should be visible. If no improvement is seen or if the acne worsens, topical treatment with two agents or systemic therapy should be considered. However, the risk of skin irritation is increased when two topical agents are combined, and therapy should be started slowly to minimize these effects. Systemic oral antibiotic treatment should generally be continued for a period of 4 to 6 months.

There is no need to wait until acne becomes severe before considering referral to a dermatologist. Moderate to severe acne that is unresponsive to conventional treatment should be referred to a dermatologist for more aggressive treatment to minimize scarring. Without treatment, acne lesions can persist for months to years.

Patient Education: Acne

Appropriate education regarding the causes and treatment of acne can help prevent disappointment in angry and discouraged patients who might become noncompliant due to a loss of trust in both the treatment and the health-care provider. In particular, patient education is needed to correct many common misconceptions about acne. For example, no connection has been found between the ingestion of specific foods and the risk of acne, despite the folklore surrounding certain foods, such as chocolate and fried foods.

Patient education is a vital component of acne treatment because of the long duration of treatment required and the potential for adverse effects, including serious ones (see Box 17.2 for key information). Patients and parents/guardians of patients younger than 18 years should be warned of the potential adverse effects of acne medications (as discussed under the section Management). For example, topical retinoids frequently cause skin dryness and irritation if not started gradually or if used incorrectly. Most patients are not willing to try them again after they experience skin irritation and the temporary flare-up of acne typically seen within 4 to 6 weeks of starting therapy. In addition, as mentioned earlier regarding maskne, the importance of frequent washing or disposing of facial masks should be stressed.

Patients should also be encouraged to read consumer information labels on skin products and to use only noncomedogenic (non–acne-causing) products, such as makeup, moisturizers, and sunscreens. Patients on oral contraceptives for acne therapy should be aware of potential drug interactions, which include a decrease in their efficacy when used in conjunction with certain antimicrobials, such as tetracyclines. In general, oral contraceptives should not be used in breastfeeding patients, given their potential to effect milk production and a theoretical risk to the infant from the transfer of hormones in breast milk.

Complementary therapies suggested for acne include marigold (*Calendula officinalis*) as a topical application (e.g., soap), which has anti-inflammatory properties, and tea tree oil (*Melaleuca alternifolia*) as a topical application twice daily. Research continues to be done on these alternative therapies to evaluate their efficacy.

ROSACEA

Rosacea is a chronic and progressive skin disorder in middle-aged and older adults that resembles acne with an erythematous, flushed discoloration of the face. Rosacea and acne may respond to the same treatments and can coexist in the same patient.

EPIDEMIOLOGY AND CAUSES

It is estimated that rosacea affects more than 16 million Americans. Despite its high prevalence, fewer than 10% are diagnosed because patients confuse the symptoms with acne, sunburn, flushing, or a temporary rash. Rosacea is most common in persons aged 30 to 60 years who are of Irish, English, Scottish, Welsh, or Eastern European ancestry. Patients sometimes have one or more close relatives

> **Box 17.2 Key Information for Patients with Acne**
>
> - Wash the face gently at least twice a day with an antibacterial soap (e.g., Dial, Lever 2000) or with a very mild soap (e.g., Dove).
> - Wait at least 30 minutes after washing the face before applying topical acne medications to minimize the chance of skin irritation.
> - Topical acne medications should not be used on sunburned or irritated skin, abrasions, cuts, or on eczematous skin. If these conditions are present, the medication can be temporarily stopped for a few days.
> - Avoid contact with the eyes, lips, angles of the nose, and the mucous membranes when applying topical acne medicines.
> - Sunscreen should be used with all acne medications, especially in sunny climates and during the summer.
> - Avoid oily makeup or oily hair conditioners and scalp products.
> - Avoid excessive handling of the face and cradling phones on the chin.
> - Avoid excessive scrubbing of the face.

with the condition. Females are three times more likely to develop rosacea than males, particularly cutaneous vascular manifestations that lead to erythema of the central face.

Rosacea is idiopathic with no recognizable causes, other than certain exacerbating triggers that may differ among individual patients. Rosacea is a lifelong condition that is usually worsened by sun exposure. Other environmental triggers include hot or cold weather, wind, overheating during exercise, excessive alcohol ingestion, hot beverages, spicy or aged food products such as cheese, emotional stress, irritating cosmetics, hot baths, saunas, hot tubs, smoking, caffeine, and excessive washing of the face. Several researchers have suggested that *Helicobacter pylori*, bacteria found in the stomach, may possibly be a cause, as well as the *Demodex* species of mite, which has been found in the hair follicles of patients with rosacea. However, these hypotheses are controversial.

PATHOPHYSIOLOGY

Rosacea is characterized by flare-ups that include three cutaneous components, which may occur individually or concurrently. The first component is vascular in nature, with persistent erythema that primarily involves the central face. This may be followed after a period of time by the development of telangiectasias or clusters of small, superficial blood vessels. In addition, flushing episodes may occur spontaneously as part of these vascular manifestations. The second component is cutaneous and involves the development of recurrent acneiform, erythematous papules and pustules around the central face. The third component consists of connective tissue hyperplasia around the central face with discrete sebaceous gland hyperplasia, consisting of persistent yellow papules particularly around the nose. In some patients, the nose may become swollen and bumpy from excess tissue in a condition called *rhinophyma* (the condition which gave the comedian W.C. Fields his trademark bulbous nose). Blepharoconjunctivitis may also result if there is ocular involvement, which is considered a distinct fourth component by some.

At present, the underlying pathogenesis of the vascular dilation characteristic of rosacea is not fully understood. Inflammation, rather than infection, appears to be the primary mechanism, as shown through several lines of indirect evidence. For example, studies have failed to show consistent differences in *H. pylori* seropositivity between patients with rosacea and unaffected control subjects. Moreover, the ability of amoxicillin-metronidazole-bismuth treatments to clear *Helicobacter* infection and improve rosacea symptoms has been attributed to the anti-inflammatory effects of metronidazole, rather than the antimicrobial effects of this regimen. This was similarly shown with tetracycline treatment of rosacea associated with *Demodex* mite infestations. Mite counts were not decreased with this treatment, although symptomatic improvement was evident. Moreover, the anti-inflammatory effects of tetracycline antibiotics have been well documented in the treatment of acne vulgaris.

CLINICAL PRESENTATION

Subjective

Patients with rosacea usually do not seek out care because they mistakenly think they have acne, a sunburn, or a temporary rash. They usually present because they become intolerant of the persistent burning, itching, or stinging sensations on the face, in particular. Patients with ocular rosacea complain of watery, irritated, or bloodshot eyes.

Objective

Initially the patient's forehead, cheek, nose, or chin may have a rosy hue without comedones. This is the central third of the face and is referred to as the "flush/blush" area. There may be inflammatory papules, pustules, and telangiectasias. Scarring is usually inapparent unless the patient also has concomitant acne. Although the lesions tend to be symmetrical bilaterally, they may appear on only one side of the face. Seborrhea may also be seen. If there has been ocular involvement resulting in blepharoconjunctivitis, there will be redness of the eyelids and conjunctiva.

With prerosacea, the clinician will note a rosy-cheeked, ruddy complexion on a patient who never develops the full clinical spectrum of the disease. There is no effective treatment for prerosacea, nor is any needed. Patients should just be observed for signs of developing rosacea and encouraged to use sunscreen.

There are four subtypes of rosacea classified by the pattern and grouping of symptoms:

- Subtype 1: erythematotelangiectatic rosacea—flushing and persistent redness, which may include visible blood vessels
- Subtype 2: papulopustular rosacea—persistent redness with transient bumps and pimples
- Subtype 3: phymatous rosacea—skin thickening usually with hyperplasia of the nose, resulting in a large, bumpy, and bulbous appearance.
- Subtype 4: ocular rosacea—ocular manifestations with dry eye, tearing and burning, erythematous eyelids, recurrent styes, and possible vision loss from corneal damage.

DIAGNOSTIC REASONING

Diagnostic Tests

There is no specific diagnostic test for rosacea; physical assessment is the key to diagnosis, as other skin conditions should be ruled out. Although there is no cure for rosacea, if treatment is started early based on an accurate diagnosis, some of the cutaneous manifestations of rosacea may be prevented.

Differential Diagnosis

Differential diagnoses for rosacea include adult acne, perioral dermatitis, seborrheic dermatitis, the "butterfly" rash of systemic lupus erythematosus, and corticosteroid-dependent facial dermatoses. Acne may be a concomitant condition along with rosacea, but acne is characterized by the presence of comedones, a lack of facial flushing or telangiectasias, and a broader distribution around the face than the limited central distribution of rosacea. Perioral dermatitis is typically seen in young females, although it may occur in females 15 to 40 years of age. Multiple acneiform papules are seen around the mouth in this condition, with a clear area spared directly around the lips. The small erythematous papules or pustules of perioral dermatitis lack telangiectasias.

Seborrheic dermatitis usually has a scaly appearance not seen in rosacea; the erythema is without acneiform lesions and may be distributed throughout the nasolabial area, eyebrows, and scalp. The "butterfly" or malar rash of systemic lupus erythematosus lacks papules and pustules, and laboratory evaluation typically verifies the presence of antinuclear antibodies. Importantly, long-term topical corticosteroid use on the face can also result in burning erythema, sometimes associated with erythematous papules and/or scaling. When topical corticosteroids are abruptly discontinued, a rebound flare-up of this condition typically occurs.

MANAGEMENT

The key to management is early diagnosis and avoidance of triggers because rosacea is a chronic condition with no known cure. Topical treatments should be the mainstay of therapy, with oral antibiotics used only for breakthrough flare-ups. Potent topical corticosteroids should be avoided because they may worsen the condition.

Topical Therapy

Metronidazole cream is the mainstay of therapy for classic facial rosacea, but it may take up to 6 to 8 weeks for a therapeutic response to be seen. If metronidazole (0.75% or 1%) is ineffective, other topical antibiotics may be used. Topical ointments such as tretinoin and azelaic acid are also recommended (see Drugs Commonly Prescribed 17.1). The same therapy is used for perioral dermatitis and topical corticosteroid–induced rosacea. For ocular rosacea, treatment begins with artificial tears and daily cleansing of the eyelashes with baby shampoo.

Systemic Therapy

Antibiotics should be reserved for flare-ups or when initiating therapy with topical medications, after which antibiotics should be discontinued. Clinicians should taper the dose as soon as possible, and patients can typically learn how to taper the dosage at home. Treatment with tetracycline, minocycline, or doxycycline typically delivers a rapid therapeutic response. Antibiotic therapy is usually effective in reducing acneiform lesions, which helps confirm the diagnosis of rosacea. These antibiotics typically work more as anti-inflammatory agents rather than as anti-infectives.

The flushing and flat telangiectasias of rosacea tend to persist and do not respond well to antibiotic therapy. In refractory cases, isotretinoin may succeed when other measures have failed. More severe cases of ocular rosacea may require oral antibiotics, and because of the potential for corneal complications, an ophthalmologist should be consulted for more severe cases.

Other Therapies

Electrocautery with a small needle may be used to destroy small telangiectasias. Larger telangiectatic vessels may require laser treatment (intense pulsed light therapy). Laser therapy followed by dermabrasion has also proven effective for more severe cases. Although mild cases of phymatous rosacea may be treated with medications, more severe cases resulting in rhinophyma may require surgical reduction to decrease the bulbous appearance of the nose. Surgical interventions for rosacea include cryosurgery and radiofrequency ablation.

FOLLOW-UP AND REFERRAL

If rosacea results in telangiectasias, patients can be referred to a dermatologist for electrodesiccation or laser treatment for cosmetic purposes. A dermatologist may also use pulsed light therapy to treat patients with rosacea causing diffuse facial erythema.

Patient Education: Rosacea

Patients should be taught about the events or circumstances that can trigger a rosacea flare-up and learn how to avoid them. The most common triggers include sun exposure, emotional stress, hot weather, wind, heavy exercise, alcohol consumption, hot baths, cold weather, spicy foods, and humidity. Sunscreen with a sun protection factor (SPF) of at least 15 should be used on all exposed skin surfaces when outdoors. Patients should stay cool on hot days and protect their face from cold air and wind by using a scarf. Caution should be used when exercising, and patients should be encouraged to exercise for shorter, more frequent intervals, using a cool towel around the neck and taking frequent water breaks. Gentle cleansing with fragrance-free facial cleansers should be encouraged. Proper use of topical creams and lotions should be stressed, along with minimal use of antibiotics.

SEBORRHEIC KERATOSIS

Seborrheic keratosis is one of the most common non-cancerous skin growths seen in older adults. It is characterized by benign wart-like growths that are usually found on the trunk but may also be seen on the hands and face. These lesions develop in both sun-exposed and sun-protected areas and are often referred to as having a "stuck-on appearance," as if they could easily be peeled or pulled off the skin. Treatment is typically not required, although some patients have them removed due to irritation of the lesions by clothing, such as a bra strap.

EPIDEMIOLOGY AND CAUSES

Seborrheic keratosis is extremely common. A predisposition for seborrheic keratosis appears to be inherited in an autosomal-dominant pattern.

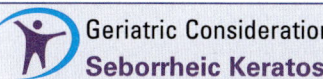
Geriatric Considerations: Seborrheic Keratosis

Seborrheic keratosis is found in approximately 90% of persons older than 60 years. In persons older than 65 years, approximately 50% develop 10 or more lesions. For some individuals, lesions may number into the hundreds. Most older adults are very nervous about developing a malignant melanoma so it is important to accurately diagnose these lesions. Diagnosis and treatment are the same for all ages and are described in the following section.

PATHOPHYSIOLOGY

Seborrheic keratosis lesions are superficial epithelial growths that originate from the horny layer of the epidermis (stratum corneum) and are the result of a benign proliferation of immature keratinocytes. Inspection of the lesions may reveal dark keratin plugs or firm, horny cysts on their surface. These are epidermal tumors, but they are not considered malignant or premalignant because they do not undergo transformation into cancerous lesions.

A condition known as Leser-Trélat sign is characterized by the sudden development of multiple seborrheic keratotic lesions, along with skin tags and acanthosis nigricans (a darkening and mild thickening of the skin in characteristic intertriginous areas). Although the skin lesions in this condition are not considered malignant, Leser-Trélat sign is associated with various types of cancer, including lung and gastrointestinal cancers, and is thus considered a neoplastic syndrome. In addition, seborrheic keratosis has also been observed in association with certain skin malignancies, such as basal cell carcinomas (BCCs), occurring at various skin sites.

CLINICAL PRESENTATION

Subjective

Although seborrheic keratosis occurs in both males and females, the typical patient is an older white female who has concerns over the outward appearance of the lesion. The patient typically complains of the unsightliness of the lesion, itching, and constant irritation from friction or clothing. The lesions are sometimes called the "barnacles of aging."

Objective

Lesions found on sun-exposed areas of the skin rarely increase in size, whereas seborrheic keratotic lesions in less visible sun-protected areas tend to be darker, have a more crumbly appearance, and may enlarge in size over time. These lesions tend to grow slowly and are round to oval in shape, occasionally appearing as smooth papules. Seborrheic keratosis is more prevalent in persons with lighter-colored skin. The lesions are typically raised, well-defined, waxy, scaly, hyperpigmented, and brownish-gray, black, or light tan (flesh-toned) in color, with a warty or "stuck-on" appearance, as if they could literally be "picked off" the skin surface. They are found most often on the trunk, face, and arms. In darker-skinned individuals, the lesions can also appear as smooth, round to oval black papules on the upper part of the face (dermatosis papulosa nigra).

DIAGNOSTIC REASONING

Diagnostic Tests

No laboratory testing is necessary to diagnose seborrheic keratosis. However, if the patient presents with an atypical lesion and the diagnosis is uncertain (especially if melanoma cannot be ruled out), the patient should be referred to a dermatologist for further evaluation, and a skin biopsy should be done for a more definitive diagnosis.

Differential Diagnosis

The diagnosis of seborrheic keratosis is based on the appearance of the lesion and on patient demographics (especially age). Skin lesions that can mimic seborrheic keratosis include any pigmented papule or nodule. The differential diagnoses for seborrheic keratosis include benign pigmented nevi, pigmented BCC, and malignant melanoma. See Table 17.1 for information about other skin lesions, including nevi, skin tags (acrochordons), and lipomas.

Actinic keratoses are precancerous lesions triggered by sun exposure that can look similar to seborrheic keratoses. These are found predominantly in older adults of Celtic (Irish, Scottish, English) descent who are light-haired (blond or red-haired) and blue-eyed. Unlike seborrheic keratosis lesions, actinic keratoses are often removed from the skin, given their risk of progression into cancer.

Pigmented nevi appear as smooth, round macules or papules that do not have a warty appearance. Nevi (moles) are also seen in younger patients, unlike seborrheic keratosis, which appears most commonly in patients aged 30 years and older. Pigmented BCCs usually have a waxy surface with dilated blood vessels. They may also be ulcerated during later stages, a feature not seen in seborrheic keratosis. Malignant melanomas can appear in younger patients; melanomas may be nodular but usually do not have a warty, stuck-on appearance. A malignant melanoma's borders can be irregular, and it can have a variegation (inconsistency) of color. Most patients with melanoma will report a history of a mole that changes in appearance over time.

MANAGEMENT

Most seborrheic keratoses do not require treatment, but removal is warranted for lesions that are symptomatic, unsightly to the patient, or become easily irritated (i.e.,

TABLE 17.1	Other Skin Lesions		
Lesion	**Description**	**Clinical Presentation**	**Management**
Lipoma	A lipoma is a benign, subcutaneous tumor that consists of adipose tissue. Lipomas are most commonly found in older adults and are usually asymptomatic. Cause is unknown.	• Rubbery, smooth, round mass of adipose tissue that is compressible and has a soft to very firm texture • May have symptoms of irritation, such as redness and tenderness • Commonly occurs on back of the neck, trunk, and forearms	• Observe for changes and rapid growth • Excision or liposuction • Referral to dermatologist if indicated
Nevus	Nevi (moles) are circumscribed areas of pigmentation. Types include congenital, acquired, atypical or dysplastic (>5 mm in diameter, with color variation and irregular borders).	• Flat or raised circumscribed area of pigmentation • Assess for suspected melanoma (check ABCDEs: Asymmetry, irregular Borders, variations in Color, Diameter >6 mm, Elevation above the surface of the skin or Evolving lesion)	• Excision • Referral to dermatologist if melanoma is suspected
Skin tag	Skin tags (acrochordons) are benign overgrowths of skin, commonly seen after middle age. Cause is unknown.	• Overgrowths of normal skin that have formed soft, polyp-like lesions that have a stalk • Usually found on the neck, axilla, groin, upper trunk, and eyelid	• Usually no intervention unless patient is bothered by the cosmetic effect or irritation • If treatment is required, may include snip excision, electrocautery, or cryosurgery • Referral to dermatologist if skin tag is located on the eyelids or face, if the patient is on high-dose corticosteroid therapy, if there is the possibility of a malignant lesion, or if the patient has a history of keloid formation, diabetes mellitus, or infection

number of melanoma deaths occur among lighter-skinned individuals who sunburn easily. Whites who are at highest risk come from Celtic (Irish, Scottish, English) backgrounds and have light hair (especially red hair), light eyes, and freckles. The ability of the skin to freckle in response to sun exposure is thought to be a marker of susceptibility to melanoma, although stronger risk factors for melanoma exist.

> ### Risk Factors: Malignant Melanoma
> ***Age***
> Risk increases with age
> ***Skin, Eye, Hair Color***
> Light-skinned
>   Blue or green eyes
>   Red or blond hair
> ***Personal History***
> History of skin cancer (any type)
>   History of dysplastic nevi
>   History of congenital nevi greater than 20 mm
>   History of blistering sunburn before age 20 years
>   History of immunosuppression
> ***Family History***
> History of melanoma
> ***Environmental History***
> Excessive outdoor exposure to UV radiation (having five or more sunburns doubles the risk for melanoma)
>   Use of indoor tanning beds

Research into the genetic components of melanoma and dysplastic nevi (precursor lesions) has found a relationship between dysplastic nevi, family history, and the development of melanoma. The finding of a dysplastic nevus (atypical mole) or any other type of skin cancer (such as BCC or SCC) is thought to increase the risk of melanoma. The number of nevi (moles) normally peaks during young adulthood (ages 20 to 25 years), then gradually decreases after the age of 50 years. Large numbers of nevi on an individual who is older than 50 years of age is considered to be a strong marker for an increased risk of melanoma. It is estimated that 7% of the white population has at least one atypical nevus, and many individuals have numerous nevi that should be monitored closely.

All melanomas should be tested for mutations in *BRAF*, a gene involved in cell growth signaling, because such mutations appear in about half of all metastatic melanomas. Although *BRAF* is the official symbol designation, the gene is also known as *B-Raf* or *v-Raf murine sarcoma viral oncogene homolog B1*. As with other proto-oncogenes, a mutation in this gene has the potential to cause normal cells to become cancerous. Identifying this mutation may be beneficial in the treatment of melanoma, because at least three small molecule inhibitor drugs, vemurafenib (Zelboraf), dabrafenib (Tafinlar), and encorafenib (Braftovi), are used to treat *BRAF* mutation–positive melanomas. These drugs are discussed in more detail in the section on malignant melanoma management.

The combination of having a first-degree relative with melanoma and the presence of one or more dysplastic nevi increases the risk of developing melanoma by up to 50% compared with the general population. Individuals with these traits tend to develop multiple primary lesions at a younger age compared with other individuals with melanomas. In addition, large-sized nevi (greater than 20 mm) are believed to be associated with increased melanoma risk. Currently, lifetime risk within the entire population is estimated at 1 in 75, with fully one-third of all cases occurring in persons younger than 45 years. However, this risk ranges widely depending on ethnic background and skin color, with a lifetime risk as high as 1 in 40 for lighter-skinned (white) individuals and as low as 1 in 1,000 for darker-skinned (i.e., black) individuals.

Although the incidence of malignant melanoma in children is low, pediatric overexposure to UV rays, especially a history of one or more blistering sunburns before the age of 20 years, has been linked to a dramatic increase in lifetime risk of developing melanoma. It is thought that the effect of accumulated sunburns, in addition to genetic predisposition, is not seen until years later. Intermittent intense sun exposures (e.g., those that may occur in occupational groups such as farmers) that result in blistering sunburns appear to be more significant in terms of increased melanoma risk than chronic sun exposure.

PATHOPHYSIOLOGY

Malignant melanoma can be divided into several subtypes:

- Superficial spreading (70% to 85%): characterized by extensive lateral or radial growth before vertical invasion
- Nodular (15% to 30%): characterized by vertical growth only
- Lentigo maligna (5%): an in situ form that may persist for years before vertical extension
- Acral lentiginous (2% to 8%): a particularly aggressive form most common in darker-skinned patients, especially when appearing on the hands or feet

In addition to these main categories, melanomas may be classified in more detail according to a combination of the strength of their association with sun exposure, the physical qualities of the malignant lesions themselves, and their physical location on the body, as summarized in the following section.

Classifications of Melanoma

1. Those related to sun exposure: cumulative solar damage (CSD)
    a. Low CSD (superficial spreading melanomas)
    b. High CSD (lentigo maligna and desmoplastic)

2. Nonsolar category
   a. Acral melanomas
   b. Some congenital nevi
   c. Melanomas in blue nevi
   d. Spitz melanomas
   e. Mucosal melanomas
   f. Uveal melanomas

A combination of UV exposure and genetic susceptibility is believed to be the most common mechanism for developing melanoma. Studies have linked UV radiation, particularly UVB rays, to genetic mutations in DNA in susceptible individuals, resulting in the development of abnormal pigmented lesions (dysplastic nevi). Genetic predisposition to melanoma appears to be the result of the presence of a mutated or absent tumor suppressor gene. Abnormalities have been mapped to chromosomes 1 and 9. In particular, mutations in chromosomal region 9p21, which encodes the tumor suppressor gene *CDKN2A* that produces the protein p16, have been observed in a large proportion of both familial and spontaneous melanomas, as well as the previously discussed mutations in the *BRAF* gene, which are seen in over half of all melanomas. Germ line mutations in the gene *CDK4* have also been observed. Individuals in these susceptible groups tend to develop melanoma at multiple primary sites at an earlier age.

Another strong genetic association is observed in the autosomal-recessive condition xeroderma pigmentosum. Persons affected with this inherited disorder lack a critical DNA repair mechanism that corrects mutations in UV light–associated cross-linked DNA nucleotides. A failure to correct these nucleotide mismatches results in multiple DNA breaks in response to cumulative UV light exposure and, therefore, a resultant high level of sun-associated skin cancers, including melanoma (as well as BCC and SCC).

Atypical nevi are precursors to malignant melanoma. They differ histologically from benign nevi in that they are disorganized and carry higher potential for transformation into malignant tissue. Initially, the tumor remains confined to the epidermis. If left untreated, it spreads into the subcutaneous fat. Microscopic lesions of superficial spreading-type melanoma have large, atypical pigmented cells of variable colors in the epidermis and the papillary dermis and lymphocytes. Nodular melanoma lesions have multiple tumor cells that form a nodule in the dermis, with invasion to the deeper dermal layers. Metastases to distant sites result when tumors invade through dermal lymphatics or blood vessels. Thus, metastasis occurs in the regional lymph nodes and occasionally at distant sites such as the bone, viscera, and especially the lungs, liver, and brain, which are the most commonly affected organs.

In the absence of metastasis, the four primary prognostic factors of melanoma are patient age, gender, tumor thickness, and tumor location. Worse prognoses are seen in older males with thicker tumors located in an axial distribution, as opposed to on the extremities. In addition, the relative importance of certain prognostic factors also depends on tumor stage. In earlier disease limited to the skin, tumor thickness and the presence of ulceration are key. However, in more advanced disease, along with the presence of ulceration, the degree of lymph nodal involvement is the most important factor.

CLINICAL PRESENTATION

Subjective

There are usually no symptoms associated with melanoma; however, some patients present with a pruritic, ulcerated, or bleeding mole. The typical patient is an adult who is concerned about a large mole that has changed in appearance. A change in characteristics of a mole is a frequent observation made by melanoma patients, whereas other patients seek care in response to a concerned family member or significant other who has advised them to have a mole checked. The patient typically will report having had the same mole for many years before its change in appearance. A family history of melanoma or skin cancer may be reported by some patients.

Objective

Most melanomas appear on sun-exposed areas of skin. The back and the neck are the most common sites in males, and the legs are more common in females. In African Americans and Asian Americans, the feet, fingers, nailbeds, eyes (uveal tract), and mucous membranes are more common sites.

Melanoma often presents as an asymmetrical lesion with an irregular border, notching, and a diameter greater than 6 mm. The tumor often exhibits variegation in color, with admixtures of blue, red, tan, brown, black, and white. Rarely, tumors may be amelanotic. Early nodular tumors, for example, are typically flat and may lack most of the typical characteristics of melanoma. As the tumor advances, however, an increase in thickness causes elevation into a firm nodule (nodular melanoma).

Atypical nevi bear many of the same characteristics of a true melanoma, including irregular ill-defined borders, color variegation, and a large size (more than 6 mm). However, the emphasis on larger lesion size as an increased risk factor for melanoma is not always accurate because early melanomas can be smaller than 6 mm in diameter. Distinguishing between malignant melanoma and benign nevi can be difficult and often requires a skin biopsy.

Nailbed or subungual melanoma may be observed in older patients and is most commonly found on the thumb or great toe. This variant of acral lentiginous melanoma may present similarly to an ungual fungal infection, because discoloration of the nailbed known as *longitudinal melanonychia* may distort the nail itself. Posterior nailbed involvement called *Hutchinson's sign* is an ominous physical finding associated with advanced disease.

DIAGNOSTIC REASONING

Diagnostic Tests

A thorough physical examination including full-body skin inspection is the initial step in diagnosis. Dermoscopy (the examination of a suspicious lesion using epiluminescence microscopy) augments the evaluation of pigmented skin and aids in the diagnosis of melanoma. Prebiopsy photographs are recommended, including a regional photo with anatomical landmarks to help with clinical correlation, as well as prevent wrong-site surgery. Suspicious lesions should be biopsied under local anesthesia by a dermatologist. Excisional biopsy is the preferred method if melanoma is suspected because a measurement of thickness can be made along with staging, as a predictor of prognosis and a guide for treatment. Thickness or depth of the melanoma is one of the critical factors in determining both prognosis and choice of therapy. The TNM (tumor, node, metastasis) system adopted by the American Joint Committee on Cancer (AJCC) provides a method to clinically stage malignant melanomas, as described in Box 17.3. In addition, this system has been developed to take into account tumor thickness, mitotic rate, ulceration, and invasiveness (localized tumor versus nodal or distant metastases) as key prognostic factors.

> **Box 17.3   TNM Malignant Melanoma Classification System**
>
> The American Joint Committee on Cancer (AJCC) has an ongoing collaborative staging system in process. The TNM (tumor, node, metastasis) system adopted by the AJCC replaces both the Clark and Breslow methods to clinically stage malignant melanomas. Assigning a stage to a melanoma will help determine treatment options.
>
> **T (Primary Tumor) Category**
>
> T0: no melanoma cells at primary site
> Tis: superficial growth; in situ or precancer
> T1, T2, T3, or T4: increasing tumor size and amount of spread
>
> **N (Lymph Nodes) Category**
>
> N0: nearby lymph nodes do not contain cancer
> N1, N2, or N3: increasing number of nearby lymph nodes affected
>
> **M (Metastasis) Category**
>
> M0: no distant cancer spread
> M1: cancer has spread to distant organs or tissues

A patient diagnosed with melanoma should be referred to a dermatologist or an oncologist for excision of the melanoma and its margins. However, if biopsy pathology reveals only atypical nevi, removal of the lesion by excisional biopsy is sufficient treatment. A patient who has dysplastic nevi should receive regular skin surveillance. Skin examinations are usually done at 6-month intervals by a dermatologist.

Subsequent testing may include a lymph node biopsy via computed tomography (CT)–guided needle aspiration. Lymphatic drainage mapping and sentinel node biopsy have been shown to identify occult metastases by employing a technique that identifies the lymph node specifically draining the area of skin that contains the melanoma. This node, called the *sentinel node,* is excised and examined for melanoma cells. If any cancer cells are present, the remaining nodes in the area are dissected. If biopsy of the sentinel node is negative, metastasis is unlikely and recurrence rates are low. If metastatic disease is suspected, however, a thorough physical examination, laboratory tests, x-ray studies, and CT scans are done to evaluate for distant metastases.

Differential Diagnosis

Differentiating between melanoma and benign or premalignant lesions can prove challenging, even for dermatologists. Although the majority of atypical nevi and melanomas fit the ABCDEs of melanoma, an occasional lesion will escape early detection. The differential diagnosis for melanoma includes pigmented skin lesions such as benign nevi, solar lentigines, and seborrheic keratoses. Seborrheic keratoses are benign lesions that are common in older adult patients. The lesions are light to dark brown and appear as soft, wart-like growths, located mainly on the trunk. In contrast, melanoma is usually located on sun-exposed areas such as the neck, the back, or the legs. Solar lentigines (liver spots) are pigmented (light to dark brown) macules that appear on sun-exposed areas such as the dorsum of the hands and arms. Benign nevi (moles) are round to oval with regular borders; most are less than 5 mm in diameter. The color is evenly distributed in a benign nevus, which is asymptomatic.

MANAGEMENT

A high index of suspicion is necessary because it is often difficult to distinguish atypical nevi from melanoma or normal nevi. If a clinician suspects possible melanoma or dysplastic nevi, referral to a dermatologist is necessary. In the United States, when a melanoma is detected early, there is an estimated 5-year survival rate of 98%. However, this survival rate falls to 62% when the melanoma extends into the lymph nodes and 18% when it metastasizes to distant organs.

There are four treatments available for melanoma, which may be used in combination: Mohs surgery (or other type of excision), chemotherapy, radiation therapy, and biological therapy. If the melanoma lesion is discovered early enough, the chance of a complete cure with excision is good. Management will depend on the staging of the lesion (see Box 17.3). In situ melanomas require excisional margins of at least 0.5 cm. Melanomas measuring less than 2 mm in thickness require at least a 1-cm circumferential surgical margin, whereas thicker tumors need at least 2-cm margins. Lymph node dissection is required when there is evidence of draining lymph node involvement on clinical examination, but its ability to improve outcomes is unclear when performed empirically. Patients younger than 40 years commonly have higher rates of positive nodes, which should be considered when determining the necessity of lymph node biopsy.

Nonmetastatic melanomas that have not spread beyond their site of origin are often curable. Melanomas with a thickness of 2 mm or more are curable in a significant proportion of patients, but the risk of lymph node and/or systemic metastasis grows with increasing thickness of the primary lesion. Some melanomas that have spread to regional lymph nodes may be curable with wide local excision of the primary tumor and removal of the affected regional lymph nodes.

In addition to excision of the lesion with its margins, patients with metastatic disease are treated with several other modalities. One of the main treatments is chemotherapy with dacarbazine (DTIC), temozolomide, carboplatin/paclitaxel, or fotemustine. Only 15% to 30% of patients respond to chemotherapy with a reduction in tumor size. Unfortunately, the response to chemotherapy is typically short term, and fewer than 5% of patients will experience a remission of their disease. If the melanoma is located on a limb, high-dose chemotherapy via isolated limb perfusion is available. In this technique, the circulation of the affected limb is isolated by a tourniquet at the root of the limb. High-dose chemotherapy is infused and is limited to the affected limb only, minimizing the adverse systemic effects from the chemotherapy.

External beam radiation to treat melanoma is usually reserved for palliative treatment. For metastatic lesions of the lung, brain, or viscera that cause pressure on tissue, radiation therapy is used to reduce the tumor's size and provide relief from pain.

Administration of biological therapy such as high-dose interferon and interleukin (IL)-2 in high-risk patients (to prevent recurrence) has shown some promise. In addition, therapies directed at specific gene mutations are used. Although melanomas that have spread to distant sites are rarely curable, *BRAF* inhibitors, including the small molecule serine/threonine protein kinase inhibitors vemurafenib (Zelboraf) and dabrafenib (Tafinlar), may be helpful. MEK inhibitors include trametinib (Mekinist) and cobimetinib (Cotellic). Trametinib is given with dabrafenib, thereby blocking both the MEK enzyme molecule and the *BRAF* molecule mutation. Combination therapy with both biological therapy and chemotherapy continues to be studied. In addition, vaccines that stimulate immune function against melanoma tumors are being developed.

FOLLOW-UP AND REFERRAL

Patients at increased risk for developing melanoma should be referred to a dermatologist for increased surveillance, including regular physical examinations and full skin and mucosal surface inspection. Ophthalmological examination may also be indicated in the metastatic patient without a readily identifiable primary tumor (e.g., a patient with melanomatous liver metastases but no primary skin tumor), given the propensity for melanoma to develop in the pigmented uveal cells of the eye. The patient who wishes to participate in clinical trials for melanoma can obtain information on current studies from an oncologist. For the patient with an inoperable melanoma or extensive distant metastases, hospice and palliative care should be offered.

Patient Education: Malignant Melanoma

Prevention of all skin cancers should start early during infancy, especially in individuals with a Celtic background or with a positive family history for skin cancer. Prevention remains the most important intervention, and early diagnosis significantly improves treatment outcomes. Early detection of melanomas is made easier to remember with the ABCDE mnemonic, as discussed earlier.

A person's risk of melanoma doubles if they have had more than five sunburns. Thus, teaching patients about the proper use of sunscreen cannot be overemphasized. Studies have shown that with daily, rather than discretionary, use of sunscreen, the risk of developing SCC was reduced by approximately 40%, the risk of developing any melanoma by 50%, and the risk of invasive melanoma by 73%. Thus, patients should avoid staying under the sun during the hottest part of the day, high-SPF sunscreens should be applied on a daily basis, and hats or headgear should be worn to protect the scalp and back of the neck. Wearing loose-fitting, long-sleeved shirts and long pants provides some protection from the sun and is equivalent to wearing sunscreen if the skin is entirely covered.

The hazards of tanning beds need to be discussed with all patients. Because more than 419,000 cases of skin cancer in the United States each year are linked to tanning beds, the FDA reclassified tanning beds from class I (no risk) to class II (moderate risk). In the United States, at least 45 states restrict minors of some age from using indoor tanning beds, and some countries (e.g., Brazil, Australia) have banned indoor tanning beds altogether, as a result of the World Health Organization declaring tanning beds a level I carcinogen.

Survivors of melanoma need to be informed of their increased risk of a second primary tumor or of recurrence of the previous lesion. Any change in an existing lesion or any new pigmented skin lesion should be reported to the patient's primary care practitioner and dermatologist. Likewise, patients should be urged to report any swelling in the lymph nodes of the neck, axilla, or groin area.

NONMELANOMATOUS SKIN CANCERS

The two most common forms of nonmelanomatous skin cancer in humans are BCC and SCC. BCC is a malignant tumor of the skin that originates in the basal cells of the epidermis. It is a slow-growing and locally invasive tumor that rarely metastasizes. It represents the beginning of a continuum of skin cancers in both severity and mortality. SCC, a malignant tumor originating from keratinocytes, can invade the dermis and occasionally metastasize to distant sites. Avoidance of excessive sun exposure is an important factor in preventing these skin cancers. In addition, screening programs are important in the early recognition and diagnosis of these cancers, because they are highly curable when discovered in their early stages.

EPIDEMIOLOGY AND CAUSES

The incidence of BCC and SCC is expected to rise in the United States over the next decade because of the increase in the older adult population and a longer overall life expectancy. More than one in three new cancers is a skin cancer, with BCC being the more common of the two nonmelanomatous skin cancers and the most common type of skin cancer overall. Each year, more than 4 million cases of BCC are diagnosed in the United States.

Rarely, BCC results from basal cell nevus syndrome, an inherited autosomal-dominant disorder. Patients with this disorder tend to have multiple sites of BCC at a younger age. It is associated with bone cysts, palmar skin pits, and frontal bossing (a protuberance of the bones of the skull, particularly those under the skin of the forehead).

SCC is the second most common skin cancer, accounting for an estimated 20% of all skin cancers. Every year in the United States, there are more than 1 million persons diagnosed with SCC. Over the past 30 years, the incidence of SCC has increased up to 200%, and as many as 8,800 individuals die of SCC annually. This increase is due in part to the use of tanning beds. One variant of the disease that affects mostly older white males is Bowen's disease, an intraepidermal SCC that can be induced by exposure to inorganic trivalent arsenic or inhaled mustard gas, in addition to chronic sun exposure.

The most important risk factor for both BCC and SCC is chronic accumulated sun exposure. Therefore, these skin cancers are typically seen in older adults. In particular, midrange UV light in the UVB part of the spectrum is believed to be more cancer-inducing than UVA rays. Individuals most at risk are those of Celtic background (Irish, Scottish, English) who are light-haired (e.g., red-haired or blond), blue-eyed, freckled, and who sunburn easily. In addition, males are twice as likely to develop BCC and three times as likely to develop squamous skin cancers compared with females.

Other conditions that increase the risk of SCC include immunosuppression, a history of exposure to ionizing radiation, exposure to arsenic and polycyclic aromatic hydrocarbons (e.g., paint thinners, organic solvents), treatment with psoralens and UV light (therapy used for psoriasis), and infection with oncogenic HPV. SCC is also seen with increased frequency in areas of skin damage due to chronic inflammation, burns, old scars, or chronic ulcers (see Risk Factors: Nonmelanomatous Skin Cancer).

Risk Factors: Nonmelanomatous Skin Cancer

Age
Risk increases with age

Sex
Male

Skin, Eye, Hair Color
Lighter-skinned, with a tendency to tan poorly and burn quickly
  Blue eyes
  Red or blond hair

Personal History
History of skin cancer
  History of basal cell nevus syndrome
  History of precancerous lesions, including actinic keratosis
  History of burn scars or areas of skin damaged by chronic inflammation or ulcers
  History of immunosuppression

Environmental History
Excessive exposure to UV radiation (sunlight)
  Exposure to arsenic, polycyclic aromatic hydrocarbons, or radiation

PATHOPHYSIOLOGY

The majority of BCCs and SCCs are the result of DNA damage in skin cells that have been exposed to many years of UV radiation from sunlight. The damage is cumulative and is mediated primarily by defects in DNA repair mechanisms in response to mutational cross-linking by UV light. Such cumulative damage is particularly important in the development of BCC, particularly within skin containing a high concentration of sebaceous glands.

Several forms of BCC are seen clinically, including nodular, sclerosing, and superficial forms. The nodulo-ulcerative type is the most common, with well-differentiated tumor cells that may extend from the dermal–epidermal interface into the dermis and subcutaneous fat. Superficial BCC appears similar to dermatitis, with erythema and scaling bordered by a fine rim. The origins of these tumors appear to be multifocal, with multiple small nodules arising from different epidermal foci. The sclerosing or morpheaform type of BCC is highly aggressive with a high rate of recurrence, presenting as a white plaque with palpable fibrosis and poorly circumscribed margins. Histologically, these tumors consist of spindle cells invading the dermal skin layer. If not treated, BCC continues to grow and invade surrounding cartilage, bone, and soft tissues. BCC rarely metastasizes to distant sites, however.

In contrast, SCC is considered more dangerous than BCC because of its faster rate of growth and tendency to metastasize. The precursor lesion of most SCC is actinic keratosis, a relatively common finding in older lighter-skinned patients. As discussed earlier, actinic keratosis results from accumulated chronic sun exposure and is found only on sun-exposed skin. Actinic keratoses are premalignant lesions involving the uppermost layer of the epidermis that have been shown in some studies to have a low potential for development into malignancy (as low as 0.1%), although other studies have suggested rates as high as 20%, especially when one considers the risk becomes additive for individuals with more than one actinic keratosis on the body, which is not unusual.

In situ SCC (Bowen's disease) involves the full thickness of the epidermis and is the earliest form of SCC. Interestingly, in contrast to BCC, more recent excessive UV light exposure, rather than cumulative lifetime exposure, correlates best with the development of squamous cell skin cancer, particularly in areas with few sebaceous glands. Invasive SCC is characterized by penetration through the epidermis and into the dermis, with a rate of metastasis of approximately 5%, primarily to the regional lymph nodes. Lesions that metastasize at a higher rate include those located on the lips, the ear, or at sites of trauma such as old scars and chronic wounds (e.g., ulcers), as well as larger lesions (more than 2 cm in diameter or more than 4 mm in depth). Patients on immunosuppressive therapy also have a higher rate of metastasis.

As observed in melanoma, any underlying condition affecting DNA repair increases the risk of developing BCC and SCC. For example, in the rare autosomal recessive condition xeroderma pigmentosum, individuals lose the ability to repair UV light–induced DNA cross-linking damage, resulting in multiple DNA breaks and malignant transformation of skin cells. UV light exposure has also been correlated with mutations of specific oncogenes and tumor suppressor genes, including *p53* (seen in more than half of all BCC and up to 90% of SCC) and the human patched (PTCH) gene. Such mutations result in dysregulated programmed cell death (apoptosis) and uncontrolled proliferation of epidermal cellular clones.

Several other mechanisms also contribute to the development of keratinocyte and basal cell skin cancers. Epidermal antigen-presenting Langerhans cells suffer direct damage from UV radiation, compromising the ability of the immune system to recognize and clear tumor antigen-expressing cancer cells. Systemic glucocorticoids also contribute to immunosuppression and have been shown in some studies to more than double the risk of developing nonmelanomatous skin cancer. In fact, intact immunosurveillance is key to the prevention of cutaneous carcinomas, as BCC is 10 times more likely to develop in chronically immunosuppressed organ transplant recipients, whereas SCC is up to 250 times more likely to occur. Although these tumors tend to develop at least 2 years after the transplant, they are more aggressive, more likely to occur at multiple sites, and begin to develop at a younger age than in nontransplanted, immunocompetent individuals.

Several types of proinflammatory cytokines have been identified in skin affected by cutaneous carcinomas, including tumor necrosis factor–alpha and IL-10. Prostaglandin synthesis also appears critical to this process, and selective cyclooxygenase-2 inhibitors have been shown to confer a protective effect against BCC and SCC in mouse models. Infection with HPV is associated with the development of anogenital SCC, particularly serotypes 16 and 18. In immunosuppressed individuals, the development of cutaneous warts and nonmelanomatous skin cancers appears to be correlated. In addition, keratoacanthoma (a fast-growing hyperkeratotic nodular lesion indistinguishable from well-differentiated SCC) has also been associated with HPV infection. However, the specific role of HPV in additional forms of keratinocyte skin cancers remains controversial, and further research to explore this relationship is ongoing.

CLINICAL PRESENTATION

Subjective

A typical patient with nonmelanomatous skin carcinoma is an adult or older patient who presents with complaints of a spot or bump that is getting larger or a sore that is not healing. Often, the lesion appears as a thick, rough patch that may bleed if scratched or scraped. Some patients mistakenly think they are warts with a raised border and crusted surface. The skin lesion may be pruritic or asymptomatic.

Objective

BCC typically appears on areas of the skin that are chronically exposed to the sun, such as the face, ears, cheeks, nose, and the neck. Nodulo-ulcerative BCC is characterized by elevated papules that have a pearly appearance, with some crusting. When the crusts are removed, a small amount of bleeding ensues. On close examination, telangiectatic blood vessels are seen on the border of the lesion. A central ulceration is seen during the later stages of BCC lesions. BCC lesions may be the same color as the patient's skin or have areas of variegated color such as blue, black, or brown.

SCC is typically found on sun-exposed areas, such as the lips, the tips of ears, the nose, the upper cheeks, the scalp (in bald males), the dorsa of the hands and forearms, and the shins in females. Smokers are prone to cancerous lesions on the lips and tongue. The most common presentation of SCC is a firm papule with a scaly (keratotic) rough surface with irregular borders. These lesions may even present as cutaneous horns, with columnar hyperkeratosis atop an erythematous base. Later, the surfaces of SCC lesions tend to bleed easily (become friable) with minor trauma and appear eroded with ulcerations. The typical lesion of Bowen's disease appears as a solitary, slowly enlarging erythematous, red-brown, hyperkeratotic plaque that has slight scaling and minimal crusting. Similar lesions in the anogenital region known as *Bowenoid papulosis* have been associated with oncogenic HPV strains.

DIAGNOSTIC REASONING

Diagnostic Tests

Suspicious lesions (if not located on the face) can be biopsied by an experienced primary care practitioner or referred to a dermatologist. Because BCC rarely metastasizes, staging of the lesions is not necessary. SCC, however, has a higher rate of metastasis and may require staging based on the pathologist's report. Other important factors that determine staging include tumor characteristics, spread to regional lymph nodes, and metastasis to other organs.

Differential Diagnosis

The differential diagnoses of nonmelanomatous skin cancer include actinic keratosis, seborrheic keratosis, atopic dermatitis (eczema), and solar lentigo. The presence of actinic keratosis lesions on patients is considered a marker for excessive sun exposure. Recognition of actinic keratosis, a precancerous skin lesion, is important because treatment during this stage is very simple. Typical actinic keratosis lesions appear on sun-exposed surfaces and are pink to red or sometimes brown. In contrast to BCC, in which only one or a few lesions are present at a time in most patients, actinic keratosis lesions are typically present in greater numbers. Lesions vary in size from 2 mm to 1 cm in diameter. These numerous lesions are also located on chronically sun-exposed areas such as the face and the head, the back of the neck, the dorsum of the hands and arms, and the upper shoulders.

In contrast to BCC and SCC, seborrheic keratosis lesions predominantly appear on non–sun-exposed areas of the body, such as the trunk in older adult patients, and do not appear erythematous or scaly. A patient with atopic dermatitis will report an atopic history and the recurrence of lesions in the same location that resolve with 1 to 2 weeks of treatment with topical corticosteroids. Solar lentigo lesions are found in older adults on sun-exposed areas of the skin; these "liver spots" appear as multiple smooth, flat, brown macules (like enlarged freckles) that are from 1 to 3 cm in size.

MANAGEMENT

Management of nonmelanomatous skin cancers is dependent on several factors: size and depth of the invasion, location, cosmetic concerns, and metastasis to other sites. Almost all cases of BCC and most cases of SCC require only simple excision under local anesthesia. Some primary care practitioners and dermatologists elect excisional biopsy at the time of initial diagnosis; this procedure is both diagnostic and curative. Alternative methods for removal of small BCC and SCC lesions include electrodesiccation and curettage, cryosurgery with liquid nitrogen, and laser surgery. SCC has an overall rate of remission of up to 90% after therapy.

Mohs microsurgery has the highest cure rate for both BCC and SCC. This precise technique involves the surgical removal and simultaneous microscopic examination of small layers of skin, with removal of only the smallest amount of tissue necessary to eradicate the tumor (until disease-free margins are confirmed). This technique involves less scarring and is particularly suited for the treatment of tumors in places of cosmetic importance, such as the face. Skin grafting may be necessary in addition to tumor removal.

In addition to surgical excision, lymph node dissection and systemic chemotherapy are used to treat large and invasive SCC lesions that have metastasized. External beam radiation is used as the primary treatment for tumors that are large or located in areas of skin that make surgery difficult, or in older or debilitated patients who are poor surgical candidates. External beam therapy is also used as adjuvant therapy in lesions with a high risk of recurrence or in cancers that have metastasized.

Topical therapies are also used for superficial forms of BCC, including imiquimod cream (used five times weekly), topical 5-fluorouracil (5-FU), and photodynamic treatment (used for both nodular and superficial forms) utilizing a photosensitizer with blue wavelength phototherapy to create reactive oxygen species. Similar approaches are being used for SCC. For example, imiquimod is used for in situ Bowen's disease. Premalignant actinic keratosis is also typically treated with topical chemotherapy (e.g., 5-FU cream) or cryotherapy with liquid nitrogen. Other treatment options include dermabrasion, shave excision, electrodesiccation and curettage, and laser therapy.

Recurrence rates for both BCC and SCC after treatment vary with tumor characteristics and the treatment modality selected. Most recurrences occur within 3 years of treatment. Mohs microsurgery is an option for recurrent lesions, as it has a particularly high cure rate for lesions that have recurred after other types of treatment. Metastasis after SCC usually occurs where there is a chronic inflammatory skin condition, such as on the ears, nose, lips, or in mucosal areas such as the mouth, nose, or genitals.

FOLLOW-UP AND REFERRAL

Referral to a dermatologist or oncologist is necessary for all suspicious skin lesions, including nonmelanomatous skin cancers. The majority of patients require only simple excision of the skin lesion, with follow-up by the dermatologist or the clinician who performed the procedure to monitor skin healing. Subsequent follow-up includes complete physical examinations with full skin examinations every 6 to 12 months or more often if there are any signs of new or changing skin lesions or recurrence of a lesion at the primary site. The patient who has been diagnosed with any type of skin cancer is at increased risk of developing more skin lesions in the future, including recurrences of the original primary lesion.

Patient Education: Nonmelanomatous Skin Cancers

Although the U.S. Preventive Services Task Force states there is insufficient evidence to recommend screening for skin cancer by clinicians, the American Cancer Society recommends skin examinations both by clinicians and patients (self-examination). Patients of all ages should be taught the importance of monthly skin self-examinations and to report any changes in preexisting skin lesions (see Table 17.2). Moreover, the importance of careful examination of the skin on an annual basis by a trained health professional cannot be overemphasized for certain patients. These include patients with a family history of melanoma, multiple nevi, a history of sunburns, frequent sun exposure, and persons who work in certain high-risk occupations or avocations, such as farmers, gardeners, and sailors. Unfortunately, research has shown that a large proportion of primary care practitioners do not routinely document findings related to the skin on physical examination.

Survivors of nonmelanomatous skin cancer should be informed of their increased risk of developing a second lesion or of recurrence of the original lesion. Thus, these patients in particular should be instructed to report any changes in existing moles or the development of new or rapidly growing lesions.

Approximately 80% of lifetime exposure to UV radiation occurs before the age of 20 years in the majority of patients. Therefore, *Healthy People 2030* has several objectives to increase the proportion of adolescents and adults who follow protective measures that may reduce the risk of skin cancer. Strategies to avoid sun exposure should be discussed with all patients at every physical examination, particularly with the parents of infants, young children, and adolescents. Patients and their families should be advised of the following preventive strategies for skin cancers in general:

- Avoid sun exposure from 11 a.m. to 4 p.m., which is typically the period of the day with the most intense UV radiation.
- Wear protective clothing (e.g., tight-weave fabric, long-sleeve shirt, and a wide-brimmed hat); males frequently get lesions on the top of the ear.
- Wear large-framed, wraparound sunglasses with 99% to 100% UV absorption.
- Apply a sunscreen with an SPF of at least 15 as directed, even on hazy days; reapply sunscreen as needed.
- Avoid the use of tanning beds and sun lamps.
- Learn the ABCDEs of malignant melanoma.

TABLE 17.2 Patient Education: Skin Self-Examination

Once a month, perform a skin self-examination. Record your initial examination, then note any changes with each subsequent examination. Use the following table as a guide.

Head	Looking in a mirror, carefully inspect your head. Using a comb or hair dryer, carefully part your hair and inspect your scalp.
Face and neck	Looking in a mirror, carefully inspect your entire face and neck, including the nose, lips, and ears.
Arms and hands	Holding up each arm, carefully inspect each arm and hand, including the underarms and back of your upper arms (a mirror may be needed). Holding up each hand, carefully inspect the front and back of each hand and wrist, including the areas between each finger and the fingernails.
Chest, torso, and front of the legs	Standing and looking in a full-length mirror, carefully inspect your chest (including breasts), torso, and front of the legs.
Back, buttocks, and back of the legs	Standing and looking in a full-length mirror, turn so that you can carefully inspect your full back, buttocks, and back of the legs (a hand mirror may be needed).
Ankles and feet	Sitting and propping each foot on a chair or stool at a comfortable height, carefully inspect the tops and bottoms of both ankles and feet, including the areas between the toes and the toenails.
Genitalia	Sitting and using a hand mirror, carefully inspect the genitalia.

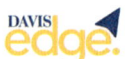 **Go to Davis Edge for practice Q&A.**

REFERENCES

Acne Vulgaris

Oge LK, Broussard A, Marshall MD. Acne vulgaris: diagnosis and treatment. *Am Fam Physician.* 2019 Oct. 15;100(8):475–484.

Actinic Keratosis

Drugs.com. Fluorouracil cream. https://www.drugs.com/cdi/fluorouracil-cream.html. Accessed 3/28/2021.

Malignant Melanoma

DiChiara T. Published 2020. The 5 stages of melanoma. Definitions and how each stage impacts treatment and survival. https://www.verywellhealth.com/melanoma-staging-what-it-means-and-reveals-3010755. Accessed 3/28/2021.

Elder DE, Bastian BC, Cree IA, et al. The 2018 World Health Organization Classification of Cutaneous, Mucosal, and Uveal Melanoma: Detailed Analysis of 9 Distinct Subtypes Defined by Their Evolutionary Pathway. *Arch Pathol Lab Med.* 2020;144(4):500. Epub 2020 Feb 14.

Skin Cancer Foundation. Skin cancer facts & statistics. http://www.skincancer.org/skin-cancer-information/skin-cancer-facts. Accessed 3/8/2021.

Swetter SM, Tsao H, Bichakjian CK, et al. Guidelines of care for the management of primary cutaneous melanoma. *J Am Acad Dermatol.* 2019;80(1):208–250. https://doi.org/10.1016/j.jaad.2018.08.055

U.S. Preventive Services Task Force. Published 2020. Screening for skin cancer. https://www.uspreventiveservicestaskforce.org/uspstf/draft-update-summary/skin-cancer-screening-1. Accessed 3/8/2021.

Nonmelanomatous Skin Cancers

American Family Physician. Screening for skin cancer: recommendation statement. *Am Fam Physician.* 2016;94(6):479–481.

Healthy People 2030. Skin cancer objectives. https://health.gov/healthypeople/objectives-and-data/browse-objectives/cancer/reduce-proportion-students-grades-9-through-12-who-report-sunburn-c-10. Accessed 3/8/2021.

Skin Cancer Foundation. Basal cell carcinoma overview. The most common skin cancer. http://www.skincancer.org/skin-cancer-information/basal-cell-carcinoma. Accessed 3/8/2021.

Skin Cancer Foundation. Squamous cell carcinoma overview. The second most common skin cancer. http://www.skincancer.org/skin-cancer-information/squamous-cell-carcinoma/. Accessed 3/8/2021.

Rosacea

Gallo RL, Granstein RD, Kang S, et al. Standard classification and pathophysiology of rosacea: The 2017 update by the National Rosacea Society Expert Committee. *J Am Acad Dermatol.* 2018;78(1):148.

National Rosacea Society. Tools for the professional. https://www.rosacea.org/physicians/tools-for-the-professional. Accessed 2/27/2021.

Seborrheic Keratosis

American Academy of Dermatology. Seborrheic keratosis: diagnosis and treatment. https://www.aad.org/public/diseases/bumps-and-growths/seborrheic-keratoses. Accessed 3/8/2021.

Wehner M, Chren M-M, Nameth D, et al. International prevalence of indoor tanning: a systematic review and meta-analysis. *JAMA Dermatol.* 2014;150(4):390–400.

RESOURCES

General

National Institutes of Health/National Center for Complementary and Integrative Health. https://www.nccih.nih.gov/health/skin-conditions-at-a-glance

Acne Vulgaris

American Academy of Dermatology. https://www.aad.org/public/diseases/acne/skin-care/tips#treatment

Malignant Lesions

American Academy of Dermatology. https://www.aad.org/public/diseases/skin-cancer/

American Cancer Society
 https://www.cancer.org/cancer/skin-cancer.html

Skin Cancer Foundation Skin Cancer Staging
 http://www.skincancer.org/skin-cancer-information/melanoma/the-stages-of-melanoma/guide-to-staging-melanoma

Section 3: EYE PROBLEMS

SECTION EDITOR

Lynne M. Dunphy, PhD, APRN, FNP-BC, FAAN, FAANP

Chapter 18

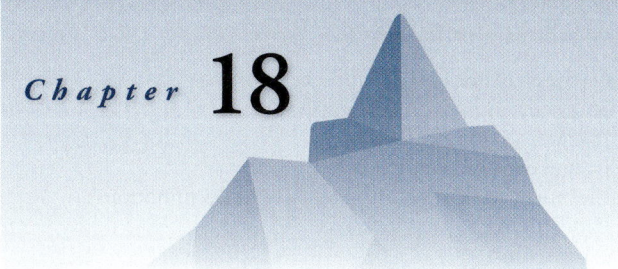

Common Eye Complaints

Benjamin G. Kuhar, DO
Lynne M. Dunphy, PhD, APRN, FNP-BC, FAAN, FAANP
Brian Oscar Porter, MD, PhD, MPH, MBA

OVERVIEW

It is important to determine the appropriate cause of a patient's eye complaints and know when to refer to an ophthalmologist. Symptoms of vision-threatening conditions, such as cataracts, retinal detachment, macular degeneration, and glaucoma, should be recognized. A careful history (see Focus on History: Eye Complaints) should also include inquiries about current medication usage, particularly ocular medications. Past medical history or family history of coexisting connective tissue disorders, rheumatoid arthritis, inflammatory bowel disease, Parkinson's disease, rosacea, and thyroid abnormalities are pertinent positives that will help the clinician formulate a diagnosis. Dry mouth (xerostomia), muscle or joint pain, and heat or cold intolerance are significant findings because they are often associated with comorbid inflammatory disorders. The physical examination of the eyes must always include visual acuity, which may be normal. Evaluation of pupillary size, symmetry, and light reflex is also an important technique that can aid in diagnosis. The examination may reveal a mechanical, infectious, and/or traumatic cause for the patient's complaint.

Focus on History: Eye Complaints

The following questions should be asked when evaluating a patient presenting with eye complaints:

- When did the symptoms start? Was the onset sudden or gradual?
- Do you have changes in vision? If yes, were the changes sudden or gradual?
- Do you have any pain?
- Are you experiencing any sensitivity to light or sound?
- Are you noticing any flashes of light or floaters?
- Did you sustain an injury to your eyes? If so, please describe.
- Do you have any discharge? If yes, please describe its characteristics.
- Do you wear contact lenses? If yes, describe the type, wearing schedule, and care.
- What current medications are you taking?
- Do you have a history of eye problems or eye surgeries?
- Have you had any new or past exposures to cosmetics, a person with an eye infection, smoking, or pollution? Have you traveled recently? What is your occupation? What type of environment do you live and work in?
- Do you have any systemic complaints (e.g., fever, genital discharge, rash, joint pain, etc.)?
- Do you have a family history of eye problems (glaucoma, macular degeneration, etc.)?

DRY EYE

Dry eye syndrome (DES), also known as *dry eye disease,* is a multifactorial disease of the tear film that results in discomfort, visual disturbance, and tear film instability with potential damage to the ocular surface. Essentially, DES occurs when the quantity and/or quality of tears fails to keep the surface of the eye adequately lubricated. DES is covered in more detail in Chapter 19.

DIFFERENTIAL DIAGNOSIS

The differential diagnosis of dry eye includes the following conditions:

- Blepharitis
- Contact lens complications
- Lifestyle causes (allergen exposure, dry climate, frequent computer use or TV watching)
- Inadequate blinking or eyelid closure (Bell's palsy, exophthalmos, ectropion, Parkinson's disease)
- Medications (e.g., oral contraceptives, antihistamines, beta blockers)

- Connective tissue diseases (e.g., Sjögren's syndrome, rheumatoid arthritis)
- Age-related changes
- Hormonal changes, particularly in menopausal and postmenopausal women
- Vitamin A deficiency

EXCESSIVE TEARING (EPIPHORA)

Excessive tearing is defined as the overflow of tears from one or both eyes and can occur continuously or intermittently. Excessive tearing may be a result of a paradoxical response to dry eye, exposure to an irritant, or an obstruction of the nasolacrimal duct. It is an especially common complaint in older patients and individuals with allergies. Excessive tearing is covered in more detail in Chapter 19.

DIFFERENTIAL DIAGNOSIS

The differential diagnosis of excessive tearing includes the following conditions:

- Allergens or environmental pollutants
- DES
- Viral or bacterial conjunctivitis
- Blocked lacrimal duct
- Ectropion or entropion
- Trauma (e.g., foreign body, corneal abrasion)
- Congenital glaucoma
- Uveitis
- Inflammatory orbital disease

EYE PAIN

One of the most important aspects in the management of eye pain and eye problems for the primary care practitioner to know is when to refer the patient to an ophthalmologist. The risks related to liability and complications, such as permanent damage to a patient's vision, are high. Table 18.1 presents conditions associated with eye pathology that require immediate referral to an ophthalmologist.

Due to the subjective nature of the pain experience, the presentation of eye pain may reflect a variety of underlying conditions. Thus, it is important to differentiate whether the pain is coming from the eye itself or from one of the surrounding structures.

DIFFERENTIAL DIAGNOSIS

The differential diagnosis of eye pain includes the following conditions:

- Conjunctivitis (concurrent with ocular itch)
- Corneal abrasions (manifesting as sharp pain), ulcerations

TABLE 18.1 Conditions Requiring Immediate Referral to an Ophthalmologist

- Patient complains of sudden vision loss or severe non-traumatic eye pain
- Sudden onset of flashing lights, floaters, or a "curtain" being drawn across the patient's vision (may suggest retinal detachment)

Physical examination reveals:

- Corneal ulceration
- Suspected herpes zoster ophthalmicus
- Hazy or opaque cornea
- Irregular pupil shape
- Elevation of fundus on funduscopic examination
- Papilledema
- Limbal flush
- Muscle paresis

Management issues at risk for ocular sequelae:

- Any condition requiring prolonged corticosteroid therapy
- Patient with ocular condition not improving on conservative therapy

- Foreign body irritation, overuse of contact lenses
- Eye strain, prolonged computer use
- Eyelid disorders (e.g., hordeolum, trauma, blepharitis)
- Uveitis (ache, photophobia)
- Orbital cellulitis (pain on eye movement with associated eyelid swelling)
- Scleritis (deep ache with eye movement)
- Episcleritis (mild pain typically without photophobia)
- Referred pain may occur from trauma, headache, sinusitis, temporomandibular disorder, herpes zoster ophthalmicus, postherpetic neuralgia, tumors, stroke, or trigeminal neuralgia

RED EYE

Red eye, a common ophthalmic problem encountered in both acute and primary care settings, is a nonuniform redness of the conjunctiva from hyperemia, which can be diffuse, localized, or peripheral or may encircle a clear cornea. Red eye is covered in greater detail in Chapter 19.

DIFFERENTIAL DIAGNOSIS

The differential diagnosis of red eye includes the following conditions:

- Conjunctivitis (diffuse, superficial)
- Hordeolum (stye)
- Dry eye (keratitis sicca)
- Subconjunctival hemorrhage (bright red, confluent)
- Corneal abrasions
- Acute angle-closure glaucoma

- Anterior uveitis
- Orbital cellulitis, scleritis, or episcleritis

See Table 19.1 for a comparison of selected characteristics that may be helpful in assessing the differential diagnosis of red eye.

VISUAL CHANGES

Patients often present to the primary care setting with symptoms related to changes in vision. Common visual disturbances include "floaters" and flashing lights. These subjective complaints usually have different causes. The visualization of floaters is usually due to liquefaction and contraction of the vitreous humor with aging. These degenerative vitreous changes are common sequelae of the aging process, called syneresis. Floaters may also result from tear-film debris or other material in the vitreous. Floaters are typically unilateral and are often seen when looking at a bright background. Floaters that appear gradually and become less noticeable over time are usually benign and require no treatment; however, floaters that appear suddenly and in excess warrant further evaluation.

Photopsia (i.e., flashing lights) is the subjective sensation of sparks or flashes of light induced by mechanical retinal stimulation. Any patient who complains of seeing flashing lights should be evaluated immediately for retinal tear or detachment. Monocular photopsia may occur secondary to migraine headaches, epilepsy, vertebral basilar insufficiency, retinitis, optic neuritis, retinal detachment, or microembolization. A common cause of photopsia is a posterior vitreous detachment (PVD), which causes a fluid-filled, optically empty space to form between the vitreous and the retina. It is commonly seen in patients aged 50 years and older with a female predilection. Photopsia typically carries a good visual prognosis.

Geriatric Considerations: Posterior Vitreous Detachment

PVD is a separation of the gel-like vitreous from the retina. It is estimated to occur in approximately two-thirds of people older than age 65 years. With aging, the gel-like vitreous inside the globe can liquefy, which places increased traction on the retina. This can cause classic symptoms of floaters from light passing through the condensed vitreous and flashes of light from retinal traction. In approximately 15% of patients, the vitreous can cause enough traction on the retina to result in a retinal tear, which is a vision-threatening condition. For this reason, PVD requires close monitoring and observation from an ophthalmologist to ensure there are no retinal tears or detachments. The prognosis is generally good for PVD, but an acute complaint of flashing lights or floaters in an older patient should warrant an urgent referral to an ophthalmologist.

DIFFERENTIAL DIAGNOSIS

The list of differential diagnoses of impaired vision is lengthy; however, a number of conditions occur commonly and should be well-known to the primary care provider:

- Refractive errors
- Cataracts
- Glaucoma
- Diabetic retinopathy
- Macular degeneration
- Retinal detachment
- Vitreous hemorrhage
- Central retinal artery or vein occlusion

More information about these differential diagnoses is covered in Chapter 20.

REFERENCES

General

American Academy of Ophthalmology. Preferred practice pattern guidelines. https://www.aao.org/about-preferred-practice-patterns. Accessed September 2018.

Bagheri N. *The wills eye manual: office and emergency room diagnosis and treatment of eye disease.* Wolters Kluwer; 2017.

Dry Eye

Akpek EK, et al. Dry Eye Syndrome Preferred Practice Pattern®. *Ophthalmology.* 2019 Jan;126(1):P286-P334. doi: 10.1016/j.ophtha.2018.10.023. Epub 2018 Oct 23. PMID: 30366798.

National Eye Institute. (2017). Facts about dry eye. https://www.nei.nih.gov/health/dryeye/dryeye. Accessed 8/31/31, 2017.

Epiphora

Patel J, Levin A, Patel BC. Epiphora. [Updated 2020 Aug 10]. In: StatPearls [Internet]. Treasure Island (FL): StatPearls Publishing; 2020 Jan. https://www.ncbi.nlm.nih.gov/books/NBK557449/

Eye Pain

Bowen RC, et al. The most common causes of eye pain at 2 tertiary ophthalmology and neurology clinics. *J Neuroophthalmol.* 2018; 38(3):320-327.

Collier SA, Gronostaj MP, MacGurn AK, et al. Estimated burden of keratitis–United States, 2010. *MMWR Morb Mortal Wkly Rep.* 2014;63:1027.

Galor A, Levitt RC, Felix ER, et al. Neuropathic ocular pain: an important yet underevaluated feature of dry eye. *Eye (Lond).* 2015;29(3):301-312.

Kaiser PK, et al. *The Massachusetts Eye and Ear Infirmary Illustrated Manual of Ophthalmology.* Saunders; 2014.

Roque MR. (2017). Scleritis. http://emedicine.medscape.com/article/1228324-overview.

Verma A. (2016). Corneal abrasion. http://emedicine.medscape.com/article/1195402.

Waldman N, Winrow B, Densie I, et al. An observational study to determine whether routinely sending patients home with a 24-hour supply of topical tetracaine from the emergency department for simple corneal abrasion pain is potentially safe. *Ann Emerg Med.* 2018;71:767.

Red Eye

Azari AA, Barney NP. Conjunctivitis: a systematic review of diagnosis and treatment. *JAMA*. 2013;310(16):1721-1729.

Cronau H, Kankanala RR, Mauger T. Diagnosis and management of red eye in primary care. *Am Fam Physician*. 2010;81(2):137-144.

Kaiser PK, et al. *The Massachusetts Eye and Ear Infirmary Illustrated Manual of Ophthalmology*. Saunders; 2014.

Varu DM, et al. Conjunctivitis Preferred Practice Pattern®. *Ophthalmology*. 2019 Jan;126(1):P94-P169. doi: 10.1016/j.ophtha.2018.10.020. Epub 2018 Oct 23. PMID: 30366797.

Visual Changes

Bond-Taylor M, Jakobsson G, Zetterberg M. Posterior vitreous detachment—prevalence of and risk factors for retinal tears. *Clin Ophthalmol*. 2017;11:1689-1695.

Johnson MW. Posterior vitreous detachment: evolution and complications of its early stages. *Am J Ophthalmol*. 2010 Mar; 149(3): 371-82.

Kaiser PK, et al. *The Massachusetts Eye and Ear Infirmary Illustrated Manual of Ophthalmology*. Saunders; 2014.

Sebag J. Vitreous aging and posterior vitreous detachment. *Vitreous: in Health and Disease*. Springer; 2014:131-150.

RESOURCES

National Eye Institute

Aging Eye

https://nei.nih.gov/sites/default/files/health-pdfsAgingAndEyeHealth_Tagged.pdf

https://nei.nih.gov/sites/default/files/nehep-pdfs/NEHEP_VisionAging_Infographic.pdf

https://nei.nih.gov/nehep/programs/visionandaging/toolkit

Blepharitis

https://nei.nih.gov/health/blepharitis/blepharitis

Dry Eye

https://nei.nih.gov/health/dryeye

Eyelid Disorders

https://www.nei.nih.gov/faqs/eyelid-disorders-chalazion-stye

Red Eye

https://nei.nih.gov/health/pinkeye/pink_facts

Chapter 19

Lid and Conjunctival Pathology

Benjamin G. Kuhar, DO

Brian Oscar Porter, MD, PhD, MPH, MBA

Lynne M. Dunphy, PhD, APRN, FNP-BC, FAAN, FAANP

BLEPHARITIS

Blepharitis is an inflammation of the eyelids and their margins. Blepharitis can be divided into types that affect either the anterior or posterior eyelid. The anterior form can be further subdivided into seborrheic or staphylococcal blepharitis. Seborrheic blepharitis is associated with greasy scaling that may be found on the eyelashes, eyelids, eyebrows, and scalp. Staphylococcal blepharitis refers to bacterial infection of the anterior eyelids, which differs from the inflammatory nature of seborrheic blepharitis. The posterior form of blepharitis typically involves inflammation and obstruction of the meibomian glands of the eyelid (meibomitis). Secondary infections may develop with any of these, and recurrences are common and frequently persistent. These various types of blepharitis may coexist with one another.

EPIDEMIOLOGY AND CAUSES

Blepharitis is a common ocular disease, affecting males and females equally and often coexisting with other ocular disease including dry eye syndrome (DES), conjunctivitis, and keratitis. Seborrheic blepharitis tends to affect patients with rosacea, psoriasis, seborrhea, eczema, allergies, and can be seen in those with trisomy 21. Poor hygiene is implicated, as well as poor nutritional status and immunosuppression. Exposure to chemical or environmental irritants, as well as the use of eye makeup and contact lenses, may also contribute to the development of this disorder. Staphylococcal blepharitis is more common in younger individuals and is most often caused by *Staphylococcus aureus*. Posterior blepharitis often is synonymous with meibomitis.

PATHOPHYSIOLOGY

Although difficult to discern without a full ophthalmological examination, the localization of blepharitis assists in identifying which structures are affected. Anterior blepharitis typically affects the eyelash follicles along the eyelid's anterior lamella, whereas posterior blepharitis involves obstruction of the meibomian glands along the tarsal plate, with subsequent inflammation. Seborrheic gland dysfunction along with accelerated shedding of skin cells appear to be the primary insult resulting in anterior inflammation, in which an oily crust envelops individual eyelash cilia (seborrheic blepharitis). Staphylococcal blepharitis also creates crusting on the anterior eyelid, but these are typically hard, fibrinous scales, rather than the greasy scales seen in seborrheic blepharitis.

CLINICAL PRESENTATION

Subjective

Blepharitis may present with complaints of eye itching, burning, tearing, redness, and foreign body sensation. Presentation may be unilateral or bilateral, and symptoms are typically worse in the morning. Further questioning regarding medication use and coexisting medical conditions can help elicit helpful information in the history.

Objective

Lid margins are typically edematous and erythematous. Closer visual inspection with a magnifying glass or Wood's lamp may reveal scaling, erythema, or crusting. Anterior blepharitis may present with scale fragments along the lid margins that are easily removed. Scales may encircle the base of the eyelash, a finding known as "collarettes." With staphylococcal blepharitis, there may be pustules at the base of the hair follicles that may crust and bleed. The lashes become thin and break easily, causing loss of eyelashes (madarosis). The eyelid and lid margins should be palpated for masses. Gentle pressure on the eyelids may express white, sebaceous discharge from the meibomian glands at the eyelid margin, indicating meibomian gland dysfunction.

DIAGNOSTIC REASONING

Diagnostic Tests

With any eye problem, it is vital to evaluate visual acuity in both eyes. In cases of unilateral disorder, visual acuity should be assessed in both the affected eye and the unaffected eye. Additionally, visual acuity of both eyes with and without corrective lenses should be documented. Any alteration in visual acuity may indicate a potentially serious underlying problem that warrants further investigation. Eyelid and conjunctival cultures are not typically necessary for simple blepharitis, but they may be warranted if the diagnosis is in doubt or the condition is worsening.

Differential Diagnosis

Persistent inflammation and thickening of the eyelid margin may indicate squamous cell, basal cell, or sebaceous cell carcinoma masquerading as chronic blepharitis. Sebaceous cell carcinoma is potentially fatal and can resemble chronic benign inflammatory disease, particularly chalazion, stye, or blepharoconjunctivitis. Other differential diagnoses include hordeolum, conjunctivitis, retained foreign body, herpes simplex infection, orbital cellulitis, and dacryocystitis (infection or inflammation of the nasolacrimal sac).

MANAGEMENT

Box 19.1 describes the management of various forms of blepharitis. Warm compresses and gentle eyelid scrubbing are the mainstay of treatment and should be directed at the base of the lashes, where the majority of bacteria and seborrhea are located. Any swelling or inflammation of the eyelid that does not resolve promptly (within 1 month) with treatment should be evaluated further.

FOLLOW-UP AND REFERRAL

Blepharitis may be difficult to treat, and recurrences are common; hordeolum, madarosis, misdirection of the eyelashes (trichiasis), scarring, and corneal infection may occur. Thus, the clinician should reevaluate the patient in 2 weeks, and if symptoms are improving, the patient should then be reevaluated in 2 months or otherwise seen sooner. If there is no resolution in 1 month, the patient should be referred to an ophthalmologist. Immediate referral for patients with blepharitis should occur in the following situations: significant visual loss, moderate to severe eye pain, and corneal involvement. Chronic redness of the eye, recurrent blepharitis, and/or a failure to respond to treatment also warrant an ophthalmology referral. Moreover, patients with chronic inflammation or thickening of the eyelid should be referred to a specialist for possible biopsy.

Box 19.1 Treatment for Blepharitis

Type	Treatment Goal	Treatment Description
Seborrheic blepharitis	This type of blepharitis may be persistent, and treatment is aimed at improving hygiene.	Eyelid cleaning with a diluted 1:1 mixture of "no-tears" shampoo (i.e., baby shampoo) and water, using a soft washcloth or cotton balls. The patient should apply warm compresses for 10 to 15 minutes, then rest for at least 1 hour. Patients should be advised that eyelid hygiene may be required for life, and symptoms may recur if treatment is discontinued. Advise the patient to discontinue the use of eye makeup and contact lenses until the condition is completely resolved. Once resolved, only new hypoallergenic makeup products and new contact lenses should be used to avoid reinfection.
Staphylococcal blepharitis	Infectious blepharitis should be treated with topical antibiotic ointments that adhere to the eyelid margins more effectively than eye drops.	Bacitracin or erythromycin 0.5% ointment can be prescribed and applied on the eyelids one or more times daily or at bedtime after gentle cleansing and using warm compresses. Treatment may continue for 7 to 10 days. The frequency and duration of treatment should be guided by the severity of the blepharitis. Staphylococcal infections resistant to this treatment warrant a referral to an ophthalmologist.
Posterior blepharitis (meibomian gland dysfunction)	Loosen and thin out meibomian gland secretions to help facilitate drainage.	Eyelid warming with hot compresses for 10 minutes in the morning and evening, followed by massage of the closed eyelid. Also continue eyelid cleansing with dilute baby shampoo. If eyelid hygiene techniques do not improve condition, topical fluoroquinolones or bacitracin can be used. If still no improvement, consider oral antibiotics (e.g., doxycycline) or referral to an eye care specialist.
Severe blepharitis	Associated with rosacea; treatment is aimed at curing the infectious process with systemic antibiotic therapy.	Oral doxycycline 100 mg by mouth twice daily or tetracycline 250 mg by mouth four times daily is appropriate. These are prescribed for several weeks and then tapered. Continue hygienic measures as described earlier.

Patient Education: Blepharitis

Patients with blepharitis should be encouraged to wash their hands often and dry them with clean towels to prevent reinfection or the transfer of bacteria or viruses to other persons. In addition, patients should be advised to avoid environmental irritants, use hypoallergenic soap and makeup, and exercise care in the use of contact lenses. The clinician should educate the patient about the chronic and recurrent nature of this disorder and the need for strict adherence to the treatment plan until the blepharitis is completely resolved. Long-term eyelid hygiene (gently cleansing with diluted baby shampoo daily) is required to control this disorder. Eye makeup should be avoided until resolution of the disorder, after which the patient should switch to hypoallergenic makeup. A blepharitis fact sheet is available from the American Academy of Ophthalmologists (see Resources).

HORDEOLUM AND CHALAZION

A hordeolum, also known as a stye, is an acute, erythematous, tender lump within the eyelid. This condition is caused by inflammation or infection of the eyelid margin affecting the hair follicles of the eyelashes (external hordeolum) or the meibomian glands (internal hordeolum), which may evolve into a chalazion. A chalazion is a granulomatous inflammation of a blocked meibomian gland that presents as a painless swelling on the eyelid. Initially, a chalazion may be tender and erythematous before evolving into a nontender lump. Blepharitis is frequently associated with a chalazion. The primary difference between a chalazion and a hordeolum is that chalazia are a result of inflammation due to glandular blockage, whereas hordeola (styes) are infectious.

EPIDEMIOLOGY AND CAUSES

Both of these eyelid disorders are common and affect males and females equally. The cause is often a blockage in a duct of the meibomian gland leading to the eyelid surface; secondary infection may be present, again, commonly with *Staphylococcus*. This ductal obstruction results in inflammation that may manifest as an external or internal hordeolum and may progress to a chalazion. Previously unresolved blepharitis, poor hygiene, immunosuppression, and underlying chronic diseases all contribute to the development of these eyelid disorders. Skin conditions, such as rosacea or seborrheic dermatitis, may also predispose a patient to the development of a hordeolum.

PATHOPHYSIOLOGY

Hordeola and chalazia are various manifestations of an inflammatory response in the eyelids, exhibiting both microscopic (accumulation of fluid and cells at the inflammatory site) and macroscopic (redness, swelling, heat, pain, and loss of function) hallmark signs of inflammation. An external hordeolum occurs with infection of the more superficial, anteriorly located glands of Zeis or Moll found at the eyelid margin. An internal hordeolum is a suppurative infection of the oil-secreting meibomian glands within the tarsal plate of the eyelid that may evolve into a chalazion. With a hordeolum, the eyelid may show a classic inflammatory reaction secondary to bacterial infection caused by stasis of these glands. Both internal and external hordeola are associated with *S. aureus* infection. Conversely, a chalazion results from a granulomatous response secondary to an obstruction of the meibomian gland and is typically painless. In a chalazion, blockage of the meibomian gland's duct results in the release of the gland's contents into the surrounding soft tissue, and a lipogranulomatous reaction ensues, producing a pea-sized nodule within the eyelid.

CLINICAL PRESENTATION

Subjective

A hordeolum typically presents as a localized, tender eyelid with associated redness and swelling without a history of trauma or foreign body. The erythema and pain are often localized to the eyelid and should not cause ocular pain or pain on extraocular movement. A chalazion commonly presents as a slow-developing, painless, firm mass, with inflammation and possible involvement of the surrounding tissue. Patients with chalazia will often report previous similar lesions in the past, given their high rate of recurrence.

Objective

As with all eye complaints, the clinician should evaluate visual acuity. Visual acuity is typically unaffected, unless the lesion is pressing on the cornea. With a chalazion, inversion of the eyelid will reveal a red, elevated, painless mass that may become quite large and press against the eye, potentially causing distortion of vision. With a hordeolum, there is erythema and localized tenderness with palpation; there may also be drainage from the lesion on the margin of the lid. Often a pustule can be located with careful inspection. Pain on eye movement is atypical in hordeola, and the presence of eyelid edema and erythema should raise concern for orbital cellulitis, which requires an urgent ophthalmology referral.

DIAGNOSTIC REASONING

Diagnostic Tests

A hordeolum and a chalazion are usually diagnosed by their appearance. Cultures are not indicated for uncomplicated first-time occurrences. If these conditions persist, referral for biopsy may be indicated.

Differential Diagnosis

As noted previously, patients with inflammation or swelling that do not resolve with conservative therapy should be referred to an ophthalmologist to rule out other conditions. Basal cell or sebaceous cell carcinoma may mimic other disorders of the eyelid, so differentiating these disorders is key. Up to one-half of potentially fatal sebaceous cell carcinomas may initially resemble benign inflammatory disorders, making this diagnosis important to consider in patients with recurrent eyelid lesions unresponsive to conservative therapy.

MANAGEMENT

Box 19.2 describes the various treatment options for hordeola and chalazia. Warm compresses can help improve drainage. Topical antibiotics are typically not effective unless there is an associated conjunctivitis.

FOLLOW-UP AND REFERRAL

Patients with vision changes or eye pain should be referred to an ophthalmologist. Recurrence of a hordeolum or chalazion is likely without proper eyelid hygiene. If there is no improvement with eyelid hygiene and warm compresses, the clinician should refer the patient to an ophthalmologist for further evaluation.

> **Patient Education: Hordeolum and Chalazion**
>
> The patient should understand the recurrent nature of the disorder, along with the need for vigilance and good treatment compliance. Setting the expectations with the patient up front about recurrence risk will help alleviate patient distress if the lesion does recur. Treatment should be initiated at the first sign of recurrence. There are no specific treatments to prevent hordeola and chalazia formation, but regular lid hygiene is thought to have a preventive role. This consists of eyelid cleansing and warm compresses, which may help thin secretions and improve glandular stasis, which predisposes to lid pathology. Infections with *S. aureus* are contagious; therefore, patients and family members should not share towels, washcloths, or eyewear such as sunglasses. The patient should use a clean cloth each time a compress is applied to the eye and should wash their hands frequently.

Box 19.2 Treatment for Hordeolum/Chalazion

Initial treatment of hordeolum	At the first sign of inflammation and pain, warm compresses should be applied to increase blood supply and potentiate spontaneous drainage. Gently scrub the eyelids with a 1:1 dilution of "no-tears" shampoo (baby shampoo) and warm water two to four times a day, or directly apply diluted baby shampoo with a cotton-tipped applicator and then rinse with warm water. Follow with gentle massage of the eyelid. The hordeolum (stye) should not be squeezed. Blepharitis, if present, should be treated. Eye makeup should be discontinued until the infection resolves. Contact lenses should not be used during treatment. Once the condition is resolved, a new pair of contact lenses and new hypoallergenic eye makeup may be resumed.
Infection or inflammation of hordeolum	Erythromycin ophthalmic ointment or sulfacetamide (Sulamyd) ophthalmic ointment can be applied four times a day or ciprofloxacin ointment (Ciloxan, Cipro) can be applied three times a day. Use a thin application to the eyelid margin with a cotton-tipped applicator.
Resistant or recurrent hordeolum	A course of oral antibiotics that is effective against *Staphylococcus* and *Streptococcus*, such as cephalexin (Keflex, Keftab), can be prescribed. At this point, referral to an ophthalmologist should be considered for incision and drainage. *Note: Basal cell carcinoma or sebaceous cell carcinoma of the eyelid can be misdiagnosed clinically and should be included in the differential diagnosis for recurrent hordeolum or chalazion.*
Chalazion (unresolved)	Warm compresses and gentle massage of the swelling in the eyelid with a 1:1 dilution of "no tears" shampoo (baby shampoo) and warm water may help to open the blocked meibomian duct. *Note: A chalazion that persists for more than 4 weeks needs referral to an ophthalmologist for incision and drainage, biopsy, or local injection directly with glucocorticoids.*

DRY EYE

DES is a multifactorial disease of the ocular surface secondary to tear film abnormalities. In a healthy eye, lubricating secretions called *basal tears* continuously bathe the cornea (the clear, dome-shaped outer surface of the eye). With every blink of the eye, basal tears flow across the cornea, nourishing its cells and providing a layer of liquid protection from the environment. When the glands near each eye fail to produce enough basal tears or when the composition of the tears changes, the health of the eye and vision are compromised. Vision may be affected because tears on the surface of the eye play an important role in focusing light.

Lacrimal disorders may be acquired or congenital. Acquired disorders may be systemic, such as Sjögren's syndrome, may reflect a more local infectious process (as in some forms of conjunctivitis), or may be related to trauma or facial nerve (cranial nerve VII) palsy. Certain medications, such as anticholinergic agents, beta-adrenergic blockers, and antihistamines, decrease tear production, as the lacrimal gland is stimulated by the parasympathetic nervous system. Other systemic medications including diuretics, antidepressants, and isotretinoin may exacerbate dry eye. Frequent instillation of any eye drop (more than four drops daily) may also worsen symptoms due to preservatives in these preparations. Mucin deficiency may also be caused by certain medications, vitamin A deficiency, chronic conjunctivitis, or as a result of the aging process. Tear production also decreases with aging, especially in females during menopause. In addition, patients who use a computer or microscope excessively may have a diminished blink rate, which can cause evaporative loss of natural tears.

EPIDEMIOLOGY AND CAUSES

DES is a common disorder affecting approximately 10% to 30% of the population, especially those older than 40 years of age. In the United States, an estimated 3.23 million females and 1.68 million males aged 50 years and older are affected. The frequency of this condition globally closely parallels that in the United States, as dry eye seems to affect all racial and ethnic groups equally.

Keratoconjunctivitis sicca (KCS) associated with Sjögren's syndrome is a type of dry eye that affects 1% to 2% of the population, with 90% of those affected being female. Approximately 1% of the U.S. population is affected with Sjögren's syndrome, and it occurs in 15% of patients with rheumatoid arthritis. Other medical conditions associated with DES include diabetes mellitus, osteoporosis, and thyroid eye disease. Lifestyle factors including alcohol consumption and current tobacco use are also associated with a higher risk of DES.

PATHOPHYSIOLOGY

The pathophysiology of DES is cyclical in nature. Tear hyperosmolarity on the cornea leads to reduced cell volume and increased stress of corneal epithelial cells,

> **Geriatric Considerations: Dry Eye Syndrome**
>
> DES is quite common in the geriatric population and should be at the top of the differential diagnosis list for older patients presenting with chronic eye irritation and fluctuating vision. Its prevalence increases from roughly 8.4% in patients younger than 60 years to 19% in patients older than 80 years, with females being affected more often than males. A thorough medication review should be conducted, as well as a review of the patient's past medical history to assess for contributing factors to DES. Even without a history of Sjögren's syndrome, rheumatoid arthritis, or other autoimmune disease, dry eyes can be a very common complaint in the older adult population.

causing them to release inflammatory mediators, which disrupt junctions between epithelial cells. This allows T cells to infiltrate the epithelium and produce cytokines such as tumor necrosis factor-alpha and interleukin-1 that cause detachment of epithelial cells and induce apoptosis. This further disrupts epithelial cell junctions, allowing more inflammatory cells to infiltrate, thereby repeating the cycle.

Tear film consists of three main components: aqueous, lipid, and mucin fractions. Each is secreted by different glands of the eye, which can be influenced by various disease states. The aqueous (water) portion of the tear film is secreted by the lacrimal gland, which is the target of Sjögren's syndrome, an autoimmune disease. A genetic predisposition to Sjögren's syndrome–associated dry eye is evidenced by a high prevalence of human leukocyte antigen (HLA)-B8 in these patients. A high level of HLA-B8 is associated with a chronic inflammatory state, in which autoantibodies (e.g., SS-A, SS-B) are produced. In addition, this condition is associated with T cell–mediated inflammation and infiltration of the lacrimal and salivary glands, with eventual apoptosis and destruction of the lacrimal glands. The result is dysfunction of the lacrimal gland, with decreased aqueous tear production, loss of response to neural stimulation, and less reflexive tearing.

Lipids secreted by the meibomian glands are an important component of tear fluid that keeps it from evaporating. The function of the meibomian glands can be altered by hormones and certain disease states, which ultimately affects tear film composition. Both androgen and estrogen receptors are located in meibomian glands, and the decline in androgens with age results in decreased lipid production from these glands, contributing to dry eye. At menopause, there is a decrease in circulating sex hormones, possibly affecting the secretory function of this gland as well. Rosacea (an inflammatory skin disease) and blepharitis (an inflammatory eyelid disease) can also disrupt the function of the meibomian glands, affecting secretion of the lipid component of tears.

Another important component of the tear film is mucin, which is secreted by goblet cells. Different disease states and genetic factors may affect the function of goblet cells, which can exacerbate dry eye. Vitamin A deficiency, Stevens-Johnson syndrome, and ocular cicatricial pemphigoid may contribute to the loss of goblet cells. Deficient functioning of mucin-synthesizing genes may be a factor in DES as well.

CLINICAL PRESENTATION

Dry eye commonly affects both eyes and often presents with eye irritation, burning, tearing, stinging, and blurry vision that are worse at the end of the day. Symptoms may be exacerbated by dry environments, wind, and prolonged staring (e.g., watching television, using computers, reading), which are associated with a decreased blink rate. The eyes can feel hot, irritated, and gritty, and may become reddened. The discomfort experienced can be out of proportion to clinical findings. The triad presentation of burning, itching, and a foreign body sensation in the eye is characteristic of DES. This symptom is frequently associated with the diagnosis of Sjögren's syndrome, a systemic disorder affecting the function of all secretory glands. In the majority of patients, DES is not vision-threatening. However, untreated or severe DES may result in inflammation, erosion, and eventually keratinization of the cornea and/or conjunctiva, which may permanently effect vision.

Subjective

A complete history (see Chapter 18, Common Eye Complaints) should focus particularly on symptom severity, duration, and exacerbating or alleviating factors. Careful questioning regarding contact lens use, current medications, and other systemic disease can be helpful in elucidating a cause. Previous eye or eyelid surgeries should be included in the history, as DES can be seen after refractive surgeries (e.g., laser-assisted in situ keratomileusis [LASIK], photorefractive keratectomy [PRK]), and eyelid surgeries. Assessment tools such as the Ocular Surface Disease Index and Dry Eye Questionnaire can be helpful in evaluating symptom severity.

Objective

For the primary care provider, examination of visual acuity must be included in the physical examination. When grossly examining the eyes, the conjunctiva may appear injected and dull, and the eyelids and surrounding tissues may be erythematous due to frequent rubbing. The lacrimal apparatus will be nontender, and in the case of KCS or Sjögren's syndrome, the mucous membranes of the mouth will also be dry. Examination of the eyes by a trained professional with fluorescein staining and a slit lamp may reveal punctuate lesions of the conjunctiva or a secondary abrasion.

DIAGNOSTIC REASONING

The complaint of dry eye is frequently a subjective finding with no obvious signs on physical examination; therefore, a clinical diagnosis will often require referral to a specialist for examination and testing. The gross external examination should rather focus on eyelid positioning, blink frequency, proptosis, and any skin or joint abnormalities indicative of coexisting autoimmune disease. Occasionally, the patient will complain of excessive tearing (epiphora) or inappropriate tearing, which may be reflexive due to poor neural control of the lacrimal apparatus from dry eyes.

Diagnostic Tests

In addition to a slit-lamp examination, tests that may be used in the work-up of dry eye include ocular surface staining, measurement of tear break-up time, the Schirmer tear production test, and quantification of tear components through analysis of tear proteins or tear film osmolarity. Laboratory tests to rule out autoimmune disease include an erythrocyte sedimentation rate, antinuclear antibodies, and rheumatoid factor. Serology for circulating autoantibodies may be indicated if specific autoimmune conditions are suspected, such as anti-SSA (anti-Ro) and anti-SSB (anti-La) for Sjögren's syndrome.

Symptom questionnaires can also be used to help establish a diagnosis of DES, assess the grade of disease severity, and evaluate the effects of treatment. At least 14 questionnaires are available; among the most commonly used and validated are the following:

- Ocular Surface Disease Index
- Dry Eye Questionnaire
- McMonnies Questionnaire
- Symptom Assessment in Dry Eye

Differential Diagnosis

The differential diagnosis of dry eye is geared toward determining its underlying cause, which can include conjunctivitis, blepharitis, contact lens complications, exophthalmos, ectropion, Bell's palsy, iatrogenic medication effects, Sjögren's syndrome, rheumatoid arthritis, age-related and hormonal changes, corneal abrasion, and vitamin A deficiency.

MANAGEMENT

The goals of treatment should be to reduce symptoms of ocular irritation, improve visual function, and prevent surface damage to the eye. This is usually attained through the use of artificial tears, warm compresses, and lid hygiene. Elimination of systemic or topical medications that may have contributed to the condition should also be considered. Such interventions alone may not be successful, however, further illustrating the importance of inquiring about causative factors. Review of the patient's environment, habits, and work practices may identify modifiable contributing factors such as reduced humidity, air drafts, or prolonged computer or smartphone use. Also, it is not unusual for patients to need adjustment of their contact lens or eyeglass prescription or a review of their ocular self-care regimen. In turn, realistic expectations and goals of treatment should be discussed with the patient, and when the complaint of dry eye is persistent and unrelieved by self-care measures, referral is warranted.

The principles of treatment for dry eye are based on the severity of the condition. The first level of treatment involves the introduction of artificial tears, lubricants, gels, and ointments. Artificial tears instilled up to four times daily, ointment at bedtime, and warm compresses are the recommended self-care regimen. The overuse of artificial tears can occasionally lead to corneal toxicity, however, due to active ingredients or preservatives in lubricant formulations. For this reason, preservative-free formulations should be used if artificial tears are needed more frequently than four times daily. Aside from lubrication and warm compresses, treatment plans should also encourage environmental and dietary modifications. Wearing wrap-around sunglasses to keep wind from drying the eye surface, using a humidifier in the home, eliminating offending medications, and scheduling regular computer, smartphone, and television breaks may help reduce the symptoms of dry eye. Because smoking is also a risk factor for DES, smoking cessation should be strongly encouraged.

A second level of care is instituted if the first level is ineffective, and at this point, ophthalmological consultation should be considered. Treatment here includes the use of specific pharmacological measures in addition to ocular lubricants and preservative-free artificial tears. These eye drops include anti-inflammatory and immunomodulatory agents such as topical cyclosporine, topical or systemic omega-3 fatty acids, or topical corticosteroids. Topical cyclosporine ophthalmic emulsion (Restasis) is used to treat chronic dry eye. It contains a very small concentration of cyclosporine, which is believed to inhibit the activation of T cells. Temporary punctal plugs may be warranted after inflammation has resolved. Punctal plugs are painlessly inserted and act as a dam that prevents tears from draining into the puncta and nasolacrimal duct. Several studies have demonstrated subjective and objective improvement with punctual plugs in the treatment of DES.

The third level of treatment is instituted when the previous levels have failed to adequately control symptoms. The therapies at this level consist of use of special contact lenses, moisture chamber goggles, systemic anti-inflammatory agents, and permanent punctal occlusion. In severe cases, surgical intervention to correct abnormalities of the lid may be necessary.

FOLLOW-UP AND REFERRAL

Supportive measures such as listening to the patient's fears associated with vision changes or the possible systemic causes of dry eye are both therapeutic and compassionate. A patient with chronic complaints of dry eye or conjunctivitis may need to be referred to an ophthalmologist. Arranging for prompt referral for accurate diagnosis and specialized treatments promotes a patient's confidence in the primary care practitioner.

Patient Education: Dry Eye

In general, the prognosis for visual acuity in patients with DES is good. However, complications of decreased visual acuity can occur, and patients need to seek medical advice if visual changes occur, the current regimen has lost effectiveness, or symptoms worsen. Box 19.3 summarizes several environmental modifications that patients can make to minimize the symptoms and recurrence of dry eye.

Omega-3 fatty acid deficiency, especially reduced levels of docosahexaenoic acid (DHA) and eicosapentaenoic acid (EPA), have been linked to DES in previous studies. However, a recent multicenter, randomized, double-blind clinical trial of 3,000 mg supplementation of omega-3 fatty acids for 1 year did not show any benefit in symptoms compared with placebo (Dry Eye Assessment and Management Study et al., 2018). Thus, the regular supplementation of omega-3 fatty acids in the treatment of DES remains controversial. Regular use of lubricating drops or ointments and consistent use of prescribed ocular medications should be stressed.

Box 19.3 Ocular Self-Care for Dry Eye

Keep home humidity between 30% and 50%.
Cleanse humidifier frequently with dilute 1:10 bleach/water solution. Rinse well with fresh water.
Wear wrap-around sunglasses, especially on windy days.
Wear goggles when swimming.
Use preservative-free artificial tear preparation.
Avoid air drafts from ceiling fans, car air vents, blow-dryer for hair, etc.
Take frequent rest periods away from computers, handheld electronic devices (e.g., smartphones), televisions, or microscopes. Make conscious effort to blink while using these devices.
Stop smoking to eliminate direct exposure to ocular irritants in tobacco smoke.

EXCESSIVE TEARING (EPIPHORA)

Epiphora is the presence of a watering eye caused by either increased lacrimation or impaired tear outflow. Good ocular surface lubrication is the sign of a healthy eye; however, an eye with uncontrolled tearing signals a malfunction with a variety of possible causes.

EPIDEMIOLOGY AND CAUSES

Epiphora, or excessive tearing, can be separated into two categories: reflexive tearing and impaired tear outflow. Reflexive tearing is a common problem and will become more widespread as the population ages. Tearing typically occurs in response to conditions such as dry eye, ocular allergy, pain, trauma, or inflammation. The eye may also water excessively as a protective mechanism secondary to irritation from contact lenses, medications, and environmental irritants. Sensitivity to preservatives in certain eye drops and contact lens solutions can also cause this relatively common problem. Additionally, eyestrain from prolonged computer or screen use (including smartphones) may lead to decreased blinking, which may then lead to compensatory and excessive tearing. Because epiphora is frequently associated with dry eye as a paradoxical and compensatory response, the epidemiological statistics are similar to dry eye, with older and allergic patients being particularly predisposed.

Reduced tear outflow, the other cause of epiphora, usually involves eyelid abnormalities or obstruction of the nasolacrimal duct system (NLDO). Anatomical abnormalities, such as ectropion, entropion, lower lid laxity, and lacrimal pump weakness due to Bell's palsy, may lead to structural and functional problems in the distribution and drainage of tears. These problems are more commonly seen in older patients. NLDO limits normal drainage into the lacrimal ducts and can significantly contribute to epiphora. NLDO can be congenital or acquired and frequently affects the pediatric population. Obstruction can be associated with thickened discharge secondary to infection, tumor, trauma, or autoimmune diagnoses.

PATHOPHYSIOLOGY

The tear film serves many important purposes, including removing ocular pathogens and contributing to the primary refractive element of the eye. Tears are made up of several components, with each playing a role in the maintenance of stable tear film. The aqueous or water portion of tear film provides hydration and is produced mainly by the lacrimal gland. The lipid component is produced by the meibomian glands of the eye and prevents tear evaporation. The mucin component helps provide further lubrication and anti-adhesive properties and is produced by goblet cells. During blinking, a suction effect draws the tear film into the lacrimal apparatus. In the case of facial nerve palsy, the loss of the blink reflex allows tearing to occur without any physiological tear pumping and drainage. This is also an issue with prolonged computer use accompanied by a decreased blink reflex; the eyes become dry and may reflexively tear. A malfunction of the lacrimal apparatus or its neural control may also cause eyes to water inappropriately.

CLINICAL PRESENTATION

Subjective

A complete history, which should include any trauma and infections that could threaten vision, should be elicited. If the patient complains that clear tears run down the cheek, it may signal that there is an obstruction of the lacrimal system. If the complaint is of "watery eyes," with tears collecting or welling up in the lower eyelid pouch, the problem may be associated with reduced tear quality or poor tear distribution. Blurred vision, diplopia, photophobia, or eye pain may indicate a more serious condition. Allergic causes for excessive tearing are common, and occasionally the source of the allergen is identified during the history. Past medical history of seasonal allergies, asthma, or other atopic diseases, as well as a family history of atopic conditions, helps in making an accurate diagnosis. The review of systems should address systemic symptoms such as fever, headache, upper respiratory complaints, sore or scratchy throat, cough or wheeze, dizziness, malaise, and skin changes.

Objective

The physical examination should include an assessment of visual acuity and careful examination of the structures in the eye and the surrounding tissues, evaluating for edema, redness, discharge, rashes, and any structural abnormalities. Careful examination for foreign bodies or corneal irritants is essential. Many primary care clinics have access to a Wood's lamp and fluorescein staining, whereas specialists will use a slit lamp to assess for damage in the anterior structures of the eye. In addition, signs of allergies such as pale, boggy mucous membranes in the nose, dry skin, or eczematous changes may be present.

DIAGNOSTIC REASONING

Diagnostic Tests

Diagnostic testing is rarely done in the primary care setting, with the exception of a Wood's lamp examination. Ophthalmologists use a variety of other tests to determine tear quality, quantity, and flow. The dye disappearance test is one such test. A drop of fluorescein dye is placed in both eyes in the inferior fornix, and the tear meniscus height is measured after 5 to 10 minutes. This is an easy test for assessing the presence of an excretory problem with excessive tearing. Other dye tests evaluate whether fluid drains properly into the inferior meatus and lacrimal sac. Lacrimal irrigation and probing can demonstrate a punctal or canalicular problem. Occasionally, computed tomography scanning of the lacrimal drainage system can be done.

Differential Diagnosis

The presentation of acute unilateral epiphora with red eye and pain suggests the presence of a foreign body or corneal abrasion. Irritating bilateral epiphora may be due to allergies, DES, environmental pollutants, or viral conjunctivitis. A blocked lacrimal duct or bacterial conjunctivitis usually manifests unilaterally. Ectropion may be unilateral or bilateral, whereas the development of lid laxity associated with aging is usually bilateral.

MANAGEMENT

Treatment of excessive tearing involves targeting the underlying cause. The treatment of tearing secondary to trauma or infection includes the use of topical antibiotics for treatment. Corticosteroid eye drops and anesthetic drops should not be used in these cases because they may disrupt healing and increase the risk of infection. If a foreign body is visualized on physical examination, it should be removed by saline irrigation using a Morgan Lens or by direct removal with a moist cotton swab. Eye rest is important, but patching is generally not recommended.

Treatment of allergic causes of excessive tearing (e.g., allergic conjunctivitis) consists of cold compresses for comfort and relief of itch, topical antihistamines, topical NSAIDs, mast cell stabilizers, and systemic antihistamines. Occasionally, consultation with an allergy specialist is necessary for allergy testing to identify trigger agents to avoid.

See Drugs Commonly Prescribed 19.1 for approved medications to treat allergic and infectious forms of conjunctivitis that typically lead to excessive tearing and watery eyes. In patients who wear contact lenses and develop excessive tearing due to a corneal abrasion with signs of bacterial conjunctivitis, an anti-*Pseudomonas* antibiotic (e.g., ciprofloxacin [Ciloxan], gentamicin, ofloxacin [Ocuflox]) should be used and the contact lens use discontinued. Clinical trial data are lacking, but it is recommended that contact lenses be avoided until the abrasion is healed and the antibiotic course is completed.

Drugs Commonly Prescribed 19.1: Conjunctivitis

TYPE OF CONJUNCTIVITIS	DRUG CATEGORY	DRUGS
Allergic Conjunctivitis		
	Mast Cell Stabilizers Block calcium channel essential for mast cell degranulation, stabilizing the cell and thereby preventing the release of histamine and related mediators	Lodoxamide 0.1% (Alomide) Nedocromil 2% (Alocril) Pemirolast 0.1% (Alamast)
	Antihistamines Combat the histamine released during an allergic reaction by blocking the action of the histamine on tissues	Emedastine 0.05% (Emadine)
	Combination Mast Cell Stabilizers and Antihistamines	Olopatadine 0.1% (Patanol) Azelastine 0.05% (Optivar) Ketotifen fumarate 0.025% (Zaditor) Epinastine 0.05% (Elestat)
	NSAIDs Mechanism of action thought to be due to ability to inhibit prostaglandin biosynthesis, thereby having analgesic and anti-inflammatory actions	Ketorolac 0.5% (Acular)
Bacterial Conjunctivitis		
Streptococcus pneumoniae, Haemophilus influenzae, Group A Streptococcus, Staphylococcus aureus, Pseudomonas	**Antibiotics** First-line therapy: Treat empirically with broad-spectrum topical agents. High levels of the agent are delivered directly to the site of infection. Level of concentration exceeds what is normally achieved in body tissues by oral or parenteral routes. Most agents available as ointments or solutions.	Topical treatment: Sodium sulfacetamide (Bleph-10, Cetamide, AK-sulf) Erythromycin ointment (E-Mycin) Azithromycin ophthalmic (AzaSite) Bacitracin (AK-Tracin, Baciguent) Ciprofloxacin (Ciloxan) Trimethoprim and polymyxin B (Polytrim) Tobramycin (Tobrex) Neomycin (Mycifradin) Ofloxacin (Ocuflox) Levofloxacin (Quixin) Besifloxacin (Besivance) Gentamicin (Genoptic, Ocumycin)
Chlamydial Conjunctivitis		
	Antibiotics Systemic antibiotics in addition to topical agents are necessary. Sexual partners should be evaluated for infection and treated simultaneously.	Systemic treatment: Oral azithromycin 1 g as single dose Doxycycline 100 mg twice daily for 7 days
Viral Conjunctivitis		
	Antibiotics Usually not recommended unless there is secondary bacterial infection. Treat with lubrication for comfort.	Ocular lubricants: Artificial tears (Refresh, Celluvisc, Murine) one to two drops four to eight times a day
	Antiviral Agents Herpes simplex conjunctivitis requires topical or systemic antiviral treatment. Note: Any patient with HSV or herpes zoster ophthalmicus (varicella zoster virus) eye disease needs to be seen by an ophthalmologist.	Topical treatment: Trifluridine (Viroptic) ophthalmic solution; may have toxic corneal reaction Systemic treatment: Acyclovir (Zovirax); start therapy within 72 hours to prevent postherpetic neuralgia

FOLLOW-UP AND REFERRAL

Any foreign body that cannot be promptly removed in the primary care setting should be referred to an ophthalmologist or an emergency department (ED) within 24 hours, given the risk of corneal abrasion and infection. Corneal abrasions that cause acute excessive tearing should also be reevaluated in 24 hours. If corneal erosion is suspected or there has been no relief in the excess tear production and the pain level is unchanged or worsened, the patient needs to be referred immediately for evaluation by an ophthalmologist. It is important to communicate this information to the patient because timely referral to a specialist is essential to avoid vision loss.

The patient with chronic epiphora should have an ophthalmological consultation to evaluate and treat. Individuals with conjunctivitis should be reevaluated after a course of antibiotic therapy or after 2 weeks of instituting pharmacological measures for allergic problems. As noted, referral to an allergist may be appropriate for further evaluation and treatment.

Patient Education: Excessive Tearing (Epiphora)

Patients need to be attentive to changes in eye pain, tearing, or discharge and should understand general expectations as to how quickly symptoms should resolve. In addition, they should be alert as to when to seek medical intervention. Vision loss is a very concerning issue, and problems of red eye with visual changes must be addressed promptly. Hygienic measures, such as washing hands, using separate washcloths, and disposing of dressings appropriately, should be stressed. Washing hands before applying eye drops or topical ointments is essential to prevent infection or cross-contamination of a bacterial infection. Patients need to know that there are surgical options to manage changes in eyelid structure that occur with aging and lead to epiphora. If the excessive tearing is paradoxically associated with dry eye, consistent use of artificial tears and lubricants should help improve their condition. If there is no response to lubrication, topical cyclosporine emulsion should eventually bring both symptoms under control, although it may take several weeks for the full effect to be realized.

RED EYE/CONJUNCTIVITIS

Conjunctivitis is an inflammation of the conjunctiva (mucous membrane) covering the sclera of the eye. The conjunctiva protects the eye against foreign materials and microorganisms, but it can become infiltrated by pathogens under certain circumstances. Although most conjunctivitis is self-limiting, some types may lead to permanent vision impairment if not promptly diagnosed and treated. The three main etiologies of conjunctivitis are viral, bacterial, and allergic. It is important for the clinician to be able to distinguish different types of conjunctivitis.

EPIDEMIOLOGY AND CAUSES

Conjunctivitis is one of the most common eye disorders, affecting all ages. A recent study showed that the rates of conjunctivitis presenting to the ED were slightly higher in females than males, although there are no specific ethnic predispositions. This study also noted a bimodal distribution of incidence rate, with the first peak among children younger than 7 years and a smaller second peak of patients in their 20s (i.e., the third decade of life). There is also seasonal variation in incidence rate, with the highest incidence of conjunctivitis occurring in the spring. Although there are many causes of conjunctivitis, the three most common types are viral, bacterial, and allergic conjunctivitis.

Viral conjunctivitis accounts for about 80% of all cases of acute conjunctivitis, with adenovirus responsible for 65% to 90% of viral cases. There are many serotypes of Adenoviridae, which can cause conjunctivitis of varying severities. For instance, a nonspecific follicular conjunctivitis is caused by serotypes 1 through 11 and 19, and a highly contagious form of epidemic keratoconjunctivitis (EKC) is caused by serotypes 8, 19, and 37. Other common causes of viral conjunctivitis include herpes zoster, herpes simplex, coxsackievirus, and enterovirus. Transmission occurs more commonly in close quarters, including schools, military barracks, nursing homes, and summer camps.

Bacterial conjunctivitis is more common in children than adults. Gram-positive bacteria make up 70% of cases of nongonococcal bacterial conjunctivitis, with gram-negative organisms comprising the other 30%. The most common causes of bacterial conjunctivitis include *S. aureus, Streptococcus pneumoniae,* and *Haemophilus influenzae. Neisseria gonorrhoeae, Moraxella catarrhalis,* and *Chlamydia* are responsible for a particularly virulent form of hyperacute bacterial conjunctivitis. Sexually transmitted conjunctivitis and ophthalmia neonatorum (vertical transmission from mother to child of eye infection during passage through the birth canal) are associated with *Chlamydia, N. gonorrhoeae,* and herpes simplex virus (HSV) type 1. Most forms of conjunctivitis, depending on the causative organism, may be transmitted by contaminated towels, washcloths, or the patient's own hands (autoinoculation).

Allergic conjunctivitis is a group of diseases that involve IgE-mediated inflammation of the eye in response to an allergen. Forms of allergic conjunctivitis include (1) seasonal (simple allergic conjunctivitis), which is usually caused by grass pollen in May and June and by ragweed pollen in August and September; (2) vernal keratoconjunctivitis, which usually occurs in warm, dry climates in individuals younger than 10 years with a

Pediatric/Adolescent Considerations: Trachoma

Trachoma, the leading cause of preventable blindness worldwide, is caused by *Chlamydia trachomatis,* specifically serotypes A through C. It is commonly found in the developing world in places without access to clean water and proper sanitation. Children are the most susceptible to infection because they are more likely to come into contact with contaminated inanimate objects and have worse facial and hand cleanliness. It is spread by direct contact with eye, nose, and throat secretions from affected individuals or from contact with fomites. Flies can also be routes of mechanical transmission. Untreated, repeated trachoma infections result in entropion—in which the eyelids turn inward, causing the lashes to touch the cornea (known as *trichiasis*). The lashes then repeatedly scratch the cornea, which can lead to permanent blindness. However, the blinding effect and more severe symptoms are often not realized until early adulthood. The global effort to eliminate trachoma has shifted from treating isolated cases to advancing socioeconomic development in high-incidence areas. This mainly consists of introducing water and sanitation programs to these endemic areas. Also, educational programs are being widely implemented for children to improve facial hygiene and cleanliness to eliminate the spread of pathogens. The trachoma eradication campaign has been widely successful thus far, but continued effort is needed to eliminate this common preventable cause of blindness.

personal or family history of atopy; or (3) atopic keratoconjunctivitis that affects patients with atopic dermatitis.

Noninfectious conjunctivitis may be drug induced as a result of chronic irritation from the use of eye medications over a prolonged period of time. Certain autoimmune phenomena such as Sjögren's syndrome or Wegener's granulomatosis (a form of vasculitis) may also involve conjunctivitis. Chronic inflammatory conjunctivitis may similarly develop secondary to irritation from contact lens use, seen most commonly with soft lenses but also occasionally with hard lenses.

PATHOPHYSIOLOGY

Bacterial and viral conjunctivitis are the result of direct transmission of pathogens onto conjunctival tissue. Conjunctivitis can occur when the eye's epithelial layer is damaged or the normal defense mechanisms against pathogens are interrupted. This leads to conjunctival inflammation and the hallmark hyperemia of the ocular and palpebral surfaces with engorged, superficial vessels. This vascular injection gives the eye the typical angry red appearance of conjunctivitis.

Conjunctivitis can also be associated with certain systemic diseases, such as thyroid disorders and reactive arthritis (formerly known as *Reiter's syndrome* [a problematic moniker named for a German doctor with ties to the Nazi party]). Allergic (atopic) conjunctivitis is mainly thought to involve an immunoglobulin E (IgE)-mediated type I hypersensitivity reaction and histamine release in response to an inciting environmental allergen. In vernal keratoconjunctivitis, there is thought to be T-cell involvement, in addition to a type I hypersensitivity reaction. Atopic keratoconjunctivitis is thought to involve a type IV hypersensitivity reaction, along with a type I reaction in response to an allergen.

CLINICAL PRESENTATION

Subjective

Symptoms of conjunctivitis vary with the cause, but cardinal symptoms include itching, watering, and redness of the eye. There may be a foreign body sensation and/or a sense of fullness around the eyes. Bacterial infections, such as with *S. aureus,* may produce thick, yellow, sticky exudates at the eyelids. This exudate is especially apparent in the morning, and patients may complain that their eyelids are "stuck together" when they wake, which is known as matting. Preauricular lymphadenopathy and corneal involvement are not typically present. Bacterial infections usually occur unilaterally, whereas viral infections can appear in both eyes at once, given their extremely contagious nature. The clinician should also inquire about sexual history and symptoms of sexually transmitted diseases. Chlamydial infections tend to present bilaterally with minimal pruritus and moderate to profuse tearing and exudate.

Adenoviral conjunctivitis typically causes a foreign body sensation, minimal pruritus and exudate, but profuse tearing. This type of conjunctivitis can often become bilateral; preauricular adenopathy is common, along with systemic symptoms typical of a viral infection, such as fever and myalgias. Other family members may be affected, as it is highly contagious. Associated symptoms of upper respiratory tract infection or gastroenteritis may point to a viral cause. Visual loss, photophobia, and severe eye pain may suggest corneal involvement, warranting referral to an ophthalmologist.

Allergic conjunctivitis usually presents bilaterally with severe pruritus and moderate tearing but no exudate. It will often accompany known allergy symptoms, making it important for the clinician to ask about a history of atopy or allergen exposures. Recurrent episodes are commonly seen, given its relationship with seasonal allergy symptoms. The complaint of extreme itchiness often helps differentiate an allergic cause from an infectious cause of conjunctivitis.

Objective

The first step in the examination is testing of visual acuity in both eyes, as well as in each eye individually. On inspection of the eyes, there will be hyperemia and tearing. The clinician needs to determine the extent of inflammation, whether it is local or diffuse, and whether it is in one or both eyes. It is important to note if the inflammation involves the cornea, which would warrant a referral. If exudate is present and is thick and copious, the cause is likely bacterial.

There may be eyelid swelling, and the clinician should examine the eyelids, lashes, and surrounding skin for abnormalities. Areas of lymphoid tissue hyperplasia that appear as dome-shaped elevations with blood vessels on their surface are called follicles; these are present in many types of conjunctivitis. If follicles are prominent in the upper tarsus, this is usually indicative of a viral etiology, such as adenovirus or *Chlamydia*. Minute elevations with vascular cores that may coalesce to form large papillae occasionally form secondary to an inflammatory process. Large papillae on the upper tarsal conjunctiva in a contact-lens wearer should raise concern for giant papillary conjunctivitis.

Preauricular nodes often reflect a viral etiology, such as HSV or adenovirus, and may also be present in *Chlamydia* and *N. gonorrhoeae* infections. These nodes are less prominent but more tender to palpation in patients with conjunctivitis of bacterial etiology. Subconjunctival hemorrhage may be seen in bacterial conjunctivitis, EKC, or enteroviral conjunctivitis.

Pupillary response should be assessed for equality and reactivity to light and accommodation, as failure of the pupil to react appropriately is indicative of a more serious problem. Patients with this sign require referral to an ophthalmologist for evaluation.

Corneal involvement, which often manifests with eye pain, decreased visual acuity, and photophobia, may be present and appear as punctate epithelial lesions. The potential for corneal involvement is increased in cases of vernal keratoconjunctivitis, adenovirus, and *N. gonorrhoeae* infection. The presence of a membranous film (pseudomembrane) that covers and adheres to the palpebral surface of the conjunctival epithelium is usually associated with EKC or infection with HSV, *S. pneumoniae,* or *N. gonorrhoeae.*

DIAGNOSTIC REASONING

Diagnostic Tests

The clinician should always check visual acuity first. A dilated pupillary examination should be performed by a trained professional in patients with hyperemia accompanied by proptosis, optic nerve dysfunction, decreased visual acuity, diplopia, or anterior chamber inflammation. Fluorescein staining may be indicated to rule out corneal involvement or keratitis, and ultraviolet illumination can be used to check for corneal abrasions, corneal dendrites (fluorescein-staining branched, tree-like lesions, which occur in HSV infection), or corneal ulceration. The clinician should use anesthetic drops before fluorescein-staining the eye. If *N. gonorrhoeae* is suspected, the conjunctivitis has failed to respond to treatment, or in cases of ophthalmia neonatorum, membranous conjunctivitis, or prolonged severe conjunctivitis, Gram stain and culture should be done on conjunctival secretions or exudate. In these cases, referral to an ophthalmologist is essential so that scrapings, cultures, and smears can be taken for further diagnostic work-up. Conjunctival biopsy is occasionally useful in refractory or atypical conjunctivitis and in cases of suspected neoplasm. When a hypopyon (a layer of white blood cells) or hyphema (a layer of red blood cells) in the anterior chamber is detected on examination, an immediate referral to an ophthalmologist is required because this may reflect infectious keratitis, endophthalmitis, or penetrating eye trauma.

Differential Diagnosis

The task at hand for the primary care practitioner is to determine which type of conjunctivitis is involved, an important first step before initiating treatment. See Table 19.1 for a comparison of selected differential diagnoses for red eye/conjunctivitis.

In allergic conjunctivitis, there is bilateral itching with a watery discharge. The patient or family may have a history of atopy. The conjunctiva and lids are swollen and reddened. This is a seasonal occurrence, most commonly seen in the fall and spring, which may be accompanied by sneezing, rhinorrhea, and a scratchy throat.

In bacterial conjunctivitis, signs and symptoms include itching, either bilaterally or unilaterally, with a moderate amount of mucopurulent (yellow-green) discharge. There is a moderate amount of conjunctival hyperemia, with a shiny red appearance of the lower lids. There is typically no focal pain or overt visual disturbances. The cornea is clear, and there is usually no preauricular adenopathy, although if present, lymph nodes may be painful to palpation. Bacterial conjunctivitis most commonly occurs in the winter and fall.

Viral conjunctivitis should also be ruled out. A patient with this type of conjunctivitis typically complains of itching, burning, and increased tearing. The conjunctiva is pink, diffuse, and peripheral. There is a watery mucoid discharge, with a moderate amount of mucoid debris. The patient may also have conjunctival edema, follicles on the palpebral conjunctiva, and eyelid edema. Preauricular adenopathy is more common with viral conjunctivitis. There are usually signs of an upper respiratory tract infection or a history of recent contact with another person with pink eye.

In iritis (inflammation of the iris), the patient presents with perilimbal conjunctival injection, mainly around the cornea; it is unilateral and without discharge. The patient may have moderate to severe pain and photophobia. Vision is blurred, the pupil is constricted, and the pupillary response to light is poor. Iritis requires prompt referral to an ophthalmologist and may be associated with an underlying systemic autoimmune connective

TABLE 19.1 Selected Causes of Red Eye

Assessment	Bacterial Conjunctivitis	Allergic Conjunctivitis	Viral Conjunctivitis	Iritis	Acute Glaucoma
Discharge	Purulent, thick; crusted lids in morning	Ropy, mucoid	Watery	Rare	None
Visual acuity	Normal	Normal	Normal	May be decreased if iritis is severe	Decreased
Pain and other sensation	Sandy, gritty, or foreign body sensation; no itching	Itching primarily	Itching, burning, gritty, or foreign body sensation	Moderate pain	Severe pain
Conjunctival abnormalities	Moderate to severe, diffuse	Mild, diffuse	Moderate, diffuse	Moderate, around cornea	Anterior chamber may appear narrow with penlight examination
Pupillary abnormalities	None	None	None	Poor light reflex	Mid-dilated; nonreactive to light or sluggish
Photophobia	No	No	No	Yes	Mild
Bilateral involvement	Sometimes	Usually	Often	No	Sometimes
Intraocular pressure	Normal	Normal	Normal	Normal	Increased
Preauricular lymph nodes	Not palpable	Not palpable	Palpable	Not palpable	Not palpable
Other symptoms and associations	Occurs most commonly in fall and winter	Rhinorrhea, sneezing, watery eyes; occurs most commonly in fall and spring	Highly contagious; associated with upper respiratory infection	Associated with autoimmune connective tissue disease	Nausea, vomiting, and headache

tissue disease. The broader diagnosis of uveitis, which may encompass iritis, iridocyclitis, and/or choroiditis, usually presents with severe eye pain, photophobia, blurred vision, injection in the limbus area, and deposits in the cornea. All of these conditions warrant an urgent referral to an ophthalmologist to avoid permanent vision loss.

In keratoconjunctivitis, the lack of adequate tear film to cover and protect the cornea and conjunctiva results in nonspecific irritation, with burning, redness, dryness, a foreign body sensation, and generalized eye pain.

Blepharitis, as discussed earlier in this chapter, is an inflammation involving the structures of the eyelid margin, with redness, scaling, and crusting. It commonly affects older adults and is usually secondary to either chronic staphylococcal infection or seborrheic dermatitis. Treatment includes warm eyelid compresses and eyelid scrubs with dilute baby shampoo two to four times per day. Chronic cases may require antibiotic ointment.

Pterygium, a conjunctival degeneration that results in an opacity that partially covers the cornea, is most commonly seen at the 3- and 9-o'clock positions. There can be associated conjunctival injection and tearing; the opacity is usually slow-growing and may eventually obstruct the vision. Pterygium is most commonly seen in persons with excessive exposure to ultraviolet light, windy conditions, or dusty surroundings. Treatment includes artificial tears to alleviate irritation, protective eyewear to be worn when outside, and surgical removal of the opacity if visual disturbance occurs.

Subconjunctival hemorrhage, the sudden onset of painless red eye without any other associated symptoms, is usually caused by trauma, excessive straining, coughing, or hypertension. No treatment is needed if the cause can be found, and the patient should be reassured that the condition resolves in 2 to 4 weeks.

The signs and symptoms of herpes zoster ophthalmicus include eye pain (which may be severe), tearing, photophobia, mucoid discharge, and moderate conjunctival hyperemia. The cornea may be clear or cloudy, and vesicles may or may not be present. Symptoms are usually the result of reactivation of a latent herpes zoster infection due to stress or other infection. Patients with herpes zoster ophthalmicus should be immediately referred to an ophthalmologist.

Signs and symptoms of corneal abrasion include sharp pain, foreign body sensation, photophobia, conjunctival hyperemia, and acute profuse tearing. The patient will usually have a history of scratching the eye, contact lens irritation, or ocular trauma. The clinician can stain the eye with fluorescein and use an ultraviolet light or slit lamp to inspect the eye for foreign objects or scratches. Treatment includes antibiotic eye drops or ointment for 5 days. Patching is not usually necessary. The patient should avoid wearing contact lenses until the abrasion heals.

With acute angle-closure glaucoma, the patient will have a sudden onset of severe pain and blurred vision, with nausea and vomiting. The patient can report seeing rainbow halos around lights. There will be corneal edema with diffuse conjunctival hyperemia. The pupil of the affected eye will be moderately dilated and completely unresponsive to light. Any patient with glaucoma should be referred to an ophthalmologist immediately. The patient who presents with acute glaucoma is usually older, with visual loss, severe pain, and possibly headache and nausea.

MANAGEMENT

Treatment depends on etiology and effect on visual acuity. Any purulent material or debris should be removed from the conjunctival area. Lubrication of the eye with artificial tears is recommended, or frequent cleansing by lavage. Pharmacological therapy for conjunctivitis depends on the identified etiology and/or suspected causative agent (see Drugs Commonly Prescribed 19.1). Although corticosteroids sometimes help with conjunctival irritation, clinicians should not routinely order topical corticosteroids, as there is a risk that their immunosuppressive effects could worsen infection.

With blepharitis or conditions that are accompanied by conjunctival discharge, the patient should be instructed to clean the lid margins with a dilute "no-tears" shampoo and discontinue wearing contact lenses, if used. Compresses are often effective for local relief; they should be warm in cases of infective conjunctivitis and cold in cases of allergic or irritative conjunctivitis. Patching of the eye is not typically warranted.

FOLLOW-UP AND REFERRAL

Given the potential for unresolved conjunctivitis to threaten vision, patients with red eye that does not resolve as expected with standard therapy should be referred to an ophthalmologist in a timely fashion for further diagnostic studies and therapeutic management. Urgent referral is warranted if there is an ulcer, keratitis, suspected HSV infection, or if the conjunctivitis worsens within 24 hours with treatment.

Patient Education: Red Eye/Conjunctivitis

The clinician should explain that secretions may remain infectious for at least 48 hours after the start of treatment. Conjunctivitis is highly contagious; therefore, the patient should take care when coming into contact with other members of the household, especially infants, children, older adults, and pets. The spread of conjunctivitis may be prevented by effective hand washing, avoiding touching the eyes, and not sharing towels or washcloths. The clinician should instruct the patient to avoid autoinoculation by not touching the medication applicator to the eye and using separate eyecups for each lavage. The patient should be taught to instill topical medication in the outer aspect of the lower eyelid. It may be best to use ophthalmic solution during the daytime and then apply a thin film of ointment before sleep. Contact lenses should be avoided until the infection is resolved.

REFERENCES

General

Bagheri N. *The wills eye manual: office and emergency room diagnosis and treatment of eye disease.* Wolters Kluwer; 2017.

Bohm KJ, Djalilian AR, Pflugfelder SC, et al. Dry eye. In: Mannis MJ, Hollan EJ, eds. *Cornea*, Vol 1. 4th ed. Elsevier; 2017: 377-396.

Kaiser PK, et al. *The Massachusetts Eye and Ear Infirmary Illustrated Manual of Ophthalmology.* Saunders; 2021.

Weisenthal RW. *2020-2021 Basic and Clinical Science Course (BCSC), Section 08 External Disease and Cornea.* American Academy of Ophthalmology; 2020.

Blepharitis

Amescua G, et al. Blepharitis preferred practice pattern®. *Ophthalmology.* 2019 Jan;126(1):P56-P93. doi: 10.1016/j.ophtha.2018.10.019. Epub 2018 Oct 23. PMID: 30366800.

Geerling G., et al. Emerging strategies for the diagnosis and treatment of meibomian gland dysfunction: Proceedings of the OCEAN group meeting, *The Ocular Surface.* 2017;15(2): 179-192.

Weisenthal RW. *2020-2021 Basic and Clinical Science Course (BCSC), Section 08 External Disease and Cornea.* American Academy of Ophthalmology; 2020.

Dry Eye

Akpek EK, et al. Dry eye syndrome preferred practice pattern®. *Ophthalmology.* 2019 Jan;126(1):P286-P334. doi: 10.1016/j.ophtha. 2018.10.023. Epub 2018 Oct 23. PMID: 30366798.

Dry Eye Assessment and Management Study Research Group, Asbell PA, et al. n-3 fatty acid supplementation for the treatment of dry eye disease. *N Engl J Med.* 2018 May 3;378(18):1681-1690. doi: 10.1056/NEJMoa1709691. Epub 2018 Apr 13. PMID: 29652551; PMCID: PMC5952353.

Foster S. Dry eye syndrome (keratoconjunctivitis sicca). (2017). http://emedicine.medscape.com/article/1210417-overview.

Jin X, Lin Z, Liu Y, et al. Hormone replacement therapy benefits meibomian gland dysfunction in perimenopausal women. *Medicine (Baltimore).* 2016;95(31):e4268. doi:10.1097/MD. 0000000000004268

Pucker AD, Ng SM, Nichols JJ. Over the counter (OTC) artificial tear drops for dry eye syndrome. *Cochrane Database Syst Rev.* 2016; 2CD009729.

Excessive Tearing (Epiphora)

Nordqvist C. (2017). Why do my eyes keep watering, and how to treat excessive eye-watering. http://www.medicalnewstoday.com/articles/169397.php.

Shen GL, Ng JD, Ma XP. Etiology, diagnosis, management and outcomes of epiphora referrals to an oculoplastic practice. *Int J Ophthalmol.* 2016;9(12):1751-1755. doi:10.18240/ijo.2016.12.08

Verma A, Singh D. (2016). Corneal abrasion treatment & management. http://emedicine.medscape.com/article/1195402-treatment.

Hordeolum and Chalazion

Bragg KJ, Le PH, Le JK. Hordeolum. [Updated 2020 Aug 8]. In: StatPearls [Internet]. Treasure Island (FL): StatPearls Publishing; 2020 Jan. https://www.ncbi.nlm.nih.gov/books/NBK441985/.

Jordan GA, Beier K. Chalazion. [Updated 2020 Aug 8]. In: StatPearls [Internet]. Treasure Island (FL): StatPearls Publishing; 2020 Jan. https://www.ncbi.nlm.nih.gov/books/NBK499889/.

Kabat AG, Sowka JW. Stye vs. stye. (2016). https://www.reviewofoptometry.com/article/stye-vs-stye. Accessed 8/31/31, 2017.

Lindsley K, Nichols JJ, Dickersin K. Interventions for acute internal hordeolum. *Cochrane Database Syst Rev.* 2017;9:CD007742.

Red Eye/Conjunctivitis

Baab S, Le PH, Kinzer EE. Allergic Conjunctivitis. [Updated 2020 Nov 18]. In: StatPearls [Internet]. Treasure Island (FL): StatPearls Publishing; 2020 Jan. https://www.ncbi.nlm.nih.gov/books/NBK448118/.

Graham R. Red eye. (2017). http://emedicine.medscape.com/article/1192122-overview.

Ramirez DA, Porco TC, Lietman TM, et al. Epidemiology of conjunctivitis in US emergency departments. *JAMA Ophthalmol.* 2017 Oct 01;135(10):1119-1121.

Scott IU, Luu K. (2017). Viral conjunctivitis (pink eye). http://emedicine.medscape.com/article/1191370-overview.

Varu DM, et al. Conjunctivitis preferred practice pattern®. *Ophthalmology.* 2019 Jan;126(1):P94-P169. doi: 10.1016/j.ophtha.2018.10.020. Epub 2018 Oct 23. PMID: 30366797.

Yeung K. Bacterial conjunctivitis (pink eye). (2017). http://emedicine.medscape.com/article/1191730.

RESOURCES

General

Digital Atlas of Ophthalmology (New York Eye and Ear Infirmary of Mount Sinai)
http://www.nyee.edu/health-professionals/digital-atlas-of-ophthalmology

American Academy of Ophthalmology
www.aao.org

Blepharitis

https://www.aao.org/eye-health/diseases/what-is-blepharitis

Chalazion

https://www.aao.org/eye-health/diseases/what-are-chalazia-styes

Dry Eye

https://www.aao.org/eye-health/diseases/what-is-dry-eye

Chapter 20

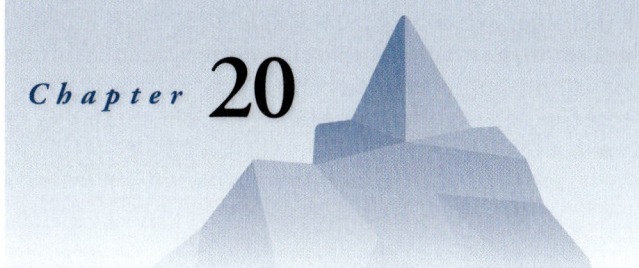

Visual Disturbances and Impaired Vision

Benjamin G. Kuhar, DO

Brian Oscar Porter, MD, PhD, MPH, MBA

Lynne M. Dunphy, PhD, APRN, FNP-BC, FAAN, FAANP

REFRACTIVE ERRORS

Normal vision is dependent on a clear image being projected through the cornea, aqueous humor, lens, and vitreous humor, and then onto the retina. All of these structures must be healthy to provide a clear retinal image, and the optic nerve must be able to transmit an accurate image to the visual cortex in the occipital lobe of the brain. Refractive errors result in blurred vision due to aberrations in how external light is reflected onto the retina.

EPIDEMIOLOGY AND CAUSES

Refractive errors that are uncorrected or incompletely corrected are a common cause of visual impairment (Table 20.1). Refractory errors include myopia (nearsightedness), hyperopia (farsightedness), astigmatism,

TABLE 20.1 Selected Causes of Impaired Vision

Diagnosis	Typical Patient Age	Subjective Assessment	Objective Assessment	Urgent Treatment and Immediate Referral Required?
Acute glaucoma	Usually aged 50 to 85 years	Sudden onset of severe eye pain, vomiting, and headache	Conjunctiva may be infected; steamy cornea; pupil may be fixed and partially dilated with narrow chamber angle	Yes
Cataracts	Older adults	Painless progressive loss of vision	Vision decreased; opaque or cloudy lens may be apparent; decreased view of the fundus	No
Chronic glaucoma	Usually older than 40 years, but may occur in younger patients	PPLV; halos seen around lights	Decreased peripheral field of vision, decreased central vision is a later sign; increased intraocular pressure and increased cup-to-disc ratio with anterior normal chamber angle	Usually not
Diabetic retinopathy	Related to length of time patient has had diabetes and any comorbid conditions	PPLV	Vision will usually not improve with pinhole test; vision varies with stages of retinopathy; dot-blot hemorrhages, microaneurysms, lipid exudates, or infarcts in nerve fiber layer may be apparent	Usually not
Macular degeneration	Older adults	PPLV; decreased central vision	Decreased central vision; blood or lipid exudates on fundal examination	Usually not
Myopia	Teenager	Painless progressive loss of vision (PPLV)	No change in fundal examination	No
Presbyopia	Older than 40 years	PPLV; may have blurred vision	No change in fundal examination	No

and presbyopia. Astigmatism is typically due to abnormal corneal curvature in different meridians. Hyperopia is commonly due to decreased refractive power of the cornea or decreased axial length of the eye. Conversely, myopia is typically due to increased refractive power of the cornea or increased axial length of the eye. Presbyopia usually occurs in the older adult population due to decreased lens elasticity and ability to accommodate.

The prevalence of hyperopia and myopia in the United States is about 25% each, and approximately 50% of the U.S. population has some degree of astigmatism. One of the objectives of *Healthy People 2030* is to increase the use of assistive and adaptive devices such as visual aids in smartphones or screen readers that might help people with vision loss, including 12.4% to 15.9% of adults over the age of 18.

Geriatric Considerations: Eye Conditions

Most eye conditions are more prevalent in the older adult population and, as such, must be screened for (also see Chapter 18). Most clinicians recommend an eye examination for screening at age 40 years if the person does not already wear eyeglasses.

- Glaucoma is a leading cause of irreversible blindness in the United States and worldwide and is more common in people ages 55 to 70 years. The necessity of screening for glaucoma cannot be overstated.
- Macular degeneration is also a leading cause of blindness affecting individuals older than age 50 years. If treated early, blindness and many complications can be avoided.
- Cataracts are likely the most common eye condition in older adults and are easily treated when diagnosed, but unfortunately, the majority of these cases are undiagnosed. Cataracts are also a leading cause of visual impairment and blindness.

PATHOPHYSIOLOGY

To transmit an external image into the eye, parallel rays of light enter the cornea; the rays are bent by the cornea and lens to converge on the retina. The macula is the pigmented portion of the retina responsible for central visual acuity and is thus the most important for vision. The patient perceives a blurred image when light rays do not converge on a common point on the retina. Light ray convergence in front of the retina causes myopia, or nearsightedness. If light rays converge posterior to the retina, the patient is hyperopic, or farsighted. If light rays focus on two separate lines rather than a single point, the patient has astigmatism.

CLINICAL PRESENTATION

Subjective

Patients with refractive errors may present with a chief complaint of poor vision or a change in vision. They may also report that their current eyeglasses are not effective or present with a complaint of recent headaches suggestive of eye strain. Refractive errors have a gradual onset and are not usually accompanied by pain or redness. Refractive errors may be found on screening during a routine physical examination. Patients may be unaware of a change in vision because they have become accustomed to it; this is especially true when the error is in only one eye.

Objective

For patients with refractive errors, visual acuity on examination with a Snellen eye chart will be worse than 20/20 and typically worse than previous examinations. A simple "pinhole test" can be administered in the primary care setting to determine whether the diminished visual acuity is the result of a refractive error or underlying organic disease. A pinhole test is performed by creating pinholes 0.5 to 2 mm in diameter in a stiff paper card. The patient is asked to look through one of the pinholes using one eye at a time. If the visual acuity improves without the use of corrective lenses, the diminished acuity is due to a refractive error, as improvement occurs because light rays are focused through the pinhole and the pinhole card blocks peripheral light waves. If there is no improvement, the diminished acuity is due to the presence of organic disease, which can be caused by a variety of conditions.

DIAGNOSTIC REASONING

The role of the primary care provider is to evaluate the patient for the need for emergent or routine referral to an ophthalmologist or optometrist. Refractory errors are not life-threatening but do require timely referral to prevent secondary injury from accidents or falls related to poor visual acuity.

Diagnostic Tests

The hallmark of diagnostic assessment of refractory errors is examination of visual acuity, which is typically done in the primary care setting, using a properly distanced Snellen eye examination wall chart or handheld printed card. Although these office-based tests can quantify refractive errors on a gross level and generally characterize the visual defect as farsightedness or nearsightedness, a more detailed examination will be required by an appropriate referral to an optometrist for corrective lenses or an ophthalmologist for more serious eye pathology.

Differential Diagnosis

A thorough history and physical examination will reveal if the vision change is acute or progressive, along with associated signs or symptoms. Vision-threatening conditions requiring emergent referral to an ophthalmologist should be ruled out. Some of these conditions include:

1. Ischemic optic neuropathy. Must rule out giant cell arteritis (GCA). An eye examination would show a pale, swollen disc with a flame-shaped hemorrhage.
2. Central retina artery occlusion. Must rule out GCA, emboli, and thrombus. An eye examination would show diffuse retinal whitening and a foveal cherry-red spot.
3. Retinal detachment. Patients experience a lot of new floaters, flashes of light in one or both eyes, and/or a dark shadow or "curtain" on the sides or in the middle of their field of vision. A dilated eye examination will show the detachment.
4. Acute third nerve palsy. Must rule out intracranial aneurysm. Extraocular changes will be visualized; these include complete ptosis, inability to adduct and supraduct the eye, and a dilated pupil.
5. Endophthalmitis. A slit-lamp examination will show conjunctival injection and corneal edema.
6. Orbital cellulitis. An examination will show lid swelling and erythema with proptosis and pain with eye movement.

MANAGEMENT

Given their ease of use, eyeglasses are the first-line management to correct refractive errors. Accurate prescriptions for such lenses may be obtained from an optometrist or ophthalmologist. Contact lenses are also available in a wide variety of types and specifications to correct for almost any type of refractive error, although their proper use and maintenance require patient training. Some patients may be candidates for and benefit from vision correction procedures, such as laser-assisted *in situ* keratomileusis (LASIK) eye surgery.

FOLLOW-UP AND REFERRAL

Accurate diagnosis and characterization of refractive errors require referral to an optometrist or ophthalmologist, who have the appropriate equipment to accurately measure refractive errors. These referrals are needed to obtain prescriptions for effective corrective lenses, as well as to screen for other common eye problems, which may contribute to decreased visual acuity. The timing of follow-up is determined by the presence of more significant eye pathology. Simple refractive errors that are adequately addressed with corrective lenses may not require more than annual follow-up to assess for a progressive component.

> **Patient Education: Refractive Errors**
>
> Patients should be encouraged to use corrective lenses for all activities that require optimal visual acuity, such as reading, driving, or operating machinery. Proper care of eyeglasses and contact lenses should be discussed with all patients.

CATARACTS

A cataract is any opacity of the lens of the eye. Cataracts may or may not be associated with visual impairment or functional consequences and may form in one or both eyes. When the optical quality of the crystalline lens is damaged, visual impairment ensues (see Table 20.1).

EPIDEMIOLOGY AND CAUSES

Cataracts are the leading cause of blindness worldwide. The World Health Organization has estimated that more than 20 million people are blind due to cataracts and that cataracts are responsible for more than 70 million cases of vision impairment and blindness worldwide. Up to 90% of these cases of blindness are found in developing nations. In the U.S.-based Framingham Eye Study, the prevalence of cataracts was 42% in adults 52 to 64 years of age and up to 91% in 75- to 85-year-olds. Cataracts are more likely to be seen in African American males and females of all age groups and are the leading cause of visual impairment in these populations. They are also the leading cause of visual impairment among Americans of Hispanic/Latino and European descent. The number of Americans with cataracts is expected to double by 2050. *Healthy People 2030* includes an objective to decrease the number of adults aged 65 years and older with visual impairment due to a cataract from 141 per 1,000 to 126 per 1,000 adults. The more well-established, consistent risk factors for cataract formation include cigarette smoking, diabetes mellitus, and excessive exposure to sunlight (i.e., ultraviolet B rays). Other studies have suggested long-term corticosteroid use, prior intraocular surgery, and trauma as additional risk factors for cataract development. Avoidance of these risk factors is key to cataract prevention, including smoking cessation and the wearing of protective eye gear, especially when engaged in high-risk activities for cataract formation or ocular injury, such as the use of tanning beds or welding.

PATHOPHYSIOLOGY

The lens is a transparent, biconvex structure located behind the iris (colored portion of the eye) and is supported by fibrous strands called zonules. The lens works in conjunction with the cornea to help focus incoming light onto the retina. The lens itself is composed of a central nucleus surrounded by a cortex, which are both encased by an outer lens capsule. The lens is avascular, deriving its metabolic needs from the surrounding aqueous humor. Early in life, the lens is pliable and can change its shape as connecting zonules anchored to ciliary bodies place varying degrees of tension on the lens through involuntary contraction and relaxation. These changes in lens shape result in accommodation, allowing objects to come into focus at varying distances based on how light rays are focused onto the retina.

The transparency of the human lens results from the highly ordered nature of its composite stratified epithelia, which contain a high density of cytoplasmic proteins called crystallins. Crystallins are water-soluble proteins that help create the refractive nature and clarity of the lens.

Aging alters the biochemical and osmotic balance required for lens transparency, as do comorbid disease processes, such as diabetes mellitus. As the lens ages, it loses both its pliability and its clarity. Crystallins undergo chemical changes that result in the formation of protein aggregates. Over time, these aggregates eventually become large enough to cause changes in the refractive index of the lens, causing a scattering of light and reducing the transparency of the lens. Healing fibrosis from ocular trauma is a primary etiology of acquired cataracts, whereas secondary cataracts may result from other sources of ocular inflammation that extend to the lens, including uveitis, corticosteroids, and radiation therapy used to treat ocular tumors.

There are three subtypes of cataracts, categorized by anatomical location. The size, density, and location of the cataract determine its effect on vision and the most appropriate method of surgical intervention and lens replacement. Some patients may have a combination of these subtypes:

1. Nuclear cataracts are centrally located opacifications, characterized by significant nearsightedness and a slow, indolent course.
2. Cortical cataracts are peripheral, asymmetric radial opacities that typically cause worse glare symptoms than other types of cataracts.
3. Subcapsular cataracts can be anteriorly or posteriorly located and are commonly associated with acute

angle-closure glaucoma and corticosteroid use, respectively. They typically progress faster than the other forms—over months rather than years.

Regardless of anatomical type, immature cataracts are those that do not obscure the red retinal light reflex on fundoscopy. In contrast, mature cataracts obscure the red reflex with significant visual impairment, and hypermature cataracts are characterized by liquefaction of the cortical lens with mobility of the nucleus.

CLINICAL PRESENTATION
Subjective

The patient with cataracts may present with visual changes and/or functional impairment; however, asymptomatic cataracts (without a perception of vision loss) may be found on routine examination. Cataracts produce a gradual, painless, and progressive loss of vision, although many patients are unaware of any vision problems due to the gradual nature on onset. For example, with monocular (asymmetrical) cataracts, reduced vision may only be apparent when the unaffected eye is covered. Age-related cataracts tend to be bilateral in nature and may manifest as blurred or distorted vision, with complaints of a glare when driving at night or in bright light. The patient may also complain of decreased color and contrast sensitivity, although loss of contrast sensitivity is not specific to cataracts.

Increased density of the lens nucleus (nuclear cataracts) typically results in impaired distance vision that may require frequent changes in a patient's eyeglass prescription. Myopia (nearsightedness) may result from nuclear cataracts. The term "second sight" refers to older adults who abandon their reading glasses related to this phenomenon; however, as the cataract worsens, so does their near vision.

The Lens Opacities Classification System III is a widely used subjective grading tool to assess cataract severity. Decision making for cataract surgery also includes assessment of visual functional status, with a specific focus on limitations in the ability of the patient to perform daily activities. These aspects can be measured with clinical history or with formal instruments or questionnaires, such as the Visual Function Index-14, which was designed to assess patient-reported visual functioning. Ultimately, when deciding whether to operate, the surgeon needs to determine whether the improvement in the patient's visual function would warrant cataract surgery.

Objective

In some patients, lens opacity will be apparent on inspection, but this is not always the case. Decreased visual acuity is the most common objective finding associated with cataracts. As with any eye complaint in the primary care setting, it is important to assess vision, extraocular movement, and pupillary size and light reactivity. If equipment allows, evaluating the intraocular pressure would be beneficial as well. Mature cataracts may eventually produce a gray or white pupillary reflex known as leukocoria, although a dense posterior subcapsular cataract may produce reduction in vision without altering the pupillary reflex. The best direct visualization of cataracts is obtained in a dilated eye examination performed by an ophthalmologist using a slit lamp.

DIAGNOSTIC REASONING
Diagnostic Tests

There is no single eye test or examination that can fully describe the effects of a cataract on a patient's visual status or functional ability, nor is there a single test that establishes the need for cataract surgery. The decision to have surgery is based on the patient's quality of life and perception of visual deficits, as well as the size and maturity of the cataract(s).

A detailed history and physical examination are vital to proper diagnosis, including visual acuity with current corrective lenses, measurement of best-corrected (distance) visual acuity, external eye examination, ocular alignment and motility, and pupillary function. More specific tests such as glare testing and contrast sensitivity testing would be done by an ophthalmologist.

A detailed ophthalmic examination would also include visual acuity testing, refraction, intraocular pressure, slit-lamp, and fundus examination to rule out other ocular comorbidities that could affect the postoperative prognosis. B-scan ultrasonography may be used if direct visualization of the retina is not possible because of dense cataract. Other tests commonly used include brightness acuity tester (BAT), as well as keratometry and biometry that help calculate the intraocular lens implant power needed for optimal visual outcomes.

Artificial intelligence (AI) for cataract detection, grading of cataract severity, and management of cataracts has made significant strides in ophthalmology care. AI algorithms have been developed for automated detection and grading of the cataract, based on either machine learning or deep learning approaches. The algorithms were developed based on slit-lamp photographs and color fundus photographs. New AI systems can provide better outreach for cataract screening, especially in rural settings.

Differential Diagnosis

The following causes of visual impairment should be ruled out in patients suspected of having cataracts: refractive errors, glaucoma, retinopathy, and age-related macular degeneration (AMD). Any sudden change in vision or sudden vision loss should be treated as an emergency and referred to an ophthalmologist immediately.

Cataracts are gradual in onset and develop over time. Macular degeneration also presents with a slow, progressive loss of vision, but this impairment is focused centrally, by virtue of its effects on the macula. In addition, macular degeneration may also manifest with symptoms of acute visual distortion (metamorphopsia), resulting from leakage of exudative fluid or bleeding from abnormally proliferative subretinal vessels. Open-angle glaucoma produces a slow and painless visual field loss that usually begins peripherally and often (although not always) presents with increased intraocular pressure and/or an increased cup-to-disc ratio (greater than 0.6) of the optic nerve. Diabetic retinopathy may also result in vision loss; fundoscopic examination will usually reveal dot-and-blot hemorrhages, microaneurysms, exudates, dilated and tortuous ocular blood vessels, and neovascularization of the disc and retina.

MANAGEMENT

There are limited options when it comes to nonsurgical treatment for cataracts, typically including eyeglasses with special tints to reduce glare, handheld monoculars for distance vision, or magnifiers for near vision. However, surgery is typically used to manage visually significant cataracts. Surgery should be discussed when changes in eyeglasses no longer correct vision sufficiently and quality of life is jeopardized. Cataract surgery is a relatively safe outpatient procedure that has been shown to be highly cost-effective, given the reduction in comorbidities and injuries associated with progressive visual impairment. Patients who are scheduled for cataract surgery may be referred to their primary care practitioner for a preoperative health assessment. However, healthy adult patients scheduled for cataract surgery under local anesthesia do not typically require preoperative medical testing.

For patients with risk factors or comorbid medical conditions, a physical examination, electrocardiogram, electrolytes, and urinalysis may be ordered. Causes for concern include the presence of diabetes mellitus, hypertension, ischemic heart disease, certain pulmonary disorders, and the use of anticoagulants. Any patient with uncontrolled diabetes mellitus is at risk of postoperative vision loss related to diabetic macular edema, which causes the retinal vessels to leak, leading to swelling of the visual center (macula). Anticoagulant therapy should be discontinued before surgery. This includes over-the-counter supplements such as high doses of fish oil or omega-3 fatty acids that have been associated with prolonged bleeding. Systemic hypertension may also place the patient at risk for intraocular hemorrhage during or after surgery.

The standard of care in cataract surgery in the United States is a small-incision phacoemulsification with foldable intraocular lens implantation. The procedure is safe and affords improved vision with decreased dependence on corrective eyewear for distance, intermediate, and near vision. Two surgical techniques are currently used—phacoemulsification and extracapsular cataract extraction. In the developed world, phacoemulsification is the most commonly performed method of cataract extraction, using ultrasound energy to emulsify a lens. In both types of surgery, an incision is made into the eye, and the central anterior lens capsule is removed. In phacoemulsification, the surgeon makes a 2- to 4-mm incision and inserts an ultrasonic vibrating needle that breaks the cataract into small pieces, which are then aspirated through the needle's central bore. The smaller incision and smaller sutures used in phacoemulsification make it the preferred method for cataract removal. In extracapsular surgery, the surgeon makes a 10- to 14-mm incision, and the entire lens nucleus is loosened from the cortex and removed through the incision. In both cases, the surgery continues with removal of the residual lens cortex and insertion of a replacement intraocular lens. The incision may be self-sealing or closed with sutures.

There is little evidence from randomized controlled studies that evaluated the optimal regimen of antibiotics and/or corticosteroids postoperatively. There is more evidence demonstrating that intracameral (i.e., injected into the eye cavity) antibiotics reduce the risk of postoperative bacterial endophthalmitis. Postoperative straining of the eyes (from reading small print, prolonged computer or smartphone use, etc.) should be avoided until the patient receives clearance from an ophthalmologist.

FOLLOW-UP AND REFERRAL

Patients need early referral and monitoring by an ophthalmologist, although education about the advances in surgical techniques and reassurance may be important aspects of care before referral. A patient who has undergone cataract removal surgery should be reevaluated by the ophthalmologist within 48 hours of the procedure. Approximately 4 weeks after surgery, the patient should be evaluated for the need for corrective lenses.

Patient Education: Cataracts

Modification of dietary intake and nutritional supplements have demonstrated minimal to no effect in the prevention or treatment of cataracts; however, there is some conflicting evidence of their utility. A Cochrane review found no evidence supporting high doses of vitamin E, vitamin C, or beta-carotene in preventing the formation or progression of cataracts. Daily lutein has shown no significant impact, and there is little research to support high-dose antioxidants. There is moderate evidence, however, that multivitamins and mineral supplements may decrease the risk of nuclear cataracts. In addition, for patients with diabetes mellitus, tight glucose control is critical to minimize the risk of cataract formation.

GLAUCOMA

Glaucoma is defined as a group of diseases characterized by progressive damage to the optic nerve, resulting in optic nerve atrophy and vision loss, most typically associated with elevated intraocular pressure (IOP) (see Table 20.1). Glaucoma is commonly classified as open-angle glaucoma and angle-closure glaucoma (classically referred to as closed-angle or narrow-angle glaucoma). These classifications are based on the anatomy of the anterior chamber. Both types of glaucoma may be present in the same eye (referred to as combined-mechanism glaucoma). Glaucoma is further differentiated as primary or secondary (associated with an ocular condition or a systemic process). There is also a congenital form of glaucoma seen in infants.

Open-angle glaucoma is the most common type and is characterized as a chronic, progressive disorder causing optic nerve damage and associated visual field loss. It typically has a good prognosis if recognized early and treated appropriately. Angle-closure glaucoma, on the other hand, may have subacute and chronic components, but it is most often associated with acute episodes of significant eye pain, redness, and acute visual loss, which, if untreated, may rapidly lead to permanent blindness.

EPIDEMIOLOGY AND CAUSES

With life expectancies increasing in most populations, the prevalence of glaucoma, is expected to increase drastically in the coming decades. More than 3 million Americans are living with glaucoma, with most being older than 40 years. Low vision or blindness affects 3.3 million Americans older than age 40 years. In 2020, about 80 million people had glaucoma worldwide, and by 2040 this is expected to be more than 111 million. *Healthy People 2030* has an objective to decrease the prevalence rate of adults over age 65 years with visual impairment due to glaucoma from 13.2 per 1,000 to 10.6 per 1,000 people. The prevalence of glaucoma is four to five times higher among black people than white people. Glaucoma is 15 times more likely to cause blindness in black patients than white patients. Primary open-angle glaucoma is the most prevalent form of glaucoma and accounts for 90% to 95% of all cases. Angle-closure glaucoma (acute glaucoma) is not as common; it affects approximately 0.1% of the population. Angle-closure glaucoma tends to occur in people aged 55 to 70 years old and is more prevalent in people of Asian and Inuit (Native Alaskan) descent. Open-angle glaucoma occurs equally in males and females, whereas angle-closure glaucoma occurs more frequently in females. Every year, glaucoma costs the U.S. economy $2.86 billion in direct costs and productivity losses.

Increased IOP, positive family history, older age, and African descent all place an individual at increased risk for glaucoma. Older African Americans have a higher prevalence of glaucoma and a more rapid progression of disease. Other risk factors for development of primary open-angle glaucoma include decreased corneal thickness and increased cup-to-disc ratio.

Glaucoma may also develop secondarily as a result of local or systemic disease, as well as medication use. The use of corticosteroid therapy (topical, inhaled, or systemic) may lead to increased IOP in about 30% of the population. Viscoelastic agents, commonly used during intraocular surgeries, can also cause abrupt spikes in IOP. Other common causes of secondary glaucoma include uveitis, trauma, and intraocular tumors. Over time, increased pressure in the anterior chamber that is uncorrected will damage the optic nerve, impair peripheral visual fields, and ultimately begin to affect central vision. Increased IOP, optic nerve atrophy, and visual field loss make up the classic triad of glaucoma. Patients older than 40 years with a family history of glaucoma should have an eye examination every 1 to 2 years.

PATHOPHYSIOLOGY

The ciliary body of the eye produces aqueous humor, which circulates from the posterior chamber, through the pupil, and into the anterior chamber. It then exits through the trabecular meshwork and uveoscleral pathway. In primary open-angle glaucoma (in which no secondary cause is identified), elevated IOP is typically caused by obstruction of the outflow channels, particularly the trabecular meshwork. The manner in which the trabecular meshwork is obstructed is a matter of debate, but it likely involves changes in the biochemical makeup of the cells that line the meshwork. Secondary glaucoma may result from increased IOP caused by ocular trauma or inflammation such as uveitis, chronic corticosteroid use, vasoproliferative retinopathy, and recurrent retinal hemorrhages.

The specific mechanism by which increased IOP leads to optic nerve atrophy is also debated. One theory is that increased IOP causes direct mechanical compression of the nerve fibers and disruption of axonal transport. Others theorize that increased IOP impairs the small-vessel circulation that provides nutrients to the optic nerve. Glutamate toxicity and processes involving apoptosis leading to axonal loss are also currently being investigated.

It is critical to recognize, however, that optic atrophy may occur in the absence of increased IOP. Traditionally, elevated IOP has been defined as greater than 21 mm Hg. Ocular hypertension has also been identified in the absence of optic nerve atrophy. Thus, other pathophysiological processes leading to progressive, irreversible vision loss also function in primary open-angle glaucoma. Increased IOP by itself must be considered only a risk factor, rather than the definitive glaucomatous etiology. Work is also under way to identify the gene products and functions associated with inherited forms of open-angle glaucoma, which typically occur before the age of 40 years, known collectively as juvenile glaucoma.

Angle-closure glaucoma, which may be either acute or chronic, is less common than open-angle glaucoma. It is caused by anatomical narrowing of the anterior chamber angle, a factor that is fundamentally determined by genetics and becomes more likely with advanced age. Specifically, angle-closure glaucoma results from the forward displacement of the iris toward the cornea, with narrowing of the iridocorneal angle resulting in an obstruction of outflow from the anterior chamber. Acute angle-closure glaucoma occurs when there is an acute closure of the iridocorneal angle with a sudden, severe rise in IOP, often well above 40 mm Hg, which is highly symptomatic. Permanent vision loss may result if this condition is not treated promptly.

CLINICAL PRESENTATION

Subjective

Generally, patients with open-angle glaucoma are asymptomatic until optic nerve damage is quite advanced. It typically has a gradual onset, with slow, painless bilateral peripheral vision loss and poor night vision. Frequent changes in refractory prescription may be a common presenting symptom. In later stages, symptoms may include seeing halos around lights and further visual loss. Acute angle-closure glaucoma has a rapid onset, with unilateral pain and pressure, blurred vision, seeing halos around lights, and photophobia, followed by loss of peripheral vision, subsequently followed by central vision loss. A headache may be present with possible nausea and vomiting. Chronic angle-closure glaucoma is as insidious in onset as open-angle glaucoma. Its fundamental mechanism relates to the anatomical narrowness of the anterior chamber angle. Often, patients have a history of vague discomfort about the eyes and intermittent blurring of vision.

Objective

In the primary care setting, the physical examination in most patients with chronic glaucoma will likely be unremarkable. Visual acuity may or may not be affected. Visual field abnormalities to confrontation will be present usually only in the later stages of severe cases. A Marcus Gunn pupil (afferent pupillary defect, with an asymmetric reaction to light in one pupil versus the other) may be present, particularly if one optic nerve has more severe damage than the other.

In acute angle-closure glaucoma, IOP rises rapidly to very high levels. The eye becomes red and painful, the cornea can become hazy, and vision is severely blurred. The pupil of the affected eye may be mid-dilated and nonreactive. Findings on fundoscopic examination may show a pale optic disc with excavated cupping and a shallow anterior chamber; there may be an increased cup/disc ratio and asymmetry on comparison with the other eye. In many cases, the clinician can detect a shallow anterior chamber and narrow angle with the flashlight test: in this test, a penlight is held at the temporal limbus of the eye, and the degree of illumination is noted. A narrow angle is suggested if the nasal half of the iris is in the shadow. Dilation of the pupil with mydriatic agents tends to narrow the angle further, which can lead to an acute attack, as can dim light or darkness and physical or emotional stress. The primary care provider should closely monitor patients with a family history of angle-closure glaucoma or hyperopia (farsightedness) accompanied by a history of eye ache, headache, and blurred vision. Urgent referral to an ophthalmologist is warranted if there is any suspicion of angle-closure glaucoma.

DIAGNOSTIC REASONING

The U.S. Preventive Services Task Force concluded that the evidence of effectiveness of glaucoma screening on clinical outcomes is lacking and that the balance of benefits and harms therefore cannot be determined. However, because of the significant economic and health implications, patients older than 40 years with a family history of glaucoma might want to be tested every 1 to 2 years. Diagnosis of primary open-angle glaucoma is based on a combination of tests showing characteristic degenerative changes in the optic nerve and visual field defects (often loss in peripheral vision). Although increased IOP was previously considered an important part of the definition of this condition, it is now known that many people with primary open-angle glaucoma do not have increased IOP and that not all people with increased IOP have or will develop glaucoma. Therefore, screening with tonometry alone may be inadequate to detect all cases of primary open-angle glaucoma.

Measurement of visual fields can be difficult. The reliability of a single measurement may be low; several consistent measurements are needed to establish the presence of defects. Specialists use dilated ophthalmoscopy or slit-lamp examination to evaluate changes in the optic nerve; however, there is variability in describing glaucomatous progression of the optic nerve. In addition, no single standard exists to define and measure progression of visual field defects. Most tests that are available in a primary care setting do not have acceptable accuracy to detect glaucoma. Multiple testing methods requiring specialized equipment and training are available, including pneumotonometry, which uses a puff of air against the eyeball to assess IOP, and the more accurate method of applanation tonometry, in which the cornea is directly observed while pressure is placed against it.

Diagnostic Tests

The diagnosis of glaucoma is not made on the basis of a single test but on the finding of characteristic degenerative changes in the optic nerve and defects in visual fields. Tonometry to measure IOP is essential, although not diagnostic. Traditionally, normal IOP is between 10 and 21 mm Hg. In chronic open-angle glaucoma, there may be normal or elevated IOP, whereas in an acute exacerbation of angle-closure glaucoma, IOP may be as high as 40 to 80 mm Hg. However, increased IOP alone is not required for the diagnosis of glaucoma because many patients with open-angle glaucoma consistently have IOPs within the normal range.

Physical diagnosis relies on gonioscopic evaluation of the anterior chamber angle by an ophthalmologist. Gonioscopy determines the angle of the eye's anterior chamber and thus enables the examiner to differentiate between open-angle and angle-closure glaucoma. Visual inspection of the angle is done using a special lens (goniolens) at the slit lamp. The two primary types of disease, open-angle glaucoma and angle-closure glaucoma, are classified according to the anatomy of the anterior chamber angle.

The appearance (e.g., color and contour) of the optic nerve and findings on visual field examination are the most important clues to diagnosis, and pathognomonic changes indicate glaucoma. Fundoscopic examination of the optic nerve reveals changes in the cup and neuroretinal rim relatively early in the disease, indicating the possibility of open-angle glaucoma. Particularly significant are the size of the cup relative to the optic nerve, any thinning or nicking of the disc rim, and the presence of disc hemorrhages. Visual field examination, which requires specialized equipment, detects defects in the field of vision that are characteristic for glaucomatous damage to the optic nerve relatively early in the disease.

Testing of visual fields using confrontational finger motions to assess the location of the patient's fields compared with the examiner's is unreliable for diagnosing glaucoma. Specialized tests can be performed by an ophthalmologist or optometrist for visual field assessment, including automated perimetry, Goldmann perimetry, or tangent screen testing. Pachymetry, which is a method of measuring corneal thickness, may also be done by an ophthalmologist, as thinner corneas are at higher risk for the development of primary open-angle glaucoma.

Differential Diagnosis

Unlike open-angle glaucoma, patients with conjunctivitis and uveitis usually have objective findings that should alert the clinician to these diagnoses. With conjunctivitis, the conjunctiva of the eye is inflamed—either red, pink, swollen, and/or irritated, with or without mucus. Uveitis symptoms may occur suddenly or develop gradually and may get worse quickly. The patient may complain of eye redness, eye pain, light sensitivity, blurred vision, floaters, or decreased vision. Medications such as corticosteroids, amphetamines, and chlorpromazine can all increase IOP. Many ocular and systemic conditions are associated with the development of glaucoma; in addition, the use of topical, systemic, and inhaled corticosteroids may increase IOP, depending on dose and duration of treatment. Any ocular complaints from patients on these medications should warrant referral to an ophthalmologist if there is concern for glaucoma.

MANAGEMENT

Once nerve damage has occurred, it is irreversible; thus, the goal of treatment is to prevent progression of damage and to protect the optic nerve from increased IOP. Adequate lowering of IOP is the only way to prevent or slow the progression of glaucoma. The goal of pressure lowering therapy is a near 30% reduction in IOP. The Collaborative Normal-Tension Glaucoma Study (CNTGS) showed that lowering IOP by at least 30% reduced the 5-year risk of visual field progression from 35% to 12%.

Ophthalmologists will often set a "target pressure," which is an estimated IOP level below which glaucomatous progression is expected to be minimized. IOP lowering is typically achieved using either medication eyedrops or surgical intervention. The goal of pharmacological therapy is to decrease and control IOP (see Drugs Commonly Prescribed 20.1), with the choice of medication regimen usually made by an ophthalmologist. Once started on pressure-lowering eyedrops, the patient is likely to stay on it for life, which is an important discussion to have with the patient.

First-line therapy typically consists of prostaglandin analogs because of their convenient once-daily dosing, efficacy, and decreased systemic absorption compared with other IOP-lowering medications. Beta blockers and alpha-agonists are alternative options that can be used in adjunct if one medication is not sufficient. Treatment compliance with multiple doses of eyedrops daily is often poor in open-angle glaucoma; however, newer topical agents require less frequent dosing (e.g., once daily for prostaglandins). The target IOP that therapy attempts to achieve is to be decided on an individual basis. If one medication is not sufficient to lower IOP, a second medication from a different class may be added. It should be noted that occasionally, localized or systemic reactions to the medication may occur, and the patients should be instructed in what to look for. Interactions with other systemic medications that the patient may be taking must be considered.

Surgical options such as laser trabeculoplasty (LTP) can be effective as primary or adjunctive therapies. In LTP, laser energy is directed at the trabecular meshwork, resulting in biomechanical changes of the meshwork cells, improving aqueous humor outflow. The pressure-lowering effects of

Drugs Commonly Prescribed 20.1: Glaucoma

DRUG	MECHANISM OF ACTION	ADVERSE EFFECTS
Cholinergic Agents		
Pilocarpine (Isopto, Pilocar, Pilostat)	Constrict pupils to open the angle and allow aqueous humor to escape	Increased salivation, increased gastric secretion, abdominal cramping
Beta Blockers		
Timolol (Timoptic), betaxolol (Betoptic), levobunolol (Betagan), carteolol (Cartrol), metipranolol (Betanol)	Reduce the production of aqueous humor	Bradycardia, bronchospasm, decreased libido, masked symptoms of hypoglycemia, exacerbation of myasthenia gravis. Contraindicated in asthma, sinus bradycardia, second- or third-degree atrioventricular block, overt congestive heart failure
Prostaglandin Analogs		
Bimatoprost (Lumigan), latanoprost (Xalatan), uveoscleral travoprost (Travatan)	Decrease intraocular pressure by increased outflow (drainage)	Can cause conjunctival hyperemia, iris pigment color changes, anterior uveitis, trichiasis (ingrowth or inversion of eyelashes)
Carbonic Anhydrase Inhibitors		
Brinzolamide (Azopt), dorzolamide (Trusopt), echothiophate (Phospholine), physostigmine (Eserine sulfate ophthalmic)	Reduce aqueous humor production	Taste disturbance, less likely to induce systemic side effects, but may occur; caution in patients with nephrolithiasis, diabetes mellitus, hepatic disease, and history of sulfonamide sensitivity
Alpha-Adrenergic Agonists		
Epinephrine and dipivefrin (Propine), apraclonidine (Iopidine), brimonidine (Alphagan P)	Inhibit aqueous humor production	Eye irritation, hypotension, vasovagal attack; avoid in patients with grade 2 or 3 heart block, congestive heart failure, chronic obstructive pulmonary disease, asthma, or pulmonary edema
Systemic Medications		
Acetazolamide (Diamox), dichlorphenamide (Keveyis), methazolamide (Neptazane)	Reduce production of aqueous humor.	Acidosis, numbness, lethargy, renal stones, cramps, taste disturbance

laser therapy may only last a few years, and occasionally, the procedure may have to be repeated.

In acute angle-closure glaucoma, medications are administered during the acute attack to rapidly lower IOP. Acetazolamide (Diamox) and IV mannitol with a topical miotic, such as pilocarpine, may be administered, followed by a more definitive laser peripheral iridotomy to create an alternate pathway for aqueous to flow into the anterior chamber. Bedrest should be maintained until the attack is broken.

FOLLOW-UP AND REFERRAL

Patients with glaucoma should be referred to and followed by an ophthalmologist. Nonetheless, as the primary care provider, the clinician needs to understand what medications the patient is receiving, as well as how often the patient should be monitored by an ophthalmologist. The clinician needs to be alert to possible signs and symptoms of exacerbation. There is always potential for loss of vision and blindness if acute glaucoma attacks are not treated promptly and consistently.

Patient Education: Glaucoma

Careful and lifelong follow-up is essential for patients with glaucoma, specifically periodic checks of IOP and eye examinations. Patients with glaucoma should understand the importance of medication compliance, potential adverse effects of medications, and changes in vision that warrant a call to their health-care provider. The clinician may need to teach the patient how best to instill the eyedrops. If vision is severely compromised, a caregiver will need to be taught as well. In addition, the knowledge that certain medications, such as systemic corticosteroids, may interfere with glaucoma control is essential. Support and counseling may also be necessary.

DIABETIC RETINOPATHY

Diabetic retinopathy is a noninflammatory disorder of the retina that develops in patients with diabetes mellitus (see Table 20.1). It is typically divided into nonproliferative diabetic retinopathy (NPDR) and proliferative diabetic retinopathy (PDR). The initial evaluation for a patient with diabetes mellitus should include a referral to an ophthalmologist for a comprehensive eye evaluation, with particular attention to the aspects relevant to diabetic retinopathy.

EPIDEMIOLOGY AND CAUSES

Diabetes mellitus is a fast-growing epidemic that is predicted to affect 642 million people in the United States by the year 2040. Approximately one-third of patients with diabetes mellitus will develop some form of diabetic retinopathy, which accounts for approximately 10% of new cases of blindness each year. Diabetic retinopathy is the leading cause of blindness among Americans aged 20 to 64 years.

The peak incidence of type 1 (autoimmune) diabetes mellitus is between the ages of 12 and 15 years; the peak incidence of type 2 diabetes mellitus is between the ages of 50 and 70 years. Diabetes mellitus type 1 occurs about equally in males and females, whereas type 2 is more common in females. The longer a patient has had diabetes mellitus, the greater the likelihood that they will develop retinopathy. An important epidemiological finding of the Wisconsin Epidemiological Study of Diabetic Retinopathy helped establish this direct association between duration of diabetes mellitus and prevalence of diabetic retinopathy. The study found that nearly 99% of patients with type 1 and 60% with type 2 diabetes mellitus developed NPDR after having the disease for 20 years. PDR was seen in about 50% of type 1 patients and 25% of type 2 patients after 25 years' duration. Contributing factors to diabetic retinopathy include poor glycemic control, pregnancy, renal disease, systemic hypertension, smoking, and elevated serum lipid levels. *Healthy People 2030* has an objective to increase the percentage of people older than 18 years with diabetes to have an annual eye examination from 62.3% to 67.7%.

PATHOPHYSIOLOGY

The key insult driving diabetic retinopathy is uncontrolled hyperglycemia. The precise mechanism by which this causes retinal damage is unclear, but there are several prevailing hypotheses that likely contribute to varying degrees. Prolonged exposure to hyperglycemia creates biochemical pathway changes, leading to an increase in glycation end products, protein kinase C pathways, and oxidative stress. Ultimately, the result of this is damage to endothelial cells and eventual pericyte loss. In addition, hematological abnormalities can contribute to the formation and progression of retinopathy, these abnormalities include increased platelet adhesion and erythrocyte aggregation.

In the case of NPDR, retinal pericytes and the microvascular endothelium are damaged early in the disease process, leading to vascular permeability and basement membrane thickening (similar to the histopathological changes seen in diabetic nephropathy). This predisposes retinal capillaries to microaneurysms and the retinal surface to thickening with deposits of proteinaceous and lipid material (hard exudates). If the macula is affected (i.e., macular edema occurs), vision may gradually blur and progress to profound visual loss if left untreated. Continued exposure to hyperglycemia leads to multiple cycles of cellular death and renewal, leading to venous beading, tortuous venous dilation, and intraluminal cellular proliferation, along with platelet, erythrocyte, and fibrinogen aggregation, which ultimately results in vascular occlusion. Upstream of such lesions, flame-shaped and blot hemorrhages occur; downstream, microvascular infarcts present as "cotton wool spots" or soft exudates on fundoscopy. Finally, the proliferative phase is characterized by neovascularization due to release of vascular endothelial growth factor (VEGF), which is produced by ischemic retinal tissue. This leads to neovascularization on the retinal surface, optic nerve, and iris. These fragile vessels may be venous or arterial in origin and may extend into the vitreous chamber, attaching to the posterior pole of the vitreous in a fine fibrous mesh. This network places stress on the retinal surface as the fibers contract. As a result, hemorrhage into the vitreous body and even retinal detachment may occur, requiring both vitrectomy and laser photocoagulation.

CLINICAL PRESENTATION

Subjective

The patient will complain of visual changes as the disease progresses, but it is usually asymptomatic in the early stages. In time, the patient will typically complain of progressive, painless visual loss.

Objective

Changes will be noted on fundoscopic examination. NPDR, microaneurysms, intraretinal hemorrhage, macular edema, and lipid deposits may be apparent. As the disease progresses, nerve fiber layer infarctions ("cotton wool spots"), venous beading and dilation, edema, and, in some cases, extensive retinal hemorrhage will be noted. The proliferative form of diabetic retinopathy is characterized by neovascularization, which may be seen on the retinal surface, optic nerve, and iris.

DIAGNOSTIC REASONING

Diagnostic Tests

A thorough eye examination should be done, including an assessment of visual acuity and documentation of the status of the iris, lens, vitreous, and fundus. Fluorescein angiography is an important imaging study that can help demonstrate retinal nonperfusion, retinal leakage, and proliferative diabetic retinopathy.

Differential Diagnosis

A history of diabetes mellitus, especially if present for more than 10 years, correlated with observable changes on fundoscopic examination, establishes the diagnosis of diabetic retinopathy. Other causes of retinopathy include hypertensive retinopathy, radiation retinopathy, and retinal venous obstruction.

MANAGEMENT

The first goal for patients at risk for microvascular complications, including diabetic retinopathy, is prevention. The most important preventive measure is tight blood sugar control. The American Diabetes Association sets an acceptable level of glycated hemoglobin or HgbA1c at less than 7%. In patients who have their blood sugar under adequate control, the incidence of diabetic retinopathy is far lower, and the onset in those who do develop this disease occurs later. All patients diagnosed with diabetes mellitus must be referred to ophthalmology upon diagnosis and are typically followed with yearly examinations.

Similarly, patients with diabetes mellitus and hypertension should strive to maintain as normal a blood pressure as possible to prevent the development of end-organ damage. Because many patients have both disorders, vigilance is especially important in this subset of patients. Angiotensin-converting enzyme inhibitors, such as lisinopril, are often used to both lower blood pressure and limit microvascular disease in diabetics.

Laser photocoagulation is recommended for patients with proliferative diabetic retinopathy and for patients with clinically significant macular edema. Patients with diabetic retinopathy should be followed by an ophthalmologist, who can decide when to treat the disorder with laser treatment (focal and panretinal photocoagulation). In certain cases, intravitreal anti-VEGF therapy can be used to decrease the neovascular stimulus and treat proliferative diabetic retinopathy and associated macular edema. Vitrectomy may be considered for patients with severe proliferative diabetic retinopathy, traction retinal detachment involving the macula, and nonclearing vitreous hemorrhage.

FOLLOW-UP AND REFERRAL

All patients with diabetes mellitus should be monitored annually by an ophthalmologist. Patients with NPDR should be followed at least yearly and patients with PDR should be seen at least every 3 to 4 months. Patients with concomitant PDR and center-involving macular edema (i.e., in which the center of the macula is affected) should be seen approximately every 4 weeks.

Glaucoma, cataracts, retinal detachment, vitreous hemorrhage, and disc edema can be seen in patients with diabetic retinopathy, even in its early stages. Cataracts especially are common in patients with diabetes mellitus. If the patient has both cataracts and significant retinopathy, delaying cataract surgery may be a consideration, as cataract surgery can sometimes worsen diabetic retinopathy.

Patient Education: Diabetic Retinopathy

Patients with diabetes mellitus, as well as those with hypertension, need to be educated regarding the need to keep their disease under optimal control to decrease the incidence of complications. Creating an alliance with the patient and family is essential in encouraging lifestyle changes. Working with the patient over time and supporting the patient are essential. Patients should be educated about the importance of ophthalmological evaluation and follow-up. Patience, advocacy, and commitment are all important qualities in working with these patients. Optimism and emphasis on the possibility for change, even if just to prevent further disease progression, are essential characteristics.

MACULAR DEGENERATION

Macular degeneration is a progressive disease of aging and is the leading cause of blindness in patients older than 50 years (see Table 20.1). Risk factors associated with macular degeneration appear in the following bulleted list.

Risk Factors: Macular Degeneration

- Caucasian
- Female gender
- Age older than 60 years
- Cigarette smoking
- Family history

Macular degeneration gene (complement factor H polymorphism)

Other risk factors that are unproven but documented in some studies include:

- High serum cholesterol/obesity
- Low serum carotenoid levels
- Exposure to ultraviolet light
- Hypertension
- Light-colored eyes
- Farsightedness
- Past cataract surgery

Age-related macular degeneration (AMD) is a condition characterized by slow, progressive atrophy and degeneration of the retina. This condition is known as nonexudative or "dry" macular degeneration. In North America, it is estimated that "dry" AMD accounts for 85% to 90% of all cases of AMD. Occasionally, new blood vessels develop under the retina in the macula, causing a sudden distortion or loss of central vision. This condition is known as exudative or "wet" AMD; it typically presents as a sudden decrease in vision that requires immediate referral to an ophthalmologist. "Wet" AMD accounts for approximately 10% to 15% of all cases of AMD in North America. There is often a progression from "dry" to "wet" macular degeneration.

EPIDEMIOLOGY AND CAUSES

The macula is the most sensitive central portion of the retina, a nerve-rich area essential for sight. For poorly understood reasons, the macula can break down with age. As the macula degenerates, central vision and fine detail perception deteriorate. Patients typically cannot read well (if at all), see facial details, or perform ordinary daily visual activities.

A recent study reported that 30% of individuals aged 75 years and older have some form of AMD, and 7% of those aged 75 years and older have an advanced form. Recent studies estimate that 8 million Americans are at risk for developing advanced AMD in the next 5 years, and 1.75 million are currently affected with the advanced form of the disease. AMD is the leading cause of blindness in the developed world in people older than 50 years. *Healthy People 2030* has an objective to decrease the number of adults older than 45 years having visual impairment due to AMD by getting dilated eye examinations from 15.6 per 1,000 adults to 12.5 per 1,000 adults.

PATHOPHYSIOLOGY

Normal aging results in a variety of changes in the macula, many of which are clinically undetectable. These changes include decreased photoreceptor density, atrophy of the retinal pigment epithelium (RPE), and lipid deposits between the RPE and a collagenous layer called Bruch's membrane. These changes may or may not be a part of AMD. The defining lesions of dry AMD are drusen, which are small, yellow, round lesions deposited in Bruch's membrane, just underneath the RPE. The deposition of drusen affects the overlying photoreceptors of the retina, causing mild to moderate vision loss, decreased contrast sensitivity, and impaired color vision. Neovascular, or wet AMD, is defined by the presence of choroidal neovascularization. The accumulation of drusen in Bruch's membrane, which characterizes dry AMD, stimulates neovascularization to develop. The new vessels may leak and disrupt the normal structure of the RPE-photoreceptor complex, leading to a more rapid form of vision loss.

Research has provided a few genetic-based clues to the pathogenesis of AMD, which suggests the interplay between genetic predisposition and other risk factors inducing inflammatory dysfunction. Growth factor, choriocapillary endothelial damage, and inflammatory cytokines are likely involved. More recently, genetic research has identified two major susceptibility genes, *CFH* and *ARMS2*. *CFH* codes for complement factor H on chromosome 1, which is strongly associated with AMD. The *CFH* mutation confers a 4.6-fold increased risk for AMD when heterozygous and a 7.4-fold increase when homozygous. The gene product and function of *ARMS2* is poorly understood. Genetic testing is available for AMD, but the usefulness of these results is controversial, as poor lifestyle choices increase AMD risk regardless of genetic predisposition.

CLINICAL PRESENTATION

Subjective

The clinician's main task is to determine whether the problem is acute and requires referral for immediate treatment or is more routine. Establishing whether the onset of the visual impairment is acute or gradual will assist the clinician in making this determination. Likewise, the severity of the vision loss is also important. Severe and sudden vision loss requires immediate referral to an ophthalmologist.

Objective

First, visual acuity must be evaluated, with the patient wearing any assistive lenses. If vision is less than 20/20, it should be checked by the pinhole test. Vision that corrects with the pinhole test implies an uncorrected refractive error. The clinician should then evaluate the external structure of the eye. The lids, conjunctivae, pupils, and extraocular movements should be checked. The use of an Amsler grid can be helpful to clue clinicians into AMD, but the best way to diagnose AMD is by visualizing the retina during a dilated eye examination. Drusen on the macula may be indicative of early macular degeneration. Clumps of pigment irregularly interspersed with depigmented areas of atrophy in the macula are more typical of a later phase of the disorder.

DIAGNOSTIC REASONING

Diagnostic Tests

Analysis of central vision may be done with an Amsler grid to locate macular blind spots and metamorphopsia. Often, patients will be sent home with an Amsler grid to self-monitor their visual changes. The test card contains white grid lines on a black background with a central dot for fixation and can be a helpful indicator of worsening macular degeneration. Measurement of contrast sensitivity with specially designed tests for low vision may reveal the degree of loss of retinal sensitivity to contrast and predict the potential success or failure of optical magnifying devices.

Differential Diagnosis

Visual impairment may be associated with a variety of conditions. The task of the clinician is to know when to refer for ophthalmological evaluation and treatment, versus which conditions can be treated in primary care. The characteristics of the associated symptoms and physical findings in the problem of visual loss require focused history and excellent physical examination skills. A recent study of primary care providers found that approximately 25% of eyes deemed to be normal based on dilated eye examination by primary eye care physicians had macular characteristics that indicated AMD revealed by fundus photography and trained raters. A total of 30% of eyes with undiagnosed AMD had AMD with large drusen that would have been treatable with nutritional supplements had it been diagnosed. Thus improved AMD detection strategies may be needed in primary eye care.

Other differential diagnoses may include vitreous hemorrhage, retinal detachment, uveitis, retrobulbar optic neuritis, and vascular occlusion, which present with severe and sudden vision loss. A gradual progression suggests a changing refractive error, cataract, glaucoma, diabetic retinopathy, or macular degeneration.

MANAGEMENT

Although there are no proven cures for AMD, there are various epidemiological studies that have shown a positive association between micronutrient intake and a decreased risk of AMD. The Age-Related Eye Disease Study (AREDS) was the first that established this link. Vitamins and supplements specifically used in this study included vitamins C and E, beta-carotene, zinc, and copper. Patients with intermediate AMD having taken these supplements showed a 25% risk reduction for progression to advanced AMD. It is strongly important for people who currently smoke to avoid high-dose beta-carotene due to an increased risk of lung cancer. Follow-up studies showed that replacing beta-carotene with lutein and zeaxanthin had similar effects on AMD progression without the increased risk of lung cancer in people who smoke.

Thermal laser photocoagulation may be used to treat certain forms of wet AMD. However, its use is of limited value due to poor outcomes and increased risk of disease recurrence. Wet AMD is commonly treated with injections directly into the eye (intravitreal) by a retinal specialist or ophthalmologist (see Drugs Commonly Prescribed 20.2). The medication injected belongs to a class of drugs called anti-VEGF therapies. These drugs reduce the growth of abnormal blood vessels and may slow leakage from blood vessels. The ideal treatment time frame with anti-VEGF has not been well established, but it is frequently given monthly or prn for specific patients. Large-scale clinical trials have demonstrated that these drugs preserved and even improved visual acuity. There are four drugs in this class: the monoclonal antibodies ranibizumab (Lucentis) and bevacizumab (Avastin), the nucleic acid VEGF inhibitor pegaptanib (Macugen), and the receptor fusion protein aflibercept (Eylea). As the number of cases increases with the growing aging population, strategies that incorporate cost-effective methods may include treatments provided by specialized nurse practitioners.

Several clinical trials are also investigating potential alternative treatments for AMD, such as submacular surgery, photodynamic therapy, and irradiation. Antioxidants and other plant chemicals (phytochemicals) have been shown to protect against the development of macular degeneration.

FOLLOW-UP AND REFERRAL

The patient should be referred to a rehabilitation service where the prognosis of the disease can be evaluated. In patients with advanced macular degeneration, daily living needs should be assessed and visual aids offered. Rehabilitation services may be sourced from ophthalmologists who provide low-vision services in their practices; optometrists who are trained to offer low-vision remediation; agencies for the visually impaired (either private or state supported); institutions that offer services for veterans; and organizations such as the American Academy of Ophthalmology, the American Optometric Association, the National Eye Institute, and Lighthouse Guild. A team approach is useful in rehabilitation, and the primary care provider is part of the team. Because the loss of vision can be especially debilitating, quality of life needs to be assessed during routine primary care visits.

Drugs Commonly Prescribed 20.2: Wet Acute Macular Degeneration

DRUG	INDICATION	DOSAGE	ADVERSE EFFECTS
Vascular Endothelial Growth Factor (VEGF)-Receptor Fusion Protein			
Aflibercept (Eylea)	Wet AMD (FDA-approved)	2-mg intravitreal injection once a month for 3 months, then every 2 months	Conjunctival hemorrhage, eye pain, cataract, vitreous detachment, vitreous floaters, increased IOP, allergic reactions (including hives, difficulty breathing, and facial swelling), retinal detachment, endophthalmitis
Anti-VEGF Monoclonal Antibody			
Ranibizumab (Lucentis)	Wet AMD (FDA approved)	0.5-mg intravitreal injection every month	Conjunctival hemorrhage, eye pain, vitreous floaters, increased IOP, hypersensitivity (severe ocular inflammation), retinal detachment, endophthalmitis
Bevacizumab (Avastin)	Wet AMD (unapproved)	1.25-mg intravitreal injection once a month (off-label use)	Eye pain, eye redness, sudden vision changes with flashes of light, photophobia, lacrimation disorder, severe headache with confusion, epistaxis, hypertension, rhinitis, proteinuria, taste alteration, dry skin, rectal hemorrhage, exfoliative dermatitis
Nucleic Acid VEGF Inhibitor			
Pegaptanib (Macugen)	Wet AMD (FDA approved)	0.3-mg intravitreal injection every 6 weeks	Watery eyes, blurred vision, visual disturbance, vitreous floaters, eye pain, cataract, conjunctival hemorrhage, eyelid and corneal edema, increased IOP, anterior chamber inflammation, hypertension, increased IOP, punctate keratitis, endophthalmitis, anaphylaxis

Abbreviations: AMD, age-related macular degeneration; FDA, U.S. Food and Drug Administration; IOP, intraocular pressure.

Vision loss increases the risk of falls and may limit the patient's ability to live independently. Depression rates are high in cases of vision loss, and screening in primary care settings for signs of depression is important. A psychosocial assessment with a multidisciplinary team should be arranged to explore resources and monitor quality of life.

Nursing Situation: Living With Severe Visual Impairment

Mr. Nesbitt is a 78-year-old widower who has been in your practice for 15 years. You have managed his hypertension and mild congestive heart failure for the past 5 years, and he has been following all your advice, including walking 1 mile every day, weather permitting. He was recently diagnosed with AMD, and his visual loss has been progressive. He has always been very active in community events since the death of his wife and spends several hours each day at the local senior center where he entertains the other seniors by playing the piano during lunchtime. He usually drives himself the 2 miles across town to the center and has been doing all of his own grocery shopping, cooking, and tending to his house and yard. He has a large garden and shares his produce with his neighbors. He tearfully admits that his children have been after him to stop driving, give up his home, and move to an assisted living facility. He says he has not had any accidents and that he stays close to the centerline when he drives and knows the route by heart. "I could get there blindfolded," he jokingly remarks. As to moving he says, "Why would I do that? I know where everything is, and I haven't had any problems. My kids can help me. If they put me in a home, I might as well be dead."

Mr. Nesbitt has two sons aged 50 and 49 years. Both of these men have jobs that take them out of town a good portion of the week. Both work in the family business started by their father. One son is divorced with two teenage boys, and the other is married with four children and one grandchild. This past week, both sons called asking you to bring Mr. Nesbitt to his senses and to take away his car keys, relating that he has had two near-misses in the past 2 weeks. They say that he refuses to listen to reason and that his explanation for the near-misses is that he "got distracted by a pedestrian jaywalking and by a school bus."

Some of the issues described in this Nursing Situation were addressed in a small study that focused on older men's experiences of living with severe visual impairment. In this study, a phenomenological approach was used to investigate the experience of severe visual impairment in eight older men with macular degeneration.

Six central themes emerged: (1) abilities and inabilities, (2) cherishing of independence, (3) creating strategies, (4) acknowledging the progression of visual impairment, (5) confronting uncertainties and fears, and (6) persisting with hope and optimism.

One interesting finding in this study was that the theme of uncertainty encompassed skepticism about their diagnosis and treatment. Acceptance of the fact that there is no successful treatment for AMD is hard for most individuals, and persisting with hope and optimism needs to be supported in the face of severe progressive visual loss and mistrust of how their case is managed. A recent study conducted patient interviews that revealed insights into nursing actions that created a sense of good nursing care in patients with wet AMD. Nurses acknowledged people as individuals and created trust by building partnerships and sharing decision making. To address each patient's concerns, nurses need to prioritize patients' narratives and participation by documenting agreements in their medical record.

A 2015 study investigated caregivers of those with advanced AMD. A high prevalence of caregiver distress related to caring for people with advanced AMD was observed. Level of dependence on the caregiver and presence of comorbid chronic illnesses were independent predictors of the caregiver's experiencing psychological distress. More than one in two caregivers reported a negative state of mind.

Patient Education: Age-Related Macular Degeneration

Recognition of the signs of advanced AMD is crucial for the success of treatment in preventing visual loss. Self-monitoring of central vision in both eyes, using an Amsler grid, may be useful in detecting subtle visual changes or distortion, as well as for monitoring changes in vision once they have been detected. A hallmark of AMD is visual difficulties in low light.

Smoking cessation and improvement of cardiovascular risk factors, such as blood pressure and obesity, are important variables in the progression of AMD. Patients should be instructed about rehabilitation resources in the community and encouraged to take advantage of programs specifically targeting AMD.

Optical aids include spectacles with and without prisms, hand magnifiers, stand-mounted magnifiers, and telescopes. As with any type of rehabilitation, time and patience are needed to determine the appropriate remedial lens for the patient. Working with the patient until they understand how to use these devices is an important part of patient education. In addition, patients may be taught skills such as folding money in such a way that the denomination is more apparent, as well as techniques for grooming and for identifying medications. The goal is to use "practical approaches tailored to the individual's specific needs" (see The Patient's Voice 20.1).

The Patient's Voice 20.1: Macular Degeneration

My mother, who is 78 years old, called me in a panic because she could not see out of one eye. The ophthalmologist agreed to see her right away. When we met with the doctor after her examination, he told us that she had been diagnosed with macular degeneration 4 years ago. She had never told a soul! "I couldn't stand the thought of being a burden." That's what she told me. If only I'd known, maybe we could have done more to slow down the disease. Now, if anything happens to her other eye, I don't know what we'll do. This will change everything about how my mother lives and will affect everyone in the family.

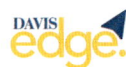 Go to Davis Edge for practice Q&A.

REFERENCES

General

Bostock-Cox B. Red flag eye conditions: A guide for the practice nurse. *Practice Nurse.* 2017;47(2):28–32.

Final Recommendation Statement: Impaired visual acuity in older adults: screening. Rockville, MD: Agency for Healthcare Research and Quality; March 1, 2016. https://www.uspreventiveservicestaskforce.org/uspstf/announcements/final-recommendation-statement-screening-impaired-visual-acuity-older-adults. Accessed 4/29/2021.

Healthy People 2030. https://health.gov/healthypeople/objectives-and-data/browse-objectives. Accessed 4/29/2021.

Patel SP. (2016). Top 10 Eye Emergencies. American Academy of Ophthalmology. https://www.aao.org/young-ophthalmologists/yo-info/article/top-10-eye-emergencies. Accessed 4/29/21.

Cataracts

American Academy of Ophthalmology Cataract and Anterior Segment Panel, Hoskins Center for Quality Eye Care. Preferred Practice Pattern® Guidelines. *Cataract in the Adult Eye.* American Academy of Ophthalmology; 2016. https://www.aao.org/preferred-practice-pattern/cataract-in-adult-eye. Accessed 4/29/2021.

Brar VS. 2020-2021. *Basic and Clinical Science Course (BCSC), Section 2 Fundamentals and Principles of Ophthalmology.* Amer Academy of Ophthalmo, 2020.

Goh JHL, Lim ZW, Fang X, et al (2020). Artificial Intelligence for Cataract Detection and Management. *Asia-Pacific Journal of Ophthalmology* 2020 Mar-Apr;9(2): https://journals.lww.com/apjoo/Fulltext/2020/04000/Artificial_Intelligence_for_Cataract_Detection_and.6.aspx. Accessed 4/29/2021.

Juthani VV, Clearfield E, Chuck RS. Non-steroidal anti-inflammatory drugs versus corticosteroids for controlling inflammation after uncomplicated cataract surgery. *Cochrane Database Syst Rev* 2017;7:CD010516. Accessed 4/29/2021.

Keel S, He M (2018). Risk Factors for age-related cataract. Clin Exp Ophthalmol 2018 May;46(4):327-328. https://pubmed.ncbi.nlm.nih.gov/29898261/. Accessed 4/29/2021.

Kessel L, Andresen J, Erngaard D, et al. Indication for cataract surgery. Do we have evidence of who will benefit from surgery? A systematic review and meta-analysis. *Acta Ophthalmol.* 2016;94:10–20. https://reference.medscape.com/medline/abstract/26036605. Accessed 4/29/2021.

Olson RJ, Braga-Mele R, Huang Chen S, et al. Cataract in the adult eye preferred practice pattern®. *Ophthalmology.* 2017;124(2): P1–P119.

Diabetic Retinopathy

Centers for Disease Control and Prevention. (2019). *Diabetes Report Card 2019.* Atlanta, GA: Centers for Disease Control and Prevention, US Dept of Health and Human Services. https://www.cdc.gov/diabetes/pdfs/library/Diabetes-Report-Card-2019-508.pdf. Accessed 4/30/2021.

Flaxel CJ, Adelman RA, Bailey ST, et al. (2020). Diabetic retinopathy preferred practice pattern. *Ophthalmology* 127(1). 66-145.Jan 1, 2020.

McCannel CA. *2020-2021 Basic and Clinical Science Course (BCSC), Section 12 Retina and Vitreous.* Amer Academy of Ophthalmo, 2020.

Solomon SD, Chew E, Duh EJ, et al. Diabetic retinopathy: A position statement by the American Diabetes Association. *Diabetes Care.* 2017;40(9):412–418. https://care.diabetesjournals.org/content/40/3/412. Accessed 4/30/2021.

Glaucoma

Primary Open-Angle Glaucoma Suspect PPP 2020. AAO PPP glaucoma Committee, Hoskins Center for Quality Eye Care. https://www.aao.org/preferred-practice-pattern/primary-open-angle-glaucoma-suspect-ppp. Accessed 4/29/2021.

Glaucoma: Facts & Figures. BrightFocus Foundation. https://www.brightfocus.org/glaucoma/article/glaucoma-facts-figures#:~:text=Glaucoma%20is%20a%20leading%20cause%20of%20irreversible%20blindness,affects%203.3%20million%20Americans%20age%2040%20and%20over. Accessed 4/29/2021.

Netland PA, Tanna AP, eds. *Glaucoma medical therapy: principles and management.* 3rd ed. Kugler; 2020.

Tanna AP. (2020). 2020-2021 Basic and Clinical Science Course (BCSC), Section 10 Glaucoma. Amer Academy of Ophthalmo. Accessed 4/30/2021.

U.S. Preventive Services Task Force. (2020). Impaired visual acuity and glaucoma in adults: Screening. Accessed 4/30/2021.

Macular Degeneration

American Academy of Ophthalmology. Retina/vitreous panel. (2019). Age-related macular degeneration. Preferred Practice Pattern® Guidelines. San Francisco, CA: American Academy of Ophthalmology. https://www.aao.org/preferred-practice-pattern/age-related-macular-degeneration-ppp. Accessed 4/30/2021.

Emsfors Å, Christensson L, Elgán C. Nursing actions that create a sense of good nursing care in patients with wet age-related macular degeneration. *J Clin Nurs.* 2017;26(17/18):2680–2688.

Rojas-Fernandez CH, Tyber K. Benefits, potential harms, and optimal use of nutritional supplementation for preventing progression of age-related macular degeneration. *Ann Pharmacother.* 2017;51(3):264–270. https://pubmed.ncbi.nlm.nih.gov/27866147/. Accessed 4/30/2021.

Refractive Errors

Chou R, Dana T, Bougatsos C, et al. Screening for impaired visual acuity in older adults: Updated evidence report and systematic review for the US Preventive Services Task Force. *JAMA.* 2016;315(9):915–933.

World Health Organization. (2007). Vision 2030 the right to sight: Global initiative for the elimination of avoidable blindness. Accessed 4/20/2021.

Causes of blindness and vision impairment in 2020 and trends over 30 years, and prevalence of avoidable blindness in relation to VISION 2020: the Right to Sight: an analysis for the Global Burden of Disease Study. *Lancet Glob Health.* Published Online December 1, 2020 https://doi.org/10.1016/S2214-109X(20)30489-7

National Eye Institute. (n.d.). Glaucoma resources. Retrieved from https://www.nei.nih.gov/learn-about-eye-health/resources-for-health-educators/glaucoma-resources

RESOURCES

American Diabetes Association—Retinopathy
http://www.diabetesforecast.org/diabetes-101/retinopathy-eye-disease

American Macular Degeneration Foundation
https://www.macular.org

Cleveland Clinic
https://my.clevelandclinic.org/health/articles/age-related-macular-degeneration

Glaucoma Research Foundation
http://www.glaucoma.org/

National Eye Institute

Age-Related Macular Degeneration
https://nei.nih.gov/health/maculardegen/armd_facts

Cataracts
https://nei.nih.gov/health/cataract

Diabetic Eye Disease
https://www.nei.nih.gov/learn-about-eye-health/resources-for-health-educators/diabetic-eye-disease-resources

Glaucoma
https://nei.nih.gov/health/glaucoma/

Refractive Errors
https://nei.nih.gov/sites/default/files/health-pdfs/Refractiveerrors.pdf

Section 4 — EAR, NOSE, AND THROAT PROBLEMS

SECTION EDITOR
Michael E. Zychowicz, DNP, ANP, ONP, FAAN, FAANP

Chapter 21

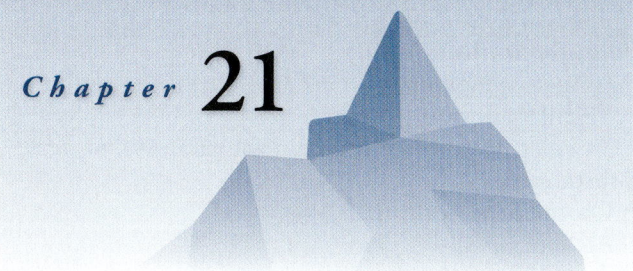

Common Ear, Nose, and Throat Complaints

Maria Colandrea, DNP, NP-C, CORLN, CCRN, FAANP
Michael E. Zychowicz, DNP, ANP, ONP, FAAN, FAANP
Brian Oscar Porter, MD, PhD, MPH, MBA

EAR PAIN (OTALGIA)

Ear pain, known as *otalgia,* is a common clinical complaint. Two separate and distinct types of otalgia exist. Pain that originates within the ear is primary otalgia; pain that originates outside the ear is secondary otalgia. Primary otalgia is typically caused by otitis externa, otitis media, mastoiditis, or auricular infections. When ear pain is accompanied by edema, erythema, otorrhea, fluid or purulence behind the tympanic membrane, or tympanic membrane perforation, simply looking in the ear and observing the pathology can make the diagnosis. When the ear canal and tympanic membrane appear normal, however, the diagnosis becomes more difficult. Otalgia may also be referred from other locations (secondary otalgia). Although many conditions can cause referred otalgia, their relationship to ear pain must be identified. Causes of referred ear pain include dental abscesses, sinus infections, temporomandibular joint disorder, head and neck cancer, and mastoiditis.

Otalgia can be bilateral or localized to one ear. Ear pain may become more prevalent in the summer months due to an increase in cases of otitis externa (swimmer's ear) or sinus infections, which can be more common during peak allergen season. Ear pain associated with acute and chronic otitis media is frequently associated with eustachian tube dysfunction that leads to signs and symptoms of pressure dysregulation in the middle ear, a condition seen especially in the pediatric population. Head and neck cancers can present with unilateral otalgia and chronic unilateral otitis media, along with weight loss and a constellation of other symptoms.

DIFFERENTIAL DIAGNOSIS

The differential diagnosis of ear pain includes the following disorders:
Primary causes of otalgia
- Otitis externa
- Acute otitis media
- Otitis media with effusion
- Eustachian tube dysfunction
- Barotrauma (pressure changes in the immediate atmosphere, such as when flying)
- Cerumen impaction
- Perforated tympanic membrane

Secondary causes of otalgia
- Dental disease
- Temporomandibular joint disorder
- Sinus disease
- Head and neck cancer
- Pharyngitis or tonsillitis
- Cervical lymphadenopathy
- Cervicalgia

IMPAIRED HEARING

Hearing loss is the decreased ability or inability to hear, which may be temporary or permanent. It may involve the middle ear, which indicates a mechanical (conductive) problem, or the inner ear, which indicates a nerve-related (sensorineural) problem. In fact, hearing loss may have both conductive and sensorineural components.

Cerumen, which can impair the effective conduction of sound waves to the middle ear, is the most common cause of reversible hearing loss. However, hearing loss is also a universal phenomenon of aging and exposure to prolonged loud noise, with an increased incidence seen in individuals with a family history of hearing loss. In particular, sensorineural hearing loss increases with age, with degenerative decline starting at age 20 years, without regard to ethnicity or gender.

DIFFERENTIAL DIAGNOSIS

The differential diagnosis of hearing loss includes the following disorders:

- Presbycusis
- Noise exposure
- Ototoxicity from medications
- Eustachian tube dysfunction
- Cerumen impaction
- Otitis externa
- Chronic middle ear infection, effusion
- Otosclerosis
- Tympanosclerosis
- Cholesteatoma
- Trauma
- Congenital disorders
- Sudden sensorineural hearing loss

TINNITUS

Tinnitus is the perception of sound in the ear, most often a buzzing or ringing. It is a symptom, not a disease. Tinnitus is most commonly caused by changes in peripheral auditory function; however, about 10% of patients with tinnitus have normal hearing. Tinnitus is characterized as subjective and objective tinnitus. Subjective tinnitus is perceivable only by the patient, whereas objective tinnitus, most commonly caused by vascular problems, is audible by the observer as well as the patient.

Tinnitus has been described in many ways, including as the sound of escaping air or running water; the sound heard inside a large seashell; and as a buzzing, ringing, or humming noise. Tinnitus has also been described as a roaring or musical sound. It may be intermittent or continuous and can occur in one or both ears. Tinnitus can also be described as pulsatile (i.e., synchronous with the heartbeat), which requires a work-up to evaluate for vascular causes. Tinnitus can be a minor irritation for some patients or a debilitating condition for others. It can be caused by different diseases or drug toxicities, and the underlying cause should be addressed to effectively reduce the tinnitus.

DIFFERENTIAL DIAGNOSIS

The differential diagnosis of tinnitus includes the following disorders:

Otological
- Hearing loss
- Ménière's disease
- Acoustic neuroma

Neurological
- Multiple sclerosis
- Head injury

Metabolic
- Thyroid disorder
- Hyperlipidemia
- Vitamin B_{12} deficiency

Psychogenic
- Depression
- Anxiety
- Fibromyalgia

Pulsatile tinnitus
- Vascular neoplasm
- Vascular anomaly
- Vascular malformation within the ear, head, or neck

Substances
- Ototoxic medications
- Alcohol

Other
- Temporomandibular joint disorder
- Arthritis of the neck
- Myoclonus

MOUTH SORES

Acute oral mucosal lesions are commonly observed in primary care settings. Although the mouth may be thought of primarily as a receptacle for food and a vehicle for speech, several anatomical structures within the oral cavity may be the focuses of disease. The oral cavity is lined by the buccal mucosa, which is rich in mucous glands. The mucous glands of the lips open into the oral cavity, and the mouth cavity communicates with the pharynx posteriorly. The floor of the mouth contains the tongue and the openings of the submandibular and sublingual salivary glands.

Specific lesions of the oral, posterior pharyngeal, and buccal mucosa may be immunogenic or inflammatory (most commonly aphthous ulcers) in etiology, trauma related, or caused by an underlying malignancy. Painful inflammatory lesions may occur in isolation, or they may be associated with a generalized disorder of other mucous membranes or the skin. The patient's medical history is important because it indicates whether the lesions are acute or chronic, single or multiple, and primary or recurrent.

DIFFERENTIAL DIAGNOSIS

The differential diagnosis of mouth sores includes the following:

- Food or drug allergies
- Chemical irritation
- Dry mouth
- Mechanical or thermal injury, such as braces or dentures
- Infections (e.g., bacterial, viral, fungal)

- Host immunosuppression
- Nutritional deficiency
- Stomatitis
- Inflammatory bowel diseases (e.g., Crohn's disease, ulcerative colitis)
- Mucocele
- Benign inflammatory lesions
- Premalignant or malignant lesions of the mouth, tongue, or posterior pharynx

HOARSENESS

Hoarseness, also known as *dysphonia,* is a common complaint, suggesting an abnormality in voice production at the level of the larynx. Dysphonia can affect patients of all ages with a higher incidence in the pediatric and older adult populations. Dysphonia is common in professionals such as singers, teachers, clergy, telemarketers, drill sergeants, and others with high vocal demands. Age-related changes in voice are natural and can be expected. However, hoarseness can also be a sign of laryngeal cancers, so screening should be considered for patients most at risk.

DIFFERENTIAL DIAGNOSIS

The differential diagnosis of hoarseness includes the following disorders:

Inflammation/irritation/trauma
- Infections (e.g., viral upper respiratory infection [URI], fungal laryngitis, sinusitis)
- Allergic rhinitis
- Throat irritants (e.g., tobacco, alcohol, environmental irritants)
- Laryngopharyngeal reflux
- Direct trauma (e.g., intubation)

Neurological diseases
- Parkinson's disease
- Amyotrophic lateral sclerosis
- Primary lateral sclerosis
- Myasthenia gravis
- Multiple sclerosis
- Guillain-Barré syndrome
- Dystonia
- Essential tremor

Autoimmune diseases
- Rheumatoid arthritis
- Wegener's granulomatosis
- Sarcoidosis
- Amyloidosis

Neuromuscular and psychiatric
- Nerve injury (e.g., vagus, recurrent laryngeal)
- Spasmodic dysphonia
- Muscle tension dysphonia
- Presbylaryngis (age-related vocal cord atrophy)
- Stroke
- Psychogenic

Vocal cord lesions
- Cyst
- Scar
- Hemorrhage
- Granuloma
- Leukoplakia
- Reinke's edema
- Nodules
- Laryngeal papillomatosis
- Squamous cell carcinoma

Medications
- Inhaled corticosteroids
- Anticholinergics
- Antihistamines
- Decongestants
- Antihypertensives

SORE THROAT

Sore throat (pharyngitis) is defined as discomfort or pain in the throat, typically more intense when swallowing. Acute pharyngitis is an inflammatory process of the posterior pharynx and/or tonsils caused by different microorganisms. Most cases of viral pharyngitis occur from a generalized URI such as the common cold (e.g., rhinovirus) or influenza. *Streptococcus pyogenes* (group A beta-hemolytic streptococci) is the most common bacterial cause of pharyngitis. Chronic pharyngitis, which occurs over 3 or more months, can be caused by many different factors. The most common causes of chronic pharyngitis are chronic tonsillopharyngitis, gastroesophageal reflux disease (GERD), submandibular sialadenitis, laryngopharyngeal reflux, and allergy. Cancer of the tonsil, base of the tongue, and hypopharynx should be ruled out, especially in patients who present with weight loss, unilateral otalgia, trismus, or a neck mass.

DIFFERENTIAL DIAGNOSIS

The differential diagnosis for sore throat includes the following conditions:

Viral
- Herpes simplex virus type 1 (oral) but may also be type 2 (genital)
- Influenza virus
- Rhinovirus
- Adenovirus
- Epstein-Barr virus
- Coxsackievirus

Bacterial
- Streptococcal pharyngitis
- *Gonococcus* (gonorrheal pharyngitis)
- *Mycoplasma* infection
- Syphilis (*Treponema pallidum*)

Fungal
- Oropharyngeal candidiasis

Inflammatory
- Tonsillitis
- Aphthous ulceration/stomatitis/mucositis
- Retropharyngeal/parapharyngeal/tonsillar abscess
- Ludwig's angina (submandibular cellulitis, postdental infection)
- Submandibular sialadenitis

Irritation
- GERD (from acid reflux into pharynx)
- Allergic rhinitis (from postnasal drip)
- Chronic sinusitis (from postnasal drip)

Head and neck cancer
- Tonsillar cancer
- Base of tongue cancer
- Hypopharyngeal cancer

Speech disorders
- Muscle tension dysphonia

Trauma
- Chemical injury
- Inhalation injury
- Intubation
- Foreign body

Structural (bone)
- Hyoid syndrome
- Eagle (stylohyoid) syndrome

Systemic disease
- Type 2 diabetes mellitus
- Hypothyroidism with history of subacute thyroiditis
- Uremia

EPISTAXIS

Commonly referred to as a *nosebleed*, epistaxis is caused by the rupture of blood vessel(s) within the nasal mucosa. Epistaxis is extremely common, with about 60% of the general population experiencing at least one significant nosebleed over their lifetime. Epistaxis most commonly occurs in children younger than 10 years and in adults older than 50 years. Males and females are affected equally by nosebleeds. The most common site of bleeding occurs in the anterior portion of the nasal septum known as *Little's area*, where Kiesselbach's plexus, the anastomoses of five arteries that supply the nasal septum, is located. Posterior epistaxis originates most often from Woodruff's plexus and is typically more challenging to control.

Epistaxis can range from minor bleeding that is easily treated with manual compression to severe bleeding requiring emergency department visits and/or hospitalization. Therefore, after the initial management of nasal bleeding, a thorough history and evaluation are essential to determine the underlying cause.

DIFFERENTIAL DIAGNOSES

The differential diagnosis of epistaxis includes the following disorders:

Trauma
- Digital manipulation
- Trauma to nose
- Forceful nose-blowing

Nasopharyngeal masses
- Nasopharyngeal carcinoma
- Juvenile nasopharyngeal angiofibroma
- Nasal polyps
- Papilloma

Medication induced
- Nasal corticosteroid sprays

Nasal structural deformities
- Deviated septum
- Perforated septum (e.g., from "snorting" cocaine)

Sinus infections/chronic allergies
- Acute sinus infection
- Chronic sinus infection
- Allergic rhinitis

Chronic illness
- Hypertension
- Cirrhosis
- Renal disease
- Cancer (especially Hodgkin's disease)

Bleeding disorders
- Hemophilia
- von Willebrand disease
- Hereditary hemorrhagic telangiectasia

SINUS COMPLAINTS

The sinuses are air-filled cavities inside the skull that communicate with the nasal cavity. There are four paired (bilateral) sets of sinus cavities, the frontal, ethmoid, sphenoid, and maxillary sinuses. The frontal sinuses are in the center of the forehead above the eyes; the ethmoid sinuses are six to 14 air cells located behind the middle turbinate; the sphenoid sinuses are located in the sphenoid bone adjacent to the optic nerve and pituitary gland; and the maxillary sinuses are located behind the cheekbones above the maxilla and are the largest sinus cavities. The purposes of these sinus cavities are to lighten the skull, warm and filter air before it passes into the lungs, produce mucus needed to moisturize the nose and remove debris, and assist in resonating the voice.

The sinuses are lined with pseudostratified ciliated columnar epithelia, and the cilia move in coordinated fashion to transport mucus from the sinus cavities toward the nose. Sinuses are susceptible to infection and are often the cause of symptomatology. Sinus complaints may derive from inflammatory, noninflammatory, infectious, or structural etiologies, and account for 30 million health-care visits per year, with sinusitis and allergic rhinitis ranking among the top five most common medical diagnoses in the United States.

DIFFERENTIAL DIAGNOSES

The differential diagnosis of sinus complaints includes the following disorders:

- Allergic rhinitis
- Nonallergic rhinitis
- Nasal polyps
- Deviated septum
- Sino-nasal tumors
- Nasal foreign body (in children)
- Acute viral rhinosinusitis
- Acute bacterial rhinosinusitis
- Chronic rhinosinusitis
- Fungal rhinosinusitis
- Dental infection
- Mucocele
- Adenoid hypertrophy
- Migraines

NECK MASSES

Neck masses can be a common finding in adults and children. They can be caused by infection, inflammation, congenital conditions, trauma, and benign or malignant processes. In children, the most common cause of neck masses is infection; however, in adults, persistent neck masses that do not resolve are often the result of a malignant neoplasm. Therefore, in the adult patient, a neck mass should be managed as a possible malignancy unless proven otherwise.

Neck masses may originate from the lymph nodes, salivary glands, thyroid gland, or develop as a cyst. Obtaining a thorough history to identify a patient at increased risk for cancer, performing a thorough head and neck examination, conducting appropriate diagnostic testing, and referring to a specialist are essential to the early detection of neck malignancies.

DIFFERENTIAL DIAGNOSES

The differential diagnosis of neck masses includes the following disorders:

- Viral or bacterial lymphadenopathy
- Metastatic head and neck carcinoma
- Thyroid mass
- Salivary gland tumors
- Sialadenitis
- Lymphoma
- Lipoma or benign skin cyst
- Thyroglossal duct cyst
- Branchial cleft cyst
- Vascular tumors
- Paragangliomas

REFERENCES

Ear Pain

Bhattacharya S, Singh A, Marzo RR. (2019). "Airplane ear"—A neglected yet preventable problem. *AIMS Public Health,* 6(3), 320–325. https://doi.org/10.3934/publichealth.2019.3.320

Earwood JS, Rogers TS, Rathjen NA. (2018). Ear pain: Diagnosing common and uncommon causes. *American Family Physician,* 97(1), 20–27.

Norris CD, Koontz NA. (2020). Secondary otalgia: Referred pain pathways and pathologies. *AJNR American Journal of Neuroradiology,* 41(12), 2188–2198. https://doi.org/10.3174/ajnr.A6808

Tambunan D, Rana M. (2020). Increasing ear pain and headache. *The Journal of Family Practice,* 69(9), 464–470.

Epistaxis

Béquignon E, Teissier N, Gauthier A, et al. (2017). Emergency department care of childhood epistaxis. *Emergency Medicine Journal: EMJ,* 34(8), 543–548. https://doi.org/10.1136/emermed-2015-205528

Chaaban MR, Zhang D, Resto V, et al. (2017). Demographic, Seasonal, and Geographic Differences in Emergency Department Visits for Epistaxis. *Otolaryngology—Head and Neck Surgery: Official Journal of American Academy of Otolaryngology-Head and Neck Surgery,* 156(1), 81–86. https://doi.org/10.1177/0194599816667295

Chen YP, Chan A, Le QT, et al. (2019). Nasopharyngeal Carcinoma. *Lancet (London, England),* 394(10192), 64–80. https://doi.org/10.1016/S0140-6736(19)30956-0

Cohen O, Shoffel-Havakuk H, Warman M, et al. (2017). Early and Late Recurrent Epistaxis Admissions: Patterns of Incidence and Risk Factors. *Otolaryngology—head and neck surgery: official journal of American Academy of Otolaryngology-Head and Neck Surgery,* 157(3), 424–431. https://doi.org/10.1177/0194599817705619

Li W, Ni Y, Lu H, et al. (2019). Current perspectives on the origin theory of juvenile nasopharyngeal angiofibroma. *Discovery Medicine,* 27(150), 245–254.

Min HJ, Kang H, Choi GJ, et al. (2017). Association between hypertension and epistaxis: Systematic review and meta-analysis. *Otolaryngology—Head and Neck Surgery: Official Journal of American Academy of Otolaryngology-Head and Neck Surgery,* 157(6), 921–927. https://doi.org/10.1177/0194599817721445

Tunkel DE, Anne S, Payne SC, et al. (2020). Clinical practice guideline: Nosebleed (epistaxis). *Otolaryngology—Head and Neck Surgery: Official Journal of American Academy of Otolaryngology-Head and Neck Surgery, 162*(1_suppl), S1–S38. https://doi.org/10.1177/0194599819890327

Hoarseness

Carroll TL. (2019). Reflux and the voice: Getting smarter about laryngopharyngeal reflux. *Otolaryngologic Clinics of North America, 52*(4), 723–733. https://doi.org/10.1016/j.otc.2019.03.015

Francis DO. (2018). Management of hoarseness. *JAMA Otolaryngology—Head & Neck Surgery, 144*(9), 838–839. https://doi.org/10.1001/jamaoto.2018.1239

Francis DO, Smith LJ. (2019). Hoarseness guidelines redux: Toward improved treatment of patients with dysphonia. *Otolaryngologic Clinics of North America, 52*(4), 597–605. https://doi.org/10.1016/j.otc.2019.03.003

Kost KM, Sataloff RT. (2018). Voice Disorders in the Elderly. *Clinics in geriatric medicine, 34*(2), 191–203. https://doi.org/10.1016/j.cger.2018.01.010

Stachler RJ, Francis DO, Schwartz SR, et al. (2018). Clinical Practice Guideline: Hoarseness (Dysphonia) (Update). *Otolaryngology—head and neck surgery: official journal of American Academy of Otolaryngology-Head and Neck Surgery, 158*(1_suppl), S1–S42. https://doi.org/10.1177/0194599817751030

Stinnett S, Chmielewska M, Akst LM. (2018). Update on management of hoarseness. *The Medical Clinics of North America, 102*(6), 1027–1040. https://doi.org/10.1016/j.mcna.2018.06.005

Zhukhovitskaya A, Verma SP. (2019). Identification and management of chronic laryngitis. *Otolaryngologic Clinics of North America, 52*(4), 607–616. https://doi.org/10.1016/j.otc.2019.03.004

Impaired Hearing

Chandrasekhar SS, Tsai Do BS, Schwartz SR, et al. (2019). Clinical practice guideline: Sudden hearing loss (Update). *Otolaryngology—head and neck surgery: official journal of american academy of otolaryngology-head and neck surgery, 161* (1_suppl), S1–S45. https://doi.org/10.1177/0194599819859885

Lee JW, Bance ML. (2019). Hearing loss. *Practical Neurology, 19*(1), 28–35. https://doi.org/10.1136/practneurol-2018-001926

Michels TC, Duffy MT, Rogers DJ. (2019). Hearing loss in adults: Differential diagnosis and treatment. *American Family Physician, 100*(2), 98–108.

Nieman CL, Oh ES. (2020). Hearing loss. *Annals of Internal Medicine, 173*(11), ITC81–ITC96. https://doi.org/10.7326/AITC202012010

Mouth Sores

Fitzpatrick SG, Cohen DM, Clark AN. (2019). Ulcerated lesions of the oral mucosa: Clinical and histologic review. *Head and Neck Pathology, 13*(1), 91–102. https://doi.org/10.1007/s12105-018-0981-8

Hargitai IA. (2018). Painful Oral Lesions. *Dental clinics of North America, 62*(4), 597–609. https://doi.org/10.1016/j.cden.2018.06.002

Maymone M, Greer RO, Burdine LK, et al. (2019). Benign oral mucosal lesions: Clinical and pathological findings. *Journal of the American Academy of Dermatology, 81*(1), 43–56. https://doi.org/10.1016/j.jaad.2018.09.061

Saikaly SK, Saikaly TS, Saikaly LE. (2018). Recurrent aphthous ulceration: a review of potential causes and novel treatments. *The Journal of Dermatological Treatment, 29*(6), 542–552. https://doi.org/10.1080/09546634.2017.1422079

Neck Masses

McSpadden RP, Orsini M, Higgins K. (2018). Tubular neck mass. *JAMA otolaryngology— Head & Neck Surgery, 144*(5), 453–454. https://doi.org/10.1001/jamaoto.2018.0019

Pynnonen MA, Gillespie MB, Roman B, et al. (2017). Clinical practice guideline: Evaluation of the neck mass in adults. *Otolaryngology—Head and Neck Surgery: Official Journal of American Academy of Otolaryngology-Head and Neck Surgery, 157*(2_suppl), S1–S30. https://doi.org/10.1177/0194599817722550

Yan K, Agrawal N, Gooi Z. (2018). Head and Neck Masses. *The Medical clinics of North America, 102*(6), 1013–1025. https://doi.org/10.1016/j.mcna.2018.06.012

Sinus Complaints

Pipolo C, Saibene AM, Felisati G. (2018). Prevalence of pain due to rhinosinusitis: a review. *Neurological Sciences: Official Journal of the Italian Neurological Society and of The Italian Society of Clinical Neurophysiology, 39*(Suppl 1), 21–24. https://doi.org/10.1007/s10072-018-3336-z

Scadding GK, Kariyawasam HH, Scadding G, et al. (2017). BSACI guideline for the diagnosis and management of allergic and non-allergic rhinitis (Revised Edition 2017; First edition 2007). *Clinical and Experimental Allergy: Journal of the British Society for Allergy and Clinical Immunology, 47*(7), 856–889. https://doi.org/10.1111/cea.12953

Schuler IV CF, Montejo JM. (2019). Allergic rhinitis in children and adolescents. *Pediatric Clinics of North America, 66*(5), 981–993. https://doi.org/10.1016/j.pcl.2019.06.004

Sur D, Plesa ML. (2018). Chronic nonallergic rhinitis. *American Family Physician, 98*(3), 171–176.

Sore Throat

Brook I. (2017). Treatment challenges of group A beta-hemolytic streptococcal pharyngo-tonsillitis. *International Archives of Otorhinolaryngology, 21*(3), 286–296. https://dx.doi.org/10.1055%2Fs-0036-1584294

Homme JH. (2019). Acute otitis media and group A streptococcal pharyngitis: A review for the general pediatric practitioner. *Pediatric Annals, 48*(9), e343–e348. https://doi.org/10.3928/19382359-20190813-01

Kundu S, Dutta M, Adhikary BK, et al. (2019). Encountering chronic sore throat: How challenging is it for the otolaryngologists? *Indian Journal of Otolaryngology and Head and Neck Surgery: Official Publication of the Association of Otolaryngologists of India, 71*(Suppl 1), 176–181. https://doi.org/10.1007/s12070-017-1191-5

Luo R, Sickler J, Vahidnia F, et al. (2019). Diagnosis and management of group A streptococcal pharyngitis in the United States, 2011-2015. *BMC infectious diseases, 19*(1), 193. https://doi.org/10.1186/s12879-019-3835-4

Mitchell RB, Archer SM, Ishman SL, et al. (2019). Clinical practice guideline: Tonsillectomy in children (Update). *Otolaryngology—Head and Neck Surgery : Official Journal of American Academy of Otolaryngology-Head and Neck Surgery, 160*(1_suppl), S1–S42. https://doi.org/10.1177/0194599818801757

Perkins C, Ray Brown F, Pohl K, et al. (2019). Implementing a guideline for acute tonsillitis using an ambulatory medical unit. *The Journal of Laryngology and Otology, 133*(5), 386–389. https://doi.org/10.1017/S0022215119000380

Shapiro DJ, Lindgren CE, Neuman MI, et al. (2017). Viral features and testing for streptococcal pharyngitis. *Pediatrics, 139*(5), e20163403.

Taylor DG. (2018). Acute sore throat: discussing antibiotics with patients. *BMJ (Clinical research ed.), 361*, k2443. https://doi.org/10.1136/bmj.k2443

Tran J, Danchin M, Steer AC, et al. (2018). Management of sore throat in primary care. *Australian Journal of General Practice, 47*(7), 485–489. https://doi.org/10.31128/AJGP-11-17-4393

Yoshida H, Kanamori M, Sakemi H. (2021). Sore throat with normal oropharyngeal examination. *The American Journal of Medicine, 134*(1), e49–e50. https://doi.org/10.1016/j.amjmed.2020.06.034

Tinnitus

Basura GJ, Adams ME, Monfared A, et al. (2020). Clinical Practice Guideline: Ménière's Disease. *Otolaryngology—Head and Neck Surgery: Official Journal of American Academy of Otolaryngology-Head and Neck Surgery, 162*(2_suppl), S1–S55. https://doi.org/10.1177/0194599820909438

Chandrasekhar SS, Tsai Do BS, Schwartz SR, et al. (2019). Clinical practice guideline: Sudden hearing loss (update) executive summary. *Otolaryngology—Head and Neck Surgery: Official Journal of American Academy of Otolaryngology-Head and Neck Surgery, 161*(2), 195–210. https://doi.org/10.1177/0194599819859883

Lewis S, Chowdhury E, Stockdale D, et al. (2020). Assessment and management of tinnitus: summary of NICE guidance. *BMJ (Clinical research ed.), 368*, m976. https://doi.org/10.1136/bmj.m976

Møller AR. (2016). Sensorineural Tinnitus: Its Pathology and Probable Therapies. *International Journal of Otolaryngology, 2016*, 2830157. https://doi.org/10.1155/2016/2830157

RESOURCES

American Academy of Otolaryngology—Head and Neck Surgery
   www.entnet.org
American Tinnitus Association
   https://www.ata.org/
Hearing Industries Association
   www.betterhearing.org
National Institute on Deafness and Other Communication Disorders
   https://www.nidcd.nih.gov/
Nurseslabs: Impaired Verbal Communication
   https://nurseslabs.com/impaired-verbal-communication
Oral Cancer Foundation
   www.oralcancerfoundation.org

Chapter 22
Hearing and Balance Disorders

Maria Colandrea, DNP, NP-C, CORLN, CCRN, FAANP
Michael E. Zychowicz, DNP, ANP, ONP, FAAN, FAANP
Brian Oscar Porter, MD, PhD, MPH, MBA

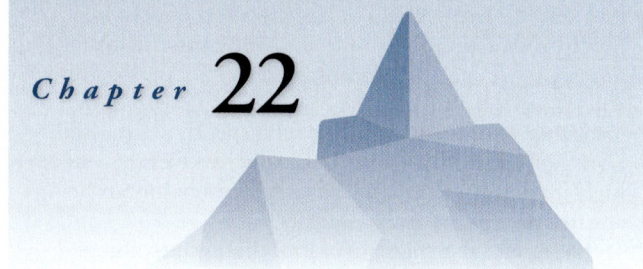

HEARING LOSS

Hearing loss is defined as a decrease in hearing threshold of 25 dB or more in one or both ears. Hearing loss, diagnosed by audiogram, can be mild, moderate, severe, or profound, and it may occur in one or both ears. Although rapid hearing loss typically triggers a patient to seek medical care, hearing loss is commonly a slowly progressive process that may not be perceptible by the patient until it interferes with communication.

EPIDEMIOLOGY AND CAUSES

The World Health Organization (WHO) reports 466 million people have hearing loss—432 million adults (93%) and 34 million children (7%). In the United States, the Centers for Disease Control and Prevention (CDC) report approximately 14.1% (27.7 million) of American adults 20 to 69 years of age have hearing loss in one or both ears.

Hearing loss of at least mild severity doubles in prevalence for every 10 years of life after age 50 years. Hearing loss affects 15% of adults between the ages of 50 and 59 years, 31% between the ages of 60 and 69 years, and 80% aged 85 years and older. Males are more likely than females to experience hearing loss, and in children, genetics and illness are common causes of hearing loss. Sudden hearing loss affects five to 27 per 100,000 people (approximately 66,000 individuals per year) in the United States, prompting patients to seek urgent medical care. It is often associated with tinnitus and/or vertigo. In turn, this is considered a medical emergency and should be treated immediately to decrease the risk of permanent hearing loss.

According to the CDC, 98% of infants born in the United States are screened for hearing loss. Of those 98%, hearing loss affects 1.7 per 1,000 infants screened. The most common causes of permanent congenital sensorineural and mixed hearing loss are congenital cytomegalovirus (CMV) (5% to 20%), structural abnormalities of the temporal bones (30% to 40%), and genetic causes (50%).

Chronic middle ear infections (otitis media) and effusions are contributing factors to the development of conductive hearing loss (CHL), especially in children. Recurrent ear infections can cause scarring that affects middle ear structures from repeated bouts of inflammation and healing. A ruptured tympanic membrane occurring as a complication of severe otitis media or from direct physical trauma can lead to hearing loss, which may improve with healing. Allergies, cerumen impaction, and other causes of eustachian tube obstruction may also contribute to CHL. Sensorineural hearing loss (SNHL) can result from increasing age, acoustic trauma (exposure to loud noises), ototoxic drugs (e.g., aminoglycoside antibiotics, aspirin, quinine), autoimmune diseases, or genetics.

PATHOPHYSIOLOGY

The conductive phase occurs when sound waves are funneled by the external ear to the external auditory canal, which causes the tympanic membrane to vibrate. The vibrations of the tympanic membrane cause the ossicles (middle ear bones: malleus, incus, and stapes) to transmit sound waves through the oval window, thereby allowing them to enter the inner ear (see Fig. 22.1). This starts the sensorineural phase, in which sound waves are passed into the cochlea, a hard shell-like, coiled organ of the inner ear that is filled with fluid and hair cells. The fluid (endolymph and perilymph) vibration in the cochlea stimulates the hair cells, which then send signals to the temporal cortex of the brain via the vestibulocochlear nerve (cranial nerve [CN] VIII). These signals are interpreted in the brain as sounds or language.

In CHL, the passage of sound waves through the ear canal, tympanic membrane, or middle ear is disrupted. This disruption of sound is often described as muffled or reverberating and can be associated with aural fullness. The conductance of sound can be disrupted by cerumen (the most common cause of CHL), fluid (e.g., middle ear effusion), infection (e.g., otitis media), foreign body, or a mass. CHL can occur at any age and may be reversible. In children, the angle of the eustachian tube is straighter and shorter, which allows for microorganisms from the nasopharynx to enter the middle ear more readily, thereby increasing the risk of otitis media or otitis media with effusion. This anatomical difference predisposes certain children to frequent ear infections, and in turn, to CHL. In infants, the most common cause of CHL or mixed hearing loss is an abnormality in ossicular bones.

In SNHL, there is abnormal functioning or damage of the otic hair cells within the organ of Corti. Damage may also occur in the central neural pathways of the ear, affecting CN VIII and the auditory cortex. After 50 years of age, otic hair cells in the organ of Corti tend to degenerate, and the stria vascularis, a capillary-fed layer of stratified epithelium that secretes endolymph and promotes the sensitization of hair cells in the cochlea, may atrophy. These changes first affect the perception of high-frequency sounds, which then progresses to affect the detection of lower-frequency tones. SNHL may also

> ### Geriatric Considerations: Hearing Loss
>
> The most common cause of SNHL is age-related hearing loss, termed *presbycusis*. The degeneration of delicate inner ear structures over time contributes to the loss of hearing as we age. Older adult patients with presbycusis will typically have a bilateral loss of hearing with difficulty localizing sounds and struggles with speech discrimination. Age-related hearing loss initially involves the loss of high-frequency sounds, with low-frequency sounds being affected as the disorder progresses.
>
> Because of the gradual onset of presbycusis, some people with age-related hearing loss may not recognize they have a deficit. This can result in delays in seeking care. It may be a significant other or a spouse who first points out the difficulty hearing. Some patients may be resistant to or delay seeking care for hearing loss due to social stigma or feeling this is simply a normal part of aging. Patients who are diagnosed with hearing loss will wait on average nearly 10 years until they obtain hearing aids. Some may attempt to adjust to their hearing loss by modifying their activities of daily living. Although presbycusis is among the top chronic conditions affecting older adult patients, only one in five seeks the care that they would benefit from.
>
> Untreated hearing loss can lead to, or increase risk for, several conditions. Older adults with untreated hearing loss can experience an increased risk for hospitalization and falls. Unmanaged presbycusis can contribute to depression, anxiety, and social isolation. Quality of life, independent function, and cognitive function can all be diminished with untreated age-related hearing loss.

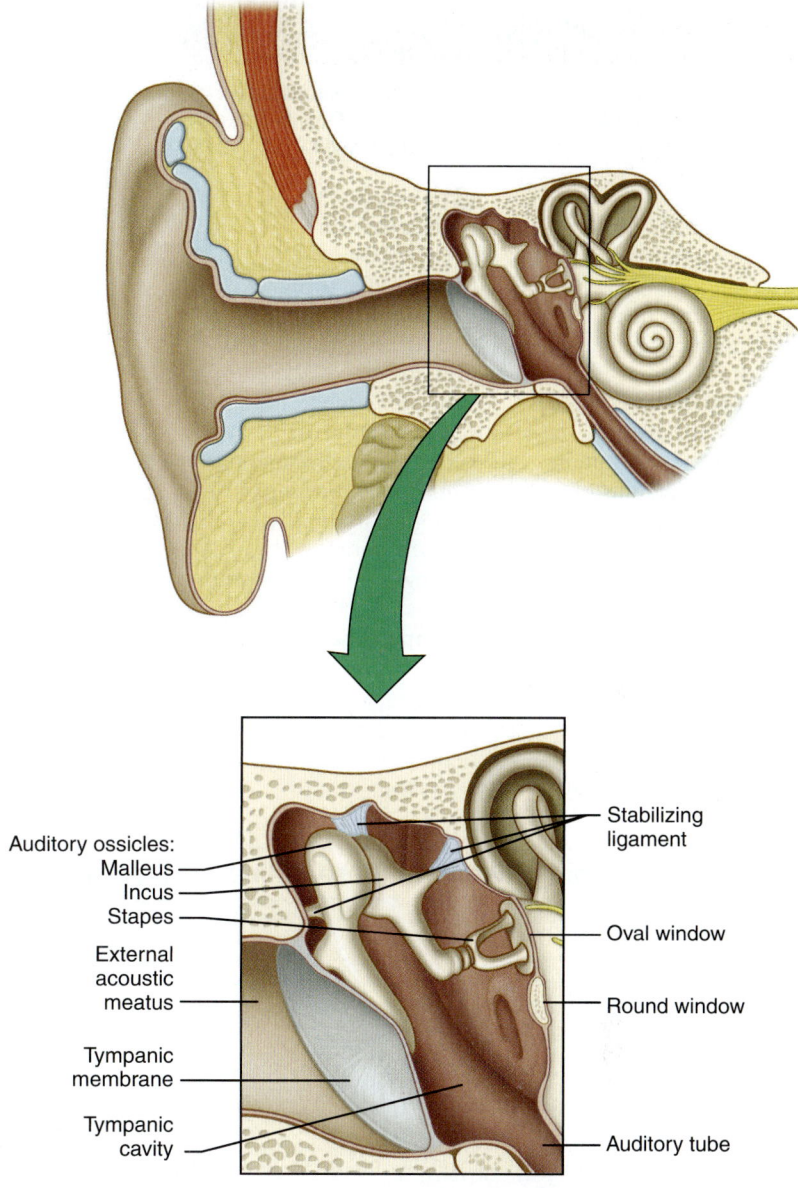

Figure 22.1 The Middle Ear

be a result of loud noise exposure or be noise induced from repeated acoustic trauma (see Table 22.1).

CLINICAL PRESENTATION

Hearing loss is a symptom that may be a component of multiple medical conditions. Patients typically present with progressive complaints of difficulty hearing, especially when viewing television or with conversations. At times, hearing loss may be associated with pain, pressure, discomfort, vertigo, or loss of balance. The patient may also complain of tinnitus, otorrhea, popping, crackling, distant sounds, or stiffness. Depending on the presentation, it is essential for the clinician to recognize if the complaint is an acute issue requiring prompt intervention or a chronic issue that can be worked up over time.

Subjective

Obtaining a thorough history of present illness, as well as obtaining information regarding medical and surgical history, medication usage, and family history can help identify the cause of the hearing loss (see Box 22.1). It is important to inquire about the duration and pattern of symptoms, including the laterality, progression, and severity of hearing loss; ototoxic medication usage; head or ear trauma; loud noise exposure; and any otological surgeries. Asking the patient about a family history of hearing loss or if family members have had ear surgeries can point toward potential genetic causes. Inquiring about associated symptoms such as tinnitus, otalgia, otorrhea, mastoid tenderness, tragal pain, vertigo, disequilibrium, and aural fullness can also help steer toward the correct diagnosis.

The review of systems should focus on the neurological system, including CN function (e.g., vertigo,

TABLE 22.1 Causes of Conductive Hearing Loss and Sensorineural Hearing Loss

Causes of Conductive Hearing Loss From Most to Least Common	Causes of Sensorineural Hearing Loss From Most to Least Common
• Cerumen • Otitis media with effusion (most common in children) • Acute otitis media • Tympanic membrane perforation • Otosclerosis • Otitis externa • Ear canal mass/middle ear mass (glomus tumor, osteomas) • Tympanosclerosis • Cholesteatoma	• Presbycusis • Noise exposure • Hereditary • Ototoxicity (drug induced) • Sudden idiopathic hearing loss • Autoimmune hearing loss • Ménière's disease • Vestibular schwannoma • Infections (meningitis, syphilis, mumps, viral labyrinthitis) • Congenital malformation of the ossicles • Temporal bone fractures

disequilibrium, unilateral tinnitus, gradual or sudden unilateral hearing loss, facial numbness, weakness or tingling, loss of taste, or dysphagia). Social and occupational history should include specific questions regarding noise or toxin exposure and any blast-related injuries, including a history of hunting and/or target shooting. A complete history of prescription and over-the-counter medication use should also be obtained.

In patients with a complaint of sudden hearing loss, rapid evaluation and treatment are essential in preserving hearing. Patients who report sudden hearing loss should receive a thorough history, physical examination, and rapid referral for otolaryngology and a same-day audiogram. Different etiologies of hearing loss may be associated with distinctive clinical characteristics. For example, presbycusis typically produces a slowly progressive, high-frequency hearing loss that is bilaterally symmetrical and is often associated with tinnitus. In contrast, ototoxicity presents first with tinnitus followed by symmetrical high-frequency hearing loss. Acoustic trauma from very loud noise exposure can cause a temporary shift in hearing that may resolve over time or cause a permanent impairment in hearing. Ménière's

---

Box 22.1 Obtaining History of Present Illness—What to ask the patient with hearing loss

History of Present Illness

- Onset of symptoms: gradual or sudden
- Location: unilateral or bilateral
- Duration: hours, days, months, years
- Severity: complete hearing loss or decrease in hearing, fluctuating hearing
- Exacerbating or relieving factors
- Noise exposure from employment or recreation (e.g., earphones, concerts, firing weapons/hunting)
- Recent ear trauma, head injury, traumatic noise exposure (e.g., blast)
- Associated symptoms: presence of tinnitus, ear fullness, vertigo, otalgia, otorrhea, fever, headache, disequilibrium
- Change in or recently added medication (including over-the-counter medications)
- Neurological symptoms: vertigo, disequilibrium, facial numbness, weakness or tingling, loss of taste, dysphagia

Past Medical History

- History of strokes, cardiovascular disease, hypertension, diabetes mellitus
- Viral diseases such as meningitis, syphilis, or recent viral upper respiratory infection
- History of sudden hearing loss
- History of eardrum rupture, head trauma, ear trauma
- Hearing loss or chronic ear infections in childhood
- History of head or neck cancer

Surgical History

- Surgical placement of pressure-equalizing ear tubes in childhood
- Otological surgeries
- Head and neck surgeries

Family History

- Family history of hearing loss or otological conditions
- Family history of head and neck cancers

Social History

- Tobacco use including chewing tobacco, snuff/dip, e-cigarettes, cigarettes, cigars: how often, quantity, type
- Alcohol use: how often, quantity, type

Pediatric Patients

- Inquire if mother had perinatal viral infections such as cytomegalovirus, rubella, herpes, toxoplasmosis, syphilis
- Birth weight less than 3.3 pounds
- Anatomical malformation of the head or neck
- Craniofacial abnormalities (e.g., cleft palate)
- Speech or learning difficulties
- Behavioral issues

disease causes fluctuating hearing loss, which is usually unilateral and associated with roaring tinnitus, aural fullness, and severe vertigo. Acoustic neuroma (vestibular schwannoma) is a rare tumor of CN VIII, causes unilateral constant or progressive hearing loss with tinnitus, and is possibly associated with disequilibrium and vertigo. With a tumor of the acoustic nerve, there may be neurological changes, such as facial numbness and/or weakness, vertigo, disequilibrium, a loss of taste, and dysphagia, in addition to hearing loss.

Objective

The physical examination should include otoscopic examination to inspect the external auditory canal and middle ear. The clinician should note any redness, foreign objects, discharge, scaling, lesions, and cerumen (ear wax). The tympanic membrane should have no perforations and should be a translucent pearly gray. Changes in the tympanic membrane may be consistent with CHL.

The clinician should perform Weber, Rinne, and Schwabach tests to determine whether hearing loss is primarily conductive or sensorineural. Unexpected findings from the three tuning fork tests must be integrated to differentiate the nature of the hearing loss. CHL occurs when sound transmission is impaired through the external or middle ear. SNHL occurs due to a defect in the inner ear that leads to the distortion of sound and misinterpretation of speech.

For clinic-based evaluation, the Weber test is done first. A vibrating 512-Hz (or higher-frequency) tuning fork is placed midline on the patient's skull. Normally, the sound should be heard equally in both ears. In SNHL, the sound in the unaffected (or less affected ear) is louder. In CHL, the sound is louder in the affected ear.

The Rinne test can also be done in the office. A vibrating tuning fork is placed on the mastoid process. When the sound fades away, the fork is promptly placed (without restriking it) over the external auditory meatus. Normally, the sound can be heard for twice as long via air conduction as via bone conduction. In SNHL, the ratio remains the same, whereas in CHL, the ratio is closer to 1:1 or even reversed.

The Schwabach test is a crude comparison of the patient's hearing to the examiner's, presuming the examiner has normal hearing. The vibrating tuning fork is placed over the mastoid process of the patient until the patient no longer hears sound, and then the examiner quickly transfers the tuning fork to their own mastoid process and compares the results. In SNHL, the patient's bone conduction is present for a shorter time on the affected side than the examiner's bone conduction; in CHL, the patient's bone conduction on the affected side persists for a longer time than the examiner's bone conduction. This test should not be performed if the examiner's hearing is not normal.

DIAGNOSTIC REASONING

Diagnostic Tests

An audiogram is recommended for those patients with subjective complaints of hearing loss. The gold standard of hearing evaluation includes pure tone audiometry with speech testing, as well as impedance (middle ear pressure) testing. Marked CHL in one ear may be difficult to exclude when testing the opposite ear. Computed tomography (CT) is used to evaluate for cholesteatomas, ossicular chain issues, chronic ear infection, or otic trauma. CT should not be used to evaluate for sudden SNHL or acoustic neuroma. Magnetic resonance imaging (MRI) scans should be ordered in patients with asymmetric hearing loss or sudden SNHL to detect tumors, such as acoustic neuromas and tympanic paragangliomas (formerly called *glomus tumors*).

For patients who present with sudden hearing loss, the clinician should first identify if it is CHL versus SNHL by examining the ear with an otoscope and using tuning forks to conduct the Weber and Rinne tests, as discussed earlier. If SNHL is identified, the patient needs immediate referral for pure tone audiometry and referral to an otorhinolaryngologist on the same day if possible or within 14 days of hearing loss onset. Audiometry is mandatory in the diagnosis of SNHL, with abnormal criteria being a hearing loss of 30 dB or more at three consecutive frequencies occurring within a 72-hour period.

Differential Diagnosis

To treat hearing loss, the etiology must be accurately identified. The differential diagnosis for hearing loss includes conditions that cause either sensorineural or conductive hearing impairment (see Table 22.2). Aging is commonly associated with sensorineural loss of hearing (presbycusis); however, other possible conditions need to be ruled out. SNHL may also have an etiology of ototoxicity, exposure to loud noises, an autoimmune disorder, an acoustic neuroma, labyrinthitis (inflammation of both the vestibular and cochlear branches of the vestibulocochlear nerve), or possibly Ménière's disease. CHL may be explained simply by cerumen accumulation or impaction (ceruminosis) or a foreign body in the external canal, otitis externa, chronic otitis media, middle ear effusion, otosclerosis, a vascular anomaly, or a cholesteatoma.

In patients who present with SNHL or have asymmetric hearing loss, MRI of the brain with fine cuts through the internal auditory canal to rule out acoustic neuroma should be performed. In idiopathic SNHL, patients typically present with unilateral hearing loss. If a patient presents with bilateral hearing loss, the clinician should be cognizant of other causes such as viral infections, autoimmune inner ear disease, ototoxic medications, head trauma, lead poisoning, genetic disorders, stroke, Cogan's syndrome (recurrent inflammation of the cornea, with fever, fatigue, weight loss, vertigo, tinnitus, and

TABLE 22.2 Common Causes, Symptoms, and Examination Findings of Conductive Hearing Loss and Sensorineural Hearing Loss

Causes of Conductive Hearing Loss From Most to Least Common	Symptoms and Examination Findings
• Cerumen impaction (ceruminosis)	• Symptoms: muffled hearing, aural fullness, decreased hearing • Examination findings: yellow, orange, or brown waxy substance in ear canal blocking visualization of the tympanic membrane; Weber test lateralizes to affected ear
• Otitis media with effusion (most common in children)	• Symptoms: usually painless, aural fullness, muffled hearing, decreased hearing • Examination findings: amber fluid behind tympanic membrane; may also visualize air bubbles; Weber test lateralizes to affected ear
• Acute otitis media	• Symptoms: pain with palpation over mastoid process, otalgia, muffled hearing, decreased hearing • Examination findings: bulging tympanic membrane with purulent material behind tympanic membrane; Weber test lateralizes to affected ear
• Tympanic membrane perforation	• Symptoms: possibly otorrhea, pain with spontaneous rupture followed by pain relief, muffled hearing • Examination findings: hole in tympanic membrane with view into middle ear chamber; disrupts vibration of tympanic membrane onto ossicles, causing Weber test to lateralize to affected ear
• Otosclerosis	• Symptoms: hearing loss • Examination findings: normal otological examination, calcifications on the ossicles (specifically, the stapes [stirrup] is not visible on examination); Weber test lateralizes to affected ear; Rinne test may show air conduction less than bone conduction with significant conductive hearing loss
• Otitis externa	• Symptoms: pain upon pulling on the helix or pressing the tragus, possible hearing loss • Examination findings: erythema, edema, and exudate within the ear canal; may have white or yellow debris or purulent drainage; can be difficult to visualize the tympanic membrane
• Ear canal mass/middle ear mass (e.g., glomus tumor, osteoma)	• Symptoms: glomus tumor with pulsating tinnitus, aural fullness, hearing loss; osteoma has hearing loss • Examination findings: red pulsating mass within the middle ear, which may extend through the tympanic membrane (glomus tumor); white, hard, round mass within the ear canal (osteoma)
• Tympanosclerosis	• Symptoms: may have hearing loss, but usually asymptomatic • Examination findings: scarring on the tympanic membrane, usually white in color
• Cholesteatoma	• Symptoms: chronic ear infection with possible erosion of the scutum (sharp bony spur at top of the tympanic membrane, formed by superior wall of external ear canal and lateral wall of tympanic cavity), tympanic membrane perforation • Examination findings: white skin debris or hard cerumen usually present in the pars flaccida (flaccid portion of tympanic membrane located above the lateral process of the malleus)
Causes of Sensorineural Hearing Loss From Most to Least Common	**Description/symptoms:** In all these situations, otoscopy is normal, Weber test lateralizes away from affected ear, and Rinne test demonstrates that air conduction is louder than bone conduction.
• Presbycusis	• Gradual, symmetrical, permanent high-frequency hearing loss that occurs in patients older than 60 years • Patient often complains of tinnitus and aural fullness.
• Noise exposure	• Exposure to loud noise typically over 85 decibels; the louder the sound, the shorter the amount of time it takes to cause hearing loss • Symptoms may be loud tinnitus and subjective decrease in hearing.
• Hereditary	• In infants, this can affect one to three per 1,000 children. • Newborn hearing screening can detect this hearing loss.

TABLE 22.2 Common Causes, Symptoms, and Examination Findings of Conductive Hearing Loss and Sensorineural Hearing Loss—cont'd

Causes of Conductive Hearing Loss From Most to Least Common	Symptoms and Examination Findings

• Ototoxicity	• Certain drugs are known to cause ototoxic effects in the cochlea:
	  • Chemotherapy (e.g., cisplatin, carboplatin)
	  • Antibiotics (e.g., aminoglycosides, macrolides, vancomycin)
	  • Aspirin (salicylates) and other NSAIDs
	  • Loop diuretics (e.g., furosemide, bumetanide)
	  • Quinine

• Sudden idiopathic hearing loss	• Considered a medical emergency that needs to be identified early to preserve hearing • Symptoms most often include sudden unilateral hearing loss that may be accompanied by vertigo, tinnitus, and aural fullness.
• Autoimmune hearing loss	• Very rare • Symptoms include fluctuating hearing loss and possibly vertigo.
• Ménière's disease	• Inner ear disorder believed to be caused by too much endolymph inside the cochlea. • Symptoms include fluctuating hearing loss associated with vertigo and lasting 20 minutes or more, roaring tinnitus, and aural fullness; usually unilateral, but can be bilateral • Episodes are recurrent and can be debilitating. • Treatment includes diuretics, antihistamines, or possibly surgery.
• Vestibular schwannoma	• Rare, slow-growing benign tumor • Symptoms include slow, progressive hearing loss that is usually unilateral and may be associated with aural fullness and/or vertigo. • Some cases present with sudden hearing loss. • Examination findings reveal normal otoscopy, though if tumor is large, may have facial paresis due to compression of facial nerve (cranial nerve VII)
• Infections (e.g., meningitis, syphilis, mumps, viral labyrinthitis)	• In meningitis, may have severe headache, fever, cranial nerve palsies, and decreased hearing • In viral labyrinthitis, may have precipitating viral upper respiratory infection causing vertigo and decreased or sudden hearing loss • Examination findings reveal normal otoscopy.

hearing loss), sarcoidosis, hyperviscosity syndrome, or a neoplastic cause.

MANAGEMENT

Management of hearing loss complaints depends on the cause of the hearing loss. Many types of CHL are reversible, but sensorineural causes tend to be irreversible. In cases of CHL caused by cerumen buildup, cerumen disimpaction may be necessary. The recommended procedure is to place a 1:1 mixture of 3% hydrogen peroxide and warm mineral oil in the external ear canal and leave it in for 1 hour followed by lavage with warm water. The water should be directed toward the canal wall during the lavage and not toward the eardrum.

Cerumenolytic agents such as 6.5% carbamide peroxide (Debrox) are effective at breaking up the impacted wax; docusate sodium liquid may also be used. However, these agents should not be used in the presence of a perforated tympanic membrane or ear infection. If the patient is scheduled for cerumen removal in the primary care clinic, advise the patient with cerumen buildup to use carbamide peroxide for 1 week before returning for ear canal irrigation as described. If not performed properly, cerumen removal may cause damage to the external auditory meatus, perforation of the tympanic membrane, or otitis media. If trauma to the ear canal occurs, a combination corticosteroid/antibiotic otic solution (e.g., Cortisporin Otic Solution; four drops three to four times daily for 5 to 7 days) should be prescribed, although not with a perforated tympanic membrane.

If hearing loss is caused by an infection, treat as appropriate, depending on whether viral, bacterial, or fungal infection is suspected. See the sections on otitis media and otitis externa in Chapter 23 for a detailed discussion.

The cause of the hearing loss in cases of sensorineural impairment must also be identified correctly to treat it properly, including diagnostic audiometry as discussed earlier. If the patient is on an ototoxic medication and develops hearing loss, dizziness, and tinnitus, the medication should be stopped. Salicylate toxicity, for example, is reversible. Likewise, in cases resulting from metabolic causes, such as hypothyroidism, the underlying disorder should be treated, rather than pursuing otic-specific treatments.

However, for SNHL related to otic inflammation, initial medical management includes prescribing systemic high-dose corticosteroids. The potential for spontaneous improvement in hearing is highest in the first 14 days of hearing loss and decreases after 14 days. Thus, prompt intervention is essential, as treatment within 14 days of the onset of SNHL has shown improvement in hearing on repeat audiogram. Prednisone 1 mg/kg/day is prescribed as a single daily dose (not divided), with a usual dose of 60 mg daily for 10 to 14 days. Equivalent doses of methylprednisolone 48 mg or dexamethasone 10 mg may also be used.

It is important for the clinician to discuss the risks of high-dose prednisone with the patient, such as elevated blood glucose and worsening control of diabetes mellitus, fluid retention, restlessness, insomnia, avascular necrosis of bone, and an increased appetite. Caution should be used in patients who have uncontrolled diabetes mellitus. If the patient has increased risk factors justifying the administration of high-dose corticosteroids or suffers from severe SNHL hearing loss, intratympanic corticosteroid injections can be performed by an otorhinolaryngologist. Intratympanic corticosteroids allow the medication to penetrate the inner ear. An audiogram should be repeated at completion of treatment.

Importantly, hearing loss can be linked to depression, anxiety, increased isolation, and frustration. In turn, hearing aids can be effective in the management and treatment of moderate to severe hearing loss and should be discussed with patients as a potential intervention, as they have shown improvements in hearing-related quality. If the patient agrees, they should be referred to an audiologist for consideration of auditory amplification. In patients with profound hearing loss or irreversible CHL, implantable amplification devices such as cochlear implants, bone-anchored hearing aids, or sound bridge implants may be an option.

FOLLOW-UP AND REFERRAL

Any patient who presents with a complaint of hearing loss without an obvious conductive cause (such as ceruminosis) should be referred to an audiologist for pure tone audiometry. As stated earlier, if a patient presents with sudden SNHL, they should be referred for a stat audiogram and to an otorhinolaryngologist for further diagnosis and treatment. Patients should also be referred to an otorhinolaryngologist if perforation of the tympanic membrane is present, as well as in cases of damage to the ossicles, tympanosclerosis, otosclerosis, tumor, chronic ear infections, cholesteatoma, and temporal bone injury. Patients who are suspected of having Ménière's disease should be referred to an otorhinolaryngologist and an audiologist for appropriate diagnostic testing and treatment. Acoustic neuromas should be referred to an otorhinolaryngologist for surgical evaluation and potential resection.

Patient Education: Hearing Loss

Patients should be counseled that middle ear problems, especially if recurrent, may progress to chronic ear problems, such as perforations or cholesteatomas, which will adversely affect hearing. In cases of presbycusis, although no specific treatment will reverse the process, it is important to educate and support the patient so that no further damage occurs; for example, exposure to excessive noise and ototoxic drugs should be avoided in these patients. Indeed, permanent hearing loss is common with a sensorineural etiology and may even occur with CHL. Thus, patients need to be counseled about follow-up with audiometry and the use of hearing aids.

Severe nerve deafness, particularly when associated with tinnitus, may produce severe depression and isolation and may even be a risk factor for suicide. Clinicians should thus inquire as to daily activities and social interaction, refer the patient to learn lip-reading if appropriate, and instruct family members to speak clearly while facing the patient. Telephone companies may also be requested to provide special audio equipment for the hearing-impaired.

As a prevention strategy in cases of hearing loss due to occupational or recreational acoustic trauma, the patient must be counseled to always use protective ear devices during excessive noise exposure. It is also important to teach the patient to equalize ear pressure when diving and to chew gum, swallow, yawn, or perform a Valsalva maneuver while pinching the nose closed to "pop" the ears when landing in airplanes. As needed (but not excessive) decongestant use may be indicated during flights and, if an upper respiratory infection is present, the patient should avoid flying and/or diving until the infection is resolved.

TINNITUS

Tinnitus is the perception of persistent sound in the ear. It is a symptom, not a disease in and of itself. Tinnitus is most often caused by changes in peripheral auditory nerve function; however, 10% of patients with tinnitus have normal hearing. Tinnitus is characterized as subjective or objective. Subjective tinnitus is perceivable only by the patient, whereas objective tinnitus is audible by the observer as well as the patient. Tinnitus can be a minor irritation for some or completely debilitating for others. Different diseases or drug toxicities can

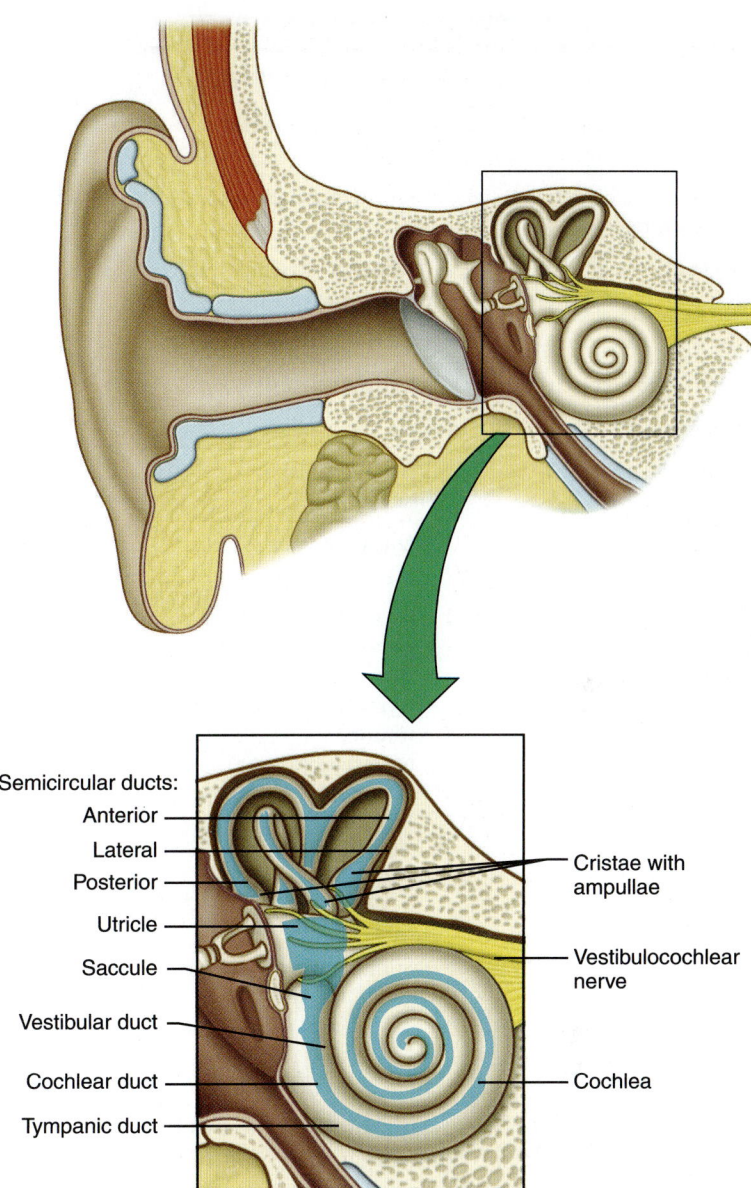

Figure 22.2 The Internal Ear

syndrome, and inner ear infection. The following sections focus on the peripheral causes of vertigo from most common to least common.

BENIGN PAROXYSMAL POSITIONAL VERTIGO

BPPV is a disorder of the inner ear with symptoms of repeated, short episodes of vertigo induced by changes in head position. Vertigo is triggered by movements of the head, especially when getting in and out of bed, turning over in bed, bending forward, or tilting the head backward. Vertigo symptoms usually last 30 to 60 seconds and up to a maximum of 2 minutes, with the average episode lasting less than 1 minute. These vertiginous episodes resolve just as spontaneously as they start. Symptoms may be described as a mild to intense sensation of the room spinning and can be associated with nausea, vomiting, or disequilibrium. Patients will have horizontal or down-beating and torsional nystagmus during an acute episode. Patients typically respond well to canalith repositioning maneuvers, as discussed later in the chapter.

EPIDEMIOLOGY AND CAUSES

BPPV is the most common cause of peripheral vertigo that occurs with changes in position of the head. The cause of BPPV is believed to be loose and free-floating otoconia that move from the utricle to the cupula of the affected semicircular canal, causing disruption of the endolymph, which sends abnormal signals from the

TABLE 22.3 Causes of Vertigo From Most to Least Common

Peripheral Causes of Vertigo	Central Causes of Vertigo
Benign paroxysmal positional vertigo	Vestibular migraines
Vestibular neuritis/labyrinthitis	Brainstem ischemia or infarction
Herpes zoster oticus (Ramsay Hunt syndrome)	Cerebellar ischemia, infarction, or hemorrhage
Ménière's disease	Chiari malformation
Labyrinthine concussion	Multiple sclerosis
Perilymphatic fistula	Episodic ataxia
Semicircular canal dehiscence	Vertebrobasilar insufficiency
Cogan's syndrome Otitis media Aminoglycoside toxicity	Central nervous system lesions • Acoustic neuroma • Meningioma • Arachnoid cyst • Cerebellopontine angle tumor • Metastatic tumor • Brainstem lesion • Arteriovenous malformation • Hemorrhage Hereditary disorders • Spinocerebellar disease

inner ear to the brain. These symptoms manifest as brief periods of vertigo and nystagmus that may be associated with nausea, vomiting, and disequilibrium.

Vertigo affects 5.6 million people per year in the United States. Of those people, up to 42% are diagnosed with BPPV. The lifetime prevalence of BPPV is 2.4%, affecting 10.7 to 140 per 100,000 and has an overall recurrence rate of up to 50%. BPPV is twice as common in females than males. The common age of onset is in the fifth or sixth decade of life; however, it is the most common vestibular disorder across all ages.

BPPV symptoms can be triggered by looking up or down, making a sudden head movement, rolling over in bed, or tilting the head. Risk factors for developing BPPV include sustained recumbent positions, sustained vibratory stimuli, sudden linear accelerations of the head, traumatic head injury, as well as associated medical conditions such as osteoporosis, diabetes mellitus, hyperlipidemia, Ménière's disease, vestibular neuritis, migraines, and hypertension. Changes in barometric pressure, lack of sleep, stress, or dehydration can also worsen BPPV symptoms.

PATHOPHYSIOLOGY

The pathophysiology underlying BPPV is related to loose, free-floating otoconia/otolith debris that enters the semicircular canals (canalithiasis). This debris or otoconia detach from the neuroepithelium of the utricular macula as a result of degeneration or insult to the vestibular system and subsequently collect near the cupula of the affected semicircular canal. These displaced otoconia cause a disruption of the flow of endolymph within the semicircular canal, which sends abnormal signals from the vestibular system to the brain.

The posterior semicircular canal is the most inferior canal, oriented vertically and intersecting with the superior canal at a 90-degree angle. The posterior semicircular canal detects movement in the coronal plane and rotation of the head around the anteroposterior axis, causing symptoms when moving the head to touch the shoulders. The anterior (superior) semicircular canal is in the vertical plane, intersecting with the posterior canal at a 90-degree angle. The anterior or superior semicircular canal detects movement in the sagittal plane, causing symptoms with movement of the head up and down (nodding). The lateral or horizontal semicircular canal head is the shortest canal, oriented horizontally, and detects movement in the transverse plane, causing symptoms with movement of the head when turning left to right.

CLINICAL PRESENTATION

Subjective

Symptoms of BPPV are characterized by acute, brief episodes (lasting less than 2 minutes) of postural vertigo without associated symptoms of hearing loss, aural fullness, tinnitus, or migraines. Symptoms can be described as feeling as if the room is spinning or the patient is spinning or whirling, with associated symptoms of loss of balance or unsteadiness, nausea, or vomiting. These symptoms are short (lasting less than 1 minute) but may occur multiple times a day. Classic movements that elicit BPPV include turning the head from side to side, rolling over in bed, making a sudden head movement, and looking up and down quickly (nodding). It is important to ask the patient to describe the dizziness symptoms to differentiate between lightheadedness and vertigo. Identifying acute versus chronic symptoms, precipitating factors, duration of vertiginous symptoms, and other associated symptoms help make the diagnosis of BPPV versus other etiologies (see Box 22.4).

Objective

The physical examination of the patient with suspected BPPV includes a neurological examination assessing CNs and a thorough head and neck examination. The examination of a patient with BPPV reveals no neural deficits

> **Box 22.4 Obtaining History of Present Illness - What to ask the patient with vertigo**
>
> **History of Present Illness**
> - Do you have a spinning or whirling sensation of your surroundings or yourself?
> - Do you feel spinning mostly when your head is moved?
> - Does the dizziness last less than 3 minutes?
> - Which position makes you dizzier?
>   - Lying down or getting out of bed? (Indicates posterior canal benign paroxysmal positional vertigo [BPPV])
>   - Turning your head or body when lying down? (Indicates horizontal canal BPPV)
> - How long does the dizziness induced by head turning last?
>   - Less than 1 minute?
>   - More than 1 minute?
> - Do you have any associated symptoms such as tinnitus, aural fullness, nausea, vomiting, headache, hearing loss?
>
> **Past Medical History**
> - Is there a history of osteoporosis, Ménière's disease, head trauma, diabetes mellitus, migraine headache, hypertension, carotid artery stenosis, stroke, transient ischemic attacks (TIAs), previous history of BPPV or canalith repositioning procedures?
>
> **Surgical History**
> - Any otological surgeries?

and a normal otological examination. A Dix-Hallpike maneuver is the gold standard test to diagnose posterior semicircular canal BPPV, which is the most common type of BPPV (85% of BPPV cases). Before performing the Dix-Hallpike test, inform the patient that it will likely elicit vertigo. The examiner may want to have a container readily available in case the patient feels nauseous and vomits.

The Dix-Hallpike maneuver is performed with the examiner standing to the left or right of the patient. The examiner will have the patient seated upright on a table with their head turned 45 degrees toward the examiner. The patient's head is then manually supported and quickly moved from the seated position to a supine position, with the head turned 45 degrees to one side, the ear angled 20 degrees toward the patient's shoulder, and the chin elevated in the air. Once in the supine position, the patient's head should be hanging off the edge of the table and supported by the clinician. The patient must be told to keep their eyes open the entire time to assess the ocular movements for latency, duration, and direction of nystagmus. The patient should stay in the supine position for about 30 seconds while being observed. The patient can then be brought back up to a seated position after 30 seconds, and the maneuver can be repeated on the patient's other side.

To confirm the diagnosis of BPPV, the nystagmus elicited by the Dix-Hallpike maneuver will be either torsional (rotary), upward-beating (toward the forehead), or a mixture of the two. The nystagmus usually has a latency period and then proceeds more quickly until it builds to a peak and then stops. Symptoms usually last from 5 to 20 seconds, and the nystagmus may fatigue after repeated Dix-Hallpike maneuvers.

In posterior canal BPPV, vertigo associated with torsional up-beating nystagmus (toward the affected ear) is seen. The maneuver can be repeated bilaterally to determine which ears are involved. Anterior canal BPPV causes a fine down-beating nystagmus that can last for a few minutes. Anterior canal BPPV can occur in patients recently treated with an Epley maneuver (a physical procedure designed to reposition canaliths in the semicircular canals) or home exercises. As described in the later section on management of BPPV, the Epley maneuver may be difficult to tolerate for patients who are not physically agile, have neck mobility limitations, or experience shortness of breath when lying down. Similarly, contraindications to performing a Dix-Hallpike maneuver include recent neck surgery or injury, severe rheumatoid arthritis, carotid sinus syncope, cervical myelopathy or radiculopathy, or vascular dissection syndrome.

If the patient has a history of symptoms compatible with BPPV but there is no nystagmus noted on the Dix-Hallpike test, the clinician should perform a supine head roll test to evaluate the lateral semicircular canal. Lateral canal BPPV is the second most common form of BPPV and differs from posterior canal BPPV symptoms as horizontal nystagmus is stimulated when turning the head from side to side while supine. The supine head roll test is performed by positioning the patient supine with the head in a neutral position. A pillow can be placed under the head to place the head and neck in approximately 30 degrees of flexion. The clinician stands at the head of the bed and informs the patient that the maneuver may elicit vertigo. The clinician quickly rotates (rolls) the patient's head 90 degrees to one side, assessing the eyes for nystagmus. In a positive test, the nystagmus can have a latency of 5 to 10 seconds and last for up to 1 minute. If no nystagmus occurs or once the nystagmus resolves, that patient's head is returned to the neutral position, and the clinician then turns the patient's head quickly to the opposite side 90 degrees, again assessing for nystagmus. A positive test elicits the symptom of vertigo with visualized horizontal nystagmus.

Two types of nystagmus can diagnose lateral semicircular canal BPPV. The geotropic type of nystagmus, which is more common, occurs when the patient is rolled to the affected side, which causes an intense horizontal nystagmus beating down toward the affected ear (geotropic = toward the ground), with less intense down-beating on the unaffected side. In this form of BPPV, the otoliths are located within the long arm of the semicircular canal (canalolithiasis). The apogeotropic type of nystagmus, which is less common, occurs when the nystagmus beats toward the upper ear (apogeotropic = toward the sky). The side that that nystagmus is beating toward is opposite the affected ear. In the apogeotropic type, the otoliths are located close to the ampulla (cupulolithiasis).

DIAGNOSTIC REASONING

Diagnostic Testing

The diagnosis of BPPV is based on history, physical examination, and a positive result on the Dix-Hallpike test or supine head roll test. There are no laboratory or imaging tests that will diagnose BPPV. Vestibular testing is not recommended for patients who meet diagnostic criteria for BPPV unless they exhibit additional vestibular signs or the symptoms are inconsistent with BPPV. In some cases where nystagmus is suspected but not clearly seen, video-oculographic recordings of nystagmus can be used to document ocular movements and slowly replay them back for evaluation. In patients who present with inconclusive BPPV symptoms or additional vestibular pathology, vestibular testing can be ordered, which includes a battery of tests to assess multiple components of the vestibular system, ocular motility, and balance.

Differential Diagnosis

The diagnosis of BPPV is made from a characteristic patient history revealing typical symptoms, including brief episodes (lasting less than 1 minute) of vertigo elicited by head movements in the absence of hearing changes, aural fullness, pressure changes, headaches, or tinnitus. These characteristics should lead the clinician to perform a Dix-Hallpike test or supine head roll test to confirm the diagnosis.

Causes of dizziness that can be confused with BPPV include orthostatic hypotension, cervical vertigo, and medication-induced vertigo. Orthostatic hypotension causes the patient to experience lightheadedness or have symptoms of syncope with changes in body position, especially going from sitting or lying flat to standing. If a patient complains of these symptoms, orthostatic blood pressure measurements should be taken to confirm. Cervical vertigo occurs in patients with degenerative cervical spine disease and may cause episodic vertigo with rotation of the head while in an upright position in the absence of nystagmus.

Other vestibular disorders that can cause vertigo include Ménière's disease, vestibular neuritis, labyrinthitis, superior canal dehiscence, vertebrobasilar insufficiency, and central positional vertigo (see Table 22.4). Ménière's disease is characterized by two or more episodes of vertigo lasting 20 minutes to 12 hours and associated with fluctuating hearing loss, roaring tinnitus, and aural fullness in the affected ear. Vestibular neuritis (inflammation of the vestibular branch of the vestibulocochlear nerve) and labyrinthitis (inflammation of both the vestibular and cochlear branches of the vestibulocochlear nerve) are closely related disorders that are typically caused by a viral illness, with a gradual onset of severe vertigo developing over hours and lasting for days to weeks. Usually described as the "worst vertigo," these disorders are present at rest and accompanied by nausea, vertigo, sweating, and pallor. Superior canal dehiscence symptoms include acute, sudden vertigo with oscillopsia elicited by loud noise, coughing, sneezing, or a Valsalva maneuver. Superior canal dehiscence is associated with conductive hearing loss. A perilymphatic fistula can occur after middle ear surgery and can cause episodic vertigo with fluctuating hearing loss.

Neurological disorders can also cause vertigo and should be ruled out. Nystagmus findings that are specific to central causes of vertigo include spontaneous nystagmus that is purely vertical or purely torsional, direction-changing nystagmus (i.e., beats to the right with right gaze and beats to the left with left gaze), and nystagmus that occurs at rest or without positional changes. Spontaneous nystagmus with fixation suppression (reducing or stopping the nystagmus by fixing the gaze on one spot) may also be a sign of a central cause. Central causes of vertigo include vestibular migraine, brainstem or cerebellar stroke, transient ischemic attacks (TIAs) of the posterior circulation, intracranial tumors, and demyelinating diseases. Vestibular migraine, in particular, is a very common central cause of vertigo, with symptoms of vertigo lasting from 5 minutes to 72 hours and associated with headache, photophobia, phonophobia, and aura. Brainstem and cerebellar strokes may generate sudden onset vertigo with neurological findings such as dysarthria (difficulty controlling speech due to paralysis or weakness of the muscles involved, such as in the tongue

TABLE 22.4 Medical Conditions that Cause Vertigo

Otological Disorders	Neurological Disorders	Other
• Ménière's disease	• Vestibular migraines	• Anxiety
• Vestibular neuritis	• Posterior circulation transient ischemic attack or stroke	• Cervicogenic vertigo
• Labyrinthitis		• Medication side effects
• Superior canal dehiscence	• Demyelinating diseases	• Postural hypotension
• Post-traumatic vertigo	• Central nervous system lesions	• Metabolic conditions
• Perilymphatic fistula	• Vertebrobasilar insufficiency	
• Inner ear lesions	• Central positional vertigo	

or larynx); dysmetria (an inability to smoothly coordinate movements due to a lack of control over the speed, range, and distance of bodily motions); dysphagia; and sensory or motor loss. If an intracranial tumor is the cause of vertigo, it will typically generate other neurological findings as determined by its location, size, and rate of growth, whereas demyelinating diseases may manifest with various combinations of motor and/or sensory deficits.

MANAGEMENT

Canalith repositioning procedures (CRPs) are very effective in the treatment of posterior and lateral semicircular canal BPPV. There are many types of CRPs, the most common of which are discussed here (see Table 22.5). Two effective CRPs for the treatment of posterior semicircular canal BPPV are the Epley maneuver and the Semont liberatory maneuver. After a BPPV diagnosis has been confirmed, the Epley or Semont maneuver can be performed to move malpositioned otolith debris from the posterior semicircular canal back into the vestibule. Before any CRPs, the patient should be instructed that vertigo, nausea, and vomiting may be elicited with treatment. The Epley and Semont liberatory maneuvers have shown similar success rates.

During the Epley maneuver, the patient is placed in an upright position on an examination table with the head turned 45 degrees toward the affected ear, as confirmed by a prior Dix-Hallpike test. The patient is then quickly placed in the supine position with their head still turned at the 45-degree angle and then hanging posteriorly over the edge of the flat surface where they are lying (i.e., a table) about 20 degrees; this supine position with the head turned and hanging backward should be maintained for 30 seconds. The patient's head is then turned 90 degrees toward the unaffected side, with the position held for 30 seconds. Next, the patient is positioned from a supine to side-lying position with their face directed toward the floor for another 30 seconds. Lastly, the patient is brought back into a sitting position. If the patient is older, has neck issues, or has mobility issues, the test can be done without lowering the head 20 degrees back below the surface of the examination table.

The Semont liberatory maneuver can be performed with the patient sitting on a table or flat surface with the head turned away from the affected side. The patient is quickly placed in a side-lying position, toward the affected ear, with the head turned up. Keep the patient in this position for at least 20 seconds or until all nystagmus has ceased. Quickly have the patient sit back up and progress through the sitting position so that they are in the opposite side-lying position with their head facedown. Keep this position for at least 30 seconds. Have the patient then sit up at a normal rate, back to the sitting position.

Lateral semicircular canal BPPV CRP treatments can be selected, based on the affected side and type (geotropic versus apogeotropic BPPV). Geotropic BPPV is the most common and treatable cause of lateral semicircular canal BPPV. The Lempert 360-degree log roll (BBQ roll) and the Gufoni maneuver both treat geotropic lateral BPPV. For the Lempert 360-degree log roll, the patient starts lying in the supine position with the head facing the affected side. The head should then turn toward the unaffected side, while the patient keeps rolling in the same direction until the head is completely prone. To complete the roll, the patent should return to a sitting position. Each position is held for 15 to 20 seconds or until nystagmus stops. The Gufoni maneuver starts with the patient in the sitting position and then going into a side-lying position on the unaffected side for about 30 seconds. The patient's head is

TABLE 22.5 Benign Paroxysmal Positional Vertigo Diagnosis and Treatment			
Canal Involved	**Diagnostic Test**	**Expected Nystagmus**	**Treatment Maneuver**
Posterior Semicircular Canal: 85% of cases	Dix-Hallpike test	Up-beating and torsional	Epley or Semont liberatory maneuver
Anterior (Superior) Semicircular Canal: 1%-2% of cases	Dix-Hallpike test	Down-beating and vertical	Epley maneuver or may resolve spontaneously
Lateral (Horizontal) Semicircular Canal: 15%-20% of cases	Supine head roll test	Canalolithiasis (most common): Geotropic (i.e., beating downward toward affected ear) occurs on both sides, though more intense on affected side	Lempert 360-degree log roll or Gufoni maneuver
		Cupulolithiasis (less common): Apogeotropic (i.e., beating upward toward unaffected ear), more intense on unaffected side	Gufoni maneuver

then quickly turned toward the ground 45 to 60 degrees and held in this position for 1 to 2 minutes. The patient sits up again with the head held toward the unaffected shoulder until fully upright, at which point the head may then be straightened.

After treatment, the patient should have less severe symptoms and should not have any postural restrictions. If nystagmus is persistent after any of these maneuvers, the examiner can repeat the maneuver or try an alternate one, depending on the type of BPPV (Table 22.6). Medications such as vestibular suppressants (e.g., antihistamines, anticholinergics, benzodiazepines) should not be prescribed for the treatment of BPPV. Benzodiazepines and drugs for motion sickness, such as meclizine (Bonine, Antivert), can cause harmful side effects and interfere with long-term neurological compensatory mechanisms. In addition, there is no evidence that these medications are effective in the management and treatment of BPPV.

FOLLOW-UP AND REFERRAL

If a clinician cannot properly evaluate the patient with a Dix-Hallpike maneuver or perform a CRP, the clinician should refer the patient to a provider who is expert in such maneuvers, which may include some primary care providers, audiologists, physical therapists, or otorhinolaryngologists. Patients with a diagnosis of BPPV who are treated with CRP should be reassessed within 1 month to evaluate for persistent resolution of symptoms. Vertigo that does not resolve with conservative BPPV management techniques should prompt clinicians to consider concurrent vestibular disorders or central causes of vertigo that may mimic BPPV. Additional history and physical examination components should be completed to evaluate for an undiagnosed central cause. In older adults who are at risk for falls, consider vestibular rehabilitation to treat instability.

Patient Education: Benign Paroxysmal Positional Vertigo

Reassure the patient that BPPV is not life-threatening and typically self-limited. Given the risk of imbalance, safety is key, and patients should be educated on precautions to reduce fall risk such as getting up slowly from a lying position, not using ladders or driving while BPPV is active. Patients should be educated to avoid vestibular suppressant medications, such as meclizine and benzodiazepines, as they pose an increased

TABLE 22.6 Summary Evaluation and Treatment for Peripheral Vertigo			
Peripheral Vertigo Cause	**Symptoms**	**Diagnosis**	**Treatment**
Benign Paroxysmal Positional Vertigo	• Seconds to minutes of acute vertigo caused by head movements • No associated hearing loss, neurological deficits, aural fullness, tinnitus • Can be recurrent and occur multiple times per day	Diagnosis made by history, including results of Dix-Hallpike maneuver and/or supine head roll test	Canalith repositioning procedures: • Epley maneuver • Semont maneuver • Lempert 360-degree log roll • Gufoni maneuver
Ménière's Disease	• Two or more episodes of vertigo that last from 20 minutes to 12 hours, with associated symptoms of fluctuating hearing loss, aural fullness, and roaring tinnitus • Episodes are recurrent.	Diagnosis made by history and presence of fluctuating low-frequency sensorineural hearing loss on audiometry	• Dietary modifications, including low salt, no alcohol use, and no tobacco use • Vestibular suppressants in acute attacks • Conservative management: diuretics, antihistamines, betahistine (Serc) • Intratympanic corticosteroid or aminoglycoside injections with severe, refractory symptoms • Surgery in severe cases
Vestibular Neuritis	• Acute, sudden vertigo lasting hours, with worsening over the first 1-2 days and then gradually improving over weeks • No associated symptom of hearing loss (the presence of hearing loss would be consistent with the related condition of labyrinthitis) • Precipitated by a viral infection	Diagnosis made by history and physical examination with positive head thrust test and negative neurological findings	• Symptom management • Vestibular suppressants for severe vertigo • May prescribe corticosteroids, although inconclusive data • Vestibular rehabilitation

risk of adverse events and do not treat BPPV effectively; moreover, they can prolong symptoms by inhibiting central compensatory mechanisms to counter vestibular dysfunction. Patients should also be educated on performing canalith repositioning procedures at home, as described in the section on management.

MÉNIÈRE'S DISEASE

Ménière's disease (Ménière's syndrome, endolymphatic hydrops) is a clinical condition defined as two or more episodes of spontaneous vertigo attacks lasting 20 minutes to 12 hours, along with fluctuating hearing loss, roaring tinnitus, and aural fullness in the affected ear. The etiology of Ménière's disease is unclear; however, it is associated with increased endolymphatic fluid within the cochlea (endolymphatic hydrops). The increased endolymphatic volume results in both vestibular (proprioceptive, balance-related) and auditory dysfunction characterized by recurrent attacks of tinnitus, vertigo, and fluctuating low-frequency hearing loss. Although Ménière's disease is not life-threatening, episodes can cause anxiety and temporary debilitation, if untreated.

EPIDEMIOLOGY AND CAUSES

Ménière's disease is estimated to affect 50 to 200 per 100,000 adults annually in the United States. Age at onset is between 40 and 60 years, with most cases developing during the fifth decade of life. The disease is rare both in young children and in adults older than 70 years of age. Some studies indicate that Americans of European descent are at an increased risk of developing the disease. Both sexes are affected nearly equally, but some studies have reported slightly higher rates in females.

There are multiple risk factors for Ménière's disease, including stress; allergies; high dietary salt, caffeine, and alcohol intake; hormonal changes; changes in barometric pressure; and exposure to high noise levels for periods of many years. There is a reported familial history prevalence of 20% with this disease, and an associated condition is migraine headache, which is also a differential diagnosis for Ménière's disease.

PATHOPHYSIOLOGY

The precise cause of Ménière's disease is not fully established, but marked edema of the membranous labyrinth is typically observed at autopsy, and endolymphatic hydrops has been established as the defining pathological finding in the disease. Theories have implicated the inflammatory response of the inner ear in a variety of insults, including blunt trauma; viral infection; allergies; reduced or negative middle ear pressure; and various vascular, endocrine, or lipid disorders. Migraine headache and autoimmune conditions, including systemic lupus erythematosus, rheumatoid arthritis, and certain thyroid disorders, also predispose to Ménière's disease. A genetic predisposition has also been identified in 8% of people affected.

Dilation of the endolymphatic system may lead to rupture of the membranous labyrinth (see Fig. 22.2). This engorgement has been associated with excessive endolymph production; decreased resorption of fluid in the endolymphatic sac; and hypoplasia of the vestibular aqueducts housing the endolymphatic ducts, which facilitate fluid flow. Resultant mixing of the endolymph and perilymph is thought to cause degeneration of both vestibular and cochlear neuroepithelial sensory hair cells, which are particularly sensitive to ionic changes from the potassium-rich endolymph. This may result in vertigo, tinnitus, and hearing loss characteristic of Ménière's disease. Compression of the vestibular portion of CN VIII by an enlarged blood vessel is yet another etiological theory for Ménière's disease.

CLINICAL PRESENTATION

Subjective

Acute episodes of Ménière's disease last anywhere from 20 minutes to 12 hours and are characterized by sudden attacks of nausea; emesis; pallor; diaphoresis; dizziness (spatial disorientation); vertigo; roaring tinnitus; and increased pressure, aural fullness, and hearing loss in the affected ear. Patients typically refer to any vestibular symptomatology as "dizziness." Rapid movement aggravates all proprioceptive symptomatology, and patients often report a history of falls or accidents during acute episodes.

The frequency and severity of attacks may decrease over time, and hearing may improve immediately after an acute attack. However, rarely, some episodes may last for more than 24 hours. Overall, low-frequency hearing loss is typically progressive, with bilateral involvement in 10% to 50% of cases. Patients may also experience motion-related imbalance without vertigo between acute attacks. Complete hearing loss in advanced cases of Ménière's disease is associated with a cessation of vertiginous episodes.

Objective

Upon inspection, otoscopic examination typically demonstrates no apparent abnormalities, unless underlying otitis media is present. Dilation of the inner ear endolymphatic system is apparent only at autopsy.

DIAGNOSTIC REASONING

Diagnostic Tests

Diagnosis of Ménière's disease is based on a careful history, neurological assessment, and response to empiric therapy, as no specific diagnostic testing exists. Diagnostic criteria require two distinct episodes of rotational vertigo lasting at least 20 minutes to 12 hours each, along with low-frequency, fluctuating SNHL; roaring tinnitus; or a perception of aural fullness.

Audiometry will confirm low-frequency SNHL and often reveal impaired speech discrimination. Both cold and warm caloric responses are typically reduced in the affected ear, as demonstrated by electronystagmography or direct patient observation, but the direction of the fast phase of nystagmus is variable. These findings are not diagnostic for Ménière's disease, however. Vestibular function tests may be used to evaluate CN VIII function, but the results could be questionable in patients taking sedative drugs of any kind (e.g., benzodiazepines).

Differential Diagnosis

Ménière's disease is a diagnosis of exclusion and is diagnosed based on symptoms. There are numerous disorders that mimic its clinical presentation that must first be ruled out. For example, otitis media is evaluated, using otoscopic examination and culture of otic fluid. If middle ear infection is present, the tympanic membrane is typically erythematous and either edematous or retracted, with altered bony landmarks and a diminished cone of light reflex. Bubbles or an air-fluid level may be seen directly behind the membrane, and mobility is reduced or absent on insufflation with a pneumatic otoscope.

Otitis media and Ménière's disease are not mutually exclusive conditions, however, as negative middle ear pressure associated with serous otitis media may be a contributing factor to Ménière's disease. Otitis media may also precipitate a viral infection of CN VIII known as vestibular neuritis (benign recurrent vertigo), which presents as recurrent vertiginous episodes lasting for several hours and may be accompanied by severe vomiting and nausea. Vestibular neuritis may also be idiopathic, but in these patients (unlike those with Ménière's disease), auditory impairment is rarely noted.

Secondary or tertiary syphilis can also affect CN VIII and is ruled out, using a variety of immunological tests specific for its causative agent, *Treponema pallidum,* such as the microhemagglutination, fluorescent treponemal antibody, and *Treponema* immobilization assays. Acute viral or bacterial infection of the labyrinth (labyrinthitis) may also present with similar symptoms (with vertigo/imbalance and hearing loss, as both branches of the vestibulocochlear nerve are affected); however, pathogenic microorganisms are not associated with Ménière's disease because it is not of infectious etiology. Discrete lesions of the central nervous system (CNS), such as tumors or infarcts of the brain and cerebellum, as well as degenerative nervous disorders such as Parkinson's disease, multiple sclerosis, and Alzheimer's disease, may be ruled out via CT and MRI if patients present with neurological deficits. Hypothyroidism may also mimic Ménière's disease and is ruled out through measurement of both free and protein-bound thyroid hormone levels (thyroxine and triiodothyronine), as well as pituitary thyroid-stimulating hormone.

BPPV is a more common diagnosis of vestibular dysfunction than Ménière's disease in older patients who complain of dizziness. It is characterized by paroxysmal vertigo accompanied by nystagmus when lying down, turning over in bed, or tilting the head backward. In contrast to Ménière's disease, BPPV does not present with hearing loss or tinnitus.

Serum glucose levels should be evaluated to rule out hypoglycemic disorders, whereas hemoglobin and hematocrit are measured to assess anemic conditions, if suspected. Lipid disorders affecting cerebral blood flow and, in turn, vestibulocochlear function may be ruled out via serum lipid studies. Other cerebral and cardiovascular disorders, such as TIAs, vertebrobasilar ischemia, or subclavian steal syndrome, may lead to CNS ischemia and vertigo, thus mimicking Ménière's disease. However, syncope (fainting) and generalized weakness are also usually observed in those conditions, which are not seen in Ménière's disease. Angiography is used to rule out such circulatory disorders, if suspected.

Another common cause of vestibular and auditory dysfunction is iatrogenic, drug-induced ototoxicity from many commonly used drugs, including aspirin; potent diuretics; quinine; tetracyclines (particularly minocycline); many cancer chemotherapies (e.g., *cis*-platinum); and aminoglycoside antibiotics, including gentamicin, neomycin, kanamycin, and streptomycin. If use of these medications is not prolonged, ototoxicity may be reversible once drug intake has stopped. Sedative side effects of many medications, as well as undesirable multidrug interactions, are a common cause of dizziness that often accompanies tinnitus, especially in older adult patients who are at an increased risk of polypharmacy-related sequelae.

In the adult patient, acoustic neuroma causing compression of the auditory portion of CN VIII is one of the most important diagnoses of auditory dysfunction to rule out because these tumors may be life-threatening if untreated. MRI and auditory brainstem response audiometry are used to detect such neoplasms.

Finally, psychiatric diagnoses should be a major consideration, if examination and laboratory findings rule out systemic disease and specific organ involvement as the cause of vestibulocochlear dysfunction. Psychiatric illness is the second most common etiology of dizziness in older adult patients after peripheral nervous system disorders. Common conditions include depression, anxiety, panic attacks, somatization disorders, alcoholism,

MANAGEMENT

The first step in management of an acute attack of Ménière's disease is to rule out all other causes of the symptoms. Acute attacks of Ménière's disease are best treated by rest with the eyes closed and protection from falling. During an acute attack, vestibular suppressants are effective in controlling acute vertiginous symptoms, including first generation antihistamines (e.g., meclizine [Bonine] 12.5 to 25 mg every 8 hours, dimenhydrinate [Dramamine] 25 to 50 mg every 6 hours, diphenhydramine [Benadryl] 25 to 50 mg every 6 hours), benzodiazepines (e.g., diazepam [Valium] 2 to 10 mg every 8 hours, lorazepam [Ativan] 1 to 2 mg every 8 hours, clonazepam [Klonopin] 0.5 to 1 mg every 8 hours), and centrally acting medications such as anticholinergics (e.g., scopolamine, atropine). It is important to note that vestibular suppressant medications should only be given during an acute attack and not as prevention for attacks, because these medications can suppress central compensatory mechanisms that counter vertigo and are not effective at preventing attacks.

Conservative treatment is reported to be effective for managing vertigo in most patients, including dietary modifications, specifically restriction of sodium, caffeine, and alcohol. Compliance with a reduced-sodium diet may reduce vertigo spells, and adherence to a caffeine-free diet may improve function; however, patients should avoid severe sodium restriction if on diuretics. Vestibular rehabilitation may specifically reduce symptoms of unilateral peripheral vestibular dysfunction, and there are a variety of patient-oriented self-management and symptom control materials that may improve symptoms in some cases.

Importantly, there is no proven cure for Ménière's disease, and current therapy is mainly palliative in nature, with a focus on reducing or coping with symptoms, although some medications can help to prevent attacks. A trial of an antihistamine, specifically betahistine 16 mg orally three times/day, can be considered to reduce the frequency and severity of vertiginous attacks. In addition, diuretics are widely used in the treatment of Ménière's disease but may have adverse effects (especially in older adult patients); moreover, strong evidence for their efficacy is lacking. Intratympanic dexamethasone may be considered for patients with vertigo that is refractory to lifestyle changes and conservative treatments, especially if an underlying autoimmune disorder is present.

If Ménière's disease progresses bilaterally, streptomycin or gentamicin inner ear ablation therapy may be appropriate to reduce unbearable vestibular symptoms. In this approach, an aminoglycoside antibiotic is administered over a course of several days to weeks to intentionally damage the neuroepithelium of the vestibular centers in the inner ear, thus reducing related symptomatology. However, the patient's hearing must be carefully monitored both during and after this treatment to avoid damage to auditory structures.

Disabling symptoms of Ménière's disease may require surgical intervention by an otorhinolaryngologist, an approach used in 5% to 10% of all cases. For patients with normal hearing ability, decompression of the endolymphatic sac may be accomplished by surgically draining excess endolymph into the mastoid or subarachnoid spaces. For patients, whose hearing ability has degenerated and is deemed unsalvageable, the cochlea itself may be decompressed (via endolymphatic sac decompression) or directly perfused with streptomycin to relieve intractable symptoms. A more radical surgery is labyrinthectomy of the affected ear, a procedure that entirely ablates vestibular function. However, these extreme interventions will also lead to hearing loss, which is a key consideration for patients and must be understood fully.

FOLLOW-UP AND REFERRAL

If symptoms do not worsen, patients may return for follow-up in 3 to 6 weeks after treatment has been initiated. However, patients should return for reevaluation immediately if disabling symptoms such as tinnitus, vertigo, nausea, or emesis persist or newly develop. Hearing loss must be carefully monitored for progression because this is a telltale sign of an underlying, potentially life-threatening acoustic neuroma, if undiagnosed. Patients often report that previously consulted clinicians failed to take this condition seriously when they first presented with symptoms. Thus, close follow-up care of the patient with Ménière's disease provides emotionally beneficial validation as well.

Progressive bilateral hearing loss may result from Ménière's disease, leading to chronic tinnitus, deafness, or disabling vertigo. Accidental injuries, including falls, related to vestibular dysfunction may occur in the work or home setting, and patients often report an increasing inability to function productively at their jobs in the face of progressive disease. Moreover, failing to diagnose an underlying acoustic neuroma is a potentially life-threatening complication.

Referral to a specialist is necessary if symptoms worsen with treatment. Advanced diagnostic procedures such as electronystagmography or specialized vestibulocochlear function tests require referral to an audiologist. A physician consultation is also needed in cases involving persistent emesis, seizures, syncope, or fever. Such referrals usually start with an otorhinolaryngologist but may also involve a neurologist. New, unexplained symptoms (which are often due to multidrug interactions or adverse effects of medications) also require referral to a specialist for diagnosis and treatment. Streptomycin ablation therapy and surgical interventions should be directed by a qualified specialist, as the risk of serious sequelae is significant, including permanent hearing loss.

Patient Education: Ménière's disease

Patients must be encouraged to stop smoking because this aggravates all otic disorders. Stress levels should be monitored and controlled through relaxation techniques. Salt intake should be reduced to a maximum of 1 g/day to lessen the severity of future attacks. Reductions in caffeine and alcohol are also recommended. Additionally, vestibular rehabilitation through the development of self-management techniques and a symptom log has been shown to be effective in some cases. All ototoxic medications should be stopped, and polypharmacy (multiple prescription and over-the-counter drug use) should be evaluated with the aid of a specialist. Polypharmacy is a particular risk in older adult patients who develop Ménière's disease or other vestibular disorders.

Patients should be instructed to return for further evaluation if symptoms worsen or acute episodes increase in frequency. Patients need to understand that treating Ménière's disease pharmacologically is difficult, and acute attacks are best managed with quiet bedrest and careful protection from falls. To avoid accidental injuries and minimize symptoms, patients should not drive, climb ladders, work near or operate dangerous machinery, walk without assistance, read, or look directly at glaring lights during these episodes. Food intake should also be reduced during acute attacks to lessen nausea and vomiting.

VESTIBULAR NEURITIS AND LABYRINTHITIS

Vestibular neuritis (VN), also known as *vestibular neuronitis,* is a vestibular disorder that is believed to be caused by inflammation of the vestibulocochlear nerve (CN VIII). Inflammation of the vestibulocochlear nerve is presumably caused by a viral infection resulting in acute, severe, and prolonged vertigo lasting from days to weeks. VN and labyrinthitis are often used interchangeably; however, labyrinthitis has the additional symptom of sudden sensorineural hearing loss and tinnitus in the affected ear, whereas VN is not associated with hearing loss. VN and labyrinthitis must be differentiated from central causes of vertigo, as symptoms can overlap.

EPIDEMIOLOGY AND CAUSES

VN and labyrinthitis account for about 10% of patients seen for dizziness in the primary care setting. The incidence is about 3.5 per 100,000 people in the United States, although it is believed that these disorders are underdiagnosed. VN and labyrinthitis affect males and females equally and usually present between 30 and 60 years of age. These disorders are more common in the spring and early summer months and may affect multiple family members, supporting the theory of a viral etiology (i.e., endemic vertigo). Viral infections that are thought to cause VN and labyrinthitis include herpes zoster, influenza, measles, mumps, polio, and hepatitis.

PATHOPHYSIOLOGY

The pathophysiology of VN and labyrinthitis is poorly understood, although they are believed to result from a viral infection causing inflammation of the vestibulocochlear nerve. Most commonly, the patient will have symptoms after a generalized viral infection; however, the viral etiology is not always known. Of note, herpes simplex virus has been identified in the vestibular ganglia of patients who have had VN; the latent herpes simplex virus is thought to remain dormant within afferent neurons, ultimately causing inflammation and atrophy of the vestibular nerve, which results in vertigo.

CLINICAL PRESENTATION

Subjective

The history and physical examination can assist the clinician in making an accurate diagnosis. The clinician should distinguish vertigo from lightheadedness and assess the timing, severity, and associated symptoms. Asking open-ended questions to allow the patient to adequately describe their symptoms is key. Patients presenting with VN or labyrinthitis will complain of sudden, sustained, and severe vertigo that lasts hours to weeks, with hearing loss also reported in labyrinthitis. Symptoms of spinning, whirling, or tilting are common, along with difficulty standing and walking, as patients may complain of veering to the affected side. Some patients also report nausea, vomiting, sweating, and/or pallor, as well as visual disturbances, such as an oscillating visual field, mild blurring, and the perception of a jumping visual image (oscillopsia).

Objective

Physical examination is very important for diagnosing VN and labyrinthitis. Performing a head and neck evaluation with an otoscopic examination is important to determine whether there is an otic infection contributing to vertigo. A focused neurological examination—assessing cranial nerves, gait, speech, and memory—should be done if neurological deficits are apparent, to evaluate for a corresponding neurological diagnosis. If the patient has a complaint of hearing loss (as in labyrinthitis), a tuning fork examination should be done to assess if the hearing loss is sensorineural or conductive (e.g., the Weber and Rinne tests, as described earlier in the section on hearing loss). The clinician should also perform a targeted oculomotor examination of the oculomotor (CN III), trochlear (CN IV), and abducens (CN VI) cranial nerves to detect ocular muscle weakness or nystagmus. In VN, the typical type of nystagmus observed in the acute phase is horizontal with a torsional component.

Performing a head impulse test (HIT) or head thrust will help identify an impaired vestibulo-ocular reflex (VOR) in patients with the complaint of vertigo. This is done with the examiner in front of the patient, holding the patient's head between their hands. The patient is asked to focus on an object in direct view (e.g., the examiner's nose); the examiner then rotates the patient's head slowly to one side and then briskly back to midline. With a normal VOR, the patient's eyes never leave the fixed object. In an impaired VOR, the eyes lag behind the head movement, known as *corrective saccade*. This positive finding will indicate which ear (i.e., vestibular nerve) is affected. For example, in a patient with a left vestibulopathy, the abnormal VOR (i.e., eye lag) will be visualized with the quick movement of the head from the left side back to midline. A positive HIT confirms the diagnosis of peripheral vertigo. In contrast, the HIT will be negative in central causes of vertigo. Contraindications to the HIT include recent cervical surgery, head and neck trauma, and severe spinal (axial) arthritis.

If a patient with a complaint of prolonged vertigo has a negative HIT, the clinician should perform an evaluation of nystagmus and a test of skew (HINTS = **H**ead **I**mpulse test, evaluation of **N**ystagmus, and **T**est of **S**kew) to evaluate for a central cause of vertigo. To evaluate for nystagmus, the patient is observed as they look straight ahead and then to the left and right without fixating on any object. Throughout these movements, the examiner assesses whether the patient has unidirectional nystagmus, which is associated with vestibulopathy. If nystagmus is observed that changes direction or is vertical, this can indicate a central cause of vertigo. Additionally, if the nystagmus is bidirectional (i.e., gaze-evoked nystagmus that changes to the side to which the patient is looking), this could indicate the patient has had a stroke.

In the test of skew, the patient looks at the examiner's nose, and the examiner covers one of the patient's eyes with a hand or opaque paddle and then quickly moves the hand or paddle to cover the patient's other eye, observing the now uncovered eye for vertical or torsional movements. This maneuver is then repeated on the other side. If the patient has any abnormal eye movements that are associated with vertical diplopia, this suggests a central cause of the patient's vertigo.

DIAGNOSTIC REASONING

Diagnostic Tests

History and examination findings can solidify a diagnosis of VN or labyrinthitis; thus, laboratory testing is not indicated. However, appropriate diagnostic testing, such as pure tone audiometry, should be performed immediately if the patient has sudden hearing loss. CT scan or MRI should not be performed in the evaluation of VN or labyrinthitis; however, imaging should be considered if a patient presents with any neurological finding. CT scan has a low sensitivity to detect posterior circulation stroke, but CT angiography is effective in evaluating patients for vestibular artery stenosis. MRI is reliable to exclude acute ischemic strokes and intracerebral hemorrhage. Vestibular testing can be done if a patient has prolonged vertigo; however, vestibular testing should not be performed during the acute phase of VN or labyrinthitis.

Differential Diagnosis

With the prolonged symptom of vertigo, differentiating between a peripheral versus central cause is important (see Tables 22.3 and 22.4). Central causes are often more serious and need prompt diagnosis and treatment. In turn, symptoms associated with central causes of vertigo, such as a history of stroke or TIA, unilateral peripheral weakness, numbness, diplopia, dysarthria, dysphagia, headaches, cranial nerve deficits, and hearing loss, should be evaluated. For example, conditions such as hypertension, diabetes mellitus, and tobacco use increase the risk for stroke and TIA.

MANAGEMENT

The management of VN and labyrinthitis includes treating severe vertiginous symptoms. Vestibular suppressants such as first generation antihistamines, benzodiazepines, and anticholinergics (as discussed previously in the section on the management of Ménière's disease) will help to suppress vertigo. These medications should not be taken for more than 3 days, as their continued use can prevent central compensatory mechanisms of vertigo. Vestibular rehabilitation can be prescribed in patients with prolonged vertigo and balance issues.

There is conflicting evidence for the treatment of VN and labyrinthitis with corticosteroids, and the risks of corticosteroids should be assessed before prescribing. If the patient presents with sudden SNHL as in labyrinthitis, corticosteroids should be considered to prevent permanent hearing loss: prednisone 1 mg/kg/day in a single dose (not divided), with the usual dose being 60 mg daily for 10 to 14 days. Equivalent doses of methylprednisone 48 mg or dexamethasone 10 mg may also be used. The potential for spontaneous improvement in hearing is highest if a patient is treated within the first 14 days of hearing loss and decreases thereafter. Therefore, prompt treatment of SNHL is essential. If herpes zoster infection is suspected, treatment with acyclovir can be used; however, antibiotics should not be used to treat VN or labyrinthitis, given their viral etiology.

FOLLOW-UP AND REFERRAL

Patients should follow up with their primary care provider if there is prolonged emesis or an inability to keep liquids down. Excessive vomiting can lead to dehydration, which may require parenteral fluids. If symptoms do not resolve, the primary care provider may refer the patient to an otorhinolaryngologist for further evaluation and treatment of SNHL and prolonged vertiginous symptoms. If the patient has SNHL, they should be referred immediately to an audiologist for pure tone audiometry. A referral should also be made to a neurologist if there are any neurological deficits that suggest another underlying disorder beyond uncomplicated VN or labyrinthitis.

Patient Education: Vestibular Neuritis and Labyrinthitis

Patients should be reassured that VN and labyrinthitis are typically benign conditions, despite their impactful symptoms. Moreover, the clinician should reassure the patient that 95% of patients fully recover. Patients should understand how long vertiginous symptoms can last, as well as new symptoms that should prompt more rapid follow-up. For example, if symptoms worsen or continue past 3 weeks, the patient should be instructed to follow up with their primary care provider. However, if the patient develops new-onset dysarthria, dysphagia, diplopia, unilateral weakness, or any other neurological deficit, they should be instructed to go to an emergency department urgently.

Safety measures should be discussed with the patient, including not operating heavy machinery, driving, or standing on ladders during vertiginous episodes. In addition, mitigation strategies should be discussed to prevent the risk of falls. Patients must also be educated to not take vestibular suppressants longer than 3 days and that vestibular suppressants should not be used prophylactically to prevent vertiginous attacks, as they are ineffective in this regard and can cause adverse effects. Once the patient is stable, vestibular rehabilitation exercises can be discussed with the patient for long-term prevention.

REFERENCES

Benign Paroxysmal Positional Vertigo

Bhattacharyya N, Gubbels SP, Schwartz SR, et. (2017). Clinical Practice Guideline: Benign Paroxysmal Positional Vertigo (Update). *Otolaryngology—head and neck surgery: official journal of American Academy of Otolaryngology-Head and Neck Surgery*, 156(3_suppl), S1–S47. https://doi.org/10.1177/0194599816689667

Domínguez-Durán E, Domènech-Vadillo E, Álvarez-Morujo de Sande MG, et al. (2017). Analysis of risk factors influencing the outcome of the Epley maneuver. *European archives of oto-rhino-laryngology: official journal of the European Federation of Oto-Rhino-Laryngological Societies (EUFOS): affiliated with the German Society for Oto-Rhino-Laryngology - Head and Neck Surgery*, 274(10), 3567–3576. https://doi.org/10.1007/s00405-017-4674-9

Johns P, Quinn J. (2020). Clinical diagnosis of benign paroxysmal positional vertigo and vestibular neuritis. *CMAJ: Canadian Medical Association journal = journal de l'Association medicale canadienne*, 192(8), E182–E186. https://doi.org/10.1503/cmaj.190334

Kim HJ, Song JM, Zhong L, et al. (2020). Questionnaire-based diagnosis of benign paroxysmal positional vertigo. *Neurology*, 94(9), e942–e949. https://doi.org/10.1212/WNL.0000000000008876

Yetiser S. (2020). Review of the pathology underlying benign paroxysmal positional vertigo. *The Journal of international medical research*, 48(4), 300060519892370. https://doi.org/10.1177/0300060519892370

Zhu CT, Zhao XQ, Ju Y, et al. (2019). Clinical Characteristics and Risk Factors for the Recurrence of Benign Paroxysmal Positional Vertigo. *Frontiers in neurology*, 10, 1190. https://doi.org/10.3389/fneur.2019.01190

Hearing Loss

Brown CS, Emmett SD, Robler SK, et al. (2018). Global Hearing Loss Prevention. *Otolaryngologic clinics of North America*, 51(3), 575–592. https://doi.org/10.1016/j.otc.2018.01.006

Carlson ML. (2020). Cochlear Implantation in Adults. *The New England journal of medicine*, 382(16), 1531–1542. https://doi.org/10.1056/NEJMra1904407

Centers for Disease Control (2019) 2017 CDC Early Hearing Detection and Intervention (EHDI) Hearing Screening & Follow-up Survey (HSFS). Retrieved at 2007 Summary of Documented Data Items (subject to change) (cdc.gov)

Cunningham LL, Tucci DL. (2017). Hearing Loss in Adults. *The New England journal of medicine*, 377(25), 2465–2473. https://doi.org/10.1056/NEJMra1616601

Dunlap PM, Holmberg JM, Whitney SL. (2019). Vestibular rehabilitation: advances in peripheral and central vestibular disorders. *Current opinion in neurology*, 32(1), 137–144. https://doi.org/10.1097/WCO.0000000000000632

Lieu J, Kenna M, Anne S, et al. (2020) Hearing loss in children: A review. *JAMA*. 324(21): 2195-2205. doi:10.1001/jama.2020.17647

Michels TC, Duffy MT, Rogers DJ. (2019). Hearing Loss in Adults: Differential Diagnosis and Treatment. *American family physician*, 100(2), 98–108.

Naples JG, Ruckenstein MJ. (2020). Cochlear Implant. *Otolaryngologic clinics of North America*, 53(1), 87–102. https://doi.org/10.1016/j.otc.2019.09.004

Nieman CL, Oh ES. (2020). Hearing Loss. *Annals of internal medicine*, 173(11), ITC81–ITC96. https://doi.org/10.7326/AITC202012010

Nieman CL, Reed NS, Lin FR. (2018). Otolaryngology for the Internist: Hearing Loss. *The Medical clinics of North America*, 102(6), 977–992. https://doi.org/10.1016/j.mcna.2018.06.013

Shan A, Ward BK, Goman AM, et al. (2019). Prevalence of Eustachian Tube Dysfunction in Adults in the United States. *JAMA otolaryngology— head & neck surgery*, 145(10), 974–975. Advance online publication. https://doi.org/10.1001/jamaoto.2019.1917

Sulway S, Whitney SL. (2019). Advances in Vestibular Rehabilitation. *Advances in oto-rhino-laryngology*, 82, 164–169. https://doi.org/10.1159/000490285

U.S. Preventive Services Task Force, Krist AH, Davidson KW, Mangione CM, et al. (2021). Screening for Hearing Loss in Older Adults: US Preventive Services Task Force Recommendation

Statement. *JAMA*, *325*(12), 1196–1201. https://doi.org/10.1001/jama.2021.2566

Ménière's Disease

Basura GJ, Adams ME, Monfared A, et al. (2020). Clinical Practice Guideline: Meniere's Disease. *Otolaryngology—head and neck surgery: official journal of American Academy of Otolaryngology-Head and Neck Surgery*, *162*(2_suppl), S1–S55. https://doi.org/10.1177/0194599820909438

Bernaerts A, De Foer B. (2019). Imaging of Meniere's Disease. *Neuroimaging clinics of North America*, *29*(1), 19–28. https://doi.org/10.1016/j.nic.2018.09.002

Espinosa-Sanchez JM, Lopez-Escamez JA. (2020). The pharmacological management of vertigo in Meniere disease. *Expert opinion on pharmacotherapy*, *21*(14), 1753–1763. https://doi.org/10.1080/14656566.2020.1775812

Gibson W. (2019). Meniere's Disease. *Advances in oto-rhino-laryngology*, *82*, 77–86. https://doi.org/10.1159/000490274

Nevoux J, Barbara M, Dornhoffer J, et al. (2018). International consensus (ICON) on treatment of Meniere's disease. *European annals of otorhinolaryngology, head and neck diseases*, *135*(1S), S29–S32. https://doi.org/10.1016/j.anorl.2017.12.006

Wu V, Sykes EA, Beyea MM, et al. (2019). Approach to Meniere disease management. *Canadian family physician Medecin de famille canadien*, *65*(7), 463–467.

Yang B, Brook CD. (2017). The Role of Allergy in Otologic Disease. *Otolaryngologic clinics of North America*, *50*(6), 1091–1101. https://doi.org/10.1016/j.otc.2017.08.005

Tinnitus

Bauer CA. (2018). Tinnitus. *The New England journal of medicine*, *378*(13), 1224–1231. https://doi.org/10.1056/NEJMcp1506631

Chari DA, Limb CJ. (2018). Tinnitus. *The Medical clinics of North America*, *102*(6), 1081–1093. https://doi.org/10.1016/j.mcna.2018.06.014

Chemali Z, Nehmé R, Fricchione G. (2019). Sensory neurologic disorders: Tinnitus. *Handbook of clinical neurology*, *165*, 365–381. https://doi.org/10.1016/B978-0-444-64012-3.00022-8

Fuller TE, Haider HF, Kikidis D, et al. (2017). Different Teams, Same Conclusions? A Systematic Review of Existing Clinical Guidelines for the Assessment and Treatment of Tinnitus in Adults. *Frontiers in psychology*, *8*, 206. https://doi.org/10.3389/fpsyg.2017.00206

Piccirillo JF, Rodebaugh TL, Lenze EJ. (2020). Tinnitus. *JAMA*, *323*(15), 1497–1498. https://doi.org/10.1001/jama.2020.0697

Tang D, Li H, Chen L. (2019). Advances in Understanding, Diagnosis, and Treatment of Tinnitus. *Advances in experimental medicine and biology*, *1130*, 109–128. https://doi.org/10.1007/978-981-13-6123-4_7

U.S. Department of Veterans Affairs Veterans Benefits Administration. (2020). Annual Benefits Report: Fiscal Year 2019. Accessed May 22, 2021. https://www.benefits.va.gov/REPORTS/abr/

Wu V, Cooke B, Eitutis S, et al. (2018). Approach to tinnitus management. *Canadian family physician Medecin de famille canadien*, *64*(7), 491–495.

Vestibular Neuritis and Labyrinthitis

Bronstein AM, Dieterich M. (2019). Long-term clinical outcome in vestibular neuritis. *Current opinion in neurology*, *32*(1), 174–180. https://doi.org/10.1097/WCO.0000000000000652

Edlow JA. (2018). Diagnosing Patients With Acute-Onset Persistent Dizziness. *Annals of emergency medicine*, *71*(5), 625–631. https://doi.org/10.1016/j.annemergmed.2017.10.012

Edlow JA. (2018). Managing Patients With Acute Episodic Dizziness. *Annals of emergency medicine*, *72*(5), 602–610. https://doi.org/10.1016/j.annemergmed.2018.06.009

Gurley KL, Edlow JA. (2019). Acute Dizziness. *Seminars in neurology*, *39*(1), 27–40. https://doi.org/10.1055/s-0038-1676857

Gurley K, Edlow JA. (2021) Diagnosis of patients with acute dizziness. *Emerg Med Clin N Am.* 39; 2021: 181-201. doi.org/10.1016/j.emc.2020.09.011

Le TN, Westerberg BD, Lea J. (2019). Vestibular Neuritis: Recent Advances in Etiology, Diagnostic Evaluation, and Treatment. *Advances in oto-rhino-laryngology*, *82*, 87–92. https://doi.org/10.1159/000490275

Lee JY, Park JS, Kim MB. (2019). Clinical Characteristics of Acute Vestibular Neuritis According to Involvement Site. *Otology & neurotology: official publication of the American Otological Society, American Neurotology Society [and] European Academy of Otology and Neurotology*, *40*(6), 797–805. https://doi.org/10.1097/MAO.0000000000002226

Tsang B, Chen A, Paine M. (2017). Acute evaluation of the acute vestibular syndrome: differentiating posterior circulation stroke from acute peripheral vestibulopathies. *Internal medicine journal*, *47*(12), 1352–1360. https://doi.org/10.1111/imj.13552

Walter AJ. (2020). Vestibular neuritis. *CMAJ: Canadian Medical Association journal = journal de l'Association medicale canadienne*, *192*(25), E686. https://doi.org/10.1503/cmaj.75014

Whitman GT. (2018). Dizziness. *The American journal of medicine*, *131*(12), 1431–1437. https://doi.org/10.1016/j.amjmed.2018.05.014

RESOURCES

General

American Academy of Otolaryngology: Head and Neck Surgery
http://www.entnet.org/

Hearing Loss

Hearing Loss Association of America
http://www.hearingloss.org/

National Institute on Deafness and Other Communication Disorders
https://www.nidcd.nih.gov/

Tinnitus

American Tinnitus Association
https://www.ata.org/understanding-facts

Chapter 23

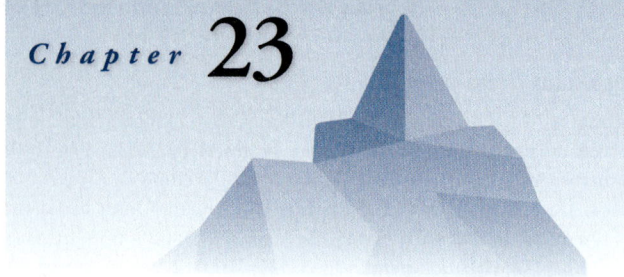

Inflammatory and Infectious Disorders of the Ear

Maria Colandrea, DNP, NP-C, CORLN, CCRN, FAANP
Michael E. Zychowicz, DNP, ANP, ONP, FAAN, FAANP
Brian Oscar Porter, MD, PhD, MPH, MBA

OTITIS EXTERNA (SWIMMER'S EAR)

Otitis externa (OE) (also called *swimmer's ear*) is an inflammation of the lining of the auditory canal and/or contiguous structures of the outer ear. The term refers to a wide spectrum of both acute and chronic inflammatory processes that may be diffuse, localized, or invasive in nature. This disorder is largely benign and self-limited, albeit painful. Of note, invasive OE (malignant OE, necrotizing OE) is a potentially life-threatening disease, which requires immediate diagnosis and management to prevent life-threatening complications.

EPIDEMIOLOGY AND CAUSES

OE has a 10% lifetime occurrence and can occur acutely (symptoms lasting less than 6 weeks) or chronically (symptoms lasting more than 6 weeks). In 98% of cases, OE is an acute illness resulting from a bacterial infection. In acute otitis externa (AOE), the most common causative bacteria are *Pseudomonas aeruginosa* (20% to 60% prevalence) and *Staphylococcus aureus* (10% to 70% prevalence). Chronic otitis externa (COE) may result from inadequately treated otitis media (OM) with continuous serous or exudative drainage from the middle ear into the auditory canal. Additionally, fungal infections are more commonly seen in COE. No ethnic or racial predispositions to OE have been documented, and males and females are affected equally.

Immunocompromised persons or individuals with chronic conditions such as diabetes mellitus are at a greater risk for developing infectious OE and, in particular, necrotizing OE. Necrotizing OE most commonly affects older males, particularly with diabetes mellitus, as well as those who are immunocompromised. Deep tissue invasion may be related to decreased polymorphonuclear neutrophil function and/or microvascular disease associated with diabetes mellitus. OE caused by fungus (otomycosis) is significantly more prevalent in the summer months, in tropical locations, and in the southeastern United States; however, in general, environmental changes are the most common risk factors for OE.

OE occurs when the protective processes within the ear canal are disrupted. Cerumen, which is bacteriostatic, is produced by cerumen glands within the proximal ear canal. Cerumen keeps the auditory canal slightly acidic and acts as a barrier to moisture. When this process is disrupted, the pH of the auditory canal shifts from acidic to alkaline, causing the auditory canal to become conducive to pathogenic colonization. In addition, an increase in temperature and/or humidity can cause infections by weakening skin barriers within the external ear canal, which may also predispose the external ear to infection. Moisture associated with swimming in hot, humid weather, especially in polluted water, is the most common cause of OE (hence, the term "swimmer's ear"). Highly chlorinated pool water can also contribute to this disorder because it can dry out the ear canal, creating a potential portal of entry for bacteria and fungi.

Inadequate cerumen (earwax) production removes another critical nonspecific barrier to infection. Manual picking of the ear, foreign bodies in the auditory canal, and the prolonged use of earplugs, hearing aids, or cotton swabs may all contribute to local irritation of the external ear, as well as predispose to infection. Other risk factors include previous ear infections, as well as skin allergies, particularly those sensitive to hair sprays and dyes that may enter the ear canal and cause contact dermatitis. In fact, dermatitis processes often precede microbial infection of the auditory canal because they create a potential portal of entry through the skin for pathogens.

PATHOPHYSIOLOGY

Pathogenic colonization of the external ear is prevented by several immune and anatomical mechanisms. The keratinizing squamous epithelia of the ear canal continually sloughs, and the hair follicles that line the outer third of the canal rhythmically sweep laterally, acting as a natural cleansing mechanism and mechanical barrier to the accumulation of matter in the auditory canal. The production of viscous, hydrophobic cerumen in the auditory canal maintains an acidic pH and repels moisture, both of which antagonize bacterial growth. In addition, the presence of competing, nonpathogenic endogenous microbial flora inhibits the overgrowth of more virulent bacteria along the auditory canal. If any of these protective mechanisms is compromised, pathogenic colonization by bacteria or fungi normally found in the auditory canal may occur, resulting in AOE.

Bacterial agents of infectious OE include *P. aeruginosa*, *S. aureus*, and group A *Streptococcus pyogenes*, which is associated with localized disease, presenting as a folliculitis, or more frequently as outer ear erysipelas. Polymicrobial infection has also been noted in up to one-third of cases of diffuse disease, and the anaerobic bacteria *Bacteroides* and *Peptostreptococcus* have been cited in up to one-fourth of cases. Commonly identified fungal agents include *Aspergillus niger* (which typically causes focal lesions but may occasionally lead to invasive disease with bony involvement in immunocompromised patients), *Malassezia pachydermatis,* and *Candida albicans.*

Additional risk factors (see Risk Factors: Otitis Externa), if not direct causes of OE, include local skin maceration; traumatic injury; stenosis of the ear canal; and hyperkeratotic processes such as eczema, psoriasis, contact dermatitis, and/or seborrheic dermatitis. The anatomy of the outer ear, which includes the tragus and conchal cartilage, serves as a physical barrier to foreign body entry into the outer ear canal. When patients excessively clean the ear with cotton swabs or other devices, it may leave small pieces of foreign matter in the canal, where they eventually disintegrate due to the canal's acidic pH, serving as a nidus of infection. This irritation in turn leads to pruritus, and excessive scratching of the ear canal only aggravates this cycle of epithelial damage and infection by creating physical access through this normally protective barrier.

Risk Factors: Otitis Externa

Anatomical risk factors

- Stenosis of the external ear canal
- Overgrowth of hair in the external ear canal
- Bony growths (exostoses)

Environmental

- High humidity
- Hot environments
- Swimming pools
- Soap or shampoo

Skin-related causes

- Eczema
- Psoriasis
- Seborrhea
- Keratosis obturans
- Other inflammatory diseases of the skin

Trauma

- Manual manipulation of the ear canal with or without foreign objects
- Cleaning the ear too much with repeated irrigations or cotton swabs
- Earplugs
- Foreign bodies
- Traumatic cerumen removal
- Ill-fitting hearing aids

Other causes

- Absence or decreased cerumen production
- Prior ear surgery
- Radiation therapy to the head and neck region
- Diabetes mellitus
- Immunosuppression
- Metabolic diseases

Necrotizing OE (formerly known as malignant OE) is the most severe infectious form of external otitis and is considered a medical emergency. Necrotizing OE is a bacterial infection that extends from the skin of the auditory canal into the soft tissues, cartilage, and bone in the temporal region or base of the skull (i.e., skull osteomyelitis). *P. aeruginosa* accounts for over 90% of cases, although invasive fungal disease in immunocompromised individuals may also extend to multiple tissues. Multiple cranial nerves may become involved, increasing morbidity, and death may result from septic thromboemboli to vessels of the brain if inadequately treated.

CLINICAL PRESENTATION

Subjective

It is critical to obtain a thorough history of present illness to identify patients who may be at increased risk for severe disease. The most common presenting complaint of patients with AOE is an acute, often severe otalgia of sudden or gradual onset. Pain may worsen at night and disturb sleep. It is exacerbated by pulling the pinna or earlobe or by applying pressure to the tragus. Chewing may also elicit otic pain. In necrotizing OE, the most common complaint is severe ear pain, often out of proportion to findings on the examination. Pain is associated with severe headache that is worse at night and disrupts sleep.

In the early stages of AOE, the affected ear may feel full or obstructed, and a temporary conductive hearing loss related to luminal occlusion on the affected side is common if there is edema, otorrhea, or debris. The affected ear may also be pruritic. Complaints of purulent discharge with or without a foul odor may be evident in bacterial disease, and systemic symptomatology such as fever or chills, although rare, may accompany cases of infectious etiology. COE usually presents with the main complaint of pruritus of the ear canal and may be associated with otorrhea. The ear canal in COE may be dry, scaly, slightly red and edematous, and there is usually an absence of cerumen.

Objective

Thorough evaluation of the head and neck with an otoscopic examination of the external ear and ear canal are critical. A classic sign of AOE is tenderness on traction of the pinna and/or applying pressure over the tragus. On otoscopic examination, the auditory canal typically appears edematous and erythematous, which may prevent full visualization of the external canal and tympanic membrane; there also may be accumulation of purulent drainage in cases of bacterial infection. Diffuse cases present with nearly complete involvement of the auditory canal, whereas localized processes are recognized as focal lesions (pustules or furuncles) anywhere along the auditory canal or external ear structures.

Otorrhea may be apparent in infectious cases. *Pseudomonas* infection produces a copious green exudate, whereas *Staphylococcus* infection presents as a yellow, crusting, purulent exudate. Fungal infections present as a fluffy white or black malodorous carpet of growth, with or without visualized fungal spores, whereas allergic reactions are characterized by scaly, cracked, and/or weepy tissue along the outer ear and auditory canal. Granulation tissue spreading out from the primary site of infection and eroding into the temporal bone, outer auricle, or through a perforated tympanic membrane is indicative of frank invasive disease.

Except in invasive disease or cases related to chronic OM, head and neck lymphadenopathy typically is not detected. Invasive disease, on the other hand, may be accompanied by tenderness of the temporomandibular joint (TMJ) and/or lymphadenopathy.

DIAGNOSTIC REASONING

Diagnostic Tests

Laboratory tests are rarely needed if symptomatology clearly fits the classic clinical picture of OE. However, any fluid from the ear may be cultured and, if microorganisms are detected, tested for antibiotic sensitivity. This may be particularly important in determining alternative treatment approaches for patients who do not respond promptly to empirical antibiotic therapy or for those with COE, particularly with purulent exudates indicative of bacterial infection. Cultures and antibiotic sensitivity testing are also important for immunocompromised patients because their disease may be caused by rare pathogens or even by endogenous, typically nonpathogenic microbial flora. Fungi and mycobacteria should be ruled out as sources of infection.

Soft tissue or bony involvement in malignant disease may be assessed by diagnostic imaging. Computed tomography (CT) will detect bony involvement, whereas magnetic resonance imaging (MRI) will be more diagnostic for soft tissue and nerve involvement. A clinical diagnosis of necrotizing OE can be confirmed with a raised erythrocyte sedimentation rate plus an abnormal CT or MRI scan. On CT, cortical bone erosion in the external auditory canal with inflammatory changes in adjacent structures may be present. In addition, there may be opacification of the mastoid air cells and middle ear from extension of the infection. It is important to remember that at least one-third of bone mineral must be lost before radiological changes become apparent. Plain films and gallium or technetium-99 bone scans may also detect bony involvement, but these imaging techniques are less desirable because they lack specificity and, in the case of x-ray films, sensitivity.

Differential Diagnosis

In the absence of visible changes in the auditory canal and tympanic membrane, otalgia from referred pain associated with other disorders must be ruled out. These disorders include TMJ dysfunction, dental disease, neurological disorders such as trigeminal and glossopharyngeal neuralgia, parotitis, or rarely, tumors of the head and neck. Chondrodermatitis nodularis chronicus helicis may also cause otalgia-like OE in older patients, manifesting as an extremely tender nodule of the inner ear helix. TMJ dysfunction and dental disease may be specifically ruled out via dental x-ray films to demonstrate alterations in joint morphology or dentition. In general, a thorough head and neck examination, complete with cranial nerve testing, will typically differentiate among the causes of ear pain (see Differential Diagnoses 23.1).

Although OE and OM may coincide, OM may be distinguished from OE by changes in the tympanic membrane that are characteristic of middle ear infection, including erythema, edema, and a significant lack of mobility on insufflation with a pneumatic otoscope. Moreover, movement of the tragus also fails to elicit pain in middle ear infection. Excessive cerumen buildup may lead to AOE because of water getting trapped behind the cerumen. OM should be suspected if continuous discharge from the middle ear is evident for more than 10 days. Otoscopic examination may rule out alternative pathologies, including other dermatological disorders such as impetigo, herpes zoster infection, and even insect bites.

Serious cranial infections requiring aggressive therapy must also be considered. Mastoiditis is characterized by fever, spontaneous rupture of the tympanic membrane, tenderness, edema, and erythema posterior to the auricle, as well as by palpable preauricular and anterior cervical lymph nodes. In addition, the mastoid process is exquisitely painful in mastoiditis. In meningitis, patients typically present with fever, diffuse headache, altered mentation, vomiting, and cervical stiffness. A recent history of upper respiratory tract infection (URI) may be a clue to these and other infectious processes, including sinusitis and OM.

Blood in the auditory canal may indicate trauma to the external ear canal or the presence of an invasive

Differential Diagnoses 23.1: Otitis Externa

Differential Diagnosis	Potential Symptoms
Acute otitis externa	- Symptoms often acute, duration of 6 weeks or less - Otalgia less than 48-hour duration - Pain with pushing on the tragus and/or pulling on the pinna - Pruritus - Aural fullness - May or may not have decreased hearing - Otorrhea - Diffuse erythema and/or edema of the ear canal
Chronic otitis externa - May result from inadequately treated otitis externa - Otomycosis (fungal otitis externa) - Cholesteatoma	- Symptoms lasting 6 weeks or more - Pruritus - Aural fullness - May or may not have hearing loss - Pain is not acute - Edema - Erythema - Otorrhea - In otomycosis, otoscopic examination may reveal brown, black, or white debris with fungal spores - Cholesteatoma often occurs in the anterior superior portion of the ear. They may present with retraction pockets in the tympanic membrane with keratin and squamous debris. May also present with white or yellow masses behind the tympanic membrane. Often associated with a chronically draining ear and hearing loss.
Necrotizing (malignant) otitis externa	- Predominately affects older, diabetic, or immunocompromised patients - Symptoms same as AOE but pain more severe and often associated with severe headaches - Deep, stabbing pain worse with head motion - Pain worse at night - Cellulitis of ear canal which can extend to auricle - Facial nerve paralysis - Fever - Dysphagia or dysphonia - Granulation tissue often seen on the inferior portion of the ear canal
Otitis media	- Absence of pain when tragus is pushed or pinna is pulled - Otalgia - Otorrhea if tympanic membrane is perforated - Bulging tympanic membrane - Edema/erythema of tympanic membrane - No tympanic membrane movement with pneumatic otoscopy - Loss of light reflex upon otoscopy - Presence of purulent fluid or amber fluid behind tympanic membrane - Hearing loss - Vertigo - Fever - Upper respiratory or allergy symptoms before presentation of otalgia

Continued

Differential Diagnoses 23.1: Otitis Externa—cont'd

Differential Diagnosis	Potential Symptoms
Inflammatory skin conditions • Eczema • Seborrheic dermatitis • Psoriasis • Lupus erythematous • Keratosis obturans • Allergic dermatitis	• Chronic pruritus • Dry skin in ear canal with xerotic scaling • Hyperkeratosis • Hyperpigmentation • Lichenification • Erythema • Often presents with other skin involvement in addition to the ear
Temporomandibular joint (TMJ) syndrome/dysfunction	• Otalgia (unilateral or bilateral) with normal ear examination • Pain radiating to neck, temple, and preauricular area • Pain with jaw movement • Crepitus over joint • Flat dental surfaces that indicate bruxism • Recent dental work • Disarticulation of the jaw with chewing or abduction of jaw
Dental pathology	• Otalgia (unilateral or bilateral) with normal ear examination • Abscess around tooth/teeth • Fever/chills
Furunculosis	• Otalgia • Otorrhea • Localized tenderness • Localized swelling • Pustular lesion
Herpes zoster oticus (Ramsay Hunt syndrome)	• Vesicles in the ear canal or on the ear • Severe otalgia • Facial paralysis or paresis • Loss of taste on the anterior tongue • Decreased lacrimation
Cancer of the ear canal or external ear	• Lesion of the external ear or ear canal that does not heal and increases in size • Bloody drainage • Erythema or granulation tissue • Pain • Facial nerve paresis in extensive cancer

tumor. Carcinoma should be considered if invasive disease is suspected or there are any lesions present within the ear canal. A biopsy of the lesion or granulation tissue will facilitate the diagnosis. Other noninfectious diagnoses that may be ruled out through biopsy include primary skin and cartilage disorders such as sarcoidosis, discoid lupus, and trauma-related perichondritis of the pinna. Perichondritis may also be of infectious origin caused by *P. aeruginosa*, as confirmed by culture. Gouty tophi may also affect the external ear, but they are usually painless. Rarer infectious conditions that should be ruled out by special stains, cultures, and antigen/antibody tests in refractory cases include tuberculous otitis and leprosy (both diagnosed by acid-fast stain for *Mycobacteria*) and syphilitic otitis (diagnosed by rapid plasma reagin [RPR] and Venereal Disease Research Laboratory [VDRL] tests and dark-field microscopy to identify the causative agent, *Treponema pallidum*).

MANAGEMENT

Treatment of OE includes pain management, medical therapy, treatment of underlying conditions as applicable, and patient education. If the ear canal is obstructed with cerumen or debris, gentle débridement is recommended, and patients should be referred to an otolaryngologist for débridement if the primary care provider lacks appropriate experience or tools to perform such a procedure. Identifying if the tympanic membrane is perforated is also important in determining medical management, as potentially ototoxic ear drops should be avoided if the provider is unsure as to the status of the tympanic membrane.

Pain Management

Because the predominant symptom of OE is pain, the patient's alteration in comfort is a primary focus of care. Medical management of the disease should focus on alleviating pain promptly, which includes the following measures:

- Local application of heat to the outer ear can offer some relief of pain.
- Some patients get relief with application of an ice pack to the outer ear.
- Nonprescription pain relievers such as aspirin or acetaminophen (325 to 650 mg by mouth [PO] every 4 hours as needed; maximum daily dose 4,000 mg/day with normal liver function) or an NSAIDs such as ibuprofen (400 to 600 mg PO every 6 to 8 hours as needed to a maximum dose of 2.4 g/day with normal kidney function and no gastrointestinal conditions) are first-line agents.
- In cases of extreme pain, acetaminophen/codeine (Tylenol #3) 325 mg/5 mg one to two tablets PO every 6 hours or acetaminophen/hydrocodone (Vicodin) 325 mg/5 mg PO one tablet every 8 hours may be prescribed for the first 24 to 48 hours, but these medications carry potential for abuse and should not be prescribed in large quantities.

Antibiotic Management

Systemic antibiotics are not recommended as initial therapy for diffuse, uncomplicated AOE unless there is extension of the infection to the auricle or the patient has risk factors such as immunosuppression or diabetes mellitus that would require systemic therapy. Diffuse bacterial OE should be treated with topical otic antibiotics, with or without an anti-inflammatory component, depending on the level of inflammation. Several preparations are available for use (see Drugs Commonly Prescribed 23.1). Occasionally, the pustules or furuncles associated with localized OE may require surgical drainage before initiating pharmacotherapy, and more serious infections refractory to topical treatment may require systemic antibiotic therapy.

Common topical otic preparations approved by the U.S. Food and Drug Administration include acetic acid/aluminum acetate, acetic acid/hydrocortisone, ciprofloxacin/hydrocortisone, ciprofloxacin/dexamethasone, neomycin/polymyxin B/hydrocortisone, and ofloxacin. Liquid ophthalmic preparations of gentamicin and tobramycin may be used in the ear to cover both *P. aeruginosa* and *S. aureus*. If the ear has extensive edema causing luminal occlusion, an absorptive 1-inch cotton wick or sponge may be inserted to facilitate delivery of otic preparations. Antibiotic drops may then be placed on the wick for the first 2 to 3 days of treatment, until swelling subsides. The patient should be reevaluated in 2 to 3 days to reexamine the ear and remove the wick. After this, drops should be placed directly into the ear canal.

For cases that are refractory to initial therapy or involve auricular cellulitis, topical antibiotics should be supplemented with systemic antibiotic treatment covering both *Staphylococcus* and *Pseudomonas*. Systemic antibiotics are also indicated in the case of specific host factors such as diabetes mellitus or in an immunosuppressed patient. Diffuse and localized OE may need to be treated with multiple various systemic antibiotic choices. If cellulitis of the periauricular skin occurs without evidence of deep tissue involvement, consider the following treatment:

- First generation cephalosporins or penicillin with relatively narrow microbial coverage, such as cephalexin (Keflex) 250 to 500 mg PO four times daily or dicloxacillin 250 to 500 mg PO four times daily.
- Second generation cephalosporins with broader spectrum microbial coverage, such as cefuroxime (Ceftin) 250 to 500 mg PO two times daily or cefdinir (Omnicef) 300 mg PO two times daily, or β-lactamase–resistant penicillins such as amoxicillin/clavulanate (Augmentin XR) 1,000 mg PO two times daily based on the amoxicillin component, which have broader-spectrum coverage.
- Ceftazidime (Fortaz) 2 g IV every 8 to 12 hours or a combination of tobramycin (1 to 1.5 mg/kg IV every 8 hours, with dosage adjusted by monitoring serum levels and renal function) and ticarcillin (3 g IV every 4 hours). These regimens, however, carry a significant risk of nephrotoxicity, ototoxicity, and bleeding diatheses.

For patients who are immunocompromised with an involved tissue infection, systemic antibiotics, in addition to topical otic antibiotics, are indicated. In these patients who may have a suspected *P. aeruginosa* and *S. aureus* infection, a quinolone such as ciprofloxacin can be given at a dose of 500 mg twice daily for adults and 10 mg/kg/dose twice daily for children (maximum 500 mg/dose) for 7 to 10 days. If necrotizing OE is diagnosed, patients will likely be admitted to the hospital and provided IV antipseudomonal therapy. Patients with invasive bony involvement may require surgical débridement of the affected area to drain abscesses and remove sequestered collagen and, therefore, should be under the care of an otolaryngologist.

For eczematous or psoriatic conditions, corticosteroid therapies such as 0.1% triamcinolone solution or cream may be applied three or four times daily to relieve symptoms. When OE has been determined to be secondary to OM, therapy should be directed toward the underlying middle ear infection. Pharmacotherapy for COE is directed by extensive antibiotic sensitivity testing after

Drugs Commonly Prescribed 23.1: Bacterial Otitis Externa

DRUG CLASS	DRUG	INDICATION	PRESCRIBING CONSIDERATIONS AND ADVERSE REACTIONS
Drugs Safe to Use with Perforated Tympanic Membrane			
Quinolones	Ciprofloxacin 0.2% and hydrocortisone 1% otic suspension (Cipro HC otic)	Treatment of moderate to severe OE Treats *Pseudomonas aeruginosa* and *Staphylococcus aureus* infection	Children older than 6 years: 4 drops in affected ear twice daily × 7 days Adults: 4 drops in affected ear twice daily × 7 days
	Ciprofloxacin 0.3% and dexamethasone 0.1% (Ciprodex otic)	Treatment of moderate to severe OE Treats *P. aeruginosa* and *S. aureus* infections	Children 6 years and older: 4 drops in affected ear twice daily × 7 days Adults: 4 drops in affected ear twice daily × 7 days
	Ofloxacin 0.3% (Floxin otic)	Treatment of moderate to severe OE Treats *P. aeruginosa* and *S. aureus* infections	Age 6 months to 13 years: 5 drops in affected ear daily × 7 days Adults: 10 drops in affected ear daily × 7 days
	Ciprofloxacin 0.2% otic (Cetraxal otic) Single-use container	Treatment of moderate to severe OE Treats *P. aeruginosa* and *S. aureus* infections	Children 6 years and older: 4 drops in affected ear twice daily × 7 days Adults: 4 drops in affected ear twice daily × 7 days
Drugs Not Safe to Use with Perforated Tympanic Membrane			
Aminoglycosides	Neomycin 0.35%, polymyxin B 10,000 units/mL, and hydrocortisone 0.5% otic solution (Cortisporin otic)	For moderate to severe infection Treats *Staphylococcus* and *P. aeruginosa* infections	Children 2 years and younger: 3 drops in affected ear three to four times a day for 10 days only Adults: 4 drops in affected ear three to four times a day for 10 days only **Limit use to 10 days only to prevent ototoxicity**
	Colistin 3 mg, neomycin 3.3 mg, hydrocortisone acetate 10 mg, and thonzonium bromide 0.5 mg (Cortisporin-TC otic)	For moderate to severe infection Treats *Staphylococcus* and *P. aeruginosa* infections	Children older than 1 year: 4 drops in affected ear three to four times a day for 10 days only Adults: 5 drops in affected ear three to four times a day for 10 days only **Limit use to 10 days only to prevent ototoxicity**
Acidifiers/antiseptics	Acetic acid 2% otic solution	Treats mild AOE or COE Treats mild bacterial and fungal infections	Children 3 years and older: 3–4 drops in the affected ear three to four times a day Adults: 5 drops in affected ear three to four times a day
	Acetic acid 2% and hydrocortisone 1% otic solution	Treats mild AOE or COE Treats mild bacterial and fungal infections	Children 3 years and older: 3–4 drops in the affected ear three to four times a day Adults: 5 drops in affected ear three to four times a day

the infectious organisms have been cultured and identified in the laboratory.

In most patients who present with COE, the condition is caused by persistent fungal infection, in which the ears are often dry and scaling. The treatment of fungal infections differs mainly in the choice of antimicrobials. Before antimicrobial administration, the auditory canal must be carefully cleaned to ensure absorption of otic medications. Medications that can be utilized to treat otomycosis include antifungal powders and otic suspensions, such as hydrocortisone/acetic acid otic (VoSol) solution or acetic acid/aluminum acetate (Otic Domeboro).

Topical fungicide preparations containing nystatin and clotrimazole creams are increasingly accepted, although these agents are not available solely as otic preparations. If such treatment is planned, a referral to an ear, nose, and throat (ENT) specialist should be considered. These creams can be placed into the external canal by a trained specialist using an operating microscope and a syringe with a blunt needle. About 1 inch of cream is needed to fill the canal, and it should be removed a week later.

Clotrimazole solution can also be used to treat fungal infections. It is available over the counter, and four drops can be placed into the affected ear twice daily for 10 to 14 days. In severe cases of COE due to fungal infection, systemic antifungals such as fluconazole, ketoconazole, or griseofulvin may be considered. Pharmacotherapy for COE is directed by extensive antibiotic sensitivity testing after the infectious organisms have been cultured and identified in the laboratory.

FOLLOW-UP AND REFERRAL

Acute OE is commonly cured after 7 to 10 days of treatment. A follow-up appointment to assess the effects of treatment may be scheduled after 1 week of therapy for uncomplicated cases. If a patient is at high risk for developing necrotizing OE, he or she should follow up in 1 to 2 days after being diagnosed with AOE. If an ear wick has been placed, the patient should return in 2 to 3 days for removal and canal cleaning. The patient should be instructed to call if symptoms do not begin to subside in 48 hours. Likewise, if a patient has OE that is not resolved with medical management or suffers from chronic or recurrent OE, referral to an ENT specialist is recommended.

Immunocompromised patients with invasive disease and any patients receiving IV antibiotic therapy require daily follow-up during hospitalization, and periodic appointments are recommended for up to 1 year after the discontinuation of treatment. Invasive OE, cellulitis, bony involvement, and all complicating cranial infections must be referred to an otolaryngologist for immediate treatment. Otherwise healthy patients with invasive disease who do not respond to treatment promptly should be monitored closely and undergo further evaluation and diagnostic procedures, as necessary. Results of CT and MRI scans remain abnormal for many months after clinical resolution of invasive disease; thus, serial nuclear medicine scans (gallium scans) may be preferable in evaluating treatment efficacy during follow-up because recurrence of infection may be as high as 10% within 6 months after treatment.

A common complication in the management of OE is dermatitis medicamentosa. Neomycin, an antibiotic commonly found in otic preparations, is known to cause skin reactions (e.g., contact dermatitis) and ototoxicity; however, these complications may be minimized by limiting the duration of pharmacotherapy. The use of neomycin-containing agents in cases in which the tympanic membrane is ruptured is controversial because neomycin may be toxic to middle ear structures if applied directly.

Patient Education: Otitis Externa

Patients should avoid getting water in the ears for at least 4 to 6 weeks after symptoms of OE subside because moisture from any source can trigger a recurrent episode of infection. Shower caps or earplugs should be worn when bathing, and swimming should be prohibited entirely for at least 1 month after an acute episode (cotton balls impregnated with petroleum jelly may be used as temporary earplugs). For persons who are particularly susceptible to repeated infections, a 2% acetic acid solution may be used prophylactically to acidify the ear canal (two to three drops in each ear twice daily and after any contact with water in which the ears become wet).

Patients should be instructed in the proper method of cleaning the ears and warned never to use swabs, sticks, or chemical agents to clean the auditory canal. Patients should understand that a small amount of earwax is necessary to prevent infection in the auditory canal and that excessive cleaning can be harmful. Clinicians should instruct patients and/or family members in how to instill topical otic drops and to finish all prescribed antibiotic treatments. Patients should lay on their side opposite to the affected ear for 5 minutes or more to allow otic drops to penetrate tissue.

The importance of keeping the ear canals dry for at least 4 to 6 weeks, both during and after an acute episode, should also be stressed. Using a blow-dryer on a low, cool setting after showers or sweating can assist to keep the ears dry. The clinician should also discuss the importance of avoiding strong jets of water from showerheads or dental water-jet systems. Alternative or complementary therapies such as candling have not been shown to be efficacious and may in fact cause harm.

OTITIS MEDIA

OM is an inflammation of the structures of the middle ear. Acute OM (AOM), also referred to as *suppurative OM* or *purulent OM,* denotes the presence of pus in the middle ear in association with local or systemic infection, manifesting with otalgia, otorrhea, and fever. OM with effusion (OME; also called *serous OM*) involves the transudation of plasma fluid from middle ear blood vessels, leading to chronic effusion in the absence of the signs and symptoms of acute infection. Recurrent OM is characterized by the clearance of middle ear effusions between acute episodes of otic inflammation. Chronic OM is present when inflammation persists for more than 3 months, typically related to tympanic membrane perforation with either intermittent or persistent otic discharge.

EPIDEMIOLOGY AND CAUSES

The incidence of OM is higher in children than in adults. An estimated 50% to 85% of children will experience at least one episode of OM by age 3 years, and almost half of these children will have three or more episodes of OM. The incidence rate of OM increases during the winter months, when the climate is colder and more time is spent indoors. Males and females are affected equally, although adults who are immunocompromised may have an increased risk of developing OM. OM tends to be uncommon in adults. Native Americans, particularly Navajos and Native Alaskans, have higher prevalence rates of OM than the general population. A smaller increase in rate is also seen in European Americans.

Differences in the anatomy of the eustachian tube in infants and young children predispose them to OM. In children, the angle of the eustachian tube is straighter and shorter, which allows microorganisms from the nasopharynx to enter the middle ear. As a child ages, the eustachian tube angle becomes more acute (narrow), decreasing the incidence of ear infections. Other anatomical abnormalities that can lead to direct blockage of the eustachian tube include hypertrophy or chronic inflammation of the adenoids (pharyngeal tonsils), cleft palate, deviated nasal septum, and nasopharyngeal tumors. Perforation of the eardrum from direct blunt trauma, swimming or diving accidents (e.g., rapid pressure changes), or sudden outward pressure or suction (such as from a kiss over the ear) may create a portal of entry for bacteria directly into the middle ear. Certain genetic conditions such as Down's syndrome (trisomy 21) also predispose individuals to middle ear infections. Both active and passive smoking have been associated with an increased risk of all forms of OM. Moreover, crowded or unsanitary living conditions, exposure to wood-burning stoves, and a family history of OM (particularly in the same household) are also contributing factors.

Additional factors contributing to eustachian tube dysfunction leading to OM or OME include allergies, sinusitis, rhinitis, and pharyngitis, all of which cause swelling of the membranous lining of the eustachian tube. However, the most significant precipitating event is a recent or concurrent URI, attributed most often to influenza type A (family Orthomyxoviridae), respiratory syncytial virus (*Pneumovirus,* in family Paramyxoviridae), or adenovirus. URIs are thought to contribute to host immunosuppression and the loss of ciliated epithelium in the eustachian tube. In turn, bacterial adherence to the membranous lining is increased.

PATHOPHYSIOLOGY

Acute Otitis Media

AOM results when bacterial infection by nasopharyngeal microorganisms follows eustachian tube dysfunction, in which the narrowest portion of the tube (the isthmus) becomes obstructed. Inflammation results primarily in response to bacterial products, including endotoxins and cell-wall components, creating in effect a middle ear abscess. Pressure from this buildup of pus may impinge on the fine blood vessels supplying the tympanic membrane, weakening its structure, reducing tensile strength, and eventually causing perforation or rupture of the eardrum to facilitate draining of inner ear fluid. Fortunately, in the absence of underlying immunocompromise, the tympanic membrane typically begins to heal spontaneously within hours and may be fully healed by 1 or 2 weeks, with complete restoration of baseline hearing capacity.

Streptococcus pneumoniae (implicated in 40% to 50% of AOM cases) is the most frequent pathogen isolated from middle ear effusions in adults. The currently available polyvalent streptococcal vaccines cover only 60% to 70% of these isolates. However, several studies have suggested the incidence of AOM infections due to *Streptococcus* strains covered by the originally developed 7-valent protein-conjugate vaccine (Prevnar-7) and the second generation 13-valent vaccine (Prevnar-13) has decreased since their introduction as recommended immunizations in pediatric populations, although the methodology of some of these studies has been criticized.

Other common organisms include nontypical *Haemophilus influenzae* (10% to 30% of cases), which are not covered by the *Haemophilus influenzae* type b (Hib) vaccine, and *Moraxella (Branhamella) catarrhalis,* the vast majority of which express the β-lactamase gene and are resistant to first-line penicillin and cephalosporin antibiotics. These organisms are thought to reach the middle ear from the upper respiratory tract via aspiration or reflux. *S. aureus* and *S. pyogenes* are far less common causative agents, particularly since the introduction of sulfonamide antibiotics, such as trimethoprim-sulfamethoxazole (Bactrim).

Up to one-half of AOM cases are attributed to viral infections originating in the nasopharynx and extending to the middle ear via the eustachian tube, including rhinovirus, adenovirus, coronavirus, influenza, and respiratory syncytial virus. In fact, nearly 40% of documented influenza cases in children younger than 3 years are complicated by AOM, adding to the impetus for widespread flu vaccination. *Mycoplasma pneumoniae* and *Chlamydia pneumoniae* are rarer causes of OM. *Chlamydia trachomatis* is typically seen only in infants younger than 6 months. In developing countries, unusual agents such as *Mycobacteria tuberculosis, Corynebacterium diphtheriae,* parasites (e.g., *Ascaris*), or fungi (e.g., *Blastomycoses, Candida, Aspergillus*) may be identified.

Recurrent OM typically results from bacterial infection due to anatomical abnormalities that repeatedly compromise eustachian tube patency. Chronic OM may also be caused by any of the bacteria associated with AOM, as well as *Escherichia coli* and *Proteus,* but *P. aeruginosa* and *S. aureus* are the most isolated pathogens in chronic suppurative OM.

Otitis Media with Effusion

OME is caused by a transudation of plasma fluid through engorged blood vessels resulting from the loss of eustachian tube patency, caused either by swelling of the membranous lining or direct anatomical blockage of the eustachian tube. Swelling of the mucosa is particularly common in the presence of an antecedent viral URI or acute allergy attack. Effective drainage of middle ear fluid is thus prevented, and negative pressure develops in the middle ear cavity, further drawing in fluid.

OME may be viral in origin but it is usually attributed to β-lactamase–producing bacterial strains that are resistant to first-line antibiotic therapies. Importantly, middle ear effusions often last for weeks to months after AOM clears; thus, OME may simply reflect part of the natural history of a resolved episode of AOM.

CLINICAL PRESENTATION

Subjective

The patient with OME will typically complain of stuffiness, fullness, and a loss of auditory acuity in the affected ear only. Pain is rare, but patients may describe aural fullness, muffled hearing (like talking in a barrel), and popping, crackling, or gurgling sounds when chewing, yawning, or blowing the nose. Very rarely, patients may experience vertigo (a sense of whirling or spinning in space) or ataxia if inner ear complications such as labyrinthitis are present. Although patients are typically afebrile, a recent history of viral URI or either allergic or vasomotor rhinitis is common.

In contrast, AOM usually presents with marked "deep" ear pain and fever, as well as unilateral hearing loss, otic discharge, and a recent history of URI. Some patients may also experience dizziness (space disorientation), vertigo, tinnitus (ringing in the ears), vomiting, or nausea. Pain typically subsides if the tympanic membrane ruptures because this relieves elevated middle ear pressure. In these cases, patients also usually complain of otic discharge. Recurrent OM is characterized by the clearance of middle ear effusions between acute episodes of inflammation.

Chronic OM typically presents with a history of repeated bouts of AOM, followed by a period of continuous or intermittent otorrhea lasting for more than 3 months. Pain is seldom a complaint, and hearing loss (related to tympanic membrane perforation) is the primary concern. Risk factors for AOM include enrollment of a child in day care, presence of tobacco smoke in the home, and residing in communities where antibiotic-resistant forms of *S. pneumoniae* are endemic.

Objective

Examination of the external ear in patients with OME is typically unremarkable; however, the mucous membranes of the nasal and oral cavities may be thickened and edematous, confirming a recent history of URI. The eardrum may be dull but usually is not bulging, and eardrum mobility typically decreases on pneumatic otoscopy. The tympanic membrane may be amber or yellow-orange, or there may be bubbles behind the tympanic membrane. In AOM, the tympanic membrane may be inflamed and pinkish gray to fiery red in color. The tympanic membrane is typically full or bulging in acute cases, with absent or obscured bony landmarks and cone light reflex.

Although the auditory canal usually shows no abnormalities, discharge from the middle ear may be present if the tympanic membrane has a perforation. Otorrhea may be purulent or mucoid, depending on the stage of inflammation; polymorphonuclear neutrophils are prominent in the early stages of bacterial infection. Otoscopic examination in chronic OM can reveal a perforated, draining tympanic membrane and possibly invasive granulation tissue. Chronic, foul-smelling otorrhea is typical of anaerobic bacterial infection, and a chronic, grayish-yellow suppuration may indicate the development of a cholesteatoma from the degenerative products of invasive epithelialization (involuted squamous epithelia and keratin debris) at the site of infection. In rare cases, bullae formed between layers of the tympanic membrane (bullous myringitis) caused by certain viruses or *M. pneumoniae* are seen. Multiple perforations of the tympanic membrane are characteristic of tuberculous otitis.

On palpation, in cases of acute infection, lymphadenopathy of the preauricular and posterior cervical nodes is common. If OM is complicated by an acute mastoiditis, tenderness over the mastoid will be elicited because the bony architecture of the middle ear is continuous with the mastoid process.

In addition to otoscopy, other examination techniques are helpful in diagnosing OM, such as pneumatic otoscopy and tuning fork examinations. Pneumatic otoscopy will demonstrate decreased or absent tympanic membrane mobility in serous, acute, or chronic OM. Tuning fork examinations can also be helpful when evaluating complaints of hearing loss associated with OM. Both the Weber and Rinne tests can provide valuable information in diagnosing a conductive hearing loss. With the Weber test, a tuning fork (512 Hz) is set to a light vibration by lightly striking the palm of the hand or elbow. The end of the tuning fork is then placed on the top of the scalp midline, asking the patient in which ear they hear the sound louder. If the sound is heard equally in both ears, there is no conductive hearing loss. If the sound is lateralized to the affected ear, it indicates a conductive hearing loss.

In the Rinne test, a tuning fork (512 Hz) is set to a light vibration by lightly striking the palm of the hand or elbow and then placing the end on the mastoid process. The patient is then asked to notify the examiner when they can no longer hear the sound. Once the patient indicates the sound is no longer audible, the tuning fork is placed 1 to 2 cm in front of the auricle and the patient is again asked to indicate when the sound ceases to be audible. In normal hearing, air conduction (AC) is greater than bone conduction (BC). Thus, if BC is greater than AC and the sound is no longer audible when the tuning fork is placed in front of the auricle, this suggests the patient has conductive hearing loss.

DIAGNOSTIC REASONING

Diagnostic Tests

Laboratory tests are rarely needed if symptomatology clearly fits the classic clinical picture of OM. A complete blood count is usually not indicated; however, patients with AOM may demonstrate a leukocytosis, particularly if they are febrile.

Cultures of tympanocentesis fluid are not indicated in serous OM and are of little practical value in acute disease unless the patient is immunocompromised or infectious complications such as mastoiditis are evident. In subacute, recurrent, or chronic cases of OM, however, cultures and antibiotic sensitivity testing are helpful in guiding alternative treatment approaches. If cultures are obtained, fungi and mycobacteria should be specifically ruled out.

Conventional sinus x-ray films and CT scans (which can reveal mucosal thickening in the middle ear space) may be helpful in evaluating patients with effusion, particularly patients with recurrent infection. Pure-tone audiometry may be helpful both before and after treatment. Tympanometry may be useful if fluid buildup behind the middle ear is suspected in the absence of other clinical signs; a flat tympanogram is consistent with restrictive disease of the middle ear cavity.

Differential Diagnosis

OM must be distinguished from OE, which is inflammation of the auditory canal and/or external ear, including the pinna and tragus. These structures are usually not affected in OM, and OE typically does not involve the tympanic membrane; however, OE may coincide with OM. Exacerbated pain on manipulation of the tragus, pinna, or earlobe is a telltale sign of external ear inflammation. Rarer infectious conditions that may cause OM, which must be ruled out by special stains, cultures, and antigen/antibody tests, include tuberculous otitis and leprosy (requiring an acid-fast stain for *Mycobacteria*) and syphilitic otitis (requiring RPR and VDRL screening tests, followed by dark-field microscopy to identify the causative agent *T. pallidum*).

TMJ syndrome/dysfunction can be similar to the pain of AOM. Patients may complain of ear pain when in fact the pain is being referred from the TMJ. Mastoiditis presenting without middle ear infection should also be considered when no physical signs of middle ear involvement are evident. Referred otalgia from TMJ dysfunction or dental abscesses may be ruled out by dental x-rays. Parotitis secondary to mumps (paramyxovirus infection) may be ruled out via serology studies (antibody titers), if suspected.

Other noninfectious causes of OM include nasopharyngeal neoplasm that must be ruled out with nasolaryngoscopy in cases of unilateral recurrent, chronic, or refractory OM. Excessive earwax buildup (cerumen impaction) with or without infection may also lead to a feeling of fullness or stuffiness in the ear, as well as pain and hearing loss. Otoscopic examination is performed before and after irrigation of the auditory canal to rule out this disorder. Barotrauma may also mimic OM, with transient middle ear effusion resulting from air travel or drastic increases in altitude, such as when driving up mountains.

MANAGEMENT

Uncomplicated cases of AOM are likely to be self-limited and may not require any specific intervention other than pain management and symptomatic relief (see Drugs Commonly Prescribed 23.2). According to American Academy of Family Physicians Clinical Practice Guidelines, treatment of nonsevere AOM in children can either be managed with close observation and follow-up or with antibiotic therapy. However, pharmacological treatment for moderate, severe, complicated, or recurrent AOM is indicated to prevent permanent anatomical changes of the middle ear and subsequent hearing loss, as changes in auditory function related to middle ear pathology can lead to sensory or perceptual alterations. In the unfortunate instance when middle ear infection leads to permanent comorbidity, loss of auditory perception may affect a patient's lifestyle, communication patterns, socialization, and self-concept. Thus, interventions should focus on moving the patient toward acceptance, identifying effective communication patterns, and recognizing support mechanisms and resources for coping with hearing loss. Fortunately, most OM cases do not reach this advanced stage.

Drugs Commonly Prescribed 23.2: Acute Otitis Media (AOM) in Children and Adults

INDICATION	DRUG	DOSE	PRESCRIBING CONSIDERATIONS
Otherwise healthy pediatric patients with mild symptoms	Acetaminophen (Tylenol)	10–15 mg/kg/dose PO every 4 hours as needed (maximum 75 mg/kg/day in infants/children)	For children ages 6–24 months, observation with the use of systemic analgesics *without* the use of antibacterial agents is an option for uncomplicated AOM based on diagnostic certainty, age, and lack of comorbid illnesses. Evaluate at 48–72 hours and discontinue medication if symptoms do not persist; if signs and symptoms of AOM persist despite systemic analgesic use for 48–72 hours, reassess and consider treatment with antibiotics.
	Ibuprofen (Motrin, Advil)	5–10 mg/kg/dose PO every 6–8 hours as needed (maximum 40 mg/kg/day in children 6 months to 11 years old)	
	Amoxicillin	High-dose: 80–90 mg/kg/day (maximum 1,000 mg/dose) PO in two divided doses for 10 days	High-dose amoxicillin is recommended as first-line treatment. Amoxicillin retains the most activity of all oral β-lactam agents against *Streptococcus pneumoniae,* including penicillin-intermediate resistant strains.
Children older than 3 months with severe illness or who failed amoxicillin treatment in the past 30 days	Amoxicillin-clavulanate (Augmentin)	Amoxicillin 90 mg/kg/day and clavulanate 6.4 mg/kg (ratio 14:1) PO in two divided doses	Use when coverage for β-lactamase–positive *Haemophilus influenzae* and *Moraxella catarrhalis* is needed.
Patients with β-lactam allergy	Of note, penicillin allergy without clinical confirmation is overreported, and the incidence of cephalosporin cross-reactivity with penicillin allergy is <2%; thus, consider allergy testing when infection resolves to confirm true penicillin allergy.		
Penicillin allergy (mild, nonanaphylactic)	Cefuroxime (Ceftin)	Suspension: 30 mg/kg/day PO in two divided doses for 10 days (maximum 1000 mg/day) Oral tablet: 250 mg twice daily for 10 days	For children older than 3 months. Due to bad taste of cefuroxime suspension, recommend tablets if possible, which can be crushed and put into a palatable fluid.
	Cefdinir (Omnicef)	14 mg/kg/day in two divided doses for 5–10 days or a single dose for 10 days	For children older than 6 months
	Cefpodoxime (Vantin)	10 mg/kg/day PO in two divided doses for 10 days (maximum 400 mg/day)	For children older than 2 months

Continued

Drugs Commonly Prescribed 23.2: Acute Otitis Media (AOM) in Children and Adults—cont'd

INDICATION	DRUG	DOSE	PRESCRIBING CONSIDERATIONS
Penicillin allergy (severe, anaphylactic) or cephalosporin allergy	Clarithromycin (Biaxin)	15 mg/kg/day in two divided doses for 10 days	For children older than 6 months. Macrolides are inferior options, due to high resistance rates and clinical failure rates.
	Trimethoprim-sulfamethoxazole (TMP-SMX; Bactrim)	TMP 6–12 mg/kg/day PO in two divided doses for 10 days (maximum 320 mg/day TMP)	For children older than 2 months. TMP-SMX is an inferior option, due to high resistance rates and clinical failure rates. Consider referral to otorhinolaryngologist for tympanocentesis.
	Azithromycin (Zithromax)	10 mg/kg/day PO on the first day and 5 mg/kg/day PO for 4 more days	Macrolides are inferior options, due to high resistance rates and clinical failure rates.
Failure of Initial AOM Treatment in Pediatric Patients			
Failure of standard-dose amoxicillin	Amoxicillin-clavulanate (Augmentin)	Amoxicillin 90 mg/kg/day PO in two divided doses for 10 days	This combination is recommended to provide a high dose of amoxicillin (for penicillin-intermediate resistant *S. pneumoniae*) and a regular dose of clavulanate (for coverage of β-lactamase–producing *H. influenzae* and *M. catarrhalis*) without excessive (greater than 10 mg/kg/day) clavulanate exposure that could lead to increased incidence of diarrhea.
Failure of high-dose amoxicillin	Ceftriaxone (Rocephin)	50 mg IM or IV for 3 days	Increased compliance if administered by healthcare provider, but requires frequent clinic visits.
	Cefuroxime (Ceftin)	30 mg/kg/day PO in two divided doses for 10 days	Due to bad taste of cefuroxime suspension, recommend tablets if possible, which can be crushed and put into a palatable fluid.
	Cefprozil (Cefzil)	30 mg/kg/day PO in two divided doses for 10 days	Available as liquid suspension or tablet.
β-Lactam (penicillin) allergy	Clarithromycin (Biaxin)	15 mg/kg/day PO in two divided doses for 10 days	Therapeutic options for these patients are limited; consider referral to otorhinolaryngologist for tympanostomy.
	Trimethoprim-sulfamethoxazole (TMP-SMX; Bactrim)	TMP 6–12 mg/kg/day PO in two divided doses for 10 days	TMP-SMX is less efficacious than amoxicillin-clavulanate.
	Azithromycin (Zithromax)	10 mg/kg/day PO on the first day and 5 mg/kg/day PO for 4 more days	Macrolides are less efficacious than amoxicillin-clavulanate; there is significant macrolide resistance in *S. pneumoniae*.
Treatment of AOM in Adults			
β-Lactamase–resistant	Amoxicillin-clavulanate (Augmentin)	Amoxicillin 875 mg twice daily for 10 days	Combination therapy is recommended as first-line treatment.
	Amoxicillin	500 mg every 8 hours OR 875 mg twice daily for 10 days	Use if amoxicillin-clavulanate is not an option.

Drugs Commonly Prescribed 23.2: Acute Otitis Media (AOM) in Children and Adults—cont'd

INDICATION	DRUG	DOSE	PRESCRIBING CONSIDERATIONS
β-Lactam (penicillin) allergy	Azithromycin (Zithromax)	500 mg PO on the first day and 250 mg PO daily for 4 more days	There is a high rate of resistance to macrolides with *S. pneumoniae*.
	Clarithromycin (Biaxin)	500 mg every 12 hours for 7 days	
Penicillin allergy without allergy to cephalosporins	Cefdinir (Omnicef)	300 mg PO twice daily for 7–10 days OR 600 mg PO once daily for 7–10 days	Do not take with aluminum or magnesium-containing antacids, iron supplements, or multivitamins.
	Cefpodoxime (Vantin)	200 mg PO twice daily for 5–10 days	Do not take with aluminum-containing antacids.
Drugs to Avoid in AOM, Unless Otherwise Indicated			
Cefaclor (Ceclor)	No activity against penicillin-intermediate resistant *S. pneumoniae*. Marginal activity against *H. influenzae* and *M. catarrhalis*.		
Cefixime (Suprax)	No activity against penicillin-intermediate resistant *S. pneumoniae*, although strong activity against *H. influenzae*.		
Ceftriaxone (Rocephin)	Routine use not recommended due to potential for increased resistance to third generation cephalosporins. May be an option in severe cases that have failed therapy, in immunosuppressed patients, or in neonates. Note: 3 days of IM/IV therapy recommended (single dose not as effective in eradicating penicillin-resistant *S. pneumoniae*)		
Cephalexin (Keflex)	No activity against penicillin-intermediate resistant *S. pneumoniae*. No activity against *H. influenzae* and *M. catarrhalis*.		
Clindamycin (Cleocin)	No activity against *H. influenzae* and *M. catarrhalis* (may be an option for *S. pneumoniae* in severe penicillin-allergic patients).		
Erythromycin (Erythrocin)	Poor activity against *H. influenzae*. Significant macrolide resistance in *S. pneumoniae*.		

Abbreviations: IM, intramuscular; IV, intravenous; PO, per os (by mouth).

In cases of OME, especially after being treated for AOM, watchful waiting is indicated, with examinations at 3-month intervals to monitor for resolution. Other treatments such as antibiotics, oral corticosteroids, and intranasal corticosteroid preparations are not recommended for the treatment of OME in a child of any age. Studies have not borne out the effectiveness of decongestants or antihistamines, although these may be of some benefit in patients with comorbid allergic rhinitis.

If the effusion is unresponsive to medical treatment and persists for longer than 12 weeks, a referral for pure tone audiometric testing and an evaluation by an otorhinolaryngologist for potential placement of tympanostomy tubes is indicated. For children with recurrent AOM with middle ear effusion, tympanostomy tubes may be considered to reduce the need for systemic antibiotics and the risk of antibiotic resistance. Once the tympanostomy tubes are inserted, topical otic drops will be used. Tympanostomy tubes are also indicated for children 6 months to 12 years of age who have had bilateral OME for 3 months or longer, with documented hearing loss. Tubes are not indicated in children with a single episode of OME lasting less than 3 months. Prolonged, recurrent AOM and OME can result in hearing impairment, speech delays leading to learning delays, poor school performance, and behavioral issues. Therefore, management and treatment of OME and chronic/recurrent AOM in the early years of a child's development are essential.

There is an increasing trend to observe uncomplicated AOM in children for the first 48 to 72 hours, rather than prescribe early antibacterial treatment, in the hopes of self-limited resolution. Antimicrobial therapy in adults with AOM is largely the norm. Selection of an agent to treat AOM requires consideration of several factors, including the patient's age, OM history, drug hypersensitivity, prior antimicrobial response, and associated illnesses. For children aged 6 to 24 months, observation and systemic analgesics without the use of antibacterial agents are an option for selected children with uncomplicated AOM based on diagnostic certainty, age, severity of illness, and assurance of follow-up. In children older than 24 months, many cases of AOM may resolve and do not require antibiotics, if the symptoms are manageable with systemic analgesics, the child has access to reevaluation at 48 hours, and symptoms do not persist. If the signs and symptoms of AOM persist for 48 to 72 hours despite using systemic analgesics, the child should be reassessed, and antibiotic treatment should be considered. Given that the majority of AOM cases occur in pediatric patients, pharmacotherapeutic approaches for AOM in both children and adults are summarized in Drugs Commonly Prescribed 23.2. It should be noted that according to the Centers for Disease Control and Prevention, approximately one-third of children with AOM do not receive the recommended first-line antibiotic (see Table 23.1).

FOLLOW-UP AND REFERRAL

Patients with AOM should be seen for follow-up in 48 to 72 hours if symptoms have not resolved; otherwise, a follow-up appointment may be scheduled several days after the completion of pharmacotherapy. Most patients experience spontaneous closure of a ruptured tympanic membrane and recovery of normal hearing within 4 weeks of treatment. Otoscopic examination should be done 4 weeks after diagnosis. If symptoms persist, consider changing the antibiotic regimen to cover β-lactamase–producing organisms. Patients with OME should be reevaluated at 4 to 6 weeks after treatment because the full clinical course of the disease may last up to several months. Evaluations at 3-month intervals or tympanometry examinations should be done if OME persists.

OME can lead to irreversible conductive hearing loss if middle ear structures are permanently damaged from effusion-related pressure changes. If AOM is poorly treated or is present in an immunocompromised patient, it may lead to OME, chronic OM, otitis interna (labyrinthitis), vertigo, ataxia, or severe acute, subacute, and chronic infections of adjacent cranial structures (e.g., including mastoiditis, etrositis [infection of the temporal bone], meningitis, and epidural, subdural, or brain abscesses). Other complications include perforation of the tympanic membrane, cholesteatoma, facial nerve palsies, lateral sinus thrombophlebitis, and otic hydrocephalus.

Although the clinical course of OME may last for several months, patients should be referred to a specialist for pure tone audiometry testing and further evaluation to rule out nasopharyngeal tumors and other anatomical eustachian tube obstructions if hearing loss persists beyond 6 weeks, extends bilaterally, or reaches more than 20 decibels. Patients with AOM may require referral to a specialist if vertigo or ataxia develops, if a ruptured tympanic membrane fails to close, if symptoms worsen after 3 to 4 days of treatment, if significant hearing loss is present, or if the patient develops chronic OM or OME.

Patient Education: Otitis Media

Measures to prevent AOM in infants and young children should be discussed with parents/caregivers at well-child visits. Preventive measures include avoidance of tobacco exposure, exclusive breastfeeding for the first 6 months of life or longer, annual influenza vaccine for all children 6 months of age and older (and all adults), Prevnar-13 for all children 6 weeks of age and older (and all adults), and pneumococcal 23-valent polysaccharide vaccine (Pneumovax-23) for high-risk children 2 years of age and older (and high-risk adults of all ages, as well as all adults 50 years of age and older), according to updated immunization schedules. Although OM is primarily a disease of infants and young children, it can also affect adults, and the same recommendations of tobacco avoidance and appropriate vaccinations apply.

Swimming should be avoided until OM clears because immersion in water may lead to OE complicating middle ear infection. The ear canal should be kept as dry as possible. Tympanic membrane perforation can be avoided by not using cotton swabs or sharp objects of any kind to clean the ears. Traumatic injuries to the middle ear should be avoided as well to prevent perforation. In all cases, especially those in which the tympanic membrane is perforated, blowing of the nose should be avoided. If the nose must be blown, it should be done

TABLE 23.1 Percentage of Patients Receiving Recommended First-Line Antibiotic by Condition, United States, 2010–2011

	Adults (20 Years and Older)	Children (0 to 19 Years)
Sinus infection	37%	52%
Pharyngitis (sore throat)	37%	60%
Middle ear infection	N/A	67%

Abbreviation: N/A, not available.
Based on the prevalence of allergy to first-line antibiotics and estimated treatment failures after first-line antibiotics, at least 80% of patients presenting with these conditions should receive first-line antibiotics. Analysis is based on National Ambulatory Medical Care Survey (NAMCS) and National Hospital Ambulatory Medical Care Survey (NHAMCS) data.
Source: Centers for Disease Control and Prevention. *Antibiotic Use in the United States, 2017: Progress and Opportunities.* Centers for Disease Control and Prevention; 2017.

as gently as possible. Nasal saline may be used to liquefy nasal secretions and facilitate drainage.

Folk remedies such as "sweet oil" instilled directly into the ear should also be avoided. Patients should be instructed to return to the clinic for further evaluation after 48 hours if symptoms of AOM have not resolved. Explain that OM per se is not contagious, but that predisposing URIs may be passed from person to person. Bedrest or reduced activity may be suggested in severe cases until fever and pain subside, and the importance of completing the full regimen of all antibiotic therapies should be emphasized. Instruct patients to keep the ear canal dry, and demonstrate the proper method of cleaning the ear canal without chemical agents, sharp objects, cotton swabs, or a finger.

REFERENCES

Otitis Externa

Chawdhary G, Pankhania M, Douglas S, et al. Current management of necrotising otitis externa in the UK: survey of 221 UK otolaryngologists. *Acta Otolaryngol.* 2017;137(8): 818–822. https://doi.org/10.1080/00016489.2017.1295468

Cohen Atsmoni S, Brener A, Roth Y. Diabetes in the practice of otolaryngology. *Diabetes Metab Syndr.* 2019;13(2):1141–1150. https://doi.org/10.1016/j.dsx.2019.01.006

Gore J. Otitis externa. *JAAPA.* 2018;31(2):47–48. https://doi.org/10.1097/01.JAA.0000529781.69812.8e

Gruber M, Sela E, Doweck I, et al. The role of surgery in necrotizing otitis externa. *Ear Nose Throat J.* 2017;96(1):E16–E21.

Hasibi M, Ashtiani MK, Motassadi Zarandi M, et al. A treatment protocol for management of bacterial and fungal malignant external otitis: a large cohort in Tehran, Iran. *Ann Otol Rhinol Laryngol.* 2017;126(7): 561–567. https://doi.org/10.1177/0003489417710473

Long DA, Koyfman A, Long B. An emergency medicine-focused review of malignant otitis externa. *Am J Emerg Med.* 2020;38(8): 1671–1678. https://doi.org/10.1016/j.ajem.2020.04.083

Morales RE, Eisenman DJ, Raghavan P. Imaging necrotizing otitis externa. *Semin Roentgenol.* 2019;54(3):215–226. https://doi.org/10.1053/j.ro.2019.04.002

Peled C, Kraus M, Kaplan D. Diagnosis and treatment of necrotising otitis externa and diabetic foot osteomyelitis—similarities and differences. *J Laryngol Otol.* 2018;132(9):775–779. https://doi.org/10.1017/S002221511800138X

Otitis Media

Brennan-Jones CG, Head K, Chong LY, et al. Topical antibiotics for chronic suppurative otitis media. *Cochrane Database Syst Rev.* 2020;1(1):CD013051. https://doi.org/10.1002/14651858.CD013051.pub2

Centers for Disease Control and Prevention. *Antibiotic Use in the United States, 2017: Progress and Opportunities.* Centers for Disease Control and Prevention; 2017.

Gaddey HL, Wright MT, Nelson TN. Otitis media: rapid evidence review. *Am Fam Physician.* 2019;100(6):350–356.

Hum SW, Shaikh KJ, Musa SS, et al. Adverse events of antibiotics used to treat acute otitis media in children: a systematic meta-analysis. *J Pediatr.* 2019;215:139–143.e7. https://doi.org/10.1016/j.jpeds.2019.08.043

Marom T, Kraus O, Habashi N, et al. Emerging technologies for the diagnosis of otitis media. *Otolaryngol Head Neck Surg.* 2019;160(3): 447–456. https://doi.org/10.1177/0194599818809337

Paul CR, Moreno MA. Acute otitis media. *JAMA Pediatr.* 2020;174(3):308–308. doi: 10.1001/jamapediatrics.2019.5664. PMID: 31985755.

Ren Y, Sethi R, Stankovic KM. Acute otitis media and associated complications in United States emergency departments. *Otol Neurotol.* 2018;39(8):1005–1011. https://doi.org/10.1097/MAO.0000000000001929

Roditi RE, Rosenfeld RM, Shin JJ. Otitis media with effusion: our national practice. *Otolaryngol Head Neck Surg.* 2017;157(2): 171–172. https://doi.org/10.1177/0194599817703056

Shirai N, Preciado D. Otitis media: what is new? *Curr Opin Otolaryngol Head Neck Surg.* 2019;27(6):495–498. https://doi.org/10.1097/MOO.0000000000000591

Sun D, McCarthy TJ, Liberman DB. Cost-effectiveness of watchful waiting in acute otitis media. *Pediatrics.* 2017;139(4):e20163086. https://doi.org/10.1542/peds.2016-3086

Venekamp RP, Schilder A, van den Heuvel M, et al. Acute otitis media in children. *BMJ.* 2020;371:m4238. https://doi.org/10.1136/bmj.m4238

Wald ER, DeMuri GP. Antibiotic recommendations for acute otitis media and acute bacterial sinusitis: conundrum no more. *Pediatr Infect Dis J.* 2018;37(12):1255–1257. https://doi.org/10.1097/INF.0000000000002009

Welling DR, Ukstins CA. Otitis media: beyond the examining room. *Pediatr Clin North Am.* 2018;65(1):105–123. https://doi.org/10.1016/j.pcl.2017.08.024

RESOURCES

General

American Academy of Otolaryngology–Head and Neck Surgery: Clinical Practice Guidelines
> https://www.entnet.org/content/clinical-practice-guidelines

Otitis Externa

American Speech-Language-Hearing Association (ASHA): Otitis externa
> https://www.asha.org/public/hearing/Swimmers-Ear/

Centers for Disease Control and Prevention: Swimming and Ear Infections
> https://www.cdc.gov/healthywater/hygiene/disease/swimmers_ear.html

Otitis Media

American Speech-Language-Hearing Association (ASHA): Ear Infections (Otitis Media)
> https://www.asha.org/public/hearing/otitis-media/

Centers for Disease Control and Prevention: Ear Infection
> https://www.cdc.gov/antibiotic-use/ear-infection.html

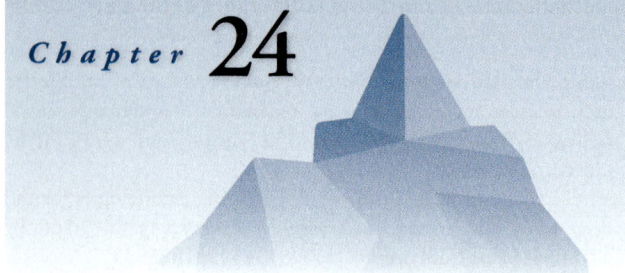

Chapter 24

Inflammatory and Infectious Disorders of the Nose, Sinuses, Mouth, and Throat

Maria Colandrea, DNP, NP-C, CORLN, CCRN, FAANP
Tiffany Ellis, MSN, ANP-C, CORLN
Michael E. Zychowicz, DNP, ANP, ONP, FAAN, FAANP
Brian Oscar Porter, MD, PhD, MPH, MBA

RHINITIS

Rhinitis is an inflammation of the nasal mucosa characterized by nasal congestion, rhinorrhea, sneezing, pruritus, and/or postnasal drainage. Its etiology is varied, but it is generally categorized as either allergic rhinitis (AR) or nonallergic rhinitis (NAR) (see Box 24.1). AR may be either seasonal or perennial. NAR may be (1) infectious (most commonly viral in origin), (2) irritant related, (3) vasomotor, (4) hormone related, (5) associated with medication use or overuse (rhinitis medicamentosa), or (6) atrophic. The most common forms are viral rhinitis and AR.

Rhinitis may be acute or chronic. Although rhinitis is often a benign and self-limited disorder, poorly controlled chronic rhinitis may contribute to sleep loss, absenteeism from work or school, secondary daytime fatigue, learning impairment, decreased overall cognitive functioning, decreased long-term productivity, and decreased quality of life. In addition, poorly controlled rhinitis may lead to the development of other related disease processes, such as acute or chronic rhinosinusitis, nasal polyps, otitis media (OM), exacerbation of underlying asthma, and sleep apnea.

Rhinosinusitis (also known as *sinusitis*) is a term that encompasses disorders affecting both the nasal passages and paranasal sinuses and has both overlapping and distinct symptoms from pure rhinitis. Symptoms of sinus involvement may include nasal congestion or obstruction, nasal drainage (which is often purulent), focal facial pressure and/or pain, and in some cases, reduced sense of smell. Headache is a commonly reported symptom; however, it is not a reliable predictor of sinus disease or infection, as headache is often related to migraine. About 2% of headaches are attributed to sinusitis, which is discussed in greater detail later in this chapter.

EPIDEMIOLOGY AND CAUSES

AR is one of the most common chronic diseases, affecting up to 60 million people in the United States across all age-groups. The incidence of seasonal AR parallels pollen production, increasing in the fall and spring, although many individuals have pollen allergies—such as to trees or grasses—that predominate in the summer months. Other forms of AR may last year-round if they are caused by perennial allergens such as dust or house mites. NAR affects 20 to 30 million patients in the United States, representing 23% of all rhinitis cases. NAR is exacerbated by nonallergic triggers including irritants, tobacco smoke, weather changes, automotive fumes, strong odors such as perfumes, hormonal changes, and age-related changes. The symptom that differentiates AR and NAR is pruritus of the nose, eyes, palate, and/or throat. Nonallergic rhinitis with eosinophilia syndrome (NARES) is an inflammatory type of rhinitis with negative allergy testing but abnormally high numbers of eosinophils confirmed on nasal mucosal biopsy.

Acute rhinitis is usually viral in etiology and self-limited, whereas chronic rhinitis may be associated with allergies, NAR, or chronic sinusitis. Rhinitis medicamentosa causes rebound nasal congestion due to prolonged use of nasal decongestants such as oxymetazoline (Afrin), phenylephrine (Neo-Synephrine), naphazoline (Clear Eyes), or xylometazoline (Triaminic) nasal spray. Atrophic rhinitis results from atrophy of the nasal mucosa because the thinning of the nasal mucosa decreases mucociliary

---

Box 24.1 Forms of Rhinitis

Allergic Rhinitis
Nonallergic Rhinitis
- Viral/infective
- Vasomotor
- Gustatory
- Nonallergic rhinitis with eosinophilia syndrome (NARES)
- Occupational
- Senile or geriatric

Other Rhinitis Syndromes
- Drug induced
- Hormone induced
- Atrophic
- Systemic/inflammatory
- Structural causes (e.g., deviated septum, nasal polyps, neoplasm, adenoid hypertrophy, foreign body)
- Rhinosinusitis

clearance, which can cause an overgrowth of bacteria stemming from colonization of the nasal passages, most commonly by *Klebsiella ozaena, Staphylococcus aureus, Escherichia coli, Streptococcus pneumoniae,* or *Proteus* species. Atrophic rhinitis can be categorized as primary or secondary. Primary atrophic rhinitis is uncommon in the United States and Europe; it occurs more commonly in developing countries with warm climates. Secondary atrophic rhinitis can occur because of surgery, radiation therapy, or inflammatory conditions. Hormonal rhinitis is seen in 20% to 30% of pregnant women and usually resolves 2 weeks after delivery.

Most forms of rhinitis appear to have no ethnic predispositions. There is a male predominance of AR and female predominance of NAR. There is also a strong correlation between AR and asthma in children and adults. Viral upper respiratory tract infections (URIs) occur more frequently in families with young children, especially those in day-care settings, whereas exposure to offending allergens is the primary risk factor for AR. The most common irritants implicated in the seasonal form of AR are pollen and mold spores. Dust mites, insect debris (e.g., from cockroaches), and animal dander are the most common offending agents for the perennial form of AR. A family history of allergic disease (e.g., atopic dermatitis, asthma) is also a risk factor for AR. Vasomotor rhinitis is aggravated by low humidity, sudden temperature or pressure changes, cold air, strong odors, emotional stress, cigarette smoke, and other nasal irritants. Use of nasal decongestants more frequently than every 3 hours and for periods longer than 3 days is the primary risk factor for rhinitis medicamentosa.

In some patients, certain medications may precipitate rhinitis. Antihypertensive agents are the most frequently cited culprits due to their vasodilatory effects. Angiotensin-converting enzyme inhibitors, beta-adrenergic antagonists, certain NSAIDs, guanethidine (Ismelin), clonidine (Catapres), hydralazine (Apresoline), prazosin (Minipress), chlordiazepoxide (Librium), amitriptyline (Elavil), or even aspirin can be contributing factors. Oral contraceptive use and hormone therapy for menopause have also been implicated as risk factors for rhinitis, along with a family history of rhinitis and septal/anatomical obstruction. In addition, ingestion of certain foods (e.g., spicy foods) may precipitate gustatory rhinitis in susceptible individuals. Illicit drug use such as cocaine snorting may also precipitate rhinitis.

PATHOPHYSIOLOGY

AR results from immunoglobulin E (IgE)–mediated type I hypersensitivity to airborne irritants affecting the eyes, nose, sinuses, throat, and bronchi. Antigen-specific IgE antibodies, elicited by repeated allergen exposure, bind to eosinophils and basophils in the bloodstream and their mucosal counterparts known as *mast cells.* These leukocytes subsequently degranulate, releasing chemo-inflammatory substances, including histamine, leukotrienes, prostaglandins, slow-reacting substance of anaphylaxis, and erythrocyte chemotactic factor, which results in increased vasodilation, capillary permeability, mucus production, smooth muscle contraction, and eosinophilia. In a small percentage of cases, food allergies (referred to in some sources as *gustatory*) may be the cause, although this should not be confused with forms of NAR that are triggered by certain foods (e.g., spicy foods).

NAR is a chronic, noninfectious process of unknown etiology without accompanying eosinophilia, characterized by periods of abnormal autonomic responsiveness and vascular engorgement unrelated to specific irritants. In addition, chemical or particulate airborne irritants may cause direct mucosal inflammation in the absence of IgE production or immune hypersensitivity. Fluctuations and reductions in estrogen levels associated with menses, hormonal birth control preparations, pregnancy, and menopause may all predispose to NAR.

Rhinitis medicamentosa is a form of NAR that results from rebound nasal congestion secondary to medication overuse. Mucosal inflammation results from the use of topical nasal decongestants such as phenylephrine (Neo-Synephrine) or oxymetazoline (Afrin) for longer than 3 days, which leads to secondary vasodilation, repeated small-vessel coagulation, and eventual fibrosis. Bacterial infection plays a role in the development of atrophic rhinitis, in which the nasal epithelia and bones progressively atrophy resulting in distinct morphological changes.

Viral rhinitis stems from an acute response caused by viral replication in the nasopharynx, resulting in varying degrees of nasotracheal inflammation. Strongly associated with viral URI (common cold), the primary etiological agents of viral rhinitis include rhinovirus, influenza virus, parainfluenza virus, respiratory syncytial virus, coronavirus, adenovirus, echovirus, and coxsackievirus. When viral sinusitis is also present, the condition is collectively referred to as *rhinosinusitis.* Most rhinosinusitis is due to viral infection, but bacterial superinfection may complicate a small percentage of these cases. Anatomical defects or obstructions anywhere along the nasopharyngeal tract may predispose to infection by impairing physiological nasal drainage.

CLINICAL PRESENTATION

Subjective

Patients with AR usually complain of a multitude of symptoms including, but not limited to, nasal congestion; headache; sneezing; sniffling; clear rhinorrhea; postnasal drip; frequent throat clearing; coughing; and pruritus that occurs in the nasal passages, conjunctivae, palate, and pharynx. Epiphora (excess tearing with stringy, watery ocular discharge) is also a common finding. Pruritus is the hallmark symptom that separates AR from other forms of rhinitis. Sneezing, coughing, and a sore or burning throat can commonly present in both viral rhinitis and AR. However, viral rhinitis is typically also accompanied by malaise, headache, sore throat, and occasionally fever. NAR symptoms are similar to those of AR with the absence of ocular, nasal, palatal, or pharyngeal pruritus. NAR symptoms may occur after being exposed to nonallergic triggers such as weather changes, tobacco smoke, diesel or automotive fumes, or strong odors such as perfumes.

Vasomotor rhinitis can be acute or chronic and be brought on by temperature changes, exercise, and strong odors. The onset of nasal congestion is rapid in vasomotor rhinitis; patients typically complain of a pronounced watery postnasal drip, as well as persistent nasal obstruction that may switch sides with each attack. Gustatory rhinitis produces acute onset of clear rhinorrhea upon eating hot or spicy foods.

Rhinitis medicamentosa may present with increased heart rate and elevated blood pressure because of the effects of sympathomimetic decongestants. Patients with atrophic rhinitis may complain of nasal congestion, a thick postnasal drip, nasal crusting, frequent clearing of the throat, anosmia (impaired olfaction), a constant foul odor in the nose, and severe epistaxis (nosebleeds). See Differential Diagnosis 24.1 for a summary of the symptoms and objective findings of multiple forms of rhinitis and other conditions that are overlapping in presentation.

Objective

In AR, the mucosa appears pale, boggy, or edematous and may take on a pale pink or bluish hue. The turbinates will be hypertrophied. Clear, watery nasal discharge is typically present; however, it is not unusual to have a yellowish color to the nasal drainage. The conjunctivae can also be inflamed (allergic conjunctivitis), with the palpebral conjunctivae being particularly edematous (chemosis), with watery discharge and red sclerae. Dark circles or "allergic shiners" under the eyes may be apparent, along with excess wrinkles under the lower eyelid (Dennie lines). In children, the palatine or pharyngeal tonsils (adenoids) may be enlarged. There may also be erythema and cobblestoning in the posterior pharynx. The external nose may have a horizontal crease across its dorsum (resulting from repetitive upward wiping of persistent nasal dripping, known as the "allergic salute"), which is more commonly seen in children. The nose may also be tender from repeated sneezing in patients with both viral and allergic rhinitis. On auscultation, wheezing breath sounds may reflect concurrent asthma associated with allergic rhinitis.

With viral rhinitis, the mucosa typically appears erythematous. Throat inspection may reveal pharyngitis, characterized by erythematous and edematous pharyngeal

Differential Diagnosis 24.1: Rhinitis

Differentials	Potential Symptoms	Objective Findings
Allergic rhinitis	Pruritus of the nose, eyes, palate and/or pharynx Sneezing Nasal congestion Postnasal drip Cough Sniffling Throat clearing	Examination Findings: Skin • May have eczemic skin rash Ocular • Injected, erythematous (red) sclerae • Watery eyes • Dark circles under the eyes ("allergic shiners") • Wrinkles under the lower eyelid (Dennie-Morgan lines) Nasal • Turbinate hypertrophy • Pale, boggy turbinates (pale pink or blue) • Watery nasal discharge but can also be slightly colored • Nasal polyps • Nasal crease (due to repeated upward wiping of nose, known as "allergic salute") Posterior Pharynx • Cobblestoning • Tonsil hypertrophy • Erythema • Postnasal drip

Differential Diagnosis 24.1: Rhinitis—cont'd

Differentials	Potential Symptoms	Objective Findings
Nonallergic Rhinitis (NAR)	Most symptoms of NAR include nasal congestion, clear rhinorrhea, sneezing (not as common), cough, sniffling, throat clearing. Additional symptoms may further differentiate various forms: Viral/infective • Pharyngitis • Otalgia • Fevers, malaise • Headache • Conjunctivitis Vasomotor • Usually triggered by environmental factors, such as strong smells or changes in weather, temperature, humidity, or barometric pressure • Absence of pruritus Gustatory • Acute, rapid congestion with clear rhinorrhea • Triggers include spicy foods, pepper, and alcohol Nonallergic rhinitis with eosinophilia syndrome (NARES) • Congestion • Clear rhinorrhea • Nasal cytology reveals increased eosinophils, but allergy testing is negative. Occupational Rhinitis • Related to exposure at work (e.g., chemicals, latex, flour) • Worse when at work and improves with time off Senile/Geriatric Rhinitis • Watery rhinorrhea • Triggered by food, odors, and other irritants in the environment	Examination Findings: Ocular • Red erythematous sclerae • Watery eyes Nasal • Hypertrophied turbinates • Erythematous turbinates • Watery nasal discharge; can also be slightly colored Posterior Pharynx • Tonsillar hypertrophy • Erythema • Postnasal drip
Atrophic rhinitis • Primarily caused by bacteria (most common is Klebsiella ozaenae) • Secondary causes: radiation, surgery, inflammatory or granulomatous diseases	Nasal crusting Nasal dryness Congestion Anterior or posterior nasal drainage	Examination Findings • Dry, crusting nasal mucosa • Mucosal atrophy • Purulent nasal drainage • Bleeding

Continued

Differential Diagnosis 24.1: Rhinitis—cont'd

Differentials	Potential Symptoms	Objective Findings
Rhinosinusitis	Nasal obstruction Facial pain/pressure Congestion Purulent rhinorrhea Localized headache Anosmia/hyposmia Dental pain Fever Cough Malaise	Examination Findings • Focal facial pain over cheeks, behind eyes • Purulent nasal discharge • Erythematous, edematous turbinates • Bleeding • Purulent nasal drip in posterior pharynx
Nasal polyposis	Nasal obstruction or blockage Rhinorrhea May have asthma symptoms and allergy to aspirin Anosmia	Examination Findings • Nasal discharge, may be clear or colored • Gray/yellow translucent polyps • Widened nasal bridge
Structural abnormalities • Septal deviation • Foreign body • Malignancy	Unilateral nasal symptoms Chronic rhinosinusitis In malignancy, unilateral epistaxis may also be present with focal headaches, and/or facial nerve paresis	Examination Findings • Deviated septum • Mass/ulcerations • Purulent nasal discharge • Epistaxis
Systemic and inflammatory causes/Granulomatous disease • Wegener's granulomatosis • Sarcoidosis	Nasal congestion Chronic rhinosinusitis	Examination Findings • External nasal collapse (saddle-nose deformity) • Nasal crusting • Epistaxis • Septal perforation
Cerebrospinal fluid leak	Salty-tasting nasal drainage Usually occurs unilaterally May occur after cranial or facial trauma, intranasal surgery, but can also occur idiopathically Symptoms may increase when bending forward	Examination Findings • Clear nasal drainage unilaterally increased with bending forward
Medications/Illicit drugs	Antihypertensives (e.g., alpha-adrenergic blockers, beta blockers, angiotensin-converting enzyme inhibitors) • Nasal congestion Cocaine (snorted) • Septal perforation • Epistaxis • Crusting • Rhinorrhea Nasal decongestants (prolonged use, especially with topical preparations) • Rebound nasal congestion and obstruction, requiring frequent use of decongestants	Examination Findings: • Erythematous or pale turbinates • Hypertrophied turbinates • Watery or colored nasal discharge

Differential Diagnosis 24.1: Rhinitis—cont'd

Differentials	Potential Symptoms	Objective Findings
Hormonal rhinitis • Pregnancy • Contraceptive use • Hormone replacement therapy • Puberty	Congestion and rhinorrhea that resolve after initial increase in hormones	Examination Findings: • Erythematous or pale turbinates • Hypertrophied turbinates • Watery or colored nasal discharge

mucosa. The nasal mucosa appears particularly friable. If the viral rhinitis is complicated by a secondary bacterial infection, the nasal discharge may be greenish-yellow or thick yellowish-white, which is indicative of purulence.

The nasal mucosa in patients with NAR or vasomotor rhinitis will range from bright red to bluish in hue, and the nasal turbinates may be hypertrophied. The mucosa in patients with rhinitis medicamentosa is also injected and edematous, with some patients presenting with pale turbinates and dry, rubbery nasal mucosa. In contrast, the mucosa in patients with atrophic rhinitis usually appears crusted with dried mucus or blood from repeated bouts of epistaxis, although the nasal passages typically remain patent.

DIAGNOSTIC REASONING

Diagnostic Tests

Laboratory tests are not typically indicated to diagnose uncomplicated cases of rhinitis. However, if an exudate is present as a colored or translucent nasal discharge, a Giemsa- or Wright's-stained smear can be prepared, along with a complete blood count (CBC) to characterize the disease process. Leukocytosis or the presence of polymorphonuclear neutrophils in the discharge reflects an infectious disorder other than a typical viral URI. Eosinophilia in the discharge is indicative of AR.

Allergy testing can be performed if the patient is refractory to medical management. Intradermal skin testing (skin prick testing [SPT]) is the gold standard to determine whether symptoms are related to an allergic reaction. SPT has up to 80% sensitivity and specificity and is considered more sensitive than serum blood testing, although the specificity of SPT has been reported to be as low as 50%. After the skin prick or intradermal injection of antigen, direct observation for possible skin reactions determines whether the patient has an allergy, in which case a wheal will form within 20 minutes. The size of the wheal produced correlates with the severity of the reaction. SPT is contraindicated in patients with severe uncontrolled asthma, severe eczema, or unstable cardiovascular disease, and test results can be altered with specific medications such as oral antihistamines, tricyclic antidepressants, and beta blockers.

Antigen-specific IgE may be measured in the serum if SPT cannot be safely performed, especially in patients who are at high risk for anaphylaxis or have comorbid conditions. Blood testing is not as sensitive as SPT, and results can vary, based on laboratory reliability. However, antigen-specific IgE results are not altered by medications, and blood testing can be performed to evaluate for food allergies in patients with a significant history of food-related anaphylaxis.

In patients with suspicion for NARES, nasal cytology will reveal elevated eosinophils in the nasal tissue upon biopsy, along with negative allergy testing (i.e., SPT and antigen-specific serum IgE levels). If a cerebrospinal fluid (CSF) leak is suspected, sending the nasal discharge for a beta-2 transferrin test is indicated, as this enzyme is found exclusively in CSF and is therefore highly specific for a CSF leak.

The diagnosis of NAR is typically based on patient history and tends to be a diagnosis of exclusion because nasal smears and skin tests are typically negative and no family history of allergic disorders is expected. Hormone-related rhinitis and rhinitis medicamentosa are diagnosed primarily through patient history once other common forms of rhinitis have been excluded. In contrast, atrophic rhinitis may be confirmed by nasal mucosal biopsy, as histopathology will demonstrate transformation of ciliated pseudostratified columnar epithelia into the stratified squamous form. In addition, the lamina propria will be decreased in thickness and vascularity. Bacterial culture of nasal secretions may be helpful if bacterial infection is expected; because the nares are normally expected to be colonized with mixed flora, positive nasal cultures will reveal a predominant bacterial organism.

Diagnostic imaging is not routinely recommended in the diagnosis of rhinitis; however, sinus imaging may be recommended if there is a concern for chronic sinusitis, neoplasm, or nasal polyps, as discussed in the following section on the differential diagnosis of rhinitis.

Differential Diagnosis

The differential diagnosis of rhinitis is typically directed toward determining the specific underlying cause, as well as ruling out other causes of nasal drainage. Acute or chronic rhinosinusitis resulting from a viral or bacterial infection will result in inflammation of the nasal mucosa and cause rhinitis. If purulence is noted, cultures or microscopic smears of sinus drainage can be done to identify the infectious organisms present. Physical examination may rule out nasal foreign bodies, nasal polyps, or a deviated septum as causes of mucosal inflammation, congestion, and nasal drainage. Cocaine snorting, inhalant abuse (i.e., sniffing, huffing), and other forms of substance abuse should also be ruled out through a detailed patient history and, if indicated, urine or serum drug screens.

In patients who report clear nasal drainage that has a salty taste, a CSF leak (most often secondary to trauma) should be ruled out. Patients at risk for CSF leak include those who have had recent sinus surgery or experienced head trauma, although CSF leaks can also occur idiopathically. In addition to the salty, clear nasal drainage, CSF rhinorrhea is typically unilateral and worsens when the patient bends forward.

Chronic inflammatory conditions such as Wegener's granulomatosis or sarcoidosis may be ruled out via biopsy, which would reveal granulomatous (histiocyte/macrophage) inflammation of the nasal mucosa. Hormonal changes associated with pregnancy or hypothyroidism may also lead to nasal vasodilation and inflammation; however, hyperthyroidism due to Graves disease has been associated with a greater risk of AR. Such conditions are ruled out through a careful physical examination, detailed patient history, and serum hormone screens.

MANAGEMENT

With all types of rhinitis, much of the treatment regimen will focus on the relief of symptoms and self-care measures, although environmental triggers must also be addressed. Viral rhinitis is mostly treated symptomatically because viral URIs are predominantly self-limited.

The following list outlines adult dosages of common medications used for symptomatic relief (see also Drugs Commonly Prescribed 24.1):

- Fever and headache may be treated with acetaminophen 325 to 650 mg by mouth (PO) every 4 hours as needed (maximum daily dose without hepatic impairment 4,000 mg/day). Aspirin is not recommended because it may increase viral shedding.
- Rhinorrhea may be treated with oral decongestants such as pseudoephedrine (Sudafed) 30 to 60 mg PO every 3 to 4 hours as needed or topical preparations such as phenylephrine (Neo-Synephrine) 0.25% to 0.5% nasal spray one to two sprays in each nostril every 3 to 4 hours as needed for no more than 3 days.
- Intranasal ipratropium (Atrovent) 0.03% two sprays in each nostril two to four times daily as needed may also relieve excessive runny nose.
- Persistent cough may be treated with dextromethorphan 15 to 30 mg PO every 3 to 4 hours as needed. In cases where sleep is disrupted because of severe cough, prescription codeine 10 to 15 mg PO every 3 to 4 hours as needed can provide consistent cough suppression.

Text continued on page 362

Drugs Commonly Prescribed 24.1: Rhinitis

DRUG	INDICATION	DOSAGE	PRESCRIBING CONSIDERATIONS
Antihistamines—First generation (generally not recommended for first-line use)			
Diphenhydramine (Benadryl)	Allergic rhinitis (AR)	Adults: 25–50 mg by mouth (PO) every 4–6 hours; maximum 300 mg/day	Use 3–5 hours before anticipated allergen exposure **Adverse effects:** May cause central nervous system (CNS) sedation; gastrointestinal (GI) upset; anticholinergic effects (e.g., dry mouth, blurred vision, confusion in older adults); additive CNS-depressant effects with alcohol, sedatives, or hypnotics *Use with caution in older adults*
Chlorpheniramine maleate (Chlor-Trimeton)	AR	Adults: 2–4 mg PO every 4–6 hours	Must use 3–5 hours before anticipated allergen exposure **Adverse effects:** CNS sedation; GI upset; anticholinergic effects (e.g., dry mouth, blurred vision, confusion in older adults); additive CNS-depressant effects with alcohol, sedatives, or hypnotics *Use with caution in older adults*

Drugs Commonly Prescribed 24.1: Rhinitis—cont'd

DRUG	INDICATION	DOSAGE	PRESCRIBING CONSIDERATIONS
Azelastine hydrochloride (Astelin)	Seasonal AR; vasomotor rhinitis	137 mcg/spray Adults: one to two sprays per nostril twice daily for AR; two sprays per nostril twice daily for vasomotor rhinitis Children: Age 5–11 years: one spray per nostril twice daily for AR Age 12 years and older: one to two sprays per nostril twice daily for AR; two sprays per nostril twice daily for vasomotor rhinitis	Intranasal spray **Adverse effects:** Bitter taste; somnolence; CNS sedation; GI upset; anticholinergic effects (e.g., dry mouth, blurred vision, confusion in older adults); additive CNS-depressant effects with alcohol, sedatives, or hypnotics *Use with caution in older adults. Only use in pregnancy if potential benefits justify potential risks to fetus*
Azelastine hydrochloride (Astepro)	Seasonal and perennial AR	137 mcg/spray (0.1%) OR 205.5 mcg/spray (0.15%) Adults: one to two sprays 0.1% or 0.15% per nostril twice daily OR two sprays 0.15% per nostril once daily for seasonal AR; two sprays 0.15% per nostril twice daily for perennial AR Children: Age 6 months to 5 years: one spray 0.1% per nostril twice daily for perennial AR Age 2–5 years: one spray 0.1% per nostril twice daily for seasonal AR Age 6–11 years: one spray 0.1% or 0.15% per nostril twice daily for seasonal or perennial AR Age 12 years and older: one to two sprays 0.1% or 0.15% per nostril twice daily OR two sprays 0.15% per nostril once daily for seasonal AR; two sprays 0.15% per nostril twice daily for perennial AR	Intranasal spray **Adverse effects:** Bitter taste; somnolence; CNS sedation; GI upset; anticholinergic effects (e.g., dry mouth, blurred vision, confusion in older adults); additive CNS-depressant effects with alcohol, sedatives, or hypnotics *Use with caution in older adults. Only use in pregnancy if potential benefits justify potential risks to fetus.*
Antihistamines—Second generation			
Desloratadine (Clarinex)	Seasonal and perennial AR	Adults: 5 mg PO once daily Children: Age 2–5 years: 1.25 mg PO once daily Age 6–11 years: 2.5 mg PO once daily Age 12 years and older: 5 mg PO once daily	**Adverse effects:** Pharyngitis, dry mouth, somnolence, headache, fatigue *Only use in pregnancy if potential benefits justify potential risks to fetus. Not recommended for nursing mothers*

Continued

Drugs Commonly Prescribed 24.1: Rhinitis—cont'd

DRUG	INDICATION	DOSAGE	PRESCRIBING CONSIDERATIONS
Loratadine (Claritin)	Seasonal and perennial AR	Adults: 10 mg PO once daily Children: Age 2–5 years: 5 mg PO once daily Age 6 years and older: 10 mg PO once daily	**Adverse effects:** Headache, mild drowsiness Less effective than first generation antihistamines; use in patients who cannot tolerate sedation
Cetirizine (Zyrtec)	Seasonal AR	Adults: 10 mg PO once daily Children: Age 2–6 years: 2.5 mg PO once daily; maximum 5 mg/day Age 6 years and older: 5–10 mg PO once daily	Somewhat more sedating than other second generation antihistamines, but less than first generation agents Less effective than first generation antihistamines; use in patients who cannot tolerate sedation **Adverse effects:** Drowsiness, somnolence, dry mouth, pharyngitis *Not recommended for pregnant women or nursing mothers*
Fexofenadine (Allegra)	Seasonal AR	Adults: 180 mg PO once daily Children: Age 2–11 years: 30 mg PO twice daily Age 12 years and older: 60 mg PO twice daily or 180 mg PO once daily	Less effective than first generation antihistamines; use in patients who cannot tolerate sedation **Adverse effects:** Headache, back pain, viral infection, dizziness *Only use in pregnancy if potential benefits justify potential risks to fetus*
Levocetirizine (Xyzal)	Seasonal and perennial AR	Adults: 5 mg PO once daily Children: Age 2–5 years: 1.25 mg PO once daily Age 6–11 years: 2.5 mg PO once daily Age 12 years and older: 2.5–5 mg PO once daily	**Adverse effects:** Sedation, mucosal dryness, urinary retention
Hydrochloride (Patanase)	Seasonal AR	665 mcg/spray Adults: two sprays per nostril twice daily Children: Age 6–11 years: one spray per nostril twice daily Age 12 years and older: two sprays per nostril twice daily	Target delivery in the nose for rapid improvement of congestion. **Adverse effects:** Bitter taste, headache, epistaxis, throat pain, nasal ulceration, somnolence *Only use in pregnancy if potential benefits justify potential risks to fetus*
Decongestants (monotherapy)			
Pseudoephedrine hydrochloride (Sudafed)	Nasal congestion	30–60 mg PO every 4–6 hours; maximum four doses/day	Should not be used for longer than 3–4 days **Adverse effects:** Can cause CNS excitation, hypertension, and palpitations *Use with caution in older patients and in those taking beta blockers* *Contraindicated in patients with diabetes mellitus, benign prostatic hyperplasia (BPH), hypertension, and cardiac disease and in those taking monoamine oxidase (MAO) inhibitors*

Drugs Commonly Prescribed 24.1: Rhinitis—cont'd

DRUG	INDICATION	DOSAGE	PRESCRIBING CONSIDERATIONS
NSAIDs and decongestants (combination therapy)			
Ibuprofen 200 mg and pseudoephedrine hydrochloride 30 mg (Advil Cold and Sinus)	Rhinorrhea, sinusitis, flu (influenza)	One to two tablets every 4–6 hours; maximum six tablets/day	Should not be used for longer than 3–4 days Take with food *Use with caution in patients with hypertension, diabetes mellitus, glaucoma, and BPH and in those taking beta blockers*
Antihistamines and decongestants (combination therapy)			
Diphenhydramine hydrochloride 25 mg and pseudoephedrine hydrochloride 60 mg (Tavist NightTime Allergy, Benadryl Allergy Decongestant)	Rhinorrhea, nasal congestion	One tablet every 4–6 hours	Should not be used for longer than 3–4 days Potentiates the effects of alcohol and sedatives *Do not use with MAO inhibitors or in patients with bronchospasm, hypertension, diabetes mellitus, or BPH*
Loratadine 10 mg and pseudoephedrine 240 mg (Claritin-D 24 Hour)	Rhinitis, sinusitis with congestion, AR	One tablet once daily	Should not be used for longer than 3–4 days Do not crush or chew *Use with caution in older patients and those taking beta blockers* *Contraindicated in patients with glaucoma, BPH, hypertension, or coronary artery disease*
Fexofenadine hydrochloride 60 mg and pseudoephedrine 120 mg (Allegra-D 12 Hour) Fexofenadine HCl 180 mg and pseudoephedrine 240 mg (Allegra-D 24 Hour)	Seasonal AR with nasal congestion	One tablet twice daily OR Extended release: one tablet once daily	Should not be used for longer than 3–4 days Avoid giving with food
Intranasal corticosteroids (monotherapy)			
Beclomethasone dipropionate (Beconase AQ)	Seasonal and perennial AR; vasomotor rhinitis; decrease nasal inflammatory reaction	42 mcg/spray Adults: One to two sprays per nostril twice daily Children: Age 6 years and older: one to two sprays per nostril twice daily	Available in aerosol and metered pump; may eliminate need for antihistamines or decongestants Must be used regularly; onset of action may require several days of use, with maximal effect after 1–2 weeks of regular use; use decongestant before application if necessary **Adverse effects:** Local irritation, increased rhinorrhea, localized fungal infection

Continued

Drugs Commonly Prescribed 24.1: Rhinitis—cont'd

DRUG	INDICATION	DOSAGE	PRESCRIBING CONSIDERATIONS
Budesonide (Rhinocort Aqua)	Seasonal and perennial AR; decrease nasal inflammatory reaction	32 mcg/spray Adults: one to four sprays per nostril once daily Children: Age 6–12 years: one to two sprays per nostril once daily Age 12 years and older: one to four sprays per nostril once daily	Aerosol; may eliminate need for antihistamines or decongestants Must be used regularly; onset of action may require several days of use, with maximal effect after 1–2 weeks of regular use; use decongestant before application if necessary **Adverse effects:** Local irritation, increased rhinorrhea, localized fungal infection Caution with CYP3A4 inhibitors (e.g., ketoconazole) *Only use in pregnancy if potential benefits justify potential risks to fetus*
Ciclesonide (Omnaris)	Seasonal and perennial AR; decrease nasal inflammatory reaction	50 mcg/spray Adults: two sprays per nostril once daily Children: Age 12 years and older: two sprays per nostril once daily	Aerosol; may eliminate need for antihistamines or decongestants Must be used regularly; onset of action may require several days of use, with maximal effect after 1–2 weeks of regular use; use decongestant before application if necessary **Adverse effects:** Local irritation, epistaxis, increased rhinorrhea, headache, pharyngitis, localized fungal infection Worsening of tuberculosis or other existing infections *Only use in pregnancy if potential benefits justify potential risks to fetus*
Fluticasone propionate (Flonase)	Seasonal and perennial AR; decrease nasal inflammatory reaction	50 mcg/spray Adults: two sprays per nostril once daily Children: Age 4 years and older to adolescence: one spray per nostril once daily	Available in metered pump; maintain regular regimen Monitor for visual changes. Onset of action may require several days of use, with maximal effect after 1–2 weeks of regular use. **Adverse effects:** Local irritation, epistaxis, increased rhinorrhea, localized fungal infection Caution with CYP3A4 inhibitors (e.g., ketoconazole) *Only use in pregnancy if potential benefits justify potential risks to fetus*
Fluticasone furoate (Veramyst)	Seasonal and perennial AR; decrease nasal inflammatory reaction	27.5 mcg/spray Adults: two sprays per nostril once daily Children: Age 2–11 years: one spray per nostril once daily Age 12 years and older: two sprays per nostril once daily	Suspension Onset of action may require several days of use, with maximal effect after 1–3 weeks of regular use. **Adverse effects:** Epistaxis, headache, nasal ulceration, pyrexia, cough, pharyngolaryngeal pain
Beclomethasone dipropionate (Qnasl)	Seasonal and perennial AR	40 mcg/spray OR 80 mcg/spray Adults: two sprays (80 mcg/spray) per nostril once daily Children: Age 4–11 years: one spray (40 mcg/spray) per nostril once daily Age 12 years and older: two sprays (80 mcg/spray) per nostril once daily	Aerosol. Onset of action may require several days of use, with maximal effect after 1–2 weeks of regular use. **Adverse effects:** Nasal discomfort, epistaxis, headache

Drugs Commonly Prescribed 24.1: Rhinitis—cont'd

DRUG	INDICATION	DOSAGE	PRESCRIBING CONSIDERATIONS
Triamcinolone acetonide (Nasacort)	Seasonal and perennial AR; decrease nasal inflammatory reaction	55 mcg/spray Adults: two sprays per nostril once daily Children: Age 2–5 years: one spray per nostril once daily Age 6–12 years: one to two sprays per nostril once daily Age 12 years and older: two sprays per nostril once daily	Available in aerosol or metered pump; maintain regular regimen. Monitor for visual changes. Onset of action may require several days of use, with maximal effect after 1–2 weeks of regular use. **Adverse effects:** Headache, epistaxis, pharyngitis, cough viral infections. It is unknown whether drug accumulates in breast milk; however, other corticosteroids are excreted in breast milk. *Nursing mothers should use with caution. Only use in pregnancy if potential benefits justify potential risks to fetus*
Mometasone furoate (Nasonex)	Seasonal AR; decrease nasal inflammatory reaction; treatment of nasal polyps in adults (18 years and older)	50 mcg/spray Adults: two sprays per nostril once daily for AR; two sprays per nostril once or twice daily for nasal polyps Children: Age 2–11 years: one spray per nostril once daily for AR Age 12 years and older: two sprays per nostril once daily	Begin 2–4 weeks before start of pollen season; maintain regular regimen. Monitor for visual changes. Onset of action may require several days of use, with maximal effect after 1–2 weeks of regular use. **Adverse effects:** Local irritation, increased rhinorrhea, viral infection, epistaxis, pharyngitis, cough, localized fungal infection Caution with CYP3A4 inhibitors (e.g., ketoconazole) *Only use in pregnancy if potential benefits justify potential risks to fetus*
Intranasal corticosteroids and decongestants (combination therapy)			
Azelastine hydrochloride and fluticasone propionate (Dymista)	Seasonal AR	137 mcg azelastine and 50 mcg fluticasone/spray Adults: one spray per nostril twice daily Children: Age 6 years and older: one spray per nostril twice daily	**Adverse effects:** Bitter taste, epistaxis, somnolence, headache.
Intranasal anticholinergics			
Ipratropium bromide 0.03% or 0.06% nasal spray (Atrovent)	Prevention of rhinorrhea associated with seasonal AR or viral upper respiratory infection	21 mcg/spray (0.03%) OR 42 mcg/spray (0.06%) Adults: two sprays (0.06%) three to four times daily OR two sprays (0.03%) two to three times daily Children: Age 5–11 years: two sprays (0.06%) three times daily Age 6 years and older: two sprays (0.03%) two to three times daily Age 12 years and older: two sprays (0.06%) three to four times daily	Does not relieve itching, sneezing, nasal blockage, or congestion **Adverse effects:** Epistaxis, pharyngitis, nasal dryness Avoid in patients with BPH and glaucoma *Only use in pregnancy if benefits outweigh the risks*

Continued

Drugs Commonly Prescribed 24.1: Rhinitis—cont'd

DRUG	INDICATION	DOSAGE	PRESCRIBING CONSIDERATIONS
Intranasal mast cell stabilizers			
Cromolyn sodium 5.2 mg (Nasalcrom)	Prevention and relief of nasal allergy symptoms	5.2 mcg/spray Adults: one spray per nostril three to four daily; maximum six sprays/nostril/day Children: Age 2 years and older: one spray per nostril three to four daily; maximum six sprays/nostril/day	Regular use required; do not use to treat sinus infection or asthma
Leukotriene receptor antagonists			
Montelukast (Singulair)	Seasonal and perennial AR	Adults: 10 mg PO once daily Children: Age 6–23 months: 4-mg oral granules once daily Age 2–5 years: 4-mg chewable tablet OR 4-mg oral granules once daily Age 6–14 years: 5-mg chewable tablet once daily Age 15 years and older: 10 mg PO once daily	Monitor with potent CYP450 inducers and with drugs metabolized by CYP2C8 **Adverse effects:** Upper respiratory infection

- Nasal saline irrigation has been shown to improve inflammation within the nose and paranasal sinuses by removing thick mucin and crusting. Nasal irrigation also improves the movement of mucus within the nasal passages and sinuses.
- Expectorants such as guaifenesin (Mucinex, Robitussin) may be helpful to reduce viscosity of mucus, causing cough. Typical doses are 200 to 400 mg every 4 hours as needed or 600 to 1,200 mg extended-release formulation every 12 hours as needed, with a maximum dose of 2,400 mg/day.

For AR, avoidance of or reduced exposure to offending allergens is the primary method of treatment because acute attacks are typically self-limited if not continually aggravated by allergens. First generation antihistamines have significant side effects, including decreased cognitive function, sedation, dizziness, and hypotension. These side effects can result in sudden cardiac death, accidental death (due to reduced dexterity and response time), and overdose. Newer generation oral antihistamines, designed to be less sedating, are now preferred over first generation antihistamines as the first-line, short-term treatment of choice for AR. These work best for early symptoms of allergy such as sneezing; watery eyes; and pruritus of the eyes, nose, and posterior pharynx. However, intranasal corticosteroids have traditionally been considered the most effective means of controlling the longer-term symptoms of AR, including nasal congestion and discharge. Meta-analyses have suggested that intranasal corticosteroids are the best overall first-line treatment for allergic rhinitis; however, intranasal corticosteroid therapy may require 2 or more weeks of continuous daily use before symptomatic relief is apparent. Systemic corticosteroids have significant side effects and tend to be discouraged for such a common condition. Leukotriene receptor antagonists, such as montelukast (Singulair) and zafirlukast (Accolate), are also approved for the chronic treatment of AR but are typically not used as first-line treatment. Figures 24.1 and 24.2 summarize the pharmacological management of intermittent versus persistent AR, respectively.

Vasomotor rhinitis is also treated symptomatically, albeit at times unsatisfactorily, with environmental humidification using a vaporizer or humidified central heating system. Avoidance of environmental triggers, if possible, is highly recommended. Rhinorrhea may be treated with systemic oral decongestants such as phenylephrine (Sudafed PE) 10 mg every 4 hours as needed, with a

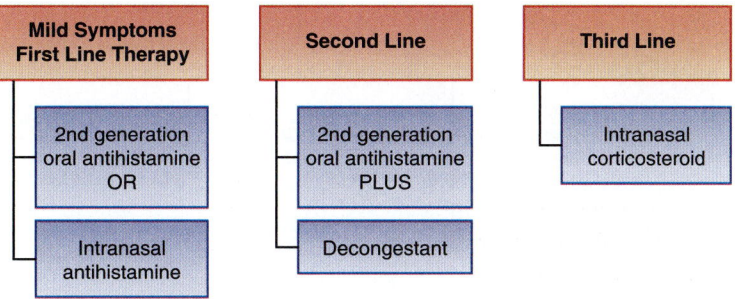
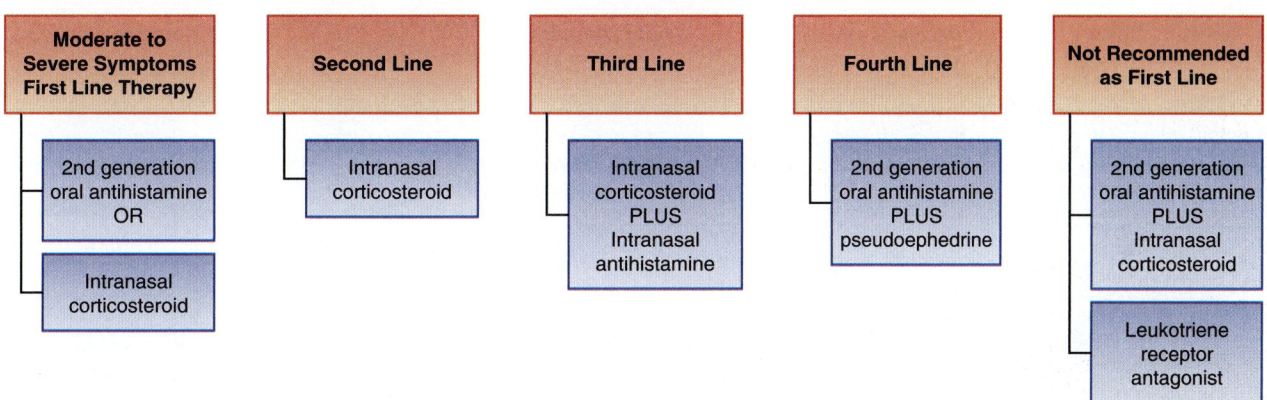

Figure 24.1 Intermittent Allergic Rhinitis: Pharmacological Management

maximum dose of 60 mg/day. Patients should be cautioned about long-term use of decongestants (particularly topical nasal preparations), however, as they can cause rebound congestion. Saline irrigation is effective in treating nasal congestion by thoroughly cleaning the nose and restoring nasal patency. This can be achieved by using a device such as a nasal irrigator or neti pot. Intranasal ipratropium bromide (Atrovent) 0.03% two sprays in each nostril two to four times daily as needed for rhinorrhea or azelastine (Astelin) two sprays in each nostril twice daily may also relieve nasal congestion and rhinorrhea symptoms.

Rhinitis medicamentosa or "rebound rhinitis" is characterized by nasal congestion without rhinorrhea after the extended use of topical vasoconstrictive medications. This condition can be remedied by immediately stopping the causative medication, although intranasal corticosteroids should be started to reduce symptoms of nasal congestion while the patient is discontinuing the offending medication. The condition typically resolves after 2 to 3 weeks. Treatment of rhinitis medicamentosa may also include a short course of systemic corticosteroids (e.g., prednisone 30 mg PO daily for 5 days), if other treatments prove ineffective.

Atrophic rhinitis may be treated with mupirocin antibiotic ointment applied intranasally two or three times daily until the nasal crusting and foul odor are eliminated. Nasal saline irrigation and saline spray may provide symptomatic relief.

Desensitizing immunotherapy ("allergy shots" or "allergy vaccines") may be an option for allergic rhinitis that is refractory to pharmacological treatment. Patients receive subcutaneous injections of purified allergen weekly at a dosage that increases with each treatment. The interval between injections is lengthened once a maintenance dose is reached. This treatment regimen may last up to 3 to 5 years, but it should not be continued past 12 months if symptoms are not improving. Cure rates may be as low as 20%, although many patients experience long-lasting relief for many years, even after allergen immunotherapy is stopped. In addition, to reduce the risk of anaphylactic reactions, antigen injections must never be given intravenously.

Occasionally, surgery is recommended if the etiology of refractory or recurrent rhinitis is anatomical, including nasal polypectomy for obstructing lesions. Similarly, if septal deviation is the cause of recurrent sinusitis, septoplasty may be recommended.

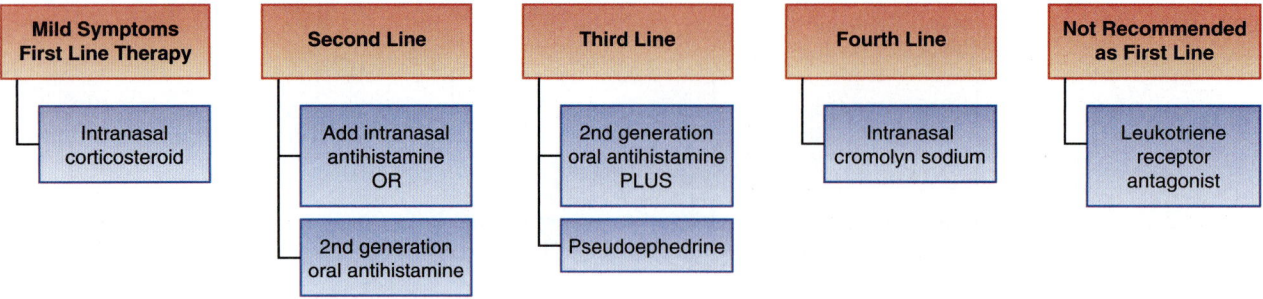

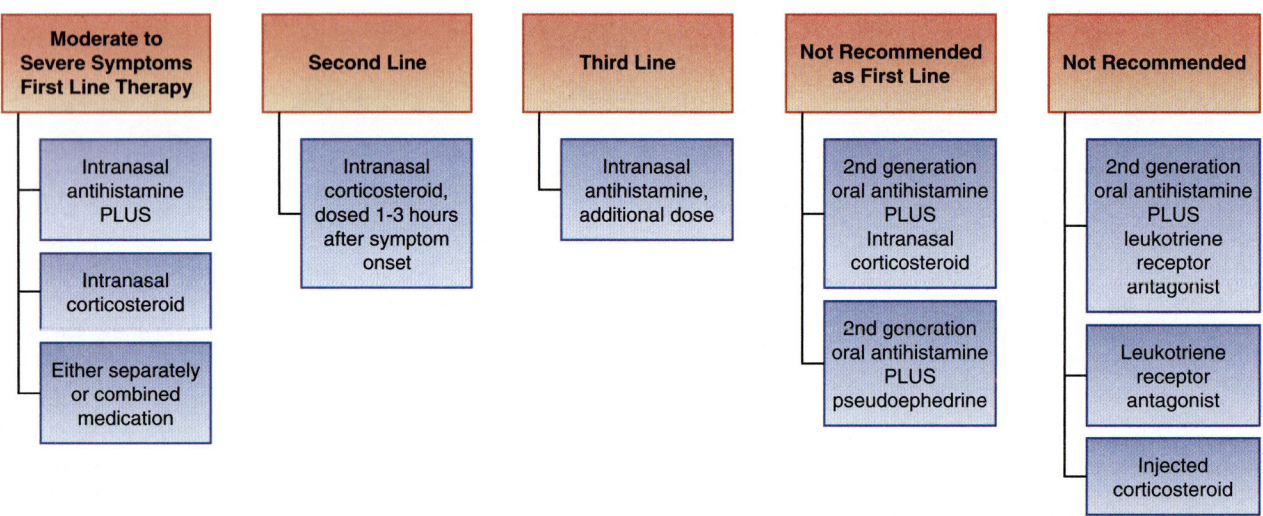

Figure 24.2 Persistent Allergic Rhinitis: Pharmacological Management

FOLLOW-UP AND REFERRAL

A return visit should be scheduled in 2 to 3 months to review patient education, adherence to the treatment plan, and effectiveness of prescribed treatments. After this, quarterly or biannual visits are recommended, depending on the patient's comfort level and general state of health.

Complications of infectious rhinitis include OM (an extension of nasal infection into the middle ear canal via the eustachian tube), acute or chronic rhinosinusitis (an extension of nasal infection into the sinuses), and repeated or disseminated respiratory infections. AR may lead to restless sleep and chronic fatigue, and asthma may complicate allergic attacks. Rhinitis medicamentosa may be complicated by physical addiction to topical nasal decongestants, as periods of relief shorten and the severity of rebound congestion increases with each use. Thus, stopping the use of nasal decongestants becomes especially difficult for the addicted patient.

Referral to an allergist may be necessary for SPT, allergen immunotherapy, or clinic-based nasal irrigation. The diagnosis and treatment of certain sequelae such as chronic sinusitis or high fever may also require referral. Otolaryngology referral is necessary if anatomical obstructions of the nasal cavity (e.g., nasal polyps, turbinate hypertrophy or a deviated septum) are causative or complicating factors. Referral to an otolaryngologist is also necessary in a patient with unilateral nasal obstruction and chronic epistaxis for direct endoscopic visualization of the nasal passages to rule out neoplasm.

Patient Education: Rhinitis

Viral rhinitis is best avoided by limiting exposure to persons with an acute URI, and all patients should be instructed to arrange for further evaluation if clear rhinorrhea becomes purulent, given the risk of bacterial superinfection with viral rhinitis. Allergic flare-ups are best prevented by avoiding exposure to environmental irritants. In turn, many preventive steps may be taken. Windows and doors should be kept closed to reduce pollen entry into the household, and high-efficiency particulate air (HEPA) filters are helpful in removing allergens and irritants from ambient air. Pet traffic from outdoors should be minimized because this may transport pollen indoors. Likewise, patients should avoid being outside on excessively sunny or windy days to minimize pollen exposure. Patients who are allergic to animal dander should bathe their pets often and restrict them from the bedroom or from the house altogether.

Patients with allergic rhinitis should be taught not only to avoid allergens but also to observe the onset, duration, and progression of symptoms, so that they can correlate their flare-ups to environmental exposures and thus better guide self-treatment. Preventive and prophylactic measures should be emphasized, particularly the importance of keeping bedrooms allergen free. Allergic attacks to mold spores can be prevented by avoiding piles of leaves during the fall months, wiping down household surfaces prone to mold growth with a diluted bleach solution, using HEPA filters, and reducing ambient humidity. Allergic attacks caused by perennial antigens such as dust or dust mites can be minimized by thoroughly cleaning or removing all carpets, drapes, curtains, and fabric-covered or stuffed furniture from the house, as well as by damp mopping, floor waxing, and dusting of all surfaces with a damp cloth. Stuffed animals, feather pillows, mattresses, and box springs should be either covered with plastic or removed and replaced with hypoallergenic pillow and mattress covers made with synthetic materials, such as polyester. Chenille bedspreads, quilts, or comforters should be avoided, and bedding should be washed weekly. The use of air-conditioning with frequent filter changes, rather than open windows, to cool automobiles or homes is recommended.

Vasomotor rhinitis is best avoided by limiting exposure to environmental triggers, and rhinitis medicamentosa can be prevented by diligently monitoring and limiting topical nasal decongestant use. Patients with all forms of rhinitis should understand the reasoning behind limiting nasal decongestant use, as well as the appropriate use of prophylactic cromolyn sodium sprays. Patients taking combination therapies, such as combined decongestants and antihistamines, must be educated on the individual ingredients in these combinations and warned of the possibility of inadvertent double-dosing with other over-the-counter (OTC) remedies with different brand names that contain the same active ingredients. It is also critical to explain that peak symptomatic relief from topical nasal corticosteroid preparations may not be evident until several weeks into therapy.

RHINOSINUSITIS

Rhinosinusitis (sinusitis) involves inflammation of the nasal mucosa and mucous membranes of one or more of the paranasal sinuses: frontal, sphenoid, posterior ethmoid, anterior ethmoid, and maxillary (see Fig. 24.3).

Rhinosinusitis is classified as (1) acute, which is characterized by an abrupt onset of infection and posttherapeutic resolution of symptoms lasting no more than 4 weeks; (2) recurrent acute rhinosinusitis (RARS) with four or more sinus infections in 1 year without persistent symptoms between episodes; or (3) chronic, which occurs with episodes of prolonged inflammation with repeated or inadequately treated acute infection, with symptoms lasting longer than 12 consecutive weeks. These classifications are based on both symptom duration as well as clinical manifestations. Rhinosinusitis can be further broken down into etiology as acute viral rhinosinusitis (AVRS) versus acute bacterial rhinosinusitis (ABRS). Differentiation between the two is important because antimicrobial therapy is not recommended for AVRS.

EPIDEMIOLOGY AND CAUSES

According to the U.S. Centers for Disease Control and Prevention (CDC), 28.9 million or 11.6% of adults are diagnosed with rhinosinusitis each year, which accounts for 11.8 million primary care visits. The cost of managing acute and chronic rhinosinusitis exceeds $11 billion per year. Rhinosinusitis affects adults more commonly between the ages of 45 and 74 years, with a higher predisposition in females than males, although there is no specific ethnic predisposition. Acute rhinosinusitis is the leading diagnosis leading to antibiotic prescribing in the primary care and emergency department setting.

Mucosal inflammation and congestion caused by a viral URI that lasts more than 7 to 10 days is a key risk factor for AVRS, particularly during the autumn, winter, and spring seasons. Smoking, exposure to air pollution, uncontrolled AR and NAR, inflammatory diseases, injury to the nose or sinuses from foreign bodies (e.g., nasogastric tubes or nasotracheal intubation) or trauma, nasal polyps, and chronic use of OTC or prescription decongestants may lead to an impaired mucociliary function and mucosal inflammation. This mucosal inflammation causes a blockage of the sinus ostia, resulting in an ideal environment for pathogenic bacterial colonization. Odontogenic causes of maxillary rhinosinusitis are seen in people with periapical and periodontal disease, dental caries, or dental abscesses.

Recurrent or persistent bacterial infection resulting from blockage of nasociliary sinus drainage via the sinus ostia has been particularly associated with chronic rhinosinusitis. Mechanical blockage may result from anatomical abnormalities such as a deviated septum, turbinate hypertrophy, nasal polyps, reduced ostial diameter, and sinus or nasal neoplasms. Some asthmatic patients also suffer from sinusitis because of their inflammation-prone, hypersensitive airways. Furthermore, genetic diseases such as mucosal immunoglobulin A (IgA) deficiency, immobile cilia syndrome (Kartagener syndrome), and cystic fibrosis also contribute to decreased mucociliary clearance and

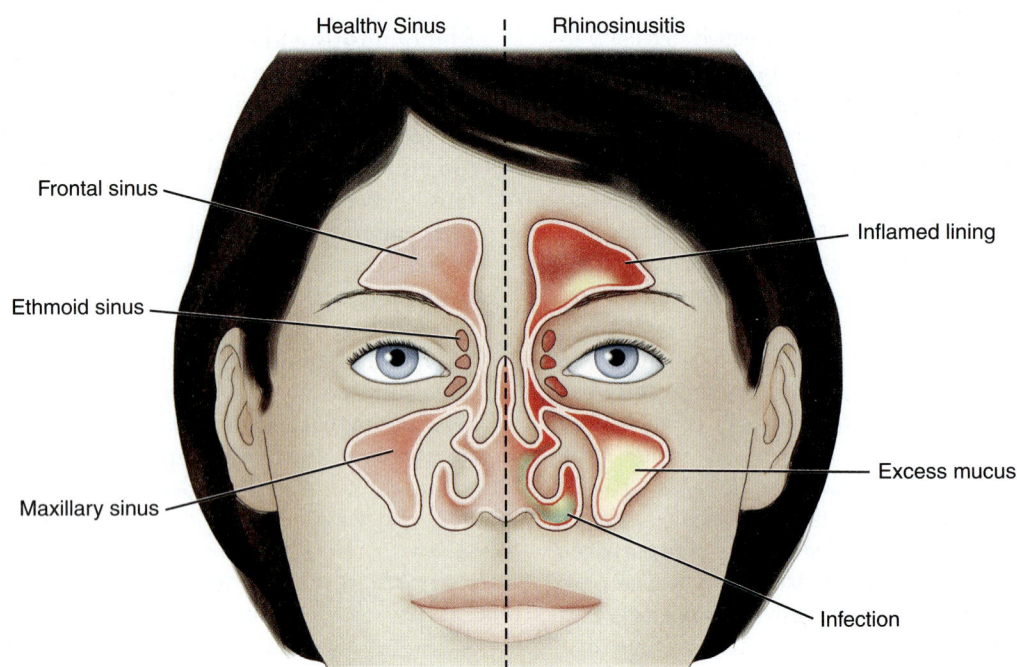

Figure 24.3 Sinus Anatomy Showing Normal Sinuses and Rhinosinusitis (Sinusitis)

persistent sinus infection. Chronic inflammatory diseases such as sarcoidosis and Wegener's granulomatosis also predispose patients to mucosal inflammation. Patients who are immunocompromised, such as those who are diabetic, have HIV infection, are malnourished, or are otherwise chronically immunocompromised, may develop severe invasive sinus disease. Complications of ABRS are rare but can be serious and even life-threatening, because of the proximity of the sinus cavities to the eyes and base of the skull. In turn, complications include brain abscess, meningitis, periorbital/orbital cellulitis, osteomyelitis of the facial bones, and cavernous sinus thrombosis.

PATHOPHYSIOLOGY

Inflammation of the nasal, paranasal, and sinus mucosa is a causative factor in acute rhinosinusitis. As the inflammation typically occurs secondary to a viral URI, allergic reaction, or other inflammatory cause, mucosal secretions from sinus goblet cells increase in volume and viscosity. The resultant mucosal edema causes obstruction of the sinus outflow tracts, inhibiting sinus drainage. The vast majority (greater than 95%) of acute rhinosinusitis cases are caused by the same viruses associated with uncomplicated URIs and are self-limiting. AVRS is most commonly caused by rhinovirus, coronavirus, adenovirus, echovirus, and coxsackievirus, as well as respiratory syncytial virus, parainfluenza virus, and influenza virus. Only 0.5% to 2% of viral rhinosinusitis progress to acute bacterial sinusitis, which means antibiotic therapy should not be routinely prescribed for rhinosinusitis.

In ABRS, the normally ciliated pseudostratified columnar epithelium lining the sinuses erodes as infecting organisms proliferate, resulting in a loss of mucociliary clearance through the sinus ostia (bony openings) and the ostiomeatal complex located in the anterior ethmoid region, which serves as a common drainage pathway for the frontal, maxillary, and ethmoid sinuses. In turn, blockage of the ostiomeatal complex and/or impairment of ciliary function is a contributing factor in rhinosinusitis. The most common bacterial pathogens isolated in acute rhinosinusitis are *S. pneumoniae, Haemophilus influenzae, Moraxella catarrhalis* (seen more commonly in children), *Streptococcus pyogenes* (especially group A beta-hemolytic *Streptococcus*), and *Staphylococcus aureus*.

The specific role of bacteria, fungi, and viruses in chronic sinusitis is hotly debated. *S. aureus*, gram-negative rods, and in up to one-half of cases, anaerobic bacteria (including *Peptostreptococcus* and *Bacteroides*) are most often implicated. Polymicrobial infection is also more common in chronic than acute sinusitis. *S. aureus* and *Pseudomonas aeruginosa* are the most common causes of cystic fibrosis–related sinusitis and nosocomial sinus infection associated with nasal or endotracheal intubation and nasogastric feeding tubes.

In the immunocompromised host, gram-negative aerobic bacteria must be considered, as well as the fungi *Aspergillus fumigatus* and *Mucor* species, both of which may cause severe, rapid, and life-threatening invasive sinusitis in diabetic or otherwise chronically immunocompromised patients. Allergic fungal sinusitis occurs more commonly in atopic individuals in which the nasal and sinus mucosa undergo an IgE-mediated type I hypersensitivity response to airborne fungal spores or fungal proliferation facilitated by obstructed sinus outflow. *Aspergillus* species and dematiaceous (brown-pigmented) molds are the most common fungi found in acute fungal rhinosinusitis. In these cases, the sinuses become filled with allergic mucin consisting of necrotic cellular debris, eosinophils, and fungal hyphae. If neither a hypersensitivity response nor an invasive sinusitis ensues, fungal colonization may result in unilateral chronic sinusitis characterized by the formation of a dense fungal ball with sclerosis of the surrounding bone.

CLINICAL PRESENTATION
Subjective

AVRS symptoms include purulent nasal drainage presenting with focal facial pain/pressure and nasal obstruction/congestion, which typically develop after a viral URI. Symptom duration is from 10 days to 12 weeks. Some patients report additional symptoms of fever, cough, sore throat, headache/pressure, anosmia/hyposmia, disturbed sleep, malaise, or fatigue. Focal pain that occurs over the cheeks and upper teeth is correlated with maxillary sinus involvement; pain over the eyebrows indicates frontal sinus involvement; and pain over or behind the eyes indicates ethmoid sinusitis. However, not every patient with acute or chronic rhinosinusitis has facial pain. Importantly, nasal obstruction or facial pain without purulent drainage is inconsistent with acute rhinosinusitis.

ABRS should be suspected if the patient has persistent symptoms of AVRS that worsen after 10 days or experiences "double worsening" in which a patient starts to improve but then gets much worse after 10 days. In addition to mucopurulent rhinorrhea, nasal congestion, and obstruction, patients may also present with a fever greater than 101°F, focal facial pain, headache, elevated white blood cell count, malaise, sore throat, and cough. Symptoms that are worrisome for complications of ABRS include ocular pain, eyelid swelling or periorbital edema, decreased eye movements, diplopia, displacement of the ocular globe, high fevers, nuchal rigidity, changes in mental status, severe headache, and/or cranial nerve palsies. Immediate referral to an emergency department is warranted for these patients, as such complications may be sight-threatening or even life-threatening.

Patients with chronic rhinosinusitis typically report a persistent cough due to postnasal drip or cold-like symptoms that last more than 12 weeks. Additional symptoms of chronic sinusitis may include headache or focal facial pressure specifically reflecting the affected sinuses, as described earlier. Fever is less common in chronic rhinosinusitis, although patients may have a history of recurrent sinus infections requiring antibiotic therapy. Other symptoms include thick mucopurulent rhinorrhea or postnasal discharge (postnasal drip), "popping" ears, toothache-like cheek pain, difficulty chewing, anosmia or hyposmia, and a foul smell emanating from inside the nasal cavity or halitosis. Immunocompromised patients may present with more subtle signs and symptoms because leukopenia may limit the inflammatory response to infection. Immunocompromised patients are at risk for chronic invasive fungal rhinosinusitis, symptoms of which include severe headache, proptosis, decreased orbital movements, visual changes, and neurological deficits.

Objective

On anterior rhinoscopy, with the aid of a nasal speculum, purulent nasal secretions (recognized by polymorphonuclear neutrophils in a Giemsa-stained nasal smear) and erythema of the nasal mucosa and turbinates are noted. Red, swollen nasal mucosa indicates infection, whereas pale, swollen mucosa with watery secretions points to an allergic etiology. Purulent secretions seen coming from inside the middle meatus are characteristic of sinusitis. Black or necrotic material may be seen in mucormycosis-related rhinorrhea in immunocompromised patients. Ethmoid sinus involvement may result in chemosis (eyelid mucous membrane edema), proptosis, conjunctival injection, extraocular muscle palsy, or orbital fixation.

On palpation, the affected sinuses are typically tender to palpation and/or percussion. Sphenoid sinusitis presents as tenderness over the vertex or mastoids, ethmoid sinusitis as retro-orbital or nasal bridge tenderness, maxillary sinusitis as cheek or dental tenderness, and frontal sinusitis as tenderness of the forehead. An examination of the oral cavity should be performed if maxillary sinusitis is suspected to rule out dental abscess as the cause. If a patient presents with periorbital swelling or ocular globe displacement, acute visual changes (e.g., decreased visual acuity, diplopia), and other neurological findings, assessment via a cranial nerve examination is warranted. Patients who have otalgia with hearing loss, aural fullness, or popping in the ears should have an otoscopic evaluation to assess for OM or OM with effusion.

DIAGNOSTIC REASONING
Diagnostic Tests

It is important for the clinician to focus on clinical signs and symptoms for the initial diagnosis of rhinosinusitis and avoid unnecessary diagnostic tests. Diagnosis of uncomplicated AVRS and ABRS can be made on the basis of symptoms alone, and neither laboratory tests nor x-ray films are indicated in uncomplicated rhinosinusitis. As stated earlier, ABRS occurs in only 0.5% to 2% of acute rhinosinusitis cases when bacteria secondarily infect an inflamed sinus cavity. Patients with ABRS tend to have symptoms that last longer (more than 10 days) or are more severe than AVRS. Collectively, purulent nasal discharge, nasal obstruction, anosmia/hyposmia, and facial pain/pressure/fullness have relatively high sensitivity and specificity for ABRS, particularly when they occur concurrently and persist for more than 10 days.

A CBC to detect leukocyte elevation may be indicated if an infectious etiology is suspected in acute sinusitis; however, leukocytosis is rarely observed in chronic sinusitis. Stains or cultures of nasal and throat secretions by swabbing are not recommended because the nasopharyngeal mucosa is widely colonized by a diverse array of endogenous, nonpathogenic microbial flora and will yield unreliable results. Allergic SPT may be necessary if the patient history suggests allergic disease (e.g., allergen exposure, seasonal attacks). These patients often demonstrate peripheral eosinophilia and elevated total or allergen-specific IgE levels. Culture with microscopic examination of sinus aspirates can assist with culture-directed, narrow-spectrum antimicrobial therapy in acute or chronic rhinosinusitis. This is typically done by an otolaryngologist using a rigid scope. If invasive fungal rhinosinusitis is suspected, sinus culture, sinus mucosal biopsy, and flexible fiber-optic rhinoscopy by an otorhinolaryngologist are indicated. Chronic sinusitis in general is characterized by a morphological change of the ciliated sinus epithelium to a hypertrophied, stratified squamous form that is evident on biopsy.

Plain sinus films are not recommended to evaluate the sinuses, as they do not adequately evaluate these anatomical structures. A sinus computed tomography (CT) scan without contrast is the gold standard to evaluate sinus structures in patients with chronic rhinosinusitis, sinusitis patients with complications such as orbital/periorbital edema or soft tissue masses (e.g., nasal polyps, intranasal or sinus masses), or in patients that have RARS. Sinus magnetic resonance imaging (MRI) is superior for soft tissue discrimination but is poor at visualizing bony structures. Thus, MRI tends to be reserved for suspected sinus neoplasia or extension of sinus disease into intracranial soft tissues.

Differential Diagnosis

Myofascial pain that is unrelated to infectious causes may mimic the pain from acute sinusitis, but pain from other myofascial disorders is typically more diffuse and does not progressively worsen. Localized odontogenic pathology may produce similar pain, but the pain will not be accompanied with nasal symptoms or focal maxillary pressure unless progressing to extension into the maxillary sinuses. Patients with migraine, cluster headache, or trigeminal neuralgia also present with facial and cranial pain in the absence of nasal symptoms and focal sinus pressure. Allergic rhinitis, vasomotor rhinitis, rhinitis medicamentosa, mechanical nasal airway obstruction, acute viral URI with persistent viral rhinitis, and chronic inflammatory conditions such as sarcoidosis and Wegener's granulomatosis may all present with nasal congestion or pain. However, if these cases are uncomplicated by sinusitis, no signs of sinus inflammation will be detected on examination (see Differential Diagnosis 24.2).

MANAGEMENT

Because most acute rhinosinusitis cases are caused by viruses rather than bacteria, antibiotics are not indicated as treatment. Overprescribing of antibiotics offers no medical benefit in AVRS, wastes financial resources, and can cause potentially harmful complications as well as antibiotic resistance in common nasopharyngeal flora. As acute rhinosinusitis is the leading cause of antibiotic overprescribing, antibiotic stewardship should be employed at all times, with antibiotics only being prescribed when bacterial infection is appropriately suspected.

Adjunctive measures may also be used to enhance mucociliary clearance, countering the main risk factor for the development of sinusitis. Saline nasal spray may be helpful in improving sinus drainage, and dedicated sinus irrigation two or more times a day with an adequate volume of saline to fully flush the sinuses has been shown to significantly relieve symptoms, even without antimicrobial therapy. Patients are instructed to infuse their sinuses using a warm isotonic or hypertonic saline-filled bulb syringe expressed into each nostril, followed by immediate drainage of the liquid over a sink to remove both infectious organisms and excess mucus. Various commercial saline sinus irrigation systems with balanced salt solutions are currently available. However, homemade preparations may be made by mixing one teaspoon of noniodized salt with 8 ounces of warm water (noniodized salt should be used, as iodine is a known mucosal irritant). A cool-mist ultrasonic humidifier (cleaned daily with a 1:10 solution of bleach and water) may also assist in thinning sinus secretions and facilitating drainage. Distilled water or water that was boiled and cooled down should be used for nasal irrigations. Well or tap water should not be used in sinus irrigation, as this increases the risk of protozoal contamination of the sinuses. Smoke and other environmental pollutants should be avoided. Fluid intake should be increased, and heated mist from a facial sauna, steam bath, shower, or hot moist towels wrapped around the face may help relieve sinus and nasal pain by liquefying secretions.

Oral analgesics may also be used for pain or fever; this includes ibuprofen (Motrin, Advil) 400 to 600 mg every 6 to 8 hours as needed or acetaminophen (Tylenol) 650 mg every 4 to 6 hours as needed. Intranasal decongestant sprays can be used for severe congestion but should not be taken for longer than 3 days at a time because long-term use can lead to rebound nasal congestion (rhinitis medicamentosa) and addiction. Phenylephrine (Neo-Synephrine) one to two upright sprays in each nostril three to four times daily as needed or the stronger oxymetazoline (Afrin) one to two upright sprays in each nostril two to three times daily as needed may be helpful in adults. Oral decongestants such

Differential Diagnoses 24.2: Rhinosinusitis

Differentials	Symptoms	Physical Examination Findings	Alarming Symptoms That Require Immediate Referral to Specialty Care or Emergency Department
Acute viral rhinosinusitis (AVRS)	Symptoms that last less than 10 days to 12 weeks Nasal blockage/congestion Nasal discharge + Facial pain/pressure + Anosmia/hyposmia Cough Fever	Nasal mucosal edema/erythema Yellow/green discharge Focal tenderness over sinuses Posterior pharyngeal erythema or drainage Injected tonsils	Periorbital edema Displaced globe Double vision Ophthalmoplegia Decreased vision Severe headache Frontal swelling Signs of sepsis Neurological signs Epistaxis Unilateral symptoms should be referred to otorhinolaryngologist
Acute bacterial rhinosinusitis	Persistent symptoms that worsen after more than 10 days or "double worsening" (initial improvement followed by worsening after 10 days) Purulent nasal discharge Nasal blockage/congestion Focal facial pressure/pain Fever	Nasal erythema Mucosal edema Purulent nasal discharge Anatomical blockage such as deviated septum, foreign body, mass	
Recurrent acute rhinosinusitis	More than four episodes per year with symptom-free intervals Symptoms same as AVRS	Same symptoms as AVRS	
Acute fungal rhinosinusitis	Thick nasal mucus Anosmia Postnasal drip Cough Nasal congestion/obstruction	Thick brown "peanut butter"–like nasal discharge Proptosis Facial deformity	
Mucormycosis	Acute rhinosinusitis Fever Congestion Severe headache Sinus pain Facial numbness Mental status change Periorbital edema Proptosis Blindness	Tissue necrosis (black eschar) of the nasal mucosa, palate or skin overlying the orbit Life-threatening and requires immediate hospitalization and referral to otorhinolaryngologist	

Continued

Differential Diagnoses 24.2: Rhinosinusitis—cont'd

Differentials	Symptoms	Physical Examination Findings	Alarming Symptoms That Require Immediate Referral to Specialty Care or Emergency Department
Invasive fungal rhinosinusitis	Profound immunosuppression Severe headache	Symptoms of chronic rhinosinusitis After months, patients may develop orbital invasion, causing visual changes and neurological complaints secondary to extension to the brain Proptosis and fixation of the globe are seen with orbital involvement May have tenderness over the maxillary sinuses and erythema overlying the malar areas	
Chronic rhinosinusitis	More than 12 weeks of the following: Two symptoms of nasal obstruction and/or purulent nasal discharge + Focal facial pain/pressure + Anosmia/hyposmia	Purulent nasal drainage Edematous/erythematous turbinates May see nasal polyps or inflammatory tissue Blood-tinged drainage	
Allergic rhinitis	See Differential Diagnosis 24.1: Rhinitis		
Nonallergic rhinitis	See Differential Diagnosis 24.1: Rhinitis		
Nasal polyposis	See Differential Diagnosis 24.1: Rhinitis		
Structural Abnormalities • Septal deviation • Foreign body • Malignancy	See Differential Diagnosis 24.1: Rhinitis		
Migraine	Aura Headache that is nonfocal, throbbing, or squeezing Vertigo Photophobia/phonophobia Nausea/vomiting	Normal examination	
Myofascial pain	Focal pain of the face Absence of purulent nasal drainage, nasal obstruction, or nasal symptoms	Tenderness over musculature	
Odontogenic causes	Absence of nasal symptoms or nasal purulence	Dental caries Swelling or purulence at the gumline	

as pseudoephedrine (Sudafed) 30 to 60 mg every 4 to 6 hours as needed give an oral alternative but tend to be less effective than topical preparations. Systemic decongestants also have a greater risk of sympathomimetic side effects, such as tachycardia and hypertension, than topical decongestants and should, therefore, also be limited to no more than 3 days of continuous use.

Expectorants such as guaifenesin 200 to 400 mg every 4 hours as needed can facilitate sinus drainage by liquefying sinus secretions. Prescription use of anti-inflammatory topical corticosteroids in nasal spray preparations such as fluticasone (Flonase), mometasone (Nasonex), or triamcinolone (Nasacort)—all calling for two sprays daily in each nostril for 2 to 3 weeks—is becoming more common as a treatment for rhinosinusitis; however, randomized controlled trials have been inconsistent regarding their effectiveness in rhinosinusitis. In fact, corticosteroid therapy has been shown to increase viral load in AVRS. Oral antihistamines should be avoided unless an allergic component is evident because they tend to dry the mucosa, thicken purulent sinus fluids, and slow mucosal drainage, although some studies have suggested their efficacy in symptomatic relief of uncomplicated viral URIs.

Although localized sinus infection may be self-limited, antibiotic and symptomatic therapy may be considered appropriate for suspected ABRS to prevent disease progression and complications. Understanding bacterial causes of ABRS is essential in prescribing the appropriate antimicrobial therapy. The most common bacterial pathogens isolated in acute rhinosinusitis are *S. pneumoniae, H. influenzae,* and *M. catarrhalis* (which is a more common pathogen in children). Empiric antibiotic therapy for 5 to 10 days, covering the most common etiological agents, should be instituted before the identification of causative organisms is confirmed because symptoms may progress while awaiting laboratory confirmation. In adults with uncomplicated ABRS, common choices include narrow-spectrum antibiotics such as amoxicillin (Amoxil) 500 mg three times a day to as high as 1 g PO twice daily or more intense coverage of potentially resistant organisms with amoxicillin-clavulanate (Augmentin) 500 mg PO three times a day or 875 mg PO twice daily. In patients who are allergic to penicillin, doxycycline (Doxy-100) 100 mg PO twice daily may be used.

Because of the increasing resistance of *S. pneumoniae, H. influenzae* (up to 50% of strains), *M. catarrhalis,* and virtually all *S. aureus* strains to first-line antibiotics, referencing local and regional antibiotic resistance histograms can reveal important community trends that guide first-line antibiotic selection. Macrolides such as clarithromycin (Biaxin), azithromycin (Zithromax), and trimethoprim-sulfamethoxazole (Bactrim, Septra) are not recommended because of high rates of resistance in *S. pneumoniae.* Drugs Commonly Prescribed 24.2 summarizes pharmacological recommendations for AVRS and ABRS.

Current treatment guidelines for ABRS in adults consider first-line therapy to be amoxicillin either with or without clavulanate, depending on whether risk factors for antibiotic resistance are present (e.g., high endemic rates of penicillin-resistant *S. pneumoniae,* antibiotic use within the past 30 days, severe infection with systemic symptoms such as fever of 102°F [39°C] or greater, age older than 65 years, hospitalization, or immunocompromised status).

As stated previously, doxycycline is usually considered first-line treatment for penicillin- or cephalosporin-allergic patients. Fluoroquinolones can also be used but should be reserved for those who have no alternative treatment options, as the serious adverse effects associated with fluoroquinolones generally outweigh the benefits for patients with ABRS. Immunocompromised patients typically require broad-spectrum coverage for gram-positive and -negative organisms and possibly empiric antifungal therapy. Acute infections that fail to clear after one course of antibiotic therapy are often treated with a second course from a separate antibiotic class for 14 days.

Only a small minority of patients require parenteral therapy for chronic rhinosinusitis. Parenteral antimicrobials are indicated in patients who are seriously ill, undergoing surgery, or in whom compliance with oral antibiotics is questionable. Sinus cultures should be obtained from patients requiring parenteral therapy. Parenteral antibiotics effective against both anaerobes and aerobes include ampicillin-sulbactam (Unasyn), ticarcillin-clavulanate (Timentin), piperacillin-tazobactam (Zosyn), imipenem-cilastatin (Primaxin), clindamycin (Cleocin), moxifloxacin (Avalox, Vigamox), the carbapenems (e.g., meropenem [Merrem], ertapenem [Invanz]), and the second generation cephalosporins (e.g., cefoxitin [Mefoxin], cefotetan [Cefotan]). If *P. aeruginosa* is suspected, the preferred antibiotics include fluoroquinolones (e.g., moxifloxacin, levofloxacin [Levaquin]), third or fourth generation cephalosporins with antipseudomonal activity (e.g., ceftazidime [Fortaz], cefepime [Maxipime]), aminoglycosides, or the carbapenems (e.g., imipenem-cilastatin, meropenem, but not ertapenem because it lacks activity against *Pseudomonas*). Risks and benefits of this treatment should be carefully evaluated, however, and consultation with an infectious disease specialist and/or pharmacist should be initiated.

Antibiotics against anaerobic organisms such as *Peptostreptococcus* and *Bacteroides* are typically required for chronic sinusitis, with regimens lasting up to 3 to 4 weeks or even as long as 6 weeks for refractory chronic cases. Antibiotic regimens include amoxicillin-clavulanate (Augmentin XR) 875 to 1,000 mg/125 mg PO every 12 hours or the second generation cephalosporin cefuroxime (Ceftin) 250 to 500 mg PO twice daily. For penicillin-allergic patients, antibiotic options include doxycycline 100 mg PO twice daily or 200 mg PO once daily and clindamycin 300 mg PO every 6 hours. For documented gram-negative infection, a fluoroquinolone (e.g., levofloxacin, moxifloxacin) should be prescribed at the doses mentioned previously. As always, a thorough risk/benefit analysis of the use of these drugs should be

Text continued on page 376

Drugs Commonly Prescribed 24.2: Acute Viral Rhinosinusitis (AVRS) and Acute Bacterial Rhinosinusitis (ABRS)

INDICATION	DRUG	DOSING	PRESCRIBING INDICATIONS
Analgesics and Antipyretics			
Pain and fever management	Acetaminophen (Tylenol)	Adults and adolescents older than 12 years of age: 325 mg two capsules/tablets every 4–6 hours while symptoms last Children 6 months–11 years: 10–15 mg/kg/dose PO every 4 hours as needed (maximum 75 mg/kg/day)	Do not exceed 800 mg in 24 hours for children and 4,000 mg in 24 hours in adults *Adverse effects: Hepatotoxicity (avoid in patients with liver disease)*
Pain and fever management	Ibuprofen (Motrin, Advil)	Adult and adolescents older than 12 years: 200 mg one to three tablets every 6–8 hours Children 6 months–11 years: 5–10 mg/kg/dose PO every 6–8 hour as needed (maximum 40 mg/kg/day)	Do not exceed 1,200 mg in 24 hours. Take with food to avoid stomach irritation/ulcerations Use cautiously in patients with cardiovascular disease, renal disease, or history of stomach ulcers or other gastrointestinal disorders *Adverse effects: Erosions/ulcerations of gastrointestinal mucosal lining; renal toxicity*
Decongestants (monotherapy)			
Nasal congestion	Pseudoephedrine HCl (Sudafed)	30–60 mg PO every 4–6 hours; maximum four doses/day	Should not be used for longer than 3–4 days Use with caution in older adult patients and those taking beta blockers Contraindicated in patients with diabetes mellitus, benign prostatic hyperplasia (BPH), hypertension, and cardiac disease and in those taking monoamine oxidase inhibitors *Adverse effects: Central nervous system (CNS) excitation, hypertension, and palpitations*
Nonsteroidal Anti-inflammatory Drug (NSAID) and Decongestant (combination therapy)			
Rhinorrhea, sinusitis, flu	Ibuprofen 200 mg and pseudoephedrine HCl 30 mg (Advil Cold and Sinus)	One to two tablets every 4–6 hours; maximum six tablets/day	Should not be used for longer than 3–4 days Take with food Use with caution in patients with cardiovascular disease, hypertension, renal disease, diabetes mellitus, glaucoma, and BPH and in those taking beta blockers *Adverse effects: CNS excitation, hypertension, and palpitations; erosions/ulcerations of gastrointestinal mucosal lining; renal toxicity*
Intranasal Decongestants			
Nasal congestion	Oxymetazoline 0.05% (Afrin)	Adults and children older than 6 years: two to three sprays in each nostril up to twice daily for maximum of 3 days	Not recommended in children less than 6 years Do not use for more than 3 days as this can cause rebound congestion (rhinitis medicamentosa) *Adverse effects: Nasal dryness, mucosal damage with long-term use; CNS depression in children*

Drugs Commonly Prescribed 24.2: Acute Viral Rhinosinusitis (AVRS) and Acute Bacterial Rhinosinusitis (ABRS)—cont'd

INDICATION	DRUG	DOSING	PRESCRIBING INDICATIONS
Oral Mucolytics			
Thick mucosal secretions (hydrates respiratory tract and thins mucus)	Guaifenesin (Mucinex, Robitussin)	Adults and children older than 12 years: 200–400 mg PO every 4 hours as needed; extended-release 600–1,200 mg PO every 12 hours as needed Children 6–12 years: 100–200 mg PO every 4 hours as needed Children 2–6 years: 50–100 mg PO every 4 hours as needed	Do not exceed 2,400 mg in 24 hours in adults Do not exceed six doses in 24 hours for children *Adverse effects: May cause drowsiness, skin rash, or gastrointestinal symptoms*
Intranasal Corticosteroids			
Nasal congestion (decreases intranasal inflammatory reaction)	Fluticasone propionate (Flonase)	50 mcg/spray two sprays per nostril daily OR one spray per nostril twice daily; maximum two sprays per nostril daily	Available in metered pump Maintain regular regimen Monitor for visual changes Onset of action may require several days of regular use. Use with caution with CYP3A4 inhibitors (e.g., ketoconazole) Only use in pregnancy if potential benefits justify potential risks to fetus *Adverse effects: Local irritation, epistaxis, increased rhinorrhea, localized fungal infection*
Nasal congestion (decreases intranasal inflammatory reaction)	Triamcinolone acetonide (Nasacort)	55 mcg/spray two sprays per nostril daily	Available in aerosol or metered pump Maintain regular regimen Monitor for visual changes Onset of action may require several days of regular use. Only use in pregnancy if potential benefits justify potential risks to fetus *Adverse effects: Headache, epistaxis, pharyngitis, cough, viral infections*
Nasal congestion (decreases intranasal inflammatory reaction)	Mometasone furoate (Nasonex)	50 mcg/spray two sprays per nostril daily	Begin 2–4 weeks before start of pollen season Maintain regular regimen Monitor for visual changes Onset of action may require several days of regular use. Use with caution with CYP3A4 inhibitors (e.g., ketoconazole) Only use in pregnancy if potential benefits justify potential risks to fetus *Adverse effects: Local irritation, increased rhinorrhea, viral infection, epistaxis, pharyngitis, cough, localized fungal infection*

Continued

Drugs Commonly Prescribed 24.2: Acute Viral Rhinosinusitis (AVRS) and Acute Bacterial Rhinosinusitis (ABRS)—cont'd

INDICATION	DRUG	DOSING	PRESCRIBING INDICATIONS
Antibiotic Therapy for ABRS: First-line Therapy for Uncomplicated ABRS			
Antibiotic therapy for patients without penicillin allergy and without risk factors for pneumococcal resistance	Amoxicillin (Amoxil)	Amoxicillin 500 mg PO three times daily or 875 mg PO twice daily	Must be renally dosed for chronic kidney disease *Adverse effects: Diarrhea, headache, allergic reaction, anaphylaxis, skin rash, nausea, vomiting,* Clostridioides difficile *colitis with prolonged use*
Antibiotic therapy for patients with penicillin allergy and without risk factors for pneumococcal resistance	Doxycycline (Doxy-100) OR Levofloxacin (Levaquin) or Moxifloxacin (Avelox) (Respiratory fluoroquinolone should only be used for those with no other alternative treatment.)	Doxycycline 100 mg PO twice daily or 200 mg PO daily OR Levofloxacin 500 mg PO once daily or 750 mg PO once daily or Moxifloxacin 400 mg PO once daily	Can cause esophageal damage as a direct result of caustic tissue injury *Adverse effects: Diarrhea, abdominal pain, candidiasis, photosensitivity, skin hyperpigmentation* Use with caution in renally impaired patients; dose must be adjusted for creatinine clearance of less than 50 mL/min *Adverse effects: Diarrhea, skin rash including severe skin rash such as Stevens-Johnson syndrome, toxic epidermal necrolysis, superinfection such as* Clostridioides difficile *colitis with prolonged use (which can be severe and life-threatening), glucose dysregulation associated with hypo/hyperglycemia, aortic dissection, liver injury, allergic reaction, exacerbation of myasthenia gravis, peripheral neuropathy, Guillain-Barré syndrome, phototoxicity, photosensitivity, skin hyperpigmentation, prolonged QT interval on ECG, tendinitis, tendon rupture, CNS effects (especially in older patients) such as restlessness, confusion, agitation, insomnia, drowsiness, hallucinations, or seizures*
Antibiotic therapy for patients without penicillin allergy and with risk factors for pneumococcal resistance	Amoxicillin-clavulanate (Augmentin)	Amoxicillin-clavulanate 2,000/125 mg PO twice daily	Must be renally dosed for chronic kidney disease *Adverse effects: Diarrhea, skin rash, nausea, vomiting,* Clostridioides difficile *colitis with prolonged use*

Drugs Commonly Prescribed 24.2: Acute Viral Rhinosinusitis (AVRS) and Acute Bacterial Rhinosinusitis (ABRS)—cont'd

INDICATION	DRUG	DOSING	PRESCRIBING INDICATIONS
Antibiotic therapy for patients with penicillin allergy and with risk factors for pneumococcal resistance	Doxycycline (Doxy-100) OR Third generation cephalosporin: Cefixime (Suprax) or Cefpodoxime (Vantin) with or without Clindamycin (Cleocin) OR Levofloxacin (Levaquin) or Moxifloxacin (Avelox) (Respiratory fluoroquinolone should only be used for those with no other alternative treatment.)	Doxycycline 100 mg PO twice daily or 200 mg PO once daily OR Cefixime 400 mg PO daily or Cefpodoxime 200 mg PO twice daily with or without Clindamycin 300 mg PO four times daily OR Levofloxacin 500 mg PO once daily or 750 mg PO once daily or Moxifloxacin 400 mg PO once daily	Can cause esophageal damage as a direct result of caustic tissue injury *Adverse effects:* Diarrhea, abdominal pain, candidiasis, photosensitivity, skin hyperpigmentation *Adverse effects:* Diarrhea, abdominal pain, nausea, dyspepsia, flatulence, acute renal failure, hypersensitivity/allergic reaction, skin rash or severe cutaneous reactions such as Stevens-Johnson syndrome, hemolytic anemia, superinfection such as Clostridioides difficile *colitis* Use with caution in renally impaired patients; dose must be adjusted for creatinine clearance of less than 50 mL/min *Adverse effects:* Diarrhea, skin rash including severe skin rash such as Stevens-Johnson syndrome, toxic epidermal necrolysis, superinfection such as Clostridioides difficile *colitis* with prolonged use (which can be severe and life-threatening), glucose dysregulation associated with hypo/hyperglycemia, aortic dissection, liver injury, allergic reaction, exacerbation of myasthenia gravis, peripheral neuropathy, Guillain-Barré syndrome, phototoxicity, photosensitivity, skin hyperpigmentation, prolonged QT interval on ECG, tendinitis, tendon rupture, CNS effects (especially in older patients) such as restlessness, confusion, agitation, insomnia, drowsiness, hallucinations, or seizures
Failure of Initial Therapy for ABRS: Use broader spectrum and different class from antibiotic for 7- to 10-day course			
ABRS infection resistant to initial antibiotic therapy	Amoxicillin-clavulanate (Augmentin) OR Third generation cephalosporin: Cefixime (Suprax) or Cefpodoxime (Vantin) with or without Clindamycin (Cleocin) OR	Amoxicillin-clavulanate 2,000/125 mg PO twice daily Cefixime 400 mg PO daily or cefpodoxime 200 mg PO twice daily with or without clindamycin 300 mg PO four times daily OR Levofloxacin 500 mg PO once daily or 750 mg PO once daily or moxifloxacin 400 mg PO once daily Doxycycline 100 mg PO twice daily or 200 mg PO once daily	Must be renally dosed for chronic kidney disease *Adverse effects:* Diarrhea, skin rash, nausea, vomiting, Clostridioides difficile *colitis* with prolonged use *Adverse effects:* Diarrhea, abdominal pain, nausea, dyspepsia, flatulence, acute renal failure, hypersensitivity/allergic reaction, skin rash or severe cutaneous reactions such as Stevens-Johnson syndrome, hemolytic anemia, superinfection such as Clostridioides difficile *colitis*

Continued

Drugs Commonly Prescribed 24.2: Acute Viral Rhinosinusitis (AVRS) and Acute Bacterial Rhinosinusitis (ABRS)—cont'd

INDICATION	DRUG	DOSING	PRESCRIBING INDICATIONS
	Levofloxacin (Levaquin) or Moxifloxacin (Avelox) (Respiratory fluoroquinolone should only be used for those with no other alternative treatment.) Doxycycline (Doxy-100)		Use with caution in renally impaired patients; dose must be adjusted for creatinine clearance of less than 50 mL/min *Adverse effects:* Diarrhea, skin rash including severe skin rash such as Stevens-Johnson syndrome, toxic epidermal necrolysis, superinfection such as *Clostridioides difficile* colitis with prolonged use (which can be severe and life-threatening), glucose dysregulation associated with hypo/hyperglycemia, aortic dissection, liver injury, allergic reaction, exacerbation of myasthenia gravis, peripheral neuropathy, Guillain-Barré syndrome, phototoxicity, photosensitivity, skin hyperpigmentation, prolonged QT interval on ECG, tendinitis, tendon rupture, CNS effects (especially in older patients) such as restlessness, confusion, agitation, insomnia, drowsiness, hallucinations, or seizures Can cause esophageal damage as a direct result of caustic tissue injury *Adverse effects:* Diarrhea, abdominal pain, candidiasis, photosensitivity, skin hyperpigmentation

carefully considered, understanding that in certain cases, they are the ideal, and possibly only, available choices.

Patients requiring two or more consecutive antibiotic courses without complete resolution of symptoms, four or more episodes in a year (i.e., RARS), or refractory chronic rhinosinusitis will likely benefit from referral to an otorhinolaryngologist for further diagnostic work-up or evaluation for sinus surgery to remove damaged mucosal tissue or to correct anatomical obstructions of the sinus ostia, such as recurrent nasal polyps. Some patients with particularly severe chronic disease have reported trying acupuncture, herbal therapies, biofeedback, and self-help groups.

Serious invasive fungal sinusitis often requires surgical débridement and inpatient IV antifungal therapy with amphotericin B (Fungizone) 1 mg/kg IV daily or, if amphotericin B is not tolerated due to rigors, chills, or hypotension, a liposomal amphotericin preparation (e.g., Abelcet 5 to 7.5 mg/kg IV daily). In contrast, allergic fungal rhinosinusitis caused by nasal polyposis calls for functional endoscopic sinus surgery and systemic corticosteroids for 2 to 4 weeks, followed by topical intranasal corticosteroid therapy. Of note, antifungal therapy is not indicated in allergic fungal rhinosinusitis, as the benefits of antifungal therapy have not been clearly demonstrated in this condition. Fungal balls associated with sinus colonization must be removed surgically because neither corticosteroids nor antifungals have been shown to be effective in relieving any resultant obstruction.

In terms of preventive care, prompt treatment of all respiratory infections can prevent acute sinusitis complications, and surgery to correct anatomical blockages of the sinus ostia (e.g., deviated septum, nasal polyps) may prevent the development of chronic sinusitis. When sinus inflammation is associated with allergy, antigenic desensitization (allergen immunotherapy) by a trained allergist should be considered. Nose drops and nasal sprays should be discarded after use during an acute episode, however, and should never be shared to avoid person-to-person transmission of infectious organisms. Regular nasal irrigation with balanced salt solutions can also restore the hydration of the nasal and sinus mucosa, both treating and preventing rhinosinusitis.

FOLLOW-UP AND REFERRAL

Patients with rhinosinusitis should be reevaluated for symptomatic improvement in 48 to 72 hours, and a return visit should be scheduled for 10 to 14 days from the initial assessment. If symptoms fail to improve with pharmacotherapy, the patient should be evaluated for antibiotic resistance, allergic contributions, or immunological abnormalities. Immunocompromised patients with sinusitis should be closely monitored on a daily basis, and consideration for inpatient monitoring may be indicated, depending on the severity of the patient's immunocompromised status.

Although complications are relatively uncommon, visual impairments, ophthalmoplegia, orbital or facial cellulitis, severe fever, aphasia, abducens palsy (cranial nerve VI deficit), seizures, altered mental status, osteomyelitis of the frontal or maxillary bones, and focal swelling over the frontal bone are all reflective of localized extension of bacterial infection. Rare but potentially life-threatening complications that require a high index of suspicion include meningitis, subdural empyema, epidural abscess, cavernous sinus thrombosis, and other intracranial or central nervous system complications.

Patients should be referred to a specialist if their sinusitis is allergic or immunological in nature, refractory to antibiotic therapy, recurrent, associated with opportunistic infectious organisms, or when the infection is adversely affecting their quality of life. In addition, when sinusitis is associated with chronic OM, bronchial asthma, nasal polyps, recurrent pneumonia, immunodeficiency, allergic fungal disease, granulomas, or multiagent antibiotic resistance, the patient should be referred to an allergist or an otorhinolaryngologist to guide further management.

Patient Education: Rhinosinusitis

Patients should be instructed to be wary of worsening rhinosinusitis symptoms after the initiation of pharmacotherapy, as this may signify antibiotic resistance. Patients should also be informed of potential complications and should be instructed to contact the practitioner at once if telltale signs such as periorbital swelling develop. The clinician should stress the importance of avoiding contact with all contributing factors (e.g., cigarette smoke, airborne allergens), as well as the exacerbating side effects of nonprescription antihistamine use due to the drying of nasal secretions. Patients should be aware of all active ingredients in OTC decongestant preparations, such as combination formulations containing antihistamines, to prevent unintentional overexposure of specific drug classes. Because of the frequency of use, patients must be aware of the full spectrum of sympathomimetic side effects associated with decongestant preparations, including the exacerbation of hypertensive and tachycardic conditions.

Patients should drink plenty of fluids to thin nasal secretions. When using saline irrigation, patients should be instructed not to use unfiltered tap water or water from a well source, because of the risk of protozoal infection. Instead, they should use distilled water or water that was decontaminated with high heat and cooled to a lukewarm temperature before intranasal use. Patients who are prescribed antibiotics should be educated on all side effects specific to the antibiotic class or agent, especially respiratory fluoroquinolones, taking into account the labeled boxed warnings for tendinitis and tendon rupture in certain patients, especially older adults. Patients should also be instructed to finish the entire course of antibiotics prescribed to minimize the risk of antibiotic resistance.

NECK MASSES

Neck masses can be a common finding in adults and children. They can result from infectious, inflammatory, congenital, traumatic, benign, or malignant processes. In children, the most common cause of a neck mass is infection; however, in adults, persistent neck masses that do not resolve are often a result of a malignant neoplasm. Therefore, in the adult patient, a neck mass should be assumed to be malignant unless proven otherwise.

Neck masses may originate from the lymph nodes, salivary glands, or thyroid gland, or develop as a cyst. Neck masses may also result from a discrete head and neck cancer via spread through the lymphatic system to the cervical lymph nodes. Obtaining a thorough history is essential in identifying patients at increased risk for cancer. In turn, to decrease morbidity and mortality associated with neck masses, conducting a thorough head and neck examination, obtaining appropriate diagnostic testing, and initiating prompt referral to a specialist are essential for the early detection and treatment of head and neck cancer.

EPIDEMIOLOGY AND CAUSES

Because neck masses in adults are most concerning for malignancy, a thorough understanding of the epidemiology of head and neck cancers is essential. According to the American Cancer Society, new cases of head and neck cancer originating from the oral cavity, pharynx, larynx, and thyroid gland are estimated at 110,910 cases per year in the United States, with deaths estimated at 16,680 people annually. Males have a higher risk of developing head and neck cancer than females, with a greater than 2:1 ratio observed. White males have a higher risk than other ethnic groups, with increased morbidity and mortality. Oral cavity and pharyngeal cancers account for most head and neck cancers, with thyroid cancers close behind (see Fig. 24.4). Tobacco use and alcohol use are the biggest risk factors for oral malignancies, as are older age and male sex. Thus, as tobacco use and alcohol use have decreased in the overall population, there has been a drop in the rate of diagnosed oral malignancies.

However, the opposite is true for oropharyngeal (OP) malignancies, which affect the tonsils and the base of the tongue; the increase in OP squamous cell carcinoma (SCC) cases is related to the prevalence of human papillomavirus (HPV). The HPV16 serotype accounts for almost 90% of cases of OP SCC, which more commonly

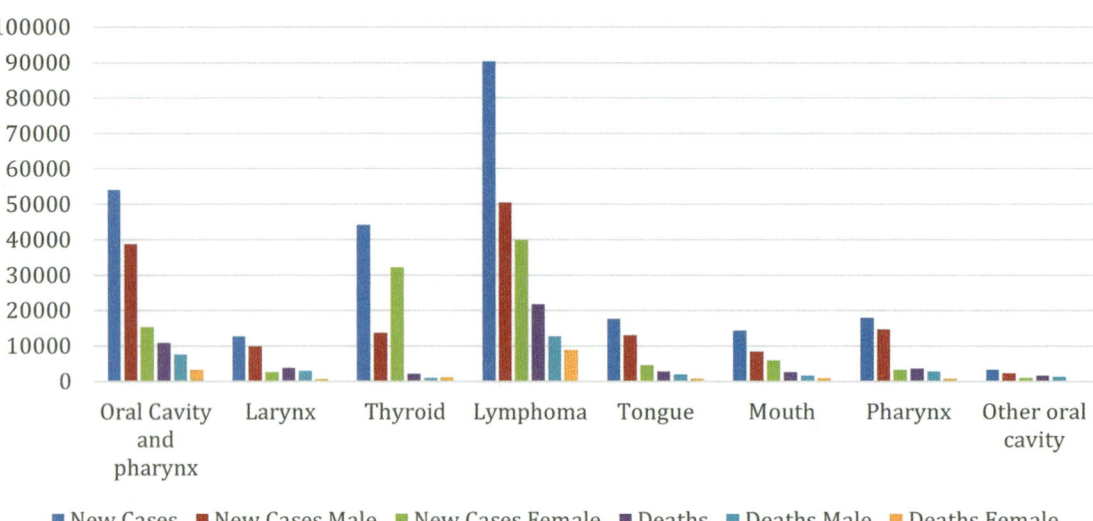

Figure 24.4 Head and Neck Cancers: New Cases and Deaths by Sex. *Data from American Cancer Society, Inc. Cancer Facts & Figures, 2021. https://www.cancer.org/research/cancer-facts-statistics/all-cancer-facts-figures/cancer-facts-figures-2021.html*

affects males and has a median age of onset of 57 years. HPV+ SCC has also been diagnosed, however, in males younger than 50 years, without the risk factors of tobacco use or alcohol use. In contrast, nasopharyngeal cancers (NPC) and salivary gland cancers (SGC) are relatively rare, with NPC estimated to occur in one in 100,000 people annually worldwide and SGC in 13.5 per 100,000 people annually worldwide.

Cutaneous lesions of the head and neck, if left untreated, can cause metastases through the local and regional lymphatic system. The two most common cutaneous nonmelanoma skin cancers (NMSC) are basal cell carcinoma (BCC) and SCC, which account for about 3 million cases per year. BCC is the most common cutaneous malignancy. Both BCC and SCC have a high survival rate. The risk of distal metastases for BCC is approximately 1%, whereas SCC has a 30% risk of distal or regional metastases. There is a higher risk of metastasis with increased size and depth of the lesion, poorly differentiated pathology, involvement of the parotid gland, immunosuppression, bony involvement, and perineural invasion (e.g., invasion of the cranial nerves). Risk factors associated with NMSC include older age, fair skin, cumulative history of sun exposure, acquired immunosuppression, and comorbid autoimmune disease.

Melanoma of the head and neck represents only 5% of skin cancers but has the highest mortality. Melanoma has an incidence in the United States of 100,350 cases annually, with 6,850 deaths. It affects males at a higher rate than females, with a 2:1 ratio and a median age of 55 years. Up to 90% of melanomas of the head and neck occur on the face. Risk factors for melanoma include fair complexion, cumulative history of sun exposure with blistering sunburns, dysplastic nevi, and a family history of melanoma.

Lymphomas of the neck are malignant tumors of the hematopoietic system, with two major classifications: Hodgkin lymphoma (HL) and non-Hodgkin lymphoma (NHL). NHL is nine times more common, affecting about 77,240 people in the United States, in comparison to HL, which affects 8,480 people. HL often presents within the lymph nodes of the neck, mediastinum, or tonsils. NHL may present within the salivary glands, paranasal sinuses, mandible, maxilla, and the lymphoid tissue of the tonsils and adenoids.

The thyroid gland is a key site of pathology to consider with a neck mass. Thyroid nodules are extremely common, affecting 65% of the general population. Ninety percent of thyroid nodules are benign and often identified incidentally with diagnostic imaging unrelated to the thyroid. Risk factors for thyroid nodules include female sex, increased age, hyperthyroidism or hypothyroidism, decreased iodine intake, radiation exposure, tobacco use, obesity, uterine fibroids, alcohol consumption, higher insulin-like growth factor-1 levels, a family history of thyroid cancer, or multiple endocrine neoplasia syndrome types 2a and 2b. Thyroid cancer is the fastest-growing cancer in the neck and the most common of the endocrine malignancies. Thyroid cancer affects females more frequently than males at a 3:1 ratio and has a 5-year survival rate of up to 99%. Papillary thyroid cancer is the most common form of thyroid cancer and has the best prognosis, followed by follicular, Hürthle cell, and medullary thyroid cancer.

Other lesions that can cause neck masses include a variety of benign pathologies, such as thyroglossal cysts, brachial cleft cysts, benign tumors of the salivary glands, lipomas, reactive lymphadenopathy resulting from viral or bacterial infections, vascular tumors, and paragangliomas.

PATHOPHYSIOLOGY

One of the most common causes of neck masses is enlarged lymph nodes, which are small kidney-shaped collections of immune tissue that constitute part of the lymphatic system. The lymphatic system works together with the circulatory system to transport excess interstitial fluid consisting of proteins and cellular metabolic waste from tissues and organs back into the circulatory system. The lymphatic system is integral to the immune system, as it filters foreign antigens such as viruses or bacteria throughout the body. There are approximately 600 lymph nodes in the human body with approximately 60 to 70 in the neck alone (see Fig. 24.5). As foreign antigens are presented to the lymphoid cells, this leads to cellular proliferation and enlargement of lymphoid follicles, which cause stretch in the lymph nodes, localized edema, and tenderness. Neutrophilic infiltrates indicate bacterial infection, whereas a lymphocytic predominance reflects viral infection.

HPV is a common virus in humans with more than 100 subtypes. HPV is associated with oropharyngeal carcinomas, especially the high-risk HPV16 and HPV18 serotypes. The HPV viral oncoproteins, E6 and E7, promote genomic DNA replication. As the virus replicates, both E6 and E7 inhibit host tumor suppressor proteins, such as p53 and retinoblastoma tumor suppressor protein, respectively. This leads to enhanced cell division and aberrant overexpression of the p16 cell cycle gene. In turn, p16 levels are used as a diagnostic biomarker for HPV-positive SCC of the oropharynx. The opposite is seen in non-HPV–related oropharyngeal SCC that is more often caused by tobacco use, in which p16 levels are not elevated. Of note, HPV16 accounts for up to 90% of oropharyngeal SCC and is also a causative agent in cervical cancer.

CLINICAL PRESENTATION

Subjective

A thorough history should be elicited in patients with a neck mass to include and potentially distinguish signs of infection versus a malignant process. For example, patients who present with symptoms of URI such as cough, rhinorrhea, nasal congestion, fever, malaise, fatigue, and pharyngitis may have an infectious etiology. Although a neck mass in adults is not a common presentation for infectious etiology, it is important to rule this out via patient history. Other symptoms related to an infectious etiology include odontalgia, a history of insect bites, recent travel, or an infection related to a cat scratch or tick bites.

The history of present illness should include eliciting duration of the neck mass and if there has been an increase or decrease in its growth or discomfort. Painful neck masses may indicate an infectious etiology, whereas a painless mass is more likely to be malignant. Symptoms that are highly suspicious for malignancy include the following: neck mass present for over 2 weeks in the absence of infectious symptoms, neck mass that is firm and fixed, neck mass that is over 1.5 cm, or ulceration of

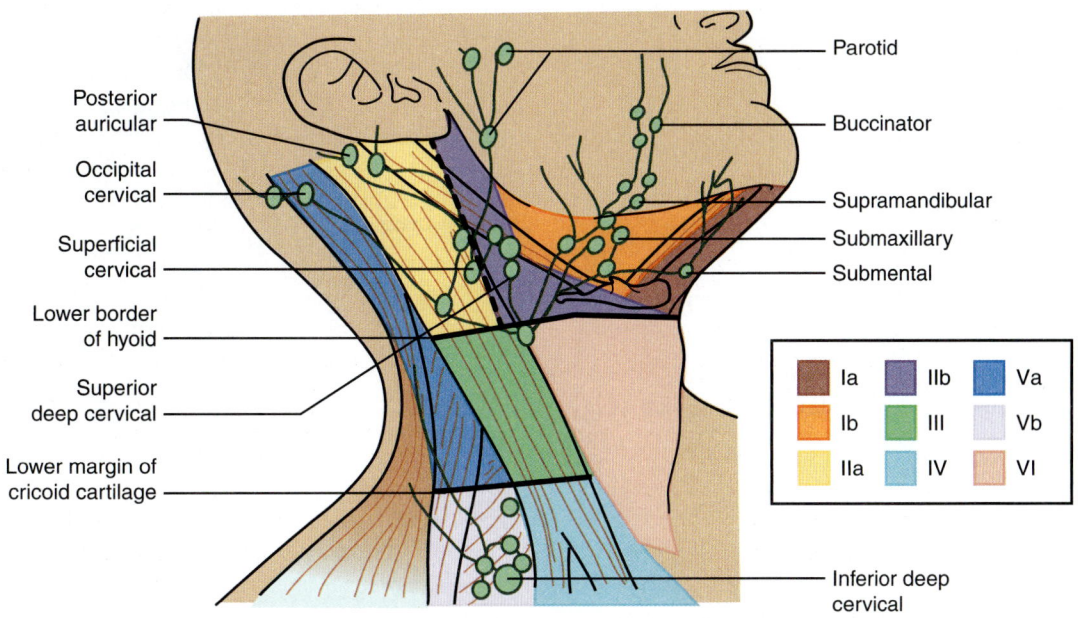

Figure 24.5 Cervical Lymph Node Levels and Corresponding Lymphatic Drainage

skin over the neck mass. Additional symptoms that are concerning for malignancy of the head and neck include pharyngitis, dysphagia, odynophagia, unilateral otalgia, recent complaint of unilateral hearing loss, dysphonia, unilateral nasal obstruction with/without epistaxis, unexplained weight loss, and cranial nerve deficits (see Box 24.2). Symptoms that are concerning specifically for cervical lymphoma include night sweats, fever, weight loss, and other areas of lymphadenopathy distant to the head and neck. Risk factors for lymphoma include immunosuppressive diseases and current or historical use of immunosuppressive medications.

In contrast, many people with thyroid nodules have no symptoms. If a thyroid nodule is larger than 2 to 3 cm, patients may have symptoms such as dysphagia, neck fullness or tightness, dyspnea, or a globus sensation (a persistent sensation of a lump in the throat). In patients with thyroid cancer that invades the laryngeal cartilage, subtle voice changes or voice fatigue may be apparent, along with odynophagia, dysphagia, and a globus sensation.

Objective

The location of the neck mass may help identify the site of the primary malignancy (see Fig. 24.5 for the lymphatic drainage pathway of the cervical lymph node chains).

Box 24.2 Symptoms Suspicious for Malignancy of the Head and Neck

- **Neck mass present for more than 2 weeks**
- **Absence of infectious symptoms**
- **Firm, fixed neck mass**
- **Size of neck mass larger than 1.5 cm**
- **Ulceration of skin over a neck mass**
- Tobacco and alcohol use
- Prolonged pharyngitis
- Dysphagia
- Odynophagia
- Dysphonia
- Otalgia
- Unexplained weight loss
- Otalgia on same side as a neck mass
- Recent hearing loss on same side as a neck mass
- Tonsillar asymmetry
- Lesions in the mouth or oropharynx
- Personal history of head and neck cancer
- Unilateral nasal obstruction or epistaxis on same side as a neck mass
- Hemoptysis or blood in saliva
- New numbness of oral cavity or cheek
- Dyspnea
- Skin lesion of the scalp, face, ears, or neck

Note: Bolded symptoms are highly suspicious, stand-alone symptoms that put patients at increased risk for malignancy.

Palpate the cervical neck using firm palpation in a systematic approach, noting the location of the neck mass, its size, mobility, and firmness. Assess the salivary glands, thyroid gland, and the skin overlying the neck mass.

A complete head and neck examination should be performed by the clinician, starting with the scalp and face, evaluating for any pigmented lesions or ulcerations to rule out cutaneous malignancy. Lesions that resemble pearly papules, irregular papules, macules, or ulcerations and have asymmetric pigmentation, borders, and shape may be a cutaneous malignancy. Examination of the cranial nerves to assess for facial sensation, symmetric facial movement, movement of the tongue and palate, and gag reflex is important to rule out perineural invasion of any tumors.

Examination of the mouth should include visual inspection with a tongue blade illuminated by a bright light, assessing the lips, gingivae, buccal mucosa, floor of the mouth, dorsal and ventral tongue, posterior pharynx, tonsils, and retromolar trigone (the area of mucosa behind the third mandibular molar that extends upward toward the maxilla) for any masses, lesions, ulcerations, or irregularities (see Fig. 24.6). Asymmetric tonsils, masses, or ulcerations may represent a tonsillar malignancy.

Palpation of the oral cavity including the tongue and its base, the tonsillar fossae, and soft palate should evaluate for firm and fixed masses. Performing bimanual palpation of the floor of mouth and submandibular glands can help evaluate these areas for submucosal masses that may not be easily visualized on inspection. Examination of the oral cavity should also encompass the dentition, assessing for signs of caries, abscess, or infection.

In a patient with a neck mass and symptoms of unilateral nasal obstruction or epistaxis, evaluation of the

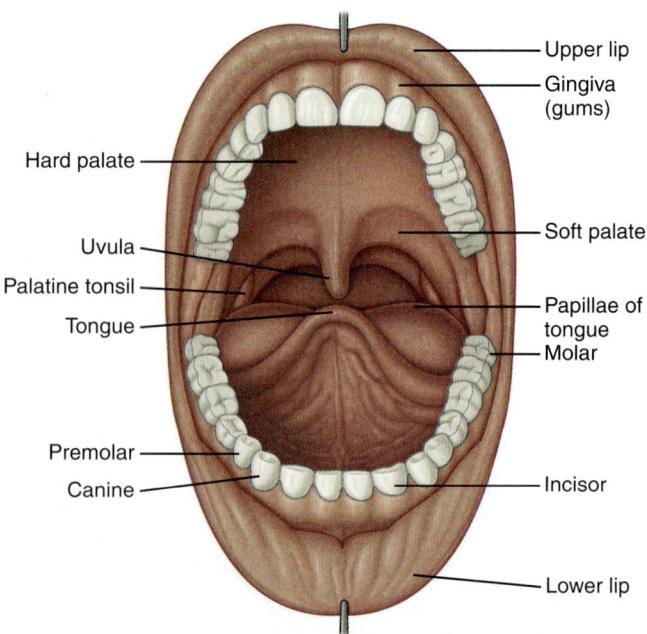

Figure 24.6 Anatomy of the Oral Cavity

nasal cavity using a nasal speculum and light should be performed to assess for masses or ulcerations. In a patient with a concurrent complaint of recent unilateral hearing loss, examination of the ear should be done using an otoscope, as this may reveal OM or OM with effusion in the presence of a nasopharyngeal mass. In a patient who presents with a neck mass and worrisome symptoms without any obvious lesion on examination, laryngoscopy and/or nasal endoscopy should be performed by a specialist to evaluate the nasopharynx, oropharynx, tongue base, hypopharynx, and larynx.

DIAGNOSTIC REASONING

Diagnostic Testing

In a patient who presents with a neck mass along with symptoms that are highly suspicious for malignancy, the clinician should order a cervical CT scan or MRI with contrast enhancement to evaluate for additional lymph node involvement, characteristics of the mass, and any abnormalities of the upper digestive and respiratory tracts. The benefits of ordering a CT scan over an MRI include greater accessibility, decreased cost, and a shorter test duration that may be better tolerated by patients. The benefits of an MRI in comparison to a CT scan include greater enhancement and therefore visualization of the soft tissues of the nasopharynx and cranial nerves. Contraindications to performing an MRI include patients who are extremely claustrophobic or who have implanted metallic devices that are not MRI compatible. Ultrasound is not ideal to evaluate a neck mass unless it is within the thyroid gland. Ultrasound can evaluate the characteristics of a neck mass but cannot adequately evaluate the upper digestive and respiratory tracts, additional lymph node involvement, or abnormalities in the surrounding structures. Ultrasound, however, is the gold standard for evaluating the thyroid gland specifically.

If a lesion is noted on the skin or within the oral cavity, nasal cavity, or ear canal, a biopsy of the lesion is indicated to obtain a tissue diagnosis. Fine-needle aspiration (FNA) should be performed to obtain a tissue diagnosis on a patient who presents with a neck mass and is at increased risk for malignancy. FNA is a procedure that can be performed under ultrasound guidance in a clinic setting by a trained provider. A small-gauge needle is inserted into the neck mass, and negative pressure is applied to withdraw cellular material into the needle. This tissue sample is then mounted on a slide and evaluated by a pathologist, as a key step in obtaining an early diagnosis of malignancy. If FNA is unsuccessful or indeterminate, performing a core biopsy of the neck mass is an option. Similar in technique to FNA, a core biopsy uses a larger needle to obtain a small portion of tissue with intact architecture and is usually performed on patients who have suspicion for lymphoma. Open biopsy is not usually recommended, as there is a potential for spread of the tumor, distal metastasis, and wound infection.

Ancillary testing can be considered if FNA, diagnostic imaging, and a comprehensive physical examination do not yield a diagnosis, although ancillary testing should be performed only when there is a concern for a specific disease process based on history. For example, white blood cell count should be obtained if infection or lymphoma is suspected. If a viral infection is suspected, laboratory testing may include HIV antibody testing, Epstein-Barr virus (EBV) antibody titer, cytomegalovirus immunoglobulin (IgM) titer, Bartonella titer (to evaluate for cat-scratch disease), or Mantoux tuberculin skin testing with purified protein derivative (PPD). If thyroid nodules are suspected, a thyroid-stimulating hormone level should be assessed. With suspicion of parathyroid carcinoma, adenoma, or hyperplasia, a parathyroid hormone level should be ordered, along with serum calcium and phosphorus levels, all of which may be elevated. If an autoimmune disease is suspected, an antinuclear antibody test can be ordered, along with an erythrocyte sedimentation rate or C-reactive protein level to evaluate for inflammation.

Differential Diagnosis

Because a neck mass in an adult is uncommon and has a high risk of malignancy, ruling out head and neck cancer should be the first priority. A comprehensive patient work-up should be expedited to obtain an early diagnosis of cancer, if present, in an effort to decrease morbidity and mortality while preserving quality of life (see Differential Diagnosis 24.3).

MANAGEMENT

A neck mass should not be considered infectious in origin in the absence of infectious symptoms; therefore, antibiotics should not be prescribed unless there is an obvious infectious etiology. If there is no resolution of a neck mass reported by the patient, diagnostic imaging (CT or MRI), FNA or other form of biopsy, and referral to an otorhinolaryngologist are indicated without delay for diagnosis and treatment because of the significant risk of malignancy.

A neck mass should be worked up until a definitive diagnosis is obtained, as the varied etiologies of neck masses drive their treatment. A cystic neck mass that is confirmed by diagnostic imaging but for which FNA is unsuccessful or nondiagnostic of an identified disorder should not be considered benign. Between 4% and 24% of cystic lesions are malignant; thus, patients should be referred to an otorhinolaryngologist for definitive diagnosis and consideration of possible surgical excision, if appropriate.

Differential Diagnosis 24.3: Neck Mass

Viral or bacterial lymphadenopathy

- Upper respiratory tract infection
- Streptococcal throat infection
- Cat-scratch disease
- Cytomegalovirus
- Epstein-Barr virus
- HIV
- Tuberculosis infection

Metastatic head and neck carcinoma

- Oral cancer
- Oropharyngeal cancer
- Hypopharyngeal cancer
- Laryngeal cancer
- Nasopharyngeal cancer
- Salivary gland cancer

Thyroid mass

- Benign nodules
- Thyroid cancer

Salivary gland benign tumors
Sialadenitis

- Submandibular gland
- Parotid gland

Lymphoma
Lipoma
Benign skin cyst
Thyroglossal duct cyst
Branchial cleft cyst
Vascular tumors
Paragangliomas
Cutaneous skin cancer

- Basal cell carcinoma
- Squamous cell carcinoma
- Melanoma

FOLLOW-UP AND REFERRAL

Patients should be reevaluated for neck mass resolution within 7 to 10 days if antibiotics are prescribed for a confirmed infectious etiology. If at any time in the examination of the patient, the clinician is not able to perform a comprehensive evaluation or needed biopsy, referral to an otorhinolaryngologist is essential to avoid a delay in diagnosis. A referral to an otorhinolaryngologist is indicated to perform nasal endoscopy or laryngoscopy to fully evaluate the nasopharynx, oropharynx, and larynx. An otorhinolaryngologist can also perform nasal, oral, or oropharyngeal biopsies as indicated. If a neck mass is large enough, FNA can be performed in the clinic with a clinical pathologist available to evaluate the cytology. If the neck mass is associated with the thyroid gland, a referral to an interventional radiologist for an ultrasound-guided biopsy is indicated.

If a skin lesion is identified and the primary care provider is unable to perform a biopsy, referral to a dermatologist for a skin biopsy is indicated. Excision of head and neck skin cancers can be performed by a dermatologist, otolaryngologist, or plastic surgeon. In some areas of cutaneous cancer such as near the eye, nose, or ear, a trained MOHS surgeon can perform micrographic surgery, as these are areas where there needs to be preservation of skin tissue or areas that have a high risk of cancer recurrence. MOHS (micrographically oriented histographic surgery) entails cutting away thin layers of skin and evaluating the tissue under the microscope until only cancer-free tissue remains. Once a patient has a history of skin cancer, they should be referred to a dermatologist for regular total body skin examinations due to an increased risk for additional skin cancers. If there is a concern for lymphoma with laboratory testing, a referral to a hematologist/oncologist to aid in the diagnosis and management is critical.

Patient Education: Neck Masses

Being transparent with the patient is essential. The clinician should explain the concern for potential malignancy with a neck mass at a comprehension level that is understandable to the patient. Providing education on potential diagnostic imaging, biopsies, referrals, and specialty examinations can help ease a patient's fears. Additionally, involving the patient in shared decision making empowers the patient to actively participate in the treatment plan. The clinician should provide education regarding head and neck malignancy risk factors, such as tobacco and alcohol use and high-risk sexual behaviors (due to the risk of HPV and HIV infection), and encouragement should be given to mitigate such risk factors. The clinician should also stress the importance of adherence to testing and follow-up appointments with specialists.

Patients with cutaneous head and neck malignancies should be educated on how to check their skin for recurrence or additional skin cancers, even at distal sites. Risk factor reduction education should be provided regarding decreasing ultraviolet (UV) radiation exposure such as use of sunblock, hats, and clothing that provide UV protection, as well as avoiding the sun for prolonged periods of time and at peak periods of sun exposure around midday.

STOMATITIS AND GLOSSITIS

Stomatitis is a generalized inflammation of the oral mucous membranes characterized by erythema and/or vesicular or ulcerative lesions. Glossitis is an acute or chronic inflammation of the tongue that shares many of the same etiologies as stomatitis. Either of the two may present alone, although glossitis often accompanies stomatitis, and clinicians often group the two conditions together under the latter designation. In general, both disorders are classified according to their etiology, which is extremely variable.

EPIDEMIOLOGY AND CAUSES

A variety of types of stomatitis are seen in adults, including oral candidiasis, aphthous stomatitis (aphthous ulcers or "canker sores"; if lesions resolve and later recur, the condition is called *recurrent aphthous stomatitis* [RAS]), secondary herpetic stomatitis/herpes labialis, Vincent's stomatitis (acute necrotizing ulcerative gingivitis or "trench mouth"), allergic stomatitis, nicotinic (cigarette-related) stomatitis, denture-related stomatitis, angular stomatitis, pseudomembranous stomatitis, and parasitic glossitis (anthracosis linguae or "black hairy tongue"). Glossitis is also a common symptom of systemic skin diseases, such as erythema multiforme or the more severe forms of Stevens-Johnson syndrome or toxic epidermal necrolysis, as well as pemphigus vulgaris. Herpetic stomatitis and RAS occur frequently, as do nicotinic and denture-related stomatitis. Other causes are less commonly seen.

Herpes simplex virus (HSV) infection is widespread in the United States. According to recent estimates, up to 20% of the adult population may be secreting herpes simplex type 1 or 2 virus at any given time, and the prevalence of HSV-specific antibodies indicative of past or dormant HSV infection is up to 30% in higher socioeconomic strata and may approach 100% in lower socioeconomic groups. In turn, prior HSV infection is the primary risk factor for all secondary manifestations of herpes simplex infection, including herpetic stomatitis and erythema multiforme (a hypersensitivity skin reaction associated with HSV infection that can involve mucosal surfaces in its more severe form, known as *erythema multiforme major*). Any factors that lead to immunosuppression in the setting of preexisting HSV infection may also be considered contributing factors. In addition, fever, physical and/or emotional stress, excess sun exposure, menstruation, common colds, gastrointestinal upset, dental work that excessively stretches the mouth, and underlying systemic illnesses are precipitating factors for herpetic stomatitis. Intercourse with multiple sexual partners and unprotected sex (i.e., failure to use barrier protection such as condoms or latex dental dams during intercourse or oral sex) increase the likelihood of HSV transmission from infected sexual partners and, therefore, predispose the patient to herpetic stomatitis.

Oral candidiasis most commonly occurs in immunocompromised adults, such as patients with HIV infection or cancer patients after chemotherapy and/or radiation therapy. If extensive, the presence of fungal lesions in the oral cavity can lead to inflammation of multiple mucosal surfaces in the mouth, constituting stomatitis. Although nicotinic stomatitis and denture-related stomatitis are common, most other forms are rare among adults. In general, mouth sores may affect adults of all ages; however, Vincent's stomatitis is specifically seen among adolescents and adults 20 to 40 years of age, whereas denture-related stomatitis primarily affects older patients.

In terms of physical risk factors for stomatitis and glossitis, chronic mouth breathing dries the tongue and oral mucosa, and hot foods or beverages may lead to thermal injury in the mouth. Chemical irritation may result from spicy, acidic, or salty foods such as potato chips or pickles, as well as from peroxide-containing mouthwashes, toothpaste, and other dental care products. Indeed, the list of predisposing factors is extensive, as described earlier. Viral, bacterial, and fungal infections; prolonged radiation or chemotherapy treatments; long-term corticosteroid or antibiotic use; chronic metabolic diseases such as diabetes mellitus; systemic autoimmune or inflammatory diseases such as systemic lupus erythematosus; emotional or physical stress; anxiety; depression; premenstrual syndrome; advanced age; low socioeconomic status; and malnourishment may all contribute to host immunosuppression and lead to the development of stomatitis and/or glossitis. In addition, pregnancy has been associated with erythema multiforme, which can involve the oral cavity mucosa in its more severe form, erythema multiforme major.

Tobacco smoking and chewing ("dipping snuff") can clearly lead to nicotinic stomatitis, whereas ill-fitting dentures, recent dental work, repeated biting during convulsive seizures, and poor oral/dental hygiene contribute to mechanical injury–related inflammation of the oral cavity and tongue. Occupational or domestic exposure to chemical irritants or allergens is a risk factor, as are gastrointestinal surgery involving the ileum and malabsorptive disorders of the ileal mucosa such as celiac sprue (gluten-associated enteropathy resulting in villous atrophy), both of which impair vitamin B_{12} absorption and thereby contribute to angular cheilitis and other vitamin deficiency–related forms of stomatitis. Anemia of any type is also a risk factor for stomatitis and glossitis. Repeated emesis secondary to bulimia may inflame the oral mucosa and erode the posterior (lingual) surfaces of the teeth because of repeated exposure to stomach acid in the vomitus. In addition, anorexia, bulimia, and off-and-on ("yo-yo") dieting may lead to malnourishment, vitamin deficiencies, or immunosuppression, all of which predispose to stomatitis and glossitis.

PATHOPHYSIOLOGY

In general, excessive dryness of the oral cavity; food and drug allergies; chemical irritation; mechanical or thermal injury; bacterial, fungal, and viral pathogens (e.g., HSV infection, coxsackievirus causing hand-foot-and-mouth disease, varicella zoster virus causing oral and lingual vesicular lesions, primary HIV infection); host immunosuppression; and nutritional deficiencies of iron, folate, niacin (vitamin B_1), riboflavin (vitamin B_2), pyridoxine (vitamin B_6), and cyanocobalamin (vitamin B_{12}) are all causes of stomatitis and glossitis via either direct mucosal injury or impaired cellular division in the rapidly proliferating mucosal surfaces of the mouth.

Aphthous ulcers are one of the most common types of oral lesions, yet their pathogenesis is poorly defined. Stress, hormonal fluctuations, inflammatory bowel disease, and antimetabolite chemotherapies all predispose a patient to aphthae. Specifically, the spirochete *Borrelia vincentii* and certain fusiform *Bacillus* bacterial species are strongly associated with Vincent's stomatitis (trench mouth), although some cases are of indeterminate etiology. If complicated by HIV infection and left untreated, this condition may progress to necrotizing stomatitis. Nicotinic stomatitis results directly from the chemical irritants in tobacco. Denture-related stomatitis results from the mechanical injury caused by ill-fitting dentures. Angular stomatitis (angular cheilitis) is symptomatic of the vitamin deficiencies discussed in the preceding text, and pseudo-membranous stomatitis has been associated with numerous chemical irritants and bacterial pathogens.

Parasitic glossitis is caused by several mycoses of the tongue, including co-infection with *Cryptococcus linguae-pilosasae* and the gram-positive bacteria *Nocardia lingualis*. The use of systemic antibiotics is well known to clear normal microbial flora from the oral cavity and, in fact, the entire gastrointestinal tract, thus facilitating fungal overgrowth caused by the lack of endogenous microbial competition. In addition, both oral and inhaled corticosteroids are known to compromise cellular immunity within the oral cavity—the main defense mechanism against fungal overgrowth and infection. HIV infection and AIDS, malignancy, chemotherapy, diabetes mellitus, and age-related decreases in natural immunity may contribute to immune suppression as well, increasing the likelihood of fungal overgrowth and viral reactivation of HSV that can result in stomatitis and/or glossitis.

Erythema multiforme is a widespread immune-mediated inflammatory reaction of the skin, which, in advanced stages, can involve the mucous membranes (erythema multiforme major), including the oral cavity. This condition may be caused by different types of infectious agents (e.g., HSV, *Mycoplasma, S. pyogenes*), drug allergies (e.g., anticonvulsants, sulfonamides, allopurinol), as well as collagen vascular disorders. However, oral involvement in erythema multiforme major, as well as its extreme forms (Stevens-Johnson syndrome, toxic epidermal necrolysis), will never be isolated to stomatitis because these are systemic, life-threatening conditions.

In contrast to these other forms of stomatitis, the etiology of pemphigus vulgaris is unknown; however, flaccid bullae typically begin in the oropharynx as superficial epidermal layers separate from their base. A similar appearing blistering disorder, bullous pemphigoid, only rarely presents with isolated oral lesions; as bullous pemphigoid progresses, however, roughly one-third of individuals may demonstrate oral involvement. Several inherited disorders of the epidermis and dermis, known collectively as *epidermolysis bullosa,* may also involve the oral mucosa in their moderate and severe forms. Finally, a wide array of autoimmune disorders such as systemic lupus erythematosus may also present with mucosal ulcerative lesions.

CLINICAL MANIFESTATIONS

Subjective

In general, patients with stomatitis may complain of excessive dryness of the mouth; halitosis; difficulty speaking or swallowing; minor to severe oral pain; or bleeding, swollen, or erythematous gums. They may also describe constitutional symptoms (including fever, malaise, headache, and weight loss) that may be secondary to infection or malnourishment. Patients with Vincent's stomatitis may complain of excess salivation. In cases of allergic stomatitis, patients may also report itching and burning in the mouth. In contrast, parasitic glossitis is usually painless, whereas anemia and niacin deficiency lead to lingual pain.

Patients with secondary herpetic stomatitis usually report a 24- to 48-hour prodrome consisting of a burning sensation in the mouth, followed by the appearance of 1- to 2-mm vesicular lesions, which start as fluid-filled bullae and then evolve into ulcerated lesions that eventually crust over the course of several days. These frequently appear around the lips at the vermilion border; however, more extensive eruptions along the inner oral mucosa may occur, particularly in immunocompromised states. Although most patients report only one to two recurrences per year, 5% to 25% of patients suffer more than one attack per month.

Objective

The mouth and the tongue (if also inflamed) often appear bright red and swollen, either at the tip and edges (characteristic of vitamin deficiencies and mechanical injury) or over the entire glossal surface. Depending on the cause of inflammation, the tongue may be ulcerated (e.g., from niacin deficiency, streptococcal infection, erythema multiforme major, or pemphigus vulgaris) or smooth and pale (e.g., from iron, folate, or B_{12} deficiencies). Vincent's stomatitis causes necrotic ulceration of the interdental gingival papillae and oral mucous membranes, characterized by a purulent gray exudate. Allergic stomatitis causes intense, shiny erythema and slight swelling of the mucosa and tongue. Nicotinic stomatitis presents with centrally erythematous white nodular elevations, and pseudomembranous stomatitis produces a membrane-like exudate coating the oral mucosa, which may appear as discrete plaques. Parasitic glossitis presents with hypertrophied (1 cm) filiform papillae that color the dorsum of the tongue dark brown or black. The lesions of pseudomembranous stomatitis cannot be scraped off with a tongue blade, whereas the lesions of parasitic glossitis are easily broken off from the mucosal surface.

Syphilis and mouth breathing result in white patches on the tongue. Inflammation and external fissuring of the corners of the mouth are characteristic of angular stomatitis (angular cheilitis). Erythema multiforme (when involving mucosal surfaces as mild or more severe "major" forms) presents with polymorphous disseminated macular, papular, nodular, vesicular, bullous, and target (bull's-eye–shaped) lesions of the skin and mucous membranes. Pemphigus vulgaris is characterized by disseminated thin-walled bullae throughout the skin and mucosa, which, when ruptured, leave raw patches.

Inspection of the oral mucosa of patients with HSV infection reveals individual or grouped vesicular lesions 1 to 2 mm in size that evolve into ulcers. These become apparent after the prodromal period of 24 to 48 hours and are characterized by pain, tingling, burning, and itching preceding vesicle formation, particularly on the gingivae, hard palate, buccal mucosa, and tongue. If observed at a later stage of healing (4 to 10 days after vesicle formation), oral lesions may appear ulcerated but crusted over. Herpes labialis presents as similar clusters of open vesicular lesions in the labial area, particularly at the mucocutaneous (vermilion) border, with erythematous bases and possibly crusting if the lesions are in an advanced stage of healing. Palpation of the oral mucosa may demonstrate edema or tenderness, aiding in the identification and characterization of oral lesions. Moreover, anterior cervical or jaw lymphadenopathy may be felt with herpes infection, as well as in cases related to autoimmune or systemic inflammatory diseases.

Back percussion over the posterior lung fields may reveal the dull tones of pulmonary consolidation characteristic of certain lung infections (e.g., tuberculosis) common to HIV infection, AIDS, or other immunocompromising disorders that often underlie the reactivation of HSV infection that leads to HSV stomatitis. Likewise, chest auscultation may reveal signs such as crackles, crepitus, or wheezing, which may reflect the presence of a systemic inflammatory disease or pulmonary infection secondary to an underlying immune disorder.

Oral candidiasis may exhibit diverse clinical patterns, and some patients exhibit more than one form. Factors that affect clinical presentation are the immune status of the host, such as the presence of HIV or a history of organ transplant, as well as the oral mucosal environment, for example, the impaired salivary function seen in Sjögren's syndrome, postradiation xerostomia (dry mouth), or age-related atrophy, and whether the person is dentate or edentulous (more common) and a nonsmoker or smoker (more common).

Pseudomembranous candidiasis, also known as *thrush,* is recognized by the development of creamy white plaques on the buccal mucosa that resemble cottage cheese or curdled milk. When these plaques are scraped off, an erythematous mucosal base is exposed. Erythematous candidiasis, in which the oral mucosa appears fiery red and the mouth feels like it has been "scalded with a hot beverage," often follows the use of broad-spectrum antibiotic therapy (due to subsequent clearance of normal oral flora) and is also associated with immunosuppression and xerostomia. Breath mints, cinnamon gum, mouthwash, or toothpaste can also cause allergic reactions in sensitive individuals, mimicking this form of candidiasis; thus, the patient's history is important in differentiating the clinical picture because treatment will vary accordingly.

Chronic hyperplastic candidiasis, or candidal leukoplakia, is the least common form of oral candidiasis. Patients have a white patch (leukoplakia) in the mouth that cannot be scraped off the mucosa. Some researchers believe that this is a candidiasis superimposed on a preexisting leukoplakia lesion. In contrast, hairy leukoplakia is associated with EBV. These white mucosal lesions also do not rub off and may appear as faint vertical streaks or thick, furrowed areas of leukoplakia. Hairy leukoplakia has been reported in organ and bone marrow transplant recipients and, on rare occasions, in immunocompetent patients. However, its presence strongly suggests HIV infection in an individual with no other signs of immune suppression. HIV patients with hairy leukoplakia frequently develop AIDS within 2 years of the onset of lesions. *Candida* may also be present in these cases without the tissue's normal inflammatory reaction to the fungus.

Other conditions leading to an inflamed appearance of the oral mucosa include systemic or local vasculitis and oral neoplasia; the latter (oral or glottic cancer) often presents as a single, painless lesion. Measles (roseola paramyxovirus infection) also leads to erythematous patches with bluish white centers on the lingual and buccal mucosa, known as *Koplik's spots.* However, this systemic infection is accompanied by a skin rash, cough, and coryza 24 to 48 hours after the appearance of these distinctive oral lesions.

DIAGNOSTIC REASONING

Diagnostic Tests

Stomatitis or glossitis may result from myriad causes, and detecting the primary underlying problem is key to effective management. A CBC may reflect bacterial infection if polymorphonuclear neutrophils are elevated or viral infection if lymphocytes and mononuclear leukocytes predominate. Biochemical tests, special cellular stains, and cultures are used to identify most causative microorganisms, along with certain serological tests such as the rapid plasma reagin test for the syphilitic agent *Treponema pallidum.* Serum levels of iron, folate, niacin, riboflavin, or cyanocobalamin may reveal nutritional deficiencies that can cause stomatitis and/or glossitis. The diagnosis of autoimmune disorders is supported by a wide array of autoreactive serologies (e.g., antinuclear antibody test for systemic lupus erythematosus, anti-SSA and anti-SSB for Sjögren's syndrome).

Herpetic stomatitis caused by HSV may be ruled out via serum levels of anti-HSV antibodies, viral culture, or a Tzanck smear of lesion scrapings, which will reveal multinucleated giant cells with intranuclear inclusions. Concurrent genital lesions are common in herpetic infection, as is also the case with Behçet's disease, a neutrophilic autoinflammatory disorder treated with topical and systemic corticosteroids, which does not appear to be infectious in etiology. Non-*Candida*–related pseudomembranous stomatitis may be distinguished from oral candidiasis by negative findings for the fungus on Gram stain or, more appropriately, a 10% potassium hydroxide wet mount of lesional scrapings, which would reveal fungal hyphae, if present. Oral candidiasis, as well as lichen planus, may resemble nicotinic stomatitis. Lichen planus may be detected by biopsy, which demonstrates hyperkeratosis, irregular acanthosis, and lymphocytic dermal band–like infiltrates. Biopsy is also indicated in the case of suspected neoplasia and should be considered for any lingual or mucosal lesions that are chronic or recurrent.

Viral culture and serological tests may rule out measles and other viral infections, including infectious mononucleosis (EBV infection), warts (papillomaviruses), prodromal primary HIV infection, and severe cases of chickenpox (varicella zoster virus infection), which may also present with vesicular lesions of the oral cavity, pharynx, and larynx.

Differential Diagnosis

Because the etiology of stomatitis and glossitis lesions is so variable, the primary goal of the differential diagnosis for mouth sores is to determine their precise cause to direct management most effectively (see Differential Diagnosis 24.4). Although the serum testing described

---

Differential Diagnosis 24.4: Common Benign Oral Lesions

Hairy Tongue/Hairy Black Tongue
- Dorsal tongue appears "hairy" and discolored
- Caused by excessive keratinization with discoloration of the papillae of the tongue
- Seen in heavy smokers, with broad-spectrum antibiotic use, xerostomia, and with poor oral hygiene
- Treatment includes brushing the tongue or use of a tongue scraper, as well as oral lubricants in the case of xerostomia
- Differential diagnosis includes candidiasis, lichen planus, and geographic tongue

Aphthous Stomatitis
- Painful ulcers with a yellow-white center and surrounding erythema that occur on the mucosa
- Likely caused by an immune response in the body, but actual cause is unknown
- Can be triggered by certain foods, hormonal changes in pregnancy or with menstruation, tobacco smoking, or nutritional deficiencies in iron, folate, or vitamin B_{12}
- For oral pain relief, use topical oral lidocaine or benzocaine; topical corticosteroids can be helpful to reduce inflammation (oral methylprednisolone [Medrol] may be required in severe cases)
- Differential diagnosis includes herpetic stomatitis, traumatic oral ulcer, and squamous cell carcinoma (SCC)

Herpes Simplex Virus
- Commonly presents as small blisters on the lips (herpes labialis)
- Can also occur as a generalized oral infection or as ulcerations on the oral palate

Torus Planus
- Bony overgrowth of normal bone; likely an inherited trait
- Easily identified, based on appearance
- Bony growths develop on the hard palate or floor of mouth and reach peak growth in adolescence
- Despite causing a change in appearance of the bones of the mouth, they usually cause no problems and require no intervention

Irritation Fibroma
- Dome-shaped soft tissue mass along the buccal mucosa, lips, or tongue
- Color is the same as the surrounding tissue
- Usually caused by accidentally biting the oral tissue or chronic dental irritation
- Avoid repeated trauma to lesion; may require surgical excision if problematic for the patient
- Differential diagnosis includes soft tissue or salivary gland tumor, mucocele, and papillomas

Geographic Tongue
- Map-like areas of the of dorsal tongue that are smooth and red with yellow-white borders
- Likely caused by hypersensitivity reaction
- Usually requires no intervention

> ### Differential Diagnosis 24.4: Common Benign Oral Lesions—cont'd
>
> - If symptomatic, topical oral (liquid formulation) corticosteroids may be considered
> - Differential diagnosis includes lichen planus and candidiasis
>
> **Mucocele**
> - Collection of saliva/mucus in the oral mucosa that usually wax and wane in size
> - Soft, round elevations that are pink, white, or light blue in color
> - Caused by trauma to the salivary ducts that allows saliva and mucus to move into the oral mucosa
> - May resolve without intervention, but can require surgical excision if problematic
> - Differential diagnosis includes salivary gland neoplasm and varicosity
>
> **Traumatic Ulcer**
> - Local area of destruction of the surface epithelium
> - Varies in size and shape based on cause of trauma
> - Often painful; topical oral lidocaine or benzocaine can be used for pain relief
> - Treatment includes removing the source of injury (e.g., denture irritation, biting injury, dental fracture)
> - Heals within 2 to 3 weeks
> - Differential diagnosis includes SCC (ulcers that do not heal within 2 to 3 weeks require biopsy), aphthous stomatitis, herpes labialis, and other bacterial or viral infections
>
> **Angular Cheilitis**
> - Fissuring of the labial commissures of the mouth
> - Often caused by *Candida albicans* or *Staphylococcus aureus*
> - Can be treated with antifungal or antibacterial creams
> - Avoid thiamine (vitamin B_1) and lip licking and encourage good oral care
> - Differential diagnosis includes oral trauma, herpes labialis, erosive lichen planus, and nutritional deficiencies of iron, riboflavin (vitamin B_2), pyridoxine (vitamin B_6), and cyanocobalamin (vitamin B_{12}); biopsy should be considered with skin changes that do not respond to therapy
>
> **Candidiasis**
> - Speckled white and red appearance with plaques that can often be scraped off to reveal an erythematous lesional base
> - Caused by fungal infection with *Candida* species
> - Most often occurs in the very young or old; with xerostomia, long-term antibiotic use or corticosteroid therapy; or forms of immunosuppression, such as HIV infection; chemotherapy; or radiation treatment of the head or neck
> - Treatment includes oral nystatin (Mycostatin) mouthwash or clotrimazole (Mycelex) troche
> - Differential diagnosis includes SCC, lichen planus, geographic tongue, leukoplakia, and hairy black tongue
>
> **Necrotizing Ulcerative Gingivitis**
> - Ulceration of the gingiva with creamy exudates
> - Also known as *trench mouth, Vincent's stomatitis,* or *Vincent's angina* when infection spreads to the throat
> - Often involves the facial and lingual surfaces, as well
> - Patient will have pain and halitosis
> - May have cervical lymphadenitis and fever
> - Treatment requires dental débridement and broad-spectrum antibiotics

earlier may be used to detect specific pathogens or nutritional deficiencies, the signs and symptoms elicited from the patient history and physical examination provide the most useful information in determining the cause of mouth sores. For example, self-induced vomiting associated with bulimic disorders should be ruled out through a careful patient history. Similarly, physical examination can rule out aphthous stomatitis, which unlike the other forms listed, produces characteristic shallow grayish nonvesicular ulcers surrounded by a ring of hyperemia and covered with a fibrinous yellow membrane.

Ludwig's angina should also be considered in the differential for patients who present with rapidly progressing gangrenous cellulitis of the soft tissues of the neck and floor of the mouth. Pregnancy epulis (pregnancy gingivitis) results from hormonal changes and may be confused with other forms of stomatitis. However, the characteristic gingival hyperplasia of this disorder is usually limited to the interdental papillae, and pyogenic granulomas may form. "Geographic tongue" (benign migratory glossitis) is a harmless, normal physical variant requiring no treatment; it may be confused with pathological forms of glossitis. It presents as continuously changing areas of loss and regrowth of filiform papillae with thickened white borders surrounded by red patches, creating a map-like appearance of the tongue.

MANAGEMENT

Most cases of stomatitis and glossitis are effectively treated with outpatient care unless severe or resulting from an underlying disease requiring inpatient care (e.g., advanced syphilis). For example, if severe dehydration secondary to oral pain and dysphagia is present, parenteral fluids may be required. The steps that can be taken to relieve the pain of stomatitis and glossitis and speed recovery are listed in Box 24.3.

> **Box 24.3 Steps to Relieve Pain and Speed Recovery for Stomatitis and Glossitis**
>
> - All behaviors or conditions contributing to lesion formation should be stopped or corrected (e.g., smoking, eating hot or spicy foods, wearing ill-fitting dentures).
> - Underlying causative infections should be treated appropriately, but pharmacological and other treatments specific to oral inflammation are primarily directed toward symptomatic relief.
> - Baking soda or saltwater rinses three or more times a day (i.e., one-half teaspoon salt or sodium bicarbonate dissolved in 8 ounces of water) may be sufficient to relieve mild discomfort. Alternatively, oral rinses of one-half strength 3% hydrogen peroxide solution (1:1 with water) may be used.
> - Liquid antacids such as attapulgite (Kaopectate Maximum Strength), aluminum hydroxide (Amphojel), or magnesium hydroxide (Maalox) may effectively relieve pain when swished and swallowed four times daily.
> - Equal amounts of antihistaminic elixirs such as diphenhydramine (Benadryl) may be mixed with liquid antacids (1:1) and used as an oral rinse to reduce inflammation.
> - Nonprescription analgesics such as acetaminophen (Tylenol) 650 mg every 4 to 6 hours may be used to relieve mouth pain.
> - A viscous solution of 2% lidocaine may be applied to oral lesions every 3 hours as a topical anesthetic or used as a gargle or swish and spit (15 mL) before meals and every 3 hours as needed.
> - Severe attacks in adults may require topical gel–based 0.1% triamcinolone (Kenalog) or fluocinonide (Vanos) applied at bedtime and, if needed, three times daily after meals.
> - Anti-inflammatory oral corticosteroid "bursts" may be appropriate in severe cases of stomatitis and glossitis, but all oral medications should be monitored for toxicity because significantly more absorption than expected may result from open oral ulcers. In addition, corticosteroids would not be indicated in immunosuppressed patients or those with viral infections, although antiviral medications such as amantadine (Symmetrel) may be appropriate.
> - For cases of HSV, ice cubes applied locally for an hour to newly formed lesions may prove helpful; likewise, drinking cool liquids and sucking on frozen juice bars may reduce discomfort.
> - Pharmacological preparations for HSV may be helpful, such as valacyclovir (Valtrex) 1 g twice daily for 2 days or famciclovir (Famvir) 500 mg twice daily for 5 days.
> - High fluid intake and antiseptic mouthwashes (without alcohol, which may be irritating and painful) may help prevent secondary bacterial infection.
>
> In cases of oral candidiasis, antifungal agents should be used in conjunction with attentive oral hygiene:
>
> - Nystatin (Mycostatin, Nilstat), a polyene antibiotic, is formulated for use as a pastille (lozenge) or suspension 400,000 to 600,000 units (of 100,000 units/mL suspension) PO (swish and swallow) four times daily. Because it is not absorbed across the gastrointestinal tract, nystatin must remain in contact with the organism and be reapplied several times a day to be effective.
> - Clotrimazole (Lotrimin, Mycelex), an imidazole agent, is not well absorbed and must be administered at least four times daily as a 10-mg troche.
> - Ketoconazole (Nizoral) 200 to 400 mg PO daily for 7 to 14 days, another imidazole, is absorbed across the gastrointestinal tract and provides systemic therapy by the oral route. It should not be used routinely for routine oral candidiasis, however, because of possible drug interactions and potential liver toxicity. Alternatively, the triazole agent fluconazole (Diflucan), given as 200 mg on the first day and then 100 mg daily for 7 to 14 days, is well absorbed systemically and only rarely causes liver toxicity, although other drug interactions, as well as drug resistance, have been documented.
> - Hydrocortisone-iodoquinol (Vytone) cream can be used to ease the discomfort of angular cheilitis. It combines the anti-inflammatory and antipruritic effects of hydrocortisone with the antifungal and antibacterial properties of iodoquinol.
> - In terms of oral hygiene, toothbrushes should be changed frequently, and a patient who wears dentures or partial dental appliances must also treat the appliances to combat the infection.

Treatment of erythema multiforme major requires eliminating exposure to the offending agent in the case of drug hypersensitivity or specific treatment of the underlying infectious agent (e.g., acyclovir for HSV infection). Specialist care by a dermatologist and close inpatient observation are required for severe cases that risk progression to Stevens-Johnson syndrome or toxic epidermal necrolysis. Vincent's stomatitis requires oral penicillin V potassium (Pen-Vee K) 250 to 500 mg every 4 to 6 hours as well as significant fluid intake of at least four to six glasses of nonacidic fruit juice or water per day.

Severe gangrenous stomatitis requires IV antibiotic treatment and débridement of wounds. Autoimmune disorders with stomatitic flares such as systemic lupus erythematosus, bullous pemphigoid, and pemphigus vulgaris are primarily treated with systemic corticosteroids. The mucosal lesions of lupus may be treated with topical or intralesional corticosteroids if located on the lips, whereas lesions of the oral cavity respond to antimalarial medications (e.g., hydroxychloroquine [Plaquenil]), provided no drug hypersensitivity manifests. However, for recalcitrant cases, increasingly potent immunosuppressive medications may be necessary. Treatment of any of these disorders typically requires specialist care and rapid referral.

Dehydration and malnutrition can result from altered eating habits due to oral pain. Secondary bacterial infections may complicate any type of ulcerative oral lesion. Recent scarification of mucosal lesions may progress to fascial space infection; tonsillar or cervical lymph gland infection; involvement of the vocal cords, bronchial tubes, rectum, or vagina; and even to sepsis. Thus, oral surgery may be needed to trim away rough, highly inflamed, infected gum tissue. Glossitis may become chronic if inadequately treated, and the severe gangrenous or necrotizing stomatitis seen in severe HIV infection may lead to death if untreated.

FOLLOW-UP AND REFERRAL

Many cases of stomatitis and glossitis can be treated by the primary care practitioner. However, depending on the underlying etiology of the condition, specialty referral may be needed. For example, difficult-to-treat and refractory cases of stomatitis and glossitis due to underlying systemic disorders, such as autoimmune conditions, require specialist referral to guide further management, such as to a rheumatologist or immunologist.

Patient Education: Stomatitis and Glossitis

The importance of proper oral hygiene and healthful nutritional habits should be stressed to all patients. Patients should be instructed to brush their teeth with a soft-bristled toothbrush at least twice daily and to floss regularly (once daily, if possible). Patients should also wear protective headgear whenever bicycling, skating, or playing contact sports to prevent cases of trauma-related tongue injury. Increased fluid intake during treatment should be encouraged, as should maintaining the recommended medication regimen while avoiding hot, spicy, salty, or acidic foods and carbonated or alcoholic beverages. Patients may be instructed to drink through a straw if lesions are particularly painful. A liquid diet may be recommended during the first 2 to 3 days of treatment if pain is severe. Milk, gelatin, yogurt, ice cream, and custard are usually well tolerated. Severe cases of Vincent's stomatitis may even call for at-home rest during the first few days of treatment.

Early treatment of viral, bacterial, and fungal infections may prevent stomatic and glossal involvement. The contagious nature of pathogen-related forms of stomatitis or glossitis should be emphasized. The most effective means of avoiding secondary manifestations of reactivated HSV infection, for example, is to refrain from behaviors that put the individual at risk of HSV infection or reinfection—most notably, unprotected sex with multiple partners and physical contact with people who have active herpetic lesions. Kissing and oral sex should be avoided if an individual is actively infected, and frequent hand washing during active flare-ups of herpetic lesions will aid in preventing autoinfection and viral transmission. It is also helpful to inform patients of the high prevalence rate of HSV infection to reduce the stigma commonly associated with herpes. Early treatment of primary or secondary HSV infection may also help prevent stomatic or labial involvement. Wearing zinc oxide–containing sunscreens on the lips and face helps to prevent herpes labialis flare-ups when exposed to excessive sunlight.

In the long term, the most effective means of avoiding stomatitis is to refrain from risky behaviors such as smoking, eating hot or spicy foods, drinking alcohol, and practicing poor dental hygiene. Avoiding exposure to affected persons, especially in the case of HSV infection, as well as avoiding exposure to allergens, chemical irritants, or foods that seem to trigger attacks, is also recommended. Care should be taken to fit all dentures and dental prostheses properly to prevent mechanical injury; for cases related to bruxism (tooth grinding), a night guard prosthesis with removable splints to reduce biting pressure on tooth surfaces may reduce damage to dentition, in turn, preventing related inflammation.

ORAL CANCER

Lesions of the mouth can be categorized as benign, premalignant, or malignant. A thorough oral assessment and the ability to decipher a benign from pathological lesion in the oral cavity are crucial components in the primary care of the mouth, as approximately 59 million Americans live in areas with shortages of dental health professionals. Many people also lack dental coverage or have an inherent fear of dental care, which prevents them from seeking regular care. Thus, the primary care provider may be the only oral health screener for many patients.

EPIDEMIOLOGY AND CAUSES

About 10.5 per 100,000 adults will develop oral cancer in their lifetime, and approximately 49,700 Americans are newly diagnosed with oral cancer each year. Worldwide, cancers of the oral cavity and pharynx are the sixth most common type of malignancy, and more than 90% of oral cancers are SCC. Rates are higher for males than for females, and specifically, they are higher for Hispanic and Black males than for White males. Rates of oral cancer also increase after 50 years of age.

Oral potentially malignant disorders (OPMD) encompass oral lesions that have the potential to transform into oral SCC. Oral leukoplakia is the most common OPMD, with a worldwide prevalence of 1% to 3%, while oral lichen planus, erythroplakia, and proliferative verrucous leukoplakia (PVL) are less frequent. The reported transformation rate of OPMD into SCC ranges from 1% in oral lichen planus to 3% in oral leukoplakia and 64% in PVL. These statistics on transformation vary according to tobacco and alcohol use, sexual practices, patient age, and anatomical size and location of the lesion.

HPV is a risk factor for several types of head and neck cancers, and the prevalence of oral HPV infection varies substantially in studies from less than 1% to greater than 50%, depending on the population studied and the specific approach used for HPV testing and data collection. HPV is transmitted through sexual contact, and HPV infection is noted in approximately 23% of OPMD cases. Although there are over 100 different variants of HPV, the HPV16 strain is most commonly associated with oral and oropharyngeal cancers.

PATHOPHYSIOLOGY

The oral cavity has a mucosal lining to protect the underlying tissue from mechanical damage, microorganisms, and chemical injury. Different regions of the mouth have distinctive cell layers to meet various demands. Masticatory mucosa contains stratified squamous keratinized epithelium tightly attached to the underlying connective tissue to protect the oral tissue while chewing and eating. The lining mucosa is made up of nonkeratinized epithelium with flexible connective tissue to allow for movement. In turn, the epithelium of the oral cavity is constantly being replaced, and some of these cell layers may thin as one ages. Consistency of the oral mucosal environment in terms of pH balance and moisture level is additionally maintained by a constant flow of saliva coating the mouth from the salivary glands. Excessive dryness of the oral cavity as a result of medications, chemotherapy, radiation, autoimmune disease, salivary gland dysfunction, food or drug allergies, chemical irritation, mechanical or thermal injury, immunosuppression, nutritional deficiencies, or bacterial, fungal, or viral pathogens alters this process and is a risk factor for the development of oral lesions.

Malignant lesions progress through a process of cellular alteration via apoptosis and proliferation, inflammation, and cellular transformation or mutation. Malignant and OPMD lesions of the oral cavity are most commonly attributed to oral carcinogens such as tobacco and alcohol. Tobacco contains chemicals such as benzo[a]pyrene and nitrosamines. These chemicals damage DNA, causing mutations that contribute to malignancy. Acetaldehyde is a carcinogenic metabolite of alcohol, and when these substances are used together, they produce a synergistic effect that increases the risk of oral carcinoma.

CLINICAL MANIFESTATIONS

Subjective

Patients with oral lesions may complain of excessive dryness of the mouth, halitosis, difficulty speaking or swallowing, minor to severe oral pain, bleeding in the mouth, and a swollen tongue or gums. They may note vesicular or ulcerated lesions present for days or months, and lesions may be recurrent or constant and worsening. Patients with underlying autoimmune disorders or vitamin deficiencies may have other systemic symptoms such as fever, weight changes, rash, paresthesias, or arthralgias. Red flag subjective symptoms, such as a lesion that is increasing in pain and size, unintentional weight loss, new or painful lumps in the mouth or neck, oral lesions that have not resolved within 2 weeks, or bleeding lesions, require prompt evaluation, especially if they occur in the setting of tobacco or alcohol abuse.

Objective

The oral cavity is easily accessible for physical examination, and a thorough evaluation should be routinely completed during patient visits, regardless of symptoms. Many malignant and OPMD lesions of the mouth are asymptomatic in their early stages and are only noted on physical examination. Physical examination findings will vary extensively, based on the location of the lesions in the mouth or on the lips and as a function of the underlying diagnosis or cause of the lesions. The mouth, lips, and tongue may appear red and swollen. Ulcerations on the tongue, lips, gums, or oral mucosa may also be observed with malignancy. Malignant oral lesions can present with any of these objective findings. Thus, some ulcerations, growths, and patchy mucosal changes may not be distinguishable as benign or malignant without a diagnostic biopsy.

DIAGNOSTIC REASONING

Diagnostic Tests

Tissue biopsy is the gold standard for the diagnosis of oral pathology. Although this is not necessary for all oral lesions, biopsy should be a consideration for lesions that are not readily distinguishable as benign in etiology, appear malignant, or are chronic or recurrent.

Differential Diagnosis

Because the etiology of oral lesions is so variable, the primary goal of the differential diagnosis is to determine their precise cause to direct management most effectively. Evaluating for the possibility of malignancy should be the first goal, followed by ruling out autoimmune disease, infections, vitamin deficiencies, and carcinogenic assaults to the mouth. Although serum testing may be used to detect specific pathogens or nutritional deficiencies, the signs and symptoms elicited from a thorough patient history and physical examination provide the most useful initial information in determining the cause of oral lesions and the need for further evaluation or treatment (see Differential Diagnosis 24.5 for common benign, premalignant, and malignant diagnoses to consider in the differential for oral lesions).

Differential Diagnosis 24.5: Common Premalignant and Malignant Oral Lesions

Lichen Planus
- White striations or erythematous erosive lesions
- Likely caused by autoimmune disease
- Linked to thyroid disorders, cancer, type 2 diabetes mellitus, hyperlipidemia, sedatives, vitamin D supplementation, and human papillomavirus (HPV) infection
- If asymptomatic, no intervention may be necessary; ulcerative types can be treated with topical oral (liquid) corticosteroids
- May be premalignant in about 1% of cases; routine monitoring for changes in these lesions is reasonable
- Differential diagnosis includes squamous cell carcinoma (SCC), candidiasis, and leukoplakia

Leukoplakia
- White lesion of the mucous membrane
- Causes may include trauma, tobacco, alcohol, vitamin A deficiency, or HPV infection
- Often asymptomatic and can go unnoticed for years
- Transformation into SCC varies in literature from 1% to 36%
- Diagnosed via biopsy
- Treatment based on biopsy results; findings of hyperkeratosis have had trials of vitamin A treatment with varying results, although biopsy results noting dysplasia or carcinoma require cancer treatment
- Encourage patient to avoid alcohol and tobacco products
- Differential diagnosis includes SCC, lichen planus, candidiasis, and hairy leukoplakia (caused by Epstein-Barr virus)

Papilloma
- Small white to pink cauliflower-like lesion of the mucosal surface
- Often found on the soft palate, tongue, or lips
- About 50% of cases are caused by HPV serotypes 6 or 11 (HPV16 is the most common cause of oral potentially malignant disorders)
- Papillomas are not necessarily premalignant, but biopsy is required to rule out HPV16 cause
- Requires surgical excision
- Differential diagnosis includes oral fibroma, tongue papillae, and verrucous carcinoma

Erythroplakia
- Red, nonulcerated area of the mucous membrane
- Often asymptomatic and varies in size and shape
- May be caused by chronic irritation, infection, tobacco, or alcohol use
- Treatment is based on biopsy results
- 90% of oral erythroplakia lesions are premalignant on biopsy
- Differential diagnosis includes trauma, chemical irritation, and oral infections; biopsy should be considered for any lesion that does not resolve within 2 weeks

Squamous Cell Carcinoma
- White or red lesion of the mouth
- Nodular or ulcerative
- Accounts for at least 90% of all oral cancers
- Can be found in all areas of the mouth
- Most common risk factors include smoking, alcohol use, and HPV infection
- Treatment requires surgical excision and possible radiation or chemotherapy
- Any oral lesion that does not resolve within 2 weeks and has no other known cause requires biopsy

MANAGEMENT

Detecting oral cancer as early as possible is the most effective approach to reducing death and morbidity from oral malignancy. The high incidence of morbidity and mortality in oral malignancy is largely attributed to the delay in diagnosis related to a lack of patient knowledge and inadequate early detection practices by health-care practitioners. Thus, any oral lesion that does not heal within 2 to 3 weeks should be referred to an oral health specialist for evaluation and biopsy.

FOLLOW-UP AND REFERRAL

Refractory cases of oral infections, persistent ulcerations, or any suspicious oral lesion that does not resolve within 2 to 3 weeks will require a biopsy and should be referred to a qualified specialist such as a dentist or otorhinolaryngologist.

Patient Education: Oral Cancer

The importance of proper oral hygiene and healthful nutritional habits should be stressed to all patients, who should be instructed to brush their teeth with a soft-bristled toothbrush at least twice daily and to floss regularly. Increased fluid intake during treatment of oral lesions should be encouraged, while avoiding oral irritants, such as hot, spicy, salty, or acidic foods, and carbonated or alcoholic beverages. A liquid or soft diet (e.g., milk, gelatin, yogurt, ice cream, custard) consumed through a straw during the first several days of treatment may be helpful in reducing the pain associated with oral lesions.

As discussed in greater detail in the patient education section for stomatitis and glossitis, patients with oral lesions should be educated to refrain from high-risk behaviors such as smoking, drinking alcohol, and having unprotected oral sex. Patients should be educated on the need for routine oral examinations, especially if participating in high-risk activity, because early malignancies may be asymptomatic.

PHARYNGITIS AND TONSILLITIS

Pharyngitis and tonsillitis denote generalized inflammatory processes of both infectious and noninfectious etiology, involving the pharynx and pharyngeal tonsils, respectively. Most virally related cases are self-limited, with spontaneous recovery, although other infectious cases may require antibiotic or antifungal therapy. Pharyngitis and tonsillitis may occur independently of one another; however, they often co-occur, sharing a common etiology, clinical course, and treatment regimen. Many cases of pharyngitis and virtually all cases of tonsillitis are contagious.

EPIDEMIOLOGY AND CAUSES

About 8% of all patient visits in the ambulatory care setting each year are for complaints of sore throat, although the etiologies vary widely. Viral pharyngitis related to respiratory tract pathogens, the most common cause, occurs most often in the colder fall and winter months. Influenza infection typically occurs in epidemics between December and April. The incidence of pharyngitis from group A beta-hemolytic streptococcal infection typically increases from 10% of cases reported in the fall to 40% in the winter and spring. Herpangina (most often due to group A and B coxsackieviruses) is known to peak in the summer and fall, and allergic pharyngitis may also peak seasonally during the summer months.

Although infectious (e.g., bacterial and viral) pharyngitis and tonsillitis tend to occur most frequently in children aged 5 to 10 years, both conditions may occur at any age. Streptococcal infection most frequently affects patients younger than 25 years; however, it may occur sporadically in older adults. Infectious mononucleosis (primarily caused by EBV) is also common in adolescents and young adults, although it is rarely seen in older adults. Pharyngitis associated with the postnasal drip of sinusitis most often affects adults. No ethnic predispositions have been reported for either pharyngitis or tonsillitis, and males and females are affected equally by both conditions.

URI is a common predisposing factor for the development of viral pharyngitis. The postnasal drip associated with URI or sinusitis may also contribute to irritant-related pharyngitis. The risk of all forms of infectious pharyngitis (i.e., viral, bacterial, and fungal) is increased in immunocompromised people who are afflicted by chronic illnesses, including diabetes mellitus and white blood cell dyscrasias such as agranulocytosis or acute leukemia. Work-related stress and excessive alcohol consumption have also been implicated as causes of decreased resistance to throat infection. In general, close living quarters, such as military barracks, schools, and day-care centers, increase the risk of person-to-person transmission of the infectious agents that cause both pharyngitis and tonsillitis.

EBV transmission resulting in infectious mononucleosis typically requires intimate person-to-person contact between susceptible people and symptomatic viral shedders (hence, its nickname of the "kissing disease"). Young adults and adolescents from higher socioeconomic backgrounds in developed countries who have not been exposed to EBV in their childhood are most susceptible. People with pharyngitis related to *Neisseria gonorrhoeae*, *T. pallidum* (causing syphilis), *Chlamydia*, or herpes usually have a history of performing oral intercourse on an infected sexual partner. Sexual abuse may be a factor in these cases as well. Bisexual and homosexual males and patients with anogenital gonorrhea are the groups most frequently affected by gonorrheal pharyngitis.

In terms of other infectious causes of pharyngitis and tonsillitis, adult cases of *Corynebacterium diphtheriae* occur almost exclusively in individuals who have not been vaccinated against this causative agent of diphtheria. Recent contact with a wild animal (especially through a bite) is the major risk factor for the development of *Francisella tularensis* infection and associated pharyngitis. Excessive antibiotic use has been associated with *Candida* fungal infection and its overgrowth in the mouth and oropharynx (thrush); tobacco and particularly marijuana smoking have also been implicated.

PATHOPHYSIOLOGY

In up to 40% of pharyngitis cases, no causative agent is identified. Definitive diagnosis of an infectious agent is difficult because the nasopharynx is a nonsterile environment that is normally colonized by an array of nonpathogenic physiological flora. However, the current literature suggests that in adults, upper respiratory tract viruses are the most common cause of infectious pharyngitis, accounting for 30% to 50% of all cases, including rhinovirus, coronavirus, adenovirus, influenza viruses A and B, parainfluenza virus, coxsackievirus (causing herpangina and hand-foot-and-mouth disease), enterovirus, and respiratory syncytial virus. Rhinoviruses and influenza viruses inflame the oral and nasopharyngeal mucosa via direct invasion and colonization, although the specific pathogenic mechanisms of other viruses are not well understood. Members of the herpes family of viruses are also common causative agents of pharyngitis, including EBV and, in immunocompromised hosts, cytomegalovirus (CMV), HSV, and reactivated herpes zoster virus. EBV, which infects pharyngeal B lymphocytes and disseminates throughout the entire lymphoreticular system, is the primary causative agent of infectious mononucleosis and accounts for 1% to 2% of all pharyngitis cases. However, CMV causes up to 20% of all infectious mononucleosis cases. Primary infection with HIV may also cause pharyngitis owing to rapid retroviral replication; thus, HIV risk factors should always be assessed.

Bacterial agents typically cause an exudative pharyngitis, which represents roughly 20% of all cases of sore throat. Group A beta-hemolytic *S. pyogenes*, which accounts for 10% to 20% of adult pharyngitis cases, invades and multiplies within the pharyngeal mucosa, causing an intense inflammatory response known as "strep throat." *Streptococcus* bacteria are characterized into groups, based on their cell wall antigenicity. Clinically relevant groups include A, B, C, D, and G. Group A is the most important cause of pharyngitis because it may lead to the most serious complications, including heart valve damage that may occur many years after systemic infection, known as *acute rheumatic fever*.

More than 80 serotypes of *Streptococcus* have been identified. The most clinically significant strain is based on the M protein, which is the major virulence factor of group A beta-hemolytic *S. pyogenes*. M protein is antiphagocytic because it blocks activation of the alternative complement pathway. An immune response to bacterial M protein stimulates long-lasting serotype-specific anti-M antibodies that adhere to individual bacteria and facilitate their phagocytosis (i.e., antibody-mediated opsonization), protecting patients against subsequent exposure to bacteria of the same M-protein serotype. The amount of time needed for patients to mount a protective immune response is unclear. In the past, it had been suggested that treatment of group A *Streptococcus* be delayed so that a protective immune response could be mounted, but this practice has since been refuted, and rapid treatment is now the standard of care to prevent subsequent complications.

S. pyogenes strains are becoming increasingly virulent, and the incidence of subsequent acute renal insufficiency due to postinfectious glomerulonephritis has increased over the past 15 years. Reports of bacteremia, deep tissue cellulitis, and systemic toxic shock–like syndrome mediated by *Streptococcal* exotoxins are also well characterized, with pharyngitis often recognized as the presenting complaint.

Other bacterial agents of pharyngitis include *N. gonorrhoeae* (especially in sexually active young adults), *H. influenzae*, *S. pneumoniae*, *T. pallidum*, *S. aureus*, *C. diphtheriae*, and *C. haemolyticum* (both species of *Corynebacteria* are associated with epiglottitis and a potentially obstructive fibrinous gray membrane adherent to the posterior pharynx). The relative importance of atypical organisms known to cause bronchitis, including *Chlamydia pneumoniae*, *C. trachomatis*, and *Mycoplasma pneumoniae*, as causative agents of pharyngitis is controversial. Studies have demonstrated markedly varied prevalence rates (0% to 20%) with these infectious agents, and nasopharyngeal colonization by these organisms may be asymptomatic.

Noninfectious etiologies of pharyngitis include trauma, allergies, collagen vascular diseases such as Kawasaki's syndrome, autoimmune blistering diseases such as pemphigus vulgaris, chemical- or drug-induced damage, and severe dehydration. Tobacco and particularly marijuana smoking are major contributing factors to noninfectious pharyngitis related to chemical irritation, and exposure to allergens such as dust and pollen increases the risk of allergic pharyngitis, which is typically associated with a personal or family history of atopy. Severe drug reactions mediated by both type I immediate hypersensitivity and type III antibody–antigen immune complex reactions may extend in their most serious forms to the oropharynx, as well as other mucosal sites. Both low humidity and mouth breathing may contribute to dehydration-induced mucosal inflammation.

In contrast, tonsillitis (which may involve the posterior pharyngeal tonsils as well as the more anterior adenoid glands) is almost exclusively a disorder of infectious etiology. It is characterized by inflammation, swelling, and purulent exudation of these lymphoid tissue collections that directly drain the colonized or infected nasopharynx. The spectrum of causative agents in this disorder is similar to that described for pharyngitis, including bacteria and upper respiratory tract viruses. Acutely, it is most often caused by group A *Streptococcus* infection, and a chronic form may also result from repeated *Streptococcus* infections. Streptococcal tonsillar infection always has the potential for progressing to peritonsillar or tonsillar abscess, which requires aggressive management (i.e., incision and drainage, followed by antibiotic therapy).

CLINICAL PRESENTATION

Subjective

Most patients with pharyngitis and/or tonsillitis report mild to severe throat pain or the sensation of a "tickle" or pruritus in the throat. Infectious mononucleosis, adenovirus, and especially group A streptococcal pharyngitis tend to cause the most painful sore throats and are accompanied by fever. Many patients also describe their throats as feeling swollen, with a "lump" in the back of the throat that persists, despite repeated swallowing. A history of dysphagia (difficulty swallowing) is also common with throat inflammation, particularly from *H. influenzae* infection, and hoarseness is often associated with *C. pneumoniae* infection.

Chills and fever are common with bacterial infection, although cough and rhinorrhea are rarely present. In contrast, laryngitis and cough are commonly associated with viral infection, but fever occurs only occasionally, because systemic symptoms are uncommon in viral pharyngitis. However, as with viral infections, streptococcal symptomatology is rapid in onset. Allergic pharyngitis, in contrast, does not present with fever but is recognized most readily by persistent postnasal drip, paroxysmal sneezing, itchy and watery eyes, rhinorrhea, and a mild sore throat that typically worsens with recumbency. However, malaise, generalized aches and pains, and headache may be reported in both conditions.

Infectious mononucleosis is infamous for its gradual onset of low-grade fever, marked fatigue, and severe sore throat. Anorexia and nausea may also be present. Influenza infection is characterized by an abrupt onset of fever ranging from 100°F to 104°F (37.8°C to 40°C), myalgias, and headache, which last for about 3 days, followed by 3 to 4 days of cough, rhinorrhea, and pharyngitis, and finally a 1- to 2-week convalescent period with persistent cough and malaise. Older adult patients with influenza may also present with gastrointestinal symptoms such as nausea, vomiting, and diarrhea. Reactivated herpes zoster infection is characterized by painful prodromes before active flare-ups. In contrast, HSV infection does not usually cause a sore throat. Gonococcal pharyngitis may be asymptomatic, and primary syphilitic lesions also tend to be painless, whereas secondary syphilis may present with a sore throat. Severe cases of tonsillitis may present with ear pain and sometimes with cough or vomiting.

Objective

On inspection, the inflamed throat typically appears erythematous, although the color may vary. Conjunctivitis is often associated with adenovirus and other respiratory viruses, whereas mucosal exudates and enlarged tonsils occur only occasionally with these causative agents. EBV-related infectious mononucleosis, however, may present with an exudative tonsillitis (in about 50% of cases), in addition to palatal petechiae and an exanthem (skin rash). The 1- to 2-mm vesicular lesions of herpes simplex infection may extend from the pharynx to the lips, gingivae, buccal mucosa, and tongue. Reactivated herpes zoster infection typically presents with 2- to 4-mm vesicular lesions unilaterally on the tongue, lip, and buccal mucosa. Herpangina presents as 1- to 2-mm oral vesicles or ulcers on the pharynx, tonsils, soft palate, pillars, uvula, and posterior buccal mucosa. Hand-foot-and-mouth disease presents with oral lesions co-occurring with an exanthem on the hands and feet. Maculopapular rashes on the extremities of young adult patients may be indicative of many types of infection, including *C. haemolyticum,* HIV, enteroviruses, or *T. pallidum* (causing syphilis).

Group A *Streptococcus* infection also usually produces a fever higher than 101°F (38.3°C); in addition, the patient may be tachycardic, and a pharyngeal exudate is usually present. Exudates and enlarged tonsils are common findings in bacterial infections, in general. Streptococcal infection produces a characteristic white to yellow exudate that may be accompanied by a sandpaper-like, scarlatiniform rash. *Mycoplasma*-related cases may be clinically indistinguishable from streptococcal infections. *C. diphtheriae* presents with a characteristic grayish pseudomembrane overlying the pharyngeal mucosa, tonsils, epiglottis, uvula, or even the nasal cavity. The nonvesicular lesions of primary syphilis are 5 to 15 mm in size and appear indurated or "healed up," extending to the lips, tonsils, or tongue. Secondary syphilitic nonvesicular lesions (2 to 10 mm) arise symmetrically on all parts of the oropharynx and mouth. *Candida* infections produce thin, white, nonvesicular, diffuse or patchy (3 to 11 mm) exudative ulcers on all parts of the oropharyngeal mucosa. In most inflammatory conditions of the throat, the pharyngeal mucosa and tonsils are edematous, particularly with group A beta-hemolytic streptococcal infection. This is true of allergic pharyngitis as well, although erythema of the pharynx is minimal.

Bacterial pharyngitis commonly presents with significant tender lymphadenopathy of the draining anterior cervical lymph nodes. This finding also occasionally occurs in viral infections such as infectious mononucleosis or primary HIV infection. However, 90% of infectious mononucleosis cases present with posterior cervical lymphadenopathy, with hepatosplenomegaly also being a common finding. Tonsillitis usually presents with readily noticeable swollen lymph glands on both sides of the jaw, located between the fauces of the posterior pharynx.

DIAGNOSTIC REASONING

Diagnostic Tests

Most cases of pharyngitis and tonsillitis are self-limited; therefore, laboratory work-up and identification of causative organisms through culture are unnecessary if the patient's clinical picture is consistent with influenza, the common cold, or irritant-induced throat inflammation. However, bacterial and viral cultures of throat swabs may be appropriate for more complicated cases or those requiring pharmacotherapy, such as with herpes virus or streptococcal infection. Herpangina and hand-foot-and-mouth disease are diagnosed via coxsackie-positive viral cultures and positive serologies.

For exudative cases of pharyngitis, the rapid (10 minute) streptococcal antigen (Rapid Strep) test is used to detect group A streptococcal antigens and diagnose infection. Increased antistreptolysin O (ASO) titers are also observed, but treatment may blunt this antibody response. Rapid streptococcal detection tests are highly specific (90%) and sensitive (80% to 90%) when used judiciously. Conducting a rapid streptococcal detection test to guide antibiotic therapy is considered appropriate for any patient with two or three of the following criteria: fever greater than 100.5°F (38.1°C), tonsillar exudate, tender anterior cervical lymphadenopathy, and the absence of cough. Patients meeting three or four of these criteria may be empirically diagnosed with group A *Streptococcus* and treated immediately. A throat swab culture of the posterior pharynx and tonsils—the current gold standard test for the diagnosis of streptococcal infection—is sent (rather than using a rapid detection test) for a patient meeting fewer of these criteria and considered to have a low pretest likelihood of streptococcal infection of less than 20%. Patients with an intermediate pretest likelihood of *Streptococcus* infection (20% to 50%) who present with sore throat and only two of the associated criteria are given the rapid streptococcal detection test first and, if positive, may avoid a throat culture. However, if the result is negative, it must be followed up by a throat culture, which typically displays greater sensitivity than a rapid detection test.

During the summer and fall, the false-positive rates of rapid streptococcal detection tests may approach 50%. In turn, the recommended diagnostic approach is less aggressive during these seasons, in comparison to the winter and spring. During the summer and fall, no testing is recommended for patients with a sore throat who meet only one of the associated criteria unless the patient is at high risk for *Streptococcus* infection (e.g., has an immunocompromising illness such as diabetes mellitus or HIV, has a history of rheumatic fever, or presents during a community outbreak of *Streptococcus* infection). If possible, household members should also be screened because treated patients may be reinfected via contact with asymptomatic carriers in the home.

Immunofluorescence staining or viral throat swab cultures are used to detect herpes virus infection. A Tzanck smear of any ulcerative exudative lesion is used to diagnose HSV and varicella zoster virus; multinucleated giant cells with ballooning degeneration represent a positive finding. Infection by the many types of herpes viruses (including HSV, EBV, and CMV) may also be diagnosed by serological tests detecting virus-specific antibodies. Convalescent titers may be necessary for proper interpretation. Nonspecific heterophile antibody tests, such as the Monospot test, are used to diagnose infectious mononucleosis related to EBV, although this test decreases in sensitivity when used at the extremes of age.

Pharyngeal, endocervical, and urethral cultures on Thayer-Martin agar can specifically detect gonorrheal bacterial growth, if suspected in high-risk patients. Syphilis is diagnosed via serology and, if the disease is in its secondary stage, by dark-field microscopy of lesional scrapings that demonstrates *T. pallidum* spirochetes. *C. pneumoniae* and *C. trachomatis* are typically evaluated via serology, although cultures and titers are not recommended initially, because the relative contribution of these pathogens to throat inflammation remains highly controversial. Suspected *Candida* infections are diagnosed via a 10% potassium hydroxide wet mount or Gram stain of pharyngeal exudates, which will demonstrate spores and budding hyphal yeast forms. These initial detection tests may be followed up by yeast cultures for speciation if needed.

A CBC may be done in any case of infectious pharyngitis. An increase in granulocytes indicates bacterial infection, and a documented lymphocytosis of the peripheral blood smear (i.e., 50% lymphocytes, of which at least 10% show atypical morphology) strongly supports a viral etiology. The presence of eosinophils in a Gram stain of nasal secretions or a nasal mucosal scraping is strongly indicative of allergic pharyngitis. Radiological evaluation of the posterior pharyngeal wall may be appropriate to detect a retropharyngeal process, if abscess formation is suspected.

Differential Diagnosis

The differential diagnosis for sore throat is initially geared toward distinguishing infectious from noninfectious cases. In the former case, the focus is then on identifying the causative organism. When challenged with an infectious agent, numerous factors contribute to patient outcomes, including host defense mechanisms, microbial virulence, the quantity of infectious inoculum, and the host's susceptibility to infection. Patients may be sicker and more febrile with bacterial infection, but this is not always the case. In addition, although the entire oropharynx may be involved during many infectious processes, certain microorganisms have a greater propensity for affecting the oral cavity, resulting in stomatitis before pharyngeal involvement develops.

Epiglottitis due to *C. diphtheriae* is an important consideration in nonimmunized (or inadequately immunized) individuals and should be ruled out carefully by history and general presentation, including an inability to swallow, with resultant drooling and an inability to speak. Importantly, examination of the oropharynx may trigger sudden glottic spasm and risk occlusion of the airway. Thus, examination of the throat should only ever take place in a facility that can support severe respiratory compromise that may result from dislodging the pseudomembrane from the posterior pharynx.

Infection with group A *Streptococcus* causes intense mucosal inflammation because of bacterial extracellular factors such as pyrogenic exotoxin and streptolysin O. A major virulence factor is the streptococcal cell wall M protein (with 80 serotypes), which has antiphagocytic properties; particular serotypes appear to correlate with the occurrence of rheumatic fever and glomerulonephritis, which can lead to acute renal failure. Streptococcal tonsillar infection (also referred to as *tonsillopharyngitis*) due to group A *S. pyogenes* always has the potential for progressing to peritonsillar or tonsillar abscess; therefore, these complications should always be ruled out when evaluating the differential diagnoses for sore throat.

Pharyngitis from postnasal drip secondary to rhinitis or sinusitis may be ruled out via nasal cavity examination and sinus x-rays. Pharyngeal or tonsillar malignancy requiring surgical removal of the affected tissues must be ruled out via biopsy if malignancy is suspected.

MANAGEMENT

Supportive and Pharmacological Management

Most cases of pharyngitis and tonsillitis in otherwise healthy patients are manageable with home care and/or antibiotics. For allergy-related forms of throat inflammation, contact with environmental irritants including tobacco smoke should be minimized, and patients may be treated symptomatically with a combination of antihistamines and decongestants, as described for allergic rhinitis. For infectious forms, patients should limit their physical activity until symptoms of pharyngitis and tonsillitis have subsided. Daily fluid intake should be increased to eight to 12 glasses (2 to 3 quarts) of fluids such as water or nonacidic juices. Bedrest is recommended if fever is present, and regular physical activity should be resumed only after 2 to 3 days of normal temperature readings. Measures to relieve throat pain are listed in Box 24.4.

Uncomplicated viral pharyngitis typically requires only symptomatic care, and antibiotics are never indicated, other than selected antiviral therapies. Influenza symptoms may be improved within the first 2 days of symptom onset by prescribing amantadine (Symmetrel) 100 mg PO twice daily for documented cases of influenza A, but this drug may also cause insomnia, dizziness, drowsiness, or difficulty concentrating. Thus, the dosage for older adult patients is reduced to once daily. Oseltamivir (Tamiflu) 75 mg PO twice daily for 5 days may be similarly given within the first 48 hours of symptom onset to reduce duration of illness and symptom severity, as well as prophylactically with once-daily dosing in high-risk individuals during peak flu season.

Many cases of bacterial pharyngitis are self-limited, such as those caused by atypical organisms. However, cases due to infection with group A *Streptococcus* or *N. gonorrhoeae* merit rapid antibiotic treatment to prevent significant sequelae in both the short and long terms. In addition, cases caused by *C. diphtheriae, H. influenzae,* or influenza virus may require hospitalization because of the risk of life-threatening complications, such as upper airway obstruction or pneumonia. Fungal infections also typically require antimycotic therapy.

Antibiotic therapy for group A streptococcal pharyngitis has been shown to shorten the clinical course of disease; reduce lymphadenopathy, fever, and pain (after 1 to 3 days of therapy); prevent suppurative complications and autoimmune sequelae such as rheumatic fever; and decrease person-to-person spread of infection. Empiric antibiotic therapy may be instituted before receiving culture results in certain clinical situations to prevent cross-reactive autoimmune phenomena including rheumatic fever and other cardiac sequelae, as well as immune complex-mediated acute renal insufficiency due to poststreptococcal glomerulonephritis. However, studies have demonstrated that delaying treatment for 48 hours in anticipation of throat culture results does not significantly affect the reduction in autoimmune sequelae provided by antibiotic therapy.

In patients with fever below 100.5°F (38.1°C) without associated tonsillar exudate or anterior cervical lymphadenopathy, neither throat swab culture nor antistreptococcal therapy is recommended because a false-positive culture may lead to unnecessary antibiotic treatment. If fever higher than 100.5°F (38.1°C) accompanies tonsillar exudate and tender anterior cervical lymphadenitis, antistreptococcal therapy should be instituted immediately because a false-negative culture could delay critical treatment. This is especially important for patients younger than 25 years. If a similar fever occurs with only one of the other two physical signs, antibiotic therapy should be instituted only for culture-positive patients. High-risk factors that favor immediate empiric treatment include a history of acute rheumatic heart fever or related cardiac damage, a scarlatiniform rash, diabetic or other immunocompromised state, documented exposure to group A *Streptococcus* within the past week, or the presence of a known streptococcal epidemic within the community.

Adults are typically given a 10-day course of penicillin V potassium (Pen-Vee K) 500 mg PO twice daily or 250 mg PO four times daily or penicillin G benzathine (Bicillin L-A) 1.2 million units intramuscular (IM) once as an alternative to prolonged oral medication. If the patient is allergic to penicillin, azithromycin (Zithromax) 500 mg

---

Box 24.4 Measures to Relieve Throat Pain

- Voice rest
- Ambient humidification with a regularly cleaned cool-mist, ultrasonic humidifier to increase ambient air moisture, which may relieve feelings of dryness or tightness in the throat
- Saline nasal sprays
- Various types of gargles taken as needed, including hot or cold double-strength tea or a warm saltwater solution (one teaspoon of noniodized salt in 8 ounces of water)
- Nonprescription throat lozenges or sprays (e.g., Cepastat, Cepacol, Chloraseptic) containing topical anesthetics such as phenol may also alleviate minor pain
- Nonprescription analgesics such as acetaminophen or aspirin (325 to 650 mg every 4 to 6 hours as needed) to relieve intermediate pain
- Viscous lidocaine (Xylocaine) throat preparations or possibly codeine preparations (30 to 60 mg PO every 4 to 6 hours as needed) for more moderate to severe pain
- Warm, moist compresses applied four times daily for at least 30 to 60 minutes at a time to relieve enlarged, tender cervical lymph glands

PO daily is recommended for 5 days. If the patient fails to respond to antibiotic therapy, tests for infectious mononucleosis and streptococcal antibiotic sensitivity should be performed. A 10-day course of amoxicillin/clavulanate (Augmentin) 40 mg/kg PO daily based on the amoxicillin component, in divided doses twice daily, erythromycin ethyl succinate (EES) 50 mg/kg PO daily in divided doses three times daily or erythromycin stearate (Erythrocin) 1 g PO daily has been shown to be effective for penicillin-resistant β-lactamase–producing organisms, whereas tetracycline (Sumycin) and trimethoprim-sulfamethoxazole (Septra, Bactrim) should be avoided.

N. gonorrhoeae infection calls for ceftriaxone (Rocephin) 125 mg IM once, along with empiric treatment for *C. trachomatis* (azithromycin 1 g PO once or doxycycline [Vibramycin] 100 mg PO twice daily for 7 days), given its propensity for co-infection. *M. pneumoniae* and *C. pneumoniae* are both treated with erythromycin 250 to 500 mg PO four times daily for 10 days, depending on the specific preparation. Extensive throat infection with *Candida albicans* (thrush, pharyngitis, esophagitis) requires antifungal treatment such as fluconazole (Diflucan) 200 mg PO once, followed by 100 mg PO daily for 2 weeks total.

Surgical Management

Surgical removal of the pharyngeal tonsils (tonsillectomy) and/or adenoids (adenoidectomy) is absolutely indicated if tonsillar inflammation leads to airway obstruction associated with any of the following: cor pulmonale (right-sided cardiac hypertrophy), dysphagia, or weight loss. Tonsillectomy may also be indicated if active flares recur more than three times a year, if the patient experiences mild dysphagia, if the tonsils remain chronically hypertrophied after a bout of infectious mononucleosis, or if the patient has a history of rheumatic fever with heart damage due to recurrent tonsillitis. However, in these situations, the indication for surgical intervention is relative and must be evaluated further. It should also be noted that lymph glands normally swell during episodes of active inflammation as part of the body's normal immune response. In turn, tonsillectomy is not indicated for colds, asthma, allergic rhinitis, focal infections, fever of unknown origin, cervical lymphadenopathy, or enlarged tonsils without obstructive symptomatology.

FOLLOW-UP AND REFERRAL

Most cases of pharyngitis and tonsillitis are self-limited, and symptoms tend to improve in 2 to 3 days. If symptoms fail to improve within this time frame, patients should return for a follow-up appointment, in which throat cultures for *Streptococcus* may be repeated on completion of therapy to confirm resolution of any infectious process. This is not recommended, however, for asymptomatic patients who have completed a 10-day therapeutic regimen for streptococcal infection or for patients whose symptoms improve within 5 days of antibiotic therapy because clinical resolution is typically the best measure of therapeutic success.

Group A *Streptococcus* pharyngeal or tonsillar infection may lead to scarlet fever or autoimmune rheumatic fever, if not treated with antibiotics or if antibiotic therapy is discontinued before a full 10-day course is completed. Patients with these complications should be referred to a specialist. In areas where group A streptococcal infection is endemic, the probability of developing rheumatic fever is 0.3%. With epidemic pharyngitis, the risk increases to 3%.

Rheumatic heart disease may develop after rheumatic fever in an adult patient with recurrent streptococcal infection or a history of poorly treated streptococcal pharyngitis as a child or young adult. This may lead to severe sequelae such as calcification of the mitral valve and/or other heart valves, as well as to the destruction of cardiac myocytes, which is attributed to cross-reacting antistreptococcal antibodies. Even when acute rheumatic fever is treated appropriately with prophylactic antibiotic therapy, 4% of patients may develop debilitating cardiac sequelae, and 1% may develop severe class IV rheumatic heart disease. Chest pain is a key indicator of cardiac complications. Hematuria resulting from poststreptococcal glomerulonephritis may occur 1 to 3 weeks after acute pharyngeal or tonsillar infection, as antibiotic therapy may not protect against this immune complex–mediated complication.

Cases caused by *C. diphtheriae,* if left untreated, may lead to epiglottitis, which can obstruct breathing and may prove fatal if the pseudomembrane dislodges from the posterior pharynx and chokes the patient as it is inadvertently swallowed. The spread of infectious organisms from the pharynx to the lungs may lead to pneumonia and severe respiratory complications. Infections of the posterior oropharynx may also ascend to the nasopharynx, leading to sinusitis and rhinitis (inflammation of the mucous membranes of the sinus and nasal cavities). The middle ear is another possible target of disseminated pharyngeal infection because the nasopharyngeal (eustachian) tube acts as a conduit for the spread of microorganisms from the nasal cavity to the middle ear canal. Indeed, OM may occur in more than 20% of adenovirus infections. A less common complication of bacterial pharyngitis is septic jugular vein thrombophlebitis, which may occur several days after the initial sore throat. Patients with this complication are typically teenagers or young adults who experience an increase in neck pain and tenderness, as well as swelling of the jaw angle.

Liver function tests (e.g., serum aspartate aminotransferase [AST], serum alanine aminotransferase [ALT], serum bilirubin, platelet count, and the Coombs autoantibody test) should be performed for all cases of suspected infectious mononucleosis to diagnose serious sequelae, including severe hepatitis (i.e., ALT or AST levels of more than 1,000 units/L; bilirubin levels greater than 10 mg/dL), hemolytic anemia, granulocytopenia, and thrombocytopenia. Airway obstruction may also occur in patients with infectious mononucleosis as a result of pharyngeal swelling. Such complications may require treatment with a corticosteroid such as prednisone (Deltasone) 60 to 80 mg PO daily in divided doses, tapered over 1 to 2 weeks. Splenic rupture related to trauma is also a serious risk for all patients with infectious mononucleosis who have marked hepatosplenomegaly (liver and spleen enlargement). Abdominal guards may be used to reduce this risk, although splenic rupture has also been known to occur spontaneously in infectious mononucleosis, without antecedent trauma.

Tonsillitis that goes untreated or fails to resolve with treatment may lead to grossly swollen suppurative cervical adenitis, OM, or a peritonsillar abscess of the surrounding throat area characterized by increasing unilateral ear and throat pain. This is characterized by ipsilateral to the affected tonsil, dysphagia, drooling, trismus, erythema, and edema of the soft palate with fluctuance on palpation. Suppurative sequelae such as these may require surgical drainage and/or tonsillectomy. Repeated attacks of acute tonsillitis may lead to a chronic condition with a recurrent sore throat and greatly enlarged tonsils, which may complicate breathing and become potentially life-threatening; these cases also require surgical intervention. In turn, all patients who develop suppurative or retropharyngeal sequelae should be referred to an otorhinolaryngologist. Surgical interventions such as tonsillectomy or abscess drainage also require surgical referral. The physical examination and treatment of *C. diphtheriae* infection are also highly risky and must be supervised by a qualified specialist, preferably in an inpatient or emergency department setting properly equipped to support upper airway patency, if needed.

Patient Education: Pharyngitis and Tonsillitis

Both pharyngitis and tonsillitis may be prevented by avoiding contact with people with actively inflamed throats, particularly with URIs. Throat swabs from household members of patients should also be cultured to identify and treat carriers simultaneously to prevent the development of clinical disease and prevent reinfection. Toothbrushes should be replaced as soon as a sore throat develops, as they may harbor causative microorganisms, and all eating and drinking utensils should be cleaned thoroughly and should not be shared. Food and washcloths also must not be shared during a period of active infection.

It is critical to keep all immunizations up to date, particularly the diphtheria-pertussis-tetanus (DTaP, Tdap) vaccine that confers immunity against *C. diphtheriae*. If a sexual partner is suspected of being infected with a sexually transmitted agent, intimate sexual contact should cease until a proper diagnosis is made and any applicable treatment has been completed. In general, oral intercourse between persons of either sex should be performed only using a form of latex barrier protection, such as a condom during fellatio or a dental dam during cunnilingus, to avoid orogenital transmission of infectious organisms. Environmental irritants such as tobacco and marijuana smoke, pollution, dust, and other allergens, as well as low-humidity environments should be avoided to prevent noninfectious forms of pharyngitis.

Warm compresses applied to relieve enlarged, tender cervical lymph nodes can be effective; however, patients must be cautioned not to burn the skin inadvertently. Although the use of aspirin during viral infections in adults has not been linked to the development of Reye's syndrome (as is the case in children), NSAIDs should be used cautiously if patients suffer from kidney disease, ulcers, or other gastrointestinal disorders. Heavy lifting and contact sports must be prohibited for all patients with infectious mononucleosis because these activities carry a high risk of splenic trauma and rupture. Patients must be instructed to finish their entire course of antibiotics, antivirals, or antifungals as prescribed to avoid complications from latent infection, such as glomerulonephritis or myocarditis. In cases involving dysphagia, patients may be instructed on how to maintain a healthy liquid or soft food diet (e.g., milkshakes, soups, high-protein nutritional supplements, and instant breakfast drinks) for several days until the pain subsides. Patients who demand prescriptions for antibiotics in the absence of a throat culture confirming disease of bacterial origin should understand the rationale for using antibacterial drugs versus other types of medication.

REFERENCES

Neck Masses

Carlson ER, Schlieve T. (2019). Salivary Gland Malignancies. *Oral and maxillofacial surgery clinics of North America, 31*(1), 125–144. https://doi.org/10.1016/j.coms.2018.08.007

Detweiler K, Elfenbein DM, Mayers D. (2019). Evaluation of Thyroid Nodules. *The Surgical clinics of North America, 99*(4), 571–586. https://doi.org/10.1016/j.suc.2019.04.001

Düzgün F, Tarhan S, Ovalı GY, et al. (2017). Is computed tomography perfusion a useful method for distinguishing between benign and malignant neck masses?. *Ear, nose, & throat journal, 96*(6), E1–E5. https://doi.org/10.1177/014556131709600601

Dyalram D, Caldroney S, Heath J. (2017). Margin Analysis: Cutaneous Malignancy of the Head and Neck. *Oral and maxillofacial surgery clinics of North America, 29*(3), 341–353. https://doi.org/10.1016/j.coms.2017.04.001

Kansara S, Bell D, Weber R. (2020). Surgical management of nonmelanoma skin cancer of the head and neck. *Oral oncology, 100*, 104485. https://doi.org/10.1016/j.oraloncology.2019.104485

Maymone M, Greer RO, Kesecker J, et al. (2019). Premalignant and malignant oral mucosal lesions: Clinical and pathological findings. *Journal of the American Academy of Dermatology, 81*(1), 59–71. https://doi.org/10.1016/j.jaad.2018.09.060

Pynnonen MA, Gillespie MB, Roman B, et al. (2017). Clinical Practice Guideline: Evaluation of the Neck Mass in Adults. *Otolaryngology-head and neck surgery: official journal of American Academy of*

Otolaryngology-Head and Neck Surgery, 157(2_suppl), S1–S30. https://doi.org/10.1177/0194599817722550

Ramadas AA, Jose R, Varma B, et al. (2017). Cervical lymphadenopathy: Unwinding the hidden truth. Dental research journal, 14(1), 73–78. https://doi.org/10.4103/1735-3327.201136

Seib CD, Sosa JA. (2019). Evolving Understanding of the Epidemiology of Thyroid Cancer. Endocrinology and metabolism clinics of North America, 48(1), 23–35. https://doi.org/10.1016/j.ecl.2018.10.002

Siegel RL, Miller KD, Fuchs HE, et al. (2021). Cancer Statistics, 2021. CA: a cancer journal for clinicians, 71(1), 7–33. https://doi.org/10.3322/caac.21654

Storck K, Brandstetter M, Keller U, et al. (2019). Clinical presentation and characteristics of lymphoma in the head and neck region. Head & face medicine, 15(1), 1. https://doi.org/10.1186/s13005-018-0186-0

Yan K, Agrawal N, Gooi Z. (2018). Head and Neck Masses. The medical clinics of North America, 102(6), 1013–1025. https://doi.org/10.1016/j.mcna.2018.06.012

Oral Cancer

Awadallah M, Idle M, Patel K, et al. (2018). Management update of potentially premalignant oral epithelial lesions. Oral surgery, oral medicine, oral pathology and oral radiology, 125(6), 628–636. https://doi.org/10.1016/j.oooo.2018.03.010

Bombeccari GP, Giannì AB, Pallotti F, et al. (2018). Oral proliferative verrucous leukoplakia: A challenge for clinical management. Head & neck, 40(7), 1605–1606. https://doi.org/10.1002/hed.25322

Bulur I, Onder M. (2017). Behçet disease: New aspects. Clinics in dermatology, 35(5), 421–434. https://doi.org/10.1016/j.clindermatol.2017.06.004

Dave A, Shariff J, Philipone E. (2021). Association between oral lichen planus and systemic conditions and medications: Case-control study. Oral diseases, 27(3), 515–524. https://doi.org/10.1111/odi.13572

de la Cour CD, Sperling CD, Belmonte F, et al. (2021). Human papillomavirus prevalence in oral potentially malignant disorders: Systematic review and meta-analysis. Oral diseases, 27(3), 431–438. https://doi.org/10.1111/odi.13322

Parakh MK, Ulaganambi S, Ashifa N, et al. (2020). Oral potentially malignant disorders: clinical diagnosis and current screening aids: a narrative review. European journal of cancer prevention: the official journal of the European Cancer Prevention Organisation (ECP), 29(1), 65–72. https://doi.org/10.1097/CEJ.0000000000000510

Qin R, Steel A, Fazel N. (2017). Oral mucosa biology and salivary biomarkers. Clinics in dermatology, 35(5), 477–483. https://doi.org/10.1016/j.clindermatol.2017.06.005

Rehan K. Demand for Dentists: Forecasting the Future of the Profession. Academy of General Dentistry. Available online at: www.agd.org/publications-and-news/newsroom/newsroom-list/2020/07/06/demand-for-dentists-forecasting-the-future-of-the-profession (Accessed April 2021).

Thomsen M, Vitetta L. (2018). Adjunctive Treatments for the Prevention of Chemotherapy- and Radiotherapy-Induced Mucositis. Integrative cancer therapies, 17(4), 1027–1047. https://doi.org/10.1177/1534735418794885

Warnakulasuriya S. (2018). Clinical features and presentation of oral potentially malignant disorders. Oral surgery, oral medicine, oral pathology and oral radiology, 125(6), 582–590. https://doi.org/10.1016/j.oooo.2018.03.011

Woo SB. (2019). Oral Epithelial Dysplasia and Premalignancy. Head and neck pathology, 13(3), 423–439. https://doi.org/10.1007/s12105-019-01020-6

Pharyngitis and Tonsillitis

Heining CJ, Amlani A, Doshi J. (2021). Ambulatory management of common ENT emergencies—what's the evidence? The Journal of laryngology and otology, 135(3), 191–195. https://doi.org/10.1017/S0022215121000554

Homme JH. (2019). Acute Otitis Media and Group A Streptococcal Pharyngitis: A Review for the General Pediatric Practitioner. Pediatric annals, 48(9), e343–e348. https://doi.org/10.3928/19382359-20190813-01

Hook EW, 3rd, Bernstein K. (2019). Kissing, saliva exchange, and transmission of Neisseria gonorrhoeae. The Lancet. Infectious diseases, 19(10), e367–e369. https://doi.org/10.1016/S1473-3099(19)30306-8

Jones GH, Burnside G, McPartland J, et al. (2018). Is tonsillectomy mandatory for asymmetric tonsils in children? A review of our diagnostic tonsillectomy practice and the literature. International journal of pediatric otorhinolaryngology, 110, 57–60. https://doi.org/10.1016/j.ijporl.2018.04.027

Klein MR. (2019). Infections of the Oropharynx. Emergency medicine clinics of North America, 37(1), 69–80. https://doi.org/10.1016/j.emc.2018.09.002

Li RM, Kiemeney M. (2019). Infections of the Neck. Emergency medicine clinics of North America, 37(1), 95–107. https://doi.org/10.1016/j.emc.2018.09.003

Marchica CL, Dahl JP, Raol N. (2019). What's New with Tubes, Tonsils, and Adenoids? Otolaryngologic clinics of North America, 52(5), 779–794. https://doi.org/10.1016/j.otc.2019.05.002

Mitchell RB, Archer SM, Ishman SL, et al. (2019). Clinical Practice Guideline: Tonsillectomy in Children (Update)-Executive Summary. Otolaryngology—head and neck surgery: official journal of American Academy of Otolaryngology-Head and Neck Surgery, 160(2), 187–205. https://doi.org/10.1177/0194599818807917

Munck H, Jørgensen AW, Klug TE. (2018). Antibiotics for recurrent acute pharyngo-tonsillitis: systematic review. European journal of clinical microbiology & infectious diseases: official publication of the European Society of Clinical Microbiology, 37(7), 1221–1230. https://doi.org/10.1007/s10096-018-3245-3

Mustafa Z, Ghaffari M. (2020). Diagnostic Methods, Clinical Guidelines, and Antibiotic Treatment for Group A Streptococcal Pharyngitis: A Narrative Review. Frontiers in cellular and infection microbiology, 10, 563627. https://doi.org/10.3389/fcimb.2020.563627

Rhinitis

Agnihotri NT, McGrath KG. (2019). Allergic and nonallergic rhinitis. Allergy and asthma proceedings, 40(6), 376–379. https://doi.org/10.2500/aap.2019.40.4251

Campo P, Eguiluz-Gracia I, Bogas G, et al. (2019). Local allergic rhinitis: Implications for management. Clinical and experimental allergy: journal of the British Society for Allergy and Clinical Immunology, 49(1), 6–16. https://doi.org/10.1111/cea.13192

Dykewicz MS, Wallace DV, Amrol DJ, et al. (2020). Rhinitis 2020: A practice parameter update. The Journal of allergy and clinical immunology, 146(4), 721–767. https://doi.org/10.1016/j.jaci.2020.07.007

Hamizan AW, Azer M, Alvarado R, et al. (2019). The Distinguishing Clinical Features of Nonallergic Rhinitis Patients. American journal of rhinology & allergy, 33(5), 524–530. https://doi.org/10.1177/1945892419850750

Liu J, Liu G, Li Z. (2018). Recent perspectives of pediatric rhinitis. *Minerva pediatrica*, 70(4), 391–395. https://doi.org/10.23736/S0026-4946.17.04819-8

Schuler IV CF, Montejo JM. (2019). Allergic Rhinitis in Children and Adolescents. *Pediatric clinics of North America*, 66(5), 981–993. https://doi.org/10.1016/j.pcl.2019.06.004

Segboer C, Gevorgyan A, Avdeeva K, et al. (2019). Intranasal corticosteroids for non-allergic rhinitis. *The Cochrane database of systematic reviews*, 2019(11), CD010592. https://www.cochranelibrary.com/cdsr/doi/10.1002/14651858.CD010592.pub2/full?highlightAbstract=allergic%7Callerg%7Ccorticosteroids%7Cfour%7Cfor%7Ccorticosteroid%7Crhinitis%7Cintranasal%7Crhiniti%7Cnon%7Cintranas

Shao Z, Bernstein JA. (2019). Occupational Rhinitis: Classification, Diagnosis, and Therapeutics. *Current allergy and asthma reports*, 19(12), 54. https://doi.org/10.1007/s11882-019-0892-0

Sur D, Plesa ML. (2018). Chronic Nonallergic Rhinitis. *American family physician*, 98(3), 171–176.

Zucker SM, Barton BM, McCoul ED. (2019). Management of Rhinitis Medicamentosa: A Systematic Review. *Otolaryngology—head and neck surgery: official journal of American Academy of Otolaryngology-Head and Neck Surgery*, 160(3), 429–438. https://doi.org/10.1177/0194599818807891

Rhinosinusitis

DeMuri GP, Eickhoff JC, Gern JC, et al. (2019). Clinical and Virological Characteristics of Acute Sinusitis in Children. *Clinical infectious diseases: an official publication of the Infectious Diseases Society of America*, 69(10), 1764–1770. https://doi.org/10.1093/cid/ciz023

Deutsch PG, Whittaker J, Prasad S. (2019). Invasive and Non-Invasive Fungal Rhinosinusitis-A Review and Update of the Evidence. *Medicina (Kaunas, Lithuania)*, 55(7), 319. https://doi.org/10.3390/medicina55070319

Dykewicz MS, Rodrigues JM, Slavin RG. (2018). Allergic fungal rhinosinusitis. *The Journal of allergy and clinical immunology*, 142(2), 341–351. https://doi.org/10.1016/j.jaci.2018.06.023

Fokkens WJ, Lund VJ, Hopkins C, et al. (2020). European Position Paper on Rhinosinusitis and Nasal Polyps 2020. *Rhinology*, 58(Suppl S29), 1–464. https://doi.org/10.4193/Rhin20.600

Gallant JN, Basem JI, Turner JH. (2018). Nasal saline irrigation in pediatric rhinosinusitis: A systematic review. *International journal of pediatric otorhinolaryngology*, 108, 155–162. https://doi.org/10.1016/j.ijporl.2018.03.001

Heath J, Hartzell L, Putt C, et al. (2018). Chronic Rhinosinusitis in Children: Pathophysiology, Evaluation, and Medical Management. *Current allergy and asthma reports*, 18(7), 37. https://doi.org/10.1007/s11882-018-0792-8

Kim R, Patel ZM. (2020). Sinus Headache: Differential Diagnosis and an Evidence-Based Approach. *Otolaryngologic clinics of North America*, 53(5), 897–904. https://doi.org/10.1016/j.otc.2020.05.019

Kwah JH, Peters AT. (2019). Nasal polyps and rhinosinusitis. *Allergy and asthma proceedings*, 40(6), 380–384. https://doi.org/10.2500/aap.2019.40.4252

Lemiengre MB, van Driel ML, Merenstein D, et al. (2018). Antibiotics for acute rhinosinusitis in adults. *The Cochrane database of systematic reviews*, 9(9), CD006089. https://www.cochranelibrary.com/cdsr/doi/10.1002/14651858.CD006089.pub5/full?highlightAbstract=acute%7Cin%7Cfour%7Cadults%7Cfor%7Crhinosinus%7Cantibiot%7Crhinosinusitis%7Cadult%7Cacut%7Cantibiotics

Patel GB, Kern RC, Bernstein JA, et al. (2020). Current and Future Treatments of Rhinitis and Sinusitis. *The journal of allergy and clinical immunology. In practice*, 8(5), 1522–1531.

Wise SK, Lin SY, Toskala E, et al. (2018). International Consensus Statement on Allergy and Rhinology: Allergic Rhinitis. *International forum of allergy & rhinology*, 8(2), 108–352. https://doi.org/10.1002/alr.22073

Stomatitis and Glossitis

Cifuentes M, Davari P, Rogers RS, 3rd (2017). Contact stomatitis. *Clinics in dermatology*, 35(5), 435–440. https://doi.org/10.1016/j.clindermatol.2017.06.007

de Campos WG, Esteves CV, Fernandes LG, et al. (2018). Treatment of symptomatic benign migratory glossitis: a systematic review. *Clinical oral investigations*, 22(7), 2487–2493. https://doi.org/10.1007/s00784-018-2553-4

Edgar NR, Saleh D, Miller RA. (2017). Recurrent Aphthous Stomatitis: A Review. *The Journal of clinical and aesthetic dermatology*, 10(3), 26–36.

Feller L, Wood NH, Khammissa RA, et al. (2017). Review: allergic contact stomatitis. *Oral surgery, oral medicine, oral pathology and oral radiology*, 123(5), 559–565. https://doi.org/10.1016/j.oooo.2017.02.007

Hargitai IA. (2018). Painful Oral Lesions. *Dental clinics of North America*, 62(4), 597–609. https://doi.org/10.1016/j.cden.2018.06.002

Ogueta IC, Ramírez MP, Jiménez CO, et al. (2019). Geographic Tongue: What a Dermatologist Should Know. Lengua geográfica: ¿qué es lo que un dermatólogo debería saber?. *Actas dermo-sifiliograficas*, 110(5), 341–346. https://doi.org/10.1016/j.ad.2018.10.022

Robinson AN, Loh J. (2019). Atrophic Glossitis. *The New England journal of medicine*, 381(16), 1568. https://doi.org/10.1056/NEJMicm1902490

Stoopler ET, France K, Ojeda D, et al. (2018). Benign Migratory Glossitis. *The Journal of emergency medicine*, 54(1), e9–e10. https://doi.org/10.1016/j.jemermed.2017.09.035

RESOURCES

Neck Masses

American Academy of Family Physicians
https://www.aafp.org/afp/2015/0515/p698.html

American Academy of Otolaryngology—Head and Neck Surgery
https://www.entnet.org/quality-practice/quality-products/clinical-practice-guidelines/evaluation-of-the-neck-mass-in-adults/

Merck Manual Professional Version
https://www.merckmanuals.com/professional/ear,-nose,-and-throat-disorders/approach-to-the-patient-with-nasal-and-pharyngeal-symptoms/neck-mass

Oral Cancer

American Cancer Society
https://www.cancer.org/treatment/treatments-and-side-effects/physical-side-effects/mouth-problems/mouth-sores.html

Pharyngitis and Tonsillitis

American Academy of Family Physicians
https://www.aafp.org/afp/topicModules/viewTopicModule.htm?topicModuleId=110
https://www.aafp.org/afp/2016/0701/p24.html

U.S. Centers for Disease Control and Prevention
https://www.cdc.gov/groupastrep/diseases-hcp/strep-throat.html

Rhinitis

American Academy of Allergy, Asthma, & Immunology
https://www.aaaai.org/Conditions-Treatments/Allergies/Hay-Fever-Rhinitis

American Academy of Family Physicians
https://www.aafp.org/afp/2018/0801/p171.html

Rhinosinusitis

American Academy of Allergy, Asthma, & Immunology
https://www.aaaai.org/Conditions-Treatments/Allergies/Sinusitis

American Academy of Otolaryngology—Head and Neck Surgery
https://www.enthealth.org/conditions/sinusitis/

U.S. Centers for Disease Control and Prevention
https://www.cdc.gov/antibiotic-use/sinus-infection.html

Stomatitis and Glossitis

Merck Manual Professional Version
https://www.merckmanuals.com/professional/dental-disorders/symptoms-of-dental-and-oral-disorders/stomatitis

The American Academy of Oral Medicine
https://www.aaom.com/index.php?option=com_content&view=article&id=131:geographic-tongue&catid=22:patient-condition-information&Itemid=120

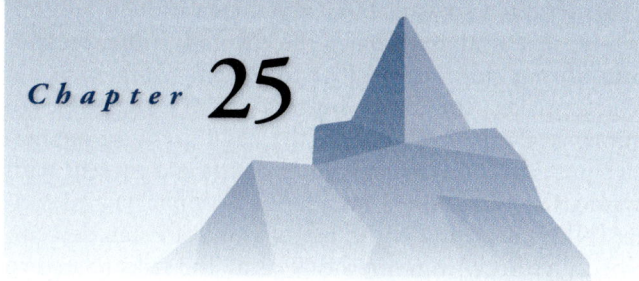

Chapter 25

Epistaxis

Maria Colandrea, DNP, NP-C, CORLN, CCRN, FAANP
Michael E. Zychowicz, DNP, ANP, ONP, FAAN, FAANP
Brian Oscar Porter, MD, PhD, MPH, MBA

Commonly referred to as a *nosebleed*, epistaxis is caused by the rupture of blood vessel(s) within the nasal mucosa. Epistaxis is a physical symptom rather than a disease, and can range from minor bleeding, which is easily treated with manual compression, to severe bleeding requiring emergency department (ED) visits and/or hospitalization. Therefore, after the initial management of bleeding, a thorough history and evaluation are essential to determine the underlying cause.

EPIDEMIOLOGY AND CAUSES

Epistaxis is extremely common, with about 60% of the general population experiencing at least one significant nosebleed over their lifetime. Epistaxis most commonly occurs in children younger than 10 years and in adults older than 50 years. Males and females are affected equally by nosebleeds. Certain risk factors increase risk for or cause nosebleeds (see Box 25.1).

Box 25.1	Risk Factors for Epistaxis

Systemic causes including chronic allergies; hypertension; and liver, cardiac, or kidney disease
 Nasal or facial trauma
 Prior nasal or sinus surgery
 Continuous positive airway pressure (CPAP) use and dry environments
 Age (younger than 10 or older than 50 years)
 Intranasal medications or intranasal illicit drug use
 Use of medications that impede platelet function or blood clotting
 Personal or family history of bleeding disorders

Systemic Causes

Chronic illness can increase risk for epistaxis. Chronic allergies can lead to chronic inflammation resulting in infection (sinusitis) of the paranasal sinuses and nasal cavity. Hypertension is significantly associated with the risk of epistaxis; however, this association does not support a causal relationship between hypertension and epistaxis. Coagulopathies with resultant bleeding may be associated with chronic disorders such as cirrhosis, renal disease, cancer (especially Hodgkin's disease), and hemophilia. Familial blood dyscrasias such as hemophilia A (factor VIII deficiency), hemophilia B (factor IX deficiency or Christmas disease), and von Willebrand disease (the most common genetic bleeding disorder), as well as hereditary hemorrhagic telangiectasia (HHT) (Osler-Weber-Rendu disease, a genetic condition causing arteriovenous malformations and telangiectasias), are examples of inherited conditions that may be complicated by significant epistaxis.

Medications

Prolonged use of intranasal sprays such as intranasal corticosteroids elevates the risk for epistaxis. Intranasal corticosteroids can thin the lining of the nasal mucosa, thereby increasing the risk of bleeding. Oral medications such as anticoagulants, NSAIDs, and salicylates may also predispose to nosebleeds by inhibiting natural clotting pathways. Inhaling substances by "snorting" can increase risk for epistaxis. Powdered drugs such as cocaine or heroin can lead to septal perforation and bleeding. Many nutritional deficiencies and febrile infectious disorders may also predispose to nosebleeds, including scurvy (caused by vitamin C deficiency) and rheumatic, scarlet, or typhoid fevers.

Environmental Factors

Excessive dryness of the nasal mucosa in poorly humidified environments or at high altitudes weakens nasal vessels, predisposing them to rupture. In addition, the use of noninvasive continuous positive airway pressure (CPAP) can lead to side effects such as mucosal dryness, sneezing, rhinorrhea, postnasal drip, nasal congestion, and/or epistaxis in the upper airways. CPAP therapy also contributes to the drying of the upper airways and inhibits the body's natural ability to hydrate the mucosa.

Trauma/Structural Issues

Trauma can result in epistaxis by causing injury to nasal vessels. The most common cause of trauma is digital manipulation (nose-picking). Fractures of the septum and facial bones, septal hematoma, insertion of nasogastric tubes or nasoendotracheal tubes, and forceful nose-blowing can all induce epistaxis. In children, foreign bodies becoming lodged in the nose are common, causing traumatic injury and resultant epistaxis.

Structural issues such as septal deviation may contribute to epistaxis through the disproportionate exposure of one side of the nose to dry environmental air, which makes the nasal mucosa more susceptible to injury. Malignant growths in the nasal cavity or paranasal sinuses may erode into blood vessels and present with epistaxis as the sole manifestation. Nasopharyngeal cancer (NPC) is prominent in populations of Asian descent, especially those from Southeast Asia. The risks related to this geographical predisposition include dietary habits, lifestyle characteristics (e.g., smoking), and exposures to harmful environmental factors. NPC is associated with a poor prognosis because the diagnosis is often delayed.

PATHOPHYSIOLOGY

The most common site of bleeding occurs in the anterior portion of the nasal septum known as *Little's area,* which contains a network of blood vessels called *Kiesselbach's plexus* that accounts for 90% of nosebleeds (see Fig. 25.1). Anterior nosebleeds tend to be easier to control because of the ability to easily apply pressure and/or quickly cauterize the area. In about 5% to 10% of patients, posterior epistaxis occurs in the area known as *Woodruff's plexus.* Posterior epistaxis can be seen in older adults with systemic illness and is often difficult to control, resulting in an ED visit or hospital admission.

The majority of nosebleeds result from local irritation of the highly vascular nasal mucosa related to trauma or inflammation, occurring most often in the absence of any

>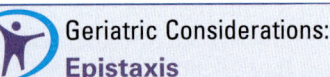
> **Geriatric Considerations: Epistaxis**
>
> A bimodal distribution exists for greatest frequency of epistaxis with a greater occurrence in children (younger than 10 years) and in older adults (older than 50 years). Older adults compared with children have a greater incidence of bleeding occurring from the posterior nasal septum. Bleeding in this area can be more severe than that involving the anterior nasal mucosa. The larger vessels of the posterior nasal septum can contribute to the epistaxis being more severe and difficult to control. A greater prevalence of ED visits or hospital management is noted with older patients who experience difficult-to-control epistaxis. In these cases, there may be greater difficulty visualizing the site of bleeding and the condition may necessitate management that is more invasive or aggressive than an anterior nosebleed. Several factors contribute to an increase in epistaxis in older people. Comorbidities such as vascular disease and hypertension, as well as medication regimens (e.g., anticoagulants), contribute to an increased incidence of nosebleed in older adults. Additionally, older people have less elastic and drier nasal mucosa, contributing to greater risk for nosebleed.

Pediatric/Adolescent Considerations: Epistaxis

Nearly three out of every four children will experience at least one episode of epistaxis. Children will experience epistaxis involving the anterior nasal septum more frequently than older adults. Epistaxis in children is typically a benign event that resolves spontaneously or with nasal compression. Dryness, chronic inflammation, and picking at nasal crust are associated with developing a nosebleed in children. Children will also have a greater rate of nasal foreign body associated with nosebleed than adults. It is rare for a child younger than 2 years to experience a nosebleed; therefore, the provider should have an index of suspicion for either abuse or coagulopathy as a potential causative factor.

In adolescent males between the ages of 10 and 20 years, juvenile nasopharyngeal angiofibroma is a rare, benign, and locally invasive nasopharyngeal tumor. This rare and highly vascularized tumor can be aggressive and grow into the sinuses, eye sockets, and skull. Early symptoms include epistaxis, nasal obstruction, chronic sinus infections, and rhinorrhea. Late-stage symptoms include headaches, facial numbness, swelling of the cheeks, droopy eyelids, protruding eyes, watery eyes, blindness, double vision, and hearing loss.

anatomical abnormality. Trauma to both nasal turbinates and the well-vascularized watershed area of Kiesselbach's plexus is the most common direct cause of nosebleed, particularly from nose-picking (epistaxis digitorum) or forcible injury related to blunt trauma. Kiesselbach's plexus marks the anastomosis of three major blood vessels of the nasal cavity: septal branch of the anterior ethmoid artery, septal portion of the superior labial branch of the facial artery, and lateral nasal branch of the sphenopalatine artery. Similarly, posterior epistaxis most commonly originates from rupture of the posterior wall and choanal branches of the sphenopalatine artery.

CLINICAL PRESENTATION

Subjective

The patient with recurrent minor anterior epistaxis typically presents with a history of several episodes over several weeks. If blood loss has been extensive, patients may report weakness or other symptoms of anemia. Bleeding from the posterior portion of the nasal cavity may be asymptomatic or may present with hemoptysis (coughed-up blood), nausea, gastrointestinal upset, hematemesis (blood-streaked vomitus), or blackened stools (melena) from the swallowed blood. Obtaining an accurate history of present illness is essential in identifying an underlying cause of the epistaxis (see Box 25.2).

Objective

Prominent blood vessels are typically seen traversing the anterior septum, and a small amount of clotted blood may be visible. If the patient is actively bleeding from the front of the nose, blood is typically bright red, and localizing the bleeding source may be difficult. The second most common site of hemorrhage after Little's area is the anterior end of the inferior nasal turbinate. Epistaxis originating deeper in the nose may produce either bright red or dark blood. Usually only one bleeding site exists, but if multiple sites or a diffuse ooze are evident, an underlying systemic bleeding disorder is likely. Anterior rhinoscopy to evaluate the anterior nose for any source of bleeding is important. This may be done with a light source and

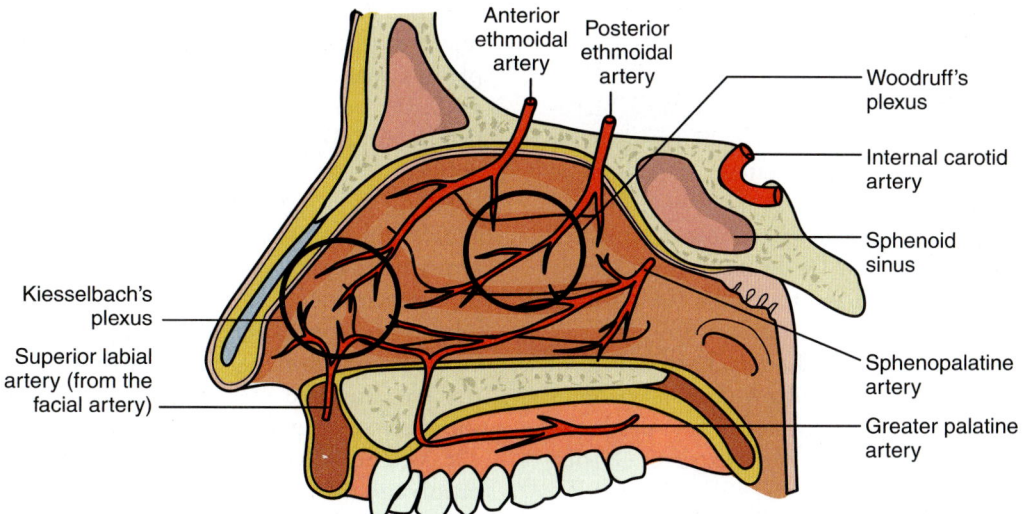

Figure 25.1 Anatomy of blood vessels in the nose. Kiesselbach's plexus is the most common site of anterior epistaxis, especially in children. Woodruff's plexus is associated with more severe but less frequent posterior nosebleeds in older adults.

> **Box 25.2 Eliciting a History of Present Illness for Epistaxis**
>
> Is the bleeding coming out the front of the nose or draining down the back of the throat?
>   Is the patient coughing up blood?
>   How long does the bleeding last?
>   Is the bleeding easily stopped?
>   What does the patient do to stop the nosebleed?
>   What types of intranasal and oral medications (both prescribed and illicit) is the patient using? What is the patient's past medical history?
>   Does the patient have a history of prior nasal/sinus surgeries or nasal/facial trauma?
>   Does the patient have a personal or familial blood coagulation disorder?
>   Other important questions to ask include whether the patient has unilateral bleeding, unilateral nasal obstruction, facial paresis, headaches, unilateral otalgia, unilateral ear infections, an anterior neck mass, or weight loss, which could suggest nasopharyngeal cancer.

speculum. An otoscope with speculum can also be used to carefully examine the interior of the nose.

If the source of hemorrhage is in the posterosuperior nasal cavity, the bleeding is termed *posterior epistaxis*. In these cases, blood loss into the nasopharynx will occur, and both clotted blood and brown to red throat discoloration may be evident. The most common sites of posterior bleeding are just under the posterior half of the inferior nasal turbinate or the roof of the nasal cavity. Patients with significant blood loss may demonstrate pallor, particularly in the face. Palpation or percussion of the paranasal sinuses may reveal tenderness if underlying sinusitis or malignancy is present.

DIAGNOSTIC REASONING

Diagnostic tests are rarely called for when nasal bleeding can be managed, and most episodes of epistaxis are not recurrent. A variety of diagnostic tests are helpful in determining the underlying cause of nasal hemorrhage. Laboratory tests exist for deficiencies of most clotting factors, but factor VIII and factor IX deficiencies are clearly the most commonly observed and tested for. Coagulation studies such as a prolonged prothrombin time (PT) or partial thromboplastin time (PTT) are characteristic of clotting factor disorders. Hemophilia A (factor VIII deficiency) and hemophilia B (factor IX deficiency) produce a prolonged PTT, whereas disorders of the extrinsic clotting pathway (factor VII deficiency) result in a prolonged PT. A complete blood count, including hemoglobin, hematocrit, and mean corpuscular volume, may offer insight into the chronicity of the condition. Radiological (x-ray) examination of the nasal cavity and paranasal sinuses may identify masses, including neoplasms or foreign bodies, as well as sinusitis if mucosal thickening or air-fluid levels are apparent. Computed tomography scan of the sinuses may also be done to detect structural and soft tissue abnormalities with greater sensitivity.

Differential Diagnosis

Differentiation among posterior epistaxis, hemoptysis (bloody sputum from a productive cough), and hematemesis (bloody vomitus) is critical. In the absence of respiratory or gastrointestinal findings, a diagnosis of posterior epistaxis can be assumed if visual evidence exists for a posterior source of bleeding (see Differential Diagnosis 25.1).

MANAGEMENT

Initial interventions for epistaxis should be geared toward stopping the bleeding and alleviating anxiety, whereas for recurrent nosebleeds, evaluation to identify an underlying cause is critical. Initial treatment of uncomplicated anterior epistaxis consists of applying firm, continuous pressure to the lower third of the nose for 5 minutes or longer. Ice packs may help. Patients should breathe through the mouth during this treatment period and must not release pressure to "sneak a peek" at the bleeding nares. To reduce vascular pressure, the patient should be seated upright with the head bent forward to prevent blood from draining into the posterior pharynx and airway (rather than hyperextending the neck with the nose pointed upward). Patients with no underlying medical problems may be treated at home, with directions to sit upright, minimize physical activity, and rest with the head elevated 45 to 90 degrees at night. Older or debilitated patients with epistaxis may require inpatient care, however, because of the increased risk of immunosuppression and anemia.

If bleeding is difficult to stop, pharmacological agents may be of some help. A small piece of cotton or nasal pledget soaked in a topical vasoconstricting agent (such as 0.25% phenylephrine, 1:1000 epinephrine, 0.1% xylometazoline, or 4% cocaine solution) should be applied to the nasal vestibule and pressed against the bleeding site for 5 to 10 minutes. Epinephrine should be avoided in hypertensive patients or those with coronary artery disease, and cocaine should be avoided in children. Oxymetazoline (Afrin) nasal spray combined with direct pressure is often effective at stopping the bleeding.

If this treatment fails, chemical cauterization of the bleeding site may be necessary. The nasal mucosa should first be anesthetized with a cotton ball soaked in 4% cocaine, 4% lidocaine, or 2% lidocaine viscous preparation and held over the bleeding site for several minutes. Alternatively, 2% lidocaine jelly may be used. A bead of chromic acid, 25% to 50% trichloroacetic acid solution, or a silver nitrate stick is then applied directly onto the bleeding vessels with firm pressure for 30 seconds,

Differential Diagnosis 25.1: Epistaxis

Trauma

- Acute bleeding after digital manipulation, blunt force to nose, forceful nasal blowing, or sneezing
- Usually unilateral

Nasopharyngeal carcinoma

- Unilateral bleeding
- Unilateral nasal obstruction
- Chronic sinusitis
- Facial numbness/paresis
- Unilateral otalgia or ear infection
- Cervical neck mass
- Weight loss

Medication-induced epistaxis

- Use of intranasal corticosteroids, illicit drugs, or oral anticoagulants

Nasal structural deformities

- Deviated septum
- Perforated septum

Juvenile nasopharyngeal angiofibroma (JNA)

- Early symptoms: epistaxis, nasal obstruction, chronic sinus infections, rhinorrhea
- Late-stage symptoms: headaches, facial numbness, cheek swelling, droopy eyelids, protruding eyes, watery eyes, blindness, double vision, hearing loss

Chronic allergies/sinus infections

- Chronic sinus infections
- Purulent drainage
- Rhinorrhea
- Nasal polyposis

Chronic medical illness or bleeding disorders (strong association with posterior epistaxis)

- Chronic illnesses: hypertension, cirrhosis, renal disease, cancer (especially Hodgkin's disease)
- Bleeding disorders: hemophilia, von Willebrand disease, hereditary hemorrhagic telangiectasia

---

which will allow for limited, shallow cautery of the bleeding site. Thermal or bipolar electrocautery may be required in cases of deeper lesions involving larger vessels; however, indiscriminate cauterization of a large area should be avoided.

If bleeding does not stop, anterior nasal packing should be placed to fill the entire nasal fossa. There are many types of nasal packing available, divided into two major categories: resorbable (i.e., packing that does not require removal) and nonresorbable (e.g., gauze dressings, polymers, and inflatable balloons). In patients on anticoagulants or with bleeding disorders or vascular disorders such as HHT, resorbable packing should be considered. Additionally, resorbable packing should be considered in young children in whom removing packing can be difficult. There are many choices of resorbable and nonresorbable packing available and utilization may be based on availability. Nonresorbable packing requires removal after a predetermined length of time, which must be communicated to the patient. Resorbable packing will require mucosal care such as intranasal saline sprays and follow-up to confirm reabsorption.

Posterior sources of bleeding require more complex treatment, and consultation with an otorhinolaryngologist may be required. Treatments include posterior nasal packing, sphenopalatine ganglion nerve block and, in extreme cases, surgical ligation of the compromised vessels. Nasal balloon-packing systems are an alternative to nasal packing, but they must not be overinflated and should be removed in a timely fashion. The patient must be monitored during the packing procedure, as some patients may experience a vasovagal response to the procedure, with syncope or a decrease in blood pressure.

Any form of nasal packing tends to be particularly painful for the patient once the local anesthetic has worn off, and analgesics should be considered. Over-the-counter (OTC) analgesics such as acetaminophen are preferred. In contrast, NSAIDs, including aspirin, should be avoided because of their capacity to impair platelet function, which may lead to further bleeding. In patients requiring nasal packing, the use of antibiotics is controversial but reasonable in patients at greater risk for infection.

All underlying medical conditions that might contribute to epistaxis should also be appropriately treated. Concurrent use of blood-thinning agents should be reevaluated in the presence of acute bleeding, and the decision to continue antithrombotic medications such as clopidogrel (Plavix), aspirin, warfarin (Coumadin), direct oral anticoagulants (e.g., dabigatran [Pradaxa], rivaroxaban [Xarelto], apixaban [Eliquis], edoxaban [Savaysa]), or any other blood-thinning agent should be discussed with a healthcare provider familiar with the prescribing indication.

FOLLOW-UP AND REFERRAL

Follow-up is not indicated for minor cases of nosebleed from local trauma or inflammation. In patients with recurrent or acute/severe epistaxis, referral to an otorhinolaryngologist to perform direct visualization of the nasopharynx is essential to evaluate acute and recurrent symptoms of epistaxis and to rule out nasopharyngeal carcinoma or HHT. In the case of acute bleeding requiring nasal packing, patients should be instructed when to follow up for timely removal. Excessive trauma during nasal packing or cauterization can result in septal hematoma, abscess, or perforation.

External nasal deformities may also result from pressure necrosis from the anterior portion of nasal packing. Balloon-packing systems may result in mucosal pressure necrosis if the balloons are overinflated. Likewise, if the anterior portion of a two-balloon system breaks, the posterior balloon may migrate posteriorly down the airway and cause obstruction.

Individuals with recurrent anterior epistaxis that causes severe blood loss or is refractory to vasoconstrictive or cauterization therapy should be referred to a specialist or ED, as appropriate. Hypovolemic or anemic patients require physician referral to evaluate the need for transfusion. Electrocautery for recurrent epistaxis caused by deep lesions should be performed only by a qualified specialist. The management of posterior epistaxis requires a specialist because treatment modalities may include ganglionic nerve blocks, posterior nasal packing, or vessel ligation. Coagulopathy-related and malignancy-related epistaxis require specialized treatment and specialty referral related to the underlying disorder.

Patient Education: Epistaxis

Patients who have been treated for epistaxis should not blow their nose and avoid sneezing, rubbing the nose, or picking the nose after an acute episode to avoid dislodging the protective blood clot. Increased environmental humidity in the home also helps prevent acute attacks, especially during the winter months. Intranasal saline and petroleum jelly applied liberally to the nares promote mucosal hydration, which helps prevent drying and cracking. If nasal probing is persistent, the patient's fingernails should be cut to avoid mucosal trauma.

OTC vasoconstrictors such as oxymetazoline or phenylephrine can be used in patients with recurrent nosebleeds that do not stop quickly. Caution should be used in patients with uncontrolled hypertension or cardiac disease. Education should be provided to the patient that the use of oxymetazoline should not exceed 3 consecutive days to avoid rhinitis medicamentosa. Additional education regarding proper nasal pinching techniques should be demonstrated to enable patients to administer self-care at home for minor episodes of epistaxis. However, the importance of maintaining nasal mucosal hydration should be stressed, as well as the need to avoid nasal probing and vigorous blowing of the nose, as preventive measures for future episodes.

The ability of certain medications to contribute to bleeding disorders (e.g., antiplatelet effects of aspirin and other NSAIDs, anticoagulant therapies such as warfarin) should also be discussed. Patients should be told not to swallow blood because this may upset the stomach, resulting in nausea, vomiting, or "gagging" (i.e., inhalation of blood into the trachea and bronchi). Patients should be instructed not to spit blood from mouth but to allow the blood to drain by gravity into a container. This prevents disruption of any clot that may be forming. Patients should not talk during episodes of active bleeding for the same reason, and alcohol and hot liquids should be avoided after an acute attack.

REFERENCES

Béquignon E, Teissier N, Gauthier A, et al. Emergency department care of childhood epistaxis. *Emerg Med J.* 2017;34(8):543–548. https://doi.org/10.1136/emermed-2015-205528

Chaaban MR, Zhang D, Resto V, et al. Demographic, seasonal, and geographic differences in emergency department visits for epistaxis. *Otolaryngol Head Neck Surg.* 2017;156(1):81–86. https://doi.org/10.1177/0194599816667295

Chen YP, Chan A, Le QT, et al. Nasopharyngeal carcinoma. *The Lancet.* 2019;394(10192):64–80. https://doi.org/10.1016/S0140-6736(19)30956-0

Cohen O, Shoffel-Havakuk H, Warman M, et al. Early and late recurrent epistaxis admissions: patterns of incidence and risk factors. *Otolaryngol Head Neck Surg.* 2017;157(3):424–431. https://doi.org/10.1177/0194599817705619

Grau-Bartual S, Al-Jumaily AM, Young PM, et al. Effect of continuous positive airway pressure treatment on permeability, inflammation, and mucus production of human epithelial cells. *ERJ Open Res.* 2020;6(2):00327–2019. https://doi.org/10.1183/23120541.00327-2019

Krulewitz NA, Fix ML. Epistaxis. *Emerg Med Clin North Am.* 2019;37(1):29–39. https://doi.org/10.1016/j.emc.2018.09.005

Li W, Ni Y, Lu H, et al. Current perspectives on the origin theory of juvenile nasopharyngeal angiofibroma. *Discov Med.* 2019;27(150):245–254.

Min HJ, Kang II, Choi GJ, et al. Association between hypertension and epistaxis: Systematic review and meta-analysis. *Otolaryngol Head Neck Surg.* 2017;157(6):921–927. https://doi.org/10.1177/0194599817721445

Tunkel DE, Anne S, Payne SC, et al. Clinical practice guideline: Nosebleed (epistaxis). *Otolaryngol Head Neck Surg.* 2020;162(1 Suppl):S1–S38. https://doi.org/10.1177/0194599819890327

Womack JP, Kropa J, Jimenez Stabile M. Epistaxis: outpatient management. *Am Fam Physician.* 2018;98(4):240–245.

Zhou AH, Chung SY, Sylvester MJ, et al. To pack or not to pack: inpatient management of epistaxis in the elderly. *Am J Rhinol Allergy.* 2018;32(6):539–545. https://doi.org/10.1177/1945892418801259

RESOURCES

American Academy of Otolaryngology—Head and Neck Surgery
https://www.entnet.org/?s=epistaxis

American Academy of Pediatrics—Clinical Practice Guideline: Nosebleed (Epistaxis)
https://pediatrics.aappublications.org/content/145/4/e20200283

Family Practice Notebook: Epistaxis
https://fpnotebook.com/ent/nose/Epstxs.htm

National Skull Base Foundation—Epistaxis Embolization
https://nsbf.us/neuro-intervention/epistaxis-embolization/

Chapter 26

Temporomandibular Disorders

Maria Colandrea, DNP, NP-C, CORLN, CCRN, FAANP
Michael E. Zychowicz, DNP, ANP, ONP, FAAN, FAANP
Brian Oscar Porter, MD, PhD, MPH, MBA

Temporomandibular joint (TMJ) disease is a collective term that refers to disorders affecting the masticatory musculature, the TMJ and its associated structures, or both. The terms *craniomandibular disorders* and *temporomandibular disorders* (TMDs) are synonymous with the more familiar term *temporomandibular joint (TMJ) disease* (most current research favors the phrase *temporomandibular disorders*). Although TMD has been traditionally viewed as one syndrome, it is actually a cluster of related disorders in the masticatory system that have many common features. The most common presenting symptom is pain in the muscles of mastication, the preauricular area, and/or the TMJ. Chewing, bruxism (clenching, grinding, or gnashing of the teeth during nonfunctional movements of the mandible), or other jaw functions tend to aggravate the pain.

EPIDEMIOLOGY AND CAUSES

It is estimated that 33% of adults are affected by TMD, 3% to 7% of whom seek medical treatment. TMD can be mild and self-limited, or it may progress to chronic pain and discomfort, which will require consultation with multiple health professionals over many years.

The incidence of TMD peaks from 20 to 40 years of age. Risk factors for TMD include being female and non-Hispanic white. Socioeconomic status does not seem to be related. There is an association between TMD and mood disorders and other psychiatric illness, as well as mechanical etiologies, such as bruxism. Various studies have indicated patients with rheumatoid arthritis have a prevalence of TMD between 53% and 94%.

PATHOPHYSIOLOGY

The TMJ is one of the most complex joints in the body. It is a synovial, encapsulated joint that is stress-bearing. The TMJ differs from other joints in the body in that its articular surfaces are covered with fibrocartilaginous tissue, rather than with chondral cartilage, as found in other joints. The articular disc separates the upper and lower joint spaces. Pain from the TMJ arises from injury to the retrodiscal tissue or the capsular ligament (see Fig. 26.1). Locking of the joint may occur secondary to jaw malocclusion and, most commonly, anterior disc dislocation. However, several variations of articular disc displacement have been noted with this condition, as joint laxity from underlying connective tissue disorders and even asymmetrical body alignment from poor posture have been cited as risk factors. Dental manipulation of the jaw and degeneration of the TMJ from rheumatoid arthritis or osteoarthritis often underlie extracapsular joint dysfunction. Misalignment of the TMJ places pressure on nearby ear structures, resulting in otalgia (ear pain), tinnitus, vertigo, hearing loss, and tongue pain.

TMJ pain may also be intracapsular in origin and involve the masticatory musculature, known as *TMJ myofascial pain syndrome* or simply *TMJ syndrome*. Like all skeletal muscles, the TMJ muscles are susceptible to muscle splinting, spasm, or inflammation. Pain that originates in the orofacial area may be referred to other locations, such as the neck, shoulders, and head. TMJ syndrome often coexists with fibromyalgia; however, pain from the masticatory musculature is usually related to mandibular dysfunction.

CLINICAL PRESENTATION

Subjective

Patients may present with several complaints that lead to the suspicion of TMD or with only a single symptom. The most common presenting symptoms are facial pain, ear discomfort or dysfunction, headache, and TMJ discomfort or dysfunction. The facial pain of TMD is usually unilateral with or without radiation to the ear, temporal region, angle of the jaw, or posterior neck. The facial pain is usually dull and may be constant or intermittent. Ear pain, fullness, and tinnitus are also common complaints of TMD that lead to referral. The typical headache of TMD is unilateral and described as a deep pain that is

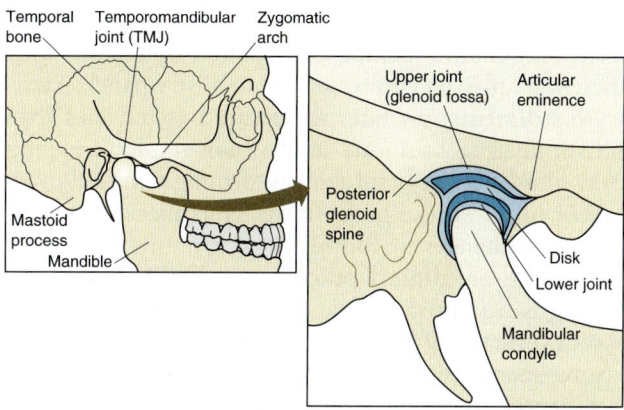

Figure 26.1 Anatomy of the temporomandibular joint.

worse in the morning; however, variants of the headache are not uncommon. TMJ dysfunction manifests as clicking, popping, jaw deviation, or jaw locking and, again, with symptoms that are worse in the morning.

Objective

Because many of the presenting symptoms of TMD may be secondary to underlying medical conditions, a complete examination should be done to exclude dental, neurological, immunological, musculoskeletal, and psychological causes. Special attention should be directed to observation of the patient's balance, possible gait problems, or unusual findings that suggest an underlying systemic disease. The muscles of mastication and the TMJ should be palpated using a bimanual technique. Muscles to be palpated include the masseter, temporalis, medial pterygoid, digastric, and mylohyoid. Tenderness, enlargement, swelling, and unusual texture of these muscles should be noted. Tenderness over the temporal artery region suggestive of giant cell (temporal) arteritis would be concerning, as would skin lesions suggestive of a herpetic etiology. Cervical muscle groups should also be palpated to differentiate craniocervical disorders. The oral examination may reveal an absence of ridges on the occlusal surface of the teeth, which appear flat. This reflects bruxism, a known risk factor for TMD.

The TMJ should be examined with the mouth closed, which will allow palpation of the lateral aspect. On opening of the jaw, assessment of mandibular range of motion and TMJ sounds and palpation of crepitus can assist with diagnosis. A mandibular opening of less than 35 mm is considered restrictive, and the mandible may deviate to one side or the other when opened (asymmetrical opening). Pain may also be elicited with mandibular movement and should be noted. Dysfunctional TMJ sounds may be described as clicking, popping, or crepitant.

DIAGNOSTIC REASONING

Diagnostic Tests

Initial testing for the diagnosis of TMD should include ruling out other underlying medical conditions. Laboratory testing should include a complete blood count with differential, platelet count, serum chemistry panel, erythrocyte sedimentation rate, rheumatoid factor, and thyroid-stimulating hormone level. Radiographic imaging (x-ray films) may be helpful in confirming a clinical diagnosis of TMD. The clinician must remember that even if anatomical changes are found, imaging results rarely have any bearing on clinical outcome in TMD. Panoramic imaging is best used to rule out any dental issues (e.g., abscesses) that may be a source of pain.

Subsequent testing should most appropriately be ordered by a dentist, otorhinolaryngologist, or oral surgeon on referral of the patient. This could include panoramic films (if not already done), computed tomography (CT) scan, or magnetic resonance imaging (MRI). CT scan provides the clearest picture of osseous structures, and when used with contrast, can help visualize the soft tissues of the head and neck; however, it is not useful in the diagnosis of disc displacement of the TMJ. MRI visualizes the soft tissues of the TMJ without radiation exposure or the need for contrast dye. MRI can be used to determine disc position and morphology. Therapeutic injections with local anesthetics or corticosteroids, synovial fluid analysis, or biopsy of suspicious areas by the specialist may be useful for differentiating TMD from similarly presenting diagnoses.

Differential Diagnosis

Because of the contributing factors and characteristic symptoms, it may be difficult to arrive at a diagnosis of TMD. Disorders of intracranial structures should be ruled out early because they may be life-threatening and require immediate attention. New or abrupt onset of pain; progressively more severe pain; interruption of sleep by pain; and systemic symptoms such as weight loss, ataxia, fever, and neurological symptoms (e.g., seizures, paralysis, vertigo) are characteristic of intracranial disorders. Differential Diagnosis 26.1 presents common differential diagnoses for TMD.

MANAGEMENT

The goals for management of TMD are similar to those of any musculoskeletal condition: reduction or elimination of pain and restoration of acceptable (mandibular) joint function. Complete resolution of TMD may not be a realistic expectation because this largely depends on the underlying cause. Initial management combines nonpharmacological and pharmacological modalities that are individualized to the patient. Nonpharmacological options include self-care,

---

Differential Diagnosis 26.1: Temporomandibular Disorder

- Sinusitis
- Dental abnormalities or infections
- Otitis media and otitis externa
- Musculoskeletal pain
- Arthritis (e.g., rheumatoid arthritis, osteoarthritis, gout, septic arthritis, psoriatic arthritis, Lyme disease)
- Parotid gland pathology
- Mastoiditis
- Giant cell arteritis
- Trigeminal neuralgia
- Postherpetic neuralgia
- Headaches (e.g., cluster, migraine, tension, vascular)
- Psychogenic pain
- Mood disorders (e.g., depression, anxiety)
- Head and neck cancer pain

biobehavioral pain management (including biofeedback, relaxation and imagery techniques, and cognitive therapy), occlusal splints (bite guards), and physical therapy.

Some of the most significant contributions toward management of TMD can be made by adjustments in dietary consistency, disease education, alteration of oral parafunctional habits (e.g., bruxism), and the application of ice (for acute symptomatology) or moist heat (for chronic symptomatology). Wearing an intraoral appliance with an occlusal splint component may be recommended, generally by a dentist. Physical therapy may be employed, primarily as an adjunct to other therapeutic modalities, in an attempt to relieve pain of musculoskeletal origin and restore normal masticatory function. Physical therapy for TMD may include electromodalities and therapeutic exercises as prescribed by a physical therapist. Biobehavioral therapy is indicated for patients with behavioral and emotional problems and/or noxious habits that accompany TMD. Stress relief and pain control methods such as counseling, hypnosis, biofeedback, and guided imagery are safe and noninvasive.

Pharmacotherapy can be beneficial in controlling the pain and inflammation associated with TMD. Careful monitoring of the patient's tolerance to prescribed medications and the effectiveness of these drugs are key. A course of 10 to 14 days of NSAIDs is the initial treatment of choice. If there is pain on palpation of the muscles of mastication, short-term use of a short-acting muscle relaxant combined with an NSAID may benefit some patients. Tricyclic antidepressants are an option for long-term use, especially if TMD is associated with anxiety or depression. For patients with rheumatoid arthritis, treatment and control of the underlying disease is recommended, but neither corticosteroids nor hyaluronic acid is recommended for long-term use in these patients. In addition, the use of opioids or benzodiazepines is discouraged in TMD because of their abuse potential. Drugs Commonly Prescribed 26.1 presents the drugs commonly used to treat TMD.

Drugs Commonly Prescribed 26.1: Temporomandibular Disorder

DRUG	INDICATION	DOSAGE	COMMENTS
Nonopioid Analgesics			
Acetaminophen (Tylenol)	TMD (acute and chronic)	1,000 mg three times daily	Increased risk of hepatic impairment with long-term use
Ibuprofen (Motrin, Advil)	TMD (acute and chronic): anti-inflammatory effect is desired	400–800 mg three to four times daily with food	Contraindicated with aspirin allergy Increased risk of gastrointestinal bleed and renal insufficiency with long-term use
Naproxen (Aleve, Naprosyn)	TMD (acute and chronic): anti-inflammatory effect is desired	220 mg every 12 hours with food	Contraindicated with aspirin allergy Increased risk of gastrointestinal bleed and renal insufficiency with long-term use
Muscle Relaxant			
Cyclobenzaprine HCl (Flexeril)	TMD (acute): to relieve muscle spasm	5–10 mg three times daily	Adverse effects include drowsiness, blurred vision, dry mouth, and dizziness Cannot drive while taking Pregnancy Category B Known abuse potential
Tricyclic Antidepressants			
Amitriptyline (Elavil)	TMD (chronic): especially helpful when underlying anxiety and/or depression are contributing factors	25 mg three to four times daily or 75 mg at bedtime Begin with low nightly dose and increase	May result in decreased orofacial pain, improvement in sleep disorders, and promotion of muscle relaxation and decreased bruxism Adverse effects include anticholinergic effects (e.g., dry mouth, constipation, urinary retention), drowsiness, and arrhythmias Contraindicated within 14 days of use of monoamine oxidase inhibitors and in acute postmyocardial infarction Monitor serum levels with concomitant use of drugs metabolized by CYP450 enzyme complex

Abbreviation: TMD, temporomandibular disorder.

For refractory cases, referral to a dentist or oral maxillofacial specialist for injection of trigger points with anesthetic agents may be beneficial. In rare cases, surgical procedures such as arthroscopy, arthrocentesis, open arthrotomy, or even reconstructive jaw surgery may be required.

For the majority of cases of TMD, subsequent management will necessarily be initiated and followed by a dentist, otorhinolaryngologist, or oral surgeon to whom the patient has been referred (see The Iceberg of TMD).

The Iceberg of TMD

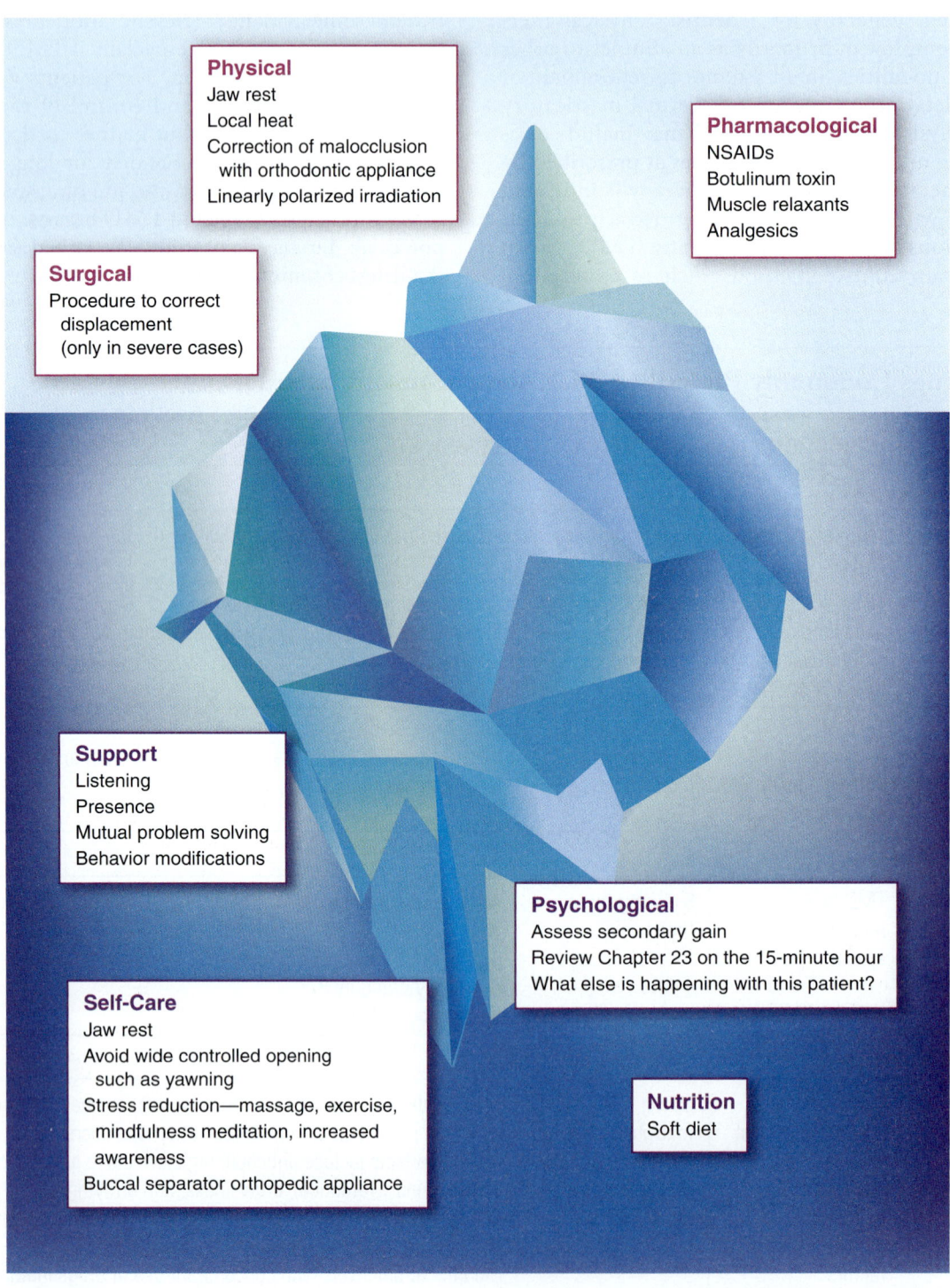

Physical
Jaw rest
Local heat
Correction of malocclusion with orthodontic appliance
Linearly polarized irradiation

Pharmacological
NSAIDs
Botulinum toxin
Muscle relaxants
Analgesics

Surgical
Procedure to correct displacement (only in severe cases)

Support
Listening
Presence
Mutual problem solving
Behavior modifications

Psychological
Assess secondary gain
Review Chapter 23 on the 15-minute hour
What else is happening with this patient?

Self-Care
Jaw rest
Avoid wide controlled opening such as yawning
Stress reduction—massage, exercise, mindfulness meditation, increased awareness
Buccal separator orthopedic appliance

Nutrition
Soft diet

FOLLOW-UP AND REFERRAL

The decision to refer a patient with TMD to a specialist should be based on the individual practitioner's knowledge level and comfort in treating TMD. If there is any uncertainty about the diagnosis, referral should be made to a dentist, otorhinolaryngologist, or oral maxillofacial surgeon who is knowledgeable in the treatment of TMD. Once other systemic conditions have been ruled out, the primary care practitioner may choose to begin initial management of TMD symptoms. Follow-up should be early and repeated (e.g., in 1 to 2 weeks initially and monthly thereafter), especially if pharmacotherapy is ordered. If initial therapy is unsuccessful or if advanced management is indicated, appropriate referrals should be undertaken.

Patient Education: Temporomandibular Disorder

Home care and patient education are integral components in the management of TMD. The majority of patients achieve relief of symptoms with conservative therapy, including self-care techniques. Patient education for the management of TMD includes the following recommendations:

- Limit overworking the jaw by eating softer foods, taking smaller bites, and not opening the mouth wide when eating; avoid foods such as apples, corn on the cob, hard breads, raw vegetables, and steak or tough meats.
- To help reduce stress, strive for a nutritionally balanced diet and an active exercise program.
- Ice packs can be used for acute pain and muscle spasm; for chronic pain, moist heat should be used following the same guidelines.
- Disengage your teeth: the rule is "lips together, teeth apart."
- Do not chew gum or ice.
- Sleep on your back with a pillow under your knees and not on your stomach. Do not use firm, full pillows under your head; orthopedic pillows can be helpful in reducing head and neck pain.
- When talking on the telephone, do not support the receiver with your shoulder.
- Prevent wide opening of the mouth when yawning.
- Do not sit with your chin resting on your hand.
- Practice good posture; if you must sit for long periods of time, stand and move around frequently to stretch your muscles.

REFERENCES

Abbasgholizadeh ZS, Evren B, Ozkan Y. Evaluation of the efficacy of different treatment modalities for painful temporomandibular disorders. *Int J Oral Maxillofac Surg.* 2020;49(5):628–635. https://doi.org/10.1016/j.ijom.2019.08.010

Beecroft E, Penlington C, Desai H, Durham J. Temporomandibular disorder for the general dental practitioner. *Prim Dent J.* 2019;7(4):62–70.

Bueno CH, Pereira DD, Pattussi MP, et al. Gender differences in temporomandibular disorders in adult populational studies: a systematic review and meta-analysis. *J Oral Rehabil.* 2018;45(9):720–729. https://doi.org/10.1111/joor.12661

Christidis N, Lindström Ndanshau E, Sandberg A, et al. Prevalence and treatment strategies regarding temporomandibular disorders in children and adolescents—a systematic review. *J Oral Rehabil.* 2019;46(3):291–301. https://doi.org/10.1111/joor.12759

Kusdra PM, Stechman-Neto J, Leão B, et al. Relationship between otological symptoms and TMD. *Int Tinnitus J.* 2018;22(1):30–34. https://doi.org/10.5935/0946-5448.20180005

Lai YC, Yap AU, Türp JC. Prevalence of temporomandibular disorders in patients seeking orthodontic treatment: a systematic review. *J Oral Rehbil.* 2020;47(2):270–280. https://doi.org/10.1111/joor.12899

Ohrbach R, Dworkin SF. AAPT Diagnostic Criteria for Chronic Painful Temporomandibular Disorders. *J Pain.* 2019;20(11):1276–1292. https://doi.org/10.1016/j.jpain.2019.04.003

Ouanounou A, Goldberg M, Haas DA. Pharmacotherapy in temporomandibular disorders: a review. *J Can Dent Assoc.* 2017;83:h7.

Pietropaoli D, Cooper BC, Ortu E, et al. A device improves signs and symptoms of TMD. *Pain Res Manag.* 2019;2019:5646143. https://doi.org/10.1155/2019/5646143

Sójka A, Stelcer B, Roy M, et al. Is there a relationship between psychological factors and TMD? *Brain Behav.* 2019;9(9):e01360. https://doi.org/10.1002/brb3.1360

Talley RL. TMJ and OSA are sisters. *Cranio.* 2019;37(5):273–274. https://doi.org/10.1080/08869634.2019.1641910

RESOURCES

American Migraine Foundation
https://americanmigrainefoundation.org/resource-library/temporomandibular-disorders/

National Institutes for Health; National Institute of Dental and Craniofacial Research
https://www.nidcr.nih.gov/health-info/tmj/more-info

The TMJ Association (TMJA)
https://tmj.org/

U.S. Food and Drug Administration (FDA)
https://www.fda.gov/medical-devices/dental-devices/temporomandibular-disorders-tmd-devices

Chapter 27

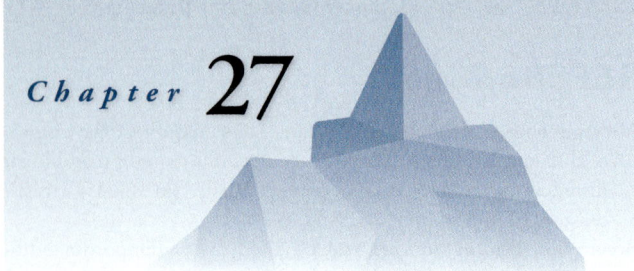

Dysphonia

Maria Colandrea, DNP, NP-C, CORLN, CCRN, FAANP
Michael E. Zychowicz, DNP, ANP, ONP, FAAN, FAANP
Brian Oscar Porter, MD, PhD, MPH, MBA

Dysphonia, or hoarseness, is an impaired voice production or altered voice quality. Hoarseness is the symptom, whereas *dysphonia* is the diagnostic term. Dysphonia suggests an abnormality in voice production at the level of the larynx. There are numerous causes of dysphonia; some are functional and others are organic.

EPIDEMIOLOGY AND CAUSES

Dysphonia affects approximately 10% of the general population. It can affect patients of all ages, with a higher incidence in the pediatric and older populations. Dysphonia is common in professions with high vocal demands such as singers, teachers, clergy, telemarketers, and drill sergeants, among others. In children, dysphonia is frequently related to viral illness or growths on the vocal cords. In adults, changes in voice are part of the natural process of aging.

PATHOPHYSIOLOGY

The larynx is made up of cartilage, extrinsic and intrinsic muscles, and mucosal lining. The muscles are innervated by the vagus nerve, which branches into the recurrent laryngeal nerve. The main functions of the larynx include the coordination of phonation, respiration, and protection of the trachea to prevent aspiration during swallowing or performing the Valsalva maneuver.

The process of phonation occurs with an exhaled column of air through the vocal cords. The forced air causes the superficial layer of the vocal cord mucosa to vibrate at different frequencies. The length and tension of the vocal cords determine the voice pitch. The sound resonates in the pharynx and sinonasal cavity, producing a voice that is unique to each person. Articulation of words is formed by the palate, tongue, lips, and teeth. Changes in voice can be related to inflammation or irritation of the vocal cords, medications, growths on the vocal cords, neurological disease, inflammatory diseases, voice overuse/strain, aging, or neuromuscular and/or psychiatric causes.

CLINICAL PRESENTATION

Subjective

The onset of dysphonia is an important key to its diagnosis. An acute, short, self-limited complaint of vocal changes is unlikely to be caused by cancer, whereas hoarseness persisting for more than several weeks is unlikely to be the result of an acute infection. Dysphonia that persists for longer than 4 weeks, without associated upper respiratory infection, requires a work-up.

Associated signs and symptoms should be ascertained. Shortness of breath, stridor, cough, hemoptysis, throat pain, difficulty swallowing, unilateral otalgia, tobacco or alcohol use, and weight loss in a patient with vocal symptoms raise concern for cancer. Chronic pain often suggests more serious underlying disease than acute onset of pain. Dysphagia or odynophagia accompanying hoarseness indicates the presence of disease affecting the pharynx or esophagus. An accompanying cough suggests irritation of the endolarynx or pulmonary disease. Fever and oral, nasal, or otologic discharge with dysphonia suggest an infectious process.

Vocal use and lifestyle should be reviewed to assess for pertinent positives and negatives associated with the specific etiology of dysphonia. Overuse of the voice can cause hoarseness, as would be seen in singers. A prolonged history of tobacco use may cause irritation or malignancy. A scratchy throat in the morning or symptoms after eating could suggest a diagnosis of gastroesophageal reflux disease (GERD) or allergies. Previous head, neck, or thoracic surgery; tracheal intubation; thoracic malignancy; or radiotherapy to the neck may all be factors affecting the laryngeal nerve, which can lead to vocal impairment. The use of asthma inhalers and chronic exposure to pollutants or allergens may contribute to hoarseness as well (see Box 27.1).

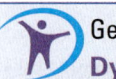

Geriatric Considerations: Dysphonia

In older adult males, the voice becomes weaker and higher pitched because of muscle atrophy and increased stiffness of tissues. In older females, the same changes occur, but the pitch of the voice becomes lower because during menopause, mucoid edema occurs in the submucosa of the vocal folds. More severe edema and polyps may occur in older females who smoke. Dysphonia is a cardinal sign of laryngeal cancer, which is seen most commonly in males 50 to 70 years of age, as well as in those with a history or current use of tobacco and alcohol.

Box 27.1 Pertinent History of Present Illness Questions

How long has your voice been hoarse?
Has your voice been hoarse before? If so, what did you do for it?
Was the voice change sudden or did it progress over time?
Is the hoarseness intermittent or do you stay hoarse all day?
Is the hoarseness worse after eating or in the morning?
Does your voice sound coarse or harsh? Or is it breathy?
Do you lose your breath during or after speaking?
Is your throat scratchy or does it hurt with speaking?
What is your occupation?
Have you had an upper respiratory infection or did you experience voice overuse before the hoarseness?
Does your voice get worse after prolonged speaking?
Did you recently have surgery? If so, what type of surgery, and were you intubated?
Do you use tobacco? Alcohol? Illicit drugs?
Can you describe your past medical history?
Have you used any medications, especially drying agents like antihistamines and decongestants?

Specific considerations in infants and children:
Does the child have a change in the way they cry?
Are they more short of breath? Is there noisy breathing?
Has the voice change been acute or chronic?
Have they had changes in swallowing or difficulty breathing with feeding?
Do you have associated symptoms of:

- Cough
- Shortness of breath
- Spitting up blood or blood-tinged sputum
- Feeling of a lump in your throat
- Sore throat
- Painful swallowing
- Difficulty swallowing
- Acid reflux
- Constant throat-clearing
- Unilateral earache, hearing loss, or ear infections
- Weight loss
- Fever or symptoms of upper respiratory infection
- Allergies, postnasal drip, or sinus drainage

Objective

A complete examination of the head and neck is necessary when evaluating dysphonia. Stridor or shortness of breath could indicate an airway obstruction and should be immediately addressed. Nasal drainage and excess mucus may indicate sinusitis. Tonsillar erythema or exudate indicates viral or bacterial infection, as does ear canal erythema or exudate. A normal ear examination, despite the complaint of otalgia, may be seen in patients with cancer of the pharynx or larynx. The clinician should inspect and palpate the oral cavity including the buccal mucosa, posterior pharynx including the tonsillar fossa, floor of the mouth, and tongue. The neck should be palpated for cervical adenopathy and thyroid nodules or abnormalities. Lymph nodes in the neck related to infection often are tender to touch and feel tense or fluctuant. Lymph nodes related to malignancies typically feel hard and fixed to underlying tissue. Neck anatomy, including tracheal alignment, should be inspected and palpated. However, with dysphonia, it is important to note that examination of the head, eyes, ears, nose, and throat may all be normal.

DIAGNOSTIC REASONING

Diagnostic Tests

The routine use of computed tomography scans or magnetic resonance imaging, as well as antibiotic therapy, are not typically recommended for the evaluation and treatment of hoarseness. However, if infection is suspected (for instance, due to an elevated white blood cell count), culture and antibiotic sensitivity tests of oral or otologic discharge can reveal the organism responsible for the infection and guide antimicrobial therapy.

If hoarseness persists for more than 4 weeks and is clearly not caused by infection, referral to an otolaryngologist for direct visualization of the vocal cords (laryngoscopy) is required. An adequate laryngeal examination should visualize the base of the tongue, epiglottis, pyriform sinuses, false vocal cords, subglottic larynx, and true vocal cords. Use of stroboscopy improves detection of small lesions by "freezing" the vocal cords (making them appear immobile) during vibration. Thyroid tumors are the most common cause of bilateral vocal cord paralysis, whereas esophageal and pulmonary tumors are common causes of left-sided vocal cord paralysis, which emphasizes the need for direct laryngeal visualization in these circumstances.

Differential Diagnosis

The differential diagnosis of hoarseness focuses on the specific causes of hoarseness, which include infection, especially viral, as the most common etiology. Overuse, vocal cord pathology (e.g., polyps, nodules, tumors), adverse effects from medicines (e.g., antihistamines, decongestants, anticholinergics), vocal cord paralysis (due to neurological defects or tumors/growths), age-related muscle atrophy, GERD, chronic tobacco and alcohol use, and chronic allergies with resultant postnasal drip are other differential diagnoses (see Differential Diagnosis 27.1).

Differential Diagnosis 27.1: Dysphonia

Inflammation/trauma/irritation

- Infections (e.g., viral upper respiratory infection, fungal laryngitis [*Candida*], sinusitis)
- Allergic rhinitis
- Irritants such as tobacco smoke, alcohol, pollen, or environmental pollutants
- Laryngopharyngeal reflux from gastroesophageal reflux disease
- Direct trauma (e.g., tracheal intubation)
- Indirect trauma (e.g., recurrent laryngeal nerve injury secondary to thyroid surgery)

Neurological

- Parkinson's disease
- Amyotrophic lateral sclerosis
- Primary lateral sclerosis
- Myasthenia gravis
- Multiple sclerosis
- Guillain-Barré syndrome
- Dystonia (aberrant muscle contraction)
- Essential tremor

Neuromuscular and psychiatric

- Nerve injury (vagus or recurrent laryngeal nerve)
- Spasmodic dysphonia
- Psychogenic
- Muscle tension dysphonia

- Presbylarynges (age-related vocal cord atrophy)
- Stroke

Autoimmune

- Rheumatoid arthritis
- Wegener's granulomatosis
- Sarcoidosis
- Amyloidosis

Vocal cord lesions

- Cyst
- Scar
- Hemorrhage
- Granuloma
- Leukoplakia
- Reinke's edema
- Nodules
- Laryngeal papillomatosis
- Squamous cell carcinoma

Medications

- Inhaled corticosteroids
- Anticholinergics
- Antihistamines
- Decongestants
- Antihypertensives/diuretics

MANAGEMENT

Management of the underlying cause of dysphonia is the key. Guidelines for the management of hoarseness recommended by the American Academy of Otolaryngology–Head and Neck Surgery Foundation, include the following:

- Assess a dysphonia complaint with a thorough history and physical examination, including the head and neck.
- If symptoms of dysphonia last longer than 4 weeks, referral to an otolaryngologist is recommended to perform laryngoscopy.
- Review current medications that may be causing the symptom (e.g., drying agents, such as antihistamines, anticholinergics, or decongestants).
- Avoid vocal excess and irritants, such as inhaled smoke, pollen, and airborne pollutants.
- If dysphonia is a result of overuse of the vocal cords, complete rest of the voice can help, although avoid whispering because this strains the larynx.
- Avoid antihistamines because they dry the mucous membranes.
- Antibiotics are not recommended to treat acute laryngitis.
- Imaging studies should not be performed before directly visualizing the larynx with laryngoscopy.
- Use of humidified air, especially at night and during dry seasons, may be helpful.
- Encourage increased oral fluids.
- Treatment with antireflux medication should not be prescribed in the absence of signs or symptoms of significant GERD and before evaluation by laryngoscopy.
- After evaluation by an otolaryngologist and confirmation that there are no pathological causes of dysphonia, voice therapy may be prescribed. Vocal therapy sessions directed by a speech language pathologist are a well-established intervention for patients of all ages who have hoarseness.
- To decrease vocal cord strain, use of an amplifying device during heavy voice use can reduce hoarseness.
- Oral steroids are not routinely recommended, and oxymetazoline (Afrin) nasal spray should be avoided due to its drying effects.

FOLLOW-UP AND REFERRAL

As noted previously, if dysphonia persists for more than 4 weeks, further evaluation by an otolaryngologist is warranted. For persistent or recurrent episodes of hoarseness, vocal hygiene and voice therapy should be considered, especially in professionals who rely on their voice and are prone to vocal overuse or strain.

Patient Education: Dysphonia

Because hoarseness is generally self-limited, the following vocal hygiene measures, which are behaviors that reduce laryngeal irritation or injury, should be recommended:

- Avoid vocal straining, chronic throat clearing, and excessive coughing, which can irritate the larynx.
- Control GERD and allergic symptoms.
- Avoid medications that cause drying effects, such as antihistamines or anticholinergics.
- Avoid alcohol and caffeine use.
- Avoid inhaled irritants such as tobacco smoke, vaping, pollen, or environmental pollutants.
- Maintain adequate fluid intake and ambient humidification.
- Voice training can help, especially in those patients with high vocal demands.
- These prevention strategies should be emphasized, especially for those at high risk of recurrence.

REFERENCES

Carroll TL. (2019). Reflux and the voice: getting smarter about laryngopharyngeal reflux. *Otolaryngol Clin North Am.* 2019;52(4):723–733. https://doi.org/10.1016/j.otc.2019.03.015

Çiyiltepe M, Şenkal ÖA. The ageing voice and voice therapy in geriatrics. *Aging Clin Exp Res.* 2017;29(3):403–410. https://doi.org/10.1007/s40520-016-0597-3

House SA, Fisher EL. Hoarseness in adults. *Am Fam Physician.* 2017;96(11):720–728.

Sood S, Street I, Donne A. Hoarseness in children. *Br J Hosp Med (Lond).* 2017;78(12):678–683. https://doi.org/10.12968/hmed.2017.78.12.678

Stachler RJ, Francis DO, Schwartz SR, et al. Clinical Practice Guideline: Hoarseness (Dysphonia) (Update). *Otolaryngol. Head Neck Surg.* 2018;158(1 Suppl):S1–S42. https://doi.org/10.1177/0194599817751030

Stinnett S, Chmielewska M, Akst LM. Update on management of hoarseness. *Med Clin North Am.* 2018;102(6):1027–1040. https://doi.org/10.1016/j.mcna.2018.06.005

Yang J, Xu W. Characteristics of functional dysphonia in children. *J Voice.* 2020;34(1):156.e1–156.e4. https://doi.org/10.1016/j.jvoice.2018.07.027

RESOURCE

American Academy of Otolaryngology—Head and Neck Surgery
http://www.entnet.org/

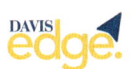 Go to Davis Edge for practice Q&A.

Section 5 — RESPIRATORY PROBLEMS

SECTION EDITOR
Jill E. Winland-Brown, EdD, APRN, FNP-BC, FAANP

Chapter 28

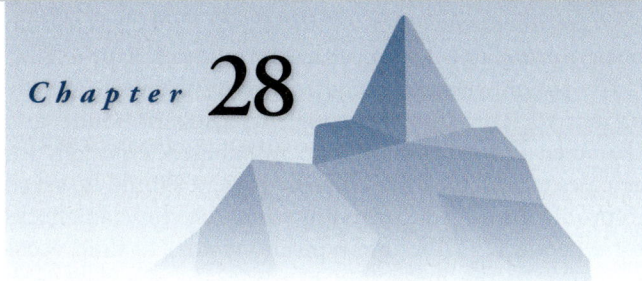

Common Respiratory Complaints

Jill E. Winland-Brown, EdD, APRN, FNP-BC, FAANP
Brian Oscar Porter, MD, PhD, MPH, MBA

COUGH

Each year, approximately 30 million Americans seek medical treatment for cough; this is more than for any other complaint. In the United States, treatment costs are estimated to be more than $1 billion annually. Cough (tussis) is the body's natural protective mechanism for clearing the airways of secretions and irritants and may be classified by its duration. An acute cough lasts for less than 3 weeks, a subacute cough lasts for 3 to 8 weeks, and one lasting longer than 8 weeks is considered chronic. Given the anxiety many patients associate with this condition, severe or persistent cough may affect psychological health.

Cough is commonly caused by the following mechanisms associated with several conditions and diseases:

- Alteration (increase or thickening) of pulmonary secretions (e.g., chronic obstructive pulmonary disease [COPD], bronchiectasis, cystic fibrosis, bronchitis, pulmonary edema, postnasal drip)
- Increased sensitivity of the cough receptors and airways (e.g., asthma) or postinfectious bronchial hyperreactivity (e.g., after a respiratory viral illness)
- Direct (aspiration) or indirect stimulation of cough receptors (e.g., gastroesophageal reflux disease [GERD])
- Infections (e.g., pneumonia, tuberculosis [TB], pharyngitis, *Pneumocystis jirovecii*)
- Progressive disease (e.g., sarcoidosis), including lung cancer, tumors (bronchogenic or mediastinal), or interstitial lung disease (ILD)
- Cardiopulmonary conditions (e.g., heart failure, cardiac tamponade, pulmonary embolism)
- Occupational and environmental exposures (e.g., air pollution, industrial dust, secondhand cigarette smoke)
- Psychogenic factors

Cough may also be an adverse side effect of certain hypertension medications that affect the bradykinin system, such as angiotensin-converting enzyme (ACE) inhibitors or angiotensin receptor blockers (ARBs). Persistent cough occurs in about 10% of patients taking ACE inhibitors or ARBs.

In extreme cases of debilitation or in certain neuromuscular conditions, the cough mechanism may be impaired, which may predispose to respiratory infection. Thus, there are times when the cough mechanism should be supported to clear the airways of unwanted irritants and times when it should be suppressed, depending on the underlying condition that initiates the cough mechanism.

DIFFERENTIAL DIAGNOSIS

Patients who present with cough require a comprehensive medical history and assessment to determine its etiology and appropriate treatment and management, given the broad scope of its differential diagnosis. One patient may present with the complaint of a dry, hacking cough of sudden onset (acute cough), whereas another may present with a persistent cough of longer duration. In turn, many patients try over-the-counter (OTC) measures for a chronic, nagging cough and delay seeking treatment altogether or only when a cough becomes productive or when there is blood in the sputum.

A diagnosis can be made about 80% of the time by taking a thorough history and eliciting the following details regarding the onset and nature of the cough:

- When did the cough first start? What factors may have prompted the cough (e.g., recent respiratory infection, exposure to noxious agents, initiation of a new medication)? Is there a seasonal pattern? Is it related to work or hobbies?
- When does the cough occur: on arising, at bedtime, during exercise, or throughout the night?
- What factors seem to stimulate the cough or make it worse? Is the cough aggravated by exposure to certain chemicals, body position, exercise, or cold air? Does the patient have any reactive airway disease?

417

- Has the patient identified any factors that seem to provide relief from the cough, such as sitting upright or avoiding exposure to certain agents? What measures have been tried to alleviate the cough?
- What is the quality of the cough: Is it dry and hacking, wet, raspy, deep, or throaty?
- Is the cough productive or unproductive? If the patient produces sputum with the cough, ask the patient to describe the amount of sputum produced per day (e.g., 1 teaspoon, 1 tablespoon), the color (e.g., yellow, gray, green, brown, clear, white, blood-tinged), and consistency (e.g., thick, ropey, frothy). When is the cough most productive (e.g., morning, evening)?
- Does the patient cough more when lying supine? Is the cough constant throughout the day and night?

In addition, it is essential to find out whether the patient has other signs and symptoms associated with the cough, such as pedal edema, dizziness, chest pain or tightness (which may indicate reactive airway disease), fatigue, dyspnea, hoarseness, fever, tachypnea, chills, heartburn, wheezing, or hemoptysis. In describing dyspnea, ask the patient to rate the degree of dyspnea on a continuous scale from 0 to 10 (similar to a pain scale) that compares today's dyspnea with previous dyspnea. Research indicates that a vertical visual analog scale is the most accurate way for a patient to rate dyspnea, and it allows the patient to keep a diary or record until their next visit.

The patient should be asked to describe in detail the onset of any associated signs and symptoms. Standard data regarding the patient's medical history should be recorded, including hospitalizations, surgeries, and major illnesses, particularly recent illnesses and respiratory allergies. The patient's lifestyle and social history should be explored, such as occupational history; hobbies; exposure to noxious agents; and use of alcohol, tobacco, and other substances. Patients should be asked about the use of marijuana, as well as e-cigarettes that contain nicotine or other extracts. The most common cause of chronic cough is cigarette smoking, which triggers the cough reflex by direct bronchial irritation.

The patient should be asked about the use of prescription and OTC drugs. Certain antihypertensive drugs such as ACE inhibitors and beta blockers can cause hyperreactive airways, producing wheezing and a cough. Other drugs such as nitrofurantoin (Macrobid, Macrodantin) and aminoglycosides (e.g., gentamicin) may cause interstitial fibrosis and associated cough. In turn, all patients taking these drugs should be monitored for changes in lung function through directed history-taking and periodic lung function tests with long-term use (e.g., for chronic prophylaxis).

Physical examination should focus on the following features related to the etiology of cough:

- Check the ears for cerumen or hairs impinging on the tympanic membrane, which may cause cough (Arnold reflex).
- Examine the nose for discharge, edema, polyps, and sinus tenderness. In the throat, look for cobblestoning of the oropharynx, which suggests postnasal drip (a frequent cause of cough).
- Palpate the neck, including both anterior and posterior cervical chains, for enlarged lymph nodes or masses.

A complete assessment of the thorax and chest should be performed to rule out cardiac or pulmonary problems. If the patient has not coughed during the visit, ask the patient to reproduce the cough to assess its sound and character. The lungs should be auscultated, especially for crackles (rales) and rhonchi. The patient should be asked to produce a forced expiration while the clinician checks for wheezes. Crackles are typically related to fluid accumulation in the lungs and generally do not clear with cough. Rhonchi, which are typically due to mucus accumulation, often clear after the patient is asked to cough, which clears the airways. The presence of heart murmurs, gallops, and carotid bruits should also be assessed, as these may reflect suboptimal cardiac function.

In most cases of cough, the underlying cause can be determined from a history and physical examination, but it may be necessary to consider the judicious use of one or more of the following diagnostic tests in conjunction with the differential diagnosis process. For example, if TB is suspected, a Mantoux purified protein derivative (PPD) tuberculin skin test (TST) should be administered and results read 48 to 72 hours later by qualified personnel at a second visit (information on interpreting PPD results is given in Chapter 30). A blood test that may be used to detect TB is the interferon-release assay, such as the QuantiFERON-TB Gold test, which only requires a single patient visit for one blood draw. A positive result on either screening test should be followed by a chest x-ray (CXR). For patients who are immunocompromised, the TST may need to be repeated because of T-cell anergy against TB antigens. The use of positive and negative control antigens alongside the TST has fallen out of favor due to their poor predictive value in interpreting TST results.

Spirometry is helpful to determine the presence of obstructive or restrictive lung disease. A CXR should be taken if there are signs and symptoms of pneumonia, TB, possible tumor, aspiration, foreign body, ILD, or if the patient is not recovering as expected. Sinus films may be useful to rule out sinusitis when the patient presents with a history of chronic postnasal drip or chronic sinus infections.

Computed tomography (CT) scanning of the chest can detect small peripheral lung nodules, evaluate coin lesions (solid, cystic, or calcified), and distinguish the chest wall from areas of pleural or parenchymal disease. Chest vessels can be distinguished from lymph nodes and other solid, nonvascular structures. The CT scan has replaced bronchography in diagnosing bronchiectasis. CT scan may help to better delineate endobronchial, parenchymal, or mediastinal masses. High-resolution chest CT scan, ventilation–perfusion scan, or pulmonary angiography is indicated when pulmonary thromboembolism is suspected. Sinus CT scans are more sensitive than sinus plain films in detecting sinusitis, although findings of sinus inflammation on imaging may not correlate with clinical symptoms.

A complete blood count (CBC) with differential is helpful in diagnosing a bacterial infection. Fungal serology should be done to identify coccidioidomycosis, histoplasmosis, or aspergillosis, if there is a positive history of exposure or if the patient is immunosuppressed (e.g., patients with AIDS).

MANAGEMENT

Because cough is a symptom, treatment should be directed toward resolving the underlying cause(s) and removing any identified triggers, rather than purely symptomatic treatment. In patients with chronic cough who are weak and debilitated, the goal is to reduce complications from uncontrolled, forceful coughing, such as fractured ribs, pneumothorax, aspiration, exhaustion, sleep deprivation, and post-tussive syncope.

With severe, acute coughing that disrupts sleep and causes pain or extreme fatigue and weakness, it may be necessary to treat with antitussives. However, because patients should be encouraged to expectorate during the day, these drugs have a limited role and should only be used on a short-term basis and only at night. Nonnarcotic agents such as dextromethorphan or pseudoephedrine/brompheniramine/dextromethorphan combination therapy may be used every 3 to 4 hours as needed. In addition, benzonatate (Tessalon) may be effective. When sleeping or eating is interrupted by persistent cough, the preferred choice is codeine, 8 to 30 mg every 3 to 4 hours, but only on a short-term basis. Patients with terminal lung cancer and patients with cystic fibrosis at the end of life should receive codeine in sufficient doses to keep them comfortable, although codeine may cause constipation.

Decongestants and antihistamines, alone or in combination, are indicated in cases of allergic rhinitis and postnasal drip. Antihistamines are useful for those who have allergic upper airway disease but should usually be avoided in patients with asthma because they may thicken secretions and inhibit expectoration, due to their anticholinergic effects. Intranasal corticosteroid sprays or aerosols such as beclomethasone (Beconase), fluticasone (Flonase), and mometasone (Nasonex) may be helpful when used consistently for a sufficient time, as prn use of intranasal corticosteroids is ineffective in producing the desired anti-inflammatory and drying effects needed to affect cough related to postnasal drip.

Expectorants are intended to decrease sputum viscosity and are used when the patient has a productive cough and needs help in clearing the airways. Suppression of a productive cough, however, may lead to complications such as obstructive pneumonia because the patient may not be able to clear the airways of sputum. Although expectorants may work in some cases, increasing the patient's water intake to 3 to 4 L/day is the most cost-effective means of helping to liquefy secretions, as long as the patient can manage the fluid volume and does not have cardiac or kidney failure or other disorder in which increased fluid intake could compromise health. Guaifenesin (Mucinex, Robitussin), which is available OTC, helps to break up mucus. Patients must be reminded to drink plenty of fluids when taking guaifenesin. Some clinicians prefer to give an expectorant during the day and a cough suppressant at night so patients may have more restful sleep.

Two popular herbal remedies that are commonly used as cough suppressants, but which have not been thoroughly researched in randomized controlled trials, are horehound and licorice. Licorice preparations have also been said to have expectorant qualities, but should be used with caution because they may increase blood pressure.

Patients who smoke tobacco or use e-cigarettes should be encouraged to stop smoking, as the smoke destroys the mucociliary structures of the airway lining and reduces the body's natural ability to clear mucus and respiratory pathogens. A chronic cough may not disappear in ex-smokers for a year or more after smoking cessation. Smoking cessation techniques are discussed in Chapter 33.

Patients with GERD whose cough reflex can be triggered by the reflux of acidic stomach contents usually respond to a course of antireflux therapy, which may include antacids, H_2 receptor blockers, or proton pump inhibitors. The benefits may not be noticed for several weeks, however.

Patient Education

Educating the patient and family about potential environmental and occupational factors that precipitate cough is essential, including exploring ways to avoid exposure to irritants. If a family member smokes, the dangers of secondhand smoke should be explained to the patient and family. Adequate hydration (increasing fluids) and adequate ambient humidification may also help reduce coughing. Breathing in the steam from a hot shower may also be effective. Simple measures such as changing air filters may also help in removing environmental irritants.

DYSPNEA

Dyspnea is one of the most common complaints for which patients seek help from health-care providers. Dyspnea, or shortness of breath, is estimated to be the third most frequent reason for seeking medical attention in the primary care setting. Although dyspnea occurs primarily in patients with respiratory and cardiac disorders, it may also occur in other conditions such as lung neoplasms with metastasis, neuromuscular myopathies, neuropathies, spinal cord lesions, diaphragmatic disorders, and panic disorders. In patients receiving hospice care, it is the second most common symptom secondary to pain.

As with pain, dyspnea is a perceived sensation that may vary among patients, which is why using a scale from 0 to 10 is recommended. Patients with dyspnea usually describe a sense of difficulty breathing or an inability to get sufficient air into or out of the lungs. Dyspnea may also be described as a feeling of breathlessness, suffocation or smothering, air hunger, or labored breathing. In many cases of dyspnea, the respiratory rate is rapid and cough may be present, depending on the underlying disease or cause of the dyspnea. Dyspnea may be caused by several different health problems. Some individuals may experience exercise-induced dyspnea or exercise-induced bronchospasm. In older patients, dyspnea is the major atypical presentation for ischemic heart disease and myocardial infarction and is considered a frequent anginal equivalent. Dyspnea in aging patients may be difficult to evaluate when there are associated comorbidities.

DIFFERENTIAL DIAGNOSIS

In the majority of cases, dyspnea is a result of cardiac or pulmonary decompensation. There are several symptoms associated with dyspnea, such as tachypnea (rapid breathing), orthopnea (dyspnea relieved in a seated or upright position), and paroxysmal nocturnal dyspnea (PND) (sudden episodes of acute dyspnea at night). The causes of dyspnea may be complex and include the following common causes and precipitants:

- **Pulmonary**: COPD, asthma, pulmonary parenchymal disease, ILD, pulmonary hypertension, severe kyphoscoliosis, exogenous mechanical factors (ascites, morbid obesity, extensive pleural effusion)
- **Cardiac**: Congestive heart failure, pulmonary venous congestion (e.g., due to mitral stenosis or regurgitation)
- **Hematological**: Severe chronic anemia
- **Psychogenic**: Anxiety and panic disorders

Dyspnea may be acute or chronic, and patients with COPD may have acute worsening of chronic dyspnea, reflecting acute episodes of infectious bronchitis. A complete work-up is needed to determine the underlying cause of dyspnea and initiate appropriate treatment. Dyspnea caused by acute anxiety may mimic cardiopulmonary decompensation, and patients with pulmonary hypertension may have episodes that resemble anxiety-related dyspnea. Onset of dyspnea at rest, accompanied by a sense of chest tightness, a feeling of suffocation, and an inability to "get air in," is a common presentation of anxiety-related dyspnea. In the absence of heart and lung disease, a history of multiple somatic complaints, emotional difficulties, no activity limitations (absence of exercise intolerance), and dyspnea unrelated to physical activity provides evidence for psychogenic dyspnea.

About 75% of dyspnea cases are caused by respiratory conditions that may be acute or chronic. The majority of other causes of dyspnea are cardiac in origin. It is important to explore with the patient the details of the onset and character of the dyspnea. The clinician should note whether the patient has dyspnea at rest or on exertion. The rate and clarity of the patient's speech during exercise can provide important clinical information regarding the patient's level of exercise tolerance. The following standard questions are designed to gauge the severity of dyspnea in an easily quantifiable manner that most patients can comprehend:

1. How many flights of stairs did the patient climb before dyspnea occurred (e.g., one-flight dyspnea)?
2. How many blocks did the patient walk before dyspnea occurred (e.g., one-block dyspnea)?
3. How many feet did the patient walk before dyspnea occurred (e.g., 100-feet dyspnea)?

Exploring when the dyspnea first occurred and what the patient was doing at the time is essential. Specific questions should be directed toward factors that either precipitate or alleviate the dyspnea. Questions should explore potential environmental exposures (e.g., recent travel) or exposure to triggering agents that aggravate the dyspnea (e.g., occupational or recreational exposure). Paying attention to other signs and symptoms that may be associated with the dyspnea, such as cough, peripheral edema, dizziness, wheeze, fever, chest pain, heartburn, leg pain, and paresthesias, is also critical.

A complete physical examination should be done, with particular attention directed to the pulmonary and cardiovascular systems. The examiner should check for tachycardia, tachypnea, fever, and hypertension, and assess mixed venous oxygen saturation (SvO_2). The quality of breath sounds (increased, decreased, or absent) should be noted, along with the presence of crackles, rhonchi, wheezes, egophony, and fremitus. Bronchial lung sounds heard at other than the normal locations (tubular sounds) are common with acute bronchitis. Assessment should include checking for third (S_3) or fourth (S_4) heart sounds (gallops), murmurs, friction rubs, jugular venous distention, pedal edema, and calf tenderness. A visual analog scale (0 = no dyspnea; 10 = worst dyspnea ever had) or the Borg scale for perceived exertion with a score of 6 to 20 (6 = no exertion; 20 = very, very hard exertion) is useful in assessing the degree of dyspnea, as previously mentioned. The scales can be used again on the patient's next visit for the clinician to compare the effects of treatment over time, as well as for patients to track their own self-management.

Diagnostic tests are guided by data from the history and physical examination, depending on the suspected causes of the dyspnea. CXRs are useful in ruling out tumors, TB, pneumonia, and other major pulmonary disorders. A CBC with differential should be done to rule out anemia and infection. A blood chemistry profile should be ordered if metabolic acidosis is suspected and to differentiate anion-gap acidosis from non–anion-gap acidosis. Oximetry to measure the saturation level of oxygen may be useful in assessing whether the patient is hypoxic. If the O_2 saturation level is less than 90%, arterial blood gas (ABG) analysis should be done. Of note, perceived levels of dyspnea have not been found to correlate well with physiological measures.

If carbon monoxide (CO) exposure is suspected, a carboxyhemoglobin (COHb) level should be obtained. COHb levels of 4% to 15% may be found in heavy smokers. Levels greater than 20% may cause dyspnea and headache, and levels greater than 40% may cause seizures and death.

Peak expiratory flow rate (PEFR) is a simple, inexpensive test that can be done with a handheld flow meter in the office or at the bedside. This test determines the degree of expiratory airflow obstruction in patients with asthma and COPD. Full spirometry is useful in determining whether the dyspneic patient has obstructive, restrictive, or mixed (obstructive and restrictive) lung disease. Diffusion capacity should be checked if ILD is suspected as the cause of dyspnea. If the patient uses a peak flow meter at home and notes an acute decrease in peak flow, they should be instructed to contact their health-care provider for further evaluation and possible treatment.

MANAGEMENT

Initial treatment is directed at helping the patient find relief from shortness of breath by removing the underlying cause and contributing factors. Subsequent management is directed at prevention and assisting the patient with the management of chronic dyspnea in conditions such as COPD or ILD. In cases of dyspnea caused by hypoxemia, supplemental oxygen may be indicated. In cases of pulmonary shunting (i.e., redirection of the pulmonary circulation away from the lung parenchyma where oxygenation takes place), the cause of the shunting must be corrected. For management of dyspnea in inflammatory respiratory disorders, see Chapter 31.

For the treatment of dyspnea related to cardiac disorders such as heart failure, refer to Chapter 35. Diuretics to relieve fluid overload may improve breathing and supplemental oxygen may be necessary in some cases.

For anxiety-related dyspnea, psychiatric referral may be needed if other measures, such as rebreathing exercises, have failed. Dyspnea caused by rapid overbreathing (hyperventilation) during anxiety attacks can often be corrected by teaching the patient breathing techniques. Until the patient masters these techniques, it may be helpful to prescribe short-term use of anxiolytics, such as buspirone HCl 20 to 30 mg/day.

HEMOPTYSIS

Hemoptysis is defined as the expectoration of blood. The patient often reports coughing up blood or sputum that is streaked or tinged with blood. In addition, hemoptysis may be manifested as fresh (bright red) or old (dark red or black) blood or, in the case of bleeding from an infected lung cavity, it may present as slow oozing or frank bleeding. In cases of profuse hemoptysis, blood clots may be expectorated. Of note, the patient should observe whether the blood is from the nasal cavity (as opposed to the airways or lungs), which may result from severe irritation or dehydration of the nasal mucosa.

DIFFERENTIAL DIAGNOSIS

About 80% of hemoptysis cases are related to inflammatory causes, such as bronchitis, bronchiectasis, pneumonia, or TB. Less common causes may include neoplasms that damage a pulmonary vessel or rupture a pulmonary artery. Use of pulmonary artery balloon catheters has increased the incidence of pulmonary artery rupture. Hemoptysis may also occur in patients with cystic fibrosis who have significant damage to the lung parenchyma. Cardiovascular causes of hemoptysis include left ventricular failure, mitral stenosis, pulmonary embolism or infarct, primary pulmonary hypertension, and aortic aneurysm. Clotting defects may also cause hemoptysis. Bleeding leading to hemoptysis may occur anywhere along the respiratory tract, including the nose, sinuses, and mouth.

About 95% of the pulmonary circulation is supplied by the pulmonary artery and its branches, which is a low-pressure system. Bronchial circulation, a high-pressure system, originates from the aorta and usually provides about 5% of the blood to the lungs, mostly to the airways and supporting structures. When bleeding occurs, it usually arises from the bronchial circulation, unless trauma or erosion has affected a major pulmonary vessel. Pulmonary venous bleeding is modest and occurs in pulmonary venous hypertension, especially in conjunction with left heart failure.

The patient usually presents with a complaint of "coughing up" blood. To most people, the presence of blood in the sputum is a frightening experience, and most patients will seek immediate medical attention. Patients should be asked about hemoptysis, including its onset, amount of blood, aggravating and alleviating factors, and the presence of other associated symptoms such as dyspnea, cough, dizziness, fatigue, and chest pain.

Bronchopulmonary bleeding may present as hematemesis (vomiting of blood). The patient may swallow blood during the night and may vomit blood on arising.

The history and physical examination for hemoptysis are similar to those conducted for cough and dyspnea. In addition, if the examiner suspects that the hemoptysis is due to a pulmonary neoplasm, the physical examination should focus on the pulmonary system and lymph node enlargement.

Further diagnostic tests may be indicated, depending on the results of the history and physical examination. Common causes of hemoptysis will direct laboratory assessments. If hemoptysis occurs in patients aged 45 years or younger, it is likely caused by mitral stenosis, TB, bronchiectasis, or a lung abscess. For patients older than 45 years, common causes of hemoptysis include bronchogenic carcinoma, bronchitis, TB, and pulmonary embolus with infarction. In massive hemoptysis (loss of more than 600 mL of blood in 24 hours, which may occur in lung cancer, TB, bronchiectasis, or lung abscess), the condition is life-threatening and constitutes a medical emergency. There may be time to do only a CXR and a CBC before emergency surgery or bronchoscopy.

For nonemergency cases in which the sputum is tinged or streaked with blood, there is time to do essential tests to identify the cause of hemoptysis. In addition to CXR and a CBC, sputum should be cultured for acid-fast bacilli if TB is suspected. For suspected pneumonia or lung abscess, sputum culture and sensitivities should be done. Patients who present with hematemesis may also have hemoptysis caused by aspiration of blood, and a CXR is indicated for these patients. Patients with a history of thromboembolism may be taking anticoagulants. In these patients, clotting times should be assessed to rule this out as a cause of the hemoptysis. Because of the exertion (forceful expiratory maneuvers) required by the patient during spirometry, the measurement of lung volumes during periods of active hemoptysis is not recommended.

MANAGEMENT

Massive hemoptysis requires immediate treatment, surgery, or bronchoscopy. Prevention of aspiration and keeping the airway open are of the utmost importance. Endotracheal intubation may be needed. Supplemental oxygen and replacement of blood loss may also be necessary, depending on the patient's blood pressure, pulse, ABG results, and hemoglobin level.

Treatment of chronic hemoptysis is directed toward the underlying cause. When the cause is inflammation, as in chronic bronchitis, TB, or bronchiectasis, the patient must be educated to stop smoking, comply with the use of prescribed medications (e.g., antibiotics, bronchodilators), perform deep-breathing and coughing exercises every 2 to 4 hours regularly, and avoid exposure to secondhand smoke and other noxious agents that might precipitate cough.

Patient Education

Education of the patient and family regarding the causes of the hemoptysis is essential. The patient should know what factors may precipitate hemoptysis and how it can be prevented. The patient should be taught to note any change in the color, amount, or consistency of blood expectorated. Any sudden increase in the volume of expectorated blood or change in the character of the hemoptysis should be reported to the health-care provider immediately for prompt medical attention.

REFERENCES

Cardenas-Garcia J, Feller-Kopman D. POINT: should all initial episodes of hemoptysis be evaluated by bronchoscopy? Yes. *Chest.* 2018;153(2):302

National Heart, Lung, and Blood Institute. Cough. (2016). http://www.nhlbi.nih.gov/health/health-topics/topics/cough/. Accessed 9/7/2020.

Papadakis MA, McPhee SJ. *Current Medical Diagnosis and Treatment.* Appleton-Lange/McGraw-Hill; 2017.

Yilmaz I. Angiotensin-converting enzyme inhibitors induce cough. *Turk Thorac J.* 2019 Jan;20(1):36-42. https://www.ncbi.nlm.nih.gov/pmc/articles/PMC6340691/. Accessed 9/6/2020.

RESOURCES

American Lung Association: Learn About Cough
https://www.lung.org/lung-health-diseases/wellness/cough/learn-about-cough

National Institute of Allergy and Infectious Disease
http://www.niaid.nih.gov

National Heart, Lung, and Blood Institute: Cough
https://www.nhlbi.nih.gov/health/health-topics/topics/cough

Chapter 29

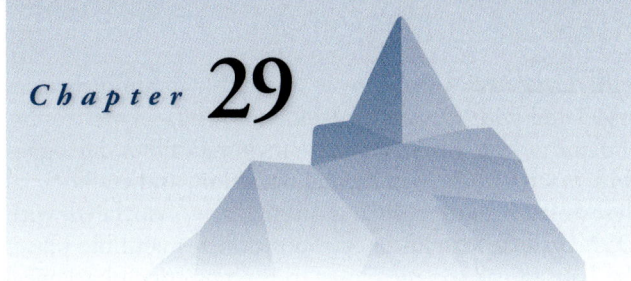

Sleep Apnea

John Suen, MD
Jill E. Winland-Brown, EdD, APRN, FNP-BC, FAANP

Sleep apnea is defined as a temporary pause in breathing during sleep that lasts at least 10 seconds. For a confirmed diagnosis, this should occur a minimum of five times an hour. The three patterns of apnea are central, obstructive, and mixed. Central apnea occurs when both airflow and respiratory efforts are absent. Central apneas are a result of an absence of neural output from the brainstem's respiratory control center, which leads to a lack of inspiratory effort. The respiratory center in the brain fails to respond to elevated carbon dioxide concentrations. In contrast, during obstructive sleep apnea (OSA), respiratory efforts persist although airflow is absent at the nose and mouth. Airflow obstruction occurs when the tongue and the soft palate fall backward and partially or completely obstruct the pharynx. Finally, many adult patients exhibit mixed apnea, in which both central and obstructive patterns occur.

Each type of apnea results in progressive asphyxiation until an arousal from sleep occurs, with a subsequent restoration of upper airway patency and airflow. A patient then usually returns to sleep quickly, resulting in another occlusion of the upper airway. Apnea and arousal cycles occur repeatedly, as many as 200 to 400 times during 6 to 8 hours of sleep in severe cases. Sleep hypopnea is a period of hypoventilation, or decreased airflow, defined as a 50% reduction in thoracoabdominal movements, with a 4% decrease in oxygen saturation lasting at least 10 seconds during sleep. OSA/hypopnea is present when the respiratory drive is intact, but the upper airway intermittently becomes obstructed during sleep.

The apnea-hypopnea index (AHI) may be used to define and quantify the severity of OSA. The AHI is obtained by dividing the total number of events (the number of apnea episodes plus the number of hypopnea episodes) throughout the entire night by the total sleep time in hours. The *respiratory disturbance index* (RDI), another commonly cited parameter, is defined as the AHI plus the average number of snoring-related arousals per hour. A diagnosis of OSA is confirmed with AHI and RDI scores as follows:

- AHI or RDI greater than or equal to 5 and less than 14 if comorbid factors such as excessive daytime sleepiness, hypertension, stroke, or heart failure are present, or
- AHI or RDI greater than or equal to 15 in the absence of comorbid factors.

In general, as the AHI increases, so does the severity of symptoms, although the condition may not become clinically significant until the AHI becomes greater than 15.

Patients with OSA may experience a number of potentially adverse physiological and neurobehavioral problems. Consequences of OSA result from daily exposure to abnormalities in breathing during sleep and may cause long-term neurobehavioral and cardiovascular morbidity. Sleep-disordered breathing is an independent risk factor for the development of hypertension and, subsequently, left ventricular dysfunction. The patient with combined coronary artery disease (CAD) and OSA may have increased cardiac risk because of the worsening relationship between myocardial oxygen demand and supply as a result of apnea-associated hypoxemia and activation of the autonomic nervous system (see Box 29.1).

Cardiac dysrhythmias, usually occurring during apneic episodes, have been reported to be a significant complication of OSA. Atrial fibrillation, a common arrhythmia, is causally associated with OSA; treating OSA will improve the effectiveness of treatment of atrial fibrillation. People with sleep apnea have a higher risk of dying from sudden cardiac arrest. In addition, sleep quality may be influenced by apnea-associated activation of the central nervous system (CNS) (arousals) and ischemia-associated arousals. Timely diagnosis and treatment of CAD, as well as sleep apnea, is necessary for these patients.

OSA is also more prevalent in patients with chronic congestive heart failure. In these patients, treating OSA often will improve the heart failure.

OSA can cause mild pulmonary hypertension, even in the absence of pulmonary disease. Sustained pulmonary hypertension, often associated with clinical evidence of right ventricular failure, has been observed in approximately 20% of OSA patients. It is hypothesized that repetitive hypoxemia during sleep may lead to vascular

Box 29.1	Possible Consequences of Sleep Apnea
Pulmonary hypertension
Systemic hypertension
Cardiac dysrhythmias
Right or left ventricular failure
Right ventricular hypertrophy
Myocardial infarction (increased risk of)
Stroke (increased risk of)
Nocturnal angina
Chronic obstructive pulmonary disease (exacerbation of)
Insulin resistance
Endothelial cell dysfunction

remodeling in susceptible patients, causing pulmonary hypertension during the day. In addition, because the patient with OSA is often obese or has pathological lung function resulting in abnormalities of daytime arterial blood gas (ABG) values, pulmonary vasoconstriction is another mechanism inducing pulmonary hypertension.

EPIDEMIOLOGY AND CAUSES

Sleep apnea is an extremely common clinical disorder; as such, it has major public health implications. Unrecognized and untreated significant OSA is estimated to be 30% in the adult male population and 15% in the adult female population, most of whom are in the most productive period of their lives, and this contributes to significant and disabling psychomotor deficits. An estimated 40 million Americans are chronically ill with various sleep disorders, and 38,000 cardiovascular deaths annually are directly attributable to OSA; yet the majority of Americans with sleep disorders remain undiagnosed and untreated. This, in turn, costs billions of dollars in accidents in the home, at the workplace, and in traffic.

OSA is most prevalent in males older than age 50 and in postmenopausal females; in this latter group, OSA may be related to hormonal changes. OSA occurs in younger people as well. In general, males usually have a significantly higher pharyngeal and supraglottic resistance than females, which makes them more susceptible to pharyngeal collapse and OSA and may contribute to the male predominance of the syndrome. Pharyngeal resistance increases with age in normal males, possibly related to greater body weight. Although it is widely believed that the risk of developing OSA increases with age in males, this assumption is far from conclusive and requires further study. Clinicians should be aware that OSA also occurs in females and that patients who present with typical signs and symptoms should be referred to sleep disorder centers.

Compared with OSA, central sleep apnea syndrome is uncommon. In most sleep laboratories, patients with central sleep apnea syndrome constitute fewer than 10% of patients tested. The division between central and OSA is not as clear-cut as it might appear, because many patients with central sleep apnea present with clinical features more suggestive of OSA. It is possible that in some patients, upper airway occlusion triggers a central, rather than an obstructive, apnea. Support for this notion comes from the finding that some patients with central sleep apnea can be successfully treated with nasal continuous positive airway pressure (CPAP).

The cause of OSA is poorly defined but appears to be multifactorial; upper airway tract malformation, oropharyngeal muscle dysfunction, and abnormal respiratory drive may play a role. A few recognized anatomical abnormalities are associated with narrowing of the upper airway and predispose patients to OSA. Conditions associated with facial dysmorphism or mandibular abnormalities associated with OSA include adenotonsillar hypertrophy, choanal atresia, micrognathia (small mandible), retrognathia, macroglossia, nasal septal deviation, and craniofacial dysostosis. Micrognathia is particularly associated with OSA because a small or retropositioned mandible places the base of the tongue closer to the posterior pharyngeal wall and interferes with the efficiency of the genioglossus muscle in keeping the tongue out of the narrowed pharynx.

There is increasing evidence that sleep apnea has a familial distribution. Relatives of a person with sleep apnea have approximately twice the normal risk of having sleep apnea. Most adult patients with OSA, however, have no specific skeletal or soft tissue lesion obstructing the upper airway, but they often have a small, congested oropharyngeal airway. Symptoms of sleep apnea are present two to six times more frequently in family members of affected patients than in a control population.

Obesity and alcohol consumption are well recognized as aggravating factors. One possible explanation for the relationship between obesity and OSA is that the upper airway is narrowed in the patient with obesity as a result of increased fat deposition in the pharyngeal walls. Fat in the neck plays the largest role. Neck (or collar) size is the best indicator of the presence of sleep apnea. Approximately 30% of snoring males with a collar size larger than 17 inches will have OSA. Neck size in females is less well investigated, but when it is greater than 16 inches, it increases the risk for sleep apnea. Another possible explanation for the relationship between neck size and apnea is that the obese patient often has a smaller lung volume, particularly functional residual capacity, than the nonobese patient; this, in turn, can indirectly influence upper airway size and contribute to upper airway narrowing. About 15% of patients with sleep apnea, however, are not obese. Any factor that interferes with the arousal mechanism, such as alcohol consumption, could lead to more profound and prolonged apneas. Both alcohol and sedative hypnotics reduce upper airway muscle tone and the arousal mechanism, potentially exacerbating OSA.

PATHOPHYSIOLOGY

Sleep is divided into two states: rapid eye movement (REM) sleep and nonrapid eye movement (NREM) sleep. NREM sleep is further divided into three stages, based on changes in the electroencephalogram (EEG) pattern:

- Normal sleep begins with stage I, which is characterized by slow eye movements, usually preceding sleep onset.
- Stage II involves further slowing of the EEG, with the presence of sleep spindles and slow eye movements.
- Stage III is manifested by low-frequency, high-amplitude delta waves with occasional sleep spindles but no slow eye movements.

accomplished by sewing pockets for one or two tennis balls in the back of patients' sleeping attire to prevent them from assuming the supine position. Commercially available devices to facilitate sleeping in the nonsupine position exist. Devices to train people to sleep in the lateral position have been described.

Devices That Maintain Upper Airway Patency

CPAP administered through a nasal mask has become the most common treatment for OSA. Nasal CPAP also effectively reduces or eliminates mixed apneas, including both the central and obstructive components. A continuous flow of air is delivered from a blower unit to a tightly fitting nasal mask held in place by head straps. Nasal CPAP acts as a pneumatic splint preventing collapse of the upper airway in all phases of respiration. The device is used for the entire sleep period every night. The optimal CPAP pressure is determined by technologists during polysomnography. Typically, 5 to 20 cm H_2O is the pressure needed to abolish apneas, snoring, and oxyhemoglobin desaturations in all positions and during REM sleep. Although CPAP use is associated with few serious complications, it does elicit patient complaints. Minor adverse effects of CPAP include feelings of suffocation, nasal drying or rhinitis, ear pain, difficulty exhaling, mask and mouth leaks, chest and back pain, and conjunctivitis. Most of these can be alleviated.

Newer automatic CPAP devices continuously adjust the positive pressure to the required levels. In the automatic CPAP mode, the positive pressure is maintained as long as ventilation remains stable; however, any respiratory disorder results in a progressive increase in pressure. If a breathing disturbance has not occurred for more than 4 minutes, the positive pressure decreases again.

For many patients who use it regularly, CPAP dramatically eliminates apneas and hypopneas, improves sleep architecture, and reduces daytime sleepiness, even for those with mild sleep apnea. The effectiveness of CPAP is limited, however, by incomplete patient compliance. About 25% of patients prescribed CPAP will not be compliant. Factors that help to improve CPAP compliance include patient education and regular follow-up with the health-care provider. CPAP is the only therapy for OSA that improves life expectancy and outcomes of hypertension and heart failure.

Oral Appliances

Oral appliances are an effective noninvasive alternative to CPAP in patients with mild to moderate sleep apnea. Although oral appliances are effective in some patients with OSA, they are not universally effective. There are major design differences in the numerous oral appliances that are now available, and this may have an effect on their success and compliance rates. A novel anterior mandibular positioner has been developed with an adjustable hinge that allows progressive advancement of the mandible. This appliance may be an effective first-line treatment for the patient with mild to moderate OSA and may be associated with greater patient satisfaction than CPAP. For these devices to treat sleep apnea effectively, the mandible should be advanced to 50% to 75% of the maximal forward protrusion of the jaw. In most patients, dental appliances lessen but do not abolish OSA and snoring. In many patients treated with an oral appliance, the RDI remains high, with more than 20 events per hour after treatment. The side effects of oral appliances include excessive salivation, dental misalignment, and pain in, or damage to, the temporomandibular joint. To assess the efficacy of the oral appliance, a follow-up sleep test is useful to determine whether further forward advancement of the mandible would be helpful.

Surgical Management

Surgery for OSA is designed either to bypass the obstructing region of the upper airway or modify the upper airway in a way that makes loss of patency less likely. Because upper airway obstruction is associated with a wide variety of structural aberrations, including nasal deformity, nasal polyps, hypertrophic tonsils and/or adenoids, craniofacial disproportion, and neoplasms, as well as with no detectable anatomical abnormalities, many different surgical procedures have been used in OSA patients.

UPPP, which is extensive excision of soft tissue in the oropharynx, was developed to improve pharyngeal function during sleep. The procedure involves a bilateral tonsillectomy and a submucosal resection of redundant tissue. A variable portion of the posterior margin of the soft palate and the uvula is also removed, and the palatopharyngeus muscle may also be resected. In the absence of weight gain or other confounding factors, a success rate of 50% has been sustained for at least 1 year postoperatively. However, even patients in whom UPPP fails to resolve OSA often have substantial reduction in snoring after surgery, despite persistent apnea. A repeat polysomnogram is necessary to assess the therapeutic outcome of surgery. The success rate in patients undergoing UPPP appears to be partly related to the location of the obstructing tissue. Patients with retropalatal obstruction removal experience better results than those with retroglossal obstruction removal. The preoperative presence of tonsils has been associated with improved success of UPPP.

The patient undergoing surgical reconstruction of the airway for OSA, such as UPPP, often has coexisting medical problems, especially cardiovascular disease, which can complicate treatment. The uncertainty regarding the proper predictive parameters for surgical success greatly limits optimal patient selection. Further, a significant number of patients have difficulty at induction and intubation for general anesthesia. Males with increased neck circumference and associated skeletal deformities should be evaluated carefully and considered for fiber-optic intubation.

Laser-assisted uvulopalatoplasty is a procedure to treat snoring in the outpatient setting. The procedure entails reshaping the palate and tonsillar pillars in one to seven serial sessions under local anesthesia. Each session lasts approximately 15 minutes and is generally well tolerated; the incidence of complications is low. The procedure is successful in reducing snoring in 90% of patients; however, the success rate in patients with OSA is not yet clear.

A variety of maxillofacial and nasal surgical procedures may be performed to normalize the bony relationships of the maxilla and mandible to minimize the likelihood of airway collapse during sleep. Many of these procedures are preceded by UPPP, and if the results are unsatisfactory, a second stage involving mandibular advancement is undertaken. These procedures require a great deal of surgical and orthodontic expertise, along with careful consultation with anesthesia services and pulmonary medicine.

Nasal surgery has been performed on patients with OSA in an effort to reduce the predisposition to collapse during sleep. A nasal septoplasty is performed if gross nasal septal deformity is present. The definitive therapy is a tracheostomy. Because of the drastic nature of this procedure, it is limited to patients with life-threatening arrhythmias or severe disability who have not responded to conservative therapy.

A novel upper airway muscle stimulator has recently been approved in the United States for severe OSA in patients intolerant to CPAP. A surgically implanted stimulator sends electrical signals to activate the genioglossus muscle (tongue) that are synchronized to respiratory activity as sensed by electrical signals from diaphragmatic muscle activation.

Central Sleep Apnea

Medical treatment may be ineffective in the patient with central sleep apnea. Some patients with central sleep apnea do respond to CPAP therapy. Implantation of a diaphragm-pacing device is an option, the efficacy of which has not been proven by long-term clinical trials. Diaphragm pacing may precipitate upper airway occlusion during sleep due to dyssynchrony between activation of the diaphragm and the upper airway and laryngeal dilators. Thus, tracheostomy is often performed concomitantly with diaphragm pacing. These difficulties, in conjunction with the resource-intensive nature of the procedure and subsequent care, have made this technique one that is infrequently employed in the clinical setting of central sleep apnea.

The use of a timed BiPAP device may normalize blood gases during sleep. BiPAP prevents development of severe pulmonary artery hypertension during sleep. It delivers a higher airway pressure during inspiration (when the airway is most likely to be occluded) and a lower airway pressure during expiration (patient exhales against less resistance). Cardiac dysrhythmias may decrease significantly. Improvement of the respiratory situation and of the hemodynamics using a timed BiPAP device may reduce the mortality rate in these patients. Bilevel systems are more expensive than conventional CPAP systems, however, and the algorithms to adjust the inspiratory and expiratory pressures are essentially empiric. Consequently, bilevel systems are typically reserved for patients who cannot tolerate CPAP, especially for those who experience difficulties with exhalation or chest pain as a result of the hyperinflation produced by the applied positive pressure.

FOLLOW-UP AND REFERRAL

In recent years, chronic obstructive pulmonary disease (COPD) and sleep apnea syndrome have been found to coexist in many patients, placing them at increased risk of respiratory insufficiency. The detection of small airway disease may be difficult in OSA patients because this syndrome is associated with various pulmonary function abnormalities resulting from obesity and upper airway obstruction. Both of these factors can be responsible for airway obstruction. Patients with both disorders frequently have marked hypoxemia, hypercapnia, and pulmonary hypertension, so they should be referred for investigation of both COPD and sleep apnea. The patient with this "overlap syndrome" is at a higher risk of developing respiratory insufficiency and pulmonary hypertension than the patient with "pure" OSA. Finally, hypoxemic stress is placed on the coronary circulation during sleep that may contribute to nocturnal mortality in the patient with COPD.

Patient Education: CPAP Use

Because CPAP is a safe and effective treatment for OSA, it is important to improve patient compliance with regular CPAP use. Only 75% of patients continue to use CPAP after 1 year, citing the noise, interference with positioning, and complaints of bed partners. Systematically collected data on family members' or significant others' learning needs and descriptions of the psychosocial effect of CPAP technology treatments on family/household function and quality of life are essential to developing a comprehensive protocol for teaching and counseling for CPAP therapy. The effect of group patient education sessions on compliance with CPAP therapy has proved to be a simple and effective means of improving treatment of OSA. Nasal discomfort and lack of perceived benefit are possible characteristics of patients with poor compliance; these patients might benefit from education sessions and emotional support. The personal contact and teaching, along with interaction with other OSA patients, may provide an atmosphere of encouragement and support.

Counseling may be needed concerning the potential loss of employment because of poor performance or poor decision making related to profound fatigue from sleep deprivation. Problems of depression, extreme sleepiness, and the effects of hypoxia on cognition pose special difficulties for teaching these patients; their family members/significant others must be educated. Problem-solving skills of family or support persons for managing equipment, overcoming psychosocial barriers to regular nightly use, and eliminating the physiological side effects of CPAP such as oral dryness are important skills and knowledge for this patient population. Home follow-up programs could help patients eliminate reported physiological adverse effects of CPAP treatments, monitor cardiac stability, and provide ongoing education and family/household function assessment as evidenced in other follow-up programs. A follow-up program would be cost-effective when quality of life is considered or compared with hospital admissions for traffic accidents or the severe cardiovascular sequelae associated with OSA.

Teaching must include nutrition counseling. Weight loss may be curative, but because 10% to 20% of body weight loss is required, many patients give up. Strict avoidance of alcohol and hypnotic medications must also be stressed. Many vehicular crashes are caused by persons with excessive sleepiness. One of the objectives of *Healthy People 2030* is to increase the proportion of adults with symptoms of OSA who seek medical evaluation. Educating patients to take corrective action is an important role of the health-care provider.

REFERENCES

American Academy of Sleep Medicine. *International Classification of Sleep Disorders*. 3rd ed. American Academy of Sleep Medicine; 2014.

Epstein LJ, Kristo D, Strollo PJ Jr, et al. Clinical guideline for the evaluation, management and long-term care of obstructive sleep apnea in adults. *J Clin Sleep Med*. 2009;5(3):263–276.

Healthy People 2030. U.S. Dept. of Health and Human Services. Increase the proportion of adults with sleep apnea symptoms who seek medical evaluation-SH02. https://health.gov/healthypeople/objectives-and-data/browse-objectives/sleep/increase-proportion-adults-sleep-apnea-symptoms-who-get-evaluated-health-care-provider-sh-02. Accessed 3/25/2021.

Kapur VK, Auckley DH, Chowdhuri S, et al. Clinical practice guideline for diagnostic testing for adult obstructive sleep apnea: an american academy of sleep medicine clinical practice guideline. *J Clin Sleep Med*. 2017;13:479.

Kryger MH, Roth T, Dement WC. *Principles and Practice of Sleep Medicine*. 6th ed. Elsevier; 2016.

Patil SP, Ayappa IA, Caples SM, et al. Treatment of adult obstructive sleep apnea with positive airway pressure: an american academy of sleep medicine clinical practice guideline. *J Clin Sleep Med*. 2019;15:335.

Strollo PJ Jr, Soose RJ, Maurer JT, et al. Upper-airway stimulation for obstructive sleep apnea. *N Engl J Med*. 2014;370:139.

RESOURCES

American Sleep Apnea Association
http://www.sleepapnea.org
American Sleep Association
https://www.sleepassociation.org/
National Sleep Foundation
http://sleepfoundation.org

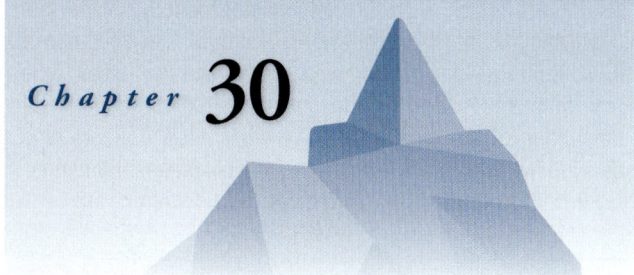

Chapter 30

Infectious Respiratory Disorders

Jill E. Winland-Brown, EdD, APRN, FNP-BC, FAANP

Nilesh Patel, DO, FAAEM, FACOEP

Janine Duran Llamzon, DNP-C, MS, AGNP-C, RN, CEN, NEA-BC

Brian Oscar Porter, MD, PhD, MPH, MBA

UPPER RESPIRATORY INFECTIONS

Upper respiratory infections (URIs) include some of the most common infectious diseases and account for millions of visits to health-care providers annually. Most URIs are caused by viruses; bacteria cause about 25% of the cases. For the typical adult, URIs are a source of discomfort, disability, and loss of productivity. For young children, the immunocompromised, and older adults, these infections may be a cause of morbidity and serious illnesses. In children and older adults, as well as adults with underlying respiratory diseases, viral URIs are frequently complicated by bacterial superinfection. Although both influenza (the flu) and the viral rhinitis or acute coryza (the common cold) are caused by viruses and have similar symptoms, flu is usually more severe, causes more hospitalizations, and accounts for tens of thousands of deaths in the United States each year.

EPIDEMIOLOGY AND CAUSES

The flu, the common cold, and acute laryngitis are some of the more frequently occurring URIs that the practitioner will need to manage.

URIs

The common cold most frequently affects children younger than 5 years. On average, children have approximately three to eight URIs per year, adolescents and adults two to four per year, and persons older than 65 years have fewer than one URI per year. Most URIs are viral in origin, with the most common agents being rhinoviruses, coronaviruses, adenoviruses, and coxsackieviruses. The incubation period for most viral URIs is 1 to 4 days. For URIs caused by bacteria, the agents are similar to those causing otitis media. In decreasing order of frequency, they include *Streptococcus pneumoniae, Haemophilus influenzae, Moraxella catarrhalis,* and *Staphylococcus aureus*. Community-acquired respiratory tract infections caused by *Streptococcus* account for more than 20 million primary care practitioner visits annually and are a major cause of work and school absenteeism.

Infections such as acute epiglottitis and respiratory syncytial virus (RSV) infection occur predominantly in infants and younger children, but may occur as life-threatening infections in adults (RSV infection can also cause severe pneumonia and lower respiratory tract disease in older institutionalized adults and adults with suppressed immune status). Acute epiglottitis is a bacterial infection that can result in complete or partial airway obstruction (Box 30-1), whereas acute laryngitis is generally associated with a viral URI and often persists for a week or more after other symptoms have cleared.

Influenza

Seasonal influenza epidemics occur each year in the United States. In 2019, the U.S. Centers for Disease Control and Prevention (CDC) reported approximately 8.5% of persons in the United States are infected annually with the flu. This is about 27 million persons per year. There were an estimated 1,400 to 3,900 flu-related deaths during the 5-month influenza season from October 2020 to February 2022, but according to the CDC, this number may be skewed due to COVID-19. Most flu-related deaths occur in older persons, particularly those with underlying pulmonary or cardiac disease. Infants and very young children also appear to be at greater risk for influenza-associated morbidity and mortality. Although influenza and colds may occur at any time, most cases occur during the winter and spring months.

Box 30.1 Acute Epiglottitis

Acute epiglottitis is a life-threatening, rapidly progressive cellulitis of the epiglottis that may cause complete airway obstruction. Epiglottitis begins as a cellulitis between the tongue base and the epiglottis; the epiglottis is then pushed posteriorly. The epiglottis becomes swollen and threatens airway patency. Epiglottitis is more common and more severe in young children, but it may occur in older children and adults.

Clinical Manifestations

Epiglottitis in adults should be suspected when odynophagia (pain on swallowing) seems severe compared with pharyngeal findings. Other findings include dyspnea, drooling, and stridor.

Diagnostic Reasoning

Direct viewing of the epiglottis with a tongue blade and lighting should *never* be attempted because immediate laryngospasm and airway obstruction may result. It is recommended that children and adults be transported to the operating room (OR) while sitting up for visualization of the epiglottis with a fiberoptic laryngoscope, with preparations made for immediate airway control, if needed. The epiglottis will appear swollen and erythematous ("cherry red"), and an uncuffed endotracheal tube should be inserted, if needed to maintain airway patency.

Management

Acute epiglottitis requires emergency care for adequate airway control. No painful or stressful procedures should be performed on these patients unless preparations are in place for a planned intubation, such as in the OR.

The patient with epiglottitis will require hospitalization for IV antibiotics such as cefuroxime (Ceftin), ceftriaxone (Rocephin), or ampicillin/sulbactam (Unasyn). Dexamethasone (Decadron) should also be administered IV and tapered as signs and symptoms resolve. Continuous pulse oximetry and careful monitoring of the patient's airway are critical. Patients who develop hypoxemia and respiratory distress require intubation.

 Geriatric Considerations: Influenza

Older adults are more prone to dying from influenza due to coexisting pulmonary and/or cardiac problems. Treatment includes rest, fluids, antipyretics, analgesics, and cough suppressants. Antiviral therapy may be indicated for compromised patients. Prevention is the best remedy, and all older adults should receive a yearly influenza vaccination.

PATHOPHYSIOLOGY

URIs

The common cold (coryza) is caused by viruses spread through direct inhalation of airborne droplets aerosolized by the infected person while speaking, coughing, or sneezing, as well as hand-to-face transmission after handling fomites serving as reservoirs of infection. Hand-to-hand transmission, however, is probably the most common mode of transmission in adults, underscoring the importance of frequent hand washing in the prevention of new cases. Numerous serotypes of rhinoviruses, adenoviruses, coronaviruses, coxsackieviruses, and parainfluenza viruses are associated with the common cold. The ability of these viruses to mutate readily ensures their ability to consistently evade host immune mechanisms. The number of rhinovirus serotypes, for instance, currently stands at more than 100. After infection, individuals develop immunity to a specific viral strain but are susceptible to repeated infection by the same parent virus that has undergone only minor changes in surface proteins or polysaccharides.

Symptoms of congestion, rhinorrhea, and sneezing result directly from inflammation and edema of upper airway mucosal surfaces. The cough reflex may be triggered by this same mucosal inflammation in the posterior pharynx. After acute infection, postviral cough may persist for as long as 6 to 8 weeks due to postnasal drip—the persistent drainage of thin mucus into the posterior pharynx resulting in direct pharyngeal irritation.

Influenza

Classic flu is caused by the orthomyxovirus influenza type A and, to a lesser extent, influenza type B. Both are enveloped RNA-based viruses. In addition to the viral rhinitis symptoms of the common cold, influenza infection causes generalized muscle aches and pains, fatigue, significant fever, and rigors (chills). Influenza infection may lead to viral pneumonia (lower airway infection), which may be further complicated by bacterial superinfection, particularly with *S. aureus.* These additional manifestations and high potential for complicated disease underscore the importance of widespread yearly vaccination against influenza.

The influenza virus frequently undergoes mutation of its major surface proteins, hemagglutinin and neuraminidase, which renders protein-specific host antibody defenses ineffective. Each year, a vaccine is developed using influenza proteins from the most likely serotype combination predicted to cause widespread infection for that year. The vaccine determination is made using complex disease modeling algorithms based on extensive CDC and World Health Organization (WHO) epidemiological data. However, despite these data, the compilation of each yearly vaccine is a "best guess" that may or may not provide adequate protection against that year's primary strain. In addition, other strains of the virus not covered by the vaccine may also cause numerous infections in any given year.

Given concerns in recent years for the potential spread of other forms of influenza, including H5N1 influenza (avian or bird flu) and H1N1 influenza (swine flu), significant efforts are also being directed toward developing safe and effective vaccines against these forms of the disease. Throughout history, the most widespread and devastating flu-related pandemics have been traced back primarily to these novel forms of the virus (in particular, avian flu). On an annual basis, however, classic seasonal influenza results in far greater morbidity and mortality each year than these other forms. For the past 40 years, widespread pandemics of avian flu and H1N1 influenza have largely been avoided through multinational public health measures. Clinical trials of an oral influenza vaccine tablet are underway, although the long-term effects of this drug are not known.

Most cases of laryngitis (inflammation of the vocal cords with extreme hoarseness and temporary voice loss) and croup (any combination of laryngotracheobronchitis with edema leading to airway obstruction with characteristic stridor) are caused by parainfluenza virus, RSV, influenza virus, coxsackievirus, rhinovirus, and adenovirus. Laryngitis may also be caused by group A beta-hemolytic *Streptococcus pyogenes, H. influenzae,* and *M. catarrhalis.* These same viral and bacterial agents, along with *Neisseria gonorrhoeae* and Epstein-Barr virus (causing infectious mononucleosis), are also common causes of pharyngitis (see full discussion in Chapter 24).

RSV and influenza A (and influenza B to a lesser degree) are the most common causes of bronchiolitis in children and adolescents, but adults tend to experience infection in the larger airways (i.e., acute bronchitis). Since the advent of widespread vaccination against *H. influenzae* type B (Hib vaccine) and *Corynebacterium diphtheriae* (DTaP vaccine), epiglottitis occurs only rarely in the United States (see Box 30.1). Bacterial tracheitis is a serious purulent infection of the subglottic trachea caused primarily by *S. aureus,* with a toxic clinical presentation requiring hospitalization and IV antibiotic therapy.

CLINICAL PRESENTATION

The onset of influenza is usually abrupt, with fever, chills, malaise, myalgia, headache, nasal stuffiness, sore throat, and sometimes nausea. A nonproductive cough is usually present and occurs early in the course of illness. The fever may be as high as 103°F (39.4°C) in adults and typically lasts 3 to 5 days. Subjective findings with the common cold include headache, myalgia, nasal congestion, watery rhinorrhea, sneezing, foul breath, and a "scratchy throat." Laryngitis results in inflammation of the laryngeal mucosa and vocal cords. Symptoms include hoarseness, aphonia, and, occasionally, pain when swallowing. Physical findings in cases of URI are usually minimal, other than typical congested facies. Cervical lymphadenopathy may also be present. Although chest auscultation in uncomplicated URI is typically normal, upper airway congestion may lead to noisy breathing, which should not be mistaken for adventitious lung sounds.

DIAGNOSTIC REASONING

Diagnostic Tests

The diagnosis of influenza tends to be more accurate during epidemics. A successful presumptive diagnosis requires appropriate symptoms at the right time of the year and knowledge of patterns of influenzal illnesses around the world. If necessary, the diagnosis can be confirmed via virology studies (e.g., nasal and pharyngeal cultures, cells from nasopharyngeal washings stained with monoclonal antibody fluorescence stains, and complement fixation studies on paired serum samples). Diagnosis of colds and laryngitis is typically based on the subjective presentation of the patient, except when the etiological agent in laryngitis is thought to be bacterial. In these situations, the practitioner should perform a throat culture to rule out group A beta-hemolytic streptococcal infection. Rapid strep tests have greater than 70% sensitivity and greater than 90% specificity. Leukocytosis found on a complete blood count (CBC) with differential may help diagnose a bacterial infection.

Differential Diagnosis

Conditions that need to be ruled out include allergic rhinitis, group A streptococcal pharyngitis, bacterial sinusitis, atypical *Mycoplasma* pneumonia, infectious mononucleosis, and possibly mumps, rubeola, and cytomegalovirus (CMV). Close attention to epidemiological patterns (e.g., current outbreak in the community) is important, and the CDC or local health department can be helpful in determining the type of disease outbreak.

MANAGEMENT

Management of influenza and the common cold is generally symptomatic and is directed toward the relief of symptoms and prevention of secondary infections. Antibiotics are not indicated for influenza or common colds, which are predominantly virally mediated, unless a secondary bacterial infection occurs.

URIs

Mucopurulent rhinitis frequently accompanies the common cold and is not an indication for antimicrobial treatment. Although antibiotics are often viewed by the layperson as a necessary treatment for a cold or the flu, these drugs have no effect on viruses and if taken injudiciously may produce resistant organisms. In the past, clinicians ordered antibiotics in about half of all URI cases, which is thought to have contributed to the current antimicrobial-resistant crisis. Health-care providers continue to prescribe antibiotics to adults and children with viral infections, at times indiscriminately. Although most cases of acute rhinosinusitis (including bacterial sinusitis) resolve without antibiotics, if symptoms persist longer than 10 days, antibiotic therapy should be considered for 5 to 7 days.

Rest, fluids, and antipyretics are also useful in controlling the discomfort associated with a cold. Oral decongestants such as pseudoephedrine (e.g., Sudafed) are widely used and may help control rhinorrhea and nasal congestion. These systemic medications should be used only for 3 days due to rebound effects and should not be used in the presence of hypertension. Nasal sprays such as phenylephrine (Neo-Synephrine) and oxymetazoline (Afrin) or ocular vasoconstrictor formulations of oxymetazoline (OcuClear, Visine LR) are rapidly effective for localized symptoms. Despite their topical delivery and lesser association with hypertension, patients should still be cautioned to use these local medications for only a few days, as chronic use leads to rebound congestion at local tissue sites (particularly the nasal mucosa). Intranasal ipratropium (Atrovent) may be effective for significant rhinorrhea associated with URIs. Nasal saline rinses and/or intranasal corticosteroids may also be considered, although the latter must be used chronically (rather than as needed) to elicit the desired therapeutic effect, which may take several days or more to develop.

Vitamin C and zinc lozenges with echinacea are currently popular alternative treatments that are sold as over-the-counter cold therapies. Despite numerous randomized trials, the evidence for the effectiveness of zinc lozenges in reducing the duration of colds is lacking. The ability of vitamin C supplements to decrease the incidence of colds or shorten their duration has also not been demonstrated, although there may be an exception for the patient who has vitamin C deficiency. Several small studies have shown that black elderberry syrup shortens the duration of flu-like illnesses by up to 4 days.

Treatment of laryngitis includes complete voice rest, steam inhalations, codeine or nonnarcotic cough suppressants for cough and pain, and a liquid or soft diet. If throat cultures are positive for group A beta-hemolytic *Streptococcus,* penicillin should be prescribed if the patient is not allergic to penicillin. Erythromycin should be used for infections associated with *M. catarrhalis* or *H. influenzae.* For particularly toxic bacterial infections such as bacterial tracheitis, blood cultures may be appropriate to rule out bacteremia. Even in the absence of systemic infection, bacterial tracheitis requires IV antibiotic therapy with nafcillin or an appropriate cephalosporin; if methicillin-resistant *S. aureus* (MRSA) is suspected, vancomycin or linezolid should be administered.

Because of impaired oral intake, all such infections other than the common cold are prone to dehydration requiring oral or IV rehydration therapy. In addition, hypoxemia based on pulse oximetry or blood gas analysis should be addressed with supplemental oxygen therapy. Bronchodilator therapy is often used as well, but randomized clinical trials do not consistently demonstrate its efficacy. For the management of croup, however, racemic epinephrine and dexamethasone are indicated, and intubation may be needed in severe cases.

Influenza

Generally, most patients with influenza should rest at home until symptoms decrease in severity. Older patients or patients with an underlying chronic illness may require hospitalization for influenza. In addition to rest and fluids, antipyretics and analgesics are recommended. Cough suppressants with codeine may be necessary for adequate tussive control.

If the practitioner is reasonably confident that the virus in question is type A influenza, the patient may benefit from an antiviral drug. Widespread amantadine (Symmetrel) and rimantadine (Flumadine) resistance among influenza A virus strains has made this class of medications less useful clinically. Therefore, amantadine and rimantadine are not recommended for antiviral treatment or chemoprophylaxis of currently circulating influenza A virus strains. The majority of currently circulating influenza viruses are susceptible to the neuraminidase inhibitor antiviral medications oseltamivir (Tamiflu), zanamivir (Relenza), and peramivir (Rapivab). Antiviral treatment is recommended as early as possible (within 48 hours of symptom presentation) for patients with confirmed or suspected influenza who have severe, complicated, or progressive illness, who require hospitalization, or who pose a risk for influenza-related complications, including pregnant women. Oseltamivir, either as a pill or in liquid form, is for the treatment of influenza in persons aged 2 weeks and older and for chemoprophylaxis to prevent influenza in patients 1 year of age and older. Zanamivir, given as a powder that is inhaled, is to treat flu in people aged 7 years and older and to prevent influenza in patients aged 5 years and older. Zanamivir is not recommended for persons with respiratory problems, such as asthma or chronic obstructive pulmonary disease (COPD). Both medications are usually prescribed for 5 days for individuals in a primary care setting, although people hospitalized with the flu may need the medication for longer than 5 days. Peramivir is a single-dose IV medication given in the emergency department (ED) for patients 2 years of age and older. These medications should not be used in place of getting an annual flu vaccination, however, which is currently recommended for all individuals aged 6 months and older without contraindications (e.g., severe allergic reaction to any component of the vaccine).

FOLLOW-UP AND REFERRAL

URIs

Most cases of the common cold and laryngitis are self-limited. Complications of a cold may include pharyngitis, sinusitis, otitis media, tonsillitis, and chest infections. Unless symptoms of these complications are present, antibiotic therapy is not indicated for URIs. The patient with laryngitis needs to maintain voice rest until hoarseness and aphonia have resided. Any vigorous use of the voice such as shouting or singing may foster the formation of vocal cord nodules.

Influenza

The duration of an uncomplicated case of influenza is 1 to 7 days, with an excellent prognosis. However, complications can occur, including acute sinusitis, otitis media, purulent bronchitis, and pneumonia. Influenza causes necrosis of some respiratory epithelium, predisposing the infected person to secondary bacterial infections. The interaction between bacteria and influenza is bidirectional, with bacterial enzymes activating influenza viruses. If a fever persists for more than 4 days, the white blood cell count rises to 12,000 cells/μL or higher, or the cough becomes productive, bacterial infection should be ruled out or verified and treated.

The most common complication of influenza is pneumonia; most fatalities result from bacterial pneumonia. The patient with influenza with superimposed bacterial pneumonia may experience gradual improvement of symptoms for 2 to 3 days and then develop cough and purulent sputum. Pneumococcal pneumonia is the most common bacterial pneumonia associated with influenza, but staphylococcal pneumonia is the most serious. Primary viral influenza pneumonia is the least common but has a high mortality rate among pregnant women and patients with rheumatic heart disease. These patients develop symptoms of influenza that increasingly worsen, and respiratory distress is often severe enough to require mechanical ventilation.

> **Patient Education: Upper Respiratory Infections**
>
> There currently is no immunization for the prevention of colds. Research has demonstrated that the best method of preventing transmission of infected droplets is through frequent hand washing, particularly in day-care facilities and congregate adult living facilities. During the cold and influenza seasons, the person with a chronic illness or compromised immune status should be advised to avoid crowded settings and other persons with apparent symptoms.

The Advisory Committee on Immunization Practices (ACIP) currently recommends an annual vaccination for all persons 6 months of age or older. Trivalent influenza vaccine provides partial immunity (in approximately 86% of patients vaccinated) for a few months to 1 year. The vaccine's antigenic configuration changes yearly. It is based on the prevalent strains of the previous year, the viruses that are currently being seen in other parts of the world during the current year, and the estimated antibody response in persons previously infected with or vaccinated against these viruses. Vaccination in October or November of each year is recommended for all persons older than 6 months and particularly for those aged 65 years and older; nursing home residents; adults and children with underlying medical conditions, including cardiac, pulmonary, malignant, and some metabolic diseases; health-care workers; and pregnant women. Medicare covers the cost of both influenza and pneumococcal vaccinations. Vaccination is also encouraged for the members of large groups who may be the principal vectors of influenza transmission in their communities, such as schoolchildren, children in day care, college students, military personnel, and employees of large companies. High-risk children have a particularly low influenza vaccination rate annually, which is of significant concern. In addition, low-income, ethnic minority populations in the United States typically have lower vaccination rates than other populations.

Recent research has shown that obtaining yearly influenza vaccination can be influenced by a health-care provider's recommendations and phone calls offering encouragement and reminders. *Healthy People 2030* set a goal of vaccinating 70% of persons aged 6 months and older. Currently, more than 49% receive the annual flu vaccine, which remains below target. Clinicians may keep informed of current epidemiological trends in influenza epidemics and changes in vaccine recommendations by accessing the CDC's flu Web site at https://www.cdc.gov/flu/index.htm.

CYSTIC FIBROSIS

Cystic fibrosis (CF) is no longer considered solely a childhood disease. It is a lifelong disease diagnosed in infancy usually by age 2 years. CF is the most common life-shortening autosomal recessive disease among European Americans. It also affects Hispanics (1:10,000 births), Native Americans (1:10,500 births), African Americans (1:15,000 births), and Asian Americans (1:30,000 births). In 10 years, more than 70% of persons in the United States with CF will be adults. Although one thinks of the lungs as being involved, it is a disease of exocrine gland function that involves multiple organ systems including the digestive system with pancreatic enzyme insufficiency, sweat glands, and the reproductive tract. Although all these systems are involved, it is progressive lung disease that results in the major cause of morbidity and mortality for most patients with CF.

EPIDEMIOLOGY AND CAUSES

Patients with CF inherit one copy of a gene mutation from each parent in the CF transmembrane conductance regulator (*CFTR*). The mutation of the *CFTR* gene results in the thick, sticky mucus that lines the body's mucosal membranes, specifically in the airways. Newborn screening for CF has been required since 2010, and CF occurs in 1 in 2,000 to 3,000 live births. In the past, children with CF were not expected to live beyond the age of 5 years. Currently, more than 50% of individuals with CF live to be adults, with the average survival age of 47 years, which is increasing rapidly with the advent of *CFTR* modulators. CF-caused hepatobiliary disease is the third leading cause for liver transplantation in adolescents or adults. Up to 25% of CF patients will develop diabetes mellitus by age 20 years, which increases to 50% as these patients age.

PATHOPHYSIOLOGY

The *CFTR* gene codes for the *CFTR* protein, which controls salt and water balance in the lungs and other tissues. CF is a result of pathogenic mutations on chromosome 7 that encodes the *CFTR* protein. There must be mutations in both copies of the *CFTR* gene to result in clinical disease; thus, genetic inheritance of this condition is autosomal-recessive. There are more than 2,000 different mutations in the *CFTR* gene, the most common of which result in the loss of a phenylalanine amino acid (abbreviated as F) at the 508th position of the *CFTR* protein (F508), accounting for two-thirds of all CF cases worldwide and 90% of cases in the United States. Each mutation leads to diverse symptoms affecting the lungs, pancreas, sinuses, liver, gallbladder, and endocrine and reproductive systems. Some prenatal findings of CF may be found on a routine prenatal ultrasonography, including a hyperechogenic bowel. Exocrine pancreatic insufficiency may result in dysfunction of the endocrine pancreas, leading to glucose intolerance and CF-related diabetes (CFRD).

CLINICAL PRESENTATION

Subjective

The majority of patients with CF develop sinus disease and they may complain of chronic nasal congestion (due to polyposis), headaches, cough from chronic postnasal drip, and sleep disturbance. If pancreatic insufficiency is present, patients may complain of steatorrhea with frequent, bulky, foul-smelling stools that may be oily. They may also have failure to thrive or be unable to gain weight because of malabsorption of fat and protein. Most men (95%) experience infertility related to defects in sperm transport. In addition, women with CF are found to be less fertile than women without CF. Patients with CF also have increased rates of fractures and kyphoscoliosis due to reduced bone mineral content.

Objective

Typical respiratory symptoms include a persistent productive cough, a chest x-ray showing hyperinflation of the lung fields, and pulmonary function tests consistent with obstructive airway disease. Patients may exhibit cough, wheezing, or dyspnea. In addition, they may be tachypneic. As the disease progresses, patients develop chronic bronchitis with acute exacerbations of increased sputum production, malaise, anorexia, and weight loss. Advanced disease will result in digital clubbing. Ten percent to 20% of infants with CF develop meconium ileus. Older CF patients complaining of abdominal pain should be evaluated for a small bowel obstruction. This distal intestinal obstructive syndrome (DIOS) occurs in approximately 15% of adult CF patients. In addition, patients with CF may exhibit venous thrombosis, anemia, or nephrolithiasis.

DIAGNOSTIC REASONING

Diagnostic Tests

In the United States, all infants are screened at birth for CF using two serial assays. If the first assay is abnormal, the infant is retested with a second assay. A serum immunoreactive trypsinogen (IRT) and DNA analysis for variants in *CFTR* are used. An abnormal IRT may be followed by another IRT on a different sample of the infant's blood, or the IRT may be followed by DNA analysis. If the infant tests positive, at 2 weeks of age, a sweat chloride test should be done to determine a positive diagnosis of CF. Sweat chloride of less than 29 mmol/L is considered normal, 30 to 59 mmol/L is considered intermediate, and greater than 60 mmol/L is abnormal. Sweat testing is done by administering pilocarpine to the skin to trigger sweat formation. It is then collected by applying plastic wrap to the skin to accumulate the sweat, which takes approximately 1 hour. Usually, two different samples are tested. If results of the DNA analysis and sweat test are inconclusive, nasal potential difference (NPD) may be measured to further evaluate for *CFTR* dysfunction, although this test is not widely available.

Differential Diagnosis

Some disorders mimic the signs and symptoms of CF:

- Immunological abnormalities, such as severe combined immunodeficiency (SCID), which has sinopulmonary infections similar to CF
- Primary ciliary dyskinesia, which leads to recurrent sinopulmonary infections in addition to male infertility
- Shwachman-Diamond syndrome, which may cause pancreatic insufficiency and is associated with chronic or recurrent hematological abnormalities

MANAGEMENT

Airway clearance techniques (ACTs) remain a staple of therapy, which may require 2 to 3 hours per day of chest physiotherapy. Percussion or vibration of the chest and back loosens mucus from airway walls. ACTs are used in conjunction with inhaled bronchodilators, mucolytics, and possibly inhaled antibiotics.

Pulmonary exacerbations (PEx) requiring IV antibiotics occur in slightly more than one-third of all CF patients annually. Antibiotics should be selected based on the bacteria identified by culture of respiratory secretions. Antibiotic choices include aminoglycosides, colistin, vancomycin, ciprofloxacin, and sulfonamides. PEx are associated with increased morbidity and mortality. They are characterized by an increased cough, sputum production, or chest congestion; increased nasal congestion or drainage; increased dyspnea on exertion with an increased respiratory rate; increased fatigue; and decreased appetite. The goal of therapy is to reduce exacerbation frequency because between 12% and 35% of patients who have an exacerbation fail to recover to at least 90% of their baseline functioning, as measured by FEV_1. IV antibiotics for at least 2 weeks are recommended as the standard treatment of PEx.

Patients with CF should be treated prophylactically with the antiviral oseltamivir, as they are at increased risk for severe consequences from influenza infection. All patients with CF older than 6 months of age should receive an annual vaccination against viral influenza using an inactivated flu vaccine.

Almost 85% of CF patients require oral pancreatic enzyme replacement therapy with all their meals and snacks. Although all the previously mentioned therapies treat the symptoms of CF, it is the *CFTR* modulators that treat the underlying cause of CF, thereby restoring partial function to the gene mutation. All patients should undergo *CFTR* genotyping to determine whether they carry one of the mutations approved for *CFTR* modulator therapy. Approximately 10% of patients with CF have two copies of rare *CFTR* mutations that do not have an approved modulator therapy (see Drugs Commonly Prescribed 30.1).

FOLLOW-UP AND REFERRAL

Patients with CF have frequent exacerbations and must be followed closely. Once the decision is made to begin *CFTR* modulators, it is a lifelong commitment, as the effects of these medications only last as long as the medication is in the patient's system. These

Drugs Commonly Prescribed 30.1: *CFTR* Modulators

CFTR MODULATOR	AGE GROUP	COMMON ADVERSE REACTIONS	INTERACTIONS/SPECIAL CONSIDERATIONS
Ivacaftor	6 months to 11 years	Elevated hepatic transaminases; cataracts; abdominal pain; nausea/vomiting; hypoglycemia; headache; dizziness	CYP3A inducers; grapefruit; Seville oranges
Lumacaftor/ivacaftor	2 to 5 years of age	Same as above, plus: dyspnea; chest tightness; flu-like symptoms	Same as above. Should be taken with fat-containing foods.
Tezacaftor/ivacaftor	6 to 11 years of age	Same as ivacaftor	Same as ivacaftor
Elaxacaftor/tezacaftor/ivacaftor	12 years of age and older	Same as ivacaftor	Same as ivacaftor

Adapted from Lomas PH, Tran QT. The changing face of cystic fibrosis. *Am Nurse J.* 2020;15(3):28–32
Rosenfelld M, Wainwright CE, Higgins M, et al. Ivacaftor treatment of cystic fibrosis in children aged 12 to <24 months and with a *CFTR* gating mutation (ARRIVAL): a phase 3 single-arm study. *Lancet Respir Med.* 2018;6(7):545.
Abbreviation CFTR, cystic fibrosis transmembrane conductance regulator

medications are expensive, and there are assistance programs available to help patients get the drugs at a reduced cost.

Patient Education

It is exhausting living with CF for both the patient and the caregiver (see the Patient's Voice 30.1). Several hours each day must be devoted to ACTs. Preventing infection with consistent hand washing is essential, as well as maintaining adequate nutrition, given the risk of malabsorption. Establishing a caring relationship with all support persons is critical. Using the Circle of Caring model, support persons may be introduced to yoga, meditation, or even counseling to assist them in caring for their loved one.

PNEUMONIA

Pneumonia is typically an acute inflammation of the lung parenchyma, usually infectious in origin. The lung tissue typically becomes consolidated as alveoli fill with exudate. Gas exchange may be impaired as blood is shunted around nonfunctional alveoli. The timely diagnosis and appropriate management of pneumonia in patients is critical because of the morbidity associated with bacterial etiologies, as well as the increased mortality among older patients and those with underlying pulmonary disease. Community-acquired pneumonia (CAP) occurs outside the hospital or is diagnosed within 2 days after hospitalization in a patient who has not resided in a long-term care facility for 2 weeks or more before the onset of the symptoms. Clinicians diagnose and treat CAP in the primary care setting. In lay terms, it is often called *walking pneumonia*. Recently, severe acute respiratory syndrome coronavirus 2 (SARS-CoV-2) has become another notable cause of pneumonia, with more than 28,000,000 infections and more than 500,000 deaths in the United States reported through February 2021.

EPIDEMIOLOGY AND CAUSES

It is estimated that in the United States, almost 5 million people develop pneumonia annually. Of these, approximately 1.3 million persons with pneumonia are admitted to hospitals, and more than 90,000 die each year. Approximately 70% to 80% of patients who develop CAP are aged 65 years or older or have a coexisting medical condition. CAP remains one of the 10 leading causes of mortality among older people in the United States and is frequently the terminal event in older adults and those debilitated by chronic diseases, particularly chronic respiratory disease. Two percent of persons older than 65 years are hospitalized for CAP annually. This population is increasing, thus making adequate treatment of pneumonia a health-care priority. Nosocomial (hospital-acquired) pneumonias account for approximately 15% of all hospital-associated infections; pneumonia is second only to urinary tract infection in terms of frequency among hospitalized patients. In addition, pneumonia is still the leading infectious cause of death worldwide in children younger than 5 years. The most common pathogens associated with CAP and nosocomial pneumonia are shown in Box 30.2.

The Patient's Voice 30.1: Cystic Fibrosis

In 1978, I was diagnosed as a baby with cystic fibrosis (CF). The messy remnants in my diaper were the impetus for my parents bringing me to the doctor. The test was simply measuring the salt concentration in my arm sweat. Years later after the CF gene was discovered and sequencing became affordable, I'd find out my CF mutations were the common ΔF508 from my Irish mom, and W1282X, common to Ashkenazi Jews such as my dad. At the time they were told to give me a comfortable life and that I may live to 10 years.

In second grade, I started experiencing serious lung infection exacerbations that would require hospitalization and IV antibiotics. Through the rest of elementary school, I would be hospitalized three to five times per year. I grew to actually like the children's hospital; my mom was a nurse on "the floor" and I liked hanging with the nurses behind the scenes. More so, I had made a bunch of friends with CF that were frequently inpatients. This was before the bacteria *Burkholderia cepacia* became the main reason we CF patients weren't supposed to hang out together. There could sometimes be four kids with CF in one room. I'd usually go hang out in the girls' rooms. We would play games and race our IV poles down the hallway, and we never wore hospital gowns. We knew how to pack for the hospital. One parent commented he could always pick out the kids with CF because they look like nothing's wrong with them. Now we're not supposed to be within the same room. Sadly, I've outlived all the hospital friends I made, but have made a few new ones I see online. We've lost some sense of community.

When I was 11, I had an upper-right lobectomy because that lobe was the most infected. After that, my exacerbations dropped quite a bit to where I only needed IV meds once every year or two on average for the last 30 years. It's a high-maintenance illness, requiring a large handful of assorted pills and 30 to 60 minutes of nebulizers twice a day, 10 to 15 enzymes with every meal, three inhalers, and 20 minutes of a vibrating vest to shake up the mucus. Despite all of this, most of my day is fairly normal. I've managed to succeed as a solar engineer, moved across the country, I was a drummer in a few bands, and exercise a few times a week. For most of my life, the thick mucus congestion was a daily nuisance, I was mostly used to it, but sometimes coughing and spitting is uncomfortable in public. At the gym, I used to duck into the bathroom so I could cough myself into a red-faced sweat to clear the airway blockage. My other troubling symptom has been chronic hemoptysis since my teens. The episodes have been very random, often when laying to bed, and sometimes at work or other inconvenient places. They became mostly a nuisance, likely hundreds of minor episodes with maybe dozens severe enough to scare me. I recently had my seventh bronchial artery embolization; this severity isn't common for people with CF, but it can happen.

I produced a lot of mucus up until 8 months ago when I started taking Trikafta, a *CFTR* modulator. It has been a life-changer in that I cough *much* less, and the mucus is thinner! It helps more than all my other meds combined. I still do the other treatments as maintenance but I feel a lot better! My FEV_1 before Trikafta was 55%, and is currently around 70% of normal now, not bad for 43 years old!

I've lived through an interesting time with CF, witnessing exciting new treatments and longer life expectancy. I've recently accepted that I'll probably live to a normal retirement age. It's been a wild ride so far.

Eric Hyman

Box 30.2 Common Causes of Pneumonia

Community-Acquired Pneumonia (CAP)	Nosocomial Pneumonia
Streptococcus pneumoniae (70% of all cases of bacterial pneumonia and 25%–35% of all CAP)	Most are caused by gram-negative bacteria.
Staphylococcus aureus	Enteric aerobic gram-negative bacilli
Klebsiella pneumoniae	*Klebsiella pneumoniae*
Moraxella catarrhalis (less common)	*Pseudomonas aeruginosa*
Atypical pneumonias:	*Staphylococcus aureus* (gram-positive)
Mycoplasma pneumoniae (second most common cause of CAP)	Oral anaerobes
Legionella pneumophila	*Legionella pneumophila* (which grow in wet mechanical environments, including cooling systems, condensers, and shower heads)
Chlamydia pneumoniae	
Fungi	
Oral anaerobes	
Viruses	

Geriatric Considerations: Community-Acquired Pneumonia

The majority of patients with CAP are older adults, in part due to their propensity for respiratory disease. Older adults may present atypically (for example, without a temperature), so a thorough examination is indicated. Diagnosis includes a chest x-ray, white blood cell count, and a Gram stain of sputum. Specific empiric antibiotic therapy is cited later. As always, prevention is the best cure. Older adults should be encouraged to stop smoking, limit alcohol intake, and receive an annual influenza vaccine and the pneumococcal vaccine per the following guidelines: https://www.cdc.gov/vaccines/vpd/pneumo/hcp/recommendations.html.

Pneumocystis jiroveci (formerly *Pneumocystis carinii*) pneumonia (PCP) remains one of the leading causes of death in patients with AIDS. However, widespread use of highly active antiretroviral therapy and antibiotic prophylaxis based on CD4 T-cell counts has led to a dramatic decline in PCP incidence over the last 15 years.

For pneumonia in general, however, other vulnerable populations include infants younger than 6 months, children younger than 5 years, patients who smoke, patients with alcohol use disorder, residents of nursing homes, young adults living in close quarters (e.g., college students and military recruits), and individuals with impaired swallowing capacity or cough reflex who are at risk for aspiration. Geographical location, the winter season, occupation, travel history, and pet or animal exposure are other factors associated with the development of pneumonia.

In January 2020, the WHO declared an outbreak of a novel coronavirus, which soon after was deemed a public health emergency on a global scale. SARS-CoV-2 is the virus responsible for coronavirus disease 2019 (COVID-19). The earliest cases in the COVID-19 pandemic were linked to a seafood market in Wuhan (Hubei Province), China, in December 2019, and the virus was thought to have originated within an animal reservoir such as bats; however, intermediate animal hosts are also suspected, although this has yet to be fully confirmed. As a betacoronavirus, SARS-CoV-2 is member of a larger family of RNA viruses, which include coronaviruses responsible for the common cold, Middle East respiratory syndrome coronavirus (MERS-CoV), and SARS-CoV-1. Both MERS-CoV and SARS-CoV-1 were responsible for earlier outbreaks, but neither proved to be as large and with as much global impact as SARS-CoV-2.

Although the initial spread of SARS-CoV-2 infection was linked to travel from endemic areas in China, person-to-person transmission via respiratory droplets rapidly became the norm, as COVID-19 quickly spread across the globe, with Europe and the United States particularly affected. As of March 2022, there have been more than 441 million cases of COVID-19 worldwide, with mortality linked to risk factors such as obesity, advanced age, and comorbid conditions. The likelihood of infectious transmission is increased with closer proximity between infected and noninfected persons, specifically less than 6 feet (2 m). Transmission also occurs via contaminated surfaces or fomites and subsequent contact with the eyes, nose, or mouth. Airborne transmission can also occur, and transmission is thought to be highest when patients with COVID-19 are symptomatic and undergo aerosolizing procedures such as airway management, nebulization, or bronchoscopy.

SARS-CoV-2 is a highly infectious virus with an initial R0 infectivity rate of more than 2.2, meaning that for every case of COVID-19 identified, greater than 2.2 more people are likely to be infected without adequate isolation measures. The R0 of SARS-CoV-2 has changed as the pandemic has progressed over the course of many months. At the height of the pandemic, the R0 was over 4 but then dropped to closer to 1 as the pandemic improved. More recently, community transmission has become the predominant mode of viral transmission.

PATHOPHYSIOLOGY

Pneumonia is an infection of the alveoli, distal airways, and interstitium of the lungs and is therefore predominantly a parenchymal disease. Pathogens such as bacteria, viruses, fungi, or parasites reach the lower respiratory tract in sufficient number or with sufficient virulence to overwhelm the innate defenses of the respiratory tract. An inflammatory response is initiated that increases capillary permeability and attracts neutrophils, lymphocytes, platelets, and fibrinogen to the site of infection. Tissue fluid extravasates into the interstitial space from the pulmonary capillary bed, forming an exudate with higher protein content than typical transudative fluid. As this exudate develops, an increasing amount of cellular debris accumulates, impeding optimal oxygen diffusion from the alveoli to capillaries with resultant hypoxemia. Vital capacity, lung compliance, residual capacity, and total lung capacity are diminished, and ventilation–perfusion mismatch occurs.

The spongy consistency of the lung tissue fills with fluid and several lineages of white blood cells infiltrate depending on the infective agent involved, including neutrophils, lymphocytes, and macrophages, as well as red blood cells and fibrin. Because of these changes, the area of pneumonia is often referred to as a *consolidative focus,* which is typically dull to percussion on physical examination. Pneumonia may be classified as lobar pneumonia, interstitial pneumonia, miliary pneumonia, or bronchopneumonia. Figure 30.1 shows some of the parenchymal changes in pneumonia. Lobar pneumonia involves an entire lobe of the lung, whereas interstitial pneumonia is a patchy or diffuse inflammatory process throughout regions of the interstitium. Miliary pneumonia consists of numerous discrete lesions resulting from hematogenous spread of infection, and bronchopneumonia is a patchy consolidation involving one or several lobes of the lung. Moreover, inflammation can also extend into the pleural space, causing a parapneumonic effusion or inflammation of the pleural membranes, known as *pleuritis* or *pleurisy.*

Possible routes of infection include aspiration, aerosolization, hematogenous spread from a distant infected site, and direct spread from a contiguous infected site. Aspiration pneumonia occurs most often in postoperative, stroke, comatose, or otherwise mentally altered patients with an impaired swallowing reflex. Although *S. pneumoniae* remains the most common causative agent in aspiration pneumonia, anaerobic bacteria and gram-negative bacilli (i.e., gastrointestinal [GI] flora) must also be considered. Hematogenous spread to the lungs can take place in endocarditis, from IV central catheter line infection, or from infection at other sites such as the urinary tract. Aerosolization, the most common means of infection, is the route by which most bacteria, *Mycobacterium tuberculosis,* fungi, and viruses reach the lungs.

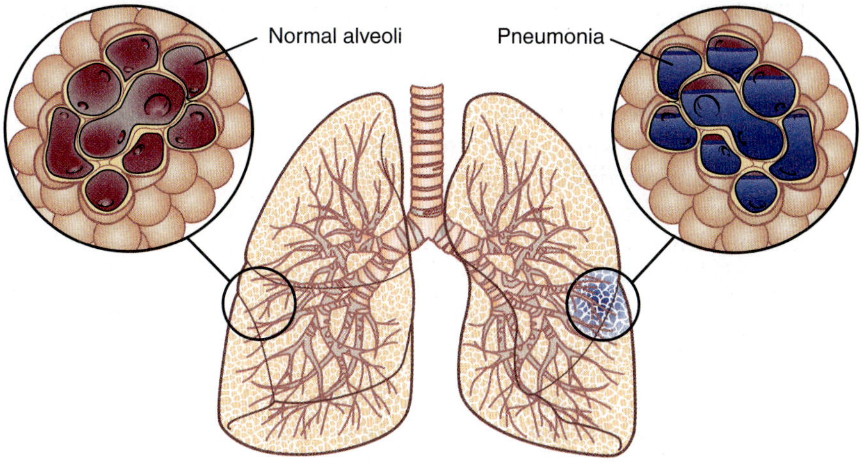

Figure 30.1 Parenchymal changes in pneumonia.

In adults, the most common organisms involved in CAP include viruses, *S. pneumoniae, M. catarrhalis, H. influenzae, Legionella pneumophila,* and MRSA. Nosocomial pneumonia may be caused by *Pseudomonas aeruginosa* and MRSA. Of note, increasing numbers of community-acquired MRSA infections are being reported, particularly among older nursing home residents, resulting in severe cases of necrotizing pneumonia.

Streptococcus Pneumoniae

The most common cause of CAP is the gram-positive bacteria *S. pneumoniae,* also referred to as *pneumococcal pneumonia. S. pneumoniae* is one of the leading causes of illness and death worldwide for young children, older adults, and persons with chronic, debilitating pathology. The pathogenesis of pneumococcal pneumonia has been extensively studied and serves as a prototype for the management of other types of bacterial pneumonia.

Pneumococcal pneumonia occurs as a result of infected mucus or inhalation of organisms that have colonized the nasopharynx. *S. pneumoniae* can be recovered from the nasopharynx of approximately 40% of healthy adults. In the normal host, the bacteria are inactivated by opsonization with immunoglobulins and complement. Persons with defects in host defense mechanisms (e.g., inadequate immunoglobulin production or deficiency, impaired phagocytic function, autoimmune disease, immunosuppression, or impaired mucociliary clearance) have far greater susceptibility.

The lower lobes are most commonly infected because of the effects of gravity. On inhalation, pneumococcus establishes itself in the alveoli, spreading rapidly through the pores of Kohn that connect adjacent alveoli. Pneumococcal pneumonia typically includes four responsive stages of infection: engorgement, red hepatization, gray hepatization, and resolution. During engorgement, alveolar capillaries become congested, bacteria and exudate pour into alveoli from alveolar capillaries, and bacteria multiply without inhibition. There is continued engorgement of the capillaries, with diapedesis of erythrocytes giving the lungs the gross appearance of liver tissue (red hepatization). As the leukocyte count increases in the exudate, it compresses the capillaries and causes the lung tissue to assume a gray color (gray hepatization). At this point, phagocytosis ensues by polymorphonuclear leukocytes. The presence of opsonizing antibody enhances the ingestion of the bacteria. The stage of resolution is reached when the pneumococci have been destroyed and macrophages are seen within the alveolar spaces, where they lyse and absorb the exudate. There may often be pleural involvement contiguous to parenchymal lesions or from spread via the lymphatics. As in the alveoli, there is an outpouring of fluid, followed by polymorphonuclear leukocytes and fibrin. The structure of the pleural space has fewer surfaces suitable for phagocytosis than do the alveoli. Control of the infection in the pleural area is more dependent on heat-stable (antigen-specific) than heat-labile (complement opsonization) antibodies.

Haemophilus Influenzae

H. influenzae, a gram-negative bacterium, is the cause of the second most common cause of CAP. It may occur in healthy individuals, as well as in patients with chronic debilitating diseases or chronic alcohol abuse. Development of *H. influenzae* pneumonia follows colonization of the upper respiratory tract. During viral infection epidemics, there is often an increase in the incidence of *H. influenzae* pneumonia.

Legionella Pneumophila

L. pneumophila, a gram-negative bacterium, was identified in 1976 as a causative agent of pneumonia (Legionnaires' disease) during an American Legion convention in Philadelphia. These bacteria thrive in aquatic environments. Sources of human infection have been associated with contaminated air-conditioning systems and showerheads. Within the hospital setting, contaminated respiratory tubing and equipment may serve as a source of *L. pneumophila.* The bacilli enter the lungs by aspiration, direct inhalation, and hematogenous dissemination. In the normal host, it is thought that the bacilli are cleared by the mucociliary process. This would explain the high incidence of the disease in patients with impaired mucociliary clearance (e.g., patients who smoke, patients with alcohol use disorder, and older adults). Legionnaires' disease may occur in explosive outbreaks if large numbers of susceptible people are exposed to an infectious aerosol. Because of the low communicability of the disease, secondary cases typically do not occur.

Staphylococcus Aureus

S. aureus rarely causes pneumonia in healthy young adults. Local pulmonary or systemic immune defenses must be compromised before the organism can produce pneumonia. *S. aureus* accounts for 2% to 9% of CAP in older adults or in patients with concomitant medical conditions, such as diabetes, chronic renal failure, bronchiectasis, or lung cancer, or with risk factors such as residence in a chronic care facility or injection drug abuse. Infections may also occur in previously healthy adults after viral influenza with residual impaired bronchopulmonary anti-infective mechanisms.

Viral Pneumonia

Viral infections account for 5% to 15% of cases of adult CAP. Most viral infections are restricted to the upper respiratory system and tend to cause self-limited symptoms. Some patients, particularly those with influenza infections, may develop pneumonia. Influenza may result in a primary viral pneumonia or, more commonly, a secondary bacterial pneumonia; secondary pneumonia is most frequently caused by *S. pneumoniae* and *S. aureus*. Viral infections are transmitted by hand-to-hand contact or by aerosols (i.e., sneezing, coughing). The frequency of influenza as a precipitating factor of both CAP and nosocomial pneumonia increases in the winter months.

Mycoplasma Pneumonia

Mycoplasma pneumonia is also known as primary atypical pneumonia or "walking pneumonia" because of the predominance of constitutional symptoms. *Mycoplasma pneumoniae* is a class of bacterial L-forms, which are the smallest known free-living organisms. Children older than 5 years and young adults are at greatest risk of developing *Mycoplasma* pneumonia. Outbreaks can occur in populations living in close proximity, such as colleges, military bases, and prisons. Because of the long incubation phase of 2 to 3 weeks and the relatively low communicability, *Mycoplasma* pneumonia tends to move through the community slowly.

Chlamydia Pneumoniae

Chlamydia pneumoniae was recognized as a pulmonary pathogen in 1983. *C. pneumoniae* is a gram-negative bacterium. Little is known about the mode of transmission and pathogenesis. The clinical features are similar to those caused by *M. pneumoniae*. Adult-onset asthma subsequent to infection with *C. pneumoniae* has been documented. Recurrent infection is common.

Anaerobic Pneumonia

Anaerobic pneumonia may occur in both the community and the hospital setting. *Prevotella melaninogenica,* anaerobic streptococci, and *Fusobacterium nucleatum* are commonly isolated anaerobic bacteria. Aspiration of oropharyngeal secretions normally occurs during sleep in healthy individuals but rarely causes disease. Individuals who are predisposed to aspiration of larger amounts of oropharyngeal secretions are at risk of anaerobic pneumonia. Alcohol use disorder is the most frequent predisposing factor; others include dysphagia, cerebrovascular accidents, seizures, and general anesthesia. Periodontal disease, which increases the number of anaerobic bacteria, is also associated with anaerobic infection. Pneumonia typically develops in dependent lung zones. Although body position at the time of aspiration determines which lung zones are dependent, anaerobic pneumonia most often develops in the posterior segments of the upper lobes and the superior and basilar segments of the lower lobes. The onset of symptoms is usually insidious. Empyema, lung abscess, or necrotizing pneumonia may be present by the time the patient seeks medical attention.

Nosocomial Bacterial Pneumonia

Nosocomial bacterial pneumonia is most frequently caused by gram-negative organisms such as *P. aeruginosa, Klebsiella pneumoniae, Escherichia coli, Serratia, Proteus,* and *Enterobacter.* However, *S. aureus* (especially MRSA), *S. pneumoniae,* and *H. influenzae* are frequently reported among older adult nursing home residents. As in CAP, bacteria invade the lower respiratory tract by aspiration of oropharyngeal organisms, inhalation of aerosols containing bacteria, or hematogenous spread from a distant body site. Patients at high risk of nosocomial bacterial pneumonia include postoperative patients (particularly those with thoracoabdominal procedures), patients with endotracheal incubation and/or mechanically assisted ventilation, and those with a depressed level of consciousness, an episode of large-volume aspiration, or an underlying chronic lung disease, as well as patients 70 years of age and older. Nosocomial pneumonia has a mortality rate of approximately 30%. Hospital-acquired pneumonia in patients on mechanical ventilation has a mortality rate of approximately 48%. Patients who develop acute respiratory distress syndrome have a mortality rate greater than 68%.

Pneumocystis Pneumonia

PCP is an AIDS-defining opportunistic infection that was once seen in as many as 65% of HIV-infected individuals and remains a major identifiable cause of death in AIDS patients. The causative agent, *P. jiroveci,* was originally classified as a protozoan named *P. carinii,* but it has since been reclassified as a fungus and renamed. Disease in adults represents reactivation of latent infection because almost all people are infected with *P. jiroveci* during the first decade of life. Most cases of PCP occur when the CD4-positive T-lymphocyte count has fallen below 200 to 250 cells/ μL. Pathologically, alveolar membranes become thickened, and mononuclear cell interstitial inflammation occurs as the disease progresses. PCP is discussed in more detail in Chapter 63.

Cytomegalic Inclusion Virus

CMV is a causative agent of pneumonia in immunocompromised patients. It is a type of herpes virus that results in latent infections and reactivation, with shedding of infectious viral particles. Pathologically, CMV produces an interstitial pneumonia that ranges from a mild disease to a fulminant course resulting in pulmonary insufficiency and death. CMV is discussed further in Chapter 63.

SARS-CoV-2 (COVID-19)

The pathophysiology of COVID-19 is incompletely understood, and much of what is known is based on knowledge related to other coronaviruses, which like SARS-CoV-2, have spike proteins on their outer coat that contribute to infectivity and transmission. SARS-CoV-2 primarily infects the upper and lower respiratory tracts and GI tract of hosts, given its propensity to attach to angiotensin-converting enzyme 2 (ACE 2) cellular receptors located in these regions. The main spike protein involved in its virulence is the S protein, which attaches to host cells and allows the virus to invade the cell. Once a patient is infected with SARS-CoV-2, the median incubation period is 5 days but can be as long as 14 days, during which patients can readily transmit the virus, with over 50% of transmission occurring during this time. Because of this high risk of infectivity, social distancing, the use of face masks, and proper hand hygiene are highly encouraged to prevent spread both from symptomatic as well as asymptomatic infected individuals. Of note, genetic changes to SARS-CoV-2 spike proteins have led to new variants of the virus with differing rates of infectivity and response to treatment and prevention measures, such as vaccination.

CLINICAL PRESENTATION

Pneumonias may be classified as two syndromes according to clinical presentation, typical and atypical, which are very similar. However, the characteristics of these clinical manifestations have some diagnostic value.

Subjective

The "typical" pneumonia syndrome is seen in pneumococcal pneumonia, as well as in pneumonia caused by *H. influenzae* and *S. aureus* (Box 30.3). The syndrome is characterized by a sudden onset of fever, cough, chest pain, and fatigue. Generally, patients with a productive cough are more likely to have a bacterial infection. Patients with pneumococcal pneumonia produce sputum that has a characteristic rusty coloration; purulent sputum may also be evident. Fever may run as high as 106°F (41.1°C), with peaks observed in the afternoon or evening. The chest pain tends to be pleuritic in nature and increases in intensity during coughing or on inspiration. Patients often feel cold; about half experience teeth-chattering, shaking, and chills. Myalgia is a common complaint and may extend to tenderness in the calves and thighs. Severe myalgia, particularly when accompanied by vomiting, strongly suggests the possibility of bacteremia. Respiratory and nonrespiratory symptoms are less commonly reported by older patients with pneumonia. Older patients may not show the typical febrile response (chills and sweats) or report pain (myalgia, headache, and chest pain). Although the older adult may present with attenuated symptoms, this should not be misconstrued as an indication that such patients are less ill.

"Atypical" pneumonia is most commonly caused by *M. pneumoniae* but can also be caused by *L. pneumophila, C. pneumoniae, P. jiroveci,* and viruses. The atypical pneumonia syndrome is characterized by a more gradual onset of dry "hacking" cough, fever, and prominence of constitutional symptoms (e.g., pounding headaches, coryza, sore throat, shaking chills, and myalgia).

Pneumonias caused by anaerobic infections usually present with subacute or chronic constitutional and pulmonary symptoms. A chronic cough that produces purulent sputum is reported by the majority of patients.

Box 30.3	Typical Pneumonia Syndrome Associated With Pneumococcal Pneumonia
Subjective Findings	**Objective Findings**
Sudden onset of fever (may be blunted in older adults)	Crackles
	Dullness on percussion
	Bronchophony, egophony, whispered pectoriloquy
Productive cough	
Rust-colored or purulent sputum	Pleural friction rub (severe consolidation)
Pleuritic-type chest pain	Decreased or absent breath sounds
Splinting	
Chills	Dense, homogenous shadows in one or more lung lobes on chest x-ray
Myalgia	

Between 30% and 60% of patients report putrid sputum. This finding is considered to be diagnostic of an anaerobic infection and is associated with the development of tissue necrosis and cavitary lesions. Patients also present with dull or pleuritic chest pain, hemoptysis, anemia, leukocytosis, and weight loss.

Patients with PCP present with fever, sweats, weight loss, nonproductive cough, decreasing exercise tolerance, and dyspnea on exertion. The median duration of symptoms is 1 month. Tachypnea is common and is worsened by activity.

COVID-19 presents with a multitude of symptoms typical of respiratory viruses, although its manifestations vary depending on the severity of illness. The most common presenting symptoms are cough (70%), fever (44%), fatigue (38%), and dyspnea (20%), followed by other respiratory, GI, and neurological symptoms, including malaise, weakness, sore throat, nasal congestion, nausea, vomiting, diarrhea, headaches, confusion, and loss of sense of taste and/or smell. Of note, patients infected with SARS-CoV-2 have a period of time (median of 5 days) during which they are presymptomatic before developing acute symptoms. Indeed, patients can remain asymptomatic throughout their entire course of infection, yet still transmit SARS-CoV-2. This varied clinical presentation makes COVID-19 difficult to diagnose without confirmatory testing.

Objective

Physical examination of a person with typical pneumonia syndrome usually reveals an acutely ill patient who complains of chest pain and often demonstrates respiratory splinting on one side of the thorax. In some patients, crackles and dullness to percussion may be the only abnormality, particularly early in the disease process. This finding may correspond with an outpouring of fluid into the alveoli. A second group of patients shows the classic signs of consolidation: egophony (increased resonance of voice sounds on auscultation), bronchophony (increased volume or persistent loudness of the patient's voice throughout the lung fields and especially toward the periphery), whispered pectoriloquy (increased loudness of whispering on auscultation), bronchial breath sounds (tubular or hollow breath sounds over the large airways), and dullness on percussion. In patients with severe consolidation, crackles may be absent or minimal, and a leathery pleural friction rub may be heard over the area of chest tenderness. Finally, a third group of patients has one or more areas of dullness, inspiratory crackles, and diminished breath sounds, which are signs of mucous plugs in the smaller bronchioles.

Objective findings in atypical pneumonia tend to be less pronounced. Fine to medium crackles may be heard early or at the very end of the inspiratory cycle. Dullness on percussion and crackles or wheezing are more likely to be observed later in the disease course. Frank consolidation, pleural friction rubs, and pleural effusions are less common than in a typical pneumonia.

Although there is no "typical" syndrome of nosocomial pneumonia, one or more of the following clinical findings are present in most patients: fever, leukocytosis, purulent sputum, and a new pulmonary infiltrate on chest x-ray. These findings must occur more than 48 hours after admission to the hospital to be considered suggestive of nosocomial pneumonia.

Auscultation of the lungs is generally negative in patients with PCP, although fine crackles may occasionally be heard. Mucocutaneous lesions such as oral thrush, hairy leukoplakia, and Kaposi's sarcoma are common and suggest the presence of underlying HIV-related immunodeficiency in previously undiagnosed individuals. Physiologically, patients manifest arterial hypoxemia.

Physical signs and examination findings of COVID-19 are nonspecific and, as with its symptoms, mimic a viral illness. Fever is one of the most common presenting signs, whereas others include tachypnea, hypoxia, tachycardia, pharyngeal erythema, tonsillar swelling, lethargy, altered mental status, signs of dehydration, crackles or wheezing on lung auscultation, and rash. Extrapulmonary manifestations of COVID-19 include acute coronary syndrome, myocarditis, thrombotic complications such as deep venous thrombosis or pulmonary embolus, stroke, encephalopathy, and acute kidney injury. With these manifestations, patients will demonstrate signs (and symptoms) consistent with these disease processes.

DIAGNOSTIC REASONING

Diagnostic Tests

Initial Testing

Although a specific etiological diagnosis is optimal in the management of CAP, limitations in diagnostic testing make this difficult. The responsible microbe is not identified in approximately 50% of patients, even when extensive diagnostic tests are performed. The three most helpful tests used in the initial establishment of a diagnosis of pneumonia include chest x-ray, leukocyte count, and Gram stain of sputum specimens.

The chest x-ray study is important for three reasons. First, it may help distinguish whether the pneumonia is bacterial or viral in nature. Lobar infiltrates strongly suggest a bacterial infection. A bacterial pneumonia will show dense homogeneous shadows involving one or more lobes. Diffuse interstitial infiltrates are suggestive of a viral, *Mycoplasma,* or *Chlamydia* infection. Lateral and anterior-posterior views are necessary to evaluate lesions lying directly behind the heart.

A second reason for a chest x-ray study is to rule out a pleural effusion, a complication occurring in approximately one-third of pneumococcal pneumonia patients. It is important to note that chest x-ray films may be normal in patients who are unable to mount an inflammatory response or early in an infiltrative process. Follow-up chest x-ray films are needed to see whether the infiltrate clears completely. Younger patients and those with only single-lobe involvement tend to have earlier resolutions.

Third, cavities may be seen on chest x-ray films in patients with pneumonia caused by anaerobes, *S. aureus*, *S. pneumoniae* serotype III, *M. tuberculosis*, aerobic gram-negative bacilli, and fungi. Cavities occur when necrotic material is discharged into airways, resulting in a necrotizing pneumonia (multiple small cavities, each smaller than 2 cm) or lung abscess (one or more cavities larger than 2 cm). Anaerobic abscesses are located in dependent segments, are most frequently seen in the right lung, and have air-fluid levels. Typical and atypical forms of tuberculosis (TB) produce unilateral, well-drained, upper lobe fibrocavitary disease. Cavities are rarely produced by *H. influenzae*, *M. pneumoniae*, viruses, and other serotypes of *S. pneumoniae*.

Although pulmonary infiltrates on x-ray films are considered suggestive of nosocomial pneumonia, findings tend to be very nonspecific. Conditions such as atelectasis, pleural effusion, pulmonary thromboembolism, and pulmonary edema may mimic nosocomial pneumonia on x-ray evaluation.

It may not always be practical or feasible to obtain a chest x-ray study, so good clinical judgment is essential. Factors that have been found to be predictive of pneumonia infiltrates on chest films include fever higher than 100°F (37.8°C), tachycardia, locally decreased breath sounds, and sputum production. Chest x-ray films may be normal when the patient is unable to mount an inflammatory response (e.g., in agranulocytosis), is in the early stages of an infiltrative process, or has PCP associated with AIDS.

To help identify patients who need hospitalization, a CBC with differential should be done. The count may aid in differentiating between bacterial and viral pneumonia. Although there is no clear distinction, total white blood cell counts of more than 15,000 cells/μL suggest a bacterial infection. A differential cell count is not a reliable indicator of causation. Leukopenia may be seen in severe infections, as well as in patients with alcohol use disorder, older adults, and malnourished individuals. Blood cultures are indicated only for patients who require hospitalization or for cases of suspected nosocomial pneumonia.

A Gram stain of sputum is a widely available diagnostic tool for practitioners at the onset of therapy. Caution needs to be exercised in the evaluation of a sputum specimen because expectorated material is frequently contaminated by bacteria that normally colonize the upper and lower respiratory tracts. Large numbers of epithelial cells (more than 25 cells per low-power field) reflect contamination of the specimen with oral contents and mandate that another specimen be collected. If the sputum has been properly collected, polymorphonuclear leukocytes can be readily seen with a Gram stain. The characteristic lancet-shaped gram-positive diplococci associated with pneumococcal pneumonia are generally seen in abundance. In contrast, Gram stains are seldom useful in patients with atypical pneumonia because sputum is scant and most organisms that cause this syndrome cannot be detected by a Gram stain. For example, acid-fast staining of sputum should be done when mycobacterial infection is suspected (see Advanced Assessment 30.1).

A sputum culture is less valuable than a Gram stain for providing a causal diagnosis in bacterial pneumonia. Approximately 50% of patients with pneumococcal pneumonia have negative sputum cultures, even when large numbers of organisms are present on Gram stain. Sputum cultures are also negative in 35% to 50% of cases of proven *H. influenzae* pneumonia. Isolation of the causative agent in atypical pneumonia is rare.

Sputum cultures may be valuable in the diagnosis of subacute and cavitary pneumonia. Mycobacteria grow well on specialized culture media, and it has been estimated that sputum cultures can detect as few as 10 acid-fast bacilli (AFB) per milliliter of concentrated sputum. For a more in-depth discussion of the use of sputum

Advanced Assessment 30.1: Sputum Staining

Sputum Stain	Organism
Gram stain	*Streptococcus pneumoniae* (gram-positive, lancet-shaped diplococci) *Haemophilus influenzae* (gram-positive coccobacilli) *Staphylococcus aureus* (gram-positive tetrads and grapelike clusters)
Acid-fast stain	Mycobacterial infection
Direct fluorescent antibody stain	Viral respiratory culture
Fluorescent antibody: sensitivity diminished with concurrent use of inhaled pentamidine	*Legionella* infection
Wright-Giemsa stain: frequent false-positive and false-negative results	PCP
Gomori's methenamine silver	Fungal growth (living and dead organisms)
Periodic acid-Schiff stain	Fungal growth (living organisms only)

cultures for the isolation of mycobacteria, refer to the section on tuberculosis.

The usefulness of fungal cultures varies with the organism and the stage of the disease. Chronic forms of coccidioidomycosis and blastomycosis may yield positive cultures in 70% to 100% of cases if multiple specimens are collected. However, positive cultures are not found in patients with histoplasmosis until the disease is in the chronic, cavitary stage. Fewer than 50% of patients with cryptococcosis have positive sputum cultures.

Expectorated sputum is usually collected in patients with a productive, vigorous cough, but may be scant in those with atypical pneumonia syndrome, in older adults, and in patients with altered mental status. If the patient is not producing sputum and can cooperate, respiratory secretions can be induced with ultrasonic nebulization of 3% saline solution. The use of more invasive procedures to induce sputum in the patient who is unable to produce a spontaneous sputum specimen carries risks that must be weighed against the potential benefits. In patients who do not require hospitalization or in hospitalized patients who are not severely ill, the need to establish an accurate microbial diagnosis may not be crucial, and empiric therapy can be started on the basis of clinical and epidemiological evidence alone. Patients who are hospitalized with CAP and are seriously ill or those who acquire a nosocomial pneumonia clearly need to have a specific causal diagnosis established. In these patients, it may be necessary to obtain specimens from the lower respiratory tract by fiber-optic bronchoscopy, transtracheal puncture, or percutaneous transthoracic lung puncture. Of these invasive procedures, fiber-optic bronchoscopy is currently the preferred technique for obtaining lower respiratory tract secretions. Specimens obtained by bronchoscopy should be tested with Gram and acid-fast stains, *Legionella* direct fluorescent antibody, and Gomori's methenamine silver stains and should be cultured for aerobic and anaerobic bacteria, *Legionella*, mycobacteria, and fungi.

Diagnostic testing for CAP caused by *S. pneumoniae* may include a pneumococcal urinary antigen test that can detect a protein common to all pneumococcal serotypes. Within 15 minutes, this test can demonstrate the presence of pneumococcus in unconcentrated urine. This can facilitate more immediate decisions about antibiotic therapy. However, the sensitivity of this test varies, and it should be used in addition to sputum and/or blood culture. Urinary antigen testing is also available for the gram-negative bacteria *L. pneumophila* (but only for serogroup 1, which may not capture all forms of the disease), as well as the fungus *Histoplasma*.

Diagnostic testing for SARS-CoV-2 is obtained via a nasopharyngeal swab for nucleic acid testing, as recommended by the CDC. With this swab, viral RNA can be detected via reverse transcription polymerase chain reaction testing (RT-PCR). Lower respiratory tract specimens can also be obtained from patients with a productive cough, from bronchoalveolar lavage, or tracheal aspirates. The sensitivity and specificity of the particular diagnostic test depends on multiple factors, including sampling technique and viral burden. False negatives may be seen in asymptomatic patients and those early in the course of the disease. The sensitivity of the RT-PCR COVID-19 test has been reported to be 60% to 80%. Thus, a single negative RT-PCR test result should not be used to exclude COVID-19, especially in asymptomatic patients or those thought to be early in the course of the disease. However, if a patient is symptomatic and has a negative RT-PCR result, it is unlikely that the patient is infected with COVID-19. Other swab-based testing is available, including rapid antigen testing, which detects specific SARS-CoV-2 antigens; however, rapid tests tend to have lower sensitivity compared with RT-PCR testing. Finally, serological testing is also available to detect COVID-19-related antibodies. Antibody testing is useful for determining immunity from previous infection, identifying asymptomatic infections, and determining the efficacy of vaccination. However, serological testing is less useful in diagnosing acute infection with SARS-CoV-2, as a patient may not have mounted a sufficient immune response early in infection. However, later in the disease course, the sensitivity and specificity of serological testing may be greater than 90% in detecting IgA, IgM, or IgG antibodies.

Subsequent Testing

If the pneumonia is severe enough to require hospitalization, at least two blood samples should be obtained for culture, as well as a CBC and serological analysis of sodium, urea, nitrogen, creatinine, and glucose. Liver and enzyme tests should be included if hepatic disease or malnutrition is suspected. Serological studies are sometimes helpful in defining the etiology of certain types of pneumonia. An IgM or IgG titer obtained by indirect immunofluorescence may be diagnostic of *M. pneumoniae* or *C. pneumoniae*. A *Legionella* antibody titer or a urinary antigen test may help confirm Legionnaires' disease.

Pulse oximetry is indicated if the patient presents with respiratory distress, dyspnea at rest, or tachypnea or if the chest x-ray film shows multilobar pulmonary infiltrates. A blood gas analysis should be performed if the patient has known carbon dioxide (CO_2) retention, exacerbations of asthma, or COPD. Typically, an Sao_2 of less than 90% or a Pao_2 of less than 60 mm Hg indicates the need for supplemental oxygen. These threshold values must be modified if the patient is chronically hypoxemic.

In COVID-19 patients, a number of laboratory tests may be abnormal, including absolute lymphocyte count (ALC), albumin, and platelet count, which all may be low; in particular, a low ALC can be a marker of severe COVID-19. Tests that are often abnormally elevated include white blood cell count, neutrophil count, lactate dehydrogenase (LDH), D-dimer, ferritin, C-reactive protein (CRP), erythrocyte sedimentation rate (ESR), liver function tests, and prothrombin time, as well as partial thromboplastin time. Elevated inflammatory markers may indicate more severe illness or the onset of cytokine storm, a complication of COVID-19. Elevated coagulation parameters such as D-dimer may be indicative of a thromboembolic process. Other laboratory tests that may be abnormally elevated include total bilirubin, creatinine kinase, and creatinine (which may be elevated in the setting of COVID-19-related acute kidney injury). Troponin and brain natriuretic peptide levels may be elevated in patients with cardiac involvement, and an arterial blood gas will reveal hypoxemia in patients with moderate to severe COVID-19.

The most commonly obtained imaging study in COVID-19 patients is a chest x-ray, which is often normal but may also have a number of findings, depending on the extent of disease. These may include bilateral ground-glass opacities, bilateral infiltrates, interstitial abnormalities, or areas of consolidation. Other imaging findings related to COVID-19 include pleural effusions, pneumothoraces, or subcutaneous emphysema. Computed tomography (CT) scan of the chest and lung ultrasound can also be utilized as diagnostic imaging. A chest CT scan will show similar findings as a chest x-ray, including ground-glass opacities and bilateral involvement. It may also show a "crazy paving pattern" due to ground-glass opacities with superimposed inter- and intralobular thickening.

Differential Diagnosis

Acute bacterial pneumonia should be differentiated from acute bacterial bronchitis. Both respiratory infections will cause fever and a productive cough. On auscultation, however, a patient with bronchitis will have clear lung sounds except for a few scattered rhonchi and possibly tubular sounds. In comparison, the patient with bacterial pneumonia will likely have crackles, abnormal breath sounds, and dullness to percussion. Cavitary forms of pneumonia need to be differentiated from pulmonary TB and systemic mycoses, particularly coccidioidomycosis and histoplasmosis. Likewise, the patient who presents with symptoms of PCP and a history of fever, weight loss, and pulmonary symptoms should be concurrently evaluated for TB, lymphomas, and brucellosis, in addition to HIV infection. Signs and symptoms secondary to central or endobronchial growth of a primary lung cancer will mimic those of a bacterial pneumonia (e.g., productive cough, fever, dyspnea, hemoptysis). The practitioner needs to be aware of any occupational or environmental hazards to which the patient is exposed. For example, workers who develop berylliosis through exposure to beryllium (found in ceramics, high-technology electronics, and alloy manufacturing) may present with an acute pneumonia or, more commonly, with a chronic interstitial pneumonia. Exposure to moldy hay can result in symptoms of pneumonia (e.g., coughing, fever, chills, malaise, and dyspnea) within 4 to 8 hours after exposure, due to a severe allergic reaction to the dust or mold on the hay. This disease (known as "farmer's lung") may become chronic.

SARS caused by SARS-CoV-1 and COVID-19 caused by SARS-CoV-2 should also be ruled out. Patients should be questioned about travel to an area with known transmission of these coronaviruses, as well as close contact with an infected person. The clinical presentation of COVID-19 was described earlier; symptoms of SARS include fever greater than 100.5°F (38°C), cough, or respiratory distress. Thus, these conditions are difficult to distinguish on the basis of clinical presentation and, rather, are differentiated primarily through exposure history and diagnostic testing. As the treatment of SARS and most COVID-19 cases is primarily supportive, identification of the specific causative coronavirus agent is critical from a public health perspective to prevent further viral transmission.

Pediatric/Adolescent Considerations: COVID-19 in Children and Adolescents

As COVID-19 first emerged, it was apparent that children were significantly less affected than adults, including demonstrating a much lower mortality rate, as the large majority of pediatric patients were asymptomatic or had only a mild illness. However, during the pandemic, a new condition emerged related to COVID-19 in children, called *multisystem inflammatory syndrome in children* (MIS-C). Initial reports of MIS-C arose in Europe and then quickly surfaced in the United States. MIS-C is a rare inflammatory condition of multiple organ systems, described as being similar to Kawasaki disease or toxic shock syndrome. The most common presenting symptoms of MIS-C are GI symptoms (e.g., abdominal pain, nausea, vomiting, diarrhea) and fever, although patients can present with a multitude of other severe symptoms including cardiac (e.g., coronary artery dilation, aneurysms, arrhythmias, ventricular dysfunction) and mucocutaneous (e.g., rash, conjunctivitis) manifestations, as well as lymphadenopathy and elevated inflammatory markers.

The case definition of MIS-C includes the following: younger than 21 years old, fever of greater than 38°C for at least 24 hours, laboratory evidence of at least one abnormal inflammatory marker (e.g., elevation in ESR, CRP, ferritin, D-dimer, LDH, procalcitonin, fibrinogen, interleukin [IL]-6, or neutrophil count; reduction in lymphocyte count or serum albumin), evidence of severe disease with multisystem involvement (two or more bodily systems: cardiac, renal, respiratory, hematological, GI, dermatological, or neurological), with no plausible alternative diagnosis and at least one of the following: positive RT-PCR, antigen test, or serology for SARS-CoV-2 or exposure to suspected or confirmed COVID-19 case within 4 weeks before

Continued

symptom onset. Many cases of MIS-C develop weeks after exposure or diagnosis of COVID-19, implicating an immune-mediated etiology versus a direct infectious response to the virus. Therapies for MIS-C are being actively studied, and typical treatments include IV immunoglobulin and aspirin, although their therapeutic benefits are unclear.

Although the pediatric population as a whole has been less affected than adults by COVID-19 in terms of number of cases and severity of illness, children have experienced other untoward effects thought to be related to the COVID-19 pandemic. Restrictions on movement and social interaction during the pandemic (e.g., social distancing, school closures, stay-at-home directives) have led to increased stress for families and children. This has been compounded by other family-based stressors including loss of health insurance, food insecurity, worsened health and wellness factors, decreased quality of education, and a reduction in community-based support programs. In turn, this has led to impaired childhood socialization and increased rates of mental health conditions and suicide in pediatric patients, especially in adolescents. Child abuse rates have also increased during the COVID-19 pandemic, including nonaccidental trauma and neglect. This may relate to heightened family stress and increased rates of substance abuse during the pandemic. Calls to poison control centers for pediatric poisonings have also increased. Moreover, access to mental health services has been curtailed in many instances due to social distancing restrictions and decreased in-person care, limiting both the treatment and follow-up of mental health disorders and addiction problems. Despite this, our knowledge of SARS-CoV-2 infection continues to evolve, as does our understanding and approach to pediatric COVID-19 patients, and the pediatric population as a whole to mitigate these challenges.

MANAGEMENT

The initial task in the management of patients with CAP is to determine whether the person can be treated on an outpatient basis or whether hospitalization is required. The use of hospital services is costly and may further impair the patient's health because of the risk of nosocomial infections. The majority of patients with CAP with no comorbidity can be treated successfully as outpatients. Most patients, even those treated initially in a hospital, prefer outpatient treatment.

The decision to hospitalize a patient with CAP may be the single most important decision during the entire course of the illness. Scoring systems are helpful in determining the site-of-care decision. The CURB-65 criteria to determine the severity of CAP is an objective, easy tool to remember. The calculator takes into account **C**onfusion, **B**UN (blood urea nitrogen), **R**espiratory rate, Systolic **B**P (blood pressure),

and age. The calculator for this may be found at https://www.mdcalc.com/curb-65-score-pneumonia-severity. Additionally, at the end of the calculation, it asks for clarification of whether this is a COVID-19 patient, given the unique considerations of that patient population. The severity of illness will help determine in what setting treatment should take place. In addition, known risk factors for CAP-associated mortality and complications are summarized in the accompanying text.

Risk Factors for CAP-associated Mortality and Complications

Age: Older than 65 years
Presence of coexisting illness:

- Chronic pulmonary disease
- Diabetes mellitus
- Chronic renal failure
- Congestive heart failure
- Chronic liver disease of any etiology
- Previous hospitalization within 1 year of the onset of pneumonia
- Suspicion of aspiration
- Altered mental status
- Postsplenectomy state
- Chronic alcohol abuse or malnutrition

Abnormal physical findings:

- Respiratory rate greater than 30 breaths/min
- Diastolic BP 60 mm Hg or below and/or systolic BP 90 mm Hg or below
- Temperature greater than 101°F (38.3°C)
- Evidence of extrapulmonary sites of disease (e.g., septic arthritis, meningitis)
- Decreased level of consciousness or confusion

Abnormal laboratory findings:

- White blood cell count less than 4×10^9/L or greater than 30×10^9/L
- Pao_2 less than 60 mm Hg or $Paco_2$ greater than 50 mm Hg on room air
- Hemoglobin less than 9 g/dL
- X-ray showing involvement of more than one lobe, pleural effusion, or evidence of rapid spreading
- Severe electrolyte or renal abnormality not known to be chronic (e.g., BUN greater than 50 mg/dL, creatinine greater than 1.2 mg/dL, sodium less than 130 mEq/L)

Antimicrobial therapy represents the mainstay of treatment for patients with suspected or confirmed pneumonia. Additional management is supportive and includes the use of analgesics for relief of chest pain and myalgia, antipyretics to control fever, increased fluid intake (typically at least 3 L over 24 hours), restricted activity or bedrest, a position of comfort (usually seated or lying upright) to facilitate breathing, and humidified air to relieve irritated nares and pharynx. Expectorants may be indicated to decrease sputum viscosity and clear airways if a productive cough is present. Although many promote the use of expectorants, the most cost-effective way to liquefy secretions for ease of coughing and elimination of secretions is hydration with water. Patients experiencing a dry, nonproductive cough may benefit from a cough suppressant with codeine if expectoration is not deemed necessary.

Patients requiring hospitalization need to have ongoing assessment for any indications of impaired respiratory status. Patients who manifest arterial hypoxemia will require supplemental oxygen therapy to attempt to maintain a Po_2 greater than 80 mm Hg. In the past, chest physiotherapy had been widely used to mobilize secretions. However, percussion and postural drainage probably offer no added benefit to the patient who has an uncomplicated pneumonia without underlying pulmonary disease.

Treatment Guidelines for Community-Acquired Pneumonia

The Infectious Diseases Society of America has recommended specific therapy for CAP (Metlay et al, 2019). Before initiating treatment, the clinician must determine whether the patient has had recent antibiotic therapy and any coexisting diseases that may be present, such as COPD or congestive heart failure. The Treatment Standards/Guidelines box summarizes the empiric treatment of the patient with CAP.

Treatment Standards/Guidelines: Empiric Antimicrobial Choices for Community-Acquired Pneumonia (CAP)

PATIENTS	STANDARD REGIMEN
No comorbidities nor risk factors for MRSA or *Pseudomonas*	Monotherapy with amoxicillin or doxycycline or macrolide antibiotic
With comorbidities, e.g., chronic heart, lung, liver, or renal disease, diabetes mellitus, alcoholism, malignancy, or asplenia	Combination therapy with amoxicillin/clavulanate or cephalosporin AND macrolide or doxycycline OR monotherapy with respiratory fluoroquinolone

Source: Metlay JP, Waterer GW, Long AC, et al. Diagnosis and treatment of adults with community-acquired pneumonia. An official clinical practice guideline of the American Thoracic Society and Infectious Diseases Society of America. Am J Respir Crit Care Med. 2019;200(7):e45–e67.

Highly penicillin-resistant *S. pneumoniae* strains are a rare cause of CAP because most *S. pneumoniae* strains remain susceptible to ceftriaxone. Preferred monotherapy for CAP includes doxycycline or a respiratory quinolone. These are the most cost-effective ways to optimally treat CAP. They are well-tolerated in oral and IV forms and are ideal for IV-to-oral switch monotherapy in terms of patient compliance, safety, and cost. Use of proton pump inhibitors (PPIs) for gastric protection should be avoided when using respiratory quinolones for CAP drug therapy because they may alter drug levels. PPIs should be stopped and a histamine$_2$ (H$_2$) receptor blocker may be used for the duration of therapy. However, there is conflicting evidence regarding the relative safety of PPIs and H$_2$ blockers.

Treatment regimens for community-acquired MRSA pneumonia should typically start with vancomycin until results of sensitivity testing are available, which may indicate susceptibility to sulfamethoxazole-trimethoprim (Bactrim). Most recently, guidelines have established linezolid (Zyvox) as an effective alternative therapy for susceptible vancomycin-resistant infections, including CAP.

Subsequent Management

Pneumonia that is associated with bacteremia, leukopenia, or multilobar involvement has an increased likelihood of complications and death. The mortality rate for patients older than 65 years with bacteremia and involvement of more than three lobes is approximately 60%. Complications are more frequently found in patients with underlying chronic diseases.

The radiographic resolution of CAP is complete in half of patients after 2 weeks and in two-thirds of patients after 4 weeks. Follow-up x-ray studies should be done within 3 to 6 months for all patients who smoke or are older than age 40 years. If an abnormality has not cleared on follow-up films, the patient should be evaluated for possible cancer or other noninfectious diagnosis.

Pleural effusion represents the most common complication seen in patients with pneumonia. Fluid can be detected radiographically in the pleural space of more than 40% of patients hospitalized with pneumonia. In most cases, the amount is so small that needle aspiration is unsuccessful. If fluid is removed, it is typically not purulent, nor can microbes be seen on Gram stain.

Fluid that is purulent and has a gram-positive stain or a pH of less than 7.1 is indicative of an empyema. *S. pneumoniae*, *S. pyogenes*, and anaerobic pneumonias are associated with most cases of empyema. It is critical that the infected material be removed from the pleural space by means of a thoracentesis, needle aspiration, or thoracotomy. If this treatment is delayed, the patient is likely to require a prolonged hospital stay. Lung abscesses develop infrequently in *S. pneumoniae* but often occur as complications of pneumonias caused by gram-negative bacteria (e.g., *Klebsiella*), anaerobic bacteria, and

S. aureus. Drainage of an abscess is essential to prevent further necrosis of lung tissue, and prolonged antimicrobial therapy is critical for the successful treatment of this complication.

Delayed resolution results from persistent infection and is seen on x-ray studies as residual consolidation. Delayed resolution occurs most often in the patient who is older, malnourished, alcoholic, or who has COPD. Progression of infiltrates despite antimicrobial therapy is a poor prognostic sign.

Distal spread of infection tends to occur in the meninges, pericardium, heart valves, and skeletal system. Although these complications occur less frequently with antimicrobial therapy, persons with compromised health status remain at risk for the development of spreading infection, which can manifest as septic arthritis, pericarditis, endocarditis, and meningitis. Patients who develop septic arthritis will experience swollen, red, and painful joints, and purulent exudate may be aspirated from the joints. Similarly, meningitis caused by *S. pneumoniae* produces purulent cerebrospinal fluid. Thus, patients with pneumococcal pneumonia who become disoriented, confused, or somnolent should have a lumbar puncture to assess for meningitis.

Treatment of COVID-19

No specific treatment is curative for COVID-19. Highly efficacious vaccines, which were rapidly developed using both established and novel delivery platforms, include vaccines from Pfizer-BioNTech, Moderna, and Johnson & Johnson (Janssen). However, the mainstay of treatment for acute COVID-19 is supportive care, particularly regarding respiratory support. Four anti-SARS-CoV-2 monoclonal antibody products are currently approved by the U.S. Food and Drug Administration (FDA) for the treatment of COVID-19 and are most effective if given early in the course of disease, although their efficacy varies against different variants of SARS-CoV-2. Many therapies are still undergoing active study in ongoing clinical trials and require additional data to support their widespread use.

Patients suspected of having COVID-19 (person under investigation [PUI]) should be evaluated and treated by a health-care provider wearing full personal protective equipment (PPE). Patients should also be wearing a face mask. Suspected COVID-19 patients should be separated from other patients by at least 6 feet and ideally in an isolation room. A PUI who is critically ill or requires aerosol-generating procedures, such as intubation, should be evaluated and treated in airborne isolation rooms (i.e., negative pressure rooms). Providers should practice vigorous hand sanitizing procedures (either using an alcohol-based hand sanitizer or hand washing with soap and water) before and after evaluation or treatment of a PUI or known COVID-19 patient.

Patients who present with mild illness and no hypoxia or respiratory distress should receive supportive care and other symptomatic treatments, such as fever control with acetaminophen or NSAIDs. For more significant disease with hypoxia, oxygen therapy is recommended. The goal oxygen saturation is greater than 90% and no higher than 96%. Clinicians can start with oxygen delivery methods such as nasal cannula or various oxygen masks if patients do not have significant work of breathing or require a higher level of respiratory support. For patients who have progressive respiratory failure, oxygen delivery via high-flow nasal cannula (HFNC) is recommended over noninvasive positive pressure ventilation (NIPPV). The risk of aerosolization is lower with HFNC compared with NIPPV and is likely low; however, all patients on either low-flow or high-flow nasal cannula should wear a face mask. FIO_2 and flow rates for HFNC can be titrated to achieve oxygenation goals as well as decrease work of breathing. If patients fail these measures or are in severe respiratory distress or failure, intubation and mechanical ventilation is required. Overresuscitation with IV fluids should be avoided, and vasopressor therapy may be needed in critical care settings. Antibiotics are not indicated unless the patient has severe illness, shock, or suspected secondary bacterial infection. Other types of supportive care may be needed in critically ill patients, including nutrition, GI prophylaxis, anticoagulation prophylaxis, and renal support.

Although the large majority of COVID-19 cases are mild and do not require hospitalization, most COVID-19-specific therapies are approved for administration in hospital settings requiring a higher level of care. Dexamethasone confers a mortality benefit to hypoxic COVID-19 patients on mechanical ventilation. Remdesivir (Veklury) is an approved IV antiviral medication that may lead to decreased symptoms and improved outcomes in hospitalized, oxygen-dependent COVID-19 patients aged 12 years and older; it is most effective early in the course of SARS-CoV-2 infection. Convalescent plasma is another consideration for treatment of COVID-19 patients early in the course of illness; this therapy consists of protective antibodies collected from recovered COVID-19 patients. Oral Janus kinase (JAK) inhibitors, such as baricitinib (Olumiant), may have a role in decreasing the severe cytokine-release inflammatory response (i.e., cytokine storm) of COVID-19. Anti-SARS-CoV-2 monoclonal antibodies (mAb), including the combination therapies bamlanivimab/etesevimab and casirivimab/imdevimab, are being used with increasing frequency to treat nonhospitalized mild to moderate COVID-19 patients, due to their emergency use authorization by the FDA. They are used for both treatment and prevention and have been shown to decrease symptom progression and viral load in patients with mild COVID-19. One of them, sotrovimab (Xevudy) is expected to retain efficacy against the highly transmissible omicron variant, which has proven more resistant to other anti-COVID-19 mAb therapies.

In summary, current recommendations support the use of anti–SARS-CoV-2 mAb for nonhospitalized patients with mild to moderate COVID-19. If patients are hospitalized, it is recommended they receive remdesivir, and if they are hypoxic, dexamethasone should be added. If the patient cannot receive dexamethasone, treatment with a JAK inhibitor may be considered. With all of these treatments, however, the mainstay of therapy is supportive care, as therapeutic recommendations are rapidly changing and may differ, depending on the specific COVID-19 variant (e.g., delta, omicron) being treated.

Many other therapies have been used in the treatment of COVID-19, but are not fully supported by current recommendations and some have trial data pending. These include vitamin C, vitamin D, IL-6 receptor antagonists, zinc, ivermectin, lopinavir/ritonavir, and hydroxychloroquine. Finally, multiple SARS-CoV-2 vaccines have been developed in record time using multiple delivery platforms (e.g., RNA vaccines, adenoviral vectors). Both single-dose and multidose regimens have been granted emergency use authorization or full approval by the FDA and are available for widespread use. The COVID-19 RNA vaccines, in particular, have shown efficacy levels of greater than 90% in the reduction in symptomatic COVID-19. For the most current COVID-19 treatment and vaccination recommendations, the CDC and WHO continuously update their guidelines, as the treatment armamentarium against COVID-19 is rapidly evolving.

Nursing Situation: Impact of COVID-19: A Nurse's Perspective

Although the priority of the medical community is to reduce transmission of, diagnose, and treat COVID-19, there are many secondary effects of the crisis that need to be addressed. This global pandemic exposed many disparate social and health determinants, and nurses play an important role in the provision of care, not only in the acute setting of COVID-19 treatment but also in managing the holistic needs of these patients and their communities.

The art of nursing focuses on two key theoretical frameworks. The first is the concept of holistic care, which is the heart of nursing. It is described as the provision of care that recognizes a person as a whole and acknowledges the interdependence among one's biological, social, psychological, and spiritual aspects. Holistic care includes medication administration, patient and family/support person education, therapeutic communication, music therapy, and other adjuncts. In holistic nursing, it is important to assess and provide therapeutic interventions to the patient's thoughts, emotions, values, spirituality, and culture.

The second framework is relationship-based care. This is a transformational and operational model that promotes safety, quality, and the patient through human and compassionate care. The goal of this framework is to continue to provide patients with an extraordinary experience through relationship-building, therapeutic touch, caring conversations, and the seamless transition of care.

The global pandemic has shown the important role of nurses in leading the COVID-19 response around the globe. Nurses have been on the front line of the crisis, as they work across all health systems from the acute hospital setting to skilled and long-term care facilities, schools, public health offices, and governmental agencies. The following are just some of the contributions nurses have made to the COVID-19 pandemic:

1. **Prevention and early detection:** Nurses play an important role in community education, especially to high-risk populations. Screening services are conducted not only to prevent the transmission of disease but also to ensure that patients are provided emotional support, abuse prevention services, and mental wellness care.
2. **Surveillance and isolation:** Nurses are critical to ensuring isolation and Standard Precautions against infectious spread are followed. Nurses conduct contact tracing, monitoring of transmission, and prevention of nosocomial infection.
3. **Acute care for COVID-19 patients:** Nurses ensure timely assessment and treatment as ordered by the provider. Nursing-driven interventions such as mindfulness, provision of assistance for activities of daily living, and coordination of family/support network communication are prioritized. Numerous patients are placed in isolation, which denies them face-to-face contact with family members or support persons. Nurses use telehealth and video conference calls to facilitate human connection.
4. **Palliative and end-of-life care:** The nurse's role is to provide comfort and relief of symptoms. Nurses offer a wide range of services such as music therapy, coordination with religious and spiritual services, management of pain, and emotional support.
5. **Teamwork and collaboration:** The safety and quality of care that patients receive during a crisis depends on physicians and nurses; the concept of teamwork is integral. The Professional Practice Environment model proposes that the relationship between nurses and physicians is a positive quality indicator to preventing medical errors, which allows optimal care. Interdisciplinary collaboration is one of the most important recommendations of this model. It is a decision-making and communication process among clinicians that satisfies the needs of the patient while still respecting the unique abilities of each professional involved in the care.

Sources: Chen SC, Lai YH, Tsay SL. Nursing perspectives on the impacts of COVID-19. *J Nurs Res*. 2020 Jun;28(3):e85. doi: 10.1097/NRJ.0000000000000389. PMID: 32398577. Frisch N, Rabinowitsch D. What's in a definition? Holistic nursing, integrative health care, and integrative nursing: report of an integrated literature review. *J Holist Nurs*. 2019 Sep;37(3):260–272. doi: 10.1177/0898010119860685. Epub 2019 Jul 1. PMID: 31257971. Soklaridis S, Ravitz P, Adler Nevo G, et al. Relationship-centred care in health: a 20-year scoping review. *Patient Exp J*. 2016;3(1):16. doi: 10.35680/2372-0247.1111.

FOLLOW-UP AND REFERRAL

Patients considered well enough for outpatient treatment do not need to be closely monitored unless symptoms worsen despite antibiotic therapy. The patient should be contacted within 24 to 48 hours of starting therapy and should be scheduled for an office visit at 1 week and 4 to 6 weeks after the initial evaluation.

As mentioned, x-ray resolution of CAP is complete in 50% of patients after 2 weeks and in two-thirds of patients after 4 weeks. Examination at the second follow-up visit should include a chest x-ray film if clinical symptoms have not resolved. Follow-up x-ray evaluations for previous abnormalities should be done for all patients who smoke, and if an abnormality has not cleared on follow-up films, the patient should be evaluated for possible lung cancer.

COVID-19 infection, in particular, has been associated with long-term complications, especially in patients who developed severe pneumonia. Commonly termed "long COVID," these sequelae can manifest in a variety of organ systems including respiratory dysfunction (e.g., shortness of breath), neurological disorders and cognitive deficits, cardiovascular and metabolic disorders, gastrointestinal and musculoskeletal weakness, mental health disorders, debilitating fatigue or pain (e.g., headaches), and anosmia (loss of smell) or parosmia (distorted smell). Treatment guidelines for these long-term consequences of COVID-19 are rapidly evolving.

Smoking cessation is essential if respiratory health is to be maintained. Patients may be most receptive to antismoking counseling while they are still ill or recovering from pneumonia. Thus, the follow-up examination provides an opportune time for patient education. Pneumococcal and influenza vaccines should also be given at this time, if indicated.

Patient Education

The primary care practitioner should prioritize educating patients and their families or support persons on current immunization guidelines to prevent pneumonia. Annual influenza vaccine is strongly recommended for all individuals older than 6 months. The 2020 guidelines of the ACIP recommend one dose of the pneumococcal 23-valent polysaccharide vaccine (PPSV23) for persons 19 to 64 years of age with chronic medical conditions or a history of cigarette smoking. Individuals older than 19 years with compromised immune systems have a different schedule that includes one dose of the 13-valent PCV13 vaccine followed by one dose of PPSV23 vaccine 8 weeks later, then another dose 5 years after that. At the age of 65 years, individuals should have one dose of PPSV23 vaccine 5 years after their previous dose, although they only need one dose after the age of 65 years. Of note, almost 69% of adults over 65 years of age have received at least one pneumococcal vaccination. The interval between vaccines depends on the order in which the vaccines are given (see the ACIP Interval Guidelines cited in the reference section).

The increasing prevalence of multiantibiotic-resistant pneumococci makes immunization of high-risk individuals of the utmost importance. Vaccine use tends to increase when efforts are made to raise awareness and promote the benefits of vaccination. However, antivaccination movements and conspiracy theorists have become increasingly active in recent years and have been particularly successful in mounting campaigns based on nonscientific and unvalidated claims, which directly countermand long-accepted public health tenets. Thus, the need for clear and consistent patient education by primary care practitioners on the benefit-risk assessment of immunization is critical for both well-understood infectious diseases and emergent ones for which new vaccines are actively being developed, such as COVID-19. In turn, clinicians may obtain current and relevant data on pneumococcal vaccines, incidence rates of CAP and hospital-acquired pneumonia, drug therapy, and other related information by contacting the CDC, the National Institute on Aging, or the National Foundation for Infectious Diseases (see Resources).

TUBERCULOSIS

TB is one of the oldest human diseases. It is an infectious disease most frequently caused by *M. tuberculosis* in humans. In early writings, TB was called "consumption" because of its tendency to cause significant wasting in its victims. During the 18th and 19th centuries, it was known as the "white plague." TB is the leading cause of death worldwide from any single infectious agent. The pandemic of HIV infection and the emergence of drug-resistant TB strains have worsened the global problem of TB. One-third of the world's population is infected with TB, although not everyone infected with the mycobacteria becomes ill. Two conditions exist: latent TB infection (LTBI) and (active) TB. Active TB may be a primary infection or secondary reactivation of LTBI. In turn, individuals with LTBI who become immunocompromised may progress to active TB. The WHO has an "End TB" strategy for implementation from 2016 to 2035 that focuses on reducing the number of deaths by 90% and reducing the disease incidence by 80%, thereby reducing the catastrophic costs related to TB.

EPIDEMIOLOGY AND CAUSES

TB had once been considered to be under such good control that eradication of the disease in developing countries was considered an obtainable goal. Worldwide, the majority of infected persons are living in developing countries; about 75% of infected persons are younger than 50 years. Each year, 1.5 million people worldwide die of the disease, with one recent report indicating 10 million individuals became ill with TB within a year. TB is the most common HIV-associated opportunistic infection in many developing countries. Currently, the highest estimated case rates of TB occur in India.

According to the CDC, in the United States the number of reported TB cases in 2019 of 8,920 was the lowest recorded since national reporting began in 1953. Of these U.S. cases, just over 30% were in U.S.-born individuals, whereas almost 70% were in foreign-born persons. According to the WHO, half of all persons with TB are located in eight countries: Bangladesh, China, India, Indonesia, Nigeria, Pakistan, Philippines, and South Africa. In the United States, TB disproportionately affects patients belonging to underrepresented racial and ethnic groups, and the prevalence is three times higher in urban than rural populations. California, Florida, New York, and Texas are the four states with the most cases of TB, which relates in part to their receiving large volumes of traffic from out of the country into the United States. These states also have a proportionally higher number of patients with AIDS, which is a risk factor for reactivation TB. African Americans continue to experience a disproportionate share of TB cases.

Overall, approximately 5% to 15% of persons infected with *M. tuberculosis* will develop clinical TB at some point during their lifetime. About 5% of infected persons will manifest the disease within 1 year of infection. The remaining persons who develop the disease will have a delayed onset of TB, typically at a period of reduced protective immunity, which can occur as a result of silicosis, diabetes mellitus, cancer, HIV infection, advanced age, or the use of immunosuppressive drugs. Susceptibility to TB is also greater during the first 2 years of life, at puberty, and during adolescence.

Outbreaks of drug-resistant TB (i.e., resistant to at least one anti-TB drug) and multidrug-resistant TB (MDR-TB) (i.e., resistant to isoniazid [INH] and rifampin [RIF]) have occurred in hospitals, prisons, shelters for the homeless, nursing homes, and residential facilities for people with AIDS.

The genus *Mycobacterium* includes the causative agents of TB and leprosy. Mycobacteria are aerobic, asporogenous, nonmotile, acid-fast staining rods. Of the 58 species of the genus *Mycobacterium,* the members of the TB complex (*M. tuberculosis, M. bovis, M. africanum,* and *M. microti*) are known to be closely related, based on DNA homology studies. The TB complex depends on host transmission for its survival. *M. tuberculosis* is the major cause of human disease, whereas disease due to *M. bovis* is rare in the United States. *M. africanum* is a common cause of TB in Africa, and *M. microti* is a pathogen found primarily in rodents.

PATHOPHYSIOLOGY

M. tuberculosis strains vary in virulence due to differences in the bacteria's genetic makeup. Similarly, persons display varying susceptibility to TB infection due to genetically conferred resistance, age, and comorbid conditions (e.g., chronic illness, immunosuppression). *M. tuberculosis* is most commonly transmitted from person to person by droplet nuclei that are aerosolized by coughing, sneezing, or speaking. Person-to-person transmission is influenced by the intimacy and duration of contact, the degree of infectivity of the patient, and the shared contact environment. Patients with acid-fast staining organisms in their sputum are most infectious to others.

When *M. tuberculosis* organisms are first inhaled, some are expelled by the ciliated epithelium of the respiratory tract, and only a small fraction reaches the alveoli, leading to primary infection. There, alveolar macrophages attempt to phagocytose and contain the bacteria; however, virulent strains can multiply rapidly and overcome these macrophages by countering their oxidative bactericidal mechanisms. Nonetheless, activated macrophages react by releasing inflammatory mediators, such as IL-12 and tumor necrosis factor-alpha, which contribute to fever, anorexia, and weight loss. Macrophages also stimulate the recruitment of T lymphocytes to the area of infection. Helper T (CD4+) and cytotoxic killer T (CD8+) lymphocytes are also integral in the effort to kill mycobacteria. Activated macrophages and T lymphocytes form granulomas, or larger tubercles, in an effort to confine bacterial growth by walling off and containing the mycobacteria.

Within these tubercles, multiplication of the organisms is inhibited by low oxygen content and a low pH. T lymphocytes release inflammatory mediators that neutralize the mycobacteria contained in the tubercle's central necrotic area known as the caseum because of its cheese-like appearance on gross inspection. In a minority of cases, highly virulent strains of *M. tuberculosis* may cause rapid infection, invading lung parenchyma, bronchioles, and blood vessels. Hemoptysis, a frequent clinical sign of active infection, may reflect the erosion of a granuloma into a pulmonary blood vessel. Old granulomas eventually calcify, identifiable as one or more Ghon complexes on a chest x-ray. Known as LTBI, viable bacteria may remain dormant in these lesions for decades, only to be reactivated when the balance between host immunity and bacterial pathogenesis is tipped in favor of the mycobacteria. This results in secondary infection known as *reactivation TB,* seen typically in chronically ill or otherwise immunosuppressed individuals. Secondary reactivation TB is typically the most lethal form of the infection.

Mycobacteria can also spread via the lymphatic system or bloodstream, resulting in disseminated infection. Extrapulmonary sites of TB infection include the lymph nodes, pleura, bones, meninges, peritoneum, pericardium, and genitourinary tract. Solid organs may be seeded at multiple tiny foci, approximately 2 mm in diameter, taking on a millet seed–like appearance on gross inspection, termed "miliary tuberculosis." Such pathological findings have been noted as far back as the 1700s. Today, the term *miliary TB* has been extended to encompass all forms of progressive, disseminated TB infection, but it is still seen most often in children younger than 1 year.

M. tuberculosis organisms are aerobic and, therefore, particularly attracted to the apical segments of the upper lung lobes where high oxygen concentrations favor their proliferation. Although the upper lung zone is the most common site of accelerated growth of the organisms, there may be later progression to distant sites in the body. The kidneys, brain, and bones are the most common sites of distant progression.

Individuals may continue to discharge mycobacteria into the environment from pulmonary tubercles until multidrug therapy is instituted to drive bacteria into a dormant state or eradicate infection completely. Although mycobacteria are almost always found in the bone marrow, liver, and spleen when disease occurs, uncontrolled multiplication of the mycobacteria in these organs is rare. Immunosuppressed individuals, particularly those with T-lymphocyte deficiencies and compromised cell-mediated immunity (e.g., persons living with HIV), are highly susceptible to TB.

CLINICAL PRESENTATION

Subjective

TB may mimic or occur concurrently with pneumoconiosis, pneumonia, bronchiectasis, sarcoidosis, lung abscess, neoplasm, or respiratory fungal infections. Onset commonly is insidious, with symptoms of anorexia, fatigue, digestive disturbances, slow weight loss, irregular menses, and lack of stamina. This pattern of symptoms at onset may continue for several weeks or even months, with a low-grade elevation of temperature that appears characteristically in the afternoon.

Pulmonary TB is characterized principally by a productive cough, purulent sputum, and repeated occurrences of coryza-like symptoms with rhinorrhea and nasal congestion. The cough progresses slowly over weeks or months to become more frequent and associated with the production of mucoid or mucopurulent sputum. The cough is usually due to sloughing of small caseous lesions with the presence of exudate in the bronchi. Sputum is characteristically yellow but is not tenacious or foul-smelling. Hemoptysis is a common symptom in patients with necrotizing or cavitary lesions. Blood usually appears as small streaks in the sputum. Dyspnea is uncommon in pulmonary TB and usually indicates extensive parenchymal involvement, massive pleural effusion, or other underlying cardiopulmonary disease.

A less frequent pattern of onset is that of an acute febrile illness with an abrupt occurrence of high fever, chills, tachycardia, and weakness, accompanied by a productive cough with myalgia, and sweating. Erythema nodosum may occur with the acute onset of symptoms. Some patients may pay little attention to milder symptoms that precede the acute episode; this is a common occurrence in people with lower health literacy, people with alcohol or substance use disorder, or older adults.

Less frequent modes of onset include pleuritic pain and hoarseness. Pleuritic pain, usually unilateral, tends to be accentuated by coughing or deep inspiration. Hoarseness is usually a result of involvement of the larynx and may be accompanied by severe pain. Constitutional symptoms tend to be general in nature and consist of night sweats, fatigue on exertion, weight loss, and malaise.

In obtaining the health history, the clinician must keep in mind the chronicity of TB and the insidious nature of the onset of symptoms. Patients should be questioned about exposure to anyone with an active case of TB. Potential sources of exposure include family and coworkers. Other significant disclosures obtained from a health history include a past diagnosis of pneumonia with recurrence, pleurisy, uncontrolled diabetes mellitus, alcoholism, malnutrition, and occupational exposures to quartz dust or silica. Additional risk factors include substance use disorder, country of origin, corticosteroid use, and gastrectomy.

Objective

A complete examination of any patient suspected of having TB should always be performed. Examination of the chest usually reveals the primary indications of pulmonary TB. Rhonchi, crackles, wheezing, and bronchial breath sounds may be heard on auscultation but may have no radiographic counterparts. Dullness on percussion is commonly associated with pneumonic lesions. Persons with long standing disease may manifest asymmetrical lung expansion, displacement of the trachea, and muscular atrophy. Although there are no specific changes related to pulmonary function, in patients with extensive parenchymal involvement, the vital capacity and other lung volumes may decrease.

Although pulmonary TB is the most common form, the clinician should be alert to any indications of extrapulmonary TB. The patient should be examined for evidence of present or past extrapulmonary TB in structures such as the genitourinary tract, lymph nodes, bones and joints, peritoneum, larynx, eyes, abdominal organs, and neurological system (Table 30.1). Physical findings may include hepatomegaly, splenomegaly, and generalized lymphadenopathy. Abnormal behavior, headaches, and seizures may indicate TB meningitis. Meningitis occurs frequently in infants and small children as a complication of early infection, but it may be seen in any age group. Bone and joint involvement, most often seen in older adults, is often accompanied by fever and may result in arthritis, osteomyelitis, and localized pain. The lower spine and weight-bearing joints are most often affected by skeletal TB. Genitourinary TB may present as recurrent urinary tract infection with no growth of common pathogens, pyuria without bacteriuria, pelvic inflammatory disease, amenorrhea, infertility, or perianal fistulas.

TABLE 30.1 Clinical Indicators of Extrapulmonary Tuberculosis

Extrapulmonary Sites	Clinical Manifestations
Genitourinary tract	Recurrent urinary tract infections with no growth of common pathogens Pyuria without bacteriuria Unexplained hematuria Irregular menses, amenorrhea, pelvic inflammatory disease, infertility Epididymitis Induration of the prostate
Bone and joints (lower spine and weight-bearing joints are most common sites)	Arthritis, osteomyelitis Fever and localized pain
Meninges	Headaches, convulsions Abnormal behavior
Peritoneum	Ascites, fever
Pericardium	Pericarditis
Lymph nodes	Hilar or mediastinal lymphadenitis Cervical and supraclavicular lymphadenopathy

DIAGNOSTIC REASONING

Diagnostic Tests

Initial Testing

The Mantoux tuberculin skin test (TST) is the most accurate and widely used method for TB skin testing. It involves injecting a small amount of mycobacterial antigen (purified protein derivative [PPD]) intradermally. Persons with previous exposure to or infection with TB organisms develop a positive cell-mediated (type IV) delayed-type hypersensitivity skin reaction as a result of previously sensitized helper T lymphocytes (CD4+) that are attracted to the testing site. Reactions of this type typically require 48 to 72 hours to develop and are classified based on the degree of skin induration at the site of injection in relation to specific population norms. Less invasive quantitative interferon-gamma release assays (IGRAs) also may be used to screen for TB. In these tests, T cells are collected by a whole blood draw and subjected to ex vivo immunostimulation assays with TB-specific antigens. Both TB screening tests only assess for past exposure to TB and do not distinguish between LTBI versus active TB infection.

The TST is easily performed in an office or clinic setting. It is useful as an epidemiological tool to identify infected (including recently infected) people for preventive therapy and contact tracing. The TST is the preferred TB screening test for children younger than 5 years. Persons for whom tuberculin testing is routinely indicated are listed in the Screening Recommendations/Guidelines.

The TST must be administered correctly to avoid false-negative or false-positive results. Factors that may contribute to an inaccurate result include improper handling of the tuberculin, improper administration technique, and inaccurate reading of test results (e.g., by an inexperienced reader). To minimize reduction in potency by adsorption, tuberculin should never be transferred from one container to another, and the skin testing material should be placed soon after the syringe has been filled. Tuberculin should be kept refrigerated and stored away from light as much as possible. The TST (0.1 mL) should be injected into the volar or dorsal surface of the forearm, away from veins and into intact skin that is free of lesions. The injection should be made just beneath the surface of the skin, with a one-quarter to one-half-inch 27-gauge needle and a tuberculin syringe. A discrete, pale elevation of the skin (a wheal) 6 to 10 mm in diameter

Screening Recommendations/Guidelines: Screening for Tuberculosis

- Persons with signs and/or symptoms of current TB
- Close contact with persons with known TB
- Persons with HIV infection
- Persons who inject illicit drugs
- Persons from medically underserved or high-risk populations
- Residents or employees in prisons or long-term care facilities
- Employees in health-care facilities
- Infants, children, and adolescents exposed to adults in high-risk categories (use of IGRAs in children younger than 5 years is not established)
- Foreign-born persons arriving within 5 years from countries that have high TB incidence or prevalence (use IGRAs for persons with recent BCG vaccination)
- Persons on long-term high-dose corticosteroid therapy (use TST rather than IGRA)
- Persons on immunosuppressive therapy (use TST rather than IGRA)
- Persons with medical conditions that increase the risk of TB: chronic renal failure, diabetes, hematological disorders, cancer of the head or neck, body weight 10% less than ideal body weight, silicosis, gastrectomy, jejunal bypass

Abbreviations: BCG, bacillus Calmette-Guérin; IGRA, interferon-gamma release assay; TB, tuberculosis; TST, tuberculin skin test.

Sources: Centers for Disease Control and Prevention. Interferon-gamma release assays (IGRAs)-blood tests for TB infection. https://www.cdc.gov/tb/publications/factsheets/testing/igra.htm#:~:text=Interferon%20Gamma%20Release%20Assays%20(IGRAs)%20are%20whole%20blood,(LTBI)%20from%20tuberculosis%20disease. Accessed 3/6/2022

Lewinsohn DM, Leonard MK, LoBue PA, et al. Official American Thoracic Society/Infectious Diseases Society of America/Centers for Disease Control and Prevention Clinical Practice Guidelines: diagnosis of tuberculosis in adults and children. *Clin Infect Dis.* 2017;64:111.

should be produced when the injection has been done correctly. If the test is improperly administered, another test dose can be given immediately, but at a site several centimeters from the original injection.

The reaction to intradermally injected tuberculin protein is a classic example of a delayed-type cellular hypersensitivity reaction. These reactions begin 5 to 6 hours after injection and are maximal at 72 hours. In older adults or in persons who are being tested for the first time, the reaction may develop more slowly and may not peak until after 72 hours. Older adults should be checked initially at 72 hours, and then 1 and 2 days later. Tests should be read 72 hours after the injection, using good lighting with the forearm slightly flexed at the elbow. Interpretation of the test result is based on the presence or absence of induration, which is determined by inspection and palpation. Erythema is not a factor in interpretation of the TST reaction. The diameter of the induration is measured transversely to the long axis of the forearm and recorded in millimeters (Table 30.2).

Factors that may cause a decreased ability to respond to tuberculin are listed in Box 30.4. The TST tends to have a strong positive predictive value but poorer negative predictive value due to the potential for anergy in immunosuppressed patients, who may have reduced delayed-type hypersensitivity responses. In addition, patients with previous exposure to bacillus Calmette-Guérin (BCG) vaccine (commonly used in developing countries in childhood) may have false-positive results on TB skin tests. These factors do not negate testing, however, because only a fraction of infected persons in these circumstances may have falsely nonreactive results. For example, because immunity from BCG vaccine wanes over time, if it has been many years since the vaccination, a TST may be performed and accurately read. To minimize the confounding of TB screening test results, however, the IGRA test is preferred in persons with a history of BCG vaccination (see subsequent discussion of IGRA).

If the lack of reaction to the TST is suspected to be a false-negative response, a repeat TST should be done. If generalized inability to respond is suspected, it may be necessary to test delayed hypersensitivity using several other antigens to which the person has had a likely exposure. Anergy should be suspected if the person fails to respond to any of the antigens. Of note, despite its use in the past, many infectious disease specialists now feel anergy testing is not useful because patients may have selective anergy to TB but not to other antigens; thus, this practice is not helpful in ruling out TB.

Persons with sensitivity to tuberculin are known as reactors. The definition of a tuberculin reaction size that is indicative of an infection with *M. tuberculosis* is influenced by the dose, dilution, and nature of the tuberculin preparation being used, immunological factors of the patient, and the relative prevalence of tuberculin sensitivity resulting from infection with *M. tuberculosis* versus other mycobacteria in the population being studied. Reactions caused by infections with mycobacteria other than *M. tuberculosis* (cross reactions) are common in many parts of the world. Generally, a reaction to *M. tuberculosis* will be

Box 30.4 Factors Contributing to Decreased Response on Tuberculin Skin Testing

Infections:
- Viral: measles, mumps, chickenpox, HIV infection
- Bacterial: typhoid fever, brucellosis, typhus, leprosy, pertussis, recent or overwhelming *M. tuberculosis* infection
- Fungal: South American blastomycosis
- Live virus vaccinations: measles, mumps, oral polio

Nutritional factors: severe protein depletion
Diseases affecting lymphoid organs: Hodgkin's lymphoma, chronic lymphocytic leukemia
Drugs: corticosteroids and other immunosuppressive agents
Age: newborns, older adults
Stress: surgery, burns, mental illness, graft-versus-host reactions

TABLE 30.2 Interpretation of Tuberculin Skin Testing

Diameter of Induration	Positive Result
>5 mm	• Persons with HIV infection or persons with risk factors for HIV infection and unknown HIV status • Persons who were recently exposed to clinically active TB • Persons with organ transplants • Persons with chest films indicating healed TB
>10 mm	• Recent arrivals to United States (<5 years) • Foreign-born persons from high-risk countries in Africa, Asia, or Latin America • Medically underserved, disadvantaged populations and high-risk racial or ethnic populations • Injection drug abusers • Residents and employees of high-risk congregate settings: prisons and jails, nursing homes and other residential settings for older adults and/or patients with AIDS, homeless shelters • Mycobacteriology laboratory personnel • Persons with medical conditions known to increase the risk for TB: diabetes mellitus, renal failure, silicosis, immunosuppressive therapy, hematological disorders (e.g., leukemia, lymphoma), gastrectomy, 10% or more below ideal body weight
>15 mm	• All other persons

larger than would be seen in a cross reaction. Guidelines for the classification of reactions to intradermal Mantoux tests have established three categories of positive reactions based on the patient's immune status, risk factors for TB exposure, and probability of cross-reaction: 5-, 10-, and 15-mm induration (see Box 30.4). A positive reaction indicates only the presence of TB infection at some point in the patient's history. In the United States, a positive TST without clinical evidence of active TB infection (i.e., negative chest x-ray findings and no symptoms) reflects latent infection that should be treated to minimize the possibility of reactivation (secondary) TB.

In addition to the TST, an IGRA may be used. The QuantiFERON-TB Gold Plus and the T-SPOT are whole blood tests that can aid in the diagnosis of TB but also do not differentiate LTBI from active TB. IGRAs are less invasive and require only a single patient visit to conduct the blood draw. Results can be available within 24 hours. Limited data are available on the use of IGRAs in children younger than 5 years and immunocompromised persons.

An additional advantage of the IGRA is that it does not result in a false-positive test result in individuals who have received the BCG vaccine against TB. Many people born outside the United States receive BCG during infancy. Originally developed from *M. bovis,* BCG has an estimated overall protection rate from TB of approximately 50%, although it appears to be more effective in locations close to the equator. Vaccination with BCG may cause a false-positive reaction on the TST due to priming of T cells from the BCG vaccine antigens. In contrast, the IGRA and T-SPOT do not react against BCG antigens and, therefore, do not typically give false-positive results due to prior BCG exposure.

Subsequent Testing

Apart from TB testing, in patients for whom there is a clinical suspicion of TB, the first diagnostic step should be a combination of a standard anterior-posterior and lateral chest x-ray film and a sputum examination for mycobacteria. The initial radiographic manifestation of a primary infection in an adult or child is usually parenchymal infiltration accompanied by ipsilateral lymph node enlargement. The parenchymal lesions may be seen in any portion of the lung but are seen most commonly in the apical and posterior segments of the upper lobes or in the superior segments of the lower lobes. Lesions may be dense and homogeneous, with lobar, segmental, or subsegmental distribution. Patients with HIV disease tend to have atypical radiographic findings; these patients tend not to have cavitations, and infiltrates are less likely to occur in the upper lobes. Cavitations are also seen infrequently in older patients and in patients who are immunosuppressed. Hematogenous TB is characterized by diffuse, finely nodular, uniformly distributed lesions on a chest x-ray film (i.e., miliary TB).

Chest x-ray films that show no change in findings over a 3- to 4-month interval can generally be interpreted as showing a past TB infection or another disease. The use of a single chest x-ray film as a guide to the nature or stability of the underlying disease is questionable. The words "old" and "fibrotic" are not accurate terms to use when interpreting a single chest x-ray film. Any persistent infiltrate in an older person should be considered suggestive of TB. This form of TB is often missed in older adults, especially among patients residing in nursing homes.

In pulmonary TB, examination of sputum provides the most convenient method of identifying the presence of mycobacteria, in terms of low cost, widespread availability, ease of performance, and reliability. The patient must be instructed to produce material brought up from the chest by coughing. A series of at least three single specimens on different days should be collected from patients who have a productive cough. When a patient is unable to produce an adequate amount of sputum, it is possible to obtain by gastric lavage the bronchopulmonary secretions that the patient has unknowingly swallowed during the night. Gastric aspiration is done after a period of fasting for 8 to 10 hours; it should be performed before the patient arises from bed. Approximately 50 mL of gastric contents is required for this test, which is best performed in the hospitalized patient.

It is possible to induce sputum production by inhalation of hypertonic saline. These specimens will be thinner and waterier than sputum produced spontaneously. Inducing sputum by this method may produce a violent and uncontrolled cough, so special conditions to filter ambient air and minimize transmission may be indicated. Occasionally, a pooled specimen collected over a period of 10 to 24 hours may be helpful if the previous methods are not effective or appropriate. This type of specimen is more subject to contamination and is best collected in an institutional setting.

Bronchial washings obtained with fiber-optic bronchoscopy may be indicated in patients who are unable to produce sputum or in those who are thought to have TB, despite negative sputum culture reports. When extrapulmonary TB is suspected, it is necessary to collect less common clinical specimens from sources such as urine; peritoneal, pericardial, and pleural fluids; bones and joints; or lymph nodes.

The detection of AFB in stained sputum smears examined by direct microscopy provides the first evidence of the presence of mycobacteria in a clinical specimen. It is estimated that 50% to 80% of patients with pulmonary TB will have positive sputum smears. The sputum smear is the easiest and quickest procedure to provide the practitioner with a preliminary confirmation of the diagnosis. The smear also provides the practitioner with a quantitative estimate of the number of bacilli being excreted by the patient. These estimates are described as rare, few, or numerous. The lowest concentration of organisms that can be detected by microscopic examination is 10 per milliliter of sputum. For direct microscopy of sputum, the most widely used method is the Ziehl-Neelsen staining method.

All clinical specimens suspected of containing mycobacteria must be inoculated onto culture media. Culture yield appears to be associated with the clinical presentation of the patient. Some research suggests patients with cavitary disease tend to have a higher rate of positive cultures than do patients with focal infiltrates. The cultures should be incubated at 37°C and examined at weekly intervals. The time from the laboratory's receipt of the specimen to the report of the culture is usually 3 to 6 weeks. In rare situations, such as repeated contaminated specimens or patients with positive Gram stains and negative cultures, guinea pig inoculation may be necessary as an in-vivo culture system.

Susceptibility of tubercle bacilli to various anti-TB drugs may be determined via either direct or indirect tests. The direct drug-susceptibility test is performed by using clinical specimens of AFB, which are inoculated directly onto a drug-containing culture medium. Growth is then compared with growth on a non–drug-containing medium. An indirect test is performed by using a subculture from the primary isolate as the inoculum. Although the direct test is preferred, because it is more representative of the bacterial population of the patient, the indirect test may be useful when the initial smear result is negative but the culture result is positive, when growth on the control medium is inadequate for a reliable test, or when a reference culture is submitted by another laboratory. In the past, the previously untreated patient with newly diagnosed TB was started on anti-TB therapy without prior drug-susceptibility testing. Recommendations for drug-susceptibility testing have been modified because of the emergence of drug-resistant bacilli and are discussed in the Management section.

Differential Diagnosis

Difficulties in a differential diagnosis arise when the tubercle bacilli cannot be isolated by smear or culture and in situations in which other diseases such as carcinoma or pulmonary mycosis are present. Small pulmonary lesions, particularly a solitary nodule or coin nodule, need to be differentiated from early carcinoma of the lung, pulmonary infarction, localized pulmonary fibrosis, and pneumonia of fungal, viral, mycoplasmal, or bacterial origin with delayed clearing or resolution. In extensive forms of pulmonary TB, bronchopneumonia and lobar pneumonia must be considered. The acute cavitary forms of TB must be differentiated from lung abscess. Other chronic pulmonary diseases that frequently are characterized by cavity formations include systemic mycotic infections, particularly coccidioidomycosis and histoplasmosis.

Pulmonary TB of hematogenous origin must be differentiated from other types of infection that may manifest in similar fashion: silicosis, berylliosis, asbestosis, sarcoidosis, diffuse interstitial fibrosis, scleroderma, metastatic neoplasms, or alveolar cell carcinoma. From the perspective of clinical manifestations, the clinician must consider other conditions that may cause prolonged or obscure fevers, such as lymphoma, brucellosis, and HIV infection.

MANAGEMENT

The development of specific chemotherapeutic agents has revolutionized the prognosis of TB infection, making the disease truly curable and preventable. Drug treatment of TB should be viewed as both a personal health measure intended to cure the ill patient and as a public health measure intended to interrupt transmission of tubercle bacilli in the community.

Initial Management

In patients in whom the clinical and radiographic findings suggest a diagnosis of TB and the sputum examination reveals the presence of mycobacteria, a working diagnosis can be made and anti-TB chemotherapy can be started. For patients in whom TB is suspected but whose sputum smear results are negative, an alternative is to begin therapy and wait for culture results. Initiating chemotherapy in the absence of a definitive diagnosis is a valid approach, but caution is needed for patients with HIV infection and multidrug resistance. X-ray findings of TB in patients with AIDS are often atypical and may be indicative of a range of diagnostic possibilities; thus, a presumptive diagnosis of TB in these patients may be more speculative.

The main goal of therapy is to eliminate all tubercle bacilli from the patient while avoiding the development of clinically significant drug resistance. Although individuals with LTBI do not have symptoms and cannot spread the TB bacteria to others, there is the possibility that the infection can become active; therefore, treatment of LTBI is essential for controlling and eliminating TB in the United States. For these individuals, combination therapy in which both rifapentine and INH are given once a week for 12 weeks is recommended. Monotherapy regimens include daily INH alone for 6 to 9 months or daily RIF (alternatively called rifampin or rifampicin) alone for 4 months.

For patients with active TB, basic principles of treatment include administering multiple drugs to which the organism is susceptible, adding new drugs to the regimen when it is suspected that treatment is not working, providing the maximum therapy in the shortest amount of time, and ensuring patient compliance. While curing the individual patient, the transmission of *M. tuberculosis* to other persons also needs to be minimized.

The current minimum acceptable duration of treatment for all children and adults with culture-positive TB is 6 months. The initial phase of a 6-month regimen should consist of a 2-month course of INH, RIF, pyrazinamide (PZA), and ethambutol (EMB) or streptomycin in children who are too young to be monitored for visual acuity. This regimen is given until the results of drug-susceptibility studies are available, unless there is little possibility of drug resistance (e.g., less than 4% primary resistance to INH in the community and the patient has had no previous treatment with anti-TB medication, is not from a country with a high prevalence of drug-resistant TB, or has no known exposure to a drug-resistant case). Although there are 10 drugs currently approved by the FDA to treat TB, the preceding four drugs are first-line anti-TB agents that are the core of most treatment regimens. The second phase of therapy should consist of INH and RIF for a total of 4 months (daily treatment or three times per week). Therapy should be prolonged if the response is slow or otherwise suboptimal.

An alternative regimen for persons who cannot take PZA (e.g., in pregnancy) consists of a 9-month regimen of INH and RIF. EMB should also be included until the results of susceptibility studies are available unless there is little possibility of drug resistance. Drug resistance is most common in patients with HIV and those recently arrived in the United States. If INH resistance is confirmed, RIF plus PZA plus EMB should be continued for a minimum of 6 months. For RIF resistance, INH plus EMB should be used for 18 months or INH, PZA, and streptomycin for 9 months. In HIV-infected patients, rifabutin should always be used because RIF interacts with protease inhibitors and nonnucleoside retroviral inhibitors.

Adverse reactions and prescribing considerations for the most typically used TB drugs are shown in Drugs Commonly Prescribed 30.2. See Box 30.5 for a discussion of drug-resistant TB, including both MDR-TB and extensively drug-resistant TB (XDR-TB).

Drugs Commonly Prescribed 30.2: Tuberculosis

	ADVERSE REACTIONS AND PRESCRIBING CONSIDERATIONS
First-line TB Drugs	All must be taken on an empty stomach to facilitate absorption—if unable to comply, may take medicine with food that does not contain fat or oils (may ease nausea).
Isoniazid (INH or H)	May cause peripheral neuropathy (pyridoxine may be given prophylactically). May be associated with increased risk of seizures in patients with epilepsy. May be hepatotoxic (potentiated by rifampin).
Rifamycins (e.g., rifampin [RIF or R], rifabutin, rifapentine)	May cause thrombocytopenia. Commonly causes rash without itching during the first few weeks, which usually resolves on its own. May cause an elevation in bilirubin, which usually resolves in 10 days; may potentiate INH hepatotoxicity.
Pyrazinamide (PZA or Z)	May cause rash. May be hepatotoxic. If the patient will not take due to tablet size, pyrazinamide syrup may be substituted.
Ethambutol (EMB or E)	Periodic vision screens required, given ocular toxicity (optic neuritis).
Streptomycin (STM or S)	Use with caution in patients with mild to severe kidney problems. Periodic hearing screens required, given aminoglycoside-related ototoxicity.
Second-line TB Drugs	Choice of agent should be guided by resistance testing.
Aminoglycosides (e.g., amikacin, kanamycin)	Use with caution in patients with mild to severe kidney problems. Chronic use may cause ototoxicity (audiological and vestibular dysfunction).
Polypeptides (e.g., capreomycin)	May cause nephrotoxicity.
Fluoroquinolones (e.g., ciprofloxacin, levofloxacin)	Commonly cause nausea, vomiting, or other gastrointestinal (GI) symptoms. May also cause tendinitis/tendon rupture. Associated with QTc prolongation.
Thioamides (e.g., ethionamide, prothionamide)	GI side effects may occur. May cause central nervous system and psychiatric effects.
Cycloserine	GI side effects may occur.
p-Aminosalicylic acid	Potential cause of drug-induced hepatitis.

> **Box 30.5 Drug-Resistant Tuberculosis (TB): MDR-TB and XDR-TB**
>
> **MDR-TB**
>
> *Multidrug-resistant TB:* Tuberculosis resistant to at least isoniazid and rifampin
>
> **XDR-TB**
>
> *Extensively drug-resistant TB:* Tuberculosis resistant to both isoniazid and rifampin, as well as fluoroquinolones and at least one injectable second-line anti-TB agent (e.g., kanamycin, capreomycin, or amikacin)
> *Principles of treatment:* Same for both MDR-TB and XDR-TB, focused on antimicrobial sensitivity testing and the selection of active agents.
> Given resistance to second-line agents, XDR-TB has a higher mortality rate due to the reduced number of effective treatment options.
> Treatment lasts a minimum of 18 months and may extend for years.

Directly observed therapy (DOT) should be considered for all patients with active TB because of the difficulty in predicting which patients will adhere to a prescribed regimen. When TB is initially diagnosed, the practitioner should explain to the patient about the disease, required treatment, and the necessity of completing the recommended therapy. If DOT is indicated, the patient and the practitioner should agree on a method that ensures the greatest degree of adherence and maintains confidentiality. DOT may require an outreach worker to go into the community and administer each dose of medication to the patient. Many patients can, however, receive the treatment at a center agreed on by the practitioner and the patient. Common community settings include TB clinics, community health centers, migrant health clinics, homeless shelters, jails and prisons, nursing homes, schools, drug treatment centers, hospitals, HIV/AIDS clinics, or occupational health clinics. In some situations, a responsible person other than a health-care worker may be able to administer the chemotherapy. Possible resources in the community include correctional facility personnel, social and welfare caseworkers, clergy, teachers, and reliable volunteers. Adequate medication adherence is critical to the complete clearance of all infectious organisms and to the prevention of drug-resistant strains of TB.

HIV infection and other factors that compromise a patient's immune system are important considerations when selecting the most effective RIF type of treatment (known collectively as *rifamycin antibiotics*). These factors are particularly important with drug-resistant TB because of the potential for rapid disease progression and death when patients receive inadequate treatment. DOT and experienced TB/HIV caregivers are considered to be critical to the effective treatment of both conditions. Given the propensity for RIF to upregulate and induce the hepatic cytochrome p450 metabolic pathway, the dosage of several antiretroviral medications must be increased when administered with RIF. However, substituting rifabutin (Mycobutin) for RIF (Rimactane, Rifadin) allows for the concurrent administration of anti-TB and antiretroviral drug regimens, with no dosage adjustments in the latter. Currently, most guidelines indicate that patients with HIV should be treated for a total of 9 months and for at least 6 months after sputum conversion. In general, intermittent anti-TB therapy is not recommended for TB/HIV–coinfected patients. See the recommendations for the treatment of TB and antiretroviral dosage adjustments in patients with HIV in Chapter 63.

Effective therapy for TB is essential for pregnant patients. Untreated TB represents a greater hazard to a pregnant patient and fetus than does treatment of the disease. Initial treatment should consist of INH and RIF. EMB (Myambutol) should also be included unless primary INH resistance is unlikely. Streptomycin should not be prescribed in pregnancy because it may cause congenital deafness in the fetus. PZA is recommended by international TB organizations for use in pregnant patients; however, in the United States, PZA is not currently recommended because it has not been determined whether there is a risk of teratogenicity. Breastfeeding does not need to be discouraged because the small concentrations of anti-TB drugs in breast milk are not adequate to produce toxicity in the newborn. TB during pregnancy is not an indication for a therapeutic abortion.

Regimens that are adequate for treating adults with pulmonary TB should also be effective in treating extrapulmonary disease. Bacteriological evaluation of extrapulmonary TB may be limited by the relative inaccessibility of the disease site to anti-infective chemotherapy. Response to treatment must often be judged on the basis of clinical and radiographic findings. Surgery may be necessary to obtain specimens for diagnosis and to treat certain complications, such as constrictive pericarditis. Corticosteroid therapy has been shown to be of benefit in preventing cardiac constriction from TB pericarditis and in decreasing the neurological sequelae of TB meningitis.

Subsequent Management

Today, the majority of patients with TB may undergo treatment while remaining in their home setting. However, there may be specific situations that mandate the need for hospitalization of the patient with TB. These include very ill patients who have no responsible person at home to provide care, patients with advanced pulmonary disease with highly positive sputum smears or severe extrapulmonary disease, or the presence of associated medical problems that require hospitalization.

Adults should have measurements of serum bilirubin, hepatic enzymes, BUN, creatinine, and a CBC including platelet count before starting chemotherapy for TB. Visual acuity and red-green color perception tests are recommended before initiation of EMB, and a serum uric acid level should be measured before starting PZA, given the potential side effect profile of these drugs. Patients should be advised to report symptoms suggestive of drug toxicity. For INH-containing regimens, symptoms of concern include anorexia, nausea, vomiting, fatigue or weakness, dark urine, icterus, rash, paresthesias of the hands and feet, fever, and abdominal tenderness. Routine monitoring of laboratory tests for evidence of hepatic failure is not recommended, but monthly questioning for symptoms of drug toxicity is indicated. Patients with known liver disease or alcohol use disorder may need to have periodic liver function tests drawn, as they are more prone to hepatic injury. Appropriate laboratory tests are indicated if symptoms of drug toxicity develop.

Periodic examination of the patient is necessary to observe for changes in symptoms, signs, body weight, and temperature. The single most important laboratory test for following the response to anti-TB therapy is the bacteriological examination of bronchopulmonary secretions. A progressive decrease in the number of AFB in weekly or biweekly specimens is a good indicator of effective chemotherapy. Periodic laboratory checks of blood, urine, visual acuity, eighth cranial nerve (vestibulocochlear) function, renal function, and hepatic function are desirable based on the severity of the illness and the drugs being administered. Patients should be questioned carefully for any symptoms of drug toxicity, as well as the level of adherence to their treatment regimen.

It is not necessary to restrict physical activity or require bedrest of most patients. Bedrest may help make patients who are experiencing fever, night sweats, anorexia, or bouts of coughing more comfortable. Patients who present with a history of fever should have a normal temperature within 2 to 3 weeks after the initiation of chemotherapy. It may be necessary to suppress the cough reflex in patients who are experiencing severe coughing. Codeine and hydrocodone are the most useful for temporary treatment of significant cough; however, if the patient is producing thick and tenacious secretions, suppression of the cough reflex is not desirable. These patients should be instructed in adequate hydration and air humidification and prescribed an expectorant. Chest pain may manifest if the patient develops pleuritis. Occasionally, chest pain may be caused by a fractured rib resulting from severe coughing. Instillation of a local anesthetic proximate to the rib fracture is preferred over the older method of strapping the chest. Coughing that results in occasional episodes of streaked or bloody sputum requires no specific treatment other than managing the cough. There may be significant hemoptysis with bronchogenic spread of TB, although this tends to be self-limited. In advanced chronic cavitary TB, fatal pulmonary hemorrhage or shock can occur if large pulmonary arteries ulcerate or a Rasmussen's aneurysm forms, which is a pulmonary artery aneurysm adjacent to or within a tuberculous cavity.

FOLLOW-UP AND REFERRAL

The response to anti-TB chemotherapy in patients with positive bacteriology is best evaluated by repeated sputum examinations. Sputum cultures should be done at least once monthly until sputum conversion is documented. After 2 months of treatment with regimens containing both INH and RIF, the majority of patients should convert to negative cultures. Patients whose sputum culture results have not become negative after 3 months of treatment should be carefully reevaluated and referred to a pulmonologist. Drug-susceptibility tests should be repeated and treatment should be administered or continued under direct observation. If organisms are found to be resistant, the treatment regimen should be modified to include at least two drugs to which the organisms are susceptible and administered via DOT. For patients whose sputum no longer contains *M. tuberculosis,* at least one further sputum smear and culture should be performed at the completion of therapy. X-ray evaluations during treatment are less important than sputum examinations. A chest x-ray film at the completion of treatment will provide a baseline comparison for any future films.

Shortness of breath in a patient without underlying pulmonary disease is suggestive of complications of pulmonary TB and requires further diagnostic inquiry. Sudden breathlessness may be a symptom of acute pleurisy with pleuritic pain, pleural effusion, spontaneous pneumothorax, a massive extension of TB infection throughout the lung, or atelectasis. In addition, patients who have coexisting emphysema or pulmonary disease may become dyspneic with only minimal involvement of the lungs.

Preventive Therapy

The American Thoracic Society has identified risk groups for whom preventive (prophylactic) therapy is indicated (Table 30.3), as patients infected with *M. tuberculosis* who do not have active disease still harbor organisms. In turn, prophylactic or preventive treatment of LTBI significantly reduces the probability of reactivation TB later in life. INH given for 6 to 9 months is effective in asymptomatic adults (300 mg/day) or children (10 to 14 mg/kg/day, up to 300 mg/day) with LTBI demonstrated by a positive TB screening test but a negative diagnostic evaluation for active disease. Concurrent pyridoxine administration (25 to 50 mg/day in adults and 1 to 2 mg/kg/day in children) may reduce the potential for neuropathic complications associated with INH, and adjustments with intermittent dosing (900 mg twice weekly) or an overall shortened duration (6 months) may

TABLE 30.3 Groups for Whom Preventive Therapy for Latent Tuberculosis Infection (LTBI) Is Recommended

Group	Comments
The following high-risk groups should be given treatment if their reaction to the Mantoux (PPD) tuberculin skin test (TST) is ≥5 mm:	
1. Persons with known HIV infection and those suspected of having HIV infection (i.e., persons with risk factors for HIV infection whose status is unknown)	Persons with HIV infection who are at high risk for TB but have negative skin tests should be considered for preventive therapy.
2. Close contacts of persons with newly diagnosed infectious TB 3. Persons with fibrotic changes on chest x-ray examination consistent with prior TB infection	Household members and other close contacts have a 2%–4% chance of developing TB within the first year of exposure to the index case. The risk for very young children and adolescents may be twice that of adults. People who do not develop TB disease within the first year will continue to be at risk for the disease throughout their life. Children should be treated, even if their initial skin tests are negative. Skin testing should be repeated after 3 months of therapy with a rifamycin antibiotic and isoniazid (INH), and if the skin test becomes positive, INH preventive therapy should be continued for a total of 9 months.
4. Recent TST converters	A skin test conversion is defined as an increase in induration of 10 mm or more within 2 years for those younger than age 35 years and 15 mm or more for those aged 35 years or older.
5. Persons with medical conditions that increase the risk of TB with a PPD result of 10 mm or greater	
• Diabetes mellitus	The TB risk for this group may be two to four times that of the general population. Particularly at risk are persons with poorly controlled insulin-dependent diabetes.
• Prolonged therapy with corticosteroids	TB that develops during corticosteroid therapy tends to be disseminated or presents in an obscure fashion. Prednisone (or equivalent) given daily at 15 mg or higher for 2–3 weeks markedly reduces tuberculin reactivity.
• Immunosuppressive therapy	Persons receiving other forms of immunosuppressive therapy are at increased risk for TB.
• Hematological and reticuloendothelial diseases	Diseases such as leukemia and Hodgkin's disease may be associated with suppressed cellular immunity and an increased risk of TB.
• Injection drug users known to be HIV-negative	Persons injecting illicit drugs may be at increased risk of TB, even if not infected with HIV.
• End-stage renal disease (ESRD)	Persons with ESRD are predisposed to developing extrapulmonary TB with disseminated disease. Because these patients may become anergic, a documented TB history or positive TST is an indication for preventive INH therapy unless they have been treated previously.
• Clinical conditions associated with substantial rapid weight loss or chronic malnutrition	These conditions include intestinal bypass surgery for obesity (which carries an increased risk for disseminated TB), postgastrectomy, chronic peptic ulcer disease, chronic malabsorption syndromes, chronic alcohol use disorder, and carcinomas of the oropharynx and upper GI tract that prevent adequate nutritional intake or absorption. The postgastrectomy state may increase the risk of developing TB even without weight loss.
Persons in the following groups who are younger than age 35 years and have a positive TST (≥10 mm):	
• Foreign-born persons from high-prevalence countries	These countries include those in Latin America, Asia, and Africa that have a high prevalence of endemic TB. Especially at risk are recent arrivals from these geographies (<5 years).

TABLE 30.3 Groups for Whom Preventive Therapy for Latent Tuberculosis Infection (LTBI) Is Recommended—cont'd	
Group	**Comments**
• Medically underserved, economically disadvantaged groups, especially high-risk racial or ethnic populations	These groups include African Americans, Native Americans, Hispanics, Asians, and Pacific Islanders.
• Residents of facilities for long-term care • Residents and staff of high-risk congregate settings (nursing homes, jails, homeless shelters)	These residents include those in correctional facilities, nursing homes, and mental health facilities. Staff of such facilities should also be considered for preventive therapy.
• Persons with clinical conditions that place them at high risk	HIV infection, substance use disorder, recent infection with *M. tuberculosis* (within the past 2 years), previous TB, silicosis, prolonged immunosuppressive therapy, low body weight (<90% of normal), ESRD, chronic malabsorption.
• Migrant farmworkers • Children younger than 4 years • Mycobacteriology laboratory personnel	
Persons with no known risk factors for TB may be considered for therapy if their reaction to the tuberculin test is ≥15 mm. This group should be given lower priority than the groups listed previously.	

Source: Adapted from Chapter 6: Treatment of tuberculosis disease. In: Core curriculum on tuberculosis: what the clinician should know, 6th edition. National Center for HIV/AIDS, Viral Hepatitis, STD, and TB prevention—Division of Tuberculosis Elimination. https://www.cdc.gov/tb/education/corecurr/pdf/chapter6.pdf.

be used for adult patients with medication adherence issues. For patients intolerant of INH or in whom INH-resistant LTBI is suspected, RIF may be used as an alternative in adults (600 mg/day for 4 months) or children (10 to 20 mg/kg/day for 6 months).

All persons with known or suspected HIV infection who have positive TST results should receive preventive therapy for TB. HIV-infected persons who are at high risk for TB but have negative skin tests should also be considered for preventive therapy. Preventive regimens are similar to those for individuals without HIV infection. However, a full course of daily INH (9 months) or RIF (6 months) is recommended, with the latter reserved for suspected cases of INH-resistant, RIF-sensitive LTBI.

Household members and other close contacts have a 2% to 4% risk of developing TB within the first year of exposure to the index case. The risk for very young children and adolescents may be twice the risk in adults. People who do not develop active TB disease within the first year will continue to be at risk for developing the disease throughout their lives. Children should be treated even if their initial TST results are negative. A TST should be repeated after 3 months of INH, and if a previously negative skin test result becomes positive, INH preventive therapy should be continued for a total of 9 months.

Persons with medical conditions such as diabetes mellitus, long-term use of corticosteroids, use of immunosuppressive therapy, injection drug use, hematological disease, end-stage renal disease, and conditions associated with rapid weight loss or chronic malnutrition are also at risk for TB. Other risk groups include foreign-born persons from high-prevalence countries (e.g., in Asia, Africa, or Latin America); medically underserved groups, especially African Americans, Native Americans, and Hispanics; and residents of long-term care facilities (e.g., prisons, nursing homes, mental health facilities).

For updates about current TB treatment recommendations, visit the Division of TB Elimination Web site at https://www.cdc.gov/tb/about/default.htm.

Patient Education: Tuberculosis

Educating the patient and family/support persons about the disease, treatment, and importance of completing the recommended treatment regimen is critical to the management of TB. The patient and support persons should be provided with reinforcement and encouragement throughout the course of therapy, and patients should be offered the option of participating in DOT, if not otherwise mandatory. For patients who are administering their own medications, strategies that may be helpful for improving adherence include use of a weekly pill dispenser, marking off each day on a calendar as medicine is taken, taking pills at the same time every day (e.g., with breakfast or during a coffee break), and asking a friend or family member to remind the patient to take their pills.

Patients are typically considered to be infectious for about 2 to 3 weeks after initiation of drug therapy. If the patient is being cared for at home, they should not go to work or school. These patients should be instructed in how to control the spread of tubercle bacilli in microdroplets by using good hygienic measures, appropriate ventilation, and avoiding close contact with others. Patients should sleep in a separate room until no longer considered infectious (hospitalized patients are kept isolated in negative air flow rooms even after treatment is started, until their sputum smears consistently test negative for mycobacteria). Patients should be taught to always cover their mouths when they cough, sneeze, or laugh. Used tissues should be placed in a plastic or paper bag and discarded. If the weather is warm enough, patients should be instructed to place a fan in an open window to blow out air that may be contaminated with TB, while opening other windows in the room to help draw in fresh air.

Patients should be asked to identify any people who may need to be tested for TB infection, including coworkers, family members, and friends. All close contacts will need to undergo TB screening and may require preventive INH therapy. Assurance should be provided to the patient and support persons by stressing that the majority of properly treated patients with TB are cured.

Challenges associated with TB and its treatment in foreign-born patients may sometimes stem from communication barriers, cultural and cognitive dissonance between practitioners and patients, and gaps in provider training. Thus, education needs to be targeted to patients, providers, and community workers.

There are excellent TB control strategies available to the public from the CDC. Patients may access these guidelines at https://www.cdc.gov and obtain easily understood written guidance. However, the problems of MDR-TB and issues of compliance with therapy among all populations remain a significant challenge for health-care providers. Practicing within a Circle of Caring enables the clinician to approach these problems in a meaningful way.

REFERENCES

Cystic Fibrosis

Farrel PM, White TB, Ren CL, et al. Diagnosis of cystic fibrosis: Consensus Guidelines from the Cystic Fibrosis Foundation. *J Pediatr.* 2017;181S:S4–S15.e1. https://pubmed.ncbi.nlm.nih.gov/28129811/. Accessed 7/20/2020.

Lomas PH, Tran QT. The changing face of cystic fibrosis. *Am Nurse J.* 2020;15(3):28–32.

Rosenfelld M, Wainwright CE, Higgins M, et al. Ivacaftor treatment of cystic fibrosis in children aged 12 to <24 months and with a *CFTR* gating mutation (ARRIVAL): a phase 3 single-arm study. *Lancet Respir Med.* 2018;6(7):545.

Sosnay PR, Siklosi KR, Van Goor F, et al. Defining the disease liability of variants in the cystic fibrosis transmembrane conductance regulator gene. *Nat Genet.* 2013 Oct;45(10):1160–1167. Epub 2013 Aug 25.

West NE, Beckett VV, Jain R, et al. Standardized Treatment of Pulmonary Exacerbations (STOP) study: physician treatment practices and outcomes for individuals with cystic fibrosis with pulmonary exacerbations. *J Cyst Fibros.* 2017;16(5):600.

Pneumonia and COVID-19

CDC. Covid Data Tracker Weekly Review. (2021 Feb 26). https://www.cdc.gov/coronavirus/2019-ncov/covid-data/covidview/index.html. Accessed 3/5/2021.

COVID-19 Treatment Guidelines—Anti-SARS-CoV-2 Monoclonal Antibodies. (Updated 2022 Feb 1) https://www.covid19treatmentguidelines.nih.gov/therapies/anti-sars-cov-2-antibody-products/anti-sars-cov-2-monoclonal-antibodies/. Accessed 3/3/2022.

Weekly Trends—COVID 19 coronavirus pandemic. www.worldometers.info/coronavirus/. Accessed 3/3/2022.

Chavez S, Long B, Koyfman A, et al. Coronavirus Disease (COVID-19): a primer for emergency physicians. *Am J Emerg Med.* 2021;44:220–229.

Freedman MS, Hunter P, Ault K, Kroger A. Advisory Committee on Immunization Practices Recommended Immunization Schedule for Adults Aged 19 Years or Older—United States, 2020. *MMWR Morb Mortal Wkly Rep.* 2020;69:133–135.

Giwa A, Desai A. Novel coronavirus COVID-19: an overview for emergency clinicians. *Emerg Med Pract.* 2020 Feb 27;22(2 Suppl 2):1–21. Update in *Emerg Med Pract.* 2020 May 01;22(5):1–28.

Ives-Tallman C, Guest B. Novel Coronavirus 2019 (COVID-19). In: Mattu A and Swadron S, eds. *CorePendium.* CorePendium, LLC; 2021. https://www.emrap.org/corependium/chapter/rec906m1mD6SRH9np/Novel-Coronavirus-2019-COVID-19. Accessed 2/27/2021.

Koslap-Petraco M. ACIP releases 2020 pediatric and adult immunization schedules. *The Clin. Advisor.* 2020 July-Aug:24–26.

Metlay JP, Waterer GW, Long AC, et al. Diagnosis and treatment of adults with community-acquired pneumonia. An official clinical practice guideline of the American Thoracic Society and Infectious Diseases Society of America. *Am J Respir Crit Care Med.* 2019;200(7):e45–e67.

Walker D, Tolentino V. COVID-19: The impact on pediatric emergency care. *Pediatr Emerg Med Pract.* 2020;17(Suppl 6-1):1–27.

Tuberculosis

Centers for Disease Control and Prevention. Tuberculosis. https://www.cdc.gov/tb/topic/basics/default.htm. Accessed 9/12/2020.

Lewinsohn DM, Leonard MK, LoBue PA, et al. Official American Thoracic Society/Infectious Diseases Society of America/Centers for Disease Control and Prevention Clinical Practice Guidelines: Diagnosis of Tuberculosis in Adults and Children. *Clin Infect Dis.* 2017 Jan 15;64(2):e1–e33.

Lönnroth K, Raviglione M. The WHO's new end TB strategy in the post-2015 era of the sustainable development goals. *Trans R Soc Trop Med Hyg.* 2016;110:148. World Health Organization: Tuberculosis. https://www.who.int/health-topics/tuberculosis#tab=tab_1. Accessed 9/13/2020.

Upper Respiratory Infections and Influenza

Healthy People 2030. https://health.gov/healthypeople/objectives-and-data/browse-objectives/vaccination/increase-proportion-people-who-get-flu-vaccine-every-year-iid-09. Accessed 3/1/2021.

Liebowitz D, Gottlieb K, Kolhatkar N, et al. Efficacy, immunogenicity, and safety of an oral influenza vaccine: a placebo-controlled and active-controlled phase 2 human challenge study. *Lancet Infect Dis.* 2020;20(4):435–444.

Lutz R. (2020, June 2) How Deadly Was the 2019–2020 Flu Season? *Contagion Live–Infectious Diseases Today.* https://www.contagionlive.com/news/how-deadly-was-the-2019-2020-flu-season. Accessed 9/2/2020.

Walker TA, Waite B, Thompson MG, et al. Risk of severe influenza among adults with chronic medical conditions. *J Infect Dis.* 2020;221(2):183.

RESOURCES

General

CDC. Advisory Committee on Immunization Practices (ACIP)–vaccine recommendations and guidelines.
https://www.cdc.gov/vaccines/hcp/acip-recs/general-recs/timing.html

Pneumonia

CURB-65 calculation score for pneumonia severity.
https://www.mdcalc.com/curb-65-score-pneumonia-severity

National Foundation for Infectious Diseases
https://www.nfid.org/

National Institute on Aging
https://www.nia.nih.gov/health/shots-safety

Tuberculosis

Centers for Disease Control and Prevention. National Center for HIV/AIDS, Viral Hepatitis, STD, and TB Prevention
https://www.cdc.gov/nchhstp/Default.htm

Latent TB infection and TB disease
https://www.cdc.gov/tb/topic/basics/tbinfectiondisease.htm

MedlinePlus: Tuberculosis
https://medlineplus.gov/tuberculosis.html

Upper Respiratory Infections

Key Facts About Influenza
https://www.cdc.gov/flu/about/keyfacts.htm

MedlinePlus: Flu
https://medlineplus.gov/flu.html

Chapter 31

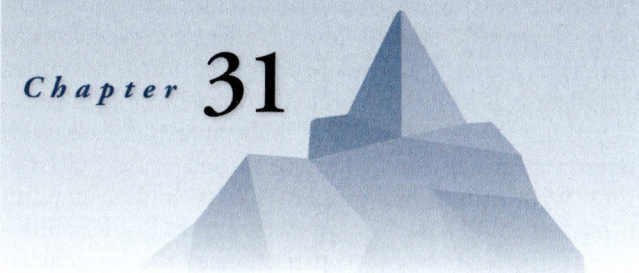

Inflammatory Respiratory Disorders

Jill E. Winland-Brown, EdD, APRN, FNP-BC, FAANP
Brian Oscar Porter, MD, PhD, MPH, MBA

ASTHMA

Asthma is a chronic, inflammatory, obstructive disease of the airways. It may occur at any age and may be characterized by wheezing due to airway spasms, tightness in the chest, breathlessness (dyspnea), and cough. The signs and symptoms may remit spontaneously or worsen in response to intrinsic (stress) or extrinsic (environmental) triggers. The severity of asthma is highly unpredictable, ranging from mild attacks to complete airway obstruction and death. Many pediatricians use the term "reactive airway disease" because the term "asthma" carries a negative connotation for some parents.

EPIDEMIOLOGY AND CAUSES

Asthma affects an estimated 300 million people worldwide, and the number is increasing rapidly. In the United States, more than 39.5 million Americans have been diagnosed with asthma at some point in their lives. It is estimated that 9.5% (6.1 million) children currently have asthma. African Americans have a prevalence rate 47% higher than European Americans. Despite newer antiasthmatic drugs, asthma is responsible for more than 134 million days of restricted activity. The economic cost of asthma is staggering. More than $56 billion annually is lost due to direct medical costs from hospital stays and indirect costs due to lost school and workdays.

There are more than 14 million ambulatory care visits related to asthma each year, along with more than 2 million emergency department visits. In the United States, 5,500 deaths each year are attributable to asthma, with a greater percentage occurring in females. Despite current prevention efforts, the incidence of asthma continues to increase each year. The prevalence of asthma in adults is 35% higher in females. In children younger than 18 years, boys have a 16% higher incidence than girls. Children aged 5 to 17 years have the highest attack prevalence rates, whereas people older than 65 years have the lowest.

The National Asthma Education and Prevention Program (NAEPP) Coordinating Committee Expert Panel 4 (EPR-4) Working Group was established in 2018 to update the 2007 Guidelines for the Diagnosis and Management of Asthma. These evidence-based practice guidelines include ways to help patients control asthma signs and symptoms and improve their quality of life. The Global Initiative for Asthma (GINA) published a report for primary care providers in 2020 delineating a comprehensive and integrated approach to asthma management. The GINA 2020 report can be obtained from https://www.ginasthma.org.

Although the pathophysiology of asthma is multifactorial and involves many inflammatory pathways, from a practical perspective, three principal triggers for exacerbations of asthma have been identified:

1. Allergens and environmental factors: allergens may include inhaled substances, such as molds, pollens, dust, animal dander, cosmetics, and tobacco smoke; food additives with sulfite preservative agents; and medications, especially beta blockers and aspirin or aspirin-containing drugs.
2. Infections: upper respiratory tract infections are common precursors to an asthma attack, particularly viral infections.
3. Psychological factors: stressful events or crises at work or home may precipitate an asthma attack, although often stressors are overlooked or dismissed.

PATHOPHYSIOLOGY

Asthma is a chronic inflammatory disease characterized by reversible hyperreactivity of the bronchi and bronchioles to a variety of stimuli. Inflammation of the airways contributes to bronchial hyperreactivity, airflow limitation, and the resultant characteristic signs and symptoms of asthma: wheezing, breathlessness, chest tightness, and cough. The stage is then set for acute bronchoconstriction, airway edema, mucous plug formation, airway narrowing, and bronchial obstruction.

Genetic predisposition, allergy, environmental factors, stress, and infectious agents are factors that play a role in the etiology of asthma. Immunologically mediated inflammation, the major pathological mechanism of this disease, involves mast cells, eosinophils, lymphocytes, neutrophils, and macrophages, which may directly infiltrate the airway at both smooth muscle and basement membrane layers. These cells release a variety of mediators that stimulate bronchoconstriction; vasodilation; edema formation; and increased mucus production, including histamine, interleukins, leukotrienes, tumor necrosis factor (TNF), bradykinin, thromboxanes, fibroblast growth factor, and prostaglandins.

The cascade of mediators in allergy-stimulated asthma is initiated when CD4+ T-helper (Th) cells bearing a Th2 phenotype (which are predominantly involved in humoral immunity and are resistant to apoptotic killing) produce interleukin-3 (IL-3), IL-4, IL-5, IL-13, and granulocyte-macrophage colony-stimulating factor in response to an allergen, which, in turn, upregulates the allergic response and airway hypersensitivity. Th1 T cells (predominantly involved in cell-mediated immunity) have been implicated to a lesser extent. Eosinophils are a rich source of leukotrienes, which directly cause contraction of bronchial smooth muscle and increase vascular permeability. Activated B lymphocytes transform into plasma cells, synthesizing large amounts of immunoglobulin E (IgE) antibody that binds to and activates tissue mast cells and eosinophils. Mast cell-bound IgE molecules become cross-linked by environmental allergens, a process that activates histamine release and additional IL-4 and IL-5 production, thereby provoking bronchial smooth muscle contraction and vasodilation.

With each acute exacerbation of asthma, inflammatory mediators incite a structural remodeling of the airways. The alveoli remain largely unaffected, because asthma is not a parenchymal disease. Rather, airway remodeling involves thickening of the bronchial and bronchiolar mucosa, submucosa, and smooth muscle layers, which contributes to the persistence of disease. Increased collagen is deposited below the basement membrane, while the loose areolar connective tissue found between epithelial and smooth muscle layers undergoes hypertrophy. Therefore, prevention of acute episodes, which minimizes remodeling, is key to the proper treatment of asthma.

Asthma is an obstructive pulmonary disease with hypoxia as the universal finding during acute exacerbations. With acute bronchospasm, residual volume increases in the lungs and peak expiratory flow rate (PEFR) diminishes. Inflammation and constriction of the bronchioles increase airway resistance, decrease inspiratory capacity and expiratory volumes, and lead to ventilation–perfusion mismatching and altered arterial blood gas (ABG) concentrations. As a result of hyperventilation, respiratory alkalosis and hypocapnia are common findings with each episode. As an acute attack resolves, narrowing in the larger airways tends to reverse first, whereas the peripheral airways remain the most constricted. If an attack progresses and fails to reverse, respiratory acidosis and an elevated arterial carbon dioxide concentration typically result, signaling impending respiratory failure. Severe, irreversible bronchoconstriction and inflammation, termed "status asthmaticus," can be fatal.

CLINICAL PRESENTATION

The clinical presentation of asthma varies and depends on whether the patient is currently experiencing an acute attack or is seeking help to manage chronic asthma. It is important to note that not all people with asthma wheeze and that not everyone who wheezes has asthma.

Subjective

During an acute attack, the patient may present with a complaint of breathlessness and may be unable to talk or may be able only to blurt out short or incomplete sentences. There may be profuse sweating and a complaint of air hunger. In patients who are severely obstructed, there may be no wheezing because only cough may be present. Thus, the patient may present, complaining of wheezing, persistent and recurrent cough, difficulty breathing, and/or tightness in the chest, particularly at night or in the early morning. Endurance problems during exercise may occur. Ninety percent of individuals with asthma report that exercise exacerbates their respiratory symptoms.

Any single symptom or combination of symptoms may occur, and symptoms are usually worse at night. The disease spectrum varies from a few mild episodes in a lifetime to daily debilitating symptoms. Food additives, particularly metabisulfite (used as a food preservative); certain dairy products; and, for some individuals, monosodium glutamate may also cause symptoms. An extreme emotional state and associated behaviors, such as excessive laughing or crying, may precipitate or exacerbate an attack.

Objective

Reversible airflow limitation and diurnal variation, as measured by PEFR, constitute objective signs and symptoms of asthma. Variability between morning and evening PEFR may reflect airway hyperresponsiveness and indicate instability and severity of asthma. Nasal discharge, mucosal swelling, frontal facial tenderness, nasal polyps, and allergic "shiners"—dark discoloration beneath both eyes—may be noted, reflecting naso-ocular signs of allergic rhinitis. The clinician should also check for manifestations of allergic skin conditions such as atopic dermatitis (eczema).

Audible inspiratory and expiratory wheezing may be present. The patient may be using accessory muscles of breathing (e.g., scalene, sternocleidomastoid) and sitting upright to facilitate respiration. Auscultation of the chest may reveal inspiratory and expiratory wheezes, if not already audible. Wheezing during forced exhalation is not considered a reliable indicator, as it may be absent between attacks and may be obscured during acute attacks due to diminished breath sounds.

DIAGNOSTIC REASONING

The essential elements to consider in making a diagnosis of asthma are listed in Box 31.1, and spirometry is recommended to confirm this diagnosis. A common feature of asthma is nocturnal awakening with one or more of the following symptoms: dyspnea, cough, and wheezing. In addition, asthma should always be considered as a possible etiology in a patient with a chronic cough.

Diagnostic Tests

To establish the diagnosis of asthma, episodic symptoms of airflow obstruction must be present, airflow obstruction must be at least partially reversible, and the provider must have ruled out any alternative diagnoses.

Box 31.1 Essential Elements to Consider When Diagnosing Asthma

History

- Cough (especially nocturnal)
- Recurrent wheeze (absence does not rule out asthma)
- Recurrent episodic dyspnea
- Recurrent chest tightness

Symptoms worsen in relation to specific factors

- Airborne chemicals or dust
- Animals with fur or feathers
- Changes in weather
- Exercise
- Gastroesophageal reflux disease
- Sensitivity to aspirin, other NSAIDs, and sulfites
- Dust mites in house (e.g., mattresses, furniture, carpets)
- Cockroaches
- Menses
- Mold/pollen
- Nighttime (patient awakens due to symptoms)
- Nonselective beta blockers
- Pollen
- Smoke (tobacco, wood, etc.)
- Strong emotional expression (laughing or crying)
- Viral infection (e.g., rhinitis, sinusitis)

Reversible (at least partially) airflow limitations with diurnal variability

- Variation in peak expiratory flow rate of at least 20% between first morning measurement (before taking inhaled, short-acting beta-agonist) and early afternoon measurement (after using inhaler)
- Exclusion of alternate diagnoses

Spirometric measurements are helpful in the diagnosis, evaluation, and management of the disease. Forced vital capacity (FVC) and forced expiratory volume in 1 second (FEV_1) are helpful measurements. Prebronchodilator and postbronchodilator pulmonary function tests (PFTs), including spirometry and diffusing capacity, to determine the response to bronchodilators are essential in the differential diagnosis and subsequent management of asthma. The diagnosis is made by demonstrating the reversibility of airway obstruction from pre- and post-bronchodilator PFTs. Reversibility is defined as a 10% or greater increase in FEV_1 after two puffs of a short-acting beta-agonist (SABA) have been inhaled. When spirometry is nondiagnostic, bronchial provocation testing may be useful with histamine, methacholine, or exercise as a trigger of airway constriction. Contraindications to spirometry may include the following:

- Hypertension or hypotension
- Rapid atrial fibrillation

- Chest pain
- Recent heart attack (myocardial infarction)
- Recent eye, chest, heart, or abdominal surgery
- Presence of cerebral, thoracic, or abdominal aneurysm
- Active pulmonary infection, including tuberculosis
- Hemoptysis

Infections often precede an asthma attack. If infection is suspected (due to a productive cough with colored sputum), a sputum test for culture and sensitivity should be done. A complete blood count (CBC) should also be done. Levels of nasal eosinophils, serum eosinophils, and IgE are assessed to determine the allergic status of the patient. Intradermal skin testing may be indicated if the allergic status is significant. When persistent asthma is present, the EPR-4 recommends that skin testing or an in-vitro radioallergosorbent test (RAST) be done to determine sensitivity to allergens to optimize treatment and prevention.

A chest x-ray (CXR) may be negative or show only hyperinflation, although CXR may also reveal thickening of bronchial walls and diminished peripheral lung vascular shadows. ABG analysis is included in the initial work-up to establish a baseline and determine the degree of hypoxemia and the need for supplemental oxygen. The results of the ABG analysis and spirometry, along with the clinical history and findings on examination, are triangulated to classify the severity of the asthma, as shown in Table 31.1.

Differential Diagnosis

Differentiating asthma from other respiratory diseases is usually not difficult, particularly with the aid of PFTs, a complete history, and laboratory test results. The key feature in the diagnosis of asthma is reversibility of the obstructive phenomenon, as expiratory airflow measurements are essential to the differential diagnosis of asthma. In contrast, nonreversible airflow obstruction may result from foreign body aspiration or viral infections, as well as a variety of underlying pulmonary conditions, such as aspergillosis, tuberculosis, hypersensitivity pneumonitis, or habitual cough. Persistent wheezing localized to one area of the lung, with paroxysms of cough, is indicative of endobronchial disease, such as foreign body aspiration, neoplasm, or bronchial stenosis. Hyperventilation syndrome, panic disorder, vocal cord dysfunction (paradoxical closure of the vocal cords upon inhalation and/or exhalation), mitral valve prolapse, recurrent pulmonary emboli, and chronic obstructive pulmonary disease (COPD) may all mimic asthma. In addition, acute left ventricular heart failure may initially present similarly to asthma (e.g., with wheezing), but the findings of moist basilar crackles, gallop rhythms, and other signs of congestive heart failure exclude the diagnosis of asthma. In addition, for some medication-sensitive patients, cough may be secondary to the use of certain drugs, such as angiotensin-converting enzyme inhibitors, beta blockers, aspirin, and NSAIDs.

TABLE 31.1 Classification of Asthma Severity

Classification	Clinical Features Before Treatment
Intermittent	- Intermittent symptoms less than 2 days per week - Nighttime asthma symptoms less than twice per month - Asymptomatic and normal peak expiratory flow (PEFR) between exacerbations - PEFR or forced expiratory volume in 1 second (FEV_1) greater than 80% predicted; pulmonary function test (PFT) variability greater than 20%
Mild persistent	- Symptoms more than 2 days per week but not daily; may be several times at night per month - PEFR or FEV_1 greater than 80% predicted; PFT variability 20% to 30%
Moderate persistent	- Symptoms daily, but not continual; nighttime symptoms more than once a week, but not nightly - Exacerbations affect activity and sleep - PEFR or FEV_1 60% to 80% predicted; PFT variability greater than 30%
Severe persistent	- Continuous daily symptoms; frequent nighttime symptoms - Frequent exacerbations - Physical activities limited by asthma - PEFR or FEV_1: less than 60% predicted; PFT variability greater than 30%

Source: National Heart, Lung, and Blood Institute; National Institutes of Health; U.S. Department of Health and Human Services. National Asthma Education and Prevention Program. Expert Panel 4 (EPR-4) Working Group.

MANAGEMENT

Upon the initial diagnosis of asthma, the clinician may want to refer the patient to an allergist or pulmonologist. An aggressive approach to asthma management is recommended to improve short-term symptoms, prevent recurrence of symptoms, and/or manage a potentially chronic problem—all with the goal of improving the patient's quality of life by achieving and maintaining long-term control of asthma symptoms. The principles of management include the following:

- Identification of factors that exacerbate the condition
- Daily monitoring of PEFR with a symptom record
- Written instructions on managing an acute asthma attack
- Intensive education and follow-up, emphasizing joint decision making by the patient and the clinician

Initial and subsequent management of asthma is aimed at first removing all identified triggers or precipitants of asthma symptoms. Acute asthma attacks are treated with SABAs, such as albuterol (salbutamol), administered via a metered dose inhaler (MDI) with a hydrofluoroalkane propellant or nebulized as an inhaled oral solution. MDIs containing chlorofluorocarbon propellants have been banned in the United States, due to their destructive effects on atmospheric ozone.

Home-based rescue therapy for bronchospasm and shortness of breath typically calls for albuterol several times a day as needed, up to every 1 to 2 hours if necessary. This has traditionally been achieved with a prescription SABA or with inhaled epinephrine (Primatene Mist), which is available over the counter. However, with the recognition that asthma is not just a problem requiring immediate relief with bronchodilation but also the treatment of pulmonary inflammation, the new GINA guidelines call for the initiation of an inhaled corticosteroid (ICS)-containing controller treatment to reduce the risk of serious asthma exacerbations and to control respiratory symptoms.

Thus, the use of a SABA should never be the sole therapy for any degree of persistent asthma. If a patient must take rescue medication more frequently or for more than three consecutive doses, they should be instructed to seek further medical care. An individualized and detailed action plan may be developed between the care provider and patient to provide specific guidance for minimizing asthma exacerbations, preventing further progression, and educating about the dangers of medication overuse and when to seek medical care if rescue treatment thresholds are exceeded.

Allergic rhinitis and atopic dermatitis often accompany a diagnosis of asthma, and concurrent treatment for these conditions is critical, because effective treatment of allergic rhinitis (e.g., with intranasal corticosteroids, as discussed in Chapter 24) is critical to prevent the triggering of acute asthma attacks. Given the "one airway, one disease" hypothesis of asthma, allergic rhinitis and asthma are both considered manifestations of allergic disease with a common pathophysiology extending throughout the entire respiratory tract, from the nares and sinuses to the bronchial airways and lungs.

The prevention of asthma exacerbations through the use of daily controller medications for those with mild to severe persistent asthma remains the mainstay of effective asthma therapy, because a reduction in exacerbations and control of daily symptoms lead to improved quality of life. The stepwise therapy approach is a guide to assist the provider in working with the patient to make individually tailored treatment decisions that adequately address symptoms while avoiding medication overuse. As a rule, the highest appropriate therapeutic step should be used to gain early control. The therapy should be "stepped up" if control is not maintained and "stepped down" if adequate control is maintained for a sufficient period of time. At each visit, the clinician should review the patient's medication delivery technique, treatment adherence, and control of asthma triggers. The stepwise approach, according to the severity of the asthma presentation, is shown in Figure 31.1.

In the management of chronic asthma, PFTs are done periodically to measure how well the patient is responding to treatment. The patient can be taught to use a handheld peak flow meter to measure the PEFR and gauge response to treatment. Several peak flow rate readings should be done when the patient is stable to establish a baseline (or "personal best"). This baseline can be used as a benchmark for guiding therapy. Once the patient's condition is stabilized, daily PEFR monitoring can be done by the patient. If the PEFR reading is less than 80% of the patient's personal best, adjustments in medications or lifestyle changes may be necessary to minimize the risk of asthma exacerbations (see Fig. 31.2).

ICSs are the treatment of choice as anti-inflammatory controller therapies, preferred above other classes of inhaled medications and theophylline. Some genetic and epidemiological studies have suggested that certain individuals (especially those of African American ethnicity) have a negative reaction to long-acting beta-agonist (LABA) bronchodilators, such as salmeterol (Serevent), especially if used as long-term therapy. Salmeterol is no longer used as a single agent because of safety concerns regarding increased morbidity and mortality if used without an accompanying corticosteroid. LABAs used in combination with an ICS (Advair Diskus, Symbicort, Dulera), however, are extremely effective at improving lung function in patients with moderate to severe asthma. See Drugs Commonly Prescribed 31.1 for a summary of medications for asthma.

Monoclonal antibody biological agents are used for more severe forms of persistent asthma, including the anti-IgE agent omalizumab (Xolair) for allergic asthma and the anti-IL-5 agent mepolizumab (Nucala), which is specifically approved for eosinophilic asthma. The addition of such therapies to an asthma regimen requires referral to an asthma specialist, such as an allergist or pulmonologist, and, in the case of omalizumab, requires close observation with dosing, given the risk of anaphylaxis.

Bronchial thermoplasty is a therapeutic strategy used for adults aged 18 years and older with severe persistent asthma who remain symptomatic despite the use of a high-dose ICS and a LABA. Bronchial thermoplasty reduces asthma attacks by delivering controlled therapeutic radiofrequency energy into the airways in a targeted fashion, heating the tissue and reducing the amount of smooth muscle present in the airway wall. As a result of less smooth muscle, less airway constriction occurs, thereby reducing asthma attacks.

Scant data exist on the prevalence of complementary therapies for asthma. Such therapies commonly used include breathing techniques, yoga, acupuncture, and herbal preparations. It is difficult to assess the safety and efficacy of these therapies, however, without well-designed clinical trials. Practitioners of herbal medicine recommend the fruit (soursop) and leaves of the graviola tree to relieve respiratory problems, such as cough and asthma,

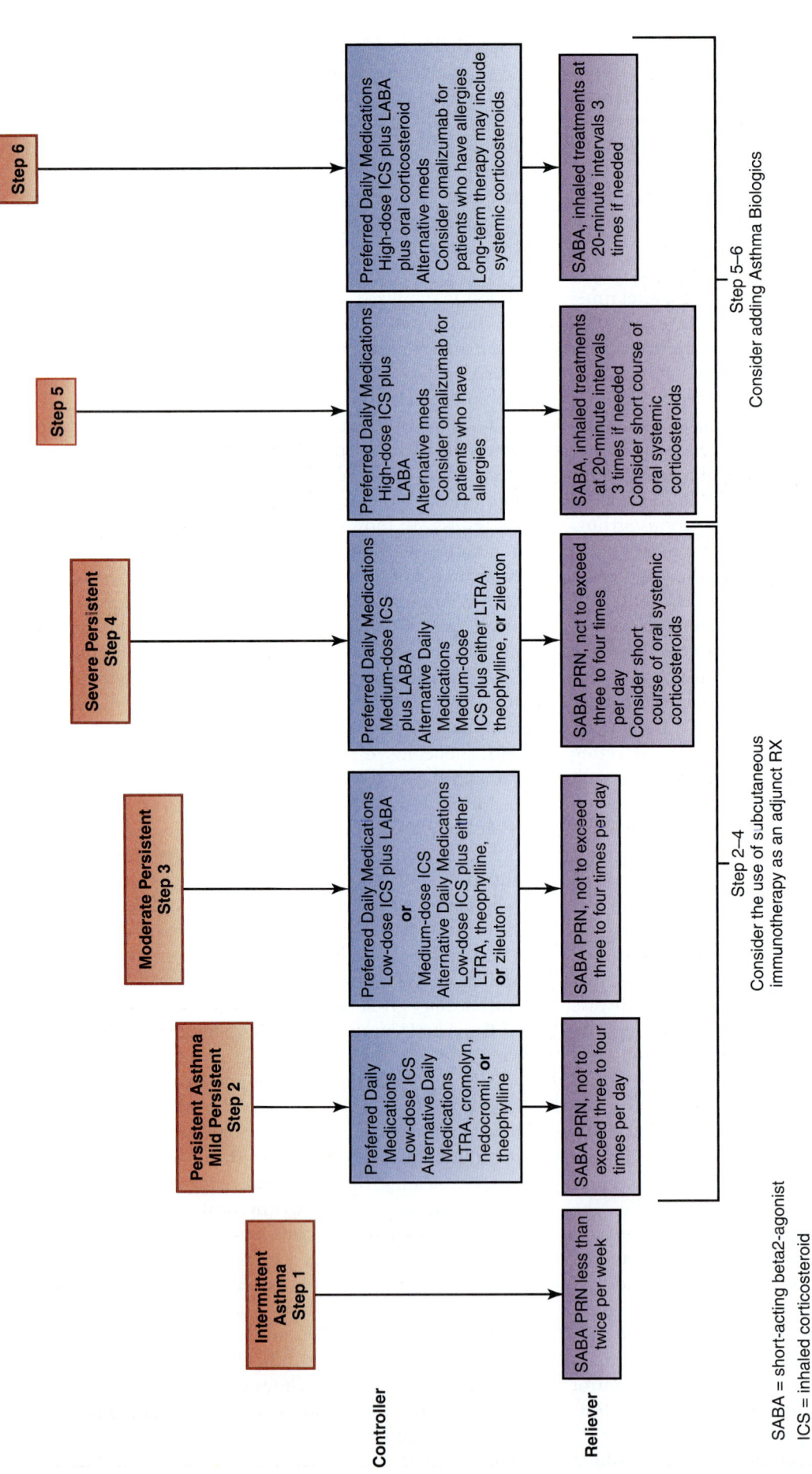

Figure 31.1 Treatment flowchart: Asthma. Adapted from the National Heart, Lung, and Blood Institute, National Asthma Education and Prevention Program. Expert Panel Report 3 (EPR-3): Guidelines for the Diagnosis and Management of Asthma, 2007 Adapted from the 2020 Focused Updates to the Asthma Management Guidelines: A Report from the National Asthma Education and Prevention Coordinating Committee Expert Panel Working Group. (updated in Feb. 2021) https://www.nhlbi.nih.gov/health-topics/asthma-management-guidelines-2020-updates. Accessed 2/14/2022 and the GINA asthma treatment strategy (www.ginaasthma.org) 2020.

Chapter 31 **Inflammatory Respiratory Disorders** 471

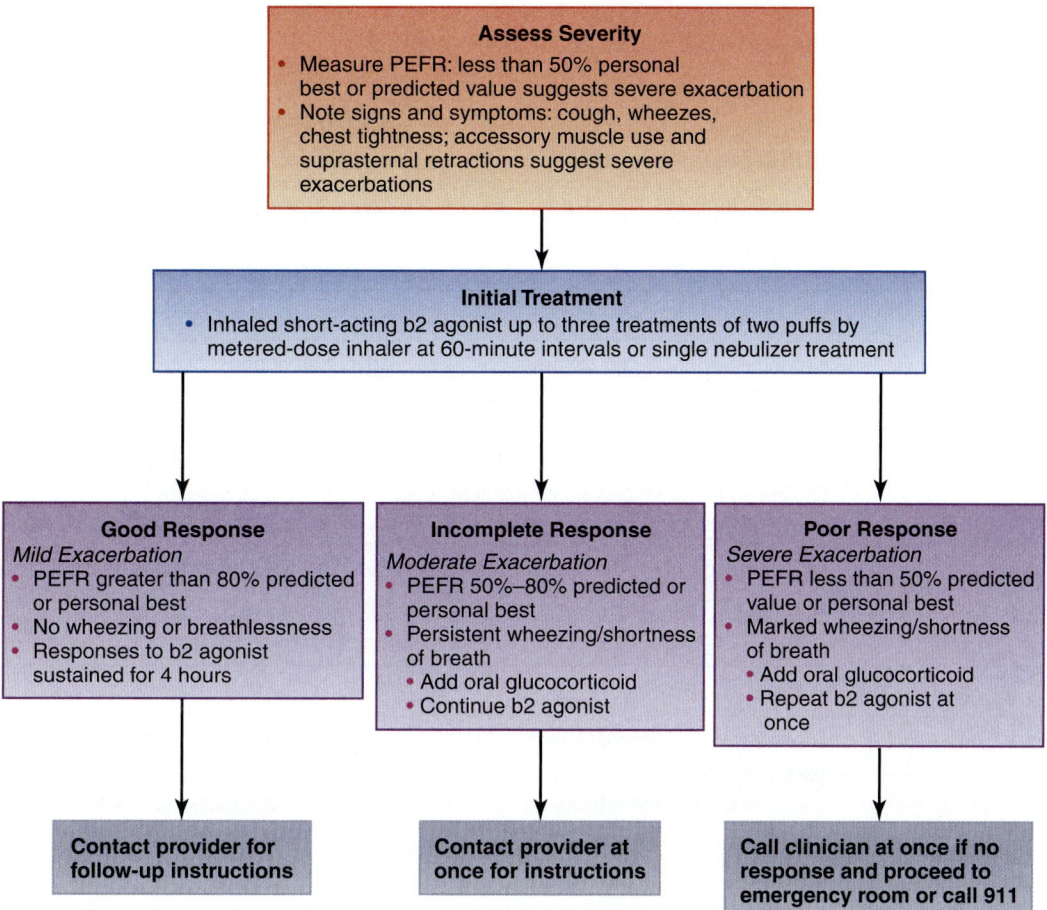

Figure 31.2 Treatment flowchart: Self-management of asthma exacerbations

Drugs Commonly Prescribed 31.1: Asthma

DRUG	INDICATION AND FORMULATION	ADVERSE REACTIONS AND PRESCRIBING CONSIDERATIONS
Short-Acting Beta-Agonists (SABAs)		
	First-line defense for acute attack; may be used prophylactically when necessary before exercise; provides smooth muscle relaxation for bronchodilation. Increased need (usage) indicates need to change treatment regimen.	Adverse reactions: tachycardia, palpitations, tremor, hypokalemia. Use with caution in older patients.
Albuterol (Ventolin hydrofluoroalkane [HFA], Proventil HFA, ProAir HFA, ProAir RespiClick inhalation powder)	Metered-dosage inhaler (MDI): 90 mcg/puff	Two puffs every 4 to 6 hours when necessary For exercise-induced asthma: two puffs 5 minutes before exercise
AccuNeb inhalation solution	Nebulizer: 2.5 mg (0.5 mL of 0.5% solution diluted to 3 mL with normal saline or 3 mL of 0.08% solution)	May be mixed with cromolyn or ipratropium solution (DuoNeb) when nebulized
Levalbuterol (Xopenex: L-isomer of albuterol)	0.63 mg in 3 mL or 1.25 mg in 3 mL	Used with a nebulizer, usually three times a day

Continued

Drugs Commonly Prescribed 31.1: Asthma—cont'd

DRUG	INDICATION AND FORMULATION	ADVERSE REACTIONS AND PRESCRIBING CONSIDERATIONS
Ventolin, Proventil	Syrup: 2 mg/5 mL	Adults: 2 to 4 mg orally three or four times a day Avoid in pediatric patients, given risk of adrenergic systemic side effects
Anticholinergics		
	Not indicated for initial treatment of acute attacks where rescue therapy is required for rapid response; may be used as daily controller therapy or for rescue therapy in limited doses under medical supervision.	Adverse reactions: tachycardia, palpitations, cardiac arrest with overuse in asthma Do not give to patients with glaucoma or benign prostatic hypertrophy
Ipratropium bromide (Atrovent HFA)	MDI: 17 mcg/puff	Two puffs four times a day; maximum 12 puffs/day
(Atrovent solution)	Nebulizer: 0.02% (500 mcg in 2.5 mL of solution)	500 mcg two to four times a day
Leukotriene Receptor Antagonists (LTRAs)		
	Long-term controller medication; prophylaxis and treatment of chronic asthma; ineffective for acute attacks	May allow gradual reduction of inhaled corticosteroids (not for abrupt substitution) Have been associated with eosinophilic granulomatosis with polyangiitis (Churg-Strauss syndrome)
Montelukast (Singulair) Others in same class: pranlukast (Onon, Prakanon), zafirlukast (Accolate), zileuton (Zyflo)	Montelukast: prophylaxis and chronic treatment with 4- or 5-mg chewable tablets, 10-mg film-coated tablet, or oral granules 4 mg/packet; may take 10 mg/night Dosing differs for each different medication type and formulation.	Monitor with potent CYP450 inducers
Inhaled Corticosteroids (ICS)		
	Long-term controller medication; prophylaxis and treatment of chronic asthma; ineffective for acute attacks	Monitor for infections and susceptibility to oral candidiasis (rinse mouth after use). Avoid excessive use.
Mometasone furoate (Asmanex Twisthaler, Asmanex HFA)	Dry powder for inhalation (DPI): 110 to 220 mcg/inhalation MDI: 100 to 200 mcg	Two inhalations twice daily
Beclomethasone (QVAR)	40 or 80 mcg/inhalation	Twice daily
Budesonide (Pulmicort, Pulmicort Flexhaler)	DPI: 90 or 180 mcg/inhalation (maximum 720 mg per day)	Twice daily
Fluticasone (Flovent)	MDI: 44, 110, 220 mcg/puff DPI: 50-, 100-, 250-mg dose	Twice daily (Not recommended for children younger than 4 years)
Combination Inhaled Corticosteroids and Long-Acting Beta-Agonists (ICS + LABAs)		
	Long-term controller medication for moderate to severe persistent asthma; prophylaxis and treatment of chronic asthma; ineffective for acute attacks	Monitor for infections and susceptibility to oral candidiasis (rinse mouth after use). Avoid excessive use.

Drugs Commonly Prescribed 31.1: Asthma—cont'd

DRUG	INDICATION AND FORMULATION	ADVERSE REACTIONS AND PRESCRIBING CONSIDERATIONS
Fluticasone and salmeterol (Advair Diskus)	DPI: 100, 250, or 500 mcg fluticasone per dose plus 50 mcg salmeterol per dose	One puff twice daily One puff daily of 500-mcg/50-mcg formulation
Budesonide and formoterol (Symbicort)	MDI: 80 or 160 mcg budesonide per dose plus 4.5 mcg formoterol per inhalation	Two inhalations twice daily
Fluticasone furoate and vilanterol (BREO Ellipta)	DPI: 100 or 200 mcg fluticasone plus 25 mcg vilanterol per inhalation	One inhalation daily
Mometasone furoate and formoterol fumarate dihydrate (Dulera)	MDI: 100 or 200 mcg mometasone plus 5 mcg formoterol per inhalation	Two inhalations twice daily
Systemic Corticosteroids		
	For long-term treatment of severe persistent asthma that cannot be controlled with other medication classes, including ICSs combined with LABAs Short courses or "bursts" effective for establishing control when initiating therapy or during a period of gradual deterioration or as a supplement to rescue bronchodilator therapy during acute attacks to prevent late-phase bronchospasm Ineffective as treatment for acute attacks	Use with caution in patients with tuberculosis, hypothyroidism, cirrhosis, or ulcerative colitis May mask or increase risk of infection; may cause hypokalemia, hypernatremia, glucose intolerance, and bone demineralization Always titrate down to minimal effective dose Use with caution in pediatric patients
Methylprednisolone (Medrol)	2-, 4-, 8-, 16-, or 32-mg tablets	7.5 to 60.0 mg once a day or every other day in a single dose or four divided doses for larger dosages, as needed for long-term control
Prednisolone (Orapred)	15 mg/5 mL solution	Short "burst" of 40 to 60 mg/day as a single dose or in two divided doses over 3 to 10 days; tapering typically necessary if given for more than 7 to 10 days to prevent adrenal insufficiency
Prednisone	1-, 2.5-, 5-, 10-, 20-, or 50-mg tablets	As stated for prednisolone
Methylxanthines		
	Long-term controller medication for moderate to severe persistent asthma (occasionally used for mild persistent asthma: Step 2); prophylaxis and treatment of chronic asthma Ineffective as treatment for acute attacks	Use with caution, as known to have multiple drug interactions with low therapeutic index; contraindicated in seizure disorders, arrhythmias, and active peptic ulcer disease
Theophylline (Theo-24)	100-, 200-, 300-, 400-mg extended-release capsules	One to two times daily Blood levels can be measured when dosed twice daily; to maintain steady state, keep serum levels between 5 and 15 mcg/mL (if on high dose, do not take within 1 hour of eating fatty foods) May have some anti-inflammatory properties

and for many other medical problems. Some literature cites the use of eucalyptus (as a decongestant/cough suppressant), lycopene (for exercise-induced asthma), vitamins B_{12} and C, and goldenseal, but research needs to be done on their effectiveness, so caution should be exercised when discussing these with patients.

Nutritional therapies have been used in the treatment of asthma, although it is also known that certain foods may precipitate an asthma flare in patients with food allergies. To treat asthma, Moses Maimonides, the noted 13th-century physician, prescribed a spicy herbal mixture of chicken broth that contained herbs such as fennel, parsley, oregano, mint, and onion. Onions and garlic have been known to have some protective effect against allergic reactions, and hydration from such a robust broth may also be a helpful component in asthma treatment. Strong coffee was a widely used treatment for asthma in 18th-century Europe and continues to be used as an effective bronchodilator today, likely a function of its methylxanthine content in the form of caffeine. Although drinking tea has never been particularly favored as an asthma treatment, tea leaves were the original source of theophylline, which means "tea leaf."

FOLLOW-UP AND REFERRAL

Therapy should be "stepped down" gradually if a review of the patient's status at 1- to 6-month intervals suggests that a reduction of treatment is warranted. Smoking cessation for patients with asthma is a must. (For more information on smoking cessation, see Chapter 33.) In addition, the patient should avoid exposure to secondhand smoke, and family members should be educated about the hazards of secondhand smoke for the patient. Regular visits to the primary care provider can be combined with appropriate referrals to specialists (e.g., allergists, pulmonologists) as necessary.

The use of immunotherapy in asthma remains controversial, and its effectiveness has not been well established. For most patients, avoidance of the allergens and triggers that cause asthma attacks, along with the appropriate use of medications, is adequate therapy. If avoidance of certain allergens is impossible or controller medications fail, referral to an allergist for immunotherapy may be indicated. However, unless the patient's symptoms are exacerbated by exposure to specific allergens, which can be confirmed by skin-prick testing, it is unlikely that immunotherapy will be effective.

Patient Education: Asthma

A list of reasonable expectations for patients with asthma should be reviewed with the patient and family, including potential triggers that might be removed or reduced in the patient's environment, as well as problematic areas such as treatment noncompliance or improper use of inhaled medications (see Box 31.2).

Box 31.2 Reasonable Expectations for Patients With Asthma

When entering into a treatment plan, the patient with asthma expects the following:

- Be able to participate fully in any activity
- Be able to sleep through the night
- Be free of severe symptoms during the day and night
- Be satisfied with asthma care
- Have the best possible pulmonary function
- Need fewer or no emergency visits or hospitalizations due to asthma
- Not miss work or school because of asthma
- Use fewer medications with minimal adverse effects

The provider is responsible for the following:

- Asking patients about their concerns and issues at each visit
- Continually teaching and reinforcing key educational points
- Ensuring ongoing and open communication with the patient and family
- Reviewing short-term goals as agreed at the initial visit
- Reviewing the asthma action plan for worsening symptoms and exacerbations
- Reviewing the daily self-management plan and steps the patient needs to take
- Supplying patients with appropriate educational materials for self-management and prevention

The patient and family should be educated about the following aspects of self-care management:

- Basic asthma facts
- When and how to use a short-acting inhaler before exercising (some patients have only exercise-induced asthma)
- How to recognize early symptoms of an exacerbation and how to initiate a predetermined plan of action
- Role of medications (long-acting controller and short-term rescue therapy) and the critical role for anti-inflammatory controller medication regimens to reduce the rate of acute attacks
- Skills for proper inhaler use, including the use of spacers, and daily peak flow meter monitoring (for patients with moderate to severe persistent asthma); spacers are universally recommended for MDIs to obtain maximum benefit (some medication delivery systems have "built-in" spacers)
- Use of a nebulizer if necessary; nebulizers may be needed if patients cannot take adequate breaths
- Environmental control for allergen reduction
- Avoidance measures for asthma triggers
- Importance of pneumococcal and annual influenza vaccination

Box 31.2 Reasonable Expectations for Patients With Asthma—cont'd

Proper medication use and the correct use of a handheld flow meter to monitor obstructive manifestations and severity should be reviewed at each visit. It should be mentioned that rescue courses of systemic glucocorticoids may be needed at times to prevent late-phase reactions in acute attacks, although recurrent attacks indicate that a greater degree of controller medication is warranted. In addition, patient and family education is essential for control of asthma triggers and recognition of warning signals. An asthma attack trigger diary may be used to assist in identifying such triggers.

Patients may ask which ICS is the most effective. Research has shown that if equipotent doses are used, the efficacy of different agents is essentially the same; the key difference is in the delivery technique. With a dry powder inhaler device, age is a factor. Providers must spend time teaching the proper technique and observing a return demonstration. One of the adverse side effects of ICSs is believed to be their effects on growth rate in children. Research has shown that this is a small but definable risk. Growth reduction is more pronounced in the first year of therapy. Daily use of ICSs can cause a small reduction in the average height of children with persistent asthma up to the age of 18 years. Nonetheless, although it must be cautioned that all individuals should be on the lowest dose of ICSs possible, this small reduction in height must be weighed against the known benefit of ICSs for asthma control.

Another question commonly asked by asthmatic patients is which pets are hypoallergenic. There are many Web sites that promote costly specialty pets that are purported to be nonallergenic, but in reality, there are no hypoallergenic pets.

Using commonsense measures such as keeping pets out of the bedroom and wiping down cats with a wet washcloth every night to help control dander may help; however, in some cases, removing pets from the home completely may be the only recourse, although asthmatic patients can still react to residual dander and hair in the environment.

The patient and family should be educated to the fullest extent possible to permit self-management and the prevention of acute fatal attacks. Although asthma is a chronic disease, patients may die of a particularly severe, acute, or persistent and refractory asthmatic attack (status asthmaticus).

The risk factors for fatal asthma are listed in Box 31.3. Patients with any of these risk factors need additional teaching time so that they can learn self-management techniques to reduce their risk to the fullest extent possible. It is extremely important that the patient be trained to use the handheld peak flow meter and learn to determine their predicted (personal best) PEFR. During exacerbations, the patient should compare a current reading to the baseline PEFR as a guide to determine how severe the attack is and to gauge medication use accordingly. The value of the green/yellow/red markers on the PEFR meter as a guide for the patient and family as to when to seek emergency help should be emphasized.

A caring relationship among the provider, the patient, and family is pivotal to effective disease management and improved quality of life. Although self-care is an essential component of treatment, a family member should be educated about how to handle an acute attack, in case the patient becomes severely hypoxic and cognitively impaired.

Box 31.3 Risk Factors for Fatal Asthma

- Comorbidity (cardiovascular or pulmonary disease, such as chronic obstructive pulmonary disease)
- Current use of, or recent withdrawal from, systemic glucocorticoids
- Difficulty perceiving airflow obstruction or its severity
- History of sudden severe exacerbations
- Hospitalization or emergency care for asthma within the past month
- Illicit drug use
- Low socioeconomic status and urban residence
- Prior intubation for asthma
- Sensitivity to the fungus *Alternaria*
- Serious psychiatric disease or psychosocial problems
- Three or more emergency visits for asthma in the past year
- Two or more hospitalizations for asthma in the past year
- Use of three or more canisters of inhaled short-acting beta$_2$-agonists per month

CHRONIC BRONCHITIS AND EMPHYSEMA (CHRONIC OBSTRUCTIVE PULMONARY DISEASE [COPD])

There are two main forms of lung disease—obstructive and restrictive. Obstructive lung diseases are those in which the expiratory flow rate is impaired. Restrictive lung diseases are those in which the lung volumes are reduced due to musculoskeletal disorders, tumors, lung resection, or interstitial lung disease (ILD). Obstructive lung diseases are further classified as reversible (such as asthma) or irreversible (such as chronic bronchitis and emphysema, which are collectively grouped together as chronic obstructive pulmonary disease [COPD]). The American Thoracic Society (ATS) defines chronic bronchitis as a clinical disorder characterized by excessive mucus secretion in the bronchial tree. It is manifested by chronic or recurrent cough (with or without sputum production) and is present on most days for a minimum of 3 months of the year, for at least 2 successive years. In addition, dyspnea with or without wheezing is present.

EPIDEMIOLOGY AND CAUSES

The ATS defines COPD as a disease state characterized by the presence of airflow obstruction due to chronic bronchitis or emphysema. Asthma is not classified as COPD but is sometimes referred to as a reversible obstructive condition, whereas emphysema is irreversible. Chronic bronchitis is usually irreversible, but it may be partially reversible if there is a bronchospastic component and a significant response to bronchodilators. It is difficult to estimate the prevalence of chronic bronchitis because there is considerable overlap of various obstructive conditions, as many patients have some combination of aspects of all three conditions—asthma, chronic bronchitis, and/or emphysema.

Whereas more than 16 million Americans have been diagnosed with COPD, an equal number are probably afflicted but not yet diagnosed. It is estimated that approximately 10% of individuals aged 40 years and older have COPD, and 52% of people with COPD are female. The CDC lists the number of adults with diagnosed chronic bronchitis in 2018 as 9 million. There were 5.7 million office visits with emphysema and other forms of COPD as the primary diagnosis, and this same primary diagnosis resulted in 923,000 emergency department visits.

The prevalence and mortality rates for chronic bronchitis and emphysema increase with age. In addition, morbidity and mortality are higher in people with lower incomes and less education. There are more than 160,000 deaths each year due to COPD, as COPD is the fourth leading cause of death in the United States and the fourth leading cause of disability. The estimated direct medical costs of COPD are more than $30 billion annually. This fact highlights the economic importance of prevention and of interventions aimed at early diagnosis and delaying disease progression. In turn, several studies have established certain predisposing risk factors for morbidity and mortality from COPD.

Risk Factors for COPD

Established risks:

- Age
- Male gender
- Cigarette smoking
- Reduced lung function
- Occupational exposures
- Air pollution
- Alpha$_1$-antitrypsin deficiency phenotypes

Probable or possible risks:

- Infections of the respiratory tract
- Allergic conditions
- Bronchial reactivity
- Climate
- Lower socioeconomic resources
- Alcohol intake
- Poor diet and inadequate nutrition
- ABO (ABH) secretor cell phenotypes
- Impaired immune function
- Familial factors

Cigarette smoking is responsible for 80% to 90% of the cases of COPD, and it is also the risk factor most amenable to modification for preventing or delaying the development of COPD. Educational intervention at an early age can help reduce smoking and some other risk factors, such as occupational exposure, exposure to air pollution and allergens, and respiratory infections. If certain genetic risk factors are present, the patient should be educated about periodic baseline testing for pulmonary function and about routine checks to prevent respiratory infections and reduce risks to the greatest extent possible. Smokers older than 40 years of age are at higher risk of developing COPD. Stopping smoking at any age has some beneficial effect for lung function, although there may be permanent damage to lung tissue.

PATHOPHYSIOLOGY

COPD is a progressive disease characterized by airflow limitation that is not fully reversible. The disease process involves a combination of the pathological mechanisms of emphysema and chronic bronchitis. In addition, hyperreactivity of the airways is a common feature. Thus, COPD is a disease of both the lung parenchyma and the small airways (bronchioles).

Emphysema is characterized by destruction of alveolar walls due to an imbalance of proteinase–antiproteinase enzymatic activity. In healthy lung tissue, protective antiproteinases counteract protein-degrading enzymes secreted by white blood cells. A genetic condition called alpha$_1$-antitrypsin deficiency may play a role in causing COPD. People with this condition have low levels of alpha$_1$-antitrypsin, a protein made in the liver. Chronic inflammation, caused by long-term cigarette smoking or chronic exposure to lung irritants, for example, repeatedly recruits white blood cells to the alveoli. In contrast to the atopic processes of asthma, the lymphocytic infiltration of COPD consists predominantly of CD8+ T cells, rather than CD4+ T cells. Neutrophil and monocyte/macrophage-derived proteinases progressively degrade the alveolar walls, overcoming antiproteinase defenses. Overdistended, hyperinflated, and less elastic alveoli are the result of recurring lung injury over time. Weak elastic recoil of alveoli leads to air trapping, increased residual lung volume, reduced expiratory flow, and retained carbon dioxide. Individuals experience hypercapnia but can maintain adequate oxygenation early in the disease process.

the establishment of advance directives, living wills, and health-care surrogates. Copies of pertinent medicolegal documents should be kept in the medical chart, as well as with patients' families and attorneys. Strategies are needed to mitigate the effects of anticipated stigma on individuals with chronic illness, as shown in Evidence-Based Nursing Practice 31.1. Interventions that increase health-care providers' awareness of anticipated stigma and stigmatizing behaviors related to COPD are needed to improve health care for this population. See the Iceberg of COPD for additional aspects of patient education.

The Iceberg of COPD

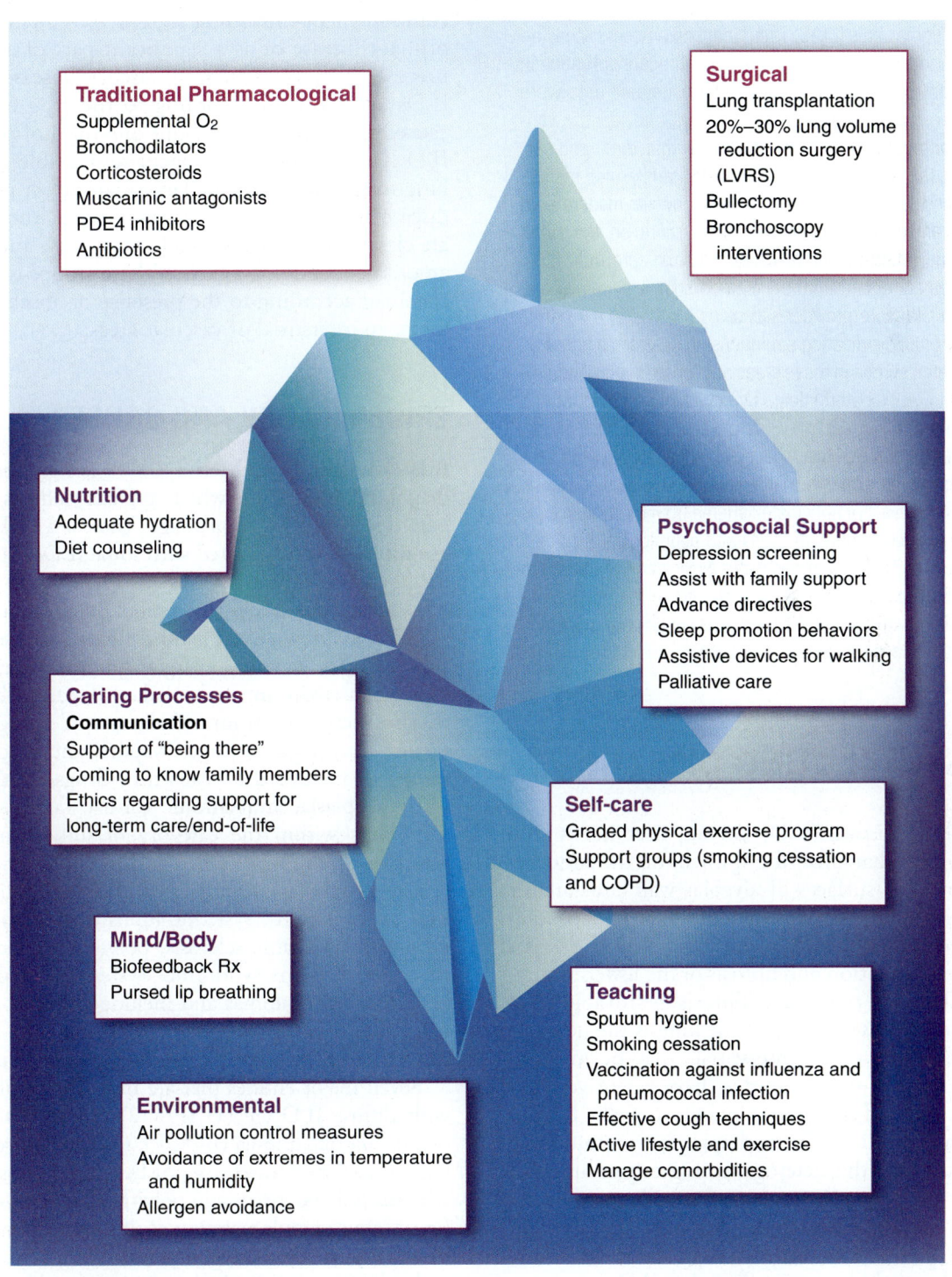

Traditional Pharmacological
Supplemental O₂
Bronchodilators
Corticosteroids
Muscarinic antagonists
PDE4 inhibitors
Antibiotics

Surgical
Lung transplantation
20%–30% lung volume reduction surgery (LVRS)
Bullectomy
Bronchoscopy interventions

Nutrition
Adequate hydration
Diet counseling

Psychosocial Support
Depression screening
Assist with family support
Advance directives
Sleep promotion behaviors
Assistive devices for walking
Palliative care

Caring Processes
Communication
Support of "being there"
Coming to know family members
Ethics regarding support for long-term care/end-of-life

Self-care
Graded physical exercise program
Support groups (smoking cessation and COPD)

Mind/Body
Biofeedback Rx
Pursed lip breathing

Teaching
Sputum hygiene
Smoking cessation
Vaccination against influenza and pneumococcal infection
Effective cough techniques
Active lifestyle and exercise
Manage comorbidities

Environmental
Air pollution control measures
Avoidance of extremes in temperature and humidity
Allergen avoidance

COPD - Chronic Obstructive Pulmonary Disease
PDE - Phosphodiesterase

> **Evidence-Based Nursing Practice 31.1**
>
> Chin, E, Armstrong, D. Anticipated stigma and healthcare utilization in COPD and neurological disorders. *Appl Nurs Res.* 2019 Feb;(45):63–68.
>
> This descriptive correlational study explored the experience of anticipated stigma and its association with health-seeking behavior in individuals with COPD or a neurological disorder. Participants with COPD (n = 38) or neurological disorders (n = 39) were recruited from specialty practices. The Chronic Illness Anticipated Stigma Scale (CIASS) and Healthcare Access Measure (HAM) were used to measure stigma and health-care utilization in this population. Sociodemographic and illness-related data were entered into a hierarchical regression analysis to identify variables that contribute to anticipated stigma from three sources. The mean scores of anticipated stigma by family and friends, coworkers, and health-care workers were low to moderate at 7.96, 11.68, and 7.94, respectively. Mean score on the HAM was 12.94, indicating moderate delay in health-care utilization. The HAM was correlated with anticipated stigma by family and friends and health-care provider subscales (r = 0.293, p = 0.010; r = 0.449, p = 0.000), indicating a relationship between higher levels of anticipated stigma in these areas and lower levels of health-care utilization. Anticipated stigma by coworkers was correlated with neurological disorders (r = .257, p = .048). In a final model, 20%, 35.4%, and 16.8% of the variance of anticipated stigma from three sources can be explained. Findings from this study describe low to moderate levels of anticipated stigma from three sources is experienced in individuals with COPD and neurological disorders and lends new understanding about the association of stigma to health-care utilization behavior in this population. Strategies are needed to mitigate the effects of stigma on health-care utilization

INTERSTITIAL LUNG DISEASE

Interstitial lung disease (ILD) encompasses nearly 200 clinical disorders that affect the epithelium, the endothelium, or both cell surfaces of alveolar wall and satellite structures, including terminal and respiratory bronchioles. ILD consists of a heterogeneous group of diseases that cause inflammation and fibrosis of the lower respiratory tract. The term "pulmonary fibrosis" is also applied to these diseases because fibrosis of the lung is the ultimate result of ILD. The term "interstitial" may be misleading in that most of these disorders have extensive alteration of alveolar and airway architecture as well. "Diffuse parenchymal lung disease" is perhaps a more appropriate descriptive term for this heterogeneous group of lung diseases because the term "interstitium" usually refers to the microscopic anatomical space bounded by the basement membranes of epithelial and endothelial cells. The entire lung parenchyma, however, is affected in ILD.

The ILDs have many common features, including similarity of patient symptoms, comparable appearance of CXRs, consistent derangements in pulmonary physiology, and typical histological features. Four infections may be associated with the cause or onset of most of the ILDs: disseminated fungus (coccidioidomycosis, blastomycosis, histoplasmosis), disseminated mycobacteria, *Pneumocystis* pneumonia, and certain viruses.

Although all of the diffuse ILDs share the common morphological characteristic of an abnormal lung interstitium, a satisfactory classification system has proved elusive as approximately 150 individual diseases have a component of interstitial lung involvement, either as a primary disease or as a significant part of a multiorgan process, such as a collagen vascular disease. Generally, ILDs are classified according to the type of agent that caused the lung injury. About one-third of patients with ILD have an identifiable agent responsible for inducing lung injury; however, the large majority of patients have disease attributable to no known cause. Therefore, ILDs are classified as those with a known cause and those with an unknown etiology; each of these groups is further subclassified according to the presence or absence of granulomas in interstitial or vascular areas.

EPIDEMIOLOGY AND CAUSES

It is estimated that about 140,000 Americans have been diagnosed with ILD, which typically affects individuals between 50 and 75 years of age. There is a slightly younger age distribution associated with some ILDs (40 to 45 years for respiratory bronchiolitis–associated ILD and 45 to 55 years for nonspecific interstitial pneumonitis).

ILDs of known cause can be divided into several major subcategories. By far, the largest group comprises occupational and environmental inhalant diseases; these include diseases resulting from inhalation of inorganic dusts, organic dusts, gases, fumes, vapors, and aerosols. Other categories include ILDs caused by drugs, irradiation, poisons, neoplasia, and chronic cardiac failure. The major subgroups within the category of unknown causes are idiopathic pulmonary fibrosis (IPF) and connective tissue (collagen vascular) disorders with ILD, including rheumatoid arthritis (RA), systemic lupus erythematosus (SLE), progressive systemic sclerosis, polymyositis-dermatomyositis, and Sjögren's syndrome. Systemic vasculitides often have tissue granulomas and include a variant of polyarteritis nodosa called allergic granulomatosis, as well as lymphomatoid granulomatosis and hypersensitivity vasculitis.

Seven major entities that are most frequently associated with diffuse ILD are (1) IPF, (2) bronchiolitis obliterans organizing pneumonia (BOOP), (3) connective tissue (collagen vascular) diseases (e.g., SLE, RA, progressive systemic sclerosis [scleroderma], and polymyositis-dermatomyositis), (4) systemic granulomatous vasculitides (Wegener's granulomatosis, lymphomatoid granulomatosis, and allergic angiitis and granulomatosis), (5) drug-induced pulmonary disease, (6) sarcoidosis, and (7) hypersensitivity pneumonitis. These entities are briefly discussed further in Box 31.4.

Box 31.4 Interstitial Lung Diseases: Primary and Secondary Forms

Interstitial Pulmonary Fibrosis (IPF): A syndrome progressing from alveolitis to interstitial inflammation to fibrosis of the lungs

Pulmonary Manifestations: Presents with dyspnea, cough, fatigue, adventitious crackles (sounding like Velcro), tachypnea, finger clubbing, abnormal pulmonary function tests (PFTs)

Management: No curative medical therapy; pirfenidone (Esbriet) and nintedanib (Ofev, tyrosine kinase inhibitor), both shown to improve lung function and approved to treat IPF; corticosteroids (e.g., prednisone), immunosuppressants, antifibrotic agents (colchicine or D-penicillamine), recombinant tumor necrosis factor (TNF)-α antagonists, and other tyrosine kinase inhibitors are being studied

Bronchiolitis Obliterans Organizing Pneumonia (BOOP): A disease characterized by masses of granulation tissue in the lumens of small airways, with patchy organizing pneumonia distal to these obstructions

Pulmonary Manifestations: Presents with cough, flu-like illness, inspiratory crackles, expiratory squeaks, restrictive ventilatory defect, and abnormal diffusing capacity; chest x-ray shows patchy alveolar infiltrates, often with a ground-glass appearance.

Management: Corticosteroids (e.g., prednisone)

Collagen Vascular Diseases

Systemic Lupus Erythematosus: Chronic, multisystem inflammatory disease of connective tissue that involves the skin, joints, serous membranes (e.g., pleura, pericardium), kidneys, hematological system, and central nervous system (CNS)

Pulmonary Manifestations: May present with pleuritis with or without effusion, diaphragmatic dysfunction with reduced lung volume, acute lupus pneumonitis, diffuse alveolar hemorrhage, diffuse interstitial disease, pulmonary hypertension, and pulmonary thromboembolism

Management: The B-lymphocyte stimulator (BLyS)-specific inhibitor belimumab (Benlysta) is approved to treat lupus; NSAIDs, corticosteroids (e.g., prednisone), disease-modifying antirheumatic drugs (DMARDs) such as hydroxychloroquine (Plaquenil) and methotrexate (Rheumatrex), and other immunosuppressive agents such as cyclophosphamide (Cytoxan) are also used; plasmapheresis and stem cell therapy have also been tried but are not approved by the U.S. Food and Drug Administration

Rheumatoid Arthritis: Chronic, systemic disease characterized by recurrent inflammation of the diarthrodial joints and related structures

Pulmonary Manifestations: Presents with abnormal PFTs with reduced diffusing capacity and restrictive lung mechanics, pulmonary nodules, BOOP, pleuritis with or without effusion, interstitial lung disease (ILD)

Management: NSAIDs, COX-2 inhibitors, corticosteroids (e.g., prednisone), methotrexate (Rheumatrex), other DMARDs, and biological response modifiers:
- Non-TNF-α antagonists (e.g., abatacept [Orencia], rituximab [Rituxan], tocilizumab [Actemra], sarilumab [Kevzara], anakinra [Kineret])
- TNF-α antagonists (e.g., infliximab [Remicade], etanercept [Enbrel], adalimumab [Humira], golimumab [Simponi], certolizumab [Cimzia])
- Janus kinase inhibitors (e.g., tofacitinib [Xeljanz], upadacitinib [Rinvoq], baricitinib [Olumiant])

Progressive Systemic Sclerosis (Scleroderma): A disorder of connective tissue characterized by fibrotic, degenerative, and occasionally inflammatory changes in the skin, blood vessels, synovium, skeletal, muscle, and internal organs

Pulmonary Manifestations: Presents with dyspnea, bibasilar crackles, reduced lung compliance, pleural thickening, pulmonary fibrosis on x-ray, abnormal PFTs, pulmonary hypertension, recurrent aspiration pneumonia

Management: Antifibrotic agents (e.g., D-penicillamine [Cuprimine]), immunosuppressants (e.g., azathioprine [Imuran], methotrexate [Rheumatrex]), and possibly stem cell therapy

Polymyositis-Dermatomyositis: A diffuse inflammatory myopathy of striated muscle, producing symmetrical weakness that is usually most severe in the proximal muscles

Pulmonary Manifestations: The three types of lung disease classically described are interstitial pneumonitis, aspiration pneumonia due to esophageal dysmotility, and pneumonia secondary to hypoventilation as a result of respiratory muscle involvement

Management: Corticosteroids (e.g., prednisone), antineoplastic agents, and immunosuppressants (e.g., cyclophosphamide [Cytoxan])

Systemic Granulomatous Vasculitis

Wegener's Granulomatosis: Characterized by a triad of (1) necrotizing granulomatous vasculitis of the upper and lower respiratory tracts, (2) glomerulonephritis, and (3) variable degrees of vasculitis of the small arteries and veins

Pulmonary Manifestations: Upper respiratory tract lesions include sinusitis, otitis media, nasal septal ulceration; pulmonary manifestations vary from focal granulomatous vasculitis to diffuse alveolitis and capillaritis that may present as alveolar hemorrhage, with PFTs revealing a restrictive pattern

Management: Immunosuppressants (e.g., cyclophosphamide [Cytoxan], azathioprine [Imuran], methotrexate [Rheumatrex]), corticosteroids (e.g., prednisone), anti-TNF-α agents, or anti-B-cell therapies

Lymphomatoid Granulomatosis: A systemic disease consisting of angiocentric lymphoid granulomatous vasculitis,

Continued

> **Box 31.4 Interstitial Lung Diseases: Primary and Secondary Forms—cont'd**
>
> primarily of the lungs, with frequent involvement of the kidneys and skin
>
> *Pulmonary Manifestations:* Presenting symptoms are usually cough and dyspnea; chest x-ray reveals multiple bilateral, ill-defined, or nodular densities that may cavitate
>
> *Management:* Cyclophosphamide (Cytoxan) and corticosteroids (e.g., prednisone); chemotherapy regimen if recurrence with malignant lymphoma; interferon treatment and stem cell therapy have also been used
>
> **Allergic Angiitis and Granulomatosis (Churg-Strauss Syndrome):** A rare disorder characterized by necrotizing angiitis of the lungs, heart, skin, and CNS, with involved organs displaying infiltration with eosinophils
>
> *Pulmonary Manifestations:* Presents with an allergic history, often with asthma; chest x-ray abnormalities may range from patchy densities to large bilateral nodular infiltrates; lung cavitation is rare
>
> *Management:* Corticosteroids (e.g., prednisone), immunosuppressants (e.g., azathioprine [Imuran], cyclophosphamide [Cytoxan]), and plasma exchange have been used
>
> **Drug-Induced Pulmonary Disease:** Iatrogenic and adverse complications of various drugs (e.g., cytotoxic agents, antibiotics, immunosuppressive drugs) can result in ILD
>
> *Pulmonary Manifestations:* Hypersensitivity pulmonary disease with dyspnea, nonproductive cough, lung crackles, tachypnea, diffuse linear streaks, and densities in lower lung zones on chest x-ray
>
> *Management:* Discontinuation of the drug or reduction in drug dosage, in conjunction with corticosteroids (e.g., prednisone)
>
> **Sarcoidosis:** A multisystem syndrome of unknown etiology, involving complex cellular immune pathways, that most frequently affects the lung
>
> *Pulmonary Manifestations:* Lung most common organ affected; PFTs reveal a restrictive pattern and small lung volumes; tissue biology demonstrates characteristic granulomas, with hilar lymphadenopathy typically seen on chest x-ray
>
> *Management:* Corticosteroids (e.g., prednisone) and other immunosuppressant drugs (e.g., hydroxychloroquine [Plaquenil] and methotrexate [Rheumatrex])
>
> **Hypersensitivity Pneumonitis (Allergic Alveolitis):** Caused by inhalation of a variety of organic dusts. These dusts can be derived from animal dander and proteins, from fungi that contaminate vegetables, wood bark, water-reservoir vaporizers, or from dairy and grain products; descriptive names for this disease underscore the frequent occupational nature of exposure (e.g., bird fancier's disease, farmer's lung)
>
> *Pulmonary Manifestations:* In the acute form of disease, respiratory and systemic symptoms develop explosively within 4 to 6 hours after dust is inhaled, consisting of dyspnea, cough, chills, fever, and malaise; symptoms typically abate within 12 hours but with each reexposure, the acute episode occurs again; the acutely ill patient is dyspneic with inspiratory crackles in the lower lung zones; chest x-ray shows fine, diffuse alveolar filling and variable interstitial streaks, and PFTs are abnormal
>
> *Management:* Avoidance of inhaled substance; corticosteroids (e.g., prednisone)

PATHOPHYSIOLOGY

ILD denotes a diverse group of conditions characterized by the common pathological finding of pulmonary fibrosis and a similar clinical presentation of restrictive lung findings (i.e., dyspnea on exertion and chronic nonproductive cough). The term "interstitial" used to describe this group of diseases is misleading because inflammation and fibrosis may affect bronchioles, alveoli, and capillary endothelia, as well as the interstitium of the lower respiratory tract. Thus, a more illustrative term for this disease is "pulmonary fibrosis." Sarcoidosis, hypersensitivity pneumonitis, pulmonary fibrosis in connective tissue disorders (e.g., SLE, RA, tuberous sclerosis, scleroderma), and occupational pulmonary diseases are all categorized as ILDs. Tissue injury and acute inflammation are believed to be the initial pathological processes. In some conditions, such as sarcoidosis, the inciting antigen is unknown, whereas occupational pulmonary diseases are caused by repeated inhalation of environmental irritants, inorganic and organic dusts, fumes, or gases. For most ILDs, including idiopathic conditions, cigarette smoking is a primary risk factor.

In the majority of ILDs, there is a perpetuation of the inflammatory process with repeated tissue injury and aberrant wound healing, resulting in remodeling of the lung architecture. Infiltration of the lung parenchyma by various combinations of immune cells mediates this process, including neutrophils, lymphocytes, plasma cells, eosinophils, basophils, mast cells, and alveolar macrophages. Cytokine production (e.g., granulocyte-colony stimulating factor, transforming growth factor–β, IL-1β, IL-8, TNF-α) drives these inflammatory and scarring (fibrotic) processes. Regions of chronic inflammation can develop granulomas consisting specifically of discrete masses of lymphocytes, macrophages, and fibroblasts. In turn, fibroblast proliferation and differentiation into myofibroblast forms (i.e., cells with both fibroblast and smooth muscle cell features) lead to fibrosis (collagen deposition) or scarring of the lungs and the development of cystic airspaces known as "honeycombing."

Such pathological pulmonary tissue becomes less compliant and increasingly rigid, with resultant impedance of ventilation and gas exchange, characteristic of a progressive, minimally reversible restrictive lung disease. Diffusion capacity of the lung for carbon monoxide (DLCO) also worsens with increasing fibrosis and thickening of the lung parenchyma. In turn, ventilation–perfusion mismatch, hypoxemia, and pulmonary vasoconstriction develop, and increased resistance to the pumping function of the right ventricle may lead to cor pulmonale (right ventriculomegaly). Hypercarbia typically manifests only in end-stage disease. Total lung capacity, functional residual capacity, residual volume, FEV, and FEV_1 are all typically decreased on PFT; however, because fibrotic lung tissue is stiffer with greater elastic recoil, rapid exhalation of a major portion of the overall expiratory volume may be seen, as reflected in a normal or increased FEV_1/FVC ratio on PFT. This is a key feature distinguishing restrictive from obstructive pulmonary disease in which the FEV_1/FVC ratio is decreased.

Interestingly, recurrent dysregulated wound healing, rather than neutrophilic or immune cell–mediated inflammation, has been cited as the primary pathophysiological mechanism in ILD, potentially explaining the ineffectiveness of anti-inflammatory and immunosuppressive treatments in many forms of ILD. Lung tissue biopsy is not required for the diagnosis of ILD, which may be made from a combination of clinical and radiographic findings (including PFTs and certain serum markers of underlying connective tissue disease). However, the extent of lung fibrosis observed histopathologically is perhaps the most accurate prognostic indicator for this condition. In turn, much investigation has shifted toward antifibroblast therapies for ILD aimed at decreasing pulmonary collagen deposition.

CLINICAL PRESENTATION

Subjective

The symptoms of ILD are similar regardless of the underlying cause, although the symptoms of lung involvement are nonspecific and can suggest many other causes, including obstructive lung disease, heart disease, or pulmonary vascular disease. The first symptom of ILD is usually progressive dyspnea on exertion or a nonproductive cough. Dyspnea in the patient with ILD is the result of increased work of breathing caused primarily by the stiffness of the lungs and excessive minute ventilation. Hypoxemia, often aggravated by exercise, may amplify the sensation of dyspnea by carotid body stimulation. The patient initially notices dyspnea only during heavy exertion, but in very advanced stages of the disease, dyspnea occurs at rest.

The patient's breathlessness has no other obvious cause such as asthma, obstructive airway disease, bronchitis, or heart failure. Although emphasis is usually on this most common presentation of patients with ILD, the provider must recognize the variability of clinical presentations. Dyspnea is a virtually constant finding in patients with IPF, but it is by no means consistent in other ILDs.

Objective

Less common but important—and sometimes misleading—presentations of ILD include the following:

- Fatigue in the absence of dyspnea
- Dry cough without other respiratory signs or symptoms
- Predominant systemic signs (e.g., fever, weight loss)
- Abnormal-appearing (90%) CXR in the absence of symptoms
- Incidental abnormalities of PFTs

Respiratory signs such as pleuritic chest pain, visceral chest pain, wheezing, or hemoptysis do not usually occur in most forms of ILD. One-half of patients have mucous hypersecretion and expectoration. This occurrence has been correlated with glandular hypertrophy in the airway mucosa and accumulated mucus in the airways. Patients with more advanced ILD may have clubbing and cyanosis. Clinical manifestations specific to the various types of ILD are discussed in Box 31.4.

DIAGNOSTIC REASONING

The occupational and environmental history is the single most helpful tool to determine whether a respiratory problem may be related to an environmental exposure (see Focus on History: Taking an Occupational and Environmental History). A careful history must include a detailed chronological account of the patient's employment activities, social activities, travel, immune status, pets, hobbies, and typical environment. A thorough review of the patient's past medical history, along with current and previous medications, is also important. The goal of these questions is to determine whether the patient has been exposed to agents known to cause ILD. Many patients have an occupational history that includes exposure to one or a variety of toxic inhalation products; this may add uncertainty to the precise onset of symptoms and may suggest the contribution of several etiological factors. The temporal relationship to the exposure may be obvious in some cases, while in others, low-grade exposure may provoke chronic illness without acute flares after exposure. The latency may be extremely long (e.g., more than 20 years for asbestosis), so it is mandatory to take a detailed occupational history, including summer jobs and hobbies, in all patients with suspected ILD. Moreover, a history of smoking is associated with an increased risk for the development of IPF. In addition, the occurrence of familial cases of IPF suggests that genetic factors may modulate responses to causative agents.

Focus on History: Taking an Occupational and Environmental History

General health history

- Does the patient think symptoms are related to anything at work?
- When was the onset of symptoms, and how was this related to work?
- Has the patient missed any days of work and why?
- Prior pulmonary problems
- Medications
- Cigarette use

Current or most relevant employment

- Job or process: title and description
- Type of industry and specific work
- Name of employer
- Years employed

Exposure information

- General description of job process and overall hygiene
- Materials used by worker
- Ventilation/exhaust system
- Use of respiratory protection
- Are other workers affected?
- Industrial hygiene samples and Occupational Safety and Health Administration data

Environmental nonoccupational factors

- Cigarettes
- Diet
- Hobbies
- Pets

Specific workplace exposures

- Fumes/dust/fibers
- Gases
- Metals
- Solvent
- Other chemicals: plastics, pesticides, corrosive agents
- Infectious agents
- Organic dusts: cotton, wood
- Radiation
- Emotional factors, stress (helpful in ruling out other causes of difficulty breathing or chest pain, such as panic attacks)

Past employment

- List jobs in chronological order
- Job titles
- Military service

Unfortunately, patients do not always know to which toxins they were exposed, and exposures to toxins may be easily overlooked, so considerable investigation may be required. For example, fungi in cooling systems or birds in the home may be a source of allergens that can elicit hypersensitivity pneumonitis. History of medication use is also critical to diagnosing ILD. Patients who have been using certain drugs (e.g., nitrofurantoin) for many years may not report them as medications on routine questioning. Mineral oil taken as a laxative or nose or ear drops also may not be reported as medications by patients.

Diagnostic Testing

Abnormalities on CXR may be the first clue to the presence of ILD; however, the patient with ILD may be asymptomatic or symptomatic with either a normal or abnormal CXR. The initial abnormality on the CXR is usually described as a ground-glass or hazy appearance of the lungs. As the disease progresses, diffuse abnormalities are found bilaterally. Pulmonary opacities (infiltrates) are usually described as containing small nodules (nodular), linear markings (reticular), or both (reticulonodular). Nodules are most commonly found in granulomatous diseases and hypersensitivity pneumonitis. The development of reticular densities is thought to be the result of edema, infiltration, or fibrosis of the septa in the periphery of the lung. A common characteristic of ILD is a progressive worsening of lung opacities, with the development of honeycomb lung. This honeycomb appearance is created by the cyst-like spaces that characterize the pathology of advanced ILD. However, many ILDs have unique radiographic presentations. For example, Wegener's granulomatosis is associated with lower-lobe cavities and nodules, whereas sarcoidosis is associated with swelling of the lymph nodes of the hilum of the lung (hilar lymphadenopathy), which contains the pulmonary arteries and their main branches, the upper lobe pulmonary veins, the major bronchi, and the proximate lymph nodes.

High-resolution computed tomography (HRCT) can evaluate ILD, as well as detect and localize pericardial and pleural fluid collections. HRCT examines only 1 mm of lung tissue at each level, thus revealing the lung parenchyma's delicate architecture. Several signs of ILD may be noted on HRCT. The most common are interface signs—the thickened and irregular appearance of the normally smooth interface of lung parenchyma with bronchi, blood vessels, and visceral pleura. Although HRCT is an exceptional tool for evaluation of parenchymal lung disease, it is important to note its limitations. It cannot be used to study the entire thorax, so conventional CT must be used to avoid missing abnormalities between images. Moreover, some HRCT findings may be difficult to interpret without a conventional CT image to use for reference.

Serological tests for antinuclear antibodies and rheumatoid factor are positive in 20% to 40% of patients, although rarely diagnostic. Antineutrophil cytoplasmic antibodies (ANCA) may be diagnostic in some settings, such as with ILD related to ANCA-associated vasculitis.

A transbronchial biopsy is the leading invasive tool for evaluating and treating patients with a wide spectrum of pulmonary disorders. In addition, the technique of bronchoalveolar lavage through a fiber-optic bronchoscope into a segmental or smaller bronchus provides a means to sample both the cellular and soluble components of the lower respiratory tract. The area beyond the bronchoscope's reach is washed with saline, which is then aspirated back through the bronchoscope, containing a small number of cells. The cells that are recovered include many from the alveoli and are representative of the cells associated with the inflammatory process. This procedure has aided in the diagnosis of ILD and in the assessment of its pathogenesis and disease activity.

PFTs measure lung volumes and airflow with a spirometer. Whether the patient is symptomatic or not, PFTs should be performed to establish the presence of disease, determine its severity, and monitor response to treatment. The sensitivity and specificity of these tests to diagnose the various ILDs, however, is low. Routine spirometry values and lung volumes are often initially normal, as are resting blood gas measurements; only after exercise may some gas exchange abnormalities become evident. The evaluation of the patient during exercise, although not constituting a direct measurement of respiration, gives more information than static measurements of lung volumes or diffusing capacity regarding ventilation, blood flow, gas exchange, and control of breathing. PFTs usually show a purely restrictive defect in most patients with ILD. Obstructive lung disease develops gradually in some patients and, more commonly, in certain forms of ILD such as sarcoidosis and hypersensitivity pneumonitis.

The compliance of the lungs decreases as lung involvement progresses. This is caused, in part, by fibrosis of the pulmonary parenchyma and the formation of cystic airspaces. DLCO is a good reflection of alveolar capillary surface area. Destruction of lung parenchyma results in a reduction in DLCO as ILD progresses. An abnormal DLCO may be the earliest evidence of ILD found on standard PFTs.

The use of the thoracoscope in combination with standard surgical instruments is known as video-assisted thoracic surgery (VATS) or video-assisted thoracoscopy. VATS provides the same access to the hemithorax as both thoracoscopy and thoracotomy. VATS procedures are particularly useful for obtaining lung biopsies in patients with diffuse ILD. With VATS, the visualization of the lung is better than it is with a limited thoracotomy because more areas of the lung can be sampled.

Transbronchial lung biopsy involves passing a forceps or needle through the bronchoscope. A specimen is obtained with forceps or aspirated through a needle. Pleural biopsy is useful in diagnosing granulomatous disease or malignancy of the pleura and may be performed if either of these two diseases is suspected. If a specific diagnosis is not made by transbronchial biopsy, an open lung biopsy may be indicated. Open lung biopsy is the most definitive way to diagnose and stage ILD so that appropriate prognostic and therapeutic decisions can be made. Depending on the age of the patient and the potential risks of the surgery in a compromised patient, empirical therapy may be initiated (see the Management section, later in the chapter).

Differential Diagnosis

In the case of a patient with unexplained dyspnea and fatigue suggestive of ILD, the differential diagnosis is nonetheless immense. Pulmonary, cardiac, hematological, renal, neuromuscular, and even endocrine diseases may present with exercise intolerance or dyspnea. A complete work-up of these systems is required to determine the correct diagnosis. Some of the conditions that give rise to dyspnea, diffuse pulmonary infiltration, and a granulomatous reaction include extrinsic allergic alveolitis, asbestosis, silicosis, berylliosis, lymphoid granulomatosis, connective tissue diseases, certain drugs, miliary tuberculosis, lymphoma, leukemias, pneumocystis pneumonia, and coccidioidomycosis.

Diseases of organ systems other than the lungs may present with ILD, so a detailed review of systems is key to the differential diagnosis. With occupational lung diseases, the physical examination is generally unrevealing for a specific cause; thus, it is more helpful in ruling out nonoccupational causes of respiratory symptoms or diseases related to cardiac or connective tissue disorders. Chronic heart disease may present as ILD with dyspnea, cough, crackles, and interstitial-type abnormalities on CXR. Malignancies of virtually any organ system may spread to the lungs as metastases and present as ILD. Patients with AIDS complicated by pneumocystis infection or lymphocytic interstitial pneumonia may first present with an insidious onset of dyspnea and fatigue, as in patients with other ILDs. Therefore, sexual orientation, multiple sexual partners, intravenous drug use, a history of sexually transmitted infections, or other possible risk factors for AIDS should be identified.

Connective tissue disease may be difficult to rule out because pulmonary manifestations occasionally precede the more typical systemic manifestations by months or years. Nonetheless, the manifestations of collagen vascular disease (e.g., rashes, Raynaud's phenomenon, fevers, arthralgias, muscle weakness) may result in important clues on history taking in a patient suspected of having ILD. For example, dysphagia or regurgitation may relate to either recurrent aspiration or collagen vascular disease, especially scleroderma.

MANAGEMENT

Management of most ILDs is difficult, and different approaches are taken, depending on the specific entity. Regardless of etiology, end-stage fibrosis is irreversible and untreatable. An extensive and aggressive diagnostic evaluation early on, even in the patient with relatively few symptoms, is recommended, as early clinical intervention in patients who are more likely to develop lung disease could be of considerable benefit for the patient. A good example is the identification and assessment of disease progression in diffuse lung disease found in systemic sclerosis.

The first course of action when working with a patient with ILD is to determine whether exposure to environmental agents or drugs is the cause and to discontinue the exposure. Therapeutic dilemmas with certain classes of drugs, such as antiarrhythmic medications, arise because discontinuation of drugs such as amiodarone may result in life-threatening dysrhythmias. However, the best chance for therapeutic success begins with the correct diagnosis.

In cases in which specific medication is used, such as prednisone or cytotoxic agents, there is usually suppression rather than cure of the primary process. Many patients with ILD are older adults, so the decision to treat them with immunosuppressive drugs should not be taken lightly because the toxicity and adverse effects of these medications can be substantial. In addition, anti-inflammatory and immunosuppressive treatments may be ineffective because of recurrent dysregulated wound healing. Antifibroblast therapies for ILD are aimed at decreasing pulmonary collagen deposition, and stem cell therapy may also be considered in some cases.

Initial Management

Corticosteroids may be initiated as therapy for ILD. A trial of corticosteroids is reasonable, even for a patient who is in an advanced stage of disease with relatively acellular and fibrotic changes in lung tissue. The best predictor of corticosteroid responsiveness and a better prognosis in ILD is an early benefit after the initial 1 to 2 months of corticosteroid therapy. The dosage and duration of corticosteroid therapy depend on the specific disorder, but in general, relatively high doses are used for the first 6 weeks (1 to 2 mg/kg/day or 60 to 100 mg/day) versus the ensuing 3 months. A period of 3 to 6 months is often required to determine the corticosteroid responsiveness of fibrosing alveolitis, although patients with sarcoidosis and cryptogenic organizing pneumonia may respond much more quickly with lower dosages. In contrast, certain disease processes, such as IPF, commonly require therapy for 12 months or longer. Moreover, the tyrosine kinase inhibitor nintedanib (Ofev) and pirfenidone (Esbriet, Pirfenex, Pirespa) may slow the progressive decline in lung function in patients with IPF.

Subsequent Management

For the patient whose disease is not well controlled with or responsive to corticosteroids, additional immunosuppressive therapy may be considered. Cyclophosphamide (Cytoxan), an alkylating drug, is a potent immunosuppressant and seems to be effective in patients with ILD in whom corticosteroids are ineffective. If improvement in the lung disease is documented after 3 months of this therapy, it should be continued for a 12-month interval. Azathioprine (Azasan, Imuran) has been used as an alternative to cyclophosphamide. Penicillamine (Cuprimine, Depen) has been used in some patients, with the rationale that it might prevent the cross-linking of abnormal collagen being synthesized in the pulmonary interstitium and prevent or retard fibrosis. Exercise tolerance may also be significantly improved with supplemental oxygen.

Because the pulmonary vascular bed is impaired by progressive fibrosis, pulmonary hypertension and cor pulmonale can develop; right-sided congestive heart failure can be difficult to control. Judicious use of diuretics is advised, as a significant decrease in intravascular volume may be deleterious for lung perfusion. Digitalis or other antiarrhythmic drugs may be required, although adequate oxygenation is probably the best treatment for heart failure in this situation. Some patients may also develop airflow obstruction and experience wheezing and coughing that may respond to bronchodilators. Because infection may occur during immunosuppressive therapy, it is important to maintain a high index of suspicion and treat infection aggressively. Prophylactic use of pneumococcal and influenza vaccines is encouraged. Finally, lung transplantation may be an option for patients with refractory disease limited to the chest. See Box 31.4 for additional therapies for ILD.

FOLLOW-UP AND REFERRAL

Reassessment of disease activity is generally performed at 3, 6, 12, and 24 months or more often if needed. Responsiveness is defined as a decrease in symptoms: radiographic improvement; physiological improvement; or no further decline in clinical, radiographic, or physiological parameters. The patient should be followed for signs of infection that are masked by immunosuppressive drugs, pneumothorax, or the development of lung cancer, which occurs in 5% to 10% of patients. The patient on corticosteroids must be monitored closely during times of illness or stress and during corticosteroid tapering or withdrawal for signs and symptoms of adrenal suppression. Such patients should be encouraged to wear a medical identification bracelet.

Given the risk of exercise-related hypoxia, the patient should be assessed for the benefit of supplemental oxygen during exercise. Patients with a collagen vascular disorder must be regularly assessed for progression or exacerbations of their chronic illnesses. For example, patients with RA require rest, joint protection, daily heat and exercise, and psychological support. Community resources such as a home-care nurse, homemaker services, and vocational rehabilitation may be considered. Self-help groups may also be beneficial for the patient. These diseases require a collaborative and integrated approach, as emphasized in the Circle of Caring model (see Chapter 1).

Specialized testing should be undertaken and the patient referred to a pulmonologist if no specific cause of dyspnea or cough can be found, if the patient's symptoms exceed the physiological or radiographic abnormalities identified, if empiric management (with bronchodilators, diuretics, smoking cessation) results in an atypical or unsatisfactory clinical outcome, if the patient needs an impairment or disability evaluation for workers' compensation or other reason, if specialized cardiopulmonary diagnostic testing (e.g., lung biopsy) is needed, or if a therapeutic immunosuppressive or cytotoxic drug trial is contemplated.

Patient Education: ILD

Patients with ILD must be educated about the nature of their illness, related diagnostic tests, and the treatment regimen for their particular type of lung disease (see Box 31.5). For example, avoidance of exposure to antigens is paramount for those with hypersensitivity pneumonitis. All patients must be advised and assisted to stop cigarette smoking to prevent further lung damage. In many cases, the most comprehensive patient education occurs within the context of a pulmonary rehabilitation program.

The need to reduce repeated hospital and intensive care unit admissions necessitates an effective pulmonary rehabilitation program. The target population for these programs has traditionally been severely disabled patients with COPD or ILD who require a broad range of comprehensive services to keep them clinically stable and out of the hospital for long periods of time. However, appropriate patients with all levels of respiratory impairment who could benefit from such programs, and not only the severely disabled, should be referred to pulmonary rehabilitation. These programs have criteria for referral that generally include the following patient characteristics: dyspnea on exertion, inability to carry out selected activities of daily living, repeated hospitalizations or the need for home-care services, time lost from work or school, and the desire/need for an educational update of self-care techniques. Moreover, the following laboratory features are inclusion criteria for pulmonary rehabilitation: reduced vital capacity in restrictive lung disease, reduced expiratory flow rate, hypercapnia, and hypoxemia at rest or during exercise.

Box 31.5 Educational Content for the Patient With Interstitial Lung Disease

- Respiratory anatomy and physiology
- Pathophysiology of interstitial lung disease
- Respiratory diagnostic tests:
  Chest x-ray
  Pulmonary function tests
  Exercise tests
  Bronchoscopy
  High-resolution computed tomography
- Self-care measures:
  Pulmonary medications
  Diet
  Fluid intake
  Smoking cessation
  Environmental control
  Awareness of early signs of infection
- Chest therapy:
  Relaxation and guided imagery
  Breathing retraining
  Controlling dyspneic episodes
  Postural drainage
- Progressive exercise conditioning:
  Walking programs
  Treadmill or bicycle exercise training
  Arm or leg range-of-motion exercises
- Respiratory equipment:
  Oxygen therapy
  Handheld nebulizer

REFERENCES

Asthma

Centers for Disease Control and Prevention. Asthma data, statistics, and surveillance. https://www.cdc.gov/asthma/asthmadata.htm. Accessed 6/16/2017.

Environmental Protection Agency. Asthma. epa.gov/asthma. Accessed 8/14/20.

Global Initiative for Asthma (GINA). (2020). The Global Strategy for Asthma Management and Prevention. https://ginasthma.org/reports/. Accessed 8/12/20.

Langton D, Sha J, Ing A, et al. Bronchial thermoplasty in severe asthma in Australia. *Intern Med J.* 2017 Jan;47(5). https://www.researchgate.net/publication/312567659. Accessed 8/14/20.

Chronic Bronchitis and Emphysema (Chronic Obstructive Pulmonary Disease)

Capriotti T, Kelley L, Galcano D. (2019). Chronic obstructive pulmonary disease: Fighting for each breath. *Clin Advis.* 2019 July/Aug:13–20.

Chin ED, Armstrong D. Anticipated stigma and healthcare utilization in COPD and neurological disorders. *Appl Nurs Res.* 2019 Feb;45:63–68.

Freedman M, Kroger A, Hunter P, et al. (2020). Recommended adult immunization schedule, U.S., 2020. *Ann Intern Med.* Clinical Guidelines, Mar. 3, 2020. https://www.acpjournals.org/doi/10.7326/M20-0046. Accessed 8/23/20.

Global Strategy for the Diagnosis, Management and Prevention of COPD. (2020). Global Initiative for Chronic Obstructive Lung Disease (GOLD). http://goldcopd.org. Accessed 8/12/2020.

494 Unit II CARING-BASED NURSING: THE SCIENCE

Leader D. A comprehensive guide to chronic obstructive pulmonary disease (COPD). Lung transplant. http://www.healthline.com/health/lung-transplant#overview1. Accessed 8/14/2020.

Potnek MF. (2019). Assessment and management of suspected chronic obstructive pulmonary disease in the primary care setting. *J Nurse Pract.* 15:701–708.

Rand Health. Rand 36-Item Health Survey. http://www.rand.org/health/surveys_tools/mos/36-item-short-form/survey-instrument.html. Accessed 8/24/2020.

U.S. Department of Health and Human Services. (2017). National Heart, Lung, and Blood Institute. COPD National Action Plan. https://www.nhlbi.nih.gov/health-pro/resources/lung/copd-national-action-plan. Accessed 8/24/2020.

Interstitial Lung Disease

American Lung Association. Introduction to pulmonary fibrosis. http://www.lung.org/lung-health-and-diseases/lung-disease-lookup/pulmonary-fibrosis/introduction. Accessed 8/20/2020.

RESOURCES

Asthma

Allergy, Asthma, and Immunology
   https://www.nhlbi.nih.gov/guidelines/asthma

American Academy of Allergy, Asthma, and Immunology
   https://www.aaaai.org

American College of Allergy, Asthma, and Immunology
   https://www.acaai.org

Asthma and Allergy Foundation of America
   https://www.aafa.org

Asthma.com (GlaxoSmithKline-sponsored Web site for asthma control test questionnaires)
   https://www.asthma.com/additional-resources/asthma-control-test.html

National Asthma Education and Prevention Program
   https://www.nhlbi.nih.gov/about/advisory-and-peer-review-committees/national-asthma-education-and-prevention-program-coordinating/EPR4-working-group

National Institute of Allergy and Infectious Disease
   https://www.niaid.nih.gov

Chronic Obstructive Pulmonary Disease

American Lung Association
   https://www.lung.org/lung-health-diseases/lung-disease-lookup/copd/living-with-copd/copd-management-tools

Clinical COPD Questionnaire (CCQ)
   https://openi.nlm.nih.gov/detailedresult?img=PMC156640_1477-7525-1-13-1&req=4. Accessed 8/24/20.

COPD Assessment Test (CAT)
   https://www.saintlukeskc.org/sites/default/files/2018-08/CAT%20%28USA%20English%29.pdf. Accessed 8/24/20.

National Heart, Lung, and Blood Institute
   https://www.nhlbi.nih.gov

RAND 36-Item Short Form Survey (SF-36)
   https://www.rand.org/health-care/surveys_tools/mos/36-item-short-form.html

Interstitial Lung Disease

American Lung Association
   https://www.lung.org/lung-health-diseases/lung-disease-lookup/interstitial-lung-disease

---

Chapter 32

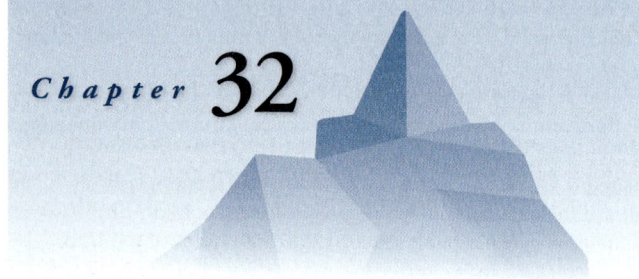

Lung Cancer

Jill E. Winland-Brown, EdD, APRN, FNP-BC, FAANP

Brian Oscar Porter, MD, PhD, MPH, MBA

Lung cancer may be preventable, is common, and may be lethal once it comes to clinical attention. It is also relatively resistant to current therapeutics. The four major histological types are (1) squamous-cell (epidermoid) carcinoma, (2) small-cell (oat-cell) carcinoma, (3) large-cell carcinoma (including giant-cell and clear-cell carcinoma), and (4) adenocarcinoma. Small-cell lung cancer (SCLC) is a very rapidly growing tumor that usually metastasizes to distant tissue while the tumor is quite small. The clinical effect of SCLC is much different from other forms of lung cancer, which is why these cancers are usually classified in terms of SCLCs and non-SCLCs (NSCLCs) (Table 32.1).

Because the lung area is so large, tumors may go undetected for some time. Early symptoms such as coughing and fatigue are nonspecific, and patients often attribute these symptoms to causes other than lung cancer. For these reasons, early-stage lung cancer (stages I and II) is difficult to detect and most patients are diagnosed at stages III and IV.

EPIDEMIOLOGY AND CAUSES

Lung cancer is the most frequent cause of cancer deaths in men and women in North America and accounts for 25% of all cancer deaths. Approximately one-fourth of all

TABLE 32.1 Cellular Classification of Lung Cancer

Major Classification	Subclassification
Small-cell lung carcinomas	• Oat-cell carcinoma • Intermediate-cell carcinoma • Combined small-cell carcinoma (with squamous-cell carcinoma or adenocarcinoma)

Non–small-cell lung carcinomas	• Squamous-cell (epidermoid) carcinoma
	   Well differentiated
	   Moderately well differentiated
	   Poorly differentiated
	• Adenocarcinoma
	   Well differentiated
	   Moderately well differentiated
	   Poorly differentiated
	   Bronchoalveolar
	• Large-cell carcinoma
	   Giant cell
	   Clear cell

patients diagnosed with lung cancer have no symptoms at diagnosis, and one-fourth of all lung cancer patients never smoked. Lung cancer is the most prevalent cancer globally, and in 2018, accounted for 2.1 million new cases and 1.8 million deaths. It is also a very expensive disease, as lung cancer care costs the United States more than $13 billion annually.

Eighty-six percent of lung cancer patients die within 5 years of diagnosis. In patients who have never smoked, the 5-year survival rate is 1%. This low survival rate may be explained by health-care professionals' lack of suspicion of lung cancer in nonsmokers, which prevents diagnosis early in the course of the disease. Lung cancer is more common in older adults with 86% of those living with lung cancer being 60 years of age or older.

The death rate for women due to lung cancer is now higher than from any other cancer because of increased cigarette smoking by women and because women may be more susceptible to the carcinogenic effects of tobacco smoke than men. In every ethnic group, men still have higher lung cancer incidence and mortality rates than women, although women are rapidly closing the gap. Although more men are diagnosed with lung cancer, more women are living with the disease. Lung cancer is the leading cause of cancer deaths in most racial and ethnic groups of women except for Native American, Filipino, and Hispanic women. New lung cancers and lung cancer deaths peak in individuals aged 55 to 65 years old. Although black men and women smoke less than white men and women, both black men and women are more likely to develop and die of lung cancer than any other racial group. Black men are 30% more likely to have lung cancer than white men. The rate for black women is approximately equal to that of white women, despite the fact that they smoke fewer cigarettes.

Smoking still causes the majority of lung cancer cases. The risk of lung cancer increases with the duration of smoking, with earlier age at onset of smoking, and with smoking unfiltered or high-tar cigarettes. Of continued note are the effects of environmental tobacco smoke (ETS), also called secondhand smoke, side-stream smoke, involuntary smoke, or passive cigarette smoke. Exposure to ETS is thought to increase the risk of dying from lung cancer by 30%. In contrast, there has not been enough research done yet on smoking marijuana or cocaine (crack) as a risk factor for lung cancer. The effects of e-cigarettes on lung cancer are also not well established, and more research needs to be done in these areas.

Lung cancer also occurs in association with occupational and environmental exposure to carcinogenic agents from sources other than smoking. Radon is the second leading cause of lung cancer deaths at almost 3,000 annually in nonsmokers. Other lung carcinogens include asbestos, radiation, certain heavy metals, and polycyclic aromatic hydrocarbons found in volcanoes, forest fires, burning coal, and exhaust fumes from cars. The combination of cigarette smoking and environmental exposure produces an additive effect, such that smokers exposed to asbestos increase their risk of lung cancer by a factor of 92 times.

PATHOPHYSIOLOGY

The bronchial walls have three layers: an epithelial lining, a smooth muscle layer, and a connective tissue layer. The epithelial lining of the bronchi contains single-celled exocrine glands (i.e., mucus-secreting goblet cells) and ciliated cells. High columnar pseudostratified epithelium lines the larger airways, changing to columnar cuboidal epithelium in the bronchioles. It is hypothesized that at sites of segmental bronchial bifurcations, airflow and mucus production are altered and the bronchial epithelium becomes susceptible to injury. Carcinogenic agents, such as tobacco smoke, are likely deposited and absorbed in these areas. Particle size in ETS is smaller than in mainstream smoke, and inhaled particles may travel to peripheral lung regions more readily. This is believed to explain the excess of peripheral adenocarcinomas seen in passive smokers.

Cigarette smoke contains tumor initiators, promoters, and cocarcinogens. DNA-mutating agents in cigarettes produce alterations in both oncogenes (a class of genes that encodes proteins involved in normal cell-growth processes) and tumor suppressor genes. Multiple genetic events occur that result in cancer, first resulting in dysregulated growth and eventually in a malignant cell. These alterations include bronchial epithelial changes that progress from squamous-cell alterations, or metaplasia, to carcinoma in situ. Repeated carcinogenic insults to the bronchial epithelium may cause increased rates of cellular replication. Healthy ciliated cells are replaced with a proliferation of basal cells, resulting in hyperplasia, dysplasia, carcinoma in situ, and invasive carcinoma.

Small-Cell Lung Cancer

SCLC, which accounts for 15% of all lung cancers, invades the submucosa and is centrally located. It typically develops around a main bronchus as a whitish-gray growth that compromises surrounding structures and eventually compresses the bronchi externally. Smoking results in SCLC more often than NSCLC. It grows more rapidly, metastasizes earlier, and is more responsive to chemotherapy than NSCLC. However, the most striking difference between small-cell carcinoma and other forms of malignant lung neoplasms is the aggressiveness of this tumor, resulting in more rapid growth and early local and distant metastases via the lymphatics and blood vessels.

There are three types of SCLC:

- Oat-cell carcinoma is composed of cells with round to oval nuclei. The tumors are soft in consistency and have shiny, gray-cut surfaces on examination.
- Intermediate cell-type SCLC is characterized by cells with larger, more vesicular, fusiform, or spindled nuclei.
- Combined cell-type SCLC is characterized by a combination of small-cell carcinoma cells and another cell type. The most important variant is the combination of small-cell and large-cell types, which is regarded as a small-cell carcinoma for treatment purposes. This variant lacks sensitivity to radiation and chemotherapy but retains the aggressiveness of "pure" small-cell carcinoma.

Non–Small-Cell Lung Cancers

NSCLCs comprise approximately 85% of all primary lung carcinomas in the United States. They include squamous-cell carcinomas, adenocarcinomas, and large-cell carcinomas, which are each described in more detail in the following sections.

Mutations in the tumor suppressor gene p53 are reported to be associated with human cancer more commonly than any other gene. A gene mutation in p53 is present in about 60% of all cases of NSCLC. The p53 gene encodes a protein with a central role in the regulation of transcriptional events in the cell nucleus, particularly in response to DNA-damaging agents, such as ionizing radiation and a variety of other carcinogens. The central regulatory role of normal p53 protein has led to its description as the "guardian of the genome." Although many efforts to improve survival have focused on expanding NSCLC indications for both radiotherapy and surgery, little progress has been made.

Squamous-Cell Carcinoma

Squamous-cell carcinoma is the second most common lung cancer, accounting for 25% to 35% of cases. It is more common in men than in women and occurs almost entirely in cigarette smokers. Squamous-cell carcinoma is named for the resemblance of cells to the epidermis of the skin. These cells usually contain the skin protein keratin and are characterized by very small cells with scant cytoplasm.

These tumors arise from the basal cells of the bronchial epithelium and usually present as masses in the segmental, lobar, or mainstem bronchi. The tumors tend to be bulky and invade cartilage and adjoining lymph nodes. On the basis of the degree of differentiation, these tumors are divided into three subtypes: well differentiated, moderately well differentiated, and poorly differentiated tumors. Well-differentiated tumors may show epithelial pearl formation, whereas poorly differentiated tumors are characterized by keratinization. Because squamous-cell carcinoma is a relatively slow-growing tumor, several years may elapse between the development of a carcinoma in situ and clinical detection. Metastases of squamous-cell carcinomas are initially to the hilar and mediastinal lymph nodes and then to the liver, adrenal glands, bones, and brain.

Adenocarcinoma

Adenocarcinoma, which represents 35% to 40% of all lung cancers, is the most prevalent carcinoma of the lung in both sexes and in nonsmokers. It forms acinar or glandular structures. Histologically, this tumor is divided broadly into well-differentiated, moderately well-differentiated, poorly differentiated, and bronchoalveolar subtypes. They arise from the bronchial epithelium and may form in lung scars or fibrous tissue. Adenocarcinoma usually presents as a NSCLC in the peripheral portion of the lungs, although rapidly progressive multifocal disease may be present at diagnosis. Although adenocarcinomas are usually slow-growing tumors, they may invade lymphatics and blood vessels early in the disease process, thus producing early metastases; nearly half are considered to be unresectable at the time of diagnosis. Areas of metastasis commonly include the brain, liver, bone, and adrenal glands. Patients with adenocarcinomas may have an associated history of chronic interstitial lung disease associated with other underlying conditions, such as scleroderma, rheumatoid arthritis, recurrent pulmonary infections, and other necrotizing pulmonary disease. Additionally, many organs of the body can develop adenocarcinomas that may metastasize to the lungs; thus, it may be difficult to determine whether an adenocarcinoma is a primary lung cancer or a metastatic tumor from elsewhere in the body.

The bronchoalveolar subtype of adenocarcinoma represents approximately 2% to 4% of all lung cancers. Often, it is associated with prior lung diseases resulting in fibrosis, including repeated pneumonias, idiopathic pulmonary fibrosis, asbestosis, scleroderma, or Hodgkin's disease. There is little correlation between this type of cancer and smoking. Bronchoalveolar carcinoma commonly arises in the periphery of the lung and grows in a scale-like fashion along the alveolar septa. Grossly, these tumors may be categorized as solitary, multinodular, or diffuse. The solitary, well-differentiated bronchoalveolar adenocarcinoma has a much better prognosis than the other forms, as diffuse and multinodular forms usually are not amenable to therapy.

Large-Cell Carcinoma

Large-cell carcinoma, also called undifferentiated carcinoma, is the least common type of lung cancer, comprising approximately 10% of cases. It is classified into two types: clear-cell carcinoma and giant-cell carcinoma. Large-cell carcinomas include all tumors that show no evidence of differentiation to small-cell carcinoma, squamous-cell carcinoma, or adenocarcinoma. They are characterized by a collection of poorly formed large cells that have abundant cytoplasm. These tumors may exhibit a gland-like structure and produce mucin.

These tumors tend to form large, bulky, somewhat circumscribed and necrotic masses in the major or intermediate-sized bronchi or in the periphery, invade locally, and disseminate widely. The giant-cell variant of large-cell carcinoma is composed of huge, multinucleated, bizarre cells that are frequently associated with an extensive inflammatory cell infiltration. These tumors are usually large, peripheral, very aggressive, highly malignant, and most often found at a late stage. These lesions are able to metastasize widely, with a predilection for the small intestine. Table 32.2 summarizes the disease characteristics of the various types of lung cancer.

CLINICAL PRESENTATION

Past history of a patient with suspected lung cancer should include an assessment of any history of chronic respiratory problems, as well as any prolonged exposure to environmental carcinogens. Habits must be explored to determine the patient's risk of developing lung cancer. Smoking history includes the age when smoking started, the average number of packs smoked per day, and the number of years smoked. The type of tobacco (cigar, cigarette, snuff, or chewing tobacco) used by the patient must also be determined. A positive family history of lung

TABLE 32.2 Disease Characteristics of Lung Cancer

Lung Cancer Type	Tumor Type	Growth Rate	Metastasis	Manifestations	Treatment
Small-cell lung carcinoma	• 15%–20% • Neuroendocrine cells: oat-cell carcinoma Combined small-cell (with squamous-cell carcinoma or adenocarcinoma)	Very rapid	Very early, via lymphatics and blood vessels	Obstruction of main bronchus; associated with paraneoplastic syndrome	• Not resectable • Treated with chemotherapy and radiation
Non–small-cell lung carcinomas	Squamous-cell (epidermoid) carcinoma • 25%–35% • Keratin-producing cells: Well differentiated Moderately well differentiated Poorly differentiated	Slow	Hilar and mediastinal lymph nodes, liver, adrenals, bone, brain	Most often in cigarette smokers; bulky mass in mainstem bronchi	• Stages I and II: resectable • Stage III: chemotherapy and radiation • Stage IV: chemotherapy (refer to Table 32.5 for staging)
	Adenocarcinoma • 35%–40% • Columnar cells: Well differentiated Moderately well differentiated Poorly differentiated Bronchoalveolar	Slow to moderate	Early and most frequently via lymphatics and blood vessels to brain, liver, bone, and adrenal glands	Forms glandular structures in scar or fibrous tissue; single distal pulmonary nodule	• Stages I and II: resectable • Stage III: chemotherapy and radiotherapy • Stage IV: chemotherapy
	Large-cell carcinoma • 5%–10% • Undifferentiated cells: Giant cell Clear cell	Rapid	Early and widespread to small intestine	Large, bulky necrotic masses in major or intermediate-sized bronchi or in periphery	• Stages I and II: resectable • Stage III: chemotherapy and radiotherapy • Stage IV: chemotherapy

cancer may indicate that the patient is at a higher risk of developing lung cancer. One study found a greater than two times higher likelihood of lung cancer in patients with a first-degree relative with lung cancer. A review of systems should reexamine all pertinent present and past symptoms that relate to the chief complaint.

Clinical manifestations of lung cancer depend on the location of the tumor and the extent of spread. Up to 25% of patients are asymptomatic at the time of diagnosis. However, if present, symptoms may be divided into four categories: intrathoracic or local–regional symptoms, nonspecific systemic symptoms, symptoms resulting from extrathoracic involvement, and paraneoplastic syndromes. Table 32.3 presents a summary of the clinical manifestations of lung cancer.

Intrathoracic or Local–Regional Signs and Symptoms

The most common signs and symptoms of local–regional disease are ambiguous and insidious; they include cough, sputum production, dyspnea, chest pain, hemoptysis, wheezing, postobstructive pneumonia, and pleural effusions. Cough resulting from bronchial irritation occurs in 60% to 75% of patients and is often initially attributed to a cold. The cough frequently goes away after a few days and returns intermittently. Cough may be produced by a small tumor acting as a foreign body and causing mucous build-up due to irritation, obstruction, or ulceration of the bronchial mucosa. Severe paroxysms of coughing may lead to cough-induced rib fractures, rupture of an emphysematous bleb, or cough syncope. The cough may be productive with bloody or rust-colored sputum, although cough and sputum production are not specific symptoms because the majority of lung cancer patients also have chronic bronchitis and emphysema due to cigarette smoking. However, a change in the character of the cough, a change in the quality and quantity of sputum, or unresponsiveness to previously effective therapy (e.g., bronchodilators, antibiotics, corticosteroids) should raise suspicion that a tumor is present.

Many patients with lung cancer experience dyspnea as a result of multiple disruptions in physiological function of the respiratory system. Dyspnea has been reported in 26% to 60% of patients presenting with NSCLC and is often an ominous development, signifying intrathoracic extension or dissemination. Some patients may have dyspnea resulting from underlying pulmonary disorders such as pulmonary fibrosis or chronic obstructive pulmonary disease (COPD). These patients may experience difficulties in airway clearance associated with excessive tracheobronchial secretions, thick tenacious secretions, muscle weakness, and chest pain. Central lung cancers cause dyspnea by means of obstruction, with or without postobstructive pneumonitis. Large pleural effusion or paralysis of the hemidiaphragm resulting from phrenic nerve involvement may also cause dyspnea. The assessment of dyspnea should include a description of the onset, duration, magnitude, and precipitating events. It is especially important to identify any interventions the patient has discovered that are helpful in relieving the dyspnea. Usually the chest radiograph in dyspneic patients demonstrates a sizable effusion, atelectasis of a lobe or the entire lung, or clear evidence of intrapulmonary dissemination of the tumor.

Chest pain with deep inspiration or coughing may be reported, as well as fatigue and anorexia. Chest pain in lung cancer may indicate local invasion of the pleura, ribs, and nerves. Pain may be dull, constant, and debilitating or intermittent and sharp, varying with the respiratory cycle. It may localize to the chest wall, or it may radiate to the midback, scapula, shoulder, or arm on the side of the tumor. The pain is usually a dull intermittent ache lasting from minutes to hours on the same side as the tumor and is not related to cough or respiration. Intercostal retractions, supraclavicular retractions, and/or use of accessory muscles on inspiration indicate obstruction to air inflow, whereas bulging interspaces on expiration are associated

TABLE 32.3 Clinical Manifestations of Lung Cancer	
Intrathoracic or local–regional manifestations	Cough Dyspnea Hemoptysis Wheezing Chest pain Stridor Hoarseness Vocal cord paralysis Hiccups Atelectasis Pneumonia Pancoast's syndrome Horner's syndrome Pleural effusion Pericardial effusion Superior vena cava syndrome
Nonspecific systemic manifestations	Weakness Fatigue Fever Anorexia Cachexia Anemia
Manifestations resulting from extrathoracic involvement	Bone pain Headache Dizziness Lymphadenopathy Central nervous system disturbances Gastrointestinal disturbances Jaundice Hepatomegaly Abdominal pain

with outflow obstruction; either may be indicative of a lung tumor. It is important to distinguish the chest pain that accompanies direct contiguous chest wall extension from painful rib metastases that are anatomically remote from the primary lesion.

Chest discomfort can be associated with atelectasis. Atelectasis develops in the patient with lung cancer secondary to mechanical obstruction of the airways, compression of lung tissue, and shallow breathing patterns. When the tumor obstructs the airway, it prevents or reduces alveolar ventilation to a region of the lung and produces atelectasis in that region. The size of the atelectatic area depends on the size of the obstructed airway and the degree of obstruction. Localized compression of lung tissue occurs with large tumors and with large pleural effusions secondary to metastases.

Hemoptysis is seen in up to 30% of patients and occurs when the tumor erodes the epithelial layer of the lung or invades a blood vessel. It occurs more often in squamous-cell carcinoma and large-cell carcinoma than in SCLC. Typically, hemoptysis consists only of blood-streaked sputum, which is sometimes erroneously attributed to chronic bronchitis. The quantity of blood is usually small, but it can become massive and life-threatening, depending on the blood vessels affected. Hemoptysis usually prompts the patient to seek medical attention and is suggestive of an endobronchial tumor. Inspection seldom reveals any changes in the chest wall. Palpation may reveal lymph node enlargement.

Auscultation may reveal wheezing if an airway is partially obstructed. Wheezing is usually monophonic and localized and does not disappear after a cough. Wheezing may be heard on both inhalation and exhalation. Absent or decreased breath sounds can be heard when normal lung tissue is replaced by tumor or when the patient has a pleural effusion. Percussion reveals diminished resonance over lung tissue affected by a large tumor, pleural effusion, or pneumonia (consolidation). Decreased tactile fremitus may be associated with pleural effusion and tumors of the pleural cavity, whereas increased tactile fremitus may indicate a lung mass.

The most frequent peripheral sign of lung cancer is clubbing of the fingers, which may be associated with generalized hypertrophic pulmonary osteoarthropathy (HPO), also known as Bamberger-Marie disease. HPO often resembles rheumatoid arthritis. The clinical syndrome consists of swelling of the soft tissues of the terminal phalanges, with curvature of the nails, pain and swelling of the joints, and periostitis of the long bones, with elevation of the periosteum and new bone formation. The incidence of HPO, which occurs almost exclusively in patients with NSCLC, has been reported from 2% to 12%. It occurs only rarely, if ever, in small-cell tumors. Its occurrence is distributed equally among the other three major cell types of NSCLC. Removal of the pulmonary lesion may give dramatic remission of the arthralgia and peripheral edema.

Physical examination evidence for surgical nonresectability includes hoarseness, facial edema, arm pain, or changes in mental or emotional status. Hoarseness suggests vocal cord paralysis caused by recurrent laryngeal nerve compression by the tumor. Facial edema suggests compression of the superior vena cava by the tumor. Superior vena cava syndrome occurs when a lung tumor, usually SCLC, presses on the superior vena cava, partially or completely occluding it and impeding venous return from the head, neck, arms, and upper chest. Symptoms are related to venous obstruction, airway obstruction, and increased cerebral venous pressure. The most common symptoms include edema of the face, neck, arms, and upper torso. The conjunctiva may also be engorged. If the compression is untreated, neurological symptoms related to increased intracranial pressure may ensue, including headache, dizziness, visual disturbances, and occasionally alterations in mental status. Associated upper airway obstruction or signs of cerebral edema are very poor prognostic signs.

Tumor compression of the cervical sympathetic nerve plexus causes Horner's syndrome, which consists of unilateral ptosis, miosis, and ipsilateral anhidrosis (lack of sweating due to extension of the tumor into the paravertebral sympathetic nerves). Horner's syndrome is often associated with radiographic evidence of destruction of the first and second ribs. Pancoast's syndrome, manifesting as arm and shoulder pain, suggests invasion of the brachial nerve plexus by a superior sulcus tumor. In addition, there may be muscular atrophy and decreased range of motion in the arm and shoulder; the patient may walk supporting the elbow of the affected arm.

Nonspecific Systemic Signs and Symptoms

Systemic symptoms of lung cancer include generalized weakness and fatigue, anorexia, cachexia, weight loss, and anemia. These nonspecific signs and symptoms are common in both SCLC and NSCLC. Weight loss, which is usually (but not always) accompanied by anorexia, occurs in more than one-half of patients, and generalized weakness occurs in one-third. Fever and anemia occur in about 20% of patients. Fever generally is not considered to be paraneoplastic in patients with lung cancer; if present, it usually is associated with a documented infection or liver metastases.

Signs and Symptoms Due to Extrathoracic Involvement

Extrathoracic metastatic spread most often occurs in the lymph nodes, brain, bones, liver, and suprarenal glands. Bone pain caused by metastases occurs in approximately 25% to 40% of patients, although pathological fractures are rare. Neurological symptoms resulting from intracranial metastases are present in 3% to 6% of patients. These include hemiplegia, epilepsy, personality changes, confusion, speech defects, gait disturbances, or only nonspecific headache. Symptoms that relate to liver involvement (right upper quadrant pain) are less common or nonspecific (e.g., nausea, weight loss, anemia). Rarely, jaundice, ascites, or an abdominal mass is the major complaint. Neck, muscle, or subcutaneous tissue masses are present infrequently. Involvement of adrenal glands often is asymptomatic, and most adrenal metastases are discovered incidentally, either during staging evaluation or at autopsy. If symptomatic, adrenal involvement presents with unilateral pain in the flank, abdomen, or costovertebral angle. Although adrenal metastases are fairly common, signs of adrenal insufficiency are rarely seen.

Paraneoplastic Syndromes

Approximately 21 identified syndromes that meet the usual definition of the term "paraneoplastic" (Table 32.4) are associated with lung cancer, and approximately 2% of patients with lung cancer seek medical advice for systemic symptoms and signs of these paraneoplastic syndromes. The major categories of paraneoplastic syndromes include endocrine, neurological, cardiovascular, skeletal, and cutaneous manifestations.

TABLE 32.4 Paraneoplastic Syndromes Associated With Lung Cancer

Type of Cancer	Associated Paraneoplastic Syndrome
Small-cell lung carcinoma	• Ectopic adrenocorticotropic hormone (Cushing's syndrome) • Inappropriate antidiuretic hormone secretion • Lambert-Eaton myasthenic syndrome • Atrial natriuretic factor secretion • Hyperpigmentation
Non–small-cell lung carcinomas	• Humoral hypercalcemia • Hypertrophic pulmonary osteoarthropathy • Nephrotic syndrome • Hypoglycemia • Gynecomastia • Nonbacterial thrombotic endocarditis
All lung cancers	• Hypercoagulable state • Disseminated intravascular coagulation • Erythrocytosis • Granulocytosis • Neurological and myopathic syndromes (dementia, limbic encephalitis, optic neuropathy, sensory neuropathy, sensorimotor peripheral neuropathy) • Dermatological syndromes (acanthosis nigricans, acquired ichthyosis, dermatomyositis)

Paraneoplastic syndromes are often the first indication of the presence of a tumor and may antedate identification of a clinically demonstrable tumor by a period ranging from months to years. SCLC is associated with paraneoplastic syndromes more frequently than the NSCLC. Most metabolic manifestations are the result of secretion of endocrine or endocrine-like substances by the tumor.

Hyperadrenocorticism, in association with ectopic secretion of adrenocorticotropic hormone, is a frequently observed hormonal syndrome in lung cancer, particularly in SCLC patients. It manifests as severe weakness, weight loss, edema, hypertension, hypokalemia, and hyperglycemia. The syndrome of inappropriate antidiuretic hormone secretion occurs in 5% to 10% of patients with SCLCs. It results from antidiuretic hormone secretion by the tumor and is associated with symptoms of water intoxication (e.g., anorexia, nausea, vomiting). Signs and symptoms include hyponatremia and low serum osmolality, characterized by mental status changes, lethargy, seizures, and confusion. Hyponatremia may also result from the secretion of atrial natriuretic factor in some patients.

Hypercalcemia may be caused by bony metastases or excessive tumor secretion of parathyroid hormone–related protein, resulting in humoral hypercalcemia of malignancy. Although squamous-cell carcinoma is most commonly associated with hypercalcemia, other histological types can cause the syndrome as well. An accompanying hypophosphatemia is also frequently found. Clinically, the hypercalcemic patient may have somnolence, irritability, confusion, or coma, as well as anorexia, nausea, vomiting, constipation, and weight loss.

Eaton-Lambert myasthenic syndrome occurs in about 6% of patients with SCLC. This pseudomyasthenic syndrome is thought to be an autoimmune disorder in which the release of acetylcholine by the motor nerve terminals is impaired. Symptoms include proximal muscle weakness (especially in the pelvis, thighs, arms, and shoulders), fatigue, peripheral paresthesia, dry mouth, dysphagia, diplopia, ptosis, difficulty chewing, and double vision.

DIAGNOSTIC REASONING

The diagnosis of lung cancer is typically made when a tumor is seen on a routine preoperative chest x-ray or a chest x-ray associated with a standard work physical. Early detection is the key to successful resection of NSCLC tumors, but mass screening programs have failed to affect mortality rates. However, *Healthy People 2030* has an objective of increasing the percentage of adults ages 55 to 80 who get screened for lung cancer from 4.5% to 7.5%.

The histological cell type and the stage of the disease are the major factors that influence choice of therapy for individuals. The currently accepted system is the 8th lung cancer tumor-node-metastasis (TNM) classification and clinical staging system presented in Table 32.5. In this

TABLE 32.5 Lung Cancer Staging

Tumor-Node-Metastasis (TNM) Stage Grouping for Lung Cancer

Occult cancer	TX N0 M0
	Tis N0 M0
Stage 0	T1 (mi) or T1a N0 M0
Stage IA1	T1b N0 M0
Stage IA2	T1c N0 M0
Stage IA3	T2a N0 M0
Stage IB	T2b N0 M0
Stage IIA	T1a to T1c N1 M0
Stage IIB	T2a N1 M0
	T2b N1 M0
	T3 N0 M0
	T1a to T1c N2 M0
Stage IIIA	T2a to T2b N2 M0
	T3 N1 M0
	T4 N0 M0
	T4 N1 M0
	T1a to T1c N3 M0
Stage IIIB	T2a to T2b N3 M0
	T3 N2 M0
	T4 N2 M0
	T3 N3 M0
Stage IIIC	T4 N3 M0
	Any T Any N M1a
Stage IVA	Any T Any N M1b
Stage IV B	Any T Any N M1c

TNM Definitions of Primary Tumor (T) Characteristics in Lung Cancer

Primary Tumor (T)	
TX	Primary tumor cannot be assessed or tumor proven by the presence of malignant cells in sputum or bronchial washings but not visualized by imaging or bronchoscopy
T0	No evidence of primary tumor
Tis	Carcinoma in situ
T1	A tumor that is 3 cm or less in greatest dimension, surrounded by lung or visceral pleura and without evidence of invasion more proximal than the lobar bronchus (e.g., not in the main bronchus)
T1 (mi)	Minimally invasive adenocarcinoma
T1a	Tumor less than 1 cm in greatest dimension
T1b	Tumor more than 1 cm but less than 2 cm in greatest dimension
T1c	Tumor more than 2 cm but less than 3 cm in greatest dimension
T2	A tumor that is more than 3 cm but less than 5 cm in greatest dimension; or involving the main bronchus without involvement of the carina; or invading the visceral pleura; or associated with atelectasis or obstructive pneumonitis (collapse) that extends to the hilar region, involving part or all of the lung
T2a	Tumor more than 3 cm but less than 4 cm in greatest dimension
T2b	Tumor more than 4 cm but less than 5 cm in greatest dimension
T3	A tumor that is more than 5 cm but less than 7 cm in greatest dimension; or has separate tumor nodule(s) in the same lobe; or of any size with direct extension to the chest wall (including superior sulcus tumors), parietal pleura, phrenic nerve, or parietal pericardium
T4	A tumor that is more than 7 cm; or has separate tumor nodule(s) in additional ipsilateral lobe(s); or of any size that invades any of the following: diaphragm, mediastinum, heart, any of the great vessels, trachea, recurrent laryngeal nerve, esophagus, vertebral body, or carina

Continued

TABLE 32.5 Lung Cancer Staging—cont'd

REGIONAL LYMPH NODES (N)	
NX	Regional lymph nodes cannot be assessed
N0	No regional lymph node metastasis
N1	Metastasis in ipsilateral peribronchial and/or ipsilateral hilar lymph nodes and intrapulmonary nodes, including direct extension
N2	Metastasis in ipsilateral mediastinal and/or subcarinal lymph node(s)
N3	Metastasis in contralateral mediastinal, contralateral hilar, ipsilateral or contralateral scalene, or supraclavicular lymph node(s)
DISTANT METASTASIS (M)	
M0	No distant metastasis
M1a	Distant metastasis: separate tumor nodule(s) in a contralateral lobe; tumor with pleural or pericardial nodules or malignant pleural (or pericardial) effusion
M1b	Distant metastasis: single extrathoracic metastasis in one organ or single nonregional lymph node
M1c	Distant metastasis: multiple extrathoracic metastases in one or more organs

Used with the permission of the American College of Surgeons. Amin, M.B., Edge, S.B., Greene, F.L., Et al (Eds.) AJCC Cancer Staging Manual, 8th Ed. Springer New York, 2017.

system, T denotes the extent of the primary tumor (ranging from TX to T4), N indicates the nodal involvement (ranging from NX to N3), and M describes the extent of metastasis (M0 to M1c). The stage of disease is based on a combination of factors including clinical (physical examination, radiological, and laboratory studies) and pathological (biopsy of lymph nodes, bronchoscopy, mediastinoscopy, paramedian sternotomy, or other type of thoracotomy).

The diagnostic approach for SCLC is the same as that for NSCLC, but the staging system is different. The TNM staging system is not typically used for SCLC staging. Although SCLC staging also focuses on disease extent, it broadly classifies the cancer as limited-stage disease (i.e., limited to one hemothorax with hilar and mediastinal nodes that can be included within a radiation therapy port) or extensive-stage disease.

Diagnostic Tests

Initial Testing

A complete blood count (CBC) should be ordered because anemia may be associated with lung cancer, along with a basic metabolic panel and hepatic panel to check for abnormalities in Na, K, Ca, and liver enzymes, as well as a prothrombin time, partial thromboplastin time, and platelet count to assess for coagulopathies. An electrocardiogram should be done, as well as baseline pulmonary function tests.

Anterior-posterior and lateral chest x-ray films remain the simplest method for identifying patients with lung cancer. The heart and other thoracic structures obscure large portions of the lung tissue, so it is important to evaluate both a frontal and a side view. The chest x-ray film may demonstrate asymptomatic lung cancer and is almost always abnormal when the patient is symptomatic. A tumor nodule must be at least 2 to 3 mm before it is visible on a chest radiograph. Associated atelectasis, postobstructive pneumonitis, abscess, bronchiolitis, rib erosion, pleural effusion, or bulky mediastinal lymphadenopathy may be identified on radiographs, raising suspicion of a primary lung malignancy. The four most common types of lung cancer usually present with slightly different chest radiographic patterns, but there is so much overlap that only biopsy and histological examination provide reliable evidence of the cell type. Mediastinal changes on radiograph may suggest lymphadenopathy or pleural effusions, and an elevated diaphragm may be seen with phrenic nerve involvement.

A chest computed tomography (CT) scan with infusion of contrast material has become widely accepted as the primary cross-sectional imaging modality for evaluation of the thorax and is recommended to stage NSCLC. The CT scan should extend inferiorly to include the liver and adrenal glands. A contrast-enhanced chest CT scan will (1) characterize the size and location of the primary tumor and its relationship to other thoracic structures, (2) identify pathologically enlarged hilar and mediastinal lymph nodes, (3) identify satellite and other ipsilateral or contralateral pulmonary nodules, and (4) identify potential metastases to the liver and adrenal glands, both being common metastatic sites. Of note, because of its earlier metastases and typical unresectability, staging for SCLC is less useful for treatment and prognosis.

Cytological evaluation of sputum, bronchial washings, bronchial brushings, and fine-needle aspirates have a high diagnostic value, but the positive and negative predictive values of each, as well as their accuracy of diagnosis, depend on sampling error, tissue preservation, processing quality, and observer experience. Sputum cytology remains a simple test with a positive predictive value that can approach 100%, but it has a sensitivity rate of only 10% to 15%. If a diagnosis can be established through collective sputum cytology, invasive tests can often be averted. Automated sputum screening may play an increasingly important role in early diagnosis. The highest yield occurs in patients with large, centrally located tumors. It is much less helpful in diagnosing peripheral lesions because relatively few cells are released from the lesion, and those that are released rarely get to the central airways. Early morning sputum samples are collected for 3 to 5 days; deep coughing is recommended because coughing dislodges cancer cells into the sputum.

Flexible fiber-optic bronchoscopy is an essential and standard technique for evaluating patients with pulmonary neoplasms. It remains the most important procedure for determining the endobronchial extent of disease. The extent and operability of the tumor are assessed by observing the site of the tumor and extent of airway involvement. When lesions are visible endobronchially, bronchial washings have a diagnostic yield of approximately 90%; bronchial brushings and bronchial mucosal forceps biopsy samples provide a tissue diagnosis in nearly 98% of visualized tumors. Fluoroscopy is used to guide these sampling procedures. Transbronchial forceps biopsies, brushings, and washings can diagnose peripheral parenchymal lesions up to 80% of the time. The visual assessment of the primary tumor can also provide a clinically useful estimate of the probability of tumor complications such as airway obstruction, postobstructive pneumonia, or hemoptysis.

Transthoracic percutaneous fine-needle aspiration biopsy is used when lung lesions cannot be visualized by bronchoscopy but are accessible percutaneously. A biopsy needle guided by CT or fluoroscopy is inserted into the lesion for aspiration of cells. This procedure is most suitable for peripheral pulmonary nodules. Pneumothorax is the most common complication, with an increased risk in patients with COPD. A positive pleural fluid cytology proves the spread of malignancy to the pleural space. Thoracentesis and pleural biopsy combined provide up to a 90% diagnostic yield in patients with malignancy.

Mediastinoscopy is an invasive procedure used for the diagnosis and staging of lung cancer. A biopsy is recommended if mediastinal lymph nodes are found on chest CT scan that are greater than 1 cm in size for the patient with clinically operable NSCLC. The patient with lymphadenopathy on chest CT scan will most likely have positive nodes on biopsy. Anterior cervical mediastinoscopy allows direct visualization and biopsy of mediastinal nodes with less risk than an exploratory thoracotomy.

Video-assisted thoracoscopic surgery is used for the staging and diagnosis of lung cancer when less invasive techniques fail to yield a diagnosis. Small thoracotomy incisions are made through which thoracoscopic instruments are inserted. Visualization of the chest and mediastinum and assessment of pleural effusions are superior to that achieved using older scopes, which may help improve diagnostic accuracy.

Thoracoscopy is useful for pleural evaluation but less useful for evaluating the inner segments of the lung. It is more than 90% sensitive for the diagnosis of pleural-based malignancies and peripheral lung nodules, with a specificity of 99%. With a thoracoscope, the mediastinum can be entered and nodes biopsied. Thoracoscopy affords the potential for more complete staging of patients with suspected mediastinal nodal spread, and it has become a valuable adjunct to cervical mediastinoscopy and anterior mediastinotomy. There is a concern, however, about seeding the thoracoscope entrance site with tumor cells.

Subsequent Testing

A head CT scan or brain magnetic resonance imaging, with and without infusion of contrast material, is recommended only in patients who have signs or symptoms of central nervous system disease. The finding of an isolated adrenal mass on ultrasonographic or CT examination requires biopsy to rule out metastatic disease, if the patient's tumor is considered to be potentially resectable. NSCLC metastasizes to the adrenal glands in 18% to 38% of cases. A bone scan should be performed only in patients who complain of bone pain or chest pain or who have elevated serum calcium or serum alkaline phosphatase levels. It is estimated that between 9% and 15% of patients with newly diagnosed NSCLC have bony metastases at presentation, with the vertebral bodies most commonly affected. Finally, the finding of an isolated hepatic mass on ultrasonography or CT examination requires a biopsy to rule out metastatic disease if the patient's tumor is otherwise considered to be potentially resectable.

Differential Diagnosis

The symptoms of lung cancer develop gradually in most cases and are often attributed by the patient to a smoker's cough or cold and by the patient's health-care provider to tracheobronchitis, pneumonia, influenza, pulmonary infarction, or lung abscess. Thus, it is common for a patient to delay seeking medical attention for several months from the first recognizable onset of symptoms. Several additional months of symptomatic treatment and antibiotic courses are typically administered before the health-care provider establishes the correct diagnosis. Much of the initial diagnostic task is to differentiate between a primary tumor and metastatic cancer, which is evaluated on biopsy. Other differential diagnoses include tuberculosis, lymphoma, *Mycobacterium avium* complex, sarcoidosis, or a foreign body aspiration that has been retained.

MANAGEMENT

The U.S. Preventive Services Task Force (USPSTF) recommends annual screening for lung cancer with low-dose computed tomography (LDCT) in adults aged 55 to 80 years who have at least a 30 pack-year smoking history and currently smoke or have quit within the past 15 years. Screening should be discontinued once a person has not smoked for at least 15 years or develops a health problem that substantially limits life expectancy or the ability or willingness to have curative lung surgery (i.e., resection).

Fewer than one-half of patients with lung cancer are candidates for resection and only a small percentage of them are cured; thus, most patients require some form of palliation. Active patient participation in therapeutic decision making respects the fundamental ethical and legal doctrine of autonomy. Whereas stage I or II NSCLC is routinely resected via thoracotomy, patient engagement in the decision-making process is especially important for the patient with unresectable NSCLC because the prognosis is often poor and symptom palliation is the central concern, as influenced by individual patient values and experiences. In turn, therapy should include efforts to slow the growth of the tumor and treat complications as they arise, but above all, symptoms should be relieved. A summary of the treatment of NSCLC is shown in Figure 32.1.

Surgery

Surgical resection offers the best chance of cure for lung cancer. Pneumonectomy (removal of a whole lung) and lobectomy (removal of a single lobe) are the most

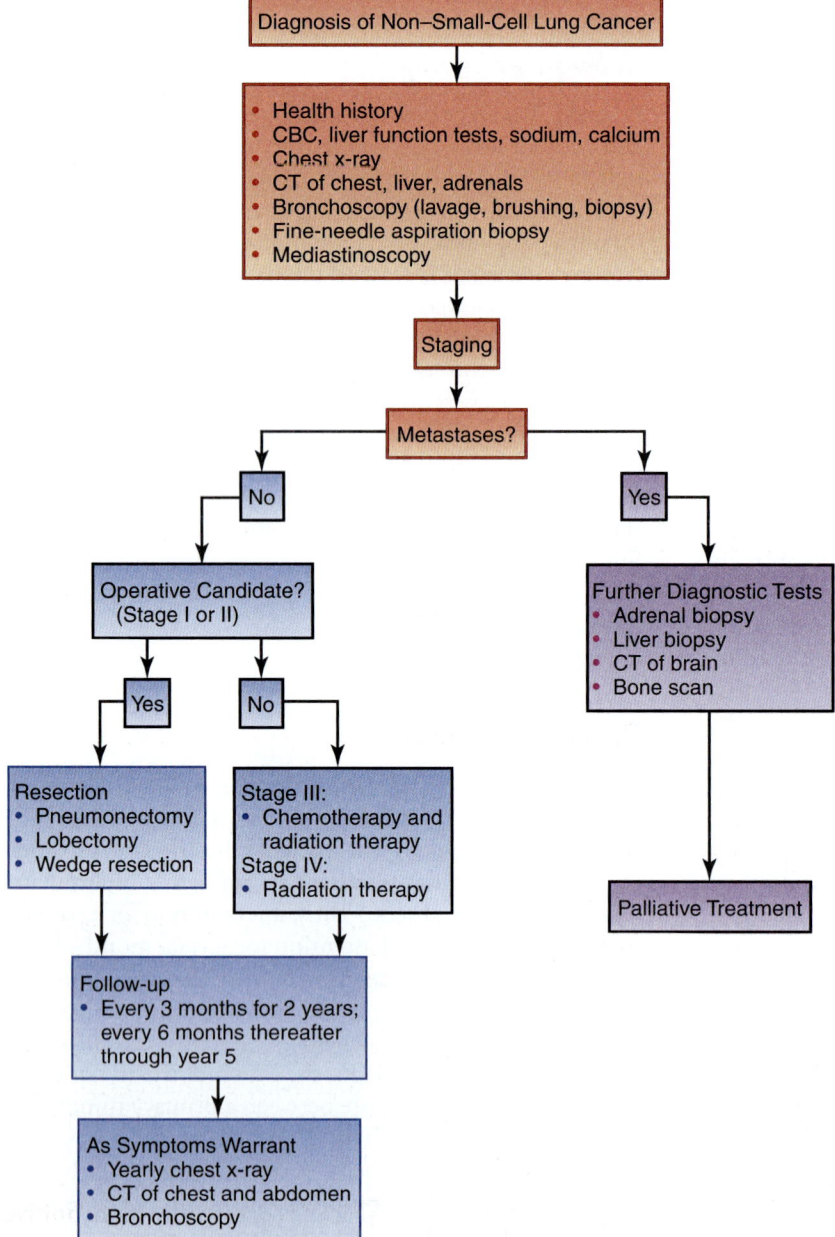

Figure 32.1 Treatment flowchart: non–small-cell lung cancer.

common of these surgical procedures. The nature of the tumor dictates the procedure, whereas pulmonary function determines whether the patient can withstand the procedure. Pneumonectomy is required when a lung-conserving operation will not allow for complete resection of the tumor, such as cases in which the tumor involves proximal structures or lymph nodes are affected. Lobectomy is the most common resection performed for lung cancer. This type of resection allows removal of the primary tumor, associated disease, and lymph node–bearing areas while leaving a significant amount of residual functional parenchyma. Survival is equivalent for patients undergoing lobectomy or pneumonectomy for all stages of disease when a complete resection is performed. For lesions close to the lobar orifice, an adequate margin of resection often cannot be achieved. In such circumstances, a portion of the main bronchus must be included with the resection. This type of resection is termed "sleeve resection," and it is performed as a parenchyma-sparing procedure, avoiding pneumonectomy.

Very limited resection in the treatment of lung cancer is reserved for patients with extremely poor lung function who can tolerate no more than minor resection because of their underlying medical condition or low pulmonary reserve. Limited resections include segmentectomy, wedge resection, or lumpectomy. Segmental resection is the removal of a lung segment, and wedge resection is the removal of a small, V-shaped wedge of lung tissue. Lesions that reside more deeply within the pulmonary tissue often are not amenable to wedge resection and may require precise, local excision with laser or electrocautery assistance (e.g., lumpectomy). These techniques are used to preserve as much lung tissue as possible, and they are performed for the removal of small tumors located close to the surface of the lung. The guiding principle of surgical therapy in lung cancer is to remove the tumor completely, leaving as much functional pulmonary tissue as possible. The aim of most operations is curative, and procedures that leave gross tumor are not warranted. Resection is abandoned if the tumor extends beyond the lung, when pleural seeding is evident, or when fixed mediastinal nodes are present.

Patients with stage I disease have a 50% to 80% 5-year survival, and patients with stage II disease have a 25% to 50% survival at 5 years. However, 75% of patients present with advanced disease and significant comorbidities. Treatment decisions should thus consider symptom control, quality of life, the patient's value or meaning of life, and the patient's perceptions and attitudes about a specific treatment.

Chemotherapy

Neoadjuvant chemotherapy involves giving antineoplastic drugs *before* surgery or radiation therapy. Adjuvant chemotherapy involves administering antineoplastic drugs *after* surgery or radiation therapy. Given that chemotherapy for advanced disease is marginally beneficial and noncurative, its use must be governed judiciously, with each treatment decision evaluated individually for each patient.

Current chemotherapeutic approaches consist initially of defining new combinations of established chemotherapeutic agents that may act synergistically. In addition, new drugs with novel mechanisms of action are also being investigated, both as single agents and, subsequently, as agents to be used in combination with established drugs. Drug developers have initiated many new studies, and it is predicted that eventually 30% of all chemotherapy drugs will be oral agents. The biological immunotherapeutic agent pembrolizumab (Keytruda), a programmed cell death 1 (PD-1) inhibitor, was the first agent approved by the U.S. Food and Drug Administration for unresectable or metastatic solid tumors with certain genetic specifications, but without regard to tissue type or location. Standard chemotherapy consists of cisplatin or carboplatin along with pemetrexed, paclitaxel, or docetaxel. Bevacizumab (Avastin), an angiogenesis inhibitor that blocks the activity of vascular endothelial growth factor A, is another option in some cases. Details on the use of these medications are beyond the scope of this text and referral to an oncologist is required to direct any chemotherapeutic regimens.

Small-Cell Lung Cancer Chemotherapy

Combination chemotherapy is capable of effecting high objective response rates in patients with SCLC. Furthermore, the simultaneous administration of multiple agents is superior to the sequential administration of the same regimen. Chemotherapy is most effective in SCLC with an 80% to 100% response in limited-stage disease (50% to 60% complete response) and a 60% to 80% response in extensive-stage disease (15% to 40% complete response). Remissions last a median of 6 to 8 months. If the cancer recurs, the median survival time is 3 to 4 months.

Non–Small-Cell Lung Cancer Chemotherapy

Chemotherapy modestly improves median survival with distant metastatic NSCLC compared with best supportive care, but it is not curative. If a patient has stage I disease, there is no agreement on the role of adjuvant chemotherapy. It is more widely used with patients with stage II and IIIA disease. Patients with stage I and N0 stage II disease treated with multidrug platinum-based chemotherapy show improved survival of 3 months at 5 years. Because of the toxicity, risks versus benefits of chemotherapy must be discussed with the patient and family. Newer drugs with less toxicity are currently being studied. With patients in advanced stages of disease, chemotherapy has been shown to improve patients' quality of life by decreasing bothersome symptoms. For patients with stage III lung cancer that cannot be removed surgically, chemotherapy is typically combined with definitive high-dose radiation treatments. In stage IV lung cancer, chemotherapy is typically the main treatment because radiation is used only for palliation of symptoms.

The newest developments in lung cancer treatment are targeted treatments. Whereas chemotherapy drugs cannot differentiate between normal cells and cancer cells, targeted therapies are designed specifically to attack cancer cells by attaching to or blocking targets that appear on cancer cell surfaces. Patients with advanced lung cancer with certain molecular biomarkers may receive treatment with a targeted drug alone or in combination with chemotherapy.

Radiation

The basic indication for radiation therapy is inoperability. In addition, it is sometimes used as prophylactic cranial irradiation to help prevent metastasis to the brain. Radiation therapy can modify the natural course of the disease, relieve distressing symptoms, and produce an apparent cure in an occasional patient. Long-term results, however, have been generally disappointing. One-year and 5-year overall survival rates range from 25% to 55% and from 4% to 10%, respectively. Radiation is used as adjunctive therapy after surgery to improve tumor control, and it is used as palliative therapy to control symptoms in other cases.

Small-Cell Lung Cancer Radiation

SCLC is quite sensitive to both radiation and chemotherapy. In limited-stage SCLC, the addition of both radiation and chemotherapy can increase the 5-year survival rate from about 11% to 20%. Most oncologists consider thoracic radiation therapy in combination with chemotherapy for limited-stage disease to be the standard of care. The major contribution of thoracic irradiation is local tumor control, and local control of the intrathoracic tumor is essential for cure. Thoracic radiation therapy reduces the risk of dying of SCLC but at the price of increased toxicity. Concurrent or alternating treatment schedules appear to improve response rates over sequential chemotherapy and radiation therapy, although toxicity is more intense with concurrent therapy.

Non–Small-Cell Lung Cancer Radiation

Radiation therapy is commonly offered to patients with inoperable NSCLC when the cancer has not spread beyond the thorax. In this case, the asymptomatic patient or the patient who is still functioning at a high level is most likely to benefit. In addition, radiation therapy is used to shrink the tumor and control symptoms in the patient with inoperable lung cancer and to prevent brain metastasis. Treating the tumor with radiation therapy may relieve hemoptysis, shoulder and arm pain, chest pain, and dyspnea. It can be used in superior vena cava obstruction to reduce the tumor size and alleviate obstruction. Although there are currently no data that demonstrate a survival advantage for postoperative adjuvant therapy in patients with completely resected stage II disease, regardless of whether the patient receives radiation therapy alone or radiation therapy and chemotherapy, most of these patients are treated with postoperative radiation therapy to decrease local recurrence. Unfortunately, prevention of local recurrence has not been shown to translate into a survival benefit. The patient with a malignant pleural effusion or with distant metastatic disease is not appropriate for definitive thoracic radiotherapy.

FOLLOW-UP AND REFERRAL

When lung cancer is first detected, the patient should be referred to a specialist for staging and treatment decisions. The patient who has been successfully treated for lung cancer needs to be routinely followed. The goal of monitoring patients with unresectable lung cancer in complete remission is to detect any symptomatic progression of their disease that may benefit from therapeutic intervention or symptom management. The large majority of patients with unresectable stage III and stage IV disease will not achieve complete remission, or, if achieved, the duration of remission will be short.

A history and physical examination should be performed every 3 months during the first 2 years, every 6 months thereafter through year 5, and then annually. For the patient treated with curative intent, there is no clear role for routine x-ray evaluation in the asymptomatic patient or for those in whom no interventions are planned. A yearly chest x-ray film to evaluate for potentially curable second primary cancers may be reasonable. CT of the chest and abdomen, bronchoscopy, CBC, and routine serum chemistries, including liver function tests, should be performed only as indicated by the patient's symptoms, as these tests do not appear to detect asymptomatic recurrent disease with a high frequency.

> **Patient Education: Lung Cancer**
>
> Assessment of learning needs and the provision of information is of paramount importance for the patient at the time of initial biopsy, between diagnosis and definitive treatment, and at discharge. These are highly stressful times for patients and they may be easily overwhelmed by the information regarding treatment options. It is important to assess what level of participation in the decision-making process the patient desires because that will help direct informational interventions and can reduce anxiety and psychological distress. This is particularly important for patients who have a choice between two treatment options or are deciding between participating in a clinical trial or receiving standard therapy.
>
> Smoking cessation, never initiating smoking, and avoidance of occupational and environmental exposure to carcinogenic substances are recommended as effective interventions to reduce the risk of a second primary lung cancer in the curatively

treated patient. For the patient with distant metastatic disease, the outlook is poor, and smoking cessation has little effect on overall prognosis but may improve respiratory symptoms. A tapering nicotine patch or other delivery system has been proven to increase the odds of smoking cessation when combined with behavioral interventions.

Additionally, patients with lung cancer who have never smoked may suffer from the stigma of lung cancer as a self-induced condition, whether accurate or not. These patients are likely to suffer from anxiety, depression, and social isolation, all of which call for increased support.

Recommendations for lifestyle modifications are the same for the patient with a history of lung cancer as for those who have no previous history of lung cancer, particularly with regard to complete avoidance of smoking. Epidemiological studies also suggest that people who consume relatively large amounts of fruits and vegetables have a lower risk of both cancer and cardiovascular disease. Antioxidant vitamins contained in fruits and vegetables prevent carcinogenesis by interfering with oxidative damage to DNA and lipoproteins; however, the use of antioxidants and/or chemopreventive agents for lung cancer (e.g., retinoic acid, beta-carotene, and selenium) is currently investigational.

When medical care for the patient with lung cancer shifts from curative to palliative, the patient and family must choose a care setting. Home or hospice care can provide familiar surroundings, feelings of normalcy, involvement of family, and a more comforting situation as the patient and family participate in readiness for the dying process. Although hospice has proven to be an extremely effective model for terminal care, referrals to hospice care are often not made until the final days of life. The difficulty lies in predicting when death will occur because Medicare reimbursement requires that a hospice patient has a life expectancy of 6 months or less. Many states now have an "open access" model that allows for patients seeking curative care to still receive hospice services.

Supportive resources for self-care should be provided as required by the individual situation. Patients will be able to manage less self-care as the disease progresses, and family members will require education with demonstration of care techniques, as well as opportunities for questions and verbalization of feelings about caring for the one who is ill. Within the Circle of Caring model, collaborative planning is essential in helping the patient and family make informed choices and live in the moment.

REFERENCES

American Joint Committee on Cancer. *AJCC Cancer Staging Manual*. 8th edition. https://cancerstaging.org/references-tools/deskreferences/Documents/AJCC%20Cancer%20Staging%20Form%20Supplement.pdf. Accessed 9/27/2020.

American Lung Association. Lung cancer fact sheet. http://www.lung.org/lung-health-and-diseases/lung-disease-lookup/lung-cancer/resource-library/lung-cancer-fact-sheet. Accessed 8/27/2020.

Centers for Disease Control and Prevention. Lung Cancer—Who should be screened for lung cancer? https://www.cdc.gov/cancer/lung/basic_info/screening.htm. Accessed 8/27/2020.

Lim W, Ridge CA, Nicholson AG, et al. The 8th lung cancer TNM classification and clinical staging system: review. *Quant Imaging Med Surg*. 2018 Aug; 8(7):709–718. https://www.ncbi.nlm.nih.gov/pmc/articles/PMC6127520/. Accessed 9/27/2020.

Office of Disease Prevention and Health Promotion. Increase the proportion of adults who get screened for lung cancer. *Healthy People 2030*. https://health.gov/healthypeople/objectives-and-data/browse-objectives/cancer/increase-proportion-adults-who-get-screened-lung-cancer-c-03. Accessed 10/17/2020.

Rigotti NA. Balancing the Benefits and Harms of E-Cigarettes: A National Academies of Science, Engineering, and Medicine Report. *Ann Intern Med*. 2018 May 1;168(9):666–667. Epub 2018 Feb 13.

Sherry V. Lung cancer: not just a smoker's disease. *Am Nurse Today*. 2017;12(2):16–20.

Thompson N, Christian A. Oral chemotherapy: not just an ordinary pill. *Am Nurse Today*. 2016;11(9):16–20.

Zhang LR, Morgenstern H, Greenland S. Cannabis smoking and lung cancer risk: pooled analysis in the International Lung Cancer Consortium. *Int J Cancer*. 2015 Feb;136(4):894–903. Epub 2014 Jun 30.

RESOURCES

American Cancer Society
 https://www.cancer.org

American Lung Association
 https://www.lung.org

Chapter 33

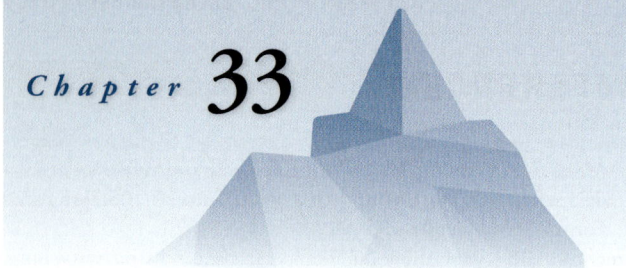

Smoking Addiction

Jill E. Winland-Brown, EdD, APRN, FNP-BC, FAANP
Brian Oscar Porter, MD, PhD, MPH, MBA

A pack-a-day smoker takes more than 70,000 cigarette puffs per year. Each puff delivers various chemicals into the lungs and bloodstream, including nicotine, an addictive substance. The act of smoking reinforces cigarette addiction by establishing secondary reinforcers, such as the sight and smell of cigarettes; the lighting procedure; and the association of cigarette smoking with a meal, a cup of coffee, or an alcoholic drink. Nicotine addiction fulfills all the criteria of a drug addiction: compulsive use, psychoactive effects, withdrawal symptoms, and drug-reinforcing behavior. Tolerance and physical dependence, manifested by an abstinence-mediated withdrawal syndrome, contribute to the strong control exerted by nicotine on smoking behavior. Although nicotine is the most likely reinforcing agent in tobacco, there are other possibilities, including tar and carbon monoxide (CO).

Tobacco use is the leading preventable cause of disease, disability, and death in the United States, particularly from cardiovascular disease, cancer, and lung disease. According to the World Health Organization ([WHO], 2020), tobacco kills up to half of its users. Table 33.1 lists the effects of cigarette smoke on the cardiovascular and respiratory systems. Cigarettes are responsible for one in every five deaths in the United States. In addition, 8.6 million people have a serious illness caused by smoking. For every person who dies from smoking, 30 more have at least one serious tobacco-related illness. Besides the premature loss of life and the reduction in quality of life of smokers, billions of dollars in medical expenses per year can be directly attributed to cigarette smoking. These statistics are even more alarming when it is recognized that more than 50 years have passed since publication of the landmark U.S. Surgeon General's 1964 Report, "The Health Consequences of Smoking." Clinicians must do more to help patients refrain from or stop smoking. One of the objectives of *Healthy People 2030* is to decrease the percentage of adolescents in grades six through 12 who smoke cigarettes, e-cigarettes, cigars, smokeless tobacco, hookah (large water pipes), or pipe tobacco from 18.3% to 11.3%. Another objective is to decrease the percentage of adults over 18 years of age who currently smoke from 13.9% to 5%. The U.S. Centers for Disease Control and Prevention (CDC) reports that in 2018, 34.2 million American adults (13.7%) were current cigarette smokers. This is down slightly from 2015. It is hoped that this will eventually decrease to less than 12%, given the available modalities to assist patients with smoking cessation.

There are also significant hazards for nonsmokers who breathe the smoke of others' cigarettes (passive smoking or environmental tobacco smoke [ETS]). ETS is defined as a combination of the smoke emitted by a burning cigarette, cigar, or pipe and the smoke exhaled by smokers. Passive smoking is associated with a modestly increased risk of lung cancers and possibly other cancers and has been classified by the U.S. Environmental Protection Agency as a known human carcinogen. According to the CDC, exposure to secondhand smoke causes more than 41,000 deaths per year in nonsmoking U.S. adults and damages the respiratory health of hundreds of thousands of children who live in homes with a parent who smokes cigarettes. It is estimated that between 150,000 and 300,000 cases of respiratory illness occurring in infants and children up to 18 months of age may be associated with exposure to ETS, which increases the risk of lower respiratory tract infections.

EPIDEMIOLOGY AND CAUSES

Substantial gains have been made in reducing smoking prevalence in the United States, although at present, almost one in five Americans still smoke. Notably, 90% of adult smokers smoked their first cigarette before age 18 years.

More than 7 million deaths per year worldwide are attributed to tobacco use. At the current smoking rate, an estimated 5.6 million people younger than 18 years will die prematurely from a disease related to smoking. At a cost of $170 billion per year in medical expenses, this problem is epidemic in proportion.

Smoking has also become an important issue in women's health. Despite widespread public education about the health risks of smoking, women continue to start smoking at high rates. Approximately 200 million of the world's 1 billion smokers are women, and about 1.5 million women die each year from cigarette smoking.

Although the reduction in overall smoking prevalence represents a major victory for public health, there are several groups within the U.S. population that continue to smoke at disproportionately high rates. These groups have been less likely to experience the benefits of tobacco control efforts. For example, low socioeconomic status and low educational attainment are now the primary predictors of smoking status in the United States and Canada. According to a 2018 NIDA survey, only 3.6% of high-school seniors smoked daily, compared with 22.4% several decades ago.

TABLE 33.1 Diseases Associated With Cigarette Smoking

Body System/Category	Disease or Condition
Cardiovascular	• Atherosclerotic cardiovascular disease (coronary artery disease [CAD]; carotid vascular disease; mesenteric, renal, iliac disease; abdominal aortic aneurysm) • Coronary artery spasm • Arrhythmias • Peripheral vascular diseases (thromboangiitis obliterans, deep vein thrombosis, pulmonary embolus)
Endocrine	• Altered hormonal secretion • Graves' disease • Antidiuresis • Goiter
Gastrointestinal	• Peptic ulcer disease (gastric, duodenal) • Gastroesophageal reflux disease • Chronic pancreatitis • Crohn's disease • Colonic adenomas
Genitourinary	• Glomerulonephritis • Benign prostatic hypertrophy • Erectile dysfunction
Rheumatologic/Musculoskeletal	• Rheumatoid arthritis • Osteoporosis
Integumentary	• Skin wrinkling • Psoriasis
Infectious	• Tuberculosis • Pneumococcal infection • Meningococcal infection
Malignancies	• Respiratory tract malignancies • Lung cancer (squamous cell, adenocarcinoma, large cell, small cell) • Laryngeal cancer • Oral cancer • Other cancers (esophageal, pancreatic, bladder, uterine, cervical, breast, renal, anal, penile, gastric, hepatic, leukemia)
Psychiatric	• Depression • Schizophrenia
Reproductive	• Premature ovarian failure • Decreased sperm quality • Pregnancy-related diseases (prematurity, premature rupture of membranes, spontaneous abortion) • Fetal-/infant-related diseases (low birth weight, impaired lung growth, sudden infant death syndrome, febrile seizures, reduced intelligence, behavioral disorders, atopic diseases, asthma)
Respiratory	• Chronic obstructive pulmonary disease (COPD) • Asthma • Eosinophilic granuloma of the lung • Respiratory bronchiolitis • Goodpasture's syndrome • Sleep apnea • Pneumothorax
Sensory/Head and Neck	• Loss of olfaction • Loss of taste • Cataracts • Periodontal disease
Pediatric	• Effects on children of parental smoking (asthma, rhinitis, otitis, pneumonia, increased risk for child to begin smoking)

> **Pediatric/Adolescent Considerations:**
> The estimated 80% of individuals who initiate smoking during adolescence and become regular tobacco users ensure an enduring supply of adult smokers. The initiation of smoking tobacco by adolescents in middle school is of great concern. Vaping and e-cigarette use are also of concern, yet the numbers seem to be decreasing. In 2017, 79.8% of eighth graders and 71.8% of 12th graders reported that they disapproved of regularly vaping nicotine. Only 14.1% of 12th graders see great risk in marijuana smoking, according to this survey, down from 17.1% the year before and down from a staggering 40.6% rate of disapproval in 1991.
>
> According to the National Institute on Drug Abuse ([NIDA], 2017), nearly one in three students in 12th grade reported use of some kind of vaping device in the past year, raising concerns about the impact on their health. Although the use of regular cigarettes and hookahs continues to decline (hookah use for tobacco has gone from 21.4% in 2013 to 7.8% in 2018), a key concern focuses on the contents of vaping e-liquid, which range from nicotine to marijuana to "just flavoring." The survey indicated that 51.8% of students said it was "just flavoring" that they vaped, 32.8% said nicotine, and 11.1% said marijuana. As first-time nicotine users, there is a risk that young people who vape may subsequently begin to smoke regular cigarettes.
>
> Beginning in adolescence, all patients should be asked if they use tobacco and should have their tobacco use status documented on a regular basis as a new vital sign (i.e., a basic, standard clinical assessment). This is the age-group that all providers should try to reach with this information, as several questionnaires measuring self-reported tobacco dependence are available.

Unlike cigarette smoking, some forms of smokeless tobacco use (e.g., plug, leaf, and snuff) have actually increased. One of these forms is "dipping snuff," which involves placement of a coarse, moist tobacco powder between the cheek and gum, which results in the direct absorption of nicotine and other carcinogens through the oral tissue. Oral cancer occurs more frequently among snuff dippers, as well as among pipe and cigar smokers, compared with nonusers of tobacco.

Another formulation for delivering nicotine is in the form of e-cigarettes, which have been available for 15 years. E-cigarettes do not produce tobacco smoke but rather an aerosol, which consists of fine particles often mistaken for water vapor. The term "vaping" is the act of inhaling and exhaling this aerosol, or vapor, produced by an e-cigarette or similar device. E-cigarettes, which resemble smoked cigarettes, and vape pens, which resemble large fountain pens, have become increasingly popular. Vaping devices include not just e-cigarettes and vape pens but also advanced personal vaporizers (also known as "mods").

Generally, a vaping device consists of a mouthpiece, a cartridge for containing the e-liquid (or "e-juice"), and a heating component for the device, which is powered by a battery. When the device is used, the battery heats up the heating component, which converts the contents of the e-liquid into an aerosol that is inhaled into the lungs and then exhaled. The e-liquid in vaporizer products usually contains a propylene glycol or vegetable glycerin-based liquid with nicotine, flavoring, and other chemicals and metals, but not tobacco. Some people use these devices to inhale tetrahydrocannabinol (THC), the chemical responsible for most of marijuana's mind-altering effects, or even synthetic drugs such as the stimulant (α-pyrrolidinopentiophenone [flakka]), instead of nicotine.

With the advent and increased use of e-cigarettes, many concerns have arisen. The U.S. Food and Drug Administration has cited the following issues with these products:

- They may increase nicotine addiction and lead adolescents to smoke conventional cigarettes.
- E-cigarettes contain known toxins.
- Sufficient clinical studies have not been conducted regarding their safety.

The use of tobacco products is a complex, learned behavior that is woven into the fiber of daily life and is linked to how the smoker deals with the world. Numerous daily activities, thoughts, and emotions serve as powerful cues to smoke. Such conditioned responses become paired with the positive neuroregulatory effects of nicotine to reinforce the addictive process. Personal characteristics such as education level, belief in one's ability to change, and coping skills are determinants of tobacco use. Similarly, environmental factors such as community norms and the level of smoking acceptance in the home, one's peer group, and the workplace influence smoking behavior.

The tobacco industry's drive for profits is the root cause of why cigarette smoking continues to thrive in the United States, despite irrefutable evidence that it is a health hazard and a form of drug addiction. Millions of dollars are spent every day on tobacco advertising. Legislative initiatives to control cigarette smoking in the United States have gained significant ground in some states such as California, but from a public health perspective, they are not as stringent nationally. Bans on smoking in the workplace and in restaurants have done little to discourage smokers from smoking in other private venues.

Initially identified in 2019, acute and potentially fatal respiratory illnesses linked to e-cigarettes and vaping have been increasingly observed, with 2,800 cases of EVALI (e-cigarette or vaping product use–associated lung injury) reported by February 2020. There were 68 deaths from this new disease (EVALI) by Feb. 2020. The majority of these patients were males younger than age 35. Some of the respiratory diseases caused by e-cigarettes include community-acquired pneumonia, acute eosinophilic pneumonia, organizing pneumonia, lipoid pneumonia, diffuse alveolar hemorrhage, hypersensitivity pneumonitis, respiratory bronchiolitis interstitial lung disease, and giant cell pneumonitis. In many states, EVALI is now a reportable disease. The increasing incidence of these diseases has led to stricter regulatory guidelines for vaping products, thereby limiting young people's exposure to them.

PATHOPHYSIOLOGY

When a cigarette is smoked, approximately 4,000 chemicals and gases are inhaled into the lungs. Many carcinogens have been isolated from cigarette smoke; 3,4-benzpyrene is the most dangerous. At least 43 other components have been identified as carcinogens, cocarcinogens, tumor promoters, tumor initiators, and mutagens. The primary active (and addictive) ingredient in tobacco is nicotine. In its purest state, nicotine is an extremely toxic, clear, oily liquid with a characteristic odor. At low doses, it acts as a stimulant; at high doses, it depresses the central nervous system (CNS).

Nicotine enters the body through a variety of routes. Inhalation of smoke from a cigar, cigarette, or pipe is perhaps the most common route. With cigarettes, some absorption of nicotine occurs through the membranes of the mouth, throat, and bronchi, as well as the alveoli of the lungs. With snuff and chewing tobacco, nicotine reaches the bloodstream by absorption through the mucosal linings of the mouth, nose, and throat.

Inhalation is the quickest and most effective delivery method of nicotine. It is estimated that 90% of the nicotine that reaches the alveoli of the lungs in each breath is absorbed into the bloodstream. Although an average cigarette contains 15 to 20 mg of nicotine, only 1 to 2 mg from each cigarette smoked is delivered to the lungs. About 25% of the nicotine is immediately carried to the brain, where it easily crosses the blood–brain barrier and affects normal brain biochemistry. In humans, 60 mg of nicotine can be a lethal dose.

Acute Effects of Nicotine Use

Outside the CNS, nicotine affects the transmission of nervous system signals by mimicking acetylcholine. It occupies receptor sites at the synapses and prevents the transmission of nerve impulses from neuron to neuron and from neuron to muscle cells. Smoking exerts its deleterious effects primarily on the cardiovascular and pulmonary systems (Box 33.1). Nicotine, a direct adrenergic agonist, causes the release of epinephrine, which increases heart rate, systemic vascular resistance, and blood pressure. Smoking directly increases coronary vascular resistance, especially at sites of atherosclerotic plaques and stenosis. Inhaled cigarette smoke also exerts

Box 33.1 Effects of Tobacco Smoke	
Cardiovascular Effects	**Respiratory Effects**
• Increased myocardial oxygen consumption • Increased heart rate • Increased systemic vascular resistance • Decreased myocardial inotropic activity • Decreased myocardial oxygen supply • Increased carboxyhemoglobin (reduced available hemoglobin) • Coronary artery vasospasm • Oxyhemoglobin dissociation curve shifted to the left	• Decreased mucociliary clearance • Bronchospasm • Cough • Sputum accumulation • Decreased circulating immunoglobulin levels • Decreased neutrophil chemotaxis • Decreased pulmonary macrophage count and adherence • Altered T-lymphocyte immunoregulatory activity • Decreased natural killer cell activity • Decreased function of alpha$_1$-antitrypsin

a negative inotropic effect on the myocardium, possibly due to the binding of CO to cytochrome oxidase and myoglobin, resulting in increased myocardial oxygen consumption and decreased oxygen delivery. These changes are accompanied by the constriction of the blood vessels beneath the skin, a reduction in motility of the bowel, and a loss of appetite.

CO, a component of tobacco smoke, is present in cigarette smoke in concentrations similar to those of automobile exhaust. CO has a binding affinity for the hemoglobin molecule that is 250 times greater than that of oxygen, thereby reducing the smoker's oxygen-carrying capacity. In heavy smokers, as much as 15% of circulating hemoglobin may be bound to CO, reducing the oxygen-carrying capacity of the blood. In addition, CO shifts the oxyhemoglobin dissociation curve to the left, inhibiting the release of oxygen. The half-life of the carboxyhemoglobin (COHb) complex is 4 to 6 hours when the individual is breathing room air. The heart's need for oxygen is increased because of the sympathetic stimulatory effect of nicotine. Because the blood's oxygen-carrying capacity is reduced, the heart must pump more rapidly to adequately supply tissues with oxygen.

The effects of smoking on the respiratory system are diverse. The irritating effect of the smoke causes hyperplasia of cells, including goblet cells, which results in increased mucus production. Hyperplasia reduces airway diameter and increases the difficulty in clearing secretions. Smoking is known to disrupt mucociliary function and the ability to clear particles from the peripheral airways, even before any abnormality in pulmonary function can be detected, because smoking may cause actual loss of ciliated cells. Smoking also produces abnormal dilation of the distal air spaces with destruction of alveolar walls. Many cells develop large, atypical nuclei, which are considered a precursor to cancer. Smoking also alters pulmonary immune defense mechanisms by depressing neutrophil chemotaxis, decreasing immunoglobulin levels, reducing natural killer cell activity, decreasing macrophage adherence, and altering immunoregulatory T-lymphocyte activity.

In the CNS, nicotine activates receptors within the brain. Stimulation of the brain is evidenced by changes in electroencephalogram (EEG) patterns, reflecting an increase in the frequency of electrical activity. This is part of a general arousal pattern signaled by the release of the neurotransmitters norepinephrine, dopamine, acetylcholine, and serotonin. Heavy tobacco use, resulting in high levels of nicotine in the bloodstream, eventually produces a blocking effect, as more and more receptor sites are filled. The result is generalized depression of the CNS. When the blood levels of nicotine reach a critical point, the brain's vomiting center may be activated.

Chronic Effects of Nicotine Use

Chronic effects of nicotine use include the development of tolerance and chemical dependence. The user will consume greater quantities of nicotine for longer periods than originally intended, further endangering their health. Dependence on nicotine is quickly established in the majority of users. Although psychological dependence may occur as well, the hallmarks of physical dependence—establishment of tolerance and presence of withdrawal symptoms—have all been demonstrated. Nicotine withdrawal symptoms include a dysphoric or depressed mood, insomnia, irritability, frustration, anger, anxiety, poor concentration, restlessness, decreased heart rate, and increased appetite.

To understand better the neuropsychopharmacological basis of why people smoke, researchers have performed positron emission tomography (PET) scans on smokers and abstainers and found that smokers had a 40% decrease in levels of a brain enzyme known as monoamine oxidase (MAO) B compared with nonsmokers. The mechanisms of (MAO) B inhibition by cigarette smoke are not known. The enzyme breaks down dopamine, a neurotransmitter associated with feelings of pleasure. Because nicotine stimulates dopamine release and dopamine produces pleasurable effects, this mechanism may play a significant role in reinforcing and motivating smoking behavior. Therefore, smoking seems to create a self-perpetuating cycle: less MAO B leads to more dopamine, which leads to more pleasure, which leads to more smoking, which leads to less MAO B, and so on. The researchers proposed that reduction of MAO B activity may synergize with nicotine to produce the diverse behavioral effects and epidemiological patterns associated with smoking.

CLINICAL PRESENTATION

Subjective

Demographic, anthropometric, physiological, and laboratory features that distinguish cigarette smokers from nonsmokers reflect both baseline differences between these groups and the effects of smoking. Smokers drink more alcohol, coffee, and tea than do nonsmokers. Their weight and blood pressures are slightly lower, and their heart rates are slightly faster than those of nonsmokers. Females who smoke are at increased risk for early menopause, decreased bone density, and osteoporosis. Smoking has also been shown to decrease fertility in those attempting pregnancy and to impair uteroplacental function, which adversely affects the fetus during pregnancy. Sudden infant death syndrome is two to four times more common in infants whose mothers smoked during pregnancy. Smokers have impaired maximum exercise performance and impaired immune systems compared with nonsmokers. A markedly increased number of pulmonary alveolar macrophages is present in smokers, and the function and metabolism of these cells are abnormal. In smokers, the ratio of high-density lipoprotein cholesterol to low-density lipoprotein cholesterol is reduced.

A causal association has been well characterized between smoking and coronary heart disease, atherosclerotic peripheral vascular disease, cerebrovascular disease, lung and laryngeal cancer, oral cancer, esophageal cancer, chronic obstructive pulmonary disease (COPD), intrauterine growth retardation, and low–birth-weight babies. In addition, smoking is considered by many to be the probable cause or contributing cause of many other conditions, including miscarriage; increased infant mortality; peptic ulcer disease; and cancers of the bladder, breast, pancreas, uterus, and kidney (see Box 33.1). Smokers are at increased risk for bone fractures, premature skin wrinkling, gingival recession, dental caries, periodontal disease, cataracts, and glaucoma. Depression is twice as common among those who smoke than in people who have never smoked and has been linked to increased smoking initiation and to failures in smoking cessation efforts. A strong association also exists between smoking and other substance abuse disorders, especially alcohol dependence. Clinical manifestations of these specific diseases, although beyond the scope of this chapter, are all directly or indirectly associated with cigarette smoking.

Objective

Smokers usually demonstrate many observable signs of tobacco addiction. The smell of tobacco smoke lingers on the individual's clothing and on their skin and hair. The breath and sputum often smell of stale tobacco, and the fingers and nails are often stained from tobacco use. Use of smokeless tobacco may manifest in periodontal disease, a condition that may lead to tooth loss, abrasive damage to the enamel of the teeth due to the effects of processed tobacco, and oral cancer. The patient may also have lumps in the jaw or neck area; color change in clumps on the inner surface of the lips; or white, smooth, or scaly patches in the mouth or throat or on the lips or tongue. Smokers may also present with red spots or sores on the lips, gums, or inside the mouth that do not heal or cause difficulty speaking or swallowing.

Signs of cardiopulmonary disease often accompany tobacco addiction. A productive cough, dyspnea, wheezing, and fatigue should alert the clinician to respiratory problems related to smoking. Frequent bouts of pneumonia, influenza, and bronchitis, as well as chronic diseases such as emphysema, interstitial lung disease, and chronic airway obstruction, often result from cigarette smoking. Cardiovascular signs of smoking including tachycardia, cardiac dysrhythmias, increased blood pressure, decreased peripheral blood flow, and angina must all be assessed to determine the risk for and extent of cardiovascular disease in smokers or those exposed to secondhand smoke.

Nicotine dependence is related to the amount and duration of smoking and can manifest as withdrawal symptoms. These signs and symptoms begin within a few hours of the last cigarette, peak 48 to 72 hours later, and return to baseline within 3 to 4 weeks of quitting. Criteria for nicotine dependence disorder are published in the *Diagnostic and Statistical Manual of Mental Disorders, Fifth Edition, Text Revision.* They include dysphoric or depressed mood, insomnia, irritability, anger, frustration, anxiety, concentration difficulties, decreased heart rate, increased appetite, and weight gain.

DIAGNOSTIC REASONING

Asking the patient about smoking status and recording this information in the medical record require only an additional 15 seconds and serve as a reminder to the clinician to discuss the problem with each smoker. Despite this, only 20% of smokers receive medical advice on smoking cessation during visits to health-care providers. The six-question Fagerström Test for Nicotine Dependence predicts the level of nicotine dependence and may help predict smoking cessation success, as well as inform nicotine replacement dosages as a function of the classification of dependence.

Diagnostic Tests

Laboratory assays of smoking-related biochemical compounds such as thiocyanate, cotinine, nicotine, and COHb in urine, blood, breath, or saliva can be performed to verify smokers' reports of smoking status or abstinence. A urine sample can be assayed for the constituents of the cigarette smoke itself or for excretion products associated with the physiological effects of smoking. Nicotine excretion in smokers correlates well with the number of cigarettes smoked and inversely with the pH of the urine. Urine metabolites of epinephrine can also be measured; however, false-positive results related to severe anxiety are possible.

CO is found in the blood of smokers and combines with hemoglobin to form COHb. A value of 2% suggests that smoking has occurred. However, environmental and occupational sources of CO must be considered. Although the COHb level increases proportionately with the number of cigarettes smoked and varies with nicotine content, clinical judgment is necessary in interpreting the data.

The measurement of mean alveolar CO partial pressure makes it possible to determine the COHb levels in the blood with a high degree of correlation. Also, by subtracting expired CO from inspired CO, it is possible to determine whether a smoker is an inhaler. Smokers have higher levels of both expired CO and thiocyanate than nonsmokers. To measure CO, the patient is instructed to inhale deeply and hold their breath for 10 to 15 seconds before expiring with full force through the inflow valve of an EC_{50} monitor. Levels of nine parts per million (ppm) or lower are considered to reflect nonsmoking status.

Cotinine is a major metabolite of nicotine and is a useful marker. A sample of at least 3 mL of unstimulated saliva is collected in a plastic cup. The presence of nicotine (as reflected in cotinine levels) in saliva can be determined in a qualified laboratory by gas chromatography and an alkali flame ionization detector, but it is difficult to distinguish the pattern of smoking based on cotinine levels. Moreover, nonsmokers exposed to secondhand cigarette smoke may also have nicotine in their saliva.

Differential Diagnosis

The most accurate way to rule out differential diagnoses is to ensure that, for every patient at every clinic visit, status of use of tobacco, e-cigarettes, or vaping is queried and documented. The cause of a smoker's cough and dyspnea must be explored to rule out other explanatory causes, such as lung cancer, interstitial lung disease, allergies, and infections. Unfortunately, many patients with symptoms of cough, dyspnea, sputum production, and changes in pulmonary function testing are not only smokers but also suffer from some form of lung disease or disorder. Smokers tend to have unique laboratory findings, such as increases in HCT, total white blood cell count, and platelet count. They may also have decreases in leukocytes, vitamin C level, serum uric acid, and albumin.

MANAGEMENT

Changes in the system of health-care delivery in the United States indicate the need to incorporate smoking cessation as a regular part of clinical care, particularly in the current managed care environment. The CDC's *Best Practices for Comprehensive Tobacco Control Programs* (2014) is an evidence-based guide that helps plan and establish effective tobacco control programs to prevent and reduce tobacco use. Clinicians must also commit to making changes in clinical culture and practice patterns to ensure that every patient who smokes is offered smoking cessation treatment at every office visit. Brief but effective interventions are essential for all tobacco users at each clinical visit. Patients who are counseled to quit are 1.6 times as likely to attempt quitting as those who receive no counseling. Clinicians aiding patients in smoking cessation should remember the five A's: Ask, Advise, Assess, Assist, and Arrange. A treatment flowchart for smoking cessation is presented in Figure 33-1.

Initial Management

When a patient is identified as a smoker, the clinician should advise them of the need to quit. This advice should be given after the patient's chief complaint has been addressed. The patient's response will determine the proper strategy to pursue. The patient must be informed of how unhealthy and dangerous smoking is. Pregnant smokers should be strongly encouraged to quit throughout their pregnancy. Because of the serious risk of smoking to the pregnant smoker and fetus, pregnant smokers should be offered intensive counseling treatment. Patients should choose a quit date, usually within the next 30 days, to allow patients to develop effective alternative behaviors to smoking. Periods of extreme stress or depression are not optimal times to attempt smoking cessation.

Smoking Cessation Programs

Most smokers move through five stages of behavioral change in their attempts at cessation: (1) precontemplation, (2) contemplation, (3) preparation, (4) action, and (5) maintenance. The first step a provider should take in initiating a smoking cessation program with a patient is to find out which stage of cessation the patient is in. By understanding the smoker's stage of behavior and readiness to change, the clinician can better assist them to achieve successful cessation.

Smokers in the *precontemplation stage* have no desire to quit in the next 6 to 12 months. These individuals usually benefit from motivational interventions that increase awareness of the adverse effects of smoking. Smokers who are seriously thinking about and expressing interest in quitting but are not yet ready to do so are in the *contemplation stage*. These smokers also benefit from motivational counseling emphasizing the negative effects of smoking. Smokers who are serious about quitting and have taken the initial steps toward cessation are in the *preparation stage*. Individuals in this stage benefit from interventions that assist them in quitting. These interventions include providing information about nicotine replacement and developing behavior modification skills.

During the *action stage*, the smoker quits smoking. The action stage lasts from several weeks to 6 months after cessation, which is a common time of relapse. Because of the likelihood of relapse during this stage, interventions should address relapse prevention, including congratulating successes and rewarding positive behavioral changes with more frequent contacts by the clinician. When a smoker has abstained from cigarettes for 6 months, the *maintenance stage* begins. Most successful quitters relapse and recycle through these stages three or four times before attaining long-term abstinence; some may take several years to move through these stages until abstinence can be maintained.

Effective smoking cessation requires behavior modification. The behavior of smoking is usually linked to a variety of triggers (e.g., stress, foods or beverages, driving). When a patient recognizes the triggers, healthy alternative behaviors can be substituted. It is crucial to develop alternative coping strategies to overcome the urge to smoke. Such strategies include deep breathing and relaxation exercises, chewing gum, exercise, drinking water, sucking on a piece of sugarless candy, and eating carrots or celery sticks.

Patients quitting smoking need support from their clinicians, families, and other people. The clinician can help the patient handle particularly difficult triggers and can treat underlying behavioral problems or mood disorders, such as anxiety or depression. The family can provide invaluable positive reinforcement to the patient during this time. If there are other smokers in the patient's household, the clinician should encourage them to quit smoking at the same time as the patient. It is difficult for a person to refrain from smoking in the long term when a spouse or other family member continues to smoke. Many patients benefit from support groups such as Nicotine Anonymous (NicA) and Quit.net. There are also online cessation programs, such as the American Lung Association's Freedom from Smoking program, the American Cancer Society's Freshstart program, Smokefree.gov, 1-800-QUIT-NOW, and Quit.net. These free online customized smoking cessation programs should be mentioned at every visit to patients who smoke.

Hypnosis

The goal of hypnosis in smoking cessation is to enable the smoker to achieve an altered state of consciousness that enhances the ability to quit. However, the hypnotic state is generally not measurably different from that associated with deep muscle relaxation. The effects of hypnosis are often short-lived. Controlled trials of hypnosis have generally not documented long-term efficacy for smoking cessation. Published quit rates range between 0% and 88%. Although it is of uncertain value, hypnosis remains a commercially popular stop-smoking method. The primary advantage of hypnosis is that it may be an attractive alternative for people who have failed to quit with other methods.

Aversion Conditioning

Aversion conditioning is based on the premise that smoking is a learned response that can be extinguished by creation of an association between smoking and a negative sensation. Among the aversion techniques

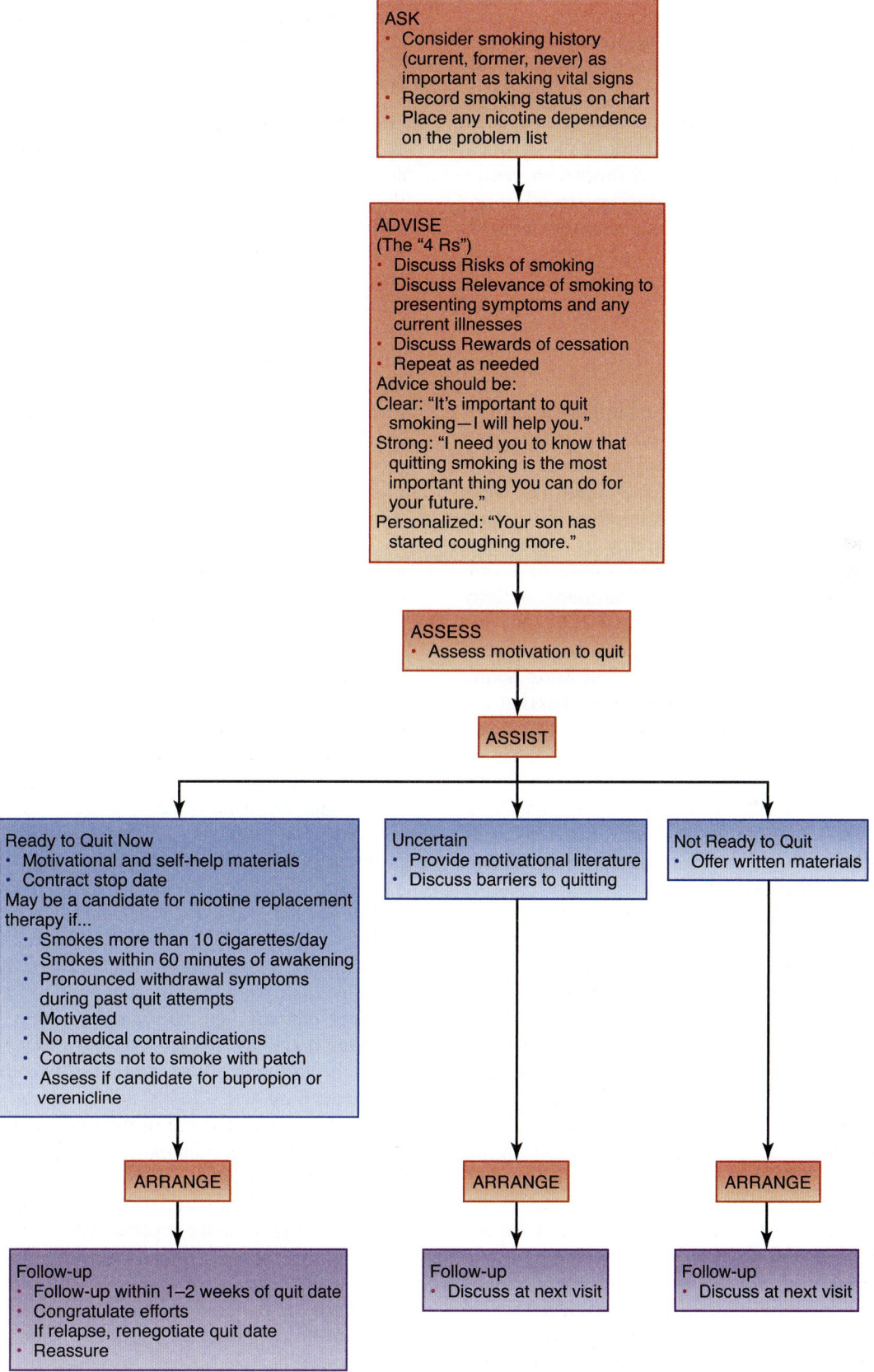

Figure 33-1 Treatment flowchart: smoking cessation strategies. *Adapted from Helping smokers quit. https://www.ahrq.gov/sites/default/files/wysiwyg/professionals/clinicians-providers/guidelines-recommendations/tobacco/clinicians/references/clinhlpsmkqt/clinhlpsmksqt.pdf (Accessed 5/5/2022)*

used for smoking cessation are electric shock, nausea-inducing drugs, hot and smoky air treatments, and rapid smoking. High quit rates have been reported in some of the early smoking cessation trials using aversion conditioning. However, these high success rates may be attributed, in part, to factors related to patient selection because arguably only the most highly motivated people are willing to undergo this type of therapy. In addition, aversion-conditioning techniques may represent a health hazard.

Subsequent Management

Pharmacological Approaches

Although some smokers may need antidepressants or anxiolytics, it is difficult to predict who will benefit from these adjunctive therapies. Bupropion (Zyban) is an antidepressant and smoking deterrent. Bupropion is a weak inhibitor of the neuronal uptake of norepinephrine and dopamine but has no effect on serotonin. Its dopaminergic and noradrenergic activities are responsible for its efficacy in smoking cessation, with the dopaminergic activity affecting areas of the brain associated with the reinforcement activity affecting nicotine withdrawal. Bupropion appears to have no effect on patient depression scores in smokers attempting to quit, so it is unlikely that the mechanism for the efficacy of bupropion in smoking cessation is through its antidepressant effects. Bupropion is well tolerated, with the most frequent adverse effects being headache, insomnia, and dry mouth. Like other antidepressant medications, bupropion is associated with a small risk of seizure and should not be given to patients with a seizure disorder. Moreover, patients with a history of severe head trauma, eating disorders, recent myocardial infarction, unstable heart disease, or active alcoholism should not take bupropion.

Bupropion for smoking cessation should be started 1 to 2 weeks before the patient's desired quit date. The initial dosage is 150 mg per day for 3 days, followed by 150 mg twice a day. It is important for steady-state plasma levels of bupropion to be reached (usually within 8 days) before smoking cessation is initiated. This dosing schedule has been found to lead to less weight gain during the medication phase. The duration of treatment is usually 7 to 12 weeks. For maintenance therapy, bupropion 150 mg twice a day for up to 6 months may be considered. Behavioral modification therapy should be provided concurrently. For heavily addicted smokers, nicotine replacement therapy (NRT) and bupropion can be coadministered.

Varenicline (Chantix) is a nicotinic acetylcholine receptor partial agonist used as a smoking cessation aid. It is recommended that therapy begin 1 week before a target quit date is set: 0.5 mg is given daily for the first 3 days, then 0.5 mg twice a day for 4 days, then 1 mg twice a day for 12 weeks. Adverse side effects include possible neuropsychiatric symptoms, particularly in those with a depressive or psychiatric history. Smoking cessation aids are listed in Drugs Commonly Prescribed 33.1.

Nicotine Replacement Therapies

Nicotine patches, gum, and lozenges are available over the counter (OTC), and nicotine nasal spray and inhalers are available by prescription (see Drugs Commonly Prescribed 33.1). Increased access through OTC availability has substantially increased the number of people attempting to quit smoking in the United States. Evaluations of the efficacy of nicotine gum through 12-month follow-up suggest that the gum improves smoking cessation rates by approximately 40% to 60% compared with control interventions. Efficacy is increased when nicotine gum use is combined with an intensive psychosocial intervention. The efficacy of the nicotine patch overall appears to be somewhat stronger than that of nicotine gum. The patch has been found to double the 6- to 12-month abstinence rate over that of placebo interventions.

The cost of nicotine patches continues to decrease each year, making them more available to smokers. Although the manufacturers of nicotine gum have developed a series of strategies for increasing access to NRT among underserved populations, it is unclear if the penetration of such programs can match the need for an effective strategy among lower-income populations and other underserved groups. Many clinics now offer nicotine patches and gum free of charge through state-sponsored smoke-free initiatives.

The gum must be correctly chewed to a softened state (until a peppery taste or a tingling sensation is felt) and then placed in the buccal mucosa. Patients should not eat for 15 minutes before or during use of the nicotine gum. Initially, one piece is chewed every 1 to 2 hours over 6 weeks, with a maximum of 24 pieces in 24 hours. Time intervals for gum use are gradually increased to 2 to 4 hours for 3 weeks, then every 4 to 8 hours for 3 weeks. Fewer than 10% of patients will become dependent on the gum, although many will require long-term use (1 to 2 years) to maintain abstinence from smoking. Nicotine absorption is decreased by acidic foods and beverages, which should be avoided during the use of nicotine gum. Irritation and trauma to the oral mucosa, teeth, and dental work can occur. Many patients experience jaw ache, gastrointestinal discomfort, hiccoughs, and increased heart rate.

Nicotine patches are applied every morning and worn continuously for 24 hours per day. Patches are usually indicated for 8 to 12 weeks to promote long-term abstinence. Patients should be instructed to change the application site daily to minimize skin irritation. The highest-dose patch should be considered if the patient smokes more than 10 cigarettes per day and has no active cardiovascular disease. Because there is a dose–response effect, researchers recommend that a higher nicotine dose is more effective for smoking cessation. Adverse effects include skin reactions, insomnia, vivid dreams, and

Drugs Commonly Prescribed 33.1: Therapies for Smoking Cessation—Prescribing Considerations

DRUG	DOSAGE	ADVANTAGES	DISADVANTAGES
Transdermal Patch		Continuous delivery	Expensive
Nicotine Patch (NicoDerm CQ, Nicotrol) (worn 24 h/day)	21 mg/day for 4 to 6 weeks, then 14 mg/day for 2 to 4 weeks, then 7 mg/day for 2 to 4 weeks Consider starting with 14-mg patch if smoking fewer than 10 cigarettes/day	Less instruction required than nicotine gum	Risk of insomnia or nightmares; if this occurs, try wearing patch for 16 h/day while awake
Gum (nicotine polacrilex)		Useful on "as-needed" basis	Requires good dentition
Nicorette	2 mg/piece; maximum 30 pieces/day 4 mg/piece; maximum 24 pieces/day	Provides oral gratification Patient control Delayed weight gain	Risk of mouth irritation Dyspnea, nausea Risk of developing dependence Complicated usage guidelines Do not use with nicotine patches or other nicotine replacement therapies
Nasal Spray		Useful on "as-needed" basis	
Nicotrol (10-mL bottle)	0.5 mg/spray; two sprays; maximum 40 doses/day for 3 months	Rapid delivery	Risk of nasal and throat irritation Runny nose Watery eyes
Inhaler			
Nicotine inhaler	13 mcg/puff; six to 16 cartridges/day for up to 6 months	Mimics smoking behavior	Risk of cough, irritation of mouth and throat
Lozenge			
Nicorette, Commit	2 mg (if first cigarette smoked 30 min or longer after waking) 4 mg (if first cigarette smoked within 30 min of waking) Maximum 20 lozenges/day, dissolve over 20 to 30 min; minimize swallowing	First-line agent; effective in combination with patch	May cause hiccoughs, heartburn, nausea
Other			
Bupropion HCL (Zyban)	150 mg/day for 3 days, then 150 mg twice daily for 7 to 12 weeks (possibly up to 6 months)	Nonnicotine, less weight gain	Risk of seizures, headache, dry mouth, insomnia
Varenicline (Chantix)	0.5 mg/day for 3 days, then 0.5 mg twice daily for 4 days, then 1 mg twice daily for 12 weeks; take with a glass of water after eating	Nonnicotine, first-line agent	Nausea Risk of serious neuropsychiatric symptoms including depression, altered mood and behavior, suicidality

myalgias. If vivid dreams or insomnia occur, the patient should be instructed to remove the patch before going to bed and then apply a new patch on arising.

The nicotine nasal spray (Nicotrol nasal spray) delivers nicotine more rapidly than the gum, patch, or inhaler and may, therefore, serve as a more effective substitute for smoking than other nicotine replacement systems. The device is similar to those used to administer nasal antihistamine sprays. The nasal spray delivers 0.5 mg of nicotine per spray. Smokers are instructed to use one to two doses per hour for up to 6 months at up to 40 doses per day. The nasal spray delivers nicotine rapidly, but less rapidly than cigarettes. Peak levels occur within 4 to 15 minutes and are about two-thirds of those associated with cigarettes. Patients may initially experience nasal and throat irritation, rhinitis, sneezing, coughing, and watering eyes. Tolerance of these effects develops in the first week. The spray may cause serious dysrhythmias, elevated blood pressure, and angina in postmyocardial infarction patients. Use of the spray is also not recommended in patients with other chronic diseases, including asthma, peptic ulcer disease, chronic nasal disorders, severe renal impairment, liver disease, diabetes mellitus, and hyperthyroidism.

Researchers have found that the use of a nicotine patch with a nicotine nasal spray is significantly more effective for long-term smoking cessation than with either alone. Studies suggest increased efficacy in the prevention of relapse with greater nicotine intake or by combining different types of nicotine replacement therapies. The combination of a nicotine patch and nicotine nasal spray may be successful not only because of the high level of substitution but also because of the opportunity to respond quickly to the smoker's cravings and physical needs. Researchers have suggested that using a patch for 5 months with a nicotine nasal spray for 1 year provides a more effective means of stopping smoking than using a patch alone.

The nicotine inhaler (Nicotrol inhaler) is a plastic rod with a nicotine plug that provides nicotine vapor when puffed on. Each active cartridge contains approximately 10 mg of nicotine and 1 mg of menthol. The menthol is added to decrease throat irritation caused by the nicotine. Although the device is designed as an inhaler, this label is a misnomer because the device does not deliver a significant amount of nicotine to the lungs; rather, the device delivers nicotine buccally. This occurs whether smokers use deep or shallow puffs. Each cartridge lasts about 20 minutes and provides the nicotine equivalent of about two cigarettes. Patients use six to 16 cartridges per day for 3 months and then taper for 6 to 12 weeks as needed. The most common adverse effects are cough and irritation in the mouth and throat.

The inhaler has the potential to assist in smoking cessation not only by providing nicotine replacement but also by mimicking the behavioral aspects of smoking. However, these devices may be problematic because they are closely related to cigarette smoking. In effect, the patient using these devices is brand switching (i.e., switching from their usual brand of cigarette to a smoke-free nicotine-delivery device), even though the effort required to obtain nicotine from the inhaler is greater than that required from a cigarette. Combining the nicotine inhaler with the nicotine patch may increase efficacy over using the patch alone because the inhaler serves to supplement the nicotine provided by the patch and mimics smoking behavior.

Nortriptyline (75 to 100 mg/day) for 12 to 14 weeks in addition to NRT has shown a trend toward higher rates of abstinence. This is a second-line therapy for those who cannot tolerate one of the first-line smoking cessation medications. Research has shown that its effect is similar to adding bupropion to NRT.

FOLLOW-UP AND REFERRAL

As with any serious medical problem, follow-up is essential after the initial intervention. A health-care worker can make a supportive phone call 1 week after the quit date, reinforced by self-help materials. Office follow-up by the clinician at 1 and 3 months after the quit date can assist the patient to cope with persistent exposure to triggers or smoking-associated situations; this support can help the patient who may have relapsed to get back on track. In the case of relapse, the patient should be assisted to set another quit date, revisit the reasons for quitting, and begin the cessation process again. It is important to assure patients that stable abstinence is commonly achieved only after five or six cessation attempts.

Patient Education: Smoking Cessation

In the past, cigarette smoking was viewed as largely a social or psychological habit. As such, the ability to quit was considered a measure of personal motivation and willpower. Motivation to stop smoking, combined with sufficient psychological resources, was seen as a driving force behind successful smoking abstinence. Thus, if smokers could be educated about the health risks of cigarette smoking, they could theoretically become sufficiently motivated and psychologically empowered to quit.

Unfortunately, the anticipated benefits of achieving smoking cessation through health education were overly optimistic. More than 80% of current smokers indicate they would like to quit but cannot. Educational programs for patients to aid smoking cessation have produced disappointing results and high long-term failure rates. Only about 4% of smokers are able to quit each year. Nonetheless, it is helpful to give the patient age-specific smoking cessation literature. Importantly, training clinicians on the emerging use and health threats of all forms of tobacco products, including e-cigarettes and other products for vaping, is critical to lay the foundation for providing effective tobacco cessation counseling to patients (see Evidence-Based Nursing Practice 33.1).

Evidence-Based Nursing Practice 33.1

SMOKING CESSATION

VanDevanter N, Zhou S, Katigbak C, et al. Knowledge, beliefs, behaviors, and social norms related to use of alternative tobacco products among undergraduate and graduate nursing students in an urban U.S. university setting. *J Nurs Scholarsh*. 2016;48(2):147–153.

The purpose of this study was to assess nursing students' knowledge, beliefs, behaviors, and social norms regarding use of alternative tobacco products (ATPs). A survey was conducted among all students enrolled in a college of nursing, both undergraduates and graduates. It assessed knowledge and beliefs about ATPs (hookahs, cigars or cigarillos, bidis, kreteks, smokeless tobacco, e-cigarettes) compared with cigarettes, health effects of ATPs, personal use of ATPs, and social norms. Nursing students demonstrated very low levels of knowledge about ATPs and their health consequences, despite high rates of ATP personal use. Nurses' lack of knowledge about the emerging use and health threats associated with ATPs may undermine their ability to provide appropriate tobacco cessation counseling. As nurses play critical roles in counseling their patients on tobacco cessation, further nursing research and education about the risks presented by ATPs are critical to reducing tobacco-related mortality.

In addition, health-care providers need to be aware of the nuances of smoking cessation. For example, individuals often experience constipation during smoking cessation, as the gastrointestinal system adjusts to withdrawal from the stimulating effects of nicotine. A bulk-forming agent such as Metamucil, increased dietary fiber, and increased fluids will alleviate the problem. A form of exercise, such as walking, is an effective and affordable stress reliever. A walking program also assists with reducing the expected mean weight gain of 5 to 7 pounds that occurs with smoking cessation. Nicotine is an appetite suppressant, and once its effects have cleared from the body, food will taste better.

It is important to understand the meaning of smoking to the individual patient and to hear the "patient's voice" (see The Patient's Voice 33.1). Smoking is an addictive behavior that for most patients has become intimately associated with daily reinforcing experiences, emotions, and coping mechanisms, despite the irrefutable evidence of its significant health risks. Assisting the patient to stop smoking involves an empowerment process that enhances the patient's motivation and self-esteem. Providers can encourage patients to identify daily stressors and assist them to reframe situations and develop alternative coping strategies. Equally important is developing enhanced self efficacy, which includes accepting and believing

The Patient's Voice 33.1

BATTLEGROUND

"What is it with you and your cigarettes, anyway?" I angrily thought to myself after yet another heated debate with my father about smoking. As usual, he had been defending cigarettes as a source of pleasure, saying he always enjoyed smoking. He was against federal attempts to regulate levels of nicotine in cigarettes or restrict access. After smoking for 60 years, he quit last year, when the severity of his lung disease nearly took his life. Why couldn't I make him understand that cigarettes were killing people?

He must have sensed my frustration or read my mind, because as his O₂ concentrator clicked off and on, he looked at me and said softly, "You know, Snicklefritz, it was cigarettes that saved my life many times during the war." My father rarely talks about The War. He was a combat infantryman, a machine gunner—part of the Fifth Division known as "Roosevelt's Red Devils." He started slowly . . .

"At night we were the point. Machine gunners never got relieved. The cold was the worst. You couldn't imagine the cold. Raining—below freezing. We would take turns sleeping. You couldn't sleep for more than an hour. You had to rely on your buddies to wake you up. You had to keep moving to keep from freezing. Many only lasted one night and had to be sent back because their feet were frozen. I think we lost more men to cold that winter than from enemy fire.

"I remember standing up one night with tracers going by my head, yelling 'Go ahead and shoot me—put me out of my misery!' My buddy had to pull me down. He said, 'Have a cigarette—calm yourself!' We had to cover our heads with raingear to keep anyone from seeing me light up and give away our positions. You can't imagine the warmth and comfort in one cigarette. We were worried about living through the night.

"There were times the warmth of a cigarette was the only thing that kept us alive. We were short of supplies that winter, but they always kept us in cigarettes. Even our K-rations came with a pack—I'll give them that."

As he talked, I tried to imagine, to understand, the inhuman conditions he was describing and the meaning cigarettes held for him. As I listened to my father's story and watched him pull his arms to his chest and cup his hands to his face, as if he were holding something as precious as life itself, I finally heard what he had been saying for years. I began to feel my anger slipping away—anger with my father for smoking all those years and for nearly dying before my 3-year-old son had a chance to come to know him.

I felt my eyes fill with tears, not for the suffering my father had experienced during the war, but for the suffering he experienced because his daughter, the nurse, never understood.

—Shirley Countryman Gordon, from "Nightingale Songs."
Publication of Florida Atlantic University College of Nursing.

in one's own ability to succeed. Providers need to ask how the patient usually deals with stress and give simple, practical alternative coping strategies. A telephone hotline with recorded messages that empower and encourage the patient can be an effective way to manage and overcome the desire to smoke. Information about the rewards of smoking cessation, such as better health status with lower blood pressure and improved circulation and lung functioning, should also be provided (positive reinforcement). Individuals who cease smoking report more energy, enhanced taste and smell, monetary savings, freedom from addiction, feeling better about themselves, and better performance in sexual and sports activities. Smokers older than 55 years should be informed that despite many years of smoking, smoking cessation will improve their health. They will enjoy a better quality of life as ex-smokers, and their risk for lung and other smoking-associated cancers will be reduced. Smokers die 5 to 8 years earlier than people who have never smoked.

Additional rewards for older adults who quit using tobacco products can be the satisfaction of being a positive role model for other family members and making a contribution to the improved health of their children, grandchildren, and others. To enhance recovery from nicotine addiction and prevent relapse, both individual and group cessation counseling and education should include a family focus with shared commitment and participation. The provider can facilitate this process by providing cessation information to both the patient and their family. In the absence of family, the clinician may focus on close friends or other social support networks for the patient.

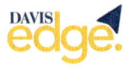 **Go to Davis Edge for practice Q&A.**

REFERENCES

American Psychiatric Association. *Diagnostic and statistical manual of mental disorders, fifth edition, text revision.* Washington, DC: American Psychiatric Publishing; 2013.

Bornemann P, Eissa A, Strayer S. Smoking cessation: What should you recommend? *J Fam Pract.* 2016;26(2):22–29B.

Butt YM, Smith ML, Tazelaar HD, et al. (2019). Pathology of vaping-associated lung injury. *N Engl J Med.* 2019;381(18):1780. Epub 2019 Oct 2.

Centers for Disease Control and Prevention. Smoking & Tobacco use. (2020). https://www.cdc.gov/tobacco/data_statistics/fact_sheets/fast_facts/index.htm. Accessed 7/7/20.

Harvey J, Chadi N. Preventing smoking in children and adolescents: Recommendations for practice and policy. *Paediatr Child Health.* 2016 May;21(4):209–214. https://www.ncbi.nlm.nih.gov/pmc/articles/PMC4934164/. Accessed 9/17/2020.

Jameson JL, Fauci AS, Kasper DL, et al, eds. *Harrison's principles of internal medicine.* 20th ed. New York, NY: McGraw-Hill; 2018.

Molero Y, Lichtenstein P, Zetterqvist J, et al. Varenicline and risk of psychiatric conditions, suicidal behaviour, criminal offending, and transport accidents and offences: population based cohort study. *BMJ.* 2015;350:h2388.

National Institute on Drug Abuse. Teens using vaping devices in record numbers. https://www.drugabuse.gov/news-events/news-releases/2018/12/teens-using-vaping-devices-in-record-numbers. Accessed 9/17/2020.

Office of Disease Prevention and Health Promotion. Tobacco use. *Healthy People 2030.* https://health.gov/healthypeople/search?query=tobacco+use. Accessed 9/17/2020.

Papadakis MA, McPhee SJ, Rabow, MW. *Current medical diagnosis and treatment 2020.* New York, NY: Appleton-Lange/McGraw-Hill; 2020.

Surgeon General's 1964 report on smoking and health. *Health.* Jan. 12, 2014. https://www.pbs.org/newshour/health/first-surgeon-general-report-on-smokings-health-effects-marks-50-year-anniversary. Accessed 9/17/20.

10 Facts on gender and tobacco. https://www.who.int/gender/documents/10facts_gender_tobacco_en.pdf. Accessed 9/18/2020.

VanDevanter N, Zhou S, Katigbak C, et al. Knowledge, beliefs, behaviors, and social norms related to use of alternative tobacco products among undergraduate and graduate nursing students in an urban U.S. university setting. *J Nurs Scholarsh.* 2016;48(2):147–153.

World Health Organization (May 27, 2020). Tobacco. https://www.who.int/news-room/fact-sheets/detail/tobacco. Accessed 7/7/20.

RESOURCES

Centers for Disease Control and Prevention: Smoking and Tobacco Use
https://www.cdc.gov/tobacco/

Smoking Cessation

1 (800) QUIT NOW 1-800 784-8669

American Cancer Society's Freshstart Program
https://www.cancer.org/healthy/stay-away-from-tobacco.html

American Lung Association's Freedom From Smoking
http://www.lung.org/stop-smoking/join-freedom-from-smoking

Centers for Disease Control and Prevention: Quit Smoking
https://www.cdc.gov/tobacco/quit_smoking/index.htm

Nicotine Anonymous
http://nicotine-anonymous.org

Smokefree.gov
https://smokefree.gov/
Quit.net

Section 6: CARDIOVASCULAR PROBLEMS

SECTION EDITOR

Jill E. Winland-Brown, EdD, APRN, FNP-BC, FAANP

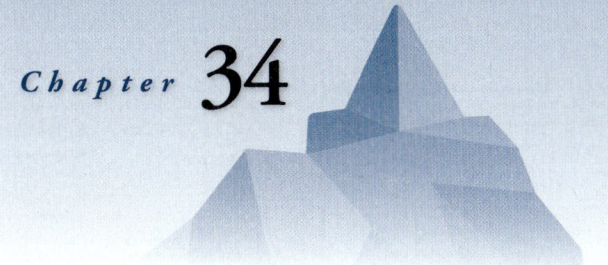

Chapter 34

Common Cardiovascular Complaints

Kathryn B. Keller, PhD, RN, CNE
Jill E. Winland-Brown, EdD, APRN, FNP-BC, FAANP
Brian Oscar Porter, MD, PhD, MPH, MBA

CHEST PAIN

Although the potential etiologies of chest pain are wide ranging, this symptom has long been a harbinger of cardiovascular disease, which remains the foremost consideration for clinicians when assessing these patients in primary care or urgent care settings. Although deaths from coronary heart disease have declined over the past 40 years, (365,914 deaths in 2017), this decrease is mainly due to advances in medical and surgical treatments, rather than lifestyle or behavioral changes. Several lifestyle changes can have a significant impact in reducing mortality risk, including smoking cessation (12% mortality reduction) and an increase in physical activity (5% mortality reduction). *Healthy People 2030* continues to stress the need for lifestyle changes to reduce coronary heart disease–related deaths. Some of the objectives related to improving cardiovascular health in adults include reducing cholesterol in adults, as well as increasing cholesterol treatment in adults; reducing the proportion of adults with hypertension (HTN) as well as increasing control of HTN in adults; and increasing aspirin use for secondary prevention of atherosclerotic cardiovascular disease. Educational initiatives continue to inform women about sex-related differences in heart attack characteristics, markedly increasing women's awareness that cardiovascular deaths constitute the leading cause of mortality in women (see Evidence-Based Nursing Practice 34.1).

 Evidence-Based Nursing Practice 34.1

CHEST PAIN

Davis LL, Maness JJ. Nurse practitioner knowledge of symptoms of acute coronary syndrome. *J Nurse Pract.* 2019 Jan;15(1):e9–e12.

Nurse practitioners (NPs) are well positioned to teach women at risk for acute coronary syndrome (ACS) to recognize symptoms and take appropriate actions should symptoms occur. However, NPs need to be knowledgeable about varied symptom presentations. This feasibility study used case vignettes of women with possible ACS symptoms to assess NP knowledge of the differential diagnosis of symptoms and actions the women should take in response to the symptoms. Findings suggest that NPs had higher accuracy in diagnosing and recommending appropriate actions for women who had abrupt-onset ACS symptoms compared with women with slow, evolving, and less typical symptoms. Highlights include the following:

- Case vignettes are used to assess provider knowledge of diagnosis/treatment of medical conditions.
- NPs were more accurate with diagnosis/treatment of cases with abrupt-onset classic heart symptoms.
- Despite accurately diagnosing ACS cases, some NPs did not believe it was necessary to call 911 (emergency response system).
- Education should highlight less common ACS symptoms in women and appropriate care-seeking actions.
- Adults with symptoms of suspected ACS should call 911 within 5 minutes of symptom onset.

DIFFERENTIAL DIAGNOSIS

Although chest pain is often associated with cardiovascular problems, it may also have pulmonary, gastrointestinal, musculoskeletal, neurological, psychogenic, or idiopathic causes. Obtaining a focused health history and performing a physical examination are essential for accurate assessment and appropriate treatment of a patient with chest pain (see Fig. 34.1). Critical components of the history include appraisal of the major symptoms and clinical manifestations of heart disease, including chest pain, dyspnea, syncope, and heart failure (HF). The clinician should ask patients in all age-groups about exercise

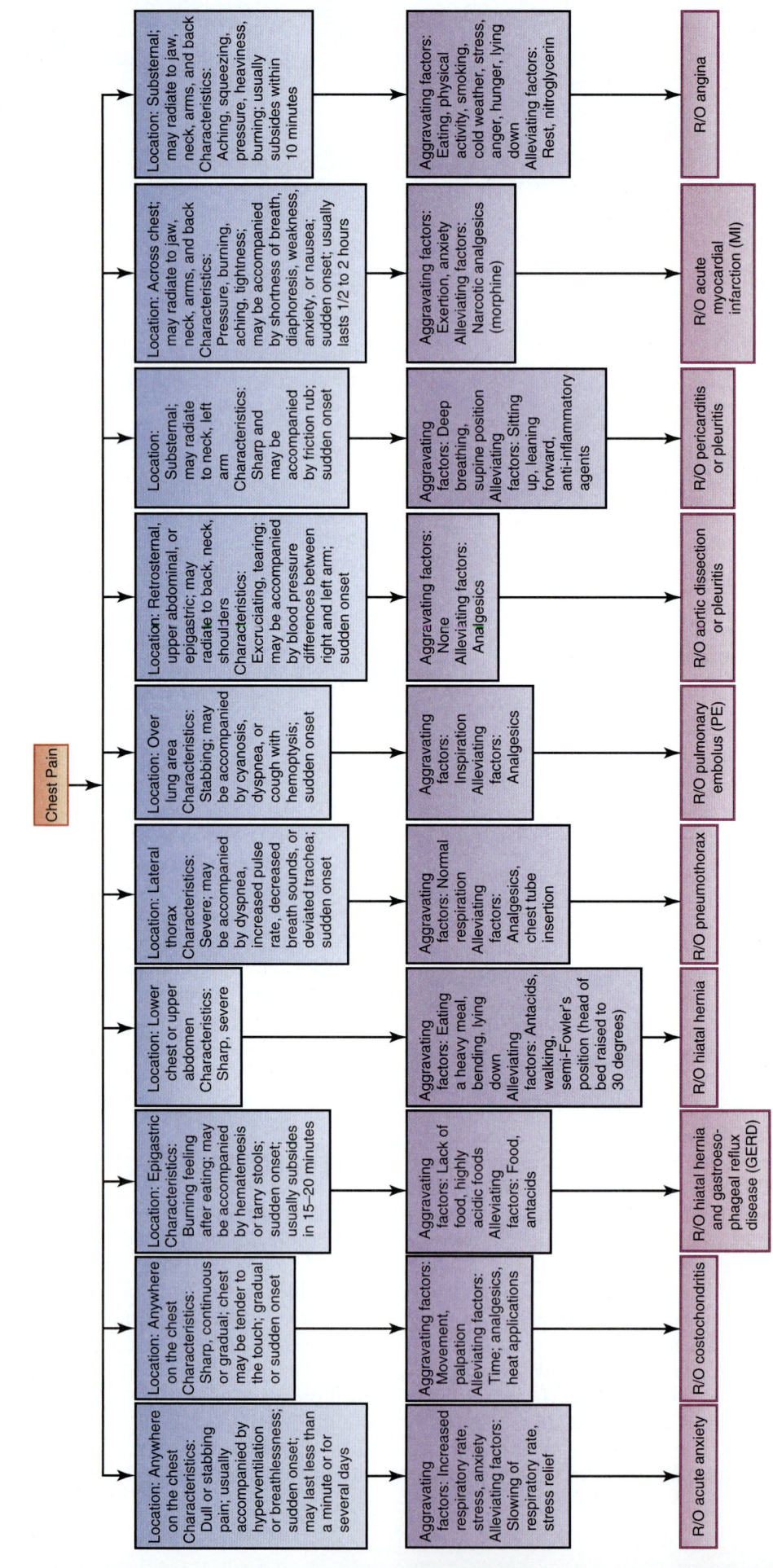

Figure 34.1 Diagnostic reasoning algorithm: chest pain.

tolerance, especially whether exercise provokes any of the aforementioned complaints. The history of present illness of the person with chest pain should assess personal risk factors for cardiovascular disease.

The clinician should obtain a complete chest pain symptom analysis including location, quality, duration, aggravating or alleviating factors, and associated symptoms or signs. In particular, localized, fleeting, and transient pain that transfers locations is rarely indicative of serious cardiac pathology. Anxiety and bereavement can cause diffuse chest pain lasting for hours. The pain of costochondritis (a type of chest wall syndrome [CWS]) is often described as localized, and it may be replicated with arm movement or pressing on the area of tenderness (point tenderness). CWS is largely a diagnosis of exclusion.

In contrast, the discomfort of angina pectoris is classically described as a diffuse, retrosternal sensation of pain, often with radiation, and a heavy, burning sensation, usually lasting more than 1 minute but less than 10 minutes. Exertional symptoms are usually more common in individuals with fixed atherosclerotic lesions. In assessing the person with known angina pectoris, it is critical to ascertain if there has been a change in the symptom pattern, as this may indicate an alteration in vessel patency such as that found in accelerated atherosclerosis or vessel spasm. The word "pain" should be used with caution in taking the history of a person with suspected myocardial ischemia because the patient may deny that pain is present but may agree that tightness, burning, fullness, or other sensations more aptly describe the complaint.

The terms "unstable angina," "preinfarction angina," and "crescendo angina" are synonyms used to describe the new onset of cardiac ischemic chest pain at rest but without evidence of acute myocardial infarction (MI). Reports of symptoms at rest are more likely to be associated with coronary artery vasospasm, a condition usually seen in patients with coronary atherosclerosis. The combination of these two mechanisms of lumen narrowing in the coronary arteries places the patient at considerable risk for acute coronary syndrome; in these cases, rapid, accurate assessment is vital to ensure appropriate disposition and treatment.

About one-third of patients with angina pectoris will have simultaneous dyspnea caused by a transient increase in pulmonary venous pressure that accompanies ventricular stiffening during an episode of myocardial ischemia. The presence of diaphoresis with chest pain is particularly worrisome, often indicating a significant drop in cardiac output during the episode and subsequent decreased perfusion of the skin. In contrast to the patient who complains of anginal pain, the patient who is experiencing an acute MI often complains of anginal-like chest pain that lasts in excess of 20 minutes but occasionally waxes and wanes during that period. The pain is frequently accompanied by dyspnea, diaphoresis, nausea, and dizziness. The pain may radiate to the neck, jaw, shoulder, or arm (left side more than right). Patients show extreme variation in the amount of pain experienced with an MI, from complaining of a "vise grip around the heart" to apologizing for seeking assistance with "just a bit of indigestion that will not clear up." In particular, women, older adults, and people with diabetes mellitus are likely to have minimal or atypical symptoms with an acute MI. A more detailed discussion of the pain of angina and MI is provided in the sections on treatment of those conditions in Chapter 35 under "Acute Coronary Syndrome."

PALPITATIONS

Palpitations are commonly reported by individuals who have or are at risk for heart disease. *Palpitations* are defined as the awareness of the beating of one's heart and may be benign or pathological in nature. When questioning the patient with palpitations, the clinician should obtain a detailed description of the sensation. If the patient reports a sensation of a strong but regular rhythmic beating of the heart after stress or exertion, this likely indicates a normal physiological response to increased catecholamine production. If there is a report of skipped or missed beats, particularly with the sensation that the heart "stopped" momentarily, this may indicate the presence of an atrial or ventricular ectopic beat. In addition, some medications, caffeine, alcohol, nicotine, and physical activity may cause palpitations.

DIFFERENTIAL DIAGNOSIS

Atrial ectopic beats are most often benign, occurring with excessive caffeine, alcohol, or tobacco use. On occasion, atrial ectopic beats occur with cardiac pathology, sometimes as a precursor to a supraventricular rhythm such as multifocal atrial tachycardia or atrial fibrillation. This is most likely in the patient with chronic obstructive pulmonary disease (COPD) or rheumatic heart disease and valvular dysfunction. Ventricular ectopic beats are somewhat more likely to indicate cardiac pathology than atrial ectopy. If the patient is at high risk for or has known heart disease, the clinician must carefully assess the complaint of palpitations because ventricular ectopy may reflect an increased risk of sudden cardiac death.

Another variation in the presentation of palpitations is the patient who complains of the sudden onset of a very rapid heartbeat or fluttering of the heart. The etiology may be an arrhythmia associated with supraventricular or ventricular tachycardia, often with equally rapid and unpredictable cessation of the rhythm or a rhythmic paroxysm. Although this type of rhythmic sensation is usually regular (with equally spaced heartbeats), such as in paroxysmal supraventricular tachycardia or ventricular tachycardia, it may also be irregular, such as in intermittent atrial fibrillation. Atrial fibrillation is the most common form of a sustained arrhythmia and increases with age.

In any case, the clinician should query the patient carefully about accompanying symptoms, such as chest pain related to decreased coronary artery filling and increased myocardial oxygen demands, as well as symptoms associated with low cardiac output.

Diagnostic testing should be directed by information obtained in the health history and physical examination. Thyroid function (thyroid-stimulating hormone and free T_4), serum chemistries, hemoglobin, and hematocrit should be evaluated to help rule out a thyroid disorder, electrolyte imbalance, and anemia, respectively, as possible, though less common, causes of palpitations. Ambulatory cardiac monitoring (Holter monitoring) done until at least one event is recorded is most helpful in ascertaining the presence of a potentially lethal cardiac rhythm disturbance. Echocardiography may be necessary to assess cardiac outflow tract patency and to help rule out valvular stenosis or hypertrophic cardiomyopathy. A diagnostic algorithm for palpitations is presented in Figure 34.2.

Intervention should be directed at the underlying cause of the palpitations. For example, if a rhythm disturbance such as recurrent supraventricular or ventricular tachycardia is the cause, treatment directed at eliminating this is warranted. In any event, the clinician should consult with a physician or cardiologist who has expertise in this area to ensure patient safety and an optimal outcome.

SYNCOPE

Syncope is a loss of consciousness that occurs abruptly as a discrete episode and usually lasts for a short period of only a few minutes. The implied pathology is decreased cerebral blood flow caused by a marked decrease in cardiac output. The incidence of syncope appears to be bimodal in nature, with occurrences peaking in late adolescence to early adulthood and then later in older adults—rising sharply after 70 years of age. Whereas some of these episodes are of noncardiac origin (e.g., fluid loss, dehydration, emotional stress), the majority are cardiovascular in origin, including the most common etiology of vasovagal or cardioneurogenic syncope. Older adult patients with syncope have an average of 3.5 chronic medical conditions, which adds to the diagnostic complexity in this population. In turn, unexplained falls in older adults should be managed as potential syncope.

Cardiac-related syncope is an ominous sign associated with high rates of mortality. A syncopal episode may be the only warning sign of impending sudden cardiac death. One of the most common cardiac causes of syncope is cardiac arrhythmias. A wide range of conduction disturbances can precede a syncopal event, including tachycardia-bradycardia syndrome (sick sinus syndrome), supraventricular and ventricular tachycardias, various forms of heart block, bradycardia, and the congenital conditions of long QT and Brugada syndromes.

DIFFERENTIAL DIAGNOSIS

Cardiac outflow tract blockage, such as the obstruction that may occur in hypertrophic cardiomyopathy or aortic valve stenosis, can also produce syncope. This is most often seen in response to increased activity or stress when the outflow tract blockage impedes the increase in cardiac output needed to meet increased oxygen demands, such as with physical activity. This leads to syncope that typically lasts for a few seconds and ends when the "rest" period of the syncopal episode rebalances the supply of oxygenated blood with demand.

Presyncope, a state of lightheadedness, feeling faint, and muscular weakness, is most often cardiovascular in origin. The etiology is usually the same as for syncope. In contrast, vertigo is the sensation of spinning that can often be reproduced by a change in head position. Vertigo is not usually caused by decreased cerebral blood flow, because an inner ear disturbance is the most common cause.

Diagnostic testing for cardiac-related syncope should be directed by the information obtained in the health history and physical examination. The work-up is similar to that for palpitations (see the preceding section and Fig. 34.2). A tilt-table test may be performed to assess for orthostatic syncope.

Intervention in cardiac-related syncope should be directed at the underlying cause. If a rhythm disturbance (as described previously) is the cause, treatment should be directed at eliminating the cardiac conduction disorder. Ablation, an internal cardiac defibrillator, and/or a permanent pacemaker may be indicated, depending on the type of arrhythmia. In any event, the clinician should consult with a cardiologist to ensure patient safety and an optimal outcome.

DYSPNEA

Dyspnea, or shortness of breath, is a highly subjective complaint, yet it is one of the most common cardiac symptoms. The challenge to the clinician is to determine its etiology. As with any complaint, the patient with dyspnea should be asked about precipitating factors, quality, duration, alleviating factors, and the length of time needed to relieve the symptom after discontinuing the precipitating event. In addition, dyspnea may be an anginal equivalent, especially in older adults and individuals with diabetes.

Patients with a chief complaint of dyspnea vary markedly in presentation; however, because this is a subjective complaint, the patient's report should be placed into context. As with the complaint of pain, the discomfort and degree of dyspnea represent the patient's reality, although correlating the complaint with physical findings may help to establish the cause of the dyspnea and thus lead to an effective intervention plan.

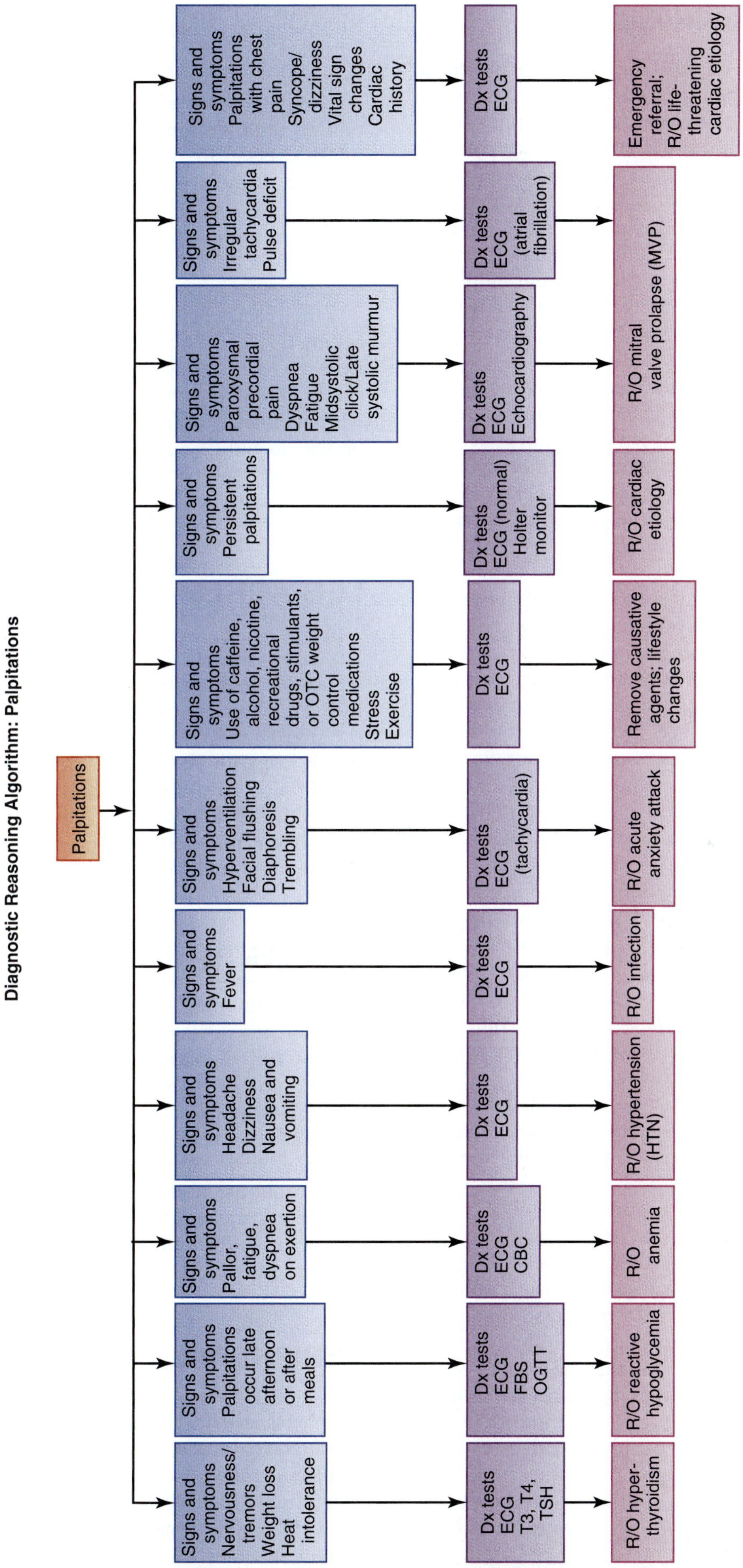

Chapter 34 Common Cardiovascular Complaints

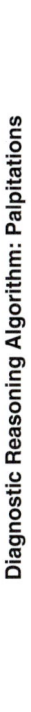

Figure 34.2 Diagnostic reasoning algorithm: palpitations.

DIFFERENTIAL DIAGNOSIS

Dyspnea has a number of possible causes. With left-sided cardiac outflow tract blockage, such as in severe aortic stenosis or obstructive cardiomyopathy, dyspnea likely arises from a decrease in cardiac output. When dyspnea is associated with recurrent myocardial ischemia, as in angina pectoris, the shortness of breath is likely caused by an increase in pulmonary vascular pressure, coupled with a transient decrease in cardiac output. In right-sided cardiac problems, such as tricuspid and pulmonic valvular dysfunction, the complaint of dyspnea usually arises from increased pulmonary pressures and resistance to cardiac emptying of the right ventricle.

Another common cause of dyspnea is pulmonary disease, such as COPD, asthma, pleural effusion, pneumothorax, pulmonary embolus, or pulmonary hypertension secondary to interstitial lung disease or pulmonary fibrosis. Other noncardiac causes of dyspnea include severe anemia and metabolic acidosis (i.e., Kussmaul's respirations), obesity, physical deconditioning, and anxiety or emotional distress.

The patient's assessment of the severity of dyspnea may differ from the clinician's assessment, based on objective findings. For example, some patients who are observed to have increased work while breathing may have little complaint of breathlessness, whereas other patients who have few objective findings may convey marked difficulty breathing. In addition, when questioned about difficulty breathing, some patients may admit to feelings of suffocation in which getting sufficient air in and out of the lungs is challenging, but others may only describe the need to take deep breaths.

In turn, dyspnea is a poorly sensitive and nonspecific marker for cardiovascular disease. Factors contributing to the complaint of breathlessness in the absence of heart disease include poor conditioning and exercise intolerance related to inactivity and obesity. The patient usually reports that the onset of this type of dyspnea accompanies increased activity and resolves rapidly when the activity ceases. In cardiovascular disease, dyspnea is usually a result of increased stiffness (i.e., reduced expansion and elasticity) in the lungs caused by increased pulmonary blood volume or pulmonary congestion. This is usually found in conditions that result in poor cardiac output, such as HF, recurrent myocardial ischemia, poorly controlled hypertension, valvular dysfunction, and heart disease.

When dyspnea is the complaint, it is essential for the clinician to assess for any change in the patient's ability to perform typical daily activities. In particular, dyspnea is often first detected by the patient as the inability to talk during exertional activities. Pinpointing the onset of symptoms and concurrent events may be helpful in determining its etiology. In addition, asking about cosymptoms such as wheezing and weight gain is crucial because dyspnea is the most common presenting complaint in HF.

Orthopnea is shortness of breath that develops when the patient is in a supine position, such as when lying faceup in bed. The patient usually compensates for this sensation by sleeping on an increased number of pillows to elevate the upper body, hence the use of the qualifying term *three-pillow orthopnea*. If the person slides off the pillows while sleeping, shortness of breath recurs, causing the person to awaken. Orthopnea is usually caused by HF as a result of increased right-sided heart pressure, which increases after the patient has been supine for a few hours, mobilizing fluid that pooled in the extremities during the more active awake hours when the patient was seated upright or standing.

Paroxysmal nocturnal dyspnea (PND) is shortness of breath that occurs 1 to 2 hours into sleep, concurrent with the redistribution of bodily fluids and a subsequent rise in left atrial pressure. The person awakens suddenly with significant difficulty breathing and usually stands or sits up until symptoms are relieved in about 10 to 30 minutes. As with orthopnea, the diagnosis of HF should be considered in patients with PND.

LEG ACHES

Leg aches associated with peripheral vascular disorders are caused by impaired blood flow to the lower extremities. Peripheral vascular disease (PVD) may affect both the arteries and veins. When the vascular disease is arterial, it is usually the result of atherosclerosis (accumulation of fatty streaks and fibrous plaques and high levels of low-density lipoproteins). Venous problems are related to venous incompetence secondary to valvular obstruction, resulting in chronic venous insufficiency and varicose veins.

DIFFERENTIAL DIAGNOSIS

Patients presenting with leg aches may have a number of disorders other than PVD; therefore, a thorough history and physical examination must be performed to rule out thrombosis, phlebitis, polycythemia, anemia, Raynaud's disease, and Buerger's disease. Because some of the contributing factors to PVD may be smoking, high blood pressure, and diabetes mellitus, these problems must be addressed and the underlying conditions managed. Both peripheral arterial disease and deep vein thrombosis are discussed in more detail in Chapter 37.

PERIPHERAL EDEMA

Peripheral edema is the accumulation of tissue fluid within the interstitial spaces of the extremities. When the edema involves the lower extremities, it is a symptom of an underlying disorder and may be caused by cardiac conditions (e.g., HF, chronic venous insufficiency, thrombophlebitis),

Chapter 34 Common Cardiovascular Complaints 527

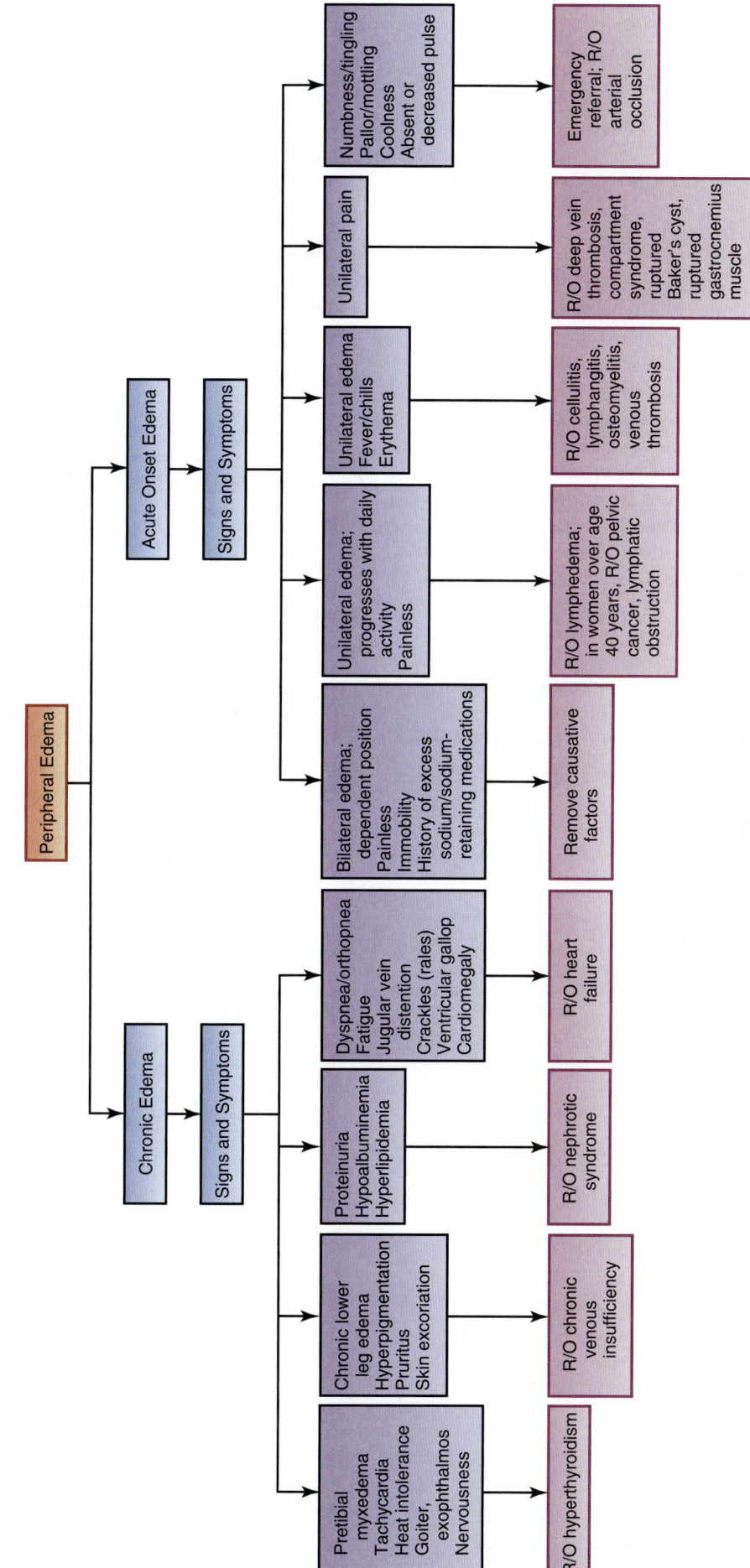

Figure 34.3 Diagnostic reasoning algorithm: peripheral edema.

renal or hepatic disease, trauma, tumors, or inflammation. Other iatrogenic causes of peripheral edema include excess dietary sodium, sodium-retaining medications (e.g., corticosteroids, NSAIDs), and arteriolar vasodilators (e.g., calcium channel inhibitors). Peripheral edema occurs equally in men and women.

DIFFERENTIAL DIAGNOSIS

Peripheral edema is usually diagnosed via patient history and physical examination, although laboratory findings may also assist in determining the cause of the edema. It is essential that the underlying cause be identified and treated, or the peripheral edema will remain, possibly causing tissue ischemia from compressed and diminished arterial circulation. Specific diagnostic tests the clinician should order include a complete blood count, urinalysis, serum chemistries, and a thyroid function profile. X-ray studies may be ordered if trauma or osteomyelitis is suspected, and a chest x-ray film should be ordered to assess the heart and lungs. A computed tomography scan may help to assess the distribution of edema and to pinpoint the extent of venous and lymphatic obstruction. An electrocardiogram is essential to assess cardiac conduction and check for arrhythmias, whereas Doppler ultrasound studies of the lower extremities may be ordered to evaluate for deep vein thrombosis. A diagnostic algorithm for peripheral edema is presented in Figure 34.3.

REFERENCES

General

Heart Disease Facts. https://www.cdc.gov/heartdisease/facts.htm. Accessed 11/10/2020.

U.S. Department of Health and Human Services/Office of Disease Prevention and Health Promotion. https://health.gov/healthypeople/objectives-and-data/browse-objectives/heart-disease-and-stroke/improve-cardiovascular-health-adults-hds-01. Accessed 11/9/2020.

Chest Pain

Davis LL, Maness JJ. Nurse practitioner knowledge of symptoms of acute coronary syndrome. *J Nurse Pract.* 2019 Jan;15(1):e9–e12.

Healthy People 2030. https://health.gov/healthypeople/search?query=cardiovascular+problems. Accessed 12/14/2020.

Dyspnea

Mittal S, Jain A, Arava S, et al. A 26-year-old man with dyspnea and chest pain. *Lung India.* 2017 Nov–Dec;34(6): 562–566. https://www.ncbi.nlm.nih.gov/pmc/articles/PMC5684818/. Accessed 12/14/2020.

Leg Aches

Nall R. (2020). Chest pain and leg pain: Are they connected? *Medical NewsToday.* https://www.medicalnewstoday.com/articles/327436/ Accessed 12/14/2020.

Palpitations

Heart Palpitations. https://www.nhlbi.nih.gov/health-topics/heart-palpitations. Accessed 11/10/2020.

Peripheral Edema

Goyal A, Cusick AS, Bansai P. (2020). Peripheral Edema. StatPearls. https://www.ncbi.nlm.nih.gov/books/NBK554452/. Accessed 12/14/2020.

Syncope

Albert JS. (2019). Syncope in the elderly. *Am J Med.* 132(10): 115–116.

Brignole M, Moya A, de Lange FJ, et al. 2018 ESC Guidelines for the diagnosis and management of syncope. *Eur.* 2018 Jan 1;39(21):1883–1948.

Shen W-K, Shelson RS, Benditt DG, et al. 2017 ACC/AHA/HRS Guideline for the evaluation and management of patients with syncope: A report of the American College of Cardiology/American Heart Association Task Force on Clinical Practice Guidelines and the Heart Rhythm Society. *Circulation.* 2017;136(5):e29–e55.

RESOURCES

American College of Cardiology
https://www.acc.org

American Heart Association (Contact AHA for local state affiliate)
https://www.heart.org/

American Medical Association (AMA)
https://www.ama-assn.org/

Chapter 35

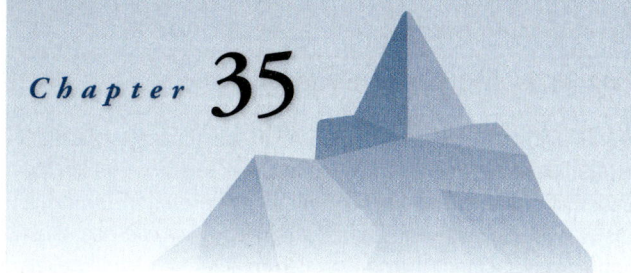

Cardiac and Associated Risk Disorders

Kathryn B. Keller, PhD, RN, CNE
Jill E. Winland-Brown, EdD, APRN, FNP-BC, FAANP
Brian Oscar Porter, MD, PhD, MPH, MBA

HYPERTENSION

Hypertension (HTN) is one of the most common chronic health problems seen in the primary care setting, affecting nearly one-half of all American adults. It is the most common reason for office visits and for persons using chronic prescription medications. Half of patients with HTN do not have effective blood pressure (BP) control. The health implications of HTN are far-reaching and widely recognized as a public health concern. *Healthy People 2030* (HP) recognizes heart disease as the leading cause of death in the United States, with stroke as the fifth leading cause. HP focuses on improving overall cardiovascular health by controlling risk factors like HTN and high cholesterol. HP aims to reduce the current rate of 29.5% of adults with HTN to 27.7%, while increasing the current rate of only 47.8% of adults who have their HTN under control to 60.8%.

EPIDEMIOLOGY AND CAUSES

With approximately 85.7 million persons currently with HTN, it is projected that by 2030, 41.4% of the population will have HTN. Historically, HTN has been more prevalent in men, particularly in African American men. As of 2017, African American women surpassed African American men with a higher prevalence of HTN. However, this gender gap is narrowing and appears to be influenced by age. For persons younger than 45 years, men are affected more often than woman, whereas in persons 65 years of age and older, more woman than men have HTN. African Americans continue to experience HTN more often and at an earlier age than European Americans or Latinos.

The prevalence of HTN continues to increase with age, particularly in industrialized societies. Data from the Framingham Heart Study suggest that even individuals who are normotensive at 55 years of age still have a 90% lifetime risk of developing HTN. There is a particular rise in systolic blood pressure (SBP) that progresses throughout life, with a difference of 20 to 30 mm Hg between early and late adulthood.

More than 95% of patients with elevated BP have primary, or essential, HTN, with no single identifiable cause. Primary HTN results from multiple genetic and environmental factors, including lifestyle and behavioral influences. It is more common in individuals whose parents or other close family members have HTN, possibly due to a diminished ability to excrete excess sodium coupled with long-term high dietary sodium intake, which predisposes to increased peripheral vascular resistance and a rise in BP.

Less than 5% of patients have secondary HTN due to a specific and potentially reversible cause, such as an identifiable cardiac, renal, or endocrinological condition or the use of vasoconstricting medications. The onset of diastolic HTN, with or without systolic elevation, after 60 years of age is unusual, and a diagnosis of new-onset secondary HTN should be considered in these individuals. In particular, renovascular disease is a common cause of new-onset diastolic HTN in this older age group.

HTN contributes to ischemic heart disease, heart failure (HF), diabetic complications, chronic kidney disease, and cerebrovascular disease. HTN is influenced by obesity, as morbidity is worsened in the setting of overweight and obesity, the prevalence of which has increased over the last 15 years, with obesity rates growing from 30.5% to 37.7% in the United States. For example, a body mass index (BMI) of greater than 30 kg/m² raises the risk of high BP and cardiovascular disease, while doubling the lifetime risk of HF compared with persons with a BMI of less than 25 kg/m².

After decades of a steady reduction in rates of HTN-related diseases, researchers have reported a recent leveling off of coronary heart disease (CHD) rates, coupled with a slight increase in end-stage renal disease (ESRD) and age-adjusted stroke rates. These changes are likely due to a number of factors, including a growing older adult population; however, the role of undetected and untreated or inadequately controlled HTN contributes significantly. Thus, primary care practitioners should be committed not only to the detection and treatment of HTN but also to its prevention.

PATHOPHYSIOLOGY

Essential Hypertension

The term *essential hypertension* describes high BP that has no identifiable etiology after a thorough clinical examination excludes possible secondary causes. The etiology and pathophysiology of essential HTN are incompletely understood. It is a complex, multifactorial disorder that involves genetic and environmental factors, diet and lifestyle practices, imbalances in vasoactive substances, and dysfunction of the arterial endothelium. Although the precise cause is unknown, endothelial dysfunction is thought to be the key pathophysiological process involved in essential HTN. The arterial endothelium is an important regulator of vascular tone, vascular structure, thrombosis, and inflammation. Endothelial dysfunction is central to many cardiovascular disorders, including HTN, atherosclerosis, and myocardial ischemia.

Vascular tone is maintained by endothelium-derived mediators such as nitric oxide, endothelin-1, and angiotensin II. Nitric oxide, a major vasodilator, counteracts the potent vasoconstrictors endothelin-1 and angiotensin II, which regulate normal vascular tone. In essential HTN, there is an imbalance in the vasodilator and vasoconstrictive substances secreted by the endothelium. Plasma levels of nitric oxide are diminished, whereas levels of endothelin-1 and angiotensin II are elevated. Reasons for this imbalance have not been elucidated, and it is not clear whether endothelial dysfunction precedes or is the result of HTN.

The role of altered sodium excretion by impaired epithelial cells in the kidney may also be a factor in the development of HTN. Renin levels are markedly abnormal in some hypertensive individuals, despite normal renal function. Individuals who secrete abnormally high levels of renin experience constant cycling of the renin-angiotensin-aldosterone cascade, which raises blood volume and BP. Low renin secretors, in general, are salt-sensitive hypertensive individuals, as ingestion of sodium increases water reabsorption into the bloodstream, which raises blood volume and BP in these patients. The cause of renin imbalance in some persons with essential HTN is unknown, but measuring plasma renin levels in patients with refractory HTN may assist in clinical diagnosis and treatment.

Other contributors include aging, sympathetic nervous system overactivity, toxins, and low numbers of renal nephrons. An often overlooked cause of essential HTN is sleep apnea with its associated activation of the sympathetic and renin-angiotensin systems. More commonly, metabolic syndrome with its resultant insulin resistance and increased insulin levels also leads to increased sympathetic activity and hypertensive states (see Box 35.1). Worldwide epidemiological evidence demonstrates that age-related HTN is uncommon in societies where individuals maintain lower body weight, consume less sodium and more potassium, and engage in greater levels of physical activity. These findings indicate that high BP is influenced by environmental and modifiable lifestyle factors (e.g., smoking, obesity, stress) and is not an inevitable consequence of aging.

Genetic and ethnic influences also play a role in the development of HTN. Persons with a family history of HTN are four times more likely to have HTN than those with no family history of the condition. Studies show that the genetic contribution to essential HTN is complex, and multiple genes are likely involved. Most genetic effects involve gene–gene interactions and gene–environment interactions. Genes that encode components of the renin-angiotensin-aldosterone system are being extensively studied. Results of this line of investigation have implicated mutations in the angiotensinogen gene and angiotensin-converting enzyme gene.

Studies of HTN in African Americans demonstrate that ethnicity is related to HTN susceptibility and plays a role in the efficacy of specific types of drugs. Morbidity and mortality due to HTN and HTN-related disorders are more common in African Americans than in European Americans and non-Hispanic Americans.

Box 35.1 Metabolic Syndrome

Metabolic syndrome refers to a cluster of specific cardiovascular-related diseases and diabetes mellitus risk factors in which the underlying pathophysiology is thought to be related to insulin resistance. Because the term *metabolic syndrome* has been imprecisely defined, the primary care practitioner should evaluate and treat all CVD risk factors without regard to whether a patient meets the criteria for diagnosis of metabolic syndrome. Nevertheless, clinicians need to be cognizant of new information pertaining to this syndrome because definitions change rapidly.

Metabolic syndrome has been characterized as a combination of atherogenic and diabetogenic factors. Increased BMI, elevated SBP, hypertriglyceridemia, hyperglycemia, and low levels of protective HDL-C are found in affected persons. Any three of these conditions occurring together usually establish the diagnosis (see Table 35.1). The etiology of metabolic syndrome is unknown; however, environmental, genetic, and behavioral factors contribute to its development, particularly physical inactivity and excess body fat. Elevated BMI is apparent as central obesity, with the affected individual demonstrating an "apple shape" or high waist circumference.

Metabolic syndrome is also a proinflammatory and prothrombotic disorder causing endothelial injury, as evidenced by elevations of the inflammatory marker C-reactive protein, increased platelet aggregation, and increased fibrinogen levels. In addition to hyperglycemia and deranged lipid metabolism, peripheral tissues are resistant to insulin. In turn, the pancreas oversecretes insulin to overcome tissue resistance, which results in hyperinsulinemia. Obesity exacerbates insulin resistance and predisposes the individual to type 2 diabetes mellitus.

Obesity is believed to contribute significantly to the development of metabolic syndrome. The National Cholesterol Education Program recommends obesity as the primary target for intervention. Abdominal obesity is defined as a high waist-to-hip ratio. Weight loss improves serum lipid profiles, reduces BP, decreases insulin resistance, and ameliorates glucose intolerance.

For further discussion of metabolic syndrome, see Chapter 60.

TABLE 35.1 Components of Metabolic Syndrome	
Risk Factor (three required for diagnosis)	**Defining Level**
Central (Abdominal) Obesity Men: Women:	Waist Circumference >40 inches >35 inches
Fasting Triglycerides	>150 mg/dL (or taking medication for high TGs)
HDL-C (cardioprotective form) Men: Women:	 <40 mg/dL (or taking medication for low HDL-C) <50 mg/dL (or taking medication for low HDL-C)
Blood Pressure	≥130/ ≥85 mm Hg (or taking medication for HTN)
Fasting Glucose	>100 mg/dL (or taking medication for hyperglycemia)

Abbreviations: HDL-C, high-density lipoprotein-cholesterol; HTN, hypertension; TG, triglycerides
Source: Adapted from American Heart Association. https://www.heart.org/en/health-topics/metabolic-syndrome/about-metabolic-syndrome.

HTN also seems to follow a more malignant course in African Americans. Compared with European Americans with HTN, African Americans have an increased risk of left ventricular hypertrophy (LVH), HF, renal failure, and sodium-sensitive low-renin HTN.

HTN has localized and systemic adverse effects. Locally, high BP creates a shearing force against the arterial walls, which injures the endothelium and accelerates development of atherosclerosis. Endothelial injury initiates a detrimental localized reaction of vasoconstriction, inflammation, platelet aggregation, and fibrin and lipid deposition—the basis of arteriosclerotic plaque formation. In turn, target organs that are damaged by HTN include the heart (LVH and coronary artery disease [CAD] resulting in angina or acute myocardial infarction [MI]), the kidneys (chronic renal insufficiency), the brain (transient ischemic attacks [TIAs], cerebrovascular accidents [CVAs], and increased risk of dementia), the eyes (retinal hemorrhages and hypertensive retinopathy), and the peripheral arteries (peripheral vascular disease).

Secondary Hypertension

Secondary HTN denotes elevated BP due to an identifiable, underlying condition. Detection of secondary HTN is critical to reverse the source of the pathological process and prevent hypertensive target organ damage (TOD). Much less common than essential HTN, secondary HTN has an overall frequency of 5% to 10% in primary care practices. Secondary HTN is often distinguished from essential HTN by certain findings, such as an age of onset younger than 30 years or being older than 50 years of age, having BP higher than 180/110 mm Hg at diagnosis, significant TOD at diagnosis, hemorrhages and exudates on funduscopic examination, renal insufficiency, LVH, accelerated or malignant HTN, and a poor response to therapy. Resistant HTN is often due to unexplored, reversible secondary causes.

Reversible causes of secondary HTN include obesity, obstructive sleep apnea, renovascular disease, chronic corticosteroid therapy, Cushing's syndrome, primary hyperaldosteronism, pheochromocytoma, coarctation of the aorta, hyperthyroid disease, parathyroid disease, and excess alcohol intake. Secondary HTN can also be drug induced, and a thorough history of the patient's medications, including herbal supplements, over-the-counter (OTC) agents, and any illicit drug use is essential. Common drugs that can cause HTN include NSAIDs, cyclooxygenase-2 (COX-2) inhibitors, sympathomimetics such as decongestants and anorectics (diet pills), oral contraceptives, erythropoietin, cocaine, amphetamines, corticosteroids, tacrolimus, cyclosporine, and herbal ephedra supplements. Licorice, smoking, and chewing tobacco also increase BP. Research has also found that smoking e-cigarettes with nicotine causes an increase in heart rate and BP in young people, and the effects remain even after a vaping session.

"White Coat" Hypertension

"White coat" HTN, with a prevalence of 13%, is a transient rise in BP experienced by a patient when in the clinical or hospital setting, most likely due to anxiety. This condition of pseudohypertension is common in primary care practice. The white coat effect can lead to an overestimation of BP and the prescribing of unnecessary antihypertensive treatment. In addition, the patient's transiently high BP can be misinterpreted as ineffectiveness of antihypertensive therapy. Approximately 30% to 40% of patients who were diagnosed with HTN based on their BP readings in a clinical office had normal "out-of-office" BP readings according to ambulatory BP measurements.

 Pediatric/Adolescent Considerations: Hypertension

Because of lifestyle behaviors, adolescents may be at risk for developing HTN in their 40s and 50s, especially if their BP is in the upper limits of normal.
Factors that may lead to this are

- Vaping, tobacco use, chewing tobacco
- Eating excessive amounts of licorice
- Being overweight/obese
- Having a poor diet; e.g., increased carbs, increased sodium
- Lack of exercise
- Having high total cholesterol (TC)
- Drinking alcohol excessively
- Taking diet pills, oral contraceptives

Clinic-based BP readings may also give an inaccurate impression due to the data collection technique and equipment used. In the primary care setting, BP should be measured in a seated position with the brachial artery positioned roughly at the level of the heart, with the BP reading taken only after the patient has been in a seated and relaxed position for 5 minutes to avoid readings immediately after the patient has entered the clinic in a rushed or stressed state. Care must also be taken to use an appropriately sized BP cuff when assessing HTN in the clinic. Obese patients or those with large arms need to have a cuff that is large enough to measure BP accurately. If the cuff used is too small, an artificially high BP reading may result. Patients with white coat HTN are more accurately assessed through the use of ambulatory BP monitoring (ABPM), which provides an automated 24-hour recording of the patient's BP during normal daily activities that can be reviewed by the clinician. Alternatively, the patient may be instructed to measure and record intermittent BP readings over several weeks with reliable, consistent equipment for later review.

Masked Hypertension

Masked HTN is defined as HTN that is present during daily life and yet absent in clinical assessment. Studies conducted by the National Institutes of Health (NIH) demonstrated that masked HTN may be present in as many as one in seven individuals with normal clinic-based BP readings. ABPM or home-based BP self-monitoring by the patient who is at high risk for masked HTN is a cornerstone of optimizing outcomes. Without active patient participation and education, however, this condition may go untreated. Risk factors identified for masked HTN include smoking, alcohol use, lack of physical activity, and work-related and physiological stressors. Patients with masked HTN have a higher incidence of cardiovascular events and subsequently a higher risk of mortality and morbidity due to missed opportunities to treat.

Malignant Hypertension

Malignant HTN (hypertensive urgency/emergency) has been noted in up to 1% of patients diagnosed with primary HTN. Malignant HTN is diagnosed when a patient presents with severely elevated BP in the range of 180/110 mm Hg or higher and evidence of acute TOD. Although these terms are often used interchangeably, *hypertensive emergency* or *hypertensive crisis* denote this process acutely. If not treated with immediate parenteral antihypertensive therapy in an acute care setting, a hypertensive emergency may prove fatal. In contrast, a significantly elevated BP alone with no evidence of TOD does not constitute an emergency and is classified as a hypertensive urgency.

Hypertensive urgencies may be treated with oral agents over a period of 24 to 48 hours to achieve stabilization.

In a hypertensive emergency, a severely elevated BP can be reduced over the course of hours with oral and/or IV medications in an inpatient setting. Acute TOD most commonly involves the neurological, cardiac, or renal systems, with evidence of TOD including the following:

- Cerebrovascular events
- Papilledema, hemorrhages, or exudates on funduscopic examination of the eye
- Acute myocardial ischemia or infarction
- HF
- Pulmonary edema
- Aortic dissection
- Acute renal failure or dysfunction, as evidenced by hematuria, proteinuria, or elevated serum creatinine
- States of catecholamine excess
- Epistaxis
- Preeclampsia or eclampsia
- Change in mental status or neurological deficits on physical examination
- Dementia

CLINICAL PRESENTATION

Subjective

The history should include a thorough investigation of cardiovascular risk factors such as age, gender, menopausal status, diet, physical activity level, alcohol and caffeine use, smoking, dyslipidemia, diabetes mellitus, family history of heart disease, and current medications. Some medications, such as NSAIDs and sympathomimetic OTC cold remedies, may exacerbate BP elevation or interfere with the antihypertensive effects of angiotensin-converting enzyme inhibitors (ACEIs) or angiotensin receptor blockers (ARBs). Culture and ethnicity should be assessed within the history as well. As noted earlier, compared with European Americans, African Americans have a higher risk of HTN, diabetes mellitus, and renal impairment, which all require aggressive management of BP and specific drug therapy.

Diagnosis of HTN is typically made after several routine outpatient visits with the patient complaining of no symptoms. Occasionally, if the BP is extremely elevated, the patient may present with a headache that occurs on awakening and is located in the occipital area. Hypertensive urgency or emergency may present with complaints related to the particular type of end-organ damage (e.g., chest pain from cardiac ischemia, blurred vision from papilledema, mental status changes from TIA).

Objective

A systematic approach should be used when assessing the person with or at risk for HTN. A patient presenting with acute, severely elevated BP requires a thorough clinical examination that includes staging of the BP elevation and investigation for evidence of TOD. This evaluation should include funduscopic examination, palpation of the chest for point of maximal impulse (PMI), auscultation of the heart, abdominal assessment for bruits or widened aortic diameter and enlarged kidneys, examination of the carotid arteries for bruits, palpation of peripheral pulses, neurological examination, electrocardiogram (ECG), urinalysis, serum creatinine measurements and complete serum chemistry, and a chest x-ray (CXR). A computed tomography (CT) scan of the head to rule out stroke may be necessary, if the patient presents with mental status changes.

Table 35.2 presents the most recent 2017 American Heart Association/American College of Cardiology (AHA/ACC) HTN classification guidelines. The assessment should include two measurements of BP in both arms, with the patient seated with both feet on a flat surface (crossing the legs may increase the SBP by 2 to 8 mm Hg) and the back supported with the arm (i.e., brachial artery) at heart level (diastolic BP [DBP] may be decreased by up to 6 mm Hg if the arm is below the level of the heart). The patient should remain quiet and not speak during the reading. As noted earlier, an appropriately sized cuff for the patient is critical because a cuff that is too large will provide a falsely low BP, whereas a cuff that is too small will provide a falsely elevated BP. When elevated BPs are detected, a bilateral assessment for confirmation should be obtained if not contraindicated (e.g., by the presence of an atrioventricular shunt or postmastectomy status). BP should be taken again after the patient has stood for at least 2 minutes, and the higher readings should be recorded.

In specific patient groups such as older adults, obese patients, and patients with arrhythmias, certain clinically meaningful findings should be noted. In older adults, the clinician should discern whether an auscultatory gap is heard. Also known as a silent gap, this transient period of absent heart sounds during manual BP measurement is associated with vascular disease and reduced peripheral blood flow, which if not recognized by the clinician (through simultaneous palpation of the radial pulse), may result in an underestimation of SBP and/or an overestimation of DBP. In addition, if severe vessel rigidity is present in the brachial artery, the BP cuff may be unable to adequately compress the calcified vessel, leading to a falsely elevated BP reading. This phenomenon is known as *pseudohypertension*. Although this may increase the BP reading by 30 mm Hg or more, it does not by itself represent a disease state.

The obese patient often has a short upper arm length relative to upper arm width; in this instance, a wrist cuff may be used with the wrist (i.e., radial artery) positioned at heart level to obtain an accurate BP reading. In patients with severe bradycardia, the clinician should deflate the cuff more slowly to prevent underestimating SBP and overestimating DBP.

A diagnosis of primary HTN should be confirmed with 24-hour ABPM or sequential home BP readings. Twenty-four–hour ABPM is indicated to rule out white coat or masked HTN, to identify hypertensive symptoms while the patient is being treated with antihypertensive medication, and to uncover apparent drug-resistant HTN.

Advanced Assessment 35.1 lists common findings associated with HTN. Evidence of TOD includes retinopathy, which may appear as arteriolar narrowing, arteriovenous nicking, hemorrhages, or exudates. A bruit may be auscultated over either carotid artery, indicating stenosis. The chest may demonstrate a displaced PMI and/or an S_4 heart sound indicating LVH. Auscultation of an S_4 heart sound is associated with the decreased elasticity of the left ventricle that occurs in LVH. The patient should also be evaluated for the presence of HF, a known sequela of longstanding HTN. An S_3 gallop, pulmonary crackles, jugular venous distention, and peripheral edema are all signs of HF. A bruit heard in the abdomen may indicate an aneurysm or renal artery stenosis. Palpation of a widened aortic pulsation is associated with abdominal aortic aneurysm. Diminished peripheral pulses and loss of sensation in the lower extremities can indicate peripheral arterial disease. Neurological examination can reveal deficits associated with TIA or a CVA.

DIAGNOSTIC REASONING

Diagnostic Tests

Diagnostic testing of a patient who has or is suspected of having HTN should focus on the evaluation of target organs and related comorbidities, as well as on excluding certain causes of secondary HTN. Additional testing may be indicated, particularly when concurrent diseases such as diabetes mellitus or hyperlipidemia are present.

The ECG is an important screening tool to assess for cardiac TOD in the hypertensive patient. It can be used to assess for the presence of left atrial enlargement (LAE), LVH, myocardial ischemia or infarction, premature ventricular

TABLE 35.2 Classification of Blood Pressure for Adults Aged 18 Years or Older

Blood Pressure (BP) Category	Systolic BP (mm Hg)	Diastolic BP (mm Hg)
Normal	<120 and	<80
Elevated	120–129	<80
Hypertension		
Stage 1	130–139 or	80–89
Stage 2	≥140 or	≥90

Source: Whelton PK, Carey RM, Aronow WS, et al. ACC/AHA/AAPA/ABC/ACPM/AGS/APhA/ASH/ASPC/NMA/PCNA guideline for the prevention, detection, evaluation, and management of high blood pressure in adults: Executive summary: A report of the American College of Cardiology/American Heart Association task force on clinical practice guidelines. *J Am Soc Hypertens.* 2018;12:579.

Advanced Assessment 35.1: Hypertension

Assessment	Common Findings
BLOOD PRESSURE MEASUREMENT	
Proper technique: • Cuff size has a bladder length of 80% and a width of at least 40% of arm circumference. • Patient in a sitting position, arm resting at level of the heart with feet on flat surface and legs uncrossed. • Rest for 5 minutes before measurement. • Average two readings at least 2 minutes apart (if >5 mm Hg difference, obtain additional readings).	SBP ≥130 mm Hg DBP ≥80 mm Hg
PHYSICAL EXAMINATION	
Height, weight, BMI	Overweight: BMI 25–29.9 kg/m^2 Obesity: BMI ≥30 kg/m^2, especially with central or truncal pattern
Waist measurement	Men: >39 inches Women: >34 inches
Funduscopy	Hypertensive retinopathy (arteriolar narrowing, arteriovenous nicking, hemorrhages, exudates, papilledema)
Carotid arteries	Bruits
Neck veins	Distention
Thyroid	Enlargement Nodules
Cardiac	Point of maximal impulse and apex displaced laterally greater than one intercostal space S_3, S_4 heart sounds Murmur or mitral regurgitation
Lungs	Crackles Bronchospasm
Abdomen	Bruits, masses, abnormal aortic pulsations Enlarged kidneys
Extremities	Absence of peripheral arterial pulsations Bruits (with peripheral arterial disease) Edema
DIAGNOSTIC TESTS	
Urinalysis	Proteinuria
Blood urea nitrogen/creatinine	Increased
Complete blood count	May show anemia
Potassium	Increased or decreased
Blood glucose	May be increased
Lipids: triglycerides, high-density lipoprotein, low-density lipoprotein	Increased
12-lead ECG	May show target organ damage, e.g., LVH, left atrial enlargement
Brain natriuretic peptide	Hormone released by the ventricle indicative of increased myocardial demand

Abbreviations: BMI, body mass index; DBP, diastolic blood pressure; LVH, left ventricular hypertrophy; SBP, systolic blood pressure.

contractions, and atrial fibrillation. LAE is one of the earliest ECG findings associated with HTN. An echocardiogram is useful to detect the presence of increased left ventricular wall thickness and hypertrophy.

Differential Diagnosis

The key to differential diagnosis is to determine the underlying etiology of the HTN, whether it is essential or secondary, for instance, and to assess the degree of HTN (and whether it is malignant or benign). A presumptive diagnosis is made if the average of at least two seated BP measurements on at least two or more visits exceeds either 80 mm Hg DBP or 130 mm Hg SBP in adults older than 18 years.

Some concurrent health problems, if inadequately treated, may also affect BP. For example, the normal pain response includes vasoconstriction and tachycardia; therefore, inadequate control of both acute and chronic pain can cause a rise in BP. In turn, adequate pain control may resolve the HTN. Certain clinical conditions may also necessitate the use of drugs that can cause or exacerbate HTN, such as cyclosporine, erythropoietin, and certain antidepressants (e.g., tricyclic antidepressants, selective serotonin-norepinephrine reuptake inhibitors). In this case, reducing the dose or stopping the causative agent of HTN should be explored, but if that is not possible, antihypertensive treatment must be chosen with care and an adequate dose prescribed, which may require referral to an HTN specialist.

MANAGEMENT

Approximately one in five adults will need medication to treat HTN. The key to HTN management is not only the reversal of HTN-related disease trends but also the prevention of TOD. The following recommendations are public health approaches to achieve a downward shift in BP distribution at the population level, thereby reducing morbidity, mortality, and the lifetime risk of an individual becoming hypertensive:

- Develop community health programs to stress reducing calories, saturated fat, and salt in processed foods.
- Encourage food manufacturers and restaurants to reduce the sodium in the food supply by 50% over the next decade.
- Increase community/school opportunities for physical activity.
- Address the diversity of racial, ethnic, cultural, linguistic, religious, and social factors in the delivery of community services to increase the community's receptiveness to the use of public health services.
- Improve opportunities for treatment and control of HTN, as health-care providers help break down barriers to the diagnosis and treatment of HTN (e.g., nursing and work-site clinics that offer health services on evenings and weekends, thereby increasing the likelihood of access to care for those who work during weekday hours).

The use of lifestyle modifications (Box 35.2) should be a part of every patient's regimen to prevent or treat elevated BP. Clinicians should work with the patient on a plan of lifestyle modification and medications as needed to lower the BP as much as is tolerated without symptoms. Patient-specific goals include the following:

- Increase awareness regarding the risks of prehypertension and the development of frank HTN. Teens and young adults with high-normal BP are at markedly increased risk of developing HTN in their fourth and fifth decades of life. Behavioral therapies such as a program of regular aerobic exercise and a diet that is low in fat and sodium and high in potassium should be initiated to help avoid HTN in otherwise healthy individuals.
- Know your own BMI, which should serve as a guide to weight loss rather than just aiming for an ideal body weight, which may prove particularly daunting for some individuals.

Box 35.2 Lifestyle Modifications to Manage Hypertension

- **Weight reduction:** Maintain normal body weight: BMI = 18.5 to 24.9 kg/m²) (lowers BP by 5 to 20 mm Hg).
- **Adopt DASH (Dietary Approaches to Stop Hypertension) eating plan:** Consume a diet rich in fruits, vegetables, and low-fat dairy products, with a reduced content of saturated and total fat (lowers BP by 14 to 18 mm Hg).
- **Dietary sodium reduction:** Reduce dietary sodium intake to no more than 100 mmol (2.4 g sodium) per day (lowers BP by 2 to 8 mm Hg).
- **Physical activity:** Engage in regular aerobic physical activity, such as brisk walking (at least 30 minutes/day on most days of the week) (lowers BP by 4 to 9 mm Hg).
- **Moderation of alcohol:** Limit consumption to no more than two drinks (1 oz or 30 mL of ethanol, e.g., 24 oz of beer, 10 oz of wine, or 3 oz of 80-proof whiskey) per day for most men and to no more than one drink per day for women and lighter-weight persons (lowers BP by 2 to 4 mm Hg).
- **Stop smoking, vaping, and/or use of other tobacco products**.
- **Understand hot tub safety:** When combined with heat, antihypertensive drugs may cause vasodilation, resulting in dizziness, lightheadedness, fainting, and reduction of cerebral blood flow, with the potential for falling and risk of injury.
- **Maintain adherence to pharmacotherapeutic plan:** When medication regimen is not followed, BP will rise.
- **Monitor for drug-induced HTN:** Drugs that may induce HTN include NSAIDs, antidepressants, glucocorticoids, oral contraceptives, hormone replacement therapy, and OTC medications that contain decongestants.

- Improving HTN control in persons already diagnosed with HTN, as many patients diagnosed and started on treatment for HTN still have a BP greater than 120/80 mm Hg (see Table 35.2 for specific diagnostic thresholds), demonstrating inadequate control.
- Reduce cardiovascular risks, in addition to BP. Many patients with HTN will have additional modifiable cardiovascular disease risk factors such as diabetes mellitus, hyperlipidemia, tobacco use, and physical inactivity/sedentary lifestyle; therefore, a comprehensive plan to treat HTN must also address these issues.

Patients with an elevated SBP up to 129 mm Hg and a DBP up to 80 mm Hg should adopt healthy lifestyle choices and have their BP reevaluated in 3 to 6 months. For patients with stage 1 HTN (SBP = 130 to 139 mm Hg, DBP = 80 to 89 mm Hg), the 10-year cardiovascular risk of heart disease or stroke should be calculated. The AHA/American Stroke Association offers a calculator to determine the risk of heart disease and stroke that is based on a patient's age, lipid profile (TC, low-density lipoprotein [LDL], and high-density lipoprotein [HDL]), current BP, and related medical history, including whether the patient is being treated for HTN and the patient has a history of stroke, angina, diabetes mellitus, peripheral arterial disease, MI, or atherosclerotic cardiovascular disease (ASCVD). This calculator can be found at http://tools.acc.org/ASCVD-Risk-Estimator-Plus/#!/calculate/estimate/.

If their calculated cardiovascular risk is less than 10%, they should institute lifestyle changes and reassess their BP in 3 to 6 months. If their risk is more than 10%, they should institute lifestyle changes and start antihypertensive medication with monthly follow-up visits until their BP is controlled. If they have stage 2 HTN (SBP of 140 mm Hg or higher, DBP of 90 mm Hg or higher), lifestyle changes should be instituted as well as antihypertensive medications from two pharmacological classes, with monthly follow-up visits until BP control is achieved.

In patients with diabetes mellitus, the American Diabetes Association continues to recommend a target SBP of less than 130 mm Hg and a target DBP of less than 80 mm Hg. For patients with chronic kidney disease and proteinuria, the therapeutic plan should be individualized with attention to balancing side effects of medications (e.g., hypotension or worsening renal disease) with recommended BP goals. Renal impairment should compel the clinician and patient to work together to maintain meticulous BP control in order to minimize the development of nephropathy. In addition to public health programs, community-affiliated programs, including parish-based, neighborhood, work-site programs, and health-promotion events should be used to assist patients, as well as those with normal BP, to make healthy lifestyle choices.

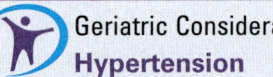

Geriatric Considerations: Hypertension

Nearly one-half of all adults aged 65 years and older develop isolated systolic HTN, defined as an SBP greater than 160 mm Hg with a normal DBP (80 mm Hg or less) as a consequence of atherosclerotic thickening of the vessels. More than two-thirds of persons older than 65 years develop HTN, and as the 2017 ACC/AHA guidelines are stricter than in the past, even more Americans are expected to meet the criteria for HTN and require treatment. Given its frequency, the development of isolated systolic HTN is often viewed as an unavoidable consequence of aging. However, clinicians should be aware that behaviorally based therapies used to prevent and treat HTN can also help minimize age-associated increases in BP.

Historically, older adults with HTN have not received the emphasis on treatment that was merited. Present-day guidelines now stress the importance of treating HTN in older adults, which results in a significant reduction in HF and cardiovascular and cerebrovascular disease. Even in persons older than 50 years of age, SBP greater than 130 mm Hg is a much more important risk factor for cardiovascular disease than elevated DBP. Even patients with a normal BP at 55 years of age still have a 90% lifetime risk of developing HTN. In a patient with a BP of 115/75 mm Hg, the risk of cardiovascular disease doubles with each incremental increase of 20/10 mm Hg.

Certain age-related physical changes predispose older adults to difficulty tolerating antihypertensive drug therapy, including the risk of postural hypotension. Because older patients benefit significantly from the control of HTN, however, the appropriate drug should be chosen in consideration of particular factors that increase the risk for postural hypotension, such as a decreased number of baroreceptors. As a result, BP should be measured with the older patient in both standing and sitting positions. In addition, older adults should be instructed to change position slowly while on antihypertensive medication.

The force of myocardial contractility decreases with age, leaving older adults more sensitive to antihypertensive medications with negative inotropic effects, such as beta blockers. Because of lower circulating blood volume, diuretics, which are particularly effective antihypertensive agents for this age group, should be used in lower doses. In general, older adults also have decreased renal excretory capacity compared with younger patients; therefore, smaller doses of medications are required. In turn, the adage "start low and go slow" should be followed, and the dose titration of antihypertensive medication should be monitored closely with every dose adjustment.

The Beers criteria are a clinical tool developed to assist clinicians in improving medication safety in older adults. The clinician should consult the Beers criteria for potentially inappropriate medication use in older adults (American Geriatrics Society 2019; see Resources).

Pharmacological Therapy

Antihypertensive drug therapy is not recommended if there is no compelling indication other than potential risk factors for HTN, for which lifestyle modifications should be instituted. In turn, monitoring for drug-induced HTN is essential before the initiation of pharmaceutical therapy, e.g., iatrogenic HTN due to the use of NSAIDs, glucocorticoids, antidepressants, oral contraceptives, hormone replacement therapy, or OTC sympathomimetic decongestants (cold medications). The use of alcohol and tobacco must also be assessed, as well as the presence of sleep apnea.

For most patients with newly diagnosed HTN, therapeutic lifestyle changes should be instituted for 1 month and, if ineffective in lowering BP after 1 month, pharmacotherapy should be added. In patients who are not African American, including those with diabetes mellitus, initial antihypertensive treatment should include any one of four classes of oral medication, which improve cardiovascular outcomes: a thiazide-type diuretic, a calcium channel blocker (CCB), an ACEI, or an ARB. Initial therapy should consist of a low dose of the chosen agent, which may be increased in dose if it is well-tolerated but BP control has not yet been achieved.

Thiazide-type diuretics are first-line antihypertensive drugs. These agents are useful in the presence of isolated systolic HTN. They are also helpful for patients with osteoporosis because they help preserve bone density. Use of thiazide-type diuretics has been shown to reduce stroke and cardiovascular-related mortality and morbidity. Chlorthalidone 12.5 to 25 mg per day is the recommended first-line thiazide diuretic drug. A second choice is hydrochlorothiazide initiated at a similar dose.

In African Americans, initial treatment may consist of either a CCB or a thiazide diuretic (ACEIs have been shown to be less effective in this population). In patients with chronic kidney disease, pharmacological treatment should be initiated to lower SBP to less than 130 mm Hg and DBP to less than 80 mm Hg. The initial agent of choice in patients with chronic kidney disease should be an ACEI or ARB.

The clinician should choose an antihypertensive therapy with the patient's concurrent medical history and comorbid conditions in mind. Examples of antihypertensive drugs that can be used in patients with concurrent diseases include choices from the following pharmacological classes:

- **Angiotensin-converting enzyme inhibitors** (ACEIs—drugs with generic names typically ending in *-pril,* such as captopril) are effective in the presence of HF and MI with systolic dysfunction to help limit the effects of myocardial remodeling. ACEIs should be used when certain comorbid conditions including renal insufficiency and diabetes mellitus are present, as these drugs may assist in preserving or enhancing renal function.
- **Angiotensin II receptor blockers** (ARBs) are helpful in antihypertensive individuals with comorbid conditions such as HF and type 2 diabetes mellitus. Because they have a higher cost than ACEIs and fewer long-term safety data, ARBs should be reserved for patients who develop a cough when taking ACEIs or are otherwise intolerant. However, some research suggests there is a risk of cross reactivity to ARBs in patients who are anaphylactic to ACEIs; thus, there are clinicians who consider both classes of medications contraindicated in these patients. Given their related mechanisms of action, an ACEI and an ARB should not be used in combination.
- **Beta blockers** (drugs with generic names ending in *-lol,* such as metoprolol) are no longer commonly recommended for the primary management of HTN but may be used in the presence of angina, post-MI (to reduce cardiac workload and enhance rhythm stability), atrial tachycardia, migraine headache (as a nonselective agent for the reduction in frequency and severity of migraine headaches), and essential tremor (as a nonselective agent).
- **CCBs** (long-acting dihydropyridine drugs that have generic names ending in *-pine,* such as amlodipine) are suggested for black patients of African or Caribbean descent who are younger than 55 years, for patients with isolated systolic HTN, and for hypertensive patients with concurrent stable angina pectoris.
- **Alpha-adrenergic antagonists** (alpha blockers) are usually effective in patients with benign prostatic hyperplasia because they facilitate bladder emptying by decreasing prostate size.
- Additional drugs may include **combination therapies** with two drugs in one tablet, such as combinations of an ACEI and a CCB, an ACEI and a diuretic, an ARB and a diuretic, a centrally acting agent and a diuretic, or more than one diuretic (see Drugs Commonly Prescribed 35.1).

After the initiation of pharmacological treatment, the BP should be reevaluated within a month. If the target BP is not attained, up-titration of the dose of the current pharmacological agent may be required. Alternatively, the addition of a pharmacological agent from another class may be added at a low starting dose. If BP goals are not obtained with the use of two BP agents, a third agent may be added, although the clinician must be aware of the risks of polypharmacy in such patients. Failure to respond to a triple-therapy regimen may require a referral to a cardiologist or HTN specialist. In addition, a more extensive evaluation for causes of secondary HTN may also be indicated in such patients.

Because small doses of two agents from different pharmacological classes may have a synergistic effect in lowering BP while avoiding the problems of higher doses of either agent given alone (see Drugs Commonly Prescribed 35.1), these combination products may be appropriate as first-line antihypertensive therapy. In particular, a very low dose (12.5 mg) of chlorthalidone has the ability to potentiate the effect of other agents, without producing negative metabolic effects.

Drugs Commonly Prescribed 35.1: Hypertension

MEDICATIONS PREFERRED WITH SPECIFIC COMORBID CONDITIONS

Diabetes mellitus*	Angiotensin-converting enzyme inhibitor (ACEI) or angiotensin II receptor blocker (ARB) For metabolic syndrome, ACEI or ARB or calcium channel blocker (CCB)
Chronic kidney disease	ACEI or ARB
Heart failure (HF)†	ACEI or ARB, mineralocorticoid receptor antagonist, beta blocker, diuretic (loop diuretic preferred) For left ventricular hypertrophy (LVH): ACEI or ARB, along with CCB
High-risk coronary artery disease (CAD)	Beta blocker or CCB for angina ACEI or CCB for asymptomatic atherosclerosis
Post–myocardial infarction (MI)	ACEI or ARB, beta blocker
Recurrent stroke prevention	Any effective antihypertensive

DRUG CLASSIFICATION	INDICATION	ADVERSE REACTIONS AND PRESCRIBING CONSIDERATIONS
Diuretics		
Thiazide diuretics: chlorthalidone (Hygroton) hydrochlorothiazide (HCTZ)	First-line diuretic to treat hypertension (HTN). Thiazide diuretics are indicated in the management of HTN, either as the sole therapeutic agent or to enhance the effect of other antihypertensive drugs in more severe forms of HTN.	Use with caution in severe renal disease, which may precipitate azotemia, and in patients with impaired hepatic function. Contraindicated in patients with anuria or known hypersensitivity to these products or other sulfonamide-derived drugs. Use with caution in patients with hepatic impairment, given the risk of hepatic coma. Hypokalemia, hyperuricemia, and rise in lipid levels may occur. May cause occasional urticaria and skin rash, postural hypotension, gastrointestinal (GI) distress, loss of appetite, impotence, and vertigo. Thiazide diuretics are less effective when creatinine is >1.8 mg/dL.
Loop diuretics: bumetanide (Bumex) furosemide (Lasix)	Loop diuretics are more potent than thiazides in promoting diuresis; however, they are less effective than thiazides in BP management. Indicated for the treatment of mild to moderate HTN and in the management of edema associated with congestive HF. Also beneficial in the management of HTN associated with hepatic and renal disease, including nephritic syndrome. Will likely remain effective in patients who have creatinine >1.8 mg/dL.	May cause hypokalemia, hyponatremia, low magnesium, dehydration, postural hypotension, tinnitus, hyperuricemia leading to gout, increased sensitivity to sunlight. Hypertensive patients who cannot be adequately controlled with thiazides will probably also be inadequately controlled with furosemide alone.
Aldosterone receptor blocker: spironolactone (Aldactone)	Weak antihypertensives. Potassium-sparing diuretics are indicated for the treatment of HTN or edema in patients who develop hypokalemia. Aldosterone antagonists block the effects of serum aldosterone and are effective at regulating Na+ and water homeostasis to maintain stable intravascular volume.	The use of potassium-sparing agents is often unnecessary in patients receiving diuretics for uncomplicated essential HTN, when such patients have a normal diet. May cause nervousness, skin rash, increased sensitivity to sunlight, confusion, irregular heart rhythm, shortness of breath, lethargy, and weakness. Hyperkalemia risk is increased with the use of ACEI or ARB. Use with caution in cases of renal impairment.

Drugs Commonly Prescribed 35.1: Hypertension—cont'd

MEDICATIONS PREFERRED WITH SPECIFIC COMORBID CONDITIONS

Beta-Adrenergic Receptor Blockers

atenolol (Tenormin) carvedilol (Coreg) metoprolol (Toprol) propranolol (Inderal)	**Not indicated** as first-line management of HTN unless compelling indications such as acute coronary syndrome (ACS) or HF are present. May be used in combination with other antihypertensive agents, especially thiazide-type diuretics. Beta blockers are a component of core measures in patients with ACS.	May cause sinus bradycardia, atrioventricular block, hypotension, shortness of breath, depression, dizziness, fatigue, vivid dreams, diarrhea, nausea/vomiting, increased triglycerides, sexual dysfunction, pruritus, skin hyperpigmentation, alopecia, xerosis, and urticaria. Use with caution in patients with chronic obstructive pulmonary disease, asthma, and peripheral vascular disease. May increase the risk of developing type 2 diabetes mellitus.

Angiotensin-Converting Enzyme Inhibitors (ACEIs)

benazepril (Lotensin) captopril (Capoten) enalapril (Vasotec) lisinopril (Zestril)	Use alone or in combination with thiazide diuretics. Effective for patients with HF, post-MI, left ventricular dysfunction, renal insufficiency, or glomerulosclerosis. Diabetes mellitus with nephropathy may likewise benefit. May be effective in the prevention of stroke. ACEIs are a component of core measures in patients with ACS.	May exacerbate hyperkalemia and carries the risk of severe angioedema of oral (e.g., tongue, lips) and upper respiratory tract structures. Avoid in pregnancy. May cause a chronic cough through effects on the bradykinin pathway. When given with an aldosterone receptor blocker, may cause orthostatic hypotension, sinus tachycardia, fatigue, dizziness, syncope, headache, or hyperkalemia. Renal adjustment is indicated in renal insufficiency. Do not dose in the presence of bilateral renal artery stenosis.

Angiotensin II Receptor Blockers (ARBs)

losartan (Cozaar) olmesartan (Benicar) valsartan (Diovan)	Use alone or in combination with other antihypertensive agents. ARBs are an alternative to ACEIs in patients who develop a chronic cough secondary to ACEI usage. Attention must be paid to the exact cause of the cough to rule out other etiologies, such as possible worsening of HF.	Avoid use in pregnancy. May exacerbate hyperkalemia, hyponatremia, angioedema, renal impairment, orthostatic hypotension, syncope, dizziness, and insomnia.

Calcium Channel Blockers (CCBs)

Dihydropyridine: amlodipine (Norvasc) felodipine (Plendil) Nondihydropyridine: diltiazem (Cardizem) verapamil (Calan)	Most potent antihypertensive agents routinely utilized. May be useful for the treatment of stable angina pectoris, especially dihydropyridines. CCBs may be effective in the management of angina from coronary artery vasospasm. Effective in reducing cardiac muscle burden and lessens myocardial demand for oxygen. Nondihydropyridines have antichronotropic effects on certain tachycardic arrhythmias (e.g., atrial fibrillation).	Use with caution in HF and second- and third-degree heart block (unless cardiac pacer is in place). Effects of CCBs are potentiated by grapefruit juice. May cause lower extremity edema. Avoid in patients with recent MI. May cause peripheral edema, headache, dizziness, flushing, palpitations, fatigue, nausea/vomiting, abdominal pain, and drowsiness. Caution in acute HF, renal, or hepatic impairment.

Continued

Drugs Commonly Prescribed 35.1: Hypertension—cont'd

MEDICATIONS PREFERRED WITH SPECIFIC COMORBID CONDITIONS

Alpha-Adrenergic Receptor Blockers

doxazosin (Cardura) prazosin (Minipress) terazosin (Hytrin)	Use with benign prostatic hyperplasia, prostatism, and dyslipidemia. May be used alone or in combination with diuretics, beta blockers, CCBs, or ACEIs.	Do not use as first-line or "solo" agents, as this is associated with higher rates of stroke and HF. Alters lipid metabolism by decreasing low-density lipoprotein and very low-density lipoprotein cholesterol. May cause mild sexual dysfunction, dizziness, lightheadedness, headache, drowsiness, fatigue, nausea/vomiting, peripheral edema, nasal congestion, and palpitations. May cause complications years later during eye surgery (e.g., cataract removal) by leading to floppy iris syndrome.

Centrally Acting Agents

alpha-methyldopa (Aldomet) clonidine (Catapres)	Effectively lower BP by decreasing central sympathetic outflow and peripheral resistance.	May cause drowsiness, impotence, dry mouth, increased respirations, increased GI motility, and miosis. Less common effects are depression and Coombs-positive anemia (with alpha-methyldopa). Abrupt withdrawal may lead to rebound HTN.

Direct Vasodilators

hydralazine (Apresoline) isosorbide dinitrate (Isordil) isosorbide mononitrate (Imdur) minoxidil (Loniten)	Good for HTN in pregnancy. Injectable hydralazine is used as a first-line agent in the treatment of hypertensive emergencies. Direct vasodilators play an important role in the treatment of severe HF.	May cause peripheral edema, headache, tachycardia, angina, hirsutism, mastalgia, and bullous rash, as well as orthostatic hypotension.

Combination Drug Therapy

ACEI-CCB: benazepril-amlodipine (Lotrel) enalapril-felodipine (Lexxel) trandolapril-verapamil (Tarka)	Effective with atrial tachycardia or fibrillation (especially the nondihydropyridine CCBs) and diabetes mellitus types 1 and 2. CCBs may be useful in Raynaud's syndrome, as well as for isolated systolic HTN and those at high risk of CAD. The nondihydropyridine CCBs (e.g., verapamil and diltiazem) have been shown to reduce cardiovascular mortality, proteinuria, and progression of diabetic nephropathy independent of ACEI use.	See information under ACEIs and CCBs.
ACEI-diuretic: benazepril-hydrochlorothiazide (Lotensin HCT) captopril-hydrochlorothiazide (Capozide) enalapril-hydrochlorothiazide (Vaseretic) fosinopril-hydrochlorothiazide (Monopril HCT) lisinopril-hydrochlorothiazide (Prinzide)	See information under ACEIs and Diuretics.	See information under ACEIs and Diuretics.

Drugs Commonly Prescribed 35.1: Hypertension—cont'd

MEDICATIONS PREFERRED WITH SPECIFIC COMORBID CONDITIONS

ARB-diuretic: candesartan-hydrochlorothiazide (Atacand HCT) eprosartan-hydrochlorothiazide (Teveten HCT) irbesartan-hydrochlorothiazide (Avalide) losartan-hydrochlorothiazide (Hyzaar) olmesartan medoxomil-hydrochlorothiazide (Benicar HCT) telmisartan-hydrochlorothiazide (Micardis) valsartan-hydrochlorothiazide (Diovan HCT)	See information under ARBs and Diuretics.	See information under ARBs and Diuretics.
Diuretic combination: spironolactone-hydrochlorothiazide (Aldactazide) triamterene-hydrochlorothiazide (Dyazide)	Used to treat fluid retention and HTN. See information under aldosterone receptor blockers and diuretics.	May exacerbate hyperkalemia, metabolic acidosis, gynecomastia, gout, renal and hepatic impairment. May cause GI disturbances. Useful in patients with refractory HTN. Use in patients with need for potassium-sparing diuretic. Do not use with potassium supplements or other diuretics. Advise patients to obtain emergency medical help if any signs of an allergic reaction occur, such as hives, difficulty breathing, swelling of face, lips, tongue, or throat. May cause numbness, muscle pain, weakness, uneven heartbeat, drowsiness, restlessness, lightheadedness, change in urination pattern, shallow breathing, tremors, confusion, nausea, stomach pain, low fever, loss of appetite, dark urine, clay-colored stools, and jaundice.

*To reduce risk for major cardiovascular events and slow progression of chronic kidney disease in adults with diabetes mellitus not on dialysis with urine albumin of <30 mg/24 hours, the blood pressure (BP) goal is <140/90 mm Hg. If urine albumin is >30 mg/24 hour, the BP goal is ≤130/80 mm Hg.
†Combined therapy should be used cautiously in those at risk for orthostatic hypotension.

Choosing the Best Drug

Certain patient characteristics, including ethnicity, may influence the choice and efficacy of an antihypertensive agent. A common perception is that the best antihypertensive effect for African Americans and older adults with HTN can be achieved by using a combination of a diuretic and a CCB. This should not be viewed, however, as a contraindication to using ACEIs or ARBs in these populations, as these classes of drugs may offer significant benefit in patients when certain concomitant diseases are present. For example, ACEIs or ARBs may be used in all groups with chronic kidney disease, although higher doses may be necessary in older adults and African Americans, and a longer period of time may elapse before improvement is seen.

An agent with once-daily dosing (i.e., 24-hour duration of action with at least 50% of activity in the past 12 hours) is recommended for chronic use to improve patient adherence and provide persistent, smooth control of HTN. In addition, with longer-acting formulas, there is less risk of hypertensive rebound resulting from a missed dose, providing protection against the risk of stroke, MI, or sudden death from cardiac arrest that may be induced by a dramatic increase in BP.

Whereas some classes of antihypertensive medications are appropriate for use in the case of certain comorbidities, in other clinical situations, some classes of medications should be used with caution or are contraindicated because they may have unfavorable effects on specific comorbid conditions (see Drugs Commonly Prescribed 35.1).

Concurrent Use of Select Concomitant Medications

NSAIDs can negate the BP-lowering effects of select antihypertensive medications, such as ACEIs and diuretics, by increasing sodium retention. In addition, the use of vasoconstricting medications such as decongestant agents (e.g., pseudoephedrine, phenylpropanolamine, caffeine) and sympathomimetic drugs of abuse (e.g., cocaine, amphetamines) can cause persistently elevated BP readings, despite pharmacological intervention. Excessive alcohol use may also prevent many antihypertensive medications from achieving their full therapeutic effect. In addition, one of the first manifestations of alcohol withdrawal is BP elevation. Nicotine and many of the chemically active, vasoconstricting substances patients are exposed to with cigarette smoke can also contribute to inadequate BP control.

FOLLOW-UP AND REFERRAL

For the patient undergoing lifestyle modification as initial treatment intervention for HTN, a follow-up visit should be scheduled every 3 to 6 months to determine effectiveness and adherence to the regimen of recommended behavioral changes. If lifestyle modifications are ineffective, pharmacological therapy should be initiated. HTN can be controlled only if patients are motivated, and using the Circle of Caring model to involve patients in their own care may assist in increasing this motivation.

After initiation of antihypertensive pharmacotherapy, a follow-up visit should be scheduled in 2 to 3 weeks for a BP check and possibly in 1 to 2 weeks for an electrolyte or side-effect check in at-risk patients. Once the BP goal is reached, visits can be scheduled every 3 months. More frequent visits may be needed if comorbid conditions exist. Serum potassium and creatinine levels should be monitored several times per year.

Patients with refractory HTN, secondary HTN, or comorbid conditions known to increase BP (either by virtue of the condition itself or due to required concomitant medications) should be referred to a cardiologist or HTN specialist for further evaluation and management. In addition, the clinician should refer patients with hypertensive emergency to an emergency department or an acute care setting for appropriate diagnostic testing, monitoring, and treatment.

Patient Education: Hypertension

Lifestyle modifications need to be stressed at each visit, particularly with vigorous promotion of tobacco avoidance. Low-dose aspirin therapy should be initiated once BP control is achieved. If aspirin therapy is started when the patient is still hypertensive, there is a potential risk of hemorrhagic stroke. Because the majority of MIs occur in the morning, aspirin should be administered at night. If a patient is on two antihypertensive medications, one should be given in the morning and one in the evening.

A patient-directed interprofessional team approach is critical to successful HTN care. This team should include representatives from nursing, pharmacy, medicine, and nutrition for the continued education of the patient and family and therapeutic monitoring during antihypertensive therapy. Education is stressed to improve patient adherence to behavioral and pharmacological therapy.

Numerous factors influence the efficacy of HTN therapy. Certain issues should be considered when HTN persists. Nonadherence to therapy is the most common reason for persistent HTN, and the most common reasons for nonadherence are (1) lack of perceived benefit of the intervention, (2) difficulty with provider follow-up, and (3) adverse effects of medication. The clinician must work with the patient to develop a plan of care that will meet therapeutic goals and fit with the patient's needs. Choosing well-tolerated drugs for intervention and continually acting as the patient's advocate and coach for lifestyle changes are critical.

Using the Circle of Caring model, the patient will be involved with the clinician in addressing diet, exercise, tobacco use, and modifiable risk factors that may be positively changed. Family may be an important component of the Circle of Caring and should be present when patient teaching occurs. Often, a successful behavioral regimen is spearheaded by a conscientious family member.

The Clin Calc Pooled Cohort Risk Assessment equation can be used to predict the 10-year risk for a first ASCVD event. If a patient's assessed risk is greater than 7.5%, it is recommended that the clinician initiate lipid-lowering therapy in addition to antihypertensive treatment. The clinician may choose to use this type of assessment tool with patients to reinforce the clinical effect of disease on their lives and to gain their commitment to make changes.

Oral contraceptives may increase BP, and the risk of HTN increases with their length of use. BP should be monitored regularly in women taking oral contraceptives. If a woman becomes hypertensive while taking oral contraceptives, the clinician should advise the patient to consider other forms of nonhormonal birth control.

The frequency of erectile dysfunction (ED) is significantly higher in men who are hypertensive than in men who are normotensive. If ED occurs, the antihypertensive medication should be discontinued and treatment restarted with another agent. Male patients should be advised that there is a lower risk of ED in men who are physically active, nonobese, and nonsmokers. Therefore, pertinent lifestyle modifications should be encouraged in all men to prevent ED.

Because some older adults develop postural hypotension with antihypertensive drug therapy, the clinician must educate these patients about avoiding abrupt positional changes while on antihypertensive medication and recommend that they sit on the edge of the bed for several minutes before arising in the morning. In addition, patients with postural hypotension should be urged to avoid volume depletion by drinking adequate quantities of water. In sum, lifestyle modifications cannot be overstressed in the treatment and prevention of comorbidities due to HTN, and teaching at every visit should reinforce the suggestions listed in Box 35.2.

DYSLIPIDEMIA

Dyslipidemia, also referred to as *hyperlipidemia*, is a general term for elevated concentrations of any or all of the different types of lipids in the plasma. A major risk factor for CVD, increased lipid levels positively correlate with an increased risk of acute coronary syndrome (ACS). The ACC/AHA guidelines recommend considering statin therapy in individuals who do not currently have CVD but who have a 7.5% or greater risk for stroke or heart attack. This risk is calculated using an equation endorsed by the ACC/AHA that includes race, gender, age, TC, HDL, BP, use of BP meds, presence of diabetes mellitus, and smoking status (discussed previously in the section on Hypertension).

The ACC/AHA recommends that the clinician begin a discussion to determine the best lipid-lowering therapy for each unique patient situation. These recommendations from the ACC/AHA are changing the way clinicians view traditional treatment guidelines, as the ACC/AHA stresses that many patients are undertreated and not receiving maximal statin therapy. Additionally, the importance of high-intensity dosing of anticholesterol medication has been emphasized.

EPIDEMIOLOGY AND CAUSES

The 2017 statistics from the U.S. Centers for Disease Control and Prevention (CDC) state that 95 million adults in the United States have TC levels higher than 200 mg/dL, with almost 29 million having levels higher that 240 mg/dL. The CDC also reports that 7% of children and adolescents aged 6 to 19 years also have a high TC. The correlation between dyslipidemia and coronary events is well documented, as elevated lipid levels present the greatest risk factor for the development of CAD. Table 35.3 shows normal and abnormal lipid values and classifications according to the Guidelines of the National Cholesterol Education Program (NCEP) of the National Heart, Lung, and Blood Institute (NHLBI) of the NIH.

Dyslipidemia can arise as a result of rare genetic disorders, such as familial hypercholesterolemia (FH). However, behavioral factors and lifestyle choices, including high dietary consumption of fats and a lack of physical activity, more often play a role. Moreover, dyslipidemia can be part of a constellation of abnormalities known as metabolic syndrome, characterized by abdominal obesity, glucose intolerance, insulin resistance, hyperinsulinemia, dyslipidemia, and HTN (see Box 35.1).

It is important to assess patients for secondary causes of dyslipidemia before instituting lipid-lowering therapy, as treatment of the primary disorder can improve or correct secondary dyslipidemia. Secondary causes of dyslipidemia include obesity, diabetes mellitus, hypothyroidism, nephrotic syndrome, ESRD, hepatic disorders, excessive alcohol consumption, estrogen administration, Cushing's syndrome (hypercortisolism), and glycogen storage disease. Certain drugs can cause lipid abnormalities such as thiazide diuretics, corticosteroids, beta blockers, anti-HIV protease inhibitors, isotretinoin, and growth hormone.

In the United States, CVD claims more than 800,000 lives each year. Approximately one in three deaths can be attributed to CVD. The Framingham Heart Study (the largest ongoing cohort study of heart disease in the United States) documented that 40% of participants with an MI had a TC level between 200 and 250 mg/dL. A patient with a TC level greater than 259 mg/dL is three times more likely to develop CAD than a patient with a level of less than 200 mg/dL. It is important to recognize that dyslipidemia is only one of many factors that increase the risk of developing CAD, and the greater the number of risk factors present, the greater the probability of developing clinically significant CAD.

PATHOPHYSIOLOGY

Dyslipidemia is a heterogeneous metabolic disorder that involves abnormal levels of lipids and lipoproteins that increase the risk of atherosclerosis. Lipoproteins are

TABLE 35.3 Serum Lipid Levels: Hyperlipidemia

Classification Level	Laboratory Value
TOTAL CHOLESTEROL (MG/DL)	
Desirable	125 to <200 mg/dL
Borderline high	200–239 mg/dL
High	≥240 mg/dL
TRIGLYCERIDES (MG/DL)	
Normal	<150 mg/dL
Borderline high	150–199 mg/dL
High	200–499 mg/dL
Very high	≥500 mg/dL
HDL (MG/DL)	
Low	<40 mg/dL
High (optimal: cardioprotective)	>60 mg/dL
LDL (MG/DL)	
For a high-risk patient, e.g., diabetic	<70 mg/dL
For general patients:	<100 mg/dL
Optimal	100–129 mg/dL
Above optimal	130–159 mg/dL
Borderline high	160–189 mg/dL
High	>190 mg/dL
Very high	

Source: Adapted from the Guidelines of the National Cholesterol Education Program of the National Heart, Lung, and Blood Institute of the National Institutes of Health. https://www.ccjm.org/content/87/4/231

molecules that carry cholesterol in the bloodstream. Lipoproteins differ in size, density, and atherogenicity and are divided into several classes: very low-density lipoprotein (VLDL), LDL, intermediate-density lipoprotein (IDL), lipoprotein (a) (Lp[a]), and HDL. Atherogenesis is mediated by the lower density lipoproteins: Lp(a), VLDL, LDL, and IDL. Small LDL particles migrate into the inflamed region of the blood vessel wall where they are oxidized and phagocytosed by macrophages to form foam cells, ultimately leading to the formation of fatty streaks and atherosclerotic plaques.

LDL cholesterol (LDL-C) is the specific type of cholesterol that constitutes the lipid core of arteriosclerotic plaque deposits. In clinical analyses, Lp(a), LDL, IDL, and VLDL are combined into the single fraction of LDL. Desirable levels of LDL are dependent on the existence of other CVD risk factors (see Table 35.3 for a classification of all lipid levels). Triglycerides (TGs) are large lipid molecules, which also contribute to atherogenesis, that are formed from fats consumed directly in the diet or formed from sugars and alcohols. To prevent cardiovascular disease, the desirable TG level is less than 150 mg/dL.

Atherogenic forms of cholesterol–lipoprotein complexes include all types of non-HDL cholesterol and TG-transporting proteins, such as LDL, IDL, Lp(a), and VLDL. TC in the blood arises both from ingested fats and from the synthesis of cholesterol in the liver. The measurement of total blood cholesterol is based on LDL-C, TG, and HDL cholesterol (HDL-C). The following equation is used to calculate TC: TC = LDL-C + TG/5 + HDL-C. The desirable level of TC in the blood without other cardiac risk factors is less than 200 mg/dL.

HDL-C is excreted from the body and, in contrast to LDL-C, is not deposited on arterial walls. HDL removes excess cholesterol from blood vessels and transports it back to the liver through reverse cholesterol transport. Once in the liver, cholesterol is excreted into the intestine as bile. HDL also plays a protective role by blocking the oxidation of LDL, which, in turn, inhibits atherogenesis. A low HDL level (40 mg/dL or less) is considered a cardiovascular risk factor, whereas a high level of HDL-C (60 mg/dL or more) is considered cardioprotective. Thus, an HDL-C level of more than or equal to 60 mg/dL is considered a "negative" or protective cardiovascular risk factor, allowing one risk factor to be counterbalanced and subtracted from the total number of CVD risk factors in the patient, for the purpose of cardiovascular risk prediction.

CLINICAL PRESENTATION

Subjective

Typically, the patient may present without symptoms when diagnosed with dyslipidemia. Often, however, problems related to CVD, such as HTN or CAD, coexist.

Objective

The clinician, on noting an abnormal lipid profile, may be the first to diagnose dyslipidemia in the unsuspecting patient. Physical examination may reveal a carotid bruit or corneal arcus. In some forms of dyslipidemia, yellowish skin deposits of cholesterol called xanthomas may develop. These deposits commonly occur around the eyelids (xanthelasma) and extensor tendons. Interestingly, even with effective lipid-lowering therapy, these deposits tend not to regress.

DIAGNOSTIC REASONING

Diagnostic Tests

The main goal of diagnostic testing for dyslipidemia is to adequately characterize the levels of various components of the plasma lipid compartment, as these levels are used to categorize disease and to set treatment goals. The ACC/AHA guidelines identify four groups of patients for whom to target primary and secondary prevention and concentrate efforts aimed at reducing CV events:

1. Patients with ASCVD
2. Patients with LDL levels greater than or equal to 190 mg/dL, such as those with FH
3. Patients with diabetes mellitus aged 40 to 75 years with LDL between 70 and 189 mg/dL and without evidence of ASCVD
4. Patients without evidence of CVD or diabetes mellitus but who have LDL levels between 70 and 189 mg/dL, along with a 10-year risk of ASCVD greater than or equal to 7.5% (as determined by a CV risk calculator)

Testing to assess these higher-risk groups of patients with dyslipidemia is critical, as it is recommended that the first two groups use high-intensity statins and the last two groups use moderate-intensity statins to achieve lipid goals.

Differential Diagnosis

Some potential causes of secondary dyslipidemia are listed in Table 35.4. Elevated TC levels may be present in CAD, type II FH, idiopathic hypercholesterolemia, obstructive jaundice, biliary cirrhosis, hypothyroidism, von Gierke disease (glycogen storage disease type I), pregnancy, uncontrolled diabetes mellitus, pancreatic disease, chronic nephritis, glomerulosclerosis, and obesity. Of note, decreased TC levels may be present in malabsorption, starvation, anorexia nervosa, liver disease, severe cell damage, HTN, chronic anemia, and drug therapy with adrenocorticotropic hormones.

Elevated TG levels may be present in liver disease, alcoholism, nephrotic syndrome, renal disease, hypothyroidism, uncontrolled diabetes mellitus, pancreatitis, gout, post-MI (increased levels may last for 1 year), metabolic diseases related to endocrinopathies, von Gierke disease

TABLE 35.4 Potential Causes of Secondary Hyperlipidemia

Causes	Lipid Abnormalities
Inactivity	HDL ↓
Alcohol abuse	TG ↑, HDL ↑, LDL ↑
Diabetes mellitus	TG ↑, HDL ↓, TC ↑
Hypothyroidism	TG ↑, TC ↑
Thiazide diuretic use (high dose)	TC ↑, LDL ↑, TG ↑
Beta blocker use (high dose)	LDL ↑, HDL ↓
Chronic renal insufficiency	TC ↑, TG ↑

Abbreviations: HDL, high-density lipoprotein; LDL, low-density lipoprotein; TC, total cholesterol; TG, triglycerides.

(glycogen storage disease type I), stress, a high-carbohydrate diet, and HTN. In contrast, decreased TG levels may be present in malnutrition, hyperthyroidism, exercise, and malabsorption syndrome.

An elevated HDL level may be associated with chronic liver disease or chronic alcohol abuse/intoxication, long-term aerobic exercise or other vigorous exercise, and elevated estrogen levels or birth control pills. A decreased HDL level may be caused by hypertriglyceridemia, hypothyroidism, end-stage liver disease, diabetes mellitus, obesity, chronic inactivity, uremia, and homozygous Tangier disease (family-based alpha-lipoprotein deficiency).

An increased LDL level may be the result of FH or secondary causes such as a diet high in cholesterol and saturated fat, nephrotic syndrome, chronic renal failure, pregnancy, porphyria, diabetes mellitus, multiple myeloma, corticosteroid use, and estrogens. A decreased LDL level may be the result of malnutrition and malabsorption syndromes.

An increased VLDL level may be caused by familial hyperlipidemia or secondarily by alcoholism, obesity, diabetes mellitus, chronic renal disease, pancreatitis, pregnancy, estrogen, birth control pills, and progestins. A decreased VLDL level may be the result of malnutrition and malabsorption syndromes.

MANAGEMENT

The primary goals of dyslipidemia treatment are (1) lowering elevated LDL, (2) lowering elevated TG, and (3) raising suboptimal levels of HDL to prevent CVD.

Dietary Modification

A cholesterol-lowering diet is recommended for all Americans. Diets very low in total fat or in saturated fat, however, may lower protective HDL-C as much as they do LDL-C. Most nutritionists advocate reducing total fat to 25% to 30% of daily calories and saturated fat to less than 7% of daily calories. The Mediterranean diet has also been shown to decrease cholesterol levels in some patients. This diet is a heart-healthy eating plan that emphasizes fruits, vegetables, whole grains, beans, nuts and seeds, and healthy fats.

Pharmacological Therapy

For years, diet has been the cornerstone of treatment for hyperlipidemia; however, recent studies have demonstrated that diet alone is often insufficient in lowering cholesterol. The 3-hydroxy-3-methylglutaryl coenzyme A (HMG-CoA) reductase inhibitors (medications with generic names ending in -*statin*) are the first-line drugs of choice in the majority of hyperlipidemic patients. Drugs Commonly Prescribed 35.2 presents information on the different levels of statin therapy along with specific dosages; statin therapies are categorized as either moderate or high intensity. Although some practitioners recommend them, evidence is less consistent to support the use of fibrates, niacin, or fish oil to treat hyperlipidemia.

Once the initial dose of a statin medication is prescribed, the clinician should consider whether to increase the dose or add another agent if the statin is ineffective or not fully effective at the initial dose (see Drugs Commonly Prescribed 35.2 for commonly used combination formulations). The clinician should caution patients about use of statins with hepatotoxic drugs or alcohol. Other adverse effects include muscle weakness and, in extreme cases, rhabdomyolysis with significant elevations in serum creatine phosphokinase (creatine kinase [CK]) and aldolase levels. Gastrointestinal (GI) complaints include dyspepsia and abdominal pain.

To determine whether a patient should be on a statin, the clinician should consider the following four questions; if any of the responses is yes, the patient is a potential candidate for statin therapy:

1. Does the patient have a history of any of the following?
   a. ACS
   b. MI
   c. Stable or unstable angina
   d. Coronary or arterial revascularization
   e. Stroke or TIA
   f. Peripheral arterial disease of atherosclerotic origin
2. Does the patient have an LDL level greater than or equal to 190 mg/dL (indicative of FH)?
3. Is the patient 40 to 75 years of age with diabetes mellitus?
4. Is the patient 40 to 75 years of age with a 10-year cardiovascular risk of greater than or equal to 7.5%?

For patients with ASCVD who are younger than 75 years, high-intensity statin therapy should be used to reduce their LDL-C levels by 50%. For patients older than 75 years, moderate-intensity therapy should be instituted. Moderate-intensity statin therapy should

Drugs Commonly Prescribed 35.2: Statin Therapy for Hyperlipidemia

DRUG	EFFECT ON LIPIDS	ADVERSE REACTIONS AND PRESCRIBING CONSIDERATIONS
HMG-CoA Reductase Inhibitors (Statins)		
High-Intensity: Atorvastatin (Lipitor) 40–80 mg Rosuvastatin (Crestor) 20–40 mg	Decreases LDL by up to 50% on average Increases HDL Decrease TGs	May cause myositis (especially in patients taking fibrates or niacin). Do not use with gemfibrozil. Take in the evening.
Moderate-Intensity: Atorvastatin (Lipitor) 10–20 mg Lovastatin (Mevacor) 40 mg–80 mg Pravastatin (Pravachol) 40–80 mg Rosuvastatin (Crestor) 5–10 mg Simvastatin (Zocor) 20–40 mg Pitavastatin (Livalo) 2–4 mg	Decreases LDL by 30%–50% on average	Do not give to patients with active or chronic liver disease. Monitor liver function tests before initiating therapy.
Combination Therapy		
Statin plus CCB: Atorvastatin + amlodipine (Caduet)	Decreases LDL Increases HDL Decreases TGs	May cause edema, dizziness, palpitations, flushing, fatigue, constipation, dyspepsia, abdominal pain, drowsiness, myopathy, elevated liver enzymes, and rhabdomyolysis with renal dysfunction. Monitor liver function before the start of therapy. May increase serum levels of digitalis, hormone concentrations from birth control pills.
Statin plus ezetimibe: Atorvastatin + ezetimibe (Liptruzet) Simvastatin + ezetimibe (Vytorin) Statin plus niacin: Lovastatin + niacin (Advicor) Simvastatin + niacin (Simcor)	Atorvastatin + ezetimibe combination lowers LDL by approximately 10% more than atorvastatin alone, but this may not translate to better patient outcomes.	May cause headache, fatigue, myalgia, extremity pain, myopathy, rhabdomyolysis, and elevated serum transaminases. Avoid fibrates, alcohol, and grapefruit juice. May potentiate vasoactive drugs. Monitor warfarin and antidiabetics. Niacin-containing combinations may cause flushing, headache, pain, pruritus, and dyspepsia.

Abbreviations: CCBs, calcium channel blockers; HDL, high-density lipoprotein; LDL, low-density lipoprotein; TGs, triglycerides.

be used for patients with diabetes mellitus aged 40 to 75 years because the goal is to reduce the LDL-C level by 30% to 49%. If these patients have a 10-year cardiovascular risk of greater than 7.5%, high-intensity therapy should be used. In addition, for patients aged 40 to 75 years without CVD or diabetes mellitus, but who have a cardiovascular risk score greater than 7.5% and an LDL level of 70 to 189 mg/dL, moderate-intensity therapy is also acceptable.

If patients do not fall into any of the previous categories, additional factors should be considered that suggest the need for statin therapy, such as family history of premature ASCVD in a first-degree relative, high-sensitivity C-reactive protein (hsCRP) greater than 2 mg/dL, presence of calcification on a coronary artery calcium scan, and an ankle-brachial index (BP ratio) of less than 0.9.

FOLLOW-UP AND REFERRAL

Because hyperlipidemia is so common, the clinician must be prepared to treat patients with this condition. If treatment goals are not reached, consultation with a cardiologist may be indicated. Consultation with a nutritionist may be recommended if the patient cannot follow or understand how to adhere to a cholesterol-lowering diet. Endocrinological referral is indicated for FH.

Patient Education: Dyslipidemia

Lifestyle counseling should occur at the initial and follow-up visits as the foundation for statin or other cholesterol-lowering pharmacotherapy and may lower the patient's overall risk of morbidity due to hyperlipidemia. It is important for the clinician to provide ongoing support and reinforcement to patients undertaking both dietary modification and pharmacological therapy for dyslipidemia. Many patients do not like to take medications and feel that dietary modification alone is sufficient to keep their cholesterol "under control." Showing patients their laboratory testing results and discussing what the numbers actually mean, in terms of their risk of having an MI, is an effective way to get the patient to focus on the potential benefits of combined dietary and pharmacotherapy.

Calculating the patient's 10-year cardiovascular risk score may facilitate the conversation about the possible need for statin therapy. The risk of having an acute coronary event may help to motivate a patient in adhering to a comprehensive diet, exercise, and drug treatment program. The ACC/AHA urges clinicians to use shared decision-making models. In turn, the Circle of Caring model encourages shared decision making and supports patients in initiating long-term lifestyle and medication changes.

- Family history of CAD
- African, Indigenous, or Hispanic descent

Modifiable:

- Hypertension (greater than 140 mm Hg SBP and/or greater than 90 mm Hg DBP, depending on age)
- Smoking
- Excessive alcohol use
- Sedentary lifestyle
- Unhealthy diet
- Hyperlipidemia
- For women: natural or surgical menopause without estrogen replacement therapy; oral contraceptive use combined with cigarette smoking

The following are contributing factors. It could be debatable that they are modifiable factors considering that the patient may alter the condition with diet, exercise, weight loss, pharmacotherapy, and stress-reduction techniques like meditation and yoga.

- Diabetes mellitus
- Obesity
- Stress

CORONARY HEART DISEASE

CHD is the leading cause of death in the United States, responsible for more than one in seven deaths per year. Every 37 seconds in the United States, one person will die of heart disease. Nonetheless, mortality from CHD has declined in recent years because of patient education regarding risk factors; early recognition and treatment of CHD symptoms; management of comorbidities such as HTN, dyslipidemia, and diabetes mellitus; and therapeutic advances such as thrombolytic drugs.

EPIDEMIOLOGY AND CAUSES

More than 18 million Americans have CHD, the incidence of which increases with age. The cost of health-care services, medicines, and lost productivity due to death from CHD costs the United States approximately $219 billion each year.

The causes of CHD are reflected in a number of risk factors that are classified as nonmodifiable, modifiable, or contributing. These risk factors are ostensibly associated with the development of ASCVD, which is the primary etiology of CHD.

Risk Factors: Coronary Heart Disease

Nonmodifiable:

- Male gender
- Increasing age

PATHOPHYSIOLOGY

The coronary arteries provide arterial blood flow that supplies oxygen and nutrients to cardiac muscle tissue to allow for optimal myocellular function of the heart. The coronary arteries dilate via the release of vasoactive substances that further augment oxygen delivery to keep pace with changing metabolic demands. In addition, the lumen of each coronary artery needs to be patent to maintain optimal tissue perfusion.

In CAD, arteriosclerotic plaque formation along the inner vessel walls hinders optimal blood flow. Coronary arteries become obstructed, stiffened, and incapable of vasodilation, which severely impedes perfusion of the myocardium. During physical exertion, when increased blood flow to the heart is required for greater myocardial contractility, coronary artery blood flow becomes insufficient for the oxygen demands of the myocardium.

This coronary insufficiency, in turn, leads to ischemia of heart muscle. Ischemia creates anaerobic conditions for the myocardium, particularly if acute occlusion of the coronary vessels results. Anaerobic metabolism yields inadequate energy (approximately 5% of normal) for myocardial demand, allowing for less than a 20-minute period of tissue viability after occlusion. Lactic acid is created as a waste product, leading to localized tissue acidosis. Because lactic acid is irritating to muscle tissue, lactic acid buildup is the source of chest pain in ischemic heart disease. Thus, if left untreated, CAD will progress to ischemia of the heart muscle, resulting in angina pectoris (i.e., chest pain due to cardiac ischemia), which can then lead to an MI if the ischemia is persistent.

Although it is the main cause of CHD, atherosclerosis (arteriosclerosis) is a systemic disease affecting all arteries of the body. *Arteriosclerosis* means "hardened arteries," which is an apt term for the rigid arteries resulting from long-term plaque formation along the vessel wall. Once CAD is diagnosed, it is likely that arteriosclerosis is present throughout all arterial systems, in addition to the heart. Likewise, if vascular disease is identified in target end organs, CAD is likely to already be present. The process of arteriosclerosis begins with endothelial injury, which can be incited by a number of etiological agents.

Free radicals, HTN, hyperglycemia, and hyperlipidemia have all been found to be agents of injury to arterial endothelial cells that can precipitate atherosclerosis. Endothelial injury provokes an inflammatory reaction that attracts T cells, macrophages, monocytes, and platelets to the site. White blood cells (WBCs) secrete inflammatory cytokines, such as interleukins and tumor necrosis factor-α (TNF-α), as well as acute phase reactants like CRP, which perpetuate the inflammatory reaction. In turn, platelets aggregate and form microthrombi along the vessel wall. Inflammation is now thought to be the major force that drives atherosclerosis. This idea is supported by the prognostic utility of hsCRP levels as a predictor of cardiovascular risk in individuals with coronary arteriosclerosis.

Inflammation of the endothelium depletes nitric oxide, a major vasorelaxant of the arterial muscle wall. This depletion results in a net vasoconstrictive effect. Other proinflammatory mediators stimulate proliferation of vascular smooth muscle within the arterial wall, which further intensifies the vasoconstrictive effect. Concurrently, macrophages within the vessel wall engulf and ingest LDL, forming foam cells. Disruptions of the arterial endothelium by inflammation, lipid-laden macrophages, platelets, and vasoconstricting mediators are the initiating events of arteriosclerosis and atherogenesis.

In the process of atherogenesis, an initial fatty streak on the arterial wall evolves over time, serving as a nidus for fibrin deposition to become a fibrous, calcified plaque. As they become lined by calcified arteriosclerotic plaque, arteries lose significant vasodilatory capacity. The lipid-rich, calcified plaque becomes brittle and unstable, easily rupturing with mechanical stress due to increased or turbulent blood flow, such as that seen with uncontrolled HTN. When disruption of the plaque occurs, this induces platelet aggregation and activation of the coagulation cascade. A thrombus forms at the site of endothelial injury that can ultimately break free (embolize), lodge in, and obstruct the lumen of narrowed arteries.

In patients who die of unstable angina or MI, pathological studies find that death occurs as a result of a ruptured plaque with associated thrombosis. Obstruction due to thrombosis is the most common cause of ischemia in *any* arterially supplied region of the body. Ischemia-prone regions of the body include the myocardium, brain, and lower extremities. Common sites of arteriosclerosis are the coronary arteries (i.e., CAD potentially resulting in ACS, including MI), cerebral arteries (potentially resulting in stroke), and peripheral arteries of the lower extremities (potentially resulting in peripheral arterial insufficiency, a form of peripheral vascular disease).

CLINICAL PRESENTATION

Subjective

In most patients, CHD develops many years before the patient is aware of its existence. Because collateral circulation develops, the patient is usually unaware that anything is wrong unless other concomitant conditions are present, such as dyslipidemia or HTN. Thus, the medical history should include a detailed description of all risk factors that may be present, which will guide further assessment for resultant problems such as angina (pertinent questions related to angina are covered in the section on Acute Coronary Syndrome).

Typically, symptoms of CHD are not reported until 75% of a coronary artery is narrowed due to atherosclerosis. Eventually, if CHD is left untreated, the patient will usually present with exertional angina, which should lead the clinician to suspect CHD. Angina is the presenting symptom in CHD in 38% of men and 61% of women. Middle-aged and older men and postmenopausal women are most prone to developing angina. Associated symptoms may include radiation of the discomfort to the left arm and jaw, nausea, shortness of breath, and lightheadedness or syncopal episodes. It should be noted that not all patients present with these typical CHD symptoms (see Differential Diagnosis on page 549).

Objective

For the patient with known or suspected CHD, the clinician should note all the peripheral pulses; auscultate for carotid bruits; note jugular venous distention; take the BP in sitting, lying, and standing positions; and examine the skin and nailbeds for evidence of decreased perfusion (e.g., prolonged capillary refill time). Because atherosclerosis is a widespread problem, patients with CHD also have a much higher incidence of peripheral vascular disease and cerebrovascular disease than other individuals. In turn, the clinician should assess for other symptoms that suggest vascular insufficiency, such as intermittent claudication or TIAs.

DIAGNOSTIC REASONING

Diagnostic Tests

An ECG, cardiac stress test, nuclear myocardial scanning, and coronary angiography may be ordered to determine the extent of CAD as an etiology of CHD and to identify which vessels are affected. Twelve-lead ECGs are discussed in detail later in this chapter in the section on Diagnostic Tests for Acute Coronary Syndrome.

An exercise ECG or cardiac stress test may be ordered to detect and evaluate potential ischemia due to CAD. In these tests, carefully controlled and supervised exercise increases myocardial oxygen demand, which evaluates the coronary arteries' ability to meet this demand for increased myocardial perfusion successfully. When the patient is unable to achieve a vigorous level of exercise to meet the required testing parameters, a dipyridamole thallium-201 nuclear stress test may be used. These tests may produce false-positive readings, however, especially in women and in the presence of certain drugs such as beta blockers and CCBs that blunt the adrenergic response or with electrolyte imbalances. A stress test is contraindicated in the presence of known acute CVD (e.g., MI, unstable angina, or HF) because the heart cannot respond to the increased demand for oxygen.

Nuclear scanning of the heart (technetium-99m ventriculography) assesses the motion of the left ventricular wall and measures the ventricle's ability to eject blood, referred to as the ejection fraction (EF) (normally 55% to 75%). When ischemia is present because of a narrowed coronary artery, the segment of the myocardium served by that particular artery exhibits diminished wall motion (hypokinesis) or contractility that is represented as pooled blood within the ventricular and atrial chambers.

Contrast-enhanced CT scan imaging of the coronary arteries is a noninvasive imaging method of assessing overall "plaque burden" (i.e., the extent to which atheromatous plaque undermines the integrity of an arterial wall). Estimating plaque burden assesses the risk of atheromatous plaque rupturing from the vessel wall and causing ischemia. This type of CT scan, also termed *CT calcium scoring*, evaluates the overall burden of calcified atherosclerotic plaque in the coronary vessels.

A diagnostic cardiac catheterization with angiography for coronary artery visualization is commonly performed after stabilizing a patient in ACS or if there is a high suspicion of ACS. Visualization of the coronary arteries confirms the diagnosis of CAD and can evaluate the extent of coronary artery stenosis. Cardiac catheterization can also be used for interventional purposes to unblock clogged coronary arteries, as discussed in the section on Management of Acute Coronary Syndrome.

Ultrasonography can be used with cardiac catheterization to add diagnostic information. Intravascular ultrasonography (IVUS) used during cardiac catheterization measures plaque burden through real-time intraluminal imaging of vessel walls. IVUS can also be used to assess plaque regression when the patient is on drug therapy for hyperlipidemia.

Because arteriosclerosis is a chronic inflammatory condition, the biomarker CRP is commonly elevated in individuals with CHD. CRP is an acute-phase inflammatory protein produced by the liver and the smooth muscle cells within arteriosclerotic coronary arteries. An elevated level of CRP, as detected by the hsCRP test with greater sensitivity (i.e., a reduced lower limit of detection) than standard CRP testing, has been shown to be an independent predictor of the risk of MI, stroke, peripheral arterial disease, and sudden cardiac death. Measurement of hsCRP adds to the total cardiac risk assessment of the patient but should not be solely relied on as a confirmatory test, given its lack of specificity, because CRP levels may be nonspecifically elevated in many different inflammatory conditions of noncardiac etiology.

Epidemiological studies show that an elevated level of the amino acid homocysteine is an independent risk factor for arteriosclerosis and CHD. Homocysteine requires folic acid, vitamin B_6, and vitamin B_{12} for its metabolism. In turn, this amino acid accumulates in the blood and injures the endothelium when there are inadequate levels of the B complex vitamins and folate for its proper metabolism. Therefore, an elevated serum homocysteine level adds to the cardiac risk assessment of a patient. Of note, reducing homocysteine levels with vitamin supplements has not been shown to reduce the risk of heart disease.

Differential Diagnosis

The key clinical finding of CHD, angina pectoris, may be produced by many causes. A thrombus, coronary artery vasospasm, aortic stenosis, aortic insufficiency, severe HTN, or idiopathic subaortic hypertrophic stenosis can also lead to angina. In addition, the differential diagnosis for CHD also includes GI, pulmonary, and cardiac problems that are not related to ischemia. For example, gastroesophageal reflux disease, esophageal spasm, or biliary colic can present with angina and other symptoms similar to MI, and by the same token, patients with CHD or MI often present with epigastric pain that is misinterpreted as "heartburn" or related pain. This misinterpretation is often the reason for a patient's delay in obtaining prompt medical evaluation for ACS, including MI.

Patients with anxiety or panic attacks often present to the emergency department with symptoms that mimic angina or an MI. For example, extreme stress can precipitate chest pain, dizziness, dyspnea, and hyperventilation, all of which mimic the symptoms of angina or an MI. Costochondritis, a musculoskeletal problem due to nonspecific inflammation of the articular joints of the chest wall (e.g., rib cage, clavicle, sternum), can also present as chest pain that may be misinterpreted as CHD by patients. However, the pain of costochondritis is typically not constant and can usually be reproduced as point tenderness by pressing on the sternum and costochondral regions of the chest.

Persons with diabetes mellitus may experience angina or MI with minor symptoms or no symptoms at all (e.g., a silent MI), given the resultant nerve-related damage that occurs with chronic hyperglycemia, which blunts cardiac-related pain. For example, some patients with CHD may experience nausea and vomiting, dyspnea, epigastric pain, diaphoresis, or dizziness with no complaint of chest pain. These symptoms are referred to as "anginal equivalents" and can be particularly common in older patients.

In addition, women experiencing angina or MI commonly present with anginal equivalents rather than with classic radiating chest pain. Historically, clinicians have underestimated the risk of CHD in women, as atypical presentations of ACS in women contribute to the lack of early recognition of cardiac symptoms by both patients and clinicians. Women classically delay seeking medical care for ischemic symptoms, which contributes to their overall higher morbidity and mortality rates with cardiac events.

Because chest pain is often the impetus for the diagnosis of CHD, the pain characteristics that drive the differential diagnoses of CHD need to be carefully assessed. For example, in a young, otherwise healthy adult, reproducible point tenderness is likely musculoskeletal chest wall pain and not ischemic in nature. In addition, pneumothorax, pneumonia, pericarditis, pulmonary embolism, mitral valve prolapse, and aortic dissection are all less common causes of chest pain that may mimic ischemic angina due to CAD. Pleuritic chest pain worsens on inspiration and is likely due to lung pathology, such as pneumonia, especially if accompanied by fever and a productive cough. Of note, the pain of pericarditis may be alleviated by having the patient sit up and lean forward. Thus, the clinician needs to have a high level of suspicion and complete a thorough cardiac risk assessment to rule out CHD, as well as a frank MI, in all patients complaining of chest pain or anginal equivalents.

MANAGEMENT

The principles of management of CHD include establishing the diagnosis, controlling symptoms, and preventing disease progression that may lead to MI or sudden death. During a cardiac catheterization, fibrinolytic agents may be infused directly into an occluded coronary artery in an attempt to restore coronary blood flow. Other therapeutic approaches include balloon angioplasty, stent placement, and coronary artery bypass graft (CABG). Presently, there are two types of stents in use, bare-metal stents and drug-eluting stents impregnated with medication (e.g., everolimus, paclitaxel, sirolimus) designed to prevent restenosis of the stented lumen. With both types of stents, dual antiplatelet therapy (DAPT) should be started for its antithrombotic effects, consisting of aspirin and a $P2Y_{12}$ receptor inhibitor (e.g., clopidogrel [Plavix], prasugrel [Effient], ticagrelor [Brilinta], cangrelor [Kengreal]). Drug-eluting stents require a longer duration of DAPT anticoagulation therapy than bare-metal stents, i.e., at least 6 months versus 1 month, respectively.

Risk Factor Modification

Risk factor modification is essential to stop the progression of CHD. This involves aggressive lowering of lipid levels (as discussed in the section on Dyslipidemia); strict glycemic control in patients with diabetes mellitus (see Chapter 59); aggressive antihypertensive therapy (discussed in the section on Hypertension); smoking cessation (see Chapter 33) and cessation of all other tobacco use (e.g., chewing/dipping, nasal "snuff" tobacco, vaping or e-cigarettes); and modifying lifestyle behaviors to include regular exercise, stress reduction, and a heart-healthy diet (i.e., less than 300 mg of cholesterol per day and 7% or less of total calories from saturated fats).

Pharmacological Therapy

Pharmacological agents are used to control the anginal symptoms of CHD and to prevent subsequent cardiovascular events (see the section on Management of Acute Coronary Syndrome). Most clinicians recommend low-dose daily aspirin (81 mg) taken at bedtime to decrease the incidence of a first MI in middle-aged men and women. Coated aspirin is recommended for individuals with gastric problems or GI intolerance. There is controversy over whether aspirin should be used concomitantly in patients on other anticoagulants and, if so, what dosage is recommended.

Complementary Therapy

Complementary Therapies 35.1 presents suggested vitamin, mineral, and herbal supplements for various cardiovascular disorders. Of note, the isolated effects of these agents have not been as rigorously tested for positive outcomes and an acceptable risk-benefit profile in CHD or other cardiovascular conditions as have the medications recommended in the Management sections of this chapter.

FOLLOW-UP AND REFERRAL

Patients need to understand the chronicity of CHD and be committed to frequent follow-ups for the control of cardiovascular risk factors. The clinician should refer the patient to a cardiologist for a cardiac stress test and any further work-up indicated by the results.

> **Patient Education: Coronary Heart Disease**
>
> At each visit, the clinician should stress cardiac risk factor modification. The lifestyle modifications listed in Box 35.2 for managing HTN are good activities to stress in patient education for overall cardiovascular health.

Complementary Therapies 35.1: Cardiac Conditions

AGENT	INDICATION	ADVERSE REACTIONS AND CONSIDERATIONS*
Hawthorn	Angina, CHF, CHD, functional cardiovascular disorders, HTN (in diabetes mellitus), orthostatic hypotension	May cause abdominal discomfort, agitation, arrhythmia, diaphoresis, dizziness, dyspnea, fatigue, headache, palpitations, sleeplessness, or rash. Caution with the following: HTN medications (increased risk of hypotension), antilipemic agents (additive effects), CCBs (additive vasodilation), cardiac glycosides, and vasodilators (additive vasodilation). Monitor BP, coagulation panel, heart rate, and lipid profile.
Magnesium	Arrhythmia, acute MI, CHD, HTN, mitral valve prolapse	May cause areflexia, asthenia, cardiac arrhythmias, cardiac arrest, drowsiness, hypermagnesemia, hypotension, loss of tendon reflexes, polydipsia, or respiratory paralysis. Caution with the following: aminoglycosides (increased risk of muscular weakness and paralysis), antibiotics (decreased effects), antidiabetic agents (increased absorption), and antihypertensive agents (additive effects). Monitor alkaline phosphatase, blood glucose, BP, calcium levels, coagulation panel, cortisol, LFTs, ECG, and parathyroid hormone.
Beta-glucan	Antioxidant, CHD, cardioprotection during CABG, hyperlipidemia, HTN	May cause dizziness, flushing, headache, HTN or hypotension, inflammatory airway disease, keratoderma, nausea, polyuria, urticaria, or vomiting. Caution with the following: antidiabetic agents (additive effects), antihypertensive agents (additive effects), and antilipemic agents (additive effects). Monitor blood glucose, BP, lipid profile, and WBC count.
Selenium	Antioxidant, cardiomyopathy, CHD prevention, circulation	May cause digitalis dysfunction, garlic-like breath odor, hepatorenal dysfunction, irritability, loss or thickening of hair and nails, metallic taste, muscle tenderness, nausea/vomiting, nervous system abnormalities, skin lesions, thrombocytopenia, tremor, or weakness. Caution with the following: barbiturates (increased sedation), HMG-CoA reductase inhibitors (decreased efficacy), and niacin (decreased efficacy).
Vitamin B_6	Angioplasty, CHD, CHD risk reduction, coronary restenosis, reduction in homocysteine level	Prolonged excessive use may cause neuropathy. Monitor vitamin B_6 levels.
Vitamin B_{12}	Angioplasty, CHD, coronary restenosis, reduction in homocysteine level, orthostatic tremor (restless legs syndrome)	Monitor vitamin B_{12} levels.
Vitamin C	Atherosclerosis, circulation, ischemic heart disease, MI risk reduction	In large doses may cause abdominal cramps, diarrhea, nausea, or skin rashes. In diabetics, may cause falsely elevated blood glucose readings. Caution with iron (increased iron levels) and warfarin (in high doses, lowers prothrombin time). Monitor vitamin C levels, although excess is typically excreted in the urine.
Vitamin E	Angina, reduced arterial elasticity, atherosclerosis, CHD, HF, dyslipidemias, intermittent claudication, deep venous thrombosis	May cause abdominal pain, blurred vision, diarrhea, fatigue, or headache. Increased risk of mortality with high doses with history of severe CHD (stroke or MI). Caution with the following: anticoagulants/antiplatelet agents (increased risk of bleeding) and chemotherapy (interferes with effectiveness). Monitor vitamin E levels, and monitor coagulation panel (with high doses); discontinue use 2 weeks before dental or surgical procedures.

Continued

Complementary Therapies 35.1: Cardiac Conditions—cont'd

AGENT	INDICATION	ADVERSE REACTIONS AND CONSIDERATIONS*
Flaxseed oil	CHD, HTN, hyperlipidemia	May cause abdominal discomfort, anaphylaxis, bleeding, bowel obstruction, constipation, diarrhea, dyspnea, hypoglycemia, hypotension, mania, nausea/vomiting, increased risk of prostate cancer, pruritus, skin rash, sneezing, stuffy nose, seizures, or watery eyes. Contraindicated with hypertriglyceridemia. Caution with the following: anticoagulants/antiplatelet agents (increased risk of bleeding), antidiabetic agents (increased risk of hypoglycemia), antihypertensives (increased risk of hypotension), antilipemic agents (decreased effects on triglycerides), furosemide (decreased absorption of furosemide). Monitor alkaline phosphatase, blood glucose, coagulation panel, inflammatory markers, lipid profile, PSA, red blood cells, and triglycerides.
Garlic	Anticoagulant, atherosclerosis, familial hypercholesterolemia, hyperlipidemia, HTN, prevention of MI, peripheral vascular disease	May cause anorexia, bleeding, burning inside the mouth, chills, constipation, diarrhea, dizziness, diaphoresis, dyspepsia, dyspnea, fever, flatulence, halitosis, hyperglycemia, or hypoglycemia.
Lycopene	CHD, HTN	May cause abdominal pain, cramps, anorexia, diarrhea, flatulence, or nausea/vomiting. Monitor androgen, lipid profile, and PSA.
Coenzyme Q10	Adjunct to statin therapy, angina, cardiomyopathy, cardioprotection during surgery, HF, CHD, hyperlipidemia, HTN, and MI	May cause bleeding, diarrhea, dizziness, dyspnea, fatigue, flu-like symptoms, GI upset, headache, heartburn, hyperglycemia or hypoglycemia, hypotension, insomnia, irritability, loss of appetite, nausea/vomiting, photosensitivity, pruritus, rash, thrombosis, or thyroid hormone alterations. Caution with antidiabetic agents (altered effects), antihypertensives (additive effects), antilipemic agents (additive effects), corticosteroids (decreased effects), and warfarin (decreased anticoagulant effects). Monitor blood glucose, BP, coagulation panel, LFTs, lipid profile, and CD4 lymphocyte T_4/T_8 ratio.
Calcium	HTN	May cause abdominal pain, arrhythmias, calcium deposits in heart and kidney, chalky taste in mouth, confusion, constipation, GI irritation, headache, irritability, MI, nausea/vomiting, nephrotoxicity, polydipsia, polyuria, renal calculi, skin reactions, or urinary incontinence. Caution with CCBs (decreased effects) and levothyroxine (decreased effectiveness). Monitor bone mineral density, calcium levels, and renal function tests.
Red yeast rice	CHD, hyperlipidemia	May cause bloating, dizziness, flatulence, GI discomfort, headache, or kidney damage. Caution with alcohol (increased risk of liver damage), gemfibrozil and niacin (increased risk of myopathy), HMG-CoA reductase inhibitors (increased risk of adverse effects), protease inhibitors (altered effects). Monitor LFTs and kidney function.

*For an extensive review and additional information on these agents, see Ulbricht C. *Davis's pocket guide to herbs and supplements.* FA Davis; 2011.

Abbreviations: BP, blood pressure; CABG, coronary artery bypass graft; CCB, calcium channel blocker; CHD, coronary heart disease; CHF, congestive heart failure; ECG, electrocardiogram; GI, gastrointestinal; HF, heart failure; HMG-CoA; 3-hydroxy-3-methylglutaryl coenzyme A; HTN, hypertension; LFTs, liver function tests; MI, myocardial infarction; PSA, prostate-specific antigen; WBC, white blood cell.

ACUTE CORONARY SYNDROME

ACS is a term used for the disorders of myocardial ischemia, such as unstable angina, MI, and variant angina (Prinzmetal's angina). The three traditional types of ACS are non–ST-elevation MI (NSTEMI), ST-elevation MI (STEMI), and unstable angina. Unstable angina due to myocardial ischemia is newly diagnosed angina or previously diagnosed angina that has changed in pattern, frequency, or severity. Unstable angina is commonly a forerunner of acute MI, which is necrosis or death of the myocardium as a result of prolonged ischemia due to an insufficient supply of oxygenated blood. Variant angina may occur in patients with normal coronary arteries who have cyclically recurring angina at rest that is unrelated to effort.

Although ACS, by definition, refers to acute conditions, stable angina is also covered in this section. Stable angina (chronic exertional angina) is a diagnosed condition of myocardial ischemia that is predictable in pattern and frequency and controlled with medication.

EPIDEMIOLOGY AND CAUSES

Each year, an estimated 605,000 Americans have a new ACS attack and almost 200,000 have a recurrent attack. Patients with a previous MI are the highest risk group for further coronary events. ACS is responsible for one-third of total deaths in individuals over the age of 35 years. This amounts to a new coronary event approximately every 40 seconds. About 20% of MIs are silent. More men than women experience MIs; however, after menopause this gap dramatically closes. The average age for a first MI is 64.5 years in men and 70.3 years in women. MIs are more common in Western societies, and African American patients have a higher incidence of MI due in part to the greater incidence of HTN in that population. The mortality rate is approximately 30% for a severe MI.

The contributing causative factors for ACS (including MI) are the same as those for CHD discussed in the previous section. In addition, tachycardia, LVH, anemia, increased platelet aggregation, and the abuse of illegal substances (particularly sympathomimetics, such as cocaine and amphetamines) all may contribute to decreased perfusion of the coronary arteries.

PATHOPHYSIOLOGY

ACS is a broad term describing a continuum of disorders that arise from coronary artery occlusion. ACS denotes high-risk forms of angina pectoris (e.g., unstable or variant angina) or an MI. In both angina and MI, decreased myocardial perfusion occurs because of coronary artery narrowing caused by thrombus formation subsequent to rupture of atherosclerotic plaque. In stable angina, which is not considered a form of ACS, coronary artery occlusion causes a brief episode of ischemia that is treatable and reversible. In contrast, in unstable angina, coronary artery occlusion causes ischemia with a high risk of MI, which can occur with prolonged ischemia. Variant angina, on the other hand, is an atypical form of angina pectoris that occurs as a result of vasospasm of otherwise normal coronary arteries.

Two types of MI are classified according to their electrocardiographic changes: NSTEMI and STEMI. NSTEMI indicates an infarction caused by a nonocclusive thrombus that partially interrupts perfusion of the myocardium and results in an infarction affecting only part of the myocardial wall, rather than its full thickness. STEMI is caused by an occlusive thrombus that leads to a complete transmural MI, which is an infarction of the full thickness of the myocardial wall. The majority of MIs are NSTEMIs. Table 35.5 describes a universal definition of MI based on pathophysiology.

TABLE 35.5	Definition of MI Based on Pathophysiology	
Type	Classification	Clinical and diagnostic Criteria
1	Spontaneous MI	Plaque rupture, ulceration, fissuring, erosion, or dissection, resulting in coronary thrombosis
2	Supply/demand mismatch	Mismatch between myocardial oxygen supply and demand, driven by a secondary process other than CAD
3	Suspected MI-related death	Cardiac death in a setting suggestive of ischemic process without definitive cardiac biomarker evidence of MI
4a	PCI-related MI	Rise in cardiac biomarkers accompanied by symptoms, ECG, angiographical, or imaging evidence of ischemia after PCI
4b	Stent thrombosis	Confirmed stent thrombosis in context of ischemia and dynamic cardiac biomarker changes
5	CABG-related MI	Rise in cardiac biomarkers accompanied by ECG, angiographical, or imaging evidence of ischemia after CABG

Abbreviations: CABG, coronary artery bypass graft; CAD, coronary artery disease; ECG, electrocardiogram; MI, myocardial infarction; PCI, percutaneous coronary intervention.
Source: Thygesen K, Alpert JS, Jaffe AS, et al. Fourth universal definition of myocardial infarction (2018). *Circulation.* 2018;138:e618–e651.

After myocardial ischemia occurs, anaerobic metabolism becomes the predominant form of energy production in the affected cardiac tissue. Anaerobic metabolism yields a low energy output that can sustain the heart tissue for a maximum of only 20 minutes. Death of myocardial tissue due to infarction occurs as energy requirements are not met, thus underscoring the importance of acute beta blocker therapy in the management of MI to decrease cardiac workload and myocardial oxygen demand. Moreover, lactic acid, a waste product of anaerobic metabolism, is noxious to surrounding cells, further disrupting cellular function.

Necrosis in the infarcted region of the myocardial wall disrupts the conduction system and decreases the strength of the heart muscle as a mechanical pump. In turn, arrhythmias and HF are common sequelae of an MI. In particular, the more damage to the heart muscle, the greater the risk of HF. Papillary muscle rupture is also a common complication that may result from an MI. Heart valve leaflets are attached to papillary muscles via string-like membranous attachments called chordae tendineae. Disrupted papillary muscles and ruptured chordae tendineae cause valvular dysfunction that manifests as a heart murmur due to turbulent blood flow. Specifically, MI of the left ventricle with papillary muscle rupture can cause dysfunction of the mitral valve, and mitral regurgitation is a common complication of left ventricular MI.

CLINICAL PRESENTATION

Subjective

As a common symptom of ACS, the patient with angina pectoris typically complains of chest discomfort that may be described as pressure, tightness, burning, or heaviness. The patient should be asked to describe the pain in terms of its quality, location, radiation, precipitating factors, alleviating factors, and associated signs and symptoms during the acute episode. Although angina pectoris is classically described as chest discomfort, the pain may radiate elsewhere, including to the arms, chest, back, neck, jaw, or teeth. Patients frequently describe the discomfort as feelings of indigestion because angina pectoris may also be accompanied by nausea or vomiting. The patient may also complain of shortness of breath and sweating, with symptoms developing either at rest or with physical activity. The patient may also be anxious, lightheaded, and tachycardic.

The pain of ACS may frequently occur after meals because of increased oxygen consumption during the meal and greater diversion of blood flow to the splanchnic circulation. Alternatively, ACS pain may be brought on by psychological stress. Rest and nitroglycerin, either via sublingual (SL) tablet or lingual spray, may relieve the symptoms of stable angina. In contrast, the pain of unstable angina tends to last longer and be of greater intensity than the pain of stable angina, whereas the pain of variant angina occurs at rest, due to spontaneous coronary vasospasm (see Table 35.6 for a description of the characteristics of the various forms of angina). Of note, patients may be in denial when experiencing angina pectoris and will often rationalize that the symptoms are caused by indigestion or overexertion.

In acute MI, the patient often complains of angina-like chest pain lasting more than 20 minutes, while occasionally waxing and waning during that period. Often, dyspnea, diaphoresis, nausea, and dizziness are also reported. Radiation of the pain to the neck, jaw, shoulder, or arm (left more often than right) is usually described. The degree of distress with these symptoms varies greatly, however, from the patient who complains of an "elephant sitting on my chest" to the patient who is apologetic for seeking assistance with "just a bit of indigestion that will not clear up." In particular, women, older adults, and persons with diabetes mellitus are likely to have minimal or atypical symptoms with an acute MI.

TABLE 35.6 Forms of Angina	
Type of Angina	*Characteristics*
Stable	Chest pain: transient episodes related to activities that increase myocardial oxygen demand Duration: typically lasts 3 to 15 minutes Associated signs and symptoms: nausea, vomiting, shortness of breath Relief: rest and/or nitroglycerin tablets
Unstable	Chest pain: more severe and brought on with less exertion; may occur at rest Duration: prolonged Associated signs and symptoms: nausea, vomiting, shortness of breath, diaphoresis Relief: not relieved by rest and/or nitroglycerin tablets; relieved by morphine
Variant (Prinzmetal's)	Chest pain: episodes unrelated to activities that increase myocardial oxygen demand Duration: cyclical; often occurs during sleep (most common in early morning hours); pain intensifies quickly and lasts longer than that of stable angina Associated signs and symptoms: palpitation, syncope, bradycardia Relief: may subside with exercise

About 20% of patients suffer a painless MI that may be detected only on a future ECG, on autopsy, or if the patient presents with other symptoms that prompt the clinician to more thoroughly evaluate for the possibility of an MI. This occurs more often in older patients or patients with diabetes mellitus or HTN. In these cases, patients may complain of dyspnea, general upper abdominal pain, exacerbation of HF, or acute confusion.

Objective

The cardiac examination in a patient suspected of having ACS should include inspection, palpation, and auscultation. As with any physical examination, the cardiac evaluation should begin with the general survey, as the clinician begins to develop a picture of the overall health status of the patient and continues to gather diagnostic clues.

In a patient with angina due to ACS, the clinician may auscultate a transient third (S_3) or fourth (S_4) heart sound, a transient mitral regurgitant murmur, and/or a carotid arterial bruit. In addition, the patient may appear dyspneic and be diaphoretic. In a patient specifically with an MI, the clinician may observe pallor, cool and diaphoretic skin, crackles on auscultation, a third (S_3) or fourth (S_4) heart sound, cardiac murmurs, edema of the extremities, and possibly jugular venous distention. In addition, the patient may have a low-grade fever. The presence of diaphoresis with chest pain is particularly worrisome, often indicating a significant drop in cardiac output during the episode of pain and subsequent decreased perfusion of the skin.

DIAGNOSTIC REASONING

Diagnostic Tests

Although chest pain can be caused by a number of conditions, assessing for ACS in the patient with angina pectoris is critical. In particular, given the life-threatening implications of an MI, the diagnostic work-up of a patient with suspected ACS must always rule out infarction. The most specific laboratory tests to rule out MI are cardiac-specific troponin I (cTnI) and T (cTnT) along with high sensitivity cardiac troponin I (hs-cTnI) assays. These troponins are cardiac proteins released from dead heart muscle, and they are essentially undetectable in the blood of healthy individuals. Troponin levels rise within the first 2 to 4 hours after an MI and remain elevated for 7 to 10 days. High-sensitivity cardiac troponin testing can provide results even sooner than traditional troponin testing. They are able to detect lower concentrations of the troponin proteins, thus facilitating more rapid identification of myocardial injury.

The muscle and brain isoforms of the creatine phosphokinase enzyme are also released from necrotic heart muscle after an MI. These isoenzymes are detected in the blood as a combined fraction of CK isoforms using the CK-myocardial band (MB) test. CK-MB levels rise within 4 to 8 hours after an MI and generally return to normal by 48 to 72 hours. The rise in CK-MB fraction also correlates better with infarct size than does troponin level.

CK-MB remains elevated in the blood for a shorter period of time than the cardiac troponins. Therefore, episodes of recurrent ischemia with resultant MI are more readily diagnosed by a rise in cardiac troponins. However, the prolonged elevation of cardiac troponins does not allow for recognition of repeat episodes of acute MI within the first few days after the initial insult. If the diagnosis of an MI remains uncertain, serum cardiac biomarkers should be measured on admission, at 6 to 9 hours after admission, and again after 12 to 14 hours.

Myoglobin is a muscle protein that rises in the blood within only a few hours after an acute MI. It is one of the earliest serum cardiac markers to rise after an MI; however, it is nonspecific for cardiac muscle death and can rise with skeletal muscle injury as well. Blood levels return to normal within 24 hours of infarction and cannot be relied on for diagnosis of MI. Other cardiac enzymes, which are rarely used in diagnostic work-ups, include serum glutamic oxaloacetic transaminase and lactate dehydrogenase; they become elevated in the serum much later in the course of an MI and are, therefore, not sensitive as indicators of an acute MI.

Other laboratory tests that should be drawn as part of a full work-up of ACS include a complete blood count (CBC), erythrocyte sedimentation rate (ESR), serum electrolyte panel, blood urea nitrogen (BUN), and serum creatinine. Leukocytosis is a nonspecific indicator of myocardial injury, as WBC counts often reach levels of 12,000 to 15,000 cells/μL. ESR, a general indicator of inflammation, also rises after an MI and remains elevated for several days.

After the patient is stabilized, echocardiography and cardiac catheterization with angiography are procedures that provide significant prognostic information. Echocardiography can be done to detect cardiac wall motion abnormalities, right and left ventricular dysfunction, valvular or septal defects, and left ventricular ejection fraction (LVEF). Echocardiography is a noninvasive procedure that is easily performed in most emergency departments; however, it is not recommended as a reliable diagnostic test of MI. When the patient is assessed via angiography, coronary artery occlusion can be estimated using the thrombolysis in myocardial infarction (TIMI) grading system. The TIMI scale grades coronary artery occlusion from grade 0, indicating complete occlusion, to grade 3, indicating full perfusion of the coronary artery with normal blood flow.

In addition, radionuclide imaging can detect reversible ischemic regions or fixed infarcted areas of the heart. Injected radionuclide tracer substances are distributed in proportion to myocardial blood flow. This type of imaging reveals a "cold spot" with decreased myocardial perfusion during the first few hours after an MI. However, it cannot distinguish an acute MI from the scarring of the myocardium due to an MI experienced in the past.

In the emergency department and urgent care settings, a 12-lead ECG is a critical tool to reveal myocardial ischemia, STEMI, NSTEMI, or cardiac arrhythmias, and should be performed promptly on presentation of a patient with suspected ACS to a clinical setting. The 12-lead ECG presents 12 leads or "views" of the heart to detect and localize myocardial damage (Figure 35.1 shows the ECG wave configuration of a normal 12-lead ECG): leads I, II, and III are the three standard limb leads; leads aV_R, aV_L, and aV_F are the augmented limb leads; V_1 through V_6 are the chest or precordial leads that view the heart in a horizontal plane. In ACS, ischemic and injured cells have an altered action potential and pathological patterns of depolarization and repolarization that lead to deviations from the normal ECG pattern. By identifying the leads that contain these ECG changes, the location of myocardial damage and the corresponding coronary artery supply can be determined (Table 35.7).

Myocardial injury is demonstrated by ST segment changes, and the ECG can delineate the location of myocardial ischemia and its corresponding coronary artery supply. With epicardial injury, injured cells depolarize normally but repolarize more rapidly than normal cells. This causes an elevation of the ST segment in

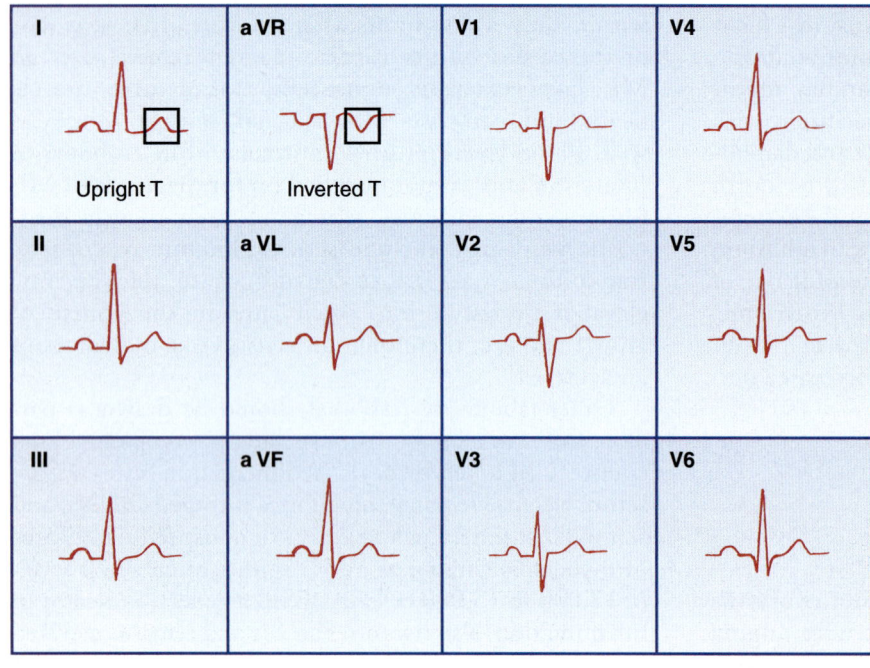

Figure 35.1 Normal 12-lead ECG.

TABLE 35.7 Localizing Myocardial Infarction via Electrocardiogram			
Location of MI	**Abnormal ECG Leads**	**Reciprocal ECG Changes**	**Coronary Arteries Affected**
Anterior	V_1–V_4	II, III, aV_F	Left anterior descending artery
Anteroseptal	V_1, V_2	None	Left anterior descending artery
Anterolateral	I, aV_L, V_3–V_6	II, III, aV_F	Left anterior descending artery Left circumflex artery
Inferior	II, III, aV_F	I, aV_L	Right coronary artery in 80% to 90% Left coronary artery in 10% to 20%
Posterior	V_1–V_3	R wave greater than S wave, depressed ST segment, elevated T wave	Right coronary artery Left circumflex artery
Lateral	I, aV_L, V_5, V_6	V_1, V_2	Left circumflex artery

Abbreviations: ECG, electrocardiogram; MI, myocardial infarction.

the leads facing the areas of injury. In endocardial and subendocardial injury, the ST segment is more likely to be depressed (usually by 1 mm or more) in the leads facing the injury. With variant angina, an ECG taken during an acute attack will indicate ST segment elevation rather than depression. However, if there is a preexisting or acute left bundle branch block (LBBB), these changes cannot be accurately assessed.

The decision to proceed with thrombolytic therapy in the setting of an acute MI is largely based on the presence of ST segment elevation in two or more ECG leads. The presence of ST segment elevation greater than 1 mm in contiguous leads (which evaluate the same anatomical area of the myocardium) usually indicates acute coronary artery occlusion, typically arising from thrombosis. In addition, clinically significant ST segment elevation is observed during reperfusion therapy for coronary artery blockage.

The various waves of electrical activity on an ECG also show changes characteristic of myocardial ischemia and infarction. Myocardial ischemia is demonstrated by enlargement and inversion of T waves due to altered late repolarization. The ischemic area also remains depolarized when adjacent areas have returned to the resting, polarized electrical state, as infarcted cells have no action potential and cannot conduct impulses through dead tissue. Thus, electrical impulses are deflected away, causing an abnormal Q wave. Because of the absence of depolarization of cells in the area of an acute MI, Q waves develop 1 to 3 days after the infarction. These abnormal Q waves are usually at least 0.04 seconds wide and 25% or greater in depth than the R wave is tall.

Figure 35.2 shows the typical ECG changes seen with cardiac damage.

At times, myocardial perfusion halts temporarily and is then reestablished in a relatively short period of time. This may be the result of a coronary vessel spasm or a sudden drop in BP, such as with severe blood or fluid loss that is eventually compensated for by peripheral vasoconstriction. In this situation, a small portion of subendocardial tissue may be damaged, whereas adjacent myocardial tissue remains viable. As a result, ECG changes are present but differ significantly from those seen in a classic transmural MI. Q waves do not form because electrically active tissue backs up the area of infarction. Because tissue injury, ischemia, and infarction occur subendocardially, rather than oriented toward the epicardium as in a transmural MI, the injury pattern is reflected in ST-segment depression.

Moreover, the ECG changes in these settings are transient, or present only during the acute event and during tissue healing. Thus, if not found during the acute presentation, a non–Q-wave MI may never be diagnosed. The terms Q-wave and non–Q-wave MI are now referred to as STEMI and NSTEMI (as previously defined). There may be a temptation to consider a non–Q-wave MI/NSTEMI as a "small heart attack" with limited long-term sequelae. However, these patients have well-demonstrated risk for future MI and other cardiac events, particularly during the next 3 to 6 months. The majority of patients with non–Q-wave MIs are adults aged 70 years or older with a history of prior MI and CHF. Figure 35.3 illustrates the difference between STEMI and NSTEMI ECG changes.

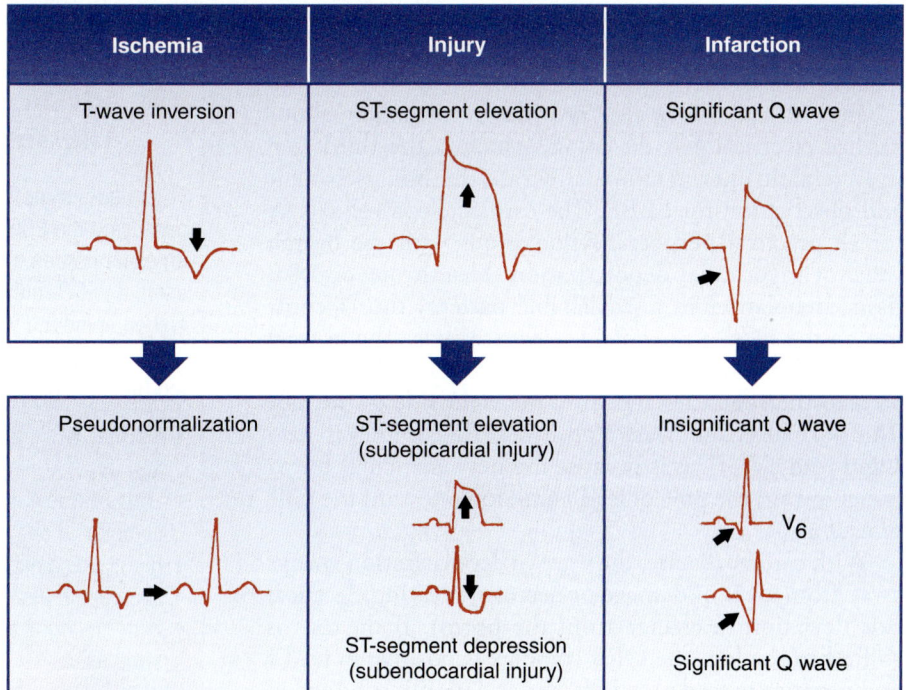

Figure 35.2 Typical ECG changes seen with cardiac damage.

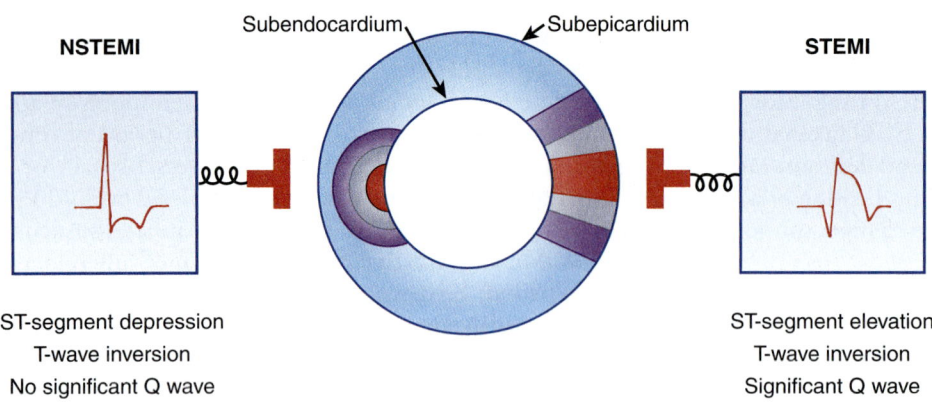

Figure 35.3 ST segment versus non–ST-segment elevation myocardial infarction.

Systematic Approach to ECG Interpretation

The identification of the abnormal ECG patterns associated with an acute MI should not overshadow the wealth of information that can be obtained from a thorough and stepwise ECG reading. If the clinician is not systematic in the approach to ECG interpretation, the risk of error and oversight of critical findings increase. For example, if the presence of an LBBB is not detected, these changes may be interpreted as Q waves in the inferior leads or ST elevations in the precordial leads.

An LBBB prevents a true evaluation of this area of the heart because the normal path of depolarization is blocked and does not travel directly down the typical electrical conduction pathway. This results in a distorted view, with the typical pattern of LBBB ECG changes. Therefore, after first determining the rate and rhythm on an ECG, observation for LBBB should be the next step. However, the clinician needs to keep in mind that an LBBB could also result from the acute ischemic process of an MI. Thus, if this is a new ECG finding, it should be noted and incorporated into the clinical picture to evaluate for possible MI.

The 12-lead ECG also provides information about cardiac electrical axis deviation, which is the third step in systematic interpretation, after rate/rhythm assessment and observation for LBBB. The cardiac electrical axis is, for all practical purposes, synonymous with the overall wave of myocardial depolarization. Healthy myocardial tissue depolarizes in a predictable pattern, thus recording on the ECG a predictable electrical axis. The normal wave of depolarization travels down the heart from the atria to the ventricles and from the right side to the left. This normal axis shows as a positive QRS complex in lead I and lead aV_F. This is because the net ventricular forces travel toward the pole of lead I and down toward the pole of lead aV_F.

With cardiac disease, the wave of depolarization swings away from areas of damage or necrosis, creating electrical axis deviation (a change from the norm). If the axis is shifted to the left, the QRS complex is positive in lead I and negative in lead aV_F. Left axis deviation is subdivided into normal left axis deviation (NLAD) and abnormal left axis deviation (ALAD). NLAD is often seen in the presence of LVH due to enlargement of the left-sided myocardium. ALAD is seen in a block of the anterosuperior division of the left bundle branch, often referred to as a left anterior fascicular block. ALAD is also seen in Q wave inferior wall MI and with a right apical pacemaker. Right axis deviation (RAD) is seen in a block of the posterior inferior division of the left bundle branch, often referred to as a left posterior fascicular block. RAD can also be caused by an extensive Q wave lateral wall MI and may be seen in hypertrophy of the right ventricle.

Axis deviation is occasionally present in the absence of cardiac disease. In pregnancy, the heart is shifted in the cavity because of the height of the diaphragm. This may cause a left axis deviation. In addition, adults with abdominal obesity may demonstrate left axis deviation. In infants and children, as well as tall, thin adults, RAD is normal. Advanced Assessment 35.2 presents a rapid quadrant-based assessment method for determining ECG axis deviation.

> **Advanced Assessment 35.2: Assessing Axis Deviation**
>
> The quadrant method is a rapid and accurate system of assessing the ECG electrical axis. Although it does not yield an exact degree measurement, such as that obtained when using an ECG ruler, this method can be used without any special equipment. First, examine leads I and aV_F for the presence of a positive or negative QRS complex. Then, apply the following rules to characterize axis deviation:
>
> - Normal axis: positive complexes (tall R wave) in leads I and aV_F
> - Left axis deviation: positive complex in lead I and negative complex in aV_F
> - Right axis deviation: negative complex in lead I and positive complex in aV_F
> - Extreme right axis deviation: negative complexes in leads I and aV_F

The 12-lead ECG may also provide information about heart chamber enlargement. Chamber enlargement, or hypertrophy, is usually a consequence of obstruction of blood flow out of the affected area of the heart, given the need for greater contractility to increase cardiac outflow. For example, left atrial hypertrophy is a common consequence of mitral valve stenosis because the atrium must generate excessive pressure to compensate for the pathologically smaller valve opening, thereby becoming enlarged as a result of forcing open a stiff, diseased valve.

The following are typical ECG findings associated with chamber enlargement:

1. Right atrial hypertrophy, also known as P pulmonale
   - Peaked P wave in leads II, III, aV_F, and V_1
   - P wave of more than 2.5 mm in leads II, III, and aV_F
2. LAE, also known as P mitrale
   - Notched P wave of more than 0.10 seconds in leads II, III, and aV_F
   - Prominent negative P terminus (latter portion) in V_1 (more than 1:1 size ratio)
3. Right ventricular hypertrophy (RVH)
   - Reversal of R-wave progression in the precordial leads
   - Although not routinely seen, RVH may be observed in patients with chronic obstructive pulmonary disease (COPD)
4. LVH, using the Estes Scoring System:
   - 3 points for any or all of the following: voltage (height) of 30 mm or more in the S wave in V_1 or V_2, 30 mm or more in the R wave in V_5 or V_6, or 20 mm or more in the R or S wave in lead I, II, III, aV_F, or aV_L
   - 1 point for secondary ST-segment/T-wave changes if the patient is taking digitalis
   - 3 points for secondary ST-segment/T-wave changes if the patient is not taking digitalis
   - 3 points for an abnormal P terminus in V_1, reflecting LAE
   - 2 points for LAD
   - 1 point for a QRS interval of more than 0.09 seconds
   - 1 point for an intrinsicoid deflection time (R-wave peak time, i.e., the time from the beginning of the QRS complex to the peak of the R wave) in V_5 or V_6 of 0.05 seconds or more
   - *Total score interpretation:* 0 to 3 = LVH unlikely; 4 = LVH likely; 5 to 13 = LVH present

Although the pathological ECG changes in ACS were discussed earlier in this section, given their relevance for the diagnosis of life-threatening conditions such as unstable angina and MI, identifying the leads that contain ECG changes to localize injury and assess for myocardial damage should actually be the *final* step in ECG interpretation. For example, if the determination of an LBBB has not been made before this last step, the ECG interpretation will be flawed. Moreover, focusing only on ischemic ECG changes in ACS may cause clinicians to overlook other important findings on this cornerstone diagnostic test, such as electrical axis deviation, conduction blocks, and underlying arrhythmias.

Of note, even if the clinician is unable to fully interpret the 12-lead ECG due to a LBBB, the clinical context of the situation needs to be considered and further diagnostic and treatment interventions rapidly implemented. For example, if an acute STEMI is suspected, additional diagnostics should be obtained such as an echocardiogram and possibly left heart catheterization with angiography, which can facilitate therapeutic intervention (e.g., angioplasty, stenting) in a timely fashion.

Differential Diagnosis

Differential diagnoses for ACS, whether presenting as angina pectoris or with further symptoms suspicious for an acute MI, include costochondritis, esophagitis, esophageal spasm, peptic ulcer, gastritis, cholecystitis, biliary tract disease, pericarditis, myocarditis, aortic dissection, pulmonary embolus (PE), pulmonary HTN, pneumothorax, anxiety, and panic disorders. Although the capacity for these other disorders to mimic the signs and symptoms of ACS is well known, a high index of suspicion for a cardiac etiology is nonetheless warranted, given the importance of ruling out life-threatening ACS.

MANAGEMENT

In ACS, the goal is to promptly diagnose and appropriately treat the underlying etiology of myocardial ischemia. In the primary care setting, the clinician can attempt to stabilize the patient with acetylsalicylic acid (aspirin, ASA) and nitroglycerin. However, the patient experiencing ACS must be transferred to a hospital-based emergency care setting as soon as possible to prevent significant morbidity and death, preferably one with access to a cardiac catheterization laboratory.

Treatment of Angina

Although not included in the definition of ACS, it is important to distinguish stable angina from unstable angina, as the former is more readily treatable than unstable angina, which is a harbinger of more severe cardiac ischemia. If a patient presents with ischemic chest pain that is relieved by nitroglycerin and rest, this implies stable angina. Chronic anginal pain is typically of short duration, usually lasting only for 3 to 5 minutes, although it may last up to 30 minutes or longer in some cases. For an acute attack of chronic stable angina, nitroglycerin may be given as an SL tablet or lingual spray. One tablet or one spray should be administered under the tongue (the spray formulation may also be delivered directly onto the tongue) every 5 minutes for a maximum of three doses until the pain is relieved. If three doses are insufficient to relieve the pain, the local emergency medical services system should be activated to immediately transport the patient to the nearest emergency department.

After the patient's chest pain has been relieved, a beta blocker and/or long-acting nitrate agent may be prescribed. Beta blockers decrease myocardial oxygen demand by interfering with the effects of the sympathetic nervous system on beta-1 receptors of the heart. Long-acting nitrates, either in a topical (e.g., Nitro-Bid ointment, Nitro-Dur patch) or oral formulation (e.g., isosorbide mononitrate or dinitrate), may be added to a beta blocker (e.g., atenolol, metoprolol, nadolol, propranolol) to increase myocardial oxygen supply through coronary artery vasodilation.

Long-acting topical nitrate formulations include the nitroglycerin transdermal patch or paste/gel/ointment, which are available in various strengths. The patch or paste must not be used continuously and should be applied for 12 to 14 hours and then removed for 12 hours to prevent the development of tolerance. The use of hydralazine is being evaluated as a way to inhibit tolerance to nitroglycerin paste. Isosorbide dinitrate is available as a long-acting oral nitrate agent, which may be taken daily as an alternative form of prophylaxis to prevent recurrent angina.

All patients with diagnosed angina should be placed on daily aspirin therapy to help prevent coronary thrombosis. ASA 81 mg (colloquially referred to as "baby aspirin") may be taken daily at bedtime, although some clinicians still order 325 mg. Enteric-coated ASA may be used in patients with concurrent gastric problems to reduce the risk of stomach irritation by delaying absorption of the tablet until it is in a less susceptible portion of the GI tract. Ticlopidine taken with food may be ordered for patients who are allergic to aspirin or those with a history of GI bleeding.

As unstable angina is defined as chest pain of new onset, a progressive nature, or a new pattern, if rest and nitroglycerin do not relieve the chest discomfort in typical fashion, the patient must be immediately transported by ambulance to the emergency department for further evaluation and to rule out an MI (Figure 35.4 presents a flowchart for the management of unstable angina). In variant angina, the ECG findings of ST-segment elevation will abate when the patient is treated with nitroglycerin and drugs that influence calcium metabolism, such as a CCB (e.g., verapamil).

Treatment of Myocardial Infarction

The location and extent of infarcted myocardial tissue and the speed with which reperfusion is supplied to the "cutoff" areas of the myocardium determine prognosis after an MI. Because the use of early reperfusion therapy increases the likelihood of survival and improves left ventricular function, the patient with a suspected MI should be assessed rapidly to provide the most appropriate care. The Iceberg of Myocardial Infarction explores many facets involved in recognizing and treating the patient with an MI.

The pharmacological treatment of ACS is directed primarily at dissolution of the intracoronary thrombus causing obstruction to blood flow by antiplatelet therapy (e.g., aspirin, glycoprotein IIb/IIIa receptor antagonists), anticoagulant therapy (e.g., heparin), and relief of symptoms by antianginal (e.g., nitroglycerin, beta blockers, supplemental oxygen therapy) and analgesic (e.g., morphine sulfate) medications. After an MI is confirmed, urgent evaluation for salvage of viable myocardial tissue is initiated through reperfusion treatments based on coronary angiographical studies. Ultimately, the goal of management is to salvage the ischemic myocardium before it becomes necrotic by reperfusing the area as soon as possible. After that, the goal of ongoing treatment shifts to preventing future attacks.

Immediate interventions for a suspected MI mirror those of unstable angina, including rest, aspirin, and nitroglycerin to relieve chest pain, to decrease heart rate, BP, and myocardial oxygen demand. Nitroglycerin can be administered sublingually as a tablet or spray. If relief is not achieved within 2 to 3 minutes after the initial dose of nitroglycerin, a second or third dose can be given at 5-minute intervals for a total of three doses. One or more inches of nitroglycerin gel (e.g., Nitropaste, Nitro-Bid) may also be used to induce vasodilation and lower BP. This topical form of nitroglycerin may be easily removed by wiping it off the skin to stop its effects. In more advanced clinical settings, an adjustable IV nitroglycerin drip may be used if appropriate nursing and medical supervision is available.

Aspirin at a dose of 162 to 325 mg should also be administered in the ambulatory care setting. Aspirin confers antiplatelet effects, whereas nitroglycerin decreases preload and coronary artery vasospasm, thus contributing to an overall beneficial effect in acute MI. The patient should initially chew and swallow one aspirin tablet. It is important that the 325 mg dosage not be exceeded, because that may negate the antiplatelet effect. This initiation of antiplatelet therapy given at the time of onset (within 70 minutes) of symptoms, before hospitalization, has been shown to lower the mortality rate in MI patients.

The patient should then be transferred to an emergency medical setting. The clinician or first health-care provider to encounter the patient should place a large-bore IV if possible and monitor the patient until the emergency medical services system can be activated. Providing supplemental oxygen via nasal cannula or face mask is no longer done routinely, as oxygen is administered only if the patient's oxygen saturation falls below 90%. Once the patient is stabilized, emergency care clinicians can determine whether the patient is a candidate for emergent reperfusion treatment with intravenous

The Iceberg of Myocardial Infarction

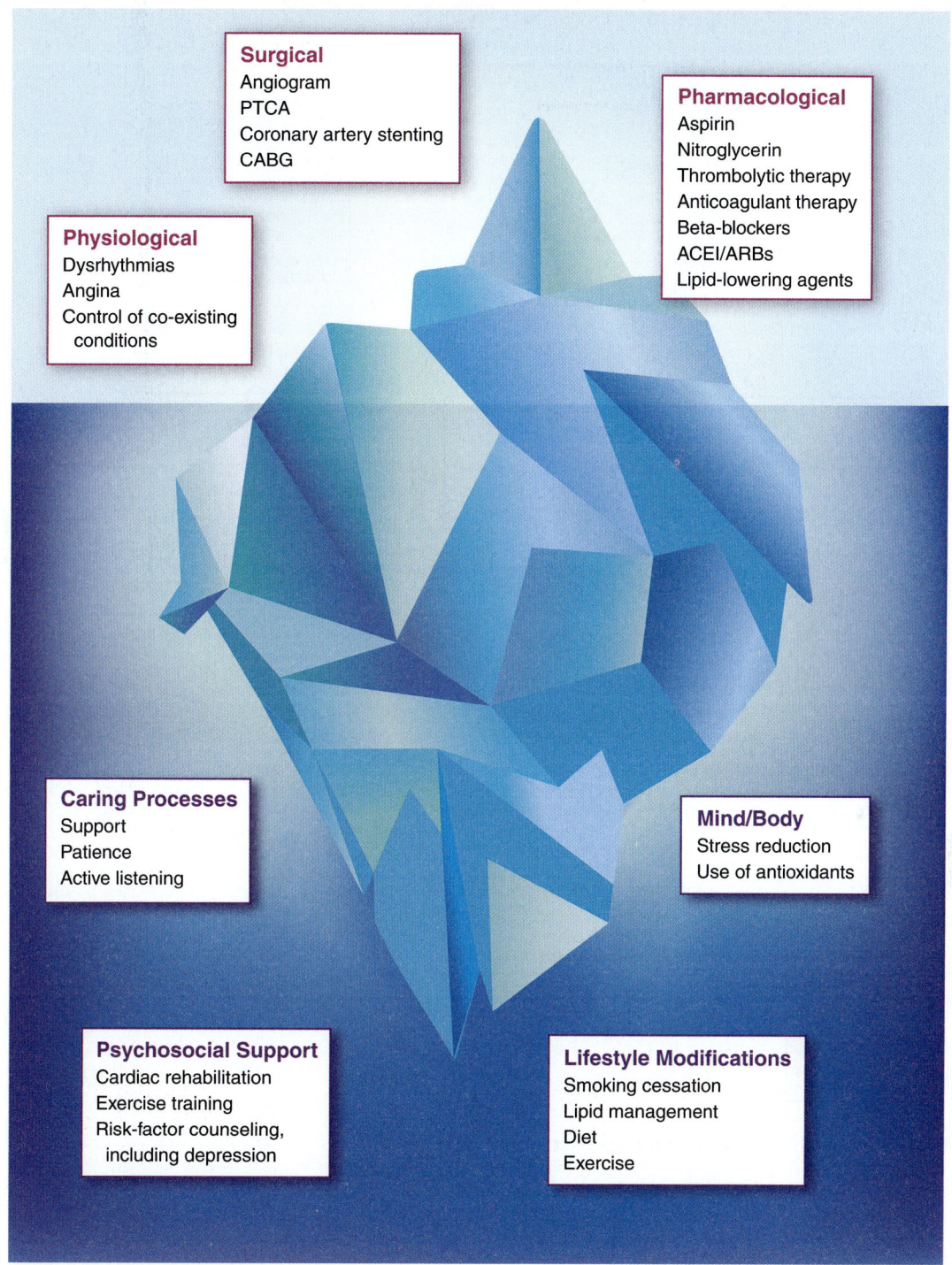

Surgical
Angiogram
PTCA
Coronary artery stenting
CABG

Pharmacological
Aspirin
Nitroglycerin
Thrombolytic therapy
Anticoagulant therapy
Beta-blockers
ACEI/ARBs
Lipid-lowering agents

Physiological
Dysrhythmias
Angina
Control of co-existing conditions

Caring Processes
Support
Patience
Active listening

Mind/Body
Stress reduction
Use of antioxidants

Psychosocial Support
Cardiac rehabilitation
Exercise training
Risk-factor counseling, including depression

Lifestyle Modifications
Smoking cessation
Lipid management
Diet
Exercise

PTCA - Percutaneous Transluminal Coronary Angioplasty
CABG - Coronary Artery Bypass Graft
ACEI - Angiotensin-Converting Enzyme Inhibitor
ARB - Angiotensin Receptor Blocker

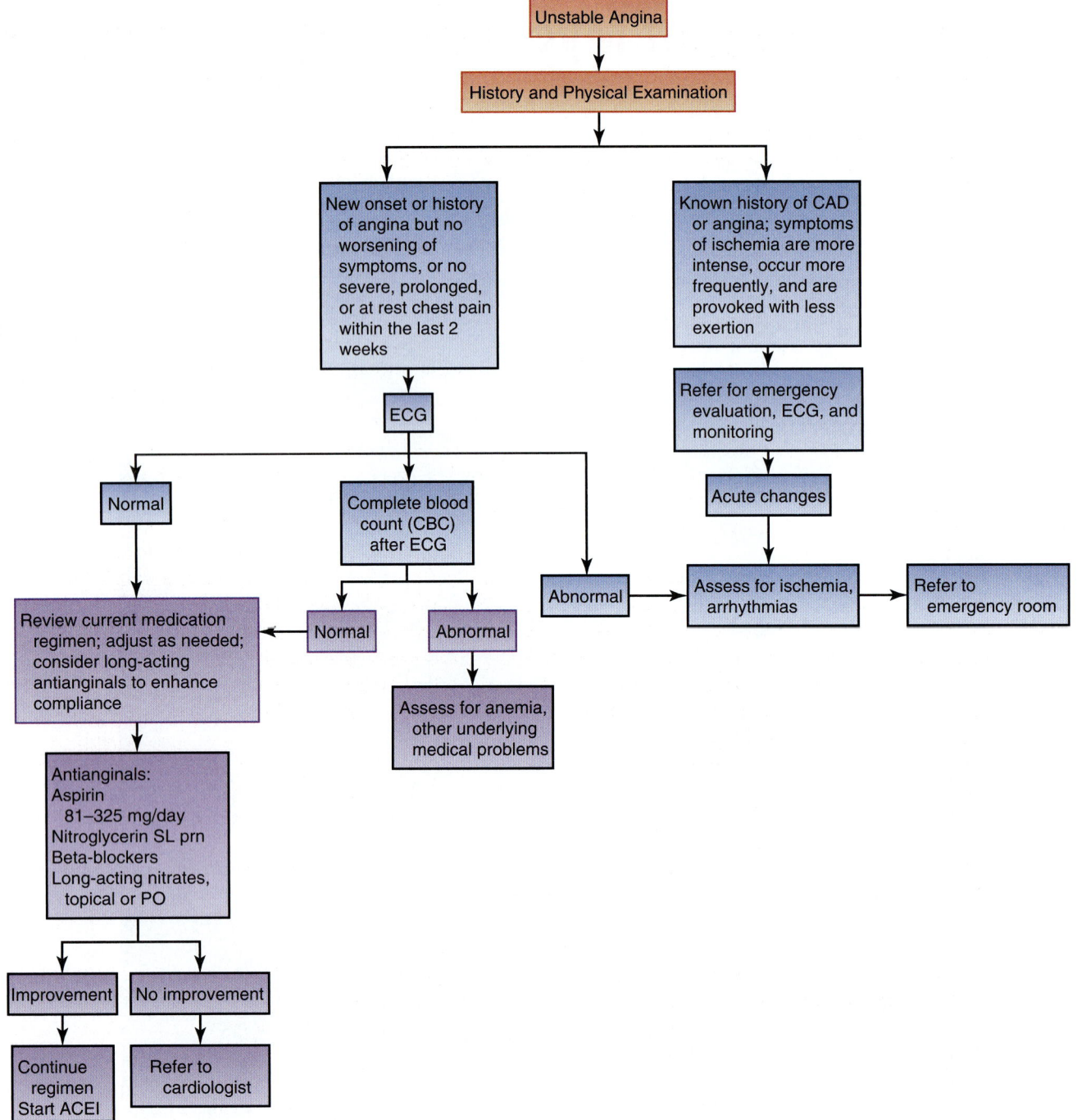

Figure 35.4 Treatment flowchart: unstable angina

thrombolytic agents or primary percutaneous coronary intervention (PCI). This approach should only be used for patients with a STEMI or with suspected acute MI in the setting of LBBB.

Thrombolytic agents, such as alteplase (recombinant tissue plasminogen activator), reteplase, or tenecteplase, are most effective when administered early in the course of an MI. The first thrombolytic agent, streptokinase, is not commonly used today because it is not a fibrin-specific inhibiting agent. For the best therapeutic effect, thrombolytics should be administered within the first 3 hours (ideally 30 minutes) of MI symptom onset, although studies have shown that thrombolytic therapy can be of benefit up to 12 hours after the initial presentation of symptoms of MI. Thrombolytic therapy can also be combined with the antiplatelet agents known as glycoprotein IIb/IIIa inhibitors, including abciximab (ReoPro), eptifibatide (Integrilin), and tirofiban (Aggrastat).

Cardiac catheterization with angiography can determine whether the patient is a candidate for reperfusion therapy, percutaneous transluminal coronary angioplasty (PTCA), coronary artery stenting, or CABG. Immediate be administered concomitantly with an ACEI or with the direct renin inhibitor aliskiren (Tekturna) in patients with diabetes mellitus, given the risk of hypotension, renal insufficiency, and hyperkalemia. Entresto can be started after an ACEI has been discontinued for 36 hours. In addition, a previous history of hypersensitivity to either component of this combination drug or angioedema to an ACEI or ARB are contraindications to its use.

Vasodilators and nitrates can be used for HF in those who cannot tolerate ACEIs. Diuretics should be added to this regimen if symptoms persist or frank volume overload develops at the first signs of ACC/AHA stage C overload (e.g., orthopnea, PND). However, over diuresis must be avoided, as this will lead to hypotension, renal insufficiency, and may interfere with the effectiveness of other medications. For mild HF, thiazide diuretics (e.g., hydrochlorothiazide) are used, and for severe HF, loop diuretics such as furosemide (Lasix) or bumetanide (Bumex) are indicated. Dosages of these agents can be increased during acute HF exacerbations to counteract fluid overload. For those patients who become refractory to traditional loop diuretics, intermittent use of a thiazide-like diuretic, such as metolazone (Zaroxolyn), may be helpful in treating volume overload. In addition, all patients should be on a sodium-restricted diet.

The sympathetic nervous system is stimulated as a compensatory mechanism in HF, causing arterial vasoconstriction and an increased heart rate, which have further detrimental effects on the weakened heart. For this reason, beta-adrenergic blockers, such as carvedilol (Coreg), have been recommended as part of the drug treatment regimen in HF and have been shown to reduce mortality. Carvedilol is also an alpha-1 adrenergic receptor antagonist and, along with its beta-adrenergic blockade, will slow heart rate and limit peripheral arterial vasoconstriction, thereby decreasing the force of afterload against the ventricles and, in turn, the work of the heart. Bisoprolol and sustained-release metoprolol are other beta blockers that have been shown to reduce mortality in HF. An additional category of HF drug is ivabradine (Corlanor), which is a sinoatrial node modulator that, when added to maximally tolerated doses of beta blockers, can assist in keeping the heart rate at 70 beats per minute or lower in symptomatic chronic HF.

Once HF has progressed to ACC/AHA stage C, the aldosterone antagonist spironolactone has been shown to be of benefit in selected patients, as described in the latest AHA updates for stage C HF therapy. In addition, patients in stage C HF should be evaluated for biventricular pacing and an implantable defibrillator, as HF is often associated with ventricular remodeling and arrhythmias, such as LBBB. These conditions lead to unsynchronized ventricular contractions. Cardiac resynchronization therapy (CRT) is an option for patients who present with a LVEF of less than or equal to 35%, a QRS greater than 120 milliseconds, NYHA class III of IV HF, or who otherwise are not optimized on medical therapy. CRT involves implantation of a biventricular pacing device, and if necessary, an implantable cardioverter-defibrillator. CRT has been shown to improve cardiac mechanics by inducing concordant contraction of both ventricles.

Implantation of an internal cardiac automated defibrillator may be considered for primary prevention in chronic HF patients (NYHA functional class II or III and ACC/AHA stage C) with ischemic or nonischemic cardiomyopathy or in a patient with an EF of less than or equal to 35%, given the patient's increased risk of sudden cardiac death due to a greater risk of sustained ventricular tachycardia and ventricular fibrillation. As noted earlier, CRT may also be used for patients with NYHA class III or IV HF with persistent symptoms who are already receiving optimal medical therapy. Left ventricular assist devices as end-stage (destination) therapy or, alternatively, as a bridge to heart transplantation may be considered for patients who have exhausted all other treatment recommendations with poor efficacy (i.e., ACC/AHA stage D HF).

Historically, digoxin has been used to treat HF. However, with the establishment of ACEIs and ARBs along with beta blockers and diuretics as first-line treatment options in HF, the use of digoxin has declined, given its narrow therapeutic index and risk for toxicity. Digoxin may still be used in conjunction with other medications in patients with severe HF (ACC/AHA stage C), although it may not be necessary in patients who become asymptomatic after treatment with ACEIs and diuretics.

IV inotropic agents that may be ordered in a monitored inpatient setting for end-stage cardiac failure (ACC/AHA stage D) include dopamine (Intropin), dobutamine (Dobutrex), and milrinone (Primacor). When inotropic support is implemented in the inpatient setting and the patient is unable to be weaned from this therapy, the decision may be made with the patient, family, and care team to discharge the patient home with end-stage HF on home inotropic support.

Controlling the ventricular rate and, when possible, eliminating the arrhythmia of atrial fibrillation if present are essential in treating HF. Atrial fibrillation may be seen in approximately one-third of HF patients and is associated with an increased risk of disease progression and death in patients with asymptomatic or symptomatic left ventricle systolic dysfunction. Because of this, anticoagulation treatment is instituted in HF to decrease the formation of thrombi in the dysfunctional heart chambers, thus decreasing the risk of cerebral thromboembolism. Long-term oral anticoagulation with warfarin (Coumadin) is usually recommended, although newer oral anticoagulant agents (e.g., the direct thrombin inhibitor dabigatran [Pradaxa], the factor Xa inhibitors rivaroxaban [Xarelto], apixaban [Eliquis], and edoxaban [Savaysa]) that do not require frequent laboratory monitoring with prothrombin time (PT)/international normalized ratio (INR) have been shown to be effective alternatives in HF patients (NYHA class II or higher) with atrial fibrillation.

In addition to optimal medical and electrophysiological therapy, self-care and other interventions for patients with HF include the following:

- Regular exercise should be encouraged for all patients with stable HF, because it improves functional status and decreases congestive symptoms, provided physical exertion does not exceed cardiac capacity and trigger an HF exacerbation.
- Cardiac rehabilitation programs that include exercise on a regular basis, although not specifically indicated for patients with HF, might benefit patients who are anxious about exercising on their own or who have low cardiac output.
- Rest with elevation of the lower extremities during the midday is recommended, with the use of elastic stockings to reduce the risk of venous thrombosis and PE.
- Dietary sodium should be restricted to 2 g per day or less.
- Limitation of fluid intake should be advised, based on the patient's HF status.
- Alcohol consumption should be discouraged; patients should drink no more than one glass of beer or wine, or a mixed drink with no more than 1 ounce of alcohol, per day.
- Patients should record their weight daily and notify the primary care practitioner of a weight gain of 3 pounds or more in 24 hours or 5 pounds or more within 1 week, as this likely reflects significant fluid retention from an HF exacerbation; in turn, an optimum body weight should be maintained.
- Immunization with influenza, pneumococcal, and COVID-19 vaccines reduces the risk of respiratory infections, as per current CDC recommendations, and should be encouraged.
- All barriers to medication adherence must be removed to assist the patient with management of the disease. Such barriers include the cost of medications, the complexity of the regimen (which typically includes multiple agents from different therapeutic classes), and adverse medication effects, including those related to polypharmacy.
- Psychological support is essential, and patient support groups have been shown to be effective in helping patients cope with the effects of chronic HF and follow a prescribed treatment regimen; rest and relaxation should be emphasized as critical components of health and wellness.
- The patient must be counseled concerning the prognosis of HF for the benefit of understanding the rationale for decisions underlying the care plan and effectively planning for the future. This must be done while maintaining hope, as the clinician should explain that a good quality of life is still possible in cooperation with the recommended treatment regimen.
- The patient should be encouraged to complete an advance directive, given the risk of cardiac arrest with HF.

FOLLOW-UP AND REFERRAL

Patients in chronic cardiac failure may be treated on an outpatient basis, in which changes in cardiac status are assessed thoroughly, including questions regarding health-related quality of life (e.g., sleep quality, sexual function, mental health status, outlook on life, appetite, and social activities). After the patient, family, and caregiver have been educated on the condition, they should be encouraged to communicate all signs, symptoms, fears, and concerns related to HF, as patients are likely to experience changes in symptoms before developing evidence of deterioration on physical examination.

The frequency of follow-up of these patients generally depends on the underlying cause of their HF, although patients are typically seen by the clinician at least every 3 months. Intensive home-care surveillance has been shown to decrease the need for hospitalization and to improve the functional status of older adult patients with HF.

Referral to a cardiologist is recommended with the onset of symptoms in HF; however, initial medical treatment should begin immediately as directed by the clinician, followed by a phone referral to a cardiologist. Increasingly in the United States, dedicated HF clinics are becoming popular referral resources.

Patients in acute HF typically require hospitalization for aggressive medical intervention, unless mild in severity. The clinician and cardiologist should work together to establish a plan of care with the patient for the long-term management of HF. The Joint Commission (an international accrediting and certifying body in healthcare quality improvement) has mandated that specific core measures of care should be met before discharge. For example, there must be an assessment of left ventricle function documenting an EF. If the EF is less than 40%, the patient should be prescribed an ACEI or ARB (which may include valsartan/sacubitril combination therapy). If the patient has had an allergic reaction to any of these drugs or otherwise cannot tolerate them, this must be documented in the patient's medical record. Additional core measures include advice and counseling on smoking cessation (as well as other tobacco use) and discharge instructions that include reconciliation of the prescribed medication regimen.

Patient Education: Heart Failure

Successful management of patients with HF requires an active partnership between the patient and all health-care providers to decrease the possibility of the patient declining in function by the disease process. This includes thorough patient education regarding the condition and encouragement for patients to take responsibility for their own personal care. In turn, the primary care practitioner should educate and facilitate the patient's achieving the self-care goals described earlier in the section on Management (see page 570), which includes discussing all of the changes a patient wants to make in self-care practices before the patient takes action.

In working with patients and their families to develop a care plan, the clinician should not lose sight of the highly influential nature of medical recommendations. The clinician should keep in mind that the family, fearing losing their loved one, will attempt to ensure the care plan is followed exactly. Therefore, the clinician should remember to "build in"—and teach the patient and family how to build in—humane adaptations to the plan of care that allow for practical flexibility under certain circumstances. For example, the clinician may stress a diuretic must be taken every morning without realizing that if a patient has an important family function one morning and chooses to take the diuretic later in the day, an inflexible mandate from the clinician may cause needless stress and guilt. The patient may be frightened of falling into distress if the clinician's orders are not followed precisely, and the family may pressure the patient for deliberately not following the plan of care. In turn, the patient may feel that participation in events that take place in the morning are forbidden and subsequently self-isolate to the detriment of the patient's social support system. Thus, it is critical that the clinician ensures patients and their families understand the rationale for the decisions underlying the care plan, as perceived restrictions may unnecessarily compromise the quality of the patient's life.

With the rising incidence of HF, researchers are increasingly evaluating patient self-care practices and their effect on clinical outcomes. Exercise training is now being recommended for most individuals with moderate to severe HF, as activity intolerance associated with chronic HF leads to a decreased quality of life. In addition, exercise training as therapy for chronic HF has been shown to reduce morbidity and mortality.

Coaching and encouraging a terminally ill patient in self-care practices may be time-consuming and can be draining for the clinician and patient. However, the clinician must maintain an authentic presence and respond to calls for assistance that are often not timed with the patient's regularly scheduled appointments, given the acute nature of HF exacerbations. To patients with chronic, progressive, and ultimately terminal illnesses, the significance of the effects of the illness on their lives is directly related to their perceptions of the attention and care being given by health-care providers. For example, a thoughtful discussion should take place with patients who are admitted to hospice care, along with their family members, regarding removal of an internal cardiac defibrillator, if present, to be consistent with do not resuscitate (DNR) orders that are typical in hospice management.

REFERENCES

General

American Geriatric Society 2021 Beers Criteria for Potentially Inappropriate Medication Use in Older Adults. *J Am Geriatr Soc*. 2019;67:674–694. https://www.pharmdlive.com/blog/2021-updated-review-of-ags-beers-criteria/. Accessed 1/22/2021.

The Framingham Heart Study. https://framinghamheartstudy.org/. Accessed 1/22/2021.

ACUTE CORONARY SYNDROME

Arslanian-Engoren C, Scott LD. Delays in treatment-seeking decisions among women with myocardial infarction. *Dimens Criti Care Nurs*. 2017;36(5):298–303.

Bularga A, Ken Lee K, Stewart S, et al. High-sensitivity troponin and the application of risk stratification thresholds in patients with suspected acute coronary syndrome. *Circulation*. 2019;140:1557–1568.

Editorial Board. 2020 American Heart Assoc. Guidelines for Cardiopulmonary Resuscitation and Emergency Cardiovascular Care. *Circulation*. 2020;142(16);suppl 2:S336. https://www.ahajournals.org/toc/circ/142/16_suppl_2#. Accessed 11/9/2020.

Jones SA. *ECG Mastery: Improving your ecg interpretation skills*. 2nd edition. FA Davis; 2020.

Little KM Recognizing and managing complications of acute myocardial infarction: good outcomes require early identification and prompt treatment. *Am Nurse J*. 2020;15(4):40–44.

Singh A, Museedi AS, Grossman SA. Acute coronary syndrome. [Updated 2020 Jul 17]. In: StatPearls [Internet]. Treasure Island (FL): StatPearls Publishing; 2020 Jan-. Available from: https://www.ncbi.nlm.nih.gov/books/NBK459157/. Accessed 9/5/2020.

Thygesen K, Alpert JS, Jaffe AS, et al. Fourth universal definition of myocardial infarction (2018). *Circulation*. 2018;138:e618–e651.

CORONARY HEART DISEASE

Benjamin EJ, Biaha MJ, Chiuve SE, et al. Heart disease and stroke statistics—2017 update: a report from the American Heart Association. *Circulation*. 2017;135(10):e146–e603.

Levine GN, Bates ER, Bittl JA, et al. 2016 ACC/AHA guideline focused update on duration of dual antiplatelet therapy in patients with coronary artery disease: a report of the American College of Cardiology/American Heart Association task force on clinical practice guidelines. *J Thorac Cardiovasc Surg*. 2016;152:1243–1275.

DYSLIPIDEMIA

ATP III Guidelines at-a-glance. https://www.nhlbi.nih.gov/files/docs/guidelines/atglance.pdf. Accessed 9/5/2020.

Drozda JP, Ferguson B, Jneid H, et al. 2015 ACC/AHA focused update of secondary prevention lipid performance measures: a report of the American College of Cardiology/American Heart Association task force on performance measures. *Circ Cardiovasc Qual Outcomes*. 2016;9:68–95.

Hirode G, Wong RJ. Trends in the prevalence of metabolic syndrome in the United States, 2011–2016. *JAMA*. 2020;323(24):2526.

HEART FAILURE

Benjamin EJ, Muntner P, Alonso A, Bittencourt MS, Callaway CW, Carson AP, et al. Heart disease and stroke statistics—2019 update: a report from the American Heart Association. *Circulation*. 2019;139(10):e56–e528.

Brown L, Boos C. Atrial fibrillation and heart failure: factors influencing the choice of oral anticoagulant. *Int J Cardiol.* 2017 Jan 15;227:863–868.

Gronda E, Vanoli E, Iacoviello M. The PARAGON-HF trial: the sacubitril/valsartan in heart failure with preserved ejection fraction. *Eur Heart J Suppl.* 2020;22(Supplement L):L77–L81. https://academic.oup.com/eurheartjsupp/article/22/Supplement_L/L77/5989597.

Healthy People 2030. Reduce heart failure hospitalizations in adults. https://health.gov/healthypeople/objectives-and-data/browse-objectives/heart-disease-and-stroke/reduce-heart-failure-hospitalizations-adults-hds-09. Accessed 9/6/2020.

Maisel AS, Daniels LB. Breathing not properly 10 years later: what we have learned and what we still need to learn. *J Am Coll Cardiol.* 2012;60(4):277–282. https://www.sciencedirect.com/journal/journal-of-the-american-college-of-cardiology/vol/60/issue/4.

O'Neal WT, Mazur M, Bertoni AG, et al. Electrocardiographic predictors of heart failure with reduced versus preserved ejection fraction: The Multi-Ethnic Study of Atherosclerosis (MESA). *J Am Heart Assoc.* 2017;6(6). https://europepmc.org/article/med/28546456. Accessed 10/1/2020.

Redfield MM. Heart failure with preserved ejection fraction. *New Engl J Med.* 2016;375:1868–1877.

Roscoe M, Lampkins A, Harper S, et al. Heart failure: a dynamic approach to classification and management. *Clinician Rev.* 2018 May/June:32–43.

Solomon SD, McMurray JJV, Anand IS, et al. Angiotensin-neprilysin inhibition in heart failure with preserved ejection fraction. *New Engl J Med.* 2019 Oct 24;381(17):1609–1620.

HYPERTENSION

Baudrand R, Vaidya A. The low-renin hypertension phenotype: genetics and the role of the mineralocorticoid receptor. *Int J Mol Sci.* 2018;19(2):546. https://doi.org/10.3390/ijms19020546.

Chazal RA, Creager MA. New quality measure core sets provide continuity for measuring quality improvement: concerns raised about conflicting blood pressure measures. *Hypertension.* 2016;67:1053–1054.

Cobos F, Haskard-Zolnierek K, Howard K. White coat hypertension: improving the patient–health care practitioner relationship. *Psychol Res Behav Manag.* 2015;8:133–141.

Davis, L. Hypertension: how low to go when treating older adults. *J Nurse Pract.* 2019;15(1):1–6.

Experimental Biology. Say no to vaping: blood pressure, heart rate rises in healthy, young nonsmokers. EurekAlert. News Release Apr 27, 2020. https://www.eurekalert.org/pub_releases/2020-04/eb-snt042320.php#:~:text=%2D%2DNew%20research%20finds%20that,even%20after%20a%20vaping%20session. Accessed 8/28/2020.

Indarawis D. Acute management of severe asymptomatic hypertension. *Clinician Rev.* 2017 Nov:40–45.

Muntner P, Carey RM, Gidding S, et al. Potential US Population Impact of the 2017 ACC/AHA High Blood Pressure Guideline. *Circulation.* 2018;137(2):109. Epub 2017 Nov 13.

Unger T, Borghi C, Charchar F, et al. 2020 International Society of Hypertension global hypertension practice guidelines. *J Hypertens.* 2020;38(6):982.

Whelton PK, Carey RM, Aronow WS, et al. ACC/AHA/AAPA/ABC/ACPM/AGS/APhA/ASH/ASPC/NMA/PCNA guideline for the prevention, detection, evaluation, and management of high blood pressure in adults: executive summary: a report of the American College of Cardiology/American Heart Association task force on clinical practice guidelines. *J Am Soc Hypertens.* 2018;12:579.

Williams B, Giuseppe M, Spiering W, et al. 2018 ESC/ESH guidelines for the management of arterial hypertension. *Eur Heart J* 2018;39:3021.

RESOURCES

General

American College of Cardiology
https://www.acc.org

American Heart Association
https://www.heart.org

Beers Criteria for potentially inappropriate medication use in older adults
https://geriatricscareonline.org/ProductAbstract/american-geriatrics-society-updated-beers-criteria-for-potentially-inappropriate-medication-use-in-older-adults/CL001

Acute Coronary Syndrome

American College of Cardiology ASCVD Risk Estimator Plus
https://www.acc.org/tools-and-practice-support/mobile-resources/features/2013-prevention-guidelines-ascvd-risk-estimator

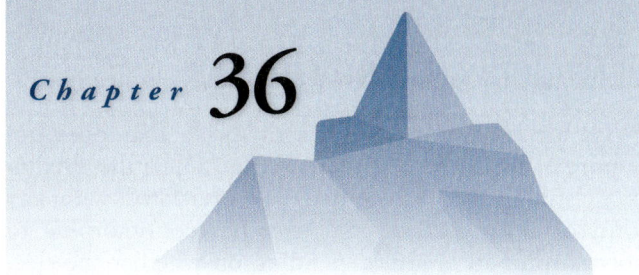

Chapter 36

Dysrhythmias and Valvular Disorders

Kathryn B. Keller, PhD, RN, CNE
Denese Sabatino, MSN, APRN, NP-C, CCRN
Jill E. Winland-Brown, EdD, APRN, FNP-BC, FAANP
Michael B. Keller, MD
Brian Oscar Porter, MD, PhD, MPH, MBA

ARRHYTHMIAS

Arrhythmias that the clinician may encounter in the clinical setting include the atrial arrhythmias of atrial fibrillation, premature atrial contractions (PACs), atrial tachycardia, atrial flutter, and supraventricular tachycardia (SVT), as well as the ventricular arrhythmias of premature ventricular contractions (PVCs) and ventricular tachycardia (VT). First-, second-, and third-degree heart blocks are other common arrhythmias. In the past, arrhythmias associated with digitalis toxicity were not uncommon, but they are seen less frequently today because of the decreased usage of digitalis preparations.

ATRIAL ARRHYTHMIAS

Atrial Fibrillation

Atrial fibrillation is one of the most common arrhythmias that clinicians will encounter in clinical practice. In many cases, atrial fibrillation initially will be associated with a rapid ventricular response and most patients will have some type of underlying heart disease. In these patients, the loss of atrial contribution to left ventricular (LV) blood volume (the atrial "kick"), along with a rapid ventricular rate, can have serious hemodynamic effects caused by diminished cardiac output. These effects may manifest as hypotension, diaphoresis, dizziness, and syncopal episodes.

The loss of mechanically effective atrial contractions in atrial fibrillation leads to stasis of blood in the atrium that predisposes an individual to the formation of embolic atrial thrombi. Thrombi that form in the left atrium tend to travel into the left ventricle and the aorta where they are propelled into the arterial circulation. A common route for a thrombus from the aorta is to the brachiocephalic artery, carotid artery, and then into the cerebral circulation. This pathway makes atrial fibrillation a risk factor for ischemic stroke because an embolus may lodge in a branch of the middle cerebral artery.

All persons with atrial fibrillation should be evaluated for their risk of stroke and potential anticoagulant therapy. While several risk stratification tools have been developed to estimate the risk of thromboembolic events, the most widely used is the CHA_2DS_2-VASc score (Table 36.1). Anticoagulation is strongly recommended in patients with nonvalvular atrial fibrillation and a CHA_2DS_2-VASc score of 2 or greater.

Premature Atrial Contractions

PACs are common, yet in most cases, they have no clinical significance. PACs are usually a benign arrhythmia that does not require pharmacological intervention unless there are underlying causes that can be corrected. They are rarely symptomatic. This arrhythmia is commonly seen in young, healthy individuals. Cardiac stimulants such as caffeine, nicotine, alcohol, or over-the-counter decongestant medications sometimes induce PACs. They may also occur in patients with right atrial dilation caused by obstructive lung disease or bilateral atrial dilation in the setting of heart failure.

Supraventricular Tachycardia

SVT is often used as a "catch-all" term that encompasses rapid arrhythmias originating just above the ventricles. There continues to be confusion over specific terminology with respect to different forms of SVT. This confusion originates from an inability to differentiate true atrial

TABLE 36.1 CHA_2DS_2-VASc Score for Stroke Risk Assessment in Atrial Fibrillation

	Condition	Points
C	Congestive heart failure	1
H	Hypertension (or treated hypertension)	1
A	Age older than 75 years	2
	Age 65 to 74 years	1
D	Diabetes	1
S	Stroke/TIA/thromboembolism	2
V	Vascular disease	1
S	Sex Female	1

Source: CHA_2DS_2-VASc/HAS-BLED/EHRA Atrial Fibrillation Risk Score Calculator. https://www.chadsvasc.org/

tachycardias or atrial flutter from paroxysmal supraventricular tachycardia (PSVT) that occurs because of electrical reentry circuits. The use of the term *paroxysmal atrial tachycardia* (PAT) further confounds the terminology issue. PAT describes a sudden onset of atrial tachycardia, yet this term is often incorrectly used for SVTs, such as atrial flutter or atrial fibrillation, whether they occur paroxysmally or not.

For the purposes of this discussion, the condition of SVT is subdivided into PSVT, which includes atrioventricular nodal reentrant tachycardia (AVNRT) and atrioventricular reentrant tachycardia (AVRT), and non-PSVT, which includes atrial tachycardia of nonreentrant origin and atrial flutter. Although atrial fibrillation can also be classified as an SVT, this rhythm is discussed separately. The two most common forms of PSVT are AVNRT and AVRT. Specifically, AVRT can be further subdivided into orthodromic and antidromic AVRT, depending on whether the pathological atrial impulse involved in abnormal heart conduction travels in the same (orthodromic) or opposite (antidromic) direction as the normal physiological cardiac impulse.

Current Advanced Cardiac Life Support treatment standards require that the clinician be able to differentiate tachycardias originating in the atrium that are included under the term *SVT*. The atrial rate differentiates atrial tachycardia from atrial flutter. This rate difference is particularly pertinent when the clinician is attempting to discern whether the arrhythmia is an atrial tachycardia with a heart block (as seen in digitalis toxicity) or an atrial flutter. Both rhythms can present with more than one observable P wave before the QRS. An atrial tachycardia rate (P-wave rate of 140 to 250 per minute) is slower than an atrial flutter rate (P-wave rate of 250 to 350 per minute). It is important for the clinician to remember that the P-wave rate needs to be counted separately from the QRS rate. Atrial flutter is less common than atrial fibrillation and most commonly occurs in older adults. Patients with atrial flutter typically have some form of structural heart disease. Given the risk of sequelae with these conditions, referral to a cardiologist may be required, and patients may need to be managed in an acute care setting.

> **Geriatric Considerations:**
> **Arrhythmias**
>
> It is crucial to diagnose arrhythmias and cardiac conditions as soon as possible, as treatment may be a lifesaver. Atrial flutter and atrial fibrillation are extremely common in older adults. In addition, clinicians should be alert to patients who have sleep apnea, as many of the possible consequences include cardiac problems. In addition to the arrhythmias above, sleep apnea may result in right or left ventricular hypertrophy, an MI, and/or nocturnal angina.

VENTRICULAR ARRHYTHMIAS

PVCs are usually a benign arrhythmia that does not require pharmacological intervention unless the rhythm progresses to VT, which may be associated with any form of heart disease. VT may be monomorphic or polymorphic in origin, depending on whether the electrocardiogram (ECG) waveforms are uniform or varied in morphology. It may be sustained or nonsustained. In patients who have had a myocardial infarction (MI), VT is a risk factor for sudden cardiac death.

HEART BLOCKS

Atrioventricular (AV) heart blocks are classified by the severity of disturbance in the impulse going through the electrical conduction system between the atria and ventricles. Heart blocks may be permanent or transient and are classified as first-, second-, or third-degree:

- A first-degree AV block is observed with a regular rhythm and only a prolonged P-R interval.
- A second-degree AV block may be classified further as type I (Mobitz I or Wenckebach) or type II (Mobitz II). Mobitz type I blocks occurs in the AV nodal area, with progressive lengthening of the P-R interval until a QRS complex (ventricular contraction) is dropped (missing on ECG) completely. Mobitz type II blocks occur within or below the bundle of His (which is itself below the AV node), with a constant normal or lengthened P-R interval and a periodic drop of a QRS complex.
- A third-degree or complete AV heart block is a form of AV dissociation. This occurs when the atria beat regularly at a normal rate but no electrical excitation is transmitted from the atria to the ventricles. In turn, the atria and ventricles contract independently at their own intrinsic rates. This complete lack of coordination between the chambers of the heart severely compromises cardiac output and can prove fatal. Third-degree heart block is further classified as third-degree at the junctional level or third-degree at the ventricular level, depending on where the block occurs anatomically along the cardiac conduction pathway.

Progression of heart block is an important clinical concept. A second-degree Mobitz type I block does not progress to Mobitz type II; rather, a Mobitz type I block typically progresses to a third-degree heart block with an idiojunctional response, in which an "escape rhythm" mediating independent ventricular contraction emanates from the AV junction and runs antegrade, without retrograde conduction to the atria. In contrast, a second-degree Mobitz type II block progresses to a third-degree heart block with an idioventricular response (i.e., a ventricular escape rhythm emanating from a point in the ventricles below the AV junction) that carries a more ominous prognosis.

If a rhythm presents with two P waves for every QRS complex (referred to as 2:1 conduction) with a normal rate, the origin of nodal or subnodal pathology must be determined. This rhythm is often referred to as *undifferentiated second-degree AV block*. If the QRS complex is narrow (0.04 to 0.10 seconds), it can be deduced that the location of the block is from the AV junctional area and, therefore, Mobitz type I in origin. However, if the QRS complex is 0.12 seconds or wider, the block could be either from the junctional area (Mobitz type I/Wenckebach area) with a preexisting bundle branch block or it could be a Mobitz type II idioventricular response from the ventricular area below the AV junction.

ARRHYTHMIAS ASSOCIATED WITH DIGITALIS

Historically, one of the most common agents used in the treatment of heart failure and supraventricular tachyarrhythmias was digitalis. Although the use of digitalis is not as common today, it is still prescribed by many clinicians and merits discussion, as it is a common cause of various degrees of AV block. There is a narrow therapeutic range for this drug, and signs of toxicity can occur before acute symptoms are recognized. Digitalis toxicity can cause almost any type of arrhythmia. Those arrhythmias most commonly seen in digitalis toxicity are atrial tachycardia with AV nodal block, accelerated junctional rhythms, atrial fibrillation with a slow or regular ventricular response, second-degree heart block—Mobitz type I (Wenckebach), and ventricular dysrhythmias. The serum digitalis level may not reflect the amount of digitalis bound to the myocardial membrane, where it cannot be measured. Thus, a normal digitalis level should not be the determining factor in assessing digitalis toxicity. The onset of atrial tachydysrhythmias, noncardiac subjective symptoms (particularly altered visual color perception), and a pertinent medication history should make the clinician highly suspicious of digitalis toxicity.

ECG patterns representing the different types of arrhythmias are shown in Figure 36.1.

EPIDEMIOLOGY AND CAUSES

Atrial Arrhythmias

Atrial fibrillation occurs in an estimated 5 million Americans 65 years of age and older. This number is expected to double over the next two decades. Most patients with atrial fibrillation have some form of heart disease. The most common form is coronary artery disease (CAD) associated with heart failure, followed by hypertension, rheumatic heart disease, and valvular heart disease. Frequently, the precipitating event is an acute illness, electrolyte imbalance, or major cardiac surgery. Other causes of atrial fibrillation include abrupt discontinuation of beta blockers, alcohol ingestion (sometimes called "holiday heart"), hyperthyroidism, acute MI, and cor pulmonale. A danger of untreated atrial fibrillation, with or without rapid ventricular response, is a significantly increased risk of embolic stroke. The risk of stroke is increased in untreated atrial fibrillation after 48 to 72 hours; therefore, it is important to diagnose and treat this arrhythmia in an expeditious manner. A beta blocker or calcium channel blocker should be given to slow AV conduction and control the ventricular rate of atrial fibrillation, and the underlying cause of the arrhythmia should be determined to aid in its successful management.

PACs typically have no clinical significance. In a healthy patient, tobacco, caffeine, alcohol, OTC decongestants, or emotional stress may cause PACs. They may also result from stretching of the myocardium, a sign associated with developing heart failure. In patients with organic heart disease, common causes of PACs are mitral valve stenosis and cor pulmonale, which result in atrial enlargement. Occasionally in patients with organic heart disease, PACs may precipitate PSVT, atrial flutter, and atrial fibrillation. The most common cause of a pause on an ECG is a blocked PAC. Assessment of whether the P wave occurs early or is on time (in a regular pattern with other P waves) can help differentiate this diagnosis from heart block. If the P wave is early, it is a premature atrial ectopic beat. If the P wave is on time, yet not coordinated with a normal ventricular contraction, heart block should be considered.

Ventricular Arrhythmias

Frequent PVCs are seen in patients with arteriosclerotic heart disease and cardiomyopathies of differing etiologies. These patients are rarely symptomatic from the PVCs and, in general, do not need to be treated specifically for this arrhythmia. In patients with frequent PVCs, however, it is worthwhile to rule out acute underlying causes of ventricular ectopy, such as hypokalemia, hypomagnesemia, hypoxia, and myocardial ischemia. Other common causes are emotional stress and chemical stimulants, such as alcohol and nicotine. Sustained VT may be associated with a prior MI, CAD, or electrolyte disturbances and is a risk factor for sudden cardiac death in the former.

Heart Blocks

A first-degree heart block (P-R interval greater than 0.20 seconds) may occur as a result of drugs that slow AV conduction or in persons with CAD. A transient second-degree AV heart block type I (Wenckebach) may be associated with an acute inferior wall MI or with heart failure. A Mobitz type II AV block is a less common type of second-degree heart block that is marked by an intermittent blocked impulse occurring at the bundle of His or along the right or left bundle branches. This

Common Arrhythmias
ATRIAL ARRHYTHMIAS

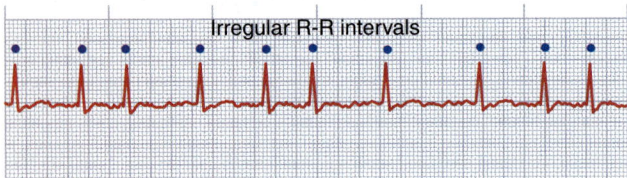

Figure 36.1a Atrial fibrillation. Fibrillatory waves distort the baseline and the R-R interval is characteristically irregular. The ventricular rate is approximately 100 beats/min.

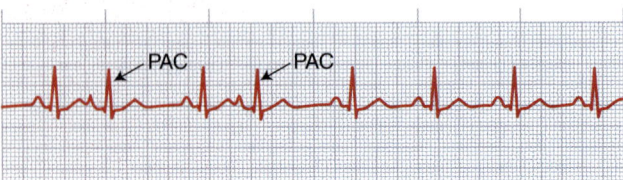

Figure 36.1b Premature atrial contractions (PACs) or atrial premature contractions (APCs). A single complex occurs earlier than the next expected sinus complex. After the PAC, sinus rhythm usually resumes.

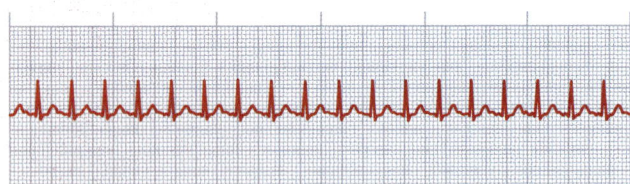

Figure 36.1c Atrial tachycardia with a rate of 180 beats/min.

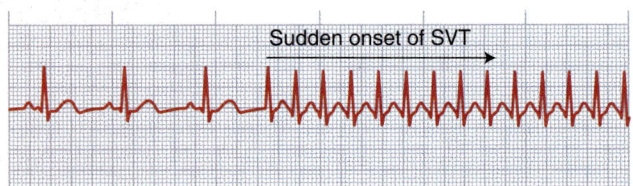

Figure 36.1d Paroxysmal supraventricular tachycardia (PSVT) or paroxysmal atrial tachycardia (PAT). Sinus rhythm that changes into atrial tachycardia at a rate of 230 beats/min.

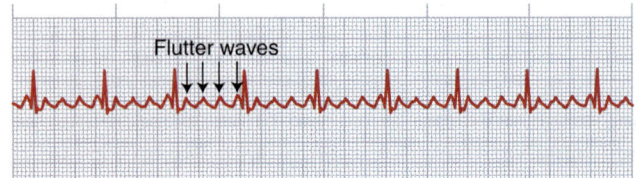

Figure 36.1e Atrial flutter. A characteristic sawtooth pattern at the baseline. Atrial flutter with a 4:1 conduction. The R-R interval is regular.

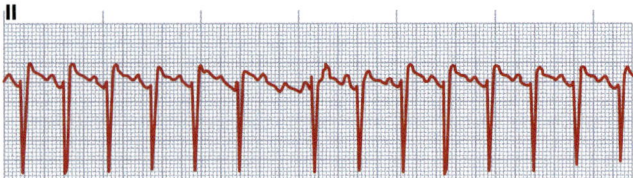

Figure 36.1f Atrial flutter with a 2:1 conduction. Initiation of carotid sinus massage temporarily slows the ventricular rate enough to unmask the flutter waves.

VENTRICULAR ARRHYTHMIAS

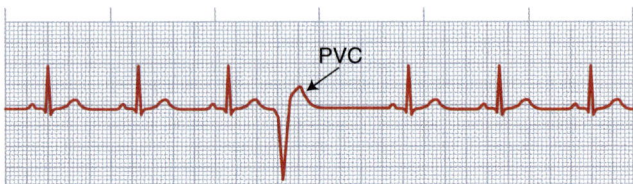

Figure 36.1g Premature ventricular contractions (PVCs). The ectopic QRS complex (the PVC) is wide, is abnormally shaped, and appears earlier than expected. The length of the compensatory pause after a PVC indicates that sinus node discharge was undisturbed. A nonconducted sinus P wave distorts the T wave (the P wave appears on time).

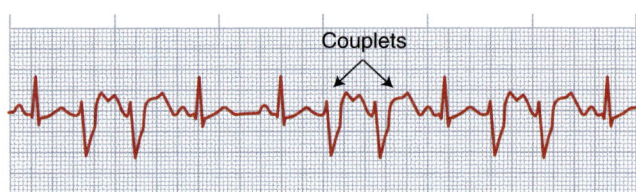

Figure 36.1h PVC couplets. Pairs of uniform PVCs originating from the same ectopic site.

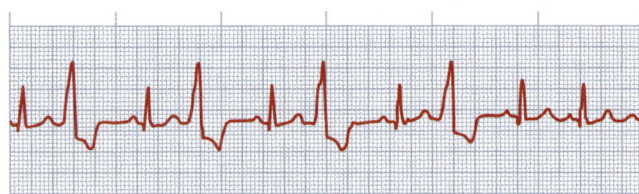

Figure 36.1i PVC bigeminy. A uniform PVC originating from the same ectopic site; occurs every other beat.

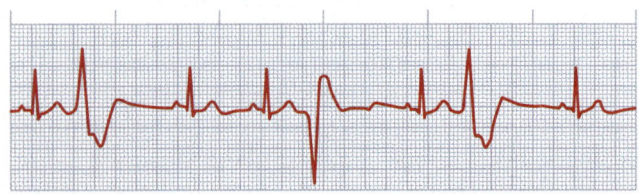

Figure 36.1j Multifocal PVCs. PVCs coming from two ectopic foci.

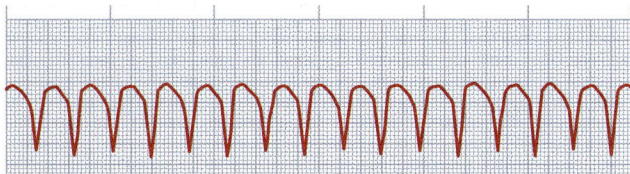

Figure 36.1k Ventricular tachycardia. The ventricular rate is approximately 160 beats/min. The QRS complexes are wide, they look alike, and the R-R interval is regular.

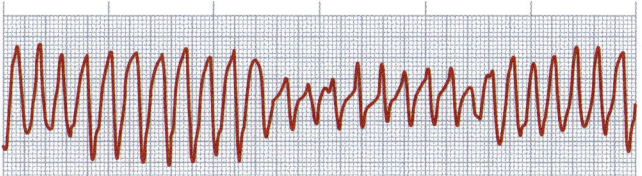

Figure 36.1l Torsades de pointes. Polymorphic ventricular tachycardia, congenital or drug-induced.

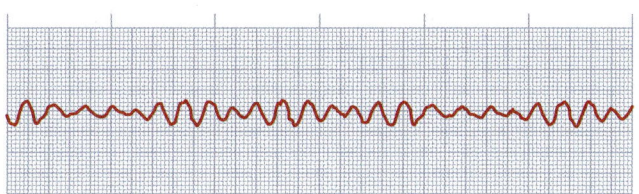

Figure 36.1m Ventricular fibrillation. Chaotic electrical activity with no ventricular contraction.

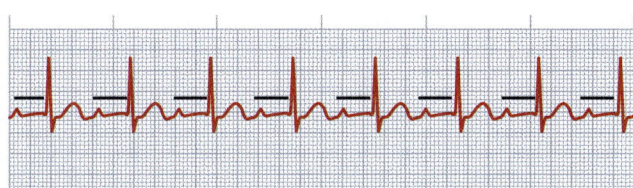

Figure 36.1n Atrioventricular (AV) heart blocks: First-degree AV block. The P-R interval is consistently prolonged at 0.20 seconds or longer, with an underlying sinus rhythm.

SECOND-DEGREE AV BLOCKS

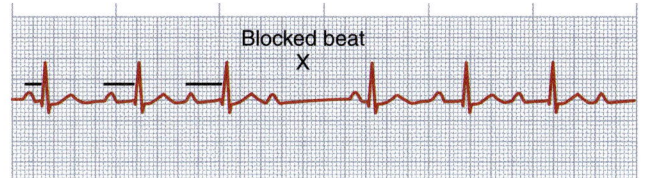

Figure 36.1o Type I (Mobitz I or Wenckebach) second-degree AV block. The P-R interval progressively lengthens with each subsequent impulse until a beat is dropped. The QRS complexes are narrow. The nonconducted P waves are easily visible.

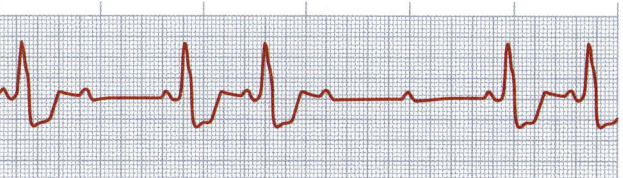

Figure 36.1p Type II (Mobitz II) second-degree AV block. The P-R interval remains fixed. The QRS complexes are wider than normal. The nonconducted P waves are visible. The conduction ratio (P waves to QRS complexes) is commonly 2:1, 3:1, or 4:1.

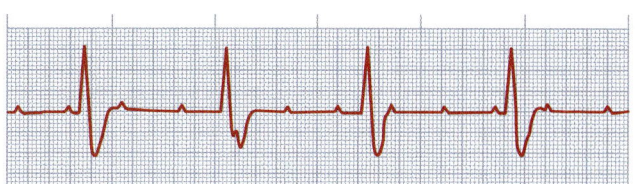

Figure 36.1q Third-degree AV block. There is no relationship between the P wave and the QRS complex. This is a third-degree AV block with a ventricular escape pacemaker.

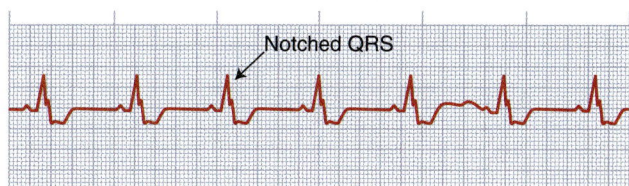

Figure 36.1r Bundle branch block (BBB). Either the left or the right ventricle will depolarize late, creating a "notched" QRS complex. In this strip, we are unable to determine whether this is a right or left BBB. An RBBB is determined in lead V_1, which will show a notched pattern in a classic rSR' (little r wave, S wave, larger R prime wave) upright QRS complex that lasts 0.12 seconds or longer. If an LBBB is present, then V_1 will retain the original formation (showing a small upright r wave with negative remaining complex) that lasts 0.12 seconds or longer. This LBBB can be confirmed in either V_5 or V_6 also by a notched appearance but does not have a set pattern to the QRS as found in the rSR' of an RBBB. It is necessary to be able to determine an LBBB in the setting of an acute MI because this will interfere with accurate 12-lead ECG interpretation of an acute injury pattern.

type of heart block may occur as the result of an anterior wall MI. As a Mobitz type II block progresses, complete heart block with an idioventricular response may follow. Insertion of a temporary pacemaker as soon as a Mobitz type II block is discovered is the standard of care. Other causes of AV block at this level are acute infections, valvular heart disease, and digitalis toxicity. Second-degree heart block is not commonly a transient arrhythmia and can progress to third-degree AV heart block at the ventricular level; therefore, it must be monitored and treated appropriately.

PATHOPHYSIOLOGY

Atrial Arrhythmias and Bypass Tracts

The mechanism of atrial fibrillation remains controversial. Cardiac disease associated with atrial enlargement is the primary cause of the rapid firing (400 to 700 beats per minute) of the ectopic foci throughout the atrium. Although electrical atrial activity is very rapid, only a small islet of myocardium is depolarized rather than the entire atrium. Because the atrium does not contract as a whole, there is no P wave. The chaotic atrial activity is seen as a wavy line between the QRS complexes and is referred to as *fibrillatory waves*. These impulses are transmitted in variable fashion from the atria to the ventricles. The ventricular response rate to atrial fibrillation may be fast or slow, depending on the refractory nature of the AV node and the degree of conduction delay within the AV node. In turn, initial therapy is usually geared toward rate control with AV nodal slowing agents, rather than toward complete resolution of the arrhythmia with antiarrhythmic medications.

Other pathological arrhythmias involve bypass tracts. Normally, electrical impulses from the sinoatrial node within the atria are conducted down the AV node to the His-Purkinje conduction system, disseminating throughout the two ventricles and leading to subsequent contraction. In addition to the AV node, some individuals have a fast-conducting accessory pathway between the atria and ventricles that bypasses the AV node. The tissue in these pathways depolarizes at a faster rate because of the presence of faster inward sodium transport channels. One of the most common and well-characterized examples of these bypass tracts is the bundle of Kent accessory tract, which is seen in individuals with Wolff-Parkinson-White (WPW) syndrome. Because conduction down this bypass pathway directly transmits a depolarizing impulse to the ventricles faster than impulses sent down the AV node, this has been termed a "preexcitation syndrome." ECG patterns in these patients demonstrate QRS fusion beats with a characteristic shape produced by the overlap of QRS complexes transmitted via each pathway in temporal proximity, hence creating a fusion complex. The first portion of the upswing in the R wave in this complex has a characteristic slanted appearance with a shallower angle than the remainder of the upward deflection, termed a "delta wave." Figure 36.2 shows a delta wave present in WPW syndrome.

The most common mechanisms of PSVT observed in symptomatic patients are AVRT (30% of cases) and AVNRT (60% of cases). The other 10% are sinoatrial reentrant tachycardia, intra-atrial reentrant tachycardia,

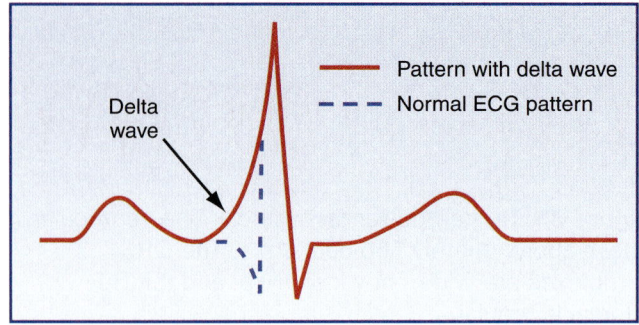

Figure 36.2 Delta wave present in Wolff-Parkinson-White (WPW) syndrome.

and permanent junctional reciprocating tachycardia. AVRT is distinguished by the dependence of the circular, reentrant impulse on an accessory conduction pathway, separate from the AV node. Thus, the fast bypass tract found in WPW syndrome is an ideal setup for development of AVRT. Normal physiology dictates that cardiac conducting tissue become refractory (i.e., resistant to depolarization and electrical conduction) for a brief period of time following transmission of an electrical impulse. Bypass pathways, such as that seen in WPW syndrome, typically have shorter refractory periods than the AV node. Once depolarizing impulses are transmitted down the AV node to the ventricles, the refractory nature of the AV node prevents retrograde conduction back up this pathway. However, the same impulse may be conducted in retrograde fashion from the ventricles back up the accessory bypass tract to the atria. In turn, this impulse may then be conducted back down the AV node, which will have recovered from its refractory state by this time, only to circle back around once again to the atria via the fast accessory pathway. This type of circular, orthodromic conduction accounts for 90% of AVRT cases, with a P wave occurring immediately after the QRS complex, rather than before it. The remaining 10% of AVRT cases are considered antidromic, with the depolarizing impulse initially conducted down the fast accessory tract, only to circle back up the slower AV nodal pathway to the atria to complete the circular movement.

In AVNRT, PSVT typically results from an interplay of two conducting pathways within the AV node itself—one fast and one slow. The key aspect of this type of PSVT is that reentry of the impulse is dependent on an AV nodal pathway, as opposed to an accessory bypass pathway. In AVNRT, the fast AV nodal conducting pathway has a refractory period that lasts longer than that of the slow AV nodal pathway. Thus, if an electrical impulse enters both pathways of the AV node simultaneously, the fast pathway will remain refractory longer. In turn, if an early PAC then enters the AV node while the fast accessory pathway is still refractory, it can depolarize the ventricles only via transmission down the slower AV nodal pathway. By the time the impulse has traveled down this open slow pathway, the fast pathway is no longer refractory, and the impulse may travel in retrograde fashion back up to the atria via the fast pathway, and then back down again to the ventricles via the slow pathway. This mechanism activates the atria and the ventricles nearly simultaneously, which places the P wave within the QRS complex, distorting its terminal portion.

Ventricular Arrhythmias

PVCs and VT may be the result of enhanced normal automaticity from catecholamines within the His-Purkinje system or abnormal automaticity anywhere in the ventricles from ischemia, injury, or electrolyte imbalances. Another mechanism for these arrhythmias is reentry through slowly conducting tissue within the His-Purkinje system or the ventricular myocardium related to catecholamines.

Heart Blocks

The mechanism of AV block is delayed conduction or nonconduction of an atrial impulse when the AV junction is not physiologically refractory. In first-degree AV block, there is not an actual block but rather a prolongation of conduction. In second-degree block, there is nonconduction of some of the atrial impulses. The P-R interval either varies as in a Mobitz type I or is fixed as in a Mobitz type II. The pathology is either in the AV node itself (Mobitz type I) or within or below the bundle of His (Mobitz type II). The QRS complex duration assists the clinician in localizing the level of the block. A narrow QRS complex is seen if the ventricular response is initiated at the level of the AV node and conducted down both bundle branches simultaneously, as seen in Mobitz type I heart block. A wider QRS complex indicates that the block is located further down the conduction system at the bundle of His or within the bundle branches. These criteria may not be helpful if the patient has a preexisting right or left bundle branch block because such a patient could present with a prolonged P-R interval and a broad QRS complex. In this case, the pathology could be either in the AV node or within or below the bundle of His. The clinician would then need to assess the P-R interval carefully for varying lengths and Wenckebach conduction patterns. If the patient's ECG has a pattern of two P waves for every wide QRS complex (2:1 conduction), the origin of pathology is difficult to determine from the ECG. However, a narrow QRS complex (0.06 to 0.10 seconds) points to a Mobitz type I block.

CLINICAL PRESENTATION

Subjective

The most common presenting symptoms of clinically significant tachyarrhythmias are fatigue, dyspnea, and palpitations. Less commonly reported symptoms are angina, changing level of consciousness, and syncope. If the patient is aware of palpitations, the clinician should have them "tap" out the rhythm in the palm of the hand. Irregular tapping at irregular intervals (i.e., an irregularly irregular heart rhythm) can differentiate this rhythm from the regular patterns of other arrhythmias.

A patient experiencing SVT will complain of dizziness, shortness of breath, and chest pain. As part of the patient's history, the clinician should ask about polyuria that is associated with SVT. Polyuria may be present in patients with PSVT or atrial fibrillation. It is thought to be related to the cardiac secretion of atrial natriuretic factor (atrial natriuretic peptide) due to changes in the heart rhythm and atrial pressure. Polyuria is particularly common in AVNRT with high atrial pressures.

A patient presenting with nonsustained VT may complain of palpitations or may present with symptoms similar to those of patients with sustained VT. Usually, patients with sustained VT will demonstrate findings compatible with a loss of cardiac output, such as decreased levels of mentation and hypotension.

In patients with heart block, the origin of the block may determine the degree of symptomatology. A patient experiencing first-degree heart block will be asymptomatic. Patients with second-degree Mobitz type I AV block that progress into third-degree block with an idiojunctional response may or may not exhibit overt signs and symptoms of bradycardia. Hemodynamic symptoms will depend on the rate of the junctional response (anywhere from 40 to 60 beats per minute), the status of the patient's LV ejection fraction, and the loss of atrial kick (up to 20% to 30% of cardiac output). A patient whose Mobitz type II heart block progresses to third-degree heart block with a ventricular response of 20 to 40 beats per minute will almost always exhibit signs and symptoms of severe bradycardia, such as hypotension and profound changes in level of consciousness, which may preclude subjective symptom complaints.

Objective

Atrial Fibrillation

Physical examination of the patient with atrial fibrillation will yield an irregularly irregular heart rhythm. In most cases of new-onset atrial fibrillation, the rate is rapid (100 to 180 beats per minute). Patients can be asymptomatic, although most present with symptoms such as palpitations, dizziness, a decrease in blood pressure (BP), or new-onset activity intolerance. A stroke can be the presenting manifestation of atrial fibrillation as a result of emboli traveling from a clot formed in the dysfunctional atrium into the cerebral vasculature.

Cannon waves may be seen, which are unpredictable expansions of the jugular pulse caused by the atria contracting against closed AV valves, which results in a reflux of blood into the jugular vein. When present in atrial fibrillation, cannon waves signify AV dissociation.

The ECG strip will show fibrillatory waves representing an atrial rate of 350 to 600 beats per minute (although unmeasurable on an ECG), with a ventricular rate of 100 to 180 beats per minute. The rhythm is irregular, and there are no discernible P waves on the ECG, with a coarse or fine fibrillatory wave (f wave) present. This is the hallmark of this type of arrhythmia and represents chaotic atrial activity.

Premature Atrial Contractions

PACs may be found on a routine ECG. The rate is usually 60 to 100 beats per minute with a regular rhythm, except when premature beats are present. The premature beats have a different P-wave configuration because of their origination outside the sinus node. The PAC P-R interval may be different from the sinus P-R interval, and the QRS complex may be normal, aberrant (i.e., wide QRS complex), or absent.

The most common cause of an electrical pause on an ECG rhythm strip is a blocked or nonconducted PAC. This occurs when the PAC comes so early that it falls in the T wave. If the AV node is still refractory, the early P wave does not conduct and a pause is seen on the rhythm strip. If the clinician looks closely at the T wave and compares it with the patient's other T waves, the early nonconducted P wave may be seen distorting that specific T wave. If the nonconducted PACs present in a bigeminal pattern, the rhythm may be mistaken for profound sinus bradycardia or sinoatrial (SA) block. Thus, the clinician should always assess for nonconducted P waves within preceding T waves in any pauses observed on the ECG.

Observation of the neck veins may help the clinician rapidly distinguish between PSVT and VT. During PSVT, the atria contract against closed AV valves, resulting in a rapid, regular expansion of the neck veins (the same mechanism as cannon waves). This physical finding has been called the "frog sign" because the rapid, regular expansion of the neck veins resembles the puffing motion of a frog, which may be noted by the patient's family members.

Supraventricular Tachycardia

The ECG of a patient in SVT will present with a rate of 150 to 250 beats per minute. If the rhythm is atrial tachycardia, P waves are ectopic and distorted and may be initiated by a PAC. The P-R interval is shortened and the QRS complex may be normal or wide due to aberrant conduction. As atrial tachycardias may be grouped within SVTs, it is important to recognize that if a patient is in atrial flutter, the atrial rate will be regular at 250 to 350 beats per minute, whereas the ventricular rate may be regular or slightly irregular. The P waves are discernible and "march out" (i.e., can be mapped out with a caliper) consistently throughout the strip in atrial flutter, while P-R intervals cannot be calculated, and the QRS complexes may have variable conduction. In atrial fibrillation, the atrial rate is not discernable and the ventricular response is grossly irregular; the QRS complex may be narrow or wide if aberrant conduction is present.

Premature Ventricular Contractions

The ECG of a patient with PVCs will usually show a rate of 60 to 100 beats per minute. The rhythm will be irregular due to the premature ventricular beat. The PVC usually obscures the P wave; however, P waves may be visible if the PVC occurs late in diastole. These P waves are not related to the ectopic beat and occur at the same regular rate of the preceding sinus P waves. The P-R interval is not measurable for the PVC, whose QRS complex is wide and bizarre. It may be observed in patterns of ventricular bigeminy (with a PVC seen with every other ventricular beat), trigeminy (with a PVC seen with every third ventricular beat), or couplets (with two PVCs occurring in a row). In the setting of an acute ischemic event, PVCs that occur close to the preceding T wave (called an *R on T phenomenon*) may precipitate ventricular fibrillation.

Ventricular Tachycardia

VT can be categorized as monomorphic or polymorphic. The ECG of a patient with monomorphic VT will show a rate greater than 100 beats per minute with a regular rhythm. The P wave will be buried in the QRS complex or may be discernible after the QRS complex because of retrograde conduction. The P-R interval is not measurable, and the QRS complex is wide and bizarre. The ECG of a patient with polymorphic VT will show a "flipping" of the ventricular axis. For example, torsades de pointes is a form of polymorphic VT in which the QT interval demonstrates prolongation before the onset of the arrhythmia. It is essential to differentiate torsades de pointes from non–torsades polymorphic VT to optimize treatment (e.g., torsades de pointes may respond to magnesium treatment).

Heart Blocks

In first-degree AV block, the pulse will usually be 60 to 100 beats per minute. The ECG rhythm is usually regular, with a P wave preceding each QRS complex and a prolonged P-R interval longer than 0.20 seconds. QRS complexes follow every P wave and are usually a normal width.

A patient with second-degree Mobitz type I AV block will usually have a ventricular rate of 50 to 70 beats per minute, although the rate may vary. The atrial rate is regular, whereas the ventricular rate is irregular. P waves precede each QRS complex, and the P-R interval progressively lengthens. The QRS complex is usually normal in width, unless a preexisting bundle branch block is present. As the P-R interval progresses, eventually the QRS complex disappears for a beat. In contrast, in a Mobitz type II AV block, the P-R interval may be prolonged or normal, but it remains constant, unlike the progressively lengthening P-R interval of Mobitz type I. The blocked P wave may occur in patterns of 2:1, 3:1, or 4:1. The width of the QRS complex indicates where the block is located. The wider the complex, the lower the block is located below the AV node. The P wave is regular and the P-R interval constant, with a wide QRS following every P wave until the QRS complex is not conducted (dropped).

With a third-degree block, the AV node (if the block is of a Mobitz type I origin) or the ventricles (if the block is of a Mobitz type II origin) generate an autonomous rhythm with a ventricular rate of 25 to 60 beats per minute. The atrial rate is 60 to 100 beats per minute. P waves are present and regular, but there is no relationship to the QRS complexes. The P-R interval cannot be calculated as it is variable, and the QRS complex is normal if the block is at the AV nodal/junctional level (Mobitz type I origin), or it is wider and longer than 0.10 seconds if the block is at the level of the ventricles (Mobitz type II origin).

DIAGNOSTIC REASONING

Diagnostic Tests

As described in the sections above, the ECG is the routine diagnostic test to determine the type of arrhythmia to direct treatment appropriately. The most definitive diagnostics are confirmed by electrical physiology studies. Electrophysiological testing using intracardiac electrocardiographic recordings and programmed atrial and/or ventricular stimulation is used in the diagnosis and management of complex arrhythmias. Electrophysiological testing can evaluate recurrent syncope of possible cardiac origin and differentiate supraventricular from ventricular dysrhythmias.

Tilt-table testing (autonomic testing) is useful in patients with arrhythmias when syncope may be due to a vasovagal (neurocardiogenic) response. After positioning the patient supine on a tilt-table with a foot support in place, the table is tilted to approximately 60 to 70 degrees, so that the patient is in a near-standing position. The patient is observed for syncope (loss of consciousness) throughout this process, due to bradycardia and/or hypotension induced by the tilting, which will occur in about one-third of patients with recurrent syncope. If no loss of consciousness is observed with this initial maneuver, the sensitivity of the test may be increased through the use of a provocative agent, such as a low-dose infusion of the beta agonist isoproterenol or a vasodilator such as nitroglycerin or adenosine. However, this may also decrease specificity of the test and thereby increase the risk of a false positive result.

Transesophageal echocardiography (TEE) is a diagnostic procedure used to rule out the presence of thrombi in the left atrium before cardioversion in atrial fibrillation. The presence of clots in the left atrium is a contraindication to cardioversion, as the sudden change to sinus rhythm may inadvertently dislodge portions of the clot from the atrium. In turn, an anticoagulation regimen of at least 3 weeks must first be completed before cardioversion, if a confirmatory TEE cannot be done to rule out atrial thrombi.

Differential Diagnosis

The clinician should consider conditions that could mimic the symptoms of arrhythmia, such as a panic attack, anxiety, valvular disorders, and syncopal episodes that are either neurogenic or cardiac in origin.

MANAGEMENT

Management of patients with arrhythmias depends on the expertise of the clinician. If the clinician is at all unsure of the management of an arrhythmia, consultation with a cardiovascular specialist is necessary.

Atrial Fibrillation

The initial goal of treatment in atrial fibrillation is to control the ventricular response and then convert the patient back to normal sinus rhythm (NSR) by using medications or electrical synchronized cardioversion. Drugs that may convert atrial fibrillation to sinus rhythm include amiodarone and disopyramide, although disopyramide is rarely used and usually requires hospital admission to initiate therapy. Although many patients with atrial fibrillation revert to NSR after cardioversion, many patients return to atrial fibrillation within a short period of time. This occurs particularly in patients with long-standing atrial fibrillation or in patients with advanced heart disease and an enlarged left atrium. Patients with new-onset atrial fibrillation or chronic atrial fibrillation with a very rapid ventricular response should be admitted to a medical unit where telemetry is available, so that their response to treatment can be carefully monitored.

Elective synchronized cardioversion is recommended if acute ischemic heart disease is present with a rapid ventricular rate (120 to 200 beats per minute) or if the patient is in clinical distress. All patients should be assessed for the risk of atrial emboli before electrical cardioversion. Typically, the patient should undergo TEE to assess for the presence of mural thrombi. Successful cardioversion (in the absence of mural thrombi) and the prevention of recurrence of atrial fibrillation depend on atrial size and the length of time the patient has been in atrial fibrillation before intervention. In addition, cardiac valvular function should be assessed for further therapeutic interventions.

Before electrical or pharmacological cardioversion is attempted, anticoagulants should be considered. Anticoagulation therapy should be initiated in all patients who remain in atrial fibrillation for longer than 48 hours or who experience atrial fibrillation of unknown duration (see Drugs Commonly Prescribed 36.1). Historically, patients have been placed on IV heparin for rapid anticoagulation

Drugs Commonly Prescribed 36.1: Antithrombotic Treatment Options for Stroke Prevention in Nonvalvular Atrial Fibrillation

AGENT	DOSING	IMPLICATIONS FOR PRACTICE
warfarin* (Coumadin)	Starting dose: 2–5 mg daily in the evening	Goal INR 2.0–3.0; higher in mechanical valve patients Antidote: vitamin K
dabigatran† (Pradaxa)	150 mg twice daily for creatinine clearance (CrCl) >30 mg/mL 75 mg twice daily for CrCl = 15–30 mg/mL Contraindicated if CrCl <15 mg/mL	Requires no laboratory monitoring. Do not cut, crush, or open pill Antidote: idarucizumab (Praxbind)
rivaroxaban† (Xarelto)	20 mg daily for CrCl >50 mg/mL 5 mg daily for CrCl = 15–49 mg/mL No dosing information for CrCl <15 mg/mL	Requires no laboratory monitoring If unable to swallow, pill may be crushed No dosing if patient is on dialysis Antidote: andexanet alfa (Andexxa)
apixaban† (Eliquis)	5 mg twice daily 2.5 mg twice daily with at least two of the following: age older than 80 years, body weight <60 kg, or creatinine >1.5 mg/mL Contraindicated if CrCl <25 mg/mL	Requires no laboratory monitoring Antidote: andexanet alfa (Andexxa)

*Pregnant women (with the exception of those who have mechanical heart valves) should not receive warfarin.
†Should not be administered to patients with prosthetic heart valves, hemodynamically significant valvular heart disease, severe kidney failure, and/or advanced liver disease.

and then started concurrently on warfarin (Coumadin), which takes approximately 5 days to achieve its full anticoagulant effect. A prothrombin time (PT) with international normalized ratio (INR) is drawn when the patient is started on warfarin, with the dose adjusted according to the patient's INR. The target INR in atrial fibrillation is between 2 and 3. The PT should be checked at regular intervals to ensure the INR remains within the appropriate range. Once a constant appropriate INR range has been achieved, the PT should be monitored monthly.

More recent therapeutic anticoagulant approaches include the subcutaneous administration of low–molecular-weight heparin (enoxaparin [Lovenox]) and the use of direct oral anticoagulants (DOACs). These DOACs, including dabigatran (Pradaxa), rivaroxaban (Xarelto), apixaban (Eliquis), and edoxaban (Savaysa), have been replacing the use of warfarin in patients specifically with nonvalvular atrial fibrillation, as they do not require dose adjustments or monitoring with PT/INR. Commonalities across all these agents include shorter half-lives, fewer drug–drug interactions, and earlier peak blood levels compared with warfarin. Comparative studies against warfarin suggest that these agents lead to a 10% reduction in mortality, fewer strokes, and fewer systemic emboli. Dabigatran has an approved antidote, idarucizumab (Praxbind), while rivaroxaban, apixaban, and edoxaban can be reversed with the antidote andexanet alfa (Andexxa). Patients in chronic atrial fibrillation who are difficult to convert to a controlled ventricular rate should be on anticoagulant therapy indefinitely. For patients refractory to these therapies, cardiac ablation therapy is an option.

A permanent implantable device is available for patients with nonvalvular atrial fibrillation. Inserted via the femoral vein, the Watchman device closes the left atrial appendage of the heart and reduces the risk of stroke. After implantation for 6 weeks, patients discontinue warfarin but remain on clopidogrel (Plavix) for 4 months, which is then discontinued as well.

Premature Atrial Contractions

Treatment of PACs is not indicated unless the patient is symptomatic or an underlying cause can be corrected. Simple measures such as stopping tobacco use, reducing caffeine intake, avoiding OTC decongestants, and improving electrolyte imbalances may reduce the incidence of PACs. If symptoms persist, Holter monitoring may be indicated, and the patient should be instructed to maintain a diary of activities, especially those associated with the onset of symptomatic PACs. The patient should be followed closely for the first 3 months to establish whether the condition is acute or chronic.

Supraventricular Tachycardia

The initial treatment for stable SVT consists of vagal maneuvers, which increase parasympathetic tone and slow conduction through the AV node. These techniques include coughing, blowing into a pinched (sealed) straw, lying on the floor while elevating one's legs against the wall, or squatting. If the clinician has experience with carotid sinus massage, this maneuver is usually effective. However, carotid massage is contraindicated in patients with carotid artery stenosis, bruits, a history of transient ischemic attacks, or in patients older than 65 years who may have an exacerbated parasympathetic response to carotid pressure. Facial immersion in cold water (the dive reflex) is another method that has been used. The clinician must never use eyeball pressure as a vagal maneuver because it may cause retinal detachment and is unpleasant for the patient.

In the case of PSVT, adenosine is the treatment of choice because it blocks electrical reentry through the AV node. If the patient has symptomatic PSVT, hypotension, ischemic pain, or severe heart failure, synchronized cardioversion is usually recommended. Pharmacological intervention may involve beta blockers and calcium channel blockers. Patients who have recurrent symptomatic and refractory PSVT will need to see an electrophysiologist for possible radiofrequency ablation of the accessory pathway. Ablation therapy is often chosen over a lifetime course of prophylactic drugs.

Premature Ventricular Contractions

Treatment of PVCs is usually not needed in healthy adults because many adults experience PVCs with no untoward effects. PVCs may be related to an MI, however; in which case, it must be determined whether the PVCs are caused by a problem with oxygenation, hypotension, electrolyte disturbances, acid–base imbalance, other medications, or an increased catecholamine state from unrelieved ischemic pain or anxiety. Typically, therapy in this case involves treating the underlying cause, such as hypoxia; pain; electrolyte imbalance; or alterations in hemodynamics with nitroglycerin, oxygen, pain medications, or beta blockers.

Heart Blocks

Treatment for a first-degree AV block is not advised because it is an asymptomatic arrhythmia. However, the clinician should assess and take note of any drugs the patient is taking that may prolong AV conduction. For a Mobitz type I second-degree AV block, treatment may not be indicated unless symptomatic. Medications such as beta blockers, calcium channel blockers, and digitalis should be considered as a cause and decreasing the dose or discontinuing these drugs should be considered. Additionally, the patient should be evaluated for an inferior wall MI, which can also present with a Mobitz type I AV block. If symptomatic bradycardia develops, a temporary or transcutaneous pacemaker may be needed, whereas a permanent pacemaker may be required for a Mobitz type II AV block. A Mobitz type II AV block may be seen in the presence of an anteroseptal wall MI. For third-degree heart block, the underlying pathological site blocking AV conduction must be identified to prevent complications. The ability to determine whether the block has an idiojunctional response versus an idioventricular response is critical in determining the appropriate intervention, as third-degree heart block is considered an emergent and potentially life-threatening condition that requires a pacemaker.

Implantable Cardioverter-Defibrillators

Implantable cardioverter-defibrillators (ICDs) are multiprogrammable antiarrhythmic devices capable of treating bradydysrhythmias, ventricular fibrillation, and ventricular tachycardia. These devices offer antitachycardic pacing, as well as low- and high-energy shocks in multiple ranges of tachycardic rates. These devices are placed under the skin of the left chest. Patients need close follow-up with a cardiologist and extensive patient education. Patients should carry a device identification card at all times. The American College of Cardiology/American Heart Association/North American Society of Pacing and Electrophysiology guidelines delineate indications for ICD therapy.

FOLLOW-UP AND REFERRAL

A cardiologist should be consulted to establish the plan of care. The cardiologist may order a Holter monitor to assess the pattern of the arrhythmia. Electrophysiological studies may be indicated to evaluate the patient for cardioablation therapy for PSVTs, such as WPW syndrome.

Patient Education: Arrhythmias

The education of a patient with atrial fibrillation should include a list of vitamin K–containing foods and both prescription and OTC drugs that interfere with warfarin (see Table 36.2). A patient on warfarin is at risk for bleeding; therefore, the clinician should provide resources for medical alert identification jewelry and instruct the patient how to assess for signs of internal bleeding, such as bruising and dark stools. These patients should also use electric shavers instead of razors with blades to avoid lacerations and nightlights for illumination to avoid traumatic accidents. Patients should be taught to check their pulse rate, and if the pulse rate is below 60 beats per minute or the patient notices bursts in the heart rate, it should be reported to the clinician.

Smartphone technology now offers several choices in phone applications (apps) that are available to detect and monitor atrial fibrillation. These apps can provide highly effective screening tools for atrial fibrillation in the primary care setting. When patients are given the ability to self-screen, this empowers them and engages them in their own self-care.

For patients who have an ICD device implanted, if they are admitted to hospice care or are on a treatment withdrawal protocol, the treating clinician should consider deactivating the ICD to avoid defibrillation in the case of cardiac arrest.

TABLE 36.2 Drugs and Foods That Interact With Warfarin

Increased Anticoagulant Effect	Decreased Anticoagulant Effect
DRUGS	
acetaminophen (Tylenol)	carbamazepine (Tegretol)
allopurinol (Zyloprim)	cholestyramine (Questran)
amiodarone (Cordarone)	ethinylestradiol/
cephalexin (Keflex)	norethisterone
ciprofloxacin (Cipro)	(Loestrin)
cisapride (Propulsid)	ethinylestradiol/
disulfiram (Antabuse)	norgestimate
erythromycin (E-Mycin)	(Ortho Tri-Cyclen)
famotidine (Pepcid)	griseofulvin (Grifulvin)
fluconazole (Diflucan)	rifampin (Rifadin)
fluoxetine (Prozac)	spironolactone (Aldactone)
gemfibrozil (Lopid)	sucralfate (Carafate)
glimepiride (Amaryl)	
glipizide (Glucotrol)	
ibuprofen (Advil, Motrin)	
levofloxacin (Levaquin)	
metronidazole (Flagyl)	
penicillin V potassium (Pen VK)	
propranolol (Inderal)	
quinidine (Quinaglute)	
ranitidine (Zantac)	
sertraline (Zoloft)	
tetracycline (Achromycin)	
trimethoprim-sulfamethoxazole (Bactrim)	
valproate (Depakene)	
FOODS AND NUTRIENTS	
cranberry juice	broccoli, Brussels sprouts, chard, collard greens, kale, mustard greens, parsley, and spinach
excessive alcohol use	canola and soybean oils
vitamin A	green tea
vitamin E	vitamin K

VALVULAR DISORDERS AND MURMURS

Heart valve disorders may be congenital or acquired and may be symptomatic or asymptomatic. Many are detected during cardiac auscultation when alterations in the normal heart rhythm, presence of extrasystoles, murmurs, or other abnormal heart sounds are heard. Mitral and aortic valve disorders are the most common of the heart valve disorders.

Heart murmurs are the sounds of turbulent blood flow that typically result from specific valvular disorders. Blood traveling through the chambers and great vessels is normally a silent event. When turbulence exists along the walls of the heart or a great vessel, a murmur occurs. Murmurs may be benign, in that the clinician simply hears the blood flowing through the heart, but no cardiac or vascular structural abnormality exists. Certain cardiac structural problems, such as valvular or myocardial disorders, can contribute to the development of a murmur; for example, murmurs arise when a heart valve fails to open (stenosis) or fails to close (insufficiency).

Types of Valvular Disorders

Table 36.3 describes the common valvular disorders, several of which are discussed in this section.

Aortic stenosis is the inability of the aortic valves to open to an optimally sized orifice. The aortic valve normally opens to 3 cm^2; aortic stenosis usually does not cause significant symptoms until the valvular orifice is limited to 0.8 cm^2. The disease is characterized by a long symptom-free period, with rapid clinical deterioration at the onset of symptoms, including dyspnea, syncope, chest pain, and other symptoms of heart failure. The clinician should assess for a systolic murmur and/or a narrow pulse pressure, which are characteristics of severe aortic stenosis. Aortic stenosis can lead to LV hypertrophic changes and subsequent LV dysfunction.

The murmur of mitral regurgitation (also referred to as *mitral insufficiency*) arises from mitral valve incompetency or the inability of the mitral valve to close properly. This allows for retrograde "regurgitant" flow from a high-pressure area (left ventricle) to an area of lower pressure (left atrium). Mitral regurgitation is most often caused by the degeneration of the mitral valve, most commonly by endocarditis, a calcific annulus, rheumatic heart disease, ruptured chordae tendineae, or papillary muscle dysfunction. In mitral regurgitation from rheumatic heart disease, there is usually also some degree of mitral stenosis. Once the person is symptomatic, the disease typically progresses in a downhill course of heart failure over the next 10 years.

Mitral valve prolapse (MVP) is the most common valvular heart problem, with an incidence of 2.4% in the general population based on two-dimensional echocardiographic criteria. In most cases, MVP is a benign condition. However, MVP with mitral regurgitation may predispose the individual to thrombi and endocarditis. In the past, the prevalence of MVP was overestimated, owing to a lack of specific diagnostic procedures. In turn, patients given this diagnosis more than 10 years earlier may not have the disorder at all and should be reevaluated with two-dimensional echocardiography for confirmation.

Types of Murmurs

Benign systolic ejection murmurs (a type of physiological murmur) are found in the absence of cardiac pathology. The term implies that the reason for the

TABLE 36.3 Common Valvular Disorders

Disorder	Murmur Characteristics	Physical Examination	Diagnostic Findings
Aortic stenosis	Harsh systolic murmur, usually crescendo-decrescendo pattern Heard best: Second right intercostal space (RICS) near apex Radiation: To carotids Other: Softens with standing	Cardiac: May have diminished S_2, slow-filling carotid pulse, narrow pulse pressure, loud S_4, heaving point of maximum impulse (PMI) Other: Anxiety, difficulty breathing, compromised mental status, cyanosis, peripheral edema, hair loss, shiny skin over shins, cool extremities, decreased systolic blood pressure, pulmonary edema	Chest x-ray: Aortic valve calcification, LV enlargement, prominent ascending aorta ECG: LV hypertrophy (LVH), sinus tachycardia, atrial fibrillation, atrioventricular (AV) conduction delay, left or right bundle branch block (LBBB, RBBB) Echocardiogram: Limited aortic valve movement, thickened LV wall Cardiac catheterization: Increased pressure gradient in systole across aortic valve, decreased size of aortic orifice, increased LV end-diastolic pressure (LVEDP)
Aortic regurgitation	High-pitched blowing diastolic murmur Heard best: Third left intercostal space (LICS) Other: May be enhanced by forced expiration, leaning forward	Cardiac: Usually with S_3, wide pulse pressure, sustained thrusting apical impulse, palpitations, dyspnea, orthopnea, paroxysmal nocturnal dyspnea (PND), syncope, signs of LV failure, peripheral edema, flushed skin, cardiomegaly Other: More common in men, usually from rheumatic heart disease; fatigue, weakness, anxiety, compromised mental status	Chest x-ray: Aortic valve calcification, LV enlargement, dilation of ascending aorta ECG: LVH, sinus tachycardia, premature ventricular contractions (PVCs) Echocardiogram: Dilated and hyperdynamic LV, enlargement of aortic root and left atrium (LA), early closure of mitral valve, diastolic fluttering of aortic valve Cardiac catheterization: Decreased aortic diastolic blood pressure (BP), increased LVEDP, reflux through aortic valve
Aortic sclerosis	Soft systolic ejection "50 over 50" murmur (found in 50% of those older than 50 years) Heard best: Second RICS in aortic valve region Other: Marker for increased risk of cardiovascular events; may precede aortic stenosis	Cardiac: May also hear normal split of S_2 heart sound	Echocardiography: Best detected by two-dimensional echocardiogram; benign thickening and/or calcification of aortic valve leaflets Often accompanied by mitral annulus calcification
Mitral stenosis	Middiastolic rumbling murmur Accentuated S_1 in early disease	Heard best at apex with the stethoscope bell with patient in left lateral decubitus position	Echocardiography often reveals LA enlargement; ECG may show P mitrale, a broad notched P wave in several leads and/or a negative component to the P wave in V_1 Atrial fibrillation is often present; chest x-ray may reveal pulmonary edema
Mitral regurgitation	Holosystolic murmur	Heard best at the apex and radiates to the axilla; accentuated with clenching fists or lying supine; an S_3 may be present on auscultation; may palpate a laterally displaced PMI	ECG may reveal left atrial abnormality and LVH Chest x-ray may reveal pulmonary edema
Mitral prolapse	Midsystolic click followed by late systolic murmur	Heard best at the apex; click occurs later in systole with maneuvers that increase volume of left ventricle (e.g., squatting or lying supine)	Echocardiography will show protrusion of mitral valve into left atrium during systole
Atrial septal defect (ASD)	Fixed splitting of S_2 during both inspiration and expiration	May palpate right ventricular heave in advanced disease (Eisenmenger's syndrome)	Transthoracic echo may visualize atrioseptal defect (ASD) directly or visualize bubbles traversing ASD while performing a bubble study ECG may present with first-degree AV block or right atrial abnormality

murmur is something other than obstruction to flow and is present with a normal BP gradient across the valve. These murmurs may be heard in up to 80% of thin adults or children if the cardiac examination is performed in a soundproof room. The most common type is a Stills murmur, which is most prevalent in children and usually resolves in adolescence but may persist into adulthood; these murmurs are best heard at the lower left sternal border. The next most common type of benign systolic ejection murmur is a pulmonary flow murmur that is best heard at the upper left sternal border. Benign systolic ejection murmurs occur in early to midsystole, leaving the two heart sounds intact. In addition, the patient with a benign systolic ejection murmur denies cardiac symptomatology and has an otherwise normal cardiac examination, including an appropriately located point of maximal impulse and full pulses. No cardiac pathology is present with a physiological murmur, so no endocarditis prophylaxis is needed.

Functional murmurs exist in the presence of no obvious valvular deformity. A hemic murmur is heard in hyperkinetic or high-volume states such as anemia secondary to fluid overload, fever, or in response to exercise. The murmur has a crescendo–decrescendo pattern and is harsh; both heart sounds are preserved. Because there is no cardiac pathology associated with this condition, it resolves when the underlying high-flow state normalizes. Functional murmurs also occur in other high flow states, including hypervolemia, sepsis, hyperthyroidism, and pregnancy. As with a physiological murmur, no structural cardiac abnormality is present, and no endocarditis prophylaxis is needed.

An aortic sclerosis murmur is also called the *50/50 murmur* because it is present in about 50% of adults older than 50 years. Its etiology is likely due to fibrotic and/or calcific changes in the aortic valve. The valve can open enough to prevent a significant pressure gradient but is restricted enough to cause the murmur. It differs from an aortic stenosis murmur in that it has an early peak and resolution, as well as having no hemodynamic significance.

EPIDEMIOLOGY AND CAUSES

Bacterial endocarditis, rheumatic heart disease, and aortic calcification are among the most common etiologies of valvular disorders that cause heart murmurs. Bacterial endocarditis is most often due to septicemia caused by *Staphylococcus aureus* or *Streptococcus viridans* (alpha-hemolytic) infection. Valvular deformities are among a spectrum of abnormalities associated with endocarditis. Injection drug users and patients with indwelling IV catheters are at risk for bacterial septicemia that can lead to endocarditis. Patients with prosthetic heart valves, heart murmurs, or valvular damage require prophylactic antibiotics to prevent endocarditis before any invasive procedures, such as dental or surgical interventions.

Rheumatic heart disease is another cause of heart valve injury. Rheumatic heart disease is a result of rheumatic fever, an infection caused by group A beta-hemolytic *Streptococcus* infection. The pathological mechanism involves antibodies developed against the bacteria. These antistreptococcal antibodies are thought to cross-react with the body's own tissues and "mistakenly" attack the heart valves in susceptible individuals. Because of the wide availability of antibiotics, rheumatic fever has become a less common etiology of valvular disease.

Calcification of the aortic valve is a common finding in older patients who present with the systolic murmur of aortic stenosis. A calcified aortic valve is often the result of longstanding arteriosclerosis. This calcification causes narrowing of the aortic valve resulting in an audible disturbance in blood flow across the valve.

In children and younger adults, aortic stenosis may also be present; it is usually caused by a congenital bicuspid (rather than tricuspid) aortic valve or by leaflet fusion in a three-cusp valve. This defect is most often found in males and is commonly accompanied by a longstanding history of becoming excessively short of breath with increased activity, such as running. The physical examination is usually normal, except for the associated cardiac findings.

Mitral valve prolapse occurs in about 2% to 4% of the population and is usually detected in young adulthood. It is more common in women younger than 20 years, whereas the incidence is equal in men and women after the age of 20 years.

PATHOPHYSIOLOGY

Normal heart valves allow unidirectional, unimpeded forward blood flow through the heart. The entire stroke volume is able to pass freely during one phase of the cardiac cycle, and there is no backflow of blood. When a heart valve fails to open to its normal orifice size, it is considered stenotic. When it fails to close appropriately, the valve is incompetent, causing regurgitation of blood flow to the previous chamber or vessel. Both of these events place the patient at significant risk for embolic disease.

CLINICAL PRESENTATION

Subjective

Patients may or may not know whether they have a heart murmur because they may be asymptomatic or, depending on the specific problem, may complain of dyspnea at rest, dyspnea on exertion, orthopnea, paroxysmal nocturnal dyspnea, fatigue, hoarseness, palpitations, weakness, chest pain, symptoms of heart failure, activity intolerance, vertigo, syncope, and peripheral edema.

Objective

Systolic murmurs are graded on a 1 to 6 scale, from barely audible to audible with the stethoscope held off the chest. Grade 4 to 6 murmurs have a palpable thrill. Diastolic murmurs are usually graded from 1 to 4 because these murmurs are not loud enough to reach grades 5 and 6. The bell of the stethoscope is most helpful for auscultating lower-pitched sounds, whereas the diaphragm is best used for hearing higher-pitched sounds. Advanced Assessment 36.1 gives more information about cardiac examination findings, including maneuvers to assess for heart murmurs, and lists the physical signs of common valvular disorders, which may underlie cardiac murmurs.

DIAGNOSTIC REASONING

Diagnostic Tests

Initially, the primary care practitioner may be the first to discover a murmur on physical examination. Depending on the associated symptoms, the primary care practitioner

Advanced Assessment 36.1: Cardiac Examination and Assessment of Heart Murmurs

Focus of Examination	Factors to Assess	Potential Clinical Correlation
Skin temperature	Variations from normal	Cool, moist skin may indicate a decrease in cardiac output Cool, dry skin may reflect environmental temperature or use of vasoconstricting substances such as sympathomimetics (e.g., caffeine, nicotine)
Skin color	Central cyanosis Peripheral cyanosis Palmar erythema Pallor	Poor blood oxygenation Excessive removal of oxygen from the blood Suggests liver impairment May be present in severe anemia (hemoglobin [Hgb] <8 g/dL)
Pulse	Rate Rhythm Character and volume	Note presence of bradycardia or tachycardia Regular, irregular, regularly irregular (extrasystoles), or irregularly irregular (likely atrial fibrillation) Normally full and rapidly filling
Blood pressure	Pulse pressure (difference between the systolic and diastolic pressure readings)	Narrow pulse pressure may be found in volume depletion and aortic stenosis Wide pulse pressure may be found in aortic regurgitation
Point of maximum impulse (PMI)	Location	Normally located at fifth intercostal space (ICS) at midclavicular line With hypertrophy, PMI shifts laterally and may span more than one ICS
Apical impulse	Sensation and quality	Normally a gentle tapping sensation Forceful and thrusting with ventricular overload Sustained in poorly controlled hypertension and aortic stenosis Double apical impulse in ventricular aneurysm
Heart sounds	S_1 (normal first heart sound)	Marks onset of systole Closure of mitral and tricuspid valves Heard just before palpation of carotid artery pulse High-pitched, click-like sound
	Variations from normal S_1	Unusually loud: mitral stenosis Unusually soft: In mitral stenosis, S_1 becomes softer as the valve calcifies and becomes more rigid and less mobile; mitral regurgitation Abnormally wide split: delayed closure of tricuspid valve (as in right bundle branch block)
	S_2 (normal second heart sound)	Marks end of systole Closure of the pulmonic and aortic valves Vibration of aortic and pulmonic valves after closure

Continued

Advanced Assessment 36.1: Cardiac Examination and Assessment of Heart Murmurs—cont'd

Focus of Examination	Factors to Assess	Potential Clinical Correlation
	Physiologically split S_2	Occurs at end of systole Widest split at peak inspiration (due to increased venous return to the heart caused by negative intrathoracic pressure), then shortens or disappears with exhalation May disappear with sitting or standing Normal finding in younger adults, which usually disappears by middle-age
	Fixed split S_2	Occurs at end of systole No closure of split with positional change Does not increase with inspiration Occurs with atrial septal defect or pulmonary stenosis
	Paradoxically split S_2	Splitting heard during expiration and disappears during inspiration Occurs when closure of the aortic valve and pulmonic valve are not synchronous (e.g., severe aortic stenosis, hypertrophic obstructive cardiomyopathy, left bundle branch block)
	S_3 (third heart sound, ventricular gallop, protodiastolic gallop)	Occurs in early diastole just after the mitral valve opens Likely produced by rapidly filling ventricles at a point when ventricular filling slows or by recoil of the heart as it is pushed against the chest Heard best by the bell of the stethoscope Generally no change with respiration, although occasionally inspiration or expiration will increase intensity Found with disorders of systolic emptying (e.g., heart failure, valvular heart disease, ischemic heart disease, hypertrophic cardiomyopathy) Has been described as sounding like the word Kentucky (**KEN**-tuh-key), in which S_3 corresponds to the final "key" syllable
	S_4 (fourth heart sound, atrial gallop, presystolic gallop, S_4 gallop)	May be caused by the tug of chordae tendineae and papillary muscles in the state of poor ventricular compliance Found with disorders of late diastolic filling (e.g., poorly controlled hypertension, angina, ischemic heart disease) Occurs just before S_1 Has been described as sounding like the word Tennessee (teh-**NEH**-see), in which S_4 corresponds to the first "teh" syllable

may refer the patient for subsequent testing or directly to a cardiologist for more invasive testing. Two-dimensional echocardiography is the definitive procedure to diagnose heart valve disorders. Additional diagnostic tests used to detect valvular lesions or structural heart changes include the ECG, chest x-ray (CXR), and cardiac catheterization. The clinician usually orders an echocardiogram, ECG, and CXR to confirm the definitive diagnosis of a murmur and then refers the patient to a cardiologist if indicated.

The ECG may reveal LV hypertrophy or atrial enlargement, depending on where the valvular pathology creates changes in resistance. The CXR may show an enlarged cardiac silhouette, an LV prominence, calcification of the aortic valve, and/or dilation and calcification of the ascending aorta. An echocardiogram is useful in demonstrating the underlying pathological process, including whether the lesion involves the aortic root or if valvular disease is present. Cardiac catheterizations can provide an accurate assessment of regurgitation and stenosis, along with LV function and pulmonary artery pressures. Coronary angiography is often indicated to determine the presence of coronary artery disease before valvular surgery.

Differential Diagnosis

The differential diagnosis of valvular heart disease can be approached from either the perspective of clinical presentation or the underlying etiology of the valvular disorder. While it is important to consider other causes of the clinical signs and symptoms associated with each type of valvular pathology, careful physical examination and an echocardiogram typically reveal the specific valvular disorder, leaving the differential diagnosis for the underlying cause of the valvular disorder to be more relevant.

Each valvular disorder presents with signs and symptoms that can overlap with a variety of cardiopulmonary diseases, most commonly other causes of heart failure. For example, the clinical presentation of aortic stenosis can mimic other causes of heart failure, syncope, and angina, such hypertrophic cardiomyopathy and CAD. In addition, other causes of LV outflow tract obstruction should be considered, including subvalvular disease secondary to thick membranous lesions or supravalvular disease secondary to anatomical deformities. The differential diagnosis for the underlying etiology of aortic stenosis includes calcific aortic deposition and congenital bicuspid aortic valve and rheumatic heart disease. The systolic murmur and bounding pulses associated with aortic regurgitation can also be seen in other disorders including sepsis, anemia, arteriovenous fistula, and thyrotoxicosis. The differential diagnosis for the underlying etiology of aortic regurgitation includes rheumatic heart disease, infective endocarditis, bicuspid aortic valve, valvulitis secondary to a connective tissue disorder, aortic aneurysm, aortic dissection, or aortic inflammation secondary to an underlying rheumatological disorder or syphilis.

The character of the murmur and clinical presentation of mitral regurgitation can overlap with that of hypertrophic cardiomyopathy, tricuspid regurgitation, aortic stenosis, or a ventricular septal defect. The differential diagnosis for the underlying etiology of mitral regurgitation can be divided into primary or functional causes. Primary causes include a myxomatous mitral valve, infective endocarditis, rheumatic heart disease, calcific deposits, valvulitis, rupture of the chordae tendinae in the setting of acute coronary syndrome, or anorectic drugs. A functional cause is mitral regurgitation that develops secondary to LV remodeling due to dilated cardiomyopathy.

The clinical signs and symptoms of mitral stenosis can overlap with those of a left atrial myxoma, tricuspid valve stenosis, LV thrombus, and can be confused with aortic regurgitation. The differential diagnosis for the etiology of mitral stenosis includes rheumatic heart disease, mitral annular calcification, infective endocarditis, or valvulitis secondary to connective tissue disease.

MANAGEMENT

Although asymptomatic patients typically require no treatment, the principle of management of valvular disorders is to help the patient maintain normal cardiac output, thus preventing the complications of heart failure, venous congestion, and inadequate tissue perfusion. Proper management of certain valvular disorders involves preventive therapy to minimize the risk of developing infective endocarditis under certain circumstances, such as dental work or surgery, to which abnormal valves are prone. In recent years, the recommendations for antibiotic prophylaxis before dental work have undergone revision and are now more selective. For current guidelines pertaining to the use of prophylactic antibiotic therapy, the clinician is advised to refer to the American College of Cardiology/American Heart Association (ACC/AHA) guidelines for the prevention of infective endocarditis (see Treatment Standards/Guidelines: Infective Endocarditis Prophylaxis).

Mitral Valve Disorders

Mitral Valve Prolapse

There is no medical treatment to correct MVP. Symptomatic management includes lifestyle changes, such as beginning a mild exercise program to reduce plasma catecholamines, lower the heart rate, decrease stress, and increase cardiac output and blood volume. Beta blockers may be prescribed for patients with MVP to help control heart palpitations. However, fatigue is a problem with this disorder, and it may be exacerbated by beta blockers.

The clinician should refer to the most current guidelines available from the ACC/AHA regarding the use of antibiotic prophylaxis. Antibiotics are no longer recommended for prophylaxis against infective endocarditis if patients are undergoing genitourinary or gastrointestinal tract procedures. Anticoagulation with aspirin (81 to 325 mg/day) is prescribed for some individuals with MVP who have also had a history of transient ischemic attack, ischemic stroke, or atrial fibrillation.

Persons with MVP and severe mitral regurgitation should be followed periodically with stress echocardiography. Surgical intervention is indicated for MVP with severe mitral valve regurgitation.

Mitral Stenosis

For symptomatic mitral stenosis, diuretics and sodium restriction should be initiated to reduce blood volume and pulmonary and systemic venous pressures, along with anticoagulation therapy with warfarin if there is a history of systemic embolism, atrial fibrillation, or a large left atrium. If the patient is in atrial fibrillation, the antiarrhythmic amiodarone or the calcium channel blocker diltiazem may be prescribed and are preferred over the use of digitalis. Surgical intervention may be required for some patients and may include mitral commissurotomy, balloon valvuloplasty, or mitral valve repair or replacement.

Mitral Regurgitation

For a symptomatic patient with mitral regurgitation, vasodilators should be initiated to reduce ventricular filling volume and to decrease systemic vascular resistance. Rate control agents and anticoagulation with warfarin should be

> **Treatment Standards/Guidelines: Infective Endocarditis Prophylaxis**
>
> While these guidelines are from 2007, they are the most widely recognized and current. Clinical evidence for infective endocarditis prevention is lacking. The guidelines below remain an expert consensus, focusing on those at greatest risk of adverse outcomes from infective endocarditis.
>
> Antibiotic prophylaxis should be given to patients undergoing the following procedures:
>
> - Dental procedures involving the gingival tissues or periapical region of a tooth and those procedures that perforate the oral mucosa
> - Invasive respiratory tract procedures that involve incision or biopsy of the respiratory mucosa
>
> Antibiotic prophylaxis is recommended for high-risk patients with any of the following:
>
> - Prosthetic heart valves
> - Previous history of infective endocarditis
> - Complex cyanotic congenital heart disease (surgically repaired or unrepaired)
> - Cardiac valvulopathy in a transplanted heart
>
> Antibiotic prophylaxis is not indicated for common valvular lesions; however, clinicians should exercise judgment in selecting the dose and duration of antibiotics in individual cases or under special circumstances. Adequate oral hygiene is an important factor in preventing infective endocarditis.
>
> **ENDOCARDITIS PROPHYLAXIS (30 TO 60 MINUTES BEFORE PROCEDURE)**
>
> *If no penicillin allergy:*
> amoxicillin oral—adults 2 g; children 50 mg/kg
> If no penicillin allergy and unable to take oral agents:
> ampicillin IM or IV—adults 2 g; children 50 mg/kg
> *If penicillin-allergic:*
> clindamycin oral—adults 600 mg; children 20 mg/kg
> OR
> cephalexin oral—adults 2 g; children 50 mg/kg
> OR
> azithromycin or clarithromycin oral—adults 500 mg; children 15 mg/kg
> *If penicillin-allergic and unable to take oral agents:*
> clindamycin IV—adults 600 mg; children 20 mg/kg
> OR
> cefazolin or ceftriaxone IM or IV—adults 1 g; children 50 mg/kg

NOTE: Cephalosporins should not be used in persons with a history of serious penicillin allergy, such as anaphylaxis, angioedema, or widespread urticaria.
Source: Wilson W, Taubert KA, Gewitz M, et al. Prevention of infective endocarditis: guidelines from the American Heart Association: a guideline from the American Heart Association Rheumatic Fever, Endocarditis, and Kawasaki Disease Committee, Council on Cardiovascular Disease in the Young, and the Council on Clinical Cardiology, Council on Cardiovascular Surgery and Anesthesia, and the Quality of Care and Outcomes Research Interdisciplinary Working Group. Circulation. 2007;116(15):1736–1754.

prescribed to control the ventricular rate and decrease the risk of embolic complications, respectively, if the patient has atrial fibrillation. Sodium restriction and diuretics will relieve symptoms of heart failure if they are present in patients with mitral regurgitation. A mitral valve replacement may be required, which can be done conventionally (via thoracotomy) or by transcatheter mitral valve replacement.

Aortic Valve Disorders

Aortic Stenosis

Presurgical management may include afterload reduction and optimizing fluid balance with medications. Aortic valve replacement or aortic valve commissurotomy may be required for aortic stenosis, which can be done conventionally (via thoracotomy) or by transcatheter aortic valve replacement.

Aortic Regurgitation

For the patient with symptomatic aortic regurgitation, diuretics can be used to treat the symptoms of heart failure. Arterial vasodilators are used to reduce LV afterload. Aortic valve replacement may be required.

FOLLOW-UP AND REFERRAL

The clinician should follow the patient at regular intervals for close monitoring, as well as whenever a new drug has been added or a dosage changed. The patient should be referred to a cardiologist if the diagnosis is unconfirmed or if symptoms are not well-managed with medical therapy.

Patient Education: Valvular Disorders and Murmurs

Valvular heart disorders require lifelong management. Patients may benefit from maintaining a diary to monitor the effectiveness of lifestyle changes and compliance with specific drug therapy in controlling symptoms of the disorder. Patients with MVP should be instructed to begin a gradual program of exercise and to avoid caffeine, decongestants, and products containing ephedrine, alcohol, chocolate, or cheese, to decrease plasma catecholamines. Provided MVP has not led to severe mitral regurgitation and subsequent congestive heart failure, patients should be encouraged to drink at least eight glasses of water a day to prevent dehydration. Patients with aortic stenosis often require activity restrictions. The patient should understand how to pace activity, note improvements in fatigue, and, ideally, accept activity restrictions. A critical part of the evaluation of a person with a heart murmur is the decision to offer antimicrobial prophylaxis. No prophylaxis is needed with benign murmurs. Patients and their primary care providers should follow current treatment guidelines for bacterial endocarditis prophylaxis.

REFERENCES

Arrhythmias

Boersma L, Ince H, Kische S, et al. Evaluating real-world clinical outcomes in atrial fibrillation patients receiving the WATCHMAN left atrial appendage closure technology. *Circ Arrhythm Electrophysiol.* 2019;12(4).

Jaakkola S, Kiviniemi TO, Nuotio I. Usefulness of the CHA2DS2-VASc and HAS-BLED scores in predicting the risk of stroke versus intracranial bleeding in patients with atrial fibrillation (from the FibStroke Study). *Am J Cardiol.* 2018;121(10);1182–1186.

Kirchhof P, Benussi S, Kotecha D, et al. 2016 ESC guidelines for the management of atrial fibrillation developed in collaboration with EACTS. *Eur Heart J.* 2016 Aug 27. https://www.acc.org/latest-in-cardiology/ten-points-to-remember/2016/09/14/14/33/2016-esc-guidelines-for-the-management-of-atrial-fibrillation#:~:text=ESC%20Guidelines%20for%20the%20Management%20of%20Atrial%20Fibrillation.,ischemic%20events%20%28Class%20IIa%2C%20Level%20of%20Evidence%20C%29. Accessed 1/26/2021.

Kusumoto FM, Schoenfeld MH, Barrett C. 2018 ACC/AHA/HRS guideline on the evaluation and management of patients with bradycardia and cardiac conduction delay: executive summary: a Report of the American College of Cardiology/American Heart Association Task Force on Clinical Practice Guidelines, and the Heart Rhythm Society. *Heart Rhythm.* 2018;16(9):e227–e279. Published online: November 6, 2018. https://www.heartrhythmjournal.com/article/S1547-5271(18)31126-3/fulltext

Ibanez B, James S, Agewall S, et al. 2017 ESC Guidelines for the management of acute myocardial infarction in patients presenting with ST-segment elevation: The Task Force for the management of acute myocardial infarction in patients presenting with ST-segment elevation of the European Society of Cardiology (ESC). *Eur Heart J.* 2018;39(2):119–177.

Page RL, Joglar JA, Caldwell MA, et al. 2015 ACC/AHA/HRS guideline for the management of adult patients with supraventricular tachycardia: a Report of the American College of Cardiology/American Heart Association Task Force on Clinical Practice Guidelines and the Heart Rhythm Society. *Circulation.* 2016;133(14):e506–574.

vvanDoorn S, Debray TPA, Kaasenbrood F, et al. Predictive performance of the CHA2DS2-VASc rule in atrial fibrillation: a systematic review and meta-analysis. *J Thromb Thrombolysis.* June;15(6):1065–1077.

Zapata J, Zimmer D, Rinard B, et al. Review of current screening and diagnostic tools for atrial fibrillation. *J Clin Med.* 2020 Jan/Feb.

Valvular Disorders and Murmurs

Jneid H, Mack MJ, McLeod CJ, et al. 2017 AHA/ACC focused update of the 2014 AHA/ACC Guideline for the Management of Patients with Valvular Heart Disease. 2017 AHA/ACC Focused Update of the 2014 AHA/ACC Guideline for the Management of Patients With Valvular Heart Disease: A Report of the American College of Cardiology/American Heart Association Task Force on Clinical Practice Guidelines. *Circulation.* 2017;135(25):e1159–e1195.

Peterson GE, Crowley AL. Antibiotic prophylaxis for infective endocarditis. a pound of prevention and an ounce of cure. *Circulation.* 2019;140:181–183.

Wilson W, Taubert KA, Gewitz M, et al. Prevention of infective endocarditis: guidelines from the American Heart Association: a guideline from the American Heart Association Rheumatic Fever, Endocarditis, and Kawasaki Disease Committee, Council on Cardiovascular Disease in the Young, and the Council on Clinical Cardiology, Council on Cardiovascular Surgery and Anesthesia, and the Quality of Care and Outcomes Research Interdisciplinary Working Group. *Circulation.* 2007;116(15):1736–1754.

RESOURCES

CHA_2DS_2-VASc/HAS-BLED/EHRA Atrial Fibrillation Risk Score Calculator
https://www.chadsvasc.org

Chapter 37

Disorders of the Vascular System

Kathryn B. Keller, PhD, RN, CNE
Jill E. Winland-Brown, EdD, APRN, FNP-BC, FAANP
Brian Oscar Porter, MD, PhD, MPH, MBA
Michael B. Keller, MD

PERIPHERAL ARTERY DISEASE

Peripheral artery disease (PAD) is an occlusive disorder of the arteries that most commonly affects the lower extremities. PAD is most frequently the result of occlusive atherosclerotic plaques that impede blood flow to the peripheral vasculature. The resulting arterial insufficiency most commonly manifests in the form of lower extremity claudication—cramping pain triggered or exacerbated by exertion and relieved by rest. Although atherosclerosis is the most common etiology of arterial insufficiency, several other disorders may precipitate lower extremity ischemia, including vasculitis, radiation exposure, arterial wall dissection, and aneurysm.

EPIDEMIOLOGY AND CAUSES

PAD is caused by atherosclerosis, blood clots, trauma, spasms of smooth muscle in the arterial walls, and congenital structural defects in the arteries. Approximately 6.5 million people older than 40 years in the United States have PAD, and the most common symptom is intermittent claudication. PAD affects males and females equally. In patients older than 60 years, 12% to 20% have PAD. Black people have an increased incidence of PAD, compared with the general population, and Hispanic people have a slightly higher incidence of PAD, compared with non-Hispanic white individuals. PAD is also nine times more common in smokers, compared with nonsmokers.

> **Risk Factors: Peripheral Artery Disease**
> - Smoking: Vasoconstriction/spasm leading to decreased circulation
> - Obesity: Increased cardiac workload
> - Inactivity: Decreased circulation
> - Hypertension: Increased fibrous tissue, which decreases stretch of arterial walls and increases peripheral vascular resistance
> - High cholesterol: Contributes to formation of atherosclerotic plaque
> - Diabetes mellitus: Increased atherosclerosis of smaller vessels
> - Age older than 60 years: Decreased vascular compliance

PATHOPHYSIOLOGY

Atherosclerosis is the most common cause of PAD. Arteriosclerotic plaques obstruct optimal arterial blood flow to the muscles of the extremities. The lower extremities are generally most affected. With increasing muscle activity, there is an increased need for arterial blood flow. For this reason, during ambulation or exercise, limitations of arterial blood flow cause ischemia, resulting in muscle pain. This cramping muscle pain is referred to as *intermittent claudication* because in the initial stages of PAD, ischemia occurs periodically and generally with exertion. Muscular activity of the extremities requires arterial vasodilation to increase blood flow. In contrast, PAD causes impairment of arterial vasodilation, thereby diminishing arterial blood flow. As the severity of PAD increases, ischemic pain may occur at gradually lower levels of exertion until pain is present at rest, an indication of severe PAD.

Arteriosclerotic plaque formation within the lower extremities is accelerated by the presence of diabetes mellitus; therefore, PAD is more common in people with diabetes. Hyperglycemia may contribute to endothelial injury of the arteries and accelerate the formation of atherosclerotic plaque. Clinical manifestations of arterial insufficiency are often apparent in the lower extremities of individuals with diabetes mellitus. Diminished circulation in the legs may lead to poor wound healing and peripheral neuropathy. The smaller-caliber arterial vessels of the most distal regions of the lower extremities are affected initially. Therefore, careful periodic physical assessment of the feet and lower extremities is recommended in people with diabetes mellitus; assessment should include inspections for pedal ulcerations, poor wound healing, and diminished peripheral pulses.

Aneurysms, another manifestation of PAD, result from weakening areas in arterial walls, which render the walls susceptible to rupture. The most common cause of this weakening is arteriosclerosis. Aneurysms appear as bulges in the arterial wall and are classified according to location. The aorta and cerebral arteries are the most common sites of aneurysms. In the aorta, a dissecting aneurysm, which is an incomplete tear in the vessel wall, may occur when elevated blood pressure leads to separation of the layers of aortic tissue.

Arteritis, a form of vasculitis, involves inflammation of arterial blood vessels. Inflammation decreases the vasodilatory capacity of arteries and may cause spasm of the arteries. This condition is often associated with autoimmune disease. Raynaud's phenomenon is a result of cold-induced vasospasm of the small blood vessels, starting in the fingers and toes, causing a characteristic blanching. A tricolor change may also occur, which appears first as blanching of the fingertips and toes, followed by cyanosis and rubor (redness).

CLINICAL PRESENTATION

Subjective

A thorough history distinguishes the cause of leg pain in more than 90% of patients. The patient with PAD will usually present with intermittent leg pain (intermittent claudication) that increases in severity with exertion. The location of the lower extremity pain depends on where the occlusion of arterial circulation is located. Aorto-iliac occlusions typically produce claudication of the thigh and buttock, whereas occlusions of the femoral artery produce pain in the upper calf. The pain is described as severe, "grabbing," and cramplike. It generally lasts minutes, is relieved by rest, and recurs with exertion. Pain at rest may signify severe PAD. The patient usually denies swelling, pain at night, or color or temperature changes of the skin.

Assessing risk factors assists in the diagnosis of PAD, as well as determining the rapidity of symptom onset. Careful attention should be paid to identifying any signs or symptoms suggesting severe arterial insufficiency, which is concerning for a limb-threatening state necessitating urgent treatment. Gradual onset of claudication is more consistent with progressive obliteration of lower extremity vessels and the formation of collateral circulation as seen with PAD, rather than an acute event such as an embolus from the heart or proximal arteries.

Objective

A classic finding in PAD is diminished or absent pulses in the affected limb. In turn, the clinician should evaluate the cervical, radial, ulnar, brachial, femoral, popliteal, dorsalis pedis, and posterior tibial pulses bilaterally. A consistent grading system should be used for pulse strength. A commonly used pulse grading system uses 0 as absent, 1+ diminished, 2+ normal, and 3+ bounding. The clinician should keep in mind that about 10% of the population has absent pedal pulses, even in the absence of PAD. Because a bruit indicates turbulence and possible atherosclerotic narrowing, the cervical, supraclavicular, abdominal, flank, and inguinal pulse sites should be assessed, using the diaphragm of a stethoscope.

To differentiate chronic venous insufficiency from PAD, the clinician can raise the patient's legs for several minutes. When the legs are dependent again, the patient with PAD will have pale, dusky red (rubor) extremities, whereas the patient with chronic venous insufficiency will have improved color in the extremities. The six P's of PAD—pain, pulselessness, paresthesia, paralysis, poikilothermia (coolness), and pallor—should be assessed to evaluate for the presence of arterial ischemia. The clinician should also perform a sensory examination to rule out peripheral neuropathy associated with ischemia in patients with diabetes mellitus.

With PAD, the affected limb may be smaller as a result of muscular atrophy. The clinician may note thinning of the skin, loss of hair over the affected area, and possible skin ulcers. The extremity may be cool and pale, and the toenails will be thickened with cornlike material (dead skin callus) under the nails. The patient will have a history of delayed wound healing. When the extremity is dependent, it will appear reddish blue. Eventually, with severe disease, the lower legs and ankles may assume a purple-black color characteristic of cyanosis and gangrene.

DIAGNOSTIC REASONING

Diagnostic Tests

If arterial insufficiency is suspected and pulses are absent, a Doppler ultrasound flow study should be performed, which can quantify the degree of ischemia. If lower extremity PAD is suspected, the ankle-brachial index (ABI), a comparison of ankle blood pressure to arm blood pressure, should be calculated during the Doppler flow study, using a blood pressure cuff. The normal ratio of ankle to brachial pressure is more than 0.9. An ABI reading of 0.6 to 0.9 indicates a moderate level of disease, and levels less than 0.5 indicate severe ischemia, as these decreased ratios reflect reduced circulation in the leg compared with the arm. Although an arteriogram is not usually ordered as an initial diagnostic test, it is often performed at the time of intervention or reserved for rare instances in which the diagnosis of PAD is uncertain.

Additional assessment tools and diagnostic procedures for PAD include the Walking Impairment Questionnaire (WIQ), treadmill exercise testing, a lipid profile, and magnetic resonance angiogram (MRA). The WIQ is used to assess the patient's ability to walk defined distances at certain speeds and to climb stairs.

Differential Diagnosis

Differential diagnoses for PAD include chronic venous insufficiency, thrombosis, phlebitis, polycythemia, anemia, Raynaud's disease, vasculitis such as Buerger's disease, aneurysms, and peripheral neuropathy.

MANAGEMENT

Treatment for PAD depends on the severity of disease, the age of the patient, and accompanying comorbidities. Initial treatment often focuses on medical management, although patients with PAD should be counseled about modification of risk factors, such as smoking, with aggressive control of hypertension, diabetes mellitus, and hyperlipidemia. The clinician should encourage the patient to walk at least 30 minutes three to four times per week. Any ulcers or traumatic lesions to the extremities warrant medical attention and close follow-up. The patient should be encouraged to keep the legs dependent to improve blood flow to the extremities. Tight bandages and stockings should be avoided.

Although drug therapy is not a substitute for exercise, some medications have been helpful in extending ambulation distances for more than 25% of patients. Patients with PAD should be started on antiplatelet therapy with aspirin (75 to 325 mg) daily or clopidogrel (Plavix) 75 mg daily. These antiplatelet agents do not provide measurable improvement in symptoms of claudication but are prescribed to reduce the risk of concomitant atherosclerotic disease, such as myocardial infarction and stroke. Although early studies suggested that ticagrelor (Brilinta) may be beneficial in PAD, a large randomized controlled trial that included almost 14,000 patients with symptomatic PAD did not demonstrate a benefit of ticagrelor over clopidogrel. A statin should also be added to the patient's medication regimen.

Current American College of Cardiology (ACC) and American Heart Association (AHA) guidelines recommend cilostazol (Pletal) 100 mg twice daily for the treatment of claudication. Cilostazol is a phosphodiesterase-3 inhibitor that causes vasodilation and inhibits platelet aggregation. Cilostazol may be ordered specifically to treat leg pain and cramping due to blockages from atherosclerosis in arteries of the lower extremities. Cilostazol should not be prescribed in patients with heart failure due to prior data indicating that other oral phosphodiesterase inhibitors increase mortality in this population.

Most patients with moderate PAD can be effectively managed with medical therapy and risk modification alone, including attention to smoking cessation, exercise, and diet. If these steps fail, however, surgical intervention and angioplasty are used selectively in patients with severe PAD. Indications for surgical or percutaneous revascularization include profound functional and occupational limitation due to claudication, disease refractory to pharmacological therapy, and critical limb-threatening ischemia. Other comorbid conditions (e.g., severe pulmonary disease, heart failure, coronary artery disease) may render revascularization futile.

FOLLOW-UP AND REFERRAL

All patients with PAD should be followed up at least every 3 months to assess the effectiveness of lifestyle changes, skin care, and management of ulcers. If ulcers are present, the patient may need to be seen on a weekly basis. Patients with PAD may be referred to a vascular surgeon for evaluation and potential surgery, including balloon angioplasty in the distal extremity or an arterial graft using a section of the great saphenous vein or synthetic graft material.

Patient Education: Peripheral Artery Disease

Patients who have been diagnosed with PAD should be counseled about the modification of risk factors. Smoking cessation must be encouraged, and hyperlipidemia must be controlled. In addition, it is essential to adequately treat hypertension and diabetes mellitus. Dietary control must include limitations on fat and salt intake.

Patients must be taught to do meticulous daily foot care that includes inspecting the feet daily for sores, ulcers, and abrasions, including the use of a mirror to check the soles of the feet. Patients should not walk barefoot and should wear well-fitting supportive shoes. They should not soak their feet and should be careful trimming their nails to avoid skin injuries. All patients should be taught to watch for signs and symptoms that might indicate progressive limb ischemia, such as increased pain, increased pallor or cyanosis, and pain at rest without exertion (rest pain).

Patients with PAD should be encouraged to perform Buerger-Allen exercises three to four times per day, in which the patient raises and lowers the extremities while lying flat, with each of five repetitions taking at least 5 minutes. In each repetition, the legs should be raised to a 45-degree angle and supported in place for 1 to 2 minutes until the skin blanches. The legs are then lowered to a level below the rest of the body (without exerting any pressure on the backs of the knees to avoid popliteal artery occlusion) for several minutes until redness appears, followed by resting the legs flat in a supine position for several minutes. These changes in position cause the veins of the legs to refill by gravity and improve overall circulation.

Additionally, exercise therapy is recommended for PAD because it stimulates collateral vessel growth in the lower extremities. Patients should be encouraged to walk a sufficient distance until moderate pain occurs, stop until pain subsides, and then resume walking. A supervised treadmill walking program three times a week over a 6-month period is part of cardiovascular rehabilitation. The grade and speed of the treadmill are gradually increased over time as the patient's activity tolerance improves.

DEEP VEIN THROMBOSIS/ CHRONIC VENOUS INSUFFICIENCY

Deep vein thrombosis (DVT) is a disorder of the venous system characterized by clot formation in the deep vessels of the venous vasculature. DVT primarily results as a complication associated with Virchow's triad—venous stasis, endothelial injury, and a hypercoagulable state. The resulting thrombus formation may lead to a variety of complications including chronic venous insufficiency and, most notably, pulmonary embolism (PE). PE is a potentially life-threatening complication of DVT in which venous thrombi propagate to the pulmonary vasculature, resulting in respiratory compromise. It is estimated that 10% to 30% of patients will die within 1 month of diagnosis of DVT/PE and that sudden death is the first symptom in about 25% of people who have a PE. Moreover, about one-third of patients who have a DVT/PE will have a recurrence within 10 years.

Chronic venous insufficiency is a disorder characterized by valvular incompetence, which manifests as lower extremity edema, skin discoloration, and ulceration as a result of poor antegrade venous flow. Although the condition is commonly a complication of DVT, it may be the result of inflammatory conditions such as phlebitis or anatomical disturbances.

EPIDEMIOLOGY AND CAUSES

DVT and PE are often complications encountered during the treatment of medical and surgical patients. Approximately 300,000 to 600,000 hospitalizations can be associated with DVT and PE each year. In the United States, it is estimated that there are more than 2 million cases per year of DVT, and up to 50,000 deaths occur annually because of PE. However, the actual number of cases is often underdiagnosed due to the silent nature of the problem. Although mortality caused by PE previously seemed to be declining, the trend over the past decade has demonstrated that mortality rates of PE are now on the rise. In particular, black people are at higher risk, as well as individuals younger than 65 years, although rates have remained stable for people older than 65 years. Multiple risk factors for DVT and PE have been identified.

Risk Factors: Deep Vein Thrombosis (DVT)—Virchow's Triad

Venous Stasis

- Possible causes include immobility, venous insufficiency, prolonged sedentary position, poststroke, postmyocardial infarction, and heart failure.

Vessel Injury

- Possible causes include trauma, surgery (especially orthopedic), and indwelling IV catheters.

Hypercoagulability

- Possible causes include high estrogen states (oral contraceptives or hormone replacement therapy), pregnancy/postpartum period, cancer, and inherited coagulation abnormalities.

Additional Risk Factors

- Abdominal/pelvic surgery: Immobility leading to venous pooling/stasis
- Obesity
- Advanced neoplasm: Coagulation abnormalities, interference with venous blood flow

Patients undergoing various types of surgical procedures, such as orthopedic, gynecological-obstetrical, urological, neurosurgical, and general surgical procedures, are at high risk for developing DVT and PE. Of these groups, orthopedic patients appear to be especially prone to thrombosis, particularly patients with hip fracture. All elective orthopedic surgical patients undergoing lower extremity surgery are at risk for DVT. The risk is greatest for patients undergoing hip surgery and knee reconstruction, for which DVT rates range from 45% to 70%.

Patients with various types of medical diseases, usually chronic, are also at high risk for venous thrombotic events. The risk of DVT in pregnancy has been reported to be five times higher than in nonpregnant patients of the same age, and it may be increased postpartum. A silent DVT may cause a postphlebitic syndrome, characterized by swelling and pain in an extremity that was previously affected by thrombophlebitis.

A frequent complication of DVT is PE, in which a thrombus located in the venous system propagates to the lungs. The mortality rate of PE is estimated to be approximately 30%, although with the availability of newer diagnostic tools such as computed tomography angiogram that can detect small peripheral emboli, it is estimated that the mortality rate of PE can be decreased to approximately 10%. Of note, more than 80% of patients who died from PE showed DVT on autopsy.

Chronic venous insufficiency usually results from venous incompetence secondary to valvular dysfunction. More than 20% of the population is affected by chronic venous insufficiency. The incidence increases with age with no evident ethnic predisposition; however, chronic venous insufficiency is more common in females than males.

PATHOPHYSIOLOGY

Blood clots can originate anywhere in the venous system, but the majority begin in the deep veins of the pelvis and lower extremities, with a significant number at or above the popliteal vein. Clots that originate in the proximal veins are potentially more dangerous because they are larger and result in more clinically significant thromboembolic events.

The causative factors in the formation of blood clots are referred to as *Virchow's triad* (see earlier discussion). Clots are likely to form when two of the three factors in the triad—venous stasis, vessel wall damage, and coagulation changes—are altered. Stasis of blood may result from immobility, edema, or anesthesia; blood tends to coagulate in and around the valve cusps of the veins, thus increasing the likelihood of clot formation. Vessel wall damage may result from trauma, surgical incision, laceration, venous wall distention (venous pooling) from immobility or anesthesia, or a previous DVT. Coagulation changes leading to activated coagulation factors as a result of damaged endothelium may be the result of surgery, trauma, injury, disease states (such as sepsis, infection, or cancer), or foreign substance invasion via IV lines or catheters. In turn, orthopedic surgery is a major risk factor for DVT, and there is a high incidence of concurrent DVT in persons with cancer of the pancreas, lungs, breast, genitourinary tract, or stomach.

In these processes, damage to the endothelium causes local activation of coagulation factors as platelets come into contact with exposed collagen found in connective tissue, including skin, bone, ligaments, and cartilage. In turn, the platelets release substances that cause vasoconstriction and accelerate clotting. Hypercoagulability predisposing to DVT may also result from exogenous estrogen use (e.g., hormonal contraception) or pregnancy due to hormonal and circulatory changes (e.g., increased venous pooling and dependent edema).

Once formed, a DVT can propagate, embolize, or lyse. When the clot propagates, it extends proximally and becomes larger, and thus more dangerous by obstructing blood flow, which causes the vein to dilate and the vessel wall to be damaged. When a clot embolizes, it may lodge itself in the arteries of the lungs, resulting in a PE. Even if a clot lyses (breaks down), it can still cause irreversible valvular damage by allowing blood to reflux in the veins. The damage sets up a cycle of pooling and hypertension known as *postphlebitic syndrome.* Patients with this syndrome experience chronic pain, swelling, and venous ulcers.

Deep venous thrombophlebitis and thromboembolism is a critical disorder of the veins of the lower extremity. The presence of a thrombus within a deep vein with an accompanying inflammatory response is termed *deep venous thrombophlebitis.* If the thrombus breaks away from the wall of the vein and travels upward toward the heart, it is termed a *venous thromboembolism.* The venous thrombus may break free from the venous wall and travel from the lower extremity to the inferior vena cava and up to the right atrium, right ventricle, and into the pulmonary arterial circulation. This may cut off blood flow to an entire lung segment, resulting in potentially fatal ventilation/perfusion (V/Q) mismatch. It is critical to diagnose DVT early because the complication of PE can be life-threatening. Signs of pulmonary embolism can be subtle or severe depending on the size of the embolus. Sudden death can result from pulmonary embolism and may not be heralded by clearly observable signs of DVT.

In addition, any abnormal communication between the right and left chambers of the heart (e.g., atrial septal defect, patent foramen ovale, ventricular septal defect) creates the potential for cerebral thromboembolism and a subsequent cerebrovascular accident (stroke). In these circumstances, the clot may bypass the lungs and cross over from the right to the left side of the heart, with the potential of embolizing into the systemic circulation, including to the brain.

Chronic venous insufficiency is a disorder of the valves within the deep veins of the lower extremities. Valves within veins assist venous blood to flow upward toward the heart, regulating unidirectional flow by preventing retrograde flow of venous blood away from the heart. Weakened venous valves do not form tight closures, however, thereby failing to prevent retrograde blood flow.

The appearance of superficial varicose veins may be associated with chronic venous insufficiency. Superficial varicose veins are benign in most cases and are treatable with conservative measures. However, under more severe circumstances, venous stasis results as excess pressure builds up in the legs, causing distention of the veins, thinning and scaling of the skin with dusky discoloration (stasis dermatitis), and eventually the formation of large venous ulcers. In addition, dependent edema and poor wound healing result.

CLINICAL PRESENTATION

Subjective

Although many lower extremity thrombi are silent, the patient may present with a complaint of pain in the calf muscle (the most common complaint), slight swelling of the calf or asymmetry of appearance, or muscle tenderness when massaging the affected area.

The patient with chronic venous insufficiency will complain of dependent edema, venous engorgement (varicose veins), and localized pain. In advanced disease, the patient may complain of a darkened color in the lower extremities, along with dryness and scaling of the skin.

Objective

The signs of DVT may be subtle. Overt signs of DVT may include tenderness and a palpable cord along the course of a vein, although more often, the only sign is a unilateral swelling of an extremity, with or without signs of inflammation. In turn, an acute DVT in the femoral or iliac veins may manifest as tenderness over the veins, swelling, and a slightly bluish skin color. The clinician may assess for warmth or heat of the affected extremity and note distention of the superficial veins. A slight fever and tachycardia may also be present. Although used in the past, a positive Homans' sign (pain on dorsiflexion of the foot) is now considered an unreliable diagnostic indicator, given its lack of specificity.

In patients with chronic venous insufficiency, the earliest detectable signs may be the presence of spider veins (superficial tangles of bluish to purple thin veins just under the surface of the skin) or varicose veins (large, dilated, and tortuous superficial veins that have an engorged, raised, ropy appearance), particularly on the lower extremities. In more advanced disease, the clinician may note a brownish hyperpigmentation of the extremities, edema, subcutaneous fibrosis, and possibly leg ulcers. When the clinician elevates an affected extremity, the sharp and deep muscle pain may be lessened. The peripheral pulses may be normal or diminished, and there may be superficial ulcers around the medial malleolus.

DIAGNOSTIC REASONING

Diagnostic Tests

If DVT is suspected, the clinician should first assess for the probability of thrombosis. This may be done, using a clinical probability assessment model, which estimates the probability of DVT, such as the Wells' criteria—a tool that computes a score indicating the probability of PE based on 10 yes/no questions (see Resources). Further diagnostic work-up is contingent on the patient's clinical likelihood of DVT. If the patient is determined to have a low clinical probability of DVT, a D-dimer level may be ordered, which has become increasingly available in primary care practices. A low Wells score and a negative D-dimer test result would indicate the absence of DVT. However, if a high or intermediate Wells score is calculated, then no screening D-dimer is needed, and further investigation is required.

The D-dimer assay can be helpful in ruling out, but not definitively confirming, the diagnosis of DVT. D-dimer is a breakdown product of fibrin and is positive in venous thrombosis and PE. However, the D-dimer assay has low specificity and cannot be solely relied on for diagnosis. If D-dimer is present, it does not prove a DVT exists because many conditions (e.g., advanced age, malignancy, recent surgery, pregnancy, infection) may cause a positive result. However, given its high sensitivity for venous thrombosis, if the D-dimer is negative, it effectively rules out the presence of DVT. A false-negative result can occur if the sample is drawn too early after thrombus formation or if testing is not done in an acute time period.

In patients with an intermediate or high clinical probability of DVT, compression ultrasonography of the femoral and popliteal regions has become the diagnostic standard (compression of the vein by the ultrasound probe in the region of the thrombus will be abnormally limited due to the clot, and obstruction in venous blood flow may be detected). The ascending venogram was long considered the gold standard for the diagnosis of venous thromboembolism; however, it is rarely used today. If pulmonary embolus is suspected, a ventilation/perfusion (V/Q) scan or a spiral (helical) computed tomography scan of the lungs and pulmonary arterial system would be indicated.

To confirm venous insufficiency if the history and physical examination are inconclusive, a venogram may be performed. This is a radiological test in which the suspected vein is injected with a radiopaque dye. Sequential films will show engorged, tortuous veins if venous insufficiency is present. In addition, plethysmography may be done to determine the changes in fluid volume of the extremities. The air-cuff plethysmography measures the changes in the circumference of a limb by recording the changes in pressure in an air-filled cuff surrounding the extremity. However, this test is rarely done because the history, physical examination, and other tests are usually adequate to confirm the diagnosis.

Differential Diagnosis

Patients with chronic venous insufficiency may exhibit some of the symptoms of DVT. Patients who suffer from chronic venous insufficiency have swelling and dilated superficial veins. They may also complain of aching or fatigue in the legs while standing or walking. Other differential diagnoses for DVT include cellulitis, lymphedema, and muscle strain.

MANAGEMENT

Deep Vein Thrombosis

The cornerstone of therapy for DVT is anticoagulation. Traditionally, patients with DVT were admitted to the hospital for initial anticoagulant treatment. Current guidelines recommend outpatient treatment for selected patients in the primary care outpatient setting who are otherwise healthy and have no significant comorbidities. If the patient exhibits a massive DVT, shows symptoms suggestive of PE, is at high risk for bleeding on anticoagulant therapy, or has significant comorbid conditions, the patient should be admitted to an acute care facility. After initial anticoagulation and discharge from the hospital, the clinician can manage therapy for a more prolonged period. A provoked DVT (such as in the setting of surgery or immobility) requires 3 to 6 months of anticoagulation. Patients experiencing an unprovoked DVT, recurrent DVT, those with cancer, or any other ongoing risk factors may require indefinite anticoagulation, with frequent reassessment of the need for ongoing anticoagulation based on weighing the benefits and risks of treatment.

The choice of anticoagulant therapy should be individualized, based on patient comorbidities, risk of bleeding, access to follow-up care and laboratory monitoring, patient preferences, and costs. Although warfarin (Coumadin) was the "tried and true" anticoagulation treatment for decades, its use requires frequent monitoring with prothrombin time and international normalized ratio (PT/INR) tests. If a patient is placed on warfarin, the starting doses recommended are from 2 to 5 mg daily for the first 2 days, before checking the first follow-up PT/INR result. However, in otherwise healthy adults, some clinicians start with doses as high as 7.5 to 10 mg daily for the first 2 days. Regardless, the warfarin dose is adjusted as needed every 2 to 3 days, based on PT/INR results, to achieve the desired level of anticoagulation.

For long-term anticoagulant therapy that does not require laboratory monitoring to judge the level of anticoagulation, several newer direct oral anticoagulants (DOACs) are recommended: dabigatran (Pradaxa) 150 mg twice daily, apixaban (Eliquis) 5 mg twice daily, edoxaban (Savaysa, Lixiana) 30 to 60 mg daily, or rivaroxaban (Xarelto) 15 mg twice daily for the first 3 weeks and then 20 mg once daily.

If anticoagulant therapy is contraindicated, filtering devices such as a vena cava filter may be used to trap emboli before they reach the lungs and cause a PE. Vena cava filters are mechanical barriers that are inserted in the inferior vena cava under percutaneous radiological guidance. Although they do not prevent clot formation, they prevent potentially fatal clot migration from the legs to the lungs.

High-risk patients without active lower limb thrombosis within the last 6 months should receive nonpharmacological prophylaxis with intermittent pneumatic compression of the lower legs in the postsurgical setting or during other episodes of significant immobilization. External pneumatic compression and gradient compression stockings are effective alternatives for decreasing lower leg thrombosis, if lower extremity trauma does not preclude their use. However, use of pneumatic compression devices on limbs with a known DVT is not recommended. Rather, patients should elevate the affected limb, apply heat, and limit activity as anticoagulant therapy is initiated.

Thrombolysis is not indicated for DVT except in cases of massive iliofemoral thrombosis. Thrombolytic agents are also indicated for patients with massive PE and associated hemodynamic instability. The role of thrombolysis in patients with smaller PEs is controversial, however, given its significant associated bleeding risk.

Chronic Venous Insufficiency

Conservative treatment of chronic venous insufficiency is effective in alleviating symptoms in 85% of patients. The degree of dependent edema can be a guide to the effectiveness of therapy. The clinician should order light exercise, support or compression stockings, weight loss, and elevation of the legs several times each day for approximately 30 minutes to facilitate venous blood return to the heart and reduce lower extremity edema. Subsequent management involves aggressively treating any ulcers and reducing factors that cause atherosclerosis. Although diuretics are not indicated in the treatment of edema caused by chronic venous insufficiency, diuretics may be prescribed for other medical problems that exacerbate lower extremity edema, such as heart failure and renal dysfunction.

Interventional cosmetic procedures may be used to reduce the appearance of dilated and tortuous varicose veins. These include venous stripping (surgical removal of varicose veins), venous ligation (tying off defective valves to reduce retrograde venous blood flow), and venous sclerosis (injection of an irritant salt solution directly into a varicose vein to cause fibrosis of vessel walls and vascular collapse).

FOLLOW-UP AND REFERRAL

Some patients with acute DVT are briefly hospitalized, with the clinician following the patient after release from the hospital. A patient on warfarin must be seen frequently, with PT/INR typically checked every 2 to 3 days for potential dose adjustments, until the target INR range is achieved, and then on a monthly basis thereafter. DOACs do not require regular laboratory monitoring. The progression of chronic venous insufficiency is typically monitored through physical examination and patient history to assess for improvement in signs and symptoms and monitor for complications, such as the development of DVT.

Patient Education: Deep Vein Thrombosis

Patients should be educated about DVT prevention and receive prophylactic measures, depending on the number of risk factors exhibited and the resulting need for hospitalization or surgery. To prevent DVT, prophylactic methods should be used for all patients at risk, including pharmacological treatments, physical or mechanical modalities, or some combination of the two.

Physical modalities that treat chronic venous insufficiency and prevent DVT by reducing venous stasis include leg elevation, passive leg exercises, and early ambulation. Although these techniques are somewhat effective, each has drawbacks and should be combined with other physical measures, such as graduated elastic compression or external pneumatic compression devices. Graduated compression stockings provide safe, simple, and inexpensive prophylaxis against DVT formation. Besides preventing stasis, they also prevent venous distention, which can initiate vessel wall damage. Pneumatic compression devices are more effective at emptying the veins, sustaining femoral blood flow velocity, and expelling the blood from behind the valve cusps in the femoral vein, thus stimulating fibrinolysis.

Education for patients recovering from DVT includes teaching about the need to avoid trauma to the affected veins. The patient should be educated regarding potential adverse effects of anticoagulant medications, including signs and symptoms of bleeding, anticoagulant-induced skin necrosis, and when to seek medical care. The patient must avoid food fads and crash diets and should not drink alcohol or take vitamin E, cold medicines, antibiotics, aspirin, cimetidine (Tagamet), thyroid hormones, or NSAIDs without first consulting the primary care provider. Immobility should be discouraged, and patients must know when to return for a follow-up PT/INR test if they are on warfarin.

Go to Davis Edge for practice Q&A.

REFERENCES

Deep Vein Thrombosis/Chronic Venous Insufficiency

Centers for Disease Control and Statistics. *Venous thromboembolism—data & statistics*. Division of Blood Disorders, National Center on Birth Defects and Developmental Disabilities, Centers for Disease Control and Prevention. https://www.cdc.gov/ncbddd/dvt/data.html. Revised 2020. Accessed 10/30/2020.

Martin KA, Molsberry R, Cuttica MJ. Time trends in pulmonary embolism mortality rates in the United States, 1999 to 2018. *J Am Heart Assoc.* 2020;9(17). https://www.ahajournals.org/doi/full/10.1161/JAHA.120.016784. Accessed 10/3/2020.

Michiels JJ, Maasland H, Moossdorff W, et al. Safe exclusion of deep vein thrombosis by a rapid sensitive ELISA D-dimer and compression ultrasonography in 1330 outpatients with suspected DVT. *Angiology.* 2016;67(8):781–787.

Youn YJ, Lee J. Chronic venous insufficiency and varicose veins of the lower extremities. *Korean J Intern Med.* 2019;34(2): 269–283. https://doi.org/10.3904/kjim.2018.230

Peripheral Artery Disease

Centers for Disease Control and Statistics. Peripheral Arterial Disease (PAD). https://www.cdc.gov/heartdisease/PAD.htm. Accessed 10/3/2020.

Duffett L, Castellucci LA, Forgie MA. Pulmonary embolism: update on management and controversies. *BMJ.* 2020; 370:m2177.

Gerhard-Herman MD, Gornik HL, Barrett C, et al. AHA/ACC Guideline on the management of patients with lower extremity peripheral artery disease: A report of the American College of Cardiology/American Heart Association Task Force on Clinical Practice Guidelines. *Circulation.* 2017;135;e726–e779.

Hiatt WR, Fowkes FGR, Heizer G, et al. Ticagrelor versus clopidogrel in symptomatic peripheral artery disease. *N Engl J Med.* 2017. Jan 5;376(1):32–40. https://www.nejm.org/doi/full/10.1056/nejmoa1611688. Accessed 10/3/2020.

Lavender ZR, Sandor PS. Oral anticoagulation: reversing the current view in bleeding events. *J Clin Med.* 2018 May;34–37.

Nead KT, Zhou M, Diaz Caceres R, et al. Walking Impairment Questionnaire improves mortality risk prediction models in a high-risk cohort independent of peripheral arterial disease status. *Circ Cardiovasc Qual Outcomes.* 2013;6:255–261. https://www.ahajournals.org/doi/pdf/10.1161/CIRCOUTCOMES.111.000070. Accessed 10/3/2020.

Radhika J, Poomalai G, Nalini S, et al. Effectiveness of Buerger-Allen exercise on lower extremity perfusion and peripheral neuropathy symptoms among patients with diabetes mellitus. *Iran J Nurs Midwifery Res.* 2020;25(4):291–295. https://doi.org/10.4103/ijnmr.IJNMR_63_19

RESOURCES

Wells' Criteria: DVT Risk Assessment Calculator
https://www.mdcalc.com/wells-criteria-dvt

Section 7: ABDOMINAL PROBLEMS

SECTION EDITOR

Debera J. Thomas, PhD, RN, ANP/FNP

Chapter 38

Common Abdominal Complaints

Debera J. Thomas, PhD, RN, ANP/FNP

ABDOMINAL PAIN

Abdominal pain is one of the most common complaints for which people seek medical attention. The causes of abdominal pain are numerous; a few are serious enough to require surgical intervention. Conditions associated with an acute abdomen can be inflammatory, metabolic, or structural; therefore, any acute abdominal pain must be evaluated quickly and precisely. Abdominal pain that occurs without any other signs or symptoms is rarely a serious problem. In instances when the exact cause of pain is not immediately evident, an empiric trial of therapy or test selection may help suggest the underlying pathophysiology, narrow the differential diagnoses, and guide further assessment and treatment. It is important to keep in mind that nongastrointestinal (GI) etiologies such as ovarian cancer, ectopic pregnancy (see Chapter 49), or myocardial ischemia (see Chapter 35) may present as abdominal pain.

One-half of patients who complain of abdominal pain do not receive an accurate diagnosis. The source of the abdominal pain may be from one of a triad of vascular emergencies: mesenteric ischemia, abdominal aortic aneurysm, or myocardial infarction. Conditions in this triad can cause severe pain and should not be excluded from the differential diagnosis.

DIFFERENTIAL DIAGNOSIS

Total patient presentation and a careful history are key when evaluating abdominal pain and determining the severity of the condition. The onset, location, duration, characteristics, any associated/aggravating factors, relieving factors, temporal factors, and severity, as well as what the pain means to the patient, are useful in the diagnostic reasoning. The presence or absence of bowel sounds is also an important diagnostic factor. Tachycardia, tachypnea, and hypertension often indicate the intensity of the pain. Many nonsurgical conditions can present with classic acute "surgical" abdomen symptoms such as intense pain, rebound tenderness, and guarding. All patients with abdominal pain should undergo rectal, genital, and pelvic evaluations. Blood found in the stool or intense pain on examination may indicate more serious conditions.

Abdominal pain can be caused by mechanical, inflammatory, and ischemic factors. The characteristics of a patient's abdominal pain often give clues as to the specific factors involved. For example, abdominal organs are sensitive to stretching and distention but not as sensitive to cutting, crushing, or tearing. *Visceral pain* is caused by distention or spasm of a hollow viscus and is usually generalized and dull. Distention of an organ capsule such as Glisson's capsule around the liver, vascular compromise, and mucosal irritations cause pain that is visceral in nature. Conversely, *parietal pain,* described as sharp and well localized, is caused by irritation of the peritoneum. Appendicitis often causes this type of pain as the peritoneum becomes involved. Abdominal pain described as *colicky,* which means that it comes and goes, may result from gallstones or renal stones. *Burning pain,* caused by irritation of the gastric mucosa by gastric contents, is associated with peptic ulcers and esophagitis.

A thorough history and physical examination are essential to narrow the list of differential diagnoses of patients with abdominal pain. First, the nature of the pain is assessed to provide clues to the mechanism of the pain. Although location of the pain is valuable information, it is important to remember that abdominal pain can be referred from other areas. Timing of the pain (onset, duration, frequency, and relationship to associated symptoms) can help eliminate some causes. The palliative and provocative aspects of the pain can give clues about the cause of the pain. For example, does moving, eating certain foods, assuming different positions, or taking medications make the pain better or worse? Associated symptoms will further narrow the list of diagnostic possibilities. Some causes of abdominal pain will necessitate a surgical referral. Any time the pain is very severe and associated with a rigid abdomen, referral to a physician is essential. Abdominal pain can be the presenting symptom of many pathophysiological processes, ranging from very mild gastritis to more serious causes such as bowel obstruction or appendicitis.

A complete blood count, serum chemistries, liver function tests, urinalysis, pregnancy test, and abdominal films will help determine the acuity of the problem. Figure 38.1 presents diagnostic algorithms for abdominal pain. Treatment of abdominal pain depends on the cause.

CONSTIPATION

Constipation, which is difficult or infrequent defecation, is a common symptom in Western society and is the most common GI disorder in the United States, particularly in older adults and sedentary individuals (see Geriatric Considerations later in the chapter). The clinician and the patient must have a similar operational definition of

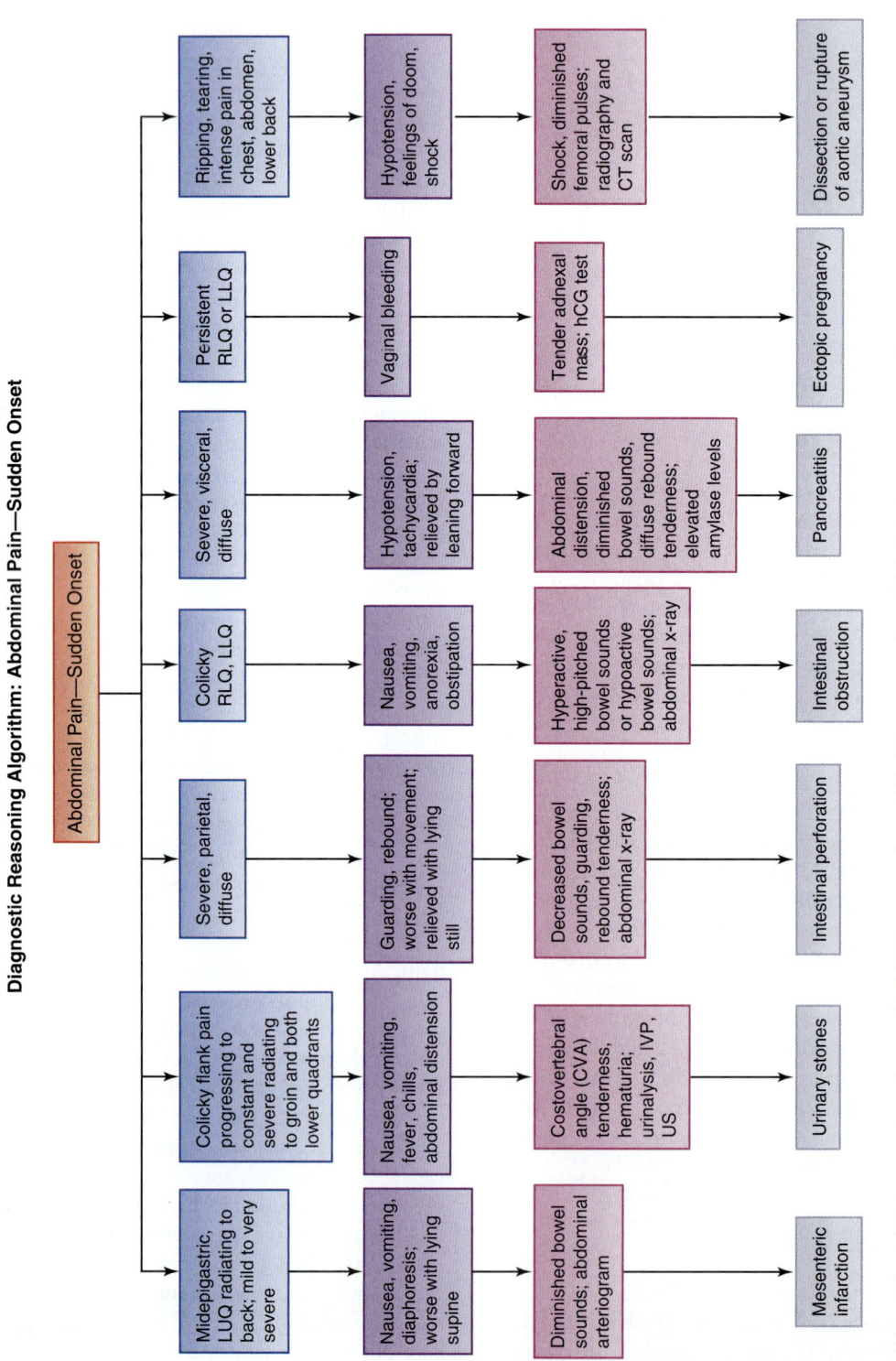

Abbreviations: IVP, intravenous polygram; LLQ, left lower quadrant; LUQ, left upper quadrant; RLQ, right lower quadrant; US, ultrasound

Figure 38.1a Diagnostic reasoning algorithm: abdominal pain–sudden onset.

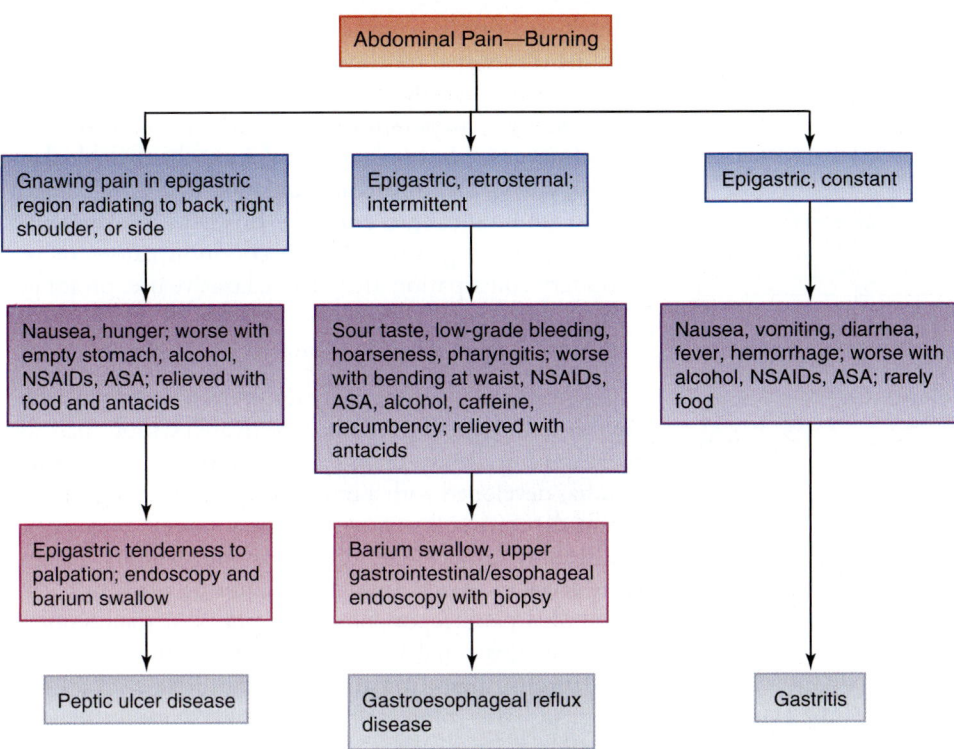

Figure 38.1b Diagnostic reasoning algorithm: abdominal pain–burning.

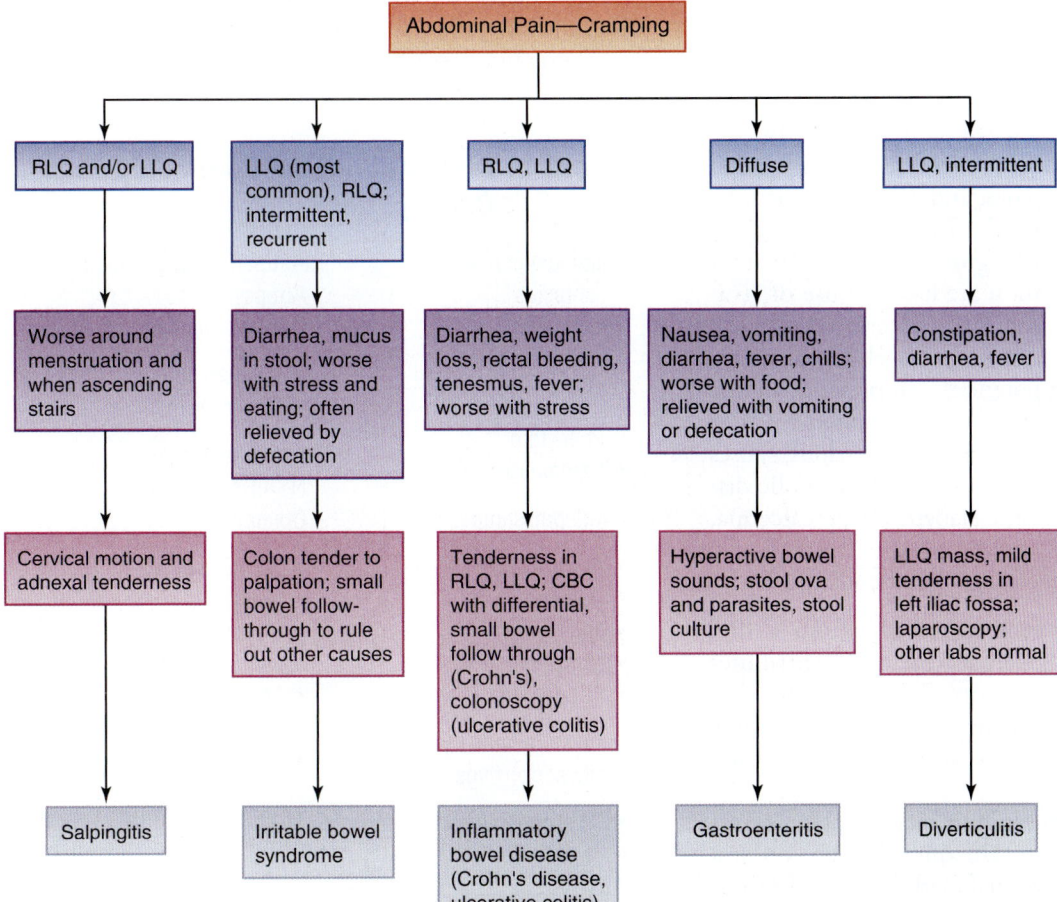

Figure 38.1c Diagnostic reasoning algorithm: abdominal pain–cramping.

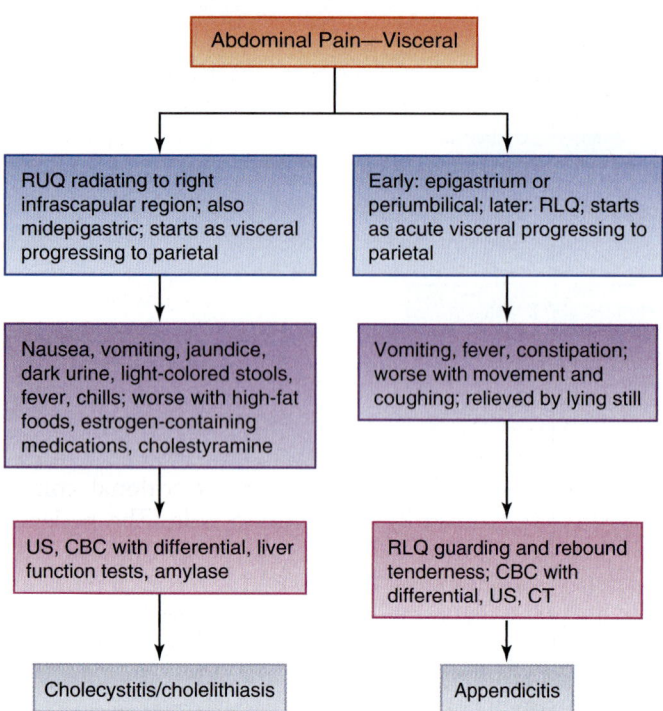

Figure 38.1d Diagnostic reasoning algorithm: abdominal pain–visceral.

constipation and what a normal bowel pattern is for that patient.

The most common cause of constipation in the United States is a lack of dietary fiber. The recommended amount is 25 g daily for women and 35 g daily for men to achieve optimal bowel health. The average American consumes only about 10 to 15 g of fiber per day. Other common causes of constipation are habitual use of laxatives, irritable bowel syndrome (IBS), decreased physical activity, a change in environment or travel, use of medications with constipating potential, suppression of the urge to defecate, and painful defecation caused by anorectal problems. Other less common but serious causes of constipation include bowel tumors and metabolic disorders such as hypothyroidism, diabetes, hypercalcemia, and depression.

Generally, there are three categories of constipation:

- *Functional constipation* generally results from a diet that is low in fiber. A sedentary lifestyle contributes as well. In addition, some people have difficulty defecating in an environment other than their own home and suppress the urge to defecate, thereby promoting functional constipation.
- *Disordered motility* is most often seen in older adults and is caused by slowed transit time. Megacolon and megarectum are also common disorders of motility, but they most frequently occur in children with conditions such as Hirschsprung disease. Other conditions that cause disordered motility and constipation include IBS and diverticular disease.
- *Secondary constipation* often is a result of medications such as opioids, analgesics, calcium channel blockers, antidepressants, antiparkinsonian drugs, cough medicine, and aluminum antacids. Box 38.1 presents a list of constipating drugs. Other common causes of secondary constipation are chronic laxative use, prolonged immobilization, and organic diseases of the lower GI system such as colorectal cancer.

Chronic constipation rarely results from a serious condition, and the patient can usually be treated symptomatically by increasing dietary fiber. Patients who have constipation that has developed with a recent disability, a change in diet, recent depressive illness, or the ingestion of a constipating medication can also be treated symptomatically. Patients who develop constipation that cannot be explained, have abdominal pain, report blood or mucus in their stool, or require a substantial increase in their laxative use require more investigation. Constipation occurs in fewer than 30% of patients with colon cancer.

DIFFERENTIAL DIAGNOSIS

An accurate description of the feces can give clues to the cause of the constipation. For example, ribbon-like stools often indicate a motility disorder but can also be caused by an organic narrowing of the distal or sigmoid colon.

Box 38.1	Medications That Commonly Cause Constipation
Aluminum-containing antacids	Antiparkinsonian drugs
Anticholinergics	Antipsychotics
Anticonvulsants	Bismuth-containing products
• Phenobarbital • Phenytoin • Carbamazepine	• Bismuth subsalicylate (Pepto-Bismol)
	Iron preparations NSAIDs
Antidepressants	Opiates
• Amitriptyline • Doxepin • Imipramine • Nortriptyline • Protriptyline	• Codeine • Morphine • Heroin • Fentanyl • Methadone • Propoxyphene • Tramadol
Antihistamines Antihypertensives	Sympathomimetics
• Calcium channel blockers • Clonidine	

If the patient complains of a progressive decrease in the diameter of the stools, this suggests an organic lesion. If steatorrhea (fatty stools) and greenish-yellow stools are associated with the constipation, the clinician should look for a small bowel or pancreatic lesion. Constipation alternating with diarrhea is often a result of IBS.

The cause of constipation is multifactorial, which can make the differential diagnosis difficult. Figure 38.2 presents various causes of constipation.

MANAGEMENT

The management of simple constipation is straightforward. Most patients respond well to education about bowel habits, activity, and dietary intervention. Some patients may require pharmacological intervention as well. Patients should be instructed to slowly increase the amount of dietary fiber to 25 to 35 g per day, with at least 12 to 15 g at breakfast. Mild exercise after the morning meal is often helpful in stimulating peristalsis and promoting defecation. Uninterrupted toilet time in the morning is also helpful. Adequate hydration is essential, and patients should be encouraged to drink at least 64 ounces of fluids daily.

Treatment with a pharmacological agent may be needed for patients who do not respond to increases in fiber, fluids, and exercise. Most drugs should be used for a short time only, and most are available without a prescription. Because these agents are available without a prescription, patients may have self-medicated for some time. By the time they seek medical attention, they may either have overused laxatives or may have a more serious underlying pathology. The only agents that are appropriate for long-term use are bulking agents. The different agents used in the treatment of constipation are listed in Drugs Commonly Prescribed 38.1. Complementary Therapies 38.1 lists the uses of vitamins, minerals, and herbs for constipation and other GI problems.

DIARRHEA

As with constipation, there is no single definition of diarrhea, but it is generally defined as an increase in the frequency, volume, or fluid content of bowel movements over what is normal for the individual. Because dietary intake of fiber in the United States is low, the average daily stool for each individual weighs about 200 g. For most individuals, if the daily stool is more than 200 g or the frequency of bowel movements is more than three times a day, the patient's condition is diarrhea.

There are several types of diarrhea, including the following:

- *Osmotic diarrhea* results when the osmotic gap between the stool and the serum is more than 50 mOsm/kg. Normally, the fecal osmolality is equal to the serum osmolality. An increasing osmotic gap implies either ingestion or malabsorption of a substance that is osmotically active. Carbohydrate malabsorption is the most common cause and includes lactose, fructose, and sorbitol. Other causes include laxative abuse and other malabsorption syndromes. Osmotic diarrhea usually responds to fasting. Celiac disease is a malabsorption syndrome related to an immune reaction to gluten in the diet. It is most common in women, and the peak incidence is in women aged 40 to 50 years. Gluten is found in food products that contain wheat, barley, and rye. The effects on the intestinal mucosa cause the villi to become flat, the crypts to hypertrophy, and an increased number of intraepithelial lymphocytes and plasma cells to appear. Complications such as collagenous sprue and intestinal ulcers, nutritional complications, and malignancy are possible. The patient will have a history of chronic diarrhea, foul-smelling stools, abdominal bloating, weakness, and fatigue. A presumptive diagnosis is based on a combination of clinical presentation and positive serology. Distal duodenal biopsy is needed to confirm the diagnosis. Treatment includes a lifelong gluten-free diet and treatment of nutritional deficiencies such as iron, folate, and vitamin B_{12}.
- *Secretory diarrhea* produces voluminous, watery stools but is unresponsive to fasting. Most cases of acute and chronic diarrhea are secretory in nature. Secretory diarrhea results from bacterial toxins (most notably from cholera and strains of *Escherichia coli*) and viruses (norovirus). However, it can also be caused by laxative abuse; bile acid malabsorption, which stimulates colonic secretion; and endocrine tumors that stimulate pancreatic or intestinal secretion.
- Diarrhea is associated with *morphological changes* within the mucosa of the intestinal wall that occur with inflammatory conditions of the intestines, and these changes can result in acute or chronic diarrhea. Both Crohn's disease and ulcerative colitis cause inflammation of the mucosa of the intestinal lumen, resulting in diarrhea.
- *Altered intestinal motility* secondary to diabetic neuropathy, dumping syndrome, or IBS can also cause diarrhea. Chronic parasitic infections with organisms such as *Giardia*, *Entamoeba histolytica,* and *Cyclospora* can cause diarrhea. Some medications such as antibiotics can induce diarrhea by disrupting the normal balance of bacteria. Probiotics have been studied in the treatment of diarrhea. The use of probiotics has been shown to decrease the incidence of antibiotic-associated diarrhea (AAD) in adults at risk but has not demonstrated effectiveness consistently in older adults. Probiotic use for travelers' diarrhea, *Clostridium difficile,* and inflammatory bowel disease (IBD) has not proved effective. Pathogenic bacteria also

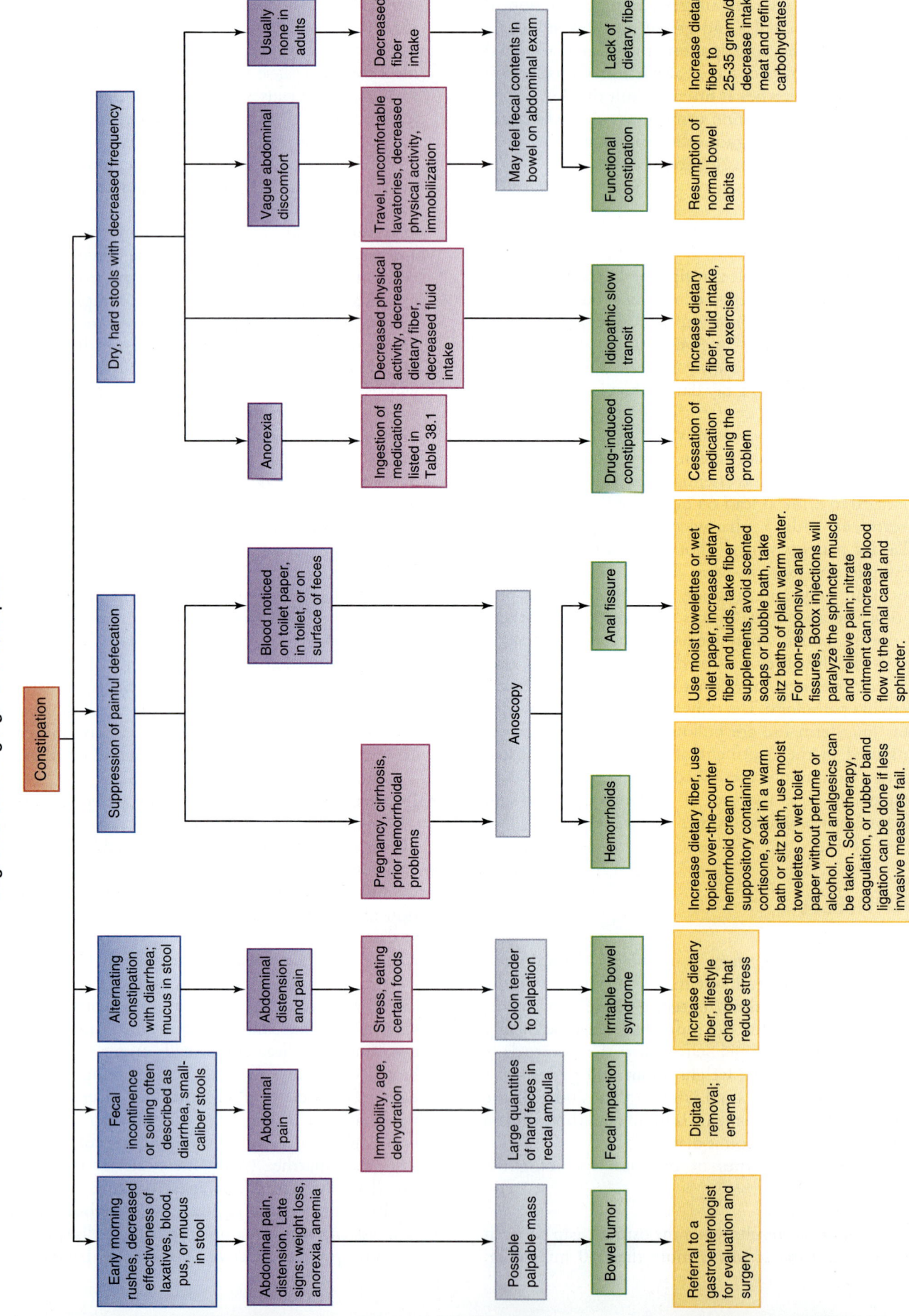

Figure 38.2 Diagnostic reasoning algorithm: constipation.

Drugs Commonly Prescribed 38.1: Constipation

DRUG	INDICATION	ADVERSE REACTIONS AND PRESCRIBING CONSIDERATIONS
Bulking agents Psyllium preparations Methylcellulose preparations	Irritable bowel syndrome Chronic constipation Diverticulitis	Causes flatulence, bloating and requires adequate fluid intake
Stool softeners Docusate sodium	Frequently used for prevention of constipation but not effective	Hepatotoxic if combined with irritant laxatives
Saline laxatives Magnesium hydroxide	Intermittent use in chronic constipation and bowel preparation	Can cause dehydration and electrolyte imbalance
Stimulant/irritant laxatives Bisacodyl Senna cascara	Acute constipation; should not be used for chronic constipation	Patient can become dependent. Also causes dehydration and electrolyte imbalance
Lubricants Mineral oil	Intermittent use in chronic constipation	Can cause lipoid (lipid) pneumonia if aspirated

Complementary Therapies 38.1: Complementary Therapies for Gastrointestinal Problems

AGENT	INDICATION	ADVERSE REACTIONS AND PRESCRIBING CONSIDERATIONS
Senna (*Cassia senna*)	Constipation	1–2 tsp dried leaves per 8 oz water taken as a tea once daily (not to be taken for longer than a few days)
Acupuncture	Heartburn	Eight to 12 treatments
Ginger	Nausea and motion sickness	250 mg daily

cause increases in GI motility and intestinal secretions. There have been promising results with the use of fecal microbiota transplantation (stool transplant) for the treatment of *C difficile* diarrhea. This procedure involves taking fecal bacteria from a healthy person and infusing this via enema into the person with the *C difficile* infection.

DIFFERENTIAL DIAGNOSIS

Differential diagnosis of diarrhea is aided by separating acute diarrhea from chronic diarrhea. *Acute diarrhea* usually has an abrupt onset and lasts less than 1 week. Nausea, vomiting, or fever may be associated with acute types of diarrhea. *Chronic diarrhea* lasts for more than 2 weeks or recurs over months or years. When diarrhea occurs suddenly in an otherwise healthy patient without signs or symptoms of other organ involvement, the most likely cause is an infectious agent, most often viral. The most frequent causes of chronic diarrhea are IBS, medications, dietary factors, IBD, and colon cancer.

A thorough history and comprehensive review of systems can elicit information that the patient may not think is important, but they can facilitate diagnosis. For example, recent travel is particularly important because viral, bacterial, and protozoan causes are endemic in many areas. Hikers and campers in the United States who drink unfiltered water are at a high risk for giardiasis. Focus on History: Diarrhea presents important information to obtain from the patient's history.

Focus on History: Diarrhea

Characteristics of Feces

- Frequency
- Amount and fluidity
- Color and characteristics: bloody, tarry, black, steatorrheic, mucous

Other History

- Diet history: intolerance to lactose or certain foods
- Recent travel
- Source of drinking water: well or city water supply
- Medication use: magnesium-containing antacids (or supplements), antibiotics, chemotherapy, immunosuppressive agents
- Medical/surgical history: diabetes mellitus, hyperthyroid, HIV, organ transplant, GI surgery
- Sexual practices: frequency of anal intercourse, number and sex of partners
- Social history: living conditions
- Family history: colon cancer, IBD

Other Factors

- Associated symptoms: abdominal pain, fever, vomiting, neurological symptoms, headache, malaise, myalgia, muscle weakness
- Exacerbating or alleviating factors

Acute viral gastroenteritis is the most common cause of diarrhea. (Gastroenteritis is discussed in detail in Chapter 39.) Other common causes of diarrhea the practitioner should consider are IBS, IBD, ingestion of magnesium-containing antacids, lactose intolerance, antibiotic therapy, laxative abuse, and AIDS. Figure 38.3 presents a diagnostic algorithm for diarrhea.

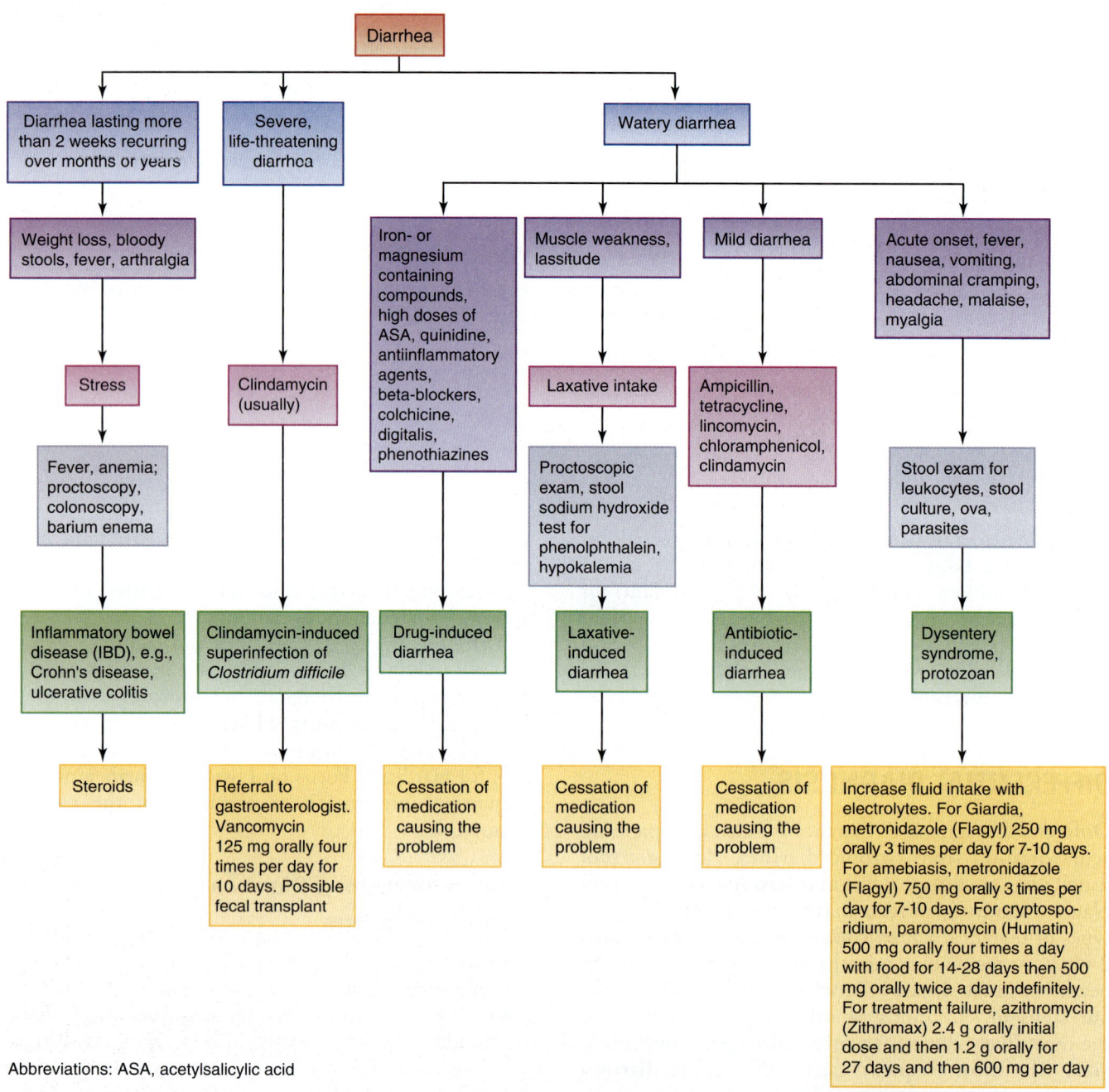

Abbreviations: ASA, acetylsalicylic acid

Figure 38.3 Diagnostic reasoning algorithm: diarrhea.

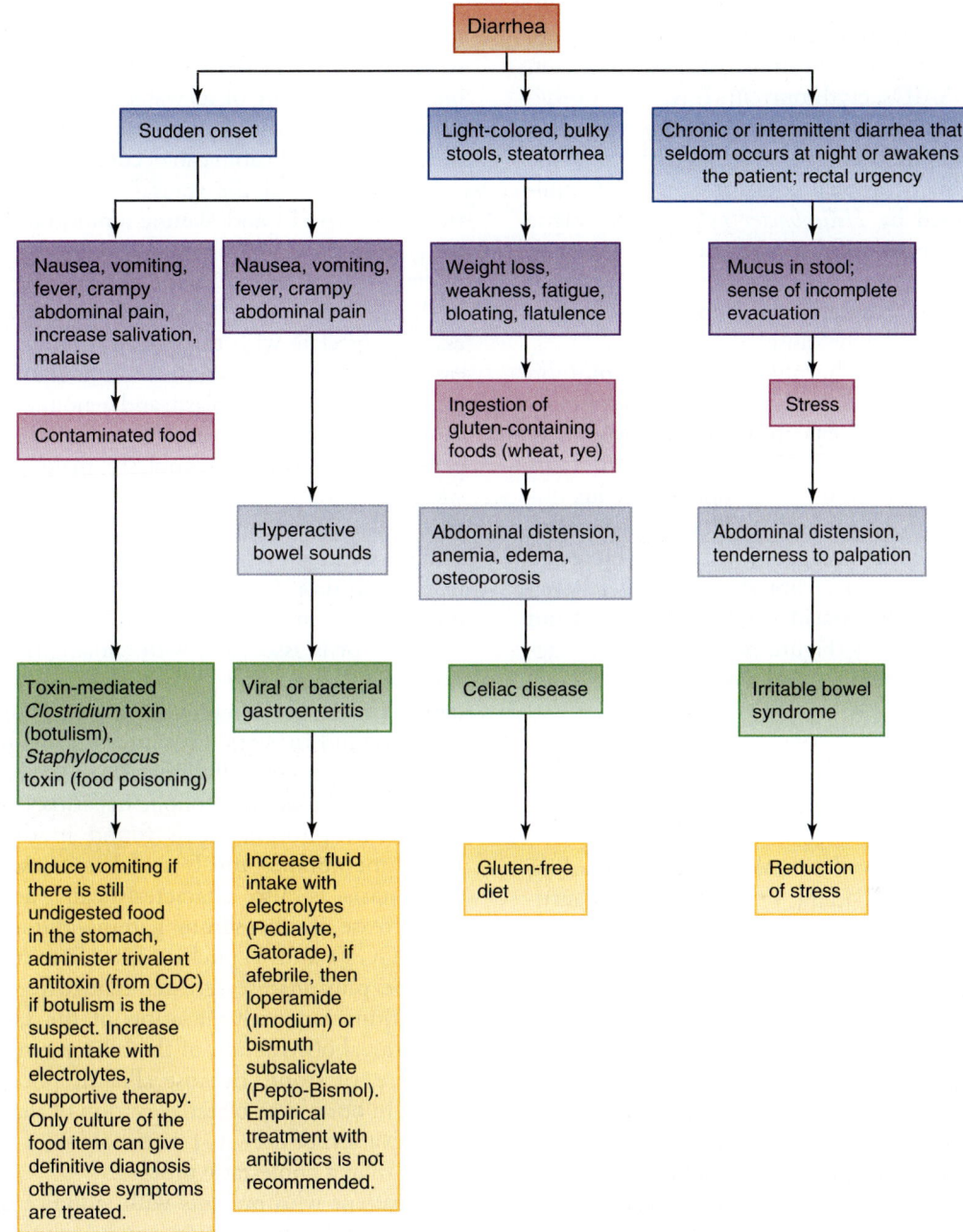

Figure 38.3—cont'd

DYSPEPSIA AND HEARTBURN

The frequency with which patients present with dyspepsia and heartburn as their chief complaints has been diminishing, probably because of the availability of over-the-counter histamine-2 receptor blockers and proton pump inhibitors. Aggressive advertising of these products by pharmaceutical companies over the past decade has led to increased self-medication for what could be a serious illness that the individual mistakes as simple heartburn.

DIFFERENTIAL DIAGNOSIS

Dyspepsia and heartburn are two different entities. *Heartburn* is occasionally described as extreme pain, and this makes it difficult to distinguish heartburn pain from that of angina pectoris or myocardial infarction. Patients with heartburn sometimes describe the pain as radiating to the back, arms, or jaw, which further complicates the diagnosis. Symptoms of *dyspepsia* include epigastric discomfort, postprandial fullness, early satiety, anorexia, belching, nausea, heartburn, vomiting, bloating, borborygmi, dysphagia, and abdominal burning. These symptoms most often have functional or organic causes. The possibility of an organic cause for dyspepsia increases as a person ages (see the following Geriatric Considerations). Patients who ingest alcohol in significant amounts or take drugs such as salicylates, corticosteroids, NSAIDs, erythromycin (E-Mycin), or theophylline (Theo-Dur, Theo-24) often have dyspepsia as a result of medication-induced gastritis. Giardiasis can cause dyspepsia with only occasional bouts of diarrhea. Nonulcer dyspepsia caused by *Helicobacter pylori* causes vague abdominal pain, a sense of fullness, nausea, and bloating, which are worse after eating. If the symptoms of dyspepsia are continuous and associated with anorexia and weight loss, gastric cancer may be the cause.

Heartburn, a retrosternal burning sensation, is common in the general population, with 7% complaining of daily symptoms, 14% having weekly episodes, and 36% experiencing heartburn at least once in their lives. The most common cause of heartburn is gastroesophageal reflux disease. Pregnant women have a high incidence of esophagitis, most often later in the pregnancy because of increased intra-abdominal pressure. Heartburn is commonly relieved by the ingestion of alkali (antacids) and is precipitated and aggravated by recumbency. Figure 38.4 provides a diagnostic algorithm for heartburn and dyspepsia.

JAUNDICE

Jaundice (icterus) is a yellow coloration of the skin, mucous membranes, and sclera, resulting from an accumulation of bilirubin in the blood. Patients who develop jaundice usually seek medical attention promptly because it is so dramatic, frightening, and difficult to ignore.

The hyperbilirubinemia that causes the jaundice can be a result of increased production, decreased uptake, decreased conjugation, or decreased excretion of bilirubin. The etiology of hyperbilirubinemia is shown in Box 38.2. Hyperbilirubinemia and jaundice in most patients result from cholestasis, either because of impaired bile formation and/or bile flow, which can be the result of extrahepatic biliary tract obstruction or hepatic parenchymal disease.

DIFFERENTIAL DIAGNOSIS

Understanding laboratory values reported for typical liver function tests is essential in determining the cause of hyperbilirubinemia and establishing a diagnosis. Icterus is not usually evident until the serum bilirubin level exceeds 2.5 to 3.0 mg/dL. The normal serum bilirubin level is 0.3 to 1.0 mg/dL. Most bilirubin is formed from the heme portion of the breakdown of red blood cells. This initial bilirubin is unconjugated and therefore not soluble in water. When measured in the serum, it is reported as indirect bilirubin. This form of bilirubin is reversibly bound to albumin and transported to the liver, where it is taken up by hepatocytes and conjugated with glucuronic acid. Conjugated bilirubin, which is water soluble, is transported from the hepatocyte into the bile. It is measured in the serum as the direct fraction of bilirubin. Only conjugated bilirubin, by nature of its water solubility, is found in the urine of patients with hyperbilirubinemia. Problems in the metabolism of bilirubin can occur at any point of the cycle.

Serum levels of the transaminases—aspartate aminotransferase (AST) and alanine aminotransferase (ALT)—are good indicators of hepatocyte damage from a variety of causes. Elevated transaminase levels reflect the activity of the disease process, but actual serum levels do not necessarily correlate with the overall severity of the liver disease, nor with the prognosis. AST is found in hepatocyte mitochondria and cytoplasm and in nonhepatic tissues such as skeletal muscle, the heart, and the brain. ALT is found primarily in hepatocyte cytoplasm, making it a much more specific marker for hepatocyte damage. Levels of AST and ALT that are below 300 U/L are nonspecific; however, some extreme elevations can be diagnostic. For example, it is uncommon for the AST to be elevated 15 times the normal value in biliary obstruction except when it occurs suddenly or is associated with cholangitis. Striking elevations of ALT and AST (greater than 1,000 U/L) occur in patients with acute viral hepatitis, toxin- or drug-induced hepatitis, and ischemic liver injury. If the ratio of AST to ALT is high, it generally indicates severe hepatic necrosis, most often caused by alcoholic hepatitis.

Alkaline phosphatase is found in the biliary canalicular membranes and is useful in assessing cholestasis. Cholestasis is also characteristically accompanied by an increase in the serum gamma-glutamyl transpeptidase (GGT) and 5'-nucleotidase. Extreme elevations in alkaline phosphatase (greater than three times normal) in conjunction with elevation of the GGT indicate a mechanical obstruction of the biliary system by a tumor, stricture, or stone. Because alkaline phosphatase is also found in bone, an isolated elevation of that enzyme without elevation of the GGT is indicative of a bone disorder rather than a cholestatic process.

A patient who presents with jaundice often has complaints of pruritus, anorexia, nausea, vomiting, fever, light-colored stools, weight loss, and fatigue. Examination may reveal right upper quadrant pain and tenderness, dark urine, and abdominal distention. Pruritus, dark urine, and light-colored stools in conjunction with the jaundice are indicative of cholestasis, either intrahepatic or extrahepatic, such as cholelithiasis, cirrhosis, or other biliary obstruction.

MELENA

Melena is defined as black, tarry stools that test positive for occult blood. The most common cause of melena is upper GI bleeding, but bleeding in the small bowel or

> **Box 38.4 Common Causes of Nausea and Vomiting**
>
> **Gastrointestinal Disorders and Problems**
>
> Gastroenteritis
> Acute gastrointestinal infections
> Food poisoning
> Gastritis, including alcoholic
> Peptic ulcer disease
> Hepatitis
> Food intolerance
> Celiac disease (celiac sprue)
> Lactase deficiency
> Ingestion of fatty foods
> Intestinal obstruction
> Appendicitis
> Cholecystitis
> Peritonitis
> Diabetic gastric atony
>
> **Central Nervous System Disorders and Problems**
>
> Increased intracranial pressure
> Migraine headache
> Meningitis
> Acute labyrinthitis
> Ménière's disease
> Altitude sickness
>
> **Other Disorders and Problems**
>
> Motion sickness
> Uremia
> Bulimia nervosa
> Diabetic ketoacidosis
> Adrenal insufficiency
> Acute myocardial infarction
> Congestive heart failure
> Gastroparesis
> Postinfectious gastroparesis
> Pregnancy
>
> **Adverse Effect of Drugs and Chemicals**
>
> Antibiotics (erythromycin, metronidazole)
> Opiates
> Estrogen
> Ipecac
> Digitalis
> Chemotherapy
> Theophylline

A careful history and documentation of signs and symptoms are often necessary to determine the cause of the nausea and vomiting. The circumstances surrounding the episode or episodes give clues to the cause. Vomiting after a meal can occur with gastritis and in digitalis toxicity. If the vomiting occurs 1 to 2 hours after eating, diseases of the biliary tract or pancreas should be suspected. Projectile vomiting without nausea is classically a sign of a neurological source such as increased intracranial pressure. If the nausea and vomiting occur in the early morning, the cause may be uremia, pregnancy, or chronic alcohol ingestion. The duration of the nausea and vomiting depends on the cause. Infectious agents in the GI tract usually cause nausea and vomiting only for 24 hours or less. Nausea as a result of pregnancy can last for weeks.

The characteristics of the vomitus are important in determining the cause. For example, repeated vomiting without bile staining is indicative of pyloric obstruction, which can be caused by scars from an ulcer or a tumor, whereas vomiting of undigested food could indicate an esophageal obstruction. The odor of the vomitus is important information to elicit from the patient in determining the cause. Odorless vomitus indicates a lack of gastric acid, possibly from esophageal stricture or achalasia. Fecal odor, on the other hand, indicates a bowel obstruction or gastrocolic fistula.

Associated symptoms can further narrow the field of possibilities. Ménière's disease or middle ear disturbances should be suspected if the patient complains of vertigo, tinnitus, or hearing loss. Nausea and vomiting often accompany migraine headaches, which are usually unilateral. Nausea and vomiting with diarrhea and abdominal pain are often caused by gastroenteritis. Figure 38.5 provides a diagnostic algorithm for nausea and vomiting.

MANAGEMENT

Management of nausea and vomiting is aimed at the underlying cause, which is covered in detail in specific chapters in this section and in other chapters of this book. Symptomatic relief, however, is useful for the comfort of the patient and in preventing complications such as dehydration and electrolyte imbalance. Drugs Commonly Prescribed 38.2 presents a list of medications commonly used for the control of nausea and vomiting

DYSPHAGIA

Dysphagia is defined as difficulty swallowing that may or may not have a component of *odynophagia,* or painful swallowing. Although dysphagia may accompany odynophagia, classic dysphagia is not usually painful. The prevalence increases with age and is common in older adults (see Geriatric Considerations).

The process of swallowing is complex and involves 50 pairs of muscles and many nerves. Swallowing has three phases: (1) The *oral phase* involves movement of the tongue and jaw, allowing for mastication and

616 *Unit* II CARING-BASED NURSING: THE SCIENCE

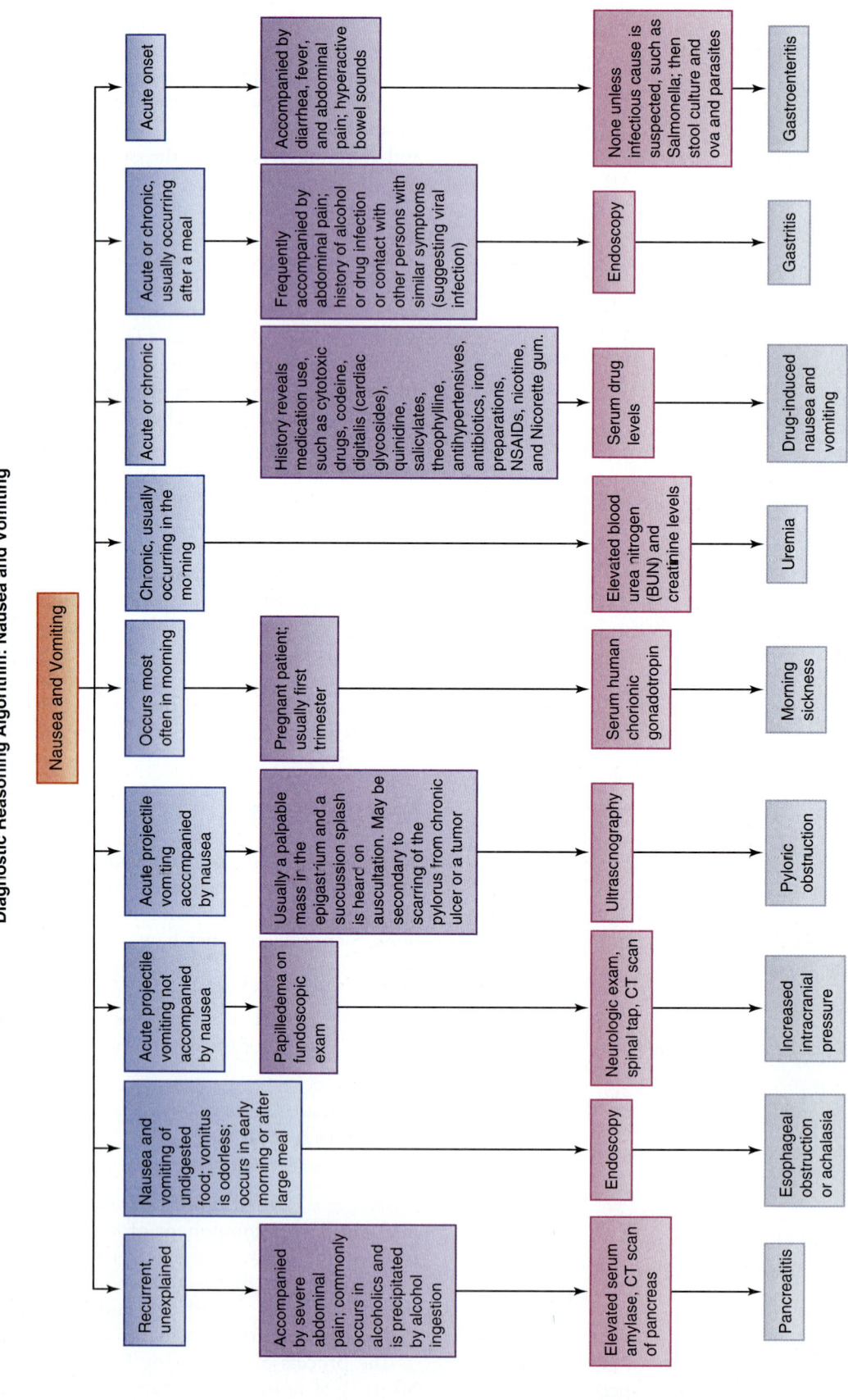

Abbreviations: CT, computed tomography; NSAIDs, nonsteroidal antiinflammatory drugs

Figure 38.5 Diagnostic reasoning algorithm: nausea and vomiting.

Drugs Commonly Prescribed 38.2: Nausea and Vomiting

DRUG	INDICATION	ADVERSE REACTIONS AND PRESCRIBING CONSIDERATIONS
Antihistamines (dimenhydrinate, promethazine, hydroxyzine, meclizine)	Motion sickness Drug-induced nausea Postoperative During labor	Sedation, dry mouth, blurred vision, headache
Antidopaminergics (prochlorperazine)	Chemotherapy- and radiation-induced nausea and vomiting Postoperative	Sedation, dry mouth, urinary retention, constipation, extrapyramidal effects
Antidopaminergics and cholinergics (metoclopramide)	Postoperative Diabetic gastroparesis	Restlessness, drowsiness, fatigue, extrapyramidal effects
Cholinergic antagonists (scopolamine)	Motion sickness	Dry mouth, blurred vision, tachycardia, constipation, sedation
Serotonin receptor antagonists (ondansetron, granisetron)	Chemotherapy- and radiation-induced nausea and vomiting	Anxiety, euphoria, depression, headache, insomnia, restlessness, weakness

 Geriatric Considerations:
Common Abdominal Complaints

Constipation

Results from:

- Decreased physical activity
- Decreased fiber in the diet
- Decreased fluid intake

Dyspepsia

Results from:

- Intake of NSAIDs
- Diabetes mellitus and diabetes medications
- Antibiotics
- High-fat diet
- Chronic kidney disease
- Hiatal hernia
- Malignancy

Dysphagia

Results from:

- Decreased esophageal motility
- Stroke
- Parkinson's disease

DIFFERENTIAL DIAGNOSIS

Dysphagia can be caused by mechanical obstruction or a functional problem that impairs motility. Mechanical obstruction can be either intrinsic (strictures, tumors, diverticular outpouchings) or extrinsic (a tumor or other growth outside the esophagus that presses inward to compress the esophageal wall). Functional dysphagia can have a neurological or muscular cause. Neurological conditions that interfere with voluntary swallowing or peristalsis are cerebrovascular accidents, Parkinson's disease, multiple sclerosis, amyotrophic lateral sclerosis, and achalasia. Eighty percent of oral phase and pharyngeal phase abnormalities have a neurological origin. Dermatomyositis is a muscular disease that causes functional problems in the upper esophagus, leading to dysphagia. Dysphagia may be the first sign of such an underlying disorder. Psychological conditions may also cause the symptoms; the term *globus hystericus* refers to a manifestation of acute anxiety disorders and panic attacks. Dysphagia may also be associated with an underlying depressive disorder.

Alterations of the swallowing process may manifest differently, depending on the underlying pathology. For example, if there is a problem in the oral phase, dribbling, spillage, pocketing of food in the mouth, or aspiration may be present. The pharyngeal phase is the first reflexive, or involuntary, phase; problems during this phase are characterized by nasal regurgitation, aspiration, and/or altered voice. This is the phase in which aspiration most commonly occurs during swallowing. Esophageal phase problems are characterized by neck pain, heartburn, and the sensation of food becoming "stuck" below the sternum.

An upper endoscopy is the first choice to evaluate chronic dysphagia and has the benefit of direct visualization and the ability to obtain a biopsy if an abnormality is found.

preparation of food into a bolus and making it ready for swallowing; (2) the *pharyngeal phase* includes the reflexive passage of the bolus from the oral cavity through the pharynx and into the upper esophagus; and (3) the *esophageal phase* is the reflexive passage of the bolus through the esophagus and into the stomach. There is often a combination of underlying factors that cause dysphagia.

A videofluoroscopic swallow study is useful in evaluating swallowing. This imaging technique videotapes the entire swallowing process and shows an outline of the structures from the oral cavity to the stomach, as well as assesses the velocity and movement of oral and hypopharyngeal structures and their temporal relationship to each other. Through observation of the ingestion of various food consistencies such as thin liquids, thick liquids, semisolids, and solids, the safest plan for oral intake can be determined.

MANAGEMENT

There are a number of approaches to treating dysphagia, depending on the cause. One approach involves muscle strengthening exercises of the facial muscles to improve the coordination of swallowing. Most approaches involve instructing the patient and family members in ways to improve safe food intake, including positioning (usually sitting upright, with the head tilted slightly forward and downward) and food-consistency modification (no thin liquids, mechanical soft diet) during food intake. However, if the risk of aspiration is severe, the clinician may have to consider elimination of oral intake. For these patients, enteral feeding is the next choice.

REFERENCES

Bascom A. *Incorporating herbal medicine into clinical practice.* Philadelphia: FA Davis; 2002.

De Wolf TJ, Eggers S, Barker AK, et al. Oral probiotic combination of Lactobacillus and Bifidobacterium alters the gastrointestinal microbiota during antibiotic treatment for *Clostridium difficile* infection. *PLoS One.* 2018;13(9):e0204253. Published 2018 Sep 28. doi:10.1371/journal.pone.0204253

Domino FJ, Baldor RA, Golding J, et al, eds. *The 5-minute clinical consult,* 28th ed. Philadelphia: Wolters Kluwer; 2020.

Huether SE. Alterations in digestive function. In McCance KL, Huether SE (eds.), *Pathophysiology: The biologic basis for disease in adults and children,* 8th ed. St. Louis, MO: Mosby; 2019: 1321–1372.

Sniffen JC, McFarland LV, Evans CT, et al. Choosing an appropriate probiotic product for your patient: An evidence-based practical guide. *PLoS One.* 2018;13(12):e0209205. Published 2018 Dec 26. doi:10.1371/journal.pone.0209205

Vernaya M, McAdam J, Hampton MD. Effectiveness of probiotics in reducing the incidence of *Clostridium difficile*–associated diarrhea in elderly patients: a systematic review. *JBI Database System Rev Implement Rep.* 2017;15:140–164.

Woo TM, Robinson MV. Pharmacotherapeutics for advanced practice nurse prescribers, 5th ed. Philadelphia: FA Davis; 2020.

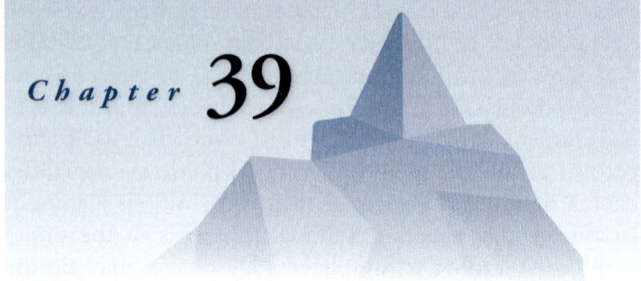

Chapter 39

Infectious Gastrointestinal Disorders

Debera J. Thomas, PhD, RN, ANP/FNP

GASTROENTERITIS

Gastroenteritis is an inflammation of the stomach and intestine that manifests as anorexia, nausea, vomiting, and diarrhea. Gastroenteritis can be acute or chronic and can be caused by bacteria, viruses, parasites, injury to the bowel mucosa, inorganic poisons (sodium nitrate), organic poisons (mushrooms or shellfish), and drugs. Chronic causes include food allergies and intolerance, stress, and lactase deficiency. Gastroenteritis caused by bacterial toxins in food is often referred to as food poisoning; it should be suspected when groups of individuals present with the same symptoms.

The symptoms and subsequent electrolyte imbalances are usually self-limiting in the healthy adult but can have serious consequences for older adults and immunocompromised or pediatric patients. The severity of the illness is indicated by the presence of dehydration secondary to profuse watery diarrhea, fever greater than 101°F (38.3°C), vomiting, or dysentery (frequent small stools containing blood and mucus). A careful history and physical examination provides clues about the causative agent and the suspected vector of transmission. Travel, dining locations, and antibiotic history should be included as part of the assessment.

EPIDEMIOLOGY AND CAUSES

Acute gastroenteritis results most often from an infectious agent. Although it is one of the most frequent diagnoses in primary care practice (about 30% of patients seen each year), the exact number of individuals affected is not known because acute gastroenteritis presents with a group of nonspecific symptoms that often go unreported or the etiology cannot be determined. The estimated annual rate for gastroenteritis is approximately one episode per adult per year in the United States and Western Europe. Foodborne and waterborne outbreaks are of particular importance and gain the attention of the news media in an effort to identify and treat all the individuals who were exposed to the harmful pathogen.

The most common mode of transmission for acute infectious gastroenteritis is the fecal–oral route from contaminated food or water. Person-to-person transfer of the disease is more common within the hospital setting, long-term care facilities, and day-care centers where there are larger groups of people capable of transmitting the disease. Groups considered at high risk for developing gastroenteritis include anyone traveling to a developing country, immunocompromised patients, anyone engaging in anal intercourse, residents of institutions or nursing homes, infants and children attending day-care centers, and individuals consuming raw shellfish and seafood.

Bacterial pathogens account for 30% to 80% of acute gastroenteritis cases and are an important cause of morbidity in tropical areas and in travelers to areas of high risk for the pathogens (traveler's diarrhea). Roughly 10% to 40% of travelers are afflicted depending on the destination and the country of origin. Areas considered high risk for developing traveler's diarrhea include Africa (South Africa excepted), South and Southeast Asia, South and Central America, Mexico, Haiti, and the Dominican Republic. Table 39.1 presents the most common bacterial, viral, and parasitic causes of gastroenteritis.

Gastroenteritis can also be caused by dietary factors such as coffee, tea, and sodas containing caffeine, medications (primarily antacids and antibiotics), and metabolic factors, including diabetes mellitus, hyperthyroidism, and adrenal insufficiency.

PATHOPHYSIOLOGY

Pathophysiological causes of gastroenteritis are numerous; however, bacterial, viral, and parasitic infections are among the most common. Almost all forms of enteric infection manifest with diarrhea. Diarrheal diseases cause an increase in the frequency of stools, less well-formed feces, and an increase in the fecal water content. The definition of diarrhea is dependent on each patient's normal bowel habits. Diarrhea is not considered a medical emergency unless it affects children or older adults who are less able to regulate their fluid intake. Diarrhea is a major cause of infant mortality in developing nations.

The gastrointestinal (GI) tract has several defenses against the development of infection. When bacterial or viral pathogens can overcome these barriers, they proliferate, causing varying degrees of gastroenteritis. The acidity of the stomach is normally maintained at a pH of 2, which creates a hostile environment for most microorganisms. The acidic barrier in the stomach protects the small bowel and colon from ingested pathogens. If the organism is resistant to the acid environment or the patient has taken medications that alter the pH, the organism may thrive and cause illness.

Another host defense mechanism is the constant peristalsis of the small bowel, which prevents the colonization of pathogens within the lumen. Patients who have small bowel stasis as a result of obstruction, diverticula, or blind loop syndrome frequently develop an overgrowth of bacteria within the stagnant segment, causing gastroenteritis resulting from the increased number of bacteria in the small bowel. In contrast, the colon is relatively stagnant; it typically harbors about 1 billion bacteria per gram of intestinal contents. Normal feces are composed primarily of water and bacteria. These beneficial bacteria protect against potential pathogens by consuming available nutrients and producing by-products that create a hostile environment to the invading pathogens.

The gut microbiome also plays a protective role. The gut becomes colonized with hundreds of bacterial species shortly after birth. The most common species are *Bacteroides, Bifidobacterium, Eubacterium, Fusobacterium, Clostridium,* and *Lactobacillus*. The normal flora of the GI tract help prevent overgrowth of pathogens. The bacterial composition, number, and diversity of the normal flora is influenced by diet, aging, chronic disease, medications, radiation exposure, genetics, pollution, and personal hygiene. The composition of the gut microbiome is believed to play a role in immunity.

The GI tract also produces specific immunoglobulins that protect against invading organisms. After exposure to certain organisms, immunoglobulins may even protect against future invasions by the same organism, much like an antigen–antibody response. IgA, a secretory immunoglobulin, may help defend against many of the bacteria that cause gastroenteritis by invading the intestinal mucosa.

Ingestion of contaminated food can result in clinical symptoms of gastroenteritis, depending on the number and virulence of the organisms in the food. Almost all bacteria are capable of producing mild diarrhea if ingested in large enough quantities. Other organisms (e.g., *Shigella, Salmonella, Campylobacter, Cryptosporidium*) have such a high virulence that only a small inoculum can produce symptoms.

Often, the incubation time of the pathogen, coupled with the presenting symptoms, will give specific clues for establishing a diagnosis. Infectious processes of the small intestine often result in watery, secretory, or a malabsorptive type of diarrhea; infections of the large intestine tend to produce bloody diarrhea and abdominal pain. Gastroenteritis with an onset of nausea and vomiting within 6 hours after exposure to the pathogen suggests food poisoning resulting from the ingestion of a preformed toxin such as that of *Bacillus cereus*. Incubation periods greater than 14 hours and the initial symptom of vomiting are highly suggestive of viral infections.

TABLE 39.1 Organisms Causing Gastroenteritis

Pathogen	Pathogenesis	Duration/Onset	Clinical Findings	Diagnosis and Treatment
Bacterial Pathogens *Bacillus cereus*	Type of food poisoning from formation of enterotoxins within food or gut; two forms, differing in duration of illness.	Duration is normally less than 24 hours. Onset is within 1 to 8 hours after exposure.	Illness begins with vomiting and proceeds to diarrhea; no fever. Commonly occurs in rice dishes; the spores are heat resistant and not affected by cooking.	No antibiotic treatment is required; oral hydration and supportive care.
Campylobacter jejuni	Found primarily in eggs and poultry but may be found in domestic animals. Organism invades the intestinal mucosa and produces a cholera-like toxin. Organism grows within ileum and jejunum.	Duration of illness is 2 to 6 days. Onset of symptoms approximately 48 hours after ingestion of pathogen.	Common cause of traveler's diarrhea from ingestion of contaminated water. Symptoms include fever, bloody diarrhea, and abdominal pain. Stool is positive for polymorphonuclear neutrophils.	Normally self-limiting. Erythromycin ethylsuccinate can be used in severe cases. Rapid antibiotic resistance is common. Stool culture requires special media. Quinoline antibiotics have been effective in increasing recovery.
Clostridium botulinum	Anaerobic gram-positive bacillus that produces seven distinct toxins. In the foodborne type the toxin is ingested with contaminated food. Once absorbed, the toxin blocks the release of acetylcholine from peripheral nerve endings. Canned foods are the primary source.	Duration of illness depends on diagnosis and treatment. Mortality rate is high. Onset is abrupt, although incubation can be as long as 4 to 8 days.	GI symptoms often precede neurological findings, which are bilateral and symmetrical, and occur in a descending fashion. Initial neurological symptoms include dry mouth, diplopia, and loss of pupillary reflex. Dysphagia and dysarthria can lead to aspiration pneumonia. Progression of neurological insult leads to paralysis of the diaphragm and death if mechanical ventilation is not employed.	Diagnosis is made by isolation of organism in suspected food, the serum, or feces. Symptoms are often confused with Guillain-Barré. Treatment is to first eliminate any unabsorbed food (toxin) by inducing vomiting or by gastric lavage, then administration of trivalent antitoxin (A, B, or E) from the Centers for Disease Control and Prevention. The antitoxin does not reverse the existing neurological symptoms but prevents progression. Little benefit if given after 72 hours. Toxin may cause serum sickness or anaphylaxis. Mechanical ventilation must be considered in an emergency.

TABLE 39.1 Organisms Causing Gastroenteritis—cont'd

Pathogen	Pathogenesis	Duration/Onset	Clinical Findings	Diagnosis and Treatment
Clostridium difficile	Gram-positive anaerobe maintained in spore form. It colonizes bowel when normal bowel flora are suppressed by antibiotics. It produces two toxins: toxin A, an enterotoxin, and toxin B, a cytotoxin causing pseudomembranous colitis and necrosis.	Duration and intensity of disease vary. Onset normally is in a hospitalized patient who has had recent antibiotic treatment.	Symptoms range from none to acute abdomen secondary to toxic megacolon with perforation; symptoms usually begin after initiation of antibiotics. Profuse, watery, or mucoid diarrhea, which may be blood-tinged, accompanied by fever, abdominal cramping and distention, white blood cells (WBCs) greater than 20,000, and ascites. Metabolic acidosis indicates severe colitis or toxic megacolon. Common cause of health-care–associated infections.	Diagnosis is confirmed with isolation of toxin A or B in the stool. Culture alone is no longer diagnostic because of the number of patients who are asymptomatic carriers. Flexible sigmoidoscopy may reveal pseudomembranous colitis. It is associated with recent abdominal surgery. It is treated with oral metronidazole (Flagyl) 250 mg four times daily for 10 days, vancomycin (Vancocin) 125 mg four times daily for 10 days. Relapse (20%) is treated with second course of previously mentioned medications. Patients with multiple relapses may require 30 days of antibiotic treatment. Avoid antimotility agents.
Clostridium perfringens	Found in soil, feces, air, and water. Outbreaks caused most often by contaminated meat. Type A enterotoxin causes mild to moderate gastroenteritis. Type C enterotoxin can be fatal.	Duration of illness is similar to mild gastritis, lasting 1 to 4 days without medical intervention. Fatal cases are less common. Onset is usually within 12 hours of ingestion of contaminated food.	Abrupt onset of diarrhea without fever. If fatal, cases have severe diarrhea with abdominal pain and distention.	Diagnosis is made by isolating organism in food or feces. Cultures usually show many clostridia in food or feces. No treatment is necessary for mild forms other than supportive care. Penicillin may be useful in severe cases.
Escherichia coli	Five identified strains classified by pathogenesis of diarrhea. All are gram-negative rods.	Dependent on strain; epidemics are due to ingestion of contaminated meat or dairy products.		
	Enterohemorrhagic *Escherichia coli* (EHEC). Most serious; produces a hemorrhagic infection; O157:H7 strain produces two toxins, which inhibit protein synthesis in intestinal cells.	Duration typically is 1 to 8 days. Onset is 24 hours after ingestion of contaminated food.	Acute onset of dysentery with 12 to 24 hours of abdominal cramps, watery diarrhea, and fever, followed by bloody stools. Can cause hemorrhagic infection of colon and can be fatal. Complications include hemolytic-uremic syndrome or thrombolytic thrombocytopenic purpura. WBCs are greater than 20,000; azotemia; dehydration. Infants and older adults are most prone to adverse effects.	Diagnosis is by isolation of *E. coli* O157:H7 in stools. Look for the source of undercooked meat. It can be transmitted in feces and dirty diapers. Treatment is supportive. Antibiotics have not proved effective.

Continued

TABLE 39.1 Organisms Causing Gastroenteritis—cont'd

Pathogen	Pathogenesis	Duration/Onset	Clinical Findings	Diagnosis and Treatment
	Enterotoxigenic *E. coli* (ETEC). Adheres to the mucosa of small bowel, releasing toxins that cause diarrhea.	Duration 2 to 4 days. Incubation period is 24 to 36 hours.	Most common cause of traveler's diarrhea from contaminated food or water. Mild fever, abdominal cramps, watery stool, nausea, and vomiting are common.	Usually self-limiting, requiring no treatment other than supportive care. It is common in developing countries.
	Enteropathogenic *E. coli* (EPEC).	Duration is 1 to 3 days; 12- to 36-hour incubation period.	Profuse, watery, foul-smelling diarrhea. It is of special concern to infants and older adults who are prone to dehydration.	Usually self-limiting. Infants and older adults may require hospitalization. It is rare in the United States.
	Enteroinvasive *E. coli* (EIEC) causes invasion and proliferation within enterocytes, much like *Shigella* infection.	Duration is 4 to 10 days; 12- to 72-hour incubation period.	It is an uncommon cause of foodborne dysentery in the United States. Patients have fever, anorexia, cramps, and watery diarrhea. Stools may be mucoid or bloody. Clinical presentation is much like that of *Shigella* infection.	May isolate leukocytes in stool. Diarrhea is self-limiting. Food poisoning of this kind is rare in the United States.
	Enteroadherent *E. coli* (EAEC) is rare and adheres to liver cells.		Mild, nonbloody diarrhea; strain is uncommon.	No leukocytes in stool.
Vibrio cholerae	Commonly found in areas with poor sanitation; food and water contaminated with feces. Enterotoxin causes hypersecretion in small intestine. Rarely found in the United States but may be endemic along the Gulf Coast.	Incubation is 1 to 3 days. Duration is 1 to 2 weeks.	Most cases in the United States are hemolytic and are transported here from contaminated foods. Diarrhea can be severe, causing septicemia, especially in immunocompromised patients, children, or older adults. Diarrhea is profuse, "rice water" and can be life-threatening. There is no abdominal cramping or fever. Patients may stool at the rate of 1 L/hr.	To diagnose *V. cholerae*, a special *Vibrio*-selective medium must be used in the stool culture. Diarrhea requires prompt replacement of fluids and electrolytes. Antibiotic: tetracycline 500 mg by mouth (PO) every 6 hours for 2 days or Bactrim DS every 12 hours for 2 days.
Vibrio parahaemolyticus	Pathogen found in seafood. Produces toxins in the gut or invades intestinal mucosa. Outbreaks frequent in summer; usually associated with improperly cooked seafood.	Incubation period 8 to 24 hours. Duration is 1 to 3 days.	Patient presents with abdominal cramping, headache, fever. Usually associated with explosive, noninflammatory, watery diarrhea, which may be bloody depending on the degree of mucosal destruction.	Stool is positive for *Vibrio*. Often diagnosed when a group of people become sick after consuming seafood. Food cultures are positive.

TABLE 39.1 Organisms Causing Gastroenteritis—cont'd				
Pathogen	**Pathogenesis**	**Duration/Onset**	**Clinical Findings**	**Diagnosis and Treatment**
Yersinia enterocolitica	Primarily transmitted via fecal–oral route; foodborne. It is rare in the United States; more common in northern Europe and Canada. Organism forms an enterotoxin and invades the intestinal epithelium.	Onset and incubation are unknown. Duration usually resolves in 1 to 3 weeks.	Symptoms include fever, abdominal pain, and bloody diarrhea. Older children may develop mesenteric adenitis, which presents with fever, right lower quadrant pain, and leukocytosis; similar to symptoms of appendicitis. Adults may present with polyarthritis, Reiter's syndrome, and erythema nodosum. *Yersinia* can cause bacteremia.	Diagnosis is made by isolation of organism in the stool. Stool also tests positive for fecal leukocytes. Treatment for severe cases is tetracycline 250 to 500 mg every 6 hours for 7 to 10 days; ciprofloxacin 500 mg PO twice daily; tobramycin 3 to 5 mg/kg per day every 8 hours.
Salmonella	One of the major causes of diarrhea worldwide. Three species: *S. typhi*, *S. choleraesuis*, and *S. enteritidis*. Found primarily in chicken, eggs, and livestock, causing 85% of community-acquired *Salmonella* outbreaks. Individuals must ingest 10,000–1 million organisms to become infected.	Duration is 2 to 5 days; onset is 8 to 48 hours after ingestion. Patients may become "chronic carriers," defined as individuals with positive stool cultures 1 year after initial disease.	Peak incidence is in summer and fall. Symptoms begin with nausea and vomiting, followed by colicky abdominal pain and bloody or mucoid diarrhea. Enteric fever results from organisms entering the bloodstream via the bowel lymphatics, causing bacteremia, headache, and myalgias. Tissue abscesses may develop. Stools may be foul-smelling.	Diagnosis is made by isolation of organism in stool. No treatment is necessary unless associated with fever and systemic disease. Treatment includes trimethoprim-sulfamethoxazole (Bactrim DS) or a quinoline, norfloxacin 400 mg or ofloxacin 400 mg PO twice daily for 7 to 10 days. Stress proper handling of food, thorough cooking, and good hand washing.
Shigella	One of the most common causes of bacillary dysentery. Several species: *S. sonnei* is isolated in 75% of cases in the United States. Because of poor hygiene and overcrowding, it is spread via the fecal–oral route and requires only a small number of organisms to produce disease. Organism causes epithelial invasion of intestinal mucosa.	Duration usually 4 to 7 days and is self-limiting. Incubation period of 1 to 2 days after exposure or ingestion of pathogen.	Initially, patients present with watery diarrhea and high fever. Later, colitis-type symptoms develop: abdominal cramps, tenesmus, urgency, frequent small stools with blood and mucus. Low-grade fever may persist for 2 to 20 days. Complications can include hemolytic-uremic syndrome and colitis.	Diagnosis is made by isolation of organism in stool or rectal swab. In severe cases, sigmoidoscopy shows mucosal hyperemia, friability, and ulceration. Treat with Bactrim DS twice daily for 3 days if infection was acquired in the United States.
Staphylococcus	Common cause of food poisoning. Caused by ingestion of enterotoxin found in improperly handled or stored foods. Enterotoxins produced by *Staphylococcus* act on receptors in the gut, which then transmit impulses to medullary centers.	Abrupt onset 1 to 8 hours after ingestion of contaminated food. Duration is usually less than 24 hours.	Abrupt onset of nausea, vomiting, colicky abdominal cramps, profuse watery diarrhea.	Definitive diagnosis is made only if contaminated food source is tested; otherwise, diagnosis is made based on short incubation and duration of symptoms.

Continued

TABLE 39.1 Organisms Causing Gastroenteritis—cont'd

Pathogen	Pathogenesis	Duration/Onset	Clinical Findings	Diagnosis and Treatment
Viral Pathogens Rotavirus	Very common cause of gastroenteritis in industrialized areas. Organism most often implicated in deaths from diarrhea. Frequently involves small bowel. A disaccharidase deficiency is common after rotavirus infections. Rotavirus is an RNA virus with four antigenic serotypes.	Incubation period 24 to 36 hours. Duration is 4 to 6 days.	Common in children younger than age 3. Peak incidence at age 6 to 24 months. Uncommon in adults because most have developed immunity. Symptoms include low-grade fever and copious watery diarrhea. Outbreaks are more common in winter months.	Diagnosis is made by electron microscopy. Serological enzyme-linked immunosorbent assay tests are available. No leukocytes found in stool.
Norwalk virus	Cube-shaped virus with seven known antigenic variants. It can cause large epidemics when spread by contaminated water. It is transmitted by the fecal–oral route. It is a common cause of absenteeism due to "viral gastroenteritis."	Incubation is 18 to 48 hours. Duration is 48 to 72 hours.	Illness can be very debilitating to some patients. Symptoms are mild and brief and include vomiting, frequent watery diarrhea, diffuse myalgias, chills, and sometimes fever. Often causes family outbreaks.	No known antiviral therapy is available. Fluid and electrolyte replacement is the treatment of choice. Virus can be isolated with electron microscopy but is costly and the disease is self-limiting.
Protozoal Pathogens Giardia lamblia	Approximately 4% of healthy U.S. citizens harbor *G. lamblia* in their intestines and are asymptomatic. *G. lamblia* is a protozoon that attaches to the mucosa of the small bowel. Patients with hypogammaglobulinemia and achlorhydria are predisposed to giardiasis. It is transmitted via oral–anal intercourse and is a common cause of traveler's diarrhea and diarrhea in children who attend day-care centers.	Incubation is 1 to 4 weeks. Duration usually 1 to 6 weeks.	Symptoms range from nonspecific complaints of bloating, flatulence, nausea, and watery, noninflammatory diarrhea to chronic diarrhea with weight loss, anorexia, and malabsorption.	Diagnosis can be made by examination of stool but is most often made by duodenal aspirate or small bowel biopsy. Stool examination is positive for trophozoites in about 50% of confirmed cases. Treatment with quinacrine hydrochloride (Atabrine) 100 mg three times daily after meals for 5 to 7 days or metronidazole (Flagyl) 250 mg three times daily for 5 to 7 days.

TABLE 39.1 Organisms Causing Gastroenteritis—cont'd

Pathogen	Pathogenesis	Duration/Onset	Clinical Findings	Diagnosis and Treatment
Entamoeba histolytica (amebiasis)	Transmitted via contaminated food and water, primarily in tropical areas with poor sanitation. Common in migrant workers and military personnel returning from the Far East. Human host becomes a reservoir after ingesting cysts from source and can transmit disease via fecal–oral route. Sexual transmission is through men who have sex with men.	Most common clinical variant is the asymptomatic cyst carrier who can be a reservoir for an undetermined length of time. Duration can be weeks to months.	Symptoms include abdominal cramps, abdominal pain, and weight loss. Diarrhea contains blood and mucus. Patients may have hepatomegaly and pain over the cecum and ascending colon. Some patients may have fever, tenesmus, and acute dysentery illness. Complications can include peritonitis, toxic megacolon, and hepatic abscess. The encysted ameba is passed into the environment, where it can survive for up to 10 days.	Diagnosis is important to distinguish amebiasis from ulcerative colitis because treatment with glucocorticoids can accelerate amebic colitis and enhance systemic invasion. Sigmoidoscopy reveals discrete rectosigmoid ulcers with normal intervening mucosa. Indirect hemagglutination test is effective in detecting invasive amebic disease but remains positive long after treatment. Treat with metronidazole (Flagyl) 750 mg three times daily for 7 to 10 days.
Cryptosporidium	Enteric protozoan parasite that invades the small bowel located just below the basement membrane. Causes two distinct syndromes—one in immunocompetent and one in immunosuppressed individuals. Common cause of waterborne outbreaks from inadequate filtration. Parasite produces an exotoxin.	Incubation is 1 to 3 weeks. Usually self-limiting but can last 1 to 2 weeks in immunocompromised patients.	Outbreaks can occur after ingestion of water contaminated with livestock waste. Also common in day-care centers and patients with AIDS. Immunocompromised patients develop severe cholera-like diarrhea, which can last for months and cause daily fluid losses of 5 to 10 L/day.	Diagnosis by isolation of parasite in stool. Commercially available immunofluorescent antibody test can also assist diagnosis. Leukocytes not present in stool. Intestinal mucosa not inflamed but with ulcerations. Suggested treatment includes paromomycin (Humatin) 500 mg PO four times daily with food for 14 to 28 days, then 500 mg twice daily indefinitely. If treatment fails: azithromycin (Zithromax) 2.4 g PO on day 1, 1.2 g PO for 27 days, and then 600 mg/day for maintenance indefinitely.

CLINICAL PRESENTATION

Subjective

Patients with gastroenteritis present with varying degrees of nausea, vomiting, diarrhea, fever, and abdominal pain and cramping. Symptoms depend on the underlying cause but can also include fatigue, malaise, anorexia, tenesmus, and borborygmus. Individuals with profuse diarrhea may complain of rectal burning and hematochezia from rectal abrasion and bleeding. Patients may complain of symptoms that suggest dysentery, including passage of numerous small-volume stools containing blood and mucus. Reports of voluminous stools are suggestive of a source in the small bowel or proximal colon; small stools accompanied by a sense of urgency suggest a source in the left colon or rectum. Bloody stools suggest mucosal damage and an inflammatory process secondary to invasive pathogens. Frothy stools and flatus suggest a malabsorption problem.

Objective

The physical examination is usually normal except for the aforementioned GI problems. Depending on the degree of dehydration, the skin turgor may be poor and mucous membranes may be dry. Vital signs may reflect dehydration, such as a fever with an increased heart rate. Older and very young patients with gastroenteritis may show signs of severe dehydration such as orthostatic hypotension and dizziness. Patients who have had prolonged illness and are malnourished may present with edema resulting from hypoalbuminemia.

DIAGNOSTIC REASONING

Diagnostic Tests

Evaluation of the history is paramount to the appropriate diagnosis and management of the patient with gastroenteritis. The patient must be questioned thoroughly about the temporal association of symptoms with the suspected pathogen. Patient history should include a thorough drug history, including over-the-counter drugs and supplements, antibiotics, antacids, laxatives, alcohol, and sugar substitutes. It is important to know the patient's travel history, surgical history, and sexual orientation and practices. The duration of the illness is important in the differential diagnosis because acute diarrhea is usually caused by infectious agents or toxins, whereas chronic diarrhea usually has a noninfectious etiology.

Laboratory diagnosis of acute gastroenteritis is not always necessary in patients with nonbloody diarrhea and no evidence of systemic toxicity. In the average, otherwise healthy adult, the disease will normally run its course without incident, and there is no need for costly evaluation. Selection of the most appropriate tests is based on information received from the history and physical examination. In patients with severe diarrhea and dehydration, stools should be examined for consistency, blood, and fecal leukocytes. Numerous fecal leukocytes in patients with acute diarrhea is indicative of diffuse colonic inflammation and is highly suggestive of an invasive pathogen such as *Shigella, Salmonella,* or *Campylobacter.* Other causes of leukocyte-positive stools include *Clostridium difficile, Yersinia, Vibrio parahaemolyticus,* and *Escherichia coli.* In patients with chronic diarrhea, fecal leukocytes suggest inflammatory bowel disease (IBD) or ischemia.

A stool culture should be done on any patient who has severe diarrhea, a fever of 101.3°F (38.5°C) or higher, the presence of bloody stools, or stools that test positive for leukocytes, lactoferrin, or occult blood because these findings are indications of a bacterial pathogen. Routine stool culture will identify the presence of *Shigella, Salmonella, Campylobacter, Aeromonas,* and *Yersinia.* In diarrheal illnesses that are suspected to be caused by eating contaminated hamburger meat, stools can be cultured for *E. coli.*

Blood cultures should be obtained from patients who show clinical signs of typhoid or enteric fever or from any hospitalized patient who has an intestinal illness with high fever. It is essential that the blood cultures be obtained before initiation of antibiotic therapy.

Stools should be examined for ova and parasites in cases of persistent diarrhea, especially if the symptoms began after travel to Russia, Nepal, the Rocky Mountains, or other mountainous regions, or after exposure to infants in a day-care center. Parasites should also be considered in men who have sex with men or any patient with HIV/AIDS who presents with diarrhea, as well as in a patient with diarrhea who lives in a community where a waterborne outbreak has occurred. If a patient has diarrhea that has lasted longer than 2 weeks and the stool is negative for fecal leukocytes, a stool examination for parasites should be considered. Patients with intestinal amoebiasis usually have no leukocytes in their stool because of the noninflamed areas of intestinal mucosa between the areas of ulceration, as well as the lytic effects of the exotoxins produced by the parasite. If parasitic infection is highly suspected but the stool culture is negative, a small bowel biopsy is indicated to identify the causative agent. Immunofluorescent antibody tests and diagnostic enzyme-linked immunosorbent assay (ELISA) tests are more sensitive than microscopic studies for identifying *Giardia* and *Cryptosporidium.*

In patients with epidemiological evidence, stool samples should be sent to the laboratory for specific enteropathogen studies that are not normally detected with routine stool culture, such as enterohemorrhagic colitis (*E. coli* O157:H7), *Vibrio cholerae,* other noncholera vibrios, and other Shiga toxin–producing *E. coli.* Routine stool culture identifies certain strains of *Yersinia* and *E. coli* O157:H7; however, some strains can be detected only by research laboratories. Any patient who develops diarrhea after initiation or completion of antibiotic therapy should have tissue culture assay or an ELISA test for *C. difficile* toxin.

Viral gastroenteritis should be suspected in patients who present with vomiting as the major symptom and in cases where foodborne or waterborne contamination is suspected and the incubation period is greater than 12 hours. Although there are commercially available test kits that identify rotaviruses, their application is limited because there is no known treatment for viral causes of illness.

Flexible sigmoidoscopy is usually reserved for patients with colitis that is unresponsive to antibiotic therapy and for patients with persistent diarrhea undiagnosed by laboratory evaluation. Tissue biopsy can help identify the offending pathogen, as well as differentiate infection from chronic inflammatory changes consistent with IBD or celiac disease.

Differential Diagnosis

The differential diagnosis of gastroenteritis, particularly in patients with persistent or chronic diarrhea and severe abdominal pain, should include irritable bowel syndrome, IBD, ischemic bowel disease (especially in patients with peripheral vascular disease), partial bowel obstruction, and pelvic abscess. Other considerations for diagnosis should include ruling out complications from diabetes mellitus, small bowel diverticulosis, Whipple's disease, chronic pancreatitis, and any surgical alteration of the GI tract that might interfere with normal absorption.

MANAGEMENT

All patients who present with diarrhea require fluid and electrolyte management, particularly children, older adults, and immunosuppressed patients. Patients who are dehydrated and able to tolerate oral fluid replacement need to drink fluids with a sodium content of 45 to 75 mEq/L (Pedialyte or Gatorade) or be provided with oral rehydration salts. In patients who are severely dehydrated or those who have chronic diseases and are hypotensive, hospitalization for IV hydration may be indicated. In otherwise healthy adult patients who are not dehydrated, sports drinks, diluted fruit juices, and broths or soups are usually adequate for fluid and sodium replacement.

Patients with diarrhea require a diet that includes calories that come from boiled starches and cereals (potatoes, pasta, rice, wheat, and oats), which will facilitate enterocyte renewal, with the addition of salt for the duration of illness. Once stools have started to become formed, the diet can be advanced as tolerated. Some authors advise avoiding dairy products; however, this is not necessary unless there is clinical evidence of lactose intolerance.

Nonspecific symptomatic treatment of acute diarrhea can decrease the occurrence by 50% and is most effective against secretory diarrhea. Antimotility drugs are the most frequently prescribed and most effective drugs for the treatment of symptomatic gastroenteritis. These agents work by slowing intraluminal peristalsis, thereby slowing the passage of fluids through the lumen, which facilitates absorption. Patients with febrile dysentery should not receive antimotility medications because slowing the intraluminal time may prolong the duration of the disease. Drugs Commonly Prescribed 39.1 lists medications commonly recommended for the symptomatic treatment of acute diarrhea.

Empiric antimicrobial therapy is recommended for patients with severe diarrhea, especially those with fever or stool positive for leukocytes. Empirical treatment for traveler's diarrhea is dependent on the location of the travel because of the different organisms prevalent in different areas. For example, *E. coli* is found in most locations, but *Salmonella* is found in South and Southeast Asia, *Campylobacter* is prevalent in Southeast Asia, and *Shigella* is prevalent in South Asia and Africa. On July 26, 2016, the U.S. Food and Drug Administration (FDA) issued an enhanced black box warning for fluoroquinolones, stating their association with disabling and potentially permanent side effects and that they should be reserved only for conditions where there are no other options available. In light of this recent warning, the antibiotic of choice for traveler's diarrhea is azithromycin (Zithromax) 1,000 mg orally once a day for 1 to 3 days. Nonantibiotic preventive therapy includes bismuth subsalicylate (Pepto-Bismol), two tablets before each meal and at bedtime for a total of eight tablets/day for the entire trip. This remedy has an approximately 60% effectiveness rate; however, patients should be informed that bismuth preparations can turn the tongue and the stool black. This can be quite alarming if unexpected.

FOLLOW-UP AND REFERRAL

Follow-up is not usually required except in those patients with the chronic forms of infectious diarrhea such as from *C. difficile*. Often, patients with serious infectious diarrhea will require home administration of IV antibiotics. Patients who require sigmoidoscopy for biopsy of intestinal mucosa for identification of the pathogen should be referred to a gastroenterologist.

Drugs Commonly Prescribed 39.1: Symptomatic Treatment of Acute Diarrhea

DRUG	INDICATION	ADVERSE REACTIONS AND PRESCRIBING CONSIDERATIONS
Bismuth subsalicylate (Pepto-Bismol)	Acute diarrhea	Not as effective as loperamide in acute diarrhea. May potentiate the effects of antidiabetic medications. Do not use with antibiotics in patients with HIV infection.
Loperamide (Imodium)	Acute diarrhea	Drug of choice for afebrile, nondysentery cases of acute diarrhea. Minimal central opiate effect.
Diphenoxylate with atropine (Lomotil)	Acute diarrhea	Prescription only. For use in afebrile, nondysentery cases of acute diarrhea. Has central opiate effects. Overdose possible. Atropine has adverse effects that may limit use.

Patient Education: Gastroenteritis

The aim of patient education is prevention of the spread of disease from patients with infectious diarrhea to other individuals. Teaching includes good hand washing and safe disposal of waste products. Any infant or child with infectious diarrhea should not attend day care until the diarrhea has stopped or the child has completed the prescribed course of antibiotics. Good hand washing technique is imperative to prevent household outbreaks of the disease.

Patients traveling in high-risk areas should be instructed to consume only safe foods and beverages there and on the airplane leaving the area. "Safe" foods include acidic foods such as unpeeled citrus fruits; dry foods such as breads and cereals; steamed foods and beverages such as coffee, tea, and cooked vegetables; foods containing high amounts of sugar such as syrups, jellies, and jams; and bottled carbonated drinks such as soda and beer. It is generally not considered safe to drink bottled water (unless bottled from a safe source) or to eat raw, uncooked vegetables, including salad. Patients with known HIV infection and any other individuals with a known debilitating illness who may not tolerate any degree of gastroenteritis should be encouraged to take antibiotic prophylaxis.

HEPATITIS

Hepatitis is a common problem throughout the world and has many causes, including infectious, drug, vascular, and metabolic etiologies. Many cases of hepatitis are subclinical. Symptoms may be "flu-like" and go unreported so that the true incidence of the disease may be underestimated. Table 39.2 lists some of the causes of acute hepatitis.

TABLE 39.2	Causes of Acute Hepatitis
Viral	Cytomegalovirus; Epstein-Barr virus; hepatitis A, B, C, D, and E viruses; herpesvirus; rubella; varicella-zoster virus; yellow-fever virus
Nonviral	Amebic abscess, bacterial abscess, Lyme disease, syphilis
Metabolic disorders	Alpha-1-antitrypsin deficiency, Wilson's disease
Vascular	Budd-Chiari syndrome, congestive heart failure, ischemia (hypotension, shock)
Drugs	Acetaminophen, allopurinol, ASA (high doses), captopril, carbamazepine, isoniazid, ketoconazole, methyldopa, NSAIDs, procainamide, sulfonamides
Toxins	Alcohol (ethanol), carbon tetrachloride, herbs, mushrooms

Acute viral hepatitis is a systemic infection that predominantly affects the liver and can lead to liver inflammation and necrosis. There are many viral agents that cause hepatitis, but the most common, and the ones that have public health concerns, are hepatitis A virus (HAV), hepatitis B virus (HBV), hepatitis C virus (HCV), hepatitis D virus (HDV), and hepatitis E virus (HEV). All are endemic to the United States except HEV, which is most common in Asian and African countries. However, although there seems to be a high prevalence of antibodies to HEV in the general population in the United States, there are few cases of acute illness reported and those that are can usually be attributed to travel to an area where HEV is endemic.

EPIDEMIOLOGY AND CAUSES

Hepatitis A

HAV is a small, single-stranded RNA virus of the picornavirus family. HAV is endemic in the United States, with periodic outbreaks. Because the symptoms of HAV are often mild and nonspecific, many cases remain undetected. Many other cases are asymptomatic, making it almost impossible to quantify the number of infections annually. The Centers for Disease Control and Prevention (CDC) reported a total of 12,474 new cases of HAV infection in 2018 with an estimated 24,900 acute infections. This was a considerable increase from the 2017 numbers of 3,366 reported cases and an estimated 6,700 acute infections, which shows an 850% increase from 2014 to 2018. Risk factors include crowded conditions, such as prisons, nursing homes, and day-care centers, and poor sanitation. Contaminated food or water is a common source of HAV. HAV can cause fulminant liver failure on rare occasions, usually in combination with an underlying liver disease.

Transmission is by the fecal–oral route and close personal contact, and there have been rare cases of HAV being transmitted via blood transfusion. People contract HAV by consuming contaminated water or ice; raw shellfish harvested from sewage-contaminated water; and fruits, vegetables, or other foods eaten uncooked that may have become contaminated in handling. The virus is killed by heating at 185°F for 1 minute. Adequate chlorination of water also kills the virus. The average incubation period is 28 days but the range is 15 to 50 days. Excretion of HAV in feces occurs up to 2 weeks before clinical illness. It is rarely found in feces after the first week of illness. Blood and stools are infectious throughout the incubation period and early illness until the aminotransferase levels peak. A person is most infectious about 2 weeks before and during the first week that symptoms appear.

Chronic HAV does not occur. There is no carrier state, and HAV usually causes no long-term damage. HAV may persist for up to 1 year with relapses before full recovery. The mortality rate is about 0.02 deaths per 100,000 cases, which has stayed the same since 2011.

Hepatitis B

HBV is a DNA hepadnavirus with eight genotypes that replicate in the liver. The CDC reported a total of 3,322 new cases of acute HBV infection in 2018 but estimated that 21,600 cases of acute hepatitis B actually occurred. The overall rate has been stable since 2011 with a slight increase in 2017. Overall, the rate of HBV has decreased since 1991, when a national strategy was implemented and vaccination was first recommended for infants and children. The risk for chronic infection decreases with increasing age; for example, 90% of infants, 25% to 50% of children aged 1 to 5 years, and 5% of adults become chronically infected. The CDC estimates that there were 862,000 individuals living with chronic HBV (CHB) in the United States in 2016.

High-risk groups include infants born to infected mothers, sexual partners of infected people, men who have sex with men, people who inject drugs, household contacts or sexual partners of people with known CHB infection, health-care and public safety workers, and patients undergoing hemodialysis. The risk of infection from a contaminated needle is 10% to 30%. The risk of contracting HBV from a blood transfusion is now rare in the United States.

Transmission is usually by direct contact with infected blood or blood products or by sexual contact. The highest concentrations of HBV are found in the blood; however, other body fluids such as semen, cervical secretions, saliva, and wound exudates contain lower concentrations of hepatitis B surface antigen (HBsAg). Parenteral exposure is the most efficient route of transmission, most often occurring in people who use injectable drugs sharing or using contaminated needles and in health-care workers by accidental needle sticks. HBV can be transmitted from contact with contaminated inanimate objects because the virus is capable of living in the open environment for approximately 1 week. HBV is not transmitted via the fecal–oral route. The incidence of HBV is highest in the 30- to 39-year-old age-group, with more men becoming infected than women. Pregnant women who are HBsAg positive may transmit HBV to their babies during childbirth. HBV is not spread through food, water, or casual contact. The average incubation period for HBV is 60 to 150 days with an average of 90 days.

The mortality rate for acute HBV infection is 0.4% to 1%, but it is higher when hepatitis D is superimposed (see Hepatitis D section). Patients with chronic hepatitis are at an increased risk for cirrhosis and hepatocellular cancer. Infection with HBV is also associated with arthritis, glomerulonephritis, and polyarteritis nodosa.

Hepatitis C

HCV is a single-stranded RNA virus with 7 genotypes and more than 67 subtypes. Genotypes 1a, 1b, 2, and 3 are the most common types in the United States. The clinical significance of the genotype is unclear, but different genotypes and subtypes have different responses to treatment. The estimated worldwide prevalence of HCV infections is 2% to 3%. This translates to 170 million people infected and approximately 3.2 million live in the United States. The CDC had a total of 3,621 reported cases of acute hepatitis C in 2018, but due to underreporting, estimates that the number is 50,300 cases. The incubation period of HCV is 35 to 72 days. Transmission of HCV is primarily by percutaneous exposure to blood and blood products. Injection drug use is the strongest risk factor. Having sex with a person who injects drugs is also a risk factor, although less robust. There is a 5% risk of maternal–neonate transmission at the time of birth, which some studies suggest is greatest in patients with high circulating levels of HCV RNA. People with HIV infection, people who currently or formerly used injection drugs, people who have received hemodialysis, recipients of blood transfusion before 1992, recipients of organ transplants and clotting factor concentrates before 1987, and health-care and public safety workers are also high risk for HCV infection. Infrequent routes of transmission include having sex with an HCV-infected person, sharing a razor or toothbrush with an infected person, and invasive health-care procedures. Anti-HCV antibodies are more common in non-Hispanic black and Mexican American people. Low family income and a lifetime history of more than 20 sexual partners are also risk factors. Rates of HCV infection are higher for men than for women, possibly due to riskier behavior. Other possible routes of transmission can be through body piercing and tattooing, although there is little evidence to date. For many patients infected with HCV, the source is never determined.

The most recent CDC data (2018) indicate that the group that is most affected by acute hepatitis C is those 20 to 29 years old, with 3.1 cases per 100,000 people. Fifty percent of those infected with HCV develop chronic infection. Because 50% of those infected with HCV develop chronic hepatitis, the prevalence of chronic hepatitis will increase in younger age groups.

Fewer than 20% of people with HCV infection are symptomatic. Most acute cases go undetected until they present with symptoms of chronic liver disease. At least 50% of patients with HCV develop chronic hepatitis. Sixty percent to 70% of those progress to chronic liver disease and 5% to 20% will develop cirrhosis over 20 to 30 years. The consequences of chronic infection are liver cancer and cirrhosis. Alcohol consumption appears to increase the chances of chronic disease and serious complications. The U.S. Preventive Services Task Force recommends screening for HCV in persons who are at high risk for the infection. They also recommend that all people born between 1945 and 1965 be offered a one-time screening for HCV infection.

Hepatitis D

HDV is an RNA virus that requires HBsAg for its replication. Only individuals with HBV are at risk for HDV. The major risk factor for HDV is injection drug use.

Transmission is by the parenteral route and should be suspected in any HBsAg-positive person with acute or chronic hepatitis. New cases of HDV are uncommon in the United States today, probably because of widespread vaccination for HBV. People can be infected with HBV and HDV simultaneously. HBV/HDV infections can resolve. When a person with CHB becomes infected with HDV, it is called superinfection. Superinfection with HDV usually leads to progression of the HBV infection, liver cirrhosis, and liver failure more rapidly than HBV infection alone. Signs and symptoms of acute HDV infection do not usually appear for 3 to 7 weeks post-infection. The most common clinical manifestations are fever, fatigue, loss of appetite, nausea/vomiting, abdominal pain, dark urine, light-colored bowel movements, joint pain, and jaundice.

Hepatitis E

HEV is a single-stranded RNA virus with four genotypes that is usually transmitted via the fecal–oral route. It is similar to HAV but not as easily transmitted. It is transmitted through fecally contaminated water and is responsible for waterborne hepatitis outbreaks; it is widespread in the developing world, but is most common in Asia, the Middle East, Africa, and Central America. Contaminated shellfish was responsible for an outbreak on a cruise ship, and there have been foodborne transmission outbreaks in China, Taiwan, and Japan. Large outbreaks have occurred in refugee camps in Sudan and Chad. There have been relatively few cases in the United States, and most have been associated with global travel. There are documented cases in Germany and Japan of HEV infection with consumption of meat from animals that are infected with the virus. The illness is usually self-limiting, but chronic HEV is possible in immunocompromised patients. Signs and symptoms occur from 15 to 60 days after infection, with the average being 40 days. The period of infectivity has not yet been determined. The mortality rate is low except in pregnant women, in whom the mortality rate is 10% to 20%. Table 39.3 lists the features of hepatitis A, B, C, D, and E.

Chronic Hepatitis

Chronic hepatitis, characterized by elevated aminotransferase (aspartate aminotransferase [AST] and alanine aminotransferase [ALT]) levels for more than 6 months, occurs in 1% to 2% of immunocompromised adults with HBV and in as many as 90% of neonates and infants with HBV. Chronic hepatitis occurs in up to 50% of people infected with HCV. Cirrhosis develops in 40% of patients with CHB, and 20% of those with chronic HCV are at high risk for developing hepatocellular carcinoma as well.

PATHOPHYSIOLOGY

Hepatitis is an inflammation of the liver. It can result from a variety of causes. Viral hepatitis usually presents in one of three clinical manifestations: anicteric, icteric, or cholestatic. Despite the presentation, the progression of the disease follows the same pattern, differing only in severity, enzymatic abnormality, and possible outcomes. The pathological lesions of hepatitis are similar to those caused by other viral infections. Regardless of the type of hepatitis causing the infection, all the liver acini cells are affected by patchy cell dropout, acidophilic hepatocellular necrosis, scarring, Kupffer cell hyperplasia, and mononuclear inflammatory infiltrate. The degree of cellular change is proportional to the severity of infection. Hepatocellular injury is mediated by cell-mediated immune response. Cytotoxic T cells and natural killer cells play an important part by killing the infected cells and releasing inflammatory cytokines. An intense immune response can decrease the chance of chronic infection; however, it does foster development of hepatocellular necrosis. Histological examination of tissue from livers infected with hepatitis demonstrates that even early in the disease process, liver regeneration has already started.

Normally, in patients infected with hepatitis, the underlying reticulin network is preserved, allowing for complete histological recovery. If extensive necrosis of the bridging acini occurs, however, the inflammatory process can damage and obstruct the bile canaliculi, causing cholestasis and obstructive jaundice. In most mild cases of hepatitis, the liver parenchyma is not damaged; HBV and HCV tend to be the more severe forms of hepatitis, with histological evidence of parenchymal inflammation and necrosis. Although the histological changes in the liver tissue are the same for each type of hepatitis, occasionally HBV can be diagnosed from the presence of "ground-glass" hepatocytes caused by HBsAg-infiltrated cytoplasm and by using special staining techniques that detect certain viral components. These findings are most often associated with CHB infection. The long-term, asymptomatic, chronic-carrier state is thought to result from an immunological tolerance to the hepatitis virus. The virus is not totally cleared by the immune system, and the hepatocellular injury is minimal, leading to a lifelong asymptomatic carrier state. This carrier state is most common in infants, whose immune system is immature and may be unable to overcome the virus. This chronic-carrier state is associated with a 10- to 100-fold risk of hepatocellular carcinoma.

HCV causes hepatocellular injury through direct cytopathic invasion by the virus. The viral load is directly proportional to the histological inflammation seen on liver biopsy. HCV is capable of rapid mutation, which allows it to elude immunity by development of resistant strains to the existing antibodies. Autoimmune hepatitis is most commonly associated with HCV, lending itself to the multiple

TABLE 39.3 Key Features of Hepatitis A, B, C, D, and E

Features	Hepatitis A Virus (HAV)	Hepatitis B Virus (HBV)	Hepatitis C Virus (HCV)	Hepatitis D Virus (HDV)	Hepatitis E Virus (HEV)
Transmission	Fecal–oral through sewage-contaminated water and shellfish; possibly through blood	Percutaneous and permucosal through infected blood and body fluids; sexual transmission	Percutaneous through infected blood and body fluids; community, many infected individuals have no known risk factors	Percutaneous, but must have co-infection with HBV	Fecal–oral
Incubation period (days)	15 to 50 (average 28)	60 to 150 (average 90)	35 to 72	21 to 49	15 to 60 (average 40)
Laboratory tests	Anti-HAV IgM (acute); anti-HAV IgG (resolving)	HBsAg (confirms), IgM anti-HBs (acute phase), IgG anti-HBs (resolving/immunity), HBeAg, anti-HBe, anti-HBc (persists in carriers)	Anti-HCV appears in 6 to 37 weeks	Anti-HDV appears late	Anti-HEV IgM detected within 26 days of jaundice; IgG antibody persists
Immunity/immunization	45% of United States population has antibodies against HAV; HAV vaccine available	5% to 15% of U.S. population has anti-HBs; HBV vaccine available	Unknown; no vaccine available	People immune to HBV are also protected against HDV	Unknown
Prevalence	Increasing incidence in adults 850% increase between 2014 and 2018	Decreasing in the United States	Increasing in 20- to 39-year-old age-group	Co-infection with HBV	Rare in United States; endemic in the developing world
Course/mortality	Does not progress to chronic state; mortality is 0% to 0.2% with fulminant hepatitis	Chronic liver disease occurs in 1% to 5% of adults and 80% to 90% in children; mortality rate is 0.3% to 1.5%	Chronic active hepatitis develops in 50% of cases; 20% develop chronic liver disease; mortality rate is the same as for HBV	Chronic liver disease develops if present in chronic HBV; mortality rate is 2% to 20% for acute icteric hepatitis	Does not progress to chronic liver disease; mortality rate is 1% to 2% but as high as 10% to 15% in pregnant women

Abbreviations: IgG, immunoglobulin G; IgM, immunoglobulin M.

extrahepatic manifestations of the disease. These patients develop autoimmune responses leading to membranous glomerulonephritis, vasculitis, dermatitis, pulmonary fibrosis, and rheumatoid arthritis. Chronic HCV occurs in approximately 60% to 70% of cases, with inflammatory changes leading to cirrhosis within 20 to 30 years.

Different drugs can cause different histopathological abnormalities in the liver. For example, acetaminophen damages hepatocytes by producing toxic metabolites that damage the cellular and subcellular structures of the liver. Hepatic injury resulting from sepsis is caused by direct bacterial invasion of the parenchyma, circulating endotoxins, and hypoxia. Cytotoxic lymphocytes attack hepatocyte membrane antigens in autoimmune chronic active hepatitis. All of these agents result in varying degrees of hepatocyte injury.

CLINICAL PRESENTATION

Subjective

The clinical presentation of viral hepatitis is extremely variable; it can range from asymptomatic infection without jaundice to a sudden severe infection and death in a few days. Table 39.4 displays the clinical findings and corresponding laboratory values for the different phases of viral hepatitis.

Prodromal Phase

During the prodromal phase, the onset may be abrupt or insidious with anorexia, nausea, vomiting, malaise, upper respiratory infection, or flu-like symptoms. The patient may also complain of myalgia, arthralgia, and easy fatigability. Many patients report an aversion for smoking if they are smokers. Nausea and vomiting occur frequently. Diarrhea or constipation may be reported. In the early stage of acute HBV, skin rashes and arthritis may be seen.

Fever is usually present but rarely exceeds 103°F (39.4°C), except in HAV, in which it may go higher. Chills may mark an acute onset. A decrease in fever often coincides with the onset of jaundice.

Abdominal pain is usually mild and constant in the right upper quadrant or epigastrium. The pain can be aggravated by jarring or exertion. It is occasionally severe enough to simulate cholecystitis or cholelithiasis.

Icteric Phase

During the icteric phase, jaundice and dark urine appear, usually 5 to 10 days after the initial symptoms, although some patients do not experience jaundice. With the onset of jaundice, the prodromal symptoms worsen and are followed by progressive clinical improvement.

Convalescent Phase

The convalescent phase is marked by an increased sense of well-being. The jaundice, abdominal pain and tenderness, and fatigability disappear and the appetite returns. CHB begins at this point in the case of chronic disease.

The acute illness usually subsides over 2 to 3 weeks. Complete clinical and laboratory recovery occurs by the ninth week in HAV and after 16 weeks in HBV. Five percent to 10% of the cases may last longer, and fewer than 1% have an acute fulminant course. Hepatitis B and C may become chronic.

Hepatomegaly is present in 50% of patients with viral hepatitis, and splenomegaly is seen in 15% of cases. Lymphadenopathy, especially in the cervical and epitrochlear areas, is commonly present. Signs of general toxemia may vary from minimal to severe. The clinical features of all the types of viral hepatitis are similar, with the exception of onset. Hepatitis A and E usually have an abrupt onset, whereas hepatitis B, C, and D have a more insidious onset, and the liver enzyme levels are higher. HCV is often asymptomatic.

DIAGNOSTIC REASONING

Diagnostic Tests

Laboratory tests are used to diagnose, identify the serological type, and determine the current status of the disease.

TABLE 39.4 Clinical Findings: Viral Hepatitis		
Stage	**Subjective and Objective Complaints**	**Laboratory Tests**
Incubation	None	HBsAg late in the stage HBeAg
Prodromal	Onset abrupt or insidious Anorexia, nausea, vomiting, malaise, upper respiratory infection (nasal discharge, pharyngitis), myalgia, arthralgia, easy fatigability, fever (HAV), abdominal pain	HBsAg in HBV
Icteric	Jaundice, dark urine, light-colored stools Continued prodromal complaints with gradual improvement	Anti-HBc Anti-HAV (IgG and IgM) Anti-HCV HBsAg becomes negative High urine bilirubin Markedly elevated ALT and AST Elevated LDH, bilirubin, alkaline phosphatase Markedly increased PT indicates increased mortality
Convalescent	Increased sense of well-being Appetite returns Jaundice, abdominal pain, and fatigability abate	Anti-HAV IgG Anti-HBs Decreased liver enzymes

Abbreviations: ALT, alanine aminotransferase; AST, aspartate aminotransferase; IgG, immunoglobulin G; IgM, immunoglobulin M; LDH, lactate dehydrogenase; PT, prothrombin time.

Hepatitis A

Two types of antibodies to HAV can be detected by radioimmunoassay and ELISA. The first type of antibody to HAV is the immunoglobulin M (IgM) antibody (IgM anti-HAV), which appears about 4 weeks after exposure, or just before hepatocellular enzyme elevation occurs, and disappears in 3 to 6 months. Detection of IgM is the diagnostic gold standard for acute hepatitis A. The second type of antibody, immunoglobulin G (IgG) anti-HAV, appears about 2 weeks after the IgM anti-HAV begins to increase and peaks after about 1 month of disease. The IgG antibody persists for more than 10 years and provides immunity. If the IgM is elevated in the absence of IgG, acute hepatitis is suspected. If IgG is elevated in the absence of IgM, this indicates previous exposure to HAV, noninfectivity, and immunity to recurring HAV infection.

Hepatitis B

Acute and CHB can be differentiated from other forms of viral hepatitis by serological markers representing the body's immunological response. The HBV is made up of an inner core surrounded by an outer capsule. The outer capsule contains HBsAg (hepatitis B *surface* antigen). The inner core contains the HBV *core* antigen (HBcAg). HBeAg (the *extracellular* form of HBcAg) is also found within the core. Antibodies to these antigens are called anti-HBs, anti-HBc, and anti-HBe.

Detection of HBsAg is diagnostic for HBV and is the first test to order when HBV is suspected. It will appear 1 to 10 weeks after exposure to the HBV and will remain positive throughout the acute phase of the illness. If HBsAg persists longer, this may indicate chronic hepatitis. HBsAg rises before the onset of clinical symptoms, peaks during the first week of symptoms, and returns to normal by the time the jaundice subsides. HBsAg indicates acute infection and infectivity. Anti-HBs appears about 4 weeks after the disappearance of the surface antigen and signifies recovery from the infection and noninfectivity, as well as immunity.

There are no tests available to detect HBcAg, but the IgM anti-HBc appears shortly after HBsAg is detected and can persist for 3 to 6 months. The anti-HBc level is elevated during the time lag between the disappearance of HBsAg and the appearance of anti-HBs; this interval is called the *core window*. During this window, anti-HBc is the only detectable marker of a recent hepatitis infection. Anti-HBs is composed of IgG and IgM antibodies. The IgM titer is diagnostic for acute hepatitis, whereas the IgG antibody is usually positive for life after infection.

HBeAg is generally not used for diagnostic purposes, but rather as an index of viral replication and infectivity. The presence of HBeAg correlates with early and active disease and with high infectivity in patients with acute HBV infection. HBeAg appears during the incubation period shortly after the detection of HBsAg. The continued presence of HBeAg predicts the development of CHB infection. Table 39.5 displays the serology testing and results for HBV infection.

Hepatitis C

The diagnosis of HCV is based on enzyme immunoassays, chemiluminescence immunoassay (CIA), microparticle immunoassay (MEIA), electrochemiluminescence immunoassay (ECLIA), or immunochromatographic assay (rapid test). These tests detect antibodies to HCV (anti-HCV). Limitations of these tests include moderate sensitivity for the diagnosis of acute HCV (false-negative result) and low specificity (50%) in healthy blood donors and some people with elevated gamma globulin levels (false-positive result). The diagnosis of HCV may be confirmed by use of a polymerase chain reaction (PCR) to detect HCV RNA. The risk of transfusion-associated HCV has decreased from 10% in the early 1990s to less than 0.1% today as a result of the testing of donated blood for HCV.

Hepatitis D

Diagnosis of HDV is via detection of anti-HDV or HDV RNA in the presence of HBV markers. Rising titers of anti-HDV indicate acute infection and are detectable early in the disease.

Hepatitis E

In a patient with acute hepatitis where other causes have been ruled out, serology can be performed, especially in

TABLE 39.5 Serological Testing for Hepatitis B

Interpretation	HBsAg	Anti-HBs	HBeAg	Anti-HBe	Anti-HBc
Acute hepatitis (confirms diagnosis)	+	−	+	−	IgM
Acute hepatitis	−	−	+ or −	−	IgM
Recovery from hepatitis (immunity)	−	+	−	+ or −	IgG
Vaccination (immunity)	−	+	−	−	−
Chronic HBV with active viral replication	+	−	+	−	IgG
Chronic HBV with low viral replication	−	−	−	+	IgG

those patients who have traveled to an area where HEV is common. Immunoassay tests for IgM anti-HEV and IgG anti-HEV are available but not FDA approved. Tests for HEV RNA are only performed in research labs. IgM anti-HEV is detected 3 to 4 weeks after exposure and peaks at about 7 weeks, and then quickly decreases and is undetectable in about 13 weeks. IgG anti-HEV is detected 3 to 4 weeks after exposure and persists.

Additional Testing

In any patient in whom hepatitis is suspected, liver enzyme levels should be checked for signs of injury. Elevated aminotransferase levels are the hallmark of all forms of acute hepatitis. AST is usually markedly elevated early in hepatitis. ALT is often very elevated early in hepatitis, as is lactate dehydrogenase. All of these hepatocellular enzymes are elevated during the acute and chronic active phases of hepatitis. AST and ALT levels fluctuate during the course of the disease for unknown reasons. Bilirubin and alkaline phosphatase are usually elevated and may remain elevated after the AST and ALT have normalized.

The white blood cell count is normal or low, especially in the preicteric phase. Large atypical lymphocytes may occasionally be seen and are similar to those found in infectious mononucleosis. Mild proteinuria is common, and there is bilirubinuria just preceding and during the icteric phase. The prothrombin time may be prolonged in severe hepatitis and signifies increased mortality risk. Liver biopsy is rarely indicated unless there is evidence of liver damage from a chronic state of hepatitis.

Differential Diagnosis

Differential diagnosis for hepatitis includes other viral diseases that affect the liver, such as infectious mononucleosis, cytomegalovirus infection, and herpes simplex virus. Drug- or toxin-induced liver damage should also be included in the differential diagnosis list, as well as conditions that cause jaundice.

MANAGEMENT

The principle of hepatitis management includes prevention of transmission and symptomatic relief. Vaccinations are available to prevent HAV and HBV. HAV vaccination is recommended for all children at 1 year. HAV vaccine is also recommended for persons traveling to countries with high to moderate rates of hepatitis A, men who have sex with men, people who use injectable drugs, persons who have chronic liver disease, and those who have occupational risk for infection.

HBV vaccine is recommended for:

- All infants
- All children younger than age 19 who have not been previously vaccinated
- People at risk by sexual exposure
  - Sexual partners of HBsAg-positive people
  - Sexually active people who have had more than one sex partner in the previous 6 months
  - Those seeking treatment for a sexually transmitted infection
  - Men who have sex with men
- People at risk for percutaneous or mucosal exposure to blood
  - People who inject drugs
  - Household contacts of HBsAg-positive people
  - Residents and staff of facilities for persons with developmental disability
  - Health-care and public safety personnel
  - Dialysis patients
  - People with diabetes aged 19 to 59 and those older than 60 years at the discretion of the provider
- Persons with chronic liver disease or HIV infection
- Travelers to areas with endemic HBV infection
  - People with HCV infection
  - People who are incarcerated

Treatment for hepatitis, no matter what the cause, is largely supportive. Patients rarely require hospitalization. Balanced nutrition with adequate calories and fluids is recommended, and avoidance of alcohol is stressed. Activity is generally restricted during the acute phase and during a relapse with gradual resumption of activity.

The American Association for the Study of Liver Diseases has developed guidelines for the treatment of CHB infection. For treatment decisions, they list four phases of CHB:

1. Immune-tolerant phase, in which the virus is replicating rapidly but there is a low inflammatory response.
2. HBeAg-positive immune-active phase, in which there are elevated ALT and HBV DNA levels and evidence of liver injury.
3. Inactive CHB phase, in which HBV DNA level is low or undetectable, ALT is normal, and there is anti-HBe present.
4. HBeAg-negative immune reactivation phase, in which those who are anti-HBe positive continue to have elevated ALT and high HBV DNA levels.

Patients with CHB should be referred to a hepatologist for treatment. The phase of CHB dictates what treatment options are most effective. Currently, there are six agents approved for treating CHB (see Drugs Commonly Prescribed 39.2). They are used alone or in combination depending on factors such as the phase of CHB, level of viral replication, ALT levels, and seroconversion to anti-HBe. The goal of therapy is to reduce HBV DNA levels to the lowest possible and normalizing ALT levels and prevent liver cell damage. Nucleotide and nucleotide analogs (NUC/A) are the preferred treatment because they can be taken orally and have a better side effect profile. Pegylated

Drugs Commonly Prescribed 39.2: Chronic Hepatitis B Infection

DRUG	DOSAGES	ADVERSE REACTIONS AND PRESCRIBING CONSIDERATIONS
Peg-INF-2a	180 g intramuscularly weekly	Fatigue, flu-like symptoms, mood disturbances, autoimmune disorders *Nucleotide and nucleotide analogues are preferred
Entecavir	0.5 or 1.0 mg orally once a day on an empty stomach	Rarely associated with resistance. Lactic acidosis
Tenofovir disoproxil fumarate	300 mg orally once a day	Nephropathy, osteomalacia, lactic acidosis
Tenofovir alafenamide	25 mg orally once a day	*Lower rate of renal and bone toxicity than tenofovir disoproxil fumarate.
Adefovir	10 mg once a day orally	Acute renal failure, lactic acidosis, diarrhea
Lamivudine	100 mg once a day orally	Lactic acidosis, diarrhea, headache, fatigue, muscle pain, depression, fever *No longer first-line treatment in the United States, but used in other countries because of lower cost.
Telbivudine	600 mg once a day orally	Peripheral neuropathy, lactic acidosis, creatine kinase elevations and myopathy, diarrhea

interferon alfa-2a (Peg-IFN-2a) intramuscularly is still used alone or in combination with a NUC/A. All of the agents used have serious side effects.

HCV causes chronic hepatitis and liver damage. The goal of treatment is to eradicate HCV RNA. With newer treatment regimens using direct-acting antiviral (DAA) medications, a cure is now possible for most patients. Treatment is dependent on the genotype, subtype, and presence or absence of cirrhosis. Patients should be referred to a hepatologist for evaluation and treatment. Drugs Commonly Prescribed 39.3 lists the medications commonly recommended in the treatment of HCV.

Response to therapy is judged by an ALT returning to normal by 12 weeks and negative viral markers (HCV RNA). After the ALT has returned to normal, treatment is slowly discontinued. Consuming alcohol increases the risk of these patients progressing to cirrhosis and liver failure, so abstinence from all forms of alcohol (including in medications) is especially important.

Hepatic transplantation is indicated for patients with advanced liver disease as a result of chronic HCV, and in fact it is the most common reason for liver transplantation in the United States.

FOLLOW-UP AND REFERRAL

Any patient diagnosed with HCV should be referred to a hepatologist for follow-up because of the high risk of chronic infection. Patients with HAV usually do not require follow-up. Patients with HBV should be seen in 1 month and should have blood drawn for HBsAg after 6 months. Persistent elevation of HBsAg indicates a chronic state, and these patients should be referred to a hepatologist.

Patient Education: Hepatitis

Patients and their intimate contacts should be given careful instructions about the cause of hepatitis, the mode of transmission, and measures to prevent the transmission. It is recommended that household contacts and sexual contacts be given passive immunity (immunoglobulin) for HAV and HBV, as well as active immunization. Hand washing and personal hygiene can help prevent the spread of the disease. Patients should also be taught not to share personal items such as toothbrushes, razors, and eating utensils during the period of infectivity. Patients with chronic hepatitis or a carrier state should be instructed to practice safe sex.

Patients who develop chronic liver disease as a result of hepatitis can contact the American Liver Foundation for information about treatment.

APPENDICITIS

The appendix is a fingerlike projection located at the apex of the cecum just below the ileocecal valve. It has no known function in humans; however, it is thought to have some immunological function, based on the

Drugs Commonly Prescribed 39.3: Treatment for HCV

DRUG	GENOTYPE	CONSIDERATIONS	ADVERSE REACTIONS
NS3/4A Protease Inhibitors			
Simeprevir 150 mg once a day orally	1 and 4	Combined sofosbuvir	Liver toxicity Fatigue, nausea, pruritus, weakness
Paritaprevir 150 mg once a day orally	1 and 4	Combined with ombitasvir, dasabuvir, and ritonavir*	Liver toxicity Fatigue, nausea, pruritus, weakness
Glecaprevir 300 mg once a day orally	1 through 6	Combined with pibrentasvir with or without ribavirin	Fatigue, headache, diarrhea, pruritus, nausea, elevated bilirubin, angioedema, fatigue
Grazoprevir 100 mg once a day orally	1 and 4	Used in combination with elbasvir	Liver injury Fatigue, weakness, nausea, insomnia, pruritus
NS5A Inhibitors			
Ledipasvir 90 mg daily orally	1, 4, 5, 6	Used in combination with sofosbuvir	Liver injury Fatigue, weakness, nausea, insomnia, pruritus
Pibrentasvir 120 mg once a day orally	1 through 6	Used in combination with glecaprevir with or without ribavirin	Liver injury, diarrhea, headache, pruritus, weakness, nausea
Ombitasvir 25 mg once a day orally	1 and 4	Used in combination with paritaprevir and ritonavir*	Liver injury Fatigue, weakness, nausea, insomnia, pruritus
Elbasvir 50 mg once a day orally	1 and 4	Used in combination with grazoprevir	Liver injury Fatigue, weakness, nausea, insomnia, pruritus
Velpatasvir 100 mg a day orally	1 through 6	Used in combination with sofosbuvir	Liver injury Fatigue, weakness, nausea, insomnia, pruritus
NS5B Nucleos(t)ide Polymerase Inhibitor			
Sofosbuvir 400 mg once a day orally	1 through 6	Used in combination with Peg-INF-2a and ribavirin or with simeprevir, daclatasvir, ledipasvir, or velpatasvir depending on the genotype	Liver injury Fatigue, weakness, nausea, insomnia, pruritus
NS5B Nonnucleos(t)ide Polymerase Inhibitor			
Dasabuvir 250 mg twice a day orally	1 and 4	Used in combination with Paritaprevir, ritonavir*, and ombitasvir	Liver injury Fatigue, weakness, nausea, insomnia, pruritus
Combination drugs			
Epclusa (sofosbuvir 400 mg/velpatasvir 100 mg)	1 through 6	Used in combination with ribavirin No need to use Peg-INF-2a	Headache, fatigue Symptomatic bradycardia. Other side effects as noted in the individual agents
Technivie (ombitasvir 12 mg, paritaprevir 75 mg and ritonavir 50 mg*)	4	Used in combination with ribavirin (No need to be used with Peg-INF-2a.)	Liver injury in those with advanced liver disease Fatigue, weakness, nausea, insomnia, pruritus
Zepatier (elbasvir 50 mg and grazoprevir 100 mg)	1a, 1b, and 4	Can be used in combination with ribavirin	Diarrhea, headache, insomnia, weakness, anemia, fatigue, pruritus Liver injury
Viekira Pak (ombitasvir 12.5 mg, paritaprevir 75 mg, ritonavir 50 mg, and dasabuvir 250 mg)	1a and 1b		Liver injury Fatigue, weakness, nausea, insomnia, pruritus

*Ritonavir has no activity against HCV but is a pharmacological booster.

amount of lymphoid tissue it contains. The appendix fills with food, just as the cecum does, but because the lumen of the appendix is smaller, it has a tendency to become obstructed. Appendicitis is the inflammation of the vermiform appendix caused by an obstruction and/or infection. It is the most common cause of acute right lower quadrant (RLQ) abdominal pain requiring surgical intervention. Acute appendicitis results in more than 300,000 appendectomies annually in the United States and represents 1 million hospital day stays.

EPIDEMIOLOGY AND CAUSES

Appendicitis can occur at any age; however, it is most common between ages 10 and 30 years. It is rare in infants and in older adults and is often associated with higher morbidity within these age groups because of delayed diagnosis and intervention. During the peak incidence years, men are twice as likely to be diagnosed with appendicitis as are women, but the occurrence in both genders tends to equalize over the life span. It is estimated that appendicitis will affect 10 in 100,000 people in the United States, with an incidence of 1.1 cases per 1,000 people per year.

Appendicitis is more common in Western countries, where people have diets that are low in fiber, high in fat, and high in refined sugars and other carbohydrates. Obstruction of the appendix by a variety of pathological processes is the cause of the majority of appendicitis. Other contributing factors include intra-abdominal tumors and positive family history. Recent roundworm infestation or viral infection of the GI tract have also been implicated.

PATHOPHYSIOLOGY

Appendicitis typically begins with dilation of the appendix, followed by obstruction and subsequent bacterial infection. When the lumen of the appendix is obstructed by hardened feces (fecalith), inflammatory processes (including parasites, viruses, or bacteria), strictures, neoplasms, or foreign bodies (including vegetable or fruit seeds or barium), the mucosa of the appendix continues to secrete fluid, which further distends the lumen, impairing the venous blood flow and leading to tissue necrosis. Left untreated, this increased distention impedes arterial inflow. Bacteria continue to proliferate and, in the absence of treatment, perforation of the appendix occurs. The incidence of perforation in patients with appendicitis is between 17% and 40%, with rates as high as 60% to 70% in older adults because of the nonspecific presenting symptoms. Gynecological disorders and gastroenteritis are the most common causes of misdiagnosis.

CLINICAL PRESENTATION

Subjective

The diagnosis of acute appendicitis is made clinically and is based primarily on the patient's history and physical examination. The historical presentations of signs and symptoms are important keys to prompt diagnosis and treatment. The classic presentation of appendicitis begins with the acute onset of mild to severe colicky, epigastric, or periumbilical pain. The pain is often vague at first, but within 12 hours, it usually shifts and localizes over the RLQ and is exacerbated by walking or coughing. In male patients, the pain may radiate into the testicles; pain (rigidity) also may be associated with abdominal muscle spasm in male or female patients. Most patients complain of nausea and anorexia after the onset of pain, which may or may not be associated with vomiting. If vomiting is present, the patient usually reports that abdominal pain was present before vomiting began. The sensation of constipation is typical, although diarrhea is present in some patients.

A mildly elevated temperature of 99°F to 100°F is common. If the patient with RLQ pain presents with shaking chills (rigors), perforation of the appendix should be suspected. An important point to remember is that the very young and older adults may have an atypical presentation, which can mimic other less acute disease processes. For example, older adults with appendicitis may present with weakness, anorexia, abdominal distention, and mild complaints of pain. A delay in the diagnosis in this age-group has led to an associated increase in morbidity and mortality.

Objective

On physical examination, the patient may or may not look sick depending on the degree of pain and other symptoms. The patient may have hypertension and tachycardia proportionate to the degree of fever and pain. When the patient is lying recumbent, they may flex the right knee upward to relieve the tension on the iliopsoas muscle, which overlies the appendix. Palpation of the abdomen early in the process may reveal diffuse tenderness over the umbilicus and midepigastric areas. As the process progresses, the tenderness localizes over the RLQ and may be accompanied by guarding. *Guarding* is defined as "the voluntary contraction of the abdominal muscles in anticipation of examination," as opposed to *rigidity,* which is caused by "the involuntary reflexive spasm of the muscles of the abdominal wall." Rebound tenderness is tested by placing the palmar aspect of the hand on the abdomen and pressing hard enough to depress the peritoneum. This may cause the patient pain, but the clinician should keep the abdomen depressed with constant pressure until the patient becomes accustomed to the pressure, and the pain decreases. Then, without warning, the clinician should remove the hand suddenly, preferably when the patient's attention is directed elsewhere. If positive for rebound tenderness, the patient will grimace in pain, which is a more reliable sign than a subjective complaint of pain. Asking the patient to cough helps to localize exactly the site from which the pain is coming. Advanced Assessment 39.1 outlines examination maneuvers that aid in the diagnosis of appendicitis.

A rectal examination can be performed, but it is open to greater subjective interpretation. Patients with appendicitis will normally perceive greater tenderness and fullness on the right than on the left during the rectal examination. The provider must keep in mind that both the bowel and the appendix are mobile organs; they can shift posteriorly or suprapubically, causing altered examination findings. Bowel sounds are a nonspecific finding—they may be present, absent, or decreased in patients with appendicitis.

Other physical examination findings can include alterations in vital signs consistent with increased pain, such as tachycardia or elevated blood pressure. Patients may be reluctant to take a deep breath for fear it will cause pain.

If there is perforation of the appendix, there may be a sudden cessation of the pain, which is considered an emergency. Findings consistent with peritonitis include diffuse abdominal tenderness with rigidity. The patient may exhibit signs of septic shock, with marked leukocytosis, fever, and hemodynamic instability.

DIAGNOSTIC REASONING

Diagnostic Tests

Laboratory findings are not diagnostic and are nonspecific, so they must be used in combination with data from the history and physical examination. A complete blood count usually reveals a mild to moderate leukocytosis (white blood cell count 10,000 to 20,000 µg/L) with a left shift. Urinalysis shows microscopic hematuria or pyuria in 25% of patients. Women should have a urine human chorionic gonadotropin test completed to rule out (ectopic) pregnancy. The lack of laboratory findings should not preclude the diagnosis of appendicitis.

No radiological examination is of diagnostic importance early in appendicitis, but x-ray studies become more important as appendicitis progresses. A chest x-ray film rules out pneumonia as a source of abdominal pain and is necessary as part of the preoperative procedure in most hospitals. Plain x-ray films of the abdomen may show evidence of a fecalith, a gas-filled appendix, small bowel ileus, a deviation in the bowel gas pattern, or a loss of the right iliopsoas shadow. Any of these findings is suggestive of appendicitis when combined with a suspect history and physical examination.

A computed tomography scan of the abdomen is helpful in ruling out other diagnostic possibilities, as well as determining whether there has been perforation of the appendix or development of a periappendiceal abscess. An abdominal ultrasound helps visualize the inflamed appendix and is also useful in ruling out other potential diagnoses. Diagnostic laparoscopy may be considered in female patients to rule out ectopic pregnancy, tubo-ovarian processes, or pelvic inflammatory disease (PID).

Differential Diagnosis

The differential diagnoses of appendicitis comprise a host of problems, which include, but are not limited to, urinary tract infection, ectopic pregnancy, ovarian cyst, pneumonia, gastroenteritis, Crohn's disease, diverticulitis, mesenteric adenitis, pancreatitis, PID, and cholelithiasis. If the diagnosis of appendicitis remains questionable after the history and physical examination have been completed and initial laboratory work has

Advanced Assessment 39.1: Physical Examination Maneuvers for Diagnosing Appendicitis

Maneuver	Examination	Comments
Rovsing's sign	Deep palpation over the left lower quadrant with sudden, unexpected release of pressure.	This causes tenderness over the right lower quadrant (RLQ) and is considered a positive finding.
Psoas sign	The patient is instructed to try to lift the right leg against gentle pressure applied by the examiner or by placing the patient in the left lateral decubitus position and extending the patient's right leg at the hip.	An increase in pain is considered positive and is an indication of the inflamed appendix irritating the psoas muscle.
Obturator sign	With the right hip and knee flexed, the examiner slowly rotates the right leg internally, which stretches the obturator muscle.	Pain over the RLQ is considered a positive sign and indicates irritation of the muscle by the inflamed appendix.
McBurney's sign	Pressure is applied to McBurney's point, which is located halfway between the umbilicus and the anterior spine of the ilium.	Pain when pressure is applied to this area is considered a positive response.

been obtained, radiographic studies are helpful in ruling out many of the processes found within the differential diagnoses. For women of childbearing age, the clinician should always obtain a pregnancy test before ordering any radiographic studies. In some cases, laparotomy or laparoscopy may be required to assist in definitive diagnosis.

Careful attention must be given to the sexual and menstrual history of all female patients because of the myriad potential gynecological problems that present with the same signs and symptoms as appendicitis. A pelvic examination and a diagnostic laparotomy are often necessary for differential diagnosis.

Many GI disorders have symptoms that mimic those of appendicitis, and watchful waiting may be indicated in some cases. If appendicitis is at all a suspicion, however, the prudent practitioner will follow these patients closely until a diagnosis has been reached.

MANAGEMENT

The treatment of appendicitis is usually surgical but emerging evidence indicates that antibiotic therapy may be considered as a first-line treatment and sole therapy in patients who are not good surgical candidates and in select patients with uncomplicated appendicitis. The incidence of appendiceal perforation ranges from 17% to 32% in patients with appendicitis; it is as high as 70% in older adults. With effective and timely treatment, the mortality rate is less than 1%; however, in the older adult population, mortality approaches 15%.

Preoperative management includes correction of fluid and electrolyte imbalances; bedrest; nothing by mouth, with placement of a nasogastric tube if indicated; and IV antibiotics. Narcotics should be avoided if possible because they mask any developing symptoms that might indicate a complication such as perforation. Laxatives are contraindicated in patients with appendicitis because they may cause the appendix to rupture. Stool softeners may be given if the patient is complaining about constipation and diarrhea is not present.

Cefoxitin or cefotetan 1 to 2 g IV every 8 hours, ampicillin-sulbactam 3 g IV every 6 hours, or ertapenem 1 g IV in a single dose are the antibiotics of choice. If there has been perforation and peritonitis is suspected, antibiotic coverage for both gram-negative aerobic and anaerobic organisms is recommended. Some of the choices include ampicillin, gentamicin, clindamycin, metronidazole (Flagyl), ampicillin-sulbactam (Unasyn), and ticarcillin/clavulanate (Timentin).

Patients are normally discharged the same day as surgery unless there are complications. Early ambulation is encouraged, with progression to full activity as soon as possible. Diet is advanced when bowel sounds return. The patient is given standard postoperative guidelines for individuals who have had abdominal surgery.

FOLLOW-UP AND REFERRAL

The patient is normally followed by the surgeon, who will see the patient 5 to 7 days postoperatively to remove the sutures. If there was perforation of the appendix and the patient must remain hospitalized, the surgeon will follow the patient until discharge.

Patient Education: Appendicitis

The patient will be given standard postoperative instructions from the surgeon, which should include advice to return to the hospital if anorexia, nausea, vomiting, abdominal pain, fever, or chills develop. Patients should be instructed to avoid heavy lifting for at least 2 weeks.

REFERENCES

Appendicitis

Fugazzola P, Ceresoli M, Agresta F. et al. The SIFIPAC/WSES/SICG/SIMEU guidelines for diagnosis and treatment of acute appendicitis in the elderly (2019 edition). *World J Emerg Surg.* 2020;15(19):1–15. https://link.springer.com/article/10.1186/s13017-020-00298-0.

Kim HK, Kim YS, Lee HH. Impact of a delayed laparoscopic appendectomy on the risk of complications in acute appendicitis: a retrospective study of 4,065 patients. *Dig Surg.* 2017;34(1):25–29.

Rushing A, Bugaev N, Jones C, et al. Management of acute appendicitis in adults: a practice management guideline from the Eastern Association for the Surgery of Trauma. *J Trauma and Acute Care Surg.* 2019;87(1):214–224.

Sceats LA, Trickey AW, Morris AM, et al. Nonopertive management of uncomplicated appendicitis among privately insured patients. *JAMA Surg.* 2019;154(2):141–149.

Snyder MJ, Guthrie M, Cagle S. Acute appendicitis: efficient diagnosis and management. *Am Fam Physician.* 2018;98(1):25–33.

Wagner M, Tubre DJ, Asensio JA. Evolution and current trends in the management of acute appendicitis. *Surg Clin.* 2018;98(5):1005–1023.

Gastroenteritis

Cani PD. Human gut microbiome: hopes, threats and promises. *Gut.* 2018;67:1716–1725.

Hvas CL, Jorgensen SMD, Jorgensen SP, et al. Fecal microbiota transplantation is superior to fidaxomicin for treatment of recurrent *Clostridium difficile* infection. *Gastroenterology.* 2019;156(5):1324–1332.

Kho ZY, Lal SK. The human gut microbiome—a potential controller of wellness and disease. *Front. Microbiol.* 2018l;9(article 1835):1–23.

Stuempfig ND, Seroy J. Viral gastroenteritis. (Updated 2020 June 25). In: StatPearls [Internet]. Treasure Island (FL): StatPearls Publishing; 2020 Jan. Available from: https://www.ncbi.nlm.nih.gov/books/NBK518995/.

Leung AKC, Leung AAM, Wong AHC, et al. Travelers' diarrhea: a clinical review. *Recent Pat Inflamm Allergy Drug Discov.* 2019;13:38–48.

White AE, Ciampa N, Chen Y et al. Characteristic of *Campylobacter* and *Salmonella* infections and acute gastroenteritis in older adults in Australia, Canada, and the United States. *Clin Infect Dis.* 2019;69(9):1545–1552.

Hepatitis

American Association for the Study of Liver Diseases. (Updated 2020 Aug 27). *HCV Guidance: Recommendations for Testing, Managing, and Treating Hepatitis C.* http://www.hcvguidelines.org.

Centers for Disease Control and Prevention. *Viral hepatitis.* https://www.cdc.gov/hepatitis/index.htm.

Centers for Disease Control and Prevention. (Published 2020 Jul). *Viral Hepatitis Surveillance, United States, 2018.* https://www.cdc.gov/hepatitis/statistics/2018surveillance/index.htm. Accessed 9/28/2020.

Hofmeister MG, Rosenthal EM, Barker LK, et al. Estimating prevalence of hepatitis C virus infection in the United States. 2013–2016. *Hepatology.* 2019;69(3):1020–1031.

Nelson NP, Weng MK, Hofmeister MG, et al. Prevention of hepatitis A virus infection in the United States: recommendations of the advisory committee on immunizations practices, 2020. *MMWR Recomm Rep.* 2020;69(No. RR-5):138.

Wander P, Epstein M, Bernstein D. COVID-19 Presenting as Acute Hepatitis. *Am J Gastroenterol.* 2020;115(6):941–942. doi:10.14309/ajg.0000000000000660.

RESOURCES

American Association for the Study of Liver Diseases (AASLD)
   https://www.aasld.org/publications/practice-guidelines-0
American Liver Foundation
   https://liverfoundation.org/
Centers for Disease Control and Prevention (CDC)
   https://www.cdc.gov/nchs/pressroom/sosmap/liver_disease_mortality/liver_disease.htm

---

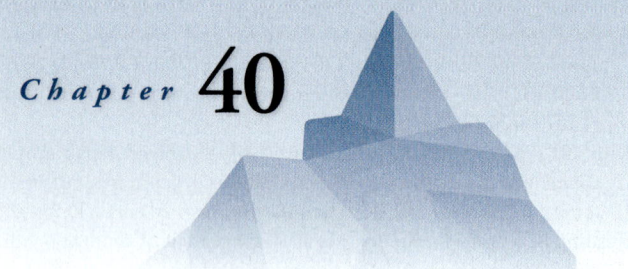

Chapter 40

Gastric and Intestinal Disorders

Debera J. Thomas, PhD, RN, ANP/FNP

GASTROESOPHAGEAL REFLUX DISEASE

Esophageal reflux is the backward flow of stomach or duodenal contents into the esophagus without associated retching or vomiting. It can occur in otherwise healthy people. If symptoms become severe or frequent or are associated with esophageal mucosal damage, the potential for serious clinical consequences becomes more likely, and the esophageal reflux is considered a disease. Gastroesophageal reflux disease (GERD) is a syndrome that results from esophageal reflux; the characteristic symptoms are caused by repeated exposure of the esophageal mucosa to the deleterious effects of gastrointestinal (GI) contents and the gradual breakdown of the mucosal barrier (see The Iceberg of GERD).

EPIDEMIOLOGY AND CAUSES

GERD can occur at any age. The prevalence of GERD is equal for the sexes and across ethnic and cultural groups in the United States; it is a common condition. Higher rates of GERD occur in individuals who are overweight or obese and have a body mass index over 25. The prevalence rate for GERD (those experiencing symptoms at least once a week) in the United States is approximately 20%. The prevalence rates in other countries are lower, ranging from 0.1% to 5% in China to 10% to 15% in the United Kingdom. In the United States, 35% to 45% of adults complain of heartburn at least once a month, and 10% of adults complain of daily symptoms. These figures may be significantly underestimated because many people with mild symptoms use over-the-counter (OTC) medications (histamine-2 blockers or proton pump inhibitors [PPIs]) or antacids. Many individuals also believe that it is normal to have symptoms from time to time and attribute them to stress or dietary indiscretion.

The primary cause of GERD is the inappropriate, spontaneous, transient relaxation of the lower esophageal sphincter (LES) as a response to an unknown stimulus. In most patients, the normal resting or baseline LES pressure is 10 to 30 mm Hg. In patients who have severe disease, the LES is incompetent, with a resting pressure of less than 10 mm Hg. An incompetent LES results in free reflux during abdominal straining, lifting, bending, and recumbency. Gastric contents are acidic, and it is this low

The Iceberg of GERD

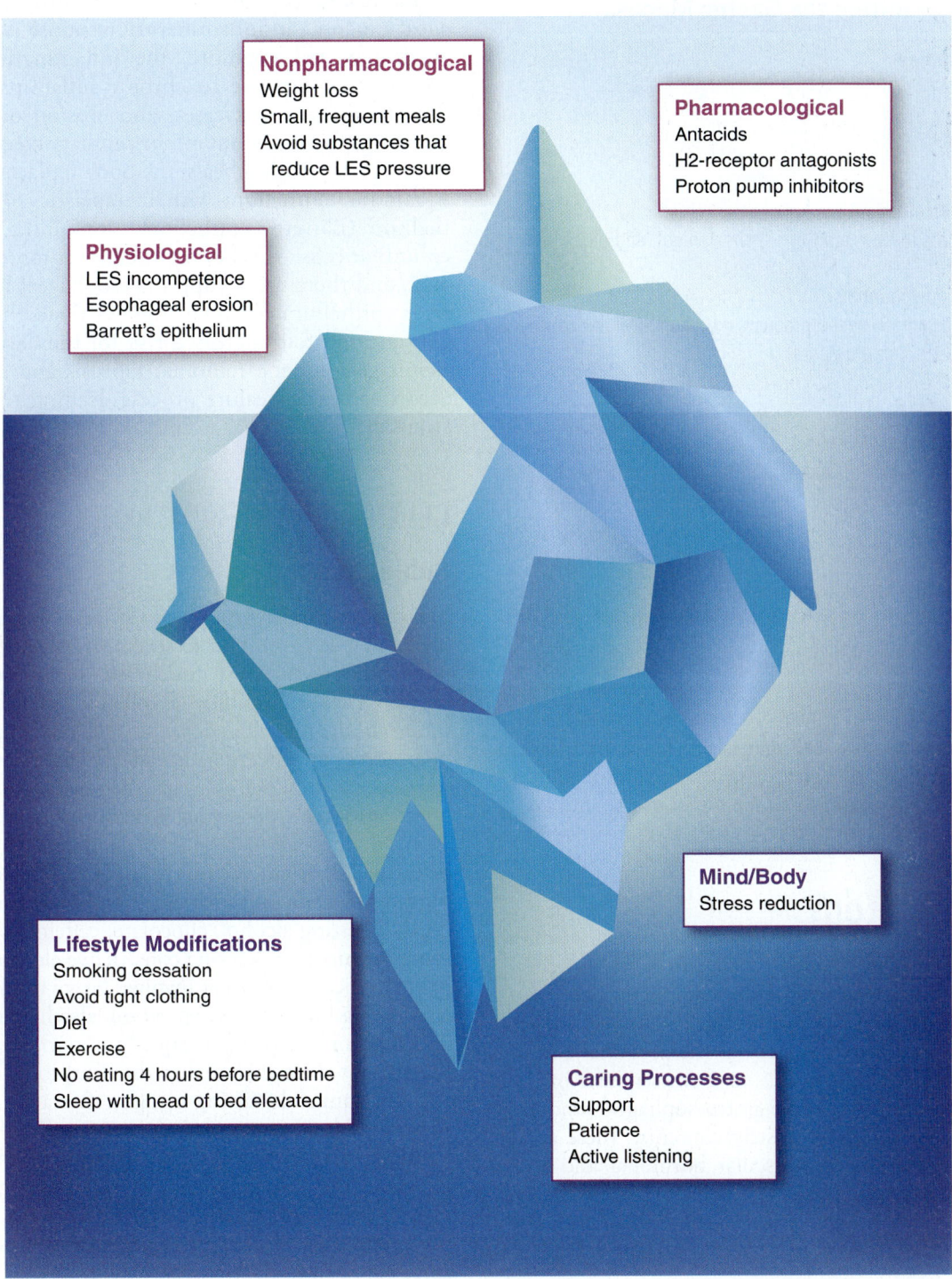

Nonpharmacological
Weight loss
Small, frequent meals
Avoid substances that reduce LES pressure

Pharmacological
Antacids
H2-receptor antagonists
Proton pump inhibitors

Physiological
LES incompetence
Esophageal erosion
Barrett's epithelium

Mind/Body
Stress reduction

Lifestyle Modifications
Smoking cessation
Avoid tight clothing
Diet
Exercise
No eating 4 hours before bedtime
Sleep with head of bed elevated

Caring Processes
Support
Patience
Active listening

pH (less than 3.9) that causes injury to the esophageal mucosa in most patients with GERD. Normally, refluxate is neutralized by swallowing salivary bicarbonate and cleared by esophageal peristalsis. The decreased rate of swallowing (by two-thirds) during sleep, coupled with recumbency, significantly increases the duration of exposure of the mucosa to acid at night.

Hiatal hernia, which displaces the LES into the thorax, is found in 75% of patients with severe erosive gastritis and 90% of patients with Barrett's esophagus but in only 25% of patients with nonerosive GERD. Delayed gastric emptying, which often worsens as people age, causes increased intra-abdominal pressure and may contribute to reflux. Obesity is also a risk factor for GERD. Several

> **Box 40.1** **Substances That Reduce Lower Esophageal Sphincter Pressure or Irritate the Gastric Mucosa**
>
> **Food Substances**
>
> Alcohol
> Caffeinated beverages (cola, tea, coffee)
> Chocolate
> Citrus fruits
> Decaffeinated coffee
> Fatty foods, fats (butter, margarine, shortening), and oils
> Onions
> Peppermint and spearmint
> Tomatoes and tomato-based products (ketchup, cocktail sauce, tomato sauce, tomato paste)
>
> **Nonfood Substances**
>
> Anticholinergic drugs
> Beta-adrenergic blocking agents
> Calcium channel blockers
> Diazepam
> Estrogen and progesterone
> Nicotine, including secondhand smoke
> Theophylline

foods and pharmacological agents are known to lower LES pressure. Box 40.1 lists the common substances that reduce LES pressure or cause direct gastric mucosal irritation.

PATHOPHYSIOLOGY

Physiologically, gastric acid is prevented from refluxing into the esophagus by the presence of two areas of high pressure in the distal esophagus. The upper esophageal sphincter is a 3-cm segment at the proximal end of the esophagus. The LES is a 2- to 4-cm segment of the esophagus just proximal to the gastroesophageal junction that prevents the reflux of gastric contents. These areas of the esophagus are under muscular, hormonal, and neural control. The anatomical placement of the LES within the abdomen supports its function, as does the acute angle (angle of His) that is formed as the esophagus enters the stomach.

Esophageal reflux occurs when the gastric volume (e.g., a large meal) or the intra-abdominal pressure is elevated (e.g., in pregnancy). It can also occur when the sphincter tone of the LES is decreased (e.g., by caffeine) or when the LES undergoes inappropriate relaxation. Gravity, saliva, and peristalsis combine to return refluxed contents to the stomach. As the esophagus becomes inflamed with repeated exposure to gastric acid, it cannot eliminate the refluxed material as quickly or efficiently, prolonging the duration of the contact with each subsequent exposure.

Because gastric contents are so irritating to the esophageal mucosa, an inflammatory response is established. With repeated exposure, the inflammation becomes chronic. In response to chronic inflammation, blood flow to the area increases, and erosion occurs. Frank bleeding is unusual, but minor capillary bleeding is common. As the erosion heals, the body replaces the normal squamous epithelium with metaplastic columnar epithelium (Barrett's epithelium) containing goblet and columnar cells. This new epithelium is more resistant to acid, and therefore it supports esophageal healing. Barrett's epithelium is a premalignant tissue, however, and confers a 40-fold increased risk for the development of esophageal adenocarcinoma. Fibrosis and scarring also accompany the healing process, leading to esophageal strictures.

CLINICAL PRESENTATION

Subjective

The most typical symptom of GERD is heartburn, ranging in degree from mild to severe. It is usually associated with other symptoms, including regurgitation, water brash (reflex salivation), dysphagia, sour taste in the mouth in the morning, odynophagia, belching, coughing, hoarseness, or wheezing, usually at night. Substernal or retrosternal chest pain may also be present, but additional questioning can determine whether the pain is activity induced, leading to the conclusion that the pain may be cardiac in origin. Factors that precipitate or worsen the symptoms, such as reclining after eating; eating a large meal; ingesting alcohol, chocolate, caffeine, fatty or spicy foods, or nicotine; wearing constrictive clothing; or working in an occupation that involves heavy lifting, straining, or working in a bent-over position, also help establish the diagnosis of GERD. It is equally important to ask what the patient does that makes the symptoms better, such as taking antacids, sitting upright after a meal, or eating small meals.

Patients with chronic GERD may present with dysphagia as their chief complaint. The dysphagia is usually present only with the first swallow of every meal and is not progressive. If the patient complains of progressive or persistent dysphagia, adenocarcinoma or the development of a stricture should be suspected.

Objective

The physical examination of the patient with GERD is usually normal. The only physical sign may be a stool positive for occult blood on rectal examination, resulting from microhemorrhages in the irritated esophageal epithelium.

DIAGNOSTIC REASONING

Diagnostic Tests

Diagnosis of GERD is usually made by history. The severity of the symptoms does not correlate well with the severity of the disease; some patients with the most severe disease have virtually no symptoms. GERD may also manifest with atypical symptoms such as adult-onset asthma, chronic cough, chronic laryngitis, sore throat, or noncardiac chest pain.

When the diagnosis of GERD is unclear or when the patient fails to respond to 4 to 8 weeks of empiric once-daily PPI therapy, the test of choice is esophagogastroduodenoscopy (EGD, also called an *upper endoscopy*). The benefit of EGD is direct visualization of the mucosa to determine the extent of tissue damage. The EGD can also detect complications of GERD such as Barrett's epithelium, esophageal stricture, and cancer. The American College of Gastroenterology (ACG) guidance for EGD in adults with GERD symptoms recommends EGD for patients with heartburn and dysphagia, bleeding, anemia, weight loss, or recurrent vomiting rather than initial empiric therapy and those who have persistent symptoms despite 8 weeks of PPI therapy. Upper endoscopy is recommended every 3 to 5 years for surveillance evaluation in anyone with Barrett's esophagus and more frequently if there is Barrett's esophagus with dysplasia.

Differential Diagnosis

The symptoms of GERD are similar to those of peptic ulcer disease (PUD), and the two conditions often coexist. Unlike GERD, however, PUD usually produces epigastric pain and tenderness on palpation. One pattern that can help differentiate GERD from PUD is that heartburn from PUD is usually relieved by food. This is not the case in GERD; instead, the symptoms are worse shortly after eating. Another possible differential diagnosis is gallbladder disease, which usually presents with epigastric or right subcostal pain. Nausea and possibly vomiting are usually associated with cholelithiasis and cholecystitis; this is not the case in gastric reflux. There may be a strong association between the ingestion of a high-fat meal and the development of the symptoms of cholelithiasis. Occasionally, GERD may present with chest pain. In these patients, the clinician must differentiate between symptoms of cardiac origin and those of GERD. If the pain is of cardiac origin (e.g., angina), the patient's history usually reveals that the pain is associated with exercise and is relieved by rest and nitrates. Patients with angina are often treated with medications (calcium channel blockers, beta-adrenergic blockers, nitrates) that decrease the LES pressure and produce a coexistent esophageal reflux, which complicates the differential diagnosis further.

MANAGEMENT

Initial Treatment

The goal of the management of GERD is to rapidly eliminate or reduce symptoms; prevent meal- or exercise-related symptoms; and prevent the complications of esophageal stricture, esophageal ulcer, Barrett's esophagus, pulmonary aspiration, and esophageal hemorrhage all in the most cost-effective way. The focus of management is patient education coupled with pharmacological intervention. The ACG conditionally recommends lifestyle modifications that include weight loss (moderate level of evidence); elevating the head of the bed 6 to 8 inches and avoidance of meals 2 to 3 hours before bedtime (low level of evidence); and avoidance of certain foods known to trigger reflux (chocolate, alcohol, caffeine, acidic [tomatoes, citrus] or spicy foods) (low level of evidence).

The ACG recommends an 8-week trial of PPIs, based on a high level of evidence. It found no difference in the effectiveness of different PPIs. A moderate level of evidence suggests that traditional PPIs should be taken 30 to 60 minutes before a meal for the best pH control. The newer PPIs can be taken on a more relaxed schedule, a conditional recommendation based on a moderate level of evidence.

For patients with mild, intermittent symptoms, lifestyle changes may relieve symptoms. For patients with mild to moderate symptoms without esophageal erosion, an 8-week course of PPI once daily before the first meal of the day is the treatment of choice (strong recommendation, moderate level of evidence). In patients with a partial response to this therapy, tailoring the dose and timing, especially for those with symptoms at night or with sleep disturbance (strong recommendation, low level of evidence), is indicated. If the patient has a partial response, changing to a twice-daily dosing schedule or switching to a different PPI may be effective (conditional recommendation, low level of evidence).

Troublesome Symptoms or Symptoms Unresponsive to 8 Weeks of PPI Therapy

Patients who have severe symptoms and have endoscopically documented erosive esophagitis or Barrett's esophagus should be treated with PPIs such as omeprazole, rabeprazole, pantoprazole, or lansoprazole once a day 30 minutes before breakfast. An 8-week course of once-daily treatment usually provides adequate control of heartburn in 80% to 90% of cases and healing of erosive esophagitis in 80%, whereas twice-daily dosing heals 95% of cases. If twice-daily dosing provides inadequate symptom relief, the patient should be evaluated with upper endoscopy. Chronic maintenance therapy with PPIs may be necessary for severe erosive esophagitis.

Patients with severe erosive esophagitis, Barrett's esophagus, or peptic stricture and those who required twice-daily PPI therapy for initial symptom control should be maintained on long-term therapy. More than 80% of patients who achieved good symptom control with initial therapy and discontinue treatment will relapse. These patients may require intermittent 2- to 4-week courses of PPI therapy.

Evidence suggests that PPIs are more effective than H_2-receptor antagonists (H_2RAs) in all cases of GERD. These agents should not be used in combination, especially with older adults. PPIs should be taken 30 to 60 minutes before breakfast to maximize effectiveness. If the patient requires twice-daily dosing, the second dose should be taken 30 to 60 minutes before dinner as well. Patients on long-term therapy should have their symptoms reevaluated every 6 months in an effort to avoid potential adverse effects such as PPI-associated pneumonia, *Clostridium difficile*, osteoporosis, and vitamin B_{12} deficiency.

Unresponsive Disease

The 5% of patients who do not respond to any of the previously mentioned treatments may require surgical intervention. However, for patients who do not respond to PPI therapy, surgical intervention is generally not recommended. For those patients who do require surgery, preoperative ambulatory pH monitoring is mandatory if they do not have evidence of erosive esophagitis. Before referring a patient for surgical intervention, other causes of refractory GERD, such as gastrinoma, proton pump resistance, pill-induced esophagitis, scleroderma-like esophagus, or patient noncompliance, should be investigated. There have been limited studies on the use of baclofen, a $GABA_B$ agonist, for the treatment of transient lower esophageal sphincter relaxation (TLESR) and PPI-refractory GERD. Baclofen has been shown to decrease the frequency of LES relaxation but may cause extreme drowsiness. Drugs Commonly Prescribed 40.1 outlines PPIs and other medication used to treat GERD.

FOLLOW-UP AND REFERRAL

GERD is a lifelong condition, and patients must be reevaluated on a regular basis to minimize the development of severe complications. Patients with mild to moderate symptoms should be instructed on appropriate lifestyle modifications and treated with PPIs for 4 to

Drugs Commonly Prescribed 40.1: Treatment for GERD

DRUG	INDICATION	ADVERSE REACTIONS AND PRESCRIBING CONSIDERATIONS
Proton pump inhibitors (PPIs): Omeprazole 20 mg orally Rabeprazole 20 mg orally Lansoprazole 30 mg orally Dexlansoprazole 60 mg orally Esomeprazole 40 mg orally Pantoprazole 40 mg orally *H_2-receptor antagonists may be effective in some patients and are less expensive	Mild, intermittent symptoms	Trial for 4–8 weeks Take 30 minutes before breakfast PPIs are generally well tolerated. Common side effects include headache, diarrhea, constipation, abdominal pain, flatulence, fever, vomiting, nausea, or rash. Serious side effects: increased risk of *Clostridium difficile* infection, serious allergic reactions, Stevens-Johnson syndrome, toxic epidermal necrolysis, reduced kidney function, pancreatitis, reduced liver function, erythema multiforme.
PPIs: Omeprazole 20 mg orally Rabeprazole 20 mg orally Lansoprazole 30 mg orally Dexlansoprazole 60 mg orally Esomeprazole 40 mg orally Pantoprazole 40 mg orally	Moderate symptoms or partial response to once-daily dosing	Twice-daily dosing or switch to a different PPI (conditional recommendation, low level of evidence) Long-term use of PPIs can cause vitamin B_{12} deficiency and risk for osteoporosis.
Optimize PPI therapy (strong recommendation, low level of evidence) Future treatment: Research is being done on transient lower esophageal sphincter inhibitors and cannabinoid receptor agonists.	Troublesome symptoms or refractory gastroesophageal reflux disease	Upper endoscopy Explore other etiologies; possible referral to pulmonary and allergy specialists (strong recommendation, low level of evidence) Refractory patients with ongoing evidence of reflux should be considered for surgery or increasing the dose of PPI.

and typically resolve on their own within 3 weeks; others can result in profuse bleeding, requiring emergency ligation.

EPIDEMIOLOGY AND CAUSES

Every year, approximately 1 million people, or 5% of the U.S. population, visit their medical provider for symptoms of hemorrhoids. Although hemorrhoids can occur at any age, their incidence increases with age.

Although the cause of hemorrhoids is not completely known or understood, they are common in countries where there is a known deficiency of dietary fiber. Thus, increased straining during defecation has been recognized as an important predisposing factor in the development of hemorrhoids. Heredity may also be a factor because 10% of the patients with hemorrhoids have a family history of the disease. Other causes of symptomatic hemorrhoids are obesity, pregnancy, prolonged sitting, and diarrhea.

PATHOPHYSIOLOGY

External hemorrhoids are dilated varicose veins originating from the inferior hemorrhoidal plexus located below the anal-rectal line. Internal hemorrhoids are a dilation of the veins within the superior hemorrhoidal plexus and are located within the distal rectum and the anal canal. Internal hemorrhoids are classified by the degree of prolapse present (Table 40.1).

The inferior hemorrhoidal plexus is prone to increased distention during defecation, which can result in rupture of a vessel and subsequent development of a perianal hematoma or thrombus within one of the vessels of the plexus. Patients who have a thrombosed hemorrhoid may present with a painful perianal lump.

TABLE 40.1 Classification of Internal Hemorrhoids

Severity	Description of the Process
First degree	Protrude into the lumen of the anal canal, usually without the sensation of protrusion
Second degree	Protrude beyond the anal canal during defecation but spontaneously reduce when defecation is completed
Third degree	Protrude beyond the anal canal during defecation but must be manually reduced after the completion of the bowel movement
Fourth degree	Protrude beyond the anal canal and are permanently prolapsed despite attempts at manual reduction

CLINICAL PRESENTATION

Subjective

External hemorrhoids may present with an abrupt onset of pain that is associated with the development of a perianal lump. Many patients complain of more intense pain after defecation or other straining maneuvers, which result in further inflammation and engorgement. Mucus discharge from the anus can lead to poor hygiene and complaints of pruritus. The natural history of a resolved hemorrhoid is the formation of external skin tags, which are asymptomatic but may be irritating and interfere with daily hygiene.

Objective

On physical examination, external hemorrhoids may not be visible at rest but usually protrude on standing or with the Valsalva maneuver. Thrombosed hemorrhoids may appear as shiny blue masses located at the anus. Evidence of hemorrhoidal skin tags may appear at the site of resolved hemorrhoids; these skin tags are fibrotic and painless.

Internal hemorrhoids most often present with rectal bleeding described as bright red streaks on the toilet paper. Patients may report that blood drips into the toilet after a bowel movement. Occasionally the bleeding is sufficient enough to cause anemia, which in any case merits further investigation.

DIAGNOSTIC REASONING

Diagnostic Tests

Initial diagnosis is made by visual inspection of the anal area. Digital rectal examination is not considered an accurate means of diagnosis because most internal hemorrhoids are soft swellings that usually are not palpable, nor are they painful unless they have thrombosed, become infected, or a fissure has developed. External hemorrhoids can usually be diagnosed at physical examination, whereas internal hemorrhoids are visible on physical examination only if they have prolapsed.

Definitive diagnosis of internal hemorrhoids requires visualization with an anoscope. Most frequently, they are identified on routine colonoscopy.

Differential Diagnosis

The differential diagnosis of hemorrhoids includes polyps, carcinoma of the anus, anorectal fistula, cryptitis, papillitis, or rectal prolapse. Proctosigmoidoscopy is an effective means of establishing the appropriate diagnosis.

MANAGEMENT

Initial treatment for symptomatic external hemorrhoids is focused on adequate pain relief with oral analgesia and sitz baths. If the hemorrhoids do not spontaneously regress, care is directed at decreasing straining with defecation and modification of toilet habits. Patients are encouraged to avoid sitting on the toilet for long periods of time, use some form of bulk-forming laxative, and increase their daily fiber intake slowly to 30 to 35 g to establish regular, formed stools. Patients who suffer from diarrhea should be treated accordingly to control frequent loose stools. Individuals who suffer from pruritus should be instructed to maintain anal hygiene. Sitz baths, witch hazel, and application of topical hydrocortisone creams are all effective in controlling pruritus. If the external hemorrhoids continue to be painful or bothersome despite treatment, referral for surgical excision should be made.

Medical treatment of internal hemorrhoids follows the same principles previously outlined, with attention toward avoiding straining during defecation, modification of diet with the addition of fiber, increasing fluids, and the addition of bulking agents. If medical treatment is not effective, other nonsurgical treatments may be employed. First-degree hemorrhoids can be treated by injection sclerotherapy or infrared coagulation. Infrared coagulation, much like electrocoagulation, uses high-intensity light to shrink the swelling. Second- and third-degree hemorrhoids are normally treated with rubber-band ligation, in which a rubber-banded ring is placed around the base of the hemorrhoid. This band acts a tourniquet, strangulating the tissue while fixing the mucosa proximal to the ligation into the muscularis. All of the nonsurgical techniques used to treat internal hemorrhoids are associated with some degree of pain and bleeding.

Large, advanced-degree hemorrhoids will most often require referral to a surgeon for a formal hemorrhoidectomy. Again, proper anal hygiene and correction of chronic constipation and diarrhea are essential to prevent the recurrence of hemorrhoids.

FOLLOW-UP AND REFERRAL

Excision of a single external hemorrhoid, evacuation of a thrombosed external hemorrhoid, and injection sclerotherapy of simple internal hemorrhoids can all be performed in the office by a trained provider. Band ligation and other specialized treatment of hemorrhoids will require referral to a gastroenterologist more familiar with these procedures. Follow-up will be based on the patient's postprocedure course. Most patients will require no further care except for instruction on proper anal hygiene and diet. The addition of a nonirritating laxative after the procedure will usually prevent the development of constipation and the associated fear of defecation.

Patient Education: Hemorrhoids

Patient education for hemorrhoids is aimed at preventing the problem through increasing fiber in the diet. Fiber should be increased to 30 to 35 g/day, but this should be done slowly to prevent bloating and gas formation. Teaching patients to read food labels can help them gain control over their nutrition. Often, patients associate salad and cereal with very high levels of fiber. This is not accurate information in most cases; for example, most breakfast cereals have only 1 to 3 g of fiber per serving, and iceberg lettuce has very little fiber as well. OTC bulking agents, such as psyllium (Metamucil), can be suggested to help eliminate constipation. It is important to teach patients the necessity of drinking 64 ounces of water a day.

ABDOMINAL HERNIAS

An abdominal hernia is the protrusion of a peritoneally lined sac through some defect or weakened area in the abdominal wall. A history of heavy physical labor or heavy lifting can elicit a hernia. There are several types of hernias, which are usually classified by the anatomical location of the protrusion.

EPIDEMIOLOGY AND CAUSES

It is estimated that up to 10% of the population has some form of hernia. Groin hernias are the most common type and are classified as indirect inguinal hernias (50%), direct inguinal hernias (25%), and femoral hernias (10%). Ventral hernias occurring through the anterior abdominal wall account for only 15% of all hernias. Ventral hernias are further broken down into epigastric hernias (5%), incisional hernias (5%), and umbilical hernias (3%).

Groin hernias are by far the most common type of hernia and occur in both males and females. Indirect inguinal hernias are the most common and occur in both sexes, although they are frequently seen in young males. Direct inguinal hernias are more common in males older than age 40 years and are caused by a congenital abnormality. Femoral hernias occur more often in females than in males and are rare in children.

The recurrence rate of hernias in general is about 10%, with direct and indirect hernias having a recurrence rate that is approximately equal. The subsequent recurrence rate of recurrent hernias is much higher at 35%.

Ventral hernias include all other hernias of the anterior abdominal wall. Epigastric hernias are much more common in males than in females and are multiple in 25% of the cases. The peak age of incidence is between ages 20 and 50 years. Umbilical hernias are considered a normal occurrence in newborn infants, with about 20% of infants being affected. These hernias are more common in males of all ages and in African Americans of either sex. The presence of an umbilical hernia is considered normal until the child reaches age 2 years. Incisional hernias are considered the only iatrogenic type of herniation. Approximately 2% to 11% of all patients undergoing abdominal surgery develop incisional hernias. Females are affected twice as often as males.

Hernias occur because there is sufficient pressure to force tissue out through a defect in the abdominal wall, as well as a potential space for that protrusion. The etiology of hernias is multifactorial, with biological, congenital, and environmental influences contributing to their development.

PATHOPHYSIOLOGY

In general, for any type of groin hernia to occur, two of the body's protective mechanisms must fail. The first is called the *shutter mechanism,* whereby the internal oblique muscle and the transversus abdominis muscles contract to overlap, strengthening the posterior wall of the inguinal canal. Second, a *closure* or *sphincter-type mechanism* causes contraction of the musculature, displacing the transversalis fascia, which in effect decreases the diameter of the deep inguinal ring.

Indirect Inguinal Hernias

Indirect inguinal hernias result when tissue protrudes through the internal inguinal ring, which in males extends the length of the spermatic cord. With continued pressure, the sac can reach the scrotum, where it is then palpable just proximal to Hesselbach's triangle. The pathophysiology of indirect inguinal hernias in most cases begins with the herniation of tissue through a still-patent vaginal process that remains after the descent of the testes. In women, the vaginal process exists within the canal of Nuck. Indirect inguinal herniation is caused by a combination of this congenital defect and a disruption in the functioning of the sphincter mechanism as a result of a variety of environmental conditions, including increased abdominal pressure and trauma to the area.

Direct Inguinal Hernias

Direct inguinal hernias occur when the transversus abdominis and internal oblique muscles are attached, forming a high arch on the inferior border that results in a faulty shutter mechanism. Any environmental factors that increase abdominal pressure enhance the chance of herniation. As with indirect inguinal hernias, the presence of this congenital defect does not explain why herniation is more common later in life.

Femoral Hernias

Femoral herniation occurs at the fossa ovalis where the femoral artery exits from the abdomen. It is presumed to be attributable to a female's larger femoral canal and smaller iliopsoas muscles. Other factors that contribute to femoral herniation are femoral engorgement during pregnancy and the size of the female pelvis.

Epigastric Hernias

Epigastric hernias occur along the midline between the xiphoid process and the umbilicus. The fibers along the linea alba are brought together in a patchwork-type closure; the defect exists within this decussation. As these fibers weaken, the contents can herniate through the abdomen. Epigastric hernias are three times more likely to occur in males than in females. Peritoneal fat, bowel, and omentum are the most common abdominal contents to protrude through the wall.

Umbilical Hernias

Umbilical hernias that develop in adulthood occur through a weakening in the abdominal wall around the umbilical ring. The herniation of abdominal contents through this defect is also dependent on environmental factors that increase intra-abdominal pressure. Of particular importance when diagnosing an umbilical hernia is to look for underlying ascites secondary to liver disease.

Incisional Hernias

Incisional hernias can occur anywhere along a surgical incision into the abdomen. They are classified into those that cannot be controlled by surgical technique and those that can be controlled by surgical technique. Controllable factors include the type of incision chosen and choice of suture and surgical techniques. Factors that are considered uncontrollable include the prior medical history of the patient, age, steroid use, nutritional status, obesity, and complications of the surgery, especially wound sepsis.

CLINICAL PRESENTATION

Subjective

In any patient presenting with an abdominal hernia, the provider must determine whether there is an abnormal increase in intra-abdominal pressure that has contributed to the herniation. A thorough history and physical examination, with special attention to the genitourinary, respiratory, and GI systems, will provide clues. All male patients who present with an abdominal hernia, regardless of age, require a prostate examination to determine whether there is any obstructive process inhibiting urinary output, which in effect increases intra-abdominal pressure. Patients should be evaluated for ascites, which also increases intra-abdominal pressure.

Patients who have respiratory difficulty, such as obstructive pulmonary disease, have an increased risk of hernia because of the increased abdominal pressure associated with coughing and the downward expansion of the diaphragm found with hyperinflated lungs.

Objective

The presentation of inguinal hernias is not always obvious and is quite often an incidental finding on routine examination. Patients may present with complaints of pain while straining or lifting heavy objects or a swelling in the groin area. In general, the physical examination for all groin hernias begins with visual inspection of both groin area and the genitalia. With the male patient standing, the spermatic cord is located on both sides and is palpated for any swelling into the scrotum. Once the inguinal canal has been palpated, three additional areas must be examined. After invaginating the scrotal sac, the examining finger follows the spermatic cord up to the external inguinal ring and the fascia of the external oblique muscle. The posterior wall is inspected for weakness or bulging, and the inguinal ring is also palpated for structural soundness. Once these areas have been examined, the provider then withdraws the finger slightly and the patient is asked to cough, which increases the intra-abdominal pressure. If the provider feels the presence of a tissue-like sac tapping against the finger, hernia is present. Other findings indicative of herniation are feeling a rush of fluid (peritoneal) under the examining finger or a patient's report of pain. In a female patient, the femoral areas are palpated while the patient increases intra-abdominal pressure by performing the Valsalva maneuver. Any bulging in the area is considered a positive finding.

Once a groin hernia has been diagnosed, the practitioner must determine whether the hernia is incarcerated or strangulated, both of which require immediate surgical attention, or whether a more chronic situation is present, which can be cared for electively. Most often, this can be determined by patient history, as well as the physical ability to reduce the hernia on examination. A strangulated hernia is a nonreducible herniation in which the blood supply to the herniated tissue is compromised. An incarcerated hernia is one that has caused a bowel obstruction as a result of the protrusion.

An indirect inguinal hernia presents as a soft swelling within the internal ring, when either provoked or unprovoked, and often descends into the scrotum. A direct inguinal hernia presents as a bulge around Hesselbach's triangle (Fig. 40.1). Direct inguinal hernias are usually painless and easily reducible. The hernia bulges anteriorly, pushing against the side of the examining finger. Femoral hernias are more common on the right side and may be accompanied by severe pain. There is a palpable bulge through the femoral ring, and the inguinal canal is empty. Normally, it is the intestine that has herniated through the abdominal wall.

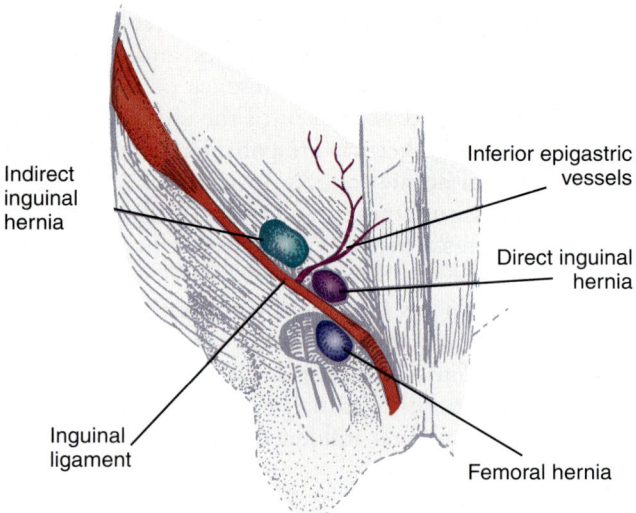

Figure 40.1 Locations of indirect and direct inguinal and femoral hernias. Anterior view of the groin, showing locations of indirect inguinal hernia, direct inguinal hernia, and femoral hernia, based on anatomical landmarks.

Epigastric hernias are normally asymptomatic and present as a small bump or bulge along the midline above the umbilicus. There may be variation in size with increasing intra-abdominal pressure. Peritoneal fat, omentum, and bowel are usually the tissues that herniate through the abdomen. The smaller hernias tend to be more painful because they involve the herniation of the preperitoneal fat, which is irritating. Larger hernias must be examined for incarceration and obstruction.

Incisional hernias manifest along the incision line of a previous abdominal operation and can be painful. Patients with incisional hernias may also have signs and symptoms of bowel obstruction, which is discussed later in this chapter.

DIAGNOSTIC REASONING

Diagnostic Tests

Hernias are diagnosed almost exclusively by physical examination findings, as described in the preceding text. On occasion, a radiographic study is necessary to determine whether an obstructive process is taking place. Other studies, such as pulmonary function testing or evaluation of a mass or lesion within the abdomen, may be indicated to assess the cause and/or extent of increased intra-abdominal pressure.

Differential Diagnosis

The differential diagnosis list for hernia is limited. It includes hydrocele, psoas abscess, femoral or inguinal adenopathy, and ectopic testis.

MANAGEMENT

When a hernia is detected, the patient should be referred to a surgeon. Despite the evolution of hernia repair over the last century, the underlying principles remain the same: reinforce the two natural defense mechanisms discussed previously; decrease the size of the inguinal ring; and strengthen the posterior wall of the canal. Repair of femoral hernias is accomplished by reducing the size of the canal, whereas repair of indirect hernia is accomplished by dissecting the hernial sac and reducing the repaired tissue. Frequently, there is not sufficient tissue to reconstruct and strengthen the posterior wall of the canal, and synthetic mesh materials are used. Laparoscopic surgery has decreased the recovery time and allowed for a single intervention for bilateral hernia repair. All ventral hernias should be repaired to decrease the possibility of incarceration.

Postoperatively, the patient may experience incisional pain, which is relieved by oral analgesics. Pain that persists for more than a few days suggests impending wound infection. Normally, there is slight postoperative swelling, ecchymosis, and erythema of the skin, up to the scrotal area in male patients. Hernia repair with significant scrotal involvement may result in increased scrotal edema, which can be relieved with ice packs, elevation, and wearing a scrotal support. In female patients, swelling is usually limited to the surgical site but may extend to the labia and vulva.

FOLLOW-UP AND REFERRAL

All patients with abdominal hernias require surgical consultation, whether emergently or electively, and appropriate referral should be made. The patient is usually seen in the surgeon's office 3 to 7 days after surgery.

> ### Patient Education: Abdominal Hernias
> After typical groin surgery, the patient can return to normal activities, including work, after about 1 week but is instructed to avoid heavy lifting or contact sports for at least 4 to 6 weeks. Patients who have undergone laparoscopic repair of groin hernias can resume regular activities, including heavy lifting, as soon as 2 days postprocedure. Patients who have had a ventral hernia repair should follow routine postoperative instruction as directed by the surgeon.

IRRITABLE BOWEL SYNDROME

IBS is a functional GI disorder characterized by abdominal pain or discomfort and a change in bowel habits. The Rome IV Diagnostic Criteria for IBS were released in June 2016 and reflect advances in basic science research and clinical trials. The official definition according to the new Rome IV Criteria is that IBS is a disorder of gut-brain interaction. IBS is linked with other functional GI disorders and is classified by a combination of GI symptoms that include motility disturbances, visceral hypersensitivity, altered mucosal and immune function, altered gut microbiota, and altered central nervous system processing. A diagnosis of IBS must include recurrent abdominal pain of at least 1 day per week for the previous 3 months and be associated with at least two of the following additional features: related to defecation, associated with a change in stool frequency, and/or associated with a change in stool appearance or form. There are three subtypes of IBS: predominant constipation (IBS-C), predominant diarrhea (IBS-D), and IBS with mixed bowel habits (IBS-M). Patients may have other symptoms such as mucus in the stool, feelings of straining, urgency, incomplete evacuation, flatulence, and abdominal distention. IBS is the most common GI problem encountered in primary care and the second leading cause of absence from work. Treatment for IBS in the United States is estimated to cost more than $20 billion.

EPIDEMIOLOGY

Traditionally, females have been affected more often than males, at a rate of 2:1. It is estimated that up to 15% of the general population is affected by symptoms that can be classified within the diagnosis of IBS, but fewer than one-third of those individuals seek medical attention. Typically, the symptoms first present in late adolescence and early adulthood but rarely in patients older than 50 years.

PATHOPHYSIOLOGY

The exact cause of IBS is unknown. IBS was once considered to have no organic cause, but several mechanisms have been identified. Normal bowel function is regulated by segmental contractions that limit the movement of bowel contents through the colon. An increase in these contractions causes constipation, and a decrease in the contractions results in frequent stooling or diarrhea. Myoelectric studies of colonic movement in individuals with IBS were inconclusive for diagnostic criteria, but the studies did demonstrate patterns of hypermotility, including high-amplitude pressure waves in patients, with pain as the predominant symptom during an acute IBS attack. Likewise, patients with IBS-D had decreased and lower-amplitude pressure waves. Studies have confirmed alterations in colonic activity during periods of emotional stress, in which motility is decreased or inhibited with depression and increased with feelings of hostility and anger.

Another major investigative focus of IBS has centered on visceral hypersensitivity. Approximately 50% of patients with IBS have perceptual abnormalities including heightened gut sensitivity, leading to a lower tolerance for abdominal pain and distention of the colon with gas and feces. Studies in which the rectums of IBS patients were distended by balloon dilation resulted in spastic contractions, leading to the characteristic symptoms seen with IBS. Patients with IBS are acutely aware of the intraluminal activities occurring with the digestive process. Sensations range from mild discomfort and tugging to frank pain. In summary, IBS patients do show evidence of abnormal colonic smooth muscle activity; however, the level at which the lesion originates is yet unknown.

Up to 10% of patients with IBS develop the disorder after bacterial gastroenteritis. It appears that patients with increased life stressors are more prone to developing IBS postinfection. Although the importance is unknown at this time, increased inflammatory cells have been found in all layers of the bowel in some patients with IBS.

Food intolerance has been identified as a trigger of symptoms in as many as 89% of patients. Specific foods reported to cause symptoms are legumes, vegetables, foods containing lactose, foods high in fat, stone fruits, and artificial sweeteners. Any food that contains fermentable oligosaccharides, disaccharides, monosaccharides, and polyols (FODMAP) worsens symptoms because of the fermentation and osmotic effects. Although some research has shown a 70% improvement in symptoms with a low FODMAP diet, it is very limited and can cause nutritional deficiencies and weight loss.

The gut microbiota in patients diagnosed with IBS show a lower microbial variety and lower numbers of *Methanobacteriales* and *Prevotella* species. Other studies have shown lower numbers of the beneficial bacteria *Lactobacillus* and *Bacteroides* with increased numbers of *Streptococcus* pathogens.

In those patients who seek medical care for symptoms of IBS, about 50% have underlying depression, anxiety, or somatization. These psychological abnormalities my affect how a person reacts to visceral sensations and to changes in bowel habits. Chronic stress may also affect the nervous system processing of visceral sensations and may alter GI motility.

CLINICAL PRESENTATION

Subjective

Patients with all three subcategories of IBS commonly present with abdominal pain they describe as originating over some area of the colon, with the left lower quadrant (LLQ) being most often affected. The pain can be sharp and burning with cramping or a diffuse, dull ache. The description of the pain usually remains constant for the individual but can vary greatly among the patient population. Pain is often precipitated by eating or stress and can be relieved with a bowel movement or passing of flatus. The pain associated with IBS is usually not significant enough to interfere with sleeping, nor is it great enough to wake the patient from sleep.

More than 50% of patients with IBS describe an overly acute sensory ability with regard to the GI tract and the digestive process. This visceral hypersensitivity is manifested by frequent complaints of abdominal distention, gas, and belching. Many of these symptoms occur 2 hours after having a meal and are often thought to be food intolerances. Patients typically complain of urgency to defecate, abdominal pain, bloating, and gas. Some patients with IBS have upper GI complaints, including dyspepsia, pyrosis, nausea, and vomiting.

The typical presentation is diarrhea alternating with constipation (IBS-M). Periods of predominant constipation can last for months, interrupted by periods of diarrhea and then back to constipation. In IBS-C, patients report that constipation that was once responsive to laxatives has become continuous and that the stool has become harder and decreased in caliber. Many patients complain of a sense of incomplete evacuation and thus repeated attempts at defecation are necessary within a short period of time. Patients with IBS-D complain of frequent, low-volume (less than 200 mL), loose stools. Diarrhea does not normally occur at night; however, it can be exacerbated by eating or stress. Many patients report the passage of large volumes of mucus within the stool. This differs from the mucus occurring with colitis because there is no associated inflammatory process nor is there any blood in the stool, other than if there is an incidental finding of hemorrhoids.

Objective

As with any illness, a thorough and detailed patient history is the key to definitive diagnosis. The physical examination is usually normal except for tenderness in some area of the colon, most often the LLQ and over the umbilicus or epigastric area in those with small bowel involvement. Digital rectal examination is normal but may reveal tenderness and exacerbate symptoms in some individuals.

There is usually no associated weight loss or deterioration in health. History of psychosocial stressors can often be correlated with the onset of symptoms. Key to diagnosis is the lack of other systemic symptoms such as fever, leukocytosis, or bloody stools, which might suggest an organic cause for symptoms.

DIAGNOSTIC REASONING

Diagnostic Tests

There are no definitive tests for IBS; rather, it is diagnosed, based on a careful history and physical examination that reveal the characteristic increase in bowel symptoms with the onset of pain, relief of pain with defecation, heightened sensation of bowel activity, or sense of incomplete defecation.

Initial laboratory testing should include CBC; erythrocyte sedimentation rate (ESR); chemistry panel including electrolytes and serum amylase; urinalysis; and stools for occult blood, ova and parasites, and cultures. Any abnormal laboratory value should prompt further investigation in the direction of the abnormal finding because most laboratory studies in the patient with IBS are normal, and any diagnostic clue as to the cause is helpful. If white blood cells (WBCs) are found in the stool, it suggests an infectious or inflammatory process, not IBS.

Colonoscopy should only be ordered if there is a specific indication such as cancer screening guidelines, blood in the stool, or positive inflammatory markers on the blood tests. Patients with IBS have no abnormalities seen on colonoscopy.

Food intolerances should be ruled out, especially in patients who present with diarrhea and gas as predominant symptoms. Lactase deficiency can be identified with a hydrogen breath test or lactose tolerance test. Other intolerances are identified by removing the most common causative agents from the diet for 3 weeks and then slowly reintroducing them to the diet one at a time.

IBS is no longer a diagnosis of exclusion; thus, the practitioner must direct diagnostic testing as information is received and lends itself toward an organic cause of the symptoms. Patients should not be subjected to endless batteries of expensive and uncomfortable tests in search of an organic disease. Laboratory findings that support a cause other than IBS include elevated ESR, anemia, leukocytosis, blood or WBCs in the stool, or stool volumes greater than 300 mL.

Differential Diagnosis

The differential diagnosis of IBS can include any of the processes in Differential Diagnosis 40.1, with emphasis on the organic GI disorders. Most of the disease processes can be ruled out with careful history and physical examination. Patients presenting with diarrhea as the dominant symptom should have thyroid function tests, 24-hour stool check for fecal fat, stool weight, stool testing for laxative content, stool analysis for microorganisms, and serology for celiac disease. Patients who present with constipation as their predominant symptom may require referral to a specialist who can measure colonic transit time. A careful medication history is necessary for either presentation.

Patients with epigastric pain must have the pain differentiated from that produced by biliary tract pain, ulcerative disease, or malignancies of the stomach and pancreas.

Differential Diagnosis 40.1: Irritable Bowel Syndrome

Food intolerance

- Lactase deficiencies
- Caffeine
- Fermentable carbohydrates
- Artificial sweeteners

Gluten intolerance/celiac disease
Fat or bile acid intolerances
Pathogen-precipitated processes

- Intestinal parasites
- Bacterial overgrowth

Medication-induced alterations in bowel motility

- Laxative abuse
- Magnesium-based antacids
- Antibiotics
- Opiate analgesics

Functional upper gastrointestinal (GI) disorders

- Dyspepsia
- Pyrosis
- Gastroesophageal reflux disease
- Peptic ulcer disease
- Cholelithiasis
- Biliary pain
- GI malignancy

Functional lower GI disorders

- Inflammatory bowel disease
- Crohn's disease
- Ulcerative colitis
- Diverticulitis
- Intestinal obstruction
- Hemorrhoids
- Lower GI malignancy
- Ascites

Endocrine disorders

- Hypothyroidism
- Hyperthyroidism
- Autonomic diabetic neuropathy

Psychological disorders

- Depression
- Anxiety

MANAGEMENT

The initial step to successful management of IBS is making the diagnosis and then identifying the symptom pattern for each individual patient. Based on the symptom pattern of each patient, therapy may include diet, education, and pharmacological and supportive interventions. The patient with IBS requires reassurance and guidance throughout the course of the disease, and a therapeutic relationship between the provider and the patient can reduce symptomatology. Patients must understand that there is no proven treatment and that the therapy is often symptomatic. Much of the recent literature suggests that there is a high degree of placebo effect with varying treatments.

A careful diet history is important in identifying foods that may precipitate symptoms. IBS is often confused with lactose intolerance and can be evaluated by removing lactose from the diet for 2 weeks and monitoring the symptoms. Other foods that are frequently identified in producing IBS syndromes include caffeine, wheat, rye, barley, legumes (and other fermentable carbohydrates), and artificial sweeteners. If any foods are identified that provoke symptoms, they should be eliminated from the diet. Patients who seem to suffer from postprandial discomfort may alleviate symptoms by eating a lower-fat diet that contains more protein. Dietary consultation can be helpful in assisting patients in developing a diet program that is palatable to them.

Diets high in fiber are beneficial regardless of predominant bowel habit. Patients are encouraged to increase their fiber intake to 25 to 30 g per day. The hydrophilic properties of fiber or bulk-producing agents help to prevent excessive hydration or dehydration of stool; thus, fiber is indicated for both diarrhea and constipation symptom presentations. Foods high in fiber include whole grains, cereals, fruits, and vegetables; however, they must be introduced slowly for IBS patients to avoid the sensation of bloating. Bulk-producing agents can be substituted for individuals who choose not to change their diet. Commercially prepared bulk-producing agents are started once a day and increased gradually to three to four times daily. Patients are encouraged to continue treatment for at least 2 months before termination to allow the bowel to adjust to the bulking agents. All patients should try to drink at least eight 8-ounce glasses of water per day. Individuals with constipation as their predominant symptom should be aware that fiber-bulking agents are not overnight laxatives, and they should not abandon this therapy because they did not get overnight results.

There is a moderate level of evidence indicating the use of probiotics is effective for patients with IBS. There are several mechanisms of probiotics in IBS proposed. Probiotics increase the mass of beneficial bacteria in the gut. Some research has shown that some *Lactobacilli* strains may induce the expression of μ-opioid and cannabinoid receptors in the intestinal mucosal barrier, thereby modulating intestinal pain. Probiotics may also reduce intestinal permeability and bacterial translocation. The probiotic that seems to have the best results in multiple clinical trials is VSL#3, one packet orally twice a day and *Bifidobacterium infantis*, one tablet orally twice a day.

Pharmacological treatment is reserved for patients with moderate to severe symptoms and is directed at specific symptoms. Antidiarrheal medications are used only as a temporary measure. When the diarrhea is severe, episodic use of loperamide (Imodium) 2 mg or diphenoxylate (Lomotil) 2.5 to 5.0 mg every 6 hours can be used as needed. Patients who anticipate stressful situations can use antidiarrheal medications prophylactically.

Patients with constipation who have not responded to a high-fiber diet, hydration, exercise, and bulking agents may benefit from intermittent use of stimulant laxatives such as lactulose or magnesium hydroxide. Long-term use of laxatives is discouraged.

Antispasmodic agents have been used successfully in controlling abdominal pain caused by intestinal spasm. Patients who suffer with postprandial pain not responsive to diet therapy can benefit from dicyclomine 10 to 20 mg three to four times a day by mouth or hyoscyamine 0.125 to 0.75 mg twice a day. Peppermint oil may be useful because of its smooth muscle relaxation properties, but it can cause heartburn and dyspepsia (see Complementary Therapies 40.1). Anticholinergics should be avoided in patients with glaucoma and benign prostatic hypertrophy because of the adverse effects and used with caution in older adults.

Complementary Therapies 40.1: Irritable Bowel Syndrome (IBS)

AGENT	INDICATION	ADVERSE REACTIONS AND CONSIDERATIONS
Acupuncture	Abdominal pain and bloating	Small studies show it may be helpful (not large studies).
Evening primrose oil Borage oil	IBS symptoms	Can help with discomfort and bloating, but claims are largely unproven
Probiotics: Lactose acidophilus *Bifidobacterium infantis*	Pain and diarrhea	Some studies have shown them to help with IBS symptoms. No adverse reactions noted
Peppermint oil	IBS-D	May make heartburn worse but can be taken in enteric-coated capsules
Hypnotherapy	IBS symptoms	Several studies have shown a 52% improvement in symptomatology.
Cognitive behavioral therapy (CBT)	IBS symptoms	60%–75% of patients showed improvement in IBS symptoms.

Tricyclic antidepressants and selective serotonin reuptake inhibitors (SSRIs) have been shown to relieve symptoms in some individuals. Individuals with IBS need reassurance and understanding that their disease is chronic. They often benefit from support groups and counseling. Psychiatric interventions that teach behavior modification and biofeedback or that can provide psychotherapy or hypnosis are helpful alternative measures for patients with refractory IBS.

FOLLOW-UP AND REFERRAL

The emotional support provided by regular follow-up appointments is important in the management of patients with IBS. A strong, honest relationship with the patient is necessary to allay fears and prevent unrealistic expectations of the patient regarding their disease. Follow-up is important to encourage preventive behaviors including high-fiber diet, regular exercise, and avoidance of foods that precipitate symptoms. Patients who are not responding to treatment should be referred to a gastroenterologist.

Patients who have IBS are often dissatisfied with treatment because no organic cause of their symptoms can be found. A second opinion is helpful in the management of these individuals; however, they must also be discouraged from continuing to search for organic causes for their symptoms. Referral for psychological intervention tends to be more helpful in patients with intermittent symptoms; those with chronic pain or intractable symptoms usually respond poorly.

Patient Education: Irritable Bowel Syndrome

Care of patients with IBS requires a positive and honest practitioner–patient relationship. Education is important in reducing the number of return visits for symptoms common to patients with IBS. The patients should understand that they have a real intestinal disorder, which is characterized by hypersensitivity to certain foods, hormonal changes, and stressors. Patients should be taught how to recognize these triggers and how to avoid or diminish their effects. Patients should understand that they have a chronic disease but that they do not have a shorter life expectancy because of it. A thorough understanding of the treatment regimen and setting realistic goals regarding treatment is the key to building a positive relationship with the patient. Patients must understand that the goal of treatment is to improve their symptoms, not cure the disease, and that improvement in symptoms can be a time-consuming process.

Dietary education is paramount to relief of the symptoms. Increasing fiber and water intake is an important component of the treatment. Teaching patients how to read nutrition labels will help them quantify the amount of fiber they are consuming daily. Patients must be encouraged to take an active role in their treatment program and understand that elimination of foods that trigger symptoms can be time-consuming and requires their careful attention.

Establishing good bowel habits is also important in the treatment of IBS. A high-fiber diet and increasing water intake to eight 8-ounce glasses per day can help in maintaining a regular bowel program. Patients who suffer with constipation should avoid laxatives and instead practice bowel training. Allowing adequate time after breakfast to sit on the toilet without straining can help establish a daily schedule.

Helping patients recognize and understand environmental stressors that trigger symptoms should be included in patient education. Involving the patient's family is important in establishing a support system. A resource available to patients for both education and support is the International Foundation for Gastrointestinal Disorders (see Resources).

CELIAC DISEASE

Celiac disease, also known as *gluten-sensitive enteropathy* or *celiac sprue,* is a gluten-sensitive autoimmune disorder that affects the small intestinal villous epithelium in individuals with a genetic predisposition and exposure to the cereal protein gluten (gliadin) in wheat, rye, and barley.

EPIDEMIOLOGY AND CAUSES

Celiac disease is a multisystem autoimmune disease caused by an immunological response to gluten. It was once considered a disease in children, but the majority of cases are diagnosed in adulthood. The estimated prevalence in adults is between 0.40% and 0.95% and the actual biopsy-confirmed prevalence is 0.5%. Serological testing indicates that 1:100 patients of Northern European descent have the disease, but only 10% have been diagnosed. It is likely that the incidence and prevalence are much higher. Risk factors for celiac disease include a family history of celiac disease, Down syndrome, HLA-DQ2 or HLA-DQ8, Turner's syndrome, or another genetic-based autoimmune disease such as type 1 diabetes mellitus and thyroiditis.

PATHOPHYSIOLOGY

Celiac disease is a disorder involving the complex interaction of genetic, immune, and environmental factors. The immune reaction is mainly T-cell-mediated, although a humoral immune reaction occurs as well. Celiac disease only develops in people with the haplotype HLA-DQ2 (95%) or HLA-DQ8 (5%). The pathogenesis remains unclear, because 40% of the population has HLA-DQ2 or HLA-DQ8. In susceptible individuals, there is an environmental trigger (gluten) that causes T-cell–mediated autoimmune injury to the intestinal epithelial cells. Antigliadin, antiendomysium, and anti-tTG IgA antibodies develop in the presence of gluten. T cells destroy the mucosal cells, causing inflammation, atrophy, and flattening of the small intestinal villi, usually in the duodenum and jejunum; however, the ileum can be involved as well. The brush border disappears, and there is a decrease in the surface area for nutrient absorption. It should be noted that patients with celiac disease have a threefold increased risk of developing non-Hodgkin's lymphoma.

CLINICAL PRESENTATION

Subjective

Many patients are asymptomatic. Patients may complain of diarrhea, weight loss, dyspepsia, and flatulence. Atypical complaints may be fatigue (resulting from anemia), joint pain, and depressed mood; in females, amenorrhea, difficulty getting pregnant, and early menopause may occur.

Objective

The physical examination may be normal. In severe cases, there may be signs of malabsorption such as muscle wasting, pallor (anemia), reduced subcutaneous fat, ataxia, and peripheral neuropathy (vitamin B_{12} deficiency). Dermatitis herpetiformis occurs as a cutaneous variant of celiac disease in less than 10% of patients. Patients presenting with dermatitis herpetiformis almost always have signs of celiac disease on intestinal biopsy.

DIAGNOSTIC REASONING

Diagnostic Tests

When a patient is suspected of having celiac disease, serological testing for anti-tTG IgA antibodies should be done. This test is inexpensive and has a high sensitivity and specificity. A total IgA should be done as well because 2% of patients with celiac disease also have an IgA deficiency and will test falsely negative. The only way to assess the extent of damage to the intestinal mucosa is through upper GI endoscopic small bowel biopsy and histological examination. This may show partial or complete villous atrophy and intraepithelial lymphocytes.

In lieu of definitive testing and in those with very mild symptoms, patients may try a gluten-free diet and evaluate for symptom improvement. For those already on a gluten-free diet, serology may be normal. In these cases, a gluten challenge can be attempted and the appearance of symptoms evaluated, as well as serological markers determined.

The clinician should consider testing for nutritional deficiencies associated with the malabsorption related to celiac disease. These include hemoglobin, iron, folate, vitamin B_{12}, calcium, and vitamin D.

Differential Diagnosis

Patients with chronic diarrhea, abdominal bloating, and flatulence are often misdiagnosed with IBS. Other diseases that can cause malabsorption of nutrients should be excluded, such as inflammatory bowel diseases (IBDs), Crohn's disease (CD), ulcerative colitis (UC), and microscopic colitis (MC). Symptoms of celiac disease mimic lactose intolerance, which should be considered.

MANAGEMENT

The treatment of choice for patients with celiac disease is a strict gluten-free diet. A referral to a dietitian or nutritionist who specializes in celiac disease is helpful. The risk of developing non-Hodgkin's lymphoma is reduced if the patient can maintain the strict gluten-free diet for more than 5 years. A gluten-free diet usually reduces symptoms and eliminates mucosal damage. For patients who do not have a robust response to a gluten-free diet, other sources of gluten intake should be investigated, such as medications. A dietitian specializing in celiac disease can assist the patient to be sure of complete removal of gluten. Some patients may require more aggressive treatment with immunomodulating agents.

FOLLOW-UP AND REFERRAL

Patients suspected of having celiac disease should be referred to a gastroenterologist for definitive diagnosis, and once that is made, they should see a dietitian specializing in celiac disease. Patients should be monitored for the development of complications or other diseases associated with celiac disease, including Addison's disease, Graves's disease, type 1 diabetes mellitus, myasthenia gravis, scleroderma, atrophic gastritis, and pancreatic insufficiency.

Patient Education: Celiac Disease

Patient education about gluten-free diets is essential to preventing the cellular changes that lead to malabsorption of nutrients. This is best done by a dietitian who specializes in celiac disease. With the expansion of gluten-free products on the market, there is concern about contamination with gluten in processing, and minimizing the use of highly processed convenience foods should be encouraged.

BOWEL OBSTRUCTION

Bowel obstruction is the consequence of any condition that inhibits the normal flow of chyme through the intestinal lumen. It can be complete or partial and can involve any segment of the large or small bowel. Bowel obstruction is considered simple when it results from a mechanical blockage or functional (paralytic ileus) when there is a disruption in motility.

EPIDEMIOLOGY AND CAUSES

Intestinal obstruction can be classified according to the onset. Acute obstruction is sudden and can be caused by torsion, herniation, or intussusception (the slipping of a proximal piece of intestine into the part below it). Chronic obstruction usually indicates a slow, gradual process, often from tumor growth or strictures. Obstructions are also classified according to the degree of obstruction, either complete or partial, and the location of the obstructing lesion. Obstructions can develop within the lumen, as in the case of foreign bodies, tumors, or intraluminal fibrosis. This type of obstruction is considered intrinsic. Conversely, they can be extrinsic or from obstruction that arises outside the intestine. For example, intussusception, torsion (volvulus), fibrosis, and hernia can all cause intestinal obstructions from outside the bowel. Another aspect in the classification of intestinal obstruction is the effect it has on the intestinal wall. A simple obstruction indicates that there is no impairment of the blood supply to that portion of the intestine. A strangulated obstruction means that the lumen is obstructed and that the blood supply is compromised. Bowel obstruction can be a complication of adhesions, which are fibrous bands of tissue that develop after a surgical procedure.

PATHOPHYSIOLOGY

There are numerous physiological alterations, resulting from an intestinal obstruction related to the onset, location of the obstruction, and the amount of intestine proximal to the obstruction. Immediately after the obstruction begins, there is distention of the intestine with sequestration of fluid and gas proximal to the obstruction. The gas is a result of bacterial fermentation and swallowed air. When the intestine begins to distend, its ability to absorb water and electrolytes decreases, and more is left in the lumen, adding to the distention. Sources of water and electrolytes include saliva, gastric juice, bile, and pancreatic juice, as well as intestinal secretions. Within 24 hours, as much as 8 L can accumulate in the intestinal lumen, leading to vomiting. Because of the vomiting and sequestration of fluid and electrolytes in the intestinal lumen, profound fluid and electrolyte imbalances result, leading to dehydration, hemoconcentration, and ultimately hypovolemic shock. The increasing distention causes pressure on the diaphragm, thereby reducing the respiratory volume and leading to atelectasis and pneumonia.

Depending on the location and stage of the intestinal obstruction, alkalosis or acidosis is possible. Alkalosis occurs early in intestinal obstruction or if the obstruction is in the proximal portion of the small bowel. This occurs because gastric juice, which is high in hydrogen ions, does not get absorbed through the intestinal lumen, resulting in loss of the ion. However, later in the course of obstruction, or if the obstruction is more distal, acidosis occurs because alkaline pancreatic secretions and bile cannot be reabsorbed. Potassium is sequestered in the intraluminal fluid, causing hypokalemia, which promotes acidosis and atony of the intestinal wall.

As pressure within the intestinal lumen increases, arterial blood flow may be compromised, leading to ischemia, necrosis, perforation, and peritonitis. Metabolic acidosis is compounded by the buildup of lactic acid that results from the decreased arterial blood flow. Venous return is reduced, leading to edema within the bowel wall. As the edema progresses, there is an increase in capillary permeability, causing fluid to be lost into the peritoneum, contributing to the hypovolemia already present.

CLINICAL PRESENTATION

Subjective

In general, patients with obstruction generally complain of a sudden onset of colicky abdominal pain accompanied by nausea and vomiting. The pain is usually intermittent and corresponds to peristaltic waves. Patients with obstruction at the jejunum or below may have emesis that has changed to a brownish, feculent type of material. They may complain of initial bouts of diarrhea, but this is soon followed by constipation.

In the later stages of obstruction, patients may have constipation and lack of flatulence. It is important to obtain information regarding previous abdominal operations, which may help in the diagnosis of intestinal obstruction. The abdominal pain of small bowel obstruction is usually centered near the umbilicus or in the epigastric area, and vomiting usually occurs early in the disease process. If the arterial circulation to the bowel is compromised, the pain becomes more constant and severe. Perforation produces severe generalized abdominal pain, as well as the classic signs of peritonitis.

Objective

The physical examination should include careful inspection for abdominal scars and the presence of hernias. The patient may show signs of dehydration, including poor skin turgor, dry mucous membranes, sunken eyeballs, and tachycardia. Blood pressure may be elevated, depending on the degree of pain and if there is evidence of strangulation and subsequent ischemia. The degree of abdominal distention depends on the level of obstruction. The more distal the obstruction, the greater the length of proximal intestine, producing greater distention. Also, if the obstruction is in the distal portion of the intestine, vomiting may occur only late in the course of the disease. The abdomen may be tender to palpation if strangulation is present. Bowel sounds are high-pitched and hyperactive; they may be accompanied by rushes, which coincide with the colicky abdominal pain. Patients with strangulation tend to have increased distention, abdominal tenderness, tympany to percussion, and hypoactive or absent bowel sounds. Sometimes a mass is palpable. If perforation has occurred, there may be a short period of pain relief, which is soon followed by increased pain, rebound tenderness, and fever, all suggestive of peritonitis.

Patients presenting with large bowel obstruction usually have a more gradual onset of symptoms, beginning with increasing constipation and abdominal distention. Large bowel obstruction is rare in patients younger than age 50 years. Lower abdominal cramps are unproductive of feces and are painful. Patients report a several-day history of no stools or flatus production. Vomiting occurs if there is an incompetent ileocecal valve or if there is a resultant superimposed small bowel obstruction. The most common cause of large bowel obstruction is carcinoma of the sigmoid colon or diverticulosis.

Physical examination findings include a distended abdomen, particularly over the transverse and descending colon, with the presence of borborygmi. Patients are normally afebrile unless diverticulitis is suspected. There is usually no abdominal tenderness or guarding unless there are areas of ischemic bowel or associated small bowel obstruction with impending cecal perforation. A mass may be palpable over the area of obstruction. Rectal examination reveals an empty vault without tenderness unless there are obstructing rectal carcinomas. The systemic manifestations of large bowel obstructions are much less serious than those caused by small bowel obstruction.

DIAGNOSTIC REASONING

Diagnostic Tests

Before diagnostic testing, patients must be thoroughly examined for any type of hernia that may be precipitating the obstruction. Diagnosis of small bowel obstruction is usually confirmed by supine and upright abdominal x-ray films that reveal a ladder-like distention of the small bowel. Upright films show multiple air-fluid levels within the loops of small bowel, which are the hallmark of small bowel obstruction. Findings indicative of other causes of small bowel obstruction are evidence of a foreign body or an actual mass suggestive of infarcted bowel. Oral contrast with small bowel follow-through can identify areas of partial obstruction. Oral barium studies are contraindicated and must be avoided unless large bowel obstruction has been ruled out.

Laboratory studies include CBC and chemistry profile but are rarely useful for the diagnosis. Leukocytosis can indicate impending ischemia or strangulation of the bowel but is not diagnostic of such. Chemistry evaluation can help with proper fluid and electrolyte replacement. Serum amylase may be elevated and can lead to the erroneous diagnosis of pancreatitis. A finding of metabolic acidosis or an elevated lactic acid level is highly suggestive of intestinal infarction.

Abdominal x-ray films of patients with large bowel obstruction usually show distention of the intestine down to the level of the obstruction. It is important to note the size of the cecum because as the diameter approaches 14 cm, the danger of perforation is imminent. If air is noted under the diaphragm, it is likely that perforation of the cecum or sigmoid colon has occurred.

Differential Diagnosis

The differential diagnosis of small and large bowel obstruction is presented in Differential Diagnosis 40.2. Volvulus, a twisting of the bowel on itself, can happen

Differential Diagnosis 40.2: Bowel Obstruction

Pseudo-obstruction
Toxic megacolon
Twisting of a loop of bowel

- Cecal volvulus
- Sigmoid volvulus

Incarcerated or strangulated hernias

- Abdominal
- Femoral
- Inguinal

Kinking of a loop of bowel

- Adhesions secondary to previous abdominal surgery

Concentric narrowing of the lumen of the intestine

- Neoplasms
- Diverticulitis
- Crohn's disease

Foreign body

- Gallstones
- Ingested objects

Intussusception
Paralytic ileus

suddenly, with loss of blood supply to the area and subsequent ischemia. Cecal volvulus presents as a large gas bubble within the midabdomen or left upper quadrant on abdominal x-ray film. A volvulus of the sigmoid colon usually occurs only in older adults. It typically appears as a "coffee bean" dilation arising from the pelvis. For both cecal and sigmoidal volvulus, a barium enema is done to reveal the precise location of the obstruction.

Colonoscopy and endoscopy are contraindicated in patients suspected of mechanical bowel obstruction because to visualize the intestine, air must be introduced into the colon and can increase the chance of perforation.

MANAGEMENT

All patients with suspected intestinal obstruction should be hospitalized and immediately referred to a surgeon. Therapy must be administered as definitive diagnosis is being obtained. Most patients with a bowel obstruction will require placement of a nasogastric (NG) tube to decrease passage of secretions, aid in decompression, and ameliorate vomiting if present. Rehydration with IV fluids and replacement of electrolytes should be done as indicated by laboratory studies. Placement of an indwelling urinary catheter is necessary to monitor urine output accurately, which is recorded on a daily intake and output sheet.

Treatment of small bowel obstruction proceeds after the aforementioned therapies have been instituted and the patient is medically stabilized. Patients with upper small bowel obstruction are prone to alkalosis and hypokalemia caused by emesis; they must be monitored carefully and given IV fluid and electrolyte replacement as necessary. All medications that can decrease intestinal motility, including anticholinergics, narcotics, and calcium channel blockers, should be discontinued. If strangulation is suspected, the patient should be started on broad-spectrum antibiotic therapy, which provides coverage for anaerobic and gram-negative organisms. Laparotomy is indicated for all patients with complete bowel obstruction.

Patients with a large bowel obstruction are rehydrated and stabilized as previously described. If the patient has evidence suggestive of sigmoidal volvulus, an initial attempt to reduce the volvulus can be made with sigmoidoscopy, but surgery is required if that attempt is unsuccessful. Patients with Crohn's disease, intestinal lymphoma, or diverticulitis with subsequent concentric narrowing of the intestinal lumen may be given a trial of medical therapy specific to the disease process in an attempt to relieve the obstruction before surgical intervention.

Obstructing carcinomas can be treated with surgical resection and anastomosis. (Colon cancer is discussed later in this chapter.) If fecal impaction has been identified as the cause, it can often be removed digitally. If the impaction is barium located within the sigmoid colon, open laparotomy is required for removal. Adhesions can be relieved by surgical intervention; however, the chances are great that they will recur. Hernia reduction is indicated if this is the determined cause of obstruction. All patients who have undergone surgical intervention as definitive therapy must be monitored for paralytic ileus postoperatively.

FOLLOW-UP AND REFERRAL

All patients with suspected bowel obstruction must be referred to a surgeon, who will manage the patient's hospitalization and postoperative care. The prognosis of appropriately treated simple intestinal obstruction is good, with a mortality rate of less than 2%. If strangulation is suspected and intervention is delayed, the mortality rate can be as high as 25%.

Because patients are usually acutely ill, postoperative teaching should be delayed until the patient is more receptive to instruction. Initial follow-up visits should be with the consulting surgeon, who will direct the patient's care until the patient is released to their primary care provider.

Patient Education: Bowel Obstruction

Follow-up of patients with bowel obstruction will be guided by the surgeon. Instructions on care of the incision, including dressing changes and signs and symptoms of infection, are provided before discharge from the hospital. Once the patient has been cleared by the collaborating surgeon, they will return to the primary care setting. Patients should be instructed to report any recurrent abdominal pain with or without vomiting, fever, or problems regarding bowel function. Laxatives should not be taken without consulting the primary care provider first. Stool softeners are prescribed as needed, and patients are encouraged to avoid foods that cause constipation. Patients should refrain from strenuous activity for at least 6 to 8 weeks.

DIVERTICULAR DISEASE

Diverticular disease is the term used to describe the inflammatory changes that occur within the diverticular mucosa of the intestine (diverticulitis), as well as the asymptomatic, uninflamed outpouchings called *diverticulosis*. Diverticula are pouchlike protrusions of the intestinal mucosa that occur most often within the descending and sigmoid segments of the colon. They decrease in frequency in the cecum and rarely are found in the rectum. Diverticula occur infrequently in the small bowel. There are two types, congenital and acquired. Congenital diverticula are situated on the antimesenteric margin of the bowel and consist of the intestinal wall layers. Acquired diverticula occur on the mesenteric margin of the bowel, where the blood vessels enter the bowel wall. A diverticulosis of the small bowel may cause malabsorption and steatorrhea. Diverticula tend to form at weakened areas of the intestinal wall, usually where arterial vessels perforate the colon. The inner layer of these pouchlike protrusions forms a narrow neck, which is continuous with the inner layer of the colon, and the sac herniates through the muscle wall. Most diverticula are asymptomatic and pose a problem only when they become inflamed or bleed. Most diverticula are found incidentally with endoscopy or barium enema (BE). Diverticula vary in diameter from 3 mm to 3 cm.

EPIDEMIOLOGY AND CAUSES

Diverticula are uncommon (less than 20%) in individuals younger than age 40, with the prevalence increasing steadily after that. The prevalence increases to 60% by age 60 years. Diverticular disease is more common in developed nations than in less-developed countries, with estimates of 5% to 45% in Western populations. The incidence is 2,200 to 3,000 per 100,000 people, occurring equally among males and females. Diverticula are a rare finding in pediatric patients.

Although there is no known cause for diverticular disease, many factors have been implicated but not definitively established through research. A lack of dietary fiber may or may not contribute to the disease as once commonly believed. Although high dietary fiber may not prevent diverticular disease, it is beneficial for preventing many other conditions such as colon cancer, obesity, and diabetes. There are a number of predisposing factors in the development of diverticular disease, including obesity, smoking, genetic predisposition, lack of physical activity, and use of such drugs as aspirin and NSAIDs. Other factors believed to contribute to the formation of diverticula include hypertrophy of the segments of the circular muscle of the colon, chronic constipation and straining, irregular and uncoordinated bowel contractions, and weakness of the bowel muscle brought on by aging.

PATHOPHYSIOLOGY

The exact cause of diverticulosis is unknown; therefore, the pathophysiology is based on the speculative findings already mentioned. Diverticula are thought to result from the increased pressure produced with the segmental contraction of the muscular portion of the wall of the colon. This increased pressure causes the herniation of the bowel wall through the weaker points in the muscle layer of the colon, normally occurring along the taeniae at the penetration site of the colonic vasculature. Inflammation occurring around the diverticular sac is often caused by the retention of undigested food and bacteria, which when formed into a hardened mass is called a *fecalith*. This mass in turn can disrupt the blood flow and lead to abscess formation. When the opening of this saclike projection becomes occluded and inflammation ensues, it can progress to the point of rupture. Acute diverticulitis is the result of this localized inflammation within the wall of the colon or peritoneum, causing the characteristic LLQ abdominal pain and tenderness. If the perforation is not localized, the patient can develop acute peritonitis and septic shock.

Fistula formation following acute diverticulitis is the result of a tract forming between the colon and other structures within the abdomen. These fistulas include colovesicular fistulas (urinary bladder), colovaginal fistulas (vagina), entero-enteric fistulas (loop of bowel), and colocutaneous fistulas (peritoneal tissue). Pericolitis is inflammation around the colon, which can result in fibrous strictures and obstruction.

Bleeding is a common complication of diverticulosis and is the most common cause of substantial lower GI bleeding. Postbleeding examinations have discovered that most bleeding occurs from uninflamed rather than inflamed diverticula.

CLINICAL PRESENTATION

Subjective

Approximately 25% of patients with diverticular disease develop symptoms. Patients with diverticulosis characteristically present with pain in the LLQ of the abdomen. Some patients report that the pain is worse after eating, which may be a result of colonic distention, and that the pain is sometimes relieved with a bowel movement or passing flatus. Elimination patterns may alternate between diarrhea and constipation, and there may be associated abdominal distention and tenderness. Diverticulitis may present with bleeding, which can be massive and is not associated with pain or discomfort.

When the diverticula become inflamed, there are the usual signs and symptoms of infection—fever, chills, and tachycardia. Patients typically present with localized pain and tenderness in the LLQ of the abdomen with associated anorexia, nausea, and vomiting. If there is fistula formation, there are symptoms associated with the particular organ involved. Patients may complain of dysuria, pneumaturia (passage of air in the urine), and/or fecaluria (passage of fecal matter in the urine) if there is fistula formation involving the bladder. Patients may be concerned about the development of hematochezia or frank bleeding from the rectum.

Objective

A physical examination reveals tenderness in the LLQ of the abdomen, and—if the patient can tolerate more vigorous examination—a firm, fixed mass may be identified in the area of the diverticula. Patients may have rebound tenderness with involuntary guarding and rigidity. Bowel sounds may initially be hypoactive or can be hyperactive if an obstructive process has developed. Examination of the rectum may reveal tenderness, and the stool is usually positive for occult blood.

DIAGNOSTIC REASONING

Diagnostic Tests

Initial laboratory testing can show mild to moderate leukocytosis, depending on whether the patient presents with diverticulitis or with a more advanced inflammatory process such as peritoneal abscess. The WBC count is usually normal in patients with diverticulosis. Hemoglobin and hematocrit may be low if there is associated rectal bleeding. If there is fistula formation between the diverticula and the bladder, urinalysis may show elevated levels of both WBCs and red blood cells, and urine culture may be positive. Patients with signs suggestive of peritonitis should have a blood culture to assess for bacteremia.

Although diverticulitis can often be diagnosed clinically, a computed tomography (CT) scan with oral contrast is a much more sensitive and accurate test to diagnose suspected diverticulitis, particularly in patients with fever, leukocytosis, or other indicators of peritonitis or sepsis. CT scan can also determine whether there is clinical deterioration by measuring the thickness of the bowel wall and assessing for the development of phlegmon over time using serial examinations. After responding to medical treatment for acute diverticulitis, the patient should have a complete colorectal evaluation (colonoscopy) 4 to 8 weeks after symptom resolution. Colon cancer can mimic symptoms of diverticulitis.

Differential Diagnosis

The differential diagnosis of diverticular disease includes IBS, carcinoma of the colon, IBD, lactose intolerance, pelvic inflammatory disease, ovarian cyst, colitis (infectious or ischemic), appendicitis, and pyelonephritis. Most often, the diagnosis can be made, using the clinical findings and initial noninvasive ultrasonography. Colonoscopy is helpful for definitive diagnosis of diverticulitis and colon surveillance for other colonic disease processes, but the American Gastroenterological Association (AGA) suggests it should not be used until after resolution of the episode of acute diverticulitis.

MANAGEMENT

With early detection and treatment of diverticulitis and the associated complications, the prognosis is good. An incidental finding of uncomplicated diverticulosis requires no further intervention and is usually managed with a high-fiber diet or daily fiber supplementation with psyllium. Treatment of a patient presenting with mild symptoms can often be managed on an outpatient basis with rest and a clear liquid diet. The AGA suggests that antibiotics should not be routinely used because acute diverticulitis is more of an inflammatory process rather than an infectious one and because of concerns about overuse of antibiotics. When antibiotics are deemed necessary, amoxicillin and clavulanate potassium 875/125 mg orally twice a day or metronidazole (Flagyl) 500 mg orally three times a day with trimethoprim/sulfamethoxazole (Bactrim DS) 160/800 mg orally twice a day for 7 to 10 days are given until the patient is afebrile for 3 to 5 days. The symptoms usually subside quickly; then the diet can be advanced to soft, low-roughage and next to high fiber as tolerated. Pain due to spasms can be managed with antispasmodics such as hyoscyamine (Levsin) 0.125 mg every 4 hours, dicyclomine (Bentyl) 20 to 40 mg four times daily, or buspirone (BuSpar) 15 to 30 mg/day.

Patients with more acute illness require hospitalization for IV antibiotics and hydration, analgesia, bowel rest, and possible NG tube placement. If the patient requires analgesia, morphine sulfate should be avoided because it increases intraluminal pressures within the colon and causes or exacerbates the presenting symptoms or perforation. An NG tube should be placed if there is evidence of ileus or if there is intractable nausea and vomiting.

The choice of antibiotics will depend on the severity of the disease process and should cover both gram-negative bacteria and anaerobic organisms. If cultures are obtained from the diverticular abscess, antibiotic coverage can be altered according to the results of the culture. Use and dosage of aminoglycosides should depend on renal function as indicated by the creatine clearance. Patients who are immunocompromised will require broader antibiotic coverage, including an anti-*Pseudomonas* agent. IV antibiotic therapy is normally continued for 7 to 10 days and may be continued orally for an additional 7 to 10 days after discharge, depending on the severity of the illness.

Patients will usually experience relief of symptoms after 72 hours of antibiotic therapy and may resume oral intake as tolerated. Once patients are able to maintain adequate nutrition and hydration, they can be discharged. A colonoscopy should be scheduled to evaluate treatment once the acute phase is resolved.

Patients whose cases are complicated by bleeding that does not subside will require angiography to locate the site of bleeding; they may also require infusion of vasopressin (Pitressin) 0.2 to 0.3 units/min via an intra-arterial catheter placed during the radiographic procedure. If the patient shows signs and symptoms of acute blood loss, transfusion may be indicated. Twenty percent of patients who have experienced diverticular bleeding bleed again within a year.

If there is no improvement or if there is clinical deterioration after 72 hours of medical treatment, surgical intervention may be indicated. Approximately 20% to 30% of patients with the diagnosis of diverticulitis require surgical management. Surgery is usually required for patients who have had several episodes of diverticulitis within 2 years or for those who have had a single episode of diverticulitis with complications. Findings such as generalized peritonitis and large abscesses that do not respond to medical treatment are indications for emergent surgical intervention. The surgical procedure of choice is colon resection. Patients who have undergone the surgical procedure will require routine postoperative care, with emphasis on pain management, pulmonary hygiene, hydration, nutrition, and wound assessment.

Localized abscesses can be drained percutaneously with the assistance of an interventional radiologist. Despite medical treatment, it is estimated that up to 40% of patients with diverticulitis continue to experience symptoms, and approximately one-half of these patients will need surgical intervention.

FOLLOW-UP AND REFERRAL

To evaluate or diagnose diverticular disease, all patients will require colonoscopy at some point during their disease process; therefore, referral to a gastroenterologist is indicated for symptoms that do not respond to treatment after 6 months. Early in the disease process, patients with diverticulitis should consult with a surgeon who can follow them and determine the necessity for emergent surgical intervention if complications should develop. Any patient who has had an acute attack of diverticulitis before age 40 will usually require surgical intervention and should be referred accordingly.

Patient Education: Diverticular Disease

Patients diagnosed with diverticular disease will need to modify their diets with an emphasis on increasing the amount of dietary fiber. Although the current research is inconclusive as to whether a low-fiber diet causes diverticulitis, most people in the United States do not get the recommended 25 to 35 g of fiber per day. Diet changes should be made slowly to avoid bloating, gas, and other GI problems that may discourage compliance. Fiber can be increased by eating bran, fresh fruits, vegetables, and whole grains. The goal of diet therapy is to avoid constipation and straining during bowel movements, which can further increase intraluminal pressures and cause complications.

Patients should also be instructed to drink at least eight 8-ounce glasses of water a day to have regular, soft bowel movements. If patients continue to have constipation despite increasing their fiber and fluid intake, a bulk-forming laxative such as psyllium (FiberCon, Metamucil) can be added.

Symptoms recur in approximately one-third of patients with diverticulitis who were initially treated with medical management. Therefore, all patients with diverticular disease should be instructed to return for follow-up if they develop signs and symptoms of infection or other associated complications of diverticulitis. Patients should understand that despite adherence to diet and medication, they may have another attack.

INFLAMMATORY BOWEL DISEASE

Inflammatory bowel disease describes a group of chronic, heterogeneous, immunological diseases that manifest in intestinal inflammation. The two most common IBDs are UC and CD, but MC is increasing in prevalence and includes collagenous colitis (CC) and lymphocytic colitis (LC). IBD is characterized by exacerbations and remissions that are experienced throughout an individual's lifetime and therefore result in significant disruption in the quality of life. The Patient's Voice 40.1 describes the impact of CD on a 39-year-old woman with a 20-year history of the disease.

UC and CD are separate diseases that share similar characteristics and causes, and the same pharmacological agents are used for both. UC involves only the mucosal surface of the colon, which ultimately results in friability, erosions, and bleeding. It occurs most often in the rectosigmoid area but can involve the entire colon but not the small bowel. CD is characterized by segmental or patchy transmural inflammation of the bowel wall involving

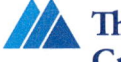

The Patient's Voice 40.1: Crohn's Disease

As a 39-year-old woman with a 20-year history of severe Crohn's disease (CD), I remain undecided as to which has been most difficult to deal with: the symptoms of the disease—uncontrolled diarrhea, bowel incontinence, malnutrition, pain, bloating, and flatulence, to name a few; the results of the symptoms—fatigue, malaise, anemia, anorexia, anxiety, embarrassment, guilt, fear, and shame; or the constant discipline necessary to incorporate lifestyle changes instrumental to the adaptation and management of this debilitating disorder—diet, stress elimination, exercise, rest, vitamin supplementation, and prescription compliance. Experience with CD has taught me that health and wellness is a personal choice and that whatever intestinal ailments or conditions one struggles with, incorporating the dietary changes necessary to promote wellness through nutrition, particularly raw, fresh fruit and vegetable juices, should be part of a comprehensive approach to achieving optimal health.

any portion of the GI tract from the mouth to the anus. Disease of the terminal ileus is present in about 80% of patients with CD, and in 20% of the cases only the colon is involved.

EPIDEMIOLOGY AND CAUSES

The incidence and prevalence of these diseases vary widely, which supports a multifactorial theory in the development of the disease. Research supports a genetic predisposition for IBD, even though less than 15% of cases are familial. A gene on chromosome 16 that encodes the protein nucleotide-binding oligomerization domain 2 (NOD2) has variants that are found in about 62% of patients with CD. Genes associated with IBD have also been found on chromosomes 10 and 7 that encode for proteins that mediate epithelial cell–cell interactions and the transport of molecules into and out of cells. Another factor is the ability of bacteria in the gut to cause inflammation related to abnormal T-cell reactions to commensal microflora and other luminal antigens. The intestinal epithelium plays an important role in the immune response, interacting with microbes and antigens and communicating with immune cells triggering the production and secretion of cytokines and chemokines. The role of the gut microbiome in the development of IBD is currently being researched.

The overall incidence of IBD is about equal in males and females; specifically, LC affects both sexes equally, but CC is 20 times more common in females. The age at onset for UC and CD is frequently in early adulthood but can be anywhere from age 10 to 40 years, whereas microscopic colitis is more common in people over 40 years of age. The incidence of both CD and UC is increasing globally and ranges from 3 to 300 per 100,000 people.

Table 40.2 compares UC and CD.

PATHOPHYSIOLOGY

Ulcerative Colitis

The inflammatory process of UC is confined to the mucosa of the colon and rectum and begins with neutrophil infiltration at the base of the crypt of Lieberkühn.

TABLE 40.2 Comparison of Ulcerative Colitis and Crohn's Disease

Feature	Ulcerative Colitis	Crohn's Disease
HISTORY		
Age at onset	Age 10–40 years	Age 15–25 years; age 50–80 years
Etiology	Unknown	Unknown
Genetic tendency	Familial tendency	Familial tendency
Nicotine use	Nonsmoker	Smoker
ASSESSMENT FINDINGS		
Serological	+ (positive) for antineutrophil cytoplasmic antibodies (pANCA)	– (negative) pANCA
Fever/malaise	With severe disease	Common
Weight loss	Uncommon	Common
Rectal bleeding	Common	Dependent on location of lesion; occurs in about 50% of cases
Abdominal pain	Usually mild	Can be moderate to severe
Abdominal mass	Negative	May be present
Perianal lesions	Absent	May develop fissures, abscesses
Fistulas	Absent	Common
Strictures	Uncommon	Common
COMMON		
Rectal involvement	Always	50% of the cases
Distribution	Confined to colon; continuous	Any portion of gastrointestinal tract; discontinuous, skipped lesions
Mucosa	Friable, granular	Cobblestone appearance
Ulceration	Crypt abscess development	Aphthous or linear ulcers
Inflammation	Surface involvement	Transmural involvement

The disease most often occurs in the rectum and sigmoid colon. The mucosa in this area is thinner and has a dark red, velvety appearance in susceptible individuals. The cytokines released from the macrophages and neutrophils during the inflammatory response are responsible for tissue damage. Ulcers form in the eroded tissue, and abscesses form in the crypts. These abscesses become necrotic and ulcerate. The muscularis mucosa becomes edematous and thickened, narrowing the lumen of the colon. Bleeding, cramping pain, and the urge to defecate result from the mucosal destruction. The characteristic stool is diarrhea that contains blood and purulent mucus. There is also a loss of the absorptive surface, leading to large volumes of watery diarrhea. Fecal leukocytes are always present with active colitis. Absence of these inflammatory changes within the deeper layers of the intestinal mucosa helps to differentiate UC from other inflammatory processes. Patients diagnosed with severe UC are at risk for a perforated colon. They require close observation and should have consultation with a surgeon.

Crohn's Disease

CD is an inflammatory process that begins in the submucosa of the intestine and gradually spreads to involve the mucosa and serosa. Any portion of the GI tract can be affected, but 80% of patients have small bowel involvement. There are abnormalities in the intestinal immune response where proinflammatory cytokines, interleukins, and tissue necrosis factor produce areas of tissue damage. Typically, some haustra segments are affected but others are not, creating a pattern called *skip lesions*. The ulcerations form longitudinal and transverse fissures, extending inflammation into Peyer's patches and the lymphoid tissue. The typical lesion is granulomatous with projections of inflamed tissue surrounded by scar tissue. It is described as a "cobblestone" appearance. With progression of the disease, fibrosis thickens the bowel wall, narrowing the lumen. Serosal inflammation causes bowel loops to adhere to one another, contributing to transmural inflammation, ulceration, and fibrosis, which can lead to obstruction, fistulas, and shortening of the bowel.

Individuals with IBD are at greater risk for developing colorectal cancer than the general population. Clinical findings suggest that carcinoma is less common in patients with CD than with UC and is attributed to the treatment of CD with colectomy.

Microscopic Colitis

Some research indicates that LC and CC may be different phases of the same disease. In LC, lymphocytes infiltrate the colonic epithelium. Lymphocyte infiltration also occurs in CC along with a thickening of the subepithelial collagen band or table (a band of collagen below the epithelial cells). Patients with CC have increased levels of immunoreactive prostaglandin E2 and nitric oxide (NO) in the colonic epithelium, which is believed to contribute to secretory diarrhea. Other processes have been implicated, such as increased mucosal secretion of transforming growth factor-1 and endothelial growth factor. Although a definitive cause for microscopic colitis has not been found, there is a strong correlation between consumption of NSAIDs and the risk of CC. Other drugs, including aspirin, ranitidine, PPIs, and ticlopidine, are associated with microscopic colitis.

CLINICAL PRESENTATION

Subjective

Individuals with mild forms of UC commonly report four or fewer loose bowel movements per day associated with abdominal cramps that are relieved with defecation, small amounts of blood and mucus in the stool, and sometimes tenesmus. Usually there are no associated systemic symptoms. With moderate disease, patients have four to six loose stools a day containing more blood and mucus. They also have systemic symptoms such as tachycardia, mild fever, and weight loss, and they may have mild edema, depending on the serum albumin level. Severe disease manifests with more frequent bloody bowel movements (six to 10 per day); abdominal pain and tenderness; and symptoms of anemia, hypovolemia, and impaired nutrition.

The most common presenting symptoms of CD are abdominal cramping and tenderness, fever, anorexia, weight loss, spasm, flatulence, and right lower quadrant (RLQ) pain or mass. Individuals may report an increase in symptomatology during periods of stress or emotional upset or after meals consisting of poorly tolerated foods such as fatty or spicy foods or milk. Stools are soft or semiliquid. Observable blood is found in the stool intermittently; when present, it occurs in a larger amount than with UC. Because of the loss of healthy bowel mucosa, there may be insufficient resorption of bile salts, causing steatorrhea (foul-smelling, fatty stools). CD can involve the entire thickness of the bowel wall, causing microperforations and symptoms of acute localized peritonitis, which can mimic appendicitis or diverticulitis. If there is fistula formation, these symptoms may dominate the clinical picture.

The most common presenting symptom for MC is protracted, nonbloody diarrhea that has been present from several months to 2 to 3 years. Forty percent of patients with CC complain of weight loss. Abdominal cramping and fecal incontinence are reported less often than diarrhea.

Several patterns of symptom onset for UC and CD are recognized: (1) gradual, with vague abdominal discomfort, malaise, cramping, and bloody, mucopurulent stools; (2) abrupt, with frequent periods of bloody diarrhea, anorexia, fever, and weight loss; and (3) abrupt and fulminating, with sudden, violent diarrhea occurring nocturnally, high fever, intense abdominal cramping, signs of peritonitis, weight loss, and anorexia. Stools may contain blood, mucus, and/or pus. Typically, CD has a more insidious and gradual onset. Individuals often experience intermittent symptoms long before presenting for medical attention. The disease is characterized by periods of acute exacerbation alternating with complete remission.

If the UC is confined to the rectal or sigmoid area, the stools can be normal or hard and dry; however, the rectum will continue to dispel mucus containing both red and white blood cells. As the disease process moves proximally, the stools become looser. Patients may report eating less to decrease the frequency of bowel movements, which leads to more pronounced nutritional deficiencies.

Objective

On physical examination, there may be tenderness in the LLQ or across the entire abdomen, often accompanied by guarding and abdominal distention. A digital rectal examination should be performed to assess for anal and perianal inflammation, rectal tenderness, and blood in the stool. Depending on the severity of the disease and the extent of potential complications, signs and symptoms of ileus and peritonitis may be found. Perirectal abscesses and fistulas are not associated with UC.

The physical examination may reveal abdominal tenderness with a tubular, tender mass in the RLQ. Fifty percent of individuals with CD have perianal involvement, including anal fissures, perianal fissures, and edematous, pale skin tags, which are often misdiagnosed as prolapsed hemorrhoids. Extraintestinal findings include episcleritis, erythema nodosum, nondeforming peripheral arthritis, and axial arthropathy, which may be more apparent than bowel symptoms and should prompt the practitioner to look for a diagnosis of CD.

CD tends to present in one of four patterns: (1) inflammation, RLQ abdominal pain, and tenderness, often presenting as appendicitis; (2) obstruction, fibrosis, and stenotic changes within the bowel, causing recurrent obstruction associated with severe colic, abdominal distention, constipation, and vomiting; (3) diffuse jejunoileitis involving the jejunum and ileum and characterized by both inflammation and obstruction, which can result in malnutrition and chronic debility; and (4) abdominal fistulas and abscesses normally occurring late in the disease process and causing fever, generalized wasting, and abdominal masses. Although CD is uncommon among children, those with CD often present with extraintestinal symptoms, especially growth retardation, fever of unknown origin, and anemia.

Generally, patients with MC have no abnormalities on physical examination. Patients with severe and prolonged disease may have signs of dehydration, malnutrition, and weight loss.

DIAGNOSTIC REASONING

Diagnostic Tests

Definitive diagnosis is made by correlating the symptoms with the history and physical examination. Results of diagnostic testing help differentiate UC from CD. Stool analysis and cultures are obtained to rule out bacterial, fungal, or parasitic infection as the cause for diarrhea. The stool is also examined for mucus and blood, which are normally present with UC.

Patients with CD who have small intestine involvement may also require evaluation for additional conditions caused by malabsorption and vitamin and mineral deficiencies, including anemia secondary to bleeding and iron deficiency and macrocytic anemia, which result from inflammation of the terminal ileum and poor absorption of folate. In addition, patients should be evaluated for hypocalcemia and vitamin D deficiency, hypoalbuminemia, and steatorrhea resulting from bile salt deficiency. Liver function tests may be helpful in screening for primary sclerosing cholangitis and other liver problems associated with IBD. Fluid and electrolyte disturbances are common in both diseases because of the extracellular fluid loss. CD may also present with an elevated WBC count and ESR, as well as a prolonged prothrombin time.

Diagnosis of acute UC is best made by sigmoidoscopy. Barium enema should not be performed because of the risk of precipitating toxic megacolon. Early in the disease, the mucous membrane is granular, friable, and edematous, with loss of the normal vascular pattern. In many patients, there may be scattered areas of hemorrhage that bleed with minor trauma. The resulting ulcerations develop after the mucosa breaks down, leaving the mucous membranes dotted with numerous bleeding and pus-oozing ulcers. Severe disease is characterized by copious amounts of purulent exudate. Colonoscopy should be avoided in individuals with severe colitis or deep ulcerations because of the risk of perforation. Although there are periods of remission, sigmoidoscopy shows some degree of friability and granulation in patients with UC. Biopsy results reveal chronic inflammation.

Plain films of the abdomen can help estimate the severity and proximal extent of the disease by demonstrating loss of haustration and the absence of formed stool within the diseased sections of bowel.

Every patient with UC requires a colonoscopy to determine the extent of the disease, but in order to avoid perforation, this is reserved for patients who have shown improvement on treatment. Ulcers suggestive of UC are shallow and confluent; they are erythematous, edematous, and friable, causing them to bleed easily. Individuals with UC usually have disease that begins in the rectum and extends proximally, without "skipped areas."

Definitive diagnosis of CD is normally based on clinical manifestations and supporting endoscopic, pathological, and radiographic evidence. The earliest manifestations of CD are aphthous and linear ulcers, which are best visualized with barium upper GI series with small bowel follow-through, depending on the location of the lesions. The ileum is stiff and nodular, and the lumen shows signs of thickening and narrowing. In advanced disease, the upper GI tract with small bowel follow-through may show the characteristic "string sign"—ileal strictures and evidence of bowel loop separation resulting from marked circumferential inflammation and fibrosis.

Colonoscopy reveals ulcers that are either minor erosions or deep longitudinal fissures. Segmental transverse fissuring creates the characteristic cobblestone appearance and is usually found above the rectum and rectosigmoid areas. Biopsies may be obtained to rule out pseudopolyposis, adenomatosis, or cancer. CT is often used in the evaluation of CD to identify bowel wall thickening or abscess formation. If an abscess is found, CT may be useful for guided drainage of the abscess.

MC is confirmed on colonoscopy with biopsy. In most patients with MC, the mucosa appears normal on colonoscopy. Biopsy in individuals with CC reveals a thick subepithelial collagenous deposit; in those with LC, there is a pronounced intraepithelial lymphocytic inflammation. An infiltrate of plasma cells, lymphocytes, and eosinophils in the lamina propria caused by chronic inflammatory may be seen on histological examination. There may be epithelial cell flattening, subepithelial blebs, and denuded epithelium. CC has the same histological features of LC, along with a thickened subepithelial collagen layer in the lamina propria.

Differential Diagnosis

Differential diagnosis of UC must begin with the exclusion of an infectious cause for the colitis before treatment is initiated. Enteric infection is ruled out through fresh stool culture for ova and parasites. Infectious colitis may be caused by *Entamoeba histolytica, Campylobacter enteritidis,* and *Shigella* species and *Chlamydia* species can cause acute colitis, which is difficult to differentiate from UC, both clinically and endoscopically. The distinction must be made because treatment with corticosteroids can be catastrophic. Obtaining a thorough travel, sexual, and antibiotic history is imperative. If the individual has had antibiotic exposure within the last 30 days, a stool sample to test for *Clostridium difficile* should be obtained. Homosexual men practicing anal intercourse should be screened for infectious proctitis as a cause of colitis. Individuals with HIV are susceptible to many opportunistic infections, which must also be considered as part of the differential diagnosis and treatment.

Older adults, patients with a history of coagulation disorders, and young females using oral contraceptives should be examined for ischemic colitis. Radiographic findings of "thumbprinting" and segmental distribution of lesions are typical of ischemic colitis. Although colon cancer rarely presents with fever and purulent diarrhea, it should be ruled out as a cause for bloody diarrhea.

As with UC, evaluation of CD must begin with ruling out infectious enteritis as the source of colitis. Enteric tuberculosis and fungal disease must also be considered in the differential diagnosis of CD. *Yersinia enterocolitica* enteritis, although a self-limiting infection, may require a 3-month follow-up examination because the initial clinical presentation is so similar to that of CD.

Although only 20% of patients with CD have disease that is limited to the colon, differentiation from UC must be made. CD is the more likely diagnosis when there is evidence of perianal disease and rectal bleeding. RLQ pain without a history of chronic bowel symptomatology may mimic appendicitis, pelvic inflammatory disease, ectopic pregnancy, ovarian cysts, or tumors; all of these must be ruled out in the differential diagnosis of CD. Both diverticular disease and ischemic colitis can present with the segmental involvement and luminal stricturing characteristic of CD.

Many drugs have been implicated in drug-induced colitis, the most common being NSAIDs and antibiotics. Many individuals who routinely take NSAIDs may have damage to the GI tract characterized by bloody diarrhea and weight loss. Some antibiotics alter the bowel flora, allowing overgrowth of pathogens such as *C. difficile,* which produces a toxin that is damaging to the bowel mucosa and can cause bloody diarrhea, abdominal pain, and weight loss. Although initial radiographic studies may be similar to those for CD, endoscopic examination reveals a more segmental distribution of lesions, and biopsy results are not supportive of inflammatory disease.

Colon cancers can cause bloody diarrhea; however, they usually do not have the associated fevers, leukocytosis, and purulent discharge. Diverticulitis can cause abdominal pain, fever, leukocytosis, obstruction, and diarrhea; however, endoscopic evaluation reveals the characteristic mucosal herniations in the bowel wall.

Patients with MC are often misdiagnosed with IBS-D. Other differential diagnoses include celiac disease, ischemic colitis, infectious colitis, hyperthyroidism CD, UC, and laxative abuse.

MANAGEMENT

Traditionally, the main target of treatment for IBD has been symptom control, but this approach fails to prevent disease progression. Symptoms do not necessarily correlate with the level of inflammation found on endoscopic examination. Early intervention primarily with immunosuppressants and/or biologics has been shown to provide better mucosal healing, induction of a steroid-free remission, and prevention of hospitalizations. Currently, treatment is directed to the therapeutic targets of mucosal healing, histological healing, and inflammatory biomarkers. These objective parameters are superior to the signs of clinical remission. The traditional mainstays of treatment for IBD continue to be used for symptom control in conjunction with immunomodulating agents and biologics.

Ulcerative Colitis

According to the new therapeutic target treatment, initial treatment should include immunomodulating drugs and/or biologics, as well as the more traditional treatments of 5-aminosalicylic acid (5-ASA) and corticosteroids. Nutrition counseling is also helpful. Patients should avoid anything that makes their symptoms worse, usually caffeine, raw fruits, vegetables, and other foods high in fiber. These foods can cause trauma to the already inflamed mucosal surface and exacerbate symptoms. Some patients may benefit from a lactose-free diet, but this is not recommended unless a trial produces symptomatic relief. A bland diet that is high in calories and protein yet low in fat can help control diarrhea and flatulence and maintain nutrition and weight. Parenteral nutrition may be necessary in individuals with severe anorexia or uncontrollable diarrhea.

Antidiarrheal medications should be avoided in the acute phase but can be helpful for patients with mild symptoms. Patients with mild to moderate diarrhea may benefit from diphenoxylate with atropine (Lomotil) 2.5 to 5.0 mg orally twice a day and up to four times per day, loperamide (Imodium) 2 mg after each bowel movement, or codeine 15 to 30 mg orally every 4 to 6 hours.

Disease that is limited to the rectosigmoid area can often be successfully treated with topical mesalamine (see Drugs Commonly Prescribed 40.3). Steroid enemas and foams (e.g., hydrocortisone [Cortifoam] 100 mg) should be administered nightly for 2 weeks. If effective, this treatment will bring about remission in 70% of initial episodes of idiopathic UC. Patients may then taper the dose over the next week to prevent the side effects associated with rapid steroid withdrawal. Mesalamine (Rowasa), a form of 5-ASA, is more expensive; it is sometimes more effective than hydrocortisone for patients with refractory or left-sided colitis and is available in enema and suppository forms. Oral preparations of 5-ASA medications (e.g., Asacol, Azulfidine) help maintain remission after the enemas have been discontinued. Sulfasalazine (Azulfidine) contains 5-ASA and sulfapyridine. It is the sulfapyridine that is responsible for many of the side effects of sulfasalazine. Other formulations of 5-ASA preparations (mesalamine) lack the sulfapyridine and have fewer adverse effects and are better tolerated for prolonged courses of treatment. Subsequent exacerbations of UC tend to show increasing resistance to therapy, requiring longer treatment regimens. Budesonide (Entocort) is an oral corticosteroid with a high first-pass loss in the liver, facilitating less systemic activity and more topical anti-inflammatory activity. An enteric-coated preparation of budesonide (Uceris) has delayed release and delivery throughout the colon.

Glucocorticoids are especially helpful in controlling the extracolonic manifestations of UC, which include peripheral arthritis, ankylosing spondylitis, erythema nodosum, anterior uveitis, and pyoderma gangrenosum. Peripheral arthritis and the skin lesions often parallel the course of the disease. Oral prednisone (Prelone), up to 40 to 60 mg in single or divided doses, must be tapered and not discontinued abruptly.

Severe or fulminant UC is manifested by 10 or more bloody stools per day, abdominal tenderness, fever, colon dilation, and tachycardia. Patients often require hospitalization for these symptoms. Patients with severe disease must be monitored closely for the development of toxic megacolon and colonic perforation. Any patient who does not show improvement after 7 to 10 days of maximized therapy should be considered for surgical intervention. Subtotal or total colectomy is often required to prevent perforation of the bowel and its complications. Some individuals may require restoration of their fluid volume and electrolytes, as well as blood transfusions, depending on the severity of the diarrhea and bleeding.

Immunosuppressive (immunomodulating) agents—azathioprine (Imuran), cyclosporine, and metabolite 6-mercaptopurine (6MP)—are used in cases of UC that are unresponsive to other medical treatment and in patients who are not surgical candidates. The long-term use of immunosuppressive agents for relapse prevention must be balanced with the increased risk of developing a malignancy. Most commonly, these agents are used to allow patients to reduce the maintenance dosage of glucocorticoids. For disease that is unresponsive to other therapies, anti–tumor necrosis factor (TNF) agents can be used. These include infliximab (Remicade) 5 mg/kg and adalimumab (Humira) administered subcutaneously 160 mg at week 1, 80 mg at week 2, and then maintenance of 40 mg every other week beginning at week 4. Anti-integrins are monoclonal antibodies that have been shown to be effective for inducing and maintaining remission in patients with UC. These include natalizumab (Tysabri) 300 mg IV over 1 hour once every 4 weeks and vedolizumab (Entyvio) 300 mg IV at weeks 0, 2, and 6 for induction and then a maintenance dose of 300 mg IV every 8 weeks. Anti-interleukin (IL)-12/23 antibody treatment with ustekinumab (Stelara) is used in patients with moderate to severe UC and CD. There is an induction dose given IV, calculated based on the patient's weight (5 to 7 mg/kg), and it is then followed every 8 weeks with a 90-mg subcutaneous injection. There has not been shown to be an increase in severe infections or malignancy with this treatment.

Individuals who progress to fulminant disease are at risk for developing toxic megacolon—an atonic and

Drugs Commonly Prescribed 40.3: Inflammatory Bowel Disease

DRUG	INDICATION	ADVERSE REACTIONS AND PRESCRIBING CONSIDERATIONS
5-Aminosalicylic Acid Agents		
Mesalamine (Asacol) Sulfasalazine (Azulfidine)	Ulcerative colitis (UC)	Research indicates that these drugs are of little value in Crohn's disease (CD). Continue to be used for UC. Headache, malaise, cramping and flatulence. Rare: pneumonitis, pericarditis, pancreatitis, interstitial nephritis
Antidiarrheals		
Loperamide (Imodium) Diphenoxylate with atropine (Lomotil)	Diarrhea First-line treatment for microscopic colitis (MC)	Do not use in acute UC. Constipation may occur. Do not use if toxic megacolon occurs
Corticosteroids		
Prednisone Budesonide (Entocort) or (Uceris)	Moderate to severe disease In severe cases of MC	Drastically suppresses clinical symptoms. This preparation is released in the ileum and induces remission in 50%–70% of cases of CD. Treatment is for 8–16 weeks, followed by a 2- to 4-week taper in 3-mg increments.
Hydrocortisone (Cortifoam, Anucort, Rectocort HC)	Initial treatment	Topical rectal application in suppository, foam, or enema. Can be very irritating to the rectal mucosa. Cost is about $800 for a 4-week supply.
Immunomodulating Drugs		
Azathioprine (Imuran) Mercaptopurine (Purinethol) Methotrexate (MTX)	Moderate to severe disease that does not respond to corticosteroid therapy (CD, UC, MC)	This class of drugs can cause bone marrow suppression, and patients are at risk for life-threatening infections.
Anti-TNF Therapies (Biological Therapy)		
Infliximab (Remicade) Adalimumab (Humira) Golimumab (Simponi) Certolizumab (Cimzia)	Moderate to severe disease	This class of drugs causes bone marrow suppression and increases the risk for life-threatening infections. These drugs are administered IV or subcutaneously.
Anti-Integrins (Monoclonal Antibodies)		
Natalizumab (Tysabri) Vedolizumab (Entyvio)	CD patients who do not respond to antitumor necrosis factor therapies CD, UC, and MC patients who do not respond to other treatments	Natalizumab can cause progressive multifocal leukoencephalopathy in immunocompromised patients. It should not be used with concomitant immunosuppressants. Vedolizumab does not have this adverse effect. Common side effects include fatigue and allergic reactions.
Anti-IL-12/23 Antibodies		
Ustekinumab (Stelara)	Moderate to severe CD and UC	Human IG_1 monoclonal antibody. No increase in severe infections or malignancy

distended, thin-walled colon. Approximately 1% to 2% of patients with UC develop this complication, which is characterized by fever, sepsis, electrolyte imbalances, hypoalbuminemia, and dehydration. Definitive diagnosis is made when radiographic measurement of the midtransverse colon shows it to be dilated to greater than 6 cm. The patient is at risk for perforation until the dilation is reduced. If medical reversal is not accomplished within 48 hours, surgical intervention is indicated, and consultation should be made early.

Patients with toxic megacolon should receive nothing by mouth, an NG tube should be placed for intermittent suction, and all antidiarrheal medications should be discontinued. Fluid and electrolyte disturbances, particularly hypokalemia, should be corrected, and total parenteral nutrition may be required until the patient is able to tolerate oral food and fluids. Broad-spectrum antibiotics for peritonitis prophylaxis and parenteral administration of glucocorticoids are indicated. Patients must be monitored closely for signs and symptoms of perforation, which may be blunted because of the large doses of glucocorticoids. Loss of hepatic dullness on percussion may be the first sign of perforation. Daily abdominal x-ray films are necessary to assess colon distention and the presence of free air within the abdomen.

Over the long term, 25% of those with UC will require surgery. Emergent total colectomy is indicated for patients who do not respond to intensive medical therapy within 48 hours or who have massive hemorrhage or perforation. Surgical intervention is sometimes done in stages for patients who are severely ill. The most common procedure is the proctocolectomy with a Brooke ileostomy; it is a curative and functional procedure. Surgical intervention is also considered in patients who require large maintenance doses of glucocorticoids or are experiencing quality-of-life issues caused by severe diarrhea or in children who are manifesting signs of growth retardation.

Crohn's Disease

Treatment of CD parallels that of UC including sulfasalazine (Azulfidine); however, 5-ASA medications have not been shown through research to be of any benefit. Glucocorticoids are used when initial treatment fails and for patients with moderate to severe disease. There is no curative therapy for CD; therefore, treatment is targeted to suppress the inflammatory process and provide symptomatic relief of complications. The patient with CD has a much greater incidence of relapse once medications are discontinued; 70% of patients started on steroid therapy must remain on the therapy to prevent relapse. Oral prednisone 40 to 60 mg/day is used as initial outpatient treatment. Once maximal response has been achieved, the dose can be tapered over 2 to 4 months. Some patients may require a daily maintenance dose of 5 to 10 mg/day. As with UC, steroids are often helpful in managing the extraintestinal manifestations of the disease. Patients with disease within the rectum may benefit from enema preparations as well.

Sulfasalazine (Azulfidine) remains a common treatment for CD; however, new research is showing that it may have little value. There is a high incidence of intolerance, including nausea, anorexia, rash, and headache. When it is used, the initial dose of sulfasalazine for treatment of mild to moderate disease of the colon or ileocolon is 500 mg twice daily; the dose can be increased to 3 to 4 g/day. Clinical improvement is usually noted in 3 to 4 weeks, at which time the medication can be tapered to 2 to 3 g/day for 3 to 6 months. Sulfasalazine interferes with folic acid absorption, so patients should receive folic acid 1 mg/day while taking this medication.

The use of metronidazole has been effective in patients who are intolerant of sulfasalazine, although metronidazole's use is also limited by adverse effects, including nausea, anorexia, metallic taste, furry tongue, and paresthesias. Although the mechanism of action is not clear, metronidazole has been effective in the treatment of perianal disease and in controlling Crohn's colitis. There is a high rate of relapse, however, once the drug has been discontinued. Other antibiotics such as ciprofloxacin, ampicillin, and tetracycline have been effective in controlling CD ileitis and ileocolitis.

The use of immunosuppressive medications has been shown to be effective in patients with CD who are unresponsive to other treatments, in individuals dependent on high-dose steroids, or in those with nonhealing fistulas. The clinical benefit of 6MP (the active metabolite of azathioprine [Imuran]) can take up to 3 months before being realized. These drugs can cause bone marrow suppression and pancreatitis; therefore, patients must be monitored frequently for leukopenia. The risk for developing malignancy is low but still must be considered. Patients remain on treatment for up to 2 years; in extremely refractory cases, treatment is continued indefinitely. Cyclosporine (Neoral, Sandimmune), an immunosuppressant drug typically used to prevent organ transplant rejection, is helpful in patients with steroid-resistant CD. Its use remains experimental, and it should be administered by practitioners who are experienced in caring for patients with complicated CD.

Other immunomodulating agents such as TNF-alpha blockers, including infliximab (Remicade), adalimumab (Humira), and certolizumab (Cimzia), are proving helpful in patients with moderate to severe CD, as is anti-IL-23 antibody (Stelara). Rapid improvement is seen when infliximab is used initially. The regimen includes an initial dose of infliximab 5 mg/kg followed by repeat doses again at 2 weeks and 6 weeks, with maximal response seen in the first 2 weeks. Adalimumab (Humira) by subcutaneous injection is prescribed at 160 mg at week 1, 80 mg at week 2, and then maintenance of 40 mg every other week beginning at week 4. The side effects include infusion-related reactions and hypersensitivity reactions as a result of the development of antinuclear antibodies. This can be reduced by concomitant administration of other immunosuppressive medications. Serious infections may develop while patients are being treated with this medication. Anti-integrins include natalizumab (Tysabri) 300 mg IV over 1 hour once every 4 weeks and vedolizumab (Entyvio) 300 mg IV at weeks 0, 2, and 6 for induction and then a maintenance dose of 300 mg IV every 8 weeks. When using anti-IL-12/23 antibodies (Stelara), there is an induction dose given IV and calculated based on the patient's weight (5 to 7 mg/kg), which is then followed every 8 weeks with a 90-mg subcutaneous injection. An increase in severe infections or malignancy has not been shown with this treatment.

Surgical intervention for CD is normally not indicated except for complications including intestinal obstruction, fistulas and abscess drainage, or perforation.

Over the long term, up to 75% of patients with CD will require surgery. Patients with fistula formation (which may be enterocutaneous, enterovaginal, or enterovesicular) should be managed with bowel rest, parenteral nutrition, and antibiotic therapy before surgery is considered. Surgery is not curative and must be reserved for complications that are resistant to medical therapy. Intestinal obstruction caused by stricture formation is often successfully treated with strictureplasty, thus avoiding multiple colon resections and the risk of short bowel syndrome. Patients with symptoms of obstruction should avoid foods that contain nuts or seeds.

As with UC, the use of anticholinergic and antidiarrheal medications should be avoided in patients with severe disease because the drugs may precipitate toxic megacolon or ileus. Loperamide (Imodium), diphenoxylate (Lomotil), and codeine may be helpful in controlling chronic diarrhea in patients with mild CD colitis.

Microscopic Colitis

The goal of management for patients with MC is similar to the other forms of IBD: symptom improvement and histological remission. Unfortunately, there is no biomarker available to assess the severity of the disease. Budesonide (Entocort EC, Uceris, Ortikos) 9 mg daily for 8 weeks and loperamide (Imodium) are the foundation of management. If symptoms are reduced after 8 weeks of treatment, then the medications are discontinued. If the patient does not respond, then the provider should consider a work-up for other causes of persistent diarrhea such as celiac disease. For symptom recurrence, resume the budesonide 4.5 mg per day for 12 months. For refractory disease, immunomodulators and biologics as outlined for CD and UC are used.

FOLLOW-UP AND REFERRAL

UC and CD are both complex illnesses with periods of exacerbation and remission requiring lifelong intervention and follow-up. Adjustment of therapy is based on symptom analysis and examination. Referral to a gastroenterologist is necessary for endoscopic evaluation and tissue biopsy. Confirmation of the diagnosis and any uncontrolled exacerbations should be referred to the gastroenterologist. Long-term use of steroids and immunosuppressive drugs dictates ongoing patient follow-up. Repeat evaluation may be indicated if symptoms of a major complication have developed. Routine colonoscopy for colon cancer surveillance is necessary in any patient with longstanding disease. Stool analysis for occult blood is not an effective means of surveillance. Individuals whose disease is not controlled with established medical therapy of low-dose prednisone should be referred to a gastroenterologist who is knowledgeable in the treatment of these chronic disease processes.

Patient Education: Inflammatory Bowel Disease

All patients need to be informed about the disease process, the treatment options, and the expected outcome of the treatment regimens. Patients must be a part of the treatment plan and must have the knowledge necessary to make informed decisions. Education about the disease, diagnostic and laboratory tests, and diet and lifestyle changes should be included in the education. Open, honest information is important in helping patients develop realistic expectations regarding treatment and outcomes.

Adequate rest and stress reduction to decrease bowel motility and promote healing are essential. Stress management techniques, such as guided imagery, should be taught, and patients can be referred for counseling if necessary. Patients should be provided with information for national organizations such as the Crohn's and Colitis Foundation that have up-to-date information and local support groups.

Dietary concerns for patients with CD include a low-residue diet when obstructive symptoms are present. Patients on a low-residue diet should avoid all foods high in fiber, including whole grain breads and cereals, all fresh fruits and vegetables, and seeds and nuts. Patients can have canned fruits and vegetables and should have only white breads. If the patient is unresponsive to medical treatment or a pediatric patient is exhibiting signs of growth retardation, oral elemental or parenteral nutrition may be necessary. Patients who are intolerant of lactose should be taught to avoid dairy foods. When patients are not in the middle of an acute attack, they can eat whatever they can tolerate.

Dietary instruction for patients with UC is the same as that for CD. If they are not having symptoms of an acute attack, patients may eat whatever they can tolerate. During an acute exacerbation, parenteral nutrition or oral supplementation for malnutrition may be necessary. Some patients will ask questions about the use of diet as a treatment. Studies to date show that diet is ineffective as a treatment or therapy for UC. Foods that can cause diarrhea and gas-producing foods should be avoided during acute attacks.

Female patients with IBD require special guidance and counseling before they attempt pregnancy. Pregnant patients must be followed closely by a gastroenterologist throughout their pregnancy.

COLORECTAL CANCER

Colorectal cancer is the third most common cancer in the United States and the second most common cause of cancer death. The majority of cases of colorectal cancer are both curable and preventable if detected early. Colorectal tumor presentation can be either symptomatic or asymptomatic and is dependent on the location of the tumor. Polyps, the most benign form of tumors, are classified as hyperplastic (nonneoplastic), adenomatous (neoplastic), or submucosal (lipomas). Adenomatous polyps are believed to be the precursors to the malignant adenocarcinomas, which comprise more than 95% of all malignant tumors of the colon. Over the past 20 years, there has been a decline in the mortality rate associated with colorectal carcinoma, which has been attributed to improvement in screening, diagnosis, and treatment. Cure rates of colorectal carcinoma are estimated to be as high as 50%.

EPIDEMIOLOGY AND CAUSES

The estimated number of new colon cancer cases in 2020 was 147,950 with an estimated number of deaths at 53,200. It is estimated that 4.3% of the population will develop colorectal cancer in their lifetime. Since 1985, the number of new cases of colorectal cancer has decreased, and the 5-year survival rate has increased.

Age is the most important risk factor for developing colorectal cancer in the United States. The risk increases steadily with age, especially after age 45 years; this cancer is rare in individuals younger than age 35 years unless they have genetic risk factors. However, almost one-half of all cases are found in patients younger than 65 years. Colon cancer affects males and females almost equally; however, males have a slightly higher incidence. The overall survival rate of patients with colorectal cancer is approximately 66% and is attributed to early detection and treatment. African American males and members of underrepresented groups have lower survival rates in comparison to national data for other groups. It is presumed—although not proved—that the lower survival rates among people of color are in part a result of inequalities in access to health care, including screening and treatment.

Studies of Seventh-day Adventists, a religious group that subscribes to a vegetarian diet, have shown that they have a lower incidence of colorectal cancer. In the past, studies have shown that people of Japanese descent have had a lower incidence of colorectal cancer; however, Japanese Americans who have adopted a diet high in fat, refined carbohydrates, and red meat have a higher incidence of this type of cancer. In general, groups that migrate from areas of low to high incidence of colorectal cancer experience a change in cancer incidence paralleling that of the new region.

Other risk factors for colorectal cancer include a family history and a personal history of adenomatous polyps (multiple polyps or individual polyps greater than 1 cm in size) or colon cancer. Twenty-five percent of patients diagnosed with colon cancer have a family history of colon cancer. The risk of developing colon cancer is directly proportional to the number of first-degree relatives affected. For patients who have one first-degree relative with colon cancer, the risk increases twofold to threefold. Disorders involving increased colon mucosal cell turnover (such as IBD and UC) have been implicated in greater risk for colon cancer. Familial adenomatous polyposis is an autosomal dominant condition that results in the development of thousands of adenomas within the colon but accounts for less than 1% of colon cancers. Other hereditary conditions that increase the chance of developing colorectal cancer include Peutz-Jeghers syndrome, Gardner's syndrome, and Turcot's syndrome. Patients with a family history or personal history of gynecological (breast, ovarian, endometrial) cancers and individuals diagnosed with Barrett's esophagus also have an increased risk of developing colon carcinoma.

Although the etiology of colorectal cancer (adenomas) is unknown, both environmental and genetic factors have been implicated. Geographical variances and a positive correlation in the incidence of disease among migrant workers both suggest that environmental factors play a role. Diets high in fat, red meat, and refined carbohydrates and low in plant fiber have been correlated with the areas of highest incidence of colorectal cancer, whereas areas with the lowest incidence of colorectal cancer have diets high in fiber and rich in vegetables and fruits. It has been theorized that the excess fat interacts with colonic bacteria to form deconjugated bile acids, which have been associated with tumor-producing activity, increased deposition of fatty acids within the cell membranes, and increased synthesis of prostaglandins, which further stimulates cell proliferation. Ketosteroids are thought to be metabolic by-products of cholesterol that induce genetic damage and have been found in higher concentrations among high-risk populations. Products of pyrolysis—decomposition of organic matter secondary to increases in temperature such as those resulting from charbroiling and frying—have also been implicated in carcinoma of the colon. Diets high in processed meats also increase the risk of colorectal cancer. Geographical areas with low levels of selenium also have higher incidence of colorectal cancer.

Conversely, diets high in fiber tend to reduce the transit time within the colon, thus decreasing exposure to potentially carcinogenic substances, altering the gut flora, and decreasing fecal pH. (Populations with the highest incidence of colorectal cancer have an associated higher fecal pH.) When fecal contents take longer to transit the bowel, the deionized bile acids and free fatty acids stay in contact with the intestinal mucosa, which has been associated with development of colorectal cancer.

Other risk factors include being overweight or obese. Physical inactivity is associated with a greater risk of developing colorectal cancer. Long-term smoking and heavy use of alcohol are also risk factors. However, moderate alcohol use, defined as no more than two drinks per day for males or one drink per day for females, may lower the risk for colorectal cancer.

PATHOPHYSIOLOGY

Most colorectal cancers are adenocarcinomas. The evolution from adenoma to invasive carcinoma can take up to 10 years. Adenomas are benign neoplasms composed of granular epithelium that are not capable of metastasis or invasion of the muscularis mucosa. They are either sessile (attached by a broad base) or pedunculated (attached by a stalk). Most smaller adenomas (less than 1 cm in diameter) are of the tubular type, and less than 1% contain carcinoma. As the polyps increase in size (greater than 2 cm in diameter), they begin to show villous changes with increasing dysplasia; the chance of one of these polyps containing cancer is about 50%.

Most adenocarcinomas of the colon form hard, nodular areas that grow irregularly. Colon cancers are staged or classified according to histological changes in the infiltrative character of the tumor. The most common classification system used today is the tumor-node-metastasis (TNM) system (Table 40.3). Histologically, colon cancers vary from well-differentiated cells that appear normal (grade 1) to highly anaplastic, poorly differentiated cells (grade 4). The accuracy of specimen collection is crucial. The most accurate method of evaluating a polyp is by removing the entire lesion for cytological examination. If the polyp is less than 7 mm in diameter, tissue for biopsy can be obtained while the polyp is destroyed through "hot" (fulguration) biopsy.

Metastatic progression of colon cancer usually involves spread by local invasion—lymphatic extension with spread to the mesenteric lymph nodes—followed by hematogenous spread through the portal system to the liver. In some patients, the cancer metastasizes throughout the peritoneal cavity and to the lungs. Rectal carcinoma spreads by direct extension through the perirectal fat to the lymph nodes and less often to the lungs and distant organs through hemorrhoidal circulation. Prognosis of colorectal carcinoma is a function of several factors, including poorly differentiated tissue histology, mucin production, aneuploidy (DNA abnormalities), tumor invasion to other organs, perforation, and venous involvement. The prognosis is not influenced by tumor size.

Colon cancers can develop as polyps within the lumen of the intestine or as a mass on the wall of the colon. Bulky polypoid tumors are more common within the right colon, whereas tumors that encircle the bowel, causing obstruction, are more common on the left side of the colon. Tumor growth is normally slow and, in most cases, is asymptomatic until the tumor becomes large. Diagnosis is usually made late in the course of the disease, often after metastasis, thereby making a surgical cure difficult. Colon cancers that produce intracellular mucin are called signet ring–type carcinomas; these tumors tend to be more aggressive in their spread.

Several types of colon cancers have been linked to specific genetic defects. Hereditary nonpolyposis colorectal cancers include two autosomal dominant conditions, Lynch syndromes I and II, that have been associated with a markedly increased risk for developing colon cancer. Although these patients have few or no adenomatous polyps, individuals diagnosed with Lynch syndrome I are at increased risk of developing colon cancer at an early age. This cancer has a propensity for the right side of the colon. Lynch syndrome II includes the features of Lynch syndrome I, as well as an increased risk of developing tumors within the ovary, uterus, urinary tract, and stomach.

CLINICAL PRESENTATION

Subjective

Signs and symptoms in patients with colorectal cancer will vary, depending on the tumor size, anatomical location, and associated complications, if any. There are few early warning signs of colorectal carcinoma; in fact, most individuals are asymptomatic. Frequently, the cancer is found incidentally during abdominal surgery or during screening sigmoidoscopy.

TABLE 40.3 Staging Classifications of Colorectal Cancer (TNM)

Stages	Tumor	Node	Metastasis	Description
Stage 0	Tis	N0	M0	Carcinoma in situ
Stage 1	T1	N0	M0	Tumor invades submucosa; greater than 80% 5-year survival
	T2	N0	M0	Tumor invades muscularis.
Stage II	T3	N0	M0	Tumor penetrates through bowel wall; 60%–80% 5-year survival
	T4	N0	M0	Tumor invades adjacent organ; no regional lymph node involvement
Stage III	T1, T2	N1 or N2	M0	Any bowel wall perforation with lymph node involvement; 20%–50% 5-year survival
	T3, T4	N1 or N2	M0	One to three pericolic or perirectal lymph nodes.
Stage IV	Any T	Any N	M1	Distant metastasis; less than 25% 5-year survival

Source: Used with permission of the American College of Surgeons, Chicago, Illinois. Original source for this information is the *AJCC Cancer Staging Manual*, Eighth Edition (2017) published by Springer International Publishing.

Patients may present with melena or bright red bleeding from the rectum, depending on the location of the tumor. A change in bowel habits, including constipation alternating with diarrhea or a change in stool caliber (described as narrowed or ribbonlike), can be signs of colon cancer. Stools streaked with blood may be mistakenly dismissed as a sign of hemorrhoidal irritation. Abdominal pain is a rare presenting symptom but may indicate obstruction resulting from tumors on the left side of the colon, which has a smaller diameter lumen, or from invasion of the bowel wall by a tumor. Patients rarely report colicky pain as a result of a right-sided colon cancer because of the larger diameter of the colon and the liquid consistency of the stool. Patients with rectal cancer may complain of tenesmus (spasm of the anal sphincter), urgency, and/or hematochezia. Patients with chronic occult blood loss from an undiagnosed tumor may experience weakness and fatigue caused by iron-deficiency anemia. Weight loss and anorexia are common with any malignant process but are usually manifested late in the disease process.

Objective

Physical examination may reveal a mass within the abdomen or an enlarged liver, which may be suggestive of metastasis. A digital rectal examination should be done even though most tumors are not palpable. The stool should be tested for occult blood, which, if positive, is pathognomonic for right-sided colon cancer. Approximately 50% of patients with a positive fecal occult blood test have either an adenoma (38%) or a neoplasm (12%). Fecal occult blood testing is positive in only 60% to 70% of patients with known large intestinal cancers; however, annual screening can reduce colorectal mortality rates by 33%.

DIAGNOSTIC REASONING

Diagnostic Tests

Although there are no definitive laboratory tests for diagnosis of colorectal cancer, a CBC should be obtained to assess for iron-deficiency anemia or anemia of chronic blood loss, either of which can be a common finding in patients with colorectal cancer. Liver function tests may reveal an elevation of the liver enzymes, especially of alkaline phosphatase, if there has been metastasis to the liver and/or bone. Usually, when there is liver metastasis, the bilirubin level tends to remain normal until late in the disease process.

The serum immune assay for carcinoembryonic antigen (CEA) was developed with the intent to provide an early means of detection for colon cancer; however, the test is too insensitive and nonspecific for screening. CEA levels have been poorly correlated with the stage of cancer; however, this test is useful for monitoring a patient's response to therapy, whether surgical or chemotherapeutic. CEA levels usually normalize after colon resection, and levels that remain elevated are associated with poor prognosis. A secondary spike in the CEA level after surgery is highly suggestive of recurrence and must be evaluated.

Colonoscopy establishes the diagnosis of colon cancer with almost 100% accuracy and is thus the diagnostic procedure of choice. Flexible sigmoidoscopy can be used for confirming lesions within the rectosigmoid area; however, full colon examination with colonoscopy is preferred. CT scan is used for evaluation of distant metastasis. Endoscopic ultrasound has been used to stage regional rectal cancers and is more accurate than CT scan in this area.

Patients with colonic polyps will require histological examination of the polyp. Polyps larger than 7 mm should be totally removed. Polyps that are less than 7 mm in size are usually not malignant and can be removed by "hot" biopsy, which destroys the polyp while obtaining the necessary tissue for cytological examination.

Differential Diagnosis

The symptoms of colorectal cancer are nonspecific; therefore, many disease processes can mimic the presenting symptoms of colon carcinoma and must be differentiated from it. Most of the inflammatory and IBD processes can be confused with colon carcinoma. Ischemic colitis, diverticular disease, IBS, IBD, or infectious colitis can form strictures within the bowel that are indistinguishable from colon carcinoma. Colonoscopy with biopsy of the lesion is the diagnostic procedure of choice. Any patient older than age 50 who presents with iron-deficiency anemia, stool positive for occult blood, change in bowel habits, or hematochezia should have a thorough evaluation to rule out the possibility of neoplasm.

MANAGEMENT

The first step in the treatment of colon cancer is the staging of the disease. The staging of the cancer is of critical importance not only for the determination of the patient's long-term survival but also for determining which patients should receive adjuvant therapy. Staging of a neoplasm first involves understanding the characteristics used to describe the histological findings: tissue of origin (adenocarcinoma, sarcoma, carcinoid), origin of specimen (colon, breast), and the degree of tissue differentiation. Staging of the carcinoma includes both the primary site and the metastatic sites and allows for the development of the most optimal treatment plan based on those findings. More than one-half of all cancers are not curable, using approved treatments available today. Many of the treatment regimens involve some form of experimental drugs or procedures; therefore, accurate staging is necessary to determine the efficacy of the treatment.

The only known cure for colon cancer is surgical resection. This is the treatment of choice for all patients who can tolerate the surgery. Even patients who have known metastasis can benefit from surgical intervention to reduce the chance of developing an intestinal obstruction or rectal hemorrhage later in the disease process. Most patients with colorectal cancer present with penetration of the mass through the bowel wall and with associated lymph node involvement. The surgeon will decide, based on the staging, what type of surgical resection is appropriate. The anatomical location of the tumor—left or right side of the colon—will dictate whether left or right hemicolectomy is performed. A wide margin of intestine (with careful ligation of the total arterial blood supply) will be resected to ensure that mesenteric and associated lymph node drainage is removed.

Lesions located within the rectosigmoid area are usually treated with anterior resection, which protects the rectal sphincter. (The rectum is the distal 8 to 11 cm of large bowel.) If the rectal lesions are small and are discovered early, they can sometimes be treated by local incision, laser photoablation, or cryosurgery. Larger lesions located within this lower portion of the large bowel usually require a combination of abdominal-perineal resection with a colostomy. Nonresectable rectal cancers can be palliated with a diverting colostomy, or, if the patient is a poor surgical candidate, laser fulguration of the tumor mass can minimize the bleeding and maintain the patency of the rectum.

Adjuvant chemotherapy for colon cancer is based on the stage of the disease (see Table 40.3). Treatment of Stage III cancer includes 6 months of chemotherapy. A combination of 5-fluorouracil (5-FU), leucovorin, and oxaliplatin is the treatment of choice for the best 5-year survival rate (73.3%) compared with 5-FU and leucovorin alone (67.4%). Stage IV metastatic cancer is treated with the same chemotherapy combination as Stage III but with the addition of a biological agent such as bevacizumab (monoclonal antibody), which improves survival but only for a mean of 2 to 5 months.

Rectal carcinomas have a lower long-term survival rate than colon cancers and are typically treated with chemoradiation of 5-FU or capecitabine. When given preoperatively, the chemotherapy sensitizes the cancer cells to the effects of the radiation therapy, leading to better outcomes. After surgery, chemotherapy with 5-FU, leucovorin, and oxaliplatin is used along with 6 months of radiation.

Twenty percent of patients with colorectal cancer have known metastases at the time of diagnosis. Patients with known metastases to the liver may have improved survival rates with resection. Some patients with liver metastases have opted for infusions of 5-FU into the hepatic artery or portal vein, which has proved superior in the treatment of hepatic disease; however, this treatment has little effect on the overall survival rate for colorectal cancer and can be extremely toxic to the patient.

Although the oncologist will manage the patient's chemoradiation therapy, the primary care practitioner will continue to work closely with the patient to treat any of the numerous adverse effects caused by the chemotherapy and the radiation therapy. The potential toxic effects of adjuvant therapy for colorectal cancer are numerous and can range from nausea, vomiting, and weight loss to cystitis and radiation proctitis. Radiation therapy to the pelvic area can cause severe GI disorders, including intractable diarrhea and even malabsorption syndromes.

FOLLOW-UP AND REFERRAL

Initial assessment and screening for colorectal carcinoma is the responsibility of every primary care provider. Patients who are known to be at higher risk for the development of colorectal cancer, such as those who have a first-degree relative with the disease, a family history of adenomas, a personal history of adenomas or colorectal cancer, or a longstanding history of IBD, require a more in-depth screening by a practitioner who is well trained in this area. Screening for high-risk patients should include colonoscopy, which is best done by an experienced gastroenterologist. The recommended screening for average- and high-risk individuals is provided in the Screening Recommendations/Guidelines feature.

Screening Recommendations/Guidelines: Colon Cancer Screening, American Cancer Society (2020)

Risk	Screening Recommendations
Average risk: Beginning at age 45 through 75 years Ages 76–85 years, screening is based on life expectancy, general overall health, and previous screening results. People over age 85 years no longer need screening.	Colonoscopy every 10 years OR Annual fecal immunochemical test (FIT) Second tier: Flexible sigmoidoscopy every 5 years Computed tomography colonography every 5 years Fecal DNA testing every 3 years
Higher risk: • Before age 60 years • Family history of a hereditary colorectal cancer syndrome	Colonoscopy every 5 years starting before age 45

Source: American Cancer Society (2020). Guideline for Colorectal Cancer Screening. https://www.cancer.org/cancer/colon-rectal-cancer/detection-diagnosis-staging/acs-recommendations.html

Follow-up is vital in the treatment of colorectal cancer. To prevent recurrence, scheduled colon surveillance is required. Early detection and removal of adenomas can improve survival rates. Close surveillance is necessary for patients who have undergone "curative resection" surgery. Recommendations include office visits every 3 months, which should include a CEA level, an annual CT of the abdomen and pelvis, and a chest x-ray film for the first 3 years postoperatively. A colonoscopy should be completed postoperatively, but if it was not performed then, a colonoscopy should be scheduled for 3 months postoperatively and then again at 1 year, with special attention to anastomotic recurrences. If the results of the examination are within normal limits, patients may continue with follow-up examinations every 3 years. Patients whose CEA levels normalize or stabilize after surgery and then spike suddenly require a thorough examination.

Patients who have undergone surgical resection for colon cancer and have a temporary or permanent colostomy may benefit from assistance from an enterostomal therapist. Consultation with a urologist for urological or sexual dysfunction resulting from surgical or radiation therapy may provide medical and social support. Patients with metastatic disease can be referred to hospice service personnel, who are trained in providing comfort and support to both the family and the patient.

Patient Education: Colon Cancer

Patient education should focus first on the prevention of colon cancer, stressing a diet that is low in fat and refined carbohydrates and high in fiber, fruits, vegetables, and complex carbohydrates. Because obesity and a sedentary lifestyle are risk factors, patients should be assisted in pursuing weight loss and exercise. The risk/benefit/cost ratio makes these preventive measures worth suggesting.

REFERENCES

General
Luthy KE, Larimer SG, Freeborn DS. Differentiating between lactose intolerance, celiac disease and irritable bowel syndrome-diarrhea. *J Nurse Pract.* 2017;13(5):348–353.

Abdominal Hernias
Almarzooqi R, Tish S, Huang LC, et al. Review of inguinal hernia repair techniques within the Americas Hernia Society Quality Collaborative. *Hernia.* 2019;23:429–438.

Charles EJ, Mehaffey JH, Tache-Leon CA, et al. Inguinal hernia repair: is there a benefit to using the robot? *Surg Endosc.* 2018;32:2131–2136.

Heniford BT, Ross SW, Wormer BA, et al. Preperitoneal ventral hernia repair: a decade long prospective observational study with analysis of 1023 patient outcomes. *Ann Surg.* 2020;217:364–374.

Bowel Obstruction
Long B, Robertson J, Koyfman A. Emergency medicine evaluation and management of small bowel obstruction: evidence-based recommendations. *J Emerg Med.* 2019;56(2):166–176.

Mellor K, Hind D, Lee MJ. A systematic review of outcomes reported in small bowel obstruction research. *J Surg Res.* 2018;229:41–50.

Celiac Disease
Bascunan KA, Vespa MC, Araya M. Celiac disease: understanding the gluten-free diet. *Eur J Nutr.* 2017;56:449–459.

Caio G, Volta U, Leffler DA, et al. Celiac disease: a comprehensive current review. *BMC Med.* 2019;17:142.

U.S. Preventive Services Task Force. Screening for celiac disease: US Preventive Services Task Force Recommendation Statement. *JAMA.* 2017;317(12):1252–1257.

Colorectal Cancer
American Cancer Society (2020). Guideline for Colorectal Cancer Screening. https://www.cancer.org/cancer/colon-rectal-cancer/detection-diagnosis-staging/acs-recommendations.html. Accessed 10/7/2021

Carethers JM. Fecal DNA testing for colorectal cancer screening. *Annu Rev Med.* 2020;71:59–69.

Centers for Disease Control and Prevention (CDC). Colorectal Cancer Screening Tests. https://www.cdc.gov/cancer/colorectal/basic_info/screening/tests.htm. Accessed 1/25/2021.

Kahi CJ, Boland R, Dominitz JA, et al. Colonoscopy surveillance after colorectal cancer resection: recommendations of the US multi-society task force on colorectal cancer. *Am J Gastroenterol.* 2016;150(3):758–768.

Ladabaum U, Dominitz JA, Kahi C, et al. Strategies for colorectal cancer screening. *Gastroenterology.* 2020;158(2):418–432.

National Cancer Institute. Colon cancer treatment (PDQ)—health professional version. https://www.cancer.gov/types/colorectal/hp/colon-treatment-pdq. Updated 7/21/2020

Provenzale D, Gupta S, Ahnen DJ, et al. NCCN guidelines insights: colorectal cancer screening, version 1 *J Natl Compr Canc Netw.* 2018;16(8):939–949.

Siegel RL, Miller KD, Goding Sauer A, et al. Colorectal cancer statistics, 2020. CA *Cancer J Clin.* 2020;70(3):145–164.

Diverticular Disease
Peery AF, Shaukat A, Strate LL. AGA clinical practice update on medical management of colonic diverticulitis: expert review. *Gastroenterology.* 2021;160(3):906–911.

Rezapour M. Ali S, Stollman N. Diverticular disease: an update on pathogenesis and management. *Gut and Liver.* 2018;12(2):125–132.

Tochigi T, Kosugi C, Shuto K, et al. Management of complicated diverticulitis of the colon. *Ann Gastroenterol Surg.* 2018;2:22–27.

Gastroesophageal Reflux Disease
Fass R, Zerbib F, Gyawali CP. AGA clinical practice update on functional heartburn: expert review. *Gastroenterology.* 2020;158(8):2286–2293.

Spechler SJ. Evaluation and treatment of patients with persistent reflux symptoms despite proton pump inhibitor treatment. *Gastroenterol Clin North Am.* 2020;49(3):437–450.

Yadlapati R, Vaezi MF, Vela MF, et al. Management options for patients with GERD and persistent symptoms on proton pump inhibitors: recommendations from an expert panel. *Am J Gastroenterol.* 2018;113(7):980–986.

Hemorrhoids

Margetis N. Pathophysiology of internal hemorrhoids. *Ann Gastroenterol.* 2019;32(3):264–272.

Mott TF, Latimer K, Edwards C. Hemorrhoids: diagnosis and treatment options. *Am Fam Physician.* 2018;97(3):172–179.

Inflammatory Bowel Disease

Lega S, Dubinsky MC. What are the targets of inflammatory bowel disease management. *Inflamm Bowel Dis.* 2018;24(8):1670–1675.

Miehlke S, Verhaegh B, Tontini GE, et al. Microscopic colitis: pathophysiology and clinical management. *Lancet Gastroenterol Hepatol.* 2019;4(4):305–314.

Shor J, Churrango G, Hosseini N, et al. Management of microscopic colitis: challenges and solutions. *Clin Exp Gastroenterol.* 2019;12:111–120.

Weisshof R, El Jurdi K, Zmeter N, et al. Emerging therapies for inflammatory bowel disease. *Adv Ther.* 2018;35:1746–1762.

Irritable Bowel Syndrome

Barbara G, Grover M, Bercik P, et al. Rome Foundation workshop team report on post-infection irritable bowel syndrome. *Gastroenterology.* 2019;156(1):46–58.

El-Salhy M, Hatlebakk JG, Hausken T. Diet in irritable bowel syndrome (IBS): Interaction with gut microbiota and gut hormones. *Nutrients.* 2019;11(8):1824.

Hadjivasilis A, Tsioutis C, Michalinos A, et al. New insights into irritable bowel syndrome: from pathophysiology to treatment. *Ann Gastroenterol.* 2019;32(6):554–564.

Ng QX, Soh AYS, Loke W, et al. A meta-analysis of the clinical use of curcumin for irritable bowel syndrome (IBS). *J Clin Med.* 2018;7(10):298.

Quigley EM. The gut-brain axis and the microbiome: clues to pathophysiology and opportunities for novel management strategies in irritable bowel syndrome (IBS). *J Clin Med.* 2018;7(1):6.

Schmulson MJ, Drossman DA. What is new in Rome IV. *J Neurogastroeterol Motil.* 2017;23(2):151–163.

Smalley W, Falck-Ytter C, Carrasco-Labra A, et al. AGA clinical practice guidelines on the laboratory evaluation of functional diarrhea and diarrhea predominant irritable bowel syndrome in adults. *Gastroenterology.* 2019;157(3):851–854.

Peptic Ulcer Disease

Dunlap JJ, Patterson S. Peptic ulcer disease. *Gastroenterol Nurs.* 2019;42(5):451–454.

Fu W, Song Z, Zhou L, et al. Randomized clinical trial: Esomeprazole, bismuth, levofloxacin, and amoxicillin or cefuroxime as first-line eradication regimens for Helicobacter pylori infection. *Dig Dis Sci.* 2017;62:1580–1589.

Kavitt RT. Lipowska AM, Anyane-Yeboa A, et al. Diagnosis and treatment of peptic ulcer disease. *Am J Med.* 2019;132(4): 447–456.

Kuna L, Jakab J, Smolic R, et al. Peptic ulcer disease: a brief review of conventional therapy and herbal treatment options. *J Clin Med.* 2019;8(2):179.

RESOURCES

American Gastroenterological Association
https://gastro.org/

Celiac Disease Foundation
https://celiac.org

Crohn's and Colitis Foundation
https://www.crohnscolitisfoundation.org/

International Foundation for Gastrointestinal Disorders
https://www.iffgd.org/

National Cancer Institute—Health Professional Version
https://www.cancer.gov/types/colorectal/hp

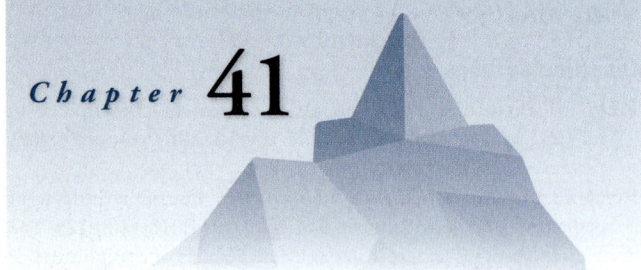

Chapter 41

Gallbladder and Pancreatic Disorders

Debera J. Thomas, PhD, RN, ANP/FNP

CHOLECYSTITIS

Cholecystitis is an acute inflammation of the gallbladder wall, which is usually the result of an impacted calculus within the cystic duct, causing inflammation proximal to the obstruction. Cholelithiasis is found in more than 90% of patients presenting with cholecystitis. Cholecystitis without gallstones, acalculous cholecystitis, is a very serious disease with high morbidity and mortality rates. It usually occurs in patients who are already critically ill because of trauma, burns, surgery, or sepsis, and who have had no oral intake or have been supplemented with hyperalimentation. Patients present with severe pain and tenderness in the epigastrium or right upper quadrant (RUQ) of the abdomen accompanied by nausea, vomiting, fever, and leukocytosis.

EPIDEMIOLOGY AND CAUSES

Cholecystitis/cholelithiasis is prevalent in Western societies. Researchers estimate that the disease affects approximately 20 to 25 million Americans or 10% to 15% of the adult population, the majority of whom are not aware they have cholelithiasis. With the increasing rates of obesity in the United States, it is anticipated that the incidence of cholelithiasis will increase exponentially. About 50% of these asymptomatic patients never require treatment. Gallstones form in people as early as in their 30s. In fact, 75% of Native American females older than 25 years have gallstones. The risk of requiring a cholecystectomy increases with age as a consequence of complications secondary to the lithiasis. By age 65, about 20% of females and 10% of males have symptoms related to gallstones that require medical attention. As many as 5,000 to 6,000 deaths each year are attributed to gallstone-related disease.

Cholesterol stones are the most common form and account for 75% of all gallstones. The remaining 25% are pigmented stones, which are categorized as black or brown depending on their chemical composition. Cholesterol stones contain between 50% and 90% cholesterol. The remainder of the stone is made of calcium salts from bilirubin pigment, carbonate, bile acids, phospholipids, fatty acids, and proteins. Risk factors for cholelithiasis are listed in the following Risk Factors section.

Risk Factors Associated With Cholelithiasis

Cholesterol stones:

- Female gender
- Obesity
- Rapid weight loss after bariatric surgery
- Pregnancy
- Increased age
- Drug induced (oral contraceptives, clofibrates)
- Cystic fibrosis
- Rapid weight loss
- Spinal cord injury
- Ileal disease with extensive resection
- Diabetes mellitus
- Sickle cell anemia

Pigmented stones:

- Hebmolytic diseases
- Increasing age
- Hyperalimentation
- Cirrhosis
- Biliary stasis
- Chronic biliary infections

After age 50, the gender distribution of cholelithiasis is equal. Pregnancy also predisposes women to cholelithiasis, presumably because of the increased abdominal pressure and increased cholesterol levels during the third trimester. Any condition that increases the development of cholelithiasis increases the chance of developing cholecystitis.

PATHOPHYSIOLOGY

More than 90% of cholecystitis cases are associated with cholelithiasis. Cholesterol stones are the most common form of gallstones. Cholesterol is insoluble in water; it is made soluble though interaction with bile salts and phospholipids, allowing it to be carried within the bile. There are two known transport systems for cholesterol within the bile, vesicular and micellar, and both are needed to maintain equilibrium of the various bile components. When this equilibrium is disturbed and the bile contains more cholesterol than can be maintained, crystallization of the cholesterol, referred to as *nucleation,* occurs. Gradual deposition of cholesterol on these crystals leads to the development of a cholesterol gallstone. Although this process seems to contribute to the formation of gallstones, not all people with cholesterol-saturated bile form stones. Thus, there is more to the process of lithogenesis than is known.

The gallbladder is of primary importance in the development of gallstones because it provides an arena for bile stasis and allows time for the slow crystallization of cholesterol, which may also be enhanced by yet unknown proteins or other materials within the bile. Biliary cholesterol is increased by ingestion of estrogen and oral contraceptives, multiparity, and inflammatory terminal ileal disease, which decreases the bile acid pool. Bile stasis, which can contribute to gallstone formation, is increased by strictures within the ductal system, parenteral hyperalimentation, fasting, and mechanical obstruction secondary to tumor or cyst formation.

The pathogenesis of pigmented stones is less understood but seems to be directly related to elevation in levels of unconjugated bilirubin. Any disease state that increases the amount of bilirubin increases the risk for pigmented lithogenesis. Black-pigmented stones are formed within the gallbladder and are commonly associated with hemolytic diseases, cirrhosis, and long-term parenteral hyperalimentation. Black-pigmented stones are more fragile and seem to crush more easily than cholesterol stones.

Brown pigmented stones are composed of alternating layers of calcium bilirubinate and calcium fatty acids. Chronic bacterial infections are believed to be partly responsible for the formation of brown pigmented stones because the enzymes the bacteria produce predispose the patient to this type of stone formation. Brown stones are typically found within the intrahepatic ducts and are rarely found within the gallbladder.

The pathophysiological changes occurring within the gallbladder before the diagnosis of acute cholecystitis are directly related to the amount of time the duct has been obstructed and the degree of inflammation that has taken place. The earliest pathological findings are erythema, edema, and a fibrinosuppurative exudate. Tissue examination reveals inflammatory infiltration, hemorrhage, and edema resulting in ulceration of the mucosa within a short period of time. The result is the development of gangrene with abscess formation. As the acute process resolves, collagen deposits develop, usually within 1 to 2 weeks. The gallbladder eventually contracts and becomes scarred, causing thickening of the wall. Often, the gallbladder becomes filled with pus preceding the development of gangrene. Perforation may occur, most often at the fundus, but it can occur anywhere there is erosion of an impacted stone. Perforation of the gallbladder allows bile to spill into the peritoneal cavity, causing bile peritonitis, abscess, and fistula formation.

CLINICAL PRESENTATION

Subjective

Acute cholecystitis causes various symptoms, ranging from generalized gastrointestinal (GI) complaints to intractable pain. Most patients complain of indigestion, nausea, and vomiting, especially after consuming a high-fat meal. Acute cholecystitis usually begins with acute, colicky-type pain. About 80% of patients report that they have experienced this type of pain before. However, the pain associated with acute cholecystitis persists, and as the inflammation progresses, the pain localizes over the RUQ or epigastrium. Patients may complain of referred pain that radiates to the middle of the back, infrascapular area, or right shoulder. The pain is increased by any movement, including respiration. If the inflammation extends to the peritoneal area, the pain worsens, the abdominal muscles become rigid, and a fever is usually evident.

Objective

Physical findings reflect the degree of inflammation present. As the pain over the RUQ becomes severe, there is often involuntary guarding of the abdominal muscles over the right side. A positive Murphy's sign is elicited when the right subcostal region is so tender that there is painful splinting with deep inspiration or when palpation over the RUQ area causes transient inspiratory arrest. The gallbladder is palpable in fewer than 50% of patients. Fever is usually low grade, 99° to 101°F (38.3°C); high fever suggests sepsis. Patients may develop mild jaundice from edema of the common bile duct. Hyperbilirubinemia should raise the suspicion of choledocholithiasis. Bowel sounds may be diminished.

In most cases, acute cholecystitis subsides spontaneously, with improvement in the first few days and resolution of symptoms after about 4 days. If symptoms persist or become more severe, the potential for perforation, gangrene, empyema, and septic shock increases. Rebound tenderness, shaking chills, or increased fever should raise suspicion that perforation has occurred. Surgical referral is indicated early in the disease process.

DIAGNOSTIC REASONING

Diagnostic Testing

During the acute presentation of cholecystitis, there is usually mild elevation of the white blood cell (WBC) count, to 15,000/μL. Serum transaminases can be elevated up to four times the normal amount; aspartate aminotransferase and alanine aminotransferase can be elevated to 300 U/L. Alkaline phosphatase is elevated two to four times greater than normal levels, and bilirubin can be as high as 4 mg/dL. Profound elevation of alkaline phosphatase and bilirubin is highly suggestive of choledocholithiasis. An elevation in amylase can be the result of passage of a stone through the common bile duct but may also indicate gallstone pancreatitis.

Abdominal x-ray films may reveal radiopaque gallstones, enlarged gallbladder, or air within the biliary system or peritoneal cavity. Abdominal ultrasound (RUQ) is usually done initially and is sensitive for cholelithiasis but less so for acute cholecystitis. It is a quick, noninvasive, reliable, and cost-effective means of identifying the presence of cholelithiasis. An obstructed cystic duct is the cause of acute cholecystitis in most patients and is best seen with hepatobiliary imaging (cholescintigraphy) using a radiographic tracer (sometimes referred to as a *HIDA scan*). A computed tomography (CT) scan is useful if gangrene or perforation of the gallbladder is suspected.

Differential Diagnosis

The differential diagnosis of acute cholecystitis in the presence of RUQ pain, nausea, vomiting, and fever includes pancreatitis, myocardial infarction, appendicitis, peptic ulcer, pneumonia, and hepatitis. Most of these potential diagnoses can be effectively ruled out via standard laboratory tests and ultrasound. Electrocardiogram can rule out myocardial infarction and is necessary as part of preoperative studies.

MANAGEMENT

Treatment of cholelithiasis depends on many variables, including age; presenting symptoms; past medical history; and size, type, and number of gallstones involved. Patients with symptomatic cholelithiasis can often be safely managed on an outpatient basis. Patients must be advised to avoid foods high in fat, which can provoke an attack. Nonsurgical options for the treatment of gallstones include dissolution of the stone by oral ingestion of ursodeoxycholic acid (ursodiol) or direct dissolution by percutaneous instillation of methyl tertiary-butyl ether. Both types of dissolution therapies are of limited value and can be used only with cholesterol stones. Recurrence rates with these treatments are almost 100%, and duration of treatment may be as long as 2 years.

Patients who are deemed poor surgical risks can also undergo extracorporeal shock wave lithotripsy along with chemical dissolution in an attempt to reduce the size of the stones. Patients who continue to have biliary colic or who have developed other complications should be hospitalized for further treatment, with prompt referral to a gastroenterologist and/or a surgeon.

Initial Management

Initial treatment begins with definitive diagnosis. For many, the diagnosis of gallstones is made as an incidental finding during medical treatment for another problem. These patients are often asymptomatic and require no further treatment except awareness of the signs and symptoms of a "gallbladder attack." Patients who are considered a poor surgical risk can be treated nonsurgically with dissolution therapy or lithotripsy. However, the recurrence rate is high and the complication rate and mortality are high in older patients. Those who remain symptomatic despite treatment or have developed other complications should be hospitalized in an attempt to reduce the risk of a life-threatening event such as gangrene, perforation, or septic shock.

Management of acute cholecystitis includes rehydration with IV fluids, antibiotics, analgesics, and GI rest. If vomiting is persistent, a nasogastric (NG) tube is inserted. A second or third generation cephalosporin (i.e., ceftriaxone 1 g IV every 24 hours) is started once the diagnosis is made. If the patient has a severe case or is septic, then a fluoroquinolone (ciprofloxacin 400 mg IV every 12 hours) plus metronidazole should added to the antibiotic coverage.

The treatment of choice for acute cholecystitis is early surgical intervention. Patients in the acute phase of the disease are usually stabilized before a cholecystectomy is scheduled; however, early surgical intervention is associated with a decreased length of stay, lower cost, and increased patient satisfaction. Patients who are considered a poor surgical risk may benefit from cholecystotomy, either operatively or percutaneously. Emergency decompression with cholecystotomy may be necessary to remove stones and purulent material before a cholecystectomy, which should be deferred for 6 to 8 weeks.

The mortality rate associated with acute cholecystitis is 5% to 10% and is usually associated with patients older than age 60 with comorbid conditions and those with septic complications. The mortality rate for cholecystectomy is less than 0.2%. Approximately 50% of patients who choose not to undergo cholecystectomy have a recurrence within 5 years, and complications are common.

Subsequent Management

The most common complications of acute cholecystitis are empyema and perforation. Perforation into the abdominal cavity can occur early in the disease process and is associated with a 30% mortality rate. Perforation may also occur into another hollow viscus or into the colon, causing draining fistulas, which may relieve the symptoms associated with cholecystitis. Surgical removal of the gallbladder with fistula repair is indicated when the patient is medically stable for surgery.

FOLLOW-UP AND REFERRAL

Patients with acute cholecystitis require referral to a general surgeon for removal of the gallbladder. Referral should be made after diagnosis of acute cholecystitis. Follow-up includes routine postoperative visits according to the surgeon. Patients who have persistent symptoms after removal of the gallbladder (postcholecystectomy syndrome) may have a mistaken diagnosis, a functional bowel disorder, retained or recurrent common bile duct stones, or spasm of the sphincter of Oddi. Patients with incidental findings of asymptomatic gallstones should be referred to a surgeon and given the option for elective surgery, medical dissolution therapy, lithotripsy, or contact solvent dissolution.

> **Patient Education: Gallbladder Disease**
>
> Patient education for individuals declining surgical intervention should include the risks and benefits of each therapy. Dietary counseling should include weight loss for those patients who are obese and the avoidance of fatty foods that provoke attacks. Patients taking oral contraceptives should be given information about alternative forms of birth control, and menopausal women taking estrogen should be counseled about alternative sources of phytoestrogens, such as soy products.

ACUTE PANCREATITIS

Acute pancreatitis is defined as acute inflammation of the pancreas and the surrounding tissues resulting from the release of pancreatic enzymes. These enzymes cause a chemical burn in the retroperitoneal spaces, which leads to systemic toxicity. The degree to which the microcirculation within the pancreas is preserved determines the histological classification of pancreatitis. If the microcirculation remains intact, the process is defined as acute interstitial pancreatitis. If the microcirculation is disrupted, it is defined as necrotizing pancreatitis. Acute pancreatitis normally resolves both clinically and histologically.

EPIDEMIOLOGY AND CAUSES

Although there are many causes of acute pancreatitis, approximately 80% of all hospital admissions for acute pancreatitis are the result of biliary tract disease (passing of a gallstone) or alcohol use disorder. See Box 41.1 for all the causes of pancreatitis. Up to 25% of patients will experience recurrence in the first several years after the initial diagnosis. More than 300,000 hospital admissions and a cost of more than $2 billion are attributed to acute pancreatitis annually.

Acute pancreatitis is usually the result of some other process, such as passing of a gallstone, excessive alcohol intake, or other type of biliary tract disease. Clinical pancreatitis is seen in up to 9.5% of patients with alcohol use disorder, and histological evidence is found in 17% to 45% of this group. Cholelithiasis is present in 60% of patients without alcohol use disorder who have pancreatitis.

PATHOPHYSIOLOGY

Pathological changes associated with pancreatitis range from acute edema and cellular infiltration to necrosis and hemorrhage. Although the exact pathogenesis is not known, temporary impaction of the sphincter of Oddi by a gallstone before its passage into the duodenum may cause edema or obstruction of the ampulla of Vater, with subsequent reflux of bile into the pancreatic ducts and injury to the acinar cells. This cascade of events causes an autodigestive process within the pancreas that can progress to shock and death without appropriate intervention.

Box 41.1 Causes of Pancreatitis

- Infection (mumps)
- Hyperlipidemia (particularly types I, IV, and V)
- Metabolic disorders (hyperparathyroidism, hypercalcemia)
- Drugs (furosemide, valproic acid, sulfonamides, thiazides)
- Endoscopic retrograde cholangiopancreatography (ERCP)
- Structural abnormalities of the pancreatic duct (stricture, carcinoma, pancreas divisum)
- Structural abnormalities of the common bile duct and ampullary region
- Surgery (particularly of the stomach and biliary tract)
- Vascular disease (atherosclerosis, severe hypotension)
- Trauma

Inflammation is confined to the pancreas in edematous pancreatitis, and the mortality rate is less than 5%.

When inflammation and tissue necrosis extend beyond the pancreas, the associated mortality rate is 10% to 50%. Pancreatic exudate containing toxins and activated enzymes permeates the retroperitoneum and causes a chemical burn that increases the permeability of the blood vessels within the peritoneal cavity. As a result, large amounts of protein-rich fluid from the circulation are sequestered in these third spaces, producing hypovolemia and shock. As these toxins and enzymes enter the systemic circulation, they can further reduce vascular tone and thus the ability to correct the hypotension and shock.

Acute pancreatitis can be classified as either mild or severe. Mild acute pancreatitis normally improves within 48 to 72 hours and does not involve other organ systems. There is minimal interstitial edema, with only occasional microscopic acinar cell necrosis. Severe, acute pancreatitis is often associated with complications and multisystem organ failure. It can be a life-threatening condition, and the patient may require monitoring in the intensive care unit (ICU).

Complications during the first few days of diagnosis are associated with hemodynamic instability: shock, renal failure, respiratory compromise secondary to adult respiratory distress syndrome (ARDS), and hypoxemia. Pancreatic necrosis with secondary gram-negative sepsis has an associated 100% mortality rate unless there is extensive surgical débridement of the infected tissue. Up to 25% of patients diagnosed with acute pancreatitis develop some degree of fluid collection within a few days of diagnosis that resolves spontaneously half of the time. Patients in whom fluid collection does not resolve may form pseudocysts, abscesses, and other necrotic collections.

Pancreatic pseudocysts take at least 4 weeks to form and resolve spontaneously after about 6 weeks in 40% of cases. If the pseudocyst does not resolve within 12 weeks after acute pancreatitis, the risk of complications in symptomatic patients (infection, bleeding, rupture) is as high as 60%, but there is little associated risk in asymptomatic patients. The decision for invasive intervention depends on the progression of symptoms and cyst size.

CLINICAL PRESENTATION

Subjective

The patient with acute pancreatitis usually presents with abrupt onset of deep epigastric pain that persists for hours to days and may radiate straight through to the back. The pain is intense and often refractory to large doses of parenteral narcotics. It is aggravated by any vigorous activity, such as coughing, and by lying supine; it improves when the patient is seated and leaning forward.

The patient appears acutely ill, often with intractable nausea and vomiting. In some cases, depending on the severity, the patient may experience sweating, weakness, and anxiety. The patient may report a history of ingestion of alcohol or a big meal before onset of symptoms or mild biliary colic preceding the episode.

Objective

On physical examination, there is severe abdominal tenderness, particularly over the epigastric area, which may be accompanied by guarding but without rigidity or rebound tenderness, and there may be milder pain in the lower abdomen without guarding or rigidity. Abdominal distention is present in approximately 20% of patients. Bowel sounds can be hypoactive or absent if associated with paralytic ileus. The rectal examination is normal, and the stool is usually negative for occult blood.

The patient is tachycardic (100 to 140 beats/min) with rapid, shallow respiration. Inspiratory effort is poor because deep inspiration causes pain. Blood pressure may be high secondary to pain or low if shock is imminent. The patient's temperature may initially be normal or subnormal but increases to 100.4° to 102.2°F (38° to 39°C) within a few hours. Mild jaundice and scleral icterus may be present. The patient's skin may be pale, cool, and clammy if shock is present.

Uncommon findings that can result from the pancreatic inflammatory process include left-sided pleural effusion, bluish discoloration over the flanks (Grey Turner's sign) or around the umbilicus (Cullen's sign), jaundice caused by impingement on the common bile duct, and epigastric mass secondary to pseudocyst development.

DIAGNOSTIC REASONING

Diagnostic Tests

The diagnosis of pancreatitis is made on the basis of the presence of abdominal pain, elevated serum amylase and/or lipase levels, and imaging findings consistent with acute pancreatitis. The gold standard for diagnosis is an elevated serum amylase level (up to three times the normal value); however, in one-third of patients with pancreatitis from alcohol use disorder, the serum amylase level may be normal. The diagnosis of pancreatitis is supported by a concurrent elevation of serum lipase. Serum amylase and lipase levels are increased on the first day of acute symptoms and return to normal in 3 to 7 days. Levels remain normal if there has been repeated prior damage to acinar cells, which renders them incapable of further enzyme secretion. The level of elevation of amylase and lipase is not indicative of the severity of the disease.

The WBC count is usually between 12,000 and 20,000 cells/μL. The hematocrit can be as high as 50% to 55% because of hemoconcentration resulting from sequestered fluids in the third spaces.

A decrease in serum calcium may indicate saponification and is indicative of the severity of the pancreatitis. Calcium levels less than 7 mg/dL (with normal serum albumin) can cause tetany and are associated with poor prognosis. Elevated C-reactive protein is correlated with pancreatic necrosis. The risk of infection is positively correlated with pancreatic necrosis and accounts for most of the deaths. Pancreatic necrosis requires surgical intervention; CT-guided aspiration of the necrotic tissue for Gram stain and culture is indicated.

Patients presenting with biliary pancreatitis have an elevation of the liver enzymes. When alanine aminotransferase is up to three times the normal limit, the positive predictive value is 95% that the pancreatitis is caused by biliary disease (gallstones). Concomitant increases in the aspartate aminotransferase, alkaline phosphatase, and bilirubin suggest gallbladder disease.

Diagnostic imaging, especially CT of the abdomen, can provide fast and accurate information for the definitive diagnosis of acute pancreatitis. Although the CT scan can be normal in 15% to 30% of patients with mild acute pancreatitis, it is the most efficient means of discerning acute pancreatitis from other potentially fatal intra-abdominal processes. CT is also helpful in monitoring the progression or resolution of pancreatic pseudocysts.

Patients with acute pancreatitis and no obvious alternative causes should undergo abdominal ultrasonography to detect the possible causes such as cholelithiasis or neoplasms. Ultrasonography can also detect dilation of the common bile duct, indicating obstruction. Endoscopic retrograde cholangiopancreatography (ERCP) with sphincterotomy and stone extraction can be performed and has been proved to decrease morbidity and mortality.

If there is evidence that the pancreatitis is severe, additional testing with IV contrast is recommended; the necrotic pancreas has damage to its microcirculation and thus is not enhanced with IV contrast. If the microcirculation remains intact, there is uniform enhancement of the pancreas. Pancreatic necrosis is associated with much higher morbidity, mortality, and infection rates.

Pancreatic infection is a complication that requires immediate diagnosis and intervention. Infection should be suspected when the patient has persistently elevated WBC counts and fever. The patient normally looks very sick. Positive blood cultures and visualization of gas bubbles within the retroperitoneum on CT support the diagnosis.

Ranson's criteria are useful for assessing the severity of acute pancreatitis. Identification of early prognostic signs may provide the best indication of a serious outcome and can alert the practitioner that the patient may require transfer to the ICU. Table 41.1 lists the 11 objective signs

TABLE 41.1 Ranson's Criteria for Assessing the Severity of Pancreatitis

At admission or at time of diagnosis:
1. Age older than 55 years
2. White blood cell count greater than 16,000/µL
3. Blood glucose greater than 200 mg/dL
4. Base deficit greater than 4 mEq/L
5. Serum lactate dehydrogenase (LDH) greater than 350 IU/L
6. Aspartate transaminase (AST) greater than 250 U/L

During the initial 48 hours:
1. Hematocrit (Hct) drop of more than 10 percentage points
2. Blood urea nitrogen (BUN) rise of greater than 5 mg/dL
3. Arterial Po_2 of less than 60
4. Serum calcium (Ca) of less than 8 mg/dL
5. Estimated fluid sequestration of greater than 6 L

Number of Diagnostic Criteria	Mortality Rate (%)
0–2	1
3–4	16
5–6	40
7–8	100

Source: Adapted from Ranson JH, Rifkind KM, Roses DF, et al. Prognostic signs and the role of operative management in acute pancreatitis. *Surg Gynecol Obstet.* 1974;139(1):69–81.

Box 41.2 Hyperamylasemia: Pancreatic and Nonpancreatic Causes

Pancreatic Hyperamylasemia
- Pancreatic pseudocyst
- Perforated duodenal ulcer
- Small bowel perforation
- Mesenteric infarction
- Mesenteric vascular thrombus
- Opiate administration
- Post–endoscopic retrograde cholangiopancreatography

Nonpancreatic Hyperamylasemia
- Salivary adenitis (secondary to mumps)
- Ruptured ectopic pregnancy
- Post–abdominal surgery
- Lactic acidosis
- Leaking aortic aneurysm
- Renal insufficiency

---

used to classify the severity of pancreatitis. Mortality rates correlate directly with the number of diagnostic criteria present. Pancreatitis is classified as severe when three or more of Ranson's criteria are met.

Differential Diagnosis

Differential diagnosis of acute pancreatitis is made by history and physical examination and supported by laboratory data and imaging studies. CT scan is useful in differentiating other intra-abdominal processes from acute pancreatitis. However, it is less helpful in identifying gallstones as a potential cause. Laboratory data are helpful in differentiating other causes of acute abdominal pain with associated hyperamylasemia. Box 41.2 differentiates hyperamylasemia resulting from pancreatic and nonpancreatic causes.

MANAGEMENT

Treatment of acute pancreatitis is aimed at limiting the severity of pancreatic inflammation, preventing further complications by interrupting the pathological processes, and managing symptoms. Mild acute pancreatitis usually resolves spontaneously in a few days; these patients can be managed conservatively as outpatients. Fasting is necessary until the symptoms of acute inflammation have subsided.

Treatment includes maintaining fluid status with parenteral fluids to prevent hypovolemia and hypotension. Pain has traditionally been controlled with meperidine (Demerol) rather than with other opiates to prevent increased pressure within the sphincter of Oddi. However, research indicates that morphine causes no more spasms in the sphincter of Oddi than meperidine. The patient is allowed nothing by mouth, and NG tube insertion should be considered when there is persistent nausea, vomiting, or evidence of ileus. The use of empiric antibiotics, H_2-receptor antagonists, and pancreatic enzyme inhibitors have not been proved effective and are not recommended.

Judicious introduction of clear liquids can be instituted once the patient is pain free, amylase and lipase levels have returned to normal range, and bowel sounds have returned. A low-fat diet may be instituted as the patient tolerates.

Patients with more severe pancreatitis tend to have sequestered larger amounts of fluid as a result of the "chemical burn" sustained by the tissues within the retroperitoneal space. These patients are usually transferred to the ICU under the care of a gastroenterologist or surgeon. Aggressive volume replacement is necessary and may require invasive hemodynamic monitoring to maintain appropriate fluid balance. Fluid resuscitation is an important part of therapy and 6 to 8 L/day may be required. Some patients may require infusion of fresh frozen plasma or serum albumin or blood transfusions, which can increase the risk of the development of ARDS. Cardiac function and fluid status can be monitored with a central line or pulmonary artery catheter. Measurement of hourly urine output is also necessary. If hemodynamic stability is not achieved through volume replacement, vasopressors may be necessary.

Daily monitoring of serum calcium, magnesium, glucose, electrolytes, total protein, albumin, amylase, lipase, and complete blood count with subsequent correction of abnormalities is required. In febrile patients, cultures of blood, urine, and sputum should be obtained, as well as CT-guided needle aspiration of necrotic areas of the pancreas with initiation of appropriate broad-spectrum antibiotic coverage as necessary to prevent increased morbidity and mortality. Arterial blood gas readings should be obtained daily, and hypoxemia treated accordingly. The patient may require assisted ventilation if hypoxemia persists or ARDS develops.

Correction of serum glucose is done with caution and should not begin until levels are greater than 250 mg/dL. Hypocalcemia is often corrected with the administration of albumin-containing fluids. Neuromuscular irritability, if present, can be corrected with a 10% solution of calcium gluconate. If there is a coexisting hypomagnesemia, correction of the magnesium level will often restore the calcium to its normal level. In patients with renal impairment, magnesium must be replaced cautiously.

Patients with severe pancreatitis must be maintained in a fasting state for prolonged periods of time, often for 2 to 4 weeks. Administration of antacids through an NG tube can help to prevent stress ulceration. The nutritional needs of the patient can be maintained with total parenteral nutrition until the gut becomes functional; enteral feedings can then be started, using the distal jejunum to reduce pancreatic stimulation. Oral feedings should not be started until all complications have been treated, the patient is free from nausea and vomiting, and amylase and lipase levels have returned to normal.

Surgical intervention is normally reserved for a pancreatic pseudocyst that has persisted for more than 6 weeks with ongoing symptomatology, necrotizing pancreatitis, pancreatic abscess, or severe hemorrhagic pancreatitis. Despite surgical intervention, the mortality rate for necrotizing pancreatitis remains high.

For pancreatitis caused by cholelithiasis, surgical intervention is determined by the presenting course of events. If biliary decompression is necessary, it can often be accomplished with ERCP. If the pancreatitis is mild, a cholecystectomy can be performed at a later time.

FOLLOW-UP AND REFERRAL

Patients with severe acute pancreatitis or those who do not respond to conservative treatment should be referred to a gastroenterologist for management. Surgical referral should be made once the diagnosis of pancreatitis is made. The patient who develops a pseudocyst requires long-term follow-up with serial CT scans to observe the resolution or growth of the cyst, which may require surgical intervention. The patient who has gallstone disease should have a cholecystectomy.

The prognosis of the patient with pancreatitis correlates directly with the severity of the inflammatory process. Patients with interstitial, or edematous, pancreatitis even with systemic complications have a mortality rate of 1% to 2%; however, patients with necrotizing pancreatitis have a mortality rate of 10% with sterile necrosis and up to 30% with infected necrosis.

In patients for whom no cause has been found, studies have suggested that half have occult gallstone disease (biliary sludge) or sphincter of Oddi dysfunction. These patients require repeated abdominal ultrasonography to detect the development of biliary sludge. Patients with hereditary hypercholesterolemia are often missed because serum triglycerides are not obtained until after several days of fasting, at which time the triglyceride level may have fallen to within normal limits.

Patient Education: Acute Pancreatitis

Patients with biliary disease as the cause of the pancreatitis should be informed of the need for a cholecystectomy, as well as the benefit of reducing their dietary intake of fat. If the etiology of pancreatitis is alcohol use disorder, the patient should be encouraged to abstain. Patients with genetic hyperlipidemia require diet instruction and information on avoidance of precipitating factors such as alcohol, estrogens, and certain drugs. These patients may benefit from lipid-lowering medications and must be taught to control their diabetes if present. If a drug is the suspected cause of the pancreatitis, it should not be restarted.

CHRONIC PANCREATITIS

Chronic pancreatitis is defined as a slowly progressive inflammatory process that results in irreversible fibrosis of the pancreas with destruction and atrophy of the exocrine and endocrine glandular tissue. There are varying degrees of ductal dilation and fibrosis. There can be intraductal formation of protein plugs, which calcify and cause further dilation and obstruction. *Chronic relapsing pancreatitis* is defined as acute attacks that occur in the setting of chronic pancreatitis and are usually precipitated by a specific event such as binge drinking or the passage of a stone.

EPIDEMIOLOGY AND CAUSES

There is little reliable information on the prevalence or incidence of chronic pancreatitis. Alcohol use disorder may account for between 70% and 80% of the cases in industrialized countries. Although there is no threshold for alcohol consumption and the development of chronic pancreatitis, there is a statistically significant increase in individuals who consume 120 g of ethanol per day (eight 12-ounce beers, 8 ounces of 100-proof whiskey, or 30 ounces of wine). Diets high in protein in combination with either high or low fat can further predispose patients to pancreatic injury from alcohol.

Other causes of chronic pancreatitis include autoimmune disease, genetic mutations, hereditary predisposition, hypertriglyceridemia, severe malnutrition (especially protein-calorie deficiency in developing countries), tropical pancreatitis, and obstruction of the main pancreatic duct caused by stenosis, stones, tumor, or cystic fibrosis. In 10% to 30% of persons with chronic pancreatitis, the cause is unknown, but patients are divided into two groups: (1) those who present with abdominal pain (usually between ages 15 and 30) and (2) older individuals (ages 50 to 70) who present, often without pain, with pancreatic calcifications, glandular insufficiency, and diabetes.

The tropical, or nutritional, form of chronic pancreatitis is almost exclusively found in tropical countries. In these countries, the disease begins in early childhood and results in death in early adulthood because of complications. This type of pancreatitis also involves large intraductal calculi and a high susceptibility to pancreatic cancer. Malnutrition has a significant role, but it is not the sole cause because many areas with comparable malnutrition do not have equal prevalence of the disease. Key features of tropical pancreatitis include abdominal pain, maldigestion leading to steatorrhea, and diabetes.

PATHOPHYSIOLOGY

The pathogenesis of chronic pancreatitis is unclear. Two characteristic findings in chronic pancreatitis are hypersecretion of protein without a subsequent increase in ductal bicarbonate secretion and inflammation. Chronic pancreatitis results in irreversible structural damage with permanent functional impairment of the pancreatic gland. For individuals who have alcohol use–related disease, ductal obstruction is thought to be caused by changes in the chemical composition of the pancreatic juice, leading to protein plugging, calcification, and subsequent pancreatic damage. Another theory postulates that continuous injury to the acinar cells causes inflammation, necrosis, and fibrosis. Analysis of pancreatic juice obtained from patients with alcohol use disorder revealed protein plugs but not always chronic pancreatitis. Proponents of the theory favoring repeated damage to the pancreatic acinar cells believe that ductal obstruction is a result of changes in the pancreatic juice that cause increased viscosity and damage to the gland itself. These changes in the enzymatic properties result in chronic inflammation and fibrosis of the gland. Biliary disease has not been identified as a causative factor in the development of chronic pancreatitis.

With the progressive inflammatory changes occurring with chronic pancreatitis, it is not uncommon to find a fibrotic common bile duct and jaundice secondary to the obstructed common bile duct. Upper GI bleeding can result from the formation of gastric varices or the development of a pseudoaneurysm in an artery within the pancreatic area. Steatorrhea and diabetes mellitus result from destruction of the pancreatic gland with subsequent endocrine and exocrine insufficiency. Steatorrhea develops as lipase and protease secretion drops below 10% of normal. Islet cell destruction reduces insulin secretion, causing glucose intolerance and diabetes.

CLINICAL PRESENTATION

Subjective

The most frequent presenting symptoms are intractable abdominal pain, weight loss, and diarrhea, but symptoms can be as mild as dyspepsia, nausea, and vomiting. Abdominal pain is usually epigastric or located in the left upper quadrant, may radiate to the back or left lumbar region, and is described as dull and constant. Pain may be absent in 5% to 10% of the cases or may represent an exacerbation of acute or relapsing pancreatitis. Pain may precede the development of other symptoms of chronic pancreatitis by years. The pain is often precipitated or aggravated by food or alcohol intake. In some patients, the pain diminishes over time (5 to 15 years) and is associated with failure or calcification of the gland. Between 10% and 20% of older adults with idiopathic chronic pancreatitis have no pain with the disease.

Weight loss may result from anorexia caused by pain and nausea, malabsorption secondary to pancreatic exocrine insufficiency, or poorly controlled diabetes mellitus. Diabetes mellitus is present in approximately 50% of patients and is often the presenting sign in individuals who have no pain associated with pancreatitis. Steatorrhea develops after the pancreas loses the ability to secrete digestive enzymes, which results in bulky, foul-smelling, fatty stools. Patients often complain of "oil leakage" from the rectum or an "oil slick" in the toilet bowl, which is indicative of pancreatic insufficiency.

Objective

Abdominal assessment in patients presenting with pain reveals mild to moderate epigastric tenderness with no rebound tenderness or guarding. A palpable abdominal mass is suggestive of a pancreatic pseudocyst. Bowel sounds may be absent in patients with paralytic ileus. Lung sounds may be diminished in the bases, which is indicative of pleural effusion.

DIAGNOSTIC REASONING

Diagnostic Tests

Diagnosis of chronic pancreatitis is normally made through evaluation of pancreatic function and radiographic visualization of structural abnormalities such as pancreatic calcification or abnormalities in the size or consistency of the pancreatic tissue. The patient usually presents with chronic abdominal pain, weight loss, exocrine insufficiency (malabsorption), and diabetes mellitus.

Tests for pancreatic function include assessment of endocrine and exocrine function. A 2-hour postprandial blood sugar level greater than 200 mg/dL or fasting glucose greater than 120 mg/dL on two occasions is diagnostic for diabetes mellitus. Glucosuria may also be present. The serum amylase level may remain within normal limits because the pancreas has lost the ability to mount a response due to the chronicity of the disease. Malabsorption is documented by a 72-hour stool analysis for fecal fat content. Although helpful for diagnosis of exocrine function, steatorrhea is not diagnostic of chronic pancreatitis because patients do not develop steatorrhea until lipase falls below 10% of normal.

Pancreatic insufficiency can be confirmed by the bentiromide (nitroblue tetrazolium–*para*-aminobenzoic acid [NBT-PABA]) test, which measures urinary excretion of pancreatic chymotrypsin, or a secretin stimulation test, which is more sensitive but is unavailable in many places. The test involves placing a tube within the duodenum and collecting pancreatic secretions after IV stimulation with secretin. Collections of normal volume and low in bicarbonate (HCO_3^-) suggest chronic pancreatitis; collections low in volume and normal HCO_3^- suggest pancreatic cancer. The detection of decreased fecal chymotrypsin or elastase helps to diagnose pancreatic insufficiency, but these tests do not have widespread availability.

Imaging studies include plain films of the abdomen, which may show intraductal stones or a calcified pancreas caused by pancreatolithiasis and mild ileus. CT and/or ultrasonography of the abdomen may show an abnormal size or consistency of the pancreas, a pancreatic pseudocyst, or dilated pancreatic ducts. Magnetic resonance cholangiopancreatography is a noninvasive procedure that is considered a safer procedure than ERCP. ERCP is associated with an increased risk of acute pancreatitis from dye injection into the pancreas. Endoscopic ultrasound can be used to visualize the pancreatic and bile ducts.

Differential Diagnosis

Differential diagnosis includes diseases that present with persistent abdominal pain such as peptic ulcer disease or mesenteric ischemia; diseases that result in weight loss and abdominal pain, including abdominal malignancies, especially cancer of the pancreas; and intestinal disorders that may present with steatorrhea. The diagnosis of chronic pancreatitis can be confirmed by visualization of the calcified pancreas on x-ray films, which will also rule out most other disease processes.

MANAGEMENT

The treatment of chronic pancreatitis is aimed at preventing further pancreatic damage, managing pain, and supplementing exocrine and endocrine function. The major cause of chronic pancreatitis is alcohol use disorder; therefore, complete abstinence is imperative. Pancreatic enzyme supplementation may relieve pain in some patients. Generally, narcotics are necessary to manage pain. Patients whose pain is not managed by analgesics or pancreatic enzyme therapy should be considered for operative treatment.

Malabsorption is managed with a low-fat diet (less than 50 g/day) and oral pancreatic enzyme supplementation. Oral supplementation should be administered 20 to 30 minutes before meals and snacks. The usual dose is 30,000 units of lipase. Non–enteric-coated pancrelipase formulations (Viokase or Cotazym) should be given with H_2-receptor antagonists to prevent degradation by gastric acids. Enteric-coated preparations of pancrelipase (Pancrease or Creon) or pancreatin (Donnazyme) are stable at an acid pH and should not be given with acid neutralizers because this will promote enzyme release within the stomach. Fat-soluble vitamin (A, D, E, and K) replacement may be required. Favorable outcomes are weight gain, decreased number of stools per day, decrease in oil seepage from the rectum, and subjective improvement in well-being.

Endocrine insufficiency is controlled with insulin supplementation. Extreme caution must be used with insulin supplementation because there is a deficiency of glucagon secretion, which can lead to prolonged hypoglycemia. Serum glucose levels of 200 to 250 mg/dL are considered acceptable and do not require treatment. The principal step in the management of diabetes associated with chronic pancreatitis is the correction of poor nutritional habits, malabsorption and malnutrition, and the elimination of alcohol use. Normal insulin requirements range from 5 to 15 units per day but may fluctuate up to 40 units per day. It is best to maintain these patients at a higher than normal glucose level to avoid hypoglycemia while avoiding significant glucosuria.

Surgical intervention may be required to drain persistent pseudocysts, for relief of pain, or to treat other complications associated with chronic pancreatitis. The goal of surgical intervention is to alleviate biliary tract disease, establish the free flow of bile into the duodenum, and remove obstruction of the pancreatic duct. Distal pancreatectomy may be necessary if the disease is located at the tail of the pancreas, and the Whipple procedure is performed when the disease is most extensive at the head of the pancreas. These procedures relieve the pain for 60% to 80% of patients.

In patients with pancreatitis from alcohol use disorder, ERCP examination often reveals alternating stricture and dilation ("chain of lakes") of the pancreatic duct. Treatment is a modified Puestow procedure (lateral pancreaticojejunostomy), which relieves pain in 70% to 80% of patients.

FOLLOW-UP AND REFERRAL

Follow-up of the patient with chronic pancreatitis depends on the complications resulting from the disease and the medical and surgical interventions employed to remedy the disease. Patients who have developed pseudocysts that have not resolved spontaneously will require periodic CT scans to monitor resolution or evolution of the cysts. Cysts that are consistently larger than 6 cm and are expanding should be referred for invasive treatment.

A nutritionist may be helpful in managing protein-calorie malnutrition. The pancreas is very nutrition-sensitive, and an improper diet can lead to atrophy and fibrosis. Follow-up with the nutritionist is often necessary for control of diabetes mellitus as well.

Patient Education: Chronic Pancreatitis

Patients should be taught about the pathophysiology of this chronic disease, common complications, and the long-term outlook. Patients with chronic pancreatitis can expect that after 5 to 10 years, the episodes of pancreatic pain diminish in frequency and may disappear as long as they follow the treatment. Patients should understand their medicine regimen, including appropriate timing of medication doses and adverse effects. Patients tend to be more compliant when they understand that the goal of treatment is to control diarrhea and gain body weight. Patients can be provided with written instructions to assist with adherence.

Patients should be cautioned against long-term narcotic analgesic use because it can result in drug dependence. If long-term narcotic use is necessary, patients may benefit from referral to a pain control clinic to learn how to relieve pain using nonpharmacotherapeutic measures.

PANCREATIC CANCER

EPIDEMIOLOGY AND CAUSES

Carcinoma is the most common neoplasm found in the pancreas. The majority (75%) of carcinomas are found in the head of the pancreas and 25% are located in the body and the tail. Carcinoma of the ampulla of Vater is far less common. Neuroendocrine tumors of the pancreas are far less common as well, with an incidence of less than 1 per 100,000 persons. Pancreatic cancer is the third most common cause of cancer deaths in the United States and the seventh leading cause of cancer deaths globally in industrialized countries. Although advancements have been made in early diagnosis, the incidence is expected to increase.

Risk factors for pancreatic cancer include increasing age, tobacco use (particularly cigarette smoking), heavy alcohol use, obesity, family history, and to a lesser extent, diabetes mellitus and chronic pancreatitis. Also implicated are arsenic and cadmium exposure.

PATHOPHYSIOLOGY

There are many types of neoplasms that occur in the pancreas and each is generally classified by its histological differentiation (epithelial or nonepithelial) and by biological behavior (benign, premalignant, or malignant). In addition, epithelial neoplasms can be exocrine or endocrine. Exocrine tumors can be classified as ductal or acinar. Pancreatic ductal adenocarcinoma (PDAC) is the most common type of pancreatic cancer and accounts for about 90% of all cases. Neuroendocrine pancreatic tumors make up between 1% and 2% of pancreatic neoplasms. They may functionally produce gastrin, insulin, glucagon, vasoactive intestinal peptide, somatostatin, growth hormone-releasing hormone, and adrenocorticotropic hormone, to name but a few, or they may be nonfunctional.

When the head of the pancreas is involved, obstruction of the common bile duct leads to painless jaundice. PDAC is rarely diagnosed in the early stages and is usually between 2 and 4 cm or larger at diagnosis. There is usually infiltration of the surrounding structures such as the duodenum, stomach, portal vein, and peripancreatic fat tissue. In addition, there is lymph node metastasis in the region.

CLINICAL PRESENTATION

Subjective

Seventy percent of patients present with vague, diffuse epigastric pain in the upper left quadrant often radiating to the back. The pain may be relieved by sitting up and leaning forward but this is a sign that the cancer has spread beyond the pancreas. Patients may complain of diarrhea due to the maldigestion and weight loss, which is a late sign. Jaundice may occur from biliary obstruction when the pancreatic head is involved.

Objective

Abdominal assessment yields little information. The patient may have abdominal tenderness on palpation. If the gallbladder is palpable, this indicates obstruction and possible neoplasm (Courvoisier sign). There may be a hard, fixed, palpable mass that is tender.

DIAGNOSTIC REASONING

Diagnostic Tests

Laboratory tests may show a mild anemia. In 10% to 20% of patients, diabetes mellitus or impaired glucose tolerance is seen. Serum amylase or lipase, liver enzymes, and bilirubin may be elevated. Carcinoma of the ampulla of Vater may cause occult blood in the stool. Although CA 19-9 has a sensitivity of 70% and a specificity of 87%, it has not been useful for early detection because increased levels are also found in cholecystitis and acute and chronic pancreatitis. 88% to 100% of patients with pancreatic neuroendocrine tumors have elevated levels of plasma chromogranin A.

CT scan (multiphase thin-cut helical) detects pancreatic masses in over 80% of patients and is used for initial diagnosis. In addition, it identifies metastasis and delineates the size and extent of the tumor. Magnetic resonance imaging (MRI) can be used as an alternative to CT. Although a positron emission tomography (PET) scan is a sensitive test for detecting pancreatic tumors, it is not used for diagnosis because of the cost. Endoscopic ultrasound is more sensitive in detecting pancreatic cancer and can be used to guide biopsy for tissue diagnosis.

Differential Diagnosis

Because symptoms and clinical manifestations are vague until the disease is advanced, differential diagnosis is difficult. Differential diagnoses include diseases that present with epigastric pain such as peptic ulcer disease; diseases that result in weight loss and abdominal pain, including abdominal malignancies; diseases of the liver and gallbladder such as cholelithiasis or hepatic duct obstruction; or pancreatitis.

MANAGEMENT

Treatment is usually surgical in nature. Radical pancreaticoduodenal resection (Whipple procedure) is usually only indicated when the cancer is limited to the head of the pancreas, periampullary area, and the duodenal area. It is not indicated for patients with peritoneal or liver metastasis. The best outcomes are obtained at centers that specialize in treating pancreatic cancer.

Adjuvant chemotherapy is increasing, particularly in nonresectable and borderline-resectable tumors; however, it remains controversial, and is used more often in the United States. Adjuvant chemotherapy, usually with gemcitabine, 5-fluorouracil, or gemcitabine with capecitabine is shown to downstage tumor burden by about 30% in patients with locally advanced cancer, often allowing for tumor resection. Chemotherapy in patients with metastatic pancreatic cancer has been disappointing, although outcomes are improving with FOLFIRINOX (5-fluorouracil, leucovorin, irinotecan, oxaliplatin). Prognosis for patients with carcinoma of the pancreas is poor with 5-year survival ranging between 2% and 5%.

REFERENCES

Cholelithiasis/Cholecystitis

Ahmed O, Rogers AC, Bolger JC, et al. Meta-analysis of outcomes of endoscopic ultrasound-guided gallbladder drainage versus percutaneous cholecystostomy for the management of acute cholecystitis. *Surg Endosc.* 2018;32:1627–1635.

Higa JT, Sahar N, Kozarek RA, et al. EUS-guided gallbladder drainage with a lumen-apposing metal stent versus endoscopic transpapillary gallbladder drainage for the treatment of acute cholecystitis. *Gastrointest Endosc.* 2019;90(3):483–492.

Reddy S, Jagtap N, Kalapala R, et al. Choledocholithiasis in acute calculous cholecystitis: guidelines and beyond. *Ann Gastroenterol.* 2021;34(2):247–252.

Talha A, Abdelbaki T, Farouk A, et al. Cholelithiasis after bariatric surgery, incidence, and prophylaxis: randomized controlled trial. *Surg Endosc.* 2019;34:5331–5337.

Pancreatic Cancer

Akirow A, Larouche V, Alshehri S, et al. Treatment options for pancreatic neuroendocrine tumors. *Cancers.* 2019;11(6):828.

Haeberle L, Esposito I. Pathology of pancreatic cancer. *Transl Gastroenterol Hepatol.* 2019;4:50. https://dx.doi.org/10.21037%2Ftgh.2019.06.02

Lai E, Puzzoni M, Ziranu P, et al. New therapeutic targets in pancreatic cancer. *Cancer Treat Rev.* 2019;81:101926.

Mizrahi JD, Surana R, Valle JW, et al. Pancreatic cancer. *The Lancet.* 2020;395(10242):2008–2020.

Ranson JH, Rifkind KM, Roses DF, et al. Prognostic signs and the role of operative management in acute pancreatitis. *Surg Gynecol Obstet.* 1974;139(1):69–81.

Rawla P, Sunkara T, Gaduputi V. Epidemiology of pancreatic cancer: global trends, etiology and risk factors. *World J Oncol.* 2019;10(1):10–27.

Salem AA, Mackenzie GG. Pancreatic cancer: a critical review of dietary risk. *Nutr Res.* 2018;52:1–13.

Singhi AD, Koay EJ, Chari ST, et al. Early detection of pancreatic cancer: opportunities and challenges. *Gastroenterology.* 2019;156(7):2024–2040.

Pancreatitis

Bollen TL. Acute pancreatitis: international classification and nomenclature. *Clin Radiol.* 2016;71(2):121–133.

Gardner TB, Adler DG, Forsmark CE, et al. ACG Clinical Guideline: chronic pancreatitis. *Am J Gastroenterol.* 2020;115(3):322–339.

Lee PJ, Papachristou GI. New insights into acute pancreatitis. *Nat Rev Gastroenterol Hepatol.* 2019;16:479–496.

Singh VK, Yadav D, Garg PK. Diagnosis and management of chronic pancreatitis: a review. *JAMA.* 2019;322:2422–2434.

RESOURCES

American Gastroenterological Association
   https://gastro.org/

The National Pancreas Foundation
   https://pancreasfoundation.org/

Acute pancreatitis causes and symptoms
   https://pancreasfoundation.org/patient-information/acute-pancreatitis/acute-pancreatitis-diagnosis-and-treatment/

Chapter 42

Cirrhosis and Liver Failure

Debera J. Thomas, PhD, RN, ANP/FNP

Cirrhosis is the result of hepatocellular injury involving the entire liver, resulting in fibrosis, nodular regeneration, and distorted hepatic architecture. Cirrhosis is considered permanent and irreversible. Fibrous bands are formed during nodular regeneration in an attempt by the liver to repair itself, and these bands give the liver a hobnailed appearance. The fibrotic changes that occur within the liver parenchyma cause disruption and compression of the vascular, biliary, and lymphatic vessels and result in many of the characteristic findings common to liver failure.

EPIDEMIOLOGY AND CAUSES

In the Western Hemisphere, cirrhosis is a leading cause of death in individuals older than age 40. The prevalence of cirrhosis in the United States is approximately 0.27% (633,323 people) and may be higher. Although there are many causes of cirrhosis (Box 42.1), chronic alcohol use disorder (AUD) and viral hepatitis remain the leading pathological insults leading to cirrhosis in the United States.

There are three consequences of AUD: fatty liver, alcoholic hepatitis, and alcoholic cirrhosis. Fatty liver is a reversible condition where large vacuoles of triglycerides accumulate in the hepatocytes. The accumulation of fat in the liver causes an inflammatory reaction in the liver called *steatohepatitis,* which is a precursor to cirrhosis. Alcoholic hepatitis results from moderate to severe AUD for years and can lead to alcoholic cirrhosis quickly even with abstinence, but it is not an obligatory phase in the development of cirrhosis.

Alcoholic cirrhosis is the most common type of cirrhosis in the United States. The incidence of AUD is increasing in the United States; an estimated 18 million people in the United States have AUD. However, only 35% of individuals with AUD develop cirrhosis.

The toxic effects of alcohol metabolism on the liver, immunological alterations, oxidative stress, and malnutrition cause alcoholic cirrhosis. Although alcoholic cirrhosis is often associated with nutritional and vitamin deficiencies, it can occur in well-nourished individuals. Studies have found no safe amount of alcohol that can be ingested daily without causing cirrhosis, which supports the theory that there are additional factors (genetic, environmental, nutritional) that may influence the development of alcoholic liver disease. Females tend to develop cirrhosis more quickly with less alcohol intake than do males, which suggests that a smaller, leaner body mass and enhanced absorption are both factors in the development of alcoholic cirrhosis.

Nonalcoholic fatty liver disease (NAFLD) is characterized by fat infiltration of the hepatocytes, primarily triglycerides, and occurs in the absence of alcohol consumption. Globally, NAFLD is responsible for 60% of all cases of chronic liver disease (CLD). NAFLD is associated with obesity in adults and children, particularly abdominal obesity, high cholesterol, high triglycerides, metabolic syndrome, type 2 diabetes mellitus (T2DM), and the gut microbiome. Some sources indicate that NAFLD may be responsible for the increase in cirrhosis because of the trends in increasing obesity and metabolic

---

Box 42.1 Causes of Cirrhosis

Alcohol
Direct hepatotoxins
- Carbon tetrachloride
- Phosphorus
- Indirect hepatotoxins
- Tetracycline
- Methotrexate
- Acetaminophen
- Mushroom toxin—*Amanita phalloides*
- Alkylated anabolic steroids
- 6-Mercaptopurine

Hepatitis B and hepatitis C virus infection
Nonalcoholic fatty liver disease
Autoimmune chronic active hepatitis
Diabetes mellitus and insipidus
Thyroiditis
Ulcerative colitis
Glomerulonephritis
Biliary cirrhosis
Primary biliary cirrhosis
Primary sclerosing cholangitis
Chronic pancreatitis
Sclerosing cholangitis
Vasculitis
Cholelithiasis
Cystic fibrosis
Genetic diseases
- Wilson's disease
- Hemochromatosis
- Galactosemia

Vascular/congestive disorders of the liver
- Budd-Chiari syndrome
- Ischemic hepatitis/shock liver
- Right-sided heart failure (chronic)

syndrome. Some patients with NAFLD go on to develop nonalcoholic steatohepatitis (NASH), which in the most severe form progresses to cirrhosis, end-stage liver disease, and hepatocellular carcinoma.

Primary biliary cirrhosis (PBC) is a disease that almost exclusively affects females aged 40 to 60 years. It is an autoimmune disease that causes destruction of the intrahepatic bile ducts, resulting in cholestasis. Autoimmune disorders such as scleroderma, Raynaud's syndrome, autoimmune thyroid disease, celiac disease, and Sjögren's syndrome have been linked to the development of PBC.

Primary sclerosing cholangitis (PSC) is most common in males aged 20 to 40 and is associated with inflammatory bowel disease (75%), as well as with the histocompatibility antigens HLA-B8, HLA-DR3, and HLA-DR4, suggesting a genetic link. It is characterized by diffuse inflammation and fibrosis throughout the biliary tree. Factors contributing to the development of PSC are anything that obstructs or inhibits the flow of bile through both the extrahepatic and intrahepatic bile ducts. Smoking is associated with a *decreased* risk of PSC.

Budd-Chiari syndrome (BCS) is a disorder resulting from hepatic vein thrombosis and outflow obstruction, which can occur anywhere from the hepatic veins to the inferior vena cava (IVC) or the right atrium. Other disease processes associated with this form of cirrhosis are coagulopathies, lymphoreticular malignancies, ischemic hepatitis resulting from profound hypotension associated with shock, and liver arteriovenous malformations characteristic of hemorrhagic telangiectasia. There are numerous causes for BCS, and definitive diagnosis is found in only approximately 65% to 75% of cases. In the Western Hemisphere, thrombosis of the hepatic veins is most often associated with myeloproliferative and coagulation disorders, as well as oral contraceptive use. Venous thrombosis is also an associated risk factor in the third trimester of pregnancy. Malignant tumors arising from within the liver or metastatic renal carcinoma can result in mechanical obstruction of the IVC, causing thrombosis within the hepatic veins and resulting in cirrhosis.

Wilson's disease (hepatolenticular degeneration) and hemochromatosis are both autosomal recessive metabolic disorders that often present with hepatocellular dysfunction and can lead to cirrhosis if left untreated. The liver is the primary organ involved in the metabolism of both iron (hemochromatosis) and copper (Wilson's disease); overload of either metal can cause cirrhosis. Hemochromatosis is diagnosed primarily in middle-aged whites, whereas Wilson's disease primarily affects persons between the ages of 3 and 55 years.

PATHOPHYSIOLOGY

Cirrhosis is the irreversible, end stage of liver injury caused by a variety of insults. Fibrotic scarring and hepatocellular changes result from chronic inflammation; obstruction; and toxic, metabolic, and congestive injuries. The morphological changes resulting from the injury are often classified according to the size of the regenerative nodules: patients may have micronodular, macronodular, and mixed forms of cirrhosis. Cirrhosis also may result from severe acute injury, as is seen with hepatitis caused by hepatitis B virus (HBV), hepatitis C virus (HCV), and chemical injury; subsequent to moderate damage sustained over months, as seen with obstructive biliary diseases; or from chronic continuous abuse, as seen in alcoholic cirrhosis.

Liver Changes in Cirrhosis

In individuals with cirrhosis, the normal lobular liver architecture is replaced by diffuse disorganization, resulting in proliferation of bands of fibrous tissue and nodular regeneration of the surviving hepatocytes. The extent to which this occurs depends on the degree of injury, the length of exposure to the injury, and the liver's reaction to the insult. The end result is a decrease in the total liver cell mass because of collagen formation or fibrosis. During the repair process, there is distortion of the microcirculation, resulting in an increased resistance to blood flow, thereby causing portal venous hypertension. As the liver attempts to repair itself, it develops a series of collateral vessels from the newly regenerated nodules to the existing portal vein and hepatic artery. These vessels, which are much less efficient than those of the normal circulation, cause portal hypertension.

Histological Classification

Histological classification of cirrhosis is useful for describing the major anatomical changes that result from the various insults. This type of classification gives no etiological information other than narrowing the scope to the injurious agents resulting in this specific histological category of injury. Moreover, it is important to remember that at any point in the disease process, a patient may exhibit varying degrees of histological change.

Micronodular (Laennec's) cirrhosis is characterized by regenerative nodules that are 1 cm in diameter or less, no bigger than normal liver lobules. Histological examination fails to identify portal tracts and hepatic venules. AUD often results in this type of cirrhosis; the theory is that continuous damage to the liver caused by alcohol exposure prevents it from regenerating. Initially, the liver becomes enlarged and fatty as changes in lipid metabolism lead to fatty infiltrates. As the disease progresses, the liver atrophies and hardens. Fibrous tissue forms in thin, regularly spaced bands throughout the liver, which in time result in a decreased liver mass.

Macronodular cirrhosis is characterized by larger nodules (diameters of 5 cm), which may occur in multiples of varying sizes and may contain central veins. These nodules are surrounded by broad fibrous bands of varying thickness, which correspond to the postnecrotic type of cirrhosis associated with chronic hepatitis. As the normal liver architecture collapses, the portal tracts converge between the fibrous scars, which is a key histological finding. Mixed cirrhosis has characteristics of both micronodular and macronodular cirrhosis.

Causes of Cirrhosis

Drug-induced liver disease can be the result of toxicity from a single drug or from a combination of the toxic effects from multiple drugs. The resultant liver toxicity may be caused by metabolism that is enhanced, altered, or the result of idiosyncratic processes, such as hypersensitivity or a genetic predisposition to liver damage. Intrinsic hepatic injury is drug-dose–dependent and influenced by environmental and genetic factors, whereas idiosyncratic drug reactions are more frequent and are not dose dependent. Patients who have hypersensitivity reactions to a drug develop hepatotoxicity secondary to the formation of drug metabolites, which are harmful to the liver.

NAFLD encompasses a variety of presentations ranging from accumulation of triglycerides in the hepatocytes with no liver damage to NASH, leading to cirrhosis or hepatocellular carcinoma. In patients with obesity, the prevalence may be as high as 75% and even higher in patients with T2DM. There is an increased risk of progression to liver damage in patients with T2DM. Although the exact pathophysiology is not well understood, there is some evidence indicating mitochondrial dysfunction that interferes with the homeostasis of fat and energy in hepatic cells. The abnormalities in the mitochondrial function alter the balance between prooxidant and antioxidant mechanisms that lead to an increase in nonmetabolized fatty acids.

Both chronic active HBV and HCV can cause severe liver injury, leading to cirrhosis and liver failure. About one-third of those diagnosed with HBV will progress to cirrhosis, and 15% of those with chronic HCV go on to develop cirrhosis. The chronic hepatitis causes repeated inflammation, resulting in fibrosis and structural change of the liver.

PBC and PSC are both chronic cholestatic liver diseases that affect adults. There is an immunological component to both diseases that causes inflammation and fibrosis, which ultimately results in bile duct destruction. Liver biopsy in patients with PBC is of limited value because the disease varies from portal tract to portal tract; biopsy is, however, helpful to validate cirrhotic changes. The beginning stages of PSC are characterized by portal infiltration of lymphocytes, plasma cells, macrophages, and eosinophils. These inflammatory changes are followed by "ductular proliferation," which is characterized by the replacement of mature bile ducts with small, ineffective ones. The inflammatory changes lead to fibrosis, and as fibrotic changes ensue, increased signs of cholestasis appear. The result of these changes is cirrhosis.

PSC can involve any part of the biliary tract from the ampulla of Vater to the small bile ducts within the liver. The lumens of these ductal systems can be narrowed or completely obstructed by fibrous scar tissue, resulting in cholestasis, which is the key functional abnormality seen in this disease. Biopsy results show fibrosis with inflammatory changes similar to those described for PSC. Bacterial infections that often occur in the area above the strictures and in the presence of longstanding disease lead to biliary cirrhosis.

The pathophysiology of liver disease caused by hereditary factors is essentially the same for both Wilson's disease and hereditary hemochromatosis (HHC). Wilson's disease results from decreased hepatic excretion of copper and excessive absorption of copper from the small intestine. There is a gradual accumulation of copper within the tissues, resulting in hepatotoxicity. Initial presentation of Wilson's disease may vary from acute hepatitis or chronic hepatitis, neuropsychiatric disease, cirrhosis, or fulminant hepatic failure in young adults. Histological examination of the initial lesions reveals hepatic steatosis, with increased glycogen deposits. These lesions eventually progress to fibrosis and finally cirrhosis.

HHC is characterized by increased intestinal absorption of iron. Liver biopsy reveals increased iron deposition, predominantly within the hepatocytes. When levels of iron exceed 20,000 mcg/g of liver tissue, fibrosis and cirrhosis usually ensue.

Vascular disorders of the liver, which include BCS and congestive hepatopathy, cause cirrhosis as the end result of necrosis. Liver biopsies show centrilobular congestion, hemorrhage, necrosis, and dilation. The resultant disruption of the hepatic circulation causes portal hypertension, fibrosis of the surrounding tissues, and ultimately cirrhosis.

CLINICAL PRESENTATION

Cirrhosis is often an incidental finding, revealed either by an asymptomatically enlarged liver or an elevation of the liver enzymes. The clinical manifestations of cirrhosis are the result of hepatocellular damage and portal hypertension. The cumulative effect of these signs and symptoms is often referred to as the "stigmata of liver disease." The onset of symptoms is usually gradual, and patients with cirrhosis may appear well and remain asymptomatic for years.

Subjective

Initial complaints generally include weakness, anorexia, weight loss, and fatigue. Malnutrition is usually evident and can be the result of anorexia or the effect of reduced bile salt excretion, resulting in fat malabsorption and deficiency of fat-soluble vitamins.

As cirrhosis advances, patients may present with upper gastrointestinal (GI) bleeding from esophageal varices, which develop secondary to portal hypertension. As the liver continues to fail, patients may present with ascites and/or encephalopathy. Patients with cirrhosis may complain of abdominal pain caused by the enlargement of the liver and stretching of Glisson's capsule or by the ascites itself.

Menstrual abnormalities, loss of libido, impotence, sterility, and gynecomastia are manifestations of increased levels of estrogen that result from the liver's inability to inactivate hormones. These symptoms may prompt individuals to seek medical attention.

Objective

Physical examination findings depend on the stage and severity of the disease process. Initial examination findings may reveal an enlarged, firm liver edge (the left lobe) that is palpable below the right costal margin; however, in patients with advanced disease, the liver may be small and difficult to palpate. Often, a firm smooth mass is palpable over the epigastric area, which is the right lobe of the liver (Riedel's lobe). Occasionally, nodular deformities may be palpable along the liver's edge. These areas of liver enlargement are dull to percussion, which can aid in measuring the expanse of the liver.

Manifestations of cirrhosis that are nonspecific but suggestive of CLD include spider nevi, which are normally found over the anterior chest; pectoral alopecia; generalized muscle wasting; Dupuytren's (palmar) contractions; parotid gland enlargement; palmar erythema; hair loss; and testicular atrophy. Patients may have dilated cutaneous veins called *caput medusae* (Medusa's head) radiating from around the umbilical area. These varicose veins are a result of the shunting of blood to the paraumbilical veins and are a manifestation of portal hypertension. Signs of vitamin and mineral disturbances are glossitis, cheilitis, and peripheral neuropathies. Fever may indicate complications such as peritonitis, cholangitis, or hepatitis.

Jaundiced sclera, skin, and mucous membranes usually develop in the later stages of cirrhosis. Hyperbilirubinemia is a consequence of the liver's inability to conjugate and excrete bilirubin. Patients with HHC may have bronze-colored skin from increased levels of iron and melanin stored in the tissue. Pruritus, although nonspecific, is often the presenting symptom in several forms of cirrhosis and can develop as a result of bile salts accumulating in the skin. Disruption in the liver's ability to synthesize clotting factors may manifest with bruising and complaints of a tendency to bleed. Peripheral edema results because of the decreased plasma osmotic pressure caused by hypoalbuminemia.

Ascites is a direct result of portal hypertension, which is a consequence of increased portal vein pressure. As liver function fails and healthy hepatic cells are replaced with fibrous nodules, blood flow through the liver is impaired, causing increased resistance and back-pressure that result in the accumulation of serous fluid within the abdomen.

An abdominal examination reveals a positive fluid wave and shifting dullness on percussion. Splenomegaly results from splenic vein congestion. Esophageal varices, another consequence of portal hypertension, may be discovered if bleeding causes hematemesis, hematochezia, and/or melena. Hemorrhoids, which result from portal hypertension, are also present and cause bright red bleeding from the rectum.

Hepatic encephalopathy can range from mild confusion to coma and is the result of increasing blood ammonia, which is toxic to the brain. Characteristics of encephalopathy include asterixis (liver flap), reversal of sleep–wake patterns, tremors, hyperactive deep-tendon reflexes, dysarthria, delirium, and drowsiness.

Patients who present with Wilson's disease may have golden brown rings of color—called *Kayser-Fleischer rings*—located within Descemet's membrane of the cornea. These rings are usually found in patients with central nervous system (CNS) involvement and are seen with a slit lamp.

DIAGNOSTIC REASONING

Diagnostic Tests

Results of initial laboratory testing vary depending on the stage of the disease process. In many patients with early-stage cirrhosis, laboratory results may be normal; however, in some patients, elevation of liver enzymes may be the only indicator of liver disease. Laboratory testing may reveal abnormalities, but these results are nonspecific unless correlated with the history and physical examination.

Alcoholic cirrhosis may manifest in different ways depending on other coexisting processes, such as malnutrition or hepatitis. A complete blood count commonly shows macrocytic anemia and, depending on the severity of the disease, pancytopenia from the overall suppression of the bone marrow. The mean corpuscular volume does not correct quickly with abstinence from alcohol and may be the only key to occult alcohol use. Anemia can represent suppression of erythropoiesis from folic acid deficiency, occult losses from the GI tract, or a combination of the two. The white blood cell and platelet counts can vary depending on whether there is infection or splenic sequestration. As the liver continues to fail and liver cell mass decreases, the prothrombin time (PT) increases as the liver loses the ability to synthesize the proteins necessary to produce clotting factors.

Blood chemistry test results may show mild to moderate increases in alanine aminotransferase (ALT) and aspartate aminotransferase (AST) levels; however, if the patient has a superimposed alcoholic hepatitis, the classic enzyme elevation of ALT/AST may be reversed, with an AST/ALT ratio ranging from 2:1 to 3:1. The levels of AST/ALT do not reflect the severity of the disease process. The gamma-glutamyl transpeptidase level is a good measurement of recent alcohol ingestion and declines rapidly with abstinence. Alkaline phosphatase levels may be markedly elevated when there is biliary obstruction; in this scenario, serum bilirubin levels can be as high as 30 mg/dL. Hypoalbuminemia is common and contributes to the development of edema.

Unless a liver biopsy is obtained, the diagnosis of alcoholic cirrhosis may be difficult to differentiate from alcoholic hepatitis, which is a reversible process. Histological examination reveals hepatocellular necrosis and evidence of Mallory bodies within the damaged cells. Depending on the stage of the disease, there is fatty infiltration and fibrosis. In early disease, there are micronodular changes, which develop into macronodular cirrhosis over time.

Abdominal ultrasound is helpful in determining the size of the liver and any ascites or nodule formation. Doppler studies, in combination with ultrasound, are used to evaluate patency of the venous system that, if disrupted, can lead to portal hypertension. Computed tomography (CT) and magnetic resonance imaging (MRI) of the liver can further characterize nodules. Any nodular findings that are suspicious for malignancy should be biopsied. If a patient presents with melena or hematemesis, an esophagogastroscopy should be performed to assess for esophageal varices or ulcerative processes.

Diagnosis of cholestatic liver disease, specifically PBC and PSC, may be made in conjunction with various autoimmune disease processes. The initial hepatic blood work-up usually shows an alkaline phosphatase level that is three to four times normal, with mild to moderate increases in the transaminases. Cholestatic liver disease can lead to prolonged PT.

Patients with PBC may also present with mild elevation of serum bilirubin and more often hypercholesterolemia. Serum immunoglobulin M levels are elevated in 50% of cases. Antimitochondrial antibodies (AMAs) are found in 95% of the patients with PBC; titers can exceed 1:500. Definitive diagnosis is made via liver biopsy, which reveals granulomatous bile duct destruction and accumulation of inflammatory cells within the portal tracts with resultant segmental necrosis of the interlobular and septal bile ducts (chronic nonsuppurative destructive cholangitis). Ultrasound evaluation of the biliary tree is negative for biliary obstruction.

Laboratory studies of patients with PSC show the typical cholestatic profile; however, unlike with patients with PBC, the AMA titer is negative. Total cholesterol levels increase as the disease progresses. Endoscopic or transhepatic cholangiography reveals characteristic beading and stricture of the intrahepatic and extrahepatic bile ducts. Liver biopsy is diagnostic for fibrous obliterative cholangitis, in which the hepatic ductal system being replaced with fibrous cords of connective tissue. The end result for both PBC and PSC is biliary cirrhosis.

Diagnosis of cirrhosis caused by vascular disorders such as BCS and other veno-occlusive diseases is normally made through imaging studies because laboratory findings are nonspecific. Serum bilirubin, transaminases, and alkaline phosphatase can be elevated as much as four times normal. A CT scan demonstrates failure of the hepatic veins to opacify, indicating an occlusive process. Pulsed Doppler studies illustrate absent hepatic flow; a normal pulsed Doppler effectively rules out BCS. Venographic studies also demonstrate narrowing and obstruction of the hepatic venous system. Histological examination reveals centrilobular congestion with associated hemorrhage and necrosis.

Wilson's disease and hemochromatosis are inherited metabolic liver diseases that result in cirrhosis if diagnosis and treatment are not made early. Diagnosis of Wilson's disease is suggested by elevated serum copper levels in conjunction with low serum ceruloplasmin levels. Once an abnormal ceruloplasmin level has been documented, a 24-hour urine check for copper should be completed. Definitive diagnosis is made through quantitative copper levels in the liver on biopsy. Most patients with Wilson's disease have histological findings consistent with hepatic steatosis, which in time progresses to fibrosis and cirrhosis.

Iron metabolism studies are used to diagnose HHC and should be collected with the patient in the fasting state. The presence of an elevated transferrin saturation level in combination with an elevated ferritin level is suggestive of HHC. Liver biopsy is necessary for definitive diagnosis. Histological studies with quantitative iron levels greater than 20,000 mcg/g are consistent with advanced disease and cirrhosis.

Differential Diagnosis

The patient who presents with cirrhosis can be a diagnostic challenge. The differential diagnosis of cirrhosis varies little between the different etiologies; therefore, the challenge is determining the cause to prevent further liver damage. The differential diagnosis of alcohol-induced liver disease includes biliary tract disease, idiopathic hemochromatosis, NAFLD, drug toxicity, and/or viral hepatitis. Ultrasound examination of the liver can often rule out an obstructive process. Patients with AUD and chronic pancreatitis frequently develop jaundice secondary to stricture of the common bile duct, which is differentiated through endoscopic retrograde cholangiopancreatography. A liver biopsy is often the only definitive test for differentiating many of the hepatobiliary diseases. Thorough history and physical examination can suggest a diagnosis, but histological study is necessary to distinguish one process from another.

Patients with AUD also have a high incidence of co-infection with hepatitis, the cause of which is often unclear; the presence of this infection can alter the typical serological findings. A hepatitis panel can reveal active or prior infection. Drug toxicity, specifically with acetaminophen, even in low doses, can alter transaminase levels and necessitates obtaining a careful drug history from each patient. Because of preexisting liver injury, patients with AUD who present with acetaminophen toxicity have significantly higher morbidity and mortality with relatively low doses of acetaminophen.

The differential diagnosis of cholestatic liver disease must include all other causes of chronic cholestasis, such as tumors, strictures, or obstructions resulting from stone formation. Autoimmune chronic active hepatitis can mimic the signs and symptoms of PBC; however, laboratory studies will show a low or negative titer for AMA. Ultrasound examination may reveal biliary duct dilation, a process consistent with both PBC and PSC, thus making cholangiography the diagnostic test of choice.

MANAGEMENT

Treatment of cirrhosis is aimed at identifying and removing the causative agent, treating the symptoms, and preventing complications.

Alcohol-Induced Liver Disease

In a patient with alcohol-induced liver disease, the most effective treatment remains abstinence. Patients who continue to ingest alcohol and present with ascites can increase their 2-year survival rate to 95% if they can completely abstain from alcohol. Those who continue to drink have a 2-year survival rate of less than 25%. The liver has a remarkable regenerative potential; despite slow progress, the patient can become functional if they are motivated to remain abstinent. Nutritional assessment with dietary supplementation to ensure adequate caloric intake (25 to 35 kcal/kg body weight per day) is imperative because many patients with alcohol-induced liver disease are also malnourished. Protein intake should be increased to 1 to 1.5 g/kg of body weight per day unless there is evidence of hepatic encephalopathy, which necessitates a reduction in protein intake. Daily vitamin and mineral supplementation is also indicated. Specifically, patients should receive a multivitamin, additional vitamin B_{12}, folate, thiamine, magnesium, and zinc supplementation if 100% of the daily requirement of these minerals is not contained in the multivitamin. Patients who continue to show clinical deterioration despite abstinence can be considered for liver transplantation, provided they have remained alcohol-free for more than 6 months.

Treatment of Complications

Many of the complications of alcohol-induced liver disease are the direct result of the development of portal hypertension and include ascites, hepatic encephalopathy, anemia, hemorrhage, spontaneous bacterial peritonitis, hepatorenal syndrome, hepatopulmonary syndrome, and hepatocellular carcinoma. Box 42.2 presents the treatment of these complications.

Irreversible, Chronic Liver Disease

Liver transplantation is the treatment of choice for irreversible CLD. Cirrhosis, hepatitis C, PBC, PSC, alcoholic liver disease, autoimmune hepatitis, and genetic disorders of the liver are diseases for which transplantation has been successful. Five-year survival rates are documented as high as 80% with advancements in surgical techniques and immunosuppressive agents such as T-cell depleting monoclonal antibodies (muromonab-CD3, alemtuzumab), calcineurin inhibitors (tacrolimus, cyclosporine), mammalian target of rapamycin inhibitors (sirolimus, everolimus), and interleukin-2 receptor antagonists (daclizumab, basiliximab). Contraindications to transplantation include malignant hepatobiliary processes, sepsis, and advanced cardiopulmonary disease. In cases of HBV and HCV, the virus can infect the new liver.

Nonalcoholic Fatty Liver Disease

Treatment of NAFLD includes mainly lifestyle modification with diet, exercise, and weight loss. Studies have shown that improvement in histology on liver biopsy was dose dependent; the greater the degree of weight loss, the greater the improvement in histopathology. Bariatric surgery may be necessary to achieve weight loss. The optimal duration of exercise has not been studied, but there are data to suggest that patients should be instructed to maintain 150 minutes/week of physical activity.

Primary Biliary Cirrhosis

Treatment of PBC is symptomatic. Pruritus is often the most aggravating manifestation of PBC. Cholestyramine (Questran) or colestipol relieves itching in patients with cholestasis by lowering serum bile acids and increasing the intestinal secretion of bile by preventing its resorption. The usual dose is 4 or 5 g, respectively, in water or juice three times daily until the pruritus has been controlled, and then the dosage is decreased to that which maintains control of the symptom. Rifampin (Rifadin) 150 to 300 mg twice daily has been beneficial in relieving pruritus in some cases; ondansetron, a $5-HT_3$ serotonin receptor antagonist, shows promise as well.

Fat-soluble vitamin deficiency occurs with the onset of steatorrhea and can be made worse with the administration of cholestyramine (a bile acid sequestrant). Vitamins A, D, E, and K can be replaced orally. Laboratory studies will reveal vitamin K deficiency as a prolonged PT. The deficiency can be treated with 5 to 10 mg daily of vitamin K by mouth; subsequent monitoring of the PT will indicate whether therapy is adequate. Because overdose of vitamin A can cause hepatotoxicity, the dosage must be individualized based on serum levels and response to treatment.

Box 42.2 Complications of Alcohol-Induced Liver Disease

Portal Hypertension and Variceal Hemorrhage

Portal hypertension is the result of disruption of the hepatocellular circulation, causing an increase in portal venous pressure. As the liver becomes progressively more cirrhotic, collateral venous circulation develops between the portal and systemic circulation to overcome the increased resistance to blood flow. The collateral circulation that forms, specifically the azygos vein, is a much weaker system and results in dilated, tortuous vessels commonly known as *varices*. Development of varices within the esophagus and submucosa of the gastric fundus predisposes patients to hemorrhage when the portal pressure gradient is greater than 12 mm Hg.

Management of this complication is as follows:

- A combination of band ligation or sclerotherapy and octreotide, which results in reduced splanchnic and hepatic blood flow to decrease portal pressure, is the most effective treatment for bleeding varices.
- Patients who have failed both endoscopic and pharmacological intervention require emergent insertion of a Sengstaken-Blakemore tube for balloon tamponade of the bleeding variceal site. The risk for aspiration, esophageal rupture, or rebleed is great, and patients normally require intensive care monitoring.
- Some patients may benefit from surgical placement of a portacaval shunt or placement of a transjugular intrahepatic portosystemic shunt. Both procedures are performed to decrease portal hypertension but are associated with a high operative mortality rate, especially if performed on an urgent basis. Prevention of future bleeding also may be accomplished using these procedures.

Ascites

Ascites, the excess accumulation of serous fluid within the peritoneal cavity, is associated with unfavorable outcomes. Ascites results from a combination of increased hydrostatic pressure (portal hypertension), decreased oncotic pressure (hypoalbuminemia), peripheral vasodilation probably mediated by nitric oxide released from the splanchnic vasculature, volume expansion resulting from a disturbance in the renin-angiotensin system with subsequent sodium and water retention, and impaired activation of aldosterone by the liver.

Ascites can be clinically observed on physical examination when 1,000 mL or more of fluid has accumulated within the abdominal/peritoneal cavities; smaller amounts are detectable with the use of ultrasound. Shifting dullness to percussion and a positive fluid wave are two findings consistent with the diagnosis of ascites.

Management of ascites includes the following:

- Initial treatment is sodium restriction of 400 to 800 mg/day with daily monitoring of weight, serum electrolytes, and renal function. The goal of treatment for the patient with ascites and peripheral edema is a daily weight loss of approximately 1 pound. For patients with hyponatremia (serum levels less than 125 mEq/L), fluid restriction of 800 to 1,000 mL/day is recommended.
- Diuretic therapy is usually required in addition to sodium and water restriction. Initial therapy is with spironolactone (Aldactone), a potassium-sparing aldosterone antagonist. Furosemide (Lasix), a loop diuretic, is added if effective diuresis has not been achieved.
- In the 10% of patients who do not respond to either of the previously mentioned treatments, large-volume paracentesis is performed. Up to 4–6 L of fluid can be removed per procedure. Intravascular volume expanders can be infused simultaneously to prevent hemodynamic instability secondary to removal of large volumes of ascitic fluid. The procedure can be performed daily until ascites is resolved, and then the patient can be maintained on diuretic therapy.

Spontaneous Bacterial Peritonitis

Spontaneous bacterial peritonitis (SBP) is a common complication of cirrhosis that can be fatal. Patients may present with abdominal pain, increasing ascites, fever, and progressive encephalopathy. Definitive diagnosis is made by paracentesis. The gold standard for the diagnosis of SBP is a total white blood cell count of greater than 300 cells/μL with a polymorphonuclear neutrophil cell count of greater than 250 cells/μL. The protein concentration is usually less than 1 g/dL. Gram-negative bacilli are the causative pathogen in 70% of patients with SBP, with *Escherichia coli* being isolated in 50% of the cases. Gram-positive organisms are isolated in approximately 25% of the cases, and infection with anaerobic organisms is rare due to the high oxygen content of the ascitic fluid. The mortality rate for untreated SBP is 50%.

Management of SBP includes empiric treatment with cefotaxime (Claforan), a broad-spectrum, third generation cephalosporin. Post-SBP prophylaxis can be accomplished with norfloxacin.

Hepatorenal Syndrome

Hepatorenal syndrome is a terminal complication frequently associated with advanced liver damage and is almost always found in patients with advanced ascites. The syndrome is characterized by oliguria, hyponatremia, azotemia, low urine sodium (less than 10 mEq/L), and hypotension. The hallmark to diagnosis is a disproportionate rise in creatinine with respect to the blood urea nitrogen. Histologically, the kidneys are normal, and diagnosis is often one of exclusion. Patients are often misdiagnosed with prerenal failure, and the only way to differentiate between the two is through insertion of a central venous catheter and assessment of venous pressures. Large-volume paracentesis, aggressive diuresis aimed at decreasing ascites, or sepsis can precipitate hepatorenal syndrome in individuals with decompensated cirrhosis and ascites.

Management of hepatorenal syndrome includes restoring the intravascular volume and avoiding any procedures that will dramatically disturb the patient's volume status, such as

> **Box 42.2 Complications of Alcohol-Induced Liver Disease—cont'd**
>
> large-volume paracentesis and aggressive diuresis. The definitive treatment of patients with hepatorenal syndrome is liver transplantation.
>
> **Hepatic Encephalopathy**
>
> Hepatic encephalopathy, also known as *portosystemic encephalopathy*, is a complex process involving a change in mental status resulting from the failure of the liver to detoxify elements of gut origin and shunting of this blood from the portal to the systemic circulation and then to the brain. Nitrogenous agents such as ammonia are believed to enter the central nervous system by way of shunted blood resulting in disturbances in neurological function. Although ammonia is thought to be the sole toxin responsible for hepatic encephalopathy, the serum levels do not correlate with the degree or presence of encephalopathy.
>
> The diagnosis of hepatic encephalopathy is made clinically and often follows an event such as increased dietary protein, GI bleeding, constipation, infection, deterioration in hepatic function, hypokalemia, azotemia, alkalosis, and hypovolemia. Physical examination findings include an altered mental status such as personality (mood) changes, decreased reaction time, and intellectual deterioration, as well as neuromuscular dysfunctions such as asterixis or metabolic flap, absence of fixed sensory or motor deficits, and hyperreflexia. Other findings include fetor hepaticus (garlic odor of the breath caused by exhalation of sulfur-containing mercaptans), hyperthermia, and hyperventilation. Obtaining a fasting arterial blood ammonia level or a spinal fluid glutamine level can be helpful in confirming the diagnosis of hepatic encephalopathy, although they are not necessary.
>
> Management of hepatic encephalopathy involves identification and treatment of factors that cause encephalopathy in patients with liver disease. For instance, gastrointestinal bleeding and diets high in protein lead to formation of ammonia and other nitrogenous compounds from the action of bacteria in the gut, which can induce or aggravate the symptoms of encephalopathy. The goal of treatment is to reduce formation of ammonia and other nitrogenous compounds. This is achieved by decreasing the numbers of colonic bacteria with the antibiotic neomycin and inducing acidification of the colon contents with lactulose (Cephulac, Heptalac), a nonabsorbable synthetic disaccharide that is fermented by intestinal bacteria. The lower stool pH binds the ammonia in the colon, rendering it nonabsorbable. Lactulose also changes the bowel flora so that there are fewer ammonia-forming bacteria.
>
> **Iron-Deficiency Anemia**
>
> Iron-deficiency anemia is a common finding in individuals with AUD. It can be treated with ferrous sulfate taken three times daily after meals. To avoid the constipating effect of iron, a stool softener can be given as well. If there is evidence of a macrocytic anemia, the patient may benefit from 1 mg of folic acid daily.
>
> **Hepatopulmonary Syndrome**
>
> Hepatopulmonary syndrome is a recently recognized pulmonary complication of cirrhosis and portal hypertension, which manifests as abnormal arterial oxygenation. The diagnosis is made when intrapulmonary dilation occurs in the absence of other morphological pathology. This syndrome is reversible with liver transplantation.

Patients with PBC often have associated osteoporosis because of an imbalance in bone remodeling. If patients have been diagnosed with PBC and have osteomalacia or osteoporosis, bisphosphonates (Fosamax, Boniva, Aclasta, Actonel) have been shown to be effective. Anyone with cirrhosis from any cause should receive calcium supplementation with 1 g per day and vitamin D_3 800 IU/day in an effort to prevent osteomalacia or osteoporosis. Patients should be instructed to eat foods rich in calcium and phosphorus and increase their exposure to sunlight.

Several immunosuppressive agents including corticosteroids, methotrexate, azathioprine, and the antifibrinogenic colchicine have been effective in reducing elevated serum alkaline phosphatase and bilirubin levels. Ursodeoxycholic acid (ursodiol), a choleretic, acts by stimulating excretion of bile by the liver, is much less toxic than the other drugs mentioned, and has been effective in reducing symptoms and improving long-term survival.

Surgical reconstruction of the biliary tract, choledochoduodenostomy, and choledochojejunostomy are palliative treatments that alleviate the symptoms of PBC. If there is notable stricture within the biliary tree, patients often do well with stenting. Liver transplantation for advanced PBC is the treatment of choice.

Hemochromatosis and Wilson's Disease

Two important but treatable inherited metabolic causes of cirrhosis are hemochromatosis and Wilson's disease. Early diagnosis and treatment are key to the management of HHC and begin with liver biopsy for definitive diagnosis. If treatment is initiated before cirrhosis ensues, the disease can be controlled with weekly phlebotomies of 1 unit (500 mL) of blood, which contains approximately 250 mg of iron. This process is continued until there is depletion of the iron stores (which can be 2 years or more). Every 2 to 3 months, iron metabolism studies monitor the patient's progress. Once the iron stores are depleted—when serum ferritin levels fall below 50 ng/mL and transferrin saturation is less than 50%—patients can be maintained with periodic phlebotomies. Patients who are exhibiting cardiac symptoms may require the use of iron-chelating agents such as deferoxamine. Administered intramuscularly, it increases the urinary excretion of iron up to 5 to 18 g annually. Phlebotomy decreases the cardiac conduction defects and lowers insulin requirements. Patients should be instructed to consume a low-iron diet that eliminates foods such as red meat, and they should avoid alcohol, vitamin C, raw shellfish, and any supplement containing iron. Patients may require specific treatment of diabetes mellitus, heart disease, arthropathy, hypopituitarism, and portal hypertension, all complications of HHC. Patients whose disease has progressed to cirrhosis must be monitored for hepatocellular carcinoma either by liver ultrasound or measurement of alpha-fetoprotein levels. Because the disease is inherited, screening of all first-degree relatives is necessary.

Wilson's disease is also an inherited disease, the early diagnosis and treatment of which can prevent the development of neurological or hepatic damage. Treatment includes both dietary and medicinal components. Limiting dietary intake of copper (legumes, animal organs, and shellfish) should become a lifelong habit. The administration of oral penicillamine (Depen) 0.75 to 2 g/day in divided doses induces the urinary excretion of chelated copper. If GI upset or hypersensitivity prohibits the use of penicillamine, trientine (Syprine) 250 to 500 mg three times daily can be substituted. Oral administration of zinc 50 mg three times daily as maintenance therapy also promotes excretion of copper in the feces. Patients who are receiving penicillamine, an antimetabolite of vitamin B_6, should receive pyridoxine (supplemental vitamin B_6) 50 mg/week. Liver transplant is the treatment of choice for patients with cirrhosis or fulminant hepatitis. Siblings and family members should be screened for the disease.

Vascular or Congestive Liver Disorders

Management of patients who present with vascular or congestive liver disorders, such as those with BCS and other hepatic occlusive diseases, is essential. Because of the many causes of BCS, initial treatment must begin with finding and treating the cause of the hepatic congestion. Hepatic vein thrombus is difficult to manage and requires a multidisciplinary approach including a hematologist, surgeon, hepatologist, and gastroenterologist. Ascites is initially managed with sodium restriction and diuretics; however, over time this is usually ineffective, and most patients will require large-volume paracentesis or shunting for symptomatic relief.

If diagnosis of acute thrombus is made early, thrombolytic therapy can be instituted and long-term anticoagulation with warfarin (Coumadin) can help prevent further thrombus formation. Surgical decompression shunting for refractive ascites can delay development of hepatic failure or cirrhosis but often results in graft thrombus. Patients with associated myeloproliferative diseases and hypercoagulopathies may benefit from low-dose aspirin therapy and chemotherapy as directed by a hematologist.

FOLLOW-UP AND REFERRAL

Any patient with advanced liver disease should be referred to a hepatologist or gastroenterologist trained to treat the disease and its complications. All patients require referral for liver biopsy to establish a definitive diagnosis. The primary care provider should be able to recognize the onset of liver disease, obtain the necessary tests, and provide results of all diagnostic testing performed by the consulting physician. Patients with end-stage liver disease should be referred to a liver transplant facility. Patient follow-up can be shared between the primary care practitioner and the consulting physician. Patients with chronic or advanced liver disease will require indefinite monitoring of their liver function tests, as well as their fluid and electrolyte status. Maintaining good nutrition is an important component of treatment of any disease process. Patients with advanced liver disease may benefit from consultation with a registered dietitian, who can review dietary restrictions and help patients understand how to achieve a balanced diet.

Patient Education: Cirrhosis

Patients with hepatic failure should be instructed to check their weight daily as a way to monitor increasing fluid retention and ascites, which may indicate a developing complication. Patients with cirrhosis have a life-threatening terminal disease; therefore, attention must be given to promoting psychological well-being. Patients should be provided with education regarding medications to prevent further hepatotoxicity, such as acetaminophen (Tylenol), vitamin A, cocaine, tetracycline (Sumycin), phenytoin (Dilantin), and ethyl alcohol. Patients with liver failure should always ask their health-care provider about the potential liver toxicity of each of their medications. Patients with hepatic encephalopathy should avoid CNS depressants, which might intensify their lethargy or fatigue. These patients may also require education about the need for self-administering enemas if they become constipated to decrease the time for bowel absorption of nitrogen-based compounds. All patients with ascites must be informed of the signs and symptoms of infection, which may indicate developing spontaneous bacterial peritonitis.

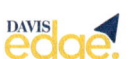 Go to Davis Edge for practice Q&A.

REFERENCES

Chalasani N, Younossi Z, Lavine JE, et al. The diagnosis and management of non-alcoholic fatty liver disease: practice guidance from the American Association for the Study of Liver Diseases. *Hepatology*. 2018;67(1):328–357.

Grant BF, Chou SP, Saha TD, et al. Prevalence of 12-month alcohol use, high-risk drinking, and *DSM-IV* alcohol use disorder in the United States, 2001–2002 to 2012–2013. Results from the National Epidemiologic Survey on Alcohol and Related Conditions. *JAMA Psychiatry.* 2017;74(9):911–923.

Lv Y, Yang Z, Liu L, et al. Early TIPS with covered stents versus standard treatment for acute variceal bleeding in patients with advanced cirrhosis: a randomised controlled trial. *Lancet Gastroenterol Hepatol.* 2019;4(8):587–598.

Masarone M, Rosato V, Dallio M, et al. Role of oxidative stress in pathophysiology of non-alcoholic fatty liver disease. *Oxid Med Cell Longev.* 2018;2081:9547613. https://doi.org/10.1155/2018/9547613.

Moon AM, Singal AG, Tapper EB. Contemporary epidemiology of chronic liver disease and cirrhosis. *Clin Gastroenterol Hepatol.* 2020;18(12):2650–2666.

Tapper EB, Parikh ND. Mortality due to cirrhosis and liver cancer in the United States, 1999–2016: observational study. *BMJ.* 2018;362:k2817.

RESOURCES

American Liver Foundation
  https://www.liverfoundation.org

Section 8: RENAL PROBLEMS

SECTION EDITOR
Debera J. Thomas, PhD, RN, ANP/FNP

Chapter 43

Common Urinary Complaints

Debbie Conner, PhD, MSN, ANP/FNP-BC, FAANP
Debera J. Thomas, PhD, RN, ANP/FNP
Brian Oscar Porter, MD, PhD, MPH, MBA

DYSURIA

Dysuria is the subjective experience of pain or a burning sensation on urination and can also be accompanied by urinary frequency, hesitancy, urgency, and strangury (slow, painful urination). Symptoms of dysuria can be secondary to several medical conditions or certain medications. For example, a light burning sensation or discomfort can be normal when associated with concentrated acidic urine. However, dysuria is most commonly associated with lower urinary tract infection. Selective serotonin reuptake inhibitors such as citalopram (Celexa), escitalopram (Lexapro), paroxetine (Paxil), fluoxetine (Prozac), and sertraline (Zoloft) may also cause dysuria. Other prescribed medications such as opiates and those used to prevent motion sickness (e.g., scopolamine) may also cause dysuria, given their anticholinergic effects on the renal system.

DIFFERENTIAL DIAGNOSIS

Dysuria is most often associated with bladder problems but rarely with renal (kidney) disease. Inflammatory lesions of the prostate, bladder, and urethra—including prostatitis in males, urethrotrigonitis in females, and bladder and urethral infections in both sexes—are the most common causes of dysuria. When caused by bladder problems, urinary frequency usually occurs secondary to diminished bladder capacity or with pain when the bladder becomes distended. Urinary frequency may be a manifestation of urinary incontinence and can occur with neurogenic bladder disorders, prostatic hypertrophy in males, or pelvic organ prolapse in females.

Other conditions associated with dysuria are bladder tumors, chronic renal failure, nephrolithiasis, and occasionally diseases of the upper urinary tract. Dysuria may also be associated with diseases outside the renal system, such as sexually transmitted diseases, vaginitis, or prostatitis. For example, female patients may present with symptoms of dysuria or external irritation from urine passing over irritated vulvar tissues. Any female who presents with dysuria should be questioned about an associated vaginal discharge or irritation. In males, dysuria frequently reflects an infection such as urethritis, prostatitis, epididymitis, or urinary tract infection. However, symptoms of dysuria may lead to other diagnoses such as urethral strictures, pelvic organ prolapse, pelvic peritonitis, cancer of the cervix or prostate, dysmenorrhea, and disorders of the prostate. Urinalysis is the easiest, least invasive, and most economical way to identify urinary tract infections and other renal problems (see Advanced Assessment 43.1). Once the underlying problem has been identified, appropriate treatment can be instituted.

Conditions associated with dysuria such as bladder tumors, chronic renal failure, nephrolithiasis, and infections of the lower and upper urinary tracts are discussed in Chapters 44 and 45. Problems associated with dysmenorrhea are discussed in Chapter 49, and conditions associated with the prostate in Chapter 50.

HEMATURIA

Hematuria is defined as blood in the urine and can be visible (gross) or occult (microscopic). Asymptomatic microhematuria has many benign causes such as infection, menstruation, vigorous exercise, viral illness, and trauma. In the primary care setting, the dipstick method to detect hematuria has a sensitivity of 95% and a specificity of 75%. Positive results should be confirmed with microscopic examination because of the possibility of a false-positive dipstick test result. On microscopic examination, hematuria is characterized by more than three red blood cells (RBCs) per high-power microscopic field (hpf). Normal urinary excretion of RBCs is 2,000,000 cells per day, which corresponds to two or three RBCs per hpf. It takes

Advanced Assessment 43.1: Urinalysis

Urinalysis Result	Finding/Abnormal Value	Common Differential Diagnosis
Appearance	Colorless	Diabetes insipidus, diuretic agents, fluid overload
	Dark	Hematuria, malignancy, stones, acidic urine
	Cloudy	Urinary tract infection, hematuria, bilirubin, mucus
	Pink/red	Hematuria, hemoglobin, myoglobin, beets, rhubarb, senna, food coloring
	Orange/yellow	Phenazopyridine (Pyridium), bile pigments
	Red/orange	Rifampin (Rifadin) (can also be reddish-brown)
	Reddish-brown/brown/black	Myoglobinuria, hemoglobinuria, bile pigments, melanin, cascara (laxative), iron preparation
	Green	Bile pigments, methylene blue, propofol, amitriptyline, indigo carmine (food dye)
	Foamy	Proteinuria, bile salts
Specific gravity	Increased	Dehydration, congestive heart failure, adrenal insufficiency, diabetes mellitus, nephrosis, increased antidiuretic hormone
	Decreased	Diabetes insipidus, pyelonephritis, glomerulonephritis, excess fluid intake
pH	Acidic	Diet, medications, acidosis, ketoacidosis, chronic obstructive pulmonary disease
	Alkaline	Diet, sodium bicarbonate, vomiting, metabolic alkalosis, urinary tract infection
Bilirubin	Positive	Jaundice, hepatitis
Blood	Positive	Kidney stones, tumors, kidney disease, trauma, infection, injury from instrumentation, coagulation problems, menses
Glucose	Positive	Diabetes mellitus, pancreatitis, Cushing's disease, shock, burns, corticosteroids, renal disease, hyperthyroidism, cancer
Ketones	Positive	Starvation, dieting (carbohydrate restricting), ketoacidosis, vomiting, diarrhea, pregnancy
Nitrate	Positive	Infection
Protein	Positive	Kidney disease, pregnancy, congestive heart failure, diabetes mellitus, cancer, nephrotic syndrome, benign cause, exercise-induced proteinuria
Leukocyte esterase	Positive	Infection
Reducing substance	Positive	Signifies presence of glucose, fructose, or galactose, lactose, pentose; may also signify certain medications (e.g., salicylates, levodopa, ascorbic acid, nalidixic acid, tetracyclines), liver disease, hyperthyroidism

only a small amount of blood to make the urine appear red, as urine will appear pink with between 20 and 30 RBCs per hpf and will become red at about 100 RBCs per hpf. There is a direct relationship between the quantity of blood found in the urine and the likelihood of pathology.

Transient hematuria occurs on a single occasion, whereas *persistent hematuria* occurs on two or more consecutive voidings. Both transient and persistent hematuria can be a sign of serious underlying disease. Urine color can vary widely from light pink to dark red and is sometimes characterized as "smoky." The color of urine depends on the amount of blood present, as well as on dietary intake, the use of certain medications, and the concentration and pH of the urine. For example, the ingestion of beets can color the urine red to pink, and medications such as rifampin (Rifadin) and phenazopyridine (Pyridium) can give urine a reddish-orange color. The presence of porphyrins, hemoglobin, or myoglobin can color the urine reddish-brown. Pus in the urine is indicative of bacterial infection somewhere along the urinary tract such as cystitis, urethritis, or prostatitis.

Rates of hematuria in the general population are usually less than 1% but can be as high as 15%. The age, sex, and activity level of the patient with hematuria should be considered during the assessment. For example, long-distance runners and other athletes can have rates of hematuria as high as 18%. However, even transient hematuria in males older than 50 years may be an indication of serious disease (see Geriatric Considerations). In general, there is a greater positive correlation between underlying malignancy and gross hematuria versus microscopic hematuria, especially in patients with a history of cigarette smoking.

> **Geriatric Considerations:**
> **Hematuria**
> - Of males older than 50 years, 2.4% with hematuria have urinary tract malignancies, typically transitional cell carcinoma.
> - In males older than 60 years, the incidence of urinary tract malignancy increases to 9%.
> - In older males with gross hematuria, the rate of associated malignancy is as high as 20%.

DIFFERENTIAL DIAGNOSIS

The causes of hematuria are grouped according to anatomical site of the blood source. For example, *isolated hematuria* (i.e., with no other abnormal components on urinalysis) may be due to bleeding anywhere from the renal pelvis to the urethra but is rarely caused by a systemic disease. RBC casts usually indicate injury to the nephron and are diagnostic of hematuria of renal origin. However, intact uniform RBCs with no casts suggest hematuria originating in the lower urinary tract. The presence of bacteria in the urine is diagnostic of an infectious origin, which is also suggested by fever. Acute cystitis and urethritis produce gross hematuria and are more common in females. The presence of both proteinuria and hematuria is suggestive of glomerular or interstitial nephritis. A drug history is important because many drugs can cause hematuria. In addition, dietary substances such as caffeine, spices, tomatoes, chocolate, aged cheeses, citrus fruits, and soy sauce may act as bladder irritants. Alcohol and cigarettes are also bladder irritants. Thus, the patient's drug and food intake history should be assessed to rule out these substances as causative agents. The drugs involved may be prescribed, over the counter, herbal or vitamin supplements, or recreational in nature.

β-Lactam antibiotics (e.g., amoxicillin with clavulanic acid [Augmentin]), sulfonamides (e.g., sulfamethoxazole/trimethoprim [Bactrim]), NSAIDs, rifampin (Rifadin), ciprofloxacin (Cipro), allopurinol (Zyloprim), cimetidine (Tagamet), and phenytoin (Dilantin) can all cause *nephritis* (typically allergic interstitial nephritis), which can result in destruction of nephrons and subsequently lead to impaired renal function and hematuria. Papillary necrosis can result from the use of anticoagulants such as warfarin (Coumadin), heparin, aspirin, and NSAIDs. Glomerulonephritis can be caused by the use of hydralazine, hydrocarbons (including glue and paint sniffing), gold, penicillamine (Cuprimine), amphetamines, NSAIDs, allopurinol (Zyloprim), and Paraquat (a type of weed killer). Urolithiasis (discussed in Chapter 44), which often presents with hematuria, can occur with the use of carbonic anhydrase inhibitors, the diuretic triamterene (Dyazide, Maxzide), sulfonamides, and vitamin D metabolites.

Menstrual history is always important in a biologically female patient with hematuria. Patients should be asked about recent strenuous or vigorous exercise (which can lead to proteinuria), streptococcal infection (which suggests poststreptococcal glomerulonephritis), a history of nephrolithiasis (which can lead to hematuria), pertinent family history (e.g., polycystic kidney disease), and recent travel to tropical areas (which suggests potential exposure to parasitic infections). Gross painless hematuria in males or females is a cardinal sign of certain malignancies such as bladder cancer.

Physical examination may reveal costovertebral angle tenderness, which could indicate pyelonephritis, renal tumor, or glomerulonephritis. An abdominal mass may indicate a neoplasm (e.g., renal cell cancer) or polycystic kidney disease. Suprapubic tenderness is suggestive of a bladder etiology, whereas urethral discharge indicates urethritis. An enlarged prostate could indicate benign prostatic hypertrophy, whereas a tender prostate would more likely be suggestive of prostatitis, and a hard prostate nodule may indicate a prostatic neoplasm.

Hematuria accompanied by colicky flank pain suggests a ureteral stone. When bleeding occurs only at the beginning or end of urination, a prostatic or urethral source is likely. Hematuria accompanied by hypertension, edema, and a sore throat or a skin infection may be indicative of poststreptococcal glomerulonephritis. Thirty percent of patients with gross hematuria are diagnosed with a malignancy of the prostate, urethra, bladder, kidney, or ureter. Differential Diagnosis 43.1 lists possible differential diagnoses of hematuria.

The most important diagnostic tool in cases of hematuria is urinalysis. One consideration of the common urine dipstick test is that it detects the presence of heme (the iron-containing nonprotein portion of the hemoglobin molecule) in the urine but not actual RBCs. If the dipstick is positive for heme but the number of RBCs on the microscopic examination is within normal limits, myoglobinuria and hemoglobinuria should be suspected.

When hematuria of renal origin is suspected, laboratory tests should include an antinuclear antibody test, immunoglobulins, cryoglobulins, antiglomerular basement membrane antibodies, a full serum chemistry panel including creatinine clearance and blood urea nitrogen, a complete blood count and platelet count, an antistreptolysin O titer (to rule out past streptococcal infection), and a Venereal Disease Research Laboratory test (to rule out syphilis). If these studies indicate a renal etiology, the patient should be referred to a nephrologist. A urine culture and sensitivity should be done on all patients with hematuria, and if bacterial infection is found, treatment with appropriate antibiotics should be instituted, with reevaluation for persistent hematuria 2 weeks after the completion of treatment.

Isolated asymptomatic hematuria is often found on a routine screening urinalysis with no apparent source determined by history or physical examination. The possibility of occult malignancy or other potentially serious etiology in this setting increases with age, and if the patient is older than 35 years, they should be evaluated for urological tumors. Patients younger than 35 years should

Differential Diagnosis 43.1: Hematuria

Origin of Pathology	Differential Diagnoses
Urethra	Urethritis (gonococcal, nongonococcal) Stricture Calculus Trauma
Prostate/male genitourinary tract	Infection (prostatitis, epididymitis) Benign prostatic hypertrophy Tumor
Kidney	Infection (pyelonephritis) Nephrolithiasis Renal cell cancer Trauma Glomerular disease (vasculitis idiopathic) Ischemia (embolism, thrombosis, papillary necrosis) Allergic interstitial nephritis (drug-induced)
Ureters	Nephrolithiasis Tumor Endometriosis in females
Bladder	Infection (bacterial, parasitic) Calculus Tumor Endometriosis in females Drugs (hemorrhagic cystitis)
Pseudohematuria	Menstrual contamination in females Phenothiazines Red food dye Beet consumption Quinine Rifampin (Rifadin) Hemoglobinuria
Systemic illness	Pyelonephritis Coagulopathies (thrombocytopenia, hemoglobinopathy, sickle cell disease)
Functional causes	Intense exercise

be monitored at least monthly for 3 months, and if the hematuria persists, a more aggressive workup is indicated.

Examination of the morphology of RBCs present in the urine, using phase-contrast microscopy, can provide clues as to the etiology of hematuria. A fresh urine sample is essential because changes in morphology occur if the urine is allowed to sit for a prolonged time after collection. Dysmorphic RBCs may indicate glomerular disease. If the hematuria persists without evidence of infection, an IV pyelogram or renal ultrasound should be done to assess kidney structure. The American Urological Association recommends cystoscopy for all patients who present with risk factors for urinary tract malignancies such as irritative voiding symptoms, current or past cigarette smoking, and certain chemical exposures, regardless of age, to rule out bladder cancer (AUA, 2016).

PROTEINURIA

The primary proteins found in urine are globulin and albumin. *Proteinuria* is usually indicative of renal pathology, most often of glomerular origin. Proteinuria can be functional as a result of acute illness, emotional stress, or excessive exercise—in which case it is a benign process or simply a resultant sign of a transient condition. However, proteinuria can also reflect more serious disease. Abnormalities in the glomerular basement membrane produce glomerular proteinuria, and damage to the proximal tubule where filterable proteins are reabsorbed can result in tubular proteinuria. Proteinuria may also develop due to the overproduction of filterable plasma proteins such as Bence Jones proteins associated with multiple myeloma. Bence Jones proteinuria (characterized by free monoclonal light chain components of immunoglobulin proteins) may also be associated with lymphosarcoma, Hodgkin's disease, and leukemia.

Intermittent proteinuria is most often asymptomatic, associated with functional disorders, and discovered incidentally through urine dipstick testing. Continuous proteinuria is associated with renal pathology. Importantly, the standard dipstick proteinuria test does not detect Bence Jones proteins or other light chain immunoglobulins, as it is most sensitive to larger proteins such as albumin, with a minimum protein detection threshold of 10 to 20 mg/dL. A false-negative reading can occur because of a diluted urine sample, alkaline pH (normal pH = 4.5 to 8 [usual range = 5.5 to 6.5]), or with Bence Jones proteinuria. Thus, the most accurate way to quantify the amount of protein in the urine is with a 24-hour urine collection. However, a spot urine albumin to urine creatinine ratio can be measured as a close approximation of the 24-hour urine collection assessment. A 24-hour urine collection with more than 150 mg of protein is considered abnormal, and a specimen with more than 3.5 g is indicative of a nephrotic process. A urine albumin to urine creatinine ratio of less than 0.2 is considered normal and corresponds to an excretion of less than 200 mg/dL of protein.

DIFFERENTIAL DIAGNOSIS

Proteinuria may occur from benign or functional causes, in which it is a resultant sign of an acute or transient condition. Such causes include orthostatic proteinuria, vigorous exercise, environmental conditions, fever, and acute illnesses. Orthostatic proteinuria occurs when the urinary protein level is elevated only when the patient has been standing for a prolonged time, but not while they have

TABLE 43.1 Proteinuria

Type of Proteinuria	Major Mechanism	Associated Disease Process
Bence Jones proteinuria	Elevated plasma concentration	Multiple myeloma (also lymphosarcoma, leukemia, Hodgkin's disease)
Tamm-Horsfall proteinuria	Increased tubular cell secretion	Normal mucoprotein in urine
Tubulointerstitial area involvement	Decreased tubular reabsorption of normal filtered protein	Pyelonephritis
Altered glomerular capillary permeability	Increase of filtered proteins	Glomerulonephritis, nephrotic syndrome
False-positive result	High-alkaline urine	Urine pH greater than 8.0

been reclining. Exercise-induced proteinuria is related more to intensity, rather than duration, of exercise and may occur in athletes such as runners or boxers, sometimes accompanied by elevated catecholamines, hemoglobinuria, or hematuria. Proteinuria caused by environmental conditions such as emotional stress, exposure to cold, prolonged lordotic posture, and excess norepinephrine levels will resolve spontaneously when the precipitating element is eliminated and subsequently avoided. Mild, transient proteinuria may result from an albumin infusion or acute illnesses such as infection with fever (given the release of inflammatory cytokines), congestive heart failure, acute pulmonary edema, head injury, or cerebrovascular accident. This type of proteinuria typically resolves as the medical condition improves. In nondiabetic patients, moderately increased albuminuria has been associated with increased cardiovascular disease risk.

When proteinuria is identified in a low-risk (nondiabetic or nonpregnant) patient, the urine should be tested for Bence Jones proteins via electrophoresis, the presence of which suggests multiple myeloma. In addition, a full serum chemistry panel should be done, including a fasting blood sugar, a lipid profile, urine culture and sensitivity, and a complete blood count with differential. If the patient's urine is positive for Bence Jones proteins, a serum protein electrophoresis should also be done.

Persistent proteinuria that is not classified as functional proteinuria requires a further workup, beginning with a 24-hour measurement of urine protein and creatinine levels. If the excretion rate of protein is more than 2 g in 24 hours, a glomerular cause is most likely, and further evaluation is warranted. If the excretion rate is more than 3.0 to 3.5 g per day, the patient by definition has nephrotic syndrome and must be referred to a nephrologist. Nephrotic syndrome can lead to acute renal failure, hypertension, and end-stage renal failure.

If renal function is normal in a patient with elevated urinary protein, the patient should be evaluated for orthostatic proteinuria. This involves having the patient collect a urine specimen upon awakening but before assuming an upright position for longer than 1 minute. After the patient has been standing or walking for 2 hours, a second specimen is collected. If the patient has orthostatic proteinuria, the first specimen will be free of protein and the second will be positive for protein. Although this condition is largely benign and self-limited, orthostatic proteinuria is not well understood, and referral to a nephrologist may be necessary, particularly if persistent. Patients with nonorthostatic proteinuria and normal renal function in whom no Bence Jones proteins have been detected should also be referred to a renal specialist for renal biopsy. Descriptions of proteinuria associated with specific disease processes involving the renal system are presented in Table 43.1.

Management of proteinuria depends on the underlying cause. Angiotensin-converting enzyme agents have been found to reduce proteinuria by decreasing intraglomerular pressure. If hyperlipidemia and/or hypertension are present, these conditions should be aggressively treated. Patients found to have chronic renal failure should also be aggressively managed by a nephrologist to prevent or delay the onset of end-stage renal disease.

REFERENCES

Chu CM, Lowder JL. Diagnosis and treatment of urinary tract infections across age groups. *Am J Obstet Gynecol.* 2018:219(1): 40–51.

Ghandour R, Freifeld Y, Singla N, et al. Evaluation of hematuria in a large public health care system. *Bladder Cancer.* 2019;5(2): 119–129. doi:10.3233/BLC-190221

Smithson A, Ramos J, Nino E. et al. Characteristics of febrile urinary tract infections in older male adults. *BMC Geriatr.* 2019;19:334. https://doi.org/10.1186/s12877-019-1360-3

Thomas B, Batuman V, Lerma EV. (2020) What is proteinuria? *Medscape.* https://www.medscape.com/answers/238158-93475/what-is-proteinuria

Tumlin JA, Campbell KN. Proteinuria in nephrotic syndrome: mechanistic and clinical considerations in optimizing management. *Am J Nephrol.* 2018;47 Suppl 1:1–2. doi: 10.1159/000481632

RESOURCES

American Urological Association
https://www.auanet.org

National Kidney Foundation
https://www.kidney.org

Chapter 44

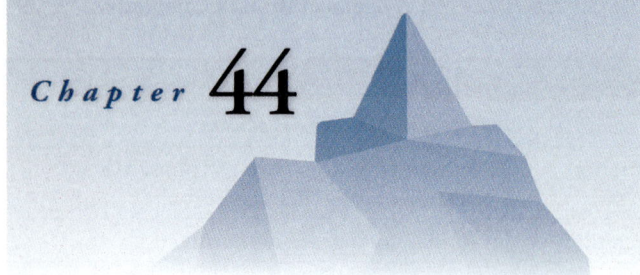

Urinary Tract Disorders

Debbie Conner, PhD, MSN, ANP/FNP-BC, FAANP
Debera J. Thomas, PhD, RN, ANP/FNP
Brian Oscar Porter, MD, PhD, MPH, MBA

URINARY INCONTINENCE

Urinary incontinence (UI) is the involuntary loss of urine from the bladder. Incontinence is so frequent in females that many patients mistakenly believe that it is an unavoidable consequence of aging. Incontinence is also common in older males as a result of an enlarging prostate. Incontinence can affect a person's quality of life and may be psychologically devastating. Ignoring incontinence or inadequate treatment of this condition can lead to social isolation, body image problems, anxiety, or depression; therefore, prompt treatment is essential (see The Iceberg of Incontinence).

EPIDEMIOLOGY AND CAUSES

UI affects more than 25 million Americans. The direct cost of treating and managing UI is reported to be more than $26 billion per year and includes costs associated with diagnostic testing, medication, and adult incontinence products such as disposable pads and undergarments. One study estimated that more than 40% of American females are affected, and there seems to be a strong association between UI and major depression. The prevalence of UI in the community population varies from 5% to 15%, depending on age and sex; more than 50% of patients in long-term care facilities have incontinence. Females are more likely than males to have incontinence, and the incidence increases with age; in fact, the risk of UI increases 14% with each decade of life. UI should not be considered a normal part of aging and can be treated.

Transient UI is characterized by sudden onset and can have several causes, including delirium, infection, pharmacological agents, or underlying systemic illnesses such as diabetes, fecal impaction, and restricted mobility. Most new-onset incontinence that occurs in the hospital resolves with appropriate treatment, but this acute transient phase can become a chronic problem if left untreated. The basic types of persistent UI are categorized as stress, urge, overflow, and functional UI. A patient may present with mixed symptoms of urge and stress incontinence. Table 44.1 provides an overview of the types of UI.

PATHOPHYSIOLOGY

The physiology of micturition involves three major components of urine storage and release: the central nervous system (CNS), the bladder, and the bladder outlet (urethral sphincters). Within the CNS, micturition is controlled by both the cortical (central) and brainstem (pontine) micturition centers. The cortical micturition center coordinates inhibitory stimuli from the frontal lobes and basal ganglia, permitting bladder relaxation and filling, as well as urethral sphincter closure to prevent urinary leakage as the bladder fills. These efferent signals originate in spinal levels T11 to L2 and are mediated by alpha-adrenergic receptors and cholinergic somatic stimulation. This maintains urethral pressure along the bladder outlet by both internal and external sphincters. Alpha-adrenergic stimulation causes muscle contraction of the internal sphincter, whereas the external sphincter is under voluntary control of striated muscle tissue (allowing patients to "hold their urine" for purposes of social appropriateness).

In contrast, bladder emptying is mediated by the parietal lobes and the thalamus, which modulate afferent proprioceptive stimuli from the distended bladder wall detrusor muscle, sensing an increase in bladder

> **Geriatric Considerations:**
> **Urinary Incontinence**
>
> Age-related changes that may affect urological functioning are as follows:
>
> - Decreased bladder capacity
> - Increased postvoid residual urine volume (greater than 50 mL).
> - Increased disinhibition of bladder contractions (i.e., overactive bladder [OAB]).
> - Increased nocturnal sodium and fluid excretion (nocturia).
> - Urinary overflow phenomenon resulting from increased urethral resistance in males related to benign prostatic hypertrophy and weakness of the pelvic floor in females.
> - Postmenopausal estrogen deficiency in females can result in decreased competence of the internal and external sphincters via atrophy of the urethral mucosal epithelium, resulting in atrophic urethritis, loss of compliance, and a diminished urethral mucosal seal.
>
> It is important to note, however, that normal aging does not cause UI.

The Iceberg of Incontinence

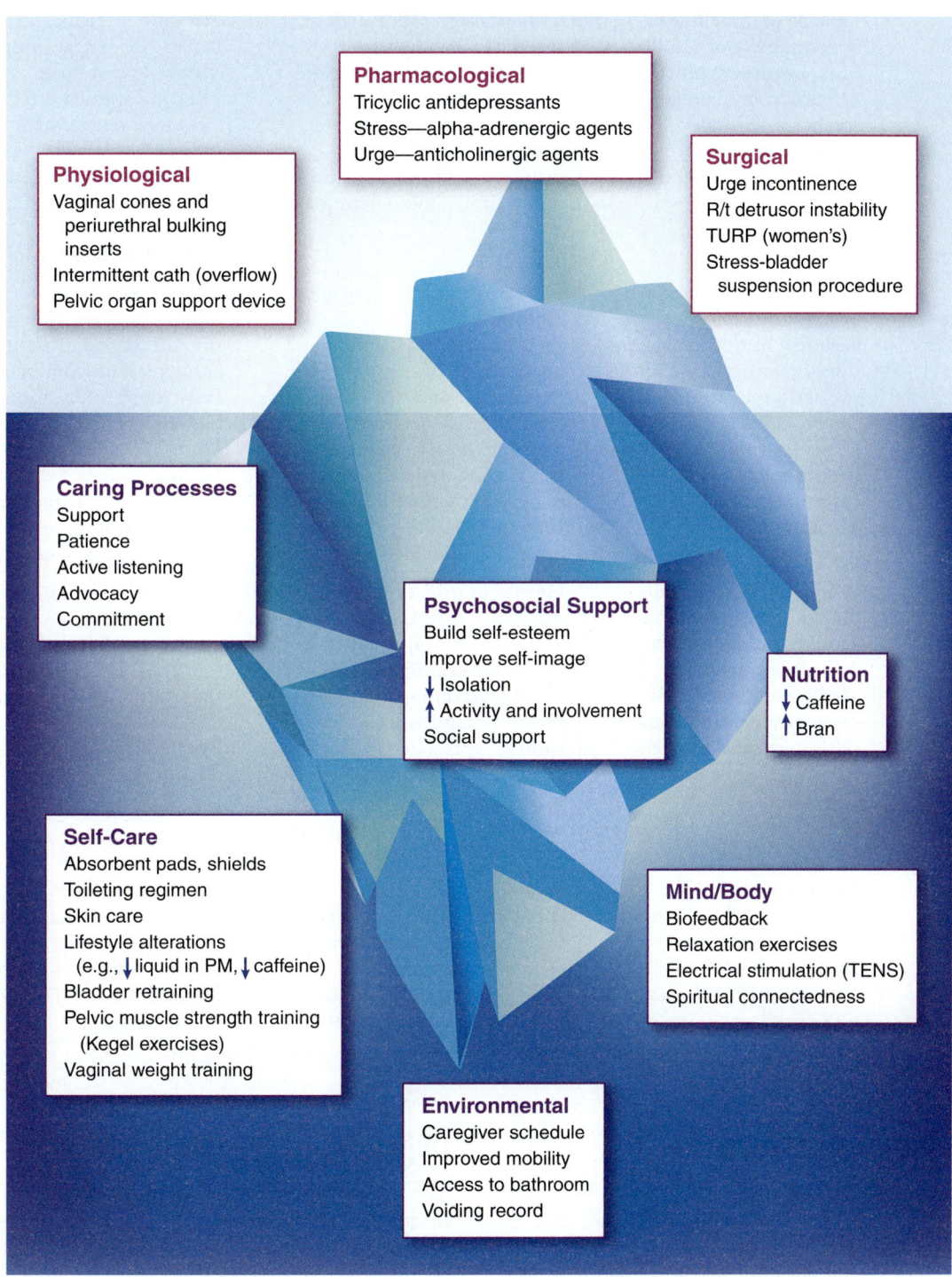

pressure that is interpreted as bladder fullness. Once the patient has the urge to void, the inhibition by the cortical micturition center ceases. In turn, the brainstem micturition center sends impulses from the pons down the spinal cord to the sacral micturition center at S2 to S4, subsequently triggering the bladder detrusor muscle to contract via cholinergic stimulation of parasympathetic M2 and M3 type muscarinic receptors found within the smooth muscle of the bladder walls. This latter action is simulated by the pharmacological agent bethanechol [Urecholine], which is used to treat urinary retention caused by an atonic or poorly responsive bladder. In addition, preganglionic sympathetic inhibition relaxes the urethral sphincter, allowing for the egress of urine.

TABLE 44.1 Types of Urinary Incontinence

Type	Cause	Assessment	Management
Stress incontinence	Leakage of urine due to hypermobility of bladder neck, intrinsic sphincter deficiency, or neurogenic sphincter deficiency Medications: sedatives, hypnotics, antispasmodics	Urine leakage with cough or sneeze History of vaginal deliveries Evidence of urine loss Pelvic examination, pad test, stress test, urinalysis with culture and sensitivity, video-urodynamics, cystometrogram	Pelvic floor reeducation with biofeedback (Kegel exercises) Weight loss, if obese Electrical stimulation Hormone replacement therapy (estrogen) Alpha-adrenergic agonist Surgical correction of hypermobile bladder neck Periurethral bulking injections
Urge incontinence	Leakage of urine due to urinary tract infection; vaginitis; bladder stones and tumors; cortical, subcortical, and suprasacral lesions; cerebrovascular accident; dementia; multiple sclerosis; Parkinson's disease; spinal cord transection Medications: diuretics, narcotics	History of dysuria, frequency, urgency, hematuria, or nocturia Evidence of a large amount of urine loss Evidence of unstable detrusor function with decreased capacity Assess perineal hygiene Pelvic examination, smear, neurological examination, urinalysis with culture and sensitivity, cystometrogram, video-urodynamics	Antimicrobial agents, antiseptics, topical estrogen, anticholinergics, smooth muscle relaxants, tricyclic antidepressants (imipramine) Pelvic floor reeducation with biofeedback (Kegel exercises) Prompted voiding and scheduled voiding Fluid intake management Removal of bladder stones Tumor resection and/or treatment
Overflow incontinence	Failure to empty bladder due to underactive detrusor activity, outlet obstruction, or diabetes mellitus Medications: anticholinergics, disopyramide, antihistamines, calcium channel blockers	History of urinary hesitancy, dribbling, decreased stream, feeling of incomplete bladder emptying, constipation Neurological examination, prostate examination (for male patients), prostate-specific antigen (for male patients), urinalysis with culture and sensitivity, serum creatinine, voiding cystometrogram, video-urodynamics	Scheduled toileting, Credé's maneuver Treatment of underlying conditions Urinary collection devices (intermittent or suprapubic) Alpha-blockers Resection of prostate, balloon dilation
Functional incontinence	Delirium, fecal impaction, lack of manual dexterity, or decreased mobility Medications: diuretics, hypnotics, alcohol, narcotics, decongestants	Fecal impaction Assess sleep patterns, mental state, hearing, vision, physical dexterity and functional ability, intake and output, toilet accessibility, infection, neurological function	Remove barriers to rapid toileting Provide barrier-free environment Bowel and bladder program Urinary collection devices Physical therapy Habit training

CLINICAL PRESENTATION

Subjective

Assessments of the urinary system should begin with a detailed medical and surgical history, including the patient's voiding history. A voiding history includes the date of incontinence onset, the number of times per day or night the patient voids, the amount of urine voided each time, the fluid-intake history including types of fluids consumed, and the characteristics of the patient's UI (e.g., "occurs when sneezing," nocturia, frequency, urgency, dysuria). Information regarding underlying medical conditions that act as risk factors such as diabetes, cancer, acute illness, and neurological disease should also be elicited.

Objective

The aim of the physical examination is to identify the underlying pathophysiological causes of incontinence, which can be multiple. The neurological assessment is important in differentiating diagnoses such as cerebrovascular accident (stroke), multiple sclerosis, and Parkinson's disease and should include an assessment of functional and cognitive ability. This provides information about limitations in mobility, self-care ability, mental status, and communication deficits, such as aphasia or language barriers.

An abdominal examination may rule out constipation, fecal impaction, masses, distended bladder, or cystitis, which can lead to incontinence. A pelvic examination will reveal the degree of pelvic floor strength, conditions such as uterine prolapse, and any problems associated with perineal structures. A rectal examination should be done to determine the sphincter tone and the presence or absence of feces that may suggest causative complications such as fecal impaction. In male patients, a prostate examination is crucial in evaluating urinary tract complaints. Inspection of the skin around the pelvic and genital area is important. For example, in female patients there may be atrophic vaginitis, and in male patients there may be abnormalities of the foreskin, penis, or perineum. In addition, the patient's skin should be evaluated for breakdown or pressure areas during the pelvic examination. Incontinence can cause skin breakdown in the perineal area and buttocks, which may lead to skin breakdown. In female patients, particularly postmenopausal females, the perineum should be assessed for dryness and atrophy of the vaginal mucosa as a result of decreased estrogen.

During the physical examination, signs of congestive heart failure (CHF) should be assessed because 50% of people with CHF experience incontinence. A cough stress test (which will allow direct observation of urine loss with a full bladder), bladder scan (ultrasound), or urinary catheterization (if necessary) to determine postvoid residual volume should be done as well. The patient or caretaker should be instructed to keep a voiding record for 3 to 7 days. The voiding record includes the time of the incontinence episode, the amount of urine, whether there was an urge to void, and the patient's activity at the time of the voiding. This record also includes an hourly record of fluid intake. For patients with a questionable history of UI, a "pad test" can be done. This involves having the patient take oral phenazopyridine (Pyridium), which will color the urine orange, and then wear a sanitary pad that can be checked at intervals for staining.

DIAGNOSTIC REASONING

Diagnostic Tests

A urinalysis and urine culture and sensitivity should be done, as well as measurements of serum electrolytes, blood urea nitrogen, creatinine, calcium (for polyuria in the absence of diuretics), and glucose. Urinary catheterization to assess postvoid residual volume is important, even on initial evaluation of the patient, unless a reliable measurement can be obtained by bladder scan. Further testing depends on whether the onset of incontinence is acute, in which case, testing related to other concurrent conditions may be warranted. Urinalysis results are often normal but may show glycosuria (in patients with diabetes), proteinuria (in patients with glomerular disease), white blood cells (WBCs; in patients with a bacterial infection), red blood cells (RBCs) (which may indicate the presence of a tumor), or nitrites or bacteria (both signs of infection). A urine culture that is positive for a predominant bacterial species (i.e., other than mixed or normal flora) also indicates infection, and specific findings can be used to guide antibiotic therapy.

Other diagnostic options include urodynamic testing and cystometry, cystometrogram, video-urodynamics, and a postvoid residual catheterization to indicate the amount of retained urine; patients requiring these tests are usually referred to a urologist. Reviewing the patient's use of medications for possible drug interactions, obtaining an accurate record of intake and output, and evaluating for other risk factors contributing to UI are also important. Patients who have indwelling catheters should be urodynamically evaluated for possible bladder retraining. Renal ultrasound may show renal pathology. A transrectal ultrasound can provide evidence of prostatic disease, and a pelvic ultrasound may demonstrate pelvic pathology. A cystogram may show abnormal sphincter pressure or bladder pathology.

Differential Diagnosis

Many older patients may normally compensate for their incontinence, but any marked alteration in status either physiologically or psychologically—such as a hospitalization—can precipitate the acute onset of incontinence. For example, the administration of IV hydration in an acutely ill or older adult may be sufficient to precipitate incontinence. Although the end point is the same for all types of incontinence (involuntary bladder emptying), the context in which this occurs may vary markedly. Thus, the primary goal of differential diagnosis is for the clinician to correctly identify the type and etiology of incontinence, which in turn drives management and treatment decisions. Normal micturition requires a complex interplay of neurological, structural, and functional components of the urinary system:

- The cerebral cortex exerts an overall inhibitory influence on the sacral spinal cord reflex. Delirium, dementia, parkinsonism, and stroke may all lead to urge incontinence without the patient's awareness. Conversely, the brainstem and suprasacral spinal cord exert a predominantly facilitating and coordinating influence that may be overcome in disorders such as stroke and multiple sclerosis, leading to overflow incontinence without awareness. This type of incontinence is referred to as neurogenic or detrusor-sphincter dyssynergy. Injuries to the sacral spinal cord, which controls reflex bladder filling and emptying, may lead to an acontractile bladder and overflow incontinence. This type of incontinence also results from the sacral nerve damage that can occur in uncontrolled diabetes mellitus.
- Local irritation and bladder or outflow obstructions may lead to urge incontinence because the smooth

muscle in the obstructed bladder can have enhanced spontaneous contractile activity. Increased outflow obstruction may be caused by anatomical obstruction by the prostate, a pelvic stricture, or cystocele, resulting in chronic urinary retention and overflow incontinence without the patient being aware that they are incontinent.
- The bladder and lower genitourinary tract must be able to store urine and empty properly for normal micturition to occur. Failure to store urine may be a result of a hyperactive or poorly compliant bladder (e.g., secondary to cystitis, stones, tumor, or a diverticulum), leading to urge incontinence. OAB is an overarching term used to describe urine storage symptoms such as urgency, frequency, and nocturia, which may or may not be accompanied by urge incontinence.
- Laxity of pelvic floor muscles, bladder outlet or sphincter weakness, and (in females) hypermobility of the urethra may cause diminished outflow tract resistance, leading to stress incontinence. Increased intra-abdominal pressure (e.g., due to pregnancy, obesity, tumors, sneezing, or coughing) can precipitate stress incontinence.

Mixed types of incontinence are common. In a patient with mixed signs and symptoms, multiple etiological factors must be considered, and a variety of interventions must be made available. The assessment and management of a patient with incontinence are best approached through the Circle of Caring (see discussion of this model in Chapter 1).

MANAGEMENT

Effective treatment of UI is largely driven by the pathophysiological basis of its etiology, as well as specific causative factors in individual patients. Understanding the mechanics of the various causes of incontinence helps clarify management.

Stress Incontinence

Stress incontinence is the involuntary loss of urine resulting from increased intra-abdominal pressure, such as that caused by coughing, sneezing, and laughing. In this condition, the bladder is unable to retain urine because of hypermobility of the bladder neck; intrinsic sphincter deficiency; neurogenic sphincter deficiency; or use of certain medications, such as sedatives, hypnotics, alpha-blockers, and/or antispasmodics that relax smooth muscle and increase urine flow. Female patients who present with stress incontinence report urinary leakage with coughing or sneezing and typically have a history of vaginal deliveries and/or hysterectomy. These physical changes may cause female patients to develop a cystocele, which can also increase their risk for stress incontinence. A detailed history guides the diagnostic work-up, which should include a pelvic examination, a pad test to determine the amount and frequency of urinary leakage, a cough stress test, urinalysis with culture and sensitivity, video-urodynamic testing, and/or a cystometrogram.

Once the diagnosis of stress incontinence has been made, treatment should be individualized and instituted to meet the patient's needs. Noninvasive treatments include pelvic floor reeducation (e.g., Kegel exercises) with biofeedback, electrical stimulation (an advanced form of biofeedback), weight loss (if the patient is obese) to decrease abdominal pressure, anti-incontinence devices or pessaries, and medications such as alpha-adrenergic agonists, which improve the muscle tone of the urinary tract. Eliminating diuretics (including caffeine) will also improve symptoms. Avoiding foods and beverages such as chocolate, coffee, tea, or carbonated drinks that can irritate the bladder is also useful. Surgical options include correction of the hypermobile bladder neck, insertion of an inflatable artificial sphincter, and periurethral bulking injections. See Drugs Commonly Prescribed 44.1 for a list of medications used for UI.

For cases in which uterine malpositioning places undue pressure on the bladder (e.g., as may be seen with uterine prolapse), vaginal cones or rings may be used to retain the uterus in a less problematic (and more physiologically correct) position. Vaginal cones can reduce the pressure on the bladder of prolapsed uterine musculature and subsequent UI. Vaginal pessaries are divided into two categories: support and space-filling. Pessaries are an effective option, particularly for older patients or those who do not tolerate incontinence medications well or have contraindications.

Surgical intervention may be appropriate if all other measures have failed or if used in conjunction with the previously discussed conservative treatment approaches. Surgery may be indicated to correct anatomical abnormalities such as a prolapsed uterus, hypermobile bladder neck, or obstructions such as an enlarged prostate or urinary tract and bladder tumors. Surgery should be used as the last treatment option unless the causative agent is diagnosed as a tumor or severe urinary tract obstruction.

Urge Incontinence

Urge incontinence, also known as detrusor instability, is the involuntary leakage of urine resulting from an inability to delay voiding. The patient has the sensation of a full bladder but is unable to store the urine long enough to reach the toilet. This failure can be caused by urinary tract infection (UTI); vaginitis; bladder stones; bladder tumors; prostate problems; stroke; dementia; multiple sclerosis; Parkinson's disease; spinal cord transection; cortical, subcortical, or suprasacral CNS lesions; and medications such as diuretics and narcotics. The patient's history and physical examination may reveal evidence of

Drugs Commonly Prescribed 44.1: Urinary Incontinence

DRUG	INDICATION	ADVERSE REACTIONS AND PRESCRIBING CONSIDERATIONS
Anticholinergic/Antispasmodic Agents		

Tolterodine (Detrol LA)
Oxybutynin (Ditropan XL, Urotrol)
Solifenacin (VESIcare)
Darifenacin (Enablex)
Trospium chloride (Sanctura XR)
Transdermal oxybutynin (Gelnique)
Fesoterodine (Toviaz)
	Urge incontinence
	Overactive bladder (OAB)
	Stress incontinence
		Contraindications:
		  Closed-angle glaucoma
		  Myasthenia gravis
		  Partial or complete gastric obstruction
		  Severe colitis
		  Urinary retention
		  Gastric retention
		Side effects:
		  Dry mouth
		  Drowsiness
		  Blurred vision
		  Urinary hesitancy
		  Urinary retention
		  Decreased gastrointestinal motility
		  Headache
		  Constipation
		  Vertigo/dizziness
		  Abdominal pain

Alpha-1 Adrenergic Blocking Agents (Used Predominantly in Males)		

Tamsulosin hydrochloride (Flomax)
Terazosin hydrochloride (Hytrin)
Doxazosin mesylate (Cardura)
	Benign prostatic hypertrophy and related urinary symptoms	Contraindications:
		  Hypersensitivity to tamsulosin terazosin, or doxazosin
		Side effects:
		  Orthostatic hypotension
		  Palpitations
		  Dizziness
		  Impotence
		  Gastrointestinal upset
		  Headache

Tricyclic Antidepressants		

Imipramine (Tofranil)
Amitriptyline (Elavil)
	OAB
	Urge incontinence
		Contraindications:
		  Hypersensitivity to tricyclic antidepressants
		  Use of monoamine oxidase inhibitors
		Side effects:
		  Dry mouth
		  Urinary retention
		  Blurred vision
		  Orthostatic hypotension
		  Sedation
		  Confusion in older adults
		  Tachycardia
		  Anxiety and nervousness
		  Sexual dysfunction
		  Constipation

Continued

Drugs Commonly Prescribed 44.1: Urinary Incontinence—cont'd

Other

Botulinum toxin (Botox) injection	OAB from neurogenic conditions OAB that does not respond to anticholinergic drugs	Side effects: Urinary tract infection Need for transient self-catheterization Dry mouth
Mirabegron (Myrbetriq)	OAB with symptoms of incontinence, urgency, and frequency	Urinary retention Blurred vision Constipation Diarrhea Memory issues Headache Joint pain Dizziness

dysuria, increased frequency or urgency, hematuria, large amounts of urine loss, unstable detrusor muscle activity with decreased urinary capacity, or nocturia. Assessment should include perineal hygiene, pelvic examination with vaginal discharge smear, a neurological examination including an assessment of mental status, and a urinalysis with a culture and sensitivity. Invasive procedures that may be needed include cystometrogram and video-urodynamics.

Treatment begins conservatively, with pelvic floor reeducation and biofeedback, if the patient is capable. Scheduled or prompted voiding by a caregiver, with management of the patient's fluid intake, may be useful for patients who have cognitive impairments or are forgetful. Medications such as antimicrobial agents may be necessary to treat underlying conditions. Other medications may include anticholinergics, smooth muscle relaxants, and tricyclic antidepressants to improve the neuromuscular function of the bladder and urethral sphincter (see Drugs Commonly Prescribed 44.1). Surgical treatment may be indicated for the removal of bladder stones or tumors.

Overactive Bladder

The term *overactive bladder* is often used interchangeably with the term *urge incontinence;* however, they are different conditions. OAB is a syndrome of symptoms that include urgency, frequency, and nocturia, all of which are associated with involuntary contractions of the detrusor muscle. Urge incontinence (the sudden intense urge to urinate and an involuntary loss of urine) may or may not be a feature of this syndrome, as about one-third of patients with OAB have urge incontinence.

OAB may also occur as a component of other types of UI, such as stress incontinence. OAB is caused by many factors, including disorders of the lower urinary tract, ingestion of alcohol or caffeine, use of a variety of prescribed drugs, or neurological conditions. This condition is most common in females and often results in anxiety and depression because of restricted daily functioning. Sexual dysfunction can occur because of the fear of urine loss during sexual intercourse. It is estimated that only about 6% to 27% of females with this condition seek treatment.

Pharmacotherapy plays an important role in management of OAB. Antimuscarinic agents or beta-adrenergic agents are commonly used drugs for OAB and are effective because they inhibit the muscarinic action of acetylcholine and prevent unwanted contractions of the detrusor muscle. These drugs can be used after or in conjunction with behavioral treatment. Botulinum toxin A injection into the detrusor muscle is effective for patients with refractory OAB. See Drugs Commonly Prescribed 44.1 for a complete list of medications used for OAB.

Overflow Incontinence

Overflow incontinence is the involuntary leakage of small amounts of urine. This is caused by an overdistended bladder in a patient who does not feel the need to void because of an atonic detrusor muscle; outlet obstruction; benign prostatic hypertrophy; diabetes mellitus; or the use of medications such as anticholinergics, disopyramide (Norpace), antihistamines, diuretics, or calcium channel blockers. The history and physical examination may indicate hesitancy, dribbling, nocturia, decreased stream, feeling of not emptying the bladder, and/or constipation. A neurological examination, prostate examination, urinalysis with culture and sensitivity, serum creatinine, voiding cystometrogram, and/or video-urodynamic testing should be done.

Management of overflow incontinence consists of treating the underlying condition, teaching scheduled toileting and Credé's maneuver, and the prescribing of medications such as alpha-adrenergic blockers (see

Drugs Commonly Prescribed 44.1). Credé's maneuver involves slowly applying downward pressure over the symphysis pubis. This is particularly helpful in patients who have a spinal cord injury or other neurological problems. It may be necessary to discontinue certain medications or to alter dosages to reduce the adverse effects causing overflow incontinence. Alternative collection devices may also be indicated, including the use of external catheters; pads; and indwelling, intermittent, or suprapubic catheterization. In the case of urinary outlet obstruction in male patients, resection of the prostate may be necessary.

Functional Urinary Incontinence

Functional UI is incontinence that occurs with a normally functioning urinary system. The leakage of urine is caused by factors outside the lower urinary tract and can be transient in nature. The causes of functional incontinence may vary from delirium or fecal impaction to lack of manual dexterity and immobility problems. Medications such as diuretics, hypnotics, narcotics, and decongestants, as well as alcohol, may also play a role. Assessment for fecal impaction, sleep pattern disturbances, mental status, hearing and vision, functional ability, fluid intake, infection (especially of the urinary tract), and neurological function is essential.

Treatment for functional UI may consist of some combination of removing barriers to effective toileting, providing education regarding a scheduled bowel and bladder program, the use of urinary collection devices, referring patients for physical or occupational therapy, and toileting habit training. Barriers to elimination may be identified when the patient cannot remove clothing or reach the toilet in sufficient time to avoid leakage. By identifying the barrier(s), interventions to resolve the problem can be developed. Some solutions include the use of hook-and-loop (Velcro) closures (which are easily managed by arthritic hands and fingers) instead of buttons and zippers if physical limitations are an issue, bedside commodes for nighttime use to eliminate the amount of time needed to get to the bathroom, or monitors for obtaining immediate assistance in getting out of bed and to the toilet.

A caregiver may be necessary to assist the patient in toileting; therefore, it is imperative to assess the caregiver's ability to provide care and determine their level of competency. Nursing research shows that caregivers want to give "good" care; however, the caregiver must be physically capable of providing this care with sufficient manual dexterity, strength, and mental cognition. Furthermore, the caregiver must be able to comprehend and follow through with instructions that may be complex and require problem-solving ability.

Identifying patients who need physical or occupational therapy to improve their functional skills may be required. Initiation of a bowel and bladder program can decrease the incidence of constipation and fecal impaction. Patients should also be encouraged to retrain the bladder to empty completely on a regular basis. For patients who cannot avoid UI, alternatives are available to keep them clean and dry. Condom catheters are effective in keeping male patients dry, and pads of various types are available for both male and female patients. Indwelling catheters, suprapubic catheters, and intermittent catheterization are options for urine collection in patients who cannot maintain bladder function or who have frequent or regular UI.

Medications used to treat incontinence are effective for patients who are unable to store urine. Pharmacological agents should be used in conjunction with other treatment modalities such as toileting and behavioral modification. Scheduled toileting along with regulation of fluid intake can have a positive effect on bladder control. Behavioral modification treatment such as pelvic floor reeducation is designed to increase pelvic floor muscular strength and endurance. Reeducation is accomplished through Kegel exercises of the targeted muscle group using biofeedback for a period of 4 to 6 weeks. Kegel exercises are the tightening and releasing of the pubococcygeal and levator ani muscles, accomplished by tightening the muscle group used to avoid defecation or urination. The patient may experience results within 2 weeks to several months of initiating the program. This treatment is noninvasive and, when appropriate, should be attempted before surgical intervention (Box 44.1).

FOLLOW-UP AND REFERRAL

Close follow-up is essential for patients with UI. This may be done biweekly at first, while the patient is being taught therapeutic exercises (e.g., Kegel exercises) or medication dosages are being adjusted. Quarterly follow-up visits may be sufficient once incontinence is under control and medication doses have been stabilized. The patient should be monitored for adverse

---

Box 44.1 Kegel Exercises: Patient Instructions

- Locate the correct muscle. To do so, try stopping your urine flow by contracting the muscle. When the urine slows or stops, you are using the pubococcygeus muscle.
- Squeeze the muscle for 2 seconds (do not hold your breath or contract your abdomen, buttocks, or thighs), then relax for 10 seconds. This is one repetition. Do 10 repetitions twice a day.
- After you have mastered the technique, begin to lengthen the time you contract the muscle. Increase the time by 1 second every few days until you are able to contract the muscle for 10 seconds at a time (and relax for 10 seconds). Continue to do 10 repetitions twice a day.

effects of medications and orthostatic hypotension. Periodic urinalysis should be done to detect any UTIs early. Female patients should have regular pelvic examinations to detect pelvic abnormalities early, and male patients should have regular rectal examinations to detect prostatic abnormalities.

> **Patient Education: Urinary Incontinence**
>
> Patient and family education is crucial in the treatment of UI. Iatrogenic causes as contributing factors to UI cannot be overemphasized. Particularly in older patients, polypharmacy is a key contributor to iatrogenic UI and may be further exacerbated by the reactionary addition of new anti-incontinence medications. Environmental assessment should include recommendations about proximity of toilet facilities. An individualized toileting schedule should be geared to each patient's pattern of incontinence. Bladder training in the form of timed voiding, working up to 3-hour intervals, is an important intervention. Good general nutritional and exercise practices are important to the upkeep of overall health. Support and encouragement are essential. Interventions geared toward preventing social isolation, setting up necessary support services, and optimism in dealing with the problem are important interventions in the primary care setting.

LOWER URINARY TRACT INFECTIONS

A lower UTI occurs when the normally sterile environment of the urinary tract system is invaded by pathogenic bacteria. Infections of the lower urinary tract can occur in the urethra, bladder, and the prostate (in males). Infection of the urethra (urethritis) and infection of the urinary bladder (cystitis) usually occur together. Female patients may be diagnosed with chronic inflammation of the bladder wall (interstitial cystitis [IC]). Prostatitis is infection of the prostate gland.

Infections can be acute, chronic, recurrent, complicated, or uncomplicated. Acute infections are characterized by the onset of UTI in a previously symptom-free individual. Infections can become chronic when unresolved after standard treatment is rendered. UTIs become chronic because of obstructions, antibiotic-resistant bacteria, or the presence of multiple strains of bacteria that are not susceptible to the antibiotic therapy prescribed. A UTI is considered recurrent when it occurs again within 2 weeks of the original infection. A complicated UTI is either an acute or chronic infection that is accompanied by factors that predispose a patient to the infection or make treatment more difficult, such as instrumentation (e.g., indwelling, suprapubic, or intermittent catheterization), underlying chronic disease, systemic symptoms, or pregnancy. An uncomplicated UTI is one that can be resolved without addressing such factors and is localized to the lower urinary tract.

EPIDEMIOLOGY AND CAUSES

Lower UTI is a common problem that affects approximately 20% of females and 1% of males each year. This condition accounts for more than 6 million visits to primary care practitioners annually. Although common in females of all ages (lifetime incidence of 50% to 60%), UTI rarely occurs in males younger than 50 years and is usually caused by urinary catheters, anatomical abnormalities of the urinary tract, unprotected anal intercourse, or vaginal intercourse with a partner who has a bacterial infection. UTI may occur at any age, but it is more prevalent in sexually active adults, very young children, or frail older adults. Females older than 65 years have approximately double the rate of UTI than the overall female population. Other populations at risk include individuals with predisposing conditions such as a suppressed immune system, pregnancy, urinary obstruction, catheter dependency, neurogenic bladder, or diabetes mellitus.

Lower UTI may be the result of other conditions within the renal system. A urethral obstruction can create stasis of urine, providing a medium for bacterial growth. Other conditions that can contribute to UTI are a descending infection from the kidney, an anatomically short urethra (in female patients), and acute infections elsewhere in the body. UTI may also occur as a result of poor or nonsterile catheterization technique or reuse of disposable catheters, poor hygiene, unprotected anal intercourse, or simply from a normal indwelling catheter, which, as a foreign body, serves as a nidus of infection.

IC is found primarily in females. An estimated 3 to 8 million females and 1 to 4 million males seeking treatment for bladder pain are diagnosed with IC, also known as bladder pain syndrome (BPS). IC/BPS is not an infection, but it may feel like a UTI. The cause of this condition is unknown, but some researchers theorize that an abnormality in the bladder surface allows potassium and urea to leak into the bladder interstitium. Other etiologies being investigated include lymphatic, infectious, neurological, autoimmune, and vasculitic mechanisms. Notably, as a noninfectious condition, IC does not respond to antibiotics.

> **Geriatric Considerations**
> **Urinary Tract Infection**
> - UTI increases with age
> - Females over age 65 years have double the rate of UTI compared with all females
> - Symptoms may be absent in older adults
> - Risk factors for UTI in males include prostatic hypertrophy and diabetes

PATHOPHYSIOLOGY

Lower UTIs usually occur as a result of contamination from the patient's own gastrointestinal tract. Bacteria may be introduced into the urinary tract from fecal contamination secondary to poor perineal hygiene, unprotected sexual (particularly anal) intercourse, and/or an anatomically shortened urethra in female patients. The use of a spermicide during intercourse (especially with diaphragm forms of contraception) alters the vaginal microenvironment, predisposing to bacterial colonization. Immunosuppressed or medically compromised patients may have difficulty suppressing bacterial growth as bacteria ascend the urethra. Patients who are dependent on catheters are at risk for introduction of bacteria into the urinary tract through contamination of the catheter.

Alkaline urine is a common complication of diabetes mellitus. The elevated pH of the urine creates a medium in which bacteria can more readily grow and proliferate. Renal stones can also create an environment that promotes bacterial growth, as the blockage causes stasis of urine or reflux. In turn, contamination can occur in the kidney when urine "backs up" due to vesicoureteral reflux, in which urine flows freely in retrograde fashion into one or both ureters, resulting in urinary stasis.

In female patients, approximately 80% to 90% of cases of uncomplicated UTI are a result of the gram-negative rod bacterium *Escherichia coli*. The second most common cause (5% to 20% of cases) of uncomplicated bacterial infection is the gram-positive coccus *Staphylococcus saprophyticus,* although this agent is rare in complicated UTI. Other gram-negative rods identified as causative pathogens in a smaller number of cases, but particularly in complicated UTI, include *Proteus mirabilis*, *Klebsiella*, *Enterobacter*, *Serratia*, and *Pseudomonas*. In addition, the gram-positive coccus *Enterococcus* has been identified. *Staphylococcus aureus* is a gram-positive coccus that can be introduced into the urinary tract through instrumentation or as a complication of renal stones. Risk of UTI in menopausal patients increases due to reduced levels of estrogen (causing thinning of the vaginal tissue) and also in individuals who have trouble with complete bladder emptying.

Fungi, particularly *Candida* species, may also be causative agents in a complicated UTI that fails to respond to antibiotic therapy, especially in the presence of an indwelling catheter. Candiduria may be asymptomatic, and fungal structures should be sought on urine microscopy because fungal colonies may be more difficult to elaborate under standard urine culture conditions, in turn leading to delays in treatment.

In up to 50% of all bacterial species associated with cystitis, genetic virulence determinants may be identified that contribute to the uropathogenicity of these organisms, such as adherence factors that allow for greater binding affinity to the uroepithelium. Another is the urease gene, expressed by certain gram-negative bacteria such as *Proteus, Klebsiella, Ureaplasma, Providencia,* and *Pseudomonas* species. This enzyme splits urea molecules within the urinary tract, creating ammonium and hydroxyl ions that produce an alkaline microenvironment. This higher pH facilitates survival of these bacteria, particularly when housed within triple phosphate (magnesium ammonium phosphate) stones, also known as struvite stones.

Cystitis is rare in males because the increased length and drier environment around the urethra contribute to less frequent bacterial colonization. In addition, prostatic fluid has inherent antibacterial properties. Thus, when UTI does occur in males, it is often associated with abnormal urethral anatomy or inadequate treatment of prostatitis. Most antibiotics do not penetrate the prostatic tissue and therefore do not eliminate prostatic infection. As a result, the bladder is reinfected from contaminated prostatic fluid, even if a lower UTI initially clears on treatment.

Two well-documented phenomena related to classic UTI are asymptomatic bacteriuria and dysuria–pyuria syndrome. In asymptomatic bacteriuria, patients experience no obvious clinical symptoms or signs of UTI (including altered mental status in older adults), yet urinalysis and urine culture yield findings consistent with bacteriuria. In contrast, dysuria–pyuria syndrome (also called "acute urethral syndrome") is characterized by painful urination with WBCs on microscopic urinalysis in the absence of a positive bacterial culture. This condition may be due to organisms such as *Chlamydia* that do not grow well under standard urinary culture conditions. Dysuria–pyuria syndrome may, however, be difficult to distinguish clinically from vaginitis due to sexually transmitted infections (STIs).

CLINICAL PRESENTATION

Subjective

The presenting signs and symptoms of UTIs vary widely in intensity and occurrence. Female patients may present with urethritis and cystitis simultaneously. The most frequently reported symptoms in both male and female patients are dysuria; urinary frequency or urgency; nocturia; hematuria; low back or suprapubic pain; UI; and cloudy, foul-smelling urine. These symptoms can occur in any combination. In older patients, altered mental status may be the sole manifestation of UTI and should create a high level of suspicion.

Urethritis in males is rare; if left untreated or treated inadequately, it can lead to complications such as urethral strictures, periurethral abscess, urethral diverticula, and fissures. Vaginal discharge in female patients and urethral discharge in male patients may suggest STI. Purulent urethral discharge may reflect *Neisseria gonorrhoeae,* whereas whitish-mucoid discharge may suggest *Chlamydia trachomatis*. If confirmed, these infections should be treated aggressively with the appropriate antibiotic therapy (see Chapter 52 for a full discussion of STIs).

Objective

Physical examination in the outpatient setting should include a "clean-catch" midstream urine sample for urinalysis. Findings on urinalysis that are associated with an infectious process in the urinary tract system include cloudy appearance; alkaline pH; hematuria; elevated levels of nitrites; leukocyte esterase (detecting pyuria of greater than 10 leukocytes per high power field [hpf]); bacterial overgrowth; and urinary sediments of RBCs, WBCs, and mucus.

Of note, Enterobacteriaceae convert urinary nitrates to nitrites, producing positive results on urine dipstick analysis if present in adequate numbers (i.e., greater than 100,000 organisms/mL). In contrast, however, *Staphylococcus* does not convert this substrate and is not detectable by this test. Moreover, false-positive urinary nitrite tests may result from the urinary tract analgesic phenazopyridine. A urine culture and sensitivity may be ordered to speciate and determine the sensitivity of the causative organism to specific antibiotic therapy.

DIAGNOSTIC REASONING

Diagnostic Tests

Diagnosis of lower UTI is made based on the subjective complaints of the patient and a clean-catch midstream urine sample showing the presence of bacteria, especially if more than 100,000 organisms/mL of the same morphology are present. Traditionally, a bacterial concentration of at least 100,000 colony-forming units (CFUs)/mL on urine culture has been used to define UTI, but UTI may result from far lower bacterial loads. UTI is currently defined as a urine sample with greater than 1,000 organisms/mL in the presence of characteristic clinical symptoms.

The method of urine collection also influences interpretation of the urine culture because the sterility of commonly performed clean-catch techniques is heavily dependent on the patient's ability to self-clean around the urethra before voiding. Sterile wipes containing iodine, chlorhexidine, or other acceptable cleaning agent must be used to wipe the urethral opening at least two to three times consecutively in a direction away from the perineum to minimize contamination by anorectal flora (e.g., normal skin flora or bacteria from vaginal discharge or fecal matter). Alcohol swabs are unacceptable cleaning agents. Straight catheterization samples obtained with sterile technique are the most reliable, whereas samples obtained from receptacles connected to indwelling catheters may prove unreliable because of repeated manipulation of the collecting bag.

Although urine culture is considered the gold standard with the greatest sensitivity for laboratory confirmation of UTI, urinalysis with microscopy is also helpful and provides rapid results. Urinalysis typically indicates pyuria (greater than 10 neutrophils/hpf on microscopic examination) and often the presence of RBCs. Hematuria is common in UTI but not with urethritis or vaginitis; however, blood in the urine is not a marker of complicated infection.

UTIs may be treated with empiric antibiotic therapy based on knowledge of the most common bacterial etiologies. However, urine culture and antibiotic sensitivity testing will aid in definitively identifying the infecting microorganism and the appropriate antibiotic therapy. Although the diagnosis of UTI is made both clinically and by urinalysis, generally urine culture and antibiotic sensitivities are indicated if complicated infection is suspected, atypical symptoms are present, or symptoms persist or recur within 1 month of the patient receiving a prior empirical course of antibiotic therapy or a new treatment regimen is desired.

IC is primarily a diagnosis of exclusion. Although somewhat controversial due to low sensitivity and specificity in some settings, a diagnostic tool for this condition is the potassium sensitivity test. This test involves slow instillation of 40 mL of sterile water into the bladder via catheterization and left for 5 minutes, after which the patient is asked to grade any discomfort on a 0 (none) to 5 scale, with 5 being the most severe. This establishes a baseline comparison. The water is then emptied and a 0.4 M potassium chloride solution is instilled into the bladder and left for 5 minutes, with any discomfort again graded by the patient. IC is suggested when there is at least a two-point increase in pain or urgency, indicating epithelial dysfunction.

Differential Diagnosis

The differential diagnosis of tumors, upper UTI (pyelonephritis), vaginitis, and STIs must be explored in cases of suspected lower UTI. Tumors of the renal system and upper UTI are discussed in Chapter 45. Vaginitis and STIs are discussed in Chapters 46 and 52. Patients with upper UTI usually show signs of sepsis such as fever and chills, have WBC casts in the urine (reflecting the passage of neutrophils through the renal tubules), or experience flank and costovertebral angle tenderness on examination characteristic of pyelonephritis. Patients with IC may present with the need to urinate frequently because of reduced bladder capacity. This may occur up to 60 times per day in extreme cases. Other symptoms include pain or discomfort in the abdominal area that holds the bladder.

MANAGEMENT

Pharmacological antimicrobial management is the mainstay of treatment. Drugs Commonly Prescribed 44.2 presents the oral agents typically used for the

Drugs Commonly Prescribed 44.2: Urinary Tract Infection (UTI)

DRUG	INDICATION AND DOSAGE	ADVERSE REACTIONS AND PRESCRIBING CONSIDERATIONS
Sulfonamides		

Trimethoprim and sulfamethoxazole (TMP-SMX) (Bactrim, Septra 80 mg TMP/400 mg SMX) (Bactrim DS) (160 mg TMP/800 mg SMX) (double strength [DS])	Precoital or postcoital prophylaxis: 100 mg trimethoprim (Trimpex) after sexual intercourse
	Acute uncomplicated UTI: One DS tablet two times daily × 3 days
	Complicated UTI: 8–10 mg/kg/day IV in two to four equally divided doses every 6, 8, or 12 hours for up to 14 days
	Pyelonephritis: One DS tablet every 12 hours for 7–14 days
		Contraindications:
		  Hypersensitivity to trimethoprim or sulfonamides
		  Allergy to sulfa
		  Folate-deficiency megaloblastic anemia
		  Pregnancy at term and lactation
		Side effects:
		  Abdominal distress
		  Nausea
		  Rash
		  Neutropenia
		Special instructions:
		  Take with a full glass of water.
		  Complete full course of therapy.

Anti-infectives		

Nitrofurantoin (Furadantin, Macrobid, Macrodantin)	UTI:
	100 mg two times daily × 5–7 days
	50–100 mg four times daily for active infection or once daily at bedtime to prevent infection
		Contraindications:
		  Hypersensitivity to nitrofurantoin
		  Renal function impairment (creatinine clearance less than 60 mL/min)
		  Anuria or oliguria
		  Pregnancy in third trimester, labor, or delivery
		  Not indicated for the treatment of pyelonephritis or perinephric abscesses
		Side effects:
		  Nausea
		  Vomiting
		  Anorexia
		  Abdominal discomfort
		Special instructions:
		  Take with food.
		  May cause urine to darken.
		  Avoid use with live vaccines.

Aminopenicillins		

Amoxicillin (Amoxil)
Amoxicillin and potassium clavulanate (Augmentin)
	Amoxicillin:
	  Mild/moderate infections: 500 mg two times daily or 250 mg three times daily × 10 days
	  Severe infections: 875 mg two times daily or 500 mg three times daily × 10 days
	Amoxicillin and potassium clavulanate
	  Mild/moderate infections: 500 mg/125 mg two times daily or 250 mg/125 mg three times daily × 10 days
	  Severe infections: 875 mg/125 mg two times daily or 500 mg/125 mg three times daily × 10 days
		Contraindications:
		  Penicillin allergy
		Side effects:
		  Hypersensitivity reactions
		  Urticarial rash
		  Nausea
		  Diarrhea
		  Superinfections
		Special instructions:
		  Complete full course of therapy.
		  May decrease effectiveness of oral contraceptives.
		  Augmentin should be given with food to decrease nausea.

Continued

Drugs Commonly Prescribed 44.2: Urinary Tract Infection (UTI)—cont'd

DRUG	INDICATION AND DOSAGE	ADVERSE REACTIONS AND PRESCRIBING CONSIDERATIONS
Cephalosporins—Second Generation		

Cefaclor (Ceclor) Cefuroxime (Ceftin)	Cefaclor: 250–500 mg three times daily × 7 days
	Cefuroxime uncomplicated UTI: 250–500 mg two times daily × 5–10 days
		Contraindications:
		  Allergy to cephalosporins
		Side effects:
		  Pruritus
		  Urticaria
		  Erythema multiforme
		  Rashes
		  Arthritis/arthralgia (with or without fever)
		  Diarrhea
		  Nausea
		Special instructions:
		  Renal dysfunction prolongs half-life.
		  May be taken without regard to meals.
		  Complete full course of therapy.

Cephalosporins—Third Generation		

Cefpodoxime (Vantin)	Cefpodoxime 100 mg two times daily × 7 days	Contraindications:
		  Allergy to cephalosporins
		Side effects:
		  Diarrhea
		  Abdominal pain
		  Nausea
		  Dyspepsia
		  Flatulence
		Special instructions:
		  Avoid antacids 2 hours before and after dose.
		  Complete full course of therapy.

Cefixime (Suprax)	Cefixime 400 mg once daily OR 200 mg two times daily × 3–7 days	
Urinary Analgesics		

Phenazopyridine (Pyridium)	Relief of pain, burning, urgency, and frequency from UTI:
	  200 mg three times daily after meals; maximum 2 days when used in conjunction with an antibacterial agent
		Contraindications:
		  Hypersensitivity to phenazopyridine
		  Renal insufficiency
		Side effects:
		  Headache
		  Rash
		  Itching
		Special instructions:
		  Take after meals.
		  May turn urine reddish-orange color and stain fabric.

Sodium salicylate/ benzoic acid methenamine (Cystex)	Relief of pain, burning, urgency, and antibacterial agent
	2 tablets every 4 hours; maximum 3 days
		Side effects:
		  Headache
		  Indigestion
		  Stomach cramps
		  Rash
		Special instructions:
		  May turn urine reddish-orange color and stain fabric.

Drugs Commonly Prescribed 44.2: Urinary Tract Infection (UTI)—cont'd

DRUG	INDICATION AND DOSAGE	ADVERSE REACTIONS AND PRESCRIBING CONSIDERATIONS
Antispasmodics		
Flavoxate (Urispas)	Relief of dysuria, urgency, frequency, and incontinence of the urinary system: 100–200 mg three to four times a day	Contraindications: 　Use with caution in patients with glaucoma and in older adults. Side effects: 　Nausea 　Vomiting 　Dry mouth 　Headache 　Drowsiness 　Blurred vision 　Vertigo

treatment of lower UTI. The first-line treatment of choice for uncomplicated lower UTI is nitrofurantoin given for 5 days. Epidemiological surveillance has revealed increasing rates of resistance in *E. coli* isolates to ampicillin and sulfonamides, whereas only a small percentage of these isolates were resistant to nitrofurantoin (Macrodantin, Macrobid), which is known to concentrate in the urine.

Nitrofurantoin is also effective against many gram-positive cocci such as *Enterococcus faecalis,* whereas other key uropathogens such as *Proteus, Enterobacter,* and *Klebsiella* may be highly resistant. Nitrofurantoin should be used as empirical therapy for uncomplicated UTI only. Fosfomycin is a broad-spectrum antibiotic also used to empirically treat uncomplicated lower UTI and has the advantage of being given as a single dose. Although the use of trimethoprim-sulfamethoxazole (TMP-SMX) as empiric therapy is no longer the first-line choice in most parts of the country, it may be indicated depending on the resistance patterns in certain areas. TMP-SMX is indicated as first-line treatment in complicated UTI in female patients who are not pregnant.

Selecting an alternative antibiotic regimen entails important considerations, such as local antibiotic resistance patterns, which are typically available from local health authorities or hospital systems. Ciprofloxacin (Cipro) and other fluoroquinolones should be reserved as an alternative antibiotic class only in cases when no other antibiotic agents are appropriate, given concerns over the development of resistant uropathogens; the risk of tendon rupture and other connective tissue abnormalities; and the potential for severe, permanent, and disabling peripheral neuropathy.

The cost-effective single-day treatment regimen with fosfomycin for uncomplicated lower UTI reduces the risk of nonadherence and the development of *Candida* vaginitis due to clearance of normal urogenital flora. Nitrofurantoin requires a longer 5-day course of therapy for maximum efficacy. Complicated UTI, on the other hand, requires at least 5 to 7 days of antibiotic therapy.

The antimicrobial effects of these medications persist for several days after the final dose is administered. In particularly severe cases of UTI (especially in high-risk groups such as older or bed-bound patients) or in cases involving urinary tract instrumentation, hospitalization and broad-spectrum IV antibiotic coverage (e.g., ceftriaxone, piperacillin-tazobactam, or ampicillin plus gentamicin) may be required until symptoms wane and urine culture and antibiotic sensitivities confirm the most appropriate narrow-spectrum antibiotic choice. The same approach may be required for upper UTI (i.e., pyelonephritis).

Empirical treatment of UTI in male patients (by definition, a complicated UTI) should be extended to at least 7 days. Nitrofurantoin and beta-lactams should be avoided.

Treatment of UTI during pregnancy is especially important because an established link exists between premature delivery and UTI (especially pyelonephritis). Empirical therapy may include ampicillin 500 mg by mouth four times daily, nitrofurantoin (Macrobid, Macrodantin) 100 mg orally two times daily, cephalexin (Keflex) 500 mg orally two times daily, or sulfisoxazole 1 g orally four times daily. Broader-spectrum regimens may include amoxicillin-clavulanate (Augmentin) 500 mg/125 mg orally two times daily or cefpodoxime (Vantin) 100 mg orally two times daily. Most clinicians will choose to treat UTI during pregnancy for 1 full week. Fluoroquinolones should be avoided, given concern for their effects on bone and cartilage formation in the developing fetus, and TMP-SMX should be avoided in the first and third trimesters of pregnancy.

Fungal UTI due to *Candida* infection is typically associated with an indwelling urinary catheter, and nearly half of all cases resolve simply with removal of the catheter. However, reinsertion of a new catheter is associated with a high rate of relapse. Antifungal treatment is typically not required for asymptomatic colonization, but if indicated in the presence of dysuria, an appropriate regimen would be fluconazole (Diflucan) 200 mg orally daily for 7 to 14 days.

The management of asymptomatic bacteriuria deserves special mention. This condition should be treated with antibiotics in pregnancy because it increases the risk of premature delivery. Although some studies suggest that treatment in girls beyond preschool age is not warranted, given the high rate of recurrent asymptomatic infection without obvious sequelae, general practice also calls for treating asymptomatic bacteriuria in young children. Treatment is also indicated in patients before they undergo a urological procedure to avoid operating on a contaminated field, after removal of a bladder catheter in place for less than 1 week, and in any patient with an underlying structural abnormality of the urinary tract, vesicoureteral reflux, or struvite stones. In contrast, treatment of this condition in adult males, nonpregnant females, older adults, patients with diabetes mellitus, and patients with spinal cord injury with indwelling urinary catheters is not warranted. Although asymptomatic bacteriuria may be a harbinger of future UTI, antibiotic therapy has not been shown to persistently eradicate bacteriuria or urinary tract colonization in these populations.

After completion of antibiotic treatment, follow-up cultures may be obtained to ensure complete eradication of the pathogen in patients with a history of recurrent infection, during pregnancy, or in those prone to complicated UTI. Chronic or recurrent UTI may be prevented through prophylactic treatment either on a daily basis or after sexual intercourse, but this should be done only after all options to eliminate the causative factors of UTI have been explored. In female patients with a prior history of recurrent UTI, postcoital prophylaxis with a single oral dose of nitrofurantoin 50 mg or cephalexin 250 mg has been shown to be highly effective. Strategies should be emphasized to decrease the incidence of infection through the guidelines outlined under Patient Education: Lower Urinary Tract Infections.

Although appropriate antibiotic treatment is often adequate to relieve dysuria, certain medications may also be prescribed for the first few days to decrease the pain and discomfort of UTI. Use of these agents should not be prolonged, however, given their significant side effect profile. Effective treatment may involve anticholinergics, which produce an antispasmodic effect, including atropine (Donnatal), hyoscyamine (Levsin, Cystospaz), propantheline (Pro-Banthine), or oxybutynin (Ditropan). However, anticholinergics may also contribute to urinary retention (especially in older adults), which is a clear risk factor for UTI, and should thus be used with caution. Analgesics may be prescribed such as phenazopyridine (Pyridium), but this alters the color of urine to orange and may cause urinary leakage secondary to anesthetization of the urethra and sphincter.

IC does not respond to antibiotics. However, this condition may be treated with pentosan polysulfate sodium (Elmiron), which tends to reduce the bladder wall inflammation. This drug has been shown to improve symptoms in 38% of patients with IC. Of note, IC is not curable, but it is controllable. If IC is left untreated, it becomes more difficult to treat and in severe cases can progress to the development of a fibrotic contracted bladder.

FOLLOW-UP AND REFERRAL

Patients with complicated or repeated UTI and those who have pyelonephritis or are pregnant should have a follow-up urinalysis or culture to assess for effectiveness of treatment. UTI that is secondary to other pathological conditions will not resolve until the primary causative factor is addressed. Thus, indwelling urinary catheters should be changed every 4 to 6 weeks with new equipment, using sterile technique.

It is important to maintain adequate hydration and to monitor urine output for signs of obstruction or renal failure. Urinary tract obstructions must be identified and removed to reduce the chances of chronic infection and renal damage that can lead to renal insufficiency and failure. It may be necessary to prescribe analgesics for the patient to reduce the pain associated with UTI. Pain-relieving medications such as phenazopyridine (Pyridium) can be effective but should be prescribed for no more than 2 days when used in conjunction with antibacterial agents.

Self-medication is usually adequate for female patients who have relatively few recurrences of UTI. If a diagnosis of recurrent bacterial UTI is confirmed, the patient should be given a supply of an antibiotic (preferably TMP-SMX or nitrofurantoin) and instructed to take it for 3 to 7 days whenever the symptoms recur. The patient should keep a diary of infections and response to treatment and review it annually with a health professional so as to track medication-associated problems. The patient should also be advised to notify the clinician if symptoms such as flank pain, fever, hematuria, or lack of response to treatment occur.

If UTI recurs frequently (e.g., monthly), prophylactic therapy should be prescribed. After a course of 10 to 14 days of a suitable antibiotic for recurrent infection, the patient should begin low-dose antimicrobial prophylaxis every other day at bedtime over a 4- to 6-month period, which has proved as effective as daily dosing. Nighttime therapy is recommended because the patient generally does not void for a prolonged period, thus giving the bacteria the opportunity to adhere to the bladder wall. If this period of prophylaxis has been effective, the patient may switch to self-medication. If the frequency of recurrence increases at this point, however, prophylaxis should be extended to every other night indefinitely. However, all lifestyle issues should be investigated first. Given inconsistencies in the literature, there remains a need for well-designed studies to evaluate whether cranberry products may reduce the frequency of UTI recurrence as another prophylactic strategy.

> **Patient Education: Lower Urinary Tract Infections**
>
> Patient education should focus on teaching the patient to prevent the recurrence of UTI by advising the patient to follow these guidelines:
>
> - Complete the full course of antibiotic therapy even if all symptoms subside early on in the course of treatment (prescribed treatment courses may be anywhere from 1 to 7 days duration).
> - Increase fluid intake to 8 to 10 8-ounce glasses of water per day; this is most important to continue flushing out bacteria.
> - Consider taking cranberry supplements (300 to 400 mg twice daily) or drink cranberry juice because this may decrease the bacteria's ability to adhere to the epithelial cells that line the bladder.
> - Wear cotton underclothes rather than nylon to avoid moisture build-up, and avoid wearing thong underwear.
> - Avoid the use of harsh soaps or feminine hygiene products that can irritate the urethra.
> - Use condoms to provide a barrier to infection from intercourse.
> - Use proper techniques for self-catheterization (if indicated) to reduce the incidence of introducing bacteria.
> - Empty the bladder frequently to avoid stasis of urine.
> - Void after sexual intercourse.
> - Take showers instead of tub baths or bubble baths to avoid chemical irritation of the urethra.
> - Keep a diary of urinary symptoms and review it annually if recurrent infections are a problem.
> - Empty the bladder completely, possibly by double-voiding (i.e., completely emptying the bladder two times in 5 minutes), especially if recurrent infections are a problem.
>
> The patient should also be educated regarding any potential adverse effects of medications, including urinary leakage associated with phenazopyridine (Pyridium) treatment or the subsequent development of vaginal yeast infections after antibiotic treatment.

UPPER URINARY TRACT INFECTION: PYELONEPHRITIS

Pyelonephritis is an infection of the kidney that is characterized by infection within the renal pelvis, tubules, or interstitial tissue that may be unilateral or bilateral. The condition may be classified as either acute or chronic. The chronic condition leads to changes in the kidney that create atrophy and scarring of the kidney and calyceal deformity that may eventually lead to renal failure.

EPIDEMIOLOGY AND CAUSES

Pyelonephritis occurs in both males and females, but it is more common in females. The incidence is higher in older adults (especially if institutionalized or hospitalized), children, and immunocompromised patients. At least 250,000 cases are diagnosed annually with a treatment cost of $2.14 billion per year in the United States. The incidence and risk of developing this disease are increased in patients with predisposing factors, including anatomical abnormalities such as ureterovesical reflux, urinary obstruction, stress incontinence, multiple or recurrent UTIs, renal disease, kidney trauma, pregnancy, prostatic enlargement, and metabolic disorders such as diabetes mellitus. Having an indwelling urinary catheter is always a prominent risk factor for pyelonephritis, especially in hospitalized older female patients. An episode of acute pyelonephritis within the prior year also puts a patient at increased risk. Most of these risk factors alter the vaginal microenvironment and predispose patients to lower UTI, as well.

In acute pyelonephritis, the actual infectious insult to the kidney may be from hematogenous seeding or urinary tract reflux, but most commonly it is an ascending infection from the bladder. Thus, it can often be attributed to an untreated lower UTI that spreads to the upper urinary system or is introduced through instrumentation. Chronic pyelonephritis usually has no specific pathological explanation if anatomical abnormalities have been ruled out.

PATHOPHYSIOLOGY

It is unclear whether lower UTI always precedes pyelonephritis, because many patients present without clinical evidence of prior cystitis. However, bacteria are believed to enter through the urethral meatus and ascend upward from the lower urinary tract (urethra and bladder) to one or both kidneys via the ureters, the bloodstream (hematogenous spread), or the lymphatic system. In female patients, pyelonephritis is typically caused by fecal flora that colonize the vaginal introitus and subsequently ascend along the urinary tract to the kidneys.

E. coli (75% to 95% of cases), *P. mirabilis*, *Klebsiella*, and *Pseudomonas* are the most common gram-negative causative agents. Between 5% and 10% of cases are caused by gram-positive organisms, including *Enterococcus*, *S. saprophyticus*, and *S. aureus* (particularly in severe infection). *S. saprophyticus* is the second most common cause of pyelonephritis in young females. *Ureaplasma urealyticum* and *Mycoplasma hominis* are rarer causative agents. In patients with normal urogenital systems, nearly all bacterial agents of pyelonephritis express virulence factors that contribute to their uropathogenicity (e.g., the *pap* and *sfa* operons, pathogenicity islands found in virulent *E. coli* strains).

In acute pyelonephritis, swelling of the renal parenchyma occurs as a result of the patchy distribution of the acute infectious process throughout the kidney. In rare instances, scarring of the renal parenchyma leading to kidney atrophy, renal hypertension, and renal failure may occur if left untreated. When the infection is severe, abscesses may develop in the renal medulla, leading to necrosis of the renal papillae. This infection can be potentially life-threatening in older adults, children, or immunocompromised patients. In addition, diagnosis and treatment in pregnancy are particularly critical because upper UTI has a clear association with premature delivery.

Chronic pyelonephritis is usually caused by a recurrent or chronic bacterial infection of the kidney, often related to the presence of instrumentation such as an indwelling catheter that serves as a nidus of infection. Patients often have other urological problems such as vesicoureteral reflux; neurogenic bladder; or urinary obstruction caused by renal tumors, stones, or prostatic hypertrophy. The persistent unresolved infection and inflammation cause fibrosis (scarring) of the tubulointerstitium, which may lead to hypertension as the body senses decreased renal blood flow or eventually chronic renal insufficiency.

CLINICAL PRESENTATION

Subjective

Acute pyelonephritis presents with a classic triad of fever, costovertebral angle pain, and nausea and/or vomiting. The fever may persist over a few hours or days and range up to 103°F (39.5°C). The patient may present with shaking, chills, nausea, vomiting, unilateral flank or localized back pain over the affected kidney, fatigue, diarrhea, or other symptoms resembling those of gram-negative sepsis. Signs of urinary urgency or frequency and suprapubic discomfort may be present. In some cases, the presentation may mimic pelvic inflammatory disease; otherwise, the patient may be largely asymptomatic and then progress to full-blown sepsis (i.e., urosepsis). In the older patient, altered mental status may be the initial manifestation of pyelonephritis.

Chronic pyelonephritis may present with the patient complaining of fatigue, nausea, decreased appetite with weight loss, nocturia, and/or polyuria. Patients may present with symptoms of renal failure resulting from asymptomatic chronic pyelonephritis that has persisted for several years. Symptoms of renal failure are discussed in detail in Chapter 45.

Objective

The physical examination will elicit marked tenderness on deep abdominal palpation and/or percussion of the affected flank and back overlying the affected kidney (costovertebral angle tenderness). Patients usually do not have a severely toxic appearance but may appear ill due to discomfort. Patients with underlying hypertension may present with blood pressure above their baseline. With severe pyelonephritis, patients may remain symptomatic for several days, even if appropriate antibiotic therapy is administered.

Patients with chronic pyelonephritis may show minimal symptoms or symptoms similar to those of acute pyelonephritis. Early signs and symptoms may be vague, and chronic pyelonephritis is usually first diagnosed when the patient presents with impaired renal function caused by damage to the kidneys.

DIAGNOSTIC REASONING

Diagnostic Tests

Diagnosis of pyelonephritis is confirmed through urinalysis, which is positive for bacteria, proteinuria, leukocyte esterase, urinary nitrites, hematuria, pyuria, and specifically WBC casts (reflecting the passage of neutrophils through the renal tubules), as well as urine culture, which typically demonstrates greater than 100,000 CFU/mL, allowing for identification of the causative organism. Any of these findings may be altered, however, if the patient is already on antibiotic therapy, and colony counts may be as low as 10,000 CFU/mL in some cases. Blood cultures may also be positive in 10% to 20% of mild to moderate pyelonephritis cases, reflecting urosepsis.

Cystoscopy with ureteral catheterization, renal ultrasound (to reveal hydroureter and/or hydronephrosis), or an intravenous pyelogram (IVP) may be indicated; however, the nuclear medicine–based dimercaptosuccinic acid (DMSA) scan is most sensitive for detecting pyelonephritis and renal scarring. Although rarely used, renal biopsy in acute pyelonephritis may reveal abscess formation with neutrophilic invasion. The area of the infection is wedge-shaped, pointing toward the medulla, and the glomeruli are spared. Findings in chronic pyelonephritis include fibrosis, scarring, and reduction of renal tissue, with calyceal clubbing, dilation, and distortion. A voiding cystourethrogram may reveal vesicoureteral reflux, which predisposes to both lower and upper UTIs.

Differential Diagnosis

It can be difficult to differentiate pyelonephritis from cystitis; however, the presence of WBC casts is diagnostic for pyelonephritis. In female patients, a pelvic examination should be performed to rule out an alternative or additional diagnosis such as pelvic inflammatory disease. Hematuria is also often present in lower and upper UTIs, but not in vaginitis or urethritis. Chronic pyelonephritis can sometimes be diagnosed through IVP, DMSA scan, or renal ultrasound, which may identify atrophied kidneys with "clubbing" of the affected calyces. A definitive diagnosis of chronic disease is made by identifying persistent pyuria and positive urine cultures. Sometimes chronic pyelonephritis is diagnosed only via kidney biopsy.

MANAGEMENT

Aggressive therapy is necessary to prevent permanent damage to the kidneys, a potential complication of upper versus lower UTI. Tissue penetration of antibiotics into the renal medulla appears more important than serum or urine drug levels. Oral antibiotics may be prescribed in mild cases of acute pyelonephritis, characterized by the absence of nausea and vomiting or signs of sepsis. Antibiotic choice should consider the local antibiogram and drug-resistance rates for the community and patient population in which the infection was likely acquired. Drugs Commonly Prescribed 44.2 presents the oral agents commonly given for lower UTI and mild to moderate pyelonephritis (not requiring hospitalization or IV therapy).

Hospitalization may be indicated, depending on the patient's ability to maintain adequate fluid intake and to tolerate oral antibiotics, along with the severity of the symptoms and evidence of bacteremia. Hospitalization of patients who are pregnant, vomiting, or dehydrated should be strongly considered. Likewise, the patient's degree of systemic illness (bacteremia or urosepsis), age, history of chronic disease, or nonadherence to therapy may lead to the assessment that hospitalization is necessary. Ninety-five percent of patients demonstrate a positive therapeutic response to IV antibiotic treatment within 48 hours and may be discharged on appropriate oral medication, once urine culture and antibiotic sensitivity results are available and subsequent antimicrobial therapy may be narrowed in spectrum. Treatment courses should typically last for 7 to 10 days for mild to moderate cases, 14 days for severe cases, or 21 days in particularly slow responders. Ample evidence has demonstrated that once common 6-week regimens led to increased adverse effects without improved treatment effectiveness. Selection of a regimen should be based on local antibiotic resistance and susceptibility results.

Second-line therapy includes ceftriaxone (Rocephin) 1 g IV daily, as well as other extended-spectrum cephalosporins or penicillins, carbapenems, monobactams (in penicillin allergy), and aminoglycosides (except in pregnant patients) such as gentamicin or tobramycin.

If the patient does not respond adequately within 48 hours, they should be reevaluated, the cultures reviewed, and an ultrasound or CT scan performed to assess the kidneys. IV antibiotics may need to be administered for up to 7 to 10 days in severe cases. During treatment, the patient must increase fluid intake, and an accurate intake and output record must be maintained for appropriate fluid management. Surgery may be indicated to remove or correct secondary causes of UTI such as urinary obstruction or anatomical abnormalities. Diagnostic studies requiring the insertion of instruments should be delayed until the urine is sterile or free of bacteria and/or pus to avoid the complications of bacteremia or septic shock. A urological anatomical evaluation should be performed for all male patients with pyelonephritis and female patients with recurrent pyelonephritis to detect any structural abnormalities that may be contributing to or causing the condition.

FOLLOW-UP AND REFERRAL

If undergoing outpatient treatment, the patient should be seen 48 hours later to assess responsiveness to therapy. Similarly, patients in the hospital should be evaluated in 48 hours for response to therapy and consideration of discharge. Follow-up urine cultures are not routinely recommended in asymptomatic patients. However, for those with recurrent pyelonephritis, reculturing 2, 6, and 12 weeks after antibiotic therapy is initiated may be done to ensure complete and lasting eradication of infection.

Further treatment decisions are based on clinical findings such as fever, pain, and the culture of causative bacteria. When a diagnosis of chronic pyelonephritis is determined, the patient should be referred to a nephrologist because of the severe damage to the kidney that can occur. As discussed previously, a renal ultrasound, renal colic CT scan, or voiding cystourethrogram may detect structural abnormalities, renal stones, or vesicoureteral reflux—all of which predispose the patient to infection. Patients should also be monitored and treated for other conditions secondary to pyelonephritis such as hypertension, chronic infection, renal insufficiency, or renal failure.

Patient Education: Upper Urinary Tract Infections

The focus should be on teaching the patient to prevent recurrence of lower UTI and pyelonephritis by following these instructions:

- Complete the full course of antibiotic therapy even if symptoms subside early on in the course of treatment.
- Prevent or reduce the incidence of lower UTIs by following the guidelines under Patient Education: Lower Urinary Tract Infections.
- Increase fluid intake to eight to 10 8-ounce glasses of water per day.
- Report any recurrence of UTI symptoms immediately.
- Consider taking cranberry supplements (300 to 400 mg twice daily) or drink cranberry juice because this may decrease the bacteria's ability to adhere to the epithelial cells that line the bladder.

NEPHROLITHIASIS

Nephrolithiasis is a condition in which stones (renal calculi) originate in the kidney. The stones form from calcium salts (approximately 75% to 85%), struvite (approximately 10% to 15%), uric acid (approximately 7%), and cystine (1% to 2%). These stones often cause acute episodes of urinary tract obstruction, infection, and severe pain in adults.

EPIDEMIOLOGY AND CAUSES

Renal calculi may occur in people aged 20 to 60 years, but the incidence peaks in those aged 20 to 30 years. Annual prevalence of renal calculi is approximately 3% to 5% and lifetime prevalence is 15% to 25%. Formation of renal calculi is more prevalent in the Southeast, West, and Midwest United States. In warm, dry climates, uric acid stones account for up to 40% of all cases.

The typical patient may report a sedentary lifestyle or occupation that involves exposure to high environmental temperatures. Calcium oxalate stones occur more often in males, whereas struvite stones are more common in females. Renal stones can occur because of obstruction, urinary stasis, infection, dehydration and urinary concentration, increased consumption of calcium or vitamin C or D, excessive excretion of uric acid, or vitamin A deficiency. Hereditary factors can also predispose the patient to kidney stone formation.

Calcium oxalate and calcium phosphate stones account for 65% to 85% of all cases of renal calculi. These types of stones are found predominantly in males and in individuals whose diet is high in salt, animal fat, animal protein, and oxalate from green leafy vegetables. Interestingly, a low-calcium diet is also a risk factor, as it leads to increased oxaluria because less oxalate is bound to calcium in the gastrointestinal tract. Vasectomy is a risk factor as well, and hypertension doubles the risk of stone formation for reasons that are as yet unclear.

Patients with calcium oxalate or calcium phosphate stones typically do not have hypercalcemia except with certain disorders such as hyperparathyroidism, sarcoidosis, and hyperuricemia, which may lead to hypercalciuria or hyperuricosuria. Loop diuretics such as furosemide (Lasix) also promote calciuria. Similarly, hypocitraturia and hyperoxaluria similarly predispose to calcium stone formation because an increased amount of calcium is available for complexing with oxalate or phosphate within the urinary tract. Inflammatory bowel disease is associated with marked hyperoxaluria. Medullary sponge kidney disease is found in 10% to 30% of persons with calcium stones.

Several other forms of renal calculi have been noted. Struvite stones are found predominantly in females; these stones are associated with UTIs. They occur when the urine is alkaline (pH greater than 7.0) and a urea-splitting organism, such as *Proteus* or *Klebsiella*, is present. Uric acid stones are formed from an increase in uric acid production or ineffective elimination of uric acid, as found in gout. This may result from dietary intake of foods high in uric acid, acidic urinary pH (e.g., type I renal tubular acidosis, significant bicarbonate loss associated with severe diarrhea), regional enteritis, hereditary factors (including a predisposition to gout), or ulcerative colitis. Uric acid stones account for approximately 15% to 20% of all cases of nephrolithiasis. Cystine stones are created because of a rare autosomal recessive disorder called cystinuria. These stones are formed when there is a metabolic error that causes a decrease in tubular reabsorption in the kidney, leading to urinary cystine concentrations greater than 250 mg/L. Cystine stones account for approximately 1% to 3% of all cases of renal stones.

PATHOPHYSIOLOGY

Renal stone formation occurs when normally soluble mineral substances supersaturate the urine and deposit out of solution as crystals, which serve as nuclei for stone-forming substances such as calcium oxalate, calcium phosphate, triple-phosphate struvite (magnesium ammonium phosphate), uric acid, or cystine. Stone formation may also be facilitated by extremes in urinary pH (alkaline or acidic). This crystal combination becomes trapped within the renal system, where it continues to attract other crystals, causing the stone to increase in size.

Stones are typically anchored at the ends of collecting ducts at sites of epithelial injury. The calculi vary in size and composition and typically grow within the renal tubules, calyces, renal pelvis, ureters, or bladder. Large stones are called staghorn calculi if they span more than one of the renal calyces. Although over the span of years their presence in the kidneys may lead to chronic renal failure, unless they fragment and pass through the urinary system, they are generally asymptomatic.

The four major types of stones and their characteristics, causes, etiology, diagnosis, and treatment are listed in Table 44.2. These forms are not mutually exclusive and share certain risk factors. Many patients have renal stones of mixed etiology. Calcium stones are light in color; their crystals characteristically resemble RBCs in shape and size or may be a larger "dumbbell" form. Formation of these stones may be secondary to hypercalcemia or they may be idiopathic. Hyperoxaluria and hyperuricosuria are more associated with calcium oxalate stones, whereas calcium phosphate stones are more associated with primary hyperparathyroidism.

Struvite stones are flat and consist of hexagonally shaped crystals that are radiopaque. They often form secondary to UTI caused by *P. mirabilis*. Staghorn calculi are more likely to be struvite stones. Uric acid stones are radiolucent and red-orange in color, with a teardrop or

TABLE 44.2 Renal Calculi

Type of Stone (Percentage of All Stones)	Characteristics	Causes	Management
Calcium (75%–80%)	Resemble RBCs in shape and size or large dumbbell form Light color	Idiopathic, hypercalcemia, or increased levels of uric acid	Thiazide diuretics Diet Cholestyramine Surgery
Struvite (15%)	Flat, hexagonal shape Radiopaque	Alkaline urine, infection with urea-splitting organisms such as *Pseudomonas*	Antibiotic therapy Surgery
Uric acid (7%)	Teardrop-shaped or flat square plates Red-orange color	Increased uric acid production, high intake of uric acid, acidic urine, regional enteritis, ulcerative colitis, or idiopathic	Allopurinol Fluid replacement Diet Surgery
Cystine (<1%)	Lemon yellow, sparkling	Hereditary (autosomal recessive cystinuria)	Force fluids D-penicillamine Tiopronin

flat square shape. Formation of these stones may be associated with a hereditary etiology of gout or with idiopathic causes. Uric acid crystals may also serve as a nidus for calcium stone formation. Cystine stone crystals are lemon yellow, hexagonal, and sparkle under light microscopy. Certain medications promote crystalluria and predispose the patient to renal stones, including topiramate, triamterene, and sulfadiazine. The protease inhibitor indinavir (Crixivan) used to treat HIV-positive patients may actually precipitate within the renal collecting system, causing direct stone formation.

The incidence of recurrence of certain stones is approximately 40% to 50% within 5 years, with an estimated one-third of patients eventually losing a kidney if the condition is untreated or inadequately treated. Complications can occur when the stone obstructs the flow of urine. This can lead to urinary retention, accumulation of uremic wastes, end-stage renal failure, and/or electrolyte imbalances. Stones can also predispose the patient to UTI and hematuria.

CLINICAL PRESENTATION

Subjective

The patient with an acute episode of nephrolithiasis may present with a variety of signs and symptoms, depending on the location, size, and type of stone. Onset is usually sudden with renal colic, which is a type of flank pain that is not relieved by changes in position or other measures. The pain may present with a referral pattern that originates in the flank or kidney area and radiates across the abdomen down into the groin, perineal area, and inner thigh. This colicky pain occasionally progresses to constant pain at a level that can be excruciating and intractable. Other symptoms of renal calculi may include nausea, urinary frequency, vomiting, diaphoresis, dysuria, hematuria, and weakness. The patient may report a history of a recent or chronic UTI, previous diagnosis with nephrolithiasis, a dietary history consistent with stone formation, or alterations in voiding patterns.

Objective

The patient may present with abdominal distention and guarding on palpation, flank tenderness on percussion, and decreased or absent bowel sounds on auscultation. Fever may be present if there is acute infection related to obstruction. Blood pressure (as well as pulse rate and respiratory rate) may be elevated because of pain.

DIAGNOSTIC REASONING

Diagnostic Tests

The diagnostic work-up should begin with a routine urinalysis, complete blood count, and blood chemistry profile. Urinalysis may be normal or it may show RBCs, WBCs, crystals, mineral casts, bacteria, pus, and an alkaline or acidic pH. Table 44.3 identifies the tests and expected results that would lead to the suspicion of renal calculi. Either gross or microscopic hematuria is observed in the majority of cases but may be absent in up to 30% of cases, depending on the time of presentation. Identification of the type of stone formation is important for the appropriate treatment to be instituted. The results of these tests should lead the clinician to continue the diagnostic work-up with noninvasive tests to identify obstructions, masses, or anatomical abnormalities.

These further diagnostic tests may include x-ray studies of the kidney, ureters, and bladder; abdominal or transvaginal ultrasonography (used for pregnant patients and those of childbearing age in whom radiation must be avoided); or noncontrast helical computed tomography scan (IV contrast dye is avoided due to potential renal toxicity). Invasive procedures may be necessary to

TABLE 44.3 Tests for Renal Calculi

Test	Rationale
Urinalysis	Shows RBCs, WBCs, crystals, casts, minerals, bacteria, pus, abnormal pH
24-hour urine	May show increased levels of creatinine, uric acid, calcium, phosphorus, oxalate, or cystine
Serum chemistry	May show increased levels of magnesium, calcium, uric acid, phosphorus, protein, and electrolytes
Serum blood urea nitrogen (BUN) and creatinine	Shows BUN elevated secondary to urinary tract obstruction; creatinine elevated secondary to damage to the kidney
Complete blood count	May show infection or septicemia
Kidney and upper bladder ultrasound	Shows calculi and/or anatomical changes
Intravenous pyelogram	Shows calculi and any abnormality in anatomic structures
Cystourethroscopy	May show calculi and/or abnormal structural defects
Computed tomography scan	Identifies calculi and other masses in the renal system

visualize or assist in removing the stone through IVP, cystourethroscopy, or other surgical procedures.

Differential Diagnosis

The differential diagnosis for renal calculi includes a variety of diseases and conditions, including appendicitis, diverticulitis, acute peritonitis, mesenteric adenitis, pancreatitis, ileus, peptic ulcer disease, abnormalities of the fallopian tubes and ovaries including ovarian cysts, ectopic pregnancy, gallbladder disease, and abdominal aneurysms. A tentative diagnosis of renal calculi is made from the history and findings on physical examination showing increased intensity of renal colic with flank pain or a pattern of referred pain coupled with flank tenderness. Because hematuria may be the only presenting sign of stone formation, malignancy (renal cell carcinoma), which is typically painless, must also be considered. The diagnosis of renal stones is confirmed by urinalysis that is positive for blood and visualization of the renal system by radiography or ultrasound.

MANAGEMENT

Treatment goals are to decrease the symptoms and complications arising from existing renal stones and to prevent subsequent recurrence. It is important, therefore, to decrease the concentration of stone-forming substances in the urine. An intake of six to eight 8-ounce glasses of water a day is essential, unless prevented by cardiac complications, such as CHF. This high fluid intake must continue indefinitely. Most stones smaller than 5 mm pass spontaneously. Rates of spontaneous passage steadily decrease for stones larger than this, and spontaneous passage is highly unlikely for renal stones larger than 10 mm.

Initially, pain management is the priority. Oral NSAIDs in dosages of 600 to 800 mg three times daily or oral narcotics such as hydrocodone-acetaminophen (Vicodin, Lortab), acetaminophen-codeine (Tylenol #3), or oxycodone-acetaminophen (Percocet) are often necessary. Intramuscular keterolac 60 mg is also effective. In some cases, intramuscular or IV narcotic analgesics may be necessary, but most studies have demonstrated that NSAIDs are as effective as oral opiates, although they are slower-acting. In addition, they have also been shown to relax ureteral smooth muscle, which may facilitate stone passage. Antispasmodics such as flavoxate or oxybutynin may also provide temporary relief, but the anticholinergic effects of these medications must be taken into account because they may lead to urinary retention. Warm compresses to the lower back, focused breathing, imagery, and diversional activities may provide minimal relief.

Certain drugs help to reduce urinary excretion of stone-forming substances. Thiazide diuretics (e.g., hydrochlorothiazide) reduce calcium excretion; allopurinol reduces uric acid production by inhibiting xanthine oxidase; and D-penicillamine affects the excretion of cystine. Importantly, loop diuretics such as furosemide (Lasix) and triamterene increase calciuria and typically worsen renal stone formation.

Noninvasive or invasive surgical interventions may be necessary if the stone does not pass spontaneously; these are presented in Table 44.4. Noninvasive procedures to treat renal calculi are aggressive and carry many of the same risks as surgery. Extracorporeal shock-wave lithotripsy (ESWL) is the least invasive technique, sending focused shock waves through the body to break apart proximal and midurethral calculi and is preferred for stones smaller than 10 mm. NSAIDs should be avoided at least 3 days before this therapy to minimize the risk of bleeding. A lithotriptic agent may also be used to dissolve the renal calculus.

Invasive procedures may be necessary to remove the stone because of its location or the failure of noninvasive procedures to destroy the stone. The procedure chosen is dependent on the location, size, and type of stone (e.g., struvite stones typically require ESWL or surgical intervention). Percutaneous ultrasonic lithotripsy is a more invasive procedure in which therapeutic ultrasound waves are applied to the kidney stone via a surgically introduced nephrostomy tract, followed by endoscopic removal of stone fragments. First and second generation lithotripters originally visualized stones via fluoroscopy or ultrasonography. However, advances in urethroscopy

TABLE 44.4 Surgical and Other Procedures for Renal Calculi Management

Procedure	Type of Procedure	Location of Calculi	Description
Lithotripsy	Invasive	Bladder or urethra	Crushing of the calculi under direct visualization using a lithotriptoscope
Percutaneous ultrasonic lithotripter	Invasive	Renal system	Ultrasound waves are applied to the stone via nephrostomy tract, with endoscopic removal of fragments
Lithotomy	Invasive	Renal system	Arthroscopic removal of the calculi
Lithonephrotomy	Invasive	Kidney	Incision of the kidney to remove the calculi
Lithotony	Invasive	Bladder or urethra	Incision of the bladder or ureter to remove the calculi
Ureteral stent	Invasive	Kidney or ureter	Stent is placed in front of the calculi to facilitate elimination
Lithotrophic	Noninvasive	Renal system	Agent used to dissolve calculi
Extracorporeal shock wave lithotripsy	Noninvasive	Renal system	Focused shock waves are applied to the outside of the body to crush the calculi

with flexible fiberoptic systems now allow for the direct visualization of stones virtually anywhere along the urinary tract from the urethra to the renal pelvis. Stones may be crushed via electrohydraulic or laser lithotripsy in conjunction with these visualization techniques. Flexible ureteroscopy combined with laser lithotripsy is now the preferred treatment for proximal ureteral stones larger than 10 mm. The patient is then able to eliminate the stones naturally after they are crushed into smaller pieces.

Lithotomy is an incision into the bladder or ureter to remove calculi or to place a ureteral stent, whereas lithotony specifically denotes arthroscopic extraction of a renal stone from the bladder. Ureteral stents may be placed within the ureters to facilitate the passage of stones through natural elimination. Lithonephrotomy is an incision into the kidney to remove a stone.

Preventive measures should be taken to reduce the incidence of recurrence. The occurrence of calcium-based stones may be reduced by increasing fluid intake (greater than 2 L/day) and taking thiazide diuretics or allopurinol. In addition, an acidic diet higher in meat content promotes calcium excretion. Hypocitraturia and hyperuricosuria may both be treated with potassium citrate supplementation. However, this may alkalinize the urine, creating another risk factor for stone formation, and care must be taken to stop this drug if urine pH is greater than 6.0. In similar fashion, appropriate treatment of UTI must be initiated to avoid recurrence of struvite stones, and the urease inhibitor acetohydroxamic acid (Lithostat) 250 mg orally three to four times daily may be given as adjunctive therapy to prevent urinary alkalinization, if infection with urease-producing organisms is confirmed.

Oxalate-containing stones may be prevented with a low-oxalate diet (see Patient Education: Nephrolithiasis). Struvite stone production may be decreased by preventing UTIs through patient education and self-care as previously discussed, maintenance of antibiotic therapy, or acidifying the urine with methenamine mandelate. Uric acid stones may be decreased through dietary modification (see Patient Education: Nephrolithiasis) or medications that facilitate uric acid excretion, such as allopurinol. Recurrence of cystine stones may be reduced through maintenance doses of D-penicillamine, tiopronin, or captopril, which bind cystine via sulfhydryl moieties.

FOLLOW-UP AND REFERRAL

Most patients with renal calculi are treated and followed on an outpatient basis. The patient may need hospitalization for secondary complications that can occur, such as severe nausea and vomiting leading to dehydration, urinary obstruction, decreased renal function, severe bleeding, intractable pain, and significant infection. The patient should be referred to a urologist and/or nephrologist for stone removal under these circumstances or if stone formation is thought to be secondary to a metabolic abnormality. Recurrences are common in up to 50% of patients within 5 years.

Patient Education: Nephrolithiasis

The patient should be instructed to increase fluid intake to six to eight 8-ounce glasses of water per day unless contraindicated (e.g., by the presence of cardiac complications, such as CHF). Increasing fluids will assist in the elimination of stones. The patient should monitor intake and output and strain the urine for passed stones. Over-the-counter drugs that contain phosphorus or calcium, such as many antacids (e.g., Tums), and most vitamin supplements, especially vitamin D_3, should be avoided. The role of vitamin C supplementation is controversial. Although some research suggests that high-dose vitamin C supplementation helps acidify the urine and facilitates stone dissolution (especially the calcium phosphate type), excess vitamin C (1 g/day) is known to undergo chemical conversion to oxalate, which may promote oxaluria and calcium oxalate stone formation. In contrast, vitamin B_6 and magnesium are both known to decrease oxaluria by facilitating oxalate metabolism. Magnesium further competes with calcium, reducing calcium-containing stone formation. In turn, supplementation of vitamin B_6 and magnesium has been shown to reduce the incidence of oxalate stones, although the ideal doses have not been established.

Patients should be encouraged to increase their activity level as tolerated because inactivity contributes to stone formation secondary to calcium shifts and urinary stasis. Dietary modification is also important. In general, caffeine, beer, and wine should be avoided. A low-oxalate diet is recommended to prevent calcium oxalate stones, in which oxalate-rich foods are excluded, including beets, black tea, chocolate and cocoa, lamb, nuts, rhubarb, and spinach. A low-phosphorus diet for calcium phosphate or struvite stones should eliminate milk products and cola drinks. A low-purine diet is often effective in reducing stones formed from excess uric acid. This diet limits the intake of purine-rich foods, such as organ meats, red meats, seafood (especially sardines, anchovies, and scallops), poultry, legumes, whole grains, and alcohol (which decreases uric acid clearance).

REFERENCES

Nephrolithiasis

Al-Mamoori F, Al-Samydal A, Aburjal T. Medicinal plants for the prevention and management of nephrolithiasis: a review. *Int J Sci Technol Res.* 2019;8(11):2700–2705.

Haas C, Wardenburg M, Shah O. Innovations in the surgical management of nephrolithiasis. In: Chapple C, Steers W, Evans C, eds. *Urologic principles and practice*. Springer Specialist Surgery Series. Springer; 2020. https://doi.org/10.1007/978-3-030-28599-9_24.

Mayans L. Nephrolithiasis. *Prim Care.* 2019;46(2):203–212.

Urinary Incontinence

Amundsen CL, Komesu YM, Chermansky C, et al. Two-year outcomes of sacral neuromodulation versus onabotulinumtoxin A for refractory urgency urinary incontinence: a randomized trial. *Eur Urol.* 2018;74(1):66–73.

Balk EM, Rofeberg VN, Aam GP, et al. Pharmacological and non-pharmacologic treatments for urinary incontinence in women. *Ann Intern Med.* 2019;170(7):465–480.

Govender Y, Gabriel I, Minassian V, et al. The current evidence on the association between the urinary microbiome and urinary incontinence in women. *Front Cell Infect Microbiol.* 2019;9 (article 133):1–10.

Hagan KA, Erekson E, Austin A, et al. A prospective study of the natural history of urinary incontinence in women. *Am J Obstet Gynecol.* 2018;218(5):502e1–502e8.

Huang C-K, Lin C-C, Tong-Long Lin, A. Effectiveness of antimuscarinics and a beta-3 adrenoceptor agonist in patients with overactive bladder in a real-world setting. *Sci Rep.* 2020;10:11355.

Lightner DJ, Gornelsky A, Souter L, et al. Diagnosis and treatment of overactive bladder (nonneurogenic) in adults: AUA/SUFU Guideline amendment 2019. *J Urol.* 2019;202:558–563.

Milsom I, Gyhagen M. The prevalence of urinary incontinence. *Climacteric.* 2019;22(3):217–222.

Peyronnet B, Mironska E, Chapple C, et al. A comprehensive review of overactive bladder pathophysiology: on the way to tailored treatment. *Eur Urol.* 2019;75(6):988–1000.

Ruju R, Linder BJ. Evaluation and treatment of overactive bladder in women. *Mayo Clinic Proc.* 2019;95(2):370–377. https://doi.org/10.1016/j.mayocp.2019.11.024.

Sung VW, Borello-France D, Newman DK, et al. Effects of behavioural and pelvic floor muscle therapy combined with surgery vs surgery alone on incontinence symptoms among women with mixed urinary incontinence. *JAMA.* 2019;322(11):1066–1076.

Vasavada, SP Urinary incontinence treatment and management. Medscape 2019. https://emedicine.medscape.com/article/452289-treatment.

Urinary Tract Infections

Alidjanov JF, Naber KG, Pilatz A, et al. Evaluation of the draft guidelines proposed by EMA and FDA for the clinical diagnosis of acute uncomplicated cystitis in women. *World J Urol.* 2020;38:63–72.

Behzadi P, Behzadi E, Pawlak-Adamska EA. Urinary tract infections (UTIs) or genital tract infections (GTIs)? It's the diagnostics that count. *GMS Hyg Infect Control.* 2019;14(doc14):1–12.

Chu CM, Lowder, JL. Diagnosis and treatment of urinary tract infections across age groups. *AJOG.* 2018;219(1):40–51.

Medina, M, Castillo-Pino, E. An introduction to the epidemiology and burden of urinary tract infections. *Ther Adv Urol.* 2019;11. https://www.ncbi.nlm.nih.gov/pmc/articles/PMC6502976/.

Pujades-Rodriguez M, West RM, Wilcox MH, et al. Lower urinary tract infections: management, outcomes and risk factors for antibiotic represcription in primary care. *EclinicalMedicine.* 2019;14:23–31. https://doi.org/10.1016/j.eclinm.2019.07.012.

RESOURCES

American Urogynecologic Society (AUGS)
https://www.augs.org/

National Association for Continence
https://www.nafc.org

National Institutes of Diabetes and Digestive and Kidney Diseases (NIDDK)
https://www.niddk.nih.gov/

Office on Women's Health
https://www.womenshealth.gov/a-z-topics/urinary-incontinence

Chapter 45

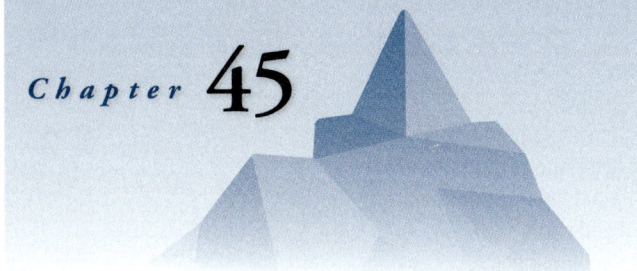

Kidney and Bladder Disorders

Debbie Conner, PhD, MSN, ANP/FNP-BC, FAANP
Debera J. Thomas, PhD, RN, ANP/FNP
Brian Oscar Porter, MD, PhD, MPH, MBA

ACUTE KIDNEY INJURY

Acute kidney injury (AKI), also known as *acute renal failure,* is the sudden and rapid deterioration of renal function resulting in the inability to maintain acid-base, fluid, and electrolyte balance and accumulation of nitrogenous wastes. AKI now has a universal definition and staging system to allow for earlier detection and management of disease. *AKI* is defined as when one of the following criteria is met: serum creatinine rises to 0.3 mg/dL (26.5 mol/L) or greater within 48 hours or 1.5-fold or greater from the reference value within 1 week, or urine output is less than 0.5 mL/kg/h for more than 6 consecutive hours. The reference serum creatinine should be the lowest creatinine value recorded within 3 months of the event.

AKI is commonly caused by intrarenal injury associated with sepsis, renal hypoperfusion, or nephrotoxins. The signs and symptoms vary with each patient and are most often attributed to uremia or its underlying cause. Persons with AKI usually do not experience the profound neurological and musculoskeletal disorders seen in patients with chronic kidney disease (CKD). Although recovery from AKI may be rapid and complete, this disorder nonetheless has a high, albeit wide-ranging, mortality rate, estimated at anywhere between 10% and 60%, depending on the patient's age, the cause of AKI, and the extent of multiorgan involvement.

EPIDEMIOLOGY AND CAUSES

It is estimated that 1% of patients admitted to hospitals have AKI at the time of admission. Between 2% and 5% of all hospitalized patients develop AKI; for patients in intensive care units, the rate is as high as 15%. Two percent to 7% of all open-heart surgery patients are estimated to develop AKI postoperatively. Fifty percent of AKI that develops in hospitalized patients is considered iatrogenic. AKI affects all ages, and both sexes are affected equally.

A major risk factor for AKI is surgery, especially for older patients or patients of any age with elevated presurgical creatinine levels. Community-based AKI occurs more frequently among vulnerable populations, such as individuals with underlying kidney disease, multiple myeloma, or diabetes mellitus. AKI is also one of the potential risks related to open-heart surgery and other cardiac procedures (e.g., cardiac catheterization) and use of IV contrast dyes. Any problem that causes decreased blood flow to the kidneys can lead to AKI: anaphylactic shock caused by drug or transfusion reactions, ingestion of nephrotoxic substances (e.g., aminoglycoside antibiotics, angiotensin-converting enzyme [ACE] inhibitors in renal artery stenosis), malignancy, sepsis, cardiac problems, aneurysms, liver cirrhosis, trauma, dehydration, or shock.

AKI is classified into three major groups based on the anatomical nature of the lesion: prerenal azotemia, intrarenal azotemia, or postrenal azotemia. Prerenal azotemia is any condition that leads to an overall decrease in renal perfusion; etiologies in this group include hypovolemia, renovascular disease, liver disease with portal hypertension, decreased cardiac output, systemic vasodilation, renal vasoconstriction, and impairment of renal autoregulation of blood flow, which is often associated with drugs such as ACE inhibitors or NSAIDs. Intrarenal azotemia includes disorders that affect the renal parenchyma itself, such as glomerulonephritis (GN), acute tubular necrosis (ATN) (often caused by ischemic insult or nephrotoxic drugs such as aminoglycosides), interstitial nephritis (often an allergic reaction to various drugs or transfusion reactions), toxic injury (from alcohol, cocaine, heavy metals, solvents and fuels, chemotherapy drugs, bowel preparations containing phosphate, and contrast dyes), and tubular obstruction. Immune-mediated phenomena may lead to AKI after acute bacterial infection, for example, thrombotic thrombocytopenic purpura (TTP) or hemolytic uremic syndrome (HUS) after *Escherichia coli* gastroenteritis. Postrenal azotemia is any etiology that might lead to an obstruction of urine flow from the kidneys, including ureteral, bladder neck, or urethral obstruction. Major causes include benign prostatic hyperplasia/hypertrophy (BPH), prostate or bladder cancer, and metastatic disease affecting the urinary tract. An important consideration in the male patient with preexisting BPH is the use of over-the-counter sympathomimetic decongestants and other cold remedies with alpha-agonist properties, which may lead to acute worsening of prostatic hypertrophy with resultant anuria.

Box 45.1 presents the major causes of AKI. Prerenal, intrarenal, and postrenal mechanisms of AKI are not mutually exclusive, and many patients present with a combination of these pathologies. Complications commonly seen as a result of AKI include intravascular volume overload; metabolic acidosis; anemia; hyperkalemia; uremic syndrome, which is characterized by nausea, vomiting, anorexia, pericarditis; and central and peripheral nervous

> **Box 45.1 Major Causes of Acute Kidney Injury**
>
> **Prerenal Acute Kidney Injury**
> - Fluid and electrolyte depletion
> - Hemorrhage
> - Septicemia
> - Cardiac failure
> - Liver failure
> - Heat stroke
> - Burns
>
> **Intrarenal Acute Kidney Injury**
> - Ischemia
> - Toxins
> - Radiocontrast agents
> - Hemoglobinuria
> - Myoglobinuria
>
> - Acute glomerulonephritis
> - Arterial or venous obstruction
> - Tubulointerstitial nephritis
> - Pyelonephritis
> - Papillary necrosis
> - Precipitation from hypercalcemia
> - Urates
> - Myeloma protein
>
> **Postrenal Acute Kidney Injury**
> - Prostatism (hypertrophy or malignancy)
> - Bladder tumor
> - Pelvic tumor
> - Retroperitoneal tumor
> - Renal calculi

system abnormalities, including altered mental status, seizures, or coma.

PATHOPHYSIOLOGY

Prerenal Azotemia

Prerenal azotemia is caused by decreased blood flow to the kidneys, usually associated with poor systemic perfusion. Etiologies include hypovolemia, altered peripheral vascular resistance, diminished cardiac output, congestive heart failure, renal artery disorders such as vasculitis, and, to a lesser extent, thromboembolic disease. Chronic liver diseases, such as cirrhosis and hepatorenal syndrome, are also recognized causes of prerenal azotemia.

The kidney's compensatory responses to hypoperfusion are autoregulation and activation of the renin-angiotensin-aldosterone axis via the release of renin. In response to renal tissue damage, these mechanisms attempt to shunt blood to undamaged nephrons in a process called *adaptive hyperfiltration*. Autoregulation depends on the body's ability to control afferent arteriole dilation and efferent arteriole constriction to maintain normal glomerular filtration rate (GFR) and creatinine clearance.

The release of renin activates the conversion of proenzyme angiotensinogen to biologically inactive angiotensin I. In turn, ACE converts angiotensin I into angiotensin II, one of the most potent vasoconstricting agents in the body. Its production results in peripheral vasoconstriction and increased sodium reabsorption via increased aldosterone production. Antidiuretic hormone (ADH) is released in response to the increased plasma sodium concentration. ADH further enhances vasoconstriction and increases water reabsorption, thereby decreasing urinary output and increasing blood volume.

These mechanisms attempt to maintain systemic and renal perfusion. However, if the adaptive mechanisms of the kidneys fail, AKI develops because of hypoperfusion. As a result, glomerular filtration and the excretion of urea decrease, along with increased sodium and water reabsorption, resulting in an overall increase in blood urea nitrogen (BUN). Thus, although adaptive hyperfiltration is initially beneficial, allowing normal serum creatinine to be maintained in the face of mild renal insufficiency, prolonged activation of this compensatory mechanism leads to progressive renal failure.

Intrarenal (Parenchymal) Azotemia

Intrarenal azotemia results from injury to renal tissue; it is usually associated with intrarenal ischemia, toxins, or both. Accounting for up to 50% of all cases, intrinsic dysfunction is considered after prerenal and postrenal causes have been excluded. The sites of injury are the glomeruli, vasculature, interstitium, and tubules.

ATN is the most common cause of intrarenal azotemia and AKI in general. In ischemic ATN, the ischemic event is prolonged hypoperfusion and ischemia of the kidneys, with a sustained mean arterial pressure (MAP) in adults of less than 75 mm Hg. When renal autoregulation fails, the sympathetic nervous system (SNS) responds by activating the renin-angiotensin system, as the kidney attempts to redirect blood flow to the remaining healthy nephrons (adaptive hyperfiltration, as explained in the preceding section). Again, however, this initial compensatory mechanism can eventually lead to progressive renal failure, because the SNS response and possible endothelin production may lead to severe afferent renal arteriole constriction. As a result, overall glomerular hydrostatic pressure, glomerular blood flow, and GFR are decreased as this process progresses.

The duration of the ischemic episode determines the amount and degree of renal cellular damage, which may continue after MAP and renal reperfusion are restored. Studies in animal models have demonstrated that a number of immunological mechanisms contribute to renal tubular injury. These include early complement activation, intracellular adhesion molecule-1 expression (which may promote neutrophilic damage to the endothelium), T cell–mediated cytotoxicity, macrophage activation, and proinflammatory cytokine expression (e.g., tumor necrosis factor-alpha, interleukin [IL]-6, IL-7, chemokines).

Renal blood flow can be reduced by 50% after an ischemic episode; this is termed the *no-reflow phenomenon*. The kidneys are unable to synthesize vasodilating prostaglandins, which usually exacerbates the ischemic injury. Blood flow is redistributed from the cortex to the medulla as a result of SNS stimulation and angiotensin II production. This further decreases glomerular capillary flow and worsens tubular ischemia because these structures are located primarily in the cortex.

With renal ischemia, the availability of nutrients and oxygen for basic cellular metabolism and the tubular transport system is diminished. There is a significant decrease in the production of adenosine triphosphate (ATP) by the mitochondria, and, with insufficient oxygen and ATP, metabolism shifts from aerobic to anaerobic. This shift corresponds with extracellular and intracellular acidosis that alters kidney function. Ischemia also causes a decrease in renal cellular potassium, magnesium, and inorganic phosphate and an increase in intracellular sodium, chloride, calcium, and reactive oxygen species. Sodium and calcium (Ca) exchange is abnormal because of low ATP, altered Ca-ATPase activity, and increased intracellular sodium. This results in an increase in intracellular calcium, which seems to increase cellular injury. The formation of free radical reactive oxygen species further exacerbates cellular damage and apoptosis (programmed cell death) during reperfusion after a prolonged renal ischemic event, an event termed *reperfusion injury*.

The glomerular basement membrane (GBM) is altered by tubular cellular edema and becomes necrotic because of prolonged tubular ischemia. Tubular obstruction occurs from sloughed necrotic cells and renal cast formation, which seems to be facilitated by a translocation of basement membrane cellular adhesion proteins called integrins to the luminal membrane. Tubular hydrostatic pressure and Bowman's capsule hydrostatic pressure (which opposes glomerular hydrostatic pressure) increase as a result of tubular obstruction, and this decreases GFR. Injury to the basement membrane increases tubular permeability, allowing tubular filtrate to leak back into the interstitium and peritubular capillaries, further decreasing tubular filtration.

Ischemic ATN is usually associated with oliguria (urine production of less than 500 mL/day in adults) because of extensive nephronal injury. Other laboratory indications of ATN include decreased urea excretion and elevated BUN, decreased creatinine clearance and elevated serum creatinine, abnormal renal handling of sodium, and an inability to concentrate urine. Urinary osmolality may approximate plasma osmolality of 300 to 350 mOsm/L, a condition called *isosthenuria*.

Toxic ATN involves exposure to toxic by-products of microorganisms or to nephrotoxic agents. Renal toxic drugs often cause allergic interstitial nephritis, characterized by eosinophilic damage. Toxic ATN begins with an event that causes injury to tubular cells. Subsequent pathophysiology is similar to that of ischemic ATN because there is tubular cell necrosis, cast formation, tubular obstruction, and altered GFR. Unlike in ischemic ATN, however, the basement membrane is usually intact and the injured necrotic areas are more localized. Other differences include improved urine production, in that nonoliguria occurs more often with toxic ATN than with ischemic ATN, as well as the extent of injury with toxic ATN, which may be less than with ischemic ATN. The healing process, therefore, can be more rapid in patients with toxic ATN.

There are several reasons why the kidney is susceptible to toxic damage. Blood continuously circulates through the kidney, repeatedly exposing the tissues to all substances carried by the blood. Also, the kidney is the major excretory organ for toxic substances, and, as these substances await transport within renal cells, they disrupt cellular function. If liver disease is present, substances that are usually detoxified by the liver can overload the kidney. The kidney also transforms many substances into metabolites that can be toxic to the kidney, and the countercurrent mechanism concentrates metabolic and urinary waste by-products and other substances that can be toxic to the kidney in increased concentrations.

Postrenal Azotemia

Bilateral (ureteral) or distal (bladder outlet or urethral) postrenal obstruction impedes urine flow and results in oliguria or frank anuria. Urine congestion increases pressure retrograde through the urinary collecting system and the nephrons, slowing the tubular fluid flow rate and GFR. Increased reabsorption of sodium, water, and urea results in decreased urine sodium, increased urine osmolality, and increased BUN. The decreased GFR results in decreased creatinine clearance and, therefore, in an increased serum creatinine level. If postrenal obstruction is prolonged, the collecting system dilates and compresses parenchymal tissue. Nephrons are injured, which results in dysfunction of the urinary concentrating and diluting mechanisms, increasing urine osmolality and urinary sodium level to approximate those of plasma. In contrast, if postrenal obstruction is temporary, there is little dilation of the collecting system or loss of renal tissue.

CLINICAL PRESENTATION

Subjective

Symptoms of AKI are not usually present until the GFR falls to approximately 10% to 15% of normal. The most common symptoms, which are secondary to the accumulation of toxic metabolites such as urea, are fatigue, malaise, nausea, vomiting, pruritus, and mental status changes. Of note, the development of uremic syndrome symptoms bears no direct correlation to the increases in BUN or serum creatinine, despite the critical role of hemodialysis in clearing the body of both identified and unidentified uremic toxins. Oliguria (approximately 400 mL or less of urine production per day) or even anuria may also be a presenting symptom of AKI but is not present in every case, as urine output depends largely on the stage of AKI and the precipitating cause. In some cases, fluid overload may be present, resulting in dyspnea and orthopnea.

A detailed history can give clues to the etiology of AKI. The patient should be questioned about any history of illicit or prescription drug use, herbal preparations, surgery, trauma, or infection as possible sources of renal insult. However, the actual diagnosis of AKI is often made by routine laboratory assessment.

There are multiple signs and symptoms of AKI in its four identified stages: initiating, oliguric, diuretic, and recovery. The initiating stage begins when the kidney is injured. This stage is variable in length from minutes to several days (e.g., renal damage caused by contrast dye may occur within 2 minutes). Decreased urine volume and other signs and symptoms of renal impairment may then become evident. These may include anorexia, lethargy, nausea, headache, muscle cramps, and fatigue. If AKI is recognized at this stage, its cause should be determined and the plan of treatment should be established in consultation with a nephrologist.

The oliguric stage usually lasts from 5 to 15 days but can persist for weeks, depending on the nature of renal damage. Renal repair begins as tubular cells regenerate. The destroyed basement membrane is replaced with fibrous scar tissue, and nephrons become obstructed with a buildup of inflammatory products. Decreases in glomerular filtration, tubular transport of substances, urine formation, and renal clearance occur. When AKI persists for weeks or longer, renal endocrine functions, such as the secretion of erythropoietin, are altered. The longer this stage persists, the poorer the prognosis.

The next phase is the diuretic stage, defined as beginning when urine output increases to greater than 400 mL per day and BUN begins to fall. This stage is considered to last until the BUN level stabilizes or is in the normal range and may take from 1 to 2 weeks.

The fourth and final stage of AKI, referred to as the recovery phase, extends from the time BUN stabilizes and urine output returns to normal to the day the patient returns to normal activity. This recovery process may take up to 10 months or more, and some patients never recover, but instead progress to CKD.

Objective

The objective manifestations of AKI depend on the stage of the disorder and may be extremely variable; however, these signs can provide an assessment of the degree of renal failure and clues as to the underlying etiology. Orthostatic vital signs, skin turgor, and distention of jugular veins should be assessed to obtain information about the patient's fluid balance. Signs of fluid depletion can point to a prerenal etiology, whereas signs of fluid overload suggest a greater degree of renal impairment. Physical assessment findings may vary depending on the etiology of AKI and should be correlated with the patient's history and laboratory findings, such as fluid volume depletion or oliguria. Findings on physical examination consistent with prerenal etiology may include dry mucous membranes, poor skin turgor, reduced jugular venous pressure, hypotension, oliguria, or weight loss, as well as uremic signs such as seizures, myoclonus, pericardial friction rub, and peripheral neuropathies.

Severe proteinuria from renal losses may lead to generalized edema (anasarca) due to the lack of intravascular oncotic pressure from hypoalbuminemia. In renal artery stenosis, an abdominal bruit auscultated in the flank or midabdominal region over the affected renal artery may be detected on physical examination, and an elevated blood renin level from the ipsilateral renal vein may be noted on specialty laboratory testing. In cases of polycystic kidney disease or hydronephrosis, the kidneys may be palpable. A pelvic or renal examination may reveal causes of outflow obstruction such as an enlarged prostate or pelvic mass.

DIAGNOSTIC REASONING

Diagnostic Tests

Elevated BUN and serum creatinine levels assist in establishing the diagnosis of AKI. GFR is difficult to measure directly and is most commonly estimated using a simplified formula for creatinine clearance (see the Diagnostic Tests section under Chronic Kidney Disease for a complete discussion). However, because acute trends are most important in the diagnosis and follow-up of AKI, direct serum creatinine levels are often used as an estimate of renal function. It is important to note that these absolute values are heavily influenced by a patient's muscle mass, age, and sex, as well as the presence of any underlying renal disease. Thus, serum creatinine levels may overestimate or underestimate renal function in certain populations (e.g., older or obese patients).

Serum electrolyte levels (sodium, potassium, chloride, bicarbonate, calcium, phosphate) should be monitored for potentially life-threatening abnormalities that may develop secondary to impaired renal function. The presence of red blood cells (RBCs), either intact or as cellular casts, may suggest a vascular or glomerular lesion, whereas white blood cells (WBCs) and WBC casts are seen in cases associated with infection and interstitial nephritis. Eosinophiluria, in particular, is characteristic of allergic interstitial nephritis due to renal toxic drugs. "Muddy-brown" granular casts and epithelial cell casts are strongly associated with ATN but are not considered specific. Moreover, their absence does not exclude intrinsic renal disease.

Serum laboratory tests, urinalysis, and microscopic examination of the urine provide important data that can help differentiate prerenal azotemia from ATN. Prerenal problems are indicated by high urinary specific gravity and osmolality, low urinary sodium caused by decreased renal blood flow, avid tubular sodium reabsorption, and decreased GFR. The kidneys interpret these changes as a state of dehydration and respond via the actions of aldosterone and ADH to maximize sodium and water reabsorption from the distal tubule and collecting duct into the peritubular capillary plasma. This results in a small amount of very concentrated urine with a high specific gravity and high osmolality. Despite maximal sodium reabsorption, the urine is concentrated because of urea or other solutes. Urinary and serum creatinine levels often show wide variation in prerenal etiologies of AKI, with a slower rate of rise than in ATN and periodic decreases in serum creatinine. Thus, significant laboratory findings in prerenal AKI include increased urine osmolality and specific gravity, decreased urine sodium and urea concentration, increased BUN, increased BUN to plasma creatinine ratio (especially a ratio greater than 20:1, because plasma creatinine is usually normal), a normal urinary sediment (seen in most cases), and oliguria. In turn, prolonged azotemia caused by a prerenal condition often leads to intrarenal failure.

Urinary sodium tends to be less than 20 mEq/L in prerenal disease, whereas in ATN, the kidneys "leak" or "spill" sodium due to failure to reabsorb this electrolyte. This results in urinary sodium values typically greater than 40 mEq/L. However, variations in water reabsorption also affect urinary sodium concentration. Thus, the fractional excretion of sodium (FENa) is easily calculated as the urinary clearance of sodium divided by the GFR, using the following simplified formula:

$$FENa = 100\% \times \frac{Sodium\ (urinary) \times creatinine\ (plasma)}{Sodium\ (plasma) \times creatinine\ (urinary)}$$

The FENa is helpful in distinguishing prerenal azotemia from ATN. The FENa is generally less than 1% in prerenal disease related to hypoperfusion because the kidneys try to preserve intravascular volume by maximally conserving sodium. A FENa of greater than 2% usually reflects ATN, as the kidney loses its ability to resorb sodium effectively, but values between 1% and 2% are considered inconclusive. Of note, FENa has little or no predictive value in the presence of diuretic therapy, because natriuresis is a mechanistic outcome of both thiazide and loop diuretics. Thus, increased urinary sodium may not exclude a prerenal etiology or implicate ATN. In addition, FENa is less helpful when ATN is superimposed on a chronic intravascularly depleted state, such as in hypoalbuminemic cirrhotic liver disease.

ATN is also characterized by the inability to concentrate urine; in turn, urine osmolality is typically lower than 450 mOsm/L, and in many cases, it can be lower than 350 mOsm/L. In contrast, the urine is highly concentrated in prerenal azotemia due to the secretion of ADH and intensified water reabsorption, producing urine osmolalities of greater than 500 mOsm/L. As renal tubular function worsens under prerenal conditions, however, this distinction tends to blur, and concentrating ability may wane as ischemic damage sets in.

If a glomerular process is suspected, detection of antinuclear antibodies, antineutrophil cytoplasmic antibodies (ANCA, as seen in Wegener's granulomatosis), antiglomerular basement membrane (anti-GBM) antibodies, or cryoglobulins and decreased complement levels can help the clinician determine whether immune-mediated disease is present.

A 24-hour urine collection is the most accurate way to measure proteinuria. A protein loss of more than 3.0 to 3.5 g every 24 hours indicates a glomerular lesion, whereas lesser amounts in the urine are more indicative of an interstitial renal disorder. Given the unwieldy nature of this test, however, and its practical challenges in the outpatient (home-based) setting, spot-urine checks for proteinuria are often used as a surrogate.

Renal ultrasound is commonly utilized to assess kidney size and rule out hydronephrosis. Ultrasound is used instead of intravenous pyelogram (IVP) to avoid the risk of radiocontrast nephrotoxicity. If hydronephrosis indicative of renal obstruction is detected, the patient should be referred to a urologist. Computed tomography (CT) scan, a retrograde pyelogram, and cystoscopy may all be useful in determining the exact location of the obstruction. A nuclear renal scan may be helpful in detecting unilateral renal artery stenosis but is less sensitive in detecting bilateral renal artery disease. Renal artery stenosis is better diagnosed via CT scan or magnetic resonance imaging/magnetic resonance angiography (MRI/MRA), although direct renal angiography is still considered the gold standard (albeit invasive) for diagnosis.

If a noninvasive work-up proves inconclusive, renal biopsy may be indicated in some cases. Most notably, biopsy is performed in cases of isolated glomerular hematuria with proteinuria to confirm acute nephritic syndrome, better characterize nephrotic syndrome or suspected vasculitis, and aid in the diagnosis of acute or subacute renal failure of unknown etiology. Percutaneous versus open biopsy techniques are chosen based on the propensity for bleeding diatheses and the difficulty in reaching the affected kidney as determined by renal imaging.

Differential Diagnosis

The main diagnostic challenge in AKI is to determine the underlying cause. This is often complicated by fluid and electrolyte alterations. Assessment of the patient involves a thorough history, physical examination, and appropriate laboratory studies. When determining whether prerenal azotemia exists, the patient's history can reveal potential episodes of poor renal and/or systemic perfusion. This may include surgery, high fever, alterations in diet or fluid status (such as a patient receiving nothing by mouth and undergoing bowel preparation repeatedly for diagnostic tests), a low-sodium diet with fluid restriction, use of diuretics and antihypertensives, anaphylactic drug or transfusion reactions, penetrating or nonpenetrating abdominal trauma, hemorrhage, burns, shock, excessive sweating and dehydration, peritonitis, malignancy, sepsis, neurogenic shock, drug overdose, acute myocardial infarction, congestive heart failure, cardiac tamponade, cardiac dysrhythmia, cardiac arrest survival, renal artery emboli, thrombus, arterial stenosis, aneurysm, renal artery occlusion, trauma, and liver cirrhosis.

Nephrotoxic agents that can cause damage to the kidneys include certain drugs (e.g., antineoplastics, anesthetics, antimicrobials, and anti-inflammatory agents), imaging contrast media, biological substances (e.g., metabolic toxins, tumor products, and heme pigments from hemoglobin or myoglobin), environmental agents (e.g., pesticides and organic solvents), heavy metals (e.g., lead, mercury, and gold), and certain plant and animal substances (e.g., toxic mushrooms and snake venoms).

Other conditions that may injure renal (parenchymal) tissue include inflammatory processes related to bacterial or viral infections; preeclampsia; immune processes such as autoimmunity, hypersensitivity, and tissue or organ transplant rejection; trauma or radiation to the kidney; and urinary tract obstruction (e.g., caused by neoplasm, stones, or scar tissue). Intravascular hemolysis related to blood transfusion reactions or microangiopathic hemolytic anemia as seen in TTP and HUS also causes damage to renal tissue. In addition, vascular and systemic disorders can cause intrarenal injury, such as renal vein thrombosis, nephrotic syndrome, Wilson's disease, malaria, multiple myeloma (due to direct proteinaceous deposition of immunoglobulin light chains into the renal parenchyma), sickle cell disease, malignant hypertension, diabetes mellitus, and systemic lupus erythematosus. Pregnancy-related disorders, such as septic abortion, preeclampsia, abruptio placentae, intrauterine fetal death, and idiopathic postpartum renal failure, can also cause damage to the kidneys.

Data that identify events or agents that may have caused renal injury, especially those related to ischemia or exposure to toxins, should be collected during the history. These may include exposure to nephrotoxins, radiological tests that require administration of contrast dye, hypersensitivity reactions to a drug or dye, recent infections, trauma, sepsis, use of antineoplastic medications with or without radiation therapy, multiple myeloma, pregnancy, or a history of cardiac, renal, or liver disease.

There is no one specific finding that pinpoints the cause of intrarenal azotemia during a physical assessment. Findings on examination must be correlated with history and laboratory findings. Differentiating prerenal problems from actual ATN is a challenge. Because prerenal problems often correspond with the onset phase of ATN and because this is a reversible phase, it is essential for diagnosis and aggressive management to begin early.

ATN is characterized by altered renal ability to conserve sodium. Clinically, ATN is seen as a urinary sodium level greater than 20 mEq/L. However, depending on the state of hydration, the serum sodium levels vary in ATN. Oliguria is usually associated with postischemic ATN, whereas either oliguria or nonoliguria may be associated with nephrotoxic ATN. Creatinine clearance is severely decreased, and plasma creatinine rises approximately 0.5 to 1 mg/dL per day in ATN. The BUN to serum creatinine ratio does not typically exceed 10:1 to 15:1 in ATN.

Response to therapy is another factor that distinguishes ATN from prerenal etiologies. The kidneys typically respond very quickly to therapy aimed at correcting an underlying prerenal problem in which no actual damage to nephrons has occurred; however, in ATN, the response to treatment of the underlying cause may be minimal depending on the degree of nephron damage. Additional therapy for ATN should be aimed at correcting alterations related to the inability of the kidneys to maintain functionality.

Postrenal azotemia results from interference with the flow of urine from the kidneys and is associated with obstruction or disruption of the urinary tract. Ureteral, bladder, bladder neck, or urethral obstruction may be the result of calculi, urinary tract or bladder neoplasms, sloughed renal papillary tissue, strictures, trauma, blood clots, congenital or developmental abnormalities, foreign objects, surgical ligation, prostatic hypertrophy, retroperitoneal fibrosis, abdominal and pelvic neoplasms, pregnancy, a neurogenic bladder, bladder rupture, or the use of drugs such as antihistamines and tricyclic antidepressants with significant anticholinergic effects or ganglionic blocking agents. The history should focus on collecting data that reflect obstruction or disruption of the urinary tract. Significant findings may include a change in urine volume, a history of prostatic disease, abdominal neoplasms, urinary tract stones, nephralgia, pregnancy, recent abdominal surgery, or paralysis (e.g., quadriplegia).

Postrenal azotemia physical assessment findings vary with etiology and need to be correlated with laboratory and history findings (e.g., nephralgia associated with passing urinary tract stones or rapidly developing hydronephrosis; bladder distention associated with prostate, bladder neck, or urethral disorders). Laboratory findings include variations in urine volume such as oliguria, polyuria, or abrupt anuria, urine osmolality (may be increased or similar to plasma osmolality), urine specific gravity, or a decrease in urinary concentration of sodium or urea, as well as a BUN to serum creatinine ratio that is normal to slightly increased. Microscopy of the urinary sediment is usually normal unless urinary tract infection (UTI) is present.

MANAGEMENT

Approximately 50% of patients with AKI are nonoliguric and have less severe signs and symptoms than oliguric patients. Frequent causes of death in the setting of severe AKI and renal failure include cardiac arrest resulting from hyperkalemia, gastrointestinal bleeding, and severe infection; thus, patients should be monitored very closely and treated appropriately on a day-to-day basis. Effective management is intrinsically tied to determining the underlying cause of the renal failure, as the etiology of AKI will drive long-term management strategies.

Prerenal azotemia secondary to absolute hypovolemia necessitates the restoration of intravascular volume. Replacement of fluids depends on the mechanism of loss. Gastrointestinal fluid loss is generally hypotonic and should be replaced accordingly; fluid loss as a result of hemorrhage usually indicates the need for administration of both saline and transfused packed RBCs. In addition, electrolyte imbalances must be managed. Hyperkalemia in AKI can be life-threatening; emergent management is required in patients with extreme elevation of potassium levels (more than 6.5 mmol/L) or in any patient with electrocardiogram (ECG) abnormalities.

With regard to parenchymal kidney damage, inflammatory diseases such as GN or Wegener's granulomatosis require immunosuppressive treatment with prednisone and cyclophosphamide to prevent irreversible renal damage. In cases of ATN caused by nephrotoxic agents, the removal of the offending agent will allow renal function to return gradually to normal. In the meantime, supportive measures may be provided to hasten the removal of toxins, such as peritoneal dialysis or hemodialysis.

Several indications exist for temporary dialysis, including fluid overload unresponsive to diuretic therapy, hyperkalemia with symptoms or ECG changes, uremic encephalopathy, severe metabolic acidosis, cardiorespiratory failure, pleuritis, pericarditis, and other forms of inflammatory serositis. Forms of dialysis include traditional intermittent hemodialysis via large-bore venous and arterial catheters; peritoneal dialysis that operates by osmotic diffusion via an indwelling dialysate within the peritoneal cavity; and continuous renal replacement therapy, which is a prolonged form of low-flow arteriovenous or venovenous hemofiltration that is indicated for hemodynamically unstable patients.

Postrenal azotemia involves identification of the level of renal or urinary tract obstruction, followed by treatment to relieve the obstruction. If the obstruction is higher in the urinary tract, such as at the vesicoureteral junction or in the ureter or renal pelvis, percutaneous nephrotomy or ureteral stent placement by a urologist is necessary. For urethral obstruction, bladder catheterization or placement of a suprapubic tube may be sufficient to relieve the obstruction. Intermittent bladder catheterization four to five times a day poses less risk of UTI than an indwelling urinary catheter and is the preferred method for urinary outflow in cases of bladder atony and neuromuscular compromise such as with spinal cord injury. However, the presence of bladder outlet or urethral obstruction, which is more likely to cause AKI, may necessitate placement of a long-term catheterization device until surgical intervention is possible.

FOLLOW-UP AND REFERRAL

After hospitalization, follow-up is necessary in about 1 week as an outpatient, and then at 1 month, 3 months, 6 months, and annually thereafter, provided there are no further complications. Serum chemistries (basic metabolic profile) and a complete blood count (CBC) should be checked at each follow-up visit. The patient should be assessed for signs and symptoms of fluid overload signifying worsening AKI, such as crackles on lung auscultation, elevated blood pressure (BP), shortness of breath, weight gain, jugular vein distention, or edema. Dietary education by the health-care provider or referral to a nutritional counselor is warranted to decrease the risk of dietary triggers that may worsen renal function and electrolyte abnormalities (e.g., a renal diet low in sodium, phosphorus, and protein).

Patient Education: Acute Kidney Injury

During the recovery stage, there is no special form of treatment other than general healthy living, with attentiveness to fluid status and BP control. However, a lack of knowledge about the causative factors of AKI is a major problem with regard to acute episodes of renal failure and may contribute to repeat episodes. Thus, patients benefit from continual education throughout their clinical pathway of treatment and recovery from AKI. Dietary education on avoiding sodium, phosphorus, and protein may be particularly important during the ongoing recovery phase, whereas follow-up care, emotional support, and prevention of additional episodes are key teaching points.

CHRONIC KIDNEY DISEASE

CKD is characterized by a progressive loss of functional nephrons, eventually leading to end-stage renal disease (ESRD). As the functional reserve of the kidneys is lost, signs and symptoms of renal failure appear. These signs may arise as sequelae of AKI, but most often CKD develops as a complication of chronic systemic disease, such as diabetes or hypertension. The time frame for the development of CKD typically ranges from months to years, whereas AKI usually occurs over days to weeks (see previous section).

EPIDEMIOLOGY AND CAUSES

According to the U.S. Centers for Disease Control and Prevention, CKD affects approximately 15% of the U.S. population or 37 million people. Nine of 10 affected adults may be unaware that they have some degree of CKD. Roughly 48% of people with severely reduced renal function are unaware that they have CKD. There are approximately 747,000 people in the United States with ESRD (a 2.6% increase since 2016), of whom 500,000 are on chronic dialysis. Men are 1.3 to 1.4 times more likely than women to have ESRD. The peak age of onset of ESRD is between 65 and 75 years, with older adults representing 38% of new patients. Older patients have both the highest incidence rates of ESRD and the highest morbidity and mortality rates.

Compared with the general population, African Americans are 3.9 times more likely to have ESRD and 6.7 times more likely to have hypertensive ESRD. It is estimated that HIV-associated nephropathy may soon be the third leading cause of ESRD (after diabetes mellitus and hypertension) in African Americans aged 20 to 64 years.

Renal disease can result from many age-related illnesses. The major underlying conditions leading to ESRD are diabetes mellitus and primary hypertension seen in approximately 70% of cases, with GN, cystic disease, and other urological diseases accounting for another 15% of cases. Renal artery stenosis and chronic ischemic renovascular disease may cause up to 20% of CKD cases in persons older than 50 years of age. Analgesic overuse (e.g., NSAIDs), cigarette smoking, collagen vascular diseases, AIDS-related nephropathies, cirrhosis, and multiple myeloma are examples of other risk factors for the development of CKD. Several hereditary renal diseases (e.g., polycystic kidney disease; Lowe syndrome, which also causes congenital cataracts; Alport syndrome, which also causes congenital deafness) can lead to CKD in children and some adults.

Overall, hypertension is present in at least 85% of patients with CKD. Hypertensive and diabetes-related CKD are forms of microvascular end-organ damage caused by these cardiovascular risk factors. Thus, these patients must also be evaluated for other forms of end-organ damage related to atherosclerotic disease, as a significant correlation exists between microvascular CKD, peripheral vascular disease, coronary artery disease, and cerebrovascular disease.

PATHOPHYSIOLOGY

The pathophysiology of renal failure varies depending on the underlying cause, although the end result is the same—a nonfunctional kidney. The most common causes of CKD are diabetic nephropathy, hypertensive nephropathy, and GN.

Diabetic Nephropathy

Diabetic nephropathy is the most common cause of ESRD and involves several mechanisms, including hyperglycemia, hormonal imbalances, and renal hemodynamic changes. Hyperglycemia leads to alterations in tubuloglomerular feedback, abnormalities in polyol (e.g., sorbitol) metabolism, and the formation of advanced glycosylation end products (AGEs) in tissues. Increases in circulating AGE peptides parallel the severity of renal dysfunction in diabetic nephropathy. Ultimately, defects in glomerular cellular metabolism lead to hemodynamic changes in the kidney.

Renal hemodynamic changes implicated in diabetes mellitus and ESRD include both glomerular hyperfiltration and glomerular hypertension. Hormonal imbalances associated with diabetes mellitus and ESRD include decreased insulin secretion, increased growth hormone and glucagon production (both of which have been shown to produce glomerular hyperfiltration in laboratory studies), and altered concentrations or responsiveness to vasoactive hormones (e.g., angiotensin II, catecholamines, and prostaglandins), which can also result in hyperfiltration. Regardless of the inciting event, factors such as hyperglycemia-induced increases in extracellular fluid volume, renal hypertrophy, and/or altered glycoregulatory or vasoregulatory hormonal actions contribute to increased pressure and flow across the glomerular membrane, resulting in glomerular hypertension.

These factors, along with associated renal vasodilation and hyperfiltration, increase transglomerular protein filtration, which leads to proteinuria and mesangial deposition of circulating proteins. As a result, mesangial expansion and glomerulosclerosis cause the destruction of nephrons, as the glomerulus eventually becomes a fibrinous scar that can no longer function. In addition, a positive feedback stimulus for compensatory hyperfiltration is initiated, with further increases in GFR and progressive renal injury. Ultimately, it is glomerular hypertension that mediates progressive nephronal destruction. Based on this glomerular hypertension–hyperfiltration hypothesis, therapies directed at lowering glomerular hypertension would be expected to protect the kidney from further progression of nephropathy.

Hypertensive Nephropathy

After diabetes mellitus, hypertensive nephropathy is the second most common cause of renal failure. The kidney is one of the major organs injured by hypertension, which results in nephrosclerosis. Benign nephrosclerosis is associated with chronic mild or moderate hypertension in which renal insufficiency develops slowly. The renal arterial vessels become thickened while their lumens narrow, resulting in decreased renal blood flow and autoregulation. Renal tubular changes correlate with the degree of reduction in renal blood flow. Signs and symptoms vary with the severity of renal injury and may include proteinuria, nocturia, urinary casts, and azotemia. Patients with benign nephrosclerosis are susceptible to AKI when a situation occurs that decreases blood flow to the kidney. Treatment is therefore focused on the control of hypertension.

Malignant nephrosclerosis is associated with marked hypertension, headache, congestive heart failure, and blurred vision. Unlike the slow progression of benign nephrosclerosis, renal failure develops rapidly in malignant nephrosclerosis. Renal arterioles and glomerular capillaries become thickened and necrotic, and renal tubules atrophy. Signs include hematuria with RBC casts, proteinuria, and azotemia. Treatment involves the immediate reduction of BP, which is necessary to prevent permanent loss of renal function and damage to other organs.

Renal artery stenosis occurs when the renal artery and its branches become thickened, stiff, and narrow due to atheromatous plaques (two-thirds of cases) or fibromuscular dysplasia (one-third of cases). The incidence of fibromuscular dysplasia is higher in women than in men, especially from 20 to 40 years of age. As the body perceives the decreased blood flow (i.e., hypoperfusion) via the stenotic renal arteries as hypovolemia, the renin-angiotensin-aldosterone axis is activated and mild to severe hypertension results from the resulting retention of sodium and water. This condition becomes critical if both renal arteries are affected or if blood flow is compromised in patients with only a single kidney, either due to a congenital defect or after live organ donation of the other kidney.

Glomerulonephritis

GN is the third most common cause of renal failure and comprises 25% to 30% of all cases of ESRD. GN is an inflammatory process that primarily affects the glomerular capillaries. It is also a major cause of ESRD. Approximately 25% of GN cases result from nonimmune mechanisms, whereas 60% to 75% stem from autoimmune mechanisms. Glomerular injury can be divided into two major categories based on pathology: *nephritis*, which is characterized by glomerular inflammation and/or necrosis, and *nephrosis*, which is characterized by abnormal permeability of the glomerular membrane. Both allow macromolecules such as albumin to pass into the urine, although to a greater degree in nephrosis. Of note, these two forms of glomerular injury are not mutually exclusive, and a single etiology can produce both forms of kidney injury.

The immunological injury that characterizes GN may occur by several different mechanisms. Anti-GBM disease is the result of direct glomerular injury occurring as a result of inflammation triggered by antibodies directed against components of the GBM. Linear deposits of immunoglobulin are seen via immunofluorescence (IF) microscopy of renal tissue and may reveal granular immunoglobulin deposits. Part of the inflammatory response that occurs is secondary to the glomerular deposition of immune complexes composed of antibodies bound to a variety of circulating antigens. The presence of these immune complexes is referred to as *immune complex disease*. Finally, pauci-immune ANCA-positive disease is characterized by the presence of serum antibodies against neutrophilic cytoplasm that are associated with the multisystem disease. Minimal or no immunoglobulin is seen by IF, however, hence the name "pauci-immune." Nonetheless, the glomerular injury is still believed to be immune mediated in nature.

The hallmark of nephrosis is increased permeability of the glomerular capillary wall to macromolecules, including serum proteins. Inflammatory changes are generally not seen but may be present. In classic forms of glomerulonephrosis, nephrotic syndrome develops, and various degrees of proteinuria may be present. In addition to hypertension, other characteristic findings include hypercholesterolemia with lipiduria and central edema from hypoalbuminemia due to albuminuria. In more than two-thirds of glomerulonephrosis cases in adults, the cause is idiopathic; in the remainder, nephrosis is secondary to systemic disease such as diabetes mellitus, lupus nephritis, or amyloidosis.

GN may also result from postinfectious inflammatory changes affecting the kidney, despite a distant location of the primary infection weeks earlier. A well-described presentation of this is poststreptococcal GN, which typically presents in a male patient aged 2 to 14 years, with puffiness of the eyelids and facial edema, and an inadequately treated sore throat 1 to 2 weeks prior (i.e., streptococcal pharyngitis or strep throat). A similar presentation may also be seen in middle-aged men, most often with diabetes mellitus and a recent history of methicillin-resistant *Staphylococcus aureus* infection.

CLINICAL PRESENTATION

Subjective

Because of the significant functional reserve of the kidneys, symptoms do not generally appear until renal function (as measured by GFR) declines to 10% to 15% of normal. At about 30% to 40% of normal GFR, biochemical evidence of renal failure may be apparent, but patients typically remain asymptomatic. Early prominent symptoms in renal failure include anorexia, lassitude, fatigability, and weakness.

The inability of the kidneys to perform their normal excretory, metabolic, and endocrine functions results in uremia, a complex syndrome that includes a variety of physiological and clinical abnormalities. Dermatological abnormalities may result in patient complaints of pruritus and dry skin, and gastrointestinal alterations may manifest as complaints of anorexia, nausea, vomiting, and hiccoughing. Neurological complaints may include emotional lability or depression, insomnia, fatigue (especially on exertion), confusion, headache, seizures, and coma. There may be an odor of urine to the breath and perspiration, complaints of shortness of breath, a metallic taste in the mouth, impotence, nocturia, and muscle cramps. The patient may present with foot drop, infection, bleeding, or gout. Often the patient is being treated for a major systemic disease such as diabetes mellitus. The primary care provider should be alert to the potential for the onset of CKD in patients who present with these signs and symptoms and have a major systemic disease.

Objective

The patient may appear pale, with a characteristic uremic frost appearance to the skin, or, conversely, hyperpigmentation may be apparent. There may be bruising and asterixis (i.e., hand-flapping on hyperextension of the wrists with complete forward extension of the upper extremities). Peripheral neuropathy and altered mental status may be present, along with peripheral edema and ascites from severe proteinuria and the resulting hypoalbuminemia, as well as auscultatory crackles in the lungs and a pericardial rub. There may be an elevated BP and a hard, rapid pulse. Some abnormalities are the result of the accumulation of toxic metabolites, whereas others are caused by an underproduction (e.g., vitamin D and erythropoietin) or overproduction (e.g., renin) of biochemically active substances produced by the kidney. Specific findings in renal artery stenosis include a bruit auscultated in the flank or midabdominal region over the affected renal artery and an elevated blood renin level from the ipsilateral renal vein.

DIAGNOSTIC REASONING

Diagnostic Tests

If a patient has a condition known to predispose them to the development of CKD, especially if that patient is in a high-risk population, biochemical monitoring (BUN, creatinine, and creatinine clearance) should be done to detect renal failure before it becomes clinically apparent. Serum creatinine can track the progression of CKD. However, the GFR, which is normally well above 90 mL/min (with values as high as 130 mL/min in healthy adults), can decrease to 40% to 50% of normal with only small changes noted in serum creatinine levels. Accurate measurement of the GFR is based on experimental calculations of renal inulin clearance. Inulin is a polymer of fructose secreted from the blood exclusively via renal glomeruli with no tubular reabsorption. Measurement of inulin clearance, however, requires a complex assay too cumbersome for regular clinical use and tends to be reserved for research purposes. GFR can be estimated in milliliters per minute using the Cockcroft-Gault formula for creatinine clearance (see Box 45.2).

It is important to realize that trends in GFR (as estimated by creatinine clearance or serum creatinine levels) are far more important in assessing renal function and stability of CKD than are the absolute values of these indices. A meta-analysis of 13 studies found that a lower GFR and a higher albuminuria level independently predict mortality and ESRD in patients with CKD. This is especially true of direct serum creatinine measurements, whose interpretation must take into account a patient's muscle mass, age, and gender. Thus, creatinine clearance is a far more informative diagnostic tool as a measure of renal function.

Although no universally agreed-on definition of CKD exists, GFR and proteinuria are often used to stratify CKD patients by disease severity. The third National Health and Nutrition Examination Survey (NHANES) defined the stages of CKD as follows:

- **Stage 1** disease is characterized by persistent albuminuria with a normal GFR greater than 90 mL/min per 1.73 m^2 of body surface area (BSA).
- **Stage 2** disease is characterized by albuminuria with a GFR between 60 and 89 mL/min per 1.73 m^2 of BSA.
- **Stage 3** disease is defined as a GFR between 30 and 59 mL/min per 1.73 m^2 of BSA.

Box 45.2 Glomerular Filtration Rate Using the Cockcroft-Gault Formula for Creatinine Clearance

- ([140 minus age] × lean body weight in kilograms) divided by (72 × stable serum creatinine in mg/dL)
- This value is multiplied by 0.85 (i.e., reduced by 15%) for women.
- Creatinine clearance values are normalized per 1.73 m^2 of body surface area (BSA) to adjust for very heavy (obese) or very thin patients by multiplying the estimated creatinine clearance value by 1.73 m^2 and then dividing the product by the total body surface area (BSA) of the patient in m^2.*

---

*Most adults have a BSA that falls within 1.6 to 1.9 m^2 (hence, the value of 1.73 m^2 representing the average adult BSA). This correction factor is sometimes not applied in clinical practice, with creatinine clearance reported in units of mL/min, rather than mL/min per 1.73 m^2 of BSA.

- **Stage 4** disease is defined as a GFR between 15 and 29 mL/min/1.73 m² of BSA.
- **Stage 5** disease is ESRD, defined as a GFR less than 15 mL/min/1.73 m² of BSA.

Routine monitoring of the patient's CBC can detect anemia secondary to erythropoietin deficiency. Monitoring of urinalysis can detect increasing proteinuria. When renal function declines further, closer monitoring of routine laboratory tests to detect dangerous electrolyte imbalances (e.g., hyperkalemia) and acidosis is required.

Numerous laboratory alterations occur in patients who develop ESRD. A CBC will usually reveal a normochromic and normocytic anemia, decreased hematocrit, increased bleeding time, capillary fragility, thrombocytopenia, and decreased immune responsiveness. Blood chemistries typically reveal some of the following abnormalities: decreased active vitamin D (calcitriol or 1,25-dihydroxycholecalciferol), elevated ammonia, BUN, serum creatinine, uric acid, sulfate, potassium, phosphate, parathyroid hormone, and glucose levels, along with insulin resistance and hyperlipidemia (particularly hypertriglyceridemia). Urinalysis may reveal proteinuria (the greater the proteinuria, the more rapid the progression of CKD) and coarse granular casts. Ketosis may artificially raise creatinine levels, and certain drugs (e.g., cimetidine, trimethoprim, cefazolin) may also alter diagnostic test results.

Twenty-four–hour urine studies (e.g., urinary protein level, creatinine clearance) may be collected, although samples are often difficult to obtain in ambulatory patients and have been largely replaced by spot urine checks. Complement levels, an antinuclear antibody test, and serum and urine protein electrophoresis may all provide data as to the underlying pathophysiology of CKD.

Renal ultrasound performed at baseline when impaired renal function is first noted is indicated in all cases of CKD. Among other pathologies, sonography may reveal decreased kidney size (less than 11 cm), polycystic kidney disease, or an obstructed ureter or bladder outlet with hydroureter and/or hydronephrosis. Renal CT scan/CT angiography or MRI/MRA may detect and localize harder to visualize structural abnormalities, renal parenchymal disease, or renal artery stenosis. Unilaterally decreased kidney size on renal imaging is highly suggestive of vascular occlusive disease and may be helpful as a screening method. Duplex Doppler ultrasonography to assess renal vascular flow has a high sensitivity and specificity for renal artery stenosis if conducted by an experienced ultrasonographer, although renal angiography remains the diagnostic gold standard for this condition. Renal biopsy is not utilized for CKD as much as for AKI, unless noninvasive diagnostic testing is unable to suggest a likely etiology.

Differential Diagnosis

The differential diagnosis of CKD is aimed at identifying the underlying etiology of renal failure, as discussed earlier. Although the terms *chronic kidney disease* and *chronic renal insufficiency* (CRI) are often used interchangeably, some authorities reserve the use of CKD to imply a dialysis-dependent state, whereas CRI denotes an earlier form of the condition not yet requiring dialysis or kidney transplantation, but that may clearly progress to CKD. The signs and symptoms and diagnostic test results commonly seen in the three stages of CKD (decreased renal reserve, renal insufficiency, and ESRD) are presented in Table 45.1.

MANAGEMENT

General principles of CKD management include (1) the determination and control of the underlying causative etiology, (2) monitoring changes in renal function, (3) conservative treatment of the physiological effects of CKD, and (4) instituting more aggressive treatment (dialysis and/or renal transplantation) as appropriate in later stages of treatment-refractory disease.

Management of Hypertension

Glucose levels and hypertension must be strictly controlled in diabetic patients, with a target hemoglobin A1c of less than 7%. For any patient with proteinuria of more than 1 g per day, the target BP is 125/75 mm Hg; for a patient with proteinuria of less than 1 g per day, the goal is a BP of no more than 130/80 mm Hg. Given the importance of maintaining renal perfusion, systolic BPs lower than 110 mm Hg should be avoided. ACE inhibitors or angiotensin II receptor blockers (ARBs) should be used for BP control in patients with diabetes mellitus, given their renoprotective effects. If monotherapy with one of these agents is insufficient to control BP, a diuretic should be added, followed by a calcium channel blocker (diltiazem or verapamil) or a beta blocker, as needed. If combination therapy using agents from these additional classes proves ineffective, an ACE inhibitor or ARB should be added (whichever class was not used initially).

For patients with renal artery stenosis, pharmacological BP management is equally as important, as definitive treatment is angioplasty or surgical repair to stent or reconstruct the stenotic vessels, along with medical therapy consisting of antihypertensives and diuretics. ACE inhibitors and ARBs are usually avoided in patients with bilateral renal artery stenosis, because their vasodilatory effect on the efferent renal arterioles (which are otherwise compensatorily constricted) effectively decreases GFR due to reduced afferent blood flow from the stenotic renal arteries to the afferent arterioles of the glomeruli. In turn, this may precipitate potentially devastating AKI or CKD.

Percutaneous angioplasty or surgical revascularization with arterial stenting should thus be considered for patients with severe hypertension refractory to

TABLE 45.1 Differentiating the Stages of Chronic Kidney Disease

Stage	Glomerular Filtration Rate	Signs and Symptoms	Management
Stage 1 Decreased renal reserve	Normal kidney function: Greater than 90 mL/min per 1.73 m^2 of BSA	• Asymptomatic • Hypertension (mild)	• Control hypertension • Observe
Stage 2 Kidney damage	Mildly reduced kidney function: 60–89 mL/min per 1.73 m^2 of BSA	• Hypertension (mild) • Increased PTH • Early bone disease • Increased BUN and serum creatinine	• Control hypertension • Observe
Stage 3 Renal insufficiency Stage 3a Stage 3b	Moderately reduced kidney function: 45–59 mL/min per 1.73 m^2 of BSA 30–44 mL/min per 1.73 m^2 of BSA	• Hypertension • Anemia due to decreased erythropoietin • Increased BUN and serum creatinine • Risk of cardiovascular events	• Refer to specialist • Evaluate serum creatinine, potassium, hemoglobin, and urinary protein every 6 months • Control blood pressure
Stage 4 Severe renal insufficiency	Severely reduced kidney function: 15–29 mL/min per 1.73 m^2 of BSA	• Moderate hypertension • Anemia • Hyperphosphatemia • Increased triglycerides • Metabolic acidosis • Hyperkalemia • Water/salt retention • Increased BUN and serum creatinine	• Refer to specialist • Control hypertension • Oral phosphate binders • Cholesterol-lowering therapy • Administration of erythropoietin (epoetin-alfa) for anemia
Stage 5 End-stage kidney disease or kidney failure	Minimal to no kidney function: Less than 15 mL/min per 1.73 m^2 of BSA or on dialysis	• Severe hypertension • Anemia • Hyperphosphatemia • Uremia	• Refer to specialist • Same management as for stage 4 • Dialysis • Renal transplant

Abbreviations: BSA, body surface area; BUN, blood urea nitrogen; PTH, parathyroid hormone.
Sources: Adapted from the UK Kidney Association, https://ukkidney.org/health-professionals/information-resources/uk-eckd-guide/ckd-stages, https://www.kidney.org/PROFESSIONALS/kdoqi/guidelines_ckd/toc.htm.

pharmacotherapy, recurrent episodes of flash pulmonary edema due to CKD-related fluid overload, or progressive renal insufficiency that fails to improve, despite effective BP control. However, individuals with particularly severe CKD (serum creatinine greater than 4 mg/dL) or chronically atrophied kidneys (less than 7 cm in length) are unlikely to respond to such interventions. Thus, revascularization is more likely to be effective in patients whose renal function rapidly declines, particularly after beginning ACE inhibitor or ARB therapy.

Management of Fluids and Electrolytes

Dietary therapy is a cornerstone of conservative management of CKD. Restriction of fluid intake (to maintain a serum sodium concentration of 135 to 145 mEq/L) and sodium intake (especially if volume expanded) may decrease secondary hypertension or congestive heart failure, although volume depletion must be avoided, given the potential for acute worsening due to renal hypoperfusion. A restricted goal of 2 g per day of sodium intake and 2 L per day of fluid intake may be needed if the patient is volume overloaded. Restricted protein intake is recommended (0.6 to 0.8 g/kg/day), although adequate caloric intake (40 to 50 cal/kg/day) should be maintained, because malnutrition is a common complication of CKD. Consultation by a skilled nutritionist is recommended at the time of diagnosis and periodically as the disease progresses and the patient's nutritional needs change. Foods rich in essential amino acids are the most effectively utilized source of nitrogen. Restriction of dietary phosphate (800 mg/day) and potassium may be necessary because of their reduced excretion and the potential for hyperphosphatemia and hyperkalemia. Strict dietary restrictions may be unnecessary in older patients because they often have low protein and sodium intake, but treatment regimens must be individualized. Low-dose sodium polystyrene sulfonate (Kayexalate) 5 mg by mouth (PO) one to three times daily with meals may be used as a potassium-binder for hyperkalemia. Oral phosphate binders such as calcium carbonate (2.5 to 20 g/day), calcium acetate (PhosLo; 1334 mg three times daily), or sevelamer (Renagel; 800 mg three times daily) are typically taken with meals when GFR falls below 30 mL/min. Sevelamer is used when CKD is complicated by iatrogenic hypercalcemia. Aluminum- and magnesium-containing salts should be avoided because of cumulative toxicity.

Given the kidneys' reduced ability to synthesize activated vitamin D in CKD and the propensity for subsequent hypocalcemia and renal osteodystrophy, oral 1,25-dihydroxyvitamin D (calcitriol 0.25 mg daily) and calcium carbonate (600 mg two times daily) supplements should be given, along with a renal-specific multivitamin (e.g., Nephrocaps). Importantly, however, this chronic treatment may result in hypercalcemia and worsen coronary artery calcification. Thus, close monitoring of serum calcium levels is critical.

If diuretic therapy is instituted for edema, dehydration must be avoided. Thiazide diuretics may be tried first, but they are far less effective at a GFR of less than 20 to 30 mL/min per 1.73 m^2 of BSA (approximated by serum creatinine levels of greater than 2.5 mg/dL); however, they provide an additive effect when used with a loop diuretic initiated for refractory edema. Potassium-sparing diuretics should be avoided because of the kidneys' reduced ability to excrete potassium.

Treatment of Anemia

Anemia should be treated with erythropoietin (80 to 120 units/kg subcutaneously per week), taking care not to induce polycythemia (goal hemoglobin = 11 to 11.5 g/dL) with its attendant risk of stroke. Dosing usually begins around 10,000 units per week but may be adjusted upward in frequency or dose as needed. Darbepoetin alfa is an alternative erythropoietic agent with a longer half-life, allowing for less frequent dosing (0.45 μg/kg subcutaneously per week). Patients with iron-deficiency anemia should take ferrous sulfate 325 mg by mouth one to three times daily with meals, with lower doses being less likely to induce constipation in older patients. For patients on hemodialysis, the IV route has been shown to work better than oral administration. Gentle transfusion with packed RBCs may be required in cases of extreme or acutely worsened anemia, but care must be taken not to induce high-output heart failure or fluid overload, as the heart typically adapts cardiac output to the chronic anemia of CKD.

Bleeding diatheses due to uremic platelet dysfunction are not uncommon in both AKI and CKD. Active bleeding in these patients should be treated with desmopressin, cryoprecipitate, estrogen, or dialysis to remove uremic toxins believed to be qualitatively inhibiting platelet function.

Management of Hypercholesterolemia

Because CKD is considered a coronary artery disease risk equivalent, hypercholesterolemia in these patients should be treated with a statin drug, with a low-density lipoprotein goal of less than 100 mg/dL. Recent evidence suggests this goal should be even lower to minimize the rate of disease progression due to atherosclerotic renovascular disease. Dietary modification to restrict cholesterol and saturated fats is also critical to adequately address hyperlipidemia, especially hypertriglyceridemia.

Ongoing Management of Symptoms

Both hypovolemia (renal hypoperfusion) and renal toxic drugs may exacerbate CKD and must always be considered when AKI or CKD is observed. A judicious trial of isotonic fluid repletion may be appropriate in patients displaying the physical stigmata of dehydration, and careful attention must be paid to the dosing of all chronic and newly started medications. All nephrotoxic agents (e.g., NSAIDs, radiocontrast dye, aminoglycoside antibiotics) should be avoided.

Other measures to relieve symptoms of pruritus (a common finding with CKD) include skin moisturizers for dry skin, menthol or phenol lotion, a trial of capsaicin cream, or the antihistamine diphenhydramine (Benadryl). Vitamin E may also be helpful in treating muscle cramps.

Management of Progressive CKD

As CKD progresses, the patient will have increased difficulties with fluid balance and may experience episodes of hyperkalemia, hypertension, acidosis, and severe uremia with altered mental status and qualitative platelet dysfunction with a tendency for bleeding diatheses. Metabolic acidosis should be treated initially with sodium bicarbonate 600 mg twice daily to titrate serum bicarbonate to the 16 to 20 mEq/L range. However, patients must display adequate respiratory function to avoid the accumulation of metabolized carbon dioxide and respiratory acidosis. The potassium and calcium levels should be monitored during treatment of acidosis, because both might fall. Hospitalization may be required for the control of fluid overload, hypertension, hyperkalemia, or infection.

A GFR of less than 10 mL/min, a serum creatinine level approaching 12 mg/dL, or a BUN of greater than 100 mg/dL all typically require more aggressive therapies, such as peritoneal dialysis or hemodialysis, to avoid life-threatening sequelae. Continuous venovenous or arteriovenous hemofiltration may be used in hemodynamically unstable patients, as an alternative to classic hemodialysis. Such therapies must be done only under the supervision of a nephrologist, however. Life-threatening indications for dialysis include pericarditis, diuretic-refractory fluid overload (e.g., pulmonary edema), medication-resistant or rapidly worsening hypertension, uremic syndrome with an attendant bleeding diathesis or neurological symptomatology, and persistent nausea and vomiting. In addition, protein malnutrition in the face of a creatinine clearance of less than 20 mL/min is considered an indication for early dialysis.

FOLLOW-UP AND REFERRAL

The course of CKD is typically punctuated by periods of rapid deterioration, often precipitated by dehydration or infection. The rate of progression to kidney failure will depend in part on the underlying renal disease. It is usually more rapid in patients with diabetic nephropathy or severe hypertension and slower in patients with polycystic kidney disease.

Patients with CKD should be referred to a nephrologist, given the progressive nature of the disease. In patients with advanced renal failure (creatinine levels greater than 10 mg/dL), mean survival time without intervention (e.g., dialysis or transplantation) is only 100 to 150 days. Vascular access for hemodialysis (arteriovenous grafts or fistulae) must be obtained 2 to 3 months in advance to permit maturation of the fistulae and allow for potential revisions. Decisions regarding dialysis and transplantation require a team approach with the primary care practitioner, nephrologist, patient, and family. Comprehensive evaluation of the patient's medical, psychological, and social contexts is necessary for successful planning and follow-up.

In general, the multiplicity of metabolic demands on the patient with CKD requires careful and close follow-up and constant adjustments in treatment. The most important cornerstone of care is the monitoring and treatment of all underlying disorders known to lead to CRF. Depending on the course of disease, at some point during follow-up, the patient may need to be hospitalized to control fluid overload, hypertension, hyperkalemia, or infection. Successful therapy depends in good part on the maintenance of a strong relationship between the healthcare provider and the patient and family.

Nowhere is the Circle of Caring approach more important than in a chronic, progressive disorder such as CKD. Interventions should be geared toward maximizing the patient's independence and reducing social isolation. Given the fact that CKD may be rapidly progressive depending on its etiology and reach its end stage in relatively young patients, clinicians and their patients may be faced with emotionally challenging situations related to the death and dying process, which necessitate a range of caring approaches.

Patient Education: Chronic Kidney Disease

For care to be effective, the patient and family must have a thorough understanding of the chronic and progressive nature of CKD, the importance of treating all underlying systemic diseases such as diabetes mellitus and hypertension, and the specifics of the treatment plan. Avoidance of infection is critical, as is maintaining a healthy, renally adjusted diet as recommended. Patients should know when and how to report bleeding, fever, decreases in urine output, or episodes of nausea and vomiting.

RENAL TUMORS

Renal tumors (neoplasms) are characterized by abnormal tissue formations on or around the kidney that may cause or contribute to renal disease. They may be primary or secondary (resulting from malignant spread), although the latter are rarely clinically relevant and are typically found during postmortem examination. Renal adenomas (benign tumors) and adenocarcinomas (malignant tumors) are rare; these tumors usually create complications requiring surgical removal.

EPIDEMIOLOGY AND CAUSES

In the United States, there are approximately 74,000 new renal tumor cases and almost 15,000 deaths each year. The incidence is higher in men (although the difference in incidence has been decreasing over time). Kidney cancer is the sixth most common cancer in men and the tenth most common in women. Age of onset is typically between 55 and 70 years and rarely occurs in people younger than 45 years. The average age of diagnosis is 64 years.

Renal cell carcinomas originating in the renal cortex are the most common (85%) type of malignant renal tumors. These tumors occur most often in the parenchyma of the kidney, with ureteral and urethral tumors occurring only rarely. Histologically, renal cell carcinomas are classified as clear cell (75% to 85%), chromophilic or papillary (15%), or chromophobic (5%). Rare forms include oncocytic and collecting duct tumors. Transitional cell carcinomas are the next most common type of renal carcinoma, comprising 5% to 8% of all tumors; these typically affect the bladder and are discussed extensively in the next section (see Bladder Tumors).

Renal cell carcinomas are curable in more than 90% of patients if they are superficial and/or localized in the renal pelvis or ureter. Tumors that are invasive, however, have only a 10% to 15% chance of being cured. In children, nephroblastoma (Wilms' tumor) is common, comprising 5% of primary tumors, whereas sickle cell disease has a known, albeit rare, association with carcinoma of the renal medulla.

Risk factors for renal cell carcinoma include obesity; exposure to asbestos, cadmium, and/or gasoline; the use of phenacetin (of which acetaminophen is a major metabolite), NSAIDs, aspirin-containing analgesics; and chronic hemodialysis for acquired polycystic kidney disease. In addition to the risk factors of hypertension and obesity, cigarette smoking has a 25% to 30% correlation with the development of renal cell carcinoma.

PATHOPHYSIOLOGY

The urinary system is lined with transitional cell epithelium, from which tumors may arise. These tumors often are asymptomatic and grow undetected until complications from the tumor present clinically. The tumors are usually encapsulated and located near the cortex unilaterally. Renal neoplasms may be diagnosed as benign or malignant, and they may be identified as either primary (originating in the kidney) or secondary (originating or spread from another source). Primary malignancies usually spread through the lymph nodes and blood vessels to the lungs, liver, and bone. Metastatic disease that spreads to the kidney, usually from the lung as the primary source, is more common than primary renal neoplasms. Metastatic lesions to the ureter typically originate via hematogenous spread from the breast or colorectal primary lesions. Direct extension into the ureter may also occur from cervical or colonic neoplasms, as well as pelvic retroperitoneal lymphoma. Benign renal neoplasms are rare but should be removed because of complications that may develop such as pain, bleeding, and urinary obstruction.

Carcinogen exposure has been associated with specific gene mutations that appear to underlie the development of various forms of hereditary renal cell carcinoma. However, definitive causal relationships between various mutational hot spots and renal cancer have not been proven. Clear cell carcinomas consistently display mutations spanning the 3p14 to 3p26 chromosomal region. In contrast, chromophilic carcinomas lack these mutations but have been associated with various trisomies, including those of chromosomes 12, 16, and 20. Chromophobic carcinomas, which arise from the intercalated cells of the collecting duct system, typically display hypodiploidy, with a wide variety of whole chromosomal deletions. The much less common oncocytic carcinomas have been associated with deletions in chromosome 11q13, but as with collecting duct tumors, no consistent chromosomal abnormalities have been identified.

CLINICAL PRESENTATION

Subjective

Symptoms vary depending on the size of the tumor. Early signs of tumor growth are silent. Approximately 60% of the time, asymptomatic patients present with gross hematuria as the only outward complaint. However, 30% of patients report dull, achy flank pain or an abdominal mass. In 10% to 15% of patients, the classic triad of flank pain, hematuria, and an abdominal mass is observed, which is often a sign of advanced disease.

Objective

Examination of the patient may reveal other signs that may present alone or in combination with hematuria. General signs of advanced disease include weight loss and fatigue. More specific signs of renal tumors include intermittent fever not associated with infection and palpable abdominal mass (which may be associated with the complaint of nephralgia, as noted previously). The spread of primary renal tumors typically involves the lungs, lymph nodes, liver, bones, and contralateral kidney, with metastasis of renal cancer indicating a poor prognosis.

DIAGNOSTIC REASONING

Diagnostic Tests

The diagnosis of a renal mass is initially confirmed by IVP with nephrotomography; however, it is often impossible to determine whether the mass is solid or cystic with these diagnostic imaging tests. Generally speaking, a cancerous tumor splays, distorts, or occludes the visualization of the collecting system and prevents normal filling and draining of the renal system. Although hematuria is common, urine cytology is not consistently reliable for diagnosing these tumors. Ureteroscopy or ultrasonography with IVP can be used to differentiate potentially neoplastic tissue from renal cyst formation by direct or indirect visualization of the entire renal system. Once tissue biopsy samples are obtained, flow cytometric analysis is used to determine the ploidy (DNA content) of the tumor, and histological analysis determines morphology and tumor grade (degree of cellular differentiation). Urine cytology samples often provide inadequate tissue for such analyses, however, and the mass must be biopsied directly. Figure 45.1 presents a flowchart for the evaluation and treatment of a renal mass.

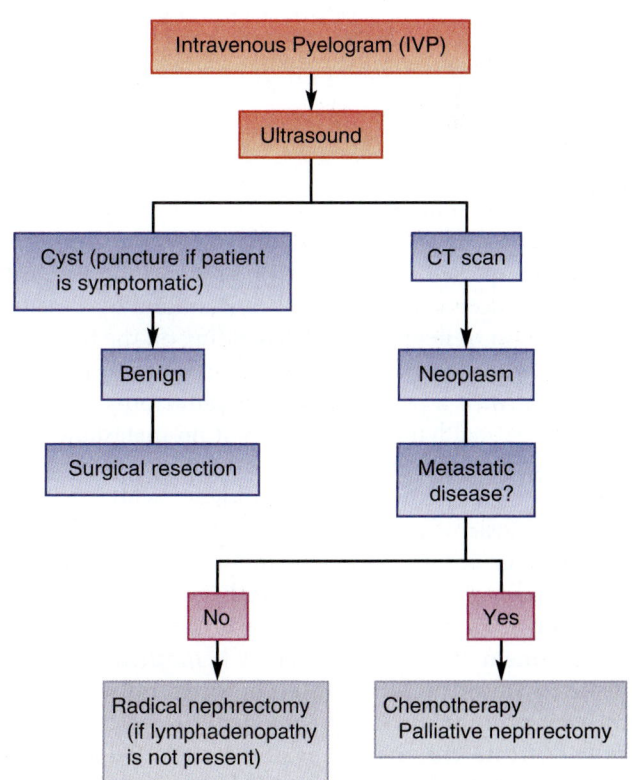

Figure 45.1 Flowchart for the treatment and evaluation of renal tumors.

MRI and CT scan are useful in the preoperative work-up and staging of metastatic lesions. It is necessary to stage the advancement of the tumor and potential for survival to initiate appropriate treatment. Staging of the neoplasm is confirmed through surgical intervention. The tumor-node-metastasis (TNM) staging of renal cell carcinoma is as follows:

- Stage I is defined as a tumor confined within the kidney capsule; it is treated by nephrectomy. The 5-year survival rate is 60% to 75%.
- Stage II is defined as the invasion of the renal capsule that is confined within the Gerota's fascia encapsulating the kidney and adrenal gland; it is treated by nephrectomy. The 5-year survival rate is 47% to 65%.
- Stage III is defined as involvement of the regional lymph nodes ipsilaterally, the renal vein, or the vena cava. The 5-year survival rate is 5% to 15%.
- Stage IV is defined as distant metastasis, with a 5-year survival rate of less than 5%.

Approximately 30% of patients with renal tumors have metastatic disease at diagnosis. The most common sites of metastasis are the lung (50% to 60%), bone (30% to 40%), regional lymph nodes (15% to 30%), brain (10%), and adjacent organs.

Differential Diagnosis

A renal cyst is differentiated from a renal tumor by biopsy. Renal calculi and renal infarction must also be ruled out, as well as (rarely) renal tuberculosis. In addition, polycystic kidney disease and hydronephrosis must be considered and may be ruled out via biopsy or imaging such as renal CT scan.

MANAGEMENT

As with any cancer, treatment of renal cancer requires immediate specialist referral to a urologist or surgical oncologist, often with additional consultation by a medical oncologist or nephrologist, depending on the patient's renal function. Treatment for a renal neoplasm is primarily surgical with a partial or total nephrectomy, with or without regional lymphadenectomy if no metastatic disease is present. Less radical surgical interventions have been suggested by a minority of urologists, who stress the poor prognosis of advanced renal tumors, regardless of surgical intervention, as well as the increased morbidity and mortality associated with radical surgery.

No universal standards have been accepted for adjunctive treatment after nephrectomy. Chemotherapy is not effective with this type of cancer; however, immunotherapy using lymphokine-activated killer cells, with or without IL-2 treatment, may be helpful for selected patients. Radiation therapy is controversial but may be used in combination with nephrectomy or for palliative effects in patients with bone metastases.

FOLLOW-UP AND REFERRAL

For follow-up of patients with a total nephrectomy, a CT scan of the abdomen and renal fossa should be done in 3 to 6 months. The patient may then be followed with renal ultrasound every 6 months for 3 years and annually thereafter, unless symptoms occur. Chest x-rays are done quarterly for a year to monitor for pulmonary metastasis.

At the time of diagnosis of the neoplasm, the patient should be referred to a urologist for a surgical evaluation and to an oncologist for potential cancer treatment. The patient should be seen by a primary care practitioner for problems not related to the cancer and to assist the patient with counseling and support regarding grief, death and dying issues, body image changes, and alterations in quality of life.

Patient Education: Renal Tumors

Patients typically require preparation for surgical intervention. Postoperatively, the focus is on pain management and promoting comfort through the use of moist heat, nonopioid analgesics or opioids for severe pain, and positioning the patient on their side with pillows and back support. Additional interventions include preventing pneumonia and atelectasis by encouraging the patient to do coughing and deep-breathing exercises, incisional care, and monitoring of bowel and bladder function.

BLADDER TUMORS

Bladder tumors are abnormal tissue masses that occur in the bladder wall lining, which is composed of transitional cell epithelium (urothelium). These tumors commonly recur despite aggressive treatment.

EPIDEMIOLOGY AND CAUSES

Bladder tumors are the most common cancer of the urinary system; they represented approximately 3% of all new cancer cases in 2018 and result in 3% of cancer deaths per year. Bladder cancer is the sixth most common neoplasm in the United States, representing almost 5% of all cancer diagnoses; it occurs in men four times more often than in women, with 90% of new diagnoses in adults 55 years of age and older, with the average age being 73 years. It is also more common among non-Hispanic white men than in other ethnic or racial groups.

There is a significant correlation between bladder tumors and risk factors including cigarette smoking, the presence of renal tumors, exposure to aromatic amine dyes known as *arylamines* (e.g., beta-naphthylamines, xenylamine, 4-nitrobiphenyl, and benzidine) and arsenic, chronic use of phenacetin-containing analgesics, use of saccharin (in rodent studies), chronic lower UTI, schistosomiasis, and recurrent nephrolithiasis. Other predisposing factors for bladder tumors include previous radiation treatment for cervical, ovarian, or prostate cancer, and prior cyclophosphamide chemotherapy.

PATHOPHYSIOLOGY

Bladder tumors are primarily transitional cell carcinomas that arise from the transitional cell uroepithelium (urothelium). Transitional cell carcinomas, in general, are the second most common form of renal carcinomas, arising from the urothelia that lines the mucosal surfaces of the collecting tubules, renal calyces, renal pelvis, ureters, bladder, and urethra. Specifically, transitional cell carcinomas account for 90% of all tumors of renal pelvic or ureteral origin. Bladder tumors may also be squamous cell carcinomas or adenocarcinomas. Transitional cell carcinomas of the bladder have the most favorable prognosis.

Bladder tumors are described as papillary (90%) or nonpapillary (10%). Papillary bladder lesions form as a small protuberance attached to a stalk. Nonpapillary lesions are more invasive and have a poorer prognosis. Primary bladder cancer tends to metastasize to the lymph nodes, liver, bones, and lungs. However, bladder cancer may also develop secondary to local extension and/or metastatic disease from adjacent organs, such as the cervix in women and the prostate in men.

Genetic analyses of transitional cell carcinomas demonstrate a loss of heterozygosity at any one of multiple chromosomal locations, including 9q (most common), 5p, 8p, 10q, 11p, and 17p—all of which may represent sites of tumor suppressor genes. Genetic predisposition also appears to be based on allelic variants of the p450 cytochrome enzyme complex. For instance, smokers with bladder cancer express p450 enzyme variants that lead to increased activation of arylamine metabolites, a required step in their contribution to bladder carcinogenesis. Along this same line, allelic variants exist for the *N*-acetyltransferase gene *NAT2,* which (along with *NAT1*) serve as the primary pathway for the metabolism and detoxification of arylamines via *N*-acetylation. Individuals with *NAT2* variants conferring a "slow-acetylation" phenotype are up to 17 times more likely to develop bladder cancer than those with a "fast-acetylation" phenotype. A similar phenomenon exists regarding the glutathione-*S*-transferase Mu 1 gene (*GSTM1*), which contributes to detoxification and secretion of carcinogenic compounds via their conjugation to glutathione. In the United States, nearly 50% of white men display deletions in both alleles of this gene, effectively eliminating any enzymatic activity from the *GSTM1* gene product.

Transitional cell carcinomas often present multifocally along the urinary tract, spreading via intraluminal seeding or intraepithelial migration via a process known as "field cancerization." Such multifocal tumors display monoclonality along their entire distribution. Squamous cell carcinoma, a less common form of bladder cancer that accounts for 7% of renal pelvis tumors, is typically associated with an underlying inflammatory process, such as chronic UTI and renal calculi. These tumors tend to be deeply invasive and have a poor prognosis.

CLINICAL PRESENTATION

Subjective

Patients with a bladder tumor are frequently asymptomatic until they have an episode of hematuria that may vary in severity from microscopic to gross amounts and may be intermittent or continuous. Other presenting symptoms may include dysuria, urinary frequency, chills, low-grade fever, weight loss, and urinary urgency. Patients with advanced disease may complain of pelvic pain and other symptoms associated with urethral obstruction.

Objective

The physical examination may be positive for a palpable mass and/or metastatic manifestations. The urinalysis shows trace to gross hematuria, possibly with elevations in protein level, RBCs, or WBCs. A CBC may indicate anemia.

DIAGNOSTIC REASONING

Diagnostic Tests

The diagnosis of a bladder tumor is confirmed by visualization of the lesion through transurethral resection of the bladder tumor. Urine cytology that is positive for transitional cell cancer can confirm the diagnosis; however, negative results do not rule out the possibility of bladder cancer. Cystoscopic evaluation can be used to confirm the suspected diagnosis, determine the location of the tumor, and aid in staging of the tumor. The cystoscopy should include a bladder washing for cytology and a mucosal biopsy. An abdominal or pelvic CT scan, with or without IVP, may be useful for determining the metastatic progress of the disease.

According to the TNM system of the American Joint Committee on Cancer, the stages of transitional cell carcinoma are as follows:

- Stage 0 tumors are confined to the mucosa.
- Stage I tumors invade the lamina propria.
- Stage II tumors invade the muscular layer.
- Stage III tumors extend to the peripelvic fat or renal parenchyma.
- Stage IV indicates metastatic disease.

Urine tumor marker tests can detect recurrent bladder tumors. The *N*-benzoyl-L-tyrosyl-*p*-aminobenzoic acid and nucleoside 5'-monophosphate tests are more sensitive in detecting recurrent tumors than urine cytology.

Differential Diagnosis

Because this disease most often presents as painless hematuria, differential diagnoses to be ruled out include renal stones, infection, trauma, other tumors such as renal cell carcinoma, arteriovenous malformations, and glomerulonephropathies. The differential diagnosis for bladder irritability includes inflammation, the passage of renal stones, neurological dysfunction, and foreign bodies in the bladder or urinary system. Visualization and biopsy may be necessary for a definitive diagnosis.

MANAGEMENT

Treatment depends on the type, size, and degree of invasion of the bladder tumor, which is classified as superficial, invasive, or metastatic. Superficial tumors (stages 0 and I) involve the bladder mucosa and submucosa; they are treated by endoscopic resection or laser resection. These tumors tend to recur, and the patient must be reexamined every 6 months. Invasive tumors (stages II and III) involve the muscle and/or perivesical fat around the bladder. These tumors are treated with radical cystectomy or with radiation and chemotherapy. Neoadjuvant chemotherapy can improve the survival rate in cases of advanced urothelial cancer. Metastatic tumors (stage IV) from the bladder involve spread to the lymph nodes, bone, or other viscera and are treated with radiation and/or chemotherapy. Treatment by TMN stage is outlined in Table 45.2.

For the majority of bladder tumors, surgical resection is the treatment of choice. Immediate referral to a urologist or surgical oncologist is critical, as well as follow-up with a medical oncologist and/or nephrologist, depending on functional renal status. Intravesical chemotherapy instilled directly into the bladder may prevent recurrence, but radiation therapy for bladder tumors is less effective than surgical and chemotherapeutic interventions.

FOLLOW-UP AND REFERRAL

All patients diagnosed with bladder cancer should be referred to a urologist or surgical oncologist for evaluation and treatment. A urinalysis and cystoscopy should be performed every 3 to 6 months because of the significant risk of recurrence of bladder tumors. Patients with invasive or metastatic disease should be referred to a medical oncologist and possibly a radiation oncologist as well, given that treatment typically involves chemotherapy and/or radiation therapy.

Home health or hospice care may be appropriate for patients who need skilled care and ongoing patient teaching, although less advanced forms of bladder cancer tend to have high cure rates. An ostomy nurse may be

TABLE 45.2 Bladder Tumor Treatment Based on TNM Staging

Stage	Description	Treatment Options	Characteristics
Stage 0	Noninvasive papillary carcinoma (Ta). Cancer has grown from urothelium toward hollow center of bladder but not into connective tissue or muscle of bladder wall. Has not spread to lymph nodes or distant sites.	• Transurethral resection of bladder tumor (TURBT) • Close follow-up every 6 months • Immunotherapy with bacillus Calmette-Guérin	Recurrence is common 5-year survival rate of 98%
Stage I	Cancer has grown into the layer of connective tissue under the urothelial lining but has not reached the muscular layer of the bladder wall. Has not spread to lymph nodes or distant sites.	• TURBT • For high-grade or large tumors, radical cystectomy recommended • If the patient is a poor surgical risk, radiation and chemotherapy recommended	5-year survival rate of 88%
Stage II	Cancer has grown into thick muscular layer of bladder wall, but has not passed through the muscle to reach the fatty tissue surrounding the bladder. Has not spread to lymph nodes or distant sites.	• Radical or partial cystectomy with lymph node resection • Radiation and chemotherapy may be done preoperatively to shrink the tumor	5-year survival rate of 63%
Stage III	Cancer has grown into the fatty tissue surrounding the bladder. May have spread to prostate, uterus, or vagina, but not growing into pelvic or abdominal wall. Has not spread to lymph nodes or distant sites.	• Neoadjuvant chemotherapy to shrink tumor preoperatively • Radical cystectomy and lymph node resection • Chemotherapy usually indicated	5-year survival rate of 46%
Stage IV	Cancer has grown through the bladder wall and into pelvic or abdominal wall. May have spread to nearby or distant lymph nodes or to sites such as the bones, liver, or lungs.	• Treatment is palliative only • Systemic chemotherapy and/or radical cystectomy or external beam radiation therapy	5-year survival rate of 12% to 15%

necessary for patients who have undergone an ileostomy or urostomy, as a result of surgical resection.

Patient Education: Bladder Tumors

It is critical for clinicians to teach the importance of ongoing follow-up care, given the potential for bladder cancer recurrence and infection of the urinary tract. This includes stressing the preventive measures of not smoking and avoiding chemical carcinogens. The possible development of associated signs and symptoms should also be discussed with patients, including nausea and vomiting, weight loss, anorexia, impotence, sterility, pain, and fatigue. Teaching ileostomy and urostomy care is indicated for patients whose bladders have been surgically removed.

Although many forms of bladder cancer have high cure rates, for terminal patients with advanced disease, death and dying issues need to be addressed and education to improve quality of life is important for both patients and their caregivers. Key emotional and mental states to be addressed include fear, anxiety, grieving, and anticipation, as well as self-image issues (including the potential loss of hair from chemotherapy or skin changes from radiation therapy). The potential loss of one's job is a critical issue for patients, whereas coping with the possible loss of a loved one is an important consideration for the patient's family.

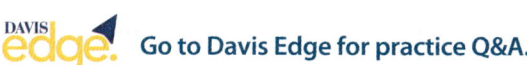
Go to Davis Edge for practice Q&A.

REFERENCES

Acute Kidney Injury

Baek SH, Chin HJ, Na KY, et al. Optimal systolic blood pressure in noncritically ill patients with acute kidney injury: a retrospective cohort study. *Kidney Res Clin Pract*. 2019;38(3)356–364. 10.23876/j.krcp.19.030g.

Chen TK, Parikh CR. Management of presumed acute kidney injury during hypertensive therapy: Stay calm and carry on? *Am J Nephrol*. 2020;51:108–115. https://doi.org/10.1159/000505447.

Moore PK, Hsu RK, Liu KD. Management of acute kidney injury: Core Curriculum 2018. *Am J Kidney Dis*. 2018;72(1):136–148.

See EJ, Jayasinghe K, Glassford N, et al. Long-term risk of adverse outcomes after acute kidney injury: a systematic review and meta-analysis of cohort studies using consensus definitions of exposure. *Kidney Int*. 2019;95(1):160–172.

Bladder Tumors

Chakraborty A, Dasari S, Long W, et al. Urine protein biomarkers for the detection, surveillance, and treatment response prediction of bladder cancer. *Am J Cancer Res*. 2019;9(6):1104–1117.

Flaig TW, Spiess PE, Agarwal N, et al. Bladder cancer, version 3.2020, NCCN Clinical Practice guidelines in oncology. *J Natl Compr Canc Netw*. 2020;18(3):329–354.

National Cancer Institute: Surveillance, Epidemiology, and End Results Program. Cancer stat facts: bladder cancer. https://seer.cancer.gov/statfacts/html/urinb.html. Accessed 10/7/2020.

Saginala K, Barsouk A, Alura J, et al. Epidemiology of bladder cancer. *Med Sci (Basel)*. 2020;8(1):15. https://www.ncbi.nlm.nih.gov/pmc/articles/PMC7151633/.

Chronic Kidney Disease

Al Kibria GM, Crispen R. Prevalence and trends of chronic kidney disease and its risk factors among US adults: an analysis of NHANES 2003–18. *Prev Med Rep*. 2020;20:101193.

CDC. Chronic Kidney. https://www.cdc.gov/kidneydisease/publications-resources/2019-national-facts.html. Accessed 11/9/2020.

CDC, Chronic kidney disease surveillance system. https://nccd.cdc.gov/CKD/detail.aspx?QNum=Q8#refreshPosition. Accessed 11/9/2020.

Myers OB, Pankratz KC, Norris JA, et al. Surveillance of CKD epidemiology in the US—a joint analysis of NHANeS and KEEP. *Sci Rep*. 2018;8:15900. https://www.nature.com/articles/s41598-018-34233-w.

United States Renal Data System. Chapter 1: CKD in the general population. USRDS annual data report: Bethesda, MD: National Institutes of Health, National Institute of Diabetes and Digestive and Kidney Diseases. Annual Data Report|USRDS. https://adr.usrds.org/2020/chronic-kidney-disease/1-ckd-in-the-general-population.

Renal Tumors

American Cancer Society (2020). Key statistics about kidney cancer. https://www.cancer.org/cancer/kidney-cancer/about/key-statistics.html.

Di Martina S, De Luca G, Grassi L, et al. Renal cancer: new models and approach for personalizing therapy. *J Exp Clin Cancer Res*. 2018;37(1):217. https://jeccr.biomedcentral.com/articles/10.1186/s13046-018-0874-4.

Escudier B, Porta C, Schmidinger M, et al. Renal cell carcinoma; ESMO clinical practice guidelines for diagnosis, treatment, and follow up. *Ann Oncol*. 2019;30(5):706–720. https://doi.org/10.1093/annonc/mdz056.

Siadat F, Trpkov K. ESC, ALK, HOT, and LOT: three letter acronyms of emerging renal entities knocking on the door of the WHO classification. *Cancers*. 2020;12(1):168. https://doi.org/10.3390/cancers12010168.

RESOURCES

American Cancer Society

Bladder Cancer
  https://www.cancer.org/cancer/bladder-cancer.html
Kidney Cancer
  https://www.cancer.org/cancer/kidney-cancer.html

National Institute of Diabetes and Digestive and Kidney Diseases

Acute Kidney Injury
  https://www.niddk.nih.gov/research-funding/research-programs/acute-kidney-injury
Chronic Kidney Disease
  https://www.niddk.nih.gov/health-information/kidney-disease/chronic-kidney-disease-ckd
Kidney Failure
  https://www.niddk.nih.gov/health-information/kidney-disease/kidney-failure

Section 9: GENDER-RELATED HEALTH PROBLEMS

SECTION EDITOR

Debera J. Thomas, PhD, RN, ANP/FNP

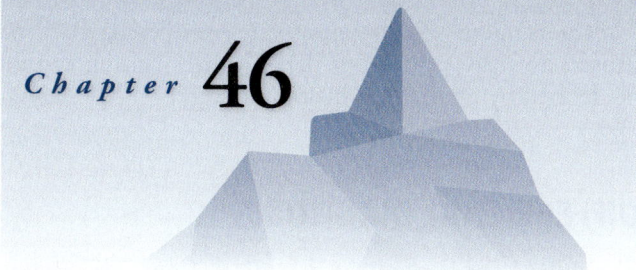

Chapter 46

Common Reproductive System Complaints

Debera J. Thomas, PhD, RN, ANP/FNP
Brian Oscar Porter, MD, PhD, MPH, MBA

Many issues that patients raise in the primary care setting relate to the male and female reproductive systems. These common complaints associated with a patient's reproductive organs (related to the interplay of genetic and hormonal developmental factors) may be separate and distinct from a patient's gender identity (psychosexual self-identification as male, female, intersex, nonbinary) or sexual orientation (sexual attraction to which individuals). Thus, the following issues and complaints commonly raised in the primary care setting may occur in patients regardless of their gender identity or sexual orientation. In addition, individuals who are transgender may experience these disorders as related to their underlying sexual anatomy, either pre- or postsurgically, if in the process of gender reassignment (see Chapter 79 for a more detailed discussion of care for the transgender person).

BREAST MASS

A breast mass is a lump in the breast. Discovering such a mass is one of the most anxiety-producing events a patient may encounter in their lifetime. Seventy percent of patients with breast cancer present with a lump in the breast; 90% of these breast masses are discovered by the patients themselves. Benign breast disorders (e.g., fibroadenoma) are referred to as *fibrocystic changes* or *fibrocystic disease* and are the most common breast lesions, diagnosed in millions of patients globally. Fibrocystic changes are extremely common and are considered a normal variant of breast tissue. In benign breast disorders, the breast masses or lumps are tender and usually bilateral. There may be a rapid fluctuation in the size of benign masses, compared with breast malignancies, which slowly increase in size. In premenopausal females, masses should be reassessed in 2 to 3 weeks during a different phase of the monthly cycle to assess for persistence or reproducibility, because the tenderness and size of a fibrocystic breast mass typically increase before menses. Fibrocystic breast disease is most common in females 30 to 50 years of age or in postmenopausal females on hormone replacement therapy. If fibrocystic breast disease is accompanied by significant pain, nipple discharge, or a palpable lump on physical examination, the patient should be evaluated for possible breast cancer. More content on breast disorders is covered in Chapter 48.

DIFFERENTIAL DIAGNOSIS

The characteristics that differentiate a breast cyst from breast cancer are tenderness, fluctuations in size, and multiplicity of lesions. It is difficult to distinguish a breast cyst from cancer, based on clinical findings alone; therefore, diagnostic testing is warranted. The first step is to rule out benign causes of a breast mass, such as infection (e.g., mastitis or cellulitis). A mammogram is usually the first test performed; however, the breast tissue in patients with fibrocystic breast disease may be too radiodense to provide a conclusive diagnosis. The American College of Radiology's *Statement on Breast Tomosynthesis* (2014) concludes that digital breast tomosynthesis (also known as 3D mammography), a diagnostic screening tool that generates a three-dimensional radiographic image of the breast, has demonstrated greater sensitivity and higher cancer detection rates than traditional mammography, with fewer patient recalls for additional testing. If a mass is present, a breast ultrasound will differentiate a cystic mass from a solid mass, although a definitive diagnosis is made via breast biopsy. Aspiration of a cystic lesion will relieve the associated breast pain and assist in the diagnosis.

MANAGEMENT

Treatment of fibrocystic breast disease consists of avoiding trauma and, for female patients, wearing a supportive bra at all times. Some research one study says eliminate caffeine from the diet and taking 400 IU of vitamin E daily can be helpful for some. For patients with severe pain, danazol (Danocrine) 100 to 200 mg twice daily is helpful. Danazol is an androgen derivative that suppresses pituitary gonadotropins and is the only treatment approved by the U.S. Food and Drug Administration (FDA) for this condition. With its androgenic side effects such as acne, edema, and hirsutism, most patients find that the treatment is more troublesome than the condition itself and prefer to try milder forms of pain relief. Some patients have experienced relief from a 3- to 6-month course of evening primrose oil. A proposed theory is that prostaglandin E-deficiency and that of its precursor gamma-linolenic acid (GLA) increase breast sensitivity, as evening primrose oil is high in GLA.

ABNORMAL UTERINE BLEEDING

A change in the pattern or volume of menstrual bleeding is a common health concern of female patients from puberty to menopause. The literature suggests that during their reproductive years, 10% to 20% of females have abnormal uterine bleeding (AUB) at least once. Patients may describe these abnormal bleeding episodes as infrequent, occurring between regular menstrual periods, prolonged in duration, and/or excessive in volume. *Acute AUB* is defined as an episode of bleeding in a nonpregnant female of reproductive age that, in the opinion of the provider, requires immediate intervention to prevent further blood loss. Chronic AUB is uterine bleeding that is abnormal in duration, volume, and/or frequency, which has been present for the majority of the past 6 months. Chronic AUB has been associated with a reduction in work productivity by as much as 30%.

Traditionally, genital bleeding in females has been vaguely defined, with inconsistent and confusing terminology. Heavy menstrual bleeding describes a patient's perception of excessive menstrual blood loss without regard to regularity, duration, or frequency of menses. In an effort to develop consistency, consensus, and clear terminology, the International Federation of Obstetrics and Gynecology Menstrual Disorders Committee developed a flexible classification system in 2011. This system, known as PALM-COEIN, classifies the causes of AUB in the reproductive years. The normal frequency of menses is every 24 to 38 days, with an average duration of 4.5 to 8 days and approximately 5 to 80 mL of blood loss per month. The determination of abnormal bleeding involves recognizing variations in frequency, regularity, duration, and volume of flow. Causes of AUB are categorized by the PALM-COEIN mnemoic, which stands for the following possible causes:

- **P**olyp
- **A**denomyosis
- **L**eiomyoma
- **M**alignancy and hyperplasia
- **C**oagulopathy
- **O**vulatory dysfunction
- **E**ndometrial disorders
- **I**atrogenic
- **N**ot yet classified

Factors of the "PALM" group are considered structural causes; however, entities of the "COEIN" group cannot be defined by imaging or histopathology.

DIFFERENTIAL DIAGNOSIS

The initial evaluation of bleeding from the vagina involves determining its source. Structural causes due to a polyp, leiomyoma, or adenomyosis can be identified via ultrasound. Anovulatory bleeding is the cause of AUB in approximately 95% of patients younger than 20 years and in 90% of perimenopausal patients who experience AUB for 2 to 3 years before the onset of menopause. In contrast, ovulatory cycles are associated with certain features such as midcycle pain, specific vaginal mucus changes, dysmenorrhea, and premenstrual breast tenderness. Approximately one-half of ovulating patients experience midcycle spotting that is self-limited. Irregular endometrial shedding may occur with the prolonged production of progesterone due to a persistent corpus luteum, resulting in AUB.

A thorough history, physical examination, pelvic examination, and selected laboratory tests will usually identify the cause of AUB. The history should include the patient's age, date of last menstrual period, birth control method, frequency of menses, amount of menstrual blood flow (e.g., the estimated number of pads or tampons used daily), duration of menses, and if there is a menstrual pattern change. In patients who report profuse acute bleeding episodes, the diagnosis of pregnancy or miscarriage (e.g., passing tissue, nausea, vomiting, breast tenderness) must be excluded. In an ectopic pregnancy, the patient may complain of abdominal pain. Complaints of fainting spells may be indicative of a ruptured ectopic pregnancy. If the patient describes bleeding only with urination or defecation, or when wiping with toilet tissue, bladder or GI disorders should be explored.

Up to 10% of patients who use oral contraceptive pills (OCPs) or other forms of hormonal contraception report irregular bleeding episodes. Any patient who presents with AUB and is 35 years of age or older should be evaluated for cervical and uterine cancers. Endometrial biopsy is an office procedure to rule out unchecked proliferation of the endometrium that can lead to hyperplasia and potentially endometrial adenocarcinoma. Similarly, a colposcopy, cervical biopsy, and endocervical curettage are used to diagnose cervical cancer. Patients older than 30 years who are positive for human papillomavirus

(HPV) and have atypical squamous cells of undetermined significance (ASC-US) or another abnormal Papanicolaou (Pap) test result should be referred for colposcopy. Patients 25 years of age and older with a low-grade squamous intraepithelial lesion should be referred for colposcopy, and any patient with ASC-H (H indicates that high-grade squamous intraepithelial lesion cannot be excluded) should also be referred for colposcopy. Trauma and foreign bodies as causes of bleeding from the vagina are seen more commonly in children. A less common cause of uterine bleeding is a blood dyscrasia that creates a tendency to bleed, such as von Willebrand's disease or thrombocytopenic purpura. This is particularly true if the patient is an adolescent and presents with heavy menstrual bleeding.

The physical examination should focus on findings pointing to possible sources of bleeding, such as an anal fissure; cervical laceration; or an enlarged, irregular, or boggy uterus, blood clots in the vaginal vault, uterine tenderness, copious blood flow, or adnexal masses or tenderness. The laboratory work-up is directed by the history and physical examination findings and usually consists of hematocrit, hemoglobin, platelet count, peripheral smear with differential, pregnancy evaluation, and Pap test. In severe bleeding, tests for partial thromboplastin time, prothrombin time, international normalized ratio, and possibly bleeding time (to detect platelet defects) are indicated. Hysteroscopy may be performed immediately before a cervical dilation and curettage of the uterus to assist in the diagnosis of polyps, exophytic endometrial cancer, or fibroids (leiomyomata) as a source of AUB. A prolactin level and thyroid function tests are ordered to rule out hyperprolactinemia and hypothyroidism, respectively.

MANAGEMENT

Management of AUB is directed toward controlling bleeding and preventing a recurrence. For teenagers, management includes observing those with mild cases and no anemia and prescribing medroxyprogesterone or an OCP. For patients of reproductive age, treatment is based on the patient's desire for fertility or contraception. For those who cannot take OCPs, medroxyprogesterone can be used. OCPs containing ethinyl estradiol are used in acute bleeding episodes. For patients with severe acute bleeding who remain hemodynamically stable, conjugated estrogen is used until the bleeding stops.

DYSPAREUNIA

Dyspareunia is painful sexual intercourse that can occur as a result of either introduction of the penis (natural or artificial) into the vagina or deep vaginal penetration. The pain a patient experiences can be a consequence of vaginal inflammation, structural (anatomical) abnormalities, vaginal atrophy, insufficient vaginal lubrication, pelvic pathology, or psychological issues.

Because patients do not often report painful sexual intercourse, it is difficult to determine the incidence of dyspareunia. A review of more than 154 studies involving over 35,973 patients experiencing chronic pelvic pain indicates that the rate of dyspareunia ranges from 1.3% to 45.7%. One study of 313 patients documented that more than 60% of subjects had experienced dyspareunia at some point in their lives. Risk factors include a history of sexual trauma, history of sexually transmitted infections (STIs), recurrent candidiasis infection, poor hygiene, menopause, psychological issues, and difficulties in intimate personal relationships.

DIFFERENTIAL DIAGNOSIS

Obtaining a thorough history requires creating a comfortable and nonjudgmental environment that normalizes the topic of sexuality, which is essential in determining the cause of dyspareunia. As noted earlier, pain may occur with initial or deep vaginal penetration and may occur with the first episode of intercourse or after a long period of pain-free sexual experiences. The patient may complain of vaginal discharge or irritation. There may be a history of unrelated pelvic pain, recent pregnancy or childbirth, pelvic or abdominal trauma, chemotherapy, radiation, or surgery. The patient may reveal difficulty using tampons or tolerating prior pelvic examinations.

On physical examination, the patient may present with signs of vulvar or vaginal mucosal irritation, inflammation, lesions, discharge, atrophy, hymenal remnants, Bartholin's cyst or abscess, or vestibulitis. Vaginismus, the involuntary contraction of perineal muscles, may occur during the speculum examination, impeding full visualization and examination of the vaginal vault and cervix. The clinician must proceed with sensitivity, allowing the patient control over the pelvic examination. The bimanual examination may reveal a pelvic mass, cervical motion tenderness, uterine prolapse, a rectocele, or cystocele.

The laboratory work-up is directed by findings from the history and physical examination and usually consists of a urinalysis, a wet mount of vaginal discharge, and cervical cultures. Urinalysis is useful in identifying any urinary tract condition that may be a contributing factor in the source of the pain. The presence of white blood cells (WBCs), red blood cells, or bacteria may indicate a UTI. Wet mount examination of vaginal discharge can reveal the presence of bacterial vaginosis (*Gardnerella vaginalis*), trichomoniasis, or candidiasis. Cervical cultures are useful in determining the presence of *Chlamydia* and gonorrhea.

MANAGEMENT

Management of dyspareunia depends on the patient's symptoms and etiology. If the cause is atrophic vaginitis, estrogens (especially vaginal estrogens) may be helpful for postmenopausal patients. A water-soluble lubricant (e.g., Astroglide, K-Y Jelly) can be used for vaginal lubrication and comfort. STIs are treated with appropriate antibiotic therapy. Progressive dilation and muscle awareness exercises such as Kegel exercises are recommended for treatment of vaginismus, hymenal strands, an anatomically narrow introitus, and scar tissue. If a psychological factor, such as sexual trauma, relationship conflicts, stress, or a restrictive sexual attitude, appears to be the cause, referral to a psychotherapist is indicated.

NOCTURIA IN MALES

Nocturia is currently defined by the International Continence Society as having to wake at night one or more times to void, each time being preceded and followed by sleep. Recording the number of times a patient urinates at night and making a reasonable estimate of the amount voided is extremely important. The frequency of urination may vary from large volumes of urine (polyuria) voided infrequently to small quantities passed at frequent intervals. Adult males normally void five to six times during the day and once or not at all during the night. As males age, nocturia is usually a sign of a prostatic problem, most often benign prostatic hyperplasia (BPH). Typically, up to 50% of males older than 50 years have BPH. Typically, 59% of males get up to urinate during the night at least twice by the age of 70 years. BPH is discussed in more detail in Chapter 50.

The occurrence of nocturia without discomfort may be due to diminished bladder capacity, overflow incontinence, or toileting habits. In males with a normal bladder, the absence of nocturia while suffering from increased frequency of urination during the day suggests a psychogenic origin. A rare finding might be a polyp or irritative lesion in the posterior urethra that is relieved by recumbence, so nocturia is not present.

Detrusor muscle instability may cause urinary incontinence, as well as nocturia. Fifty percent of male patients in nursing homes are incontinent, whereas 15% to 30% of older adult males in the community have urinary incontinence, which may be caused by decreased bladder capacity, increased residual urine (from an inability to empty the bladder fully), or involuntary bladder contractions. Moderate dribbling of urine may indicate overflow from a partially incompetent outlet and can be a congenital or acquired anomaly. Less common causes of incontinence are spinal cord disease, multiple sclerosis, tumors, trauma, syphilis, and diabetic neuropathy. Microorganisms that can cause nocturia and incontinence include *Klebsiella pneumoniae, Proteus mirabilis, Enterobacter, Staphylococcus,* enterococci (*Streptococcus* bacteria associated with the intestines), or *Pseudomonas.*

Medications, such as methyldopa, phenothiazines, diazepam, excessive vitamin D, and diuretics, may also cause nocturia, as well as precipitate or aggravate incontinence. Drugs that cause urinary retention include alpha-adrenergic agents, androgens, and sympathomimetic agents, such as ephedrine and pseudoephedrine. In turn, urinary retention can lead to nocturia and incontinence.

DIFFERENTIAL DIAGNOSIS

Nocturia may occur as a result of primary disease of the urinary tract or from metabolic diseases such as diabetes mellitus or diabetes insipidus; it may also be associated with cardiovascular disorders, fluid shifts into the lower limbs, polypharmacy, and emotional tension. Documentation of the pattern of urination during a 24-hour period is vital to a diagnosis of nocturia. Although a patient may complain if they awaken frequently to urinate, the precipitating events and activities of the day may also give a hint as to the cause. For example, alcohol intake before sleep may increase the number of times someone urinates at night and may also increase urine volume.

Urgency, a desire to urinate, can be constant or intermittent. Urgency and frequency of urination often occur together. Urgency is frequently the result of prostatic disease or bladder infection. Stress incontinence is involuntary loss of urine during physical activity or upon exertion, such as due to a cough, laughing, lifting a heavy object, changing positions, or with exercise. Incontinence is further discussed in Chapter 44. *Hesitancy* refers to difficulty in initiating a urine stream. Oliguria is a decrease in urinary output and can be caused by a decrease in the production of urine secondary to acute glomerulonephritis or other renal disease, as well as conditions that drastically decrease cardiac output. Dribbling can be symptomatic of disease; it may occur at night or during the day and usually indicates the presence of a urethral stricture, prostatic obstruction, or less commonly, a neurological disorder.

MANAGEMENT

Treatment of nocturia depends on identifying the cause. A simple urinalysis is performed to rule out UTI. A prostate-specific antigen blood test and a digital rectal examination are done to rule out a prostatic problem in male patients, such as BPH. The results of these tests may indicate a need for further diagnostic testing. Specific aspects of patient education are discussed under the particular condition causing the nocturia.

ETONOGESTREL IMPLANT

The progestin-only etonogestrel implant (Nexplanon) is a highly effective (greater than 99%) form of birth control consisting of a flexible 4-cm single hormone-containing rod that is inserted subdermally in the upper arm. The implant contains 68 mg of etonogestrel released slowly over 3 years. The implant can be inserted at any time if the patient is not pregnant; however, backup contraception should be used if insertion occurs more than 5 days after the start of menses. Risks of this contraceptive method outweigh its benefits for patients with the following conditions: cirrhosis, liver tumors, systemic lupus erythematosus, and unexplained vaginal bleeding. Use of the implant is contraindicated in patients with breast cancer.

ORAL CONTRACEPTIVE PILLS

OCPs contain either a combination of estrogen and progestin or progestin only (commonly called the *mini-pill*). The most popular OCPs are the 4-week-cycle combination pills. Combination OCPs have a failure rate of 0.3% when used correctly, but the failure rate is 8% with typical use due to a degree of nonadherence to prescribed usage instructions. The combination OCPs are taken each day for 3 weeks, with inert (placebo) pills taken during the fourth week (to facilitate adherence to an easy-to-remember, once-daily pill regimen). During the nonhormonal (fourth) week, withdrawal uterine bleeding occurs. Combination extended-cycle OCPs contain 84 active and seven inert pills (Seasonale, Seasonique, LoSeasonique) and result in menses only every 3 months (four times a year), because hormonal suppression is taken continuously for 12 weeks, followed by a 1-week placebo period, during which bleeding occurs. Combining ethinyl estradiol (EE) and levonorgestrel constitutes a form of OCP (e.g., Amethyst, Aviane, Falmina, Levlen, Orsythia, Vienva) that is taken 365 days a year and results in no menstruation.

Combination estrogen-progestin OCPs are categorized as monophasic, biphasic, triphasic, or quadriphasic. They confer different doses of hormonal exposure during the month that all suppress ovulation, thereby preventing pregnancy. Estrogen in the pill inhibits implantation of the egg by altering normal maturation of the uterine lining, while the progestins in the pill slow ovum transport and uterine motility. Progestins also cause the cervical mucus to become thick and scanty, slowing sperm transport and capacitation. In addition, the pH of the genital tract is altered, and the cervical and uterine environment becomes hostile to sperm.

EE is currently the most popular estrogen used in OCPs in the United States. The progestins currently used include desogestrel (in Mircette, Cyclessa, Ortho-Cept, Desogen), levonorgestrel (in Alesse, Nordette, Seasonale, Trivora, Triphasil), norethindrone (in Estrostep, Norinyl 1/35, Ortho-Novum 1/35 and 7/7/7, Necon 1/35, Modicon, Ovcon 35, Loestrin 1.5/30, Tri-Norinyl), norgestimate (in Ortho-Cyclen, Ortho Tri-Cyclen), drospirenone (in Yasmin), and *dL*-norgestrel (in Lo/Ovral, Low-Ogestrel).

All progestins, even in low doses, offer excellent cycle control and minimal metabolic changes. Progestins have variable estrogenic, androgenic, and progestational effects. The third generation progestins (e.g., desogestrel, drospirenone, norgestimate) are the least androgenic and are preferred for patients with acne or hirsutism. However, there have been studies with conflicting results that suggest that patients taking a contraceptive containing drospirenone are at a 1.5-fold increased risk for developing blood clots (Wu CQ, 2013).

The amounts of estrogen and progestin in combined OCPs have been greatly reduced since their inception. The lower the effective dose, the lower the rate of adverse effects; the lowest acceptable dose is guided by the ability of the pill to prevent breakthrough bleeding, which is an undesirable adverse event. Estrogen content is usually 20 to 35 mcg of EE per tablet, with no more than 50 mcg in formulations available in the United States. Progestin content ranges from 0.1 to 3 mg. Both the estrogen and progestin doses may either be constant in a cycle pack (with monophasic contraceptives) or variable (with multiphasic contraceptives). The ratio of estrogen to progestin in combination pills can range from 1:5 or 1:50; most commonly, the ratio is 1:10 to 1:30. In a normal menstrual cycle, the physiological ratio of these endogenous hormones is 1:10 (early follicular phase), 1:5 (preovulation phase), or 1:30 (luteal phase). Multiphasic OCPs are used to replicate these hormonal ratios; however, they may be associated with a higher incidence of breakthrough bleeding than monophasic pills.

Eligibility Criteria for Combined Oral Contraception

In the presence of certain medical conditions, the risks associated with combined oral contraception are considered unacceptable or outweigh its benefits. These conditions include current breast cancer, being less than 21 days postpartum, severe cirrhosis of the liver, current or past history of deep vein thrombosis (DVT), major surgery with prolonged immobilization, vascular disease, having diabetes mellitus for more than 20 years, diabetic retinopathy, and a history of migraine with aura. Other conditions in which risks typically outweigh the advantages of the use of OCPs include a history of breast cancer with no disease for 5 years or less, a low-yet-identifiable risk for DVT, or OCP-related cholestasis.

Progestin-Only Pill

The progestin-only pill (or mini-pill) contains progestin exclusively and has a reported failure rate of 1% to 4%—slightly higher than that of combined OCPs.

Progestin-only pills contain either 0.35 mg of norethindrone (e.g., Ortho Micronor, Nor-QD) or 0.075 mg of *dL*-norgestrel (e.g., Ovrette) and are taken continuously, beginning on the first day of the menstrual cycle. The progestin inhibits ovulation inconsistently but causes thickening of the cervical mucus (creating a hostile environment for sperm), alters ovum transport (leading to a higher risk of ectopic pregnancy), and inhibits implantation of the ovum. The advantages of the mini-pill are that it is safe during lactation and may increase the flow of milk and it can be used by patients older than 35 years and by those with sickle cell disease or myomas. The progestin-only pill is also less likely than combination OCPs to cause headaches, high blood pressure, depression, cramps, premenstrual syndrome, or elevations in glucose.

Disadvantages of the mini-pill include contraceptive failure and ectopic pregnancy. Irregular menstrual bleeding (e.g., amenorrhea, breakthrough bleeding, prolonged flow) is common in progestin-only users and may necessitate frequent pregnancy tests. Absolute contraindications include pregnancy and breast cancer. Conditions in which the risks of progestin-only OCPs typically outweigh their benefits include cirrhosis of the liver, diabetes mellitus for more than 20 years, diabetic retinopathy, nephropathy, neuropathy, vascular or cardiovascular disease, a history of stroke, or unexplained vaginal bleeding.

Instructions for Use of OCPs

OCPs should be started either with the onset of menses (same-day start) or on the first Sunday of the week during which menses starts (Sunday start). With a Sunday start, a backup nonhormonal contraceptive method (e.g., condom, abstinence) should be used for at least 7 days, unless Sunday is the first day of menses. There is also a quick-start method in which most patients with a negative urine pregnancy test can begin using OCPs immediately at any point in their menstrual cycle. This method improves adherence, although backup contraception should be used for 7 days.

The effectiveness of OCPs is dependent on patient adherence. Each pill must be taken at the same time every day. Once the start date is established and the pack is started, there is no waiting needed or menstrual impact in starting a subsequent pack, and as soon as the initial pack is completed, the second pack is started on the next day. Patients may need suggestions as to how to take the pill on time and every day, such as coordinating with brushing one's teeth in the morning, at a consistent mealtime, or at bedtime—as long as it is at the same hour, every day. For patients who experience nausea when taking OCPs, taking them at bedtime can minimize this adverse effect.

Standard (nonextended cycle) combination OCPs are provided in 28-day pill packs, color coded by dose and time, which include 21 active and seven inert tablets. Some manufacturers include iron supplements in the seven inert (placebo) pills, but some eliminate the seven inert pills and simply provide a 21-day dose pack. To keep a patient adherent and on time, it is usually best to recommend the habit of taking one pill a day, without stopping for the last 7 days, to prevent forgetting when to restart again.

Missed Doses of OCPs

If the patient forgets to take one or more doses of OCPs, the following guidelines are recommended:

- One dose late (less than 24 hours) or one dose missed (24 to 48 hours): Take the missed dose as soon as remembered and then the next dose at the usual time. No additional contraception is needed.
- Two or more doses missed (more than 48 hours): Take the missed dose as soon as possible, and discard any other missed pills; continue taking the remaining pills at the regular time. Use a backup form of birth control or avoid sexual intercourse until the remaining pills have been taken for 7 consecutive days. If the OCP dose was missed in the last week of the hormone containing pills (days 15 to 21), then omit the hormone-free interval and begin the next new cycle. If unable to start a new pack, then backup contraception should be used until the new pack has been taken for 7 consecutive days. Emergency contraception should be considered if the dose was missed in the first week of the cycle and unprotected sex occurred in the 5 days prior.

Some patients experience breakthrough bleeding with missed pills or the doubling of pills. Some practitioners do not advocate using the methods outlined here but instead tell their patients to discontinue the pack, use a barrier method, and restart with a new pack when regular menses begins. If menses does not occur as usual, a pregnancy test must be performed.

Special Considerations With OCPs

Patients need special instructions when starting OCPs if they had a recent full-term delivery, are nursing, had a recent abortion or miscarriage, have infrequent or irregular menses, or are using other medications. Many patients inquire about starting or restarting OCPs postpartum. The U.S. Food and Drug Administration (FDA) package inserts for OCPs indicate that because the postpartum period lends itself to a higher risk of thromboembolism, as a class of medications, OCPs should be started no earlier than 4 to 6 weeks after delivery in nonnursing mothers. Ovulation rarely takes place before 4 weeks postpartum with a full-term pregnancy; however, if a patient is using drugs (e.g., bromocriptine [Parlodel]) to suppress lactation, ovulation may occur earlier, so they will need an additional form of contraception before initiating OCPs.

Similarly, many patients who are breastfeeding inquire about starting OCPs. Because estrogen decreases the amount and quality of breast milk, OCPs are not recommended for lactating patients. Conversely, progestins promote breast milk production, so progestin-only OCPs may be used in patients who are breastfeeding and desire contraception. However, combination estrogen and progestin oral contraceptives should not be prescribed until at least 6 weeks postpartum.

Because ovulation is a possibility within 14 days after either a recent abortion or miscarriage, OCPs should be started either immediately or no later than 7 days after a first-trimester (5 to 13 weeks) abortion. After a midtrimester abortion, OCPs should be started in the same manner as after a full-term pregnancy. If a patient is not pregnant (as confirmed by a pregnancy test), OCPs may be started at any time, with backup contraception used throughout the first cycle of pills. If OCPs are started within 5 days of normal menses, no backup contraceptive method is necessary. In patients with amenorrhea or infrequent menstrual cycles, discontinuation of OCPs may cause an anovulatory or fully amenorrheic state, if their history includes secondary amenorrhea, oligomenorrhea, or irregular menstrual cycles. These patients should therefore consider another method of birth control.

Noncontraceptive Benefits of OCPs

The combination OCPs are an effective and reversible form of birth control, relatively inexpensive, and the least invasive method of correcting painful and irregular menstrual cycles. Additional benefits include reduced blood loss, resulting in a lower incidence of anemia; less risk of ectopic pregnancy and salpingitis; fewer ovarian cysts; reduction in dysmenorrhea; reduction in risks of ovarian and endometrial cancers; improvement of acne; decreased risk of developing myomas in long-term (greater than 4 years) users; and a beneficial effect on bone mass. These benefits reduce the need for costly hospitalizations. In addition, excessive facial and body hair is often reduced in OCP users, although hair loss is not usually related to OCP use and should be referred to a dermatologist for evaluation.

Adverse Effects of OCPs

If a patient taking OCPs complains of any of the adverse effects typically associated with OCPs (e.g., nausea, abdominal bloating, hair changes, weight gain, leg pain, cramps, swelling), switching the patient to a pill with a lower estrogen dose or one with a less androgenic progestin formulation will often relieve the problem. Although switching to a lower estrogen dose or different progestin component may relieve abdominal bloating, bowel irregularity can also be a source of bloating and should be evaluated. If a patient complains of nausea, they should be instructed to take the pill with food or at bedtime. If the nausea or bloating persists or worsens, the patient may need to consult a gastroenterologist.

The benefits and safety of OCPs are dependent on adherence but are also affected by other factors such as smoking. There is an increased risk of cardiovascular disease and thromboembolic disease in patients older than 35 years who smoke more than 15 cigarettes a day while taking OCPs. Patients older than 40 years who are nonsmokers may safely continue low-dose OCPs. The use of OCPs is safest throughout the menstrual lifetime of patients who are of normal weight, are nonsmokers, have normal blood pressure and cholesterol levels, do not have diabetes mellitus, and have no family history of heart disease.

The Nurses' Health Study, Nurses' Health Study II, and the Women's Health Initiative (WHI) are long-term prospective studies examining the effects of OCPs and menopausal hormone therapy on cardiovascular risk, thromboembolic risk, and cancer risk. These studies generated safety data, demonstrating that OCPs have a wide range of adverse effects. Overall, the constant presence of low-level hormones creates a pregnancy-like environment in the female body. Thyroid hormone and cortisol levels may be elevated, progestins may alter the lipid profile, and estrogens can decrease glucose tolerance (thus, patient with diabetes mellitus should be monitored closely if using OCPs). Estrogen-related increases in clotting factors result in an increased risk of thromboembolism; thus, patients who will be undergoing surgery and postoperative bed confinement should discontinue OCPs at least 4 weeks before surgery.

The risk of developing hypertension in OCP users increases with the duration of use and in older adult patients. If a patient develops hypertension while taking OCPs, the pills should be stopped and another form of contraception adopted. However, if a patient is younger than 40 years, does not smoke, and has mild hypertension that is controlled with medication, OCPs may be used as long as blood pressure is closely monitored. The use of OCPs is not recommended in patients with a history of migraines with aura because OCPs can precipitate migraine or vascular headaches or make existing migraines worse. Another form of contraception should be used if headaches increase in severity or frequency.

Patients taking OCPs (particularly pills with 50 mcg or more of estrogen) are at a higher risk of myocardial infarction. The risk is further increased in patients who smoke; are obese; or have hypertension, diabetes mellitus, or hyperlipidemia. Similarly, the risk of thromboembolic disease is increased in users of OCPs, particularly formulations that are higher in estrogen. Leg pain, cramps, and swelling usually disappear after three cycle packs, but severe extremity pain, especially if unilateral, can indicate a thrombosis and requires immediate discontinuation of the OCP and rapid medical evaluation.

Other adverse effects of OCP use are increased risks of cervical dysplasia and cancer in long-term (greater than 5 years) users who have also had persistent cervical HPV infection. There is also some evidence that there is a higher incidence of benign liver tumors or gallstones conferred by OCPs, which is usually associated with higher hormonal dosages, longer-term use, and older patient ages. It is unclear whether OCPs contribute to breast cancer. FDA packaging inserts imply an association related to duration of use and medical history. Fibrocystic breast discomfort has been found to be less frequent in OCP users. Breast swelling and tenderness are common premenstrual complaints, and low-dose OCPs seem to decrease this complaint, as does reducing caffeine intake, avoiding smoking, and reducing sodium intake.

Because the cervical mucus is affected by the progestin component in OCPs and estrogen can cause cervical mucorrhea, it is not uncommon for OCP users to experience mucus-generating irritations of the genital tract, including *Candida* infections of the vagina and vulva. Antibiotic therapy may also cause this condition.

Patients who use OCPs may have increased pigmentation of the face and forehead. Combination pill users find this darkening on the areolae and perineum as well. Weight gain may or may not be an OCP effect; although weight gain may also be tied to overeating, lack of exercise, fluid retention, thyroid problems, or poor nutrition, a gain of 2 to 5 pounds after starting OCPs is not uncommon. To metabolize OCPs properly, certain vitamins are needed as micronutrients, which may not be effectively stored in the body. Thus, patients should be instructed to take a daily multivitamin and vitamin C supplements while taking OCPs to prevent deficiency of these nutrients, which can impact how OCPs are processed.

Discontinuing Use of OCPs

When combination OCPs are discontinued, 90% of patients resume ovulation and menses within 3 months. A pregnancy test should be done to ensure the patient is not pregnant if normal cycles are not established after 3 months. If a patient does not wish to become pregnant, another form of contraception should be used when OCPs are discontinued. If a patient becomes pregnant while using OCPs, most studies show no increased incidence of congenital birth defects. However, it is best not to use OCPs if a patient suspects they are pregnant; but instead, a patient should use another method of birth control until a state of pregnancy is definitively established or not.

CONTRACEPTIVE PATCH

The transdermal contraceptive patch (Xulane) is a highly effective form of combined hormonal contraception and has potential advantages over OCPs. The patch contains EE and norelgestromin and is applied weekly. Because of the patch's continuous transdermal delivery, hormone levels are constant, without peaks and troughs. Moreover, the transdermal administration bypasses the liver, so there is no first-pass hepatic metabolism, and it is possible to achieve effectiveness at lower doses of hormones. Because the patch is applied only once every 7 days, compliance is also enhanced. About 20 to 35 mcg of EE and 150 mcg of norelgestromin are released from the patch on a daily basis. Because it is a combined hormonal contraceptive, the mechanism of action is the same as that of OCPs. The effectiveness is 99% if used perfectly and 91% in typical use, although obesity decreases the effectiveness of the patch.

Eligibility and Contraindications for Use

Because the patch is a combined hormonal contraceptive, the eligibility criteria for its use are the same as that for OCPs. The contraindications to the contraceptive patch are also the same as those for combined OCPs: history of thromboembolism, an estrogen-dependent tumor, or abnormal liver function. In addition, if a patient has sensitive skin or exfoliative dermatitis, they may not be a candidate for the patch. Some patients may experience skin sensitivity to a component of the transdermal system and should not use the patch.

Instructions for Use of the Patch

The patch should be initiated on either the first day of menses or on the Sunday after the start of menses; however, if the Sunday start is 5 days after the beginning of menses, then a form of nonhormonal contraception (e.g., condom, abstinence) is necessary for the first 7 days.

The patient should be instructed to apply the patch to the buttock, abdomen, upper arm, or upper torso but avoid the breast. The patch should be changed in 7 days, and at the same time the old patch is removed, the new patch should be applied to a different site. It is important to inform the patient that lotions should not be used at the site of the patch and an occlusive dressing cannot be used at the patch site. The patch is changed every 7 days for 3 weeks and then is followed by a patch-free week, which triggers withdrawal uterine bleeding.

If there is a delay in removing and replacing the patch during the second or third patch cycle, the patient should apply a new patch as soon as possible. If the new patch is applied within 48 hours of the intended patch change day, then there will be an adequate release of hormones, and the patch change day may remain the same. If the new patch is placed after this 48-hour time period, however, the day the new patch is applied becomes the new patch day, and intercourse should be avoided or a backup contraceptive method should be used for 7 days after application of the new patch.

If a patch becomes detached for less than 24 hours, it can be reapplied to the same location; however, if it has lost its stickiness, it cannot be used and should be replaced with a new patch. If the patch is detached for longer than 24 hours, then a new patch should be applied as soon as possible, and this becomes the new patch change day; again, an additional form of nonhormonal contraception (e.g., condom, abstinence) should be used for the next 7 days.

Adverse Effects of the Patch

As with OCPs, the transdermal patch has similar adverse effects, particularly on coagulation factors. Although both OCPs and the patch have an increased risk of VTE, patch users have a higher risk over OCP users, particularly in those with diabetes mellitus. This greater risk is attributed to the higher overall EE concentrations conferred by the patch, because it does not undergo first-pass metabolism by the liver.

The most commonly reported adverse effects were breast tenderness, headache, application site reactions, nausea, and dysmenorrhea; however, fewer than 2% of users discontinued the patch because of these side effects. Breakthrough bleeding during the first two cycles after initiating patch contraception is also very common.

CONTRACEPTIVE VAGINAL RING

The contraceptive vaginal ring (e.g., NuvaRing, Annovera) is a combined hormonal contraceptive containing both estrogen and a progestin and has the same benefits as OCPs and the transdermal patch but has the advantage that it is left in place for 3 weeks. Like the patch, the vaginal ring also has the advantage of consistent hormone release without peaks and troughs; rather, hormone levels peak immediately after insertion and then slowly decrease over the 3-week cycle. Also, there is no first-pass loss of active hormones in the liver because, as they are absorbed vaginally, the EE concentration is lower than with OCPs.

The contraceptive vaginal ring is a flexible ring measuring 54 mm in diameter and 4 mm in cross section. Different brands have specific hormone combinations (e.g., NuvaRing releases 15 mcg of EE and 120 mcg of etonogestrel per day, Annovera releases 13 mcg of EE and 150 mcg of segesterone acetate per day). The mechanism of action is the same as the other combined hormonal contraceptives with the addition of thickening the cervical mucus and preventing the penetration of sperm. Vaginal rings have the same effectiveness rating as the patch: 99% if used perfectly and 91% with typical use. Several medications decrease the effectiveness of the ring, such as rifampin, rifampicin and rifamate, griseofulvin, certain HIV medications, and the herb St. John's wort.

Eligibility and Contraindications for Use

Because the ring is a combined hormonal contraceptive, the eligibility criteria for its use are the same as those for OCPs and the transdermal patch as outlined by the CDC.

Instructions for Use of the Ring

The patient should be instructed to insert the ring on the first day of menses, but some patients will not like the idea of insertion while they have their period. Alternatively, the ring can be inserted at any point during their menstrual cycle, provided there is no possibility that the patient could be pregnant; this is referred to as the *quick-start method.* Nonhormonal backup contraception (e.g., condom, abstinence) should be used for the first 7 days if the ring is not inserted within the first 5 days of menses.

Insertion of the vaginal ring is similar to insertion of a diaphragm. The patient should be in a comfortable position, press the sides of the ring together, and insert it into the vagina as high as possible. The higher the insertion, the less the likelihood of discomfort or the ring falling out. The ring is left in position for 3 weeks and then removed. During the 3 weeks, the patient should be instructed to periodically check to ensure the ring is still in place. After one ring-free week, a new ring is inserted on the same day of the week and at the same time that the old ring was removed. If the ring is left in place for more than 3 weeks but less than 5 weeks, it should be removed and a new one inserted after a week-long ring-free interval to allow for withdrawal bleeding. If the ring is left in place for longer than 5 weeks, then the ring should be replaced with a new one immediately and nonhormonal backup contraception (e.g., condom, abstinence) should be used until the new ring has been in place for 7 days.

If the ring is removed or falls out, it can be rinsed in cool water and reinserted within 3 hours. If the ring is out of the vagina for more than 3 hours and it is during the first 2 weeks of the cycle, the ring can be reinserted as soon as possible, and backup contraception should be used until it has been in place for 7 days. If the removal occurs during week 3 of the cycle, it should be discarded. The patient then has the option of either inserting a new ring and beginning the 3-week cycle with backup contraception for the first 7 days or, alternatively, waiting for a 7-day ring-free period before inserting a new ring, using backup contraception during the ring-free week and for 7 days after the insertion of the new ring. Of note, upon removal of the vaginal ring, fertility is restored rapidly, with a median time to ovulation of 19 days postremoval.

Adverse Effects of the Ring

The adverse effects of the contraceptive vaginal ring are the same as those for OCPs, although there is some evidence for a slightly increased risk of VTE in ring users compared with those using OCPs. In addition to similar side effects seen with other forms of hormonal contraception, the ring may also lead to local vaginal symptoms such as vaginitis, increased wetness, and leukorrhea.

MEDROXYPROGESTERONE ACETATE INJECTIONS

Depot medroxyprogesterone acetate (DMPA) is available in several long-acting forms of contraception. Depo-Provera Contraceptive Injection consists of deep intramuscular (IM) injections of 150 mg, whereas Depo-SubQ Provera 104 consists of subcutaneous injections of 104 mg. Each type of injection is given every 3 months. These injections have efficacy rates of 94% to 99.7%. The initial injection is typically given on day 5 of menses but may be given at any time if the patient is not pregnant (including immediately postpartum). If the injection is given after day 7 of the start of menses, the patient needs to abstain from intercourse or use a nonhormonal backup method of birth control (e.g., condom) for 7 days after the injection. If the patient wishes to become pregnant, they should be counseled that it may take an average of 9 to 10 months for fertility to return after stopping the injections, because of the long-acting effects of these depot formulations.

Use of DMPA is contraindicated if the patient is pregnant or has breast cancer. Risks outweigh the benefits of using DMPA in patients with the following conditions: undiagnosed vaginal bleeding, current or past breast cancer, thromboembolic disorders, cerebrovascular disease, hepatic tumors (benign or malignant), active hepatic disease, papilledema, retinal vascular lesions, sudden-onset vision loss, diabetic nephropathy, retinopathy, neuropathy, diabetes mellitus with vascular involvement, ischemic heart disease, multiple risk factors for atherosclerotic cardiovascular disease, severe hypertension (persistent values of 160/100 mm Hg or more), and systemic lupus erythematosus with positive antiphospholipid antibodies or severe thrombocytopenia. The use of DMPA is associated with an increase in weight and percent body fat over that of OCPs. In 2004, the FDA issued a product label boxed warning on the long-term use of DMPA because of the possibility of loss of bone mineral density. However, it is unclear whether there is an increase in fracture risk later in life, and the World Health Organization concluded that there is no reason to restrict DMPA's use in patients aged 18 to 45 years.

BARRIER METHODS

Barrier methods of contraception that prevent contact between sperm and the ovum include male and female condoms, the diaphragm, and the cervical cap. Some barrier methods have the dual advantage of preventing pregnancy and STIs. The most common STIs are caused by herpes simplex virus, HPV, HIV, *Neisseria gonorrhoeae*, and *Chlamydia*. Preventing HPV infection also reduces the risk of cervical cancer. Adverse effects and challenges with the use of barrier methods include messiness, handling of the genitalia, precoital interruption of spontaneity, and allergy or contact dermatitis to component materials or lubricants. In turn, the use of barrier methods requires motivation on the part of both partners. Condom use is promoted, based more on the general principles of preventing STIs, rather than on epidemiological data for all STIs because protection against HPV transmission is not 100% effective. HPV can be found in many genital areas (e.g., genital tract skin and mucous membranes). Hence, condoms do not protect the vulva from microscopic HPV particles on the skin.

Male Condom

The male condom is the most commonly used barrier method of contraception and is most effective at preventing pregnancy when combined with a spermicide such as nonoxynol-9. However, condoms containing nonoxynol-9 have not been shown to reduce the rate of STI transmission, and some studies have demonstrated higher rates of HIV transmission associated with nonoxynol-9 use in condoms, which is associated with an increased risk of vaginal lesions. Thus, the World Health Organization currently recommends that nonoxynol-9 should not be used by women at high risk for HIV infection.

Condoms are available in various sizes, colors, flavors, strengths, and states of lubrication. The tip should extend one-half inch beyond the penis to collect the ejaculate. Care must be taken during withdrawal of the penis to prevent the condom from coming off and spilling the semen. Other adverse effects include contact irritation, allergic reactions, unappealing oral sex experience, and accidental breakage of the condom. With typical use, failure rates for condoms used without spermicide are approximately 18%, and when used with a spermicide, the contraceptive failure rate is equivalent to that of OCPs. However, these considerations regarding contraceptive effectiveness are separate from requirements for STI prevention, as barrier methods are the most effective means of preventing transmission of STIs.

Female Condom

The female condom is a disposable device made of seamless polyurethane. It fits loosely inside the vagina and covers the perineum. There are flexible rims on both ends. The inner rim sits on the closed end and is compressed for placement into the vagina over the cervix, which prevents direct contact with bodily secretions. The condom is soft, lubricated by spermicide, relatively inexpensive, and may be purchased over the counter. However, many patients state that it is difficult to use. Adverse effects include irritation and allergic reactions. The failure rate of the female condom is 5% (with perfect use) to 21% (with typical use) and comparable to the efficacy of cervical barrier devices, such as the diaphragm. *Perfect use* refers to the use prescribed for research subjects, and *typical use* connotes everyday use in a nonresearch real-world setting.

Diaphragm

A diaphragm is a latex hemisphere with a flexible rim that fits over the cervix. The failure rate is 6% (with perfect use) to 12% (with typical use) when used with spermicidal jelly. This method allows the patient control over contraceptive decision making and has no systemic side effects. The largest size that covers the cervix comfortably should be used. Once the device has been fitted, the patient should insert and remove the diaphragm and then return for a recheck after 1 week of practice while using a backup contraceptive method. Before insertion, one teaspoon of spermicide is placed in the cup, and a small amount is spread around the rim. The diaphragm must be left in place for 6 hours after intercourse; if additional intercourse is desired, additional spermicide must be inserted into the vagina. The diaphragm should not be left in place for more than 24 hours. There is also a single-size contoured diaphragm (Caya) available in the United States. Instead of the metal rim typically found in diaphragms, this device uses a nylon rim that is more comfortable and flexible. Although it fits most patients who have used 65- to 80-mm diaphragms, a test fit should be done for patients who have never been fitted before for a diaphragm.

Once removed, the diaphragm is washed with mild soap, dried, and stored. Before the diaphragm is used again, it should be held up to the light to check for holes, tears, and breaks. The patient should be instructed to urinate before inserting and after removing the diaphragm to reduce the risk of urinary tract infections (UTIs). Under normal circumstances, the diaphragm is fitted during the annual gynecological visit; however, if the patient has pelvic surgery, pregnancy, or a weight change of 10 to 20 pounds, the diaphragm must be refitted. This may not be necessary for the single-size contoured diaphragm.

Cervical Cap

The cervical cap is a cup-shaped plastic or rubber device that fits snugly around the cervix, with a failure rate of 23% (with typical use) and 8% (with perfect use) but is less effective in multiparous patients. As with the diaphragm, the cap is used with a spermicide. Because the cap is smaller than the diaphragm, it may be more difficult to insert and remove. The advantage of the cervical cap is that it can be used in patients who are unable to use a diaphragm because of a relaxed anterior vaginal wall or in those who have recurrent UTIs with the use of a diaphragm. The cervical cap should be left in place for at least 6 hours after intercourse but for no more than 48 hours. Patients with a history of PID, abnormal Pap tests, severe cervicitis, or an abnormally shaped cervix should not use the cervical cap. Adverse effects of the cervical cap are similar to those associated with the diaphragm: allergic reactions, contact irritation, and displacement.

Vaginal Contraceptive Sponge

A vaginal contraceptive sponge is a one-size-fits-all disposable sponge of polyurethane treated with a spermicide that protects against pregnancy but not against STIs. The sponge device most commonly available over the counter in the United States must be thoroughly wet with two tablespoons of water before being inserted into the vagina. The failure rate for the sponge is approximately 12% for nulliparous patients and up to 24% for parous patients. Adverse effects include displacement, contact irritation, and a slight risk of toxic shock syndrome (one case per 2 million sponges). It should be left in place for 6 hours after intercourse but not for more than 30 hours. It is not recommended for use during menses or in the puerperium (up to 6 weeks after childbirth).

Contraceptive Foam, Cream, Film, Jelly, and Suppository

Nonoxynol-9 is the most common spermicide contained in contraceptive foams, creams, films, jellies, and suppositories. These products have an overall contraception failure rate of 2% to 30% when used correctly. The advantages of these forms of contraception are that they are available without a prescription, easy to use, readily available, and relatively inexpensive. Nonoxynol-9 may have some virucidal and bactericidal activity, but it does not offer any protection against HIV and has not been shown to reduce rates of STIs. Other disadvantages of these products are that they can cause contact irritation and allergic reactions.

FERTILITY AWARENESS METHODS

Fertility awareness methods are techniques that can be used for both preventing and achieving pregnancy. Abstaining from sexual intercourse during the days of the menstrual cycle when the ovum is most vulnerable to fertilization is one way of avoiding pregnancy. Likewise, if achieving pregnancy is the desired outcome, engaging in sexual intercourse at this time is desirable.

There are several fertility awareness methods that can be used to predict the best time for abstinence. The calendar method is based on the assumptions that the ovum is viable for 24 hours after ovulation, spermatozoa are viable for 48 hours after coitus, and ovulation occurs 12 to 16 days before menses. The patient records the length of their cycle for several months and establishes their fertile period by deducting 18 days from the shortest cycle and 11 days from the previous longest cycle to determine the ovulation period of each cycle. During each subsequent menstrual cycle, abstinence should occur during this calculated fertile period if pregnancy is not desired. The patient must have regular menstrual cycles to use this method effectively.

Other fertility awareness methods include the basal body temperature (BBT) method, the cervical mucus method, and the symptothermal method. When several techniques are used in combination, the period of abstinence can be reduced and the effectiveness increased for preventing pregnancy or achieving pregnancy (if this is the goal).

In the BBT method, the patient measures BBT daily. Abstinence is observed from menses to 3 days of elevated temperature. Although this method does not predict ovulation effectively, it can be used to learn the pattern of temperature changes over time. The lengthy abstinence period required plus abstinence in anovulatory cycles make this a less-favorable method for many. In the cervical mucus method, a patient learns to recognize and interpret changes in the amount and consistency of cervical mucus that occur in response to changes in estrogen and progesterone levels associated with the menstrual cycle. Abstinence begins in menses (and every day thereafter to reduce the risk of confusing mucus with semen) until the first day that slippery, copious cervical mucus is detected. Abstinence is observed every day thereafter until 4 days after the last day mucus is present or after the peak mucus day, because ovulation typically occurs within 2 days of the peak day of mucus production. In the symptothermal method, the fertile period is determined by calendar calculation and cervical mucus changes to predict the fertile period; changes in mucus and basal temperature are used to pinpoint the end of this period. This method is difficult to learn but is the most effective natural method to prevent pregnancy.

The greatest obstacle to acceptance of these techniques is the need to avoid sexual relations for many days in each cycle. Some patients use a barrier method during fertile times for greater acceptance and to reduce the failure rate. Self-administered ovulation prediction kits are also available for the detection of hormonal changes in urine, which reduce the required abstinence period to just several days per cycle.

POSTCOITAL CONTROLS

Postcoital controls are another method of birth control. There are three types: withdrawal, postcoitus douche, and emergency contraception. The simplest, most effective, and most practical method of preventing implantation after unprotected sex is the use of emergency contraception. Emergency contraception is available over the counter by several brand names. Plan B One-Step, Take Action, Next Choice One Dose, and My Way are all available in the United States and contain levonorgestrel 1.5 mg in a one-tablet regimen to be taken within 72 hours of unprotected sex or levonorgestrel 0.75 mg taken as explained and then again as a second tablet taken 12 hours after the first. Available only by prescription, ulipristal (Ella) emergency contraceptive contains 30 mg of ulipristal and prevents pregnancy by blocking progesterone receptors. It should be taken as soon as possible after unprotected intercourse but is considered effective if taken up to 5 days afterward.

STERILIZATION

Sterilization is a permanent method of birth control. After the risks and benefits of sterilization are reviewed with the patient, informed consent must be obtained. Up to 10% of patients who undergo sterilization procedures later request reversal of sterilization, particularly for patients younger than 30 years of age.

Male sterilization consists of vasectomy performed on an outpatient basis in which the vas deferens (ductus deferens) leading from each testis is surgically ligated. The procedure typically takes 20 minutes to perform under local anesthesia. Complications include hematoma (5%), sperm granuloma, and spontaneous reanastomosis of the vas deferens. After vasectomy, the patient is not considered sterile until two sperm-free ejaculates have been produced. Semen analysis should be performed 8 to 16 weeks after the procedure. About 15 to 20 ejaculations are required postvasectomy to determine absolute sterility.

Female sterilization can be performed in several ways. A mini-laparotomy is usually performed postpartum, where the fallopian tubes are brought up through a small incision. Usually a small section of each tube is removed, or the entire tube can be removed. The procedure can also be performed laparoscopically through a small incision. Both of these require general anesthesia. Salpingectomy can also be done at the time of a Caesarean section.

ABORTION

An elective abortion is one of the most common gynecological procedures in the United States and has been legal since 1973. In accordance with the landmark *Roe v. Wade* Supreme Court decision, the state may not interfere with the practice of abortion in the first trimester. To protect the health of the mother, a second-trimester abortion may be performed. Since abortion was legalized in the United States, the maternal mortality rate has fallen significantly. Although legislative initiatives and judicial challenges restricting abortion access at the state level are ongoing, these have often been declared unconstitutional.

The primary method used for elective abortion in the first trimester is vacuum aspiration under local anesthesia, which involves dilation of the cervix and vacuum aspiration of the products of conception. Second-trimester abortion (after 13 weeks) can be done with dilation of the cervix and evacuation of the pregnancy (D&E) or with medication (medical abortion). A D&E is most often used because it has fewer complications than a medical abortion. A D&E is a surgical procedure that can be performed under either local or general anesthesia. Because the fetus may be too large to remove by suction alone, forceps are inserted through the cervix, and the fetus is removed. Agents used in medical abortion include hypertonic saline solution that is instilled into the amniotic cavity or prostaglandins that induce labor. The prostaglandins used most often are PGE_2 as a vaginal suppository and 15-methyl $PGF_{2\alpha}$ as an IM injection. They are given at 2- to 3-hour intervals until evacuation of the fetus is observed. Both instillation of hypertonic saline and prostaglandin administration are difficult for the patient. Abortions are rarely performed after 20 weeks, because the lower limit of fetal viability with neonatal intensive care unit intervention is considered to be 24 weeks of gestational age, although some procedures are performed past 20 weeks gestational age for medical reasons, such as severe congenital defects in the fetus.

Complications from abortions increase as gestational age increases and include retained products of conception and unrecognized ectopic pregnancy. Currently, most abortions (90%) are performed before 12 weeks of gestation, and there is an overall maternal mortality rate of one in 100,000 cases. Patients should be counseled to obtain an abortion as early as possible in the pregnancy, if this is their choice, to minimize any related complications.

In September 2000, the FDA-approved mifepristone (RU486), a synthetic antiprogestational-antiglucocorticoid pill, as an oral abortifacient. Mifepristone is used to induce an abortion during the first 9 weeks of pregnancy and is given as a single dose of 200 mg, which has a success rate of 85%. If it is followed in 36 to 48 hours with a prostaglandin vaginal suppository, the success rate in terminating pregnancy is more than 95%. Adverse effects include nausea, vomiting, bleeding, and abdominal pain.

Patient Education: Contraception and Family Planning

Contraception is not just a method; it is a life decision and part of the family planning process. There is no ideal method for every patient, but because so many options are available today, contraception can be tailored for each person's lifestyle, motivation, and participation with sexual partner(s). Research in reproductive biology may provide less invasive and more effective contraceptive methods in the future. However, at present, maximum effectiveness still depends on consistent and accurate use; thus, the human element is the primary source of error.

Every patient should consider contraception as part of their overall personal health maintenance, regardless of the desired form (including the choice of abstinence). The health regimen should include an annual gynecological examination (for physiologically female patients), balanced nutrition, smoking and alcohol cessation, weight control, mental health, exercise, and risk reduction. Fertility control and health and wellness work hand in hand for the patients and their future life plans.

FERTILITY PROBLEMS

Fertility is the quality of producing ova, fertilized ova being able to implant in the uterine lining, and implantation being sustained. Although the medical techniques that facilitate fertility continue to advance, chance continues to play a large role in achieving pregnancy. *Infertility* is defined as the failure to achieve pregnancy despite regular unprotected sexual intercourse for at least 12 months. Over a 12-month period, studies have shown an 85% cumulative probability of achieving pregnancy in normal fertile couples who are not using contraception. Infertility occurs in 10% to 15% of reproductive-aged couples in the United States. A female patient younger than 35 years is considered infertile if pregnancy does not occur after 1 year of unprotected intercourse. This time frame is shortened to 6 months in female patients aged 35 years and older. Male patients are considered infertile if they do not produce and deliver enough quality sperm to initiate a pregnancy. Given that infertility may arise from causes in both males and females, the full spectrum of causes in both sexes is discussed in this section.

Infertility is divided into two categories. *Primary infertility* refers to a female patient who is unable to bear a child, either due to failure to become pregnant or to carry a pregnancy to a live birth. *Secondary infertility* applies to a female patient who has delivered at least one child but subsequently fails to become pregnant or to carry a pregnancy to a live birth. *Sterility* is a term applied when there is an irreversible factor preventing reproduction. Cycle fecundability is the probability of a successful pregnancy occurring in a single menstrual cycle, and cycle fecundity is the probability that a live birth will occur in a single cycle.

EPIDEMIOLOGY AND CAUSES

On average, 30% of fertile couples will achieve pregnancy within 1 month of unprotected intercourse, 80% within 6 months, and 85% within 12 months. At age 25 years, the age at which couples are the most fertile, the average length of time needed to achieve pregnancy is 5.3 months. The average 20- to 30-year-old American couple has intercourse one to three times a week, a frequency that should be sufficient to achieve pregnancy if all other factors are satisfactory. Primary infertility occurs in about one of 12 couples (8.3%).

The American Society for Reproductive Medicine (ASRM) estimates there are more than 6 million females between the ages of 15 and 44 years with infertility problems in the United States. However, fertility is determined by factors affecting both partners, including age; underlying disease; and exposure to toxins, drugs, and radiation. A major difference between male and female reproductive potential is that females have a finite reproductive life span (approximately 35 years), whereas males, after puberty, have the capacity to reproduce for the rest of their lives. Nevertheless, aging does affect fertility and sexual function in both males and females.

One in seven couples aged 30 to 34 years is infertile, which increases with age to one in five couples aged 35 to 39 years and one in four couples aged 40 to 44 years. These declines reflect the natural aging process and emphasize the need for rapid evaluation and treatment of infertility, especially in a female patient older than 35 years. Infertility can be multifactorial and may result from factors affecting the male or female patient, or a combination of both. Although not well-defined, infertility is thought to result from male factors in 20% of cases, female factors in 38%, and a combination of factors in both in 27% of cases; the cause of infertility may be unidentified in up to 15% of couples.

Male fertility involves pretesticular, testicular, and/or post-testicular factors. Pretesticular conditions account for 2% to 5% of infertility and include diseases of the pituitary gland and hypothalamus, as well as factors that affect the hypothalamic-pituitary axis. Testicular defects in spermatogenesis account for up to 80% of male infertility cases, and post-testicular causes, including sperm transport disorders, account for 5% of cases. Ten percent to 20% of cases in males are idiopathic. Female causes of infertility include ovulatory disorders (25%), endometriosis (15%), pelvic adhesions (12%), tubal obstruction or related abnormalities (22%), and hyperprolactinemia (7%). An important factor that affects fertility in females is delaying pregnancy until after the age of 35 years. With increasing age, the risk grows that one or more physiological processes necessary to achieve pregnancy will be inadequate. By the age of 40 years, only about 5% of females are able to achieve pregnancy without reproductive assistance.

In general, infertility is caused by one of four conditions: the inability to produce healthy gametes (sperm or eggs); the failure of healthy gametes to come into close physical proximity, thus preventing fertilization; the inability of the fertilized egg to attach to the uterine lining successfully; and the inability of a female patient to carry a pregnancy to term postimplantation. Couples should be referred for an infertility evaluation if they have been unable to achieve pregnancy after 1 year of regular unprotected intercourse. If the female patient is between 35 and 40 years of age, the couple should be referred for evaluation after 6 months of unprotected intercourse. Immediate evaluation is encouraged in female patients older than 40 years because of the rapid increase in follicular atresia that occurs after the age of 37 years.

PATHOPHYSIOLOGY

Numerous processes are essential to normal fertility in females. One of the ovaries must produce a mature follicle and release a mature ovum. There must be no obstruction between the ovary and fallopian tube, and the movements of the fimbria must facilitate transfer of the ovum to the fallopian tube. The quality of the cervical mucus must be favorable to ensure survival of the spermatozoa and its transport to the uterus and fallopian tube. Fertilization usually takes place in the fallopian tube, and the tube must be patent to allow the fertilized ovum to travel to the uterus, as it develops into a growing blastocyst. The follicle that released the ovum will become a corpus luteum and must produce a large amount of progesterone, an adequate amount of estrogen, and inhibin A to prepare the endometrium for implantation of the blastocyst and to sustain normal growth and development.

In males, normal fertility requires that the testes must produce an adequate number of morphologically normal, motile sperm. Genital tract secretions from the seminal vesicles and prostate gland must be normal, and because sperm travels from the testis through the epididymis and vas deferens to the urethra, the male genital tract must not be obstructed. In addition, the ejaculated spermatozoa must be deposited in the female genital tract in such a manner that they reach the cervix and enter the uterus where they may contact oocytes either within the uterus or, more commonly, within the fallopian tubes.

Fertility can be affected by structural problems in the fallopian tubes, uterus, endometrium, and cervix, as well as by systemic and genetic factors. *Tubal infertility* refers to conditions originating in the fallopian tubes. The most common cause of tubal infertility is uterine infection that extends into the fallopian tubes. Pelvic inflammatory disease (PID), most commonly caused by infection with *Neisseria gonorrhoeae* or *Chlamydia trachomatis,* can lead to the formation of scar tissue that can inhibit transport of sperm to the ovum and/or the ovum to the uterus. Obstruction can then lead to development of hydrosalpinges, which are collections of fluid within the fallopian tubes. These significantly interfere with the success of in vitro fertilization (IVF), possibly because components in the hydrosalpinx fluid are toxic to developing embryos. In addition, obstruction may result from tubal endometriosis, pelvic tuberculosis, and adhesions from previous pelvic surgery.

Uterine anatomical abnormalities have not been consistently identified as causal sources of infertility because many patients with abnormal uteri are able to become pregnant and carry pregnancies to term. However, septate uteri, synechiae (severe endometrial scarring), and uterine polyps are more common in infertile patients. Similarly, uterine leiomyomata or fibroids (benign smooth muscle monoclonal tumors) are the most common type of pelvic tumors in females and have been observed in greater frequency in infertile patients. This may be due to less sustainable oocyte implantation lower in the uterus that is more likely to occur with intracavitary or submucosal leiomyomata.

Other factors also exist that can affect fertilization and pregnancy. Endometriosis occurs when endometrial tissue is found outside the uterus. These tissue implants can occur in multiple areas, including the abdomen, bowel, bladder, fallopian tubes, ovaries, the outer surface of the uterus, the cervix, and more rarely in distant organs such as the lungs. Endometriosis is more common in infertile patients and may compromise fertility in a number of ways. The endometrial tissue can irritate surrounding organs and cause the development of adhesions and scar tissue. In addition, direct damage to ovarian tissue can occur from endometrial implants or subsequent surgical removal. Cytokines and cellular growth factors produced by endometrial implants can also interfere with ovulation, fertilization, or oocyte implantation.

Fertility may also be affected by cervical stenosis, which can be a congenital condition or may occur after trauma or infection, with subsequent scarring. Cervical stenosis and alterations in cervical mucus may impair the entry of sperm into the uterus. Problems can also occur after implantation of the fertilized oocyte. If development of the corpus luteum is impaired, inadequate progesterone production can occur and delay endometrial maturation. Alternatively, despite the presence of adequate progesterone, the endometrium may not be adequately responsive to this hormone. However, the significance of luteal phase defects as a direct cause of infertility is not well understood.

Systemic factors also exist that affect the ability to initiate or maintain pregnancy. Hypercoagulable states such as antiphospholipid antibody syndrome, systemic lupus erythematosus, and other autoimmune and connective tissue disorders are known to be associated with early first-trimester miscarriages, which are most likely due to immunological rejection of the developing embryo or microthrombosis of placental vessels, leading to placental insufficiency. Genetic defects have been associated with infertility in males and females, the most common being Turner's syndrome (karyotype: 45 chromosomes, XO) in females and Klinefelter's syndrome (karyotype: 47 chromosomes, XXY) in males. Other genes and gene products capable of affecting fertility if mutated include *KAL1* (Kallmann's syndrome), which leads to congenital hypothalamic hypopituitary hypogonadism, fragile X syndrome, gonadotropin-releasing hormone (GnRH) receptor, follicle-stimulating hormone (FSH) receptor, *DAX1, FGFR1,* and *GPR54.*

In males, primary hypogonadism is the most common identifiable cause of infertility. In addition, infertility may be a result of congenital disorders (including chromosomal disorders such as Klinefelter's syndrome and fragile X syndrome), azoospermia from cryptorchidism (failure of testicular descent from the abdominal cavity during in utero development), defects in androgen production (e.g., 5-α-reductase deficiency) or receptor activity, as well as Y chromosome deletions, especially in the long arm at the Yq6 region. Acquired disorders such as testicular infection (e.g., viral orchitis from the mumps paramyxovirus, echovirus, or arbovirus), drugs toxic to sperm (e.g., alkylating immunosuppressants such as cyclophosphamide, antiandrogens such as spironolactone, ketoconazole), radiation exposure, tobacco smoking, and hyperthermia have all been associated with decreased male fertility, as well as underlying systemic disease such as chronic renal insufficiency and cirrhosis. Antisperm antibodies have also been identified in some infertile males that presumably affect fertility, but it is unclear whether these antibodies form spontaneously or as a result of testicular injury that compromises the testicular–blood barrier. Antisperm antibodies of the IgE class have also been identified in females that can lead to allergic reactions and subsequent infertility.

Disorders affecting the hypothalamic-pituitary-gonadal axis may also affect fertility. A failure of hypothalamic GnRH secretion and/or pituitary gonadotropin production may result from congenital defects (e.g., Kallmann's syndrome) or acquired conditions, such as secreting or nonsecreting pituitary macroadenomas, prolactinomas, craniopharyngiomas, or infiltrative processes such as sarcoidosis, histiocytosis, or tuberculosis.

Sperm transport may be inhibited anywhere along the male reproductive tract, either directly via functional effects on the spermatozoa or due to physical obstruction. Intrauterine exposure of male fetuses to estrogen may lead to epidydimal developmental defects. In adults, infection (e.g., epididymitis caused by *Neisseria gonorrhoeae, Chlamydia trachomatis,* or tuberculosis) and certain chemical toxins (e.g., chlorohydrin) may affect spermatozoa function within the epididymis. The vas deferens may similarly be affected by infection, intentional ligation (surgical vasectomy), inspissation of mucoid secretions (Young's syndrome), or congenital absence due to defects in cAMP-regulated chloride ion channels (cystic fibrosis).

Erectile dysfunction and ineffective ejaculation may result from spinal cord damage, neurological disease, or defects in autonomic function caused by diabetes mellitus. Although secretions from the prostate and seminal vesicles contain several components (e.g., fructose) that contribute to sperm viability and motility, defects in glandular secretion have not been causally related to infertility. Varicoceles (venous dilation of the pampiniform plexus proximal to the testicle) are also more common in infertile males, but they may also be present in males with normal fertility. Although no definitive evidence exists, varicoceles are thought to impair spermatogenesis via increased testicular temperature, hypoxia, or vascular stasis with delayed clearance of serum metabolites that are toxic to sperm.

CLINICAL PRESENTATION

Subjective

The typical presentation of infertility involves patient(s) presenting to the primary care provider with the complaint of an inability to become pregnant, despite the desire to have a child. The assessment of people seeking evaluation and treatment of infertility should begin with a comprehensive history. A detailed medical, social, and family history should be obtained from the patient(s), as well as a thorough review of systems. In some cases, the history alone will reveal the etiology. The history should include information about diet; exercise; occupation; presence of stress or depression; allergies; past illnesses, injuries, and surgeries; current medications; use of illicit drugs; and exposure to radiation, chemotherapy, or toxic environmental substances such as pesticides, lead, iron, zinc, or copper.

The duration of infertility and whether it is primary or secondary should be determined in the patient(s). In females, the onset of menses and characteristics of the menstrual cycle; presence of premenstrual symptoms; prior use of contraception; frequency and timing of sexual intercourse; sexual history; characteristics of any vaginal discharge; and history of cervicitis, pelvic infections, surgery, and trauma should be obtained. Relevant information to obtain from male patients includes a history of mumps, orchitis, trauma, diabetes mellitus, herniorrhaphy, use of anabolic steroids, and problems with urination or libido. Males should also be questioned about exposure to heat (e.g., from ambient temperatures or tight clothing). Finally, although diethylstilbestrol (DES) has not been used in the United States since 1978, both individuals should still be queried about maternal use during pregnancy, because intrauterine exposure can affect fertility.

Objective

Patients should have a complete physical examination that includes body habitus, body mass index (BMI), fat distribution, and identification of characteristics that may suggest developmental delays, genetic abnormalities, or androgen excess. Female patients should have a pelvic examination that includes inspection of the external genitalia, vagina, and cervix, as well as palpation of the uterus and adnexa. The male examination should include inspection of the external genitalia, evaluation of the scrotum for varicocele or hernia, and measurement of testicular size to determine decreased volume (less than 15 mL in an adult male is considered abnormal) and testicular length (less than 3.6 cm in an adult male is considered abnormal).

DIAGNOSTIC REASONING

Diagnostic Tests

Infertility testing can be costly, time-consuming, and emotionally distressing, as diagnostic testing ranges from simple to complex. Table 47.1 outlines fertility tests and results that determine capability of reproduction. Testing should always follow a comprehensive history and physical examination. The patient should understand when ovulation occurs (typically 12 to 14 days before the start of the next period), the signs of ovulation, and the most effective times for intercourse. Data should be obtained to confirm the timing of intercourse and the length of time a patient has been having unprotected intercourse.

In female patients, a basic test of ovulatory function can be done by serial measurements of BBT, which can aid in identifying follicular, ovulatory, and luteal phase abnormalities. With additional documentation of coitus, serial BBT charts can help identify when ovulation is likely to occur and if intercourse is occurring at the ideal time to achieve pregnancy. One proposed schedule for intercourse based on serial BBT charts is every other day beginning 3 to 4 days before and continuing for 2 to 3 days after the expected time of ovulation.

In males, semen analysis is the single most important diagnostic study and should be done early in the evaluation and always before invasive testing of a female partner. The most important parameters in semen analysis are sperm concentration (count), motility, and morphology. A normal sperm count is between 40 and 300 million/mL of semen, and according to the ASRM, a sperm count under 15 million/mL indicates infertility. The normal range for total motility (i.e., proportion of motile spermatozoa) is 40%, and at least 25% of spermatozoa must demonstrate progressive forward mobility. Morphology is the size and shape of sperm, and between 4% and 14% of spermatozoa must have a normal appearance to be considered adequate. Low sperm counts, decreased mobility, and low normal morphology may all adversely impact fertility. Semen pH is also important, as a low semen pH is correlated with decreased fertility.

Cellular debris and agglutination are of concern for antibody-mediated autoimmune destruction of sperm. Antibodies may be detected and are considered concerning if they coat more than 50% of spermatozoa. The presence of immature germ cells may represent a maturation defect, and the presence of leukocytes in ejaculate (greater than 1 million/mL of semen) reflects infection within the reproductive tract. Although a semen culture is often performed, it is usually not diagnostically useful.

It is important to note that an absence of sperm may also be due to spermatic duct obstruction, rather than a lack of sperm production by the testes. Patients lacking sperm in the semen should be referred to urology to rule out retrograde ejaculation, congenital absence of the vas deferens, or other forms of obstruction. A postejaculatory urine specimen will reflect retrograde ejaculation if sperm is present, whereas an absence of sperm may reflect obstruction or impaired spermatogenesis. Evaluation of the male partner may include at least two semen analyses to confirm or rule out a seminal deficiency.

The female infertility evaluation also includes assessing the hypothalamic-pituitary axis to determine ovulatory function. Progesterone levels are measured at different

TABLE 47.1 Fertility Tests and Favorable Clinical Findings

Gender	Test	How Obtained	Favorable Clinical Findings
Male	Semen analysis	48–72 hours after abstinence from ejaculation	Normal amount of ejaculate (3–5 mL; range 1–7 mL) No agglutination of sperm (agglutination suggests infection or autoimmunity) Normal seminal fluid Sperm count greater than 20,000,000 cells/mL with at least 50% motility 2 hours after ejaculation and more than 60% normal-appearing spermatozoa
	Karyotyping (in males with severe oligospermia or azoospermia)	Blood/bone marrow sample	Chromosomal abnormalities not detected
Female	Basal body temperature measurement	Oral temperature taken daily before arising, throughout several menstrual cycles	Biphasic pattern with persistent temperature elevation for 12–14 days before menses
	Postcoital mucus test	Vaginal examination within 8 hours after unprotected intercourse, during time of presumed ovulation	Cervical mucus suggestive of ovulation Microscopic ferning pattern present Watery, slippery, abundant mucus Spinnbarkeit is present, suggesting normal mucosal consistency (the act of pulling out a string of cervical mucus and measuring how far it can be stretched before breaking). Presence of normal live and motile sperm in cervical mucus
	Serum progesterone measurement	Blood sample	3–4 ng/mL in early luteal phase 10 ng/mL at midluteal phase
	Serum luteinizing hormone (to predict ovulation)	Blood sample	6.17–17.2 IU/L at ovulation
	Karyotyping (in patients with ovarian failure or repeated spontaneous abortions)	Blood sample/bone marrow	Chromosomal abnormalities not detected Evidence of normal pelvic anatomy and tubal functioning
	Immunoassay tests	Semen and male/female serum	Absence of sperm-specific antibody reaction
	Hysterosalpingogram	Dye injected through cervix into uterus, followed by fluoroscopic visualization of the spread of dye through fallopian tubes; done during first half of menstrual cycle before ovulation	Patency of fallopian tubes and absence of abnormalities in uterine cavity and fallopian tubes
	Laparoscopy	Direct visualization of pelvic structures via insertion of fiberoptic camera through a small abdominal incision	Normal pelvic structures and absence of signs of infection, adhesions, endometriosis, or lesions

points during the luteal phase to confirm ovulation. Elevated levels of progesterone are noted when ovulation has occurred. In addition, luteinizing hormone (LH) levels can be measured in the serum and with home urine tests to help predict ovulation. A normal surge should occur 1 to 2 days before ovulation, which can help determine the optimal timing of intercourse. Home urine tests have an 85% sensitivity rate but are not as sensitive as serum testing that is done during a formal fertility evaluation. Due to variations in renal clearance of LH, urine testing may not detect the LH surge.

Examination of vaginal discharge for increased volume and clear, slippery mucus that stretches into strings (spinnbarkeit) is a strong indicator of a preovulatory estrogen effect. The progesterone challenge test, in which medroxyprogesterone acetate 10 mg is given daily for

5 days and the induction of uterine bleeding is monitored in the week after treatment, confirms adequate production of estradiol (estrogen). An FSH level should be drawn on day 3 of the cycle to check for adequate ovarian reserve, as this hormone will be elevated in the setting of decreased ovarian hormone production; in turn, a value of less than 15 IU/mL is suggestive of adequate ovarian reserve. A prolactin level should also be checked with amenorrhea and/or galactorrhea to rule out hyperprolactinemia and/or the presence of a prolactinoma. Hyperprolactinemia can be treated with a dopamine agonist, such as bromocriptine, pergolide, or cabergoline.

The endocrinological evaluation of male patients includes serum LH, FSH, and testosterone levels. Elevated LH and FSH levels and a low testosterone level are consistent with primary hypogonadism, whereas normal to low LH and FSH reflect secondary hypogonadism. In male patients with low testosterone and normal to low LH levels, prolactin should be measured to rule out a prolactinoma.

If the results of both the male and female infertility work-ups are negative, further evaluation may be necessary. Magnetic resonance imaging (MRI) and a hysterosalpingogram (fluoroscopic radiographic imaging) are done to evaluate the structure and function of the cervix, uterus, fallopian tubes, and ovaries. Laparoscopy is more sensitive for detecting tubal abnormalities than hysterosalpingogram alone; however, the performance of the hysterosalpingogram itself (flushing the fallopian tubes with oil-based contrast medium) may improve tubal patency and increase the likelihood of future pregnancy.

MANAGEMENT

The goal of management is to assist the patient(s) in achieving pregnancy before or during the natural age-related decline in female fertility. Several lifestyle changes can increase the chances of pregnancy. Female patients should limit caffeine intake to no more than 250 mg (e.g., two cups of coffee) per day. Studies show that consumption of more than 300 mg caffeine daily can delay pregnancy and increase the risk for miscarriage and preterm labor. Caffeine intake in males does not seem to affect fertility. Likewise, alcohol affects fertility in females, and intake should be limited to no more than four drinks per week. Increasing sexual intercourse to two to three times a week is also advisable. These measures should be recommended before any other interventions.

If the patient's BMI is less than 20 kg/m^2 or greater than 27 kg/m^2, attempts should be made to achieve an ideal body weight and BMI within this range. Loss of 5% to 10% of body weight in obese, anovulatory patients with polycystic ovary disease (PCOS) can restore ovulation within 6 months and should be a first-line intervention. For patients with PCOS, in addition to weight loss, insulin-sensitizing drugs such as metformin have been shown to improve fertility. A low percentage of body fat resulting from eating disorders (e.g., anorexia nervosa, bulimia) or from extreme exercise can lead to anovulation through GnRH or gonadotropin suppression and must be addressed; pulsatile GnRH therapy may restore ovulation in patients with these conditions.

If an ovulatory defect has been identified during fertility testing, treatment depends on the specific cause of the problem. In 70% to 85% of cases, the ovaries and prolactin level are normal, and the pituitary gland is intact. This type of anovulation is called *normogonadotropic, normoestrogenic anovulation* (i.e., World Health Organization class 2 anovulation). In these patients, clomiphene citrate (Clomid), a selective estrogen receptor modulator (SERM) with both agonist and antagonist effects on the estrogen receptor, may effectively induce ovulation. Ovulation occurs in up to 80% of properly selected patients, and pregnancy rates approach 40%. The risk of multiple gestation with clomiphene is 5% and manifests almost exclusively as twins. Of note, clomiphene citrate has also been shown to improve semen parameters in male patients with infertility.

Dosing includes a 50-mg dose of clomiphene daily on days 5 through 9 of a patient's menstrual cycle. Ovulation can be expected to occur 5 to 10 days after the last dose. If ovulation is not achieved during the first cycle of therapy, the dose may be increased in 50-mg increments to a maximum of 200 to 250 mg daily for 5 days. After the first treatment cycle, a pelvic examination should be done to rule out ovarian enlargement or hyperstimulation. Ovarian enlargement and abdominal discomfort may result from follicular growth and the formation of multiple corpus lutea. Other adverse effects include hot flashes, nausea and vomiting, vision problems, headache, and dryness or loss of hair. Clomiphene citrate should not be used for more than six cycles because it is unlikely to work after that many attempts.

Tamoxifen is another SERM that works with fewer antiestrogen effects, but it has no added fertility benefit over clomiphene citrate. Aromatase inhibitors such as letrozole (Femara) and anastrozole (Arimidex) have shorter half-lives than the SERMs and fewer antiestrogen effects, producing fewer follicles and lower estradiol levels, reducing the risk of multiple gestation and miscarriage. These agents may be used for patients who do not respond to clomiphene.

Patients who have not had success with SERMs or aromatase inhibitors may respond to ovarian stimulation with injectable gonadotropins. This treatment requires much closer monitoring, and it has a higher cost and a higher risk of multiple gestation; it is, however, considered the most effective medication to use with intrauterine insemination. Intrauterine insemination (IUI) just before ovulation (based on LH measurements) is often effective when other methods have failed. IUI may be tried before IVF because it is often effective and less expensive than IVF. IUI done high in the uterus is more effective than intracervical injection, which approximates normal intercourse. With high IUI, the probability of pregnancy is improved through concurrent treatment with clomiphene for three to six cycles, and if this fails, IUI with gonadotropin injections for at least three cycles can be tried.

The most technically complex and typically final options for infertility are assisted reproductive technologies (ART), which include IVF and embryo transfer or, if the fallopian tubes are patent and normal, gamete intrafallopian transfer (GIFT) or zygote intrafallopian transfer (ZIFT). GIFT and ZIFT are done in less than 1% of cases. In some cases of tubal occlusion (e.g., patients with a low success rate of tubal repair of less than 30%), IVF appears to be preferable to surgery because of the more rapid pregnancy rate. IVF has the highest pregnancy rate in the shortest amount of time, but it is also the costliest intervention at $50,000 to $100,000 per attempt. Some studies show an improvement in success rates with intratubal transfer of embryos over transcervical transfer, although this finding is inconsistent. The Society for Assisted Reproductive Technology has Internet resources with valuable information for both providers and patients.

The pregnancy rate with IVF varies significantly between fertility clinics due to the complexity of the techniques required, whereas the pregnancy rate with GIFT is more consistent. The mean live delivery rates per egg retrieval cycle with IVF and GIFT are approximately 21% and 28%, respectively. Ectopic pregnancy occurs in about 4% to 5% of these pregnancies, whereas the rate of fetal abnormalities is slightly increased with a relative risk of 1.32 (95% confidence interval).

It is also possible to achieve pregnancy with IVF, donor sperm and embryo transfer using donor eggs, with a higher success rate than with regular IVF and embryo transfer (47% per retrieval). The eggs generally come from young fertile females (e.g., sisters of the recipient or anonymous volunteer donors). The recipient's uterus can be prepared for optimal uterine receptivity by replacement doses of estradiol and progesterone. There are many ethical considerations associated with ART, some of which are presented in Box 47.1.

Less frequently used is a procedure done during a laparoscopy called *ovarian drilling*. The procedure is performed in patients who have PCOS and have failed to ovulate with metformin or clomiphene. During laparoscopy, a laser or electrosurgical needle is used to puncture the ovary several times. This procedure may help patients respond better to clomiphene. Cervical stenosis can be treated with catheter dilation of the cervix for several days and concurrent antibiotic prophylaxis (doxycycline 100 mg by mouth [PO] twice daily). Patients with systemic clotting disorders may also benefit from aspirin and heparin anticoagulation therapy to improve the likelihood of pregnancy and decrease the chance of pregnancy loss.

Male infertility from hypogonadotropic hypogonadism may be treated with human choroinic gonadotropin (hCG) injections 1500 to 2000 IU administered

Box 47.1 Ethical Considerations of Assisted Reproductive Technologies

In vitro fertilization (IVF) has been a welcome solution for many patients who have been unable to achieve pregnancy. Recently, advances in the application of IVF technology have spurred the emergence of even more new avenues of achieving pregnancy and parenting. With hormone therapy and donor egg embryos, patients past menopause can achieve pregnancy. Other options include cryopreservation, fertilization of donor gametes (donor eggs, sperm, or both), IVF with the use of a gestational carrier, embryo adoption, and the use of surrogacy. All of these options are complicated by the introduction of a third party into the reproductive process and by ethical considerations. Some of the issues raised in connection with these techniques include the following:

1. Is it a constitutional right for individuals or couples to be able to use donor gametes or to contract with a surrogate to carry their embryo to treat their infertility?
2. With a multiple pregnancy rate approaching 20% in patients undergoing IVF procedures, the potential (less than 3%) of having a grand multiple gestation forces some to consider embryo reduction (selective abortion) to avoid an adverse obstetric and/or fetal outcome.
3. If excess embryos are frozen for storage, how long can and should they be stored? What should be done in cases of death of patient(s), divorce, or when patients choose not to claim their embryos?
4. Do providers have the right to decide who can participate in using donor gametes, embryos, gestational carriers, and surrogates? What about single patients, homosexual couples, or donor arrangements crossing generational lines (e.g., a daughter being a donor for a mother)?
5. Does the use of assisted reproductive technologies take into consideration the best interests of all parties involved, including those of the resultant offspring? For example, what are the effects on a child of knowing or not knowing the identity of one or more gamete donors?
6. How can the potential for consanguinity (having a close ancestor in common) be controlled in the case of gamete and/or embryo donation?
7. Does the existence of new technologies make it more difficult to accept childlessness by increasing pressure on patients to follow every avenue in an attempt to reproduce?
8. To what extent should health insurance policies cover these modes of treating infertility at a time of growing health-care costs?

subcutaneously or IM three times per week for at least 6 months. hCG acts similarly to LH. If this treatment does not work, human menopausal gonadotropin 37.5 to 75 IU three times per week is added that contains FSH. In turn, this treatment can last more than a year. This combination therapy is typically needed for Kallmann's syndrome (congenital hypogonadotropic hypogonadism).

Recombinant LH/FSH is also available. Pulsatile GnRH treatment delivered via IV pump is also available for hypothalamic hypogonadotropic hypogonadism.

Sperm autoimmunity may be treated in the male partner with high-dose corticosteroids (prednisone 40 to 80 mg PO daily) for up to 6 months, but this regimen may be poorly tolerated. Thus, intracytoplasmic sperm injection (ICSI) is an important IVF alternative with a clinical pregnancy rate of up to 20%. Retrograde ejaculation may be treated with IUI, traditional IVF, or ICSI as well. Repair of varicoceles to increase fertility is controversial and is usually recommended only with large defects or in younger males, because prolonged damage to the testes—indicated by testicular atrophy, epithelial damage, and severe oligospermia or azoospermia—is unlikely to be reversed by surgical ligation of the varicocele. Reversal of male vasectomy can result in successful pregnancy in a female partner in up to 50% of cases. In cases of obstruction along the reproductive tract, sperm may be retrieved for ICSI via direct microsurgical aspiration from the epididymis or the seminiferous tubules of the testes. In all cases of congenital reproductive tract defects, such as an absent vas deferens, genetic counseling is required before microsurgical aspiration and ICSI, given the risk of passing genetic defects, such as the cystic fibrosis gene, Klinefelter's syndrome (an extra X chromosome in males), or deletions in the Y chromosome, onto these individuals' offspring.

FOLLOW-UP AND REFERRAL

After a thorough examination and counseling regarding the frequency and timing of intercourse, patients who wish to proceed with testing and/or treatment need to be referred to a reproductive endocrinologist or clinic that specializes in infertility, and this is usually done after a year of unprotected intercourse. Infertile patients need a great deal of support and advocacy, as well as education and assistance in decision making. However, options must be presented in a nonjudgmental way to facilitate patients' own decision making. Providing anticipatory guidance for the battery of diagnostic tests to which patients are subjected during infertility evaluation is critical. Providing referral to other sources of assistance is another way in which the clinician supports the infertile person or couple. One important source of information is RESOLVE, a national organization composed of self-help groups that provide support and information about infertility.

Patient Education: Infertility

An important component of care for infertile people is emphasizing and teaching self-care. Patients who experience infertility often describe feeling a loss of control over their lives. Identifying and using successful coping strategies help the patient regain this sense of control. Stress-reduction techniques, such as exercise, relaxation techniques, and meditation, may be especially useful both for those with general concerns about fertility and for those concerned over specific diagnostic or treatment procedures. Infertility can become an all-encompassing concern, resulting in alterations in health and recreation patterns and a loss of interest in other aspects of life. It should be emphasized that one can be creative, productive, and successful in other areas of life even if unable to produce children. In addition, other options such as adoption can also be discussed as viable options for raising children and expanding one's family. The emotional issues surrounding infertility illustrate the need for an emphasis on family-centered care, because infertility has far-reaching implications for many family members.

PREMENSTRUAL SYNDROME AND PREMENSTRUAL DYSPHORIC DISORDER

Premenstrual syndrome (PMS) and premenstrual dysphoric disorder (PMDD) occur during the luteal phase of the menstrual cycle. Symptoms may be mild and cause little disruption in daily life; moderate, causing interference in some aspects of life; or severe, resulting in symptoms that significantly impair a patient's ability for daily activities and impact the patient's life, work, and relationships.

PMS is defined as a cyclical recurrence of a constellation of physical and psychological symptoms that arise during the second, or luteal, phase of the menstrual cycle and resolve 1 to 3 days after the onset of menses. The most common symptoms of mild PMS are headache, bloating, breast tenderness, and irritability. Both somatic symptoms (e.g., depression, angry outbursts) and physical symptoms (e.g., breast pain, bloating) are present in patients with PMS. Although the severity may vary each month, the symptoms are generally mild, of short duration, and manageable. If symptoms related to the luteal phase lead to economic or social dysfunction (e.g., work absenteeism, decreased work productivity, relationship problems) and have occurred for at least three consecutive cycles, a diagnosis of PMS can be made.

In contrast, PMDD is a severe mood disorder where patients experience symptoms during most of their menstrual cycles. In addition, the symptoms cause significant distress and interfere with usual activities and quality of life. Other symptoms include mood swings, sudden sadness, anger, irritability, depressed mood, tension, anxiety, difficulty concentrating, food cravings, loss of interest in usual activities, low energy, feeling overwhelmed, breast tenderness, bloating, weight gain, joint pain, and alterations in sleep (see Box 47.2).

> **Box 47.2 Common Symptoms of Premenstrual Syndrome**
>
> **Core Symptoms**
> - Irritability, anger
> - Tension, anxiety
> - Dysphoria, depression
> - Labile mood, mood swings
>
> **Other Symptoms**
> - Headache
> - Food craving
> - Anger
> - Backaches
> - Tender breasts
> - Clumsiness
> - Crying
> - Dizziness
> - Feeling faint
> - Fatigue
> - Fluid retention
> - Forgetfulness
> - Bloating
> - Hostility
> - Joint swelling
> - Confusion
> - Migraine

EPIDEMIOLOGY AND CAUSES

PMS is a common problem. During the reproductive years, up to 75% of females will experience minor physical and emotional symptoms for 1 to 2 days before the onset of menses. Between 20% and 40% of females will experience clinically significant PMS, and 5% to 8% of females will experience symptoms that severely disrupt their daily lives and meet criteria for a diagnosis of PMDD. PMS and PMDD can affect individuals across the full range of reproductive years, and there do not appear to be significant geographical, ethnic, or cultural differences or predispositions. Family history appears to be a risk factor for the development of PMS, and social and environmental factors such as lower levels of education and smoking are also implicated.

Lifestyle habits, including nutrition and stress, are related to PMS as the possibility of physical influence. Although no association between cyclical hormone changes and PMS has been found, it has been suggested that some patients may have an abnormal response to normal cyclical hormonal changes. Cyclical changes in levels of estrogen and progesterone appear to impact levels of the neurotransmitter serotonin, and treatment with selective serotonin reuptake inhibitors (SSRIs) has been an effective treatment option. In addition, patients with a personal history of anxiety or depression also appear to have an increased risk of developing PMDD.

PATHOPHYSIOLOGY

The influence of cyclical ovarian hormones on various neurotransmitters capable of influencing mood and emotional state has been documented, including β-endorphins and γ-aminobutyric acid (GABA). In fact, there is a lower concentration of the progesterone metabolite allopregnanolone, which potentiates GABA receptor function, in patients experiencing PMS. However, the majority of evidence supports a deficiency in the tryptophan-derived neurotransmitter serotonin as the primary factor in the pathogenesis of PMS. Serum serotonin levels and serotonin uptake by platelets are both reduced during the luteal phase of the menstrual cycle in patients with PMS. Moreover, the serotonin agonist fenfluramine and SSRIs both improve PMS symptoms, whereas tryptophan depletion and the serotonin antagonist metergoline both worsen the syndrome.

Fluctuations in ovarian steroids are believed to underlie these abnormalities in neurotransmitter levels, as demonstrated by the efficacy of GnRH treatments (e.g., leuprolide) that suppress ovarian hormones and relieve the symptoms of PMS. Interestingly, the concentrations of serum estrogen and progesterone do not differ between patients experiencing PMS and controls; thus, it is the cyclical nature of the sex hormones and the individual response to hormonal changes that appear to be key.

Several subcategories of PMS have been suggested, which are synonymously termed categories of premenstrual tension (PMT). PMT-A is categorized by the symptoms of anxiety, irritability, and nervous tension. PMT-B is categorized by fluid retention, abdominal bloating, mastalgia, and weight gain. PMT-C is categorized by premenstrual cravings for sweets, increased appetite, and food binges. PMT-D is categorized by depression, withdrawal, insomnia, forgetfulness, and confusion. Although these categories have some overlap, they may be helpful in differentiating severity of PMS and focusing on where to target interventions.

CLINICAL PRESENTATION

Subjective

A thorough medical, social, sexual, reproductive, and family history should be completed for all patients presenting with PMS symptoms. It is important to ask about family history of PMS or PMDD, personal history of depression or anxiety, and current symptoms including duration and severity. Patients should also be asked about dietary habits, drug and alcohol consumption, exercise, and social and occupational history. Increased age and parity may increase the possibility of PMS and are therefore important factors to consider when assessing for symptoms that are associated with PMS.

A 3-month symptom diary that includes the severity and timing of symptoms in relation to menses should be completed by the patient. The diary should also include treatments the patient has tried and the effect of these treatments on symptoms. In addition, notation should be made of the effects the patient's PMS symptoms have had on family members and colleagues. The patient may also find this diary to be a useful tool when exploring expectations concerning evaluation and therapy.

The examination of a patient presenting with PMS symptoms should include a neurological examination and screenings for depression and anxiety. Premenstrual cognitive symptoms that may be reported include crying spells, depression, hostility, anxiety, irritability, relationship conflicts, feelings of inadequacy, increased or decreased libido, and an inability to cope with ever recurring symptoms. These symptoms often persist for years, and patients tend to delay seeking help from a health-care professional until adverse events are linked with these alterations in mood. This delay in seeking help could come from a fear of being labeled a hypochondriac or mentally unstable. A recent crisis, threat, or ultimatum from a significant other may precipitate a perceived need for professional help, and often patients seek help out of a sense of desperation.

Other changes perceived as "positive" have been reported by patients during the premenstrual period, including increased libido, more energy, more creative ideas, and increased ability to accomplish tasks. Although patients most often initially present with physical symptoms, mood alterations are the most incapacitating and distressing.

Premenstrual symptoms occur in one of four cyclical patterns that can be discerned from a detailed patient symptom diary:

1. Symptoms appear at midcycle, disappear, and then reappear the week before menstruation.
2. Symptoms begin at midcycle, with subtle changes that gradually escalate until menses.
3. Symptoms appear the week before menses and intensify until menstruation ensues.
4. Symptoms appear in the first or second luteal weeks and do not disappear until the end of menstruation.

Objective

Multiple physical signs and symptoms may be reported ranging from mild to severe and may vary from month to month. The following is a list of reported signs and symptoms organized by bodily system:

- Gastrointestinal (GI): abdominal bloating (occurring in 90% of patients), nausea, vomiting, constipation, increased thirst
- Respiratory: colds, hoarseness, rhinitis, asthma, sinusitis, sore throat
- Urological: oliguria, urethritis, cystitis
- Ophthalmological: conjunctivitis, vision changes, glaucoma, eye infection
- Mammalogical: breast tenderness (in more than 50% of patients), swelling, heaviness
- Dermatological: acne, boils, urticaria, spot bruising, recurrence of herpes
- Neurological: headaches/migraines (in more than 50% of patients), aggravation of epilepsy, vertigo, syncope, fainting, paresthesia of the hands or feet
- Musculoskeletal: backache, joint pain, edema of extremities
- Constitutional: fatigue (affecting more than 90% of patients), weight gain
- Miscellaneous: palpitations, pelvic or lower abdominal pain, cold sweats, hot flashes, food cravings, compulsive eating

DIAGNOSTIC REASONING

Diagnostic Tests

The most commonly accepted method to diagnose PMS uses a diary during at least two menstrual cycles (three is preferred). If the intensity of symptoms increases at least 30% in the 6 days before the onset of menses (compared with days 5 to 10 of the cycle) and if the symptoms occur in two consecutive months, the patient is likely experiencing PMS. This is a rather subjective method of diagnosis because patients are asked to assess the percentage of increase in symptoms subjectively, and there is no objective means of comparison with other patients. Once symptoms are determined to be associated with the luteal phase of the menstrual cycle and the abatement of symptoms is noted to occur during other parts of the cycle, a presumptive diagnosis of PMS can be made.

A complete physical examination, including a gynecological examination, is necessary to assess the health of patients with PMS symptoms. This will enable the provider to rule out other possible causes of the symptoms. Diagnostic tests that may be useful in eliminating other illnesses as possible etiologies include a complete blood count, urinalysis, and blood glucose assessment, as well as thyroid-stimulating hormone, FSH, and prolactin levels. Depression and anxiety scales are also important assessment tools and should be used routinely when evaluating a patient for PMS. These help the practitioner rule out depression during the follicular stage of the menstrual cycle versus objectively associating mood and depressive symptoms with the luteal phase of the menstrual cycle.

Differential Diagnosis

One of the most important assessment parameters in making a diagnosis of PMS is that symptoms occur only during the postovulatory luteal phase of the menstrual cycle. If symptoms appear during the preovulatory follicular phase, this may reflect a mood or anxiety disorder. It is important to note that there is a lifetime incidence of psychiatric disorders, especially depression, of nearly 80% of patients diagnosed with PMS. Differential diagnoses include cyclothymic disorder; a dysfunctional marital/intimate partner situation; depression; bipolar disorder; menopausal transition; poor diet; endocrine abnormalities (e.g., hypoglycemia, diabetes mellitus, hypothyroidism, hyperprolactinemia, hyperandrogenism); alcoholism and drug abuse; and tumors of the brain, breast, and ovaries. The possibility of these conditions should be clinically correlated and ruled out before making a definitive diagnosis of PMS. To avoid missing a diagnosis or providing the wrong diagnosis, the primary care practitioner should be wary of diagnosing PMS without sufficient evaluation for other potential conditions.

MANAGEMENT

The main principle of management is to assist the patient in developing strategies to gain control over symptoms, alleviate signs and symptoms as much as possible, and normalize the patient's life experience. Once an accurate diagnosis of PMS is made, appropriate interventions can be individualized. There are two principles to consider when developing a plan of care. First, PMS is a chronic disorder that may last until menopause. Second, patients have different symptoms and symptom severity and will respond differently to various treatments. Treatment plans should address the chronicity of the problem and provide management options that can be modified as needed. In addition, cognitive behavioral therapy (CBT) should be included for patients with mood disorders, depression, and negative thoughts about self and circumstances.

Lifestyle Changes

Lifestyle changes are considered a first-line treatment for PMS and PMDD and include dietary changes, regular aerobic exercise (which has been shown to decrease depression), and relaxation. Dietary interventions that have been identified as effective include a reduction in salt, sugar, alcohol, and caffeine, as well as an increase in complex carbohydrates. It is hypothesized that carbohydrates are involved in the serotonergic pathway, and an increase in serotonergic activity caused by increased complex carbohydrate consumption may help to relieve symptoms. In one trial, a cohort of patients was given a carbohydrate-rich beverage during the late luteal phase of the menstrual cycle, and a control group was given an isocaloric control beverage. The patients who drank the carbohydrate-rich beverage reported lower adverse mood symptom scores, whereas the control group reported no effect on mood.

Aerobic exercise can cause an increase in endorphin levels and, thereby, improve mood. Epidemiological studies comparing the severity of premenstrual symptoms in patients who exercise to those who do not have suggested that those who exercise have fewer symptoms. This is especially true for premenstrual depression. Moreover, it appears that the benefits are independent of the intensity of exercise; therefore, low levels of exercise intensity may also be beneficial. Relaxation techniques have also proven beneficial; activities as simple as sitting quietly for 20 minutes twice a day and deep breathing while listening to relaxing music have been shown to reduce mood symptoms of PMS twice as effectively as no active therapy.

Medications

Calcium and magnesium supplements have been shown to help control the emotional and physical symptoms of PMS. In several large clinical trials, 1,000 mg of calcium per day decreased all PMS symptoms as well as any other medication or treatment. Patients taking magnesium also experienced a reduction in total symptoms. This effect is thought to be due to the reversal of lower-than-average mononuclear blood cell magnesium concentrations in patients with PMS. Other dietary supplements including vitamin B_6, folic acid, and vitamin E have been explored, but studies are limited, or results are inconclusive. However, adverse effects of most vitamins used at recommended doses are minimal, and a daily supplement may be helpful in some patients.

Beyond mineral and vitamin supplementation, SSRIs such as fluoxetine, sertraline, paroxetine, and citalopram are considered first-line pharmacological treatment options and have demonstrated effectiveness in relieving tension, irritability, and dysphoria. The recommended starting daily doses of SSRIs are as follows: fluoxetine 20 mg, sertraline 25 to 150 mg, escitalopram 10 to 20 mg, paroxetine 10 to 20 mg, and citalopram 20 to 30 mg. These medications are relatively inexpensive and have minimal adverse effects overall. The most common adverse effects include nausea, headache, jitteriness, and a decrease in libido. Lowering the dose of the SSRI may eliminate some of these adverse effects. If a therapeutic response is not reached within several menstrual cycles at initial lower doses, the dose may be increased. Although SSRIs are generally administered daily, these drugs have been shown to be effective when administered only during the luteal phase, which has the advantage of lower treatment costs and minimizing adverse effects. Other antidepressants including clomipramine (a tricyclic antidepressant) and venlafaxine (a serotonin-norepinephrine reuptake inhibitor [SNRI]) have also been used. However, these medications have more adverse effects and are not recommended over SSRIs, as their effectiveness in PMS and PMDD has not been well established.

Benzodiazepines such as low-dose alprazolam have been used during the luteal phase in patients who fit the strict diagnostic criteria of PMDD and have not had symptom relief from SSRIs. However, the risk of drug dependence is high with benzodiazepines, and the International Society for Premenstrual Disorders does not consider benzodiazepines to be an evidence-based treatment for PMDD.

Combination estrogen-progesterone oral contraception is second-line treatment and should be considered before initiating treatment with GnRH agonists. When used continuously, ovulation is suppressed, which suppresses symptoms. Although it is commonly believed that combination OCPs help relieve PMS symptoms, research has shown that there is little difference in symptomatology in users and nonusers. The only regimen that has been shown to improve both physical and psychological symptoms of PMS and PMDD in randomized controlled trials is a combined OCP containing ethinyl estradiol 30 mcg with drospirenone. Patients should be screened for the risk of DVT before the initiation of OCP therapy.

Patients who do not respond to the preceding measures are candidates for a trial of ovulatory suppression therapy with danazol 200 to 800 mg daily. Danazol is a GnRH agonist and a nortestosterone hormone derivative with progestin-like effects that induces ovarian suppression. It works by continuously suppressing pituitary gonadotropin secretion of LH and FSH. It must be given continuously because pulsatile administration leads to LH and FSH secretion. When this therapy is used, "add back" hormonal treatment is also used to provide some of the hormones suppressed by the GnRH agonist, with estrogen and progestin given in low doses. Danazol has several undesirable adverse effects, such as weight gain, increased facial hair, and acne. For patients on GnRH agonist therapy, long-term alendronate is given to help prevent bone mineral density loss.

Fluid retention is commonly reported during the luteal phase of the menstrual cycle and accounts for some of the physical symptoms of PMS. Spironolactone 100 mg once daily during the luteal phase has been shown to significantly reduce physical and psychological symptoms of PMS versus placebo. With the use of spironolactone, participants reported improvement in irritability, depression, swelling, breast tenderness, and food cravings. Other classes of diuretics, such as thiazides, do not demonstrate effective reduction of PMS symptoms.

NSAIDs administered during the luteal phase significantly reduce the physical symptoms of PMS. Naproxen sodium 500 mg twice daily, started 1 week before the onset of menses and continued through the first few days of bleeding, is effective for both PMS symptoms and dysmenorrhea. This treatment is not recommended for patients with renal impairment, GI disorders, or inflammatory bowel disease. As with any NSAID, GI distress and bleeding may occur. Although they are not first-line therapy for patients with PMDD, NSAIDs may be beneficial for patients with moderate symptoms, especially if associated with dysmenorrhea, headaches, or musculoskeletal symptoms. NSAIDs are a relatively inexpensive and safe form of therapy for younger patients and may provide the help they need to function normally during this stage of the menstrual cycle.

Apart from medications, surgical oophorectomy is an option for patients who have failed to improve on GnRH agonist therapy for at least 6 months. This option is limited to patients who no longer desire pregnancy and would likely need therapy for several more years.

People have used many folk remedies and complementary therapies for centuries to treat menstrual symptoms with varying degrees of success. Complementary Therapies 47.1 presents some of these therapies for PMS and other health issues.

FOLLOW-UP AND REFERRAL

The first follow-up visit should be in 2 months to evaluate the data collected by the patient between visits to assess symptom patterns, enabling the diagnosis of PMS to be made and to begin treatment. Frequent visits may be required after that time to evaluate the effectiveness of treatments and encourage patients to continue to examine and develop treatment plans. Eventually, once symptoms have been controlled, yearly follow-up visits should be sufficient.

Referrals to a specialist may be required, depending on findings from diagnostic tests and the physical examination. The use of certain treatments for severe PMS, such as GnRH agents, is managed by a gynecologist. For patients with PMDD, referral to a mental health practitioner may be needed to manage CBT, SSRIs, and hormonal contraceptives.

Patient Education: Premenstrual Syndrome

It is important to listen to and evaluate the concerns of patients when they present with symptoms typically associated with PMS. PMS must not be identified with weakness on the part of the patient but rather recognized as a disease entity that must be investigated and treated. It may take time and energy to manage symptoms and help the patient maintain a good quality of life. When a patient is able to reduce the symptoms of PMS, whether severe or mild, it helps them to function at a higher level.

MENOPAUSE

According to the North American Menopause Society (NAMS), menopause is the permanent cessation of menses resulting from loss of ovarian follicular function. It is defined as the final menstrual period (FMP) and is reached when there have been 12 consecutive months of amenorrhea. Menopause most often occurs due to

Complementary Therapies 47.1: Female Health

PROBLEM	THERAPY	DOSAGE	COMMENTS
Premenstrual syndrome	Evening primrose oil	250 mg orally up to three times daily, 2–3 days before menses	May decrease breast tenderness. Common side effects include headache and gastrointestinal (GI) symptoms.
	Calcium	1,200–1,600 mg orally daily	May reduce luteal phase symptoms. Should be taken in divided doses and with recommended daily dose of vitamin D (400 IU daily).
	Vitamin B_6	40–100 mg orally daily	Common side effects include numbness, paresthesia, and unsteady gait. Patients with Parkinson's disease or taking levodopa should consult their provider before starting.
	Vitamin C	1,500–3,000 mg orally daily	Take in divided doses for better absorption and to avoid diarrhea.
	Essential oils: chamomile, basil, lavender, marjoram	Use as directed on label	Aromatherapy
Menopausal symptoms	Black cohosh	40–200 mg orally daily	Not recommended for more than 6 months
	Chaste tree berry	Extracts or tinctures to provide 20 mg of crude fruit or 30–40 mg of fruit decoction	Possible adverse GI effects; contraindicated in pregnancy
	Vitamin B complex	50 mg orally daily	High levels of estrogen related to hormone fluctuations can deplete vitamin B_6, resulting in anxiety, irritability, and depression.
	Vitamin C	1,500–3,000 mg orally daily	Take in divided doses for better absorption and to avoid diarrhea.
	Vitamin E	400–800 IU orally daily	Can interfere with anticoagulant therapy; avoid if taking anticoagulants; consult with provider before starting.
Breast tenderness	Chaste tree berry	As above	As above
	Evening primrose oil	As above	As above
Candidiasis (yeast infection)	Vitamin C	3,000–6,000 mg orally daily	Take in divided doses for better absorption and to avoid diarrhea.
Decreased sexual desire	Essential oils: jasmine, neroli (bitter orange tree), rose, sandalwood, ylang-ylang, clary sage, patchouli	Use as directed on label	Aromatherapy; aphrodisiac

aging and represents the permanent decline of sex hormone levels. In addition to aging, menopause can also be induced surgically (i.e., bilateral oophorectomy) or medically (e.g., due to chemotherapy or pelvic irradiation, rendering the ovaries nonfunctional) at any age.

The average age of menopause is 51.5 years, and 95% of patients will experience their FMP between the ages of 45 and 55 years. Perimenopause is the time period before menopause when hormonal, physical, and emotional changes occur and fertility begins to decline. The menopausal transition begins with the onset of changes in the menstrual cycle. This is known as the early menopausal transition and can precede menopause by several years. The late menopausal transition is recognized by the onset of vasomotor symptoms and a greater than 60-day interval between periods. The menopausal transition ends with the FMP. The postmenopausal period is the period of time after menopause.

Menopause is not a disease state, but it does signal permanent changes in the hormonal, emotional, and reproductive lives of patients. Some may experience an increased awareness of the significance of menopause. They may have philosophical and personal beliefs about managing menopause and treating their symptoms, and because, on average, 30 years of a patient's life will be lived after menopause, they may need help to understand menopause and age-related changes so that they can make informed decisions about how best to manage this stage of life. The management of menopause has received a great deal of attention in recent years. As the average life span for females lengthens—currently at 84 years—it is evident that menopause does not signal the end but rather the beginning of another phase of life recognized by its own issues, challenges, and opportunities.

EPIDEMIOLOGY AND CAUSES

Perimenopause includes three phases in a female patient's reproductive life span: the early and late menopausal transition; menopause (FMP); and the postmenopausal period (12 months after the FMP). The menopausal transition signals the nearing of menopause and can begin up to 10 years before the FMP, usually between the ages of 38 and 42 years. The onset may be abrupt or insidious. During this time, ovulation becomes less frequent, and the number of ovarian follicles is decreased, as they become less likely to mature. There may be a small increase in the level of FSH. The beginning of this phase is marked by persistent changes in the menstrual cycle, usually with shorter cycle length and/or increased menstrual bleeding. Immediately before menopause, in the late menopausal transition, menses may occur after a short luteal phase or after an estradiol peak without ovulation. In approximately 70% of patients, menses will then become lighter and occur less often until ceasing completely. Ten percent of patients will simply stop menstruating suddenly with few or no symptoms, and 20% will experience heavier and often unpredictable bleeding. FSH levels measured at this time will be greater than 25 IU/L. All patients who experience cessation of menses before age 40 years should be assessed for primary ovarian insufficiency. If the FSH level is greater than 40 IU/L, the patient should be referred to an endocrinologist for further evaluation.

In patients with heavy bleeding, there is risk for anemia, and other causes should be considered. In addition to menopause, abnormal uterine bleeding (AUB) in this age group can be caused by endometrial hyperplasia, cancer or polyps, uterine leiomyomata, or systemic clotting disorders.

PATHOPHYSIOLOGY

Menopause is the permanent cessation of menses and ovarian function. To fully understand menopause, knowledge of normal ovarian development is required. Oocyte development is characterized by germ cell differentiation and the formation of primordial ovarian follicles. This process begins during embryonic development, and at 20 weeks' gestation the fetus will have as many as 6 to 7 million oocytes. FSH drives this process by stimulating granulosa cell formation in ovarian follicles and inducing LH receptor formation, which will eventually allow for ovulation to occur later in life in response to surges in LH at the time of menarche. In a sexually mature ovulatory female, follicular release of an oocyte leads to transformation of the follicle into a corpus luteum cyst, which produces less estrogen and increasing amounts of progesterone that will subsequently support the uterine lining and facilitate implantation of the oocyte and maintenance of pregnancy.

Follicular atresia and oocyte destruction begin during late fetal development and are normal, continuous processes that occur until menopause. At birth, the number of oocytes will have decreased from its peak of 6 to 7 million to 1 to 2 million, and to approximately 300,000 at the onset of puberty. Animal and human studies have shown that reduction in oocyte number may be driven by reductions in FSH, decreased androgen production by ovarian thecal cells (reducing substrate for estrogen production via androgen aromatization), the upregulation of proapoptotic genes such as *Bax,* and the downregulation of antiapoptotic genes such as *bcl-2* in both oocytes (primarily a fetal process) and follicular granulosa cells (primarily in adults). Although follicular atresia occurs continuously throughout a patient's reproductive lifetime, it increases rapidly after 37 years of age.

The perimenopausal period, which is 2 to 8 years before and 1 year after the FMP, is characterized by waxing and waning of ovarian function, as reflected in both ovulatory and anovulatory (estrogen-only) menstrual cycles of unpredictable duration and intensity, extended periods of estrogen deficiency, and heightened FSH and LH secretion with occasional follicular development and estradiol production. Over time, estrogen feedback to the hypothalamic-pituitary axis declines. In some patients, estrogen positive feedback no longer leads to an LH surge capable of triggering ovulation, whereas in others, estrogen negative feedback fails to suppress LH production during the follicular phase. Moreover, the failure of the corpus luteum cysts after ovulation leads to a decrease in progesterone and increased exposure to unopposed estrogen, which accounts for the increase in AUB and endometrial hyperplasia observed during this period.

Factors that influence the timing of menopause have been the subject of much research. Whereas age at menarche has steadily declined over recent decades (having been linked to nutritional status, environmental factors, and general health), the average age at menopause has remained remarkably constant since ancient times. Today, several factors are known to lower the age at menopause, including smoking (which decreases the age of onset of menopause by 2 years on average), nulliparity, menstrual regularity and a shorter cycle length, a family history of early menopause, increased galactose (a monosaccharide component of lactose) intake, concurrent type 1 diabetes mellitus, and certain genetic variants in the estrogen receptor and galactose-1-phosphate uridyl transferase gene. Menopause occurring past age 55 years is defined as late menopause.

With the depletion of ovarian follicles that are able to respond to gonadotropins, both follicular development and cyclical estrogen production cease during menopause. FSH levels rise as the body tries unsuccessfully to stimulate follicular production of estrogen. FSH levels higher than 40 IU/mL signal the approach of menopause, even though occasional menstrual bleeding may still happen. LH concentration is also elevated, but menopausal levels are difficult to distinguish from LH elevations seen during preovulatory gonadotropin surges in the normal menstrual cycle. Persistently high LH levels lead to continued androgen production by ovarian thecal cells, namely androstenedione, contributing to some of the undesirable physical changes experienced by postmenopausal individuals such as increased facial hair. Biochemical studies have revealed that gonadotropins in older females have a longer half-life (contributing to their increased serum levels) and also contain higher levels of carbohydrates that tend to render them less biologically active. Moreover, although residual oocytes and differentiating follicles have been identified in postmenopausal patients, the follicles are typically atretic and eventually become cystic in the absence of viable oocytes.

Without a follicular source, circulating levels of estrogen fall significantly during menopause—particularly the active form estradiol, produced from the aromatization of testosterone. High gonadotropin levels stimulate the ovarian stroma to produce the less potent hormone estrone, rather than estradiol, while androstenedione produced by the adrenal glands is converted to estrone by aromatization in the periphery, particularly within adipose tissue, which contains significant levels of the aromatase enzyme. In addition, serum levels of the hormone inhibin B also decline, closely correlating to the rise in FSH, implying an inhibitory action of inhibin B on FSH. Estrone and androstenedione levels remain relatively constant as the patient ages, whereas testosterone levels decline.

Obese females with larger amounts of adipose tissue typically display higher levels of circulating estrogens; however, they are still subject to vasomotor symptoms triggered by estrogen deficiency. Patients who are thin tend to experience vaginal dryness and other symptoms associated with low estrogen levels, whereas obese patients are at greater risk of experiencing symptoms associated with unopposed estrogen, such as AUB, endometrial hyperplasia, and endometrial neoplasms. In turn, patients who do not experience the vasomotor symptoms of estrogen deficiency during menopause, such as hot flashes, should be monitored yearly for endometrial pathology with vaginal ultrasound and biopsy as appropriate.

CLINICAL PRESENTATION

Subjective

Most patients go through menopause without experiencing symptoms debilitating enough to seek medical attention but may report them during their annual gynecological examinations. Information gathered during the examination should include a medical, social, sexual, surgical, and family history. Several factors may influence the timing of menopause and should be noted in the health history: genetic abnormalities, family history, surgical removal of the ovaries or uterus, smoking, and history of chemotherapy or radiation treatments. Although removal of the ovaries results in immediate surgical menopause, sparing the ovaries during a hysterectomy may still hasten the cessation of follicle stimulation and ovulation by 1 to 2 years. Family history is significant as there is a similarity in menopausal age between mothers and daughters. Patients who smoke and those with chronic disease may experience earlier menopause, and menopause can be induced during and after chemotherapy and radiation treatment by virtue of their effects on ovarian function.

About 20% of patients will seek health-care attention for one or more symptoms related to menopause. The most common symptom of menopause is hot flashes (vasomotor symptoms), as more than 80% of females will experience them to varying degrees. Over 50% of females will experience vasomotor symptoms for longer than 7 years. Vasomotor symptoms are caused by thermoregulatory dysfunction in which inappropriate peripheral vasodilation, cutaneous blood flow, and perspiration lead to a rapid loss of heat and a fall in core body temperature, causing an involuntary reaction of chills or shivering. Hot flashes can occur during the day and at night, causing night sweats that interrupt sleep. Sleep disturbances and insomnia are reported in 32% to 45% of all menopausal females, and nighttime hot flashes and night sweats can make sleep disturbances significantly worse. Sleep disturbance has been linked to mood disorders including depression, irritability, anxiety, and fatigue. It is important to note that during the menopausal transition, patients are at increased risk for developing depression, and those with a history of depression may experience worsening of symptoms at the onset of menopause.

Other symptoms of menopause include vaginal dryness, joint pain, diminished libido, and cognitive changes. Estrogen is essential to the health of vaginal tissue, and menopause can cause changes in the epithelium that lead to dryness and atrophy. Lack of estrogen leads to decreased blood flow to the vaginal mucosa and vulva, leading to thinning of the vaginal epithelial lining, decreased vaginal rugae (transverse ridges in vaginal mucous membranes), loss of elasticity, and decreased vaginal mucus. Vaginal dryness is progressive, affecting 21% of patients in the late menopausal transition and up to 45% of patients 3 years after the FMP. The severity of symptoms will vary, as some patients may experience mild symptoms such as itching, and others may experience severe dryness that can lead to bleeding. Vaginal dryness and atrophy can also result in sexual dysfunction. A decrease in estrogen influences peripheral blood flow responses to sensory stimulation, affecting the timing and degree of the vasocongestive response during sexual activity. Symptoms may include diminished sexual responsiveness, dyspareunia, decreased sexual activity, a decline in sexual desire, and relationship changes.

Vaginal atrophy may contribute to the symptoms of both stress and urge incontinence in the menopausal patient, particularly atrophy of the urethral epithelium with atrophic urethritis, loss of compliance, and irritation interfering with adequate seal of the urethral meatus. Atrophy of the bladder trigone (outlet tract) and decreased responsiveness of alpha-adrenergic receptors at the bladder neck and urethral sphincter may also contribute to incontinence symptoms.

Objective

Estrogen receptors are found throughout the body, and a thorough physical examination may demonstrate signs of estrogen deficiency in the menopausal patient. The physical examination of patients in any stage of menopause should include measurement of height and weight and inspection of skin, hair, and vaginal tissue. Many patients gain weight during the menopausal transition and may have a more difficult time shedding visceral fat. Although weight gain during this time is most likely due to aging, there is some evidence that menopause may change body composition and fat distribution.

Estrogen also helps maintain bone health, and because there is an escalation of bone loss during the menopausal transition, a decrease in height can be an early indicator of low bone mass. Because low bone mass can also affect the teeth, an examination should be done to assess oral health. It is significant that during the climacteric (i.e., the period including perimenopause, menopause, and postmenopause), patients may lose 2% to 5% of bone mass per year. Skin function is also impacted by falling estrogenic activity, and during menopause there is a rapid decline in skin collagen and skin thickness. These changes lead to dry skin, wrinkling, and atrophy of the vaginal tissue. Menopause can also cause development of facial hair that has the appearance of peach fuzz, as well as abnormal hair growth on the chin.

DIAGNOSTIC REASONING

A diagnosis of menopause can be made based on a history of amenorrhea and the presence of menopause-associated symptoms in age-appropriate patients. If these symptoms are present within this context, laboratory testing is not necessary. If the age of the patient and history are not consistent with age-related estrogen deficiency, however, other causes of amenorrhea and menopausal symptoms must be considered.

Diagnostic Tests

Several tests are appropriate for patients presenting with amenorrhea. Initially, a quantitative β–hCG test should be done. An elevated level could reflect intrauterine pregnancy, molar pregnancy, ectopic pregnancy, or even certain germ cell tumors. Serum FSH and LH levels may be checked and will be elevated in menopause. FSH levels between 10 and 25 IU/mL suggest relative ovarian resistance consistent with menopausal transition. FSH levels of greater than 40 IU/mL are consistent with complete cessation of ovarian function. LH levels are a less sensitive indicator of hormonal and ovarian function. Although they do rise during the menopausal transition, they may also be elevated during the midcycle surge and in cases of chronic anovulation.

Patients younger than 40 years presenting with amenorrhea and menopausal symptoms may be given a progesterone challenge test, in which medroxyprogesterone acetate 10 mg is given daily for 5 days and the induction of uterine bleeding is monitored in the week after treatment. If no bleeding occurs, a measurement of serum estradiol may be helpful. Normal estradiol levels range between 40 and 300 pg/mL. A level greater than 30 pg/mL may indicate some degree of residual ovarian function. Levels less than 30 pg/mL indicate cessation of ovarian function. All patients experiencing menopause at younger than 40 years will require additional testing to assess cause.

Patients taking combination OCPs should have hormone levels drawn between cycle days 5 and 7 of the placebo-pill week to assess accurate FSH and estradiol levels. This would be appropriate for menopause-aged patients who are taking the pill for contraception and want to know when it is safe to discontinue. Those on progestin-only contraceptive pills can have levels drawn at any time because progesterone does not affect FSH and estradiol levels.

Patients who present with amenorrhea and have no vasomotor symptoms may have overproduction of estrogen and should be assessed via pelvic ultrasound to rule out endometrial hyperplasia. Menopausal status can also be determined by vaginal cytological examination. On microscopic examination, parabasal cells will predominate, indicating a lack of epithelial maturation resulting from low estrogen levels.

Differential Diagnosis

The differential diagnoses for patients presenting with menopausal symptoms include pregnancy, spontaneous abortion, anovulation, endometrial hyperplasia, patient should be instructed to take these drugs on an empty stomach in the morning and wait at least 30 minutes before eating or drinking. The patient must remain upright for 30 minutes after taking these medications. If heartburn or difficulty swallowing occurs, the patient should be instructed to stop the medication and seek medical attention, given the risk of pill esophagitis with these medications.

Raloxifene HCl (Evista) is a SERM that may be used as first-line therapy for the prevention and treatment of postmenopausal osteoporosis. It protects patients from bone loss associated with decreased levels of estrogen. It has an agonistic effect on bone and an antagonistic effect on breast and uterine tissue. Breast tenderness, spotting, and other symptoms that can occur with the initiation of ET do not occur with raloxifene. A common adverse reaction to raloxifene is hot flashes that may improve over time. To date, raloxifene has not demonstrated an increased risk of breast or uterine cancer.

A newer classification of drugs used to prevent bone loss are receptor activator of nuclear factor-kappa B ligand antagonists. The first FDA-approved drug in this category is the monoclonal antibody denosumab (Prolia), which is appropriate for patients with a previous fracture and/or multiple risk factors for osteoporotic fractures. Appropriate patients also include those who have failed to respond to other options, cannot tolerate bisphosphonates, have hypocalcemia, are receiving aromatase inhibitor treatment for breast cancer, or have renal insufficiency. Denosumab is administered subcutaneously two times per year.

Calcitonin nasal spray can also be used to decrease bone resorption in postmenopausal patients and can be used alone or in conjunction with hormonal therapy. It is the drug of choice for patients who cannot take HT, bisphosphonates, or raloxifene (Evista). The dose of calcitonin is 100 IU/day subcutaneously or 200 IU intranasally daily.

Bone mineral density can also be increased with administration of daily subcutaneous injections of teriparatide (Forteo, Parathar), a parathyroid hormone (parathormone) analog. It is administered subcutaneously in 20 mcg per day doses. A serious adverse effect is an increased risk of osteosarcoma when teriparatide is administered in high doses (based on studies in rats).

Vitamin D and calcium should be taken as supplements by most female patients. The recommendation is 1,200 to 1,600 mg of daily calcium and 400 to 1,000 IU of vitamin D (ergocalciferol, vitamin D_2) to maintain bone health. Calcium supplements can be either calcium citrate or calcium carbonate. Some sources indicate that calcium citrate is better absorbed from the GI tract.

Bioflavonoids are thought to have estrogenic activity. One study showed that grapefruit juice increased the bioavailability of administered estradiol and estrone. Black cohosh, blue cohosh, ginseng, and wild yam have all demonstrated estrogenic effects. These compounds may result in endometrial hyperplasia, however, if unopposed with progesterone in patients with intact uteri.

FOLLOW-UP AND REFERRAL

When therapies recommended for the treatment of menopausal symptoms do not offer adequate relief, a referral to a gynecologist is recommended. In addition, a referral should be initiated for all patients with abnormal bleeding or suspected abnormalities, especially carcinoma. Abnormal bleeding in perimenopausal or postmenopausal periods requires further evaluation with pelvic vaginal ultrasound to check for endometrial hyperplasia and endometrial biopsy to rule out abnormal pathology. Normal postmenopausal endometrium should be less than 4 mm in thickness; measurements over 4 mm require further work-up.

Estrogen-progestin therapy usually treats AUB, but intermittent ovulation may require low-dose OCPs. In patients who smoke or patients with contraindications to OCPs (e.g., history of thromboembolism, breast, or uterine cancer) and no significant symptoms of estrogen deficiency, progestin therapy with medroxyprogesterone acetate 5 to 10 mg daily for 2 weeks per month can induce withdrawal bleeding and prevent endometrial hyperplasia. A menopausal patient with depression who does not respond to lifestyle changes and medications should be referred to a mental health specialist for counseling. Patients who are not responsive to therapy for insomnia may be referred to a sleep disorder clinic.

Patient Education: Menopause

Educating patients about menopause is challenging. Because menopause is an event that occurs with normal aging, it is important to educate patients about generally expected age-related changes versus changes that are specific to menopause. Patients should be steered toward evidence-based resources, such as NAMS. Patients in perimenopause should be reminded that it is still possible to get pregnant, and a pregnancy test should be done for all perimenopausal patients presenting with amenorrhea. Patients should receive counseling about safe methods of birth control until menopause has been achieved.

The patient plays a key role in menopause treatment decisions, and adequate education about the risks and benefits of various therapies is necessary. Before initiating HT, patients should be screened for cervical, breast, and colon cancer as appropriate. In addition, a serum chemistry panel, lipid panel, blood pressure assessment, FSH, and thyroid hormone levels should be checked. All patients experiencing abnormal vaginal bleeding should have an endometrial biopsy before starting HT to rule out abnormal uterine pathology.

Patients undergoing menopause may have deep feelings and significant emotional investment about what is happening to their bodies. The primary care practitioner must assess and evaluate these feelings to understand better how to assist the patient. Studies show that fear, lack of knowledge about menopause, and the lack of an informed decision-making process are some of the factors underlying a patient's reluctance to seek treatment for menopausal symptoms. There is considerable conflicting information in the media and among clinicians about HT, and patients will benefit from clarification of the risks and benefits of all the treatments for menopausal symptom relief.

REFERENCES

Family Planning

Abufaraj M, et al. The impact of hormones and reproductive factors on the risk of bladder cancer in women: results from the Nurses' Health Study and Nurses' Health Study II. *Int J Epidemiol.* 2020;49(2):599–607.

Burchardt NA, et al. Oral contraceptive use by formulation and endometrial cancer risk among women born in 1947–1964: The Nurses' health Study II, a prospective cohort study. *Eur J Epidemiol.* 2020: doi: 10.1007/s10654-020-00705-5

CDC. (Updated 2020). Summary chart of U.S. medical eligibility criteria for contraceptive use. https://www.cdc.gov/reproductivehealth/contraception/pdf/summary-chart-us-medical-eligibility-criteria_508tagged.pdf. Accessed 1/26/21.

Constantine GD, Kessler G, Graham S, et al. Increased incidence of endometrial cancer following the Women's Health Initiative: an assessment of risk factors. *J Womens Health.* 2019;28(2):237–243.

Cooper DB, Patel P, Mahdy H. Oral contraceptive pills. (Last updated 2021 Feb 15). StatPearls. https://www.ncbi.nlm.nih.gov/books/NBK430882. Last updated 2/15/2021. Accessed 4/19/2021.

Curtis KM, Jatlaoui TC, Tepper NK, et al. U.S. selected practice recommendation for contraceptive use, 2016. *MMWR Recomm Rep.* 2016;65(4):1–66.

Curtis KM, Tepper NK, Jatlaoui TC, et al. U.S. medical eligibility criteria for contraceptive use, 2016. *MMWR Recomm Rep.* 2016;65(No. RR-3):1–104. https://www.cdc.gov/mmwr/volumes/65/rr/pdfs/rr6503.pdf

Kortsmit K, Williams L, Pazol K, et al. Condom use with long-acting reversible contraception vs non–long-acting reversible contraception hormonal methods among postpartum adolescents. *JAMA Pediatr.* 2019;173(7):663–670. doi:10.1001/jamapediatrics.2019.1136

Mack N, Crawford TJ, Guise JM, et al. Strategies to improve adherence and continuation of shorter_term hormonal methods of contraception. Cochrane Database of Systematic Reviews 2019;4(article CD004317). DOI: 10.1002/14651858.CD004317.pub5

Makins A, Cameron S. Post pregnancy contraception. *Best Pract Res Clin Obstet Gynaecol.* 2020;66:41–54. https://doi.org/10.1016/j.bpobgyn.2020.01.004

Mofidfar M, O'Farrell L, Prausnitz MR. Pharmaceutical jewelry: earring patch for transdermal delivery of contraceptive hormone. *J Control Release.* 2019;301:140–145.

Peragallo Urrutia R, Polis CB, Jensen ET, et al. Effectiveness of fertility awareness-based methods for pregnancy prevention: a systematic review. *Obstet Gynecol.* 2018;132:591–604.

Sriprasert I, Archer DF. Transdermal contraceptive delivery systems. In: Shoupe D, ed. *The Handbook of Contraception. Current Clinical Practice.* Humana, Cham. https://doi.org/10.1007/978-3-030-46391-5_4

Vargas SE, Midoun MM, Guillen M, et al. A qualitative systematic review of women's experiences using contraceptive vaginal rings: implications for new technologies. *Perspect Sex Reprod Health.* 2019;51(2):71–80.

Whitaker AK, Chen BA. Society of Family Planning guidelines: postplacental insertion of intrauterine devices. *Contraception.* 2018;97(1):2–13.

Women's Preventive Services Initiative. (2019 Dec). Recommendations for preventive services for women final report to the U.S. Department of Health and Human Services, Health Resources & Services Administration, December 2019. The American College of Obstetricians and Gynecologists. https://www.hrsa.gov/womens-guidelines/index.html

Wu CQ, Grandi SM, Filion KB, et al. Drospirenonecontaining oral contraceptive pills and the risk of venous and arterial thrombosis: a systematic review. *BJOG.* 2013;120:801-10.

Fertility Problems

Mintziori G, Mousiolis A, Duntas LH, et al. Evidence for a manifold role of selenium in infertility. *Hormones.* 2020;19:55–59. https://doi.org/10.1007/s42000-019-00140-6

Nassan FL, Arvizu M, Minguez-Alarcon L, et al. Marijuana smoking and outcomes of infertility treatment with assisted reproductive technologies. *Hum Reprod.* 2019;34(9):1818–1829.

Rooney KL, Domar AD. The relationship between stress and infertility. *Dialogues Clin Neurosci.* 2018;20(1):41–47. doi:10.31887/DCNS.2018.20.1/klrooney

Schisterman EF, Sjaarda LA, Clemons T, et al. Effect of folic acid and zinc supplementation in men on semen quality and live birth among couples undergoing infertility treatment: a randomized clinical trial. *JAMA.* 2020;323(1):35–48. doi:10.1001/jama.2019.18714

Shah SA, Tibble H, Pillinger R, et al. Hormone replacement therapy and asthma onset in menopausal women: national cohort study. *J Allergy Clin Immunol.* 2021;147:1662–1670.

Shreffler KM, Greil AL, Tiemeyer SM, et al. Is infertility resolution associated with a change in women's well-being? *Hum Reprod.* 2020;35(3):605–616.

Menopause

Biehl C, Plotsker O, Mirkin S. A systematic review of the efficacy and safety of vaginal estrogen products for the treatment of genitourinary syndrome of menopause. *Menopause.* 2019;26(4):431–453.

Chester RC, Kling JM, Manson JE. What the Women's Health Initiative has taught us about menopausal hormone therapy. *Clin Cardiol.* 2018;41(2):247–252.

Harris MG. Sexuality and Menopause: unique issues in gynecologic cancer. *Semin Oncol Nurs.* 2019;35(2):211–216.

O'Keeffe LM, Kuh D, Fraser A, et al. Age at period cessation and trajectories of cardiovascular risk factors across mid and later life. *Heart.* 2020;106:499–505.

Panay N, Anderson RA, Nappi RE, et al. Premature ovarian insufficiency: an International Menopause Society White Paper. *Climacteric.* 2020;23(5):426–446.

Scavello I, Maseroli E, Di Stasi V, et al. Sexual health in menopause. *Medicina (Kaunas).* 2019;55:559.

Simon JA, Davis SR, Althof SE, et al. Sexual well-being after menopause: an International Menopause Society White Paper. *Climacteric.* 2019;21(5):415–427.

Ulin M, Ali M, Chaudhry ZT, et al. Uterine fibroids in menopause and perimenopause. *Menopause.* 2020;27(2):238–242.

Premenstrual Syndrome and Premenstrual Dysphoric Disorder

Carlini AV, Deligiannidis KM. Evidence-based treatment of premenstrual dysphoric disorder: a concise review. *J Clin Psychiatry.* 2020;81(2):1–2.

Frey Nascimento A, Gaab J, Kirsch I, et al. Open-label placebo treatment of women with premenstrual syndrome: study protocol of a randomized controlled trial. *BMJ Open.* 2020;10:e032868. doi: 10.1136/bmjopen-2019-032868

MoradiFili B, Ghiasvand R. Pourmasoumi M, et al. Dietary patterns are associated with premenstrual syndrome: evidence from a case-control study. *Public Health Nutr.* 2020;23(5):833–842.

RESOURCES

American Society for Reproductive Medicine
http://www.asrm.org

Caya. For providers. How Caya works.
https://www.caya.us.com/providers Accessed 4/19/21.

Fertilitext
http://www.fertilitext.org

International Council on Infertility Information Dissemination
http://www.inciid.org

International Menopause Society
https://www.imsociety.org/#

Internet Health Resources: Infertility Resources
http://www.ihr.com/infertility

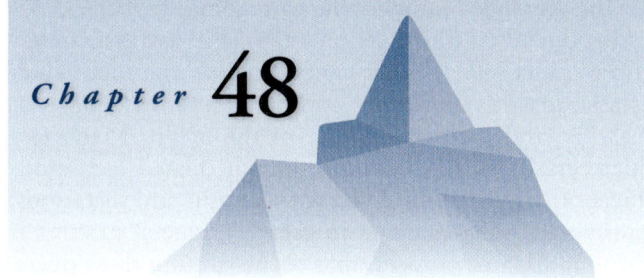

Chapter 48

Breast Disorders

Megan Pratt, DNP, APRN, FNP-BC, GS-C
Debera J. Thomas, PhD, RN, ANP/FNP
Brian Oscar Porter, MD, PhD, MPH, MBA

OVERVIEW

The term *breast* is used throughout this chapter and in practice to reference the mammary glands, whereas the term "chest" is the anatomical location between the neck and abdomen. Some individuals refer to their breasts as their chest. Transgender people, nonbinary individuals, and patients who have had a postmastectomy or surgical alteration may prefer to use the term *chest*. Mastalgia, palpable breast mass, and nipple discharge are common presenting breast symptoms. A detailed history and physical examination should be completed to help determine the cause.

Mastalgia, or breast pain, is a commonly reported symptom. Although benign in the large majority (90%) of cases, mastalgia can be a worrisome symptom to the patient. It should be determined whether mastalgia is cyclic or noncyclic and whether it is true breast pain or related to nonbreast pathology, such as chest wall pain. Cyclic mastalgia is common and generally occurs 1 to 2 weeks before menses. Mild cyclic mastalgia is a normal physiological condition related to hormonal changes throughout the menstrual cycle. Medications including oral contraceptives, hormone replacement therapy, antidepressants, and some cardiovascular agents (e.g., digoxin, spironolactone) have been associated with mastalgia.

Fibrocystic breast changes are commonly noted in patients with mastalgia. Although mastalgia is usually not an indication of underlying malignancy, focal breast pain should be evaluated with diagnostic imaging for an underlying pathology. Ultrasound can be used alone for diagnostic evaluation of focal breast pain in patients younger than 30 years of age, although it should be used in combination with mammography in patients aged 30 years and older. Mastalgia can typically be treated with acetaminophen and NSAIDs.

Palpable breast masses are a common reason patients seek primary care services, and although most are benign, this is the most common presenting symptom for breast cancer. A detailed history and physical examination should be completed to establish the level of suspicion for breast cancer. The characteristics, duration (change in size over time or in relation to menses), and associated symptoms of palpable breast masses should be assessed.

Specifically, a clinical breast examination is recommended in patients presenting with a breast mass. Benign breast masses generally have discrete margins and are smooth and mobile, whereas malignant breast masses generally have nondiscrete margins and are hard and immobile. Abnormal findings should be documented, based on their position on a clock face and distance from the nipple. Diagnostic imaging is generally warranted and is determined, based on examination findings, age, and risk factors for breast cancer. Imaging results, differential diagnoses, and breast cancer diagnoses are further discussed in this chapter.

Nipple discharge is most likely related to benign breast pathology or physiological state. When collecting a patient history, it is important to ask the patient to characterize the discharge, identify if it is unilateral or bilateral, and determine whether there are associated symptoms, such as a breast mass or pain. If the nipple discharge is spontaneous, unilateral, clear, serous, bloody, or associated with a mass, breast pathology should be considered, and an ultrasound and diagnostic mammogram should be ordered. Cytology of nipple discharge is not recommended, and referral to a surgeon for duct excision should be considered regardless of imaging results.

Physiological nipple discharge tends to be milky and bilateral, and a pregnancy test should be ordered to rule out this common cause. If negative, further assessment of galactorrhea (milky nipple discharge) should be performed by reviewing medications (especially medications that inhibit dopamine) and assessing the patient for endocrinopathies (check thyroid-stimulating hormone and prolactin levels). Though rare, galactorrhea in men may be associated with testosterone deficiency (hypogonadism).

MASTITIS

Mastitis is a general term that refers to inflammation of the breast. The terminology for the various types of mastitis can be confusing because there are overlapping definitions and contradictions in the literature. For this discussion, there are three general categories: puerperal mastitis, nonpuerperal mastitis, and periductal mastitis. Each category is defined further by an explanation of the cause of the mastitis.

Puerperal mastitis (lactational mastitis) is a cellulitis that develops in the lactating or nonlactating breast after childbirth. Epidemic puerperal mastitis, seen most commonly during the preantibiotic era, is a hospital-acquired infection that involves multiple ducts and results in inflammation of several nonadjacent breast lobes. The most common contagion for epidemic puerperal mastitis is *Staphylococcus aureus*, which is typically spread from neonate to mother, as well as via cross-transmission in the nursery. With the progression of rooming-in and the introduction of antibiotics, epidemic puerperal mastitis has become a rare occurrence. Sporadic puerperal mastitis is an acute process that is far more common in patients who breastfeed rather than bottle feed their infants, due to prolonged engorgement of milk ducts. It usually occurs in the second to sixth week postpartum; however, it has been reported in patients even after breastfeeding for 1 year. It is hypothesized that the higher occurrence of mastitis in the earlier postpartum period is due to the prevalence of nipple and feeding problems at that time, which are a risk factor for the disease and are more likely to occur in first-time breastfeeding mothers.

Nonpuerperal mastitis is a rare disease found in patients who are immunocompromised, have undergone radiation therapy, or have had an autoimmune disorder. It is common in late adolescence or early adulthood, although it can also occur in neonates. Nonpuerperal mastitis is a ductal abnormality or a local manifestation of a systemic problem. Several pathological pathways may be involved, including squamous metaplasia of the lactational ducts (the most common cause in nonpuerperal mastitis), periareolar abscesses, and cellulitis. Mastitis can also be caused by several obscure pathogens or by a foreign substance in the breast, such as silicone from implants. This disease usually presents as a palpable mass and arises from a known infectious process, such as tuberculosis (TB) or syphilis. Nonpuerperal mastitis must always be evaluated for the presence of underlying carcinoma.

Periductal mastitis has been referred to and cross-referenced under several other names, such as mammary duct ectasia, mastitis obliterans, plasma cell mastitis, comedomastitis, and secretory disease of the breast. Mammary duct ectasia is a condition in which dilated lactiferous ducts of the breast are filled with keratin and secretions, causing the milk ducts to thicken. Periductal mastitis is the inflammatory process that occurs around these ducts. Some degree of ductal dilation normally occurs with aging, and researchers have suggested that periductal mastitis seen in younger patients represents a different disease from the more chronic clinical presentation seen in older patients. The primary event leading to periductal mastitis is controversial. Some hypothesize that duct ectasia precedes the inflammatory process, whereas others claim the inverse. The disease is characterized by dilation of the subareolar ducts, as the ducts become thick walled and surrounded by plasma cells. Inside the ducts there are pasty, lipid-rich, yellow-brown secretions. The periductal regions become fibrotic and inflamed, which may be caused by rupture and leakage of the ducts themselves. Fat necrosis is often evident. Menopausal and postmenopausal patients and patients who smoke are at greater risk of developing periductal mastitis.

EPIDEMIOLOGY AND CAUSES

The incidence of mastitis in breastfeeding patients in the United States has been reported to be between 2% and 10%. Studies done in other countries report an incidence between 18% and 24%, with the majority of cases occurring in the first 6 weeks postpartum.

There are a multitude of factors that contribute to puerperal mastitis. Cracked, abraded, or otherwise damaged nipples provide a portal of entry for infecting microorganisms. Patients who are having latch-on and positioning difficulties during feeding increase their risk for both nipple skin disruption and milk stasis, which can lead to mastitis. A slow milk ejection reflex, breast engorgement, failure to empty the breast adequately, waiting too long between feedings, supplemental feedings, the use of pacifiers, wearing a tight and restrictive bra, sleeping positions that constrict the breast, and weaning also contribute to the risk of developing mastitis. Each of these situations can lead to blocked ducts and milk stasis, and unresolved milk stasis provides a medium for bacterial overgrowth.

The causative organism of sporadic puerperal mastitis is *S. aureus* in at least 50% of reported cases. *S. aureus* is frequently found on the skin and cultured from the neonate's mouth. Methicillin-resistant *S. aureus* (MRSA) is becoming increasingly common, and risk factors for MRSA should be considered. Other organisms implicated in this infection are *Escherichia coli,* group A and group B *Streptococcus,* and *Mycobacterium tuberculosis.* Tuberculosis mastitis occurs in populations in which TB is endemic. Physiological stress and psychological stress are both significant risk factors that increase the likelihood of puerperal mastitis. Fatigue, improper nutrition, and life stress are predictors of breast infections, as these circumstances lead to lower maternal immune defenses and an increased likelihood of the condition.

Periductal mastitis/mammary duct ectasia is seen primarily in perimenopausal and postmenopausal patients. The peak incidence is between 40 and 49 years of age, but it can occur at any time after menarche. The inflammatory process has been observed on microscopic examination in 30% to 40% of patients older than 50 years; however, clinical disease occurs much less frequently. The actual incidence and cause of the disease are unknown. Duct ectasia has a reported incidence of 5.5% to 25%, as demonstrated on postmortem examinations. An important (and modifiable) risk factor for periductal mastitis is tobacco use. The mechanism by which smoking increases its incidence is suggested to be due to direct damage of the ducts and inflammation. Inverted nipples have been suggested to be a source of duct obstruction, which could lead to ectasia, but they have not been shown to be a risk factor. Diabetes mellitus and obesity have also been associated as risk factors. Bacteria are isolated in 62% to 85% of cases, including *S. aureus, Pseudomonas aeruginosa, Enterococcus, Bacteroides,* and *Proteus.* Periductal mastitis and duct ectasia may have an autoimmune etiology, but this has not been well characterized.

PATHOPHYSIOLOGY

The causative mechanism of the various forms of mastitis (puerperal, nonpuerperal, and periductal) has been discussed in the preceding text. However, the pathophysiology of the infectious process in the most common form, puerperal mastitis, is a classic example of a breakdown in the body's protective outer epithelial barrier. This results in entry of bacteria from the infant's mouth or the mother's skin into the breast through cracked nipple skin or the nipple pores. With one or more lobes of the breast seeded, infection develops. Moreover, the symptoms of the disease, which include pain, tenderness, and fatigue, contribute to further decreases in effective feeding practices and adequate emptying of the breast, thus worsening the infection. Milk of a mastitic breast has a higher-than-normal sodium and chloride content, and it is not unusual for an infant to refuse to nurse from that breast.

Because the infection of puerperal mastitis is located primarily in the extraductal tissue, breastfeeding generally poses no harm to the infant, provided skin breakdown has not resulted in frank bleeding from the nipples and there is no evidence of purulent nipple discharge. Purulent material may be present within the ducts, however. In addition, although bilateral infection is possible, mastitis is usually unilateral and localized to the upper outer quadrant of the affected breast. The incidence of mastitis progressing to a subareolar breast abscess has been reported to be as high as 4% to 11% in patients treated for the disease. It is much higher for those who do not seek treatment for mastitis.

CLINICAL PRESENTATION

Subjective

The clinical presentation is acute in nature. The patient's first complaint is fatigue, followed by the onset of flu-like symptoms and breast tenderness. The involved breast segments may be red and warm. Patients describe the affected area as being tender to palpation or painful. A fever of at least 100°F (37.8°C) can be expected with myalgia, malaise, and chills. Nausea and vomiting can accompany these symptoms.

Many patients with periductal mastitis are asymptomatic. Others present with breast tenderness or pain, a breast mass, nipple discharge, nipple retraction, a nonpuerperal breast abscess, or a mammary fistula. The pain is usually subareolar and noncyclical. The nipple discharge varies in color and may contain occult blood. It is most frequently green and sticky and occurs spontaneously. The mastitis can be unilateral or bilateral. Nipple retraction and noninflammatory masses occur more commonly in older patients, whereas pain and abscesses tend to occur in younger patients. Periductal mastitis and duct ectasia account for 3% to 12% of benign breast lumps. The pain is usually focused behind the areola and tends to be more severe in younger patients.

Objective

On examination, varying degrees of erythema and edema of the affected breast may be noted. The erythema is most commonly in a V-shaped distribution and may or may not feel hard. Sometimes there is purulent nipple discharge. There may or may not be a palpable blocked duct.

DIAGNOSTIC REASONING

Diagnostic Tests

Milk cultures are rarely done in first-occurrence cases of mastitis because they are costly and may delay treatment. They are warranted with a recurrence or failure of initial treatment. A breast milk culture can be obtained by manual expression of a midstream, clean-catch specimen. Washing the nipple with water and sterile gauze prepares the breast. The first 2 to 3 mL of milk expressed should be discarded. The specimen needs to be fresh when sent to the laboratory. Breast milk is rarely found to be sterile and normally contains leukocytes. A normal leukocyte (white blood cell [WBC]) count is 1,000 to 4,000/mL.

With patients symptomatic for mastitis, there are three diagnostic categories when cytology and cultures are performed on breast milk samples. Milk stasis is present with a WBC count of less than 10^6 cells/mL and a bacterial count of less than 10^3 colony-forming units (CFU)/mL. Noninfectious breast inflammation is present with a WBC count of more than 10^6 cells/mL and a bacterial count of less than 10^3 CFU/mL. A WBC count of more than 10^6 cells/mL with a bacterial count of more than 10^3 CFU/mL is indicative of infectious mastitis. With the help of a milk culture and antibiotic sensitivities, appropriate antibiotic treatment can be initiated for infectious mastitis. There are occasionally situations in which a patient develops chronic puerperal mastitis. These patients may have anatomical strictures of some lactiferous ducts, which lead to chronically plugged ducts. Long-term antibiotic therapy and attentive breastfeeding management can improve the outcome of this condition.

Ultrasound examination of the breast or a mammogram may be helpful in making the diagnosis of periductal mastitis. The mammogram shows tubular dilated ducts. Calcification may be present in the lumen and walls of the affected ducts. Intense periductal mastitis may simulate carcinoma on a mammogram. Because carcinoma and mastitis can coexist, a biopsy may be warranted with such findings. In older patients, the mass from the duct ectasia can be difficult to differentiate from carcinoma. Both masses can be hard, irregular, and either fixed or not fixed to the surrounding tissue, with skin or nipple retraction potentially seen with the former. When the nipple discharge is bilateral and multiple ducts are involved, the likelihood of malignancy is reported to be remote. Another diagnostic tool is needle aspiration and the culture of areas of inflammation. Fine-needle aspiration (FNA) may show polymorphonuclear neutrophils, plasma cells, lymphocytes, and multinucleate giant cells.

Differential Diagnosis

The first point to consider when presented with a patient symptomatic for puerperal mastitis is to identify whether milk stasis or plugged ducts have led to an infectious process versus a potentially more serious underlying pathophysiological mechanism, such as breast cancer. The clinical presentation is invaluable in this judgment. There are documented cases of breast cancer in patients who are lactating or pregnant, and reports differ on infants rejecting a breast later diagnosed with cancerous disease. Inflammatory breast cancer is a rare disease, but it can present with some of the same symptoms as classic puerperal mastitis. The patient with inflammatory breast cancer may have a red, swollen breast and sometimes (but rarely) a fever. The patient commonly has no palpable breast mass and may or may not have peau d'orange (breast skin resembling an orange peel in texture). When inflammatory cancer is present, symptoms do not respond to antibiotic treatment as mastitis generally does. With any suspicion of a cancerous process, the patient must be referred for biopsy and a definitive diagnosis.

Breast engorgement is often mistaken for mastitis but does not have the accompanying systemic symptoms of infection (e.g., fever, erythema, myalgia). If the infant has signs of poor "latch-on" during feeding (e.g., infant showing sunken cheeks, clicking sounds signifying breaking of suction, contact between the upper and lower lips at the corners of the mouth while feeding, etc.), this can also predispose the mother to mastitis. Galactoceles (milk retention cysts), which may result from plugged lactiferous ducts, appear hard and red and may be quite painful with breast soreness, as opposed to the shooting pains of mastitis; however, galactoceles lack the systemic signs of mastitis. Hard, tender breasts with shooting pains but without redness or fever may be more associated with fungal infection.

MANAGEMENT

The basic principle of management in puerperal mastitis is to decrease contributing factors to the inflammation and infection while generally improving breastfeeding management. Flu-like symptoms should always be treated as mastitis in postpartum patients unless proven otherwise. With a first occurrence, the diagnosis can be made from clinical symptoms alone and empirical treatment initiated. If there is no response to antibiotic treatment or if there is recurrent mastitis, further diagnostics are indicated.

It is vital that the infant continue to breastfeed to avoid milk stasis. Because the infection is extraductal, there is no risk to the infant in continuing to breastfeed, except in mothers with HIV due to the potential for viral transmission. Massage of the breasts during feeding helps to better drain the breast, and additional pumping may be needed, particularly if the infant is not nursing effectively on the affected side. Pumping in addition to frequent infant feeding decreases the duration of symptoms (it is recommended to feed or pump every 6 hours) and sequelae of disease, notably the development of breast abscesses. Breastfeeding management should include correction of any latch-on or positioning difficulties and aggressive discovery and care of cracked or sore nipples.

Bedrest is imperative during the acute phase of the illness. The patient should be assisted with any household duties and rest in bed with their infant. Moist heat to the affected breast can be useful before feeding and pumping to increase milk expression. A cold compress to the affected breast may provide comfort between feedings. Pain and other uncomfortable symptoms can be treated with nonsteroidal analgesics, such as acetaminophen or ibuprofen. Stress management techniques should be implemented.

Empirical antibiotic therapy is recommended to treat the infection. Without treatment, only 15% of patients recover without recurrent infection or breast abscess. Approximately 50% improve with breast pumping alone as treatment, and more than 95% recover completely with combination therapy of breast pumping and antibiotics. The patient must be instructed to continue pharmacological therapy for the duration of the prescription to avoid partially treated disease and the development of antibiotic-resistant organisms.

The best response is expected when antibiotics are started within the first 24 hours of symptom onset. Broad-spectrum antibiotics such as dicloxacillin (Dynapen) 500 mg or cephalexin (Keflex) 500 mg orally four times daily are considered when MRSA is not present. In addition, antibiotic sensitivities should be obtained from a breast milk culture in recurrent or nonresponsive cases to help focus therapy. For patients with a beta-lactam allergy, clarithromycin (Biaxin) 500 mg orally twice daily for 10 to 14 days is recommended. If community-acquired, methicillin-resistant *S. aureus* (CA-MRSA) is suspected, then clindamycin (Cleocin) 300 mg orally three times daily or trimethoprim-sulfamethoxazole (Bactrim, Septra) 800 mg/160 mg (one double strength (DS) tablet) twice daily may be given for 10 to 14 days. Doxycycline (Doxy 100) 100 mg orally twice daily for 10 to 14 days can be used if the patient is not breastfeeding or pregnant.

In the management of periductal mastitis, broad-spectrum antibiotics (as described earlier) have been successful. They treat the periareolar inflammation associated with this condition and reduce pain. If a mass is present, it must be biopsied to rule out carcinoma. In the presence of a suspicious nipple discharge, a ductal excision is necessary to confirm the diagnosis. The wound infection rate after breast biopsies where periductal mastitis and/or duct ectasia are present is high. The infection rate is 2% after biopsies with no evidence of this disease but 10.2% when it is present. This appears to be unrelated to trends in culture results. Symptomatic treatment includes nipple and areolar hygiene, and some clinicians recommend no oral nipple stimulation (in contrast to puerperal mastitis).

Notable sequelae of this type of mastitis are breast abscesses and fistulae. Nonpuerperal breast abscesses are seen more frequently than those associated with lactation. The incidence of periareolar abscess is 10% in patients with symptomatic duct ectasia. The bacteria cultured are usually *S. aureus* and anaerobes. Surgical excision and broad-spectrum antibiotic coverage constitute the treatment of choice. Needle aspiration of the abscess may be performed if the risk of malignancy is low, but this treatment frequently needs to be done repeatedly.

Abscess is also one of the more common sequelae of puerperal mastitis. It can occur when the disease progresses either with or without treatment. The patient presents with worsening local symptoms and may or may not have systemic manifestations. A breast ultrasound can be useful to confirm the diagnosis. Most abscesses are surgically incised and drained under anesthesia. Biopsy of the cavity has been recommended to check for the presence of carcinoma. A drain is put in place, and broad-spectrum parenteral antibiotics should be started with anaerobic coverage, pending culture results, because polymicrobial infection is common. The drain may be covered with sterile gauze, because it is not unusual for breast milk to leak around the drain due to severed lactiferous ducts. There are occasions when a puerperal breast abscess is treated with recurrent needle aspiration, but this is not the treatment of choice.

A recurrence of mastitis may develop for several reasons, including inadequate antibiotic therapy. When a recurrence is evident, a breast milk culture is indicated, as well as further exploration of the patient's breastfeeding management. Chronic mastitis should be treated with an antibiotic that provides coverage of MRSA.

After antibiotic therapy, infection of the nipples with *Candida albicans* is not unusual. Topical antifungal treatment for the patient and concomitant oral nystatin for the infant is necessary. Fungal (*Candida*) mastitis may develop, which is characterized by fiery pain shooting up the ductal system; oral antimycotic treatment is indicated in this situation.

FOLLOW-UP AND REFERRAL

The patient may benefit from referral to a board-certified lactation consultant for professional evaluation and assistance with infant feeding. The lactation consultant evaluates and corrects problems related to the infant's feeding, which may be causing or contributing to the occurrence of infection. If a patient's symptoms are not resolved after reasonable treatment attempts or if there is no change in the size or condition of a breast lump presumed to be a plugged duct after 48 hours of care and treatment, the patient must be referred for further diagnostic evaluation.

> **Patient Education: Mastitis**
>
> Appropriate patient teaching and breastfeeding management in the early postpartum period can be the best prevention tool for puerperal mastitis. Early and frequent infant feedings with correct infant latching and positioning are necessary. No harsh substances such as soaps or lotions should be put on the nipples. Correct bra sizing, rest, and instructions to eat a healthy, well-balanced diet high in antioxidants can all help with disease prevention.
>
> Patients with periductal mastitis and duct ectasia require significant emotional support, as these conditions can simulate breast cancer. The fear of breast cancer in perimenopausal and menopausal patients is high, and patients must be reassured that a cancer diagnosis has been considered and ruled out after an appropriate work-up. Because of the connection between periductal mastitis and cigarette smoking, smoking cessation should be discussed at each visit.

BREAST CANCER

Cancer of the breast is the second most common cancer in American women (behind skin cancer) and accounts for approximately 30% of all cancers in women in the United States. The U.S. Centers for Disease Control and Prevention (CDC) statistics indicate that 250,520 women were diagnosed with breast cancer in 2017 (most recent data available) and that 42,000 women and 510 men died from breast cancer that year. Breast cancer is second only to lung cancer as the leading cause of cancer death among women and is the main cause of death in women aged 40 to 44 years. During the 1980s, there were yearly increases in breast cancer incidence rates, probably as a result of an increase in screening; however, this rise has slowed over the past few years, currently increasing by 0.3% per year. Mortality rates have been decreasing since 1990, most likely because of earlier detection and advances in breast cancer treatment.

EPIDEMIOLOGY AND CAUSES

In general, the lifetime risk of a woman getting breast cancer is one in eight, and the lifetime risk of dying from breast cancer is one in 39. In North America, the lifetime odds of a woman getting breast cancer is 14% for non-Hispanic white women, 14% for African American women, 11% for Hispanics, and 14% for Native Americans. The risk of breast cancer increases with age; it is low in females in their second and third decades of life but rises with each subsequent decade, with the median age for breast cancer diagnosis at 64 years. Increasing age and other risk factors (see Risk Factors: Breast Cancer) that have been associated with the development of breast cancer explain only 50% of cases, and all females have the potential for the development of breast cancer. Recommendations from the American Cancer Society (ACS) and the U.S. Preventive Services Task Force (USPSTF) for systematic breast cancer detection are presented in Screening Recommendations/Guidelines: Breast Cancer.

> **Risk Factors: Breast Cancer**
>
> - Female sex
> - White race
> - Ashkenazi Jewish descent
> - Advanced age (older than 50 years)
> - Personal history of atypical hyperplasia or lobular carcinoma *in situ*
> - Personal history of breast or ovarian cancer
> - Family history of breast or ovarian cancer in a first-degree relative (parent, sibling, or child)
> - *BRCA1* or *BRCA2* gene mutation
> - Residing in North America or Northern Europe
> - Prior breast biopsy, regardless of results
> - Early menarche (before age 12 years)
> - Late menopause (after age 55 years)
> - Nulliparity or first live birth at a late age (after age 35 years)
> - Long-term use of postmenopausal hormonal therapy, especially combined hormonal therapy
> - Exposure to high-dose radiation
> - Higher education and socioeconomic status
> - High-fat diet
> - Overweight and obesity
> - Alcohol consumption (two or more drinks per day)
> - Physical inactivity
> - Cigarette smoking, especially during adolescence
> - Exposure to pesticides and other chemicals

PATHOPHYSIOLOGY

Breast cancer is a disease of various cell populations, with different growth rates, cell surface markers, and tendencies to metastasize. It is often considered a systemic disease at the time of first diagnosis because many patients with "early" breast cancer already have established but clinically occult micrometastases, reflecting the importance of adjuvant hormonal therapy (e.g., tamoxifen, anastrozole). Invasive breast cancer is often preceded by carcinoma *in situ* lesions of either ductal or lobular distribution. However, a malignant breast mass may be present for many years before the initial diagnosis, and it is not uncommon for invasive disease to be identified at the time of diagnosis, rather than a premalignant lesion. Breast cancers spread by contiguous lymphatic and/or vascular channels. The most common sites of metastasis are the regional lymph nodes, lung, skin, bone, liver, and brain.

The development of frank breast cancer may also be preceded by a variety of benign breast conditions

Screening Recommendations/Guidelines: Breast Cancer

The American Cancer Society (ACS) (2020) recommends the following:

For women of average risk:

- Screening mammogram beginning at age 45 years and performed annually in women 45 to 54 years. Women should have the opportunity to begin screening at age 40 years.
- Biennial screening for women aged 55 years and older with the opportunity to screen annually
- Continue screening as long as overall health is good and life expectancy is at least 10 years.

For women who are at high risk for breast cancer:

- Breast magnetic resonance imaging (MRI) and mammogram every year, typically starting at age 30 years

The USPSTF (2016) recommends the following:

For women of average risk:

- Biennial screening mammography for women aged 50 to 74 years
- Screening mammography before age 50 years should be an individual choice.
- No recommendation for women older than 75 years

Note: For average-risk women at any age, clinical breast examinations and self-breast examinations are not recommended for breast cancer screening (ACS and USPSTF).

---

characterized by multicentric proliferation of breast tissue. Several genetic mutations have been recognized in both precancerous and cancerous lesions, including genes affecting cellular proliferation, DNA mismatch repair, and the conversion of procarcinogens to carcinogenic compounds. Two of the most widely publicized breast cancer susceptibility genes are the tumor suppressor genes *BRCA1* and *BRCA2*, first cloned in the mid-1990s. These gene are involved in the repair of double-stranded DNA breaks and genetic mutations in females. A decrease in function of these genes increases susceptibility not only to breast cancer but also to cancers of the ovary, pancreas, and prostate. However, *BRCA1/BRCA2* mutations are rare, accounting for only one-fifth of familial breast cancer cases. In turn, the study of breast cancer genetics—including the identification of new breast cancer susceptibility genes—is an active area of research.

The Knudsen hypothesis of malignant transformation is often credited with explaining the pathogenesis of breast cancer. In this model, at least two sequential genetic "hits" or mutations that interfere with DNA repair are thought to underlie malignant transformation of normal breast tissue, which ultimately loses its capacity for programmed cell death (apoptosis). In familial cancers, the first of these hits is thought to be the inherited germ line mutation, and the second mutation may be induced by an environmental carcinogen or related to one of many other predisposing risk factors.

CLINICAL PRESENTATION

Subjective

History and risk assessment in relation to breast cancer should include the patient's age, ethnicity, education, and socioeconomic status. The clinician should assess for a breast lump or area that feels denser (with or without pain), tenderness, dimpling, nipple retraction, nipple ulceration, nipple discharge, erythema, peau d'orange, change in breast shape, breast enlargement, alteration in the venous pattern of breast tissue, or one or more enlarged and palpable axillary lymph nodes. The date of onset, location, and duration of any change in the patient's breast and a history of prior trauma to the breast should also be assessed.

The assessment should also include any systemic symptoms, especially those that may indicate metastases to the skeleton (bone pain, fracture), spinal cord (localized radicular back pain, lower extremity weakness, paresthesias, paralysis, bladder/bowel dysfunction), brain (headache, seizure, mental status changes, vision and speech defects, sensory loss/muscle weakness, ataxia, persistent nausea/vomiting), bladder or bowel (incontinence), lungs (chest pain, dyspnea on exertion, shortness of breath, cough), and liver (abdominal pain or distention, jaundice, weakness, fatigue, nausea/vomiting, appetite, weight loss, lower extremity edema).

The medical history should assess for illnesses, especially previous breast cancer; benign or preinvasive breast conditions; other cancers such as ovarian cancer; prior radiation exposure; medications; allergies; dietary and other health habits (e.g., fat intake, alcohol consumption, cigarette use and other forms of smoking, weight gain, exercise); and past surgical history, especially breast biopsy and/or surgery. Questions should be asked regarding the patient's gynecological and obstetric history, including age at menarche, age at menopause, last menstrual period, pregnancy history (age when first full-term pregnancy occurred, abortions, miscarriages), and any use of hormonal therapy. The patient's frequency of mammograms and date of last mammogram, results of previous mammograms (noting any abnormalities), and the results of related diagnostic tests must also be sought. Family history questions should elicit information regarding first-degree relatives with a history of breast cancer (note age at diagnosis and bilaterality of disease as risk factors) and a family history of ovarian cancer, which is associated with breast cancer.

Objective

A thorough physical examination with a focus on the breasts, as well as the axillary and supraclavicular lymph nodes, should be performed. Inspection should assess the contour, asymmetry, and skin and nipple changes of the breast. In premenopausal patients, this assessment should be done during the follicular phase of the menstrual cycle, when hormone levels are low and less likely to affect breast tissue. Examination of the breasts includes inspection and palpation in the upright and supine positions. The size, location, mobility, and consistency of any palpable breast mass or dense area, as well as associated lymph nodes chains, should be documented. Any breast or nipple findings noted on inspection (including the characteristics of any nipple discharge) should also be recorded.

Clinical manifestations of breast cancer include those abnormalities already stated, although some patients may present only with an abnormality detected on a mammogram, because pain and tenderness are present in fewer than 10% of patients with breast cancer. The Patient's Voice 48.1 illustrates the individuality of symptoms due to breast cancer and the impact on different patients' life experiences.

DIAGNOSTIC REASONING

Diagnostic Tests

A diagnostic mammogram is necessary in any patient with a palpable breast mass, suspicious nipple discharge, or a suspicious area on a screening mammogram. Most radiologists will request an ultrasound be completed in combination with a diagnostic mammogram. A spot compression flattens and isolates a lesion. A diagnostic mammogram determines the need for subsequent testing and whether other suspicious nonpalpable areas are present in one or both breasts.

Suspicious findings on a mammogram include (1) asymmetry with definitive borders or discernible masses; (2) architectural distortion (a "pulling in" of breast structures) not resulting from previous surgery; (3) a nodule that is more radiodense, irregularly shaped, or has unclear margins, compared with surrounding breast tissue; (4) calcifications that are irregularly shaped, clustered, and of varying sizes; (5) skin changes such as thickening or retraction; (6) spiculations (needle-like densities); and (7) axillary and/or intramammary lymph nodes more than 2 cm in diameter.

Additional studies that may be scheduled to further delineate a breast abnormality include ultrasound, ductal lavage, and galactography (ductography). An ultrasound, which differentiates solid from fluid-filled masses, may distinguish between benign and malignant breast disease. It may better visualize abnormalities in patients with dense breast tissue (e.g., patients younger than 30 to 35 years of age) and is used in place of mammography in pregnant patients, given the risks of radiation exposure with the latter. Genetic testing for the *BRCA1*

 The Patient's Voice 48.1

A BREAST MASS

It was on my 48th birthday that I noticed a slightly tender enlargement in my left breast. I had consistently checked my breasts for years during my period. I had no family history of breast cancer and never experienced breast tenderness or lumps on a regular basis. Even before my one pregnancy at age 34, I had never experienced significant breast soreness. My nurse practitioner saw me the next day and stated that she could feel something. She sent me for a mammogram. I had one 2 years earlier, so I was sent to the same place. Two days later, I was told there are "changes," and I was referred to a surgeon. I did not know what that meant, except I knew it could be serious. I wanted to do everything they told me to do. I wanted to get better. I had a biopsy and then shortly after, a "lumpectomy." I was told I was very lucky because although the biopsy was positive for cancer, they said my "nodes" were cancer free. I was told I would need radiation therapy, because I only had the lump removed. I experienced too much stress and fear at that time in my life. My yoga classes were very important to me then because they helped me relax and heal. I have been going for 7 years since the surgery and now teach yoga too. I know I was lucky and grateful that my nurse practitioner could see me the day after I felt the lump. Waiting is so stressful.

ANOTHER PATIENT'S VOICE

I went for my annual mammogram and later got the call; I was referred to a breast specialist and had a biopsy. On my 45th birthday, I got the news that I had bilateral breast cancer. I have had a bilateral mastectomy and almost a year of treatment, first chemo and now radiation. I have a young son and husband. This will be the first Christmas since my diagnosis, and I am grateful to be here. Having this diagnosis made me rethink the important things in life. I have slowed down and appreciate all the people in my life. I know people say this, but the diagnosis of breast cancer has really been a gift. I appreciate the small things, like a beautiful sunset, the gentle breeze on my face, and the love of family and friends. I don't take life for granted anymore!

and *BRCA2* genes is expensive and done only in patients with a high suspicion of a familial breast–ovary cancer syndrome who have undergone extensive pretest (and post-test) counseling.

Mammography views with the Eklund technique are used in a patient with a breast implant to provide views unobstructed by the implant; in this process, the breast implant is pushed back against the patient's chest wall, while the breast tissue is pulled forward and compressed for mammography. Galactography (ductography) is used in the presence of serous or bloody nipple discharge without a palpable mass to visualize an intraductal lesion; however, it cannot distinguish between benign and malignant diseases.

After diagnostic imaging, suspicious areas noted on a mammogram or ultrasound must be submitted for biopsy for a definitive tissue diagnosis of breast cancer. A mammogram may not always result in a visible lesion; therefore, all clinically suspicious palpable masses must be submitted for biopsy, whether or not they are visualized with mammography. Thus, the patient should be referred to a surgeon for further evaluation at this point. One or more of the following breast mass biopsy techniques may be done in the outpatient setting, usually under local anesthesia:

- *FNA.* FNA may be performed by a specialist or primary care practitioner experienced in the procedure. A 21- or 22-gauge needle is used to aspirate a cyst or extract cells from a palpable solid lesion for analysis. It is easy to perform and provides rapid results with little trauma to the tissue. It is highly reliable when used as an adjunct to the clinical examination and mammogram. On the negative side, interpretation of FNA material requires an experienced cytopathologist, may yield false-negative results due to sampling variability, and does not differentiate *in situ* from invasive cancer. A stereotactic or ultrasound-guided FNA biopsy can be performed on nonpalpable lesions.
- *Core-needle biopsy.* A large-gauge cutting needle is used to provide a large core of tissue from the lesion for histological examination. The results of a core-needle biopsy are as accurate as those of a surgical biopsy, but the procedure is less invasive with better cosmetic results. A stereotactic or ultrasound-guided core-needle biopsy can be performed on nonpalpable lesions.
- *Incisional biopsy.* This procedure may be done when a mass is very large and cannot be removed without a surgical procedure. In this type of biopsy, a wedge of tissue is removed for histological examination.
- *Open surgical excisional biopsy (lumpectomy).* This procedure involves the entire removal of a palpable mass or nonpalpable lesion (after stereotactic or ultrasound-guided biopsy or mammographic needle localization). To qualify as a lumpectomy, lesions suggestive of cancer should be removed with a surrounding margin of at least 1 cm of normal tissue. X-ray films of needle-localization specimens are obtained to confirm removal of the mammographically detected abnormality, and a postexcision mammogram should be done to confirm complete excision. The open surgical excisional biopsy provides complete pathological assessment of the suspicious lesion but may result in poor cosmesis.

If there is suspicion of inflammatory breast cancer or Paget's disease (discussed later in the chapter), a skin biopsy or nipple biopsy should be done at the time of the breast mass biopsy.

Prognosis

Preinvasive breast cancers include ductal carcinoma *in situ* (DCIS) and lobular carcinoma *in situ* (LCIS). DCIS has malignant potential but infrequently disseminates; therefore, approximately 98% of patients are cured with local–regional therapy (total mastectomy or breast-conserving surgery and radiation therapy). The addition of tamoxifen (Nolvadex) decreases the incidence of subsequent invasive disease. LCIS has a propensity for bilaterality, multicentricity, and a 25% to 40% risk for development of a subsequent invasive cancer. It is managed with close surveillance, a bilateral mastectomy, or chemoprevention (e.g., long-term tamoxifen therapy).

Invasive breast cancers have the potential to disseminate through lymphatic and vascular channels to other organs. Most of these cancers are adenocarcinomas. Approximately 80% are infiltrating ductal carcinomas, and 10% are invasive lobular carcinomas. Their prognosis is similar. Invasive lobular carcinoma differs in its slightly greater tendency toward bilaterality and metastasis to meningeal and serosal surfaces. Other histological subtypes are pure mucinous, tubular, medullary, and papillary carcinomas. These subtypes have a slight to somewhat better prognosis, due to a smaller risk of dissemination. Paget's disease of the breast and inflammatory breast carcinoma are rare. Paget's disease of the breast, which manifests clinically as unilateral eczema of the nipple, is nearly always associated with DCIS or invasive ductal carcinoma. Inflammatory breast carcinoma has the poorest prognosis of all breast cancers.

Prognostic factors, or tumor-related features, are biological assessments done on the breast tissue specimen. They serve as guides for the oncologist in determining systemic adjuvant therapy for the breast cancer patient. In addition to the histological types of invasive breast cancer, lymph node status (0, 1–3, 4–9, or 10 or more affected nodes [range of good to poor prognosis]), tumor size (1 cm or less in diameter [good prognosis]), and histological differentiation (range of well-differentiated [low grade, good prognosis] to poorly differentiated [high grade, poor prognosis]) are the standard predictors of risk of recurrence and survival. High-grade tumors are poorly differentiated and carry a worse prognosis, whereas lower grade, well-differentiated tumors carry a more favorable prognosis.

With reference to these factors, patients with breast cancer have an excellent prognosis if they have the following features: DCIS, negative lymph nodes with an invasive tumor size less than 1 cm in diameter, and special histological subtypes of breast cancer (e.g., pure tubular) less than 3 cm in diameter. Patients who have potentially high recurrence rates and who would, therefore, greatly benefit from systemic therapy, have the following features: positive regional lymph node(s) or invasive tumors more than 2 cm in diameter, even with negative lymph nodes. Breast cancer patients who have a tumor that is poorly differentiated have an increased risk of recurrent disease, but they may also have a greater response to chemotherapy.

Hormone receptor status—for example, the presence or absence of estrogen receptors (ER) and progesterone receptors (PR)—is another important prognostic factor, especially in guiding the oncologist in the selection of hormonal therapy. Patients with breast cancer respond more favorably if ER levels are high and if both ER and PR are present. Also, a positive status of the pS2 protein (an ER-regulated secretory protein expressed mainly by ER-positive tumors) is indicative of a better prognosis in patients with either negative or positive lymph nodes.

Other prognostic factors such as those indicative of the proliferative capacity of the tumor (e.g., mitotic index, thymidine labeling index, S-phase fraction, ploidy, Ki-67 level), nuclear grade, tumor necrosis, tumor microvessel density, peritumoral lymphatic vessel invasion, cathepsin D protease level, and the expression of proto-oncogenes (*ERBB2* [*HER-2/neu*, c-erbB-2] and c-*myc*) and the *p53* tumor-suppressor gene may all be helpful in predicting response to treatment. For example, the overexpression of c-*erB-2* may predict that a breast cancer patient will be resistant to certain chemotherapy agents and possibly to hormonal therapy. It may also predict a shorter disease-free interval.

Reference to these additional prognostic factors, along with the standard ones, may be valuable in determining the need for systemic therapy in patients who have an intermediate prognosis, such as node-negative patients with invasive tumors 1 to 2 cm in diameter. In turn, referral to a breast cancer specialist is required.

Staging

After the diagnosis of breast cancer is confirmed, the stage (i.e., Stage 0, I, II, III, IV) of the disease is evaluated (Table 48.1). Certain laboratory tests may reflect distant metastasis. A complete blood count may show an abnormality of WBCs and platelets, and a low hematocrit may indicate bone marrow infiltration and occult metastatic disease. Liver enzymes and abnormal calcium and phosphorus levels may indicate occult liver metastasis and/or bone metastasis. Abnormalities in tumor markers (e.g., CEA, Ca 27.29) may indicate occult metastatic disease. If a tumor marker is abnormal, it may be useful in assessing response to treatment and disease progression or recurrence. Radiological examinations can also assist in detecting distant metastasis. A chest x-ray abnormality may indicate lung metastasis, and abnormal findings on a bone scan/skeletal survey or liver scan (if warranted by signs, symptoms, or laboratory tests) may reflect specific sites of metastasis.

Differential Diagnoses

Several differential diagnoses for breast cancer should be considered. With breast cancer, a palpable mass is usually persistent, unilateral, solitary, discrete, firm, irregularly shaped, and nontender, and it may or may not be fixed to the skin or underlying tissue. Breast distortion and skin changes such as diffuse erythema, edema, peau d'orange, dimpling, nipple retraction, or nipple ulceration are also indicative of cancer. If present, nipple discharge is spontaneous, persistent, unilateral, localized to a single duct, watery or sticky, and clear, sanguineous, serosanguineous, or serous in color. Lymph nodes suggestive of a malignancy are typically large, firm, and fixed (matted).

Fibrocystic changes (e.g., cystic breast disease, chronic cystic mastitis, or mammary dysplasia) may be difficult to distinguish from breast cancer by palpation alone. Fibrocystic changes are so common that they are considered a normal variant of breast tissue. However, if accompanied by significant pain, nipple discharge, or palpable physical examination findings that raise suspicion for breast cancer, the condition is termed *fibrocystic disease*. Cystic areas are unilateral or bilateral, somewhat more diffuse, 1 mm to many centimeters in diameter, soft, and mobile; they may also be tender and painful due to stromal edema, dilation of ducts, and accompanying inflammation. These cysts are hormonally regulated and may be worse during the premenstrual phase; this variation with menses usually distinguishes fibrocystic changes from fibroadenomas and breast cancer. Aspiration of clear fluid with complete disappearance of the cyst on follow-up examination or the appearance of a fluid-filled cavity on ultrasound confirms the diagnosis. These changes are most common in patients 30 to 55 years of age.

Fibroadenomas are benign, solid masses of fibrous and glandular tissue that are often confused with breast cancer. These masses may be isolated or multiple and are typically firm, nodular, well-defined, freely mobile, and possibly tender. Growth of these benign tumors is hormonally stimulated; thus, they may grow rapidly during pregnancy, lactation, or hormonal manipulation. These are most common in younger patients and are not associated with an increased risk of breast cancer if in their simple form. However, complex fibroadenomas (i.e., with cysts greater than 3 mm in size, calcification on mammography, or histological evidence of sclerosing adenosis or papillary apocrine changes) have been associated with a greater risk

TABLE 48.1 Tumor/Node/Metastasis (TNM) Staging of Primary Breast Cancer

STAGE	TNM STAGING	DESCRIPTION
	TX, NX, MX	Primary tumor (T), regional lymph nodes (N), or distant metastasis (M) respectively cannot be assessed (X)
0	Tis, N0, M0	Carcinoma *in situ* or Paget's disease of nipple with no tumor
I	T1, N0, M0	Tumor less than or equal to 2 cm; no regional lymph node metastasis; no distant metastasis
IIA	T0, N1, M0	No evidence of tumor; metastasis to moveable ipsilateral axillary lymph node(s); no distant metastasis
	T1, N1, M0	Tumor less than or equal to 2 cm; metastasis to moveable ipsilateral axillary lymph node(s); no distant metastasis
	T2, N0, M0	Tumor greater than 2 cm and less than or equal to 5 cm; no regional lymph node metastasis; no distant metastasis
IIB	T2, N1, M0	Tumor greater than 2 cm and less than or equal to 5 cm; metastasis to moveable ipsilateral axillary lymph node(s); no distant metastasis
	T3, N0, M0	Tumor greater than 5 cm; no regional lymph node metastasis; no distant metastasis
IIIA	T0, N2, M0	No evidence of tumor; metastasis to ipsilateral axillary lymph node(s) fixed to one another or to other structure; no distant metastasis
	T1, N2, M0	Tumor less than or equal to 2 cm; metastasis to ipsilateral axillary lymph node(s) fixed to one another or to other structure; no distant metastasis
	T2, N2, M0	Tumor greater than 2 cm and less than or equal to 5 cm; metastasis to ipsilateral axillary lymph node(s) fixed to one another or to other structure; no distant metastasis
	T3, N1 or N2, M0	Tumor greater than 5 cm; metastasis to ipsilateral axillary lymph node(s) (N1) or axillary lymph node(s) fixed to one another or to other structure (N2); no distant metastasis
IIIB	T4, Any N, M0	Tumor of any size with direct extension to chest wall (excluding pectoral muscle) and/or edema (including peau d'orange) or ulceration of the skin or satellite skin nodules confined to the same breast, or inflammatory carcinoma; any nodal status as described above; no distant metastasis
IV	Any T, N3, M0	Any tumor status as described above; metastasis to ipsilateral internal mammary lymph node(s); no distant metastasis
	Any T, Any N, M1	Any tumor or nodal status as described above; distant metastasis, including metastasis to ipsilateral supraclavicular lymph nodes

Source: Used with permission of the American College of Surgeons. Amin, M.B., Edge, S.B., Greene, F.L., Et al (Eds.) AJCC Cancer Staging Manual, 8th Ed. Springer New York, 2017.

of breast cancer when accompanied by proliferation of surrounding glandular tissue.

Hamartomas composed of stromal and epithelial tissue and tubular adenomas consisting of ductal tissue are less common benign tumors of the breast that may present similarly on physical examination but are not considered cancerous. Fat necrosis or panniculitis is another benign condition and is typically trauma induced. The mass associated with panniculitis is firm and possibly tender, often with calcification seen on mammography. Diabetic mastopathy results in a breast lump with a dense mammographic appearance but benign histology consisting of keloidal scar tissue and lobular, lymphocytic inflammation. This is most often seen in patients with type 1 diabetes mellitus who also suffer from other end-organ microvascular damage such as retinopathy or neuropathy.

Intraductal papilloma is a benign condition with a small, usually solitary and nonpalpable mass in one mammary duct, with an associated spontaneous sanguineous or serosanguineous nipple discharge. If large enough to palpate, the mass is most often close to or beneath the areola, soft, mobile, 1 to 3 cm in size, poorly delineated, nontender, and sometimes associated with skin dimpling. It is most common in patients 35 to 55 years of age. Solitary papillomas are not considered premalignant; however, diffuse papillomatosis characterized by the formation of multiple papillomas carries with it a greater risk of eventual breast cancer.

Duct ectasia is a benign condition involving inflammation of a subareolar duct, which may produce subareolar erythema and swelling, a mass with nipple retraction and/or skin dimpling, dull nipple pain, tenderness, burning, and/or itching. Nipple discharge is pasty and straw colored, cream colored, green, or brown. It is most common in perimenopausal or postmenopausal patients who have had children and have nursed.

Ductal hyperplasia without atypia is distinguished from ectasia, in that it is the most common benign breast lesion clearly associated with an increased risk of breast cancer. Epithelial cell proliferation along the basement membranes of the ducts, although benign histologically, varies in size and shape. Atypical ductal hyperplasia is associated with an even greater risk of breast cancer (up to sixfold in patients with a strong family history of breast cancer), especially in premenopausal patients. It is characterized by a loss of apical-basal cellular organization within ductal tissue. Atypical lobular hyperplasia is even more concerning because it is qualitatively equivalent to LCIS, which is considered a precursor lesion to invasive breast cancer.

Sclerosing adenosis, most common in patients 35 to 45 years of age, is a benign proliferation of the breast epithelium with increased fibrous and glandular tissue, with hard, pea-sized nodules throughout the affected area. There is mild to moderate pain and swelling premenstrually. The presence of this condition has also been associated with an increased risk of breast cancer. *Radial scars* are another benign histological finding consisting of a fibroelastic core from which ducts and lobules radiate outward. If large, these lesions may appear similar to a spiculated carcinoma on mammography and are indeed associated with an increased risk of breast cancer.

Mastitis is a typically benign infectious condition of the breast that presents with erythema, induration, pain, possible purulent nipple discharge, fever, chills, and myalgia, and it may or may not progress to an abscess. It is more common during lactation, although different presentations of mastitis exist (i.e., puerperal, nonpuerperal, periductal), as described earlier in this chapter.

MANAGEMENT

The patient diagnosed with breast cancer is referred to cancer specialists, such as a surgical oncologist, medical oncologist, and/or radiation oncologist, for comprehensive treatment of the disease (Table 48.2). The choice of treatment is influenced by such factors as tumor stage, ER and PR levels and other prognostic factors, patient age, menopausal status, and the patient's general health. When detected at an early stage, invasive breast cancer that is treatable with surgery, radiation therapy, chemotherapy, and/or hormonal therapy may be highly curable.

Surgical Management

The initial surgical management of Stage I and Stage II breast cancer includes one of several types of surgery. Breast-conserving surgery may include a partial mastectomy, lumpectomy, wide excision, segmental mastectomy, or quadrantectomy with a separate axillary node dissection and radiation therapy to the breast. A modified radical mastectomy is a total mastectomy with axillary node dissection, as opposed to a simple mastectomy, which leaves most or all of the axillary nodes intact. Breast-conserving surgery removes a portion of the breast tissue, whereas a total mastectomy removes all but approximately 2% to 3% of the breast tissue. The survival rates for these two surgical treatment options are equivalent.

The type of initial surgery for a particular patient usually depends on the location and size of the tumor, breast size, characteristics of the disease on mammography, patient age, and the patient's feelings regarding breast preservation. Breast-conserving surgery may not be an option if there is a tumor beneath the nipple; a large tumor-size to breast-size ratio; multicentricity; extensive intraductal carcinoma; diffuse malignant-appearing calcifications on the mammogram; or contraindications to radiation therapy such as pregnancy, collagen vascular disease, or prior radiation therapy to the breast or chest wall.

After a mastectomy, the patient may choose immediate or delayed breast reconstruction with a submuscular saline implant or expander, a transverse rectus abdominis myocutaneous flap, or a latissimus dorsi flap. Skin-sparing breast surgery may be appropriate for simple mastectomies in which the nipple and areola are removed and breast tissue is extracted through the resultant opening while sparing the majority of the breast skin and axillary lymph nodes; this is only appropriate if followed by immediate breast reconstruction, in which the nipple and areola are recreated from transplanted skin usually taken from another part of the patient's body.

Depending on the type of breast surgery, adverse effects may include wound infection, seroma, bleeding or hematoma, phantom breast syndrome (pain, numbness, or nipple pruritus), paresthesias, muscle atrophy, arm or shoulder weakness or stiffness, lymphedema, phlebitis, or a winged scapula (protruding scapula resulting from intraoperative injury to the long thoracic nerve).

A technique of lymphatic mapping and sentinel lymph node biopsy, eliminates the need for an axillary lymph node dissection in some patients and thus avoid some of the associated adverse effects. The sentinel node (the first lymph node along a lymphatic drainage pathway) is identified after peritumoral injection with a radioisotope or vital blue dye. If the sentinel node is negative for metastatic disease, a complete axillary lymph node dissection is not indicated.

Radiation Therapy

Radiation therapy is indicated for local–regional control of the primary breast cancer or palliation of metastatic disease. After breast-conserving surgery, primary treatment includes external beam radiation to the entire breast with or without a boost (interstitial radioactive implant

TABLE 48.2 Management of Invasive Breast Cancer

Stage	Surgery/Radiation Therapy	Adjuvant Therapy
I	Breast-conserving surgery with separate axillary node dissection and radiation therapy (RT) to the breast *or* modified radical mastectomy (MRM)	Suitable estrogen receptor (ER)-negative patients: adjuvant chemotherapy ER-positive patients: adjuvant chemotherapy or tamoxifen 20 mg daily
II	Breast-conserving surgery with separate axillary node dissection and RT to the breast *or* MRM Consider RT to the chest wall and regional nodes for patients at high risk of local-regional recurrence, including those with known residual disease or four or more involved nodes	*Node-negative patients:* ER-negative or ER-positive patients with large tumors: adjuvant chemotherapy ER-positive patients: adjuvant chemotherapy or tamoxifen 20 mg daily *Node-positive patients:* Premenopausal and postmenopausal (ER-negative) patients: adjuvant combination chemotherapy with or without tamoxifen Postmenopausal patients with positive hormone receptors: tamoxifen alone
IIIA	*Inoperable cases:* MRM with or without RT or radical mastectomy (removal of breast tissue, all axillary lymph nodes, and underlying chest muscle) with or without RT RT may be given because of the high risk of local recurrence; postoperative external beam RT to chest wall, with or without boost as necessary for positive or close margins	Combination chemotherapy with or without hormonal therapy Neoadjuvant therapy: chemotherapy may be given preoperatively if primary resection is not feasible or technically difficult
IIIB	Biopsy for diagnosis and ER/progesterone receptors (PR) If good response to chemotherapy or hormonal therapy: local therapy with surgery and/or RT If poor response to chemotherapy or hormonal therapy: palliative RT	Chemotherapy/hormonal therapy: combination chemotherapy with or without hormonal therapy *or* tamoxifen (if ER/PR positive)
IV	Biopsy for diagnosis and ER/PR receptors External beam RT or palliative mastectomy to control local disease	If visceral disease is minimal or absent and ER/PR-positive: hormonal therapy (as initial therapy) For premenopausal patients: tamoxifen or oophorectomy For patients who relapse after period of response or prolonged stability on initial hormone therapy: megestrol 40 mg four times daily or anastrozole 1 mg daily or letrozole 2.5 mg daily If visceral disease present or ER/PR-negative: combination chemotherapy
Inflammatory Breast Cancer	Refer to options for Stages IIIB or IV	Refer to options for Stages IIIB or IV

or further external-beam radiation) to the primary site. After a modified radical mastectomy, radiation therapy to the chest wall and regional lymph nodes is considered in patients at high risk of local or regional recurrence, including those with known residual disease or four or more involved lymph nodes.

Patients undergoing an axillary lymph node dissection generally do not require radiation therapy to the axilla. Internal mammary lymph nodes may be treated, and patients with four or more positive lymph nodes may require supraclavicular radiation therapy to reduce the risk of supraclavicular lymph node recurrence. A pregnant patient with breast cancer can begin radiation therapy after delivery. Potential adverse effects of radiation therapy include fatigue, edema, breast pain or tenderness, skin reactions, brachial plexopathy, radiation pneumonitis, and myocardial damage if the left breast is treated. Secondary malignancies, such as sarcomas, leukemias, and lung cancer, are rare, although patients who smoke have an increased risk of lung cancer in the ipsilateral lung.

Breast surgery or radiation therapy may make subsequent mammograms difficult to interpret. Masses (postoperative fluid collections and scarring), edema, skin thickening, and calcifications may be seen on these mammograms, especially during the first 6 months after treatment. During the next 6 to 12 months, slow resolution of these changes takes place, and stability occurs within 2 years.

Systemic Treatment

Systemic treatment options include chemotherapy, biological therapy (e.g., monoclonal antibodies), and hormonal endocrine therapy. There are many variables to consider in selecting these therapies, including cancer stage, subtype (e.g., ER and/or PR positive, HER2 negative, triple negative), risk of tumor recurrence, and other risks of specific treatments.

Neoadjuvant therapy is increasingly being used; it is the systemic treatment of breast cancer preoperatively. Neoadjuvant therapy can be chemotherapy, but it can also include endocrine therapy in certain patients. Neoadjuvant chemotherapy is associated with better clinical response rates and increases the likelihood for successful breast-conserving surgery; however, it has not been shown to improve overall survival rates.

Chemotherapy

Antineoplastic chemotherapy as adjuvant therapy is indicated for the eradication of micrometastatic disease that may be present at the time of the original diagnosis. It should be initiated within 6 weeks (preferably less) of surgery (radiation therapy would follow the chemotherapy). Combination chemotherapy is the standard of care for the treatment of primary breast cancer because it can overcome the potential for drug resistance.

Some of the more common potential adverse effects of chemotherapy include myelosuppression, nausea and vomiting, anorexia, mucositis, alopecia, fatigue, and neurotoxicity. Less common toxicities include hemorrhagic cystitis (alkylating agents), cardiomyopathy (anthracyclines), thromboembolic events, and early menopause (in premenopausal patients). Paclitaxel (Taxol) and docetaxel (Taxotere) may also produce myalgia and rare allergic reactions; docetaxel may cause cumulative fluid retention and symptomatic pleural effusions. A rare complication of antineoplastic chemotherapy may be the development of secondary leukemia.

Hematopoietic growth factors (erythropoietin, granulocyte colony-stimulating factor [Neupogen], granulocyte-macrophage colony-stimulating factor [Leukine], and oprelvekin [Neumega]) may help prevent or reduce some chemotherapy-related complications related to myelosuppression. Cytoprotective agents such as amifostine (Ethyol) and dexrazoxane (Zinecard) help reduce side effects and aim to protect against toxic cardiac adverse effects. Pamidronate (Aredia), a second generation aminobisphosphonate, is used in cases of osteolytic bone metastases to prevent pathological fractures, cord compression, the need for radiation therapy or surgery to the bone, and hypercalcemia, and it significantly reduces bone pain. Pregnant breast cancer patients may receive antineoplastic chemotherapy during their third trimester or after delivery.

Biological Therapy

In HER2-positive breast cancers, the cancer cells have a growth-promoting protein (the kinase HER2) on their surface. Biological monoclonal antibody therapies have been developed to target this protein. Trastuzumab (Herceptin) and pertuzumab (Perjeta) are given separately or combined in the treatment of early stage to advanced breast cancers. Margetuximab-cmkb (Margenza) is a monoclonal antibody used in combination with chemotherapy to treat advanced breast cancer. Antibody-drug conjugates, consisting of a monoclonal antibody linked to a chemotherapy drug, include ado-trastuzumab emtansine (Kadcyla) and fam-trastuzumab deruxtecan-nxki (Enhertu) and are used postoperatively or in advanced disease. Kinases (such as HER2) are enzymatic proteins that relay signals by chemically modifying other molecules; therefore, kinase inhibitors (e.g., lapatinib [Tykerb], neratinib [Nerlynx], tucatinib [Tukysa]) may also be used in the management of HER2-positive breast cancers. Potential adverse effects include cardiomyopathy, anemia, leukopenia, diarrhea, hand-foot syndrome, lung disease, liver disease, and infection.

Hormonal Therapy

Two-thirds of breast cancers are either ER positive or PR positive. Hormonal therapy effective for these cancers includes the use of antiestrogens (e.g., tamoxifen), progestins (e.g., megestrol acetate), luteinizing hormone–releasing hormone (LHRH) agonists (e.g., leuprolide), and aromatase inhibitors (anastrozole and letrozole). Tamoxifen is the most commonly prescribed of these agents, and the treatment period is 5 years. Because of its antiestrogenic effect, it is beneficial in breast cancer patients whose tumors have positive hormone receptors, with its greatest effect in those who have both ER-positive and PR-positive tumors. However, tamoxifen also exhibits an estrogenic effect on the endometrium; therefore, it may increase the incidence of endometrial cancer. Potential adverse effects include mild nausea, hot flashes, menstrual irregularities, vaginal discharge, vaginal dryness and irritation, benign ovarian cysts, thromboembolic events, and ophthalmological toxicities. CDK4/6 inhibitors, mTOR inhibitors, and PI3K inhibitors are all targeted therapies utilized to increase the effectiveness of hormonal therapy.

Local Recurrent Disease

Local recurrent disease is usually indicative of widespread recurrence, especially in postmastectomy patients. Some patients initially treated with breast-conserving surgery and radiation therapy who later develop a local recurrence in the ipsilateral breast may be cured with surgery and/or radiation therapy. Prolonged survival is more likely if there is a chest wall recurrence less than 3 cm in diameter, axillary and internal mammary (but not supraclavicular) lymph node recurrence, and a disease-free interval of more than 2 years after initial therapy. Treatment options for recurrent disease include surgery, radiation therapy, chemotherapy, and/or hormonal therapy. Surgery and/or radiation may be used for a local or visceral recurrence.

In asymptomatic patients with positive or unknown ER/PR tumor status and absent or minimal visceral disease limited to only one organ, treatment options for recurrent disease include tamoxifen in premenopausal and postmenopausal patients or oophorectomy (or LHRH agonists to suppress ovarian function) in premenopausal patients. In the event that a patient had an initial response to hormonal therapy but had a subsequent relapse, another type of hormonal therapy may be prescribed, such as tamoxifen, anastrozole, letrozole, megestrol, androgens, LHRH agonists (for premenopausal patients), or aminoglutethimide. A subset of patients with recurrent disease may respond to hormonal therapy withdrawal for approximately 10 months before switching to another form of hormonal therapy.

Patients with recurrence presenting as visceral disease with negative ER/PR tumor status should receive chemotherapy. The choice of regimen takes specialized knowledge and relates to the initial treatment combination. For example, if a patient relapses a year or more after receiving adjuvant treatment with the commonly used CMF regimen of cyclophosphamide [Cytoxan], methotrexate [Trexall], and fluorouracil [Adrucil], this same regimen may be readministered. However, if a patient relapses after treatment with an anthracycline (e.g., doxorubicin [Adriamycin], mitoxantrone [Novantrone])-containing regimen, they may be retreated with agents from other chemotherapeutic categories. Recurrent breast cancer treatment may also be palliative in nature, such as the use of radiation therapy to relieve the pain of bone metastases.

FOLLOW-UP AND REFERRAL

Depending on the breast cancer patient's risk for both local and distant recurrence, a history and physical examination should be done according to the following schedule: every 3 to 6 months during the first 3 years (more frequently during adjuvant therapy), every 6 months for the next 2 years, and annually after the fifth year (more frequently for patients at very high risk of recurrence).

A baseline mammogram should be done 3 to 9 months after tumor excision and at the completion of all treatment. Thereafter, it should be done at least annually, even if asymptomatic, to detect a recurrence in the ipsilateral breast of patients who had breast-conserving surgery or to detect a second primary tumor in the contralateral breast of all breast cancer patients. Further testing such as bone scans, chest x-ray films, computed tomography scans, and liver function tests are ordered for symptomatic patients according to their presentation and suspected location of recurrence. Patients treated with tamoxifen should have routine pelvic examinations. If abnormal uterine bleeding occurs, further evaluation is warranted, given the risk of endometrial cancer.

The 5-year relative survival rate for patients with localized breast cancer is 99%, with regional spread it is 86%, and with distant metastases, it declines to 27%. The 10-year survival rate for localized breast cancer is 84%, and 15-year survival declines to 80%.

Patient Education: Breast Cancer

The primary care practitioner may be involved at various phases of the patient's care, for example, at prediagnosis, diagnosis, treatment, and post-treatment. Therefore, the clinician is in a valuable position to teach the patient and support people about breast cancer prevention and detection and to reinforce information about a breast cancer diagnosis and treatment options (including both the benefits and potential complications of treatment). For example, primary and secondary breast cancer screening recommendations should be reviewed and discussed with the patient, because if diagnosed at an early stage, breast cancer may be curable with standard treatment (see Evidence-Based Nursing Practice 48.1).

The breast cancer patient needs to learn how to prevent potential postsurgical and/or radiation therapy complications, such as lymphedema. In this situation, the patient should be taught range-of-motion exercises for the involved arm and shoulder. The need to avoid infections, injuries, strains, and constriction of the ipsilateral arm is stressed. Antineoplastic chemotherapy and other forms of breast cancer treatment can be teratogenic; therefore, the patient must be advised to use effective contraception during treatment.

The breast cancer patient should be taught about the pharmacological and nonpharmacological management of the adverse effects of potential chemotherapy, radiation therapy, or hormonal therapy. For example, the patient may be instructed to take medications such as ondansetron (Zofran) and dexamethasone (Decadron) to prevent delayed chemotherapy-induced nausea and vomiting or to perform techniques such as relaxation with guided imagery to prevent or minimize these

> **Evidence-Based Nursing Practice 48.1**
>
> **BREAST CANCER**
>
> Kenison TC, Silverman P, Sustin M, et al. Differences between nurse practitioner and physician care providers on rates of secondary cancer screening and discussion of lifestyle changes among breast cancer survivors. *J Cancer Surviv.* 2015;9:223–229.
>
> This study examined the frequency of cancer screening and discussion of healthy lifestyles across provider types: surgical and medical oncologists, primary care physicians, and nurse practitioner (NP) survivorship specialists. The researchers surveyed breast cancer survivors regarding the type of provider they saw most, lifestyle changes since cancer diagnosis, cancer screening, and discussion of self-care practices. The response rate was 78.7% with 759 breast cancer survivors completing the survey. There were no differences across providers in the rates of cancer screening. However, a larger proportion of patients seeing an NP reported they discussed physical activity (78.6%; $p<0.001$) compared with any other provider. Discussion of nutrition and weight management showed a similar pattern (NP 70.0%, oncologist 36.5%, surgeon 25.7%, radiation oncologist 48.7%, and primary care physicians 35.5%). The extent of self-reported lifestyle change was basically the same across these groups of patients working with different types of providers. Thus, the researchers suggest using providers specializing in lifestyle modification to achieve better outcomes in self-reported lifestyle change.

symptoms. Patients may also be advised regarding the purchase of a breast prosthesis, mastectomy bra, or wig, as per their personal preferences.

The patient diagnosed with breast cancer may face many physical and psychosocial challenges, such as an alteration in body image and sexuality, a significant role change at home or work, anxiety, denial, anger, and depression. The primary care practitioner is in a prime position to counsel and support the patient and significant others and to direct them to the many breast cancer resources available to the public that offer individual and group counseling, among other services.

REFERENCES

Breast Cancer

American Cancer Society. (Last revised 2020 Nov 17). American Cancer Society recommendations for the early detection of breast cancer. https://www.cancer.org/cancer/breast-cancer/screening-tests-and-early-detection/american-cancer-society-recommendations-for-the-early-detection-of-breast-cancer.html. Accessed 1/25/2021.

American Cancer Society. (Last revised 2020 Jan 13). Lifetime risk of developing or dying from cancer. https://www.cancer.org/healthy/cancer-causes/general-info/lifetime-probability-of-developing-or-dying-from-cancer.html. Accessed 1/25/2021.

American Cancer Society. (Last revised 2020 Jan 13). Targeted drug therapy for breast cancer. https://www.cancer.org/cancer/breast-cancer/treatment/targeted-therapy-for-breast-cancer.html#:~:text = Pertuzumab%20(Perjeta)%3A%20This%20monoclonal,into%20a%20vein%20(IV). Accessed 1/25/2021.

Bevers TB, et al. Breast cancer screening and diagnosis version 3.2018. *JNCCN.* 2018;16(11):1362–1389.

Cancer stat facts: Female breast cancer. National Institutes of Health, National Cancer Institute: Surveillance, Epidemiology, and End Results Program. https://seer.cancer.gov/statfacts/html/breast.html. Accessed 1/25/2021.

Kenison TC, Silverman P, Sustin M, et al. Differences between nurse practitioner and physician care providers on rates of secondary cancer screening and discussion of lifestyle changes among breast cancer survivors. *J Cancer Surviv.* 2015;9:223–229.

National Cancer Institute. (Updated 2020 Sept 2). Breast cancer treatment (PDQ)—Health professional version. https://www.cancer.gov/types/breast/hp/breast-treatment-pdq. Accessed 1/25/2021.

U.S. Preventive Services Task Force. (Published 2016; currently under revision). Breast cancer: Screening. https://www.uspreventiveservicestaskforce.org/uspstf/recommendation/breast-cancer-screening. Accessed 1/25/2021.

Mastitis

Angelopoulou A, et al. The microbiology and treatment of human mastitis. *Med Microbiol Immunol.* 2018;207:83–94.

Barker M, Adelson P, Peters MDJ, et al. Probiotics and human lactational mastitis: a scoping review. *Women and Birth.* 2020; 33(6):e483–e491.

RESOURCES

Breastcancer.org
    https://www.breastcancer.org
National Breast Cancer Foundation
    https://www.nationalbreastcancer.org/breast-cancer-facts
National Cancer Institute
    https://www.cancer.gov/types/breast
Susan G. Komen Breast Cancer Foundation
    https://ww5.komen.org/

Chapter 49

Vaginal, Uterine, and Ovarian Disorders

Megan Pratt, DNP, APRN, FNP-BC, GS-C
Debera J. Thomas, PhD, RN, ANP/FNP
Brian Oscar Porter, MD, PhD, MPH, MBA

AMENORRHEA

Menarche usually occurs between ages 11 and 14 years, and the average age in the United States today is 12.8 years. Absence of menstruation is considered amenorrhea and can be primary or secondary. *Primary amenorrhea* is defined as the failure to menstruate by age 16 years. Because there are a number of causes that can be treated immediately, it is recommended to evaluate patients who have not reached menarche by age 15 years or within 3 years of thelarche (breast budding). *Secondary amenorrhea* is the absence of menstruation for 3 or more consecutive months in a female who has achieved menarche.

EPIDEMIOLOGY AND CAUSES

Primary amenorrhea occurs in about 0.3% of females and may result from hypothalamic or pituitary failure, ovarian failure, or chromosomal or enzymatic abnormalities. Amenorrhea is a manifestation of a pathological process and is not a diagnosis in itself. Causes of primary amenorrhea include congenital defects of gonadotropin production; genetic disorders (Turner syndrome); congenital central nervous system (CNS) defects such as hydrocephalus; congenital anatomical malformations of the reproductive system (e.g., absence of the vagina or uterus); abnormal outflow tract (e.g., vaginal aplasia, imperforate hymen); and acquired CNS lesions, including trauma, infection, and tumors. Females without a uterus or vagina usually have normal ovarian function in which skeletal growth and secondary sex characteristics develop in the proper sequence, but menses does not occur. In cases of uterine hypoplasia, the uterus does not respond to hormonal stimulation during puberty.

If a female patient is not pregnant (with pregnancy being the most common cause of amenorrhea), secondary amenorrhea is usually associated with anovulation caused by neuroendocrine dysfunction. Secondary amenorrhea occurs in approximately 1% to 3% of females, with a higher incidence among college students (3% to 5%) and athletes (5% to 50%). Amenorrhea reflects a disruption in the normal physiological or anatomical function of the hypothalamus, pituitary gland, ovaries, or uterine/vaginal outflow tract. Hormones produced by these structures play major roles in ovulation; any slight change in production may result in anovulation and the absence of menstruation. Females taking anabolic steroids (e.g., weightlifters, bodybuilders), elite athletes with low body fat (e.g., marathon runners), and those with anorexia nervosa may present with secondary amenorrhea.

PATHOPHYSIOLOGY

The hypothalamic-pituitary-ovarian-uterine axis needs to function in a coordinated manner for menstruation to occur. The most frequent cause of primary amenorrhea is dysfunction of the ovaries resulting from gonadal dysgenesis. This may be caused by various chromosomal abnormalities that result in a depletion of oocytes and ovarian follicles, subsequently impairing the regulated cycle of menses. Turner syndrome, characterized by an XO (single X chromosome) genotype, is one of the most common chromosomal disorders. In this condition, the ovaries are replaced by fibrous tissue (known as *streak ovaries*), which has a very limited or absent capacity for estrogen production.

In addition, primary ovarian insufficiency (i.e., menopause occurring before age 40 years), polycystic ovary syndrome (PCOS) characterized by concurrent hyperandrogenism, and estrogen- or androgen-secreting tumors may all cause amenorrhea. Secondary amenorrhea is nearly universally a hormonal problem because, by definition, female sexual development has already occurred. By far, the most common cause of secondary amenorrhea involves the expected hormonal changes associated with pregnancy, that is, increased progesterone production needed to maintain the pregnant uterus.

Under normal conditions, the hypothalamus produces gonadotropin-releasing hormone (GnRH) in a pulsatile fashion. In response to GnRH, the anterior pituitary gland produces the gonadotropins follicle-stimulating hormone (FSH) and luteinizing hormone (LH). In response to FSH and LH, the ovaries produce estrogen and progesterone, which subsequently drive secondary sexual development and cyclic menstruation. Factors such as stress, weight changes, nutritional deficiencies, strenuous exercise, and infiltrative CNS lesions including hypothalamic tumors (e.g., lymphoma, histiocytosis) and sarcoidosis may all disrupt the normal pulsatile release of GnRH. Pulsatile production of GnRH may also be affected by rare pituitary tumors including macroadenomas and microadenomas, which cause hyperprolactinemia and account for 20% of secondary amenorrhea cases. Amenorrhea may occur before or after the treatment (e.g., surgical resection) of such tumors, depending on the underlying production of pituitary gonadotropins. Functional hypothalamic amenorrhea (which may be primary or secondary) is characterized by an absence of histological CNS pathology, despite an underproduction or overproduction of GnRH that leads to a decrease in gonadotropin surges and results in amenorrhea. In contrast, a complete absence of hypothalamic GnRH production may occur congenitally, inherited in an autosomal-dominant, autosomal-recessive, or X-linked fashion.

Whereas acquired endometrial scarring known as *Asherman's syndrome* is essentially the only anatomical uterine etiology of secondary amenorrhea, nearly 25% of primary amenorrhea cases are due to structural abnormalities that prevent menstrual outflow, including imperforate hymen, vaginal agenesis, absent or abnormal uterus, or the presence of a transvaginal septum between the hymen and the cervix. Such conditions may not be connected to any specific event or environmental exposure. However, some conditions may result from biochemical abnormalities in hormone receptor functioning, manifested on either an XX or XY genetic background. Thus, an advanced work-up of patients with primary amenorrhea should also include karyotyping to confirm that the patient is an XX genetic female.

Primary amenorrhea often is the presenting symptom in patients with complete androgen insensitivity syndrome (testicular feminization syndrome). This syndrome occurs when the external genitalia of an XY fetus are unable to respond to testosterone because of a receptor defect and thus fail to undergo differentiation into a phenotypically male form. Internally, however, the testes produce functional Müllerian inhibiting factor, causing the regression of all internal female reproductive organs, thus leading to primary amenorrhea. Individuals with this syndrome have a male genotype (XY) but appear outwardly female on clinical examination. A congenital lack of 5-alpha-reductase enzymatic activity causes a similar phenomenon of external sexual ambiguity in which XY males do not undergo full secondary sexual development at puberty, because testosterone cannot be converted into its more potent metabolite dihydrotestosterone (DHT).

CLINICAL PRESENTATION

Subjective

Amenorrhea is a symptom and is usually the reason the patient seeks health care. Other subjective data from the patient usually are obtained during the history. The detailed history must include a complete menstrual history including age at menarche, date of last menstrual period and last normal menses, cycle regularity, and flow, as well as an obstetrical history, including number of pregnancies, lactation information, and birth control methods. Other components include developmental data to evaluate for short stature or growth hormone or thyroid deficiency; nutritional history including anorexia; diet; stress factors; sports activities; family history (especially mother's age of onset of menopause); symptoms that may arise from systemic disorders (e.g., diabetes mellitus, thyroid disorders); the presence or absence of secondary sex characteristics; and any medications being taken, such as antihypertensive medications or oral contraceptive pills (OCPs). Cyclic pelvic pain in a young teen or preteen could indicate Müllerian outflow tract obstruction.

Objective

The physical examination should include a neurological examination to assess for headaches and visual field abnormalities to rule out a pituitary tumor; olfactory testing to screen for Kallmann syndrome (a genetic form of hypothalamic hypogonadotropic hypogonadism with an absent sense of smell); a pelvic and rectal examination to assess for the presence of a vagina, condition of the hymen, and presence of a uterus; the existence of skin lesions, acne, needle marks, and skin darkening (to rule out adrenal insufficiency); and a breast examination to check for galactorrhea, which may be a sign of hyperprolactinemia.

DIAGNOSTIC REASONING

Diagnostic Tests

A urine pregnancy test should be the first test performed in the patient with amenorrhea. It is inexpensive, easy to perform, and should be done despite what the patient conveys regarding sexual history. If the test is positive, a serum beta-human chorionic gonadotropin level for approximate staging of pregnancy should be drawn. Other tests include baseline blood chemistry profiles to evaluate for renal or hepatic disease, thyroid function tests, and tests for estrogen, FSH, LH, and prolactin levels.

Tests for secondary amenorrhea include androgen studies of total testosterone and dehydroepiandrosterone-sulfate, which are specifically done in female patients who have clinical signs of hyperandrogenism such as acne and hirsutism; prolactin and FSH levels, which evaluate the hypothalamic-pituitary-ovarian axis; and a progesterone (progestin) challenge test, which indirectly provides information regarding outflow tract patency. A progesterone challenge test, which is only administered once a negative pregnancy test result is obtained, consists of giving medroxyprogesterone acetate (Provera) 10 mg or micronized progesterone (Prometrium) 400 mg daily for 7 to 10 days. This should induce withdrawal bleeding or spotting 7 to 10 days after the last dose of progesterone. If withdrawal bleeding occurs, this indicates intact pituitary-gonadal function, and amenorrhea is probably the result of anovulation. The test is negative if no withdrawal bleeding occurs, which suggests low levels of estrogen (e.g., premature ovarian failure, hypothalamic pituitary failure) or a nonpatent outflow tract as the etiology of amenorrhea.

Differential Diagnosis

Differential diagnoses for amenorrhea include pregnancy (intrauterine or ectopic); menopause; premature ovarian failure; genetic and chromosome-related problems; and hyperprolactinemia related to tumor, stress, or thyroid dysfunction. Outflow tract abnormalities include Asherman's syndrome, which is characterized by endometrial adhesions and scarring as a result of endometriosis or previous aggressive dilation and curettage (D&C) procedures on the uterus; uterovaginal malignancies; cervical stenosis; and imperforate hymen.

MANAGEMENT

The goal of management for amenorrhea is to initiate or restore menses while determining the cause. Treatment of amenorrhea is dependent on its etiology and the patient's wishes. For primary amenorrhea, estrogen therapy is indicated for patients to develop secondary sex characteristics and to prevent osteoporosis.

For a patient with secondary amenorrhea whose progestin challenge test is negative, treatment consists of oral estrogen 1.25 to 2.5 mg daily for 21 to 25 days, along with oral progesterone 10 mg daily during the last 5 to 10 days of the estrogen doses. The patient should experience bleeding if the endometrium is responsive to estrogen and the outflow tract is patent.

For a patient with secondary amenorrhea who is anovulatory and has adequate endogenous estrogen, the common practice is to administer periodic or cyclic progesterone 10 mg PO daily for 10 days each month. These patients must experience withdrawal bleeding for at least 3 months to prevent endometrial hyperplasia or endometrial carcinoma related to unopposed estrogen. If the patient is anovulatory and wants to become pregnant, ovulation may be induced with clomiphene citrate (Clomid) 50 mg PO on days 5 to 9 of the cycle after the induction of bleeding with progesterone.

If the patient requires contraception, hormonal contraceptives are beneficial for monthly cycle regulation. For patients with hyperprolactinemia, bromocriptine (Parlodel) is the drug of choice. If hypothalamic failure is established, GnRH may be given in a pulsatile fashion. GnRH is given as a combination with estrogen and calcium because these patients are hypoestrogenic and at high risk for osteoporosis. In patients with thyroid dysfunction, thyroid hormone replacement therapy should be initiated, and amenorrhea should be corrected.

Surgical intervention is possible for patients with endometrial scarring (Asherman's syndrome) from endometritis. Diagnosis and treatment are accomplished in the same procedure, through hysteroscopic inspection and the lysis of adhesions. After this procedure, antibiotics are given, and a small Foley catheter is placed in the uterus to be left in for 1 week. When the catheter is removed, an intrauterine device is inserted and left in place for 2 months while the patient receives cyclic estrogen and progesterone to build up the endometrial lining. This treatment usually restores normal menses and fertility, but complications of pregnancy are common, including spontaneous abortion.

FOLLOW-UP AND REFERRAL

Patients with primary amenorrhea should be referred to a gynecologist. Patients with secondary amenorrhea may need to be referred to a gynecologist and/or an endocrinologist if their initial treatment is unsuccessful. If a CNS problem is detected, computed tomography (CT) scanning or magnetic resonance imaging (MRI) should be performed to rule out pelvic pathology. Before prescribing any medications, the gynecologist may also consider an endometrial biopsy for patients who are at high risk for endometrial hyperplasia and adenocarcinoma (those with diabetes mellitus, hypertension, and/or obesity). Pelvic ultrasound may also be used to measure endometrial thickness and rule out ovarian masses. Once the work-up is completed, the patient should be evaluated annually.

Pediatric/Adolescent Considerations: Amenorrhea

Frequently, teenagers and their parents are apprehensive when menses does not start "on schedule," and reassurance and watchful waiting may be all that are needed. A female patient should be evaluated if menstruation does not occur by age 15 years or 3 years after breast budding. Patients should be taught about their medication regimen and the importance of taking medicines exactly as prescribed. Patients must be aware of the need to notify their health-care provider if they take any new medications, given the potential for drug–drug interactions with many hormonal therapies. Patients should be encouraged to maintain a healthy diet and exercise regimen, because having inadequate body fat from excessive exercise or caloric restriction can result in amenorrhea.

DYSMENORRHEA

Dysmenorrhea is painful menses. It may be primary with no pelvic pathology, or it may be secondary, which is usually accompanied by pelvic pathology.

EPIDEMIOLOGY AND CAUSES

Primary dysmenorrhea usually begins 1 to 2 years after the onset of menstruation, is associated with ovulatory cycles, and lasts for 1 or 2 days each month. There is no associated pathology in this condition, which 50% to 75% of females experience at some point in their lives. The menstrual pain associated with primary dysmenorrhea may lessen for some patients as they age or after the birth of children, or it can last until menopause.

Secondary dysmenorrhea is caused by a physical condition. Females who experience this type of dysmenorrhea tend to be older than those who have primary dysmenorrhea; it sometimes begins when they are in their third or fourth decade of life. Menstrual pain is the predominant symptom, as in primary dysmenorrhea. Possible conditions responsible for secondary dysmenorrhea include endometriosis, pelvic inflammatory disease (PID), fibroids (uterine leiomyomas), adenomyosis, and endometrial polyps. Secondary dysmenorrhea is most common in females 40 to 50 years of age.

It is estimated that each year, more than 140 million lost work hours are a result of dysmenorrhea. It is the most common gynecological complaint and the main cause of missed work, school, or other activities. An estimated 42 million females in the United States experience painful menstrual symptoms each month. Risk factors for primary dysmenorrhea include obesity, low body mass index (BMI), long menstrual cycles, menarche occurring before 12 years of age, nulliparity, cigarette smoking, and a positive family history for dysmenorrhea. Risk factors for secondary dysmenorrhea include endometriosis, pelvic infection, and sexually transmitted infections.

PATHOPHYSIOLOGY

Dysmenorrhea is caused by the production of prostaglandins and leukotrienes, chemical substances that are released when uterine tissue breaks up and is sloughed off during menstruation. Prostaglandin F_2 (PGF_2) and PGE_2 are two of the most important mediators. Elevated uterine levels of these arachidonic acid metabolites, and more specifically an increased ratio of PGF_2 to PGE_2, have been directly correlated with increases in subjective pain with menstruation. Increased prostaglandin levels found in uterine tissue, but not in plasma, cause dysrhythmic uterine contractions and increased resting tone by stimulating smooth muscle tissue to contract, which compromises blood supply and oxygenation to uterine muscle, thus causing possibly severe pelvic pain known as "cramps."

These uterine contractions may last for several minutes at a time, producing maximal pressures of up to 400 mm Hg, with resting pressures as high as 80 mm Hg. In turn, if uterine muscle tone is consistently higher than systemic arterial pressure, uterine ischemia ensues, resulting in the production of anaerobic metabolites that stimulate small type C pain fibers. In turn, pain relief has been directly correlated with decreases in uterine contraction pressure.

Because smooth muscle is found in the stomach, intestines, and blood vessels, as well as in the uterus, excessive smooth muscle stimulation accounts for the nausea, diarrhea, and headache that often accompany dysmenorrhea. Cramps facilitate the release of menstrual tissue, and because the cervical opening is usually widened after childbirth or years of menstruation, cramps may lessen in the older patient. In contrast, intensified cramps are associated with anovulatory menstrual cycles—a common phenomenon in young females, affecting up to one-half of adolescents within 2 to 4 years after the start of menses.

CLINICAL PRESENTATION

Subjective

The patient's description of the pain is an important factor. The type, severity, and duration of pain should be noted. A patient with dysmenorrhea may present with sharp stabbing pain and cramping, low back pain, nausea and possible vomiting, bowel changes, and fatigue. The pain of primary dysmenorrhea usually starts within 24 hours of menses and may last for 48 to 72 hours. Patients with secondary dysmenorrhea may have slightly varying description of symptoms, with some menstrual cycles being more painful than others, and the level of discomfort may be progressive. Secondary dysmenorrhea may have an onset of pain a week or more before the onset of menses, which may continue for a few days after the cessation of flow. Patients may state that they are immobilized by their period every month for the first day. Patients may describe the pain as so severe that at times they cannot do anything except stay in bed with a heating pad on their abdomen. Patients may lose their appetite and eat very little during this time. They may also complain of pain during intercourse.

Objective

A physical examination that reveals no signs of pathology with a history of consistent symptoms for 1 to 2 days each month will usually substantiate the diagnosis of primary dysmenorrhea, because the clinical presentation is fairly typical. If there is a complaint of painful vaginal intercourse, a diagnosis of secondary dysmenorrhea, possibly related to endometriosis, should be explored during the pelvic examination.

DIAGNOSTIC REASONING

Diagnostic Tests

Laboratory studies in the evaluation of dysmenorrhea are ordered to rule out potential causes of pelvic pain. They include a quantitative ß-hCG level, complete blood count (CBC), urinalysis, erythrocyte sedimentation rate, and stool for occult blood. Serum cancer antigen-125 (CA-125) levels are known to be elevated in patients with endometriosis (a common cause of dysmenorrhea), as well as ovarian pathology; however, this test is not sufficiently sensitive to serve as a reliable screening tool.

Imaging studies are the choice for initial evaluation of suspected pelvic disease. Gynecological consultation with visualization of pelvic organs via ultrasound is the initial procedure for the evaluation of pelvic pathology. If such testing does not produce a definitive diagnosis, it should be followed up by laparoscopic exploration to directly visualize pathological conditions such as endometriosis.

Differential Diagnosis

The ultimate goal of the differential diagnosis of dysmenorrhea is to exclude underlying pelvic pathology to differentiate between primary and secondary dysmenorrhea. This includes diagnosing conditions that may produce or mimic dysmenorrhea such as endometriosis, ovarian cysts, ectopic pregnancy, urinary tract infection, vaginitis, abnormal uterine bleeding (AUB), uterine leiomyomas, appendicitis, lower back pain, trauma from sexual assault, and PID. Endometriosis is the most common cause of secondary dysmenorrhea and should be suspected when dysmenorrhea is accompanied by a complaint of painful vaginal sexual intercourse.

MANAGEMENT

The principle of management for primary dysmenorrhea is to relieve the menstrual pain as much as possible. For secondary dysmenorrhea, the goal is to identify the underlying cause. For pain relief, NSAIDs or aspirin every 4 hours, starting 1 or 2 days before menstruation, is helpful because of the antiprostaglandin activity. Dietary changes such as the avoidance of caffeine during the first few days of menstruation have been shown to be helpful. Exercise may be of some benefit because it raises levels of ß-endorphins, which are neurotransmitters in the brain associated with pain relief. In contrast, cigarette smoking has been linked to increasing the duration and severity of dysmenorrhea.

Interestingly, in clinical studies, placebo treatments have been shown to improve symptoms of dysmenorrhea, albeit often only transiently. However, the NSAID ibuprofen (Advil, Motrin) 400 to 800 mg PO three to four times daily as needed remains the mainstay of dysmenorrhea therapy and is considered the most effective over-the-counter (OTC) pain reliever for cramps. Several studies have demonstrated that if ibuprofen fails to relieve a patient's symptoms, it is appropriate to try an alternative NSAID agent such as naproxen (Naprosyn, Aleve), indomethacin (Indocin), fenoprofen (Nalfon) 300 to 600 mg PO two to three times daily as needed, or mefenamic acid (Ponstel) 500 mg PO initially and then 250 mg four times daily for up to 3 days. The latter agent not only inhibits new prostaglandin formation but also inhibits the activity of preformed prostaglandins. In contrast, acetaminophen (Tylenol) appears to be less effective in treating dysmenorrhea because it does not inhibit prostaglandin formation and is not an anti-inflammatory agent.

Application of a hot-water bottle or heating pad to the abdomen or use of hot baths may help relieve discomfort and in some studies has been shown to be as effective as NSAID therapy. However, interestingly, the combination of heat therapy and NSAIDs together has been shown to be counterproductive. Acupuncture, transcutaneous electrical nerve stimulation therapy, and specific herbal teas (e.g., mint tea, certain ayurvedic preparations) have all been shown to decrease uterine spasms in small clinical trials. Relaxation or yoga-type exercises may also help relieve pain. Dietary restriction of both caffeine and salt is also recommended, and vitamin E, vitamin B_1, vitamin B_6, magnesium, and vitamin D have been found to reduce symptoms. There is some evidence that vitamin E therapy 400 IU/day beginning 2 days before the onset of menstruation and for 5 days total for two cycles decreases dysmenorrhea. Other research indicates that ingestion of a single high oral dose of vitamin D has a favorable effect on dysmenorrhea.

For some patients, even prescribed prostaglandin inhibitors are ineffective. Combined estrogen-progestin oral contraceptive agents may be considered for these patients because they relieve cramping by inhibiting arachidonic acid production and ovulation and, in turn, hindering high levels of prostaglandin production. These therapies may be given daily as 21-, 63-, or 105-day continuous courses, each followed by 7 days off medication, before repeating the cycle. Longer cycles of OCPs and other hormonal agents decrease the frequency of menstruation occurring during the off-therapy week.

If no relief is achieved after NSAIDs and OCPs, ultrasonography and exploratory laparoscopy may be appropriate to rule out pelvic pathology. If endometriosis (the most common cause of secondary dysmenorrhea) is found, a GnRH analog may be prescribed in continuous fashion to inhibit menses (see the section on the treatment of endometriosis).

FOLLOW-UP AND REFERRAL

Patients with dysmenorrhea should have follow-up care because treatment is typically chronic and requires further evaluation to confirm persistent symptom relief or to conduct additional diagnostic studies for continued symptoms. The prognosis for primary dysmenorrhea is good with the use of antiprostaglandins, with 70% to 80% relief of symptoms in some cases.

Patient Education: Dysmenorrhea

Patients should be educated that aspirin and other NSAIDs can significantly reduce prostaglandin levels associated with painful menstruation if started 1 to 2 days before menstruation begins. Education about changes in exercise and diet may also be useful. Dietary supplementation with omega-3 fatty acids has been shown to help provide relief in adolescents. Patients should be encouraged to stop smoking and decrease alcohol intake. Patients can also be told that symptomatic treatment with a warm bath or locally applied heat may be helpful.

ENDOMETRIOSIS

Endometriosis is a painful, chronic disease characterized by the presence and proliferation of abnormally located endometrial tissue, which responds to hormonal changes in the female body. Abnormally located endometrial tissue has been found outside the uterus, usually in the abdomen; on the ovaries, fallopian tubes, and the ligaments that support the uterus; as well as in the area between the vagina and rectum; on the outer surface of the uterus; and in the lining of the pelvic cavity. Other sites for these endometrial growths may include the bladder, bowel, vagina, cervix, vulva, and within abdominal surgical scars. Rarely, endometrial tissue may be located in the lung, arm, thigh, brain, or other non–reproductive tract locations.

This tissue reacts to hormonal changes in the same way as uterine endometrial tissue during the menstrual cycle. The bloody discharge produced by such tissue typically has no outlet, and the presence of such discharge may cause severe pain with each menstrual cycle, either during ovulation, menstruation, or both. The accumulation of the discharge may form dense fibrous tissue, leading to adhesions, infertility, and the destruction of ovarian tissue.

EPIDEMIOLOGY AND CAUSES

Endometriosis affects an estimated 10% to 15% of all females of reproductive age and 70% of females with chronic pelvic pain. Females in all levels of society and of all races may be affected, although females of Japanese descent are twice as likely to have endometriosis as those of European descent. The highest level of occurrence is reported in females 25 to 29 years of age, and the lowest incidence is found in those older than 44 years; however, the disease can be found at any age, including in adolescence. Most patients see up to five health-care providers before the correct diagnosis is made.

The cause of endometriosis is unknown. The retrograde menstruation and implantation theory suggests that during menses, some amount of menstrual tissue backs up through the fallopian tubes, implants in the abdomen, and proliferates in response to ovarian steroids. In turn, conditions that lead to genital tract obstruction and impede menstrual outflow contribute to reflux through the fallopian tubes. However, this theory does not explain all of the possible sites of endometriosis, and some experts believe that all females experience some degree of menstrual tissue backup. Direct transplantation may account for endometriosis that develops in uterine surgical scars after a cesarean section or hysterectomy. Another theory suggests that endometrial tissue is distributed from the uterus to other parts of the body through either the lymphatic or hematological circulatory systems. The coelomic (peritoneal) metaplasia theory suggests that undifferentiated cells lining the peritoneal cavity are triggered to differentiate into endometrial tissue by hormonal irregularities. There may also be a genetic predisposition to endometriosis. In addition, research by the Endometriosis Association has recently linked dioxin exposure to the development of endometriosis.

PATHOPHYSIOLOGY

In addition to the etiological theories discussed in the preceding text, a link to immune system dysfunction and the pathogenesis of endometriosis have also been suggested. Reduced T-cell and natural killer cell function is thought to impair the ability of the body to recognize and destroy abnormally implanted endometrial tissue via immunosurveillance. Interestingly, however, an increased number of peritoneal leukocytes and macrophages have been identified within ectopic endometrium. Increased levels of cytokines and chemokines produced by these cells have been identified, including interleukin-1 (IL-1), IL-6, IL-8, tumor necrosis factor, and RANTES (regulated upon activation normal T cell expressed and presumably secreted). These mediators act as growth factors for ectopic endometrium, and vascular endothelial growth factor stimulates capillary proliferation into this tissue. Patients with endometriosis are also more likely than controls to suffer from autoimmune inflammatory diseases.

Any pelvic organ may be a possible site of endometriosis. The cyclical production of ovarian sex hormones allows for the proliferation and maintenance of these implants. Thus, endometriosis occurs primarily during a female's active reproductive phase, rather than during premenstrual, immediately postmenarchal, or postmenopausal phases. This bleeding may cause severe pelvic pain, dyspareunia, infertility, and debilitation. In addition, inflammation of pelvic tissues may lead to adhesions and cyst development.

Endometriosis may be progressively staged from minimal (Stage I: isolated implants without adhesions), mild (Stage II: superficial implants less than 5 cm in aggregate without adhesions), moderate (Stage III: multiple superficial and invasive implants with or without tubo-ovarian implants), to severe (Stage IV: multiple superficial and invasive implants with large ovarian endometriomas and dense adhesions).

CLINICAL PRESENTATION

Subjective

The primary symptom of endometriosis is recurrent abdominal and/or pelvic pain, which may range from very mild to completely incapacitating. Some patients may complain only of premenstrual spotting. However, for those with pain, it may be associated with menstruation (dysmenorrhea) or may occur slightly before the menstrual period begins. Pain may be experienced as generalized abdominal or pelvic pain or pain associated with sexual intercourse (dyspareunia), urination, or defecation. Fatigue, diarrhea, constipation, or nausea may accompany the pain.

A careful menstrual history should be taken, with significant attention to any complaints of pain. A history of allergies, chemical sensitivities, and recurrent yeast (*Candida*) infections may be present. Complaints of infertility should be noted, as infertility is associated with endometriosis in 30% to 40% of cases.

Objective

On physical examination, tenderness in the posterior fornix during pelvic examination is the most common symptom. Lateral deviation of the cervix may be due to internal scarring, and bimanual examination may reveal palpable nodules on supporting ligaments and affected ovaries. However, a definitive diagnosis cannot be made via history and physical examination alone.

DIAGNOSTIC REASONING

Diagnostic Tests

Direct visualization and pathological testing of endometrial implants through laparoscopy provide the preferred diagnostic method, because most implants are located on the pelvic organs. A CBC may be done to diagnose anemia associated with blood loss resulting from endometriosis, and an elevated white blood cell count may also show evidence of an infection. This would tend to make endometriosis less likely, although it would not exclude the presence of abnormally located endometrial tissue. Serum CA-125 levels are more likely to be elevated with advanced (Stages III to IV) endometriosis, but this serum marker is not particularly sensitive and is an inadequate screening tool.

Differential Diagnosis

The clinical manifestations of endometriosis are associated with many genitourinary disorders. The pain experienced is often discounted by the patient or clinician because pain is a frequent (and presumed normal) accompaniment to menstruation, thereby contributing to the delay in diagnosis. Pelvic and abdominal pain can also be caused by gastroenteritis, appendicitis, ovarian cysts, fibroids, or ectopic pregnancy, and these diagnoses must be ruled out. In addition, specific differential diagnoses of the uterus that must be considered include adenomyosis and endometrial polyps.

Adenomyosis is the presence of ectopic endometrial glands and stroma within the musculature of the uterus, which induces hypertrophy and hyperplasia of the myometrium in response to estrogen (and possibly progesterone). It may be microscopic or nodular on gross inspection, but endometrial biopsy is typically negative because changes are primarily in the myometrium. Adenomyosis seems to be more associated with childbearing, but the pathogenesis is unknown. Although one-third of patients are asymptomatic, adenomyosis may present with AUB, dysmenorrhea, and menorrhagia—just as with endometriosis. Abdominal ultrasound may be able to distinguish this diagnosis, but laparoscopy is necessary to diagnose endometriosis.

Endometrial polyps are hyperplastic pedunculated or sessile growths of endometrial glands and stroma at the endometrial surface, ranging from millimeters to centimeters in size. They are common in middle-aged patients, and metrorrhagia (irregular uterine bleeding) occurs in 50% of cases. Less frequently, menorrhagia (abnormally heavy uterine bleeding), postmenopausal bleeding, uterine prolapse through the cervical os, and breakthrough bleeding on hormonal treatments can occur. A definitive diagnosis is made on microscopy (after D&C, biopsy, or hysterectomy), and sonohysterography (instillation of saline into the uterus before ultrasound) is preferred to transvaginal ultrasound (TVUS) for noninvasive evaluation (although it is not diagnostic). Curettage guided by hysteroscopy, rather than done blindly, is preferred for detecting polyps.

MANAGEMENT

Currently, there is no cure for endometriosis. Management is linked to relieving or reducing pain, shrinking or slowing endometrial growths, preserving or restoring fertility, and preventing or delaying recurrence of the disease. In patients with mild disease or those who are perimenopausal and will soon stop ovarian cycling and the consequent hormonal fluctuations that trigger bleeding endometriosis, expectant management (observation) is an important option.

Medication administration should begin with the onset of menstruation to avoid the possible influence of medications on pregnancy. With consistent reevaluation of symptom reduction, the risks associated with medications can be minimized. Prescription pain medications may be necessary to control symptoms, although conservative management calls for using the least potent medications first.

Pain relief is often achieved with NSAIDs and other prostaglandin inhibitors, although NSAIDs are usually sufficient only for disease with minimal pain. Typical medications include ibuprofen 400 to 600 mg four times daily, naproxen sodium (Aleve) 220 mg four times daily, and mefenamic acid (Ponstel) 250 mg four times daily to 500 mg three times daily. Oral contraceptives may also provide adequate relief for patients with mild disease. Studies indicate that low-dose drospirenone/ethinyl estradiol 3 mg/20 mcg OCPs used either continuously or cyclically are effective in reducing pelvic pain resulting from endometriosis, although any of the combination OCPs and other hormonal contraceptives discussed in Chapter 47 can be used. Breakthrough bleeding may occur and is treated with conjugated estrogen 1.25 mg daily for 1 week or estradiol 2 mg daily for 1 week.

For patients with moderate to severe disease, other hormonal therapies may help relieve symptoms. Drugs such as nafarelin nasal spray (0.2 to 0.4 mg twice daily), long-acting leuprolide acetate (3.75 mg intramuscularly [IM] once a month), or goserelin (3.6 mg subcutaneously once a month) are GnRH analogs that suppress ovulation by suppressing pituitary gonadotropin secretion with continuous exposure and, thus, ovarian estrogen secretion. These drugs are used for 3 to 6 months, although the optimum length of therapy is unclear. Adverse effects of these medications are vasomotor symptoms (e.g., hot flashes), vaginal dryness, dyspareunia, decreased libido, insomnia, breast tenderness, headache, depression, and bone demineralization, which can be mediated by "add back" therapy with norethindrone 5 to 15 mg daily. Of note, it is critical to document a negative pregnancy test before starting hormonal therapy.

Another hormonal treatment for endometriosis is danazol (Danocrine) 200 to 400 mg twice daily, which is used for 6 to 9 months. Danazol is a testosterone derivative that acts like progesterone and suppresses menstruation. Adverse effects are androgenic in nature and include weight gain, acne, hirsutism, muscle cramps, lower high-density lipoprotein (HDL) levels, and decreased breast size. Danazol must not be taken when pregnant due to potential harm to the fetus. It should be started during a menstrual cycle, and patients should be using effective birth control during treatment. Danazol may decrease the effectiveness of hormonal contraceptives; thus, patients should be instructed to use barrier contraception in addition to a hormonal method.

Progesterone alone, in the form of medroxyprogesterone acetate 100 mg IM every 2 weeks for four doses and then every 4 weeks, can be given to inhibit endometrial tissue growth and initiate deciduation and atrophy of the endometrium. Oral therapy with medroxyprogesterone 10 mg three times daily or norethindrone 5 mg daily can also be used for 6 to 9 months. These treatments provide 80% of patients with complete or partial symptom relief. Oral estrogen can be added to control breakthrough bleeding. Aromatase inhibitors that decrease estrogen production are still investigational. Regimens may be developed that combine these drugs with progestins or GnRH analogs.

Laparoscopy is used to ablate endometrial implants, which greatly reduces pain. Some patients require removal of ovarian endometriomas along with the ablation of implants, and this procedure improves fertility. For female patients who no longer desire to have children, a total abdominal hysterectomy and bilateral salpingo-oophorectomy (TAH-BSO) will treat endometriosis definitively, but in those with deep implants, TAH-BSO may not be sufficient.

Medical treatment alone is inappropriate for moderate to severe disease, and in addition, does not improve fertility in these patients. Only surgical interventions have been shown to improve fertility. For example, some reviews have shown that with observation alone, pregnancy rates with mild, moderate, and severe endometriosis are 50%, less than 25%, and only 5%, respectively. With surgery, pregnancy rates rise to 50% and 39% in patients with moderate and severe disease, respectively. However, *in vitro* fertilization methods are usually needed postoperatively for patients with severe disease in whom hysterectomy can be avoided. Infertile patients who are trying to improve their chance of pregnancy typically benefit from laparoscopic ablation of endometrial implants.

Alternative therapies are gaining acceptance in the treatment of endometriosis. Visualization techniques, patterned breathing, and massage therapy may each have their place in the treatment of this disorder. Dietary therapy and therapy to maximize function of the immune system may also be useful. Treatment must be evaluated for an appropriate match between patient and therapeutic choice. Financial issues may also be of concern, as hormonal therapies are significantly more expensive than dietary changes or massage therapy (see Complementary Therapies 49.1).

FOLLOW-UP AND REFERRAL

The signs and symptoms of endometriosis are related to the menstrual cycle, and follow-up visits should be timed to allow prescribed treatments to have already affected symptoms associated with the next menstrual cycle. The patient should be referred to a gynecologist experienced in laparoscopic diagnosis and the treatment of endometriosis if the most conservative medical treatments are insufficient to ameliorate symptoms.

Complementary Therapies 49.1: Women's Health Problems

PROBLEM	THERAPY	DOSAGE	COMMENTS
Premenstrual syndrome	Evening primrose oil	250 mg orally up to three times daily 2–3 days before menses	May decrease breast tenderness. Common side effects include headache and gastrointestinal (GI) symptoms.
	Calcium	1,200–1,600 mg orally daily	May reduce luteal phase symptoms. Should be taken in divided doses and with recommended daily dose of vitamin D (400 IU daily)
	Vitamin B_6	40–100 mg orally daily	Common side effects include numbness, paresthesia, and unsteady gait. Patients with Parkinson's disease or taking levodopa should consult their provider before starting.
	Vitamin C	1,500–3,000 mg orally daily	Take in divided doses for better absorption and to avoid diarrhea
	Essential oils: chamomile, basil, lavender, marjoram	Use as directed on label	Aromatherapy
Menopausal symptoms	Black cohosh	40–200 mg orally daily	Not recommended for more than 6 months
	Chaste tree berry	Extracts or tinctures to provide 20 mg of crude fruit or 30–40 mg of fruit decoction	Possible adverse gastrointestinal (GI) effects; contraindicated in pregnancy
	Vitamin B complex	50 mg orally daily	High levels of estrogen related to hormone fluctuations can deplete vitamin B_6, resulting in anxiety, irritability, and depression.
	Vitamin C	1,500–3,000 mg orally daily	Take in divided doses for better absorption and to avoid diarrhea
	Vitamin E	400–800 IU orally daily	Can interfere with anticoagulant therapy; avoid if taking anticoagulants; consult with provider before starting
Breast tenderness	Chaste tree berry Evening primrose oil	As above As above	
Candidiasis (yeast infection)	Vitamin C	3,000–6,000 mg orally daily	Take in divided doses for better absorption and to avoid diarrhea
Decreased sexual desire	Essential oils: jasmine, neroli (bitter orange tree), rose, sandalwood, ylang-ylang, clary sage, patchouli	Use as directed on label	Aromatherapy; aphrodisiac

Patient Education: Endometriosis

Each patient must receive appropriately formulated educational materials about endometriosis, including its signs and symptoms and both short-term and long-term consequences on the patient's reproductive, sexual, and mental health, as this is usually a lifelong condition (see The Patient's Voice 49.1).

LEIOMYOMAS (UTERINE FIBROIDS)

Leiomyomas (leiomyomata) are commonly called *uterine fibroids*. Fibroids are the most common benign tumor of the uterus and arise from smooth muscle cells in the myometrium. Most are small and asymptomatic.

> **The Patient's Voice 49.1: Endometriosis**
>
> I had very painful menstruation from day 1. As long as I can remember, every month I was in bed doubled over in pain. Nothing seemed to relieve the intensity of the pain... even taking birth control pills. My periods were not heavy, but I always had pain and even a little spotting, especially after my period every month. About 1 year after the delivery of my third child, I began experiencing great discomfort with intercourse. My gynecologist suggested that since I was almost 40 years old, a surgical intervention was needed. He explained that laparoscopy or laparotomy and eventual hysterectomy was the usual treatment for women with severe pain. My first surgery did reveal that I had endometriosis... a small amount... but my surgeon said that some of the locations of the endometriosis made it even more painful. I had a difficult time with the hysterectomy... a lot of pain. But, since they removed my uterus, the pain I had for almost 27 years is finally gone. Why did it take so long for someone to give me relief?

EPIDEMIOLOGY AND CAUSES

Leiomyomas are extremely common. Their prevalence increases in females between 30 and 50 years of age and decreases with menopause. By age 50 years, 50% of African American and Asian American females have leiomyomas and about 30% of European American females have them.

The cause of leiomyomas is unknown, but clearly there is a hormonal link. Females before menarche do not have leiomyomas, and they shrink after menopause, implicating estrogen as a growth factor. If a pregnant female has a fibroid, it dramatically increases in size during pregnancy, but decreases after delivery. Risk factors for the development of leiomyomas include nulliparity, age between 30 and 50 years, obesity, and a sedentary lifestyle. Interestingly, smoking seems to decrease the risk for developing fibroids.

PATHOPHYSIOLOGY

Leiomyomas develop from a single neoplastic smooth muscle cell with abnormal chromosomal patterns. Leiomyomas are classified by their location within the uterine wall and can be subserosal, submucosal, and/or intramural. Pedunculated fibroids may also grow out from the surface of the uterus or into the cavity of the uterus. Rarely, a leiomyoma can be intraligamentous, cervical, or parasitic (deriving its blood supply from an organ to which it becomes attached). Most uterine fibroids are surrounded by compressed but otherwise normal myometrium. When leiomyomas outgrow their blood supply, they can become necrotic and ulcerate.

CLINICAL PRESENTATION

Subjective

Most leiomyomas are asymptomatic. When symptoms are present, AUB is the most common clinical presentation. The patient may also complain of pain, particularly with intercourse. If the fibroid is large enough, it can cause pressure on the bladder, resulting in urinary frequency, urgency, and possibly dysuria. A complaint of abdominal or genital heaviness is also common with large fibroids.

Objective

Pelvic examination will reveal one or more uterine masses. Leiomyomas are usually firm and nontender. If there are multiple fibroids (which occurs in most cases), the uterus will feel irregular and nodular in shape.

DIAGNOSTIC REASONING

Diagnostic Tests

Because most patients with leiomyomas have AUB, a CBC is ordered to evaluate for anemia, as hemoglobin is typically decreased due to the increased amount and frequency of menstrual bleeding. Occasionally, compensatory polycythemia may be present. A pregnancy test should be done to rule out intrauterine or ectopic pregnancy. An endometrial biopsy may be done and will be normal, which helps rule out other diagnoses. Pelvic ultrasound or MRI will confirm the diagnosis of a leiomyoma, but TVUS is used most often. Occasionally, hysterography or hysteroscopy is used to confirm cervical or submucosal myomas.

Differential Diagnosis

Differential diagnoses include other disorders that cause uterine enlargement and AUB, including pregnancy (intrauterine or ectopic), adenomyosis (presence of endometrial glands and stroma in the myometrium), endometriosis, an ovarian neoplasm, a tubo-ovarian inflammatory mass, uterine cancer, and possibly diverticulitis.

MANAGEMENT

No treatment is necessary for patients with asymptomatic or very small leiomyomas. If the patient is severely anemic, measures should be undertaken to stop the prolonged, heavy menstrual periods and boost hemoglobin. Medroxyprogesterone acetate 150 mg IM given every 28 days or danazol 400 to 800 mg PO daily will usually slow or stop the bleeding. Patients should be instructed to take OTC iron preparations (ferrous sulfate, ferrous gluconate, or ferrous fumarate) 300 mg daily. Folic acid 400 mcg daily will help boost red blood cell production as well.

The goal of conservative medical management is to shrink the leiomyomas. Oral contraceptives may be effective for some patients, but for others, the estrogen in OCPs causes enlargement of leiomyomas, so frequent monitoring is important. GnRH agonists are given with continuous exposure to decrease LH and FSH levels, thereby producing a hypoestrogenic effect that usually causes leiomyomas to shrink. This is frequently used before fertility treatment or surgery, because the risk of surgical complications is increased with large tumors. The GnRH agents that are used are leuprorelin (Lupron) depot injection of 3.75 mg every 28 days for 3 months or a single dose of 11.25 mg IM. Treatment lasts 8 to 12 weeks and is very costly. Because these drugs induce a menopausal state, the adverse effects reflect those of menopause (see Chapter 47), and they are approved only for short-term use (up to 3 months maximum). These medications are contraindicated in patients with undiagnosed AUB and in those who are breastfeeding. There are other medication classes (selective estrogen reuptake modulators [SERMs], selective progesterone receptor modulators, aromatase inhibitors) that may shrink fibroid volume; however, use of these agents is considered off-label, as there are only limited data to support their use. Insertion of a levonorgestrel-containing intrauterine contraceptive device (e.g., Mirena) has been shown to significantly decrease bleeding with fibroids that are associated with menorrhagia. However, although devices like Mirena may improve dysmenorrhea, they have no impact on fibroid size. Intrauterine contraceptive devices are contraindicated in patients with an irregularly shaped uterus or submucosal fibroids and should eventually be removed after several years.

There are several surgical approaches for problematic leiomyomas. Myomectomy is surgical removal of the myoma and is done when preservation of fertility is desired and the tumor is larger than 12-week gestational size. Hysterectomy (with or without removal of the ovaries) is the definitive treatment for very large fibroids, particularly when bleeding is heavy and the patient is markedly anemic. Few adverse effects occur as a result of hysterectomy, although infection, bleeding, and damage to surrounding organs are always possibilities with any surgical procedure. Other possible consequences of hysterectomy and oophorectomy include depression, sexual dysfunction, and severe menopausal symptoms.

Uterine artery embolization is a relatively new alternative to surgery. Embolization of the uterine arteries produces end-organ ischemia, necrosis, and subsequent shrinkage of the uterus. This procedure is effective in reducing menorrhagia, pain, and uterine volume in 80% of patients. However, a large number of patients report severe pelvic pain, fever, malaise, nausea, and vomiting resulting from the infarcted uterine tissue.

FOLLOW-UP AND REFERRAL

Any patient with severe bleeding, marked anemia, and palpable leiomyomas should be referred to a gynecologist for evaluation and treatment. Patients with small uterine myomas should be reexamined at 3- to 6-month intervals or more often if symptoms increase. If menorrhagia is present, hemoglobin and hematocrit should be monitored frequently.

> **Patient Education: Leiomyomas (Uterine Fibroids)**
>
> Patients with leiomyomas should be reassured that this condition does not increase their chances of developing uterine cancer. If increased bleeding is a problem, the patient should be instructed to take an iron supplement daily and to increase dietary intake of iron-rich foods, as well as immediately report any symptoms of shortness of breath, palpitations, or increased fatigue or pain.

PRECANCEROUS LESIONS AND CANCER OF THE CERVIX

As a precursor of cervical cancer, cervical intraepithelial neoplasia (CIN) has been explored and studied more than any other premalignant lesion of the genital tract. The accessible anatomical location of the upper vagina and cervix facilitates the early detection of premalignant and cancerous lesions of the cervix. In addition, the development and increased use of colposcopy to identify sites of potential dysplasia and assist in directing cervical biopsy have positively affected patient outcomes in the management of CIN and cervical cancer.

EPIDEMIOLOGY AND CAUSES

Several terms have been used to describe premalignant lesions of the cervix. These changes are described on a continuum from mildly atypical to the potential to progress to invasive carcinoma. The grades of severity of premalignant lesions are CIN 1 (mild dysplasia), CIN 2 (moderate dysplasia), and CIN 3 (severe dysplasia to carcinoma *in situ*). With regard to the degree of dysplasia, mild involvement includes one-third of the cervical epithelium, moderate involvement includes two-thirds of the epithelium, and severe involvement includes the full thickness of the epithelium. Carcinoma *in situ* is considered the most advanced premalignant change.

With the increased prevalence of Papanicolaou (Pap) test screening in the United States, mortality rates due to cervical cancer have dramatically declined. The American Cancer Society (ACS) estimates that there will be 14,100 new cases of invasive cervical cancer and that more than 4,280 patients will die of the disease in 2022. Most cases of cervical cancer are found in patients younger than 50 years, although more than 20% of cases are found in those older than 65 years. Hispanic females in the United States have the highest incidence of cervical cancer, followed by African American females. Indigenous females have the lowest risk.

Precancerous dysplasia, or CIN, occurs more often in younger patients, with the incidence peaking in the early third decade of life. About 12% of females will have cervical dysplasia by 20 years of age. At the time of this publication, the American College of Obstetricians and Gynecologists (ACOG) recommends that cervical cancer screening should begin at age 21 years in all females, regardless of sexual history, whereas the most recent ACS guidelines recommend screening start at age 25 years.

The cause of CIN and cervical cancer remains unknown; however, studies implicate several factors. In particular, sexually transmitted human papillomavirus (HPV) is believed to support the development of premalignant and malignant cervical lesions. There are more than 150 genotypes of HPV, and at least 13 have been associated with various anal/genital lesions (e.g., condylomata or genital warts). Two specific genotypes, HPV-16 and HPV-18, have been most frequently (66%) associated with neoplasia (i.e., higher grades of dysplasia and cervical cancer). HPV-31 and HPV-45, and to a lesser extent HPV-33, HPV-52, and HPV-58, account for another 15% of cervical cancer cases. Condom use is promoted, based more on the general principle of preventing sexually transmitted infections rather than on epidemiological data, as protection against HPV transmission is not 100% effective. For example, HPV can be found in many genital areas, including genital tract skin and mucous membranes; hence, condoms do not protect the vulva from exposure to microscopic HPV particles on penile skin.

Although flat HPV cervical lesions are strongly associated with cellular transformation to CIN, most HPV infections are asymptomatic, and patients may be unaware of their HPV status. In addition, females who have a history of early intercourse (by the age of 15 years), begin to have children at an early age, and/or have a history of multiple sexual partners are at greater risk for developing carcinoma of the cervix.

Risk Factors: Cervical Neoplasia

History

- Early intercourse
- Multiple sex partners (more than two)
- Early childbearing
- Sex work
- Immunosuppression
- Prior exposure to radiation
- Intrauterine diethylstilbestrol (DES) exposure
- OCP use
- Cigarette smoking
- Vitamins A, B, and C and folic acid deficiencies

Male Partner

- History of genital cancer, especially penile carcinoma
- Sexually transmitted infections (STIs), especially penile or urethral condylomas
- CIN or cervical cancer in a previous female partner
- Low socioeconomic status
- Multiple sex partners

Infections

- STIs
- HPV infection (especially serotypes 16 and 18)
- Herpes simplex infection
- HIV infection
- *Chlamydia trachomatis* infection
- Cytomegalovirus infection

PATHOPHYSIOLOGY

The normal cervical transformation zone includes columnar epithelium and squamous cell metaplasia. The squamocolumnar junction (SCJ) of the cervix is viewed via a colposcope, which magnifies the epithelium of the transformation zone. Colposcopic examination of this landmark site is important because this area is most vulnerable to neoplastic changes.

Examination of the exocervix reveals where the cervical glandular and columnar epithelium (which is grapelike in appearance) meets the native squamous epithelium distal to the external os in young adult females. After childbirth, this area may enlarge and move further from the cervical os. The junction usually recedes after menopause into the endocervical canal. Throughout reproductive life, squamous metaplasia, a physiological process in which squamous tissue replaces columnar tissue, occurs. This process is most active during fetal development, adolescence, and pregnancy.

The SCJ is first delineated *in utero;* however, metaplasia is an estrogen-dependent process that accelerates during puberty and pregnancy. SCJ cells are more vulnerable and especially prone to damage at these times in a person's reproductive life. An abnormal transformation zone in the SCJ is caused by neoplastic squamous epithelium, thus explaining why exophytic tumors are the most common presentation of cervical cancer.

HPV infection may alter the morphology of the cervical epithelium, leading to nuclear enlargement and multinucleation of epithelial cells, hyperchromasia, and perinuclear cytoplasmic halos. Cellular findings of HPV infection on biopsy can be histologically similar to dysplasia, and misdiagnosis can occur. However, the diagnosis of HPV does not imply clinical disease. Thus, treatment is limited only to symptomatic patients (e.g., those with condylomas) or those with evidence of neoplasia (e.g., positive colposcopy findings). Vaccines against specific HPV serotypes (e.g., Cervarix, Gardasil) have been developed to prevent HPV infection and, therefore, reduce the risk of developing HPV-associated cancers in both females and males, including cervical cancer and penile cancer. Gardasil 9 is the only HPV vaccination available in the United States, although Cervarix and the older quadrivalent Gardasil vaccine are used in other countries. HPV vaccines also protect against genital warts and cancers of the anus, vagina, and vulva, which are also associated with HPV infection. All people should be vaccinated at 11 to 12 years of age but can be vaccinated up to the age of 26 years.

In worldwide studies, epitheliotropic HPV infection has been identified in greater than 99% of cervical neoplasias. Certain viral serotypes (e.g., HPV-6, HPV-11) that undergo episomal replication (i.e., independent replication of viral genetic material without integration into the host genome) typically lead to a condylomata acuminata or a histologically low-grade squamous intraepithelial lesion (LSIL in The Bethesda system [TBS]), which correlates to CIN 1. In contrast, oncogenic forms of the virus (e.g., HPV-16, HPV-18, HPV-58, HPV-52, HPV-31, HPV-45) that integrate into host DNA are more likely to contribute to malignant transformation, including high-grade squamous intraepithelial lesion (HSIL), which usually corresponds to CIN 2 or CIN 3, invasive squamous cell carcinoma, and adenocarcinoma. However, infection alone is insufficient for the development of squamous cervical neoplasia and most cervical cancers. In turn, most females infected with HPV do not develop high-grade cervical abnormalities or cancer. Research indicates that patients with persistent infection with HPV (of 1 to 2 years) are most likely to develop high-grade CIN or CIN 3 +.

The HPV E6 protein degrades the cell cycle inhibitory protein p53, and the HPV E7 protein interacts with the retinoblastoma protein Rb, which leads to dysregulated cell cycle progression. E7 protein also leads to upregulation of the inflammatory cytokines IL-6 and IL-8, both of which contribute to cervical cancer progression. The HPV serotypes HPV-16 and HPV-18 most strongly correlate with invasive squamous cell carcinoma, with HPV-18 portending a worse prognosis. It is clear, however, that HPV infection alone is insufficient to cause cervical neoplasia, and further insult by cigarette smoking, immunosuppression, or other risk factors appears necessary.

Although squamous cell carcinomas comprise 80% of all cervical cancers, at least 15% are attributed to adenocarcinoma, with another 3% to 5% being of a mixed adenosquamous phenotype. The incidence of adenocarcinoma of the cervix has steadily increased in patients younger than 35 years of age since the 1970s, but this may be due to improved screening detection and early treatment of squamous cell disease. However, a greater association of adenocarcinoma with oral contraceptive use seems to imply the importance of underlying hormonal mechanisms in its pathogenesis. Far rarer forms of cervical cancer include neuroendocrine tumors, small cell carcinomas, and rhabdomyosarcomas.

CLINICAL PRESENTATION

Subjective

Patients with premalignant cervical lesions may present with one or more of the following: a history of one or more epidemiological risk factors associated with the development of cervical cancer, a concurrent vaginal infection with symptoms, no recent gynecological care, and no cervical cytology screening for a prolonged period of time.

Females with invasive carcinoma may describe a brownish discharge or a history of abnormal vaginal bleeding occurring spontaneously or after intercourse. Female patients with a history of postcoital bleeding or irregular vaginal bleeding that cannot be explained should be referred to a gynecologist for further evaluation. Typically, only with extensive disease spread will other symptoms manifest (e.g., weight loss, decreased appetite, back pain).

Objective

The key to early detection and diagnosis of premalignant and malignant cervical lesions is a thorough pelvic examination, which includes a speculum examination and Pap smear testing (either for screening purposes as per recommended guidelines or due to suspicious signs or symptoms). Patients with abnormal cervical cytology (obtained by Pap smear) are usually asymptomatic, with normal cervical, vaginal, and abdominal findings on physical examination. However, even if cervical cytology findings are normal, any cervical or vaginal lesion that appears abnormal, friable, raised, or has the appearance of a condyloma requires a referral for colposcopy and potential biopsy, as the location of dysplasia directs the treatment.

DIAGNOSTIC REASONING

Diagnostic Tests

The ACS has developed cervical cancer screening guidelines that are supported by the American Medical Association, National Cancer Institute, American Nurses

Association, ACOG, and the American Academy of Family Physicians. However, an issue that is the subject of ongoing debate is the mandated frequency for performing cervical cytology screening. Currently, the ACS recommends the following:

- Screening should begin at 25 years of age. Primary HPV testing (approved for stand-alone testing) done every 5 years until the age of 65 years is the preferred screening strategy. If an FDA-approved primary HPV test is unavailable, cotesting of HPV in combination with cytology (Pap test) every 5 years or cytology (Pap test) alone every 3 years are also acceptable approaches.
- Patients with suppressed immune systems have a higher risk of cervical cancer. Any patient with a history of HIV infection, organ transplant, long-term corticosteroid use, or *in utero* exposure to DES may need to be screened more often.
- Patients 65 years of age and older who have had documented adequate negative screening for the prior 10 years and with no serious precancerous (CIN 2 or CIN 3) lesions in the past 25 years can discontinue screening.
- Screening is not necessary after total hysterectomy with removal of the cervix, unless the surgery was performed as treatment for cervical cancer or precancer. Patients who have had a hysterectomy but have an intact cervix should continue with screening as outlined earlier.

Although the Pap test is the standard test of cervical cytology, a newer FDA-approved dual-stain test may improve screening sensitivity. The dual-stain test detects the p16 and Ki-67 proteins, which serve as predictive biomarkers for the progression of HPV infection to precancerous lesions over the next 5 years. A complete cervical cytology report should include a statement on the adequacy of the specimen for examination, a general categorization, and a descriptive diagnosis. Results are typically described as follows:

- Satisfactory but limited (less than optimal; may be secondary to partially obscuring inflammation)
- Unsatisfactory (not acceptable for diagnostic evaluation and may require repeat testing or follow-up)
- Within normal limits
- Other (may require follow-up care; the report will have an additional notation if further action is required)

A protocol for the triage and referral of patients with abnormal cervical cytology results is presented in Table 49.1.

TABLE 49.1 Advanced Practice Nursing Interventions: Pap Test Results and Treatment Protocols	
The Bethesda System Category	**Treatment Protocol**
Normal cytology	Repeat Pap test as recommended in current guidelines by age (21–29 years: every 3 years; 30–65 years: every 3 years or every 5 years with HIV cotesting).
Unsatisfactory for evaluation	Repeat Pap test in 2–4 months. If HPV positive and older than 30 years, colposcopy is acceptable
Infection *Trichomonas vaginalis* Fungal organisms morphologically consistent with *Candida* spp. Shift in flora suggestive of bacterial vaginosis Bacteria morphologically consistent with *Actinomyces* spp. Cellular changes consistent with herpes simplex virus Cellular changes consistent with cytomegalovirus	Treat infections that present with symptoms or are identified with cytology results, or test to confirm organism.
Squamous Cell Abnormalities	
Low-grade squamous intraepithelial lesion (LSIL) indicates mild dysplasia (CIN 1) High-grade squamous intraepithelial lesion (HSIL) indicates moderate or severe CIN 2 or CIN 3 but does not necessarily indicate the presence of cervical cancer. Squamous cell carcinoma	Watchful waiting Refer to gynecologist Colposcopic examination likely
Glandular Cell Abnormalities	
Atypical glandular cells (AGC) AGC-NOS AGC-EC/EM—may favor neoplasia AIS (adenocarcinoma *in situ*) Adenocarcinoma	Refer to gynecologist Further endometrial evaluation likely

CIN: cervical intraepithelial neoplasia.

factors are unlikely if the patient has a normal semen volume. Some of the physical, nonpsychogenic causes of ED are listed in Box 51.1.

Medications are a common cause of ED, either directly or through adverse effects. Loss of erection can be caused by central sympatholytic agents, such as methyldopa, clonidine, and reserpine, whereas alpha blockers cause few problems with erection. However, beta-adrenergic blocking agents and spironolactone are known to contribute to physical impairments in achieving erection and can cause a loss of libido. Certain drugs, such as calcium channel blockers, can increase prolactin secretion and thereby cause ED. Selective serotonin reuptake inhibitors (SSRIs) are known to cause ED. Some drugs of addiction can decrease testosterone levels and lead to ED. In addition, zinc deficiency seen in malabsorption or malnourishment syndromes may also cause ED.

PATHOPHYSIOLOGY

To understand ED, knowledge of normal erectile physiology is necessary. Normal sexual function in males has five phases: libido, erection, ejaculation, orgasm, and detumescence. For an erection to occur, there must be an intact autonomic and somatic nerve supply to the penis and the pudendal arteries. Erection begins with neurological and vascular stimulation and is maintained by increased arterial blood flow, increased venous resistance, and relaxation of the smooth muscle of the sinusoids in the corporal bodies of the penis. Additional rigidity of the penis is accomplished by contraction of the bulbospongiosus and ischiocavernosus muscles. The process is initiated by neurotransmitters, vasoactive intestinal peptide, acetylcholine, prostaglandins, and possibly nitric oxide, although the exact mechanism is unknown.

In addition to the increase in arterial blood flow, efflux of blood is reduced. As erectile tissue expands, the peripheral veins are compressed against the enveloping tunica albuginea, which effectively impedes drainage of blood from the cavernous sinuses. The less turgid corpus spongiosum allows the urethra to dilate during ejaculation.

With continued sexual stimulation, the urethral meatus dilates, and sperm move to the ejaculatory duct. Seminal fluid is added to the sperm cells by the seminal vesicles and prostate gland. At the time of vaginal penetration, male secretions produced by the bulbourethral glands and the glands of the penile urethra combine with female cervical secretions. The bulbourethral fluid serves to neutralize the acidity of any urine residue in the urethra and helps to neutralize the acidity of the vagina. In addition, this fluid provides some lubrication for the tip of the penis, thereby promoting the survival of sperm. The sperm cells move by emission into the prostatic urethra, where they become activated by seminal fluid and are motile. In the male, orgasm is concomitant with ejaculation, which is brought about by sympathetic activity transmitted along the hypogastric nerve and lateral pelvic plexus and then through the prostatic and cavernous plexuses. Ejaculation is the strong rhythmic contraction of the vas deferens, seminal vesicles, epididymis, prostate, urethra, and penis. Retrograde ejaculation is prevented by partial bladder neck closure, mediated by sympathetic nerves. Orgasm is a sensory phenomenon in which rhythmic muscular contractions are perceived as pleasurable.

Postcoital resolution, or detumescence, results from sympathetic outflow to the genital area. The periarterial muscle increases its tone, thereby reducing blood flow to the erectile tissues of the penis. A refractory period of variable duration follows, during which time another erection cannot occur.

An understanding of vascular disease as a cause of ED is essential, as continual high blood flow into the vascular system of the penis is necessary to maintain an erect state. Atherosclerosis can cause a failure of the vascular system to fill; therefore, risk factors for this type of ED include heart disease, cigarette smoking, diabetes mellitus, aging, dyslipidemia, and hypertension. Trauma can also damage the pudendal and cavernous arteries from, for example, prolonged bicycling, and thereby cause a failure to fill. Leriche syndrome, with impedance of blood flow into the penis, occurs as the result of obstruction of the distal

---

Box 51.1   Nonpsychogenic Causes of Erectile Dysfunction

Neurological Diseases
- Anterior temporal lobe lesions
- Disease of the spinal cord
- Loss of sensory input (secondary to diabetes mellitus, polyneuropathies), tabes dorsalis (disease of dorsal root ganglia)
- Disease of nervi erigentes (secondary to complete prostatectomy, retrosigmoid operations, aortic bypass)

Vascular Disease
- Leriche syndrome

Endocrine Disorders
- Testicular failure (primary or secondary)
- Hyperprolactinemia

Penile Disorders
- Failure of detumescence
- Priapism
- Penile trauma
- Peyronie's disease

Medications
- Phenothiazines
- Thioridazine
- Imipramine
- Methyldopa
- Guanethidine
- Reserpine
- Spironolactone
- Alcohol
- Heroin
- Methadone
- Estrogen
- Beta blockers
- Thiazide diuretics
- Antihypertensives

aorta at the bifurcation of the common iliac arteries. Presenting symptoms of this syndrome are claudication and ED, either separately or in combination.

Because resistance to the efflux of blood from the penis is necessary to maintain an erection, anything that impairs this ability is considered a failure-to-store defect. It can result from insufficient relaxation or fibrosis of the corporeal smooth muscle. Adrenergic agonists and/or psychological stress can cause insufficient relaxation of the corporeal smooth muscle, whereas atherosclerosis and penile trauma can result in fibrosis. Priapism, persistent painful erection, is usually idiopathic but can be associated with sickle cell anemia, chronic granulocytic leukemia, or spinal cord injury. The persistent erection disrupts this vascular network and can lead to fibrosis and subsequent failure to store.

In addition to the inability to achieve or maintain an erection, ED may also involve abnormal functioning of several other sexual processes. Premature ejaculation seldom has an organic cause. It is usually related to anxiety about the sexual situation, performance-related fears, or an emotional disorder. Psychological disorders such as depression, bipolar disorder, anxiety disorders, and relationship dysfunction may all cause ED.

The absence of emission may be caused by three organic disorders: retrograde ejaculation, sympathetic denervation, and androgen deficiency. Retrograde ejaculation may occur after surgery on the bladder neck, or it may develop spontaneously in a male patient with diabetes. A postcoital urine sample can be analyzed to confirm the diagnosis. Smooth muscle contractions may not occur at the time of ejaculation as a result of the loss of autonomic innervation of the prostate and seminal vesicles after sympathectomy. An androgen deficiency may lead to an absence of secretions from the prostate and seminal vesicles. If libido and erectile function are normal, the absence of orgasm is almost always due to a psychiatric disorder.

Various penile diseases and anatomical abnormalities may also cause ED. Structural causes of ED include micropenis, Peyronie's disease, scarring of the corpora cavernosa, phimosis, hypospadias, and postsurgical sequelae. Peyronie's disease results from localized fibrotic thickening of the tissue around the corpora cavernosa. Fibrous plaque may be palpated along the penile shaft, usually on the dorsum, although plaque may be present on any part of the corpora cavernosa. Inelasticity produces a curvature of the penile shaft on erection that may be very painful. There is a high correlation between Peyronie's disease and Dupuytren's contracture of the palmar fascia.

CLINICAL PRESENTATION

Subjective

Because male sexual dysfunction can manifest in many ways and because the causes are numerous, a careful history is essential for the correct diagnosis of ED and subsequent treatment. Impotence is a very personal complaint, and discussion requires a trusting relationship between patient and clinician and sufficient time during the visit for the patient to voice their concerns. They may complain of a loss of sexual desire, an inability to obtain or maintain an erection, premature ejaculation, an absence of emission, or an inability to achieve orgasm. Frequently, the patient has a combination of these symptoms. It is essential to determine whether the patient has normal erections, particularly during sleep or early in the morning. If an erection does occur, an organic cause is most likely not the cause of the ED. In 25% of cases, medication use may be the cause of ED. The use of alcohol, tobacco, and recreational drugs increases the risk of sexual dysfunction.

A physical examination, including a thorough genital examination to rule out any abnormalities of the penis itself, is critical. The testes should be palpated for size or abnormal masses. If their length is less than 4 cm, hypogonadism should be considered. Evidence of feminization such as gynecomastia and abnormal body hair distribution should be assessed. All pulses should be palpated, including the penile pulse, which can be felt by pressing both corpora between the thumb and forefinger and palpating to either side of the midline. If there is an indication of a vascular etiology from either the patient's history or physical examination, an aortogram may be indicated.

A neurological examination to evaluate the erectile reflex, including anal sphincter tone, perineal sensation, and the bulbospongiosus reflex, should be part of the physical examination. The reflex can be evaluated by squeezing the glans penis and noting the degree of anal sphincter constriction. An examination for signs of peripheral neuropathy, including distal muscle weakness and loss of tendon reflexes in the legs, is indicated, along with tests that will reveal any impairment of vibratory, position, tactile, or pain sensation.

DIAGNOSTIC REASONING

Diagnostic Tests

Initially, laboratory tests that rule out the various causes of ED should be done. These tests include a fasting blood sugar to rule out diabetes mellitus, a lipid profile to rule out dyslipidemia, thyroid-stimulating hormone (TSH) level, and a testosterone level. If the testosterone level is below 300 ng/dL, a serum prolactin level is warranted. Laboratory tests for patients with established ED should include a complete blood count, a blood chemistry profile (including fasting glucose or glycosylated hemoglobin levels), a TSH level, and a prostate-specific antigen (PSA) in males as young as 40 years of age if they have a family history of prostate cancer. Most males older than

55 years will have some abnormal laboratory findings or risk factors, but these may not necessarily be the cause of the ED.

Several specialized tests can be done, but usually only if the cause of the ED is not apparent after the standard testing regimen. The most useful of these additional tests are the nocturnal penile tumescence and rigidity (NPTR) test and color Doppler sonography of the penis. NPTR testing is useful to assess the patient's physical ability to achieve an erection. Sensors are placed at the base and tip of the penis and record the circumference and rigidity of the penis during sleep. Typically, the test is done from 1 to 3 nights. Males usually have erections during rapid eye movement sleep. A physiological cause of ED is indicated if there is an absence or impairment of erections during sleep. This test is self-administered in the patient's home; however, it can be used in the clinical setting to determine erectile response to sexual stimuli.

There are, however, two medical conditions that cause ED in sexual situations yet still allow normal erectile activity during NPTR. The first is disruption of the afferent nerves that amplify the erectile response to external sexual stimuli but are bypassed in nocturnal erectile activity. The second is called *pelvic steal syndrome*, which may occur in physiological states when the patient is awake but not when they are asleep. This condition involves partial blockage of the iliac vessels, which causes erections to occur only when the patient is at rest. Loss of erection ensues, however, with gluteal muscle activity during thrusting.

Color Doppler sonography is used to assess vascular causes of ED. It measures the integrity of arterial influx in the cavernous artery during erection by measuring the peak systolic blood flow velocity in this artery.

Differential Diagnosis

Differential diagnosis of ED requires consideration of fibrosis secondary to trauma, severe urethritis, late-stage syphilitic lesions, penile infiltration with lymphogranuloma venereum, benign and malignant tumors, and congenital penile curvature. Urethral strictures produce an indurated area that may be identified by careful palpation along the penile urethra. A stricture can be identified more easily by detecting resistance to the passage of a small urethral probe or catheter (urethral sound). Occasionally, strictures may be recognized by the presence of an indolent, firm, tender mass that may involve the skin over the penile shaft. Restricted erection may cause ventral curvature of the penis, periurethral inflammation, and, in severe cases, purulent urethrocutaneous fistula.

MANAGEMENT

A number of options are available for the treatment of ED. If an organic cause cannot be found, these patients will most likely benefit from behaviorally based sex therapy. Pharmacological treatments including hormonal therapy are presented in Drugs Commonly Prescribed 51.1. Nonpharmacological interventions including vacuum constriction devices, vasoactive therapy, penile prostheses, and penile revascularization are discussed in the sections that follow.

Drugs Commonly Prescribed 51.1: Erectile Dysfunction

DRUG	ADVERSE REACTIONS	PRESCRIBING CONSIDERATIONS
Hormonal Therapy		
	Sodium retention with dependent edema, increased risk of bleeding, pain at injection site, mild gynecomastia, mood swings, lipid abnormalities	Do not use in patients with serious liver, kidney, or cardiac disease; prostate or breast cancer; or in those with mercury allergy. Peak and trough effects may lead to aggression, feelings of well-being, energy, and increased libido within 72 hours of injection; as peak level falls, patient may experience depressed mood and loss of libido.
Oral agents: Fluoxymesterone (Halotestin) Methyltestosterone (Android, Methitest, Testred, Virilon)	Same as for parenteral agents Not used as much as transdermal or parenteral formulations because of difficulty in achieving adequate blood levels due to significant first-pass metabolism in the liver	Oral agents are not generally recommended because of hepatotoxicity and unreliable androgenic effects.

Continued

Drugs Commonly Prescribed 51.1: Erectile Dysfunction—cont'd

DRUG	ADVERSE REACTIONS	PRESCRIBING CONSIDERATIONS
Transdermal testosterone patch: (Androderm, Testoderm)	Local irritation; burn-like blistering or irritation of skin where transdermal patch is applied	NOT to be applied to the scrotum Should be applied to the arm, back, abdomen, or thigh; may cause local irritation
Transdermal testosterone topical gel or solution: AndroGel 1%, 2.5–5 g packets Testim 1% gel, 5–10 g packets Axiron solution, 60–120 mg	Burn-like blistering or irritation of skin where gel is applied Problems with urination	Apply to the axilla, upper arm, or shoulder but NOT the scrotum; may transfer to partner during intimate skin-to-skin contact
Testosterone implantable pellets: Testopel, 150–450 mg	Infection at implantation site and pellet extrusion	Produces steady blood levels; must be implanted in subcutaneous tissue every 3–4 months Less flexibility in dose adjustment
Testosterone buccal system: Striant, 30 mg	Mouth or gum irritation Allergic reactions Swelling of ankles or legs Breathing disturbances, including those associated with sleep Liver damage	Insertion twice daily in the morning and evening provides continuous systemic delivery of testosterone
Vasoactive Therapy		
Oral agents: Sildenafil (Viagra) Vardenafil (Levitra) Tadalafil (Cialis) Avanafil (Stendra)	Headache, flushing, dyspepsia, nasal congestion, and visual color changes Back and lower limb pain for all PDE_5 inhibitors	None of these agents should be used in patients taking nitrates or alpha-adrenergic blockers, given risk of severe hypotension. Must wait 24 hours before giving nitrate medication after sildenafil or vardenafil and 48 hours for tadalafil
Injectables: Alprostadil (Caverject, Edex)	Penile pain, prolonged erection, penile fibrosis, injection site hematoma, numbness, yeast infection, and priapism May also cause upper respiratory infection, headache, dizziness, and hypotension	Taking along with anticoagulants or heparin may increase risk of bleeding Should not be used in patients with sickle cell anemia, penile fibrosis, coagulopathy, severe cardiovascular disease, myeloma, leukemia, penile deformity, morbid obesity, or penile implants Can be used only once every 24 hours and a maximum of three times a week Patient should be instructed to choose injection site along side of proximal one-third of penis, alternate injection sites, and avoid visible veins during injection.
Transurethral suppositories: Alprostadil (Muse)	May cause urethral irritation	As above Should not be used if partner is pregnant unless a condom is used Suppository is inserted in penis to approximately 1 inch after the patient urinates, and button on top of applicator is pushed to release suppository; gentle rocking motion will separate suppository from applicator. After applicator is removed, patient should massage penis firmly for approximately 10 seconds while standing; erection will begin in 5–10 minutes.

Hormonal Therapy

For male patients with documented testosterone deficiency who do not have prostate cancer, benign prostatic hypertrophy (BPH), breast cancer, or cardiovascular disease, testosterone therapy is the treatment of choice. However, testosterone therapy should not be used in patients with high blood pressure or clotting disorders, and it may increase the severity of sleep apnea. Testosterone therapy can be administered by several delivery methods, including injections, oral medication, topical patches, or topical gels.

Vacuum Constriction Devices

Most vacuum devices work in similar ways, using a process that takes about 2 minutes. The patient inserts their penis into the cylinder, then uses the pump to create a partial vacuum. This causes venous blood to enter the corpora cavernosa, initiating tumescence and rigidity. Once a sufficient erection is achieved, a latex constriction ring is placed around the base of the penis to help maintain the erection. This is a noninvasive procedure and complications are rare. Vacuum constriction devices are now available over the counter and cost between $300 and $500.

Vasoactive Therapy

The development of drugs that decrease the breakdown of 5-cyclic guanosine monophosphate (cGMP) has revolutionized ED treatment. cGMP is the intracellular second messenger of nitric oxide, which is the primary vasodilator and neurotransmitter involved in the erectile response. The first of these drugs was sildenafil citrate (Viagra). Sildenafil is an orally active cGMP-specific phosphodiesterase inhibitor. It results in increased blood flow necessary for successful penile erection. The standard dose is sildenafil 50 mg taken orally at least 1 hour before sexual activity. Contraindications that can cause severe hypotensive effects with sildenafil are listed in Drugs Commonly Prescribed 51.1. Other medications in this class include vardenafil (Levitra, Staxyn), avanafil (Stendra), and tadalafil (Cialis). Phosphodiesterase-5 (PDE_5) inhibitors do not affect libido and do not initiate an erection without sexual stimulation.

Vasoactive prostaglandins have been shown to be an effective treatment for ED. Alprostadil (Caverject) 5 to 40 mcg is injected directly into the base and lateral aspect of the penis, using a tuberculin syringe. Erection occurs within 20 minutes and lasts for approximately 30 to 60 minutes. Prolonged erection (priapism) occurs rarely, and the patient should be instructed to seek medical attention if this occurs. Alprostadil is also available in a transurethral suppository in dosages of 125, 250, 500, or 1,000 mcg. Suppositories produce an erection in about 5 to 10 minutes (see Drugs Commonly Prescribed 51.1 for instructions for use).

Penile Prostheses

Several prosthetic devices that can be surgically implanted into the penis are available in a variety of sizes and diameters. They are placed directly in the corporal bodies. Penile prostheses may be rigid, semifirm, hinged, or inflatable. The inflatable devices are more natural appearing; however, there is more opportunity for mechanical failure. Implantation of a prosthesis, which is a highly reliable but invasive form of therapy, may help patients who have failed therapy with other methods. It is very expensive and not without the risks that accompany surgery. Implantation may be covered by some insurance plans. Most patients desiring implants prefer spontaneity and, therefore, choose this invasive treatment. Significant problems associated with implants are infection, erosion, and occasional mechanical failure (in less than 5% of patients). The most common types of implants are nonhydraulic (using semirigid rods) and hydraulic (using inflatables). Both types of implants involve surgical placement of two cylinders inside the corpus cavernosum. Healing takes 4 to 6 weeks, after which the patient may have intercourse.

Penile Revascularization

The experience with penile revascularization is limited, and some patients fail to have a sufficient erection even after the procedure. Patients with arterial disorders may be candidates for these procedures, which may include endarterectomy and balloon dilation, or arterial bypass. For patients with venous disorders, ligation of the deep dorsal vein or emissary vein or ligation of the crura of the corpora cavernosum may be effective.

In younger patients, several conditions may warrant penile revascularization surgery. Males younger than 45 years of age whose impotence is caused by severe pelvic trauma are the best candidates for this surgery. In patients with impotence of sudden onset, the possibility that trauma to the peritoneum or pelvis may have led to vascular injury should be considered. A congenital shunt should be ruled out in any patient who reports that they have never had a full erection.

Low-Intensity Shock Wave Therapy

Low-intensity shock wave therapy (LIST) has met with success in Europe in patients with severe ED who are unresponsive to treatment with PDE_5 inhibitors such as sildenafil (Viagra), tadalafil (Cialis), and vardenafil (Levitra). It is believed that LIST promotes the release of angiogenic factors that lead to revascularization of the penis. LIST is not yet approved in the United States, although research is ongoing, and some physicians offer this procedure off-label to refractory patients.

FOLLOW-UP AND REFERRAL

Hormonal therapy should be guided by a clinician experienced in the evaluation and monitoring of patients on hormonal therapy. For example, patients on testosterone therapy should undergo monitoring prostate examinations and PSA screening tests, given the theoretical risks of BPH and prostate cancer associated with testosterone exposure. Blood levels of the hormone being supplemented (e.g., serum testosterone) and other regulatory hormones along the hypothalamic-pituitary-gonadal axis (e.g., luteinizing hormone, which stimulates testosterone secretion) should also be followed to prevent the sequelae of medication overexposure. However, interpretation of these hormone levels requires expert knowledge of reproductive endocrinology and is influenced by the timing of both the hormonal treatments and the monitoring blood draws.

Common psychogenic causes of ED include performance anxiety and relationship problems. Thus, referrals to sex therapy and/or couples counseling may be particularly helpful for some patients, especially in combination with other therapies. In addition, all of the invasive surgical interventions described in this section require appropriate referrals to a qualified urologist or pelvic surgeon.

> **Patient Education: Erectile Dysfunction**
>
> The primary role of the provider in educating the patient with ED is to stress the importance of management of chronic conditions such as hypertension, diabetes mellitus, and stress. Guided imagery, regular exercise, and yoga may be recommended as modalities to reduce stress. Tight control of blood pressure and blood sugar levels should be encouraged as a way to limit further deterioration of erectile function. In addition, counseling for the psychogenic causes of ED is essential.
>
> Instructions regarding topical hormone formulations should include warnings regarding the possibility of transfer to sexual partners during intimate contact, as well as the general risk to females and children from unintended exposure to medications affecting the hormonal axis. The risks of hormonal overexposure (e.g., cardiac events) should also be reviewed, including BPH, an increased risk of obstructive sleep apnea, polycythemia, peripheral edema, and both cardiac and hepatic dysfunction.

EPIDIDYMITIS

Epididymitis is inflammation of the epididymis, the coiled structure connecting the sperm-producing rete testis to the vas deferens that allows for maturation of sperm. This inflammation results in scrotal pain, swelling, and induration of the posterior-lying epididymis, with eventual scrotal wall edema and involvement of the adjacent testicle, possibly with reactive hydrocele formation. Concurrent involvement of the ipsilateral testicle results in a painful inflammatory epididymal-testicular complex, termed *epididymo-orchitis*.

EPIDEMIOLOGY AND CAUSES

There is a predisposition to epididymitis when the patient has a history of unprotected intercourse, a new sexual partner, a history of urinary tract infection (UTI) with dysuria, or urethral discharge. Symptoms may also occur after heavy lifting or straining. Younger sexually active males or older males with UTI are the patients who most commonly present with epididymitis. It may also (rarely) occur in prepubertal males, which likely heralds a structural abnormality in the genitourinary tract.

The causes of epididymitis in patients younger than 35 years are usually sexually transmitted diseases such as *Chlamydia* or *Neisseria gonorrhoeae* infections. There is usually a difference in the type of discharge, as *Chlamydia* infection produces a serous urethral discharge, whereas gonorrhea produces a purulent discharge.

Causes of epididymitis in patients 35 years of age and older include coliform bacteria (such as *Escherichia coli*, which is the most common cause) and sometimes *Pseudomonas aeruginosa* or *Staphylococcus aureus*. Epididymitis is often associated with a distal urinary tract obstruction in males older than 35 years or with coliform infections in males engaging in insertive anal intercourse. Tuberculous epididymitis will present with sterile pyuria and nodularity of the vas deferens, as well as pain. Another cause of epididymitis is sterile urinary reflux following transurethral prostatectomy. A granulomatous reaction following bacille Calmette-Guérin intravesical therapy for superficial bladder cancer may also cause epididymitis.

Rare causes of epididymitis include syphilis, brucellosis, blastomycosis, coccidioidomycosis, and cryptococcosis. When nonbacterial epididymitis and epididymo-orchitis occur, the cause is unclear but may be secondary to retrograde extravasation of urine.

PATHOPHYSIOLOGY

UTI and prostatitis, in particular, predispose to the development of epididymitis. Other risk factors include transmission of pathogens via indwelling urethral catheters or urinary instrumentation or as a consequence of transurethral prostate surgery. A urethral stricture of any type may also be a risk factor. Epididymitis caused by sexually transmitted diseases (STDs) is transmitted through the urethra and may be accompanied by symptomatic or asymptomatic urethritis.

Other causes include immunosuppression, trauma, or reflux of urine from the urethra through the vas deferens, causing chemical inflammation and edema within the epididymis that leads to ductal obstruction. Predisposing factors for subacute presentations of epididymitis in otherwise healthy postpubertal male patients include heavy physical activity, prolonged bicycle or motorcycle riding, and sexual activity. These patients may have negative urinalyses and often do not experience dysuria.

CLINICAL PRESENTATION

Subjective

The major complaint of patients with epididymitis is scrotal pain that often radiates along the spermatic cord or to the flank. The pain may appear relatively acute over several hours. Many patients experience pain at the tip of the penis and complain of urethral discharge or other symptoms of UTI, such as frequency of urination, dysuria, cloudy urine, or hematuria. Initially, only the lowermost tail section of the posterior-lying epididymis will be painful, tender, and indurated. Elevation of the testes and the epididymis will relieve the discomfort. Patients with sensory neuropathy as a result of diabetes mellitus may have only minimal pain despite severe infections or abscesses; older adult patients may also present without significant pain. Fever and chills occur with severe infection or abscess formation.

Objective

Physical examination in epididymitis reveals scrotal swelling, and the testis may be indistinguishable from the epididymis. The scrotum wall will be thick and indurated, and a reactive hydrocele may occur. In addition to nodularity of the vas deferens and tenderness of the epididymis, patients with the nonsexually transmitted variety of epididymitis will have pyuria. Rectal examination reveals a tender prostate.

DIAGNOSTIC REASONING

Diagnostic Tests

Initially, urinalysis in epididymitis will show pyuria and leukocytosis. A Gram stain of the urethral discharge may reveal gram-negative intracellular diplococci that are diagnostic of *Neisseria gonorrhoeae*. Culture of the penile discharge may be consistent with *Chlamydia* or gonorrheal infection. If no organisms are visible on the urethral smear but white blood cells (WBCs) are evident, the diagnosis is usually nongonococcal urethritis, in which *Chlamydia* is the most likely pathogen. A complete blood count shows increased WBCs with a left shift of the differential to more immature forms. An ultrasound of the scrotum can confirm the diagnosis of epididymitis.

Differential Diagnosis

The differential diagnoses for epididymitis include epididymal congestion after a vasectomy, testicular torsion, torsion of the appendix testis, mumps, orchitis, testicular tumor, and testicular trauma. An epididymal cyst, spermatocele, hydrocele, or varicocele should also be ruled out as part of the differential diagnosis. In epididymitis, the pain often improves when the scrotum is elevated above the level of the pubic symphysis (Prehn's sign).

MANAGEMENT

Initial treatment of epididymitis includes bedrest with scrotal elevation and ice packs, along with appropriate antibiotic therapy; in severe cases, a spermatic cord block with local anesthetic may be necessary to relieve the pain. In patients younger than 35 years with sexually transmitted epididymitis, treatment is a one-time dose of ceftriaxone (Rocephin) 250 mg intramuscular (IM) in addition to doxycycline (Vibramycin) 100 mg twice daily for 10 days. If the patient is allergic to cephalosporins or tetracyclines, a fluoroquinolone such as ofloxacin 300 mg PO twice daily or levofloxacin 500 mg PO daily can be given for 10 days. It is important to treat the sexual partner as well. Patients with nonsexually transmitted forms of epididymitis may be treated with ciprofloxacin 750 mg PO twice daily, ofloxacin 200 to 300 mg PO twice daily, or trimethoprim-sulfamethoxazole (Bactrim, Septra) one double-strength tablet PO twice daily for 2 to 3 weeks. For the septic or toxic hospitalized patient, ceftriaxone 1 to 2 g IV or IM given every 24 hours is the preferred treatment. An aminoglycoside, such as gentamicin 1 mg/kg IV or IM given every 8 hours (adjusted to the patient's renal function, after a loading dose of 2 mg/kg), may also be administered.

For patients with noninfectious epididymitis, treatment consists of NSAIDs, rest, and scrotal support. Antibiotic therapy is reserved for patients who are refractory to conservative treatment to treat possible occult infection or fastidious organisms that are difficult to culture from urethral swabs or penile discharge. Acetaminophen with codeine (Tylenol #3) may be used for moderate to severe pain.

Surgical procedures may be needed, depending on the severity of the case. An aspiration of the hydrocele may assist in examination of the scrotal contents and relieve discomfort. A vasostomy to drain the infected material may be done as well. Scrotal exploration should be done if there is uncertainty in differentiating epididymitis from testicular torsion. Drainage of abscesses, epididymectomy, or orchiectomy may be considered in severe cases that do not respond to antibiotics. The activity of the patient after these procedures is limited to bedrest for a minimum of 1 to 2 days.

FOLLOW-UP AND REFERRAL

Patient monitoring with office visits should continue until there are no signs of infection. Early treatment of prostatitis may prevent the development of epididymitis. Vigorous rectal examination of patients experiencing acute prostatitis should be avoided because this can lead to epididymitis. The prognosis is good if epididymitis is treated promptly. Pain improves in 1 to 3 days, but induration may last several weeks and take several months to resolve completely.

Complications of epididymitis include infertility or decreased fertility, recurrent epididymitis, abscess formation, or Fournier's gangrene (fulminant necrotizing fasciitis of the perineum and/or genitalia, due to synergistic polymicrobial infection)—all of which are possible if treatment is delayed or inadequate.

> **Patient Education: Epididymitis**
>
> The patient should be instructed to limit activity and immobilize the scrotal contents, which will relieve pain and aid in treating the infection. The patient will need to wear an athletic supporter and avoid sexual contact and physical activity as long as pain persists. Patient education includes stressing the need to complete the full course of antibiotics, even after the patient becomes asymptomatic.

TESTICULAR TORSION

Testicular torsion is the twisting or rotation of the testes, resulting in acute ischemia. It is a urological emergency. The torsion may vary from 90 to 360 degrees about the spermatic cord. An even more common phenomenon is torsion of the testicular appendix or appendiceal torsion, in which a small vestigial remnant of the Müllerian duct located on the anterosuperior portion of the testis twists about its base.

The average-sized adult testis is approximately 4.5 cm x 3 cm x 2.7 cm. Within the scrotum, each testis is surrounded by the tunica albuginea, a tough layer of connective tissue, as well as the tunica vaginalis, which is a potential space formed by a membranous sac covering the anterior two-thirds of the testicle. A cryptorchid testis that fails to descend into the scrotal sac is most prone to torsion.

EPIDEMIOLOGY AND CAUSES

Testicular torsion can occur at any age, from newborn to old age; however, two-thirds of cases occur between the ages of 10 and 20 years, with the peak incidence at 14 years of age. Testicular torsion is possible but rare in older males. Torsion of the appendix testis is more common in children aged 7 to 14 years.

Testicular torsion is usually an idiopathic and spontaneous occurrence. There is a history of trauma in 20% of cases, with one-third of patients having had prior episodic testicular pain. One initiating factor of torsion appears to be the contraction of the cremaster muscle, which may occur during sleep in approximately 50% of patients. The contraction of the cremaster muscle may also be stimulated by trauma, exercise (most frequently in runners), extreme cold (torsion is more common in winter months), and sexual stimulation. Paraplegics are also at high risk for developing testicular torsion, probably as a result of constant pressure while sitting. Other factors contributing to testicular torsion are alterations in testosterone levels and cremasteric contractions during the nocturnal sex response cycle, as well as congenital abnormalities of the tunica vaginalis or the spermatic cord.

PATHOPHYSIOLOGY

If the base of the testis is inadequately fixed to the tunica vaginalis via the gubernaculum, the testis may twist around the spermatic cord under several of the conditions listed in the preceding paragraphs. Arterial inflow becomes compromised, and venous outflow is obstructed, resulting in ischemia of the testis. This is exquisitely painful and may lead to necrosis if it is not treated emergently. Irreversible cellular damage may result in as little as 6 to 12 hours. Even if the testis is salvaged, fertility may be permanently compromised, owing to a disruption of the blood–testis immunological barrier. This exposes germ cell antigens to the systemic circulation, resulting in sperm-specific antibodies that lead to permanent destruction of spermatozoa.

CLINICAL PRESENTATION

Subjective

The most common symptom of testicular torsion is acute onset of pain accompanied by swelling. Torsion of the appendix testis also presents with pain, but it may be more gradual in onset. The patient may have pain for several days before seeking medical attention.

Objective

The most common clinical sign of testicular torsion is the absence of the cremasteric reflex. The testicle may also be high in the scrotum, with a transverse, rather than longitudinal, lie known as a "bell-clapper" deformity. Elevation of the testis does not relieve testicular pain, as is sometimes observed in epididymitis (Prehn's sign). However, this physical finding is insufficiently specific to distinguish between these two disorders. Occasionally, with torsion of the appendix testis, there may be a small lump that is palpable on the superior pole of the testis. If the skin is pulled tautly over it, the lump may appear blue ("blue dot sign"). This "blue dot" results from infarction and necrosis of the appendix testis and is present in about one-fifth of cases.

DIAGNOSTIC REASONING

Diagnostic Tests

Testicular torsion is diagnosed by history and presenting manifestations. The only initial assessment required is a physical examination. Color Doppler ultrasonography or radionuclide scanning can be used to diagnose both testicular torsion and appendiceal torsion. Doppler ultrasound can detect an absent or reduced pulse with torsion and an increased flow with an inflammatory process, although Doppler ultrasound is reliable only in the first 12 hours following torsion. A radionuclide testicular scintigraphy with technetium 99-m (99m-Tc) pertechnetate will show absent or decreased vascularity in patients with testicular torsion; increased vascularity will be evident in patients with an inflammatory process, including torsion of the appendix testis.

Differential Diagnosis

Differential diagnoses for testicular torsion include epididymo-orchitis, an incarcerated or strangulated inguinal hernia, an acute hydrocele, a traumatic hematoma, idiopathic scrotal edema, a torsion appendix testis, an acute varicocele, a testicular tumor, or Henoch-Schönlein purpura. Scrotal abscesses and leukemic infiltrates are also important considerations in the differential diagnosis and must be ruled out. Some pathological findings associated with testicular torsion include venous thrombosis, tissue edema, necrosis, and arterial thrombosis.

MANAGEMENT

Compression of the testicular vessels leads to ischemic necrosis of the testes within 6 hours. Failure to recognize the torsion and intervene immediately results in the loss of the testicle in 80% of cases, with subsequent atrophy of the testis in 10% or more. Resolution with the maintenance of fertility occurs in only 10% of patients.

Upon diagnosis, immediate referral of the patient to the emergency department is indicated, as testicular torsion is a urological emergency. In the emergency department, manual reduction may be successful. Manual reduction of the testis is classically done with gentle external rotation of the testis toward the thigh, because most cases of torsion occur with medial rotation away from the thigh. However, retrospective studies have demonstrated lateral testicular torsion in up to one-third of cases. Relief of pain, resolution of the "bell-clapper" deformity, and a restoration of arterial blood flow are used as the primary indications of effective reduction of testicular torsion. Reduction is followed by surgical exploration. Any testis that is not clearly viable is removed. Surgical exploration via a scrotal approach—with detorsion, evaluation of testicular viability, orchidopexy (permanent anchoring of the testis in the scrotum) of the viable testicle, and orchidectomy (removal) of the nonviable testicle—is the preferred surgical intervention. Surgery should be done within 4 hours after the onset of symptoms to preserve the testicle; after 12 hours the viability of the testicle is diminished.

For a patient with torsion of the appendix testis, surgery may also be performed, but recovery is quicker than that of testicular torsion. Conservative medical treatment may be initiated with rest, ice, and NSAIDs, but recovery is much slower, and pain may persist for weeks to months. The dead appendiceal tissue is usually reabsorbed, however, and fertility is preserved.

FOLLOW-UP AND REFERRAL

Testicular salvage is directly related to the duration of torsion; the salvage rate is 85% to 90% if torsion has persisted for less than 6 hours. The salvage rate becomes less than 10% if the duration of the torsion is greater than 24 hours. Depressed spermatogenesis occurs in 80% to 94% of individuals and may be related to the duration of ischemic injury.

Patient Education: Testicular Torsion

As many as two-thirds of testes salvaged may atrophy in the first 2 to 3 years post-torsion. The possibility of testicular atrophy in a salvaged testis, along with depressed sperm counts, necessitates patient education and understanding of these potential sequelae. Patients should be taught to seek immediate care when experiencing testicular pain to prevent permanent sequelae.

HYDROCELE

A hydrocele is a collection of peritoneal fluid within the scrotum around the testes, between the parietal and visceral (adjacent to the testis) layers of the tunica vaginalis—the two-layered sac that surrounds the testis and spermatic cord. A hydrocele forms when secretion of fluid into this potential space exceeds its reabsorption. These collections may range from only a few milliliters of fluid to enormous volumes measured in liters.

EPIDEMIOLOGY AND CAUSES

The incidence rate of hydrocele is about 1% in adult males. Most hydroceles occur in males older than 40 years. Causes of an acute hydrocele include nonspecific acute epididymitis, tuberculous epididymitis, trauma to the testes, tumor of the testes, or sequelae as complications of radiation therapy. Exstrophy of the bladder (protrusion of the bladder through the abdominal wall) may increase the risk for hydrocele formation. Patients with Ehlers-Danlos syndrome have an increased risk for hydrocele, as do patients with a ventricular peritoneal shunt for dialysis or peritoneal dialysis.

PATHOPHYSIOLOGY

A basic knowledge of scrotal anatomy is required to understand the pathogenesis of a hydrocele. The processus vaginalis originates as a diverticulum of the peritoneal sac that lines the abdomen, just inferior to the testis. During development, as the testis descends into the scrotum, it brings this diverticulum down with it, eventually becoming engulfed by it. The sac surrounding the testis (now called the *tunica vaginalis*) remains connected to the peritoneal sac via the processus vaginalis. Typically, throughout infancy and childhood, the connecting portion of the sac between the tunica vaginalis and the processus vaginalis gradually closes, breaking communication with the peritoneal sac.

Hydroceles in infants typically result from a patent processus vaginalis that fails to close during in utero development, allowing for the free flow of fluid between the peritoneal sac and the tunica vaginalis. These hydroceles have been directly correlated with the risk of indirect inguinal herniation, in which gut contents bulge through a patent processus vaginalis. A noncommunicating hydrocele results from complete closure of the processus vaginalis, trapping peritoneal fluid within the tunica vaginalis. This type of hydrocele may be self-limited in adults. A hydrocele of the spermatic cord forms when the distal processus vaginalis closes, but the midportion surrounding the cord remains patent and filled with fluid. The proximal portion may be opened or closed.

Rapidly forming hydroceles may result from reactive inflammatory processes within the scrotum such as testicular or appendiceal testicular torsion, epididymitis, and even testicular cancer. A chronic hydrocele may result from gradual fluid accumulation within the tunica vaginalis in young males, caused by an imbalance in fluid secretion, conduction, and reabsorption.

CLINICAL PRESENTATION

Subjective

Patients with a hydrocele typically present with swelling in the scrotum or inguinal canal. If the size of the scrotum fluctuates, a communicating hydrocele could exist. Hydroceles are usually painless, although patients report a sense of heaviness in the scrotum. If pain is present, it may radiate to the lower back.

Objective

The scrotum is transilluminated with a penlight in a darkened room during the physical examination. The trapped fluid appears light pink, yellow, or red. The hydrocele can be illuminated to show the full size and shape, which assists in the diagnosis. The testes themselves do not transilluminate, nor do hematomas. Swelling may be noted in the groin or in the upper scrotum.

DIAGNOSTIC REASONING

Diagnostic Tests

A detailed description of the events that precipitated finding the hydrocele should be obtained. Details of any trauma incurred will assist in the evaluation. If a hydrocele cannot be confirmed, the patient should be referred for an inguinoscrotal ultrasound, which can distinguish the presence or absence of bowel within the inguinal ring. A testicular nuclear scan is used to distinguish testicular torsion. Abdominal x-ray studies may be useful in distinguishing an incarcerated hernia from a hydrocele but are rarely needed.

Differential Diagnosis

The differential diagnoses for a hydrocele include indirect inguinal hernias (because of the location of the hydrocele), orchitis (inflammation or infection of the testes), epididymitis (an inflammatory process that can produce symptoms that mimic those of a hydrocele), or a varicocele (a mass of varicose veins in the spermatic cord within the scrotum). Pain is more likely to be present with epididymitis. Traumatic injury to the testes must be ruled out by history and physical examination. Torsion of the testicle or torsion of the appendix of the testes must also be ruled out. Exploratory surgery is indicated for the definitive diagnosis of a patent processus vaginalis in a communicating hydrocele. A scrotal mass of any type requires further evaluation for testicular or scrotal cancer.

MANAGEMENT

For adults, no treatment of a hydrocele is required unless complications are present or the clinician suspects a significant underlying cause, such as a testicular tumor. If the hydrocele is painful, large, unsightly, or uncomfortable, however, several treatments are available. For example, a variety of outpatient surgical procedures are used to treat hydroceles. The Jaboulay-Winkelmann surgical procedure is for thick hydrocele sacs that form when the hydrocele has wrapped itself posteriorly around the cord structures. The Lord procedure is used for a thin hydrocele sac, in which a radial suture is used to gather the hydrocele sac posterior to the testis and the epididymis. The hydrocele can be surgically drained and the tunica vaginalis resected. Sclerotherapy (injection of a sclerotic irritant into the tunica vaginalis to induce scarring and adhesions between the adjacent layers of the tunica) and endoscopic procedures can also be performed to alleviate hydroceles. Aspiration of hydroceles is usually not done because the fluid rapidly reaccumulates; however, it may be helpful for a postoperative hydrocele.

FOLLOW-UP AND REFERRAL

Patient monitoring for a hydrocele should be at 3-month intervals until the decision is made for or against surgery. Postoperatively, patient monitoring should be at 2- to 3-week intervals initially, followed by 2- to 3-month intervals until there is resolution.

Postoperative traumatic hydroceles are common and usually resolve spontaneously. Other possible complications seen with postoperative hydroceles include injury to the vas deferens or vessels in the spermatic cord, suture granuloma, surgical hematoma, or wound infection.

Patient Education: Hydrocele

For patients with a hydrocele, education regarding an explanation of the disease process and management plan is appropriate, along with reassurance of the overall benign nature of the condition (depending on the underlying cause).

VARICOCELE

A varicocele is an abnormal degree of venous dilation of the pampiniform plexus in the spermatic cord above the testes, which usually results in pain and engorgement of the testis.

EPIDEMIOLOGY AND CAUSES

There is no ethnic predisposition or age differentiation among patients with varicoceles. The overall incidence rate is 8% to 20%. In males evaluated for infertility, however, the rate of varicocele increases to 30% to 40%. A weakened vessel wall in the spermatic vein or excessive pressure in these vessels is the leading cause of varicoceles.

PATHOPHYSIOLOGY

The pathophysiology of a varicocele results from vascular engorgement of the internal spermatic vein. A varicocele almost always appears on the left or bilaterally, because the left spermatic (gonadal) vein empties into the left renal vein, whereas the right spermatic vein empties into the inferior vena cava. One of the longest veins in the body, the left spermatic vein, empties into the left renal vein at a perpendicular angle. Compared with the right renal vein, the left renal vein has a higher intravascular pressure owing to its anatomical positioning between the aorta inferiorly and the superior mesenteric artery. In turn, if the valves of the left renal vein become incompetent because of this increased pressure, retrograde blood flow causes back pressure to be transmitted to the pampiniform venous plexus, which overlies the testis. In contrast, a unilateral right-sided varicocele may result from serious pathology that causes increased pressure within the inferior vena cava, such as a tumor or thrombus.

CLINICAL PRESENTATION

Subjective

The patient may present with pain and engorgement of the testes. The recognition of a varicocele is usually secondary to a problem with fertility, however. A patient with a varicocele often describes the sensation of palpating the affected portion of the scrotum as feeling like a "bag of worms" due to engorgement of tortuous blood vessels.

Objective

On physical examination, with the patient in an upright position, tortuous veins located posterior to and above the testis can be assessed. The engorged veins may extend up into the external inguinal ring. Venous dilation can be increased by having the patient perform the Valsalva maneuver in a recumbent position, which reduces blood flow back to the heart. The reverse is also true; in the recumbent position, the venous distention will abate if the patient is not bearing down. In more advanced cases, testicular atrophy with impaired circulation may be present.

DIAGNOSTIC REASONING

Diagnostic Tests

A system of grading has been established to better define varicocele. A Grade 1 varicocele is palpable only when the patient performs the Valsalva maneuver. A Grade 2 varicocele is palpable when the patient is standing. A Grade 3 varicocele may be assessed with light palpation and visual inspection.

Sperm count and motility are significantly decreased in patients with a varicocele approximately 65% to 75% of the time. There is evidence of a progressive decline in fertility in patients with varicoceles. Scrotal ultrasound, venography (showing testicular venous reflux from a varicocele), and thermography (showing an increase in temperature at the varicocele) all help to confirm the diagnosis.

Differential Diagnosis

The differential diagnoses for a varicocele include hydrocele, spermatocele, testicular tumor, epididymal cyst, and renal tumor. A diagnostic priority is questioning the patient thoroughly for any contributing factors and the time course of the finding. It is essential to note whether the onset of the testicular abnormality has been rapid or has resulted from a gradual increase in the varices or other structures surrounding the testicles, as this will point the clinician in the diagnostic direction of acute or chronic pathologies. Of note, in an older patient, the development of a varicocele may be a late sign of a renal tumor.

MANAGEMENT

After a varicocele has been diagnosed, referral to a surgeon is indicated, although most patients do not require surgery because the majority of varicoceles are minor. Surgical treatment of a varicocele involves ligation of the internal spermatic vein, which usually results in decompression of the varicocele and improvement in the quality of semen, as well as a decrease in pain. The surgery can be laparoscopic, approached anteriorly via an inguinal or subinguinal approach, approached posteriorly via a lumbar approach, or even microsurgically. Embolization with coils is a second-line therapy and appears to have a higher complication rate, owing to possible migration of the coils. Testicular atrophy is a definite indication for treatment. Conservative treatment in older patients with only minor pain, for whom fertility is no longer an issue or who have normal fertility, may consist of NSAIDs and scrotal support. Treatment of varicoceles has not consistently improved sperm count or fertility in controlled trials.

FOLLOW-UP AND REFERRAL

Complications of varicoceles (if not corrected) include infertility and testicular atrophy. Referral to a urologist is recommended for affirmation of the diagnosis and further explanation of treatment options. Any patient with recent onset of a varicocele, infertility, pain, or testicular atrophy should have a urological consultation to rule out more serious pathology and to optimize the treatment plan.

Patient Education: Varicocele

Education for the patient should include an explanation of the disease process, signs, symptoms, and potential complications. The patient should be taught how to monitor growth and symptoms of the varicocele, especially if it is right sided. To relieve pain, the patient should be encouraged to wear a scrotal support; for some patients, wearing more supportive jockey shorts (briefs) rather than loose boxer shorts is sufficient to relieve discomfort.

TESTICULAR CANCER

Primary testicular neoplasms may arise from any testicular or adnexal cell component. Each testis is covered externally by two layers of fascia: the outer layer called the *tunica vaginalis* and the deeper albuginea layer, which extends internally and divides the testis into 250 to 300 lobules. Each lobule contains seminiferous tubules (the sites of spermatogenesis) and interstitial cells that produce androgens, including testosterone. The epididymis lies along the external surface of each testis and is the site of sperm maturation and storage. Tumors of the germ cells and the seminiferous tubules are the most common testicular carcinomas.

EPIDEMIOLOGY AND CAUSES

Although testicular malignancies comprise only 1% to 2% of all neoplasms in males (1 out of every 263 males will develop testicular cancer), the psychologically and physically debilitating effects of testicular cancer affecting males aged 15 to 35 years deserve mention because testicular cancer is the most common solid malignancy in this age-group. Fortunately, it is also one of the most curable of all solid cancers.

In the United States, there are 5.9 new cases of testicular cancer per 100,000 males diagnosed each year. It is less common in African Americans than in the overall population, at 1.7 cases per 100,000 males. In adult males, germ cell cancers comprise 90% to 95% of all testicular cancers, and in young males they represent 60% to 75%. The peak age of onset is between 20 and 40 years, with an average age at diagnosis of 33 years. Although testicular cancer is mainly a disease of younger males, 7% of cases occur in males aged 55 years and older.

No clear cause-and-effect relationships have been identified for testicular cancer. Prior cryptorchidism is the only undisputed risk factor for this type of cancer, with 10% of testicular tumors associated with this condition. Importantly, one-fourth of these tumors occur in the contralateral, descended testis. In addition to cryptorchidism, a personal history of previous testicular cancer and a family history of testicular cancer also appear to confer a greater risk.

Other possible risk factors that have been identified for testicular cancer include higher social status, being unmarried, and living in a rural area. Weak associations demonstrate that hormonal imbalances associated with *in utero* exposure to estrogen may increase the risk for testicular cancer later in life. One study of mothers who used diethylstilbestrol during the first trimester found a 2.5- to fivefold increase of testicular cancer in their sons.

PATHOPHYSIOLOGY

A primary testicular neoplasm may arise from any testicular adnexal cell component. These are divided into germinal (90% to 95%) and nongerminal (sex cord–stromal) tumors. For treatment purposes, germinal tumors are further divided, based on histology, into seminomas and nonseminomas (e.g., embryonal carcinomas, teratomas, choriocarcinomas, and yolk sac tumors), which are epithelial in nature. In contrast, far rarer are the sex cord–stromal tumors, which consist primarily of Leydig cell variants that produce estrogen due to increased aromatase activity, and Sertoli cell tumors, which may also present with estrogenic overload.

Only a small number of molecular markers have been consistently associated with testicular cancers, for example, an isochromosome of chromosome 12p, activating mutations in *c-kit*, increased *p53* levels, and telomerase expression. Abnormal DNA ploidy is also common in germ cell tumors. Although certain genetic alterations differ in germ cell tumors found in prepubertal males, all germ cell tumors are believed to arise from pluripotential primordial germ cells. One exception to this is the relatively rare spermatocytic seminoma, the pathogenesis of which appears to be fundamentally different, based on unique molecular markers.

Except for spermatocytic seminomas, all germ cell tumors may be preceded by a premalignant condition known as *intratubular germ cell neoplasia of unclassified type* (ITGCNU) or testicular carcinoma *in situ*. It is found adjacent to 90% of germ cell tumors, implying that genetic mutations lead to gonadal dysfunction and subsequent malignancy over a large area of tissue—a phenomenon known as a *field defect*. At least one-half of the cases of untreated ITGCNU will progress to invasive malignant disease within 5 years, predictably spreading to the retroperitoneal draining lymph nodes. Patients with a history of cryptorchidism are recommended to have an empiric testicular biopsy between the ages of 18 and 20 years to evaluate for ITGCNU.

CLINICAL PRESENTATION

Subjective

Typically, the patient with testicular cancer presents with a hard lump or nodule on the testis that is felt while performing a testicular self-examination. Generally, testicular cancer presents as a painless enlargement of the testis. The patient may also note scrotal swelling, heaviness in the scrotum that may be interpreted as pain, a sensation of fullness, or a previously small testis that has enlarged to the size of a normal testis or the contralateral testis.

Objective

During routine physical examinations (e.g., a sports physical), a scrotal nodule or swelling is most commonly detected in males with testicular cancer. A firm, nontender mass within the confines of the tunica albuginea is typically palpable and distinct from the spermatic cord structures. Acute or chronic epididymitis or epididymo-orchitis may result in a delay in the diagnosis of testicular cancer in about 10% of cases. Gynecomastia may be present in 5% of patients with testicular malignancies. Hydroceles may develop secondary to testicular cancer and are seen in 5% to 10% of patients.

As many as 10% of patients with testicular cancer will be asymptomatic, and another 10% will present with manifestations of metastasis. Symptoms of metastases may include respiratory symptoms (e.g., cough) due to lung metastases, low back pain and nerve root or psoas muscle irritation due to retroperitoneal metastasis, or lower extremity swelling from obstruction of the vena cava.

DIAGNOSTIC REASONING

Diagnostic Tests

Several biochemical markers can aid in the diagnosis of testicular carcinoma, but their main use is in following disease progression or remission after treatment by monitoring for trends in blood levels. These tests include alpha-fetoprotein (AFP) and human chorionic gonadotropin (hCG). AFP levels are elevated by pure embryonal carcinoma, teratocarcinoma, yolk sac tumor, or a combinations of these three malignancies, but not by pure choriocarcinoma or seminoma. However, AFP may also be elevated in benign liver disease, telangiectasis (capillary dilatation), tyrosinemia, and malignancies of the liver, pancreas, stomach, and lung. Heavy marijuana smoking can also elevate levels of AFP.

Levels of hCG are elevated by all choriocarcinomas and occasionally with seminomas; however, hCG is also elevated in liver, lung, pancreatic, and stomach malignancies, as well as with kidney, breast, and bladder tumors. Forty percent to 60% of patients with an embryonal carcinoma and 5% to 10% of patients with seminomas have detectable levels of hCG (usually under 500 ng/mL). In general, elevated AFP, hCG, or lactate dehydrogenase is a poor prognostic sign in testicular cancer, and prognosis worsens with the degree of elevation. Elevated placental alkaline phosphatase (PLAP) may be the marker of choice for seminomas in 70% to 90% of patients. Patients with recurrent or disseminated seminomas have elevated PLAP levels. However, PLAP is not entirely specific because it may also be elevated by heavy tobacco smoking.

Scrotal ultrasound is also a useful diagnostic tool for testicular cancer because the mass can usually be seen clearly originating within the testis. Using an echotexture (hypoechoic) pattern, ultrasound will show that the mass appears distinct from the surrounding normal testicular tissue. Uniformly cystic or fluid-filled masses are not likely to be testicular cancer, which is a solid tumor. However, ultrasound is not accurate for staging and should not replace orchiectomy as the procedure of choice. Magnetic resonance imaging is not usually more informative than scrotal ultrasound or pelvic/abdominal computed tomography (CT) for staging and identifying enlarged retroperitoneal lymph nodes that signify the need for nodal dissection. Positron emission tomography scanning is usually used only to identify residual masses after treatment.

Chest x-ray studies, with both posterior-anterior and lateral views, are important for the identification of metastasis and to rule out the spread of malignancy above the diaphragm. A CT scan is able to characterize pelvic retroperitoneal and mediastinal lymphadenopathy, as well as detect metastases to the abdominal viscera.

Differential Diagnosis

A definitive diagnosis of testicular cancer may be made with trans-inguinal scrotal exploration and biopsy and/or radical orchiectomy (excision of the testicle and spermatic cord). Trans-scrotal open or cutaneous biopsy and trans-scrotal orchiectomy are contraindicated because of the potential for anatomical trespassing into the various lymphatic drainage systems. Testicular cancer is typically a painless mass in the testis, but the differential diagnosis includes epididymitis, hernia, hydrocele, hematoma, spermatocele, syphilitic gumma, and varicocele.

MANAGEMENT

The main principle of management for testicular cancer is a radical orchiectomy, which is also the major diagnostic tool because the whole testis is removed for biopsy. Testicular cancer is highly treatable, with fewer than 450 deaths per year in the United States at present. Treatment, however, leaves the patient with a high probability of being infertile. Sperm banking (semen cryopreservation) should be done before radiographic diagnostic studies, if desired. Many of these patients have gonadal dysgenesis with a low baseline sperm count and morphology problems, but sperm banking works well in general, and future children fathered with this banked sperm do not have higher rates of congenital defects.

Testicular carcinoma is divided into two main categories when considering treatment. The first category, nonseminomas, includes embryonal cell carcinomas (20%), teratomas (5%), choriocarcinomas (less than 1%), and mixed cell types (40%). The second category is seminomas (35%). Staging depends on the type of tumor (nonseminoma vs. seminoma). In addition, the American Joint Committee on Cancer classifies tumors, using the TNM(S) system. The size of the tumor (T), the spread to nearby lymph nodes (N), any metastasis (M), and serum markers (S) are considered in this system of staging (see Table 51.1 for testicular tumor staging criteria).

Seventy-five percent of nonseminomas can be cured with orchiectomy alone, usually with a modified retroperitoneal lymph node dissection. This is done to preserve the sympathetic innervation so the patient will still have ejaculatory function. The serum markers are monitored postorchiectomy, and those patients whose levels return to normal have an excellent prognosis. For patients with nonseminomas that have metastasized or who have significant lymph node involvement (greater than 3 cm), combination chemotherapy is used after orchiectomy. Commonly used chemotherapeutic agents include cisplatin (Platinol), etoposide (VePesid), and bleomycin (Blenoxane) or paclitaxel (Taxol). If the serum tumor markers do not normalize after chemotherapy, salvage chemotherapy is needed, which may include cyclophosphamide (Cytoxan) or ifosfamide (Ifex)–based protocols, with mesna (Mesnex) to protect against hemorrhagic cystitis.

The 5-year relative survival rates from the Surveillance, Epidemiology, and End Results (SEER) program for patients with localized testicular cancer is 99%; with regional disease it is 96%, and with distant disease it is 73%. The rate for all SEER stages combined is 95%.

Seminomas are chemosensitive and have a strong therapeutic response. They are also extremely sensitive to radiation therapy. All patients with seminomas should have radical orchiectomy surgery. Then, depending on the stage of the cancer, irradiation and chemotherapy will be used. For patients with Stages I and IIA (retroperitoneal disease less than 10 cm), surgery and radiation are the treatments of choice and are associated with a 5-year survival of 98% and 92% to 94%, respectively.

More advanced Stage II (retroperitoneal disease greater than 10 cm) and Stage III seminomas receive primary chemotherapy either with etoposide and cisplatin or a combination of cisplatin, etoposide, and bleomycin. If enlarged lymph nodes (more than 3 cm in diameter) persist after chemotherapy, a retroperitoneal lymph node resection is done. In 40% of cases, there is residual carcinoma in these lymph nodes. Ninety-five percent of patients with Stage III seminoma have a complete response to orchiectomy and chemotherapy.

As with all chemotherapeutic agents, the precautions are specific for each type of agent. Cisplatin causes ototoxicity, nephrotoxicity, and neurotoxicity. Etoposide may

TABLE 51.1 Staging and Classification for Testicular Carcinoma

Nonseminoma Germ Cell Tumor Staging

Stage A		Lesion confined to testis
Stage B		Regional lymph node involvement in the retroperitoneum
Stage C		Distant metastasis

MD Anderson System for Staging Seminomas

Stage I		Lesion confined to testis
Stage II		Spread to retroperitoneal lymph nodes
Stage III		Supradiaphragmatic nodal or visceral involvement

American Joint Committee on Cancer TNM(S) staging system
(T = tumor, N = lymph node involvement, M = metastasis, S = serum tumor marker)

Stage 0	pTis N0 M0 S0	Tumor only in the seminiferous tubules with no other part of the testicle involved (pTis) No lymph node involvement and no metastases Serum tumor marker levels normal
Stage I	pT1–pT4 N0 M0 SX	Local spread beyond seminiferous tubules and possibly outside the testicle (pT1–pT4) No lymph node involvement and no metastases Serum tumor marker levels not assessed or not available
Stage IA	pT1 N0 M0 S0	Tumor beyond the seminiferous tubules but within the testicle (pT1) No lymph nodes and no metastases Serum tumor marker levels normal
Stage IB	pT2–pT4 N0 M0 S0	Tumor beyond the testicle and in nearby structures (pT2–pT4) No lymph nodes and no metastases Serum tumor marker levels normal
Stage IS	Any pT N0 M0 S1–S3	Tumor may or may not have spread beyond testicle (Any pT) No lymph nodes and no metastases At least one serum tumor marker higher than normal (S1–S3)
Stage II	Any pT N1–N3 M0 SX	Tumor may or may not have spread beyond testicle (Any pT) One or more nearby lymph nodes positive (N1–N3) No metastases Serum tumor marker levels not assessed or not available
Stage IIA	Any pT N1 M0 S0 or S1	Tumor may or may not have spread beyond testicle (Any pT) At least one nearby lymph node involved (but less than five) and no lymph node greater than 2 cm No metastases Serum tumor markers normal (S0) or one tumor marker slightly elevated (S1)
Stage IIB	Any pT N2 M0 S0 or S1	Tumor may or may not have spread beyond testicle (Any pT) At least one lymph node greater than 2 cm but less than 5 cm OR spread outside the lymph node OR more than five positive lymph nodes No metastases Serum tumor markers normal (S0) or one tumor marker slightly elevated (S1)
Stage IIC	Any pT N3 M0 S0 or S1	Tumor may or may not have spread beyond testicle (Any pT) At least one lymph node greater than 5 cm (N3) No metastases Serum tumor markers normal (S0) or one tumor marker slightly elevated (S1)
Stage III	Any pT Any N M1 SX	Tumor may or may not have spread beyond testicle (Any pT) May or may not have positive lymph nodes Spread to distant parts of the body Serum tumor marker levels not assessed or not available

Continued

TABLE 51.1 Staging and Classification for Testicular Carcinoma—cont'd

American Joint Committee on Cancer TNM(S) staging system
(T = tumor, N = lymph node involvement, M = metastasis, S = serum tumor marker)

Stage IIIA	Any pT Any N M1a S0 or S1	Tumor may or may not have spread beyond testicle (Any pT) May or may not have positive lymph nodes Spread to distant lymph nodes or lungs (M1a) Serum tumor markers normal (S0) or one tumor marker slightly elevated (S1)
Stage IIIB	Any pT N1–N3 M0 S2	Tumor may or may not have spread beyond testicle (Any pT) One or more nearby lymph nodes positive (N1–N3) No metastases At least one serum tumor marker much higher than normal (S2)
OR		
Stage IIIB	Any pT Any N M1a S2	Tumor may or may not have spread beyond testicle (Any pT) May or may not have positive lymph nodes Spread to distant lymph nodes or lungs (M1a) At least one serum tumor marker much higher than normal (S2)
Stage IIIC	Any pT N1–N3 M0 S3	Tumor may or may not have spread beyond testicle (Any pT) One or more nearby lymph nodes positive (N1–N3) No metastases At least one serum tumor marker extremely elevated (S3)
OR		
Stage IIIC	Any pT Any N M1a S3	Tumor may or may not have spread beyond testicle (Any pT) May or may not have positive lymph nodes Spread to distant lymph nodes or lungs (M1a) At least one serum tumor marker is extremely elevated (S3)
OR		
Stage IIIC	Any pT Any N M1b Any S	Tumor may or may not have spread beyond testicle (Any pT) May or may not have positive lymph nodes Metastasis to other locations outside of lymph nodes or to lungs (M1b) Serum tumor marker levels may or may not be elevated

Source: American Joint Committee on Cancer (AJCC) TNM staging system used with permission of the American College of Surgeons. Original source for this information is the *AJCC cancer staging manual*. 8th ed. Springer International Publishing; 2017.

cause thrombocytopenia. Bleomycin causes pulmonary fibrosis, while the alternative drug carboplatin (Paraplatin) can cause ototoxicity. Cyclophosphamide and ifosfamide may cause hemorrhagic cystitis, and patients must be well hydrated to flush the bladder and minimize this risk. Patients receiving these chemotherapeutic agents should also receive mesna (a cytoprotective antioxidant agent) to reduce the risk of hemorrhagic cystitis. Ondansetron (Zofran), dronabinol (Marinol), metoclopramide (Reglan), and similar medications may be used to control nausea.

FOLLOW-UP AND REFERRAL

Follow-up is extremely important for patients with testicular malignancies. In the first year after orchiectomy for testicular cancer, the National Comprehensive Cancer Network recommends a history and physical examination every 3 to 6 months with an abdominal/pelvic CT scan at 3, 6, and 12 months. In years 2 to 3 post-orchiectomy, a history and physical examination and CT scan should be done every 6 to 12 months, and in years 4 to 5, the history and physical examination should be done annually with a CT scan done every 1 to 2 years.

If the patient had adjuvant chemotherapy or radiation therapy after orchiectomy, a history and physical examination should be done every 6 to 12 months with an abdominal/pelvic CT scan done annually. A history and physical examination should be done annually thereafter with an annual CT scan starting in year 3.

This level of monitoring is critical, as nonseminomatous tumors are more likely (50% to 70%) to metastasize than seminomas (25%). Patients who have been cured of testicular cancer in one testicle have a 2% to

4% chance of developing cancer in the remaining testicle. If cancer develops in the other testicle, it is almost always a new cancer, however, and not a metastasis from the first episode. Patients with HIV are also at a much higher risk of developing cancer in the remaining testicle.

Patient Education: Testicular Cancer

Although testicular cancer patients may be reassured of the high rate of cure associated with this disease, patients should also be fully informed of the risks of chemotherapy, radiation therapy, and surgical interventions. For example, adverse effects of chemotherapy include hair loss, immunosuppression, loss of appetite, nausea, and vomiting. Radiation therapy can cause extreme fatigue and interfere with sperm production; it can also cause diarrhea, vomiting, and skin reactions at the treatment site, as well as nephritis or enteritis. Complications from retroperitoneal lymph node dissection include loss of seminal emission and/or hypoalbuminemia.

Open discussions and reassurance are extremely important in patients diagnosed with testicular cancer. Concerns over quality of life after testicular cancer are extremely important to most patients. The patient must be able to cope with the way testicular cancer affects their self-image. Patients who are concerned about their appearance after losing a testis can be educated about the availability of prostheses that simulate the weight and feel of a testicle. A low sperm count may also occur after the loss of a testis, so patients (and, if given permission, their partners) should also be educated about the risk of infertility associated with the primary disease and its treatments, as well as options such as sperm banking. Although surgery to remove lymph nodes does not compromise the patient's ability to have an erection or reach orgasm, it can interfere with ejaculation. Some patients naturally regain the ability to ejaculate, while others require medication. Thus, patients should also be educated about sterility and hormonal supplements.

REFERENCES

Epididymitis

Sieger N, Di Quilio F, Stolzenburg JU. What is beyond testicular torsion and epididymitis? Rare differential diagnoses of acute scrotal pain in adults: a systematic review. *Ann Med Surg (Lond).* 2020;55:265–274.

Zhao H, Yu C, He C, et al. The immune characteristics of the epididymis and the immune pathway of the epididymitis caused by different pathogens. *Front Immunol.* 2020;11:article 2115.

Erectile Dysfunction

Allen MS, Walter EE. Erectile dysfunction: an umbrella review of meta-analysis of risk-factors, treatment, and prevalence outcomes. *J Sex Med.* 2019;16(4):531–541. https://doi.org/10.1016/j.jsxm.2019.01.314

Irwin GM. Erectile dysfunction. *Prim Care.* 2019;46(2):249–255.

Kessler A, Sollie S, Challacombe B, et al. The global prevalence of erectile dysfunction: a review. *BJU Int.* 2019;124(4):587–599.

Pizzol D, Demurtas J, Stubbs B, et al. Relationship between cannabis use and erectile dysfunction: a systematic review and meta-analysis. *Am J Mens Health.* 2019;13(6):1557988319892464. https://journals.sagepub.com/doi/pdf/10.1177/1557988319892464

Retzler K. Erectile dysfunction: A review of comprehensive treatment options for optimal outcome. *J Restor Med.* 2019;8(1). https://journal.restorativemedicine.org/index.php/journal/article/view/129

Sokolakis I, Hatzichristodoulou G. Clinical studies on low intensity extracorporeal shockwave therapy for erectile dysfunction: a systematic review and meta-analysis of randomised controlled trials. *Int J Impot Res.* 2019;31:177–194.

Hydrocele

Hegde S, Jadhav V, Shankar G. Not a hydrocele! *J Pediatr.* 2018;197:311. https://doi.org/10.1016/j.jpeds.2018.01.011

Kafka M, Strohhacker K, Aigner F, et al. Incidental testicular pathologies in patients with idiopathic hydrocele testis: is preoperative scrotal ultrasound justified? *Anticancer Res.* 2020;40:2861–2864.

Zawaideh JP, Bertolotto M, Giannoni M, et al. Tension hydrocele as an additional cause of acute scrotum: case series and literature review. *Abdom Radiol (NY).* 2020;45:2082–2086.

Testicular Cancer

Gilligan T, Lin DW, Aggarwal R, et al. Testicular cancer, version 2.2020, NCCN Clinical Practice Guidelines in Oncology. *J Natl Compr Canc Netw.* 2019;17(12):1529–1553.

Miller KD, Nogueira L, Mariotto AB, et al. Cancer treatment and survivorship statistics, 2019. *CA Cancer J Clin.* 2019;69(5):363–385. https://doi.org/10.3322/caac.21565

NIH, National Cancer Institute. (Updated 2020 May 21). Testicular cancer treatment (PDQ)—health professional version. https://www.cancer.gov/types/testicular/hp/testicular-treatment-pdq#link/_713_toc. Accessed 10/9/2020.

Sachdeva K. Testicular cancer follow-up. (Updated 2019 Sept 11). http://emedicine.medscape.com/article/279007-followup. Accessed 10/9/2020

Stephenson A, Eggener SE, Bass EB, et al. Diagnosis and treatment of early stage testicular cancer: AUA Guideline. *J Urol.* 2019;202:272–281.

U.S. Preventive Services Task Force. Final recommendation statement: testicular cancer screening. https://www.uspreventiveservicestaskforce.org/Page/Document/RecommendationStatementFinal/testicular-cancer-screening. Accessed 10/9/2020.

Testicular Torsion

Hyun GS. Testicular torsion. *Rev Urol.* 2018;20(2):104–106.

Jacobsen FM, Rudlang TM, Fode M, et al. The impact of testicular torsion on testicular function. *World J Mens Health.* 2020;38(3):298–307.

McDowall J, Adam A, Gerber L, et al. The ultrasonographic "whirlpool sign" in testicular torsion: valuable tool or waste of valuable time? A systematic review and meta-analysis. *Emerg Radiol.* 2019;25:281–292.

Varicocele

Kohn TP, Ohlander SJ, Jacob JS, et al. The effect of subclinical varicocele on pregnancy rates and semen parameters: a systematic review and meta-analysis. *Curr Urol Rep.* 2018;19(7):53. https://doi.org/10.1007/s11934-018-0798-8

Su, JS, Farber NJ, Vij SC. Pathophysiology and treatment options of varicocele: an overview. *Andrologia.* 2021;53:e13576. doi: 10.1111/and.13576

RESOURCES

Erectile Dysfunction

WebMD
  https://www.webmd.com/erectile-dysfunction/default.htm

Testicular Cancer

American Cancer Society
  https://www.cancer.org/cancer/testicular-cancer.html

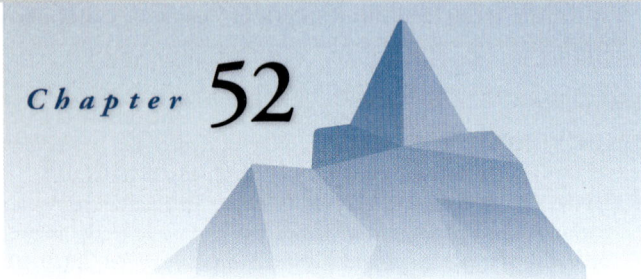

Chapter 52

Sexually Transmitted Infections

Deborah Lowell Shindell, PhD, FNP-BC, CNE
Debera J. Thomas, PhD, RN, ANP/FNP
Brian Oscar Porter, MD, PhD, MPH, MBA

Sexually transmitted infections (STIs) are caused by viruses, bacteria, and parasites and can occur in the throat, eyes, anal and perianal areas, external genitalia, vestibular glands, vagina, cervix, uterus, or adnexa. STIs are spread through sexual intercourse or intimate person-to-person contact. An STI typically occurs when the mucous membranes of these areas are exposed to specific pathogens. Common STIs include herpes simplex virus (HSV), HIV, human papillomavirus (HPV), *Chlamydia trachomatis, Neisseria gonorrhoeae, Trichomonas vaginalis,* and *Treponema pallidum* (the causative agent of syphilis). Less common STIs include chancroid (*Haemophilus ducreyi*), donovanosis or granuloma inguinale (*Klebsiella granulomatis*), *Mycoplasma genitalium,* and lymphogranuloma venereum. In addition, hepatitis B virus (HBV), hepatitis C virus (HCV), molluscum contagiosum, pediculosis pubis, scabies, and methicillin-resistant *Staphylococcus aureus* are known to be transmitted through sexual contact. Some common vaginal infections, such as *Candida* infections and bacterial vaginosis (BV), may be related to sexual activity by causing a change in the vaginal pH. They are not considered STIs, based on transmissibility, however. Table 52.1 presents the causative pathogens for common STIs.

EPIDEMIOLOGY AND CAUSES

STIs are the most prevalent communicable diseases in the United States after upper respiratory infections, and the number of STI cases continues to increase. The Centers for Disease Control and Prevention (CDC) publishes annual STD Surveillance Reports, but there is a 1- to 2-year lag in publication of these data. The Surveillance Report for 2017 to 2018 notes a significant increase in the three most commonly reported STIs: *Chlamydia*, gonorrhea, and syphilis. There were more than 1.7 million cases of *Chlamydia,* which is a 3% increase over the previous reporting period. This represents the highest number ever reported. Gonorrhea cases increased 5% with more than 580,000, which is the highest number reported

 Pediatric/Adolescent Considerations: STI

- STIs disproportionally affect adolescents and young adults between the ages of 15 and 24 years.
  - Increased sexual encounters with multiple partners concurrently
  - Risk-taking behaviors, i.e., failure to use barrier method of contraception
- This age-group accounts for almost 50% of the 26 million STIs in the United States. (CDC, 2018).
- States with *no* mandated abstinence education had lower rates of STIs.
- Rates of STIs are highest in populations with limited access to confidential family planning services.
- Adolescents have an increased biological susceptibility to infection.

since 1991. After historically low national rates of syphilis in the early 2000s, both primary and secondary syphilis infection rates are now steadily rising in the United States, with the number of syphilis cases in 2017 to 2018 being the highest reported since 1991, at more than 115,000. Included in this number is congenital syphilis, of which more than 1,300 cases were reported, demonstrating the largest rate increase of any type of syphilis, having risen 183% between 2014 and 2018. This increase parallels the increased rate of syphilis detected in females overall, as well as in females of childbearing age.

High-risk groups also include men who have sex with men (MSM) and people of color. Overall, it is estimated that one in five Americans is infected with an STI other than HIV, indicating the risk is high in all age-groups. Perhaps even more alarming is that the United States has the highest STI rate of any nation in the industrialized world.

Four common STIs (*Chlamydia,* gonorrhea, syphilis, and *Trichomonas*) can be treated with antibiotics and cured. Viral STIs (e.g., HSV, HPV, HIV), although chronic, can be treated and managed. Untreated or

Text continued on page 872

TABLE 52.1 Selected Sexually Transmitted Infections

Pathogen	Clinical Presentation	Diagnostic Reasoning	CDC Treatment Recommendations (2015)
Bacterial vaginosis	Pain, itching, strong fishy odor, thin gray discharge	Vaginal intercourse may predispose due to pH changes, but bacteria not transmitted between partners (overgrowth of vaginal microflora). Recent history of antibiotic use, IUD, or douching increases likelihood. Amsel Criteria–at least 3 of the 4 indicators are present: clue cells on saline smear; pH greater than 4.5; thin, gray, homogeneous discharge; + whiff test	Metronidazole oral 500 mg twice a day for 7 days OR Metronidazole gel 0.75% 5-g applicator intravaginally once a day for 5 days OR Clindamycin cream 2% one 5-g applicator intravaginally once a day at bedtime for 7 days
Chancroid (*Haemophilus ducreyi*)	Painful, irregularly shaped, deep red ulcer with red halo and undermined edges Found on the penis, labia, fourchette, and vaginal walls Painful inguinal adenopathy with buboes (fluctuant abscesses) Females may have multiple lesions and may be asymptomatic.	Risk factors: co-infection with HIV, HSV, or syphilis Test patients for HIV at time of diagnosis. Definitive diagnosis is obtained with culture (no FDA-approved PCR test available in United States).	Azithromycin 1-g orally single dose OR Ceftriaxone 250-mg intramuscular injection single dose OR Ciprofloxacin 500 mg orally twice a day for 3 days OR Erythromycin base 500 mg orally four times a day for 7 days
Lymphogranuloma venereum (LGV) *Chlamydia trachomatis*	Primary lesion: small painless erosion that heals quickly Inguinal stage: inguinal lymphadenopathy; may have headache, fever, and polymyalgia Late stage: anorectal swelling, perirectal abscesses, fistulae, swelling and ulcerations on labia	Risk factors: history of travel and sexual contact in endemically infected area Diagnosis is confirmed with serological LGV complement fixation test; suspected if titer is higher than 1:16 and diagnostic if titer is less than 1:64	Doxycycline 100 mg orally twice a day for 21 days OR Erythromycin base 500 mg orally four times a day for 21 days

Continued

TABLE 52.1 Selected Sexually Transmitted Infections—cont'd

Pathogen	Clinical Presentation	Diagnostic Reasoning	CDC Treatment Recommendations (2015)
Genital herpes simplex virus (HSV)	Multiple painful vesicular or ulcerated lesions that may last 12 days in the initial outbreak or 4–5 days in recurrent outbreaks Flu-like symptoms (common with first outbreak), adenopathy, and tingling at the site before outbreak	NAAT (PCR assays for HSV DNA) Type-specific serology testing is available and useful when developing plan of care.	First episode: Acyclovir 400 mg orally three times a day for 7–10 days OR Acyclovir 200 mg orally five times per day for 7–10 days OR Valacyclovir 1 g orally twice a day for 7–10 days OR Famciclovir 250 mg orally three times a day for 7–10 days Recurrent episodes: Acyclovir regimens 400 mg orally three times a day for 5 days 800 mg orally twice a day for 5 days 800 mg orally three times a day for 2 days OR Valacyclovir regimens 500 mg orally twice a day for 3 days 1 g orally once a day for 5 days OR Famciclovir regimens 125 mg orally twice a day for 5 days 1 g orally twice a day for 1 day 500 mg orally once and then 250 mg orally twice a day for 2 days Suppression (prophylactic) therapy: Acyclovir 400 mg orally twice a day OR Valacyclovir 500 mg orally once a day OR Valacyclovir 1 g orally once a day OR Famciclovir 250 mg orally twice a day Evaluate after 1 year for recurrent episodes
Anogenital warts 90% caused by HPV type 6 or 11	Flat, papular, or pedunculated growths around the vaginal introitus, under the foreskin, or on the shaft of the penis May be asymptomatic, painful, or pruritic	Visual inspection with biopsy if indicated	Watchful waiting for up to 1 year if socially acceptable Active treatment can include provider- and/or patient-administered treatment. Provider-administered treatments include cryotherapy and/or tricholoroacetic acid (TCA) 80%–90% solution and/or surgical removal. Patient-administered treatments include imiquimod 3.75% or 5% cream OR podofilox 0.5% solution OR sinecatechins 15% ointment (no single treatment is definitively better than the other).

TABLE 52.1 Selected Sexually Transmitted Infections—cont'd

Pathogen	Clinical Presentation	Diagnostic Reasoning	CDC Treatment Recommendations (2015)
Syphilis (*Treponema pallidum*)	Primary: painless ulcer at initial site of contact (chancre), adenopathy Secondary: maculopapular rash on the palms and soles, flu-like symptoms, mucocutaneous lesions, lymphadenopathy Tertiary/late: cardiac, neurological, ophthalmic, auditory, and gummatous lesions Neurosyphilis: (confusion, unstable gait, depression/irritability, emotional liability, partial paralysis. Cardiovascular syphilis: angina, MI, aortic regurgitation Ophthalmic syphilis: uveitis, retinitis Otosyphilis: hearing loss, tinnitus, vertigo	Risk factors: test all patients for HIV and other common STIs Definitive diagnosis: dark-field microscopy positive for spirochetes Presumptive diagnosis: 1. Nontreponemal test (VDRL or RPR) 2. Confirmation with treponemal test (FTA-ABS, TP-PA)	Treatment is driven by staging. Primary and secondary or early latent (less than 1 year since infection): Benzathine PCN G 2.4 million units intramuscularly one time If PCN allergy: Doxycycline 100 mg orally twice a day for 14 days OR Tetracycline 500 mg orally four times a day for 14 days OR Ceftriaxone 1 g intramuscularly or IV daily for 8–10 days Late latent, latent of unknown duration, or tertiary stage with normal cerebrovascular fluid examination: Benzathine PCN B 2.4 units intramuscularly once a week for 3 doses If PCN allergy: Tetracycline 400 mg orally four times a day for 4 weeks OR Doxycycline 100 mg orally twice a day for 4 weeks Neurosyphilis and ocular syphilis: Aqueous crystalline penicillin G 3–4 million units IV every 4 hours for 10–14 days (or continuous infusion) Alternate therapy if compliance is assured: Procaine PCN 2.4 million units intramuscularly daily PLUS Probenecid 500 mg orally four times a day for 10–14 days If PCN allergy: Desensitize and treat with PCN as earlier described OR Ceftriaxone 2 g intramuscularly/IV once a day for 10–14 days
Trichomoniasis (*Trichomonas vaginalis*)	Most infected people have minimal or no symptoms. Some infected females may have diffuse, frothy, malodorous, or yellow-green discharge and vulvar irritation. Infected males may have symptoms of urethritis, epididymitis, or prostatitis.	Vaginal pH greater than 5; cervical smear wet mount shows motile protozoa and WBCs Strawberry cervix may rarely be noted on speculum examination. NAAT testing is highly sensitive. In males, obtain penile-meatal swab. Rapid testing is available.	Metronidazole 2 g orally for one dose OR Tinidazole 2 g orally for one dose OR Metronidazole 500 mg orally twice a day for 7 days Avoid alcohol consumption during treatment with metronidazole, which may result in flushing, nausea, vomiting, and headaches.

Continued

TABLE 52.1 Selected Sexually Transmitted Infections—cont'd

Pathogen	Clinical Presentation	Diagnostic Reasoning	CDC Treatment Recommendations (2015)
Urethritis (*Neisseria gonorrhoeae*) (most common) Nongonococcal urethritis (NGU) *Chlamydia trachomatis, Mycoplasma genitalium*	May be asymptomatic Dysuria, urethral pruritus, mucoid or purulent discharge	Microscopic examination of urethral secretions will show WBCs and GNID or MB/GV purple intracellular diplococci. Test all patients for *C trachomatis*; test males with NGU for HIV and syphilis. May lead to reactive arthritis in males or females In males, complications of NGU include epididymitis and prostatitis. No FDA-approved test available for *M genitalium*	Treat with drug regimens recommended for *N gonorrhoeae* and *C trachomatis M genitalium* responds better to azithromycin than doxycycline.
Gonorrhea (*Neisseria gonorrhoeae*)	Usually asymptomatic; sexual partner may have an infection requiring treatment Females may report purulent, yellow, or green vaginal discharge; bleeding or pain with intercourse; and pelvic pain; may have inflammation of Skene's and Bartholin's glands Males may report inflammation of the urethra, discharge, and dysuria.	Gonococcal culture and NAAT Females: endocervical swab Males: urethral swab	Primary therapy: Ceftriaxone 250 mg intramuscularly for one dose PLUS Azithromycin 1 g orally for one dose Alternative therapy (less effective): Cefixime 400 mg orally for one dose PLUS Azithromycin 1 g orally for one dose If cephalosporin allergy: gemifloxacin 320 mg orally in a single dose PLUS Azithromycin 2 g orally for one dose Follow CDC guidelines for complicated or refractory gonorrhea. Consider EPT.
Chlamydia trachomatis	Asymptomatic infection is common. Females may report dysuria and mucopurulent vaginal discharge. Males may report purulent urethral discharge, dysuria, or pain/swelling of testicle(s).	NAAT Females: vaginal swab Males: urethral or rectal swab or first-catch urine specimen	Primary therapy: Azithromycin 1 g orally in a single dose OR Doxycycline 100 mg orally twice a day for 7 days Alternate therapy: Erythromycin base 500 mg orally four times a day for 7 days OR Ofloxacin 300 mg orally twice a day for 7 days OR Levofloxacin 500 mg orally once a day for 7 days

Section 10: MUSCULOSKELETAL PROBLEMS

SECTION EDITOR

Michael E. Zychowicz, DNP, ANP, ONP, FAAN, FAANP

Chapter 53

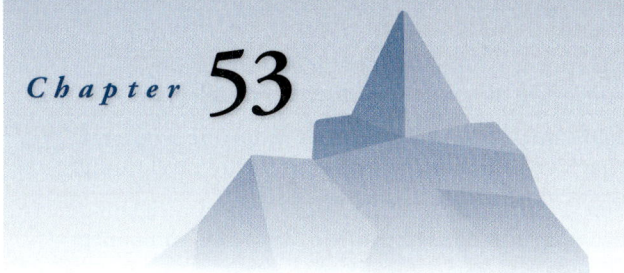

Common Musculoskeletal Complaints

Michael E. Zychowicz, DNP, ANP, ONP, FAAN, FAANP

OVERVIEW

Musculoskeletal injury, pain, and dysfunction are some of the most common reasons for visits to a primary care provider. Musculoskeletal problems in general are the most frequent cause of disability in workers, and population surveys show a greater than 50% prevalence of musculoskeletal disorders among older Americans.

Musculoskeletal complaints can be a challenge for the nonorthopedic health-care provider. A clinician should rely upon their knowledge of anatomy and physiology when approaching the patient with a musculoskeletal complaint. Many acute musculoskeletal complaints are self-limiting, requiring only conservative measures such as protection (immobilization), rest, ice or heat, compression, elevation, and medication as appropriate. Some conditions, however, if left untreated, can lead to a cycle of progressive joint instability, disability, and a higher risk of subsequent injury if recovery is not complete. It is essential to rule out any urgent or emergent musculoskeletal conditions (see Table 53.1). Delayed recognition of certain diagnoses may lead to permanent disability or death. A systematic, thorough, and accurate patient history and physical examination are essential to a correct diagnosis and the identification of urgent or emergent conditions.

The History

When obtaining a musculoskeletal history of present illness, the clinician should consider using a common mnemonic to guide obtaining a structured and complete history of present illness (e.g., PQRST or OLDCARTS). The findings will help guide a clinician's diagnostic reasoning. Precipitating events leading up to the onset of the complaint, such as trauma or injury, must be documented. Knowing what physically occurred during an injury can help a clinician anticipate or suspect a specific tissue injury. For example, anterior cruciate ligament (ACL) injuries commonly occur when a person's foot is firmly planted, the knee is extended, and the person pivots at the same time. The chronology of the complaint gives important diagnostic clues and may be divided into onset (e.g., abrupt), duration, characteristics, and temporal factors (chronic, intermittent, migratory).

If the patient complains about a specific anatomical area, that area should be further evaluated. Certain pain patterns often suggest specific diagnoses. For example, pain over the greater trochanter suggests hip trochanteric bursitis. A history of hand numbness that awakens the patient at night suggests carpal tunnel syndrome, even with no physical findings. Foot pain that begins the first thing in the morning when the patient puts their foot on the floor is suggestive of plantar fasciitis or early rheumatoid arthritis (RA). Crepitus (joint noises or palpable grinding during joint motion) may be due to articular surface abnormalities, a meniscus tear, and arthritis. Crepitus not associated with pain or limitation of motion is generally of no clinical significance.

The location, number, and distribution of involved joints should be noted. Articular disorders are classified, based on the number of involved joints: monoarticular (one joint), oligoarticular (two to four joints), or polyarticular (more than four joints). Disorders such as gout or osteoarthritis are frequently monoarticular, but pathology such as RA or polymyalgia rheumatica can affect several joints. Nonarticular disorders can be classified as either focal or widespread.

Past or current medical history, which may contribute to the patient's complaint, should be noted. If the problem is a chronic condition, ask the patient why they are addressing it now. A review of systems may provide useful diagnostic information, eliciting systemic features of diseases such as fever (systemic lupus erythematosus [SLE], infection). Musculoskeletal complaints may be associated with other organ systems, for example, the nervous system (Lyme disease, vasculitis), the eye (sarcoidosis, Reiter's syndrome), and the gastrointestinal tract (scleroderma, inflammatory bowel disease). See Focus on History: Musculoskeletal Problems.

TABLE 53.1 Potentially Urgent and Emergent Musculoskeletal Findings

Clinical Manifestations	Differential Diagnoses
History Significant trauma Constitutional signs and symptoms (fever, weight loss, malaise)	Soft tissue injury, internal derangement, fracture Infection, sepsis, systemic rheumatic disease
Hot, swollen, painful joint	Infection, systemic rheumatic disease, gout, pseudogout
Physical Examination Weakness – Focal	Compartment syndrome, entrapment neuropathy, mononeuritis, motor neuron disease, radiculopathy
Weakness – Diffuse	Myositis, metabolic myopathy, paraneoplastic syndrome, degenerative neuromuscular disorder, toxin, myelopathy, transverse myelitis
Neurogenic pain (burning, numbness, paresthesia) – Asymmetrical	Radiculopathy, reflex sympathetic dystrophy, entrapment neuropathy
Neurogenic pain – Symmetrical	Myelopathy, peripheral neuropathy
Claudication pain pattern	Peripheral vascular disease, giant cell arteritis (with jaw pain), lumbar spinal stenosis

Focus on History: Musculoskeletal Problems

Questions to ask:

1. Have you injured yourself?
2. Describe exactly how your injury occurred.
3. Specifically, where does it hurt? Does the pain radiate? Is it localized or diffuse?
4. Do you have numbness or tingling?
5. Is there loss of function?
6. Is there swelling?
7. When did the pain first occur?
   - How bad is it on a scale of 1 to 10?
   - What relieves it?
   - What makes it worse?
   - What time of day does it occur?
   - Does the pain awaken you at night?
8. Is there joint stiffness?
   - Does activity make it worse or better?
9. Do you have any other symptoms (or systemic processes)?
   - Do you have a fever?
   - Do you have a rash?
   - Do you have general fatigue?
   - Have you recently been traveling or camping?
   - Have you recently been immunized?
   - Have you recently been treated with antibiotics?
   - Do you have a history of upper respiratory infection? Sexually transmitted infection? Chronic disease?
   - Have you had any treatment (e.g., steroids)?
10. Describe your daily activities—work, hobbies, home.

The patient history should be obtained in the usual fashion, but there are some additional symptoms to consider when analyzing a musculoskeletal complaint.

During the initial patient encounter, in addition to the usual history of present illness, the clinician should explore the following symptoms of the joints:

- Clicking
- Limited motion
- Deformity
- Stiffness
- Weakness
- Pain
- Locking or buckling

Frequently, complaints of a clicking sound or sensation are of no consequence. Clicking often accompanies movement, and this is typically not a worrisome symptom if the patient has no pain associated with it. There are, however, some pathologies that have clicking associated with their dysfunction. A chronically dislocating joint or a subluxing joint/tendon can lead to clicking. Other pathologies that can cause clicking include temporomandibular joint (TMJ) disorder, meniscus tear of the knee, and degenerative joint disease of almost any articular joint.

Patients who complain of limited joint motion may be experiencing degeneration or damage to an articular cartilage surface that is inhibiting motion. Small tears of cartilage in a joint can block motion at a joint. Soft tissue edema at a joint or a joint effusion can diminish joint motion. When a patient experiences pain with motion, they may self-limit joint motion (pain inhibition). Scarring and contractures of a joint can lead to limited motion. During an acute injury, a tendon can completely tear or pull away from its attachment at a joint. When this occurs, the patient will not be able to move the joint in the direction that the tendon would normally produce movement. It is essential for the provider to understand, generally, what muscles and tendons produce movement at joints and in which directions.

Deformity following a trauma can be due to a tendon rupture, joint dislocation, or even a fracture. Rheumatic nodules, tophaceous gout, or certain tumors can also cause deformity. Spinal deformity may be due to scoliosis or kyphosis following vertebral compression fractures. Osteoarthritis (OA) is accompanied by degenerative joint changes that can leave the patient with joint deformity. These include osteophytes, loss of joint cartilage, and joint instability due to laxity of the joint supporting structures.

A complaint of stiffness can lead the clinician to consider several causes. The clinician should inquire if the stiffness is intermittent or constant and if other symptoms such as pain and swelling are also present. If intermittent, ask what brings the stiffness on and how long it lasts. RA generally manifests as stiffness that can last for more than an hour. This can occur in the morning or after a period of inactivity during the day. An early sign of RA includes stiffness of the small joints of the hands. By contrast, stiffness from OA typically lasts less than an hour, resolving faster than with RA. Stiffness can return after activity or at the end of the day for those with OA. Other causes for stiffness can include injury to joint cartilage, bursitis, lupus, gout, or a tumor.

When evaluating a complaint of weakness, be sure to differentiate this from fatigue. The clinician should inquire about any injury that preceded the weakness and if any pain is present. Pain inhibition will limit a patient's ability and desire to move a body part or use full strength in an attempt to protect the body part and avoid pain. A ruptured tendon following an injury will lead to a full loss of strength.

The pattern of weakness, especially for those who have not had an injury, can be useful in the diagnostic reasoning process. A patient may have weakness of the proximal muscles, distal muscles, or generalized weakness. Proximal weakness may be a symptom of an acquired myopathy (e.g., polymyositis) or a genetic myopathy (e.g., Duchenne muscular dystrophy). A nonmyopathic cause for proximal weakness is myelopathy. Distal weakness can also be due to an acquired myopathy (e.g., sarcoidosis) or genetic myopathy. Peripheral neuropathy is one potential cause for distal weakness from a nonmyopathic cause. Some pathology presents with generalized weakness involving both proximal and distal weakness. Myasthenia gravis and Guillain-Barré syndrome are examples of disorders that can lead to both proximal and distal weakness.

Many patients presenting with a musculoskeletal complaint will experience pain. A sudden onset of pain can accompany joint infection; gout; or injury; and trauma such as sprain, strain, or fracture. Patients with tendonitis, tumor, bursitis, or osteoarthritis can demonstrate a gradual onset of pain. Pain pattern is an important aspect to explore. Pain that is bad in the morning may accompany RA; however, pain that gets worse as the day progresses may accompany OA. Patients with pain from neuropathy or radiculopathy have a characteristic pain distribution. The clinician should understand if the pain affects only one specific joint or multiple joints. This is particularly important for clinicians to come to a diagnosis in those patients who have pain without an injury.

When a patient complains of their joint physically locking in place and they are unable to move the joint, the clinician needs to consider the mechanical conditions that can cause this to occur. First, a loose piece of joint tissue (loose body) can float in the synovial fluid within the joint and become wedged between the movable bones at the joint, causing the joint to lock in place. A loose body is often from a free-floating piece of cartilage and/or bone. A patient may also have a torn piece of cartilage, which is still partially attached to the bone but is moving freely. This torn piece of cartilage can get wedged between the bones at a joint in the same way a loose body can. Dislocations and subluxations can lead to joint locking. Additionally, a patient with a trigger finger can experience locking of movement of the finger. This is due to a nodule on a flexor tendon of a finger that gets stuck when a patient flexes and/or extends the affected finger.

Buckling is a symptom that is described as a joint giving out or giving way. Pain and muscular inhibition can cause a joint to give out. This can similarly occur when a patient has an effusion of a joint. Ligament, tendon, or cartilage tears may also lead to giving way of a joint.

The Physical Examination

Guided by the history, the physical examination helps further narrow down differential diagnoses in the clinician's diagnostic reasoning process. This can assist in distinguishing between mechanical problems, soft tissue conditions, and noninflammatory or inflammatory joint diseases. A general guide to the physical examination is provided in Advanced Assessment 53.1.

A general musculoskeletal examination would include an assessment of the patient's general appearance and their gait and posture. How does the patient's body build look? The clinician should evaluate if the patient's build is appropriate for their developmental age or if there is cachexia or obesity. The clinician should evaluate for symmetry of body parts and any abnormal body contour or alignment. Gait should be assessed for an unusual pattern such as antalgic, ataxic, Trendelenburg, or steppage gait. Evaluation of posture may reveal lordosis, kyphosis, or scoliosis.

To perform a visual inspection, the body parts to be examined need to be fully exposed. At times, this may necessitate the patient being undressed and draped. The examiner should begin a regional examination by carefully inspecting the affected part. The examiner should look for signs of trauma, ecchymosis, erythema, skin

> ### Advanced Assessment 53.1: Physical Examination for Musculoskeletal Disorders
>
> 1. Inspection
>   Does the affected extremity have any edema, erythema, ecchymosis, overlying skin lesions, previous scars from surgery, deformities?
> 2. Palpation at, above, and below the affected joint
>   Crepitus of the joint, crepitus at a fracture, joint effusion, diffuse or point tenderness, edema, skin temperature?
> 3. Range of motion (ROM)
>   Active ROM: Degree of motion at a joint, done without assistance from provider, performed in all motion planes for the joint
>   Passive ROM: Degree of motion of a joint in planes of motion; patient's body part is moved by the provider
>   Assess for less than normal ROM. Which directions are affected, and is there a difference between active and passive motion?
> 4. Strength examination
>   a. 0/5: no muscle twitching or movement (paralyzed limb)
>   b. 1/5: muscle twitching but no movement
>   c. 2/5: patient can actively move the extremity but cannot move against gravity
>   d. 3/5: patient can move the extremity against gravity but not against resistance
>   e. 4/5: patient has weakness of the extremity against resistance
>   f. 5/5: patient has full strength of the extremity
> 5. Joint stability
>   a. Stress testing: Evaluate for pain and/or joint laxity relative to opposite side. Performed by stretching or bending a joint in a direction that stretches specific ligaments (e.g., lateral collateral ligament)
>   b. Joint play: Evaluate for pain and/or increased or decreased mobility relative to opposite side. Clinician performs passive directional movement of the bones at a joint (e.g., attempt to slide the humeral head anteriorly or posteriorly).
> 6. Special tests
>   Many special tests can be performed to assess for specific pathology. Examples include:
>   a. Shoulder—Empty can test and Neer/Hawkins impingement tests (bursitis or rotator cuff)
>   b. Knee—McMurray test (meniscus), Lachman test (anterior cruciate ligament)
>   c. Cervical spine—Spurling's test (radiculopathy, herniated disc)
>   d. Lumbar spine—straight-leg/reverse straight-leg-raise test (radiculopathy, herniated disc)
>   e. Ankle—Thompson squeeze test (Achilles tendon rupture)
> 7. Neurovascular examination
>   a. Assess for sensory loss of the affected body part. Is there a pattern for the sensory loss?
>   b. Palpate peripheral pulses.
>   i. Upper extremity: radial, brachial
>   ii. Lower extremity: dorsalis pedis, posterior tibial, popliteal
>   c. Assess skin temperature and capillary refill.
>   d. Note peripheral edema.
>   Grade on a scale of 0–4.
>   e. Perform extremity reflex testing at the following locations to check specific spinal nerves:
>   i. L4: knee
>   ii. S1: Achilles tendon
>   iii. C5–C6: biceps
>   iv. C7: triceps

lesions, abrasions, lacerations, and edema. The uninvolved side should be examined and compared with the involved side. Take note of any obvious masses or nodules, deformity, edema, and muscle or skin atrophy.

After visual inspection, the next step in the physical examination is palpation. The clinician must use a systematic, purposeful method when performing palpation. Consider the specific underlying anatomy that is being palpated and any corresponding pain, as this will guide the examiner in determining specific pain generators or injured tissues. Palpate the affected body part for warmth and edema, which may accompany an infection, inflammatory condition, or injury. Bony enlargements at joints can accompany OA. Enlargement of the distal interphalangeal joints or Heberden's nodes is indicative of hand OA, whereas swelling of the proximal interphalangeal or metacarpophalangeal joints may indicate RA. Evidence of tender points and trigger points, as well as the absence of inflammation or swollen joints, increases the likelihood of a soft tissue problem. If the patient is guarding painful joints or body parts, the painful part can be examined last.

ROM testing is an important part of the physical examination. ROM testing measures the degree of movement of a joint or body part. Just like inspection and palpation, ROM testing should be performed on both the affected and the unaffected body part to assess for symmetry. Performance of ROM testing can be passive, active assistive, or active. In passive ROM testing, the examiner moves the joint or body part; the patient does not actively participate in the movement. In active-assistive ROM testing, the examiner assists the patient in movement of the joint or body part; the patient participates in the movement but not significantly.

During ROM testing, the examiner is assessing for degree and symmetry of motion or if any pain and crepitus are present. Frequently, active ROM testing is performed initially, and then passive ROM testing is used to further assess if the patient has a deficit in motion. Passive motion will give an indication if the patient is unable to move the joint due to pathology physically blocking the joint or if there is decreased motion due to pain or lack of strength. After ROM testing, strength testing of the affected joint is conducted, followed by a neurovascular examination assessing reflexes, sensations, and pulses.

Identifying the anatomical location of the musculoskeletal complaint is important, in most cases, to ensure the appropriate management plan is put in place. The primary care provider should distinguish between conditions arising from articular and nonarticular structures (see Box 53.1). Articular structures include the synovium, synovial fluid, articular cartilage, intra-articular ligaments, joint capsule, and juxta-articular bone. Disorders of these structures are characterized by deep or diffuse pain, limited ROM on active and passive movement, swelling (caused by synovial proliferation, effusion, or bony enlargement), crepitation, instability, "locking," or deformity. Nonarticular (or periarticular) structures are identified as supportive extra-articular ligaments, tendons, bursae, muscle, fascia, bone, nerve, and overlying skin. Nonarticular disorders are characterized by painful and active but not passive ROM, point or focal tenderness in regions distinct from articular structures, and physical findings far from the joint capsule. Crepitus and instability are not likely to be associated with these disorders.

Two general assessments that could be included in the evaluation are to ask the patient to rise from a chair without holding on. If the patient cannot do this, there may be an abnormality of the joints, nerves, or muscles, which requires further examination, usually by a specialist. The patient's gait and balance should also be assessed by asking the patient to walk a few steps across the room.

All maneuvers described should take less than 2 minutes and should be included in the "general" physical examination. Note any endocrinopathies (irregular heart rhythms, weight gain, and thyromegaly) and possible malignancy (severe pain, weight loss, or palpable masses). Extra-articular abnormalities, such as oral/nasal ulcers; iritis; rash; nodules; pericardial or pulmonary rub; enlargement of liver, spleen, or lymph nodes; or neurological abnormalities, suggest a systemic disease.

Diagnostic Tests

Laboratory Tests

Laboratory tests, with orthopedic complaints, can at times be misleading and produce false-positive and false-negative results. For example, many people with RA have normal blood tests and x-ray findings, particularly early in the disease, when aggressive treatment might be most effective. Some tests may be useful to research laboratories in the identification and understanding of pathogenic mechanisms, but may not add any meaningful benefit to the clinician in the diagnosis and management of the patient. A review of associated laboratory tests is presented here.

- Complete blood count (CBC)—the presence of anemia may be a clue to inflammation, and leukopenia is seen in conditions such as severe infection, autoimmune disorders (e.g., lupus), or diseases affecting the bone marrow (e.g., leukemia).
- Erythrocyte sedimentation rate (ESR) and C-reactive protein (CRP)—elevated ESR or CRP values are nonspecific indicators of inflammation. A highly elevated value indicates an increased likelihood of inflammatory rheumatic disease, infection, or malignancy. ESR increases with age, as does CRP, and some people (as many as 5% to 10% of the general population) have elevated values with no explanation. Up to 40% of patients who present with RA have normal ESR and CRP levels. In patients with giant cell arteritis and polymyalgia rheumatica, the ESR is almost always markedly elevated and is therefore diagnostically useful.
- Rheumatoid factor (RF)—25% of patients with RA never have an elevated RF. This value may also be elevated with other inflammatory conditions (e.g., SLE, subacute bacterial endocarditis, vasculitis, viral infection).
- Fluorescent antinuclear antibody (ANA) test—this test is positive in 99% of patients with SLE; however, it is also positive in 5% to 10% of normal blood donors, meaning that only one in 100 people with a positive ANA has SLE. A positive ANA can also occur with certain drugs (procainamide, hydralazine); it may be transiently positive in people with a severe infection; and it is positive in a high percentage of people with other inflammatory rheumatic conditions, including RA (30% to 50%), scleroderma (20% to 50%), polymyositis (10% to 30%), and idiopathic pulmonary fibrosis (10% to 20%). Other antibody tests are more specific for certain inflammatory disorders.
- Lyme borreliosis antibodies—Lyme disease is identified serologically by antibodies to the Lyme *Borrelia* organism. Between 5% and 10% of asymptomatic individuals have a positive Lyme borreliosis titer. A test for Lyme disease is not appropriate in patients with unexplained arthritis unless there are other risk factors such as living in an endemic area and frequent outdoor activities.

Box 53.1	Comparison of Articular and Nonarticular Structures
Articular Structures	**Nonarticular Structures**
Synovium and synovial fluid	Supportive extra-articular ligaments
Articular cartilage, intra-articular ligaments	Bone
Joint capsule	Nerve, overlying skin
Juxta-articular bone	Muscle, tendons, fascia

- Uric acid—serum uric acid is frequently elevated in people with gout. Alcohol and diuretics may cause moderately elevated uric acid levels. When a patient experiences a gouty flare-up of joint pain, frequently at a big toe, there is often a reduction in serum uric acid. A normal finding of serum uric acid during a gouty flare-up can be interpreted as a false-negative finding. A definitive diagnosis of gout, in particular during a gout flare-up, requires identification of uric acid crystals in synovial fluid of the affected joint (see Chapter 60 for a detailed discussion of gout).
- Screening panels—these tests are available from all national laboratories and are marketed as "rheumatology screening panels" to rule out an inflammatory rheumatic disease. The simplest include RF, ANA, and uric acid, although more elaborate tests are available. These panels can be a source of potential false-positive findings.

Imaging Tests

A handful of imaging studies are available to assist in evaluating patients with musculoskeletal conditions. These include conventional radiography such as standard x-rays, fluoroscopy, arthrography, and myelography. Advanced imaging studies include computed tomography (CT), magnetic resonance imaging (MRI), diagnostic ultrasound, and nuclear imaging studies. The best imaging to perform for a particular patient presentation should be based upon (1) the imaging that will be best to assess for specific suspected pathology, (2) limiting unnecessary exposure to radiation, (3) reducing potential false-negative/positive results, (4) evidence or guidance from professional organizations, and (5) cost-effectiveness. Common imaging studies used in the diagnosis of musculoskeletal disorders include:

- Radiography (plain x-ray films) is commonly used as an initial screening imaging study for patients with musculoskeletal conditions. X-ray images may help to direct further imaging such as MRI or CT. Radiography can reveal the following:
  - Joint erosions or narrowing of joint spaces
  - Tissue calcifications and cystic masses
  - Significant osteoporosis
  - Bone lesions or tumors
  - Deformity of bones or joints
  - Fractures, dislocations, or subluxation

For patients with typical acute mechanical low back pain (see Chapter 54, Spinal Disorders), a plain radiograph adds little to the management decisions and exposes the patient to significant radiation. Although radiographs may confirm the diagnosis of OA at a joint, the clinician should remember that radiographic evidence of arthritis lags behind symptoms of OA.

- Diagnostic ultrasonography may be useful in the detection of nerve entrapments, inflammation, nerve or muscle subluxation, or chondral defects. Some soft tissue injury, such as ligament tears, can be visualized. The clinician can use ultrasound to visualize fluid collection from pathology such as bursitis, infection, synovitis, or cystic masses. Point-of-care ultrasound has expanded in availability. This relatively low-cost and portable imaging technique can be extremely useful for the clinician; however, the tool is highly dependent on the user's ability to identify underlying anatomy.
- CT is an imaging tool that uses x-ray and computer technology to produce axial, sagittal, or coronal cross-sectional images of the body. In musculoskeletal care, CT is useful for imaging disc herniation, loose bodies in a joint space, or soft tissue tumors. CT is superior to MRI for imaging bone and fracture patterns. Although CT is generally less expensive and faster to perform than MRI, there is substantial radiation exposure to the patient with a CT scan. To enhance detail of tissues on the image, contrast can be used. The contrast can be injected via IV, injected into a joint space, or instilled into the spinal canal.
- MRI is useful in musculoskeletal care to assess soft tissue injury, evaluate cartilage, and image intervertebral disc. MRI is also useful to image bone marrow edema and inflammation due to pathology such as tumor, infection, or stress fracture. The ability of MRI to capture tissue hydration makes this tool effective in evaluating spinal disc degeneration. Joint and IV contrast can also be used with MRI to enhance the detail of imaged tissues.
- A bone scan may be used to evaluate physiological and metabolic tissue changes from injury or disease. By assessing bone metabolism, a bone scan can be useful to assess conditions such as osteomyelitis, avascular necrosis, stress fractures, and bony tumors or metastases. Unfortunately, the tool has low specificity and low-resolution anatomic detail, so the provider needs to correlate the imaging with patient history and physical findings.
- An electromyogram and nerve conduction study (EMG/NCS) may be used to evaluate for injury, irritation, or dysfunction of nerves. These can assist in the identification and confirmation of possible neurological abnormalities including conditions such as carpel tunnel syndrome and radiculopathy. EMG/NCS can be useful in providing clarification of the origin of neurological symptoms, helping differentiate between a peripheral nerve problem and a spinal nerve problem. For example, a patient with pain, numbness, and tingling of the hand could potentially have those symptoms emanating from the carpal tunnel or the cervical spine.

Differential Diagnosis

Differential diagnoses of musculoskeletal problems include the following:

- Trauma
- Infection

- Metabolic or circulatory disorders
- Tumors
- Synovial conditions
- Congenital or developmental problems
- Degenerative disorders
- Inflammatory disorders

The differential diagnoses may be narrowed by an identification of the underlying pathological process, the injury that occurred, and the exact site of the complaint. These help determine whether there is a need for immediate diagnostic or therapeutic intervention, or continued observation.

Joint symptoms of one and up to several joints may be due to trauma, infection, crystal-induced inflammation (gout, pseudogout), or primary inflammatory arthritis (including spondyloarthropathies and atypical presentation of RA). If both active and passive ROM are limited, soft tissue contracture, synovitis, or a structural abnormality of the joint is possible. In acute monoarthritis, it is essential that infection of a joint be diagnosed or excluded, and this can be done only via joint aspiration and synovial fluid analysis and culture (see Advanced Assessment 53.2). Chronic monoarticular symptoms with little or no joint effusion are frequently from OA.

Polyarthritis has an extensive list of differential diagnoses. The presence of prolonged morning stiffness, systemic symptoms, Raynaud's phenomenon, rash, or sicca symptoms and manifestations of other organ involvement suggest a rheumatic disease. The specific evaluation is guided by the clinical manifestations and should screen organ symptoms that can be involved without overt signs, such as the lung, heart, liver, kidney, and bowel, for potential involvement.

The combination of point tenderness, reduced active ROM, and preserved passive ROM suggests soft tissue disorders, including bursitis, tendinitis, or muscle injury.

Tendinitis and bursitis generally involve one joint region, and physical examination is usually diagnostic. Common syndromes include de Quervain's tenosynovitis, olecranon bursitis, medial and lateral epicondylitis, bicipital and rotator cuff tendinitis, rotator cuff tear, trochanteric bursitis, patellar bursitis and prepatellar bursitis, anserine bursitis, plantar fasciitis, posterior tibial tendinitis, and Achilles tendinitis.

Inflammatory disorders may be infectious or idiopathic. These are identified by the presence of all or some of the four cardinal signs of inflammation (erythema, warmth, pain, or swelling); systemic symptoms (fatigue, weight loss, morning stiffness, fever); or laboratory evidence of inflammation (elevated ESR or CRP, anemia of chronic disease, hypoalbuminemia, or thrombocytosis). Noninflammatory disorders tend to be related to trauma (meniscus tear), ineffective repair or degeneration (OA), neoplasm, or pain amplification (fibromyalgia). There may be pain without swelling or warmth, absence of inflammatory or systemic features, minimal or absent morning stiffness, and normal (for age) laboratory testing (see Box 53.2).

Generalized arthralgias and/or myalgias without physical findings have extensive differential diagnoses. Often, a definitive diagnosis is difficult to determine at the initial presentation. Common causes include fibromyalgia or polymyalgia rheumatica; viral and bacterial infections such as mononucleosis, Rocky Mountain spotted fever, and Lyme disease; an overuse syndrome (tendon strain associated with repetitive motion injuries or muscle fatigue); neuropathy; hypothyroidism; or psychogenic causes. More than one syndrome may occur concomitantly. For example, bursitis may coexist with pain from fibromyalgia. If the inflammation from the bursitis is overlooked, the patient may not receive the treatment indicated for that concomitant acute disorder. In addition, certain medications (e.g., some diuretics,

Advanced Assessment 53.2: Synovial Fluid Analysis

	Normal	Grade I: Noninflammatory	Grade II: Inflammatory	Grade III: Infectious
Visual analysis	Clear, straw colored	Clear or slightly bloody and turbid	Turbid	Turbid, gray, or yellow
Viscosity	Normal	Decreased	Decreased	Decreased
WBCs per mm^3	30–150	Less than 2,500	2,500–25,000	Greater than 50,000
PMNs (%)	<20	20–50	50–70	70–90
Protein (g/dL)	1–4	1–5	3–6	3–7
Examples		OA, SLE, mechanical derangement	RA, gonococcal arthritis, rheumatic fever, gout, pseudogout, Reiter's syndrome	Septic arthritis, tuberculosis

Abbreviations: OA, osteoarthritis; PMNs, polymorphonuclear leukocytes; RA, rheumatoid arthritis; SLE, systemic lupus erythematosus; WBCs, white blood cells.

Box 53.2 Examples of Disorders of Inflammation Versus Noninflammation

Inflammatory Musculoskeletal Disorders	Noninflammatory Musculoskeletal Disorders
Infectious Crystal induced Immune related (rheumatoid arthritis, systemic lupus erythematosus)	Ineffective repair (osteoarthritis) Pain amplification (fibromyalgia) Trauma
Idiopathic	Neoplasm

some of the statin drugs, ciprofloxacin, and clofibrate [Atromid-S]) also may cause myalgia (Fig. 53.1). If the history and physical examination do not provide a diagnosis, symptomatic management and reassessment over several weeks may be more productive initially than laboratory testing or diagnostic imaging.

ACUTE MUSCULOSKELETAL INJURY

Musculoskeletal injuries are among the most common injuries seen across many nonorthopedic settings including primary care, emergency/urgent care, school health, and occupational health, among others. Patients of all ages are susceptible to injury. Fitness classes and field sports are the most common culprits associated with musculoskeletal injuries in the younger population. Racket sports, walking, and low-intensity sports are associated with injuries in older adults. Frequently, the lower extremities are involved, especially the knees and ankles. Older patients tend to have more overuse injuries, such as metatarsalgia, plantar fasciitis, and meniscal knee injuries. Younger patients tend to have more patellofemoral syndromes and stress fractures. Knees and ankles are among the most common sites injured in high school athletes.

The importance of performing a thorough and complete physical examination for musculoskeletal injuries cannot be overemphasized. The signs of a musculoskeletal injury may include one or more of the following: tenderness, swelling, deformity, and abnormal range of motion. Sprains and strains are by far the most common types of injuries; however, other life-threatening injuries must be identified quickly. This is facilitated by completing a rapid initial survey, which can be accomplished in 90 seconds by an experienced practitioner. After this primary survey, a more thorough secondary survey can be performed, during which fractures and more minor injuries are typically identified. Additionally, musculoskeletal sequelae can be associated with or caused by problems in other systems—neurological, endocrine, nutritional, or psychological. A thorough history and physical examination are required to rule out other bodily system involvement.

Pediatric/Adolescent Considerations: Musculoskeletal Injury

The skeleton of a child is generally different from that of an adult. In addition, how their body is affected by and responds to an injury is different. One key difference is children's bone tends to be softer and more porous than adults because more space is occupied by haversian canals. This soft and somewhat flexible quality allows bone to bend before it breaks and leads to different fracture patterns in children in comparison to adults. Children can develop greenstick, bowing, or buckle fractures due to the somewhat soft and flexible bone. Avulsion fractures are also more common in adolescents. This occurs during an injury where a fragment of bone is pulled off by an attached ligament or tendon. In children, the tendons and ligaments are stronger than their softer bone, leading the bone to avulse before the tendon or ligament tears. In adults, we tend to see more ligament and tendon tears due to adult bone being stronger in relation to the tendons or ligaments.

Children will also have open growth plates, which eventually close as the child progresses through adolescence and puberty. Growth plates in females will usually close at about 14 or 15 years of age, whereas growth plates in males will close at about 16 or 17 years. Children can break through these growth plates, potentially affecting continued growth of the injured limb. Surgical repair of a musculoskeletal injury near a growth plate (e.g., ACL reconstruction) requires special surgical techniques to avoid damage to the growth plate.

Because children's bones have greater growth activity than adults, fracture healing can be slightly faster, decreasing the amount of time in an immobilizer. Children's bone growth can also help correct some angulation that may occur with a fracture, whereas adult bone does not have the same potential.

Strains and Sprains

A strain involves microscopic and macroscopic stretching or tearing of muscle and/or tendon fibers. These injuries require more than just muscle contraction to occur; excessive stretching or stretching while the muscle is being activated is required for a strain injury to occur. The injury usually occurs within the muscle's normal range of motion. The portion of the muscle that is often injured is at the muscle–tendon junction. Muscles that cross multiple joints or have a complex architecture are more susceptible to strains. Muscles most frequently

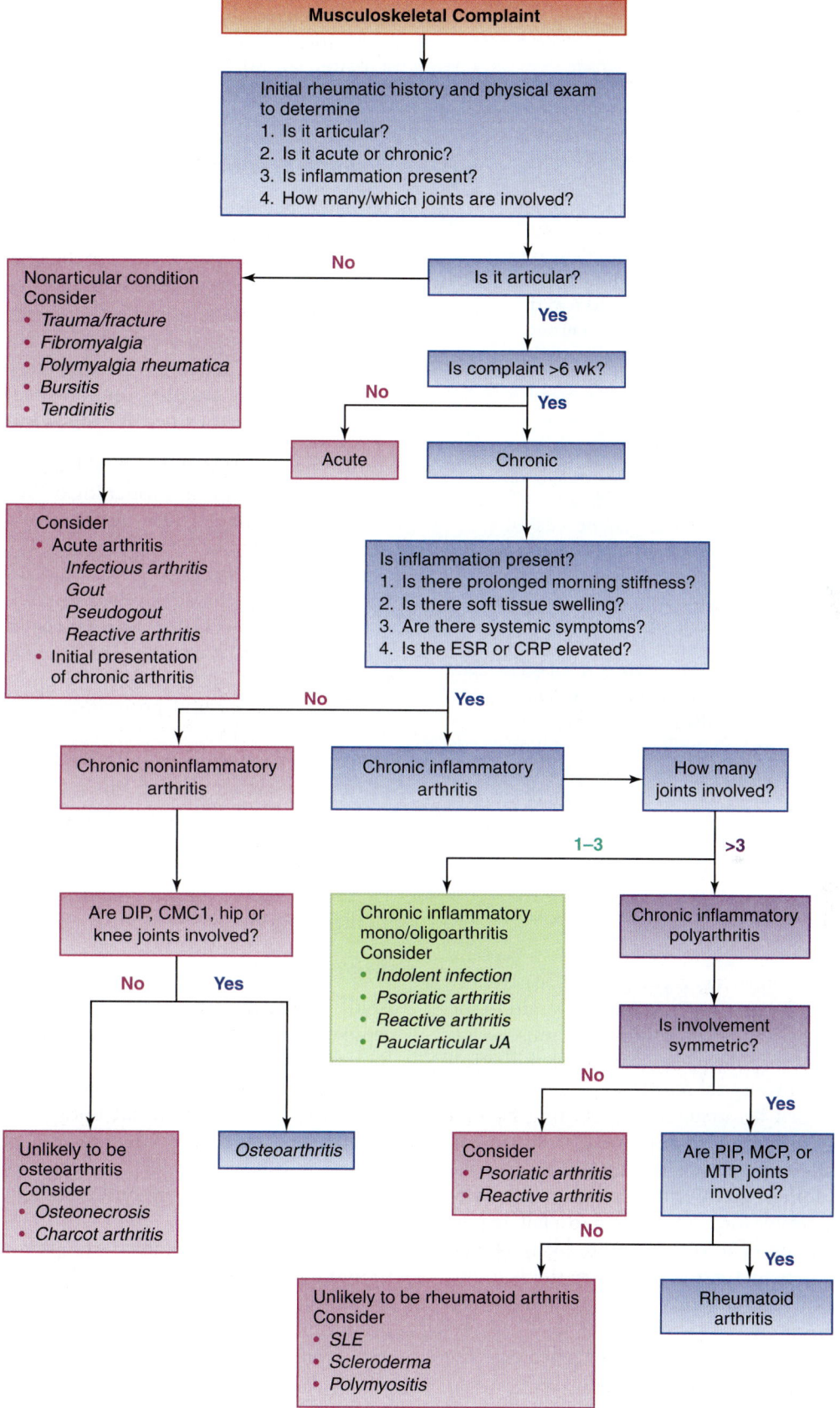

Figure 53.1 Diagnostic reasoning algorithm: articular and musculoskeletal disorders. Abbreviations: MCP, metacarpophalangeal joint; MTP, metatarsophalangeal joint; PIP, proximal interphalangeal joint; SLE, systemic lupus erythematosus. *Source:* Kasper DL, et al, eds. *Harrison's principles of internal medicine.* 16th ed. New York, NY: McGraw-Hill; 2005.

> ### Geriatric Considerations: Musculoskeletal Injury
>
> Physiological musculoskeletal changes that accompany the aging process lead to decreased muscle strength, decreased bone density, diminished flexibility and elasticity of tendons and ligaments, and decreased resilience of articular cartilage. These age-related changes increase risk for injury in older adults. Falls are the most common injuries that occur in people older than 65 years and account for more than 3 million emergency department visits annually. Diminished mobility, medication management, decreased visual acuity, and decreased strength all contribute to increased risk for a fall and musculoskeletal injury. Sprains, strains, and fractures are common sequelae following a fall in older adults.
>
> Prevention of falls and subsequent sequelae is a key component of managing older patients. This can be accomplished through modification of the home environment. Exercise can also reduce risk for falls and injury by increasing muscle strength, coordination, and bone density. In addition, fall risk can be reduced through a thorough medication review and elimination of alcohol use and smoking.
>
> Frequently, older patients who have a musculoskeletal injury will require immobilization of the injured body part. At times, older adults may take longer to recover from an injury. The clinician must balance the need for adequate length of time to immobilize a patient against the knowledge that older patients will develop significant joint stiffness from prolonged immobility. The clinician also needs to consider the potential effects of medication management on the older patient. Some pain medications, such as skeletal muscle relaxers or opiates, can increase the risk for falls, whereas NSAIDs can increase the risk for gastrointestinal (GI) bleeding and gastric ulceration.

injured include the hamstring, rectus femoris, gastrocnemius, and adductor longus muscles. A severe strain to the rectus femoris, hamstring, or abdominal wall muscles has been shown to have a poor prognosis for rehabilitation and may benefit from surgical repair.

A sprain is caused by stretching or twisting beyond the normal range of motion of a ligament. A sprain can be difficult to differentiate from a strain during physical examination, and often they occur together. A history of overuse and/or excessive force, as opposed to a fall, hyperextension, or twisting of a joint, is more likely related to a strain. If bony tenderness at the injury site is found during the physical examination, x-rays are indicated to rule out fractures.

A high suspicion of fracture is required when evaluating a patient for a strain or sprain, especially if the patient has tenderness over a bone after an injury. Minor fractures (such as a torus fracture) may be misdiagnosed as a sprain or strain because a child does not complain or have the ability to verbally communicate their injury, and the parents or guardians are unaware of an injury. Older adults can have blunted pain perception, especially in the extremities, secondary to neuropathy, increasing the risk of a clinician missing a fracture. The clinician should be aware of this when considering obtaining x-rays on these patients.

Shoulder Sprains

Acromioclavicular joint (AC) sprains often occur in young males with a direct blow to the shoulder. These are typically associated with a fall directly onto the shoulder while the arm is adducted, causing trauma to the AC joint, although the injury may occur because of indirect trauma. The patient will present with pain, especially on adduction or abduction past 90 degrees, point tenderness over the AC joint, swelling, and possible deformity.

AC sprains are classified as follows into six grades:

1. AC ligament strain; x-rays will appear normal
2. Slight disruption and widening of AC joint; slight elevation (less than 100%) of the clavicle in relation to the acromion; coracoclavicular (CC) ligament strain but remains intact
3. AC and CC ligaments fully disrupted; complete superior dislocation (100%) of the clavicle in relation to the acromion
4. AC and CC ligaments fully disrupted; clavicle is displaced superior and posterior; trapezius and deltoid are usually torn
5. AC and CC ligaments fully disrupted; complete superior dislocation (greater than 100%) of the clavicle in relation to the acromion; trapezius and deltoid are usually torn
6. AC and CC ligaments fully disrupted; the distal clavicle is dislocated inferiorly under the coracoid or under the acromion

Ankle Sprains

Ankle ligaments provide mechanical stability, proprioceptive information, and directed motion for the joint. Recurrent ankle sprains can lead to functional instability and loss of normal ankle kinematics and proprioception, which can result in recurrent injury, chronic instability, early degenerative bony changes, and chronic pain (see Advanced Assessment 53.3). Acute ankle sprains can result in lost days of work and inability to participate in sports.

For the foot and ankle, the physical examination should include inspection and palpation. Swelling in the area of the medial and lateral malleoli should be assessed by comparing the landmarks with those of the opposite foot. The location of a deformity helps to localize the injury. The ankle and foot anatomy should be palpated purposefully to localize the specific areas of tenderness. Compare the active and passive ROM with the opposite uninjured extremity. It is important to note and investigate any crepitus after an injury that is associated with pain, as it may be associated with a fracture. The anterior

Advanced Assessment 53.3: Assessing Ankle Ligaments—Special Tests

Test	Comments
Anterior drawer test—evaluate anterior talofibular ligament (ATFL) stability; position ankle at 20 degrees of plantar flexion	Stabilize the tibia with one hand, grasp the hindfoot with the other hand and slide foot forward. Should have slight motion with firm endpoint. Asymmetric motion and no firm endpoint indicate chronic ankle laxity or significant injury to the ATFL.
Varus stress test—test the stability of the calcaneofibular ligament (CFL); the ankle is placed in neutral position	Stabilize the tibia with one hand, grasp the calcaneus with the other hand, and invert the hindfoot. Should have a firm endpoint. Asymmetrical motion and no firm endpoint indicate chronic laxity of the CFL.

drawer test can be performed to test the stability of the anterior talofibular ligament, and the varus stress test should be performed to test the stability of the calcaneofibular ligament (see Advanced Assessment 53.4).

DIFFERENTIAL DIAGNOSIS

Sprains and strains may occur in the context of an injury. A trauma, such as from a car accident or other significant precipitating factor, may be identified as the initiating event for a sprain. In some cases, a trivial movement may precipitate the injury.

Differentiating between a strain and a sprain involves a careful patient history and physical examination. Patients who present with a sprain usually have some degree of swelling, pain, and disability. In severe sprains, deformity of the joint may be noted.

Sprains can be classified into three degrees of severity (see Table 53.2).

The patient with a sprain often has a history that includes a sudden injury or fall that resulted in acute pain and swelling that worsens over the next few hours and an inability to move the joint. Redness and bruising over the affected joint are usually noted, and both active ROM and passive ROM of the joint are decreased, with pain

Advanced Assessment 53.4: Assessing Knee Ligaments—Special Tests

Test	Comments
Valgus stress test—assess medial collateral ligament (MCL) stability.	Place patient supine on examination table. Test is performed first with knee fully extended then with 25–30 degrees of flexion. Examiner stabilizes the medial distal tibia with one hand, with other hand on lateral side of knee, applies gentle pressure attempting to angle the knee medially (valgus). If the knee opens in a valgus direction more than the opposite knee, the patient has MCL laxity and potentially a complete or partial MCL tear.
Varus stress test—assess lateral collateral ligament (LCL) stability	Place patient supine on examination table. Test is performed first with knee fully extended and then with 25–30 degrees of flexion. Examiner stabilizes the lateral distal tibia with one hand, places other hand on medial side of knee, and applies gentle pressure, attempting to angle the knee laterally (varus). If the knee opens in a varus direction more than the opposite knee, the patient has LCL laxity and potentially a complete or partial LCL tear.
Lachman test—anterior cruciate ligament (ACL)	With the patient supine and the knee flexed 20–30 degrees, with one hand, grasp the lower leg just below the knee joint. The examiner should stabilize the leg with the thumb on the tibial tubercle. With the other hand, grasp the distal femur, placing the thumb over the quadriceps tendon, while the rest of the examiner's hand encircles the thigh above the patella. The knee should be relaxed so that the examiner feels the full weight of it. Simultaneously apply pressure to the tibia, attempting to move it forward while pushing backward on the femur. Feel for any anterior movement of the tibia. Should have very slight motion with a firm endpoint. Asymmetric or excessive motion and no firm endpoint indicate ACL laxity or rupture.
Posterior drawer test or sag sign—posterior cruciate ligament (PCL)	With the patient supine, flex the knee to 90 degrees with the foot supported. Wrap both hands around the proximal tibia, placing the thumbs on the medial and lateral tibial plateaus. Normally, the anterior tibial plateau sits 1 cm anterior to the femoral condyles. If the PCL is injured, the proximal tibia falls back, and the area available to the thumbs decreases. Next, place pressure on the proximal tibia, attempting to push it posteriorly. Normally, there should be slight motion with a firm endpoint. Asymmetric or excessive motion and no firm endpoint indicate PCL laxity or rupture.

TABLE 53.2 Ankle Sprains

Classification	First Degree	Second Degree	Third Degree
Type of pain	Stretching, minor tearing of ligament fibers	Partial tearing of ligament fibers	Complete tear of ligament
CLINICAL MANIFESTATIONS			
Pain	Minimal	Mild to moderate	Severe
Swelling	Mild	Moderate	Significant; occurs rapidly, usually within the first 30 minutes
Ecchymosis	Mild	Moderate	Severe; occurs rapidly, usually within the first 30 minutes
ROM	Full, mildly uncomfortable	Slightly limited, painful	Limited; loss of function
Point tenderness	Mild	Point tenderness	Severe
Joint stability	Stable	Mild joint laxity	Abnormal
Weight-bearing	Able to bear weight	Painful or unable to bear weight	Unable to bear weight
Management	RICE Active ROM Partial weight-bearing activity Return to sports in 2–3 weeks with ankle support	RICE Active ROM Non–weight-bearing activity as tolerated Gradual return to sports with Aircast or taping	Refer to orthopedic specialist; surgery may be required Cast for 4–6 weeks No weight-bearing; rehabilitation Return to sports in 4–8 weeks with support
Complications	Recurrent sprains within 1 month if not fully rehabilitated	Recurrent sprains Joint instability Traumatic arthritis	Persistent instability Traumatic arthritis

Abbreviations: RICE, rest, ice, compression, elevation; ROM, range of motion.

usually elicited upon moving the joint. Radiographs to rule out fracture are warranted when there is an obvious deformity, bone tenderness, and inability to put weight on a joint.

In contrast, strains affect the muscles or tendons that connect a muscle to a bone. Minor strains usually do not cause swelling or redness. Patients may complain of a "pulled muscle" and are usually able to use the affected limb, although ROM may be limited.

In severe strains, the entire muscle, tendon, or interface between the muscle and tendon (myotendinous junction) may be torn, causing inflammation, swelling, weakness, and loss of function. Surgery may be needed to repair a torn muscle or tendon.

The primary care provider should be alert to the possibility of muscle strains and sprains that mimic potentially serious conditions. For example, a patient with acute coronary syndrome with chest pain or shoulder pain may be misdiagnosed as having costochondritis (chest wall pain) or impingement syndrome (shoulder and arm pain). Costochondritis, also called *anterior chest wall syndrome,* is an inflammation of one or more costochondral junctions that manifest with chest wall pain. The pain may be sharp and acute or dull and persistent. It is the most frequently occurring nontraumatic type of chest pain in adolescents and young adults. Pain is located over the costochondral and costosternal areas of the anterior chest and is caused by inflammation of the costochondral junctions, manifesting only with pain in the absence of erythema, heat, or swelling. Repetitive minor trauma is currently believed to be the most likely etiology.

MANAGEMENT

After appropriate stabilization and 2 to 3 days of rest and elevation of the affected body part, the injury site can be examined more easily. The pain and swelling typically will be reduced, which will facilitate a better physical examination. Injuries that had negative x-rays initially but were extremely painful or suspicious for fracture can be reradiographed in 10 to 12 days and read with an appropriate technique to maximize the chances of observing a hidden, or occult, fracture. Because of the healing process, the fracture line can be more easily visualized at that time.

Evidence-based criteria to guide when diagnostic imaging is or is not appropriate should be used by the clinician to avoid unnecessary resource utilization, as well as reduce unnecessary exposure to radiation from imaging tests. One widely available resource for diagnostic imaging appropriateness criteria was developed by the American College of Radiology (https://www.acr.org). The Ottawa Ankle Rules constitute another example that lists criteria to be met for ordering a foot and/or ankle x-ray (see Advanced Assessment 53.5). These guidelines are commonly used to determine the utility of radiography in diagnosing a fracture in the assessment of ankle and foot injuries. However, these guidelines should not be used for pregnant patients, children younger than 6 years, and those who have head injuries or who otherwise cannot follow directions.

PRICE Therapy

Protection, rest, ice, compression, and elevation (PRICE) are the mainstay of treatment for musculoskeletal strains and sprains:

- Protection of the injury involves both prevention and protection. *Protection* may refer to preventing the injury from occurring or making it less severe by wearing protective gear, such as helmets, wrist pads, and kneepads.
- *Rest* means no use of the affected limb or joint for minor injuries or sprains for 1 to 2 days, followed by slowly increasing use of the limb as tolerated by the patient. If the patient's activity causes pain to the injury site, activity needs to be reduced to levels that do not cause pain. However, mild discomfort after activity is considered normal during the rehabilitation phase. Generally speaking, the amount of limb rest needed depends on the severity of the injury.
- Ice, a potent anti-inflammatory, should be applied to the injured site in repeated cycles of 20 to 30 minutes on and 20 to 30 minutes off, three to five times per day. Ice should not be applied directly to the skin, but rather over fabric or other material that transmits cold but minimizes the risk of thermal damage to the skin. The time of application "on" the injured site should be reduced in older patients, and "off" periods are critical for all patients to prevent frostbite. Ice therapy for 24 to 48 hours after the injury is recommended, as well as during the rehabilitation phase, if mild pain after activity occurs. After that period, warm and moist heat to the region is advocated to increase circulation to the area, which promotes reabsorption of blood and edema that have collected at the injury site.
- Compression by elastic wrap or other splinting material is used to provide counterpressure at the site of injury to help tamponade bleeding to the region. This will help decrease the amount of swelling and blood collection at the injury site. The influx of blood causes localized inflammation, which leads to leaking of plasma and other substances into the injured area. The compression wrap must always include the distal portion of the extremity (i.e., the foot or hand) to prevent a tourniquet effect.
- Elevating the affected limb above the level of the heart will decrease bleeding into the tissue surrounding the injury and help reduce pain. After the first 48 hours, when bleeding into the area has stopped, elevation of the affected body part will facilitate reabsorption of blood and tissue fluid at the injury site.

Pain Management

The use of NSAIDs for pain management is also recommended in conjunction with PRICE therapy. Muscle relaxants such as cyclobenzaprine (Flexeril) may be indicated for the management of acute painful musculoskeletal conditions associated with muscle spasm. They reduce tonic somatic muscle activity at the level of the brainstem.

Fractures

A fracture is a break in the continuity of a bone. Fractures are usually associated with a blunt force. Fractures are classified as open or closed, depending on whether they communicate with the external environment (i.e., through broken skin). Open fractures have an increased incidence of infection and must be aggressively treated. Many need to be surgically irrigated. Fractures can also be partial or complete. A partial fracture involves disruption of only a portion of the cortex, whereas a complete fracture involves circumferential disruption of the cortex. Complete fractures are unstable, and inappropriate initial stabilization can lead to additional injuries to the muscles or neurovascular structures.

When assessing the patient, the clinician should ask about the mechanism of injury. Fractures can occur at locations other than the obvious site of injury. The force can be transmitted to proximal or distal areas of body, causing fractures at distant sites. A person who fell off a roof and landed on their feet may have an obvious

---

Advanced Assessment 53.5: Ottawa Ankle and Foot Rules

If a patient meets any of the following criteria, a radiograph should be performed:

- An ankle radiograph is indicated when ankle pain is present **AND** there is (1) tenderness over the posterior 6 cm or tip of the medial or lateral malleolus **OR** (2) the patient is unable to take four weight-bearing steps both immediately and in the examination room.
- A foot radiograph is indicated when midfoot pain is present **AND** there is (1) tenderness over the navicular or the base of the fifth metatarsal **OR** (2) the patient is unable to take four weight-bearing steps both immediately and in the examination room.

Source: Murphy J, Weiner DA, Kotler J, et al. Utility of Ottawa Ankle Rules in an aging population: evidence for addition of an age criterion. *J Foot Ankle Surg.* 2020;59(2):286–290.

calcaneus (heel bone) fracture, but in addition, fractures of the hips, pelvis, and back must also be ruled out.

The general goal of fracture management is to align the bones in a near-normal plane, allowing the fracture ends to heal together and return to normal function. The initial phase of fracture biology starts with hematoma formation. This starts to bridge the fractured fragments. The inflammatory phase follows, and granulation tissue forms on the fracture surfaces. During this process, the hematoma is reabsorbed, which provides the first continuity between the fragments. This occurs approximately 10 to 14 days after the injury. During this time, the bone surrounding the fracture line becomes less dense due to reabsorption of necrotic bone. This makes the fracture line easier to identify.

A callus forms on both the periosteal and endosteal surfaces of the bone, acting as a biological splint. Calcification of the healing fracture and bone then begins. First, calcium phosphate is deposited, and then the bone undergoes osseous metaplasia. It takes approximately 2 to 4 weeks for the callus to be visible on x-rays. The callus is then slowly reabsorbed, and the fracture surfaces develop a firm bony union. During this phase, the calcified region undergoes organization, and the margins begin to smoothen. The process ends with remodeling and then consolidation. In a healthy adult, the whole process takes approximately 2 months for smaller long bones (such as the humerus) and up to 4 months for large bones (such as the femur).

Shoulder Fracture

Fractures of the humerus, clavicle, and acromion are common. A fracture of the clavicle or acromion typically occurs from a moderate fall (such as from a bicycle or down the stairs) or from blows during a contact sport. Acromion fractures are less common than clavicle fractures. Patients with clavicle fractures complain of sharp shoulder pain and are reluctant to move the upper extremity. It is important to verify that no neck pain or upper extremity paresthesias are present. These fractures usually best heal spontaneously after proper immobilization; they rarely require surgery. There are a variety of humeral fracture patterns. These may occur from a fall, a direct blow to the arm, or a twisting injury. Treatment for humeral fractures ranges from immobilization through use of a simple sling to surgical repair.

Proximal Femoral (Hip) Fracture

Hip fractures are among the most common adult fractures, accounting for at least one-half of all hospital days related to fracture care in the United States. There is approximately a 25% 1-year mortality rate after a hip fracture. Hip fractures can generally be classified as intracapsular fractures, which affect the femoral neck, or extracapsular if they affect the proximal femur distal to the femoral neck. Extracapsular fractures between the femoral neck and the lesser trochanter are considered intertrochanteric, and those in the 5-cm section distal to the lesser trochanter are considered subtrochanteric. The incidence of hip fractures doubles for each decade of life after age 50 years, with females affected twice as often as males.

Risks for hip fractures include increasing age, previous fracture, visual impairment, institutionalization, and osteoporosis. Pain in the hip area after trauma, such as a fall or motor vehicle collision, especially in patients older than age 50 years, should give rise to the suggestion of a fracture. However, neither a lack of trauma nor a longstanding history of hip pain rules out a fracture. In some cases, a fracture may occur as a pathological fracture secondary to an underlying neoplasm or chronic corticosteroid usage. Patients with a suspected hip fracture should be evaluated urgently and may be admitted to the hospital.

Patients with a suspected hip fracture should be asked if an injury occurred and if so, how the injury occurred and whether the fall was witnessed by anyone other than the patient. A loss of consciousness for any period of time necessitates a cardiac and neurological referral, as well as referral for orthopedic care. The clinician should determine the patient's mental status and try to obtain a realistic assessment of the preinjury functional status.

Physical examination typically reveals an externally rotated and shortened injured leg when a hip fracture is present. Any motion to this extremity will produce severe pain at the affected groin. The pelvic bony prominences should be examined for tenderness because pubis ramus fractures may also be present or may be confused with the hip injury. It is important to check for lower-extremity pulses and neurological function. The entire limb should be examined for associated fractures at sites such as the

---

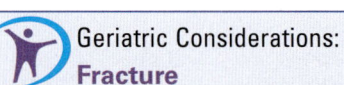

Geriatric Considerations: Fracture

Hip and distal radius fractures are among the most common fractures affecting older patients. These fractures are anticipated to have a higher incidence rate as the population continues to age. In the United States, nearly 650,000 distal radius fractures occur annually. The two primary types of hip fractures are femoral neck (intracapsular) and intertrochanteric, both of which occur most frequently in older adults who have sustained a fall at home or a similar low-energy trauma. The Fracture Risk Assessment Tool can be useful for a clinician to estimate the risk for a future fracture in a patient, especially older patients. The risk is elevated for osteoporotic insufficiency fracture with older patients, as well as potential complications, disability, and mortality. Nearly 4.5 million people globally are disabled annually after they suffer a fractured hip. Aside from osteoporosis, other risks for the development of fractures in older adults include medication and polypharmacy, urinary incontinence, impaired cognition, falls, and neuromuscular conditions.

middle or distal femur, tibia, or ankle. An anteroposterior view of the pelvis and "shoot-through" lateral views of the affected hip can provide definitive radiographic evidence to confirm the diagnosis. In many cases, surgical repair of the fracture is the treatment of choice.

Knee Fracture

A knee fracture is most likely to occur with direct trauma and result in acute onset of pain. Fractures in leg bones around the knee include those of the patella, tibial plateau, fibular head and shaft, and distal femur. Most, but not all, knee fractures are the result of significant trauma; fractures of the knee are often present in conjunction with injury to associated structures. Most fractures around the knee are associated with a large effusion. If the joint is aspirated, the presence of hemarthrosis is clinically indicative of a fracture with associated bleeding into the joint and fat globules that have come from the fractured bone. Swelling and significant pain on movement will be present. It is important to evaluate for any neurovascular compromise that may be present in the lower leg. Radiography should be obtained, and immediate referral to an orthopedic surgeon is indicated. Patellar fractures are usually the result of a direct blow from a blunt object or can be attributed to a fall or motor vehicle collision (MVC). The patient with a patellar fracture is usually unable to flex the knee. Marked joint effusion is usually present.

Ankle Fracture

Ankle fractures can result from excessive force in rolling or twisting the ankle. A person can also have an ankle fracture result from a direct blow to the ankle or after jumping/falling from a height and landing on the feet. A stress fracture of the ankle can result from modest increase in activities such as running, ballet, or gymnastics. Fractures of the ankle may involve the distal tibia and medial malleolus, distal fibula and lateral malleolus, and the talus.

The patient with an ankle fracture will have pain, swelling, inability to bear weight, and decreased range of motion. Evidence-based guidelines, such as the Ottawa Ankle Rules, should be used to guide decision making for when an ankle x-ray is appropriate after an ankle injury. Obvious bony disruption is usually noted on x-ray images; however, fractures may occasionally not be fully visualized for 1 to 2 weeks after the injury.

Stress Fractures

Stress fractures are common in patients who experience bone pain after initiating or increasing high-impact activity. Stress fractures are a result of repeated subtle bone trauma over a period of time that causes a gradual loss of bony substance. New bone is fragile until it calcifies. The cortex, temporarily weakened, is then susceptible to fracture. Common sites for stress fractures are the legs and feet.

Physical examination typically reveals point tenderness over the injured bone. Ecchymosis and soft tissue swelling may be present. Often, the patient has altered their gait to compensate for the pain and swelling, potentially causing additional knee or back pain. Resistive motion of the joint is often painless. Radiographs often appear negative until 2 to 3 weeks after the injury has occurred, and the body is attempting to heal itself. X-rays may then reveal a periosteal reaction or a hairline radiolucency. Bone scans or CT scans may be helpful in diagnosing or confirming these diagnoses if needed. Although an MRI is typically not used to diagnose a stress fracture, it would show nonspecific inflammation and edema of the bone at the stress fracture site.

Differential Diagnosis

One goal of differential diagnosis in musculoskeletal trauma is to distinguish more serious bony fractures from strains and sprains. Each of these injuries is treated differently. As joint swelling and tenderness are common presentations of such injuries, it is critical to consider a variety of rheumatological and infectious disorders, such as a septic joint, RA, or OA. An appropriate history that seeks to characterize any preceding musculoskeletal trauma will typically differentiate among these conditions.

Radiographic (x-ray) studies are the mainstay of orthopedic care, and it is critical that the clinician order the correct x-ray for the injury suspected. Many x-ray studies include views of several joints and bones, but given the specialized nature of individual x-ray views, the clinician should focus on the area the specific x-ray examination is intended to visualize. Each x-ray examination uses a specific technique to ensure that the correct joint angles, bony structures, and other information are included to allow the practitioner to rule out pathology to a specific region. If a patient has pain in the foot and the ankle, an ankle x-ray may miss foot pathology, and a foot x-ray may miss ankle pathology. Advanced Assessment 53.6 presents guidance on reading an extremity x-ray film.

Many clinicians order routine comparison x-rays of the uninjured extremity, especially in children with open growth plates. This may be helpful on rare occasions to compare a potentially injured growth plate to a "normal" uninjured growth plate. This practice is controversial because it may expose a growing child to unnecessary radiation. A thorough examination is usually enough to secure a location of injury and clinical diagnosis. When examining an infant or a child who will not move or bear weight on an extremity, the clinician should palpate the entire extremity while observing the patient's facial expressions. When the injury is palpated, the patient's face will reveal discomfort, which will assist the clinician in localizing the injured site before ordering the appropriate radiographic studies. An x-ray is excellent at visualizing bone, whereas MRI excels in visualizing joint and soft tissue injuries.

> ### ✚ Advanced Assessment 53.6: Reading an Extremity X-Ray
>
> - Conduct a thorough history and determine the mechanism of injury before ordering radiographic studies. This will help determine the location and type of injury to expect. The area of injury should be examined, as this will focus attention on the area of suspicion on the x-ray. It is good practice to review the x-ray image after the examination, even if it was originally viewed before examining the patient.
> - When viewing the image, follow the bony outer cortex of the injured body part, looking for any defects such as thinning, thickening, and disruptions/breaks. The cortex should be smooth and crisp, appearing fairly uniform in color (density) and thickness; any area of haziness or any defect needs to be further scrutinized. Software used to view x-rays usually has a manual ability to adjust contrast and brightness, which may help in viewing certain images.
> - Visualize the inner trabecula of the bone, looking for fairly uniform appearance in density, evidence of fracture, any bone lesions, or tumors.
> - Visualize adjacent bones at joints for alignment, abnormal angulation, fragments of bone in the joint space, subluxation, or dislocation.
> - When looking at the joint space, consider if there is any evidence of degenerative joint disease including increased density of or cysts in the bone just under the joint cartilage, decreased space at the joint, and bone spurs at the edges of the bones that make up the joint.
> - Look at the soft tissue surrounding the area of concern. Injuries will cause soft tissue swelling. This may help focus your attention on the injured area. Using the contrast and brightness of the image viewer software may help visualization of soft tissue.
> - Several regions of the body, especially near joints, have certain "special" signs to look for that may reflect an occult injury. These usually correspond to bleeding or edema at or near a joint with a fracture. More commonly, the patient will have the image taken at a diagnostic imaging center. It may be useful to confer with the radiologist at the imaging center to discuss the x-rays as needed.

Differential diagnoses for a fracture include reflex sympathetic dystrophy. Also known as *Sudeck atrophy* and *causalgia,* this post-traumatic syndrome has three clinical stages—early, dystrophic, and atrophic. Early in the condition, a constant aching or burning occurs in the affected limb. Motion or external stimulation increases the symptoms, usually out of proportion to the stimulus. In the dystrophic stage that follows, the skin of the affected extremity becomes glossy and cold, and range of motion is limited. Finally, the atrophic stage is marked by skin atrophy and contracture. No correlation exists between incidence or symptom severity and the extent or type of the original musculoskeletal injury. Thus, early diagnosis of this syndrome is difficult, especially after an apparently trivial injury. Early diagnosis is extremely important, however, because the earlier treatment is initiated, the better the response, which is aimed at restoration of limb function through physical therapy. Antidepressant therapy and prednisone may also be beneficial.

Management

Initial fracture care involves stabilization of the bone ends to avoid further injury or damage to neurovascular structures. Immediate temporary splinting should be instituted. Patients with severely angulated long bone fractures should be immobilized and transferred to an emergency department (ED) for definitive management, either closed reduction or open reduction with possible internal fixation. Rule of thumb says splints should be applied in such a way as to immobilize the joints above and below the fracture site to avoid motion of the bone ends involved. Commercially available metal and plastic splints are used for this purpose.

After radiographic assessment and confirmation of a nondisplaced fracture, a well-fitting and durable splint can be applied. During immobilization, the clinician must consider the fact that fracture sites will continue to swell in the first 24 to 48 hours. In turn, placing a rigid circumferential cast on the patient in the first 24 to 48 hours can potentially lead to vascular compromise and limb-threatening compartment syndrome if edema is present. To avoid this, a splint can be placed on only half of the limb and can be adjusted or molded to allow optimal stabilization of certain fractures. The skin should be padded to avoid local necrosis or skin ulceration, and the splint should be secured by an elastic bandage. This type of splint allows the extremity to swell without affecting distal circulation.

Even with the proper x-ray technique, some fractures are not visible initially and will not appear until 7 to 10 days after the injury. At that time, the fracture margins absorb and will widen the radiolucent line at the fracture site. New bone will also be produced beneath the periosteum at the margins of the fracture, which will accentuate the fracture line. This will allow visualization of fractures that were not identified initially. If a fracture is suspected but not visible at the initial visit, the injury should be treated as a fracture and reexamined clinically and radiographically in 7 to 10 days. The patient should be informed of the rationale for this treatment. It is good practice to always add this to the patient's discharge instructions in writing and to have the patient sign their understanding.

Oblique fractures typically heal more quickly than transverse ones. Children tend to heal more quickly than adults, and older patients heal even more slowly. Radiological evidence of abundant organized callus formation at the fracture site with bone ends that have remained stable on serial films suggests stabilization of the fracture. Limited physical and weight-bearing activity for the affected limb is recommended until full strength is returned.

Follow-Up and Referral

The patient should be examined by an orthopedic provider (nurse practitioner [NP], physician assistant [PA], doctor of medicine [MD], or doctor of osteopathy [DO]) within a week after a fracture and application of a cast or splint to reassess neuromuscular status. In addition, the patient should be instructed to report any of the following signs and symptoms, which may reflect compartment syndrome—intense pain, hypoesthesia (a dulled sensitivity to touch), paresthesia (numbness, prickling, or tickling), muscular weakness, swelling and color change of the digits (fingers or toes), or paralysis. A patient with these signs should be referred to an orthopedic surgeon immediately. Follow-up visits with an orthopedic specialist and an x-ray of the injured area to monitor bone consolidation will often occur at 3 and 6 weeks. An assessment of bone healing will be performed. A cast can be removed when adequate healing has occurred, at approximately 6 weeks; however, this is dependent on patient age, comorbidities, and speed of healing.

> **Patient Education: Musculoskeletal Trauma**
>
> Educate the patient about the fracture healing process. After a fracture occurs, it begins to heal. A callus is formed at the fracture site. Calcium is deposited to aid in rebuilding the bone. During the healing, there may be a time when the fracture is stronger than the surrounding bone. Later, they became equal in strength, and the previously fractured bone is neither more nor less likely to fracture again. Healed bones are able to break anywhere. This includes at the site of a prior fracture.

Bone mineral density measurements may be able to predict the risk of fragility fractures (e.g., distal radius, proximal humerus, hip, and vertebra). This would help identify patients who would benefit from medication, education, and prevention strategies.

To avoid musculoskeletal injury, good physical conditioning is important. Consistent activity and exercise will strengthen muscles and reduce the chance of injury. This is essential to recover from a fracture, as well as prevent a future fracture.

MUSCLE CRAMPS

Muscle cramps may be described as sudden, involuntary, painful contractions of a muscle that last from seconds to several minutes. Cramps may occur spontaneously while at rest or may be precipitated by a brief muscle contraction. The cause is usually related to hyperexcitability of the motor neurons supplying the muscles. In many cases, the reason for episodic, recurrent muscle cramps may remain unclear, even after complete diagnostic evaluation. Muscle cramps may also occur related to vigorous exercise and during sporting events and may be caused by dehydration.

DIFFERENTIAL DIAGNOSIS

The initial history should elicit whether the cramps occur with exercise or at rest. In pregnant females and children, leg cramps tend to occur at rest and are most often benign, requiring no treatment (see Differential Diagnosis 53.1). Certain medications (e.g., some diuretics, some of the statin drugs, and clofibrate [Atromid-S]) may cause muscle cramping. Leg pain and cramps in adults that are precipitated by exercise and relieved by rest are usually caused by peripheral vascular disease. Blood chemistry tests may be necessary, including serum enzymes, to rule out causes such as dehydration (from diarrhea or sweating).

Differential Diagnosis 53.1: Muscle Cramps

Symptom	Possible Diagnosis
Cramp-like symptoms	Intermittent claudication related to ischemia; drug induced (such as statin-induced myopathy)
Contracture	Thyroid disease, McArdle's disease
Tetany	Hypoglycemia, hypomagnesemia, respiratory alkalosis, hypokalemia
Dystonia	Occupational (such as writer's cramp) Drug induced (antipsychotics, antiparkinsonian), metabolic/neurological
True cramps	Ordinary (nocturnal), dehydration, drug induced (nifedipine, beta agonists), lower motor neuron, hemodialysis (volume and electrolyte shifts), heat induced (volume depletion, hyponatremia)

Source: Swash M, Czesnik D, de Carvalho M. Muscular cramp: causes and management. *Eur J Neurol.* 2019;26(2):214–221.

PARESTHESIAS

Paresthesia is the sensation of numbness, prickling, or tingling experienced with central and peripheral nerve lesions. Frequently, the patient's understanding and use of the terms will differ from the clinician. It is necessary to clearly establish the character of the patient's complaint. During the history, the provider should differentiate between the lack of use of a limb due to the sensation of tingling and numbness and the total loss of sensation. It is also important to ascertain whether the loss or altered sensation ascends onto the abdomen or thorax.

The location of the paresthesia may be focal or generalized. It may also be nonspecific, as in multiple sclerosis, in which the initial presentation may be bilateral diminution of sensation or paresthesia in the upper or lower extremities. It can also be unilateral, as in stroke or transient ischemic attack, in which unilateral extremity or face paresthesias may occur.

Paresthesias may be the result of anatomical or mechanical peripheral nerve injuries, such as entrapment and compression neuropathies. These are most likely to occur at sites that are more susceptible to damage due to an increase in pressure and mechanical forces. Entrapment and compression neuropathies can include the median nerve at the wrist (carpal tunnel syndrome), radial nerve of the forearm, ulnar nerve at the elbow, and peroneal nerve at the knee.

A characteristic set of signs and symptoms, such as radiculopathy, is caused by compression or injury of spinal nerve roots, which may be due to spondylosis (degeneration of the vertebrae) or disc herniation. Radiculopathy includes weakness, numbness, and tingling that typically occur along the distribution of the affected nerve root. More commonly, affected nerves are cervical nerve roots C5 to C8, lumbar nerves L3 to L5, and sacral nerve S1 (see Advanced Assessment 53.7). Patients who present with paresthesias should undergo a detailed neurological assessment to determine whether sensory or motor deficits are present. MRI is indicated when paresthesia is accompanied by motor or sensory deficit or hyporeflexia to rule out spinal cord compression. Any change in bowel or bladder function (e.g., cauda equina syndrome) constitutes an emergency and needs immediate assessment by a spine specialist.

Other causes of paresthesias include chlorinated hydrocarbon exposure, respiratory alkalosis, and the use of certain drugs, such as carbonic anhydrase inhibitors (which are used in the treatment of glaucoma).

DIFFERENTIAL DIAGNOSIS

In addition to the causes described in the previous section, other causes of paresthesias include brachial plexus injury, thoracic outlet syndrome, and peripheral polyneuropathy.

Brachial plexus injuries include a broad array of neurological dysfunction ranging from a momentary paresthesia to a completely flail extremity. The mechanism of injury is equally diverse, from high-energy motor vehicle crashes, falls from a height, and gunshot wounds to lower-energy injuries such as most athletic injuries. The symptoms are severe. Burning upper arm and shoulder pain that radiates down the arm, followed by weakness affecting C5 and T1 (thoracic) nerve root distributions. The patient is often seen holding the arm on the affected side, which hangs limp at the side.

Thoracic outlet syndrome involves a compression of the brachial plexus and/or subclavian vessels as they exit the narrow space between the superior shoulder girdle and the first rib. These structures can be affected individually or in combination. Females aged 20 to 50 years are most commonly affected. Etiology may be secondary to congenital abnormalities such as cervical rib, abnormally long transverse process of C7, or an anomalous fibromuscular band in the thoracic outlet. Post-traumatic fibrosis of the scalene muscles is also a possibility.

Peripheral polyneuropathy is a distal sensorimotor paresthesia, or "stocking-and-glove" pattern paresthesia, with diminished or variable deep tendon reflexes. Diabetes mellitus is a frequent cause. Early symptoms may respond to a regimen with tighter glucose control. A rapid onset of motor polyneuropathy is seen in Guillain-Barré syndrome, in which an ascending weakness occurs after a viral illness. Other etiologies include alcohol use disorder, vitamin B deficiencies, vitamin B_6 excess, Sjögren's syndrome, AIDS, hypothyroidism, amyloidosis, and renal failure.

MYOFASCIAL PAIN

Myofascial pain is a type of muscle pain that is believed to be caused by the development of "trigger points" within a muscle. A trigger point is an area of local irritation that,

Advanced Assessment 53.7: Paresthesias and Affected Nerve Roots

Nerve Root	Paresthesia
C6 (sixth cervical)	Thumb: dorsal and lateral aspects
C7 (seventh cervical)	Fingers: index and middle
C8 (eighth cervical)	Fingers: fifth and ulnar half of fourth Hand: ulnar side
L4 (fourth lumbar)	Thigh: anterior, just above knee
L5 (fifth lumbar)	Foot: dorsal aspect Great toe: dorsal aspect
S1 (first sacral)	Foot: lateral aspect Small toe: lateral aspect

when activated, causes referred pain in a characteristic pattern. Trigger points may be felt as hyper-irritable taut bands under the skin in areas where muscles lie close to the surface.

DIFFERENTIAL DIAGNOSIS

Although myofascial pain is a common cause of nonarticular rheumatic pain, it is often misdiagnosed. Trigger points are not visualized on routine imaging studies and cannot be objectively substantiated. Myofascial pain and fibromyalgia may occur together (see Chapter 63).

Treatment includes identifying and eliminating aggravating factors. Techniques include trigger point injections, dry needling, and massage therapy. Trigger point injections involve saline, an anesthetic, or a corticosteroid injected into the trigger point. Dry needling includes a needle without medication inserted to deactivate the trigger point. Massage therapy focuses on releasing the trigger points with specialized manual techniques.

Muscle relaxants can be effective in decreasing muscle spasticity, pain, and disability in patients with myofascial pain. Patients need to be aware that this class of drugs is for short-term use because the risk/benefit ratio for prolonged use of muscle relaxants is poorly established. Because muscle relaxants can cause drowsiness and dizziness, patients need to avoid hazardous activities, such as driving or operating machinery, while using these medicines. Patients should also avoid taking them with alcohol or other central nervous system depressants to prevent additive effects. Dry mouth is another side effect of this anticholinergic class of drugs, so frequent mouth rinsing is recommended to prevent dental disease.

Topical application of creams such as capsaicin and lidocaine patches may also help relieve pain. Some patients achieve relief with NSAIDs or cyclooxygenase-2 inhibitors. Tricyclic antidepressants, such as amitriptyline, and antiepilepsy drugs are sometimes used in cases that do not respond to other treatments. Narcotic analgesics should be used with caution due to the risk for addiction, misuse, abuse, and diversion.

REGIONAL MUSCULOSKELETAL COMPLAINTS

NECK PAIN

Discomfort and limited ROM arising from the structures in the neck are common complaints. The pain may originate from any of the musculoskeletal structures, including muscles, ligaments, tendons, intervertebral discs, vertebrae, nerves, and vasculature. Pain referred to the neck from the TMJ, pleura, or mediastinum may also be seen. Causes of neck pain are generally structural (mechanical) in nature and most often are the result of injury, degenerative changes, or muscle strain or spasm. Stress, sedentary occupations, and improper biomechanics are frequently found to be contributing factors. Questions regarding these factors should be asked during the history taking. The onset (rapid or insidious), location (arm, shoulder, head, or back), and character (sharp, dull, or aching) of the pain are essential in the differential diagnosis. Of note is neck pain (in the absence of trauma) that begins insidiously, progressively worsens, and is unimproved with rest. This may be due to vertebral infection or malignancy in the vertebrae. These conditions will often awaken a person from sleep with the unrelenting nature of the pain.

Physical examination of the neck begins with inspection for position of the head and contour of the neck (e.g., flattening due to muscle spasm), any obvious deformities (e.g., torticollis), and any guarding of painful areas by the patient. Palpation of the neck must be done purposefully, checking for any areas of tenderness, muscle spasm, and lymphadenopathy. Lymph nodes in the supraclavicular and axillary regions can be included in the examination. Enlarged nonmobile nodes, in the absence of infection, may indicate malignancy. The vascular structures of the neck and the thyroid should be evaluated. Evaluation of ROM includes flexion, extension, rotation, and side bending to determine limitations and any pain-producing movements. The neck examination typically includes an assessment of the upper extremities. This includes an assessment of biceps, triceps, wrist, and hand strength (see the Wrist and Hand Pain section later in this chapter). Abnormalities in sensation of any dermatome and altered deep tendon reflexes of the arms may indicate cervical nerve root compression. Spurling's maneuver can be used to assess cervical nerve root compression (see Advanced Assessment 53.8). Laboratory studies such as ESR, CRP, RF, ANA, or others as indicated are useful if systemic or bone disease is suspected.

Advanced Assessment 53.8: Spurling's Maneuver

To perform Spurling's maneuver, follow this procedure:

1. With the patient's neck in extension, rotate neck to the affected side.
2. Apply downward pressure on the head.
3. Assess for patient complaint of, or accentuation of, radicular limb pain or paresthesia (a positive finding).

DIFFERENTIAL DIAGNOSIS

It is often difficult to differentiate which specific soft tissues of the neck are injured. A common cause of neck pain is cervical muscle sprain or strain. This can involve an injury to the facet joints or any of the ligaments or muscles of the neck. Flexion/extension injuries that occur in MVCs, often called *whiplash,* are common neck injuries seen in primary care. Patients presenting with neck pain after an MVC should be carefully evaluated for a variety of injuries including neurological dysfunction, muscle strain, dislocations, fractures, and ligamentous tears.

A spasm is rigidity or spasticity caused by involuntary painful muscle contraction that does not relax. When a muscle is chronically in spasm, blood flow is reduced, and ischemia and pain often result. The goal in treating muscle spasm is to induce the muscle to relax, allowing for restoration of blood flow, removal of metabolic by-products, and the influx of nutrients.

Degenerative changes affecting the cervical vertebrae are called *spondylosis.* These changes may cause thinning of the intervertebral discs, hypertrophy of ligaments, and formation of bony spurs called *osteophytes.* Spondylosis is often a normal result of aging and is often asymptomatic. In some individuals, however, osteophytes may impinge on spinal nerve roots and cause radicular signs and symptoms of numbness, tingling, burning, and/or weakness in an extremity. These conditions and differential diagnoses are discussed in more detail in Chapter 54.

BACK PAIN

About 85% of the adult population experiences lower back pain at some point in their lives. Common causes of lower back pain include lumbar strain and sprains, nerve impingement, nerve compression, radiculopathy, and fractures. Additional causes include infection, tumors, and systemic inflammatory disorders. Less than 20% of people with acute lower back pain will evolve to have chronic lower back pain.

The most common causes of acute lower back pain are lumbar strain and sprains (discussed in more detail in Chapter 54). Strain occurs when the muscles or ligaments of the lower back are stretched, causing microscopic tears. Sprains are caused by the overstretching or tearing of ligaments. Lumbar strain and sprains usually occur from improper use, overuse, or trauma to the muscles and connective tissue of the lower back. Similarly, fractures of the vertebrae occur most often as a result of trauma, although they may occur spontaneously or with low-intensity injury in individuals with decreased bone density (e.g., osteopenia or osteoporosis).

Fractures usually present with an acute onset of pain that radiates around the body and is exacerbated with movement. These can occur due to trauma or with minimal injury in those with osteoporosis. If no accident or trauma is involved, the patient will usually complain of a time-sequence history of symptoms that may be gradual or sudden and may be localized in the lumbosacral area or radiating. If disc herniation or spinal nerve irritation is present, the patient may complain of radiation of pain into the leg, sensory or reflex changes, and motor weakness. Difficulties with bowel or bladder function may signal an emergency surgical situation. Lesions or tumors that compress the spine may present similarly due to localized effects on the spinal cord. For example, the patient with cauda equina syndrome typically presents with leg weakness, saddle area anesthesia, bowel or bladder incontinence or retention, and impotence. Similarly, symptoms of radiculopathy may include pain, numbness, and a tingling sensation that radiates down the spinal nerve distribution, for example, from the lower back and down the leg in lumbar radiculopathy (sciatica).

Malignancies and localized infections (e.g., spinal abscess) may cause back pain and neurological symptoms such as weakness or decreased sensation due to swelling and resultant mass effects, which compromise spinal cord or nerve root function. Radiculopathy is a condition caused by spinal nerve root compression, injury, or inflammation, most commonly due to vertebral disc herniation or spinal stenosis (narrowing of the vertebral canal). For example, lumbar disc herniation involves compression of at least one lumbar nerve root.

Initial examination should include inspection of the spine, lower extremities, and gait. The back, spine, and legs should be inspected for asymmetry, atrophy, lesions, and trauma, and leg length should be measured from the front (anteriorly), laterally, and posteriorly. The inspection should include standing, sitting with the knees and hips bent at 90 degrees, and lying in a prone position.

The clinician should purposefully palpate anatomical landmarks of the lower back, primarily including the vertebrae and muscles. Range of motion (ROM) includes forward flexion, lateral bending, and extension and rotation of the lumbar spine. The clinician evaluates for pain and limitations in ROM and strength. The clinician may need to stand behind the patient during ROM to stabilize the hips at the iliac crest and balance the patient. With the patient in a supine or seated position and the examiner's hands stabilizing the patient's pelvis as needed, hip flexion and extension, internal and external rotation of the hip, and knee flexion/extension should be evaluated for symmetric ROM, pain, and strength.

The clinician should perform an appropriate neurovascular evaluation of the back and lower extremities. Vascular examination should include palpation of the dorsalis pedis and posterior tibial pulses in both lower extremities, as well as capillary refill of the toes. The clinician should perform a neurological examination of the lower extremities that will detect the small deficits produced by disc disease and the large deficits produced by such problems as compression of the cauda equina due to spinal tumors. The lower extremities should be evaluated and compared for symmetry of sensation, which may help localize the level of nerve root lesions. Nerve root compression tests including the straight-leg-raise test can be used to evaluate lumbar nerve root impingement or irritation (see Advanced Assessment 53.9), as palpation of the spine cannot confirm the diagnosis of radiculopathy. A positive straight-leg-raise test result is reproduction of pain when the leg is raised 70 degrees or less.

Vertebral disc herniation resulting in radiculopathy of lumbar spinal nerves L4 to L5 and L5 to S1 is a particularly common source of acute back and leg pain. This may or may not be due to trauma. L4 to L5 and L5 to S1 radiculopathy (sciatica) may be objectively assessed in terms of dermatome sensory deficit, myotome muscle weakness, and deep tendon reflex deficits. The clinician should assess for the inability of the patient to walk on the toes or heels and the inability to dorsiflex the great toe, which may relate to specific lumbar spinal nerve involvement. Lower back pain is typically less severe than pain radiating down one leg with disc herniation.

DIFFERENTIAL DIAGNOSIS

Lower back pain has a number of potential causes. Several differential diagnoses for back pain include the following:

- Ankylosing spondylitis: back pain and stiffness over several months; pain relief with exercise; reduced mobility of spine; painful or ankylosed sacroiliac joints; and reduced chest wall expansion. It occurs most often with an insidious onset after age 40 years.
- Cauda equina syndrome: acute urinary or rectal incontinence, with or without paraplegia
- Dissecting aortic aneurysm: sudden onset of severe lower back pain in older adults; pain that is not relieved with rest; pallor, diaphoresis, and confusion may be present; possible asymmetrical pulses and blood pressure in extremities
- Gallstones: pain follows ingestion of a fatty meal and radiates around trunk to right scapula; belching, bloating, and stomach acid are present, along with right upper quadrant pain
- Gynecological disorders: vaginal discharge; pain worse around menstruation or ovulation
- Herniated disc: often preceded by years of recurrent episodes of localized back pain; leg pain overshadows back pain
- Infection: unremitting or progressive pain at rest; tender spinous process at level of involvement; fever; history of drug use; diabetes; immunosuppression or suspected systemic infection; previous genitourinary or spinal surgery
- Musculoskeletal strain: often no precipitating event; pain is over lower back and muscles without sciatica; aggravated by sitting, standing, and certain movements; alleviated with rest. Palpation localizes pain, and muscle spasms may be seen. Insidious onset; progressive improvement
- Prostatitis: constant low back pain; pain in the lower abdomen and or testicles; hematuria, urinary hesitancy or frequency; sexual dysfunction or painful ejaculation
- Pyelonephritis: ill-appearing patient with nausea and vomiting; back and flank pain excruciating with direct percussion
- Sciatica: pain radiating into the buttocks, thighs, and/or below the knees as the result of L5 or S1 nerve root irritation, compression, or disc prolapse
- Spinal fracture: pain felt near the site of injury; history of major trauma to the back or (in older adults) a history of strenuous lifting or a minor fall
- Spinal stenosis: gradual onset in older adults, often mimics intermittent claudication, except pain is usually in buttocks, thigh, or calf, worsens with exertion and back extension (leaning backward or walking downhill), and is relieved with sitting, walking uphill, or leaning forward; weakness and/or bowel and bladder dysfunction may be present.
- Spondylolisthesis: systemic inflammatory condition of the vertebral column and sacroiliac joints; most frequently affects males aged 20 to 30 years; chronic low back pain, worse in morning; excessive thoracic kyphosis is present.
- Tumor: unremitting or progressive pain at rest, night pain; tender spinous process at level of involvement; variable neurological findings; weight loss, fever, or other systemic symptoms; known or suspected malignancy

The initial history and physical examination can lead to the diagnosis in cases in which a specific cause can be identified. In the absence of systemic pathology or identifiable spinal pathology, a precise determination of the cause of a patient's pain cannot be made in many cases. It is important to identify patients who require more extensive, urgent, or emergency evaluation. Once emergent causes and systemic disease are ruled out, medical treatment for lower back pain is dictated by the identified or suspected underlying pathology (see Chapter 54).

Advanced Assessment 53.9: Straight-Leg-Raise Test

To perform this test, follow this procedure:

1. The patient is placed in a supine position.
2. Grasp the heel of the leg to be tested and raise the straightened leg by flexing the hip.
3. Assess for pain or reproduction of symptoms before the end of the normal range of motion (less than 70 degrees).

As with any patient complaint, diagnostic testing varies, depending on the history and physical examination findings. Laboratory tests including CBC, urinalysis, ESR, and CRP may be helpful in determining an infectious or inflammatory etiology. Additional laboratory tests such as autoantibody panels may help rule out autoimmune disorders, although positive tests may be nonspecific. Of note, ankylosing spondylitis is characterized by inflammatory back pain in the absence of RF (in contrast to RA) with most patients demonstrating elevations in acute phase reactants such as CRP and expression of the human leukocyte antigen (HLA)-B27 genetic haplotype.

In addition to laboratory tests, imaging modalities and procedures may be helpful in making a diagnosis. X-ray is a convenient technique to visualize bony structures if a fracture (traumatic or spontaneous), degeneration, or misalignment is suspected. A CT scan produces a three-dimensional image that is often more helpful than an x-ray in identifying bone detail, spinal stenosis, or tumors. Ultrasound can show ligament, tendon, and muscle tears, or may be used to identify an intra-abdominal etiology (e.g., gallbladder dysfunction, abdominal aneurysm). Bone scans can be used to measure abnormal metabolic activity seen with tumors, infection, and fractures.

MRI is better than a CT scan in imaging soft tissue injuries. These include conditions such as nerve impingement, tumor, infection, disc herniation, disc rupture, or trauma to ligaments, tendons, muscles, or blood vessels. MRI is also appropriate for patients who are surgical candidates or who have evidence of systemic disease. Electromyography (EMG) and nerve conduction studies may be used to diagnose radiculopathy.

SHOULDER PAIN

Pain and dysfunction localizing in and around the shoulder girdle are common presenting musculoskeletal complaints. Shoulder pain affects patients of various ages and activity levels. Although shoulder pain can be referred from the neck, chest, or diaphragmatic region, it is most commonly caused by a local process. The shoulder girdle includes three large bones (clavicle, scapula, and humerus) and four joints (sternoclavicular, AC, glenohumeral, and thoracoscapular). The glenohumeral joint is a ball-and-socket joint, like the hip. The two joints differ significantly in that the hip is a more substantial weight-bearing joint and the glenohumeral is a very shallow joint, maximizing mobility. The two chief presenting complaints are usually related to pain and/or instability. Symptoms of decreased motion, power, or function can accompany complaints of pain or instability, but they are rarely the chief complaints.

Common conditions affecting the shoulder include acute injuries, including fractures, dislocations, and acute tendon rupture; chronic or repetitive injuries include impingement syndromes, chronic rotator cuff tears, degenerative joint disease, inflammatory conditions, or idiopathic pathology. Although there have been many technological advances in diagnostic aids, most shoulder disorders can be diagnosed with careful history, clinical examination, and plain radiographs.

When obtaining the history of present illness, the practitioner should ask about the precipitating injury and onset of pain, the location of pain, and the factors that aggravate or alleviate it. The relationship of the pain to the time of day, active or passive movement, and body position is significant. The patient's age, occupation, activities, medical history, and social factors may also be important in making a diagnosis. Patients with acute symptoms usually have an injury, such as a fracture, dislocation, or rotator cuff tear. For patients with chronic shoulder pain, activities related to the onset of symptoms may be useful to the diagnosis.

Instability, another common complaint, occurs most frequently in younger adults and can be classified by the frequency of symptomatic episodes, as well as the direction and degree of instability:

- Frequency: acute injuries may be a first-time dislocation or a recurrent episode.
- Degree: partial (subluxation) with spontaneous reduction or complete (dislocation).
- Location: anterior, posterior, inferior, or multidirectional. Most traumatic dislocations are anterior. Multidirectional instability should be considered in patients who present with recurrent episodes of subluxations or dislocations and no history of significant trauma.

The physical examination of the shoulder should begin with inspection of the shoulder for swelling, color, edema, and symmetry. The shoulder should be inspected anteriorly and posteriorly, particularly to observe scapular winging. This is followed by palpation for tender areas, crepitus, temperature, and deformity.

Range of motion testing should be performed to assess flexion, extension, adduction, abduction, and internal and external rotation. Both active and passive ROM movements should be tested while comparing the painful shoulder to the unaffected side. It is important to determine whether there is a discrepancy between active and passive ROM. Equal losses of active and passive ROM can be secondary to soft tissue contracture, as in frozen shoulder, or the result of joint incongruity from trauma or arthritis. With a rotator cuff tear, a patient may have diminished active ROM, but passive ROM may remain full but painful.

Pain with abduction from 45 to 120 degrees (painful arc) indicates supraspinatus tendinitis and subacromial bursitis, which are early rotator cuff injuries. Muscle and bursae involvement produces pain only on active motion, whereas pain with passive ROM may involve tendons, bursae, or restricted joint movement and is generally indicative of more pathology. In an acute anterior dislocation, pain is severe, and ROM is limited. The patient will usually hold the arm slightly abducted and externally rotated.

Muscle strength should be assessed and compared with the opposite shoulder. Pain can affect the accuracy of muscle testing. Tears of the rotator cuff or neurological injury can produce weakness. Functional status should also be assessed, although this may be affected by motivation and ability to adapt to impairment. The level of functional disability will depend on the normal intensity of activities that the patient performs. Resistive muscle testing, reflex testing, and an assessment of the neurosensory and neurovascular status complete the examination.

Shoulder pain can be referred at times from other areas of the body. If referred pain is suspected, the clinician should consider evaluating for cardiac, pulmonary, abdominal, neurological, or spinal causes. Pain caused by bony malignancy is usually gnawing, constant, progressively worsening, and unrelated to movement or an injury. The pain may wake the person from sleep at night or not be relieved with rest. Malignant tumor is usually evident by a lytic lesion in the bone on x-ray film.

Plain x-ray films, including the anteroposterior projection (AP) view and an axillary lateral view, are sufficient to reveal most bony pathology including fractures and dislocations. Additional views may include a transthoracic lateral, which images the glenohumeral joint at a 45-degree posterior oblique, or a 60-degree anterior oblique (Y view). A new view—the apical oblique—is suggested to reveal shoulder instability. This view is simple to obtain and painless for the patient.

In addition to the standard x-ray studies, there are other tests used in diagnosing shoulder pain. MRI without contrast is usually sufficient for patients with intractable shoulder pain. For suspected dislocations, MRI, arthrography, and (if nerve involvement is suspected) EMG are indicated. Although the standard x-ray studies will often be normal, they should be done to rule out structural abnormalities, especially if there is history of trauma or if the problem is persistent. C-spine films and chest films may also be necessary if involvement in those areas is suspected. Laboratory studies should be done in accordance with the patient's history and suspected differential diagnoses.

DIFFERENTIAL DIAGNOSIS

A summary of common differential diagnoses for shoulder pain is provided in Differential Diagnosis 53.2. A precise differential diagnosis is often obtained by evaluating the patient's chief complaint in the context of its chronicity and the patient's age. Patients younger than 30 years, for example, commonly present with traumatic injuries or instability such as glenohumeral dislocations

Differential Diagnosis 53.2: Shoulder Pain

Musculoskeletal problems	Adhesive capsulitis (frozen shoulder) Rotator cuff syndrome Impingement Calcific tendinitis Subacromial bursitis Degenerative arthritis: glenohumeral, acromioclavicular
Trauma	Fractures: humerus, clavicle, acromion Acromioclavicular joint sprains Rotator cuff tear Dislocation: glenohumeral Nerve injuries: compression
Neurovascular problems	Reflex sympathetic dystrophy (shoulder–hand syndrome) Thoracic outlet syndrome Cervical root compression Brachial plexus injury
Systemic disease	Inflammatory disease Cancer

and AC joint separation. Impingement syndromes and rotator cuff tears are more commonly seen in middle-aged patients. These must be distinguished from frozen shoulder, which produces a global loss of passive and active ROM. Glenohumeral dislocations are much less common in older patients and must be treated with a high index of suspicion for a concomitant rotator cuff tear. Patients older than 55 years are more likely to have rotator cuff tears or degenerative arthritis. Fractures and dislocations related to falls also occur in this age-group.

ELBOW PAIN

The elbow is comprised of the radius, ulna, and humerus, making the radioulnar, ulnohumeral, and radiocapitellar joints. The motion of the elbow and forearm includes flexion, extension, supination, and pronation. The elbow is generally more stable than the shoulder. Much of the tendinous attachment at the elbow attaches to muscles that move the fingers, hand, and wrist. Because of this, some painful elbow conditions will be exacerbated by moving the fingers, hand, and wrist.

Examination of the elbow begins with inspection for symmetry, deformity, edema, erythema, and ecchymosis. The clinician should take time to palpate skeletal anatomical landmarks of the elbow as well as the ligamentous and tendinous attachments for discomfort. It is not unusual for a student or novice clinician to reference an anatomical chart when performing palpation with any of the body joints. ROM is performed to evaluate symmetry, pain, crepitus, and ease and degree of motion.

The varus and valgus stress test for instability of the collateral ligaments can be performed, similar to stress testing for the knee. The test is performed with the elbow at 20 degrees of flexion. The examiner stabilizes the elbow with one hand, with the other hand holding the wrist, and then applies gentle pressure, attempting to angle the elbow medially (valgus) to stress the medial ligamentous structures. Applying elbow pressure laterally stresses the lateral collateral ligaments of the elbow. If the elbow opens in a direction more than the opposite elbow, the patient may have laxity of the medial or lateral ligamentous structures. Strength should be assessed with resisted motion of flexion and extension of the elbow; resisted supination and pronation of the forearm; and resisted flexion and extension of the wrist. Identify any areas of weakness or increased pain that may correlate with muscle or tendon injury.

DIFFERENTIAL DIAGNOSIS

Elbow pain has a few more common causes. Some differential diagnoses for elbow pain are:

- Olecranon bursitis
- Ulnar nerve compression
- Arthritis
- Medial or lateral epicondylitis
- Biceps tendon rupture
- Fracture
- Medial or lateral ligament injury
- Infection

Elbow complaints in adults frequently occur because of overuse. A commonly seen complaint is lateral epicondylitis. Although this condition is often called "tennis elbow," it frequently occurs in patients who do not play tennis. It is associated with repeated extension of the wrist and pronation and supination of the forearm, particularly against resistance. This occurs in movements such as using hand tools and turning doorknobs. This common complaint is associated with pain in the lateral elbow that radiates into the forearm. There is pain and weakness with gripping objects ("coffee cup" sign). Tenderness is present at, and just distal to, the lateral epicondyle. Wrist extension against resistance produces the increased pain.

Rest, ice, NSAIDs, and physical therapy are generally effective. Corticosteroid injections and wrist splinting may be considered in some cases and have been shown to be effective for short-term relief of lateral epicondylitis. There is some controversy about the long-term benefit of steroid injection in comparison to placebo. Use of a padded elbow strap may ease pain by exerting counterpressure on the soft tissue below the lateral epicondyle, reducing strain at the muscle insertion of the lateral elbow. Physical therapy is more efficacious than steroid injection if symptoms persist longer than 6 weeks. Ergonomic assessment of computer keyboard position or other workstation corrections may be helpful. Surgery is reserved for cases that are refractory to conservative treatment.

Medial epicondylitis is less common and presents as medial elbow pain. This condition is often referred to as "golfer's elbow." It is a result of overuse or strain of the muscle group arising from the medial epicondyle, which is used in wrist flexion. Diagnosis can usually be made via clinical examination; findings include medial elbow pain with resisted wrist flexion, tenderness to palpation at or just distal to the medial epicondyle, and pain with resisted forearm pronation. Treatment is the same as for lateral epicondylitis.

Olecranon bursitis is a common cause of pain and swelling in the posterior aspect of the elbow. This may occur after a direct injury to the elbow, such as a fall, or it can follow prolonged direct pressure. Alternatively, gout, RA, or infection can lead to bursitis. ROM is generally normal, but caution is needed to rule out septic bursitis. Monitor for fever, redness, heat, and warmth at the site. Synovial fluid aspiration can provide evidence of infection. Radiography is indicated if there is suspicion for bone infection.

Empiric treatment with antibiotics is not recommended. If cellulitis, constitutional symptoms, or abrasions are present, aspiration and culture are warranted with possible referral to an orthopedic specialist. If none of these symptoms are present, the bursitis is likely caused by inflammation and can be treated with NSAIDs, ice for 15 to 20 minutes several times a day, and rest. An elbow pad can be used to protect the elbow.

Many elbow conditions are diagnosed with physical examination alone. X-rays or advanced imaging may be indicated, based upon suspected differential diagnoses or identified injury. Laboratory studies may be indicated if suspicions arise for a systemic cause for elbow pain such as infection, gout, or RA.

WRIST AND HAND PAIN

Pain in the wrist and hand can be disabling as it interferes with many activities of daily living (ADLs) and a patient's ability to interact with the surrounding environment. The clinician should examine the hands for inflammation, angulation, or enlargement of the interphalangeal joints of the fingers. Assess the hands and wrists for deformity, nodules, or edema. Symmetry should be assessed with the hands in both the closed and open positions. The clinician should take time to carefully and purposefully palpate the bones of the hand and wrist as well as each of the interphalangeal joints of the fingers when assessing complaints of pain.

ROM of the fingers and wrists should be assessed as follows:

- Have the patient make a fist with the thumb across the knuckles.
- Have the patient extend and widely spread the fingers.
- Have the patient touch each finger with the thumb of the same hand.
- With the palms facing down, deviate the wrist laterally and medially.
- Have the patient flex and extend the wrist.

The aforementioned motions can be done actively to assess for deficit. If a deficit is noted, passive motion can be performed. The same motions can be performed against manual resistance to assess strength. The examination should include a thorough neurovascular assessment.

Allen's test, Phalen's test, the Tinel's test, and/or Finkelstein's test (see Advanced Assessment 53.10) are used to assess the wrist and hand. When assessing and/or treating a patient with an injured hand, the patient should remove all rings as soon as possible. Inflammation secondary to most injuries will precipitate edema, making ring removal difficult. A tight-fitting ring may cause arterial compression and ischemia if not removed. Usually soap or lubricant jelly will be sufficient to remove the ring. If this does not work, other techniques may be used (see Therapeutic Procedure 53.1).

DIFFERENTIAL DIAGNOSIS

Wrist injuries are common after falling on an outstretched hand. Patients present after trauma with pain and swelling in the distal forearm or wrist. Pain, numbness, or tingling may be present if the median or ulnar nerve is affected. The mechanism of injury can often provide important clues to the diagnosis. A radiograph of the wrist (including AP, lateral, and oblique views) may be necessary to rule out a fracture. Common fractures are the Colles fracture of the distal radius and the navicular (scaphoid) fracture of the anatomical snuffbox. It is not unusual to have a navicular fracture missed on radiography. An orthopedic referral should be provided when the presenting complaints are pain and tenderness to palpation at the anatomical snuffbox after a trauma to the wrist.

A common wrist ligament injury is an ulnar collateral ligament tear at the base of the thumb. Often referred to as *gamekeeper's thumb* or *skier's thumb*, this condition is related to chronic repetitive valgus stress or an acute hyperabduction of the metacarpophalangeal joint. Surgery is often necessary to repair a tear in this area; however, in some cases repair can be managed with simple immobilization. Therefore, when the presenting complaints are pain and trauma to the proximal thumb, consideration of an orthopedic referral for further evaluation and stress testing is appropriate even if the x-ray result is negative.

Advanced Assessment 53.10: Tests for Wrist and Hand Problems

Test	Comments
Allen's test	*Purpose:* Assesses patency of radial and ulnar arteries and the arterial arch. *Procedure:* Compress the radial and ulnar arteries at the wrist with examiner's fingers. Have patient rapidly open and close their hand several times, and then have the patient open the hand. Hand should be pale or white. Release pressure from one artery. The hand should flush, indicating patency. Perform again, releasing pressure from the opposite artery.
Phalen's test	*Purpose:* Assesses for median nerve compression. *Procedure:* Have the patient maintain forced flexion of the wrist for 1 minute or more, with the dorsal surface of each hand pressed together. If the patient complains of pain, numbness, or paresthesias in fingers, the test is considered positive.
Tinel's test	*Purpose:* Assesses for median nerve compression. *Procedure:* Percuss the median nerve at the wrist over the carpal tunnel. If the patient complains of pain, numbness, or tingling in the digits, the test is considered positive.
Finkelstein's test	*Purpose:* Assesses for de Quervain's disease. *Procedure:* Have patient place thumb across the palm and make a fist with fingers over the thumb. Test is positive if moving the wrist into ulnar deviation causes pain at the radial border of the wrist.

HIP PAIN

Hip pain is characterized by discomfort deep within or around the hip. The hip joint, or femoroacetabular joint, is the largest joint in the body and is subject to stress from ambulation and weight-bearing. It may suffer injury from trauma or chronic mechanical stress. Pain in and around the hip can often be felt in the groin or the buttock. It can also be referred to the thigh or knee. Conversely, pain may be referred to the hip if irritation to the femoral, sciatic, or obturator nerve roots occurs. This pain may be the result of herniation of a lumbar disc, spinal stenosis, retroperitoneal tumor, or femoral hernia.

The history should ascertain if the pain is focal, as with bursitis, or diffuse, as with synovitis. The presence

Therapeutic Procedure 53.1: Removing Rings

	STRING TECHNIQUE
Equipment: 2–0 or 3–0 nylon suture (string technique), rubber tourniquet (tourniquet technique), lubricant (tourniquet technique), mechanical ring cutter (ring cutter technique)	1. In a distal direction, wrap 2–0 or 3–0 nylon suture tightly around the finger just distal to the ring. 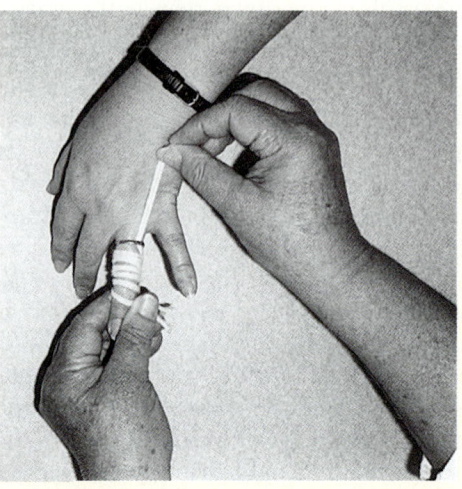 2. Slip the proximal end of the string under the ring. 3. Pull the proximal end of the suture over the ring and firmly retract it distally over the axis of the finger. As each coil of the suture unwinds, it pulls the ring slightly over the coiled suture until it is free. 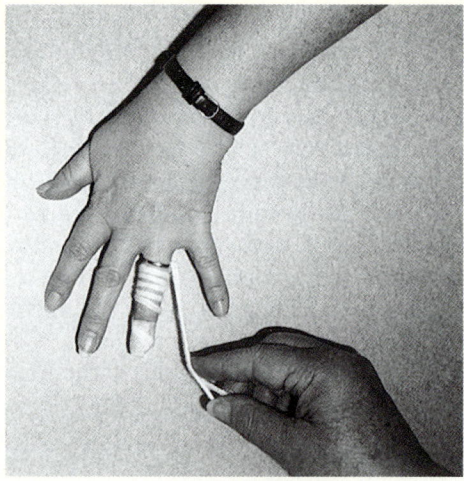
TOURNIQUET TECHNIQUE	**MECHANICAL RING CUTTER TECHNIQUE**
1. Carefully wrap the finger with a rubber tourniquet, starting at the fingertip and working up to the edge of the ring.	1. Advise patient that the ring will be cut and obtain their consent.
2. Have the patient lie supine on the examination table, with the arm pointed straight upward at the ceiling for about 5 minutes. 3. As soon as the patient lowers the arm, remove the tourniquet, apply copious amounts of lubricant, and slide the ring off.	2. Follow the manufacturer's directions. Postprocedure: Give ring to patient, or secure as per institution policy and document.

of stiffness should raise the suspicion of degenerative disease. Inquire about trauma, involvement of other joints, infection, fever, and relation of pain to activity.

Physical examination of the hip must first assess position at rest, especially if there has been an injury. A fracture of the femoral head results in external rotation and flexion, and an internally rotated shortened leg may be a posterior dislocation. These patients should not have the hip manipulated until radiographic studies have ruled out fracture or dislocation. Performing palpation of the joint allows recognition of focal tenderness and swelling. The clinician should palpate anterior, lateral and posterior over the muscle, bone, ligaments, joints, lymph nodes, and blood vessels. Attempt to identify any specific areas of pain or enlarged lymph nodes.

The ROM examination begins with assessment of gait, if possible. Next, the extremity should be put through passive ROM testing to detect crepitus, pain, limitation of movement, muscle spasm, flexion contracture, or guarding. Flexion and extension need to be performed with the knee straight as well as flexed. Abduction, adduction, and internal and external rotation are assessed. Femoral and pedal pulses (posterior tibial, dorsalis pedis) should be palpated for strength. Auscultate the femoral pulse as indicated for bruits. Neurological testing for sensation and deep tendon reflexes concludes the general examination.

DIFFERENTIAL DIAGNOSIS

Possible causes for hip pain include pathology in the hip joint, the surrounding muscles, the soft tissues, or the neurovascular structures. Consider the patient's age when formulating differential diagnoses because certain problems are more prevalent in different age-groups. In adults, common problems include OA, RA, fractures, referred pain, bursitis, and avascular necrosis. Cancer is a possible differential diagnosis with hip pain. Initially, no signs may be present with malignancy; however, tenderness and palpable swelling may develop later over bony prominences. Intractable pain that is not improved with rest and possibly wakes the patient from sleep, systemic symptoms, and pathological fractures may eventually occur.

The location of the patient's pain can give valuable clues about the etiology. If the patient's pain is located in the groin or inguinal fold, intra-articular hip pathology such as osteoarthritis should be considered in the evaluation. If the patient's pain is along the anterior or lateral hip and thigh, radicular lower back pain is a possibility. Trochanteric bursitis, now referred to as *greater trochanteric pain syndrome*, may be considered if the pain is more localized over the posterior lateral hip. If the patient's pain is posterior, radicular lower back pain or muscle strain (gluteus, proximal hamstring) is a possible diagnosis. Vascular insufficiency of the aortoiliac area may result in hip and buttock pain as well. Avascular necrosis appears as abrupt hip pain followed by progressive, intermittent episodes. Pain is worsened with motion and activity and often is worse at night. A limp, along with limited abduction and internal rotation, is present. Some avascular necrosis can be seen on x-ray; MRI is the gold standard test needed for diagnosis; and an orthopedic referral is indicated. Avascular necrosi often occurs as a serious complication of hip trauma, but it may occur unrelated to trauma. It can be related to alcohol use disorder, chronic prednisone use, or as a side effect of HIV medication management.

Diagnostic testing should include hip x-ray films. Other x-ray studies, such as spine or sacroiliac films or weight-bearing films, may be indicated in special circumstances. MRI, CT, ultrasonography, and joint aspiration are other diagnostic techniques to be considered, depending on the history, physical examination, and differential diagnoses.

KNEE PAIN

The knee joint is a complex, modified hinge joint consisting of three bones, three articulations, five major tendons, four major ligaments, and two menisci. The lateral and medial articulations are between the femoral and tibial condyles. The femoral condyles and the tibial plateaus are capped anteriorly by the patella and cushioned by the menisci, whereas the ligaments, muscles, tendons, and bursae provide stability. The intermediate articulation exists between the patella and the femur. The knee is a relatively weak joint that gains its strength from the strong ligaments that attach the femur to the tibia. There are five intrinsic ligaments that assist in strengthening the articular capsule. The cruciate ligaments connect the femur and tibia within the articular capsule, crossing each other in the form of an X.

The arrangement of the articulations allows a combination of rolling, gliding, and rotation, in addition to flexion and extension. Although it is attached to the lateral tibia, the fibula does not articulate with the knee joint. As a major weight-bearing joint, the knee is susceptible to many injuries. Torsion is limited in the joint, and any motion that extends beyond the defined range results in a ligamentous injury. Because the knee joint depends on the integrity of the ligaments to provide stability, an injury to the knee ligaments may result in disability.

DIFFERENTIAL DIAGNOSIS

The knee joint is a common site for discomfort due to injury and trauma, degenerative disease, or rheumatological conditions. Acute pain in the knee may be related to any of the following:

- Fractures
- Meniscal injuries

- Ligamentous injuries
- Musculotendinous strains
- Extensor mechanism injuries
- Contusions
- Dislocation
- Infection

Many knee complaints in adults are the result of overzealous exercise and sports activity. Obtaining a history of the mechanism of injury is key in diagnosing many knee conditions. A history of a twisting injury sustained with the foot planted on the ground and clicking or joint locking (inability to extend the knee completely) along with localized pain and tenderness along the joint space are characteristic of meniscal pathology. Some patients report that manipulating or pushing on the knee enabled them to "unlock" the knee if they experienced locking. The patient should be asked if they heard or felt a "pop" when the injury occurred. A loud pop during activity and sudden pain can accompany an acute ligament injury. Investigate actual or perceived knee instability that may accompany subluxation, effusion, or ligament instability.

Fractures can affect any portion of the knee's bony anatomy. Fractures may present with pain, swelling, and deformity after an injury. Palpate for point tenderness of the bone itself, and obtain appropriate radiographs as indicated. Patellar fractures can occur after a direct injury or rapid deceleration after running. A major trauma is usually the cause for fractures of the tibia and femur. Dislocations of the patella frequently reduce themselves after an injury when the knee is extended by the patient or an assistant.

Patients with ligamentous injuries have acute pain, swelling, and possible instability. Strains of various musculotendinous structures around the knee also cause acute pain and swelling, but most do not result in instability. An injury to the extensor mechanism may result in sudden weakness or collapse of the knee, causing the patient to fall. Such injuries also leave the patient unable to straighten their knee. Direct blows to the knee can result in a contusion, causing localized pain, edema, ecchymosis, and tenderness.

Chronic knee pain can result from an injury that did not fully heal. This can also result from noninjury–related pathology or degeneration. Some conditions that cause chronic knee pain include the following:

- Arthritis
- Tumors
- Sepsis
- Cartilage or meniscus injuries
- Overuse injuries

Patellofemoral dysfunction, which is an overuse syndrome, encompasses a continuum of disorders, including chondromalacia patellae and patellofemoral arthralgia. Pain typically occurs when climbing stairs or when standing up after a period of sitting. Pain is often reproduced by placing direct pressure on the patella, pushing it against the femur, when the patient is supine with knee extended. X-ray imaging may reveal irregularity of the patella undersurface. Management is conservative including NSAIDs, possible use of a neoprene knee sleeve, and quadriceps-strengthening exercises.

Tumors are often characterized by night pain and often can be palpated or identified on radiograph. Sepsis arthritis of the knee joint manifests as joint pain, decreased motion, swelling, warmth on palpation, erythema, and edema. The patient may have systemic symptoms of fever and chills. Patellofemoral syndromes, tendonitis, bursitis, and articular cartilage injuries are frequently bilateral, chronic, and due to overuse. Walking after being seated for a while and changing position from seated to standing can both lead to increased pain.

Physical examination of the knee can begin with an inspection of the patient's knees bilaterally while standing. Inspect medial, lateral, anterior, and posterior, looking for symmetry and evidence of edema, ecchymosis, erythema, deformity, abrasions, skin lesions, and changes in the color of the skin. Assess the popliteal space for swelling that may occur with popliteal aneurysm, Baker's cyst, and tumors. A popliteal artery aneurysm will likely feel pulsatile. It is important to assess motion in both the standing and seated or supine positions. Note any altered gait, pain, locking, or giving way of the knee. As the patient lies supine or is seated on the examination table, palpate the joint line, muscles, tendons, ligaments, and bones to localize tenderness.

An effusion may be identified with a bulge sign. With the patient lying supine, massage the medial knee toward the head, and then stroke the lateral aspect of the knee toward the medial aspect. A bulge sign or effusion is indicated if fluctuance (or bulging) occurs over the medial aspect. Palpate for crepitus while the knee is passively flexed and extended. Meniscal injury may be accompanied by pain with palpation of the medial or lateral joint line. Muscle testing of the quadriceps and hamstrings should be performed.

A complete physical examination may be indicated if systemic disease, associated with knee pathology, is suspected. Many specialized assessment techniques can be used to evaluate the knee. Most are specific and technique driven, requiring practice to master them. The Lachman test should be done on most patients with knee pain; it is 94% specific and is helpful in diagnosing ACL injury. The McMurray and Apley tests are indicated in diagnosing meniscal tears. The anterior drawer test has a low sensitivity and high specificity for confirming ACL pathology, so a positive test strongly suggests a problem, but a negative test does not rule out an ACL tear. The posterior drawer test is used to diagnose posterior cruciate ligament injury. The collateral ligament stress test, also known as the *valgus* and *varus* stress tests, evaluates the integrity of the medial collateral ligament (MCL) and the lateral collateral ligament (LCL), respectively. The

Fairbanks test, also known as the *patellar apprehension test,* can identify recent dislocation or instability of the patella (see Advanced Assessments 53.11 and 53.4).

Diagnostic testing includes the use of radiographs if mechanical injury or trauma is suspected. Specific weight-bearing views and sunrise or skyline views can be performed. MRI is helpful in diagnosing a soft tissue pathology such as a torn meniscus or cruciate ligament injury.

ANKLE PAIN

Most ankle pain is the result of ankle injury that results in ligamental damage (a sprain) (see earlier section *Ankle Sprain p. 866*). A sprain occurs at the ankle when the ligaments are overstretched, and injury results. Repeated ankle sprains may result in chronic tendon laxity (see Advanced Assessment 53.3). Ankle pain may be referred pain secondary to disc herniation at the level of L5 to S1. Signs and symptoms include a sensory deficit over the malleolus, weak eversion, and a decreased Achilles reflex.

DIFFERENTIAL DIAGNOSIS

In addition to sprains, ankle pain has several differential diagnoses. Nerve entrapment may occur secondary to ankle fracture, dislocation, or traction injury. If the tibial nerve is affected, there would be a loss of ankle plantar flexion, toe flexion, and weak ankle inversion.

Posterior impingement syndrome is commonly seen in ballet dancers. It manifests with pain and swelling of the posterior ankle and worsens with plantar flexion or dorsiflexion of the great toe. A lateral ankle x-ray may reveal a finding of os trigonum.

Peroneal tendon subluxation may occur secondary to trauma; it will present with lateral pain and a "snapping" over the posterior distal fibula. Pain will increase with active eversion of the dorsiflexed foot, and there may be palpable/visible movement of tendons. Tibial tendon dysfunction may be a cause of medial ankle pain.

Achilles tendon rupture causes significant pain and difficulty weight-bearing. Closed tendon ruptures usually result when a sudden excessive load is applied to the musculotendinous unit with failure occurring at either the tendon's substance (torn fibers) or its insertion into the bone. A tendon rupture can occasionally occur spontaneously in healthy individuals from relatively minor trauma. Achilles tendon rupture is also a potential side effect of fluoroquinolones. Physical examination will usually reveal swelling, tenderness, and bruising over the rupture. Palpation over the tendon may reveal a gap where the tendon is ruptured. The tendon's continuity can be tested by performing the Thompson's test. To do this, have the patient (1) lie prone, (2) bend the knee to 90 degrees, and (3) squeeze the calf. The test is positive if squeezing the calf does not produce plantar flexion of the ankle, indicating a complete rupture of the tendon. A patient can have a partially torn Achilles tendon but a negative Thompson test because some tendon fibers remain intact. Treatment is either surgical repair or immobilization in a cast with the ankle plantar flexed for several weeks.

Advanced Assessment 53.11: Assessing the Meniscus and the Patella—Special Tests

Test	Comments
McMurray circumduction test—to test for meniscal tear	Flex the knee to the maximum pain-free position. Hold that position while externally rotating the lower leg, and then gradually extend the knee while placing slight valgus pressure on knee. Maintain the tibia in external rotation during the maneuver. This maneuver stresses the medial meniscus and elicits a click and/or pain medially at the knee with a meniscus tear. The same maneuver is performed while rotating the lower leg internally and placing varus pressure on the knee. This will stress the lateral meniscus. Pain-free flexion beyond 90 degrees is necessary for this test to be useful.
Apprehension sign—to test patellar instability	Have the patient supine with the quadriceps relaxed. The knee is extended with 30 degrees of flexion. Displace the patella laterally and then medially. With instability, this maneuver excessively displaces the patella to an abnormal position on the lateral femoral condyle. The patient may perceive pain and become apprehensive.
Bulge sign—to assess for effusion	Apply lateral pressure to the area adjacent to the patella. Medial bulge will appear if fluid is in the knee joint.
Ballottement test—to assess for effusion	First, inspect the suprapatellar region. A large knee effusion may be visible. Subtle knee effusions can be demonstrated by "milking down" the joint fluid from the suprapatellar pouch. Hold the fluid in place with one hand by placing one hand flat above the patella and ballot (or press down vertically) the patella. Excessive fluid will create a spongy feeling as the patella is pushed down.

FOOT PAIN

Foot pain is a common problem among adults. The foot contains 26 bones, 33 joints, and more than 100 ligaments. Foot pain is frequently related to inflammation after trauma, an overuse injury, a deformity, or ill-fitting shoes. The feet are subjected to numerous forces: for example, when an individual is standing, forces exerted on the foot are equivalent to four times the individual's body weight. Any alteration in ability to use the feet for any reason, such as pain secondary to hammertoe or corns and calluses, will have a significant effect on the health and well-being of the patient. Acute pain should prompt the clinician to consider infection, sprain, or fracture. A stress fracture of the foot commonly presents with second and third distal metatarsal pain. Acute foot pain is less common than chronic pain. A patient with bilateral foot pain can potentially have a systemic illness, such as vascular disease or diabetes, causing the symptoms.

General treatment measures for foot pain include the use of footwear with roomy toes, supportive arches, and low heels. Heel lifts, cushioned inner soles, and arch supports can provide significant relief when used appropriately. Referral to a podiatrist or foot and ankle surgeon may be necessary.

DIFFERENTIAL DIAGNOSIS

Differential Diagnosis 53.3 presents common differential diagnoses for foot pain and their treatment.

Forefoot Problems

Common problems in the forefoot are calluses, corns, plantar warts, bunions, neuromas, and stress fractures. The history of patients with calluses, corns, and warts would reveal discomfort related to pressure, whereas stress fractures have an acute onset of pain frequently at the second

Differential Diagnosis 53.3: Foot Pain

Differential Diagnosis	Management
Forefoot	
Hallux valgus or bunion	Avoid pressure on the tender bunion; use NSAIDs; use protective pads, orthotic devices, appropriate footwear with roomy forefoot; if no relief, consider surgical consultation
Corns and calluses with keratinized skin	Moleskin protection; gentle rubbing with pumice or shaving lesion; separating toes with cushions or orthotics; if unrelieved, consider surgical consultation
Sesamoiditis of the first metatarsophalangeal joint	Protect the injured part by limiting weight-bearing, wearing protective padding or taping, and avoiding high-heeled shoes; use NSAIDs.
Neuromas	Shoe modification: wide toe box, metatarsal bar, and soft inner soles; NSAIDs; and in severe cases, corticosteroid injections to reduce inflammation
Stress fractures	Rest and efforts to disperse weight-bearing away from the fracture such as stiff-soled shoe, metatarsal bar, walking cast
Infection	Treatment with appropriate antibiotic therapy
Peripheral neuritis	Investigate pathology; treatment depends on underlying cause.
Midfoot	
Pes planus	No treatment if asymptomatic; if symptomatic: flexible arch support or custom orthotics, heel-cord stretching, and toe exercises such as picking up objects with toes and spreading toes
Hindfoot	
Achilles tendinitis	Initial treatment: rest, ice, use of NSAIDs, and heel lifts. Heel-cord stretching exercises. Immobilization for persistent or severe pain. Corticosteroids are contraindicated.
Plantar fasciitis	Heel lifts, padded heel cups, and orthotic devices. Acute treatment is rest, ice, NSAIDs, and local corticosteroid injections. Heel-cord stretching exercises and use of a nighttime dorsal splint to maintain ankle dorsiflexion and toe extension may be beneficial; surgical release of the plantar fascia is the measure of last resort.

or third metatarsal heads. The hyperkeratotic lesions of calluses and corns may be indistinguishable from each other, but plantar warts can be distinguished by the punctate bleeding associated with the wart. Physical examination findings in patients with stress fractures include point tenderness and swelling over the involved bone. An interdigital neuroma causes pain and numbness in the third and fourth intermetatarsal spaces with radiation into the toes. Interdigital neuromas may be accompanied by a tender nodule in the intermetatarsal space. A bunion or hallux valgus is a deformity of the first metatarsophalangeal joint associated with the lateral angulation of the toe. This presents as a painful swelling on the dorsomedial aspect of the first metatarsal head. Foot–shoe incompatibility may produce toe deformities such as hammertoe or mallet toe.

Midfoot Problems

A common midfoot problem is pes planus (flat foot). This is likely to produce pain and stiffness in the midfoot region, often associated with degenerative arthritis or laxity of the posterior tibial tendon. Tenderness to palpation usually occurs along the medial plantar border of the sole with flat foot. Flattening of the medial longitudinal arch of the foot and often a valgus deflection of the heel are indicative of this condition. Another midfoot condition involves fibromas of the plantar fascia at the undersurface of the foot. This may cause discomfort to the undersurface of the midfoot.

Hindfoot Problems

Common hindfoot conditions include plantar fasciitis, infracalcaneal bursitis, and posterior heel problems such as Achilles tendinitis and posterior bursitis. The history of individuals with plantar fasciitis includes subcalcaneal pain. This can often radiate to the arch of the midfoot while the person is running, walking, or even simply standing. The pain is often worse in the morning with the first step out of bed. Plantar fasciitis findings typically include tenderness along the medial plantar aspect of the calcaneus, with forced dorsiflexion of the digits increasing the pain. Infracalcaneal bursitis produces an aching sensation at the plantar surface of the calcaneus that becomes worse the longer the heel is bearing weight. The pain associated with Achilles tendinitis is at or proximal to the insertion of the Achilles tendon onto the calcaneus. In this condition, the physical examination reveals swelling, pain with palpation, and erythema. The pain is increased with dorsiflexion of the ankle, and crepitus may be palpated.

REFERENCES

General

Armstrong AD, Hubbard MC, eds. *Essentials of musculoskeletal care.* Enhanced 5th ed. Rosemont, IL: American Academy of Orthopedic Surgeons. Surgeons; 2018.

Kliegman RM, St. Geme JW, Blum NJ, et al., eds. *Nelson textbook of pediatrics.* 21st ed. Philadelphia, PA: Elsevier; 2020.

Miller MD, Thompson SR, eds. *DeLee, Drez, & Miller's orthopaedic sports medicine: Principles and practice.* 5th ed. Philadelphia, PA: Elsevier; 2020.

Acute Musculoskeletal Injuries

Aicale R, Tarantino D, Maffulli N. Overuse injuries in sport: a comprehensive overview. *J Orthop Surg Res.* 2018;13(1):309. https://doi.org/10.1186/s13018-018-1017-5

Arnold MJ, Moody AL. Common running injuries: evaluation and management. *Am Fam Physician.* 2018;97(8):510–516.

Berry SD, Kiel DP, Colón-Emeric C. Hip fractures in older adults in 2019. *JAMA.* 2019;321(22):2231–2232. https://doi.org/10.1001/jama.2019.5453

Bhandari M, Swiontkowski M. Management of acute hip fracture. *N Engl J Med.* 2017;377(21):2053–2062. https://doi.org/10.1056/NEJMcp1611090

Chen ET, Borg-Stein J, McInnis KC. Ankle sprains: evaluation, rehabilitation, and prevention. *Curr Sports Med Rep.* 2019;18(6):217–223. https://doi.org/10.1249/JSR.0000000000000603

Leggit JC. Sports medicine: fractures, sprains, and other musculoskeletal injuries. *FP Essent.* 2019;482:23–26.

Mauck BM, Swigler CW. Evidence-based review of distal radius fractures. *Orthop Clin North Am.* 2018;49(2):211–222. https://doi.org/10.1016/j.ocl.2017.12.001

Peterson AR, Moreno MA. Ankle sprains in youth. *JAMA Pediatrics.* 2018;172(11):1108. https://doi.org/10.1001/jamapediatrics.2018.2948

Vuurberg G, Hoorntje A, Wink LM, et al. Diagnosis, treatment, and prevention of ankle sprains: Update of an evidence-based clinical guideline. *British Journal of Sports Medicine.* 2018;52(15):956. https://doi.org/10.1136/bjsports-2017-098106

Ankle Pain

Gribble PA. Evaluating and differentiating ankle instability. *Journal of Athletic Training.* 2019;54(6):617–627. https://doi.org/10.4085/1062-6050-484-17

Lau BC, Moore LK, Thuillier DU. Evaluation and management of lateral ankle pain following injury. *JBJS Reviews.* 2018;6(8):e7. https://doi.org/10.2106/JBJS.RVW.17.00143

Murphy J, Weiner DA, Kotler J, et al. Utility of Ottawa Ankle Rules in an aging population: evidence for addition of an age criterion. *The Journal of Foot and Ankle Surgery: Official Publication of the American College of Foot and Ankle Surgeons.* 2020;59(2):286–290. https://doi.org/10.1053/j.jfas.2019.04.017

Nicolette GW, Edenfield KM, Michaudet C, et al. Foot and ankle conditions: chronic lateral ankle pain. *FP Essent.* 2018;465:24–29.

Papaliodis DN, Vanushkina MA, Richardson NG, et al. The foot and ankle examination. *The Medical Clinics of North America.* 2014;98(2):181–204. https://doi.org/10.1016/j.mcna.2013.10.001

Unruh L, Palter J, Dyer S. Adolescent with ankle pain. *Annals of Emergency Medicine.* 2020;76(3):301–338. https://doi.org/10.1016/j.annemergmed.2020.03.001

Xu A, Giunta Y, Jadav S, et al. Young female with ankle pain. *Annals of Emergency Medicine.* 2020;76(4):392–412. https://doi.org/10.1016/j.annemergmed.2020.04.011

Back Pain

Achar S, Yamanaka J. (2020). Back pain in children and adolescents. *American Family Physician.* 102(1):19–28.

Busse JW, Sadeghirad B, Oparin Y, et al. (2020). Management of acute pain from nonlow back, musculoskeletal injuries: a systematic review and network meta-analysis of randomized trials. *Annals of Internal Medicine.* 173(9):730–738. https://doi.org/10.7326/M19-3601

Koumtouzoua S, Higgins S. (2021). Evaluating and managing the patient with back pain. *The Medical Clinics of North America.* 105(1):1–17. https://doi.org/10.1016/j.mcna.2020.08.014

Pakpoor J, Raad M, Harris A, et al. (2020). Use of imaging during emergency department visits for low back pain. *AJR. American Journal of Roentgenology.* 214(2):395–399. https://doi.org/10.2214/AJR.19.21674

Popescu A, Lee H. (2020). Neck pain and lower back pain. *The Medical Clinics of North America.* 104(2):279–292. https://doi.org/10.1016/j.mcna.2019.11.003

Qaseem A, McLean RM, O'Gurek D, et al. (2020). Nonpharmacologic and pharmacological management of acute pain from non-low back, musculoskeletal injuries in adults: a clinical guideline from the American College of Physicians and American Academy of Family Physicians. *Annals of Internal Medicine.* 173(9):739–748. https://doi.org/10.7326/M19-3602

Elbow, Wrist, and Hand Pain

Alrabaa RG, Dantzker N, Ahmad CS. (2020). Injuries and conditions affecting the elbow flexor/pronator tendons. *Clinics in Sports Medicine.* 39(3):549–563. doi: 10.1016/j.csm.2020.02.001.

Chin TY, Chou H, Peh W. (2019). The acutely injured elbow. *Radiologic Clinics of North America.* 57(5):911–930. https://www.radiologic.theclinics.com/article/S0033-8389(19)30051-X/fulltext

Hanlon DP, Mavrophilipos V. (2020). The emergent evaluation and treatment of elbow and forearm injuries. *Emergency Medicine Clinics of North America.* 38(1):81–102. https://doi.org/10.1016/j.emc.2019.09.005

Leow M, Teo W, Low TL, et al. (2019). Hand assessment for elderly people in the community. Orthopedic Nursing, 38(1):25–30. https://doi.org/10.1097/NOR.0000000000000515

Patrick NC, Hammert WC. (2020). Hand and wrist tendinopathies. Clinics in Sports Medicine, 39(2):247–258. doi: 10.1016/j.csm.2019.10.004

Sanderson M, Mohr B, Abraham MK. (2020). The emergent evaluation and treatment of hand and wrist injuries: An update. *Emergency Medicine Clinics of North America.* 38(1):61–79. https://doi.org/10.1016/j.emc.2019.09.004

Schickendantz MS, Yalcin S. (2020). Conditions and injuries affecting the nerves around the elbow. *Clinics in Sports Medicine.* 39(3):597–621. doi: 10.1016/j.csm.2020.02.006

Sharawat IK, Panda PK, Bolia RK, et al. (2020). Slowly progressive elbow swelling. *The Journal of Pediatrics.* 220:262–263. https://doi.org/10.1016/j.jpeds.2019.12.043

Wagner ER, Gottschalk MB. (2019). Tendinopathies of the forearm, wrist, and hand. Clinics in Plastic Surgery, 46(3):317–327. https://doi.org/10.1016/j.cps.2019.02.005

Young AL. (2018). Common conditions of the hand for the nurse practitioner: how to diagnose, how to manage, and when to refer to a hand surgeon. *Plastic Surgical Nursing: Official Journal of the American Society of Plastic and Reconstructive Surgical Nurses.* 38(1):34–37. https://doi.org/10.1097/PSN.0000000000000212

Foot Pain

Charen DA, Markowitz JS, Cheung ZB, et al. (2019). *Overview of metatarsalgia. Orthopedics.* 42(1):e138–e143. https://doi.org/10.3928/01477447-20181206-06

Del Toro D, Nelson PA. (2018). Guiding treatment for foot pain. *Physical Medicine and Rehabilitation Clinics of North America.* 29(4):783–792. https://doi.org/10.1016/j.pmr.2018.06.012

Hogan KK, Prince JA, Hoch MC. (2020). The evaluation of the foot core system in individuals with plantar heel pain. *Physical Therapy in Sport: Official Journal of the Association of Chartered Physiotherapists in Sports Medicine.* 42, 75–81. https://doi.org/10.1016/j.ptsp.2019.11.011

Oh-Park M, Kirschner J, Abdelshahed D, et al. (2019). Painful foot disorders in the geriatric population: a narrative review. *American Journal of Physical Medicine & Rehabilitation.* 98(9):811–819. https://doi.org/10.1097/PHM.0000000000001239

Pelly T, Holme T, Tahir MA, et al. (2020). Forefoot pain. *BMJ (Clinical research ed.).* 371, m3704. https://doi.org/10.1136/bmj.m3704

Tu P. (2018). Heel pain: diagnosis and management. *American Family Physician.* 97(2):86–93.

Hip

Gómez-Hoyos J, Martin RL, Martin HD. (2018). Current concepts review: evaluation and management of posterior hip pain. *The Journal of the American Academy of Orthopaedic Surgeons.* 26(17):597–609. https://doi.org/10.5435/JAAOS-D-15-00629

Karkenny AJ, Tauberg BM, Otsuka NY. (2018). Pediatric hip disorders: slipped capital femoral epiphysis and Legg-Calvé-Perthes disease. *Pediatrics in Review.* 39(9):454–463. https://doi.org/10.1542/pir.2017-0197

LaPorte C, Vasaris M, Gossett L, et al. (2019). Gluteus medius tears of the hip: a comprehensive approach. *The Physician and Sports Medicine.* 47(1):15–20. https://doi.org/10.1080/00913847.2018.1527172

Lynch TS, Bedi A, Larson CM. (2017). Athletic hip injuries. *The Journal of the American Academy of Orthopaedic Surgeons.* 25(4):269–279. https://doi.org/10.5435/JAAOS-D-16-00171

Nakano N, Yip G, Khanduja V. (2017). Current concepts in the diagnosis and management of extra-articular hip impingement syndromes. *International Orthopaedics.* 41(7):1321–1328. https://doi.org/10.1007/s00264-017-3431-4

Saltychev M, Pernaa K, Seppänen M, et al. (2018). Pelvic incidence and hip disorders. *Acta Orthopaedica.* 89(1):66–70. https://doi.org/10.1080/17453674.2017.1377017

Speers CJB, Bhogal GS. (2017). Greater trochanteric pain syndrome: a review of diagnosis and management in general practice. *The British Journal of General Practice: The Journal of the Royal College of General Practitioners.* 67(663):479–480. https://doi.org/10.3399/bjgp17X693041

Zuckerbraun BS, Cyr AR, Mauro CS. (2020). Groin pain syndrome known as sports hernia: a review. *JAMA Surgery.* 155(4):340–348. https://doi.org/10.1001/jamasurg.2019.5863

Knee Pain

Bunt CW, Jonas CE, Chang JG. (2018). Knee pain in adults and adolescents: the initial evaluation. *American Family Physician.* 98(9):576–585.

Burnett WD, Kontulainen SA, McLennan CE, et al. Knee osteoarthritis patients with more subchondral cysts have altered tibial subchondral bone mineral density. *BMC Musculoskeletal*

Disorders. 2019 Jan 5;20(1):14. doi: 10.1186/s12891-018-2388-9. PMID: 30611224; PMCID: PMC6320646.

Chughtai M, Newman JM, Akil S, et al. (2018). Knee pain and the use of various types of footwear—a review. *The Journal of Knee Surgery*, 31(10):952–964. https://doi.org/10.1055/s-0038-1626735

Davenport M, Oczypok MP. (2020). Knee and leg injuries. *Emergency Medicine Clinics of North America.* 38(1):143–165. https://doi.org/10.1016/j.emc.2019.09.012

de Oliveira Silva D, Pazzinatto MF, Priore L, et al. (2018). Knee crepitus is prevalent in women with patellofemoral pain, but is not related with function, physical activity and pain. *Physical Therapy in Sport: Official Journal of the Association of Chartered Physiotherapists in Sports Medicine.* 33:7–11. https://doi.org/10.1016/j.ptsp.2018.06.002

Flores DV, Mejía Gómez C, Pathria MN. (2018). Layered approach to the anterior knee: normal anatomy and disorders associated with anterior knee pain. *Radiographics: A Review Publication of the Radiological Society of North America, Inc.* 38(7), 2069–2101. https://doi.org/10.1148/rg.2018180048

Marriott C, George C. (2018). Knee pain in an athletic young man. *BMJ (Clinical research ed.).* 362, k3355. https://doi.org/10.1136/bmj.k3355

Roger C, Gouron R, Klein C. (2020). Chronic anterior knee pain. *The Journal of Family Practice.* 69(2):E7–E9.

Slotkin S, Thome A, Ricketts C, et al. (2018). Anterior knee pain in children and adolescents: overview and management. *The Journal of Knee Surgery*, 31(5):392–398. https://doi.org/10.1055/s-0038-1632376

Muscle Cramps

Eichner ER. (2018). Muscle cramping in the heat. *Current sports medicine reports.* 17(11):356–357. https://doi.org/10.1249/JSR.0000000000000529

Gauer R, Meyers BK. (2019). Heat-related illnesses. *American Family Physician.* 99(8):482–489.

Giuriato G, Pedrinolla A, Schena F, et al. (2018). Muscle cramps: a comparison of the two-leading hypothesis. *Journal of Electromyography and Kinesiology: Official Journal of the International Society of Electrophysiological Kinesiology.* 41, 89–95. https://doi.org/10.1016/j.jelekin.2018.05.006

Katzberg HD. (2020). Case studies in management of muscle cramps. *Neurological Clinics.* 38(3):679–696. https://doi.org/10.1016/j.ncl.2020.03.011

Maughan RJ, Shirreffs SM. (2019). Muscle cramping during exercise: causes, solutions, and questions remaining. *Sports Medicine (Auckland, N.Z.).* 49(Suppl 2):115–124. https://doi.org/10.1007/s40279-019-01162-1

Swash M, Czesnik D, de Carvalho M. (2019). Muscular cramp: causes and management. *European Journal of Neurology.* 26(2):214–221. https://doi.org/10.1111/ene.13799

Myofascial Pain

Barbero M, Schneebeli A, Koetsier E, et al. (2019). Myofascial pain syndrome and trigger points: evaluation and treatment in patients with musculoskeletal pain. *Current Opinion in Supportive and Palliative Care.* 13(3):270–276. https://doi.org/10.1097/SPC.0000000000000445

Casale R. (2018). Myofascial pain: so common, and yet not understood. *Current Opinion in Supportive and Palliative Care.* 12(3):372. https://doi.org/10.1097/SPC.0000000000000367

Dommerholt J, Chou LW, Finnegan M, et al. (2019). A critical overview of the current myofascial pain literature—February 2019. *Journal of Bodywork and Movement Therapies.* 23(2):295–305. https://doi.org/10.1016/j.jbmt.2019.02.017

Hubbard MJ, Hildebrand BA, Battafarano MM, et al. (2018). Common soft tissue musculoskeletal pain disorders. *Primary Care.* 45(2):289–303. https://doi.org/10.1016/j.pop.2018.02.006

Weller JL, Comeau D, Otis J. (2018). Myofascial pain. *Seminars in Neurology.* 38(6):640–643. https://doi.org/10.1055/s-0038-1673674

Neck Pain

Barreto TW, Svec JH. (2019). Chronic neck pain: nonpharmacologic treatment. *American Family Physician.* 100(3):180–182.

Childress MA, Stuek SJ. (2020). Neck pain: initial evaluation and management. *American Family Physician.* 102(3):150–156.

Corwell BN, Davis NL. The emergent evaluation and treatment of neck and back pain. *Emergency Medicine Clinics of North America.* 38(1):167–191. https://doi.org/10.1016/j.emc.2019.09.007

Martel JW, Potter SB. (2019). Evaluation and management of neck and back pain. *Seminars in Neurology.* 39(1):41–52. https://doi.org/10.1055/s-0038-1677044

Mohamed F, Raal F. (2019). A pain in the neck. *BMJ (Clinical research ed.),* 367, l6008. https://doi.org/10.1136/bmj.l6008

Vijiaratnam N, Williams DR, Bertram KL. (2018). Neck pain: what if it is not musculoskeletal? *Australian Journal of General Practice.* 47(5):279–282. https://doi.org/10.31128/AFP-10-17-4358

Paresthesias

Emami SA, Sahebkar A, Javadi B. (2016). Paresthesia: a review of its definition, etiology and treatments in view of the traditional medicine. *Current Pharmaceutical Design.* 22(3):321–327. https://doi.org/10.2174/1381612822666151112145348

Ferrante MA, Ferrante ND. (2017). The thoracic outlet syndromes: Part 1. Overview of the thoracic outlet syndromes and review of true neurogenic thoracic outlet syndrome. *Muscle & Nerve.* 55(6):782–793. https://doi.org/10.1002/mus.25536

Gutkowska O, Martynkiewicz J, Urban M, et al. (2020). Brachial plexus injury after shoulder dislocation: a literature review. *Neurosurgical review.* 43(2):407–423. https://doi.org/10.1007/s10143-018-1001-x

Gwathmey KG, Pearson KT. (2019). Diagnosis and management of sensory polyneuropathy. *BMJ (Clinical research ed.).* 365, l1108. https://doi.org/10.1136/bmj.l1108

Hixson KM, Horris HB, McLeod TV, et al. (2017). The diagnostic accuracy of clinical diagnostic tests for thoracic outlet syndrome. *Journal of Sport Rehabilitation.* 26(5):459–465. https://doi.org/10.1123/jsr.2016-0051

Illig KA, Rodriguez-Zoppi E, Bland T, et al. (2021). The incidence of thoracic outlet syndrome. *Annals of Vascular Surgery.* 70, 263–272. https://doi.org/10.1016/j.avsg.2020.07.029

Noland SS, Bishop AT, Spinner RJ, et al. (2019). Adult traumatic brachial plexus injuries. *The Journal of the American Academy of Orthopaedic Surgeons.* 27(19):705–716. https://doi.org/10.5435/JAAOS-D-18-00433

Ramdharry G. (2018). Peripheral nerve disease. *Handbook of Clinical Neurology.* 159, 403–415. https://doi.org/10.1016/B978-0-444-63916-5.00026-4

Siao P, Kaku M. (2019). A clinician's approach to peripheral neuropathy. *Seminars in Neurology.* 39(5):519–530. https://doi.org/10.1055/s-0039-1694747

Shoulder Pain

Aerni G, Tirabassi J. (2020). Shoulder conditions: traumatic instability and laxity. FP essentials, 491, 22–26.

Bakhsh W, Nicandri G. (2018). Anatomy and physical examination of the shoulder. Sports medicine and arthroscopy review, 26(3): e10–e22. https://doi.org/10.1097/JSA.0000000000000202

Cotter EJ, Hannon CP, Christian D, et al. (2018). Comprehensive examination of the athlete's shoulder. Sports health, 10(4):366–375. https://doi.org/10.1177/1941738118757197

Mahon HS, Christensen JE, Brockmeier SF. (2018). Shoulder rotator cuff pathology: common problems and solutions. Clinics in sports medicine, 37(2):179–196. https://doi.org/10.1016/j.csm.2017.12.013

RESOURCES

American Academy of Physical Medicine and Rehabilitation
http://www.aapmr.org

American Academy of Physical Therapy
http://www.aaptnet.org

American Academy of Orthopaedic Surgeons
http://www.aaos.org

American Association of Clinical Endocrinologists (AACE)
http://www.aace.com

American Orthopedic Foot and Ankle Society
http://www.aofas.org

Association of Hip and Knee Surgeons
http://www.aahks.org

Ergonomics. Occupational Safety and Health Administration
https://www.osha.gov/SLTC/ergonomics/

Ergonomics and Musculoskeletal Disorders, Centers for Disease Control and Prevention/National Institute of Occupational Safety and Health
https://www.cdc.gov/niosh/topics/ergonomics/default.html

Muscle Spasms. Cleveland Clinic.
https://my.clevelandclinic.org/health/diseases/15466-muscle-spasms

Musculoskeletal Disorders. Centers for Disease Control and Prevention/National Institute for Occupational Health and Safety.
https://www.cdc.gov/niosh/programs/msd/default.html

Orthogate: The Gateway to the Orthopedic Internet
https://www.orthogate.org/patient-education/shoulder/acromio-clavicular-joint-separation

Physical Therapy Association
http://www.apta.org

Symptoms of Peripheral Neuropathy. The Foundation for Peripheral Neuropathy.
https://www.foundationforpn.org/what-is-peripheral-neuropathy/symptoms/

Trigger Points: Diagnosis and Management. *American Family Physician*
https://www.aafp.org/afp/2002/0215/p653.html

Work-Related Musculoskeletal Disorders (WMSDs). Canadian Centre for Occupational Health and Safety
https://www.ccohs.ca/oshanswers/diseases/rmirsi.html

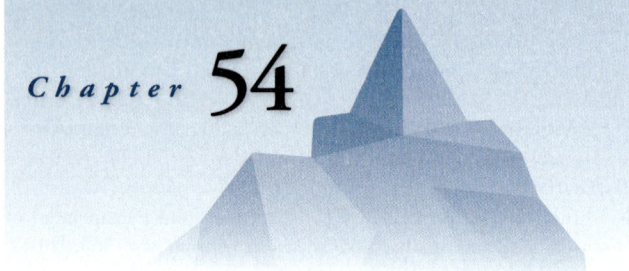

Chapter 54

Spinal Disorders

Michael E. Zychowicz, DNP, ANP, ONP, FAAN, FAANP

CERVICAL MUSCLE SPRAIN AND STRAIN

Cervical strain is an injury to the muscles and tendons of the neck, whereas a cervical sprain is an injury to the ligaments of the cervical spine. These two conditions typically occur together and rarely take place in isolation. These are common and largely self-limited conditions. It is often difficult to differentiate between sprain and strain injuries to the neck by either physical examination or more sophisticated imaging modalities. After ruling out associated neurological dysfunction, fracture, and instability, the treatments for a neck sprain or strain are essentially the same.

Whiplash describes an acceleration–deceleration injury of the neck with rapid flexion and extension usually resulting in cervical strain and sprain. This is a common sequela of motor vehicle crashes (MVCs). Despite no apparent instability, these injuries may cause prolonged disability due to a combination of relatively severe ligamentous/muscle injury, comorbid pathology, and a potential nonorganic psychosocial factor.

EPIDEMIOLOGY AND CAUSES

Neck pain is more common in middle-aged females and usually resolves within 2 months. Mechanical disorders of the cervical spine are common causes of neck pain. In addition to an acute injury, people can develop a cervical strain/sprain from nontraumatic causes including poor ergonomics at work, sleep position, and poor posture while standing and sitting. The annual prevalence of cervical pain is as high as 37% with a lifetime prevalence of nearly 50%. Neck pain is among the top five most common causes of disability in the United States. Approximately 30% of people with neck pain will have concurrent back pain. Additional factors in developing neck pain include prior episode of neck pain, sedentary lifestyle, obesity, smoking, and diminished overall health. Comorbid psychopathology can be a risk factor in the development of acute and chronic neck pain.

It has been estimated that 85% of all neck injuries presenting to primary care providers result from automobile accidents. The extent of injury and pain naturally depends on several factors including the patient's preinjury physical condition, as well as physics (e.g., speed and direction) of the MVC. Approximately 90% of people will develop neck pain within 24 hours of the whiplash injury. The natural history of hyperextension cervical muscle strain is that a majority of people will get better within the first year. Only 4% have permanent disability stopping them from returning to work.

Roughly 95% of sports-related neck injuries result in cervical strain/sprain. More of these cervical sprains/strains occur in males and people younger than 18 years. Cervical strain from sports occurs most frequently from football, weightlifting, aerobic exercise, use of trampolines, and diving. Cervical strain/sprain can also occur with other trauma and physical abuse.

The relationship between occupational factors and cervical pain is difficult to study because exposure to those factors is usually difficult to quantify. Workers may be exposed to multiple risk factors both on the job and at home. Most work-related cervical injuries are diagnosed as a sprain or strain, and certain occupations appear to have a predisposition to cervical symptoms. Workers who are occupational drivers, laborers, health-care workers, and office and computer workers are at risk of developing mechanical neck pain. Significant psychosocial work-related risk factors for developing neck pain include secondary gain, perceiving one does not have support at work, and poor job satisfaction.

PATHOPHYSIOLOGY

Cervical sprain is a clinical condition describing a nonradiating and often nonfocal pain in the neck frequently associated with diminished neck motion and stiffness. The degree of injury can range in severity. A patient may experience a minor tear of muscle, ligament, or tendon fibers, or a severe significant injury with a complete disruption of structures, muscle spasm, bleeding, inflammation, and neurological injury.

Whiplash injuries are most commonly caused by rear-end MVCs when a stationary car is struck from behind by another vehicle. The occupants of the stationary car are usually relaxed and unaware of the impending collision. The sudden acceleration of the struck vehicle pushes the back of the car seat against the person's torso. This force pushes the torso and shoulders forward while the head remains static but moves posteriorly, causing hyperextension of the neck. Often, the patient will experience a subsequent hyperflexion of the neck, resulting in a classic flexion-extension injury. This injury is most common in Western societies and metropolitan areas where there are more automobiles.

Normal posture should be effortless and painless. Abnormal forward posture of the head results in chronic strain on the posterior structures of the neck. A variety of daily activities may result in chronic abnormal posture, such as the prolonged use of a computer with a screen below eye level, a faulty sitting position, or the use of bifocal glasses. A variety of factors extraneous to the muscles also can affect muscle tension, including fatigue, pain, anger, emotional stress, anxiety, and depression.

CLINICAL PRESENTATION

Subjective

Obtaining a thorough history is essential to ensure serious pathology (e.g., meningitis), which causes neck pain, is not missed. Inquire about aggravating and alleviating factors. Ask if the pain interferes with activities of daily living or ability to work. Pain is the most common presenting symptom, although the associated complaint of a headache, usually occipital, which may persist for months, is not unusual. The pain is usually located in the middle to lower part of the posterior neck. The pain may cover a small or large area. Ask the patient about any radiation of the pain into the shoulders or upper extremities. The pain may radiate toward the shoulders but usually will not radiate down into the arm. The pain associated with a cervical strain is most often dull and aching and is exacerbated by neck motion and alleviated by rest or immobilization. Ask the patient about any numbness or tingling into the upper extremities.

The pain may come after a trauma or may be spontaneous in onset; pain after trauma often persists longer than sprains of spontaneous onset. Nonradicular, nonfocal neck pain is most common and may be noted anywhere from the base of the skull to the cervicothoracic junction. Pain is often worse with motion and may be accompanied by paraspinal spasm and discomfort in the region of the trapezius muscle. Pain may be accompanied by fatigue, sleep disturbance, irritability, and difficulty concentrating. Work tolerance may be impaired.

Cervical pain from an MVC may not appear for about 12 to 14 hours after the collision. The patient is often unaware at first of having been injured but later begins to feel stiffness in the neck. The pain at the base of the neck increases and is made worse by head and neck movement. Pain patterns should be evaluated carefully to differentiate muscular pain from radicular symptoms that typically radiate down the upper extremities. For the patient who experienced a whiplash injury that caused neck pain, inquire about blurred vision, attention or concentration deficit, sleep disturbance, dizziness, headache, or memory impairment.

Objective

Inspect head and neck position, as well as the curve of the cervical spine. A patient may slightly tilt their head and neck to one side to decrease tension on muscles and ligaments to decrease pain. With paraspinal muscle spasm, there may be a flattening of the cervical spinal curve.

Purposefully palpating the soft tissue and bony structures of the neck is essential while attempting to identify any specific pain generators. Frequently, there is tenderness to palpation over both the anterior and posterior structures of the cervical spine, specifically the paraspinal muscles, spinous processes, interspinous ligaments, or medial border of the scapula. Bony point tenderness—for example, at the spinous processes—should raise suspicion for a fracture. Attempt to identify any trigger points or muscle spasm of the neck with palpation.

Physical examination may show decreased neck range of motion (ROM) with pain or poor quality of movement. Identify the directions of movement that are decreased and painful. Also identify if the patient experiences radicular symptoms with neck range of motion, which may be indicative of nerve root irritation. Active motion of the cervical spine against any type of resistance frequently causes increased pain. The shoulder examination, as well as the remainder of the physical examination, is typically normal.

With typical cervical muscle strain or spasm, a patient will not experience any neurological deficit. Assess strength, reflexes, and sensation of the upper extremities to identify neurological deficit. For patients with radicular symptoms, a Spurling's test, relief sign, cervical distraction test, and Valsalva maneuver can assist in identifying nerve root injury. Patients who have cervical myelopathy with neck pain may exhibit upper extremity weakness and numbness along with loss of dexterity, hyperreflexia, and difficulty ambulating. Lhermitte's sign, Hoffman's sign, Babinski's sign, and clonus are useful tests to evaluate for cervical myelopathy.

DIAGNOSTIC REASONING

Diagnostic Tests

Similar to low back pain (LBP), imaging is frequently not necessary for those patients who initially present with nontraumatic onset of neck pain without any evidence of "red flags" and will typically not alter initial treatment. The Canadian C-spine rules can be utilized to assist decision making about obtaining neck radiographs for those patients who have experienced some type of trauma causing neck pain. Evidence of neurological deficit with neck pain merits further diagnostic testing, such as radiographs and/or magnetic resonance imaging (MRI).

Hyperextension cervical injuries may cause only soft tissue damage; however, plain x-ray films of the cervical spine should be obtained. It is important to include radiographic studies so that suspected fractures or dislocations, facet fractures, odontoid fractures, or spinous process fractures that might otherwise be missed in the neurologically intact patient can be identified or ruled out.

All seven cervical vertebrae must be visualized. Anterior displacement of the pharyngeal air shadow indicates soft tissue swelling and possible fracture or disruption of the intervertebral disc or anterior longitudinal ligament and requires further evaluation. The width of the prevertebral soft tissue at the level of C3 should not exceed 7 mm in normal adults. Muscle spasm may cause the normal lordotic curve of the neck to straighten or reverse. This limited finding can also be noted in nearly 10% of normal adults without neck pain. Age-related degenerative disc disease may be noted on x-ray, most frequently at C5 to C6 or C6 to C7. In a patient with severe pain, the screening radiographs should be examined for signs of instability.

Differential Diagnosis

The diagnosis of cervical muscle strain is based on the history of localized neck pain and a compatible physical examination demonstrating localized pain, muscle spasm, and a normal neurological examination. Trauma to the cervical spine may result in major neurological damage with paralysis; if the history reveals a significant trauma, a thorough evaluation with appropriate diagnostic imaging should be performed. Because of the significant consequences of potential damage to the spinal cord, referral to an orthopedic surgeon or neurosurgeon should be sought. Potential differential diagnoses include the following:

- Cervical disc herniation
- Cervical spine tumor
- Cervical spine infection
- Vertebral dislocation or subluxation
- Inflammatory conditions of the cervical spine
- Malingering, secondary gain, or nonorganic cause for pain

MANAGEMENT

Reassurance is a cornerstone of treatment in uncomplicated cases. A decrease in activity allows the injured tissues to heal. Nonnarcotic analgesics such as NSAIDs are helpful in making the patient more comfortable. NSAIDs should be used at the lowest effective dose and for the shortest time necessary. Use of NSAIDs can lead to serious gastrointestinal disease, such as ulcers, gastritis, and hemorrhage. Anti-inflammatory creams, lidocaine patches, NSAID gels, and other topical medications may be helpful for some patients.

Short-term use of muscle relaxants may be helpful if muscle spasm is noted on physical examination. Drowsiness and dizziness are common side effects. Patients should be cautioned not to drive or operate machinery while taking them and to avoid alcohol or other central nervous system (CNS) depressants to prevent additive effects. Generally, opioids should be avoided because of their potential for abuse. Short-term use of opioids can be considered for those patients with severe neck pain.

Neck pain and mobility can be improved with physiotherapy. The goal of therapy is to maximize function of the cervical spine. Physical therapy modalities may take the form of cold (ice) initially or heat (warm bath) to help relieve pain and muscle spasm. Activity should be encouraged as determined by the severity of the symptoms. Cervical traction may also be used to diminish pain and spasm if no improvement is seen with heat and medication. Aerobic activity, such as walking, should be started as soon as possible. Once improvement is seen, a course of isometric exercises should begin. Encourage an early return to work and activities.

FOLLOW-UP AND REFERRAL

Usually, the course of cervical muscle strain is one of progressive improvement with complete resolution of symptoms over several weeks. Recovery is usually complete without any lasting impairment; however, a small percentage of patients may continue to experience cervical spine pain despite treatment. Patients with recurrent neck pain may be resistant to therapies that are beneficial in management of acute neck pain episodes, and therefore they may require chronic pain assessment and management strategies. Narcotic abuse and dependency can be a problem for patients with chronic pain; consider referring the patient to a pain specialist or clinic where a variety of evaluation and treatment modalities are available.

Referral to a spine specialist is recommended for any patient who has red-flag signs or symptoms, a neurological deficit, intractable pain, a trauma history, and/or an x-ray examination revealing instability or fracture. If a patient fails to improve with conservative management over 6 to 8 weeks, imaging studies and potential referral to a spine specialist are appropriate. A referral to another member of the interprofessional health-care team (e.g., chiropractor or physical therapist) may be appropriate to manage symptoms, provide pain relief, and provide instruction about a home exercise program. A physiatry or pain management referral may be appropriate for those with neck pain that is resistant to conservative management and has no surgical pathology to be addressed. Additionally, some patients may have mental health conditions, such as depression or anxiety, that are present before or after the onset of neck pain. These patients may benefit from referral to a mental health provider to help address the mental health condition that may contribute to increased risk for chronic pain.

Patient Education: Cervical Muscle Sprain/Strain

Knowing how a healthy neck works can help patients understand their cervical spine problems and how to care for them. It is important for patients to understand the concepts behind their treatments to receive the greatest benefits. They must also learn appropriate body mechanics to help protect the cervical spine from further damage by preventing its misuse or overuse. Stress from home or work can also lead to muscle tension and other symptoms, so the patient may need professional guidance in relieving or controlling these stressors.

Instruct the patient to carefully introduce activities as they begin to recover from the pain episode. Gradual stretches and regular walking are good activities. Over-the-counter NSAIDs may be used if not contraindicated or taking prescription NSAIDs. Provide information on safe exercises or consider referral to a physical therapist. Encourage patients to make exercise a regular part of their lifestyle. Inform patients to contact the health-care provider if symptoms persist, worsen, or progress; if significant pain persists and is intractable; or if there is no improvement with conservative management.

In all patients, preventing recurrence of neck pain is an important consideration. For some patients, actual fear causes them to avoid many activities (fear avoidance). Provide reassurance that most patients will recover within a matter of weeks.

CERVICAL SPONDYLOSIS

Spondylosis (also called *degenerative arthritis*) is a blanket term for a group of chronic degenerative processes that affect the vertebrae, intervertebral discs, spinal connective tissue structures (e.g., ligaments), and facet joints. Degeneration can cause pain, stiffness, weakness, and disability. Spondylosis can occur in the lumbosacral and cervical regions of the spine. Cervical spondylosis is a common cause of neck pain in older patients.

EPIDEMIOLOGY AND CAUSES

Cervical spondylosis is fairly common and affects males more often than females. Degenerative changes on standard x-ray are found in 50% of the population at age 55; however, 80% to 90% will have degenerative changes on MRI evaluation. The peak prevalence is between

40 and 60 years of age. Spondylosis can be asymptomatic, meaning that a finding on x-ray study does not necessarily account for the patient's pain. Spondylotic changes are cumulative over time, and they generally lag behind findings on imaging, but the onset of symptoms can be accelerated by trauma, poor body mechanics, postural changes, or disc injury.

PATHOPHYSIOLOGY

Changes in the intervertebral discs caused by aging include a loss of water and elasticity, which can make the disc vulnerable to injury and surrounding ligaments less able to support the surrounding structures. As a result of these changes, the disc may degenerate, dehydrate, and/or herniate. Pain from the disc can contribute to the patient's overall discomfort. A herniating disc may impinge on a spinal nerve root and cause radiculopathy, a characteristic pattern of numbness and tingling caused by compression of the cervical nerve roots. Facet hypertrophy and hypertrophy of the uncinate processes can compress the spinal nerves as they exit the foramina, which may also lead to cervical radiculopathy. The pain and numbness typically occur in a dermatomal pattern of the affected nerve root. The most commonly involved nerve roots are C6 and C7, which produce pain and paresthesias into the radial border of the lower arm, thumb, and the pointer and middle fingers.

Facet joint arthritis can contribute to the pain. As degeneration progresses, the facet joints may undergo changes including posterior hypertrophy and thickening of the ligamentum flavum. Both changes may cause a narrowing of the spinal canal. If the secondary bony changes of cervical spondylosis encroach on the spinal cord, a pathological process called *myelopathy* develops. If this process involves both the nerve roots and spinal cord, it is called *myeloradiculopathy*. Regardless of its etiology, cervical radiculopathy causes shoulder and/or arm pain, as well as weakness, loss of reflexes, numbness and/or tingling ("pins and needles"). Fewer than 5% of patients with cervical spondylosis develop myelopathy, and they are usually between ages 40 and 60.

CLINICAL PRESENTATION

Subjective

Common symptoms include neck pain that may radiate to the shoulders, neck stiffness, cervical muscle spasm, and decreased range of motion. Symptoms are generally exacerbated with motion. Paresthesias, arm pain, arm numbness, arm weakness, and/or loss of deep tendon reflex that follows a dermatomal pattern of an affected nerve root can occur in patients who experience radiculopathy from nerve root compression or irritation. Symptoms of radiculopathy in patients with spondylosis could be due to neuroforaminal stenosis as a result of the degenerative changes that are present. Myelopathy is a result of spinal cord inflammation, edema, and mechanical compression, and it may present in patients with spondylosis. Many patients with spondylotic myelopathy have a gradual insidious onset of subtle symptoms including unsteady gait or imbalance, fine motor deficits, diminished dexterity, and neck and shoulder pain. Some patients may attribute these subtle symptoms simply to the aging process. Radiculopathy can also be present with myelopathic symptoms.

Objective

In general, patients with cervical spondylosis will experience increased neck discomfort with range of motion. Range of motion can be limited due to degenerative changes of the spine or pain inhibition.

For patients with radicular symptoms, testing may reveal findings of weakness in shoulder abduction (which indicates involvement of the C5 nerve roots), biceps weakness (indicating C6 involvement), and triceps weakness (indicating C7 involvement). Cervical muscle spasm can lead to a straightening of the cervical spinal curve (see Advanced Assessment 53.7). There may be weakness and loss of reflexes corresponding with the affected nerve root compression. The Spurling maneuver frequently worsens the patient's radicular pain whereas the cervical traction test and shoulder abduction test (relief sign) lead to decreased radicular pain.

Myelopathic physical examination findings include weakness, gait disturbances, balance problems, and difficulty performing fine motor tasks. Patients may experience sensory loss or decreased range of motion of the neck. Upper motor neuron signs such as Lhermitte's sign, clonus, hyperreflexia, Hoffman's sign, and Babinski's sign may be elicited. Patients may also experience loss of bowel and bladder dysfunction including hesitancy, urgency, or frequency.

DIAGNOSTIC REASONING

Diagnostic Tests

Diagnostic imaging of the cervical spine, including anterior-posterior and lateral radiographs, is used to initially assess degenerative or arthritic changes to the cervical spine. If the clinician is concerned about vertebral instability, lateral flexion and extension views of the neck can be obtained. If there are symptoms of myelopathy, radicular pain is severe and intractable; if there is motor deficit, sensory loss, or hypo/hyperreflexia, MRI is indicated. An MRI will help identify spinal abnormalities including spinal cord compression, neuroforaminal stenosis, disc herniation, and degeneration of the discs or facet joints. If a patient is unable to obtain an MRI, a standard CT or CT myelogram may be utilized. An electromyogram and nerve conduction velocity (EMG/NCV) test can be utilized to further evaluate and confirm cervical radiculopathy.

Differential Diagnosis

Differential diagnoses include:

- Vertebral fractures
- Cervical stenosis
- Cervical disc pathology
- Brachial plexus lesions
- Parsonage-Turner syndrome
- Multiple sclerosis
- Guillain-Barré syndrome
- Amyotrophic lateral sclerosis
- Brain tumor

MANAGEMENT

In the management of patients with spondylosis, it can be difficult to identify a specific pain generator and thus provide targeted treatment. Many patients with spondylosis without neurological symptoms can be managed with a nonsurgical approach. This can include over-the-counter or prescription analgesics. Short-term muscle relaxers may provide benefit if muscle spasm is present. Short-term rest, topical heat, physical therapy, and/or massage therapy may provide symptomatic relief. Consideration should be given to a possible underlying or mental health condition, such as anxiety, depression, or post-traumatic stress disorder (PTSD), which may contribute to the pain intensity and longevity.

If radiculopathy is present with or without neck pain, a conservative trial of cervical traction may be warranted. Short-term rest, topical heat, and/or massage therapy may provide symptomatic relief. Physical therapy to strengthen the neck musculature and teach proper body mechanics may be helpful. Treatment may also include pain relievers, such as NSAIDs, and muscle relaxers for muscle spasm. If these conservative measures do not work and radicular symptoms persist, a trial of oral steroids may be tried. Steroid epidural injections are an intermediate treatment for radiculopathy. These injections are done under fluoroscopic guidance by a physiatrist or radiologist.

FOLLOW-UP AND REFERRAL

For patients with spondylosis without neurological symptoms, if conservative measures do not improve symptoms after 6 to 8 weeks, a surgical consultation with a spine specialist should be considered to explore surgical options for the patient's pain. These may include consideration of cervical disc arthroplasty or cervical fusion. Referral to a nonsurgical pain management specialist can be considered as well.

Referral to a surgical spine specialist is reasonable when a patient with neck pain and radiculopathy has unsuccessfully engaged in conservative management for 6 to 8 weeks without symptom improvement. If surgical intervention is unnecessary or not an option, referral to a nonsurgical pain management specialist should be considered. At times, patients will experience neurological deficit along with the pain associated with radiculopathy. A surgical referral should occur sooner than the recommended 6 weeks if the patient with radiculopathy is also experiencing loss of motor strength, loss of reflexes, progressive sensory deficit, unremitting pain, and/or muscle atrophy. Surgical intervention may include cervical fusion, foraminotomy, or laminectomy, depending on underlying pathology.

Patients with symptoms of myelopathy should be referred to a surgical spine specialist for consideration of surgical intervention. Although some patients with mild myelopathic symptoms can be treated with conservative measures such as spinal injections and physical therapy, this management decision should made in consultation with a surgical spine specialist.

Patient Education: Cervical Spondylosis

Most (75% to 90%) patients with cervical spondylosis improve with conservative treatment. The remaining subset of patients will experience no change in their symptoms or a worsening of symptoms. Patients should be counseled that in the absence of myelopathy, conservative treatment is recommended as a first-line therapy and that surgery is indicated for intractable worsening pain, spinal cord and nerve root compression, and myelopathy. Patients should be instructed to report any worsening of their symptoms or development of myelopathy to their health-care provider.

LOW BACK PAIN

Low back pain (LBP), strictly speaking, is not a disease but a symptom that patients experience. LBP can be a result of spinal pathology, degeneration, or injury to the structures of the back. These may include conditions such as degenerative disc disease, strain of the paravertebral muscles, or disc herniation. LBP arising from the anatomical structures of the spine is often referred to as *mechanical LBP*.

Mechanical or nonspecific low back pain can be located solely in the back or have some radiation to the sacrum, buttocks, and hip. This is sometimes referred to as *axial back pain* because it affects only the axial skeleton. Pain radiating down the leg(s) along a dermatome, frequently accompanied with back pain, is considered lumbar radiculopathy.

Nonspinal pathology—for example, pancreatitis or endometriosis—can result in referred LBP as well. Localizing or identifying a specific pain generator or cause for LBP in patients can be difficult. Absence of an identifiable pathoanatomical cause for a patient's LBP can be referred to as *nonspecific LBP*. Nearly 80% of people who are evaluated in a primary care setting for back pain have no specifically identifiable cause for their pain, and thus they are diagnosed with nonspecific LBP. The treatment for mechanical and nonspecific LBP is generally the same with similar outcomes whereas the treatment for nonspinal causes of LBP primarily addresses the underlying nonspinal pathology.

EPIDEMIOLOGY AND CAUSES

The global disease burden of back pain is significant and is the leading cause of disability in the world. LBP occurs in up to 84% of adults at some point in their lives. Approximately 90% of patients with acute LBP will recover from their pain with improved activity tolerance within 1 month. Acute LBP (ALBP) is considered back pain that persists for less than 6 weeks, but subacute LBP (SLBP) will last 6 to 12 weeks. Chronic low back pain (CLBP), defined as pain lasting longer than 12 weeks, affects more than 20% of the global population. CLBP symptoms are typically recurrent and episodic but may be unremitting. Approximately 2% of patients with ALBP have lumbar radiculopathy, sciatica with or without a disc herniation (see next section on herniated disc).

LBP is one of the most frequent reasons that patients visit primary care providers and is the most common reason for loss of work time and disability in adults younger than 45 years. Most symptoms are of limited duration, with 85% of patients demonstrating significant improvement and returning to work within a month. Repetitive episodes, however, are common. The overall incidence of LBP is equal in males and females, but females report more LBP after age 60. These women are at risk for osteoporosis and subsequent vertebral compression fracture. In addition, a female patient's likelihood of experiencing LBP is increased after two or more pregnancies.

Occupations that require hard labor and heavy exertion have been associated with increased risk of LBP. Lifting, pulling and pushing, twisting, slipping, sitting for an extended period, and exposure to prolonged vibration (such as driving or riding in a motor vehicle for long periods of time, as truck drivers do) have been attributed to the development of LBP. In addition, patients who view their occupations as boring, repetitious, or dissatisfying have been associated with a higher rate of LBP and more time away from work, indicating a possible psychological component in some patients. LBP is the most frequent cause of lost workdays in the United States.

There is a higher risk of LBP in obese people and in tall people. Poor posture can lead to or contribute to LBP in patients. Many studies have shown decreased strength of abdominal and spinal muscles in patients with LBP. Physical fitness and conditioning have been found to have a preventive effect on low back injuries. Smoking has been shown to increase one's risk of LBP. Aging increases the risk for CLBP. Psychosocial factors such as depression, anxiety, and alcoholism, among others, have been reported with higher frequency in patients with chronic LBP.

The cause of ALBP is not always clear, but it may be related to ligamentous or muscular strain resulting from either a specific traumatic episode, repetitive strain, or incompetence of soft tissue structures. Degeneration of the intervertebral disc and spondylosis of the lumbar spine, a physiological event of aging, modified by such factors as injury, repetitive trauma, infection, heredity, and tobacco use, may lead to CLBP.

PATHOPHYSIOLOGY

The lumbosacral spine supports the upper body in a balanced, upright position while allowing locomotion. In a static, upright position, maintenance of erect posture is achieved through a balance among the expansile pressure of the intervertebral discs, the stretch placed on the anterior and posterior longitudinal and facet joint ligaments, and the sustained involuntary tone generated by the surrounding lumbosacral and abdominal muscles. The balance of the spine is also related to the reciprocal physiological curves in the cervical, thoracic, and lumbosacral areas of the vertebral column. The balance in curvature results in an individual's posture. Proper alignment is also influenced by structures in the pelvis and lower extremities. Movement of the lumbar spine is associated with a lumbar pelvic rhythm that results in the simultaneous reversal of the lumbar lordosis and rotation of the hips. During flexion and extension of the lumbar spine, tension is produced in the paraspinal, hamstring, and gluteal muscles; the fasciae that surround the muscles; and the ligaments that support the vertebral bodies and discs. In addition to the normal stressors placed on these structures with lowering and raising of the torso, stresses are increased to an even greater degree when an individual is required to lift a heavy object.

Although it is clear that force and stress applied to the spine can potentially lead to injury and pain, the traditional "injury model" of explaining LBP is being reconsidered by some researchers—in particular, because it doesn't fit with all presentations of back pain. In a study by do Carmo Silva Parreira, et al (2015) of 1,172 patients, approximately one-third were unable to identify a specific injury, trigger, or activity that caused their back pain to start. Moving away from having an identifiable cause or pathology for the onset of back pain can be frustrating for both clinicians and patients.

The most common cause of ALBP involves lumbar strains and sprains that often occur together and account for nearly 70% of patients with mechanical LBP. Strain occurs when the muscles or ligaments of the lower back are stretched, causing microscopic tears. Sprains are caused by the overstretching or tearing of ligaments. LBP may also occur during motion if the stress is greater than the supporting structures can sustain or if the components of the lumbosacral spine are abnormal. Although the precise pathophysiology of uncomplicated lumbar strain (back strain) is not well characterized, damage may occur in lumbosacral spinal structures if the amount of force generated exceeds the stress capacity of the spine for an individual patient. If the lumbosacral spine is in a mechanically disadvantaged position (e.g., rotated or flexed), the force may not need to be that great to cause a disruption of annular fibers of the intervertebral discs. These fibers may tear when stressed, which in turn can contribute to the cascade of disc degeneration.

Several other spinal conditions exist that can produce LBP. Spinal stenosis results in spinal cord or spinal nerve impingement with associated back and lower extremity pain or heaviness on extension of the spine or walking. Extending the spine further narrows the canal and neuroforamen, causing neurogenic claudication symptoms, whereas leaning forward can open the neuroforamen and spinal canal, leading to a reduction in symptoms. Lumbar spondylosis typically has several degenerative characteristics that can lead to back pain including disc degeneration, osteophytes (bone spurs) at the articular sites of the vertebrae such as the facet joints, and possible stenosis of the neuroforamen from osteophytes or ligament hypertrophy that may also result in nerve impingement and pain.

Repeated or excessive spinal hyperextension, such as from gymnastics or football, can place stress on the pars interarticularis of the vertebra. The pars is the posterior bony plate connecting the superior and inferior articular facets of an intervertebral joint. A stress fracture or acute fracture of the pars interarticularis can occur from repeated hyperextension of one or both pars interarticularis. A fracture involving one pars is fairly stable, but a bilateral fracture of the pars can potentially lead to anterior or posterior slippage of a vertebra in relation to its neighboring vertebra, known as *spondylolisthesis*. Spondylolisthesis may be acquired from an injury or can be a congenital condition. Either of these conditions may result in nerve impingement with lower back and extremity pain. Although spondylolysis may be asymptomatic, this condition may progress to spondylolisthesis.

CLINICAL PRESENTATION

Although LBP is a common symptom that may result from many causes, specific characteristics of the pain as well as its accompanying signs and symptoms relate to the underlying etiology.

Subjective

The patient with an acute onset of LBP caused by lumbar strain or sprain will usually present with localized discomfort that occurs shortly after the lumbar tissue has been mechanically injured. The most commonly reported histories include lifting and/or twisting while carrying a heavy object, prolonged sitting, MVCs, falls, or operation of a vibrating machine. LBP, however, may be precipitated by something as minor as a sneeze or cough. Remember that many patients will experience nonspecific back pain with no identifiable cause of injury. Patients may have difficulty standing erect and often change position frequently for comfort. The pain often radiates into the buttocks and posterior thigh. The injury may also be accompanied by paravertebral muscle spasms, with the sudden onset of recurrent pain.

Initial assessment of a patient with activity intolerance resulting from LBP consists of a focused medical history, including a history of the present illness and past medical, family, occupational, and social history. A review of systems, especially description of any injury, is essential and may alert the provider to possible "red flags" warranting immediate attention (see Table 54.1).

Some questions to consider while evaluating the patient's responses include the following:

- Is there evidence of a serious systemic disease potentially causing the pain?
- Is there a neurological compromise that might require surgical evaluation?

TABLE 54.1 Red Flags When Assessing a Patient With Low Back Pain

Suspect Fracture	Suspect Malignancy	Suspect Infection	Suspect Cauda Equina Syndrome
• Recent trauma or injury • Older age (older than 60–70 years) • History of osteoporosis • Use of corticosteroids	• Prior history of cancer (most common: breast, lung, or prostate cancer) • Older than 50 years or younger than 20 years • Persistent bone pain • Progressive pain at night—may wake patient from sleep • Pain at rest • Unintended weight loss • Failure of back pain to improve with therapy	• New onset of back pain with fever • Recent infection • Recent spinal procedure • IV drug use • Immunocompromised • Pain at rest • Pain at night—may wake from sleep • Potential exposure to person with tuberculosis (Tb) or endemic area	• Saddle anesthesia • New-onset fecal incontinence • New-onset bladder incontinence or urine retention • Progressive sensory loss • Progressive weakness

- Is there any social distress or psychological pathology that may amplify or prolong pain?

Focus on History: Low Back Pain

For the patient who complains of LBP, focus the history by asking questions that will obtain the following information:

1. Mode and timing of onset
   - Abrupt or insidious?
2. Characteristics:
   - Specific location of pain
   - Course (progressive, decreasing, increasing, fluctuating, episodic)
   - Associated limb and/or neurological symptoms (pain, paresthesias, numbness, weakness, atrophy, cramps, fasciculations)
   - Provoking or aggravating factors
   - Relieving factors
   - Severity
3. Effects of activities
   - Posture
   - Coughing, sneezing, straining
   - Exercise, exertion, rest
   - Sleep
4. History
   - Similar or different pains recently or in the past
   - Prior treatment and effect (medications, types of surgery, nonpharmacological management, lifestyle and work modifications, litigation, or workers' compensation issues)
5. Associated symptoms
   - Urinary problems (frequency, urgency, retention, incontinence)
   - Bowel problems (incontinence or constipation)

Most patients with CLBP will have centralized back pain possibly with some radiation to the buttocks. Some patients may have a radicular component to their condition with some degree of radiating leg pain. Patients with mechanical LBP typically find their pain is aggravated by activities such as bending, stooping, or twisting. Recall that mechanical LBP is simply defined as pain arising from the anatomical structures of the spine, so the pain pattern may vary slightly, depending on the affected structure(s). There may be stiffness and a history of intermittent radiculopathy, but discomfort in the lower back remains the predominant symptom. This may be relieved with lying down or a good night's sleep. Although pain can be severe enough to awaken the patient at night, pain that wakes a person from sleep should be considered a possible "red flag" for underlying pathology such as spinal metastasis of cancer or vertebral osteomyelitis. Psychosocial indicators should be assessed because they can be barriers to recovery in all cases of LBP, both acute and chronic. Consider factors such as fear avoidance, financial problems, anxiety, depression, job dissatisfaction, PTSD, or poor coping behaviors that can contribute to prolonged disability and greater risk for chronic pain.

Objective

The objective examination of a person with back pain starts with observation. What does the patient's posture look like? Is there a loss of, or excessive thoracolumbar spinal curve that may signal muscle spasm, spondylolisthesis, or kyphosis from lumbar compression fractures? Does the patient have an obvious scoliosis or asymmetry of the shoulders and/or pelvis? Patients may exhibit a side or forward list from muscle spasm. Always palpate the patient's back anatomy with a purpose to attempt to narrow down any specific anatomic pain generators (i.e., paraspinal muscle or spinous process). There is often diffuse tenderness in the lower back. Some patients will have one or a few specific pain generators that are identifiable on examination, but others with nonspecific back pain may not have an identifiable anatomical pain generator.

ROM of the lumbar spine usually elicits discomfort. For the patient with acute LBP, a clinician should be considerate of the mechanical stretch, stress, and compression that occur with range of motion. Pain with flexion may come from stretching injured ligaments and muscles whereas pain with extension may come from facet arthritis or degenerative disc disease. The degree of lumbar flexion and the ease with which the patient can extend the spine are helpful parameters by which to evaluate progress. Pain with lateral bending may come from compressing facet arthritis, degenerative disc disease, or the stretching of injured ligaments and muscles.

When examining all patients with back pain, the clinician needs to assess deep tendon reflexes, motor strength, and sensation in the lower extremities. Such assessments will give information about potential spinal nerve root involvement. In most cases of uncomplicated LBP, the motor and sensory functions of the lumbosacral nerve roots and reflexes of the lower extremities are normal. A negative straight-leg raise reduces the potential for disc herniation in most cases. Although not characteristic, nonorganic findings (i.e., Waddell's sign) such as widespread sensitivity to light touch, LBP with placing axial pressure on top of the head, nonanatomical pain symptoms, a negative distracted straight-leg raise that was previously positive, nonanatomical regional weakness or sensory changes, and inappropriate grimacing or exaggerated pain behaviors may be seen (see Advanced Assessment 54.1).

DIAGNOSTIC REASONING

Diagnostic Tests

Patients with back pain may want an x-ray of their back to feel reassured about their condition. When weighing the appropriateness and necessity of obtaining an x-ray, the clinician also needs to be aware of the radiation exposure

Advanced Assessment 54.1: Assessing the Lower Back—Special Tests

Test	Comments
Straight-leg-raise (SLR) test places the L5 and S1 nerve roots and the sciatic nerve under tension.	With the patient supine and relaxed, have them attempt to elevate the leg to 90 degrees of hip flexion. Note if the patient develops pain in the back, buttocks, or leg. It is considered a positive SLR when the pain radiates below the level of the knee while the hip is raised less than 60 degrees. Record the degree of elevation at which pain occurs. If the patient only experiences back/buttock pain, this is considered a negative test. The SLR test is very sensitive, but not very specific. To increase specificity, raise the leg until pain is felt below the knee and then lower the leg about 5 degrees, which should eliminate the pain. Then have patient dorsiflex the ipsilateral foot while the leg is raised. This should cause more traction on the sciatic nerve and reproduce the pain symptoms.
Reverse straight-leg raise places the L1–L4 nerve roots under tension.	With the patient prone, lift the hip into extension while keeping the knee straight. Increased pain radiating down the leg suggests compression of the upper lumbar nerve roots.
Prone rectus femoris test places the L1–L4 nerve roots under tension.	With the patient prone, maintain the hip in a neutral position while flexing the knee. Increased radicular pain suggests compression of the upper lumbar nerve roots.

that comes with lumbar spine x-rays. To put this in perspective, the amount of radiation exposure a patient has with a two-view AP and lateral lumbar spine x-ray is equivalent to more than 100 chest x-rays of radiation.

In cases of CLBP, anteroposterior and lateral radiographs often show age-appropriate changes, such as anterior osteophytes and reduced height of intervertebral discs on the lateral view. Patients with nonspecific LBP typically only need radiographs when they have failed to improve after 6 to 8 weeks of conservative therapy. Exceptions to this include (1) if the patient has a suspected pathology that the clinician would manage differently than nonspecific LBP or (2) if the patient has red flag signs or symptoms. Red flags should lead the clinician to consider pathology such as a fracture; a malignancy; a spinal infection; or a progressive, severe neurological deficit from cauda equina syndrome (CES). For patients with red flags, the clinician should not wait to order an initial x-ray with appropriate follow-up imaging and referral as warranted for further investigating and managing specific pathology.

Although x-rays are a good initial imaging test to visualize bony abnormalities, fractures, tumors, and disc degeneration, an MRI or CT scan can be used as a follow-up test as needed to further evaluate spinal structures. MRI is generally better at imaging soft tissue (i.e., disc, nerves, spinal cord, soft tissue infection) whereas CT scan is better at providing detailed imaging of the bone.

An EMG/NCV can be a useful test to confirm or provide clarity about a patient's x-ray abnormalities in relation to neurological symptoms with back pain and to help localize a patient's pathology. If a clinician suspects cancer or infection as the cause of the patient's back pain, initial laboratory work should include complete blood count with differential, C-reactive protein (CRP), and erythrocyte sedimentation rate (ESR).

Differential Diagnosis

Nonspecific LBP is a diagnosis of exclusion, which means that the clinician should rule out red flag conditions, systemic disease, and pathology that may be causing referred pain.

Differential diagnoses for LBP include the following (see Differential Diagnosis 54.1):

- Lumbar strain/sprain
- Ankylosing spondylitis
- Fracture of the vertebral body
- Herniated nucleus pulposus
- Lumbar spondylosis
- Lumbar spondylolysis
- Lumbar spondylolisthesis
- Spinal stenosis
- Extraspinal causes
- Inflammatory arthritis
- Intervertebral disc infection or vertebral osteomyelitis
- Metastatic tumors, myeloma, lymphoma

MANAGEMENT

Reassure the patient that most episodes of ALBP are mild and self-limited; almost 90% resolve within 6 weeks. Symptom control is considered an adjunct to helping the patient overcome specific activity intolerance. Multiple approaches are required to address the biopsychosocial aspects of LBP and the ways that it can interfere with the lives of patients and families. The practitioner should use the most current clinical practice guidelines to appropriately manage acute and chronic conditions in conjunction with the patient's preferences for care and management.

The Iceberg of Low Back Pain

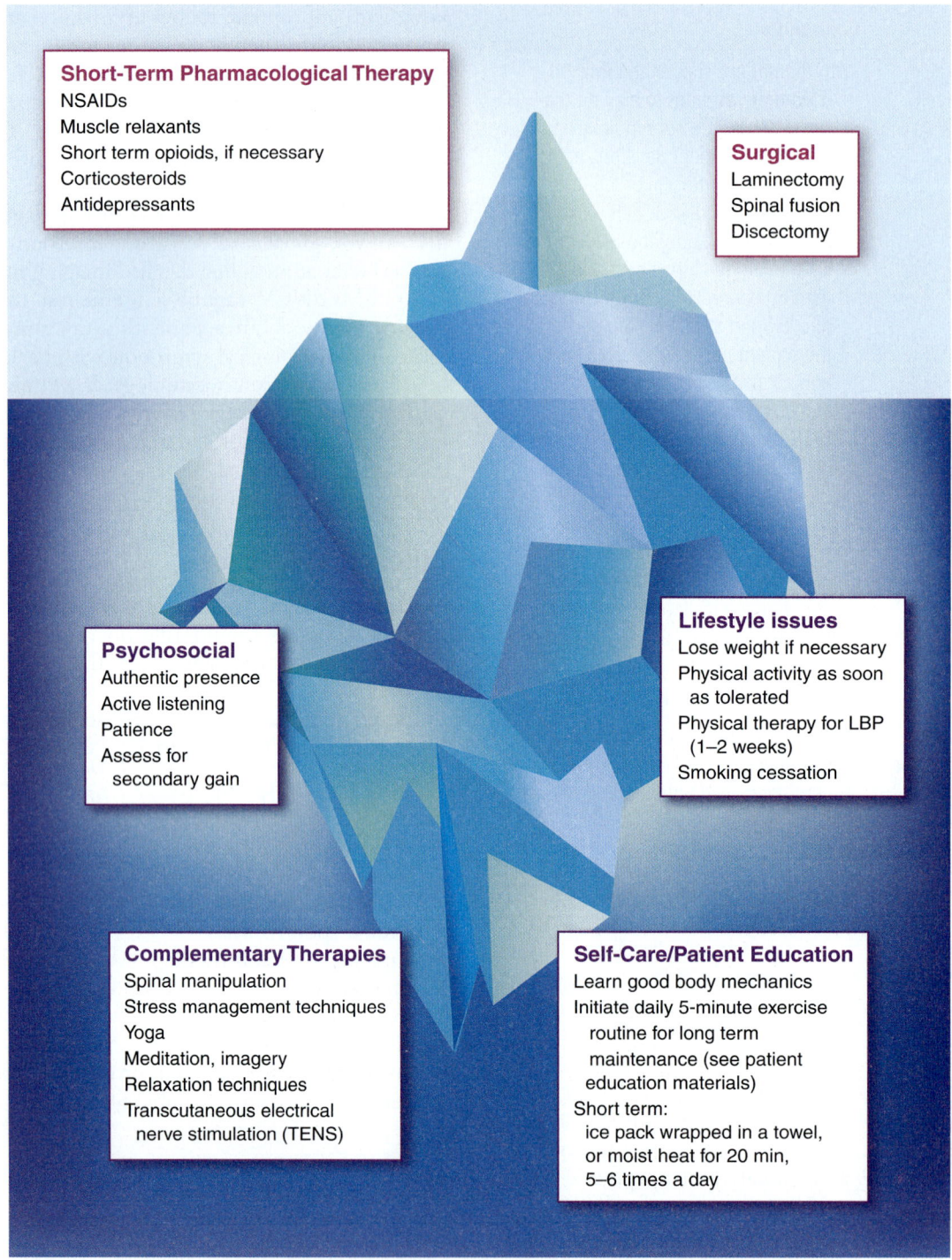

Short-Term Pharmacological Therapy
NSAIDs
Muscle relaxants
Short term opioids, if necessary
Corticosteroids
Antidepressants

Surgical
Laminectomy
Spinal fusion
Discectomy

Psychosocial
Authentic presence
Active listening
Patience
Assess for secondary gain

Lifestyle issues
Lose weight if necessary
Physical activity as soon as tolerated
Physical therapy for LBP (1–2 weeks)
Smoking cessation

Complementary Therapies
Spinal manipulation
Stress management techniques
Yoga
Meditation, imagery
Relaxation techniques
Transcutaneous electrical nerve stimulation (TENS)

Self-Care/Patient Education
Learn good body mechanics
Initiate daily 5-minute exercise routine for long term maintenance (see patient education materials)
Short term:
  ice pack wrapped in a towel, or moist heat for 20 min, 5–6 times a day

Nonpharmacological Management

The initial approach to management of LBP is the utilization of a nonpharmacological approach. There is sufficient evidence to support the following:

- Avoiding bedrest if possible, no more than 1 to 2 days if needed
- Physical therapy or gentle home exercise program
- Activity as tolerated
- Cognitive behavioral therapy or mindfulness-based activities
- Tai chi
- Yoga
- Superficial heat
- Acupuncture
- Spinal manipulation or chiropractor

Differential Diagnosis 54.1: Low Back Pain

Diagnosis	Spondylolisthesis	Muscle Strain	Scoliosis	Herniated Nucleus Pulposus	Osteoarthritis	Spinal Stenosis
Age	20	20–40	30	30–50	Greater than 50	Greater than 60
Pain location	Back	Back (unilateral)	Back	Leg and back (unilateral)	Back (bilateral)	Back & leg (unilateral or bilateral)
Pain onset	Insidious	Acute	Insidious	Acute (prior episodes)	Insidious	Insidious
Pain increases	When standing, bending	When standing, bending	When standing, bending	When sitting, bending	When standing	When standing, walking, extending
Pain decreases	When sitting	When sitting	When sitting	When standing	When sitting, bending	When sitting, bending forward
Straight-leg raising	Negative	Negative	Negative	Positive	Negative	Positive or negative
X-ray (plain film)	Will usually see pathology	Straightening of vertebral curve with muscle spasm	Lateral curve of spine	Usually negative	Will usually see loss of disc height and bone spurs	May see spondylosis and foraminal stenosis

- Multidisciplinary rehabilitation
- Shoe inserts or lifts for patients with leg length discrepancies greater than 2 cm
- Massage, traction, transcutaneous electrical nerve stimulation (TENS) unit, ultrasound, and lumbar supports have little or no evidence in the literature to demonstrate their benefit.

Pharmacological Management

The oral medications used to control the discomfort of LBP primarily include NSAIDs and skeletal muscle relaxants. Even though acetaminophen has been used often for acute back pain, there is evidence that its benefit is no greater than a placebo's. NSAIDs are effective for reducing pain in patients with LBP. Health-care providers need to be aware that NSAIDs can lead to serious gastrointestinal disease such as ulcers and hemorrhage. NSAIDs also affect renal prostaglandins and may cause fluid retention and edema, so it is also important for patients to monitor for weight gain. The risk of fluid retention and edema may be significant in older patients and in those with congestive heart failure. In addition, there is the potential for nephrotoxicity. Patients with gastrointestinal, cardiac, and/or renal problems should use this drug cautiously. Using the lowest possible effective dose for the shortest period can help to prevent potential complications. Older adults can be more sensitive to the adverse effects of NSAIDs, so it is important to use caution when prescribing NSAIDs for this age-group.

There is evidence demonstrating skeletal muscle relaxants are more effective than placebos but no evidence that they are better than NSAIDs in relieving symptoms of acute LBP. Skeletal muscle relaxants are moderately superior to placebos for short-term relief of LBP. Patients need to be aware that this class of drugs is for short-term use because the risk/benefit ratio for prolonged use of muscle relaxants is not known. Muscle relaxants cause drowsiness and dizziness, so patients need to avoid hazardous activities when taking them. This class of drug is a CNS depressant, so patients need to avoid taking muscle relaxants with alcohol or other CNS depressants because the combined use will cause additive effects. Dry mouth is another side effect from this antimuscarinic class of drugs, so frequent mouth rinsing may be needed to prevent dental disease.

Opioid analgesics may be used on a time-limited basis for severe pain. Opioid analgesics do not enhance a patient's ability to return to full activity sooner than NSAIDs. In addition, the adverse effects of opioid analgesics can be substantial, including the risk for physical dependence, misuse, or abuse.

Oral steroids provide no benefit for patients with ALBP. Limited evidence exists demonstrating effectiveness of topical lidocaine patches in comparison to placebos.

Activity

It should be stressed that rest has been proven to have little to no effect on the resolution of LBP. Bedrest should be avoided if possible and limited to 1 to 2 days if needed. Patients should do whatever activities are tolerable. Weight loss, physical activities, and exercise for 30 minutes a day (walking or biking with lumbar flexion and/or extension exercises) are also important. Deconditioning is a real phenomenon that occurs faster with increasing age. Lack of activity leading to deconditioning becomes a vicious cycle. Reassurance is always appropriate after ruling out more serious causes of back pain. Patients should also be encouraged to quit smoking.

FOLLOW-UP AND REFERRAL

The course of LBP is typically one of gradual improvement, usually over a 1- to 2-week period. For most people, recovery is usually complete without any lasting impairment. The small percentage of patients who do not make a complete recovery may continue to experience intermittent or constant chronic LBP. Patients experiencing CLBP must be evaluated and treated in a manner that takes into account the special needs and difficulties of individuals with chronic pain. Patients with more severe symptoms can have sleep disturbances and limited vocational and avocational activities and recreation. Mood, sexuality, and concentration can be adversely affected. Deconditioning can be the result of reduced activities, making both symptoms and any occupational dysfunction worse. Suggest a modified work schedule and more recreational activities that improve general conditioning. Narcotic abuse and dependency can be a problem for patients with chronic pain; refer the patient to a pain management center where a variety of evaluation and treatment modalities are available.

In all patients, preventing recurrence of back pain is an important consideration. For some, this is an actual fear causing them to avoid many activities (fear avoidance). Patients with recurrent back pain may be resistant to therapies that are beneficial in management of acute back pain episodes, and therefore they may require chronic pain assessment and management strategies. This may include the use of complementary therapies such as acupuncture or acupressure. Acupuncture is moderately effective for pain relief with CLBP.

Referral to a spine specialist is recommended for any patient who has red-flag signs or symptoms, a neurological deficit, intractable pain, a trauma history, and/or x-ray examination revealing instability or fracture.

Patient Education: Low Back Pain

Instruct the patient to carefully introduce activities back into their day as they begin to recover from the pain episode. Gradual stretches and regular walking are good activities. Application of heat for ALBP/SLBP is beneficial for functional status and short-term pain relief. Over-the-counter anti-inflammatory medications may be used if not contraindicated or taking prescription NSAIDs. Provide information on safe back exercises such as modified sit-ups and low back stretches. Encourage patients to make them a regular part of their lifestyle. Patients should call if symptoms persist, worsen, or progress; significant pain persists beyond 1 week; or there is no improvement with home management.

HERNIATED LUMBAR DISC (HERNIATED NUCLEUS PULPOSUS)

A herniated lumbar disc may result in sciatica or lumbar radiculopathy and accompany LBP. Between 5% and 15% of people with back pain will have an accompanying disc herniation. A disc herniation occurs when disc material is displaced outside the margins of the intervertebral disc space. This herniated disc material may include the two major components of the disc (nucleus pulposus and annulus fibrosis) in addition to fragments of cartilage, osteophytes, and apophyseal bone.

The radiculopathy that a patient with a disc herniation experiences is characterized by leg pain, numbness, and/or weakness in one or both lower extremities. The pain results in part from direct mechanical compression of the spinal nerve root and in part from chemical irritation of the nerve root by disc components that have herniated. Just like LBP, radiculopathy is a symptom of underlying pathology. Although disc herniation is a common cause of radiculopathy, radiculopathy is not specific to only disc herniation.

EPIDEMIOLOGY AND CAUSES

A herniated nucleus pulposus is most commonly seen in patients aged 40 to 50 years. This is rarely a condition seen in childhood or adolescence. Disc herniation occurs most commonly at the L4 to L5 or L5 to S1 levels with subsequent irritation of the L4, L5, or S1 nerve root. Herniations at more proximal levels constitute only 5% of all lumbar disc herniations. Approximately 2.5% of females and nearly 5% of males will experience this sciatica during their life. Approximately 9% of the global population will experience a symptomatic disc herniation. The global economic impact of disability for those experiencing a disc herniation, including time away from work, is substantial.

Risk factors include age-related degenerative changes (it is often difficult to distinguish between normal aging of the spine and pathological changes), cigarette smoking, a narrowed lumbar vertebral canal, obesity, osteoporosis, stress, and muscle tension. Causes include trauma (sudden or over time); frequent lifting without proper utilization of body mechanics; and vibration, such as driving and/or riding in a motor vehicle for prolonged periods of time.

PATHOPHYSIOLOGY

An intervertebral disc is located between each vertebra and is connected to the horizontal cartilage surface of the vertebral body called the *end plate*. The discs have a strong outer layer, the annulus fibrosus, which is made of concentric rings of type 1 collagen, proteoglycan, and water. The annulus exhibits high-tensile strength and extensibility. The inner nucleus pulposus, which is a gel-like material, is composed of type 2 collagen, proteoglycan, and water. The nucleus is in the center of the annulus, has a great deal of compressibility, and redistributes itself as different stresses are placed on the disc, acting like a shock absorber. Together the nucleus and annulus contribute to the degree of flexibility in the spine. Healthy discs contribute to nearly 25% of overall spine length.

Although the annulus is good at keeping the nucleus within the center of the disc, the forces from a significant trauma can overwhelm the annulus, allowing a portion of the nucleus to herniate through the annular fibers. A patient's annulus may be weakened and fissured as a result of age-related degeneration and dehydration. Annular weakness and fissuring can allow for easier herniation of the nuclear material through the fibers of the annulus even with relatively benign activities.

Even though a disc can herniate in nearly any direction, even superior or inferior into the vertebra, it typically occurs in a posterior-lateral direction. This is because (1) the annulus is typically weaker and thinner in that direction and (2) the posterior longitudinal ligament is thickest in the midline, helping to block midline herniations. The location and amount of disc material in the canal and/or neuroforamen will determine the symptoms. Most discs will rupture more to one side than the other, producing unilateral nerve root irritation and compression with subsequent unilateral symptoms. The distribution of the symptoms is determined by the vertebral level of disc herniation and the affected spinal nerve.

Over time, patients may experience a reduction or elimination of symptoms from a disc herniation. Some patients may have a corresponding reduction in size of the disc herniation, based upon diagnostic imaging. This spontaneous regression or resorption of the disc herniation is noted in the literature and is believed to be driven by the inflammatory response that accompanies a disc herniation. The inflammation that causes irritation of the nerve roots, which clinicians attempt to suppress, may be the same inflammation that aids the body in resolving a disc herniation.

CLINICAL PRESENTATION

Subjective

The onset of symptoms may be abrupt or insidious. Unilateral radiculopathy is frequently accompanied by LBP. If a patient has back pain with radiculopathy, the leg pain is typically far worse than the back pain. The pain is often severe and exaggerated by sitting, walking, standing, coughing, and sneezing. Most often, the pain radiates from the buttock to the posterior or posterolateral leg, following a dermatomal distribution to below the level of the knee, possibly to the ankle or foot. Patients with a disc herniation typically cannot find a position of comfort. Lying on their side in a fetal position or on their back with a pillow under the knees may afford some relief. Upper or midlumbar radiculopathy (L1 to L4 nerve root compression) refers pain across the dermatomal distribution to the anterior and medial aspects of the thigh and often does not radiate below the knee. Complaints of burning, numbness, weakness, or paresthesias may accompany the pain. A small percentage of patients with a midline posterior disc herniation will only have back pain and no leg pain. Conversely, a small percentage of patients with a central disc herniation can experience CES, a surgical emergency characterized by bilateral leg pain and weakness, saddle anesthesia, and bowel and/or bladder dysfunction.

Objective

The herniation can press on, or irritate, a lumbar nerve root or traversing spinal nerve, which produces the symptoms of sciatica. There may be paraspinal muscle spasm and flattening of the lumbar curve. A lumbar "list" is present when the patient's trunk is tilted laterally away from the affected side, attempting to take the pressure off the spinal nerve. With a positive flip sign, the patient has leg pain and spinal extension when the symptomatic leg is straightened at the knee. The patient leans back with a flip sign in an attempt to reduce stretch and irritation of the aggravated spinal nerve.

Motor and sensory function of the lumbosacral nerve roots and the deep tendon reflexes must be evaluated. Assess peripheral sensation for dermatomal distribution of any sensory loss and pain. Patients with a disc herniation may have unilateral and asymmetric loss of strength and deep tendon reflexes along a specific spinal nerve distribution. Injury to each of the nerve roots manifests in fairly common examination findings; however, there is variability from patient to patient in which typical findings arise and the degree to which they are present (see Advanced Assessment 54.2).

The straight-leg-raise test is performed on the involved and uninvolved limbs with the patient in the supine position. This test places stress on the L5 and S1 nerve roots, evaluating for pathology irritating

Advanced Assessment 54.2: Common Findings of Nerve Irritation From Disc Herniation

Spinal Nerve	Findings
L4 nerve	Weakness with knee extension, ankle dorsiflexion, or inversion; decreased or absent patella reflex; decreased sensation of the anterior-medial thigh, knee, and foot; pain from the low back and hip down the posterolateral thigh and anterior lower leg to the medial foot; difficulty rising from a squatting position
L5 nerve	Weakness with great toe extension and dorsiflexion or inversion of the ankle; no reflex loss; sensory loss to the anterolateral lower leg, dorsum of the foot and first three toes; pain from the sacroiliac (SI) joint and hip to the lateral thigh and leg; difficulty with heel walking; possible foot drop
S1 nerve	Weakness with great toe flexion and ankle plantar flexion or eversion; decreased or absent Achilles reflex; decreased sensation from the posterior calf to the lateral heel, foot, and toes; pain from the SI joint and hip down the posterolateral thigh and leg to the heel; difficulty with toe walking

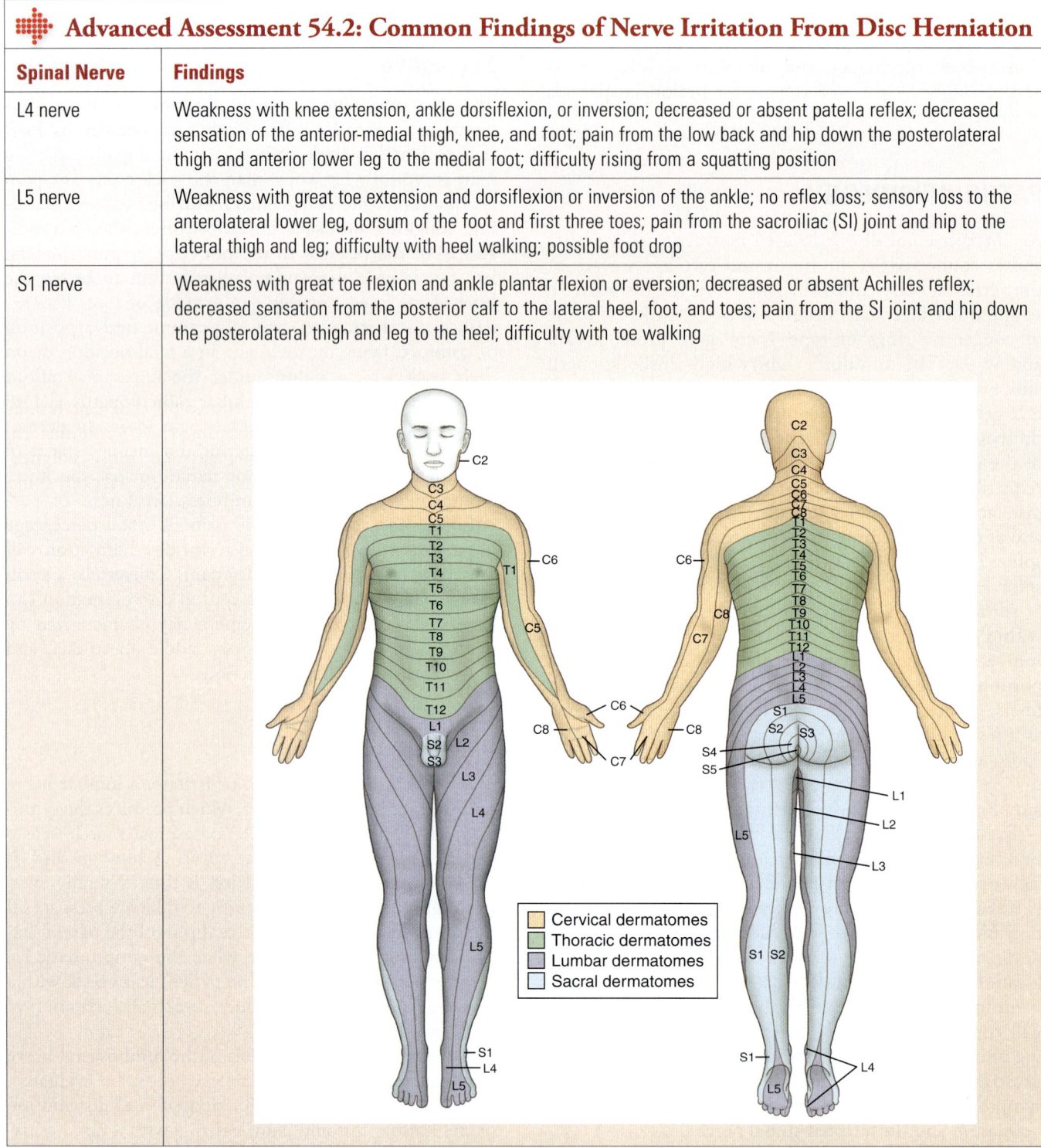

these nerves. Ipsilateral pain on straight-leg raising is common with a variety of lumbar spine differential diagnoses including disc herniation, but a positive crossed straight-leg-raising test (pain in the involved leg or buttock that occurs when lifting the uninvolved leg) is highly specific for nerve root entrapment. To stretch the upper lumbar nerve roots, a reverse straight-leg-raise test should be performed (see Advanced Assessment 54.1).

DIAGNOSTIC REASONING

Diagnostic Tests

Imaging is generally not necessary for patients who have lumbar radiculopathy with or without back pain and (1) who do not have evidence of red-flag findings and (2) who have not had any conservative management. Imaging typically does not change the initial management for patients with uncomplicated radiculopathy and back pain. Additionally, two-view lumbar spine x-rays come with a large amount of radiation, exposing a patient to radiation equivalent to more than 100 chest x-rays.

Obtaining x-rays of the lumbar spine is appropriate after a patient demonstrates little to no improvement after 6 weeks of conservative treatment. An x-ray will show any vertebral pathology, the amount of disc space, and the spinal curve; however, it will not show discs, muscles, ligaments, nerves, or other soft tissues. A follow-up imaging study to further evaluate the cause of radiculopathy and back pain is MRI without contrast to evaluate the soft tissues of the spine including the discs and nerves.

Patients suspected of having an infection or tumor should be initially screened with plain radiographs without delay followed by MRI. MRI should also be considered for patients with neurological symptoms, specifically weakness, loss of deep tendon reflex, or bilateral symptoms.

For patients with radiculopathy and back pain with a low-velocity trauma preceding the pain, for those with osteoporosis, and for those who are older or take long-term steroids, the pain may be from a disc herniation, but could also be due to a vertebral insufficiency fracture. An x-ray initially is useful to evaluate for an obvious vertebral fracture. Further evaluation of the fracture with a CT scan may be necessary if there is concern of retropulsion of fracture fragments causing the radiculopathy. On the other hand, an MRI would be superior at visualizing the disc and ligaments.

In cases of progressive neurological deficit, such as loss of reflexes or strength or signs of potential CES along with radiculopathy, an MRI should be obtained. An x-ray may also be appropriate and might provide some additional diagnostic information. CT can be a useful imaging tool if an MRI is contraindicated.

Interestingly, MRI imaging studies on populations of asymptomatic adults older than 50 years demonstrate that 30% to 40% have evidence of lumbar disc herniation and that 60% have a disc bulging, allowing potential false-positive findings. The clinical implication of this is that not all disc herniations cause pain, and even though a patient has a disc herniation and pain, the potential exists that the herniation is not truly the cause of the pain.

An EMG/NCV is typically not utilized to provide an initial diagnosis for disc herniation. This test can, at times, be useful to help clarify a confusing clinical picture. The test can help differentiate a central spinal cause of a patient's pain versus pain from peripheral nerve entrapment or peripheral neuropathy, thereby assisting the clinician to rule in or rule out a possible false-positive finding on MRI.

Differential Diagnosis

The following is a list of differential diagnoses:

- CES
- Demyelinating conditions
- Extraspinal nerve entrapment
- Hip or knee arthritis
- Lateral femoral cutaneous nerve entrapment
- Spinal stenosis
- Thoracic cord compression
- Trochanteric bursitis
- Vascular insufficiency

MANAGEMENT

Control of symptoms, relief of pain, and improved mobility are all goals of management. Most episodes improve with conservative treatment. Slightly more than one-third of people with symptoms from a disc herniation will have a substantial improvement in their symptoms within 2 weeks of symptom onset. Nearly 90% of disc herniations resolve without residual problems at 3 months. The core of effective nonsurgical management consists of medication, physical therapy, home exercises, traction, spinal manipulation, and epidural steroid injections.

As with back pain, the patient with a disc herniation should engage in activities as tolerated with no more than 1 to 2 days of bedrest if needed. The patient may have difficulty finding a comfortable position and may need to take frequent rest breaks when resuming activity. NSAIDs can be given for pain and to reduce nerve inflammation, with the usual precautions observed. Generally, all NSAIDs are equally effective. For a patient experiencing paraspinal muscle spasm, a short course of a muscle relaxer can be used. If the pain is severe in the acute phase, a short course of an opioid analgesic may be considered. Although not recommended as first-line therapy for ALBP, opioids are sometimes used for short-term relief of severe back pain; however, the potential for abuse and addiction is high with prolonged use. In addition, the use of opioids for long-term pain relief is similarly controversial because this practice may lead to abuse and diversion of prescribed medications.

Although a short course of oral steroids has been utilized by clinicians for management of pain from a disc herniation, there is increasing evidence that oral steroids may have no effect on pain improvement but moderately improve patient function. Epidural steroid injection may reduce leg pain for patients with disc herniation and provide short- or long-term pain relief.

Several regenerative or restorative options seem promising and are being studied, including gene therapy, growth factor or cell-based therapy, and tissue engineering.

Persistent numbness, progression of neurological deficits, and weakness can occur despite treatment. Absolute indications for surgical intervention include progressive neurological deficit, progressive weakness, and alteration in bladder function. Relative indications for surgical intervention include intractable and intolerable pain, typically after at least 4 to 6 weeks of conservative management. Various surgical options exist including open discectomy, microscopic discectomy, and endoscopic discectomy.

FOLLOW-UP AND REFERRAL

After an initial evaluation, the patient should return in 7 to 10 days for follow-up evaluation of pain and function. The patient should be monitored every 2 to 4 weeks until they return to normal function or require referral to a spine specialist. A progressive walking program should be initiated after pain is controlled (usually within 7 to 10 days). It is best to start with short walks initially, up to four times per day, lengthening the walks as tolerated. The patient should return to full activity as soon as possible but avoid high-risk activities such as heavy lifting and long car rides.

Referral to a spine specialist is indicated for the development or progression of neurological deficit and weakness or persistent intractable pain. Patients suspected of having CES, a surgical emergency, must be referred to an emergency department with emergent consultation with a spine surgeon. Absolute indications for surgical intervention include progressive neurological deficit, progressive weakness, and alteration in bowel and/or bladder function. Relative indications for surgical intervention include intractable and intolerable pain, typically after at least 4 to 6 weeks of conservative management. Various surgical options exist including open discectomy, microscopic discectomy, and endoscopic discectomy.

Referral to another member of the interprofessional patient care team (e.g., chiropractor or physical therapist) can be made as appropriate for the patient situation and patient desire. Referral to a chronic pain specialist is appropriate for patients who are not candidates for surgical intervention but go on to develop chronic pain. Opioid addiction is a real possibility for patients, necessitating a possible referral to a substance use disorder clinic.

Patient Education: Herniated Lumbar Disc

Patients should be reassured that most disc herniations resolve without residual pain or disability within 3 to 6 weeks. Cessation of smoking, weight reduction, good posture and body mechanics, and adherence to an exercise regimen are all ways to improve health and prevent recurrence. Modification of the work environment may be necessary.

LUMBAR SPINAL STENOSIS

Spinal stenosis occurs when there is a narrowing of one or more levels of the spinal canal (central spinal stenosis) or the neuroforamen (neuroforaminal stenosis). Although this occurs most frequently in the lumbar spine, it can occur at any level within the spine. Stenosis leads to subsequent compression of the spinal cord, nerve roots, and vasculature. This progressive disorder can potentially be asymptomatic for decades in some patients. Symptomatic patients will present with back pain with neurogenic claudication of the extremities with possible impaired ambulation.

EPIDEMIOLOGY AND CAUSES

Up to 30% of the U.S. population may have radiographic evidence of spinal stenosis after age 60 years. A portion of this population will not have symptoms. Generally, more males will experience spinal stenosis before age 70 and more females in the older-than-70 age-group. Patients acquire spinal stenosis mostly due to degenerative disease (spondylosis), but some have a congenital cause of stenosis. Patients can also have a combination of acquired and congenital. Congenital stenosis usually presents symptoms earlier (20 to 30 years of age) than degenerative stenosis. For people older than 65 years, spinal stenosis is the leading cause for spinal surgery. Approximately 135 out of 100,000 people in the United States will have surgery to address their spinal stenosis.

PATHOPHYSIOLOGY

Lumbar spinal stenosis is defined as narrowing of the spinal canal and/or neuroforamen with compression of the spinal cord, nerve roots, and/or vasculature. It may be congenital or acquired. It is most frequently acquired and results from many of the changes that accompany spondylosis, including enlarging osteophytes at the facet joints, hypertrophy of the ligamentum flavum, and protrusion or bulging combined with loss of height of the intervertebral discs. Other conditions that may lead to or contribute to spinal stenosis include vertebral compression deformities, spinal tumors or cysts, or calcium deposits. Congenital stenosis can be due to genetic disorders such as achondroplasia or may simply be idiopathic. Lumbar spinal stenosis may produce symptoms by directly compressing the spinal cord, nerve roots, or nutrient arterioles that supply the nerve roots, leading to back pain, leg pain, and neurogenic claudication.

CLINICAL PRESENTATION

Subjective

Onset of symptoms typically occurs over a longer period of time; however, onset may follow a lifting incident or minor trauma. Often there is neurogenic claudication, or pseudoclaudication, causing radicular complaints (with or without associated back pain) in the calves, buttocks, and upper thighs of one or both legs. For spinal stenosis primarily affecting the neuroforamen, the patient's pain may follow a specific dermatomal distribution, whereas central stenosis generally has a wider distribution of limb pain. Symptoms can progress from a proximal to distal direction.

Walking or prolonged standing is a common cause of pain and weakness in the legs and buttocks. A vague aching or heaviness in the legs, muscle cramping, or leg weakness may also be present. The patient may experience motor or sensory deficit. Some may experience symptoms of myelopathy, which can include pain in the back or legs; numbness, tingling, or weakness; altered balance and coordination; decreased fine motor skills; difficulty walking; altered reflexes; and altered bowel or bladder function.

Leg pain when walking can occur during neurogenic claudication, as well as vascular claudication. The clinician should differentiate neurogenic claudication from possible vascular claudication, which can be due to peripheral artery disease (PAD). In cases of vascular claudication, the pain typically stops soon after the patient stops walking, whereas neurogenic claudication usually takes a bit longer. With more advanced PAD, a patient may have constant leg pain and weakness, cool skin, difficulty with wound healing, or skin discoloration.

The patient may obtain short-term relief of leg pain from neurogenic claudication by leaning forward (manifested as "stooping"). When grocery shopping, the patient will lean or hang over the cart, often referred to as a *positive shopping cart sign*. Relief after sitting is variable, depending on the degree of neural compression. Patients who sleep flat on their back with their spine extended might wake after several hours with back and leg pain. This complaint of pain after lying flat, again, needs to be further evaluated for both neurogenic and vascular claudication. Those with spinal stenosis will typically not experience leg pain from neurogenic claudication while riding a bike; however, those with PAD will likely experience leg pain from vascular claudication during this activity. Because biking is typically a forward-leaning activity, this opens the spinal canal, reducing the chance for neurogenic leg pain. Spondylolisthesis (degenerative or spondylolytic), vascular insufficiency, osteoarthritis of the hips, and obesity are often associated with spinal stenosis.

Objective

Range of motion of the lumbar spine will likely be decreased with underlying arthritis and spondylosis. Muscle weakness of the legs is a subtle phenomenon. This may be best elicited after walking on a treadmill. Proprioception can be impaired; there may be a positive Romberg test. In this test, the patient stands with the feet together and is asked to shut the eyes. The test is positive if the patient sways or loses balance. There may be sensory changes, which can be assessed with pin-prick, light touch, or tuning fork vibration. These may be segmental and may involve more than one spinal level. Reflexes are often diminished with nearly one-half of patients with spinal stenosis having a diminished Achilles reflex. Some patients will have lumbar scoliosis. Typically, patients will have a negative straight-leg raise. Having the patient stand upright while leaning backward slightly for 30 seconds may cause symptoms with neurogenic claudication. The clinician may need to provide balance support while the patient is leaning backward. With bowel or bladder symptoms, sphincter tone may be decreased. However, because many older patients have concomitant prostate problems or urinary incontinence, genitourinary evaluation may be necessary to differentiate these processes.

DIAGNOSTIC REASONING

Diagnostic Testing

Patients presenting with signs and symptoms of spinal stenosis should have imaging studies. Radiographs may provide some evidence of spinal stenosis. Anteroposterior and lateral view radiographs (up to T10 in the lateral view) may show pathology indicative of spinal stenosis, including significant narrowing of the intervertebral disc, hypertrophy of facet joints, neuroforaminal osteophytes, or spondylolisthesis. There may be osteopenia or an old fracture of the vertebral body.

Because radiographs are not useful in assessing the spinal cord, nerve roots, and soft tissue of the spine, an MRI is the diagnostic imaging study of choice to evaluate for spinal stenosis. MRI is considered superior to CT for visualizing neuroanatomy and soft tissue of the spine as well as identifying potential causes of stenosis such as a disc bulge or herniation. CT is superior in imaging bony structures of the spine and delineating osseous causes of stenosis. CT scan should be considered when an MRI is contraindicated.

EMG/NCV can be useful to help rule out differential diagnoses or provide clarification with comorbid conditions. This may include conditions such as peripheral neuropathy. EMG/NCV is not necessarily useful, however, in the primary diagnosis of spinal stenosis.

Differential Diagnosis

The following is a list of differential diagnoses:

- Abdominal aortic aneurysm
- Arterial insufficiency
- Diabetes mellitus
- Folic acid or vitamin B_{12} deficiency
- Infection
- Tumor

MANAGEMENT

Pharmacological management of symptoms from mild to moderate spinal stenosis may include intermittent use of NSAIDs. Prolonged use of NSAIDs can cause renal failure, hepatotoxicity, and gastrointestinal ulcer disease, and it can exacerbate existing cardiac disease. Some clinicians will utilize oral corticosteroids or antidepressants for pain from spinal stenosis; however, the efficacy is not clear in the literature. If a patient is experiencing paraspinal muscle spasm along with pain, short-term use of a muscle relaxer may provide some relief. Gabapentin or pregabalin may provide some relief of neuropathic pain. Short-term and cautious opioid use can provide benefit to some patients with intolerable and insufficient pain control. Lumbar epidural corticosteroid injection may provide some short-term immediate relief for approximately 50% of patients and more sustained relief for approximately 25%.

A physical therapy or home exercise program is beneficial for those with mild to moderate symptoms. A program that focuses on flexibility and core strengthening to improve overall conditioning, as well as improving flexion of the spine, is ideal. Flexion of the spine increases intraspinal volume, thereby decreasing pain. Examples of lumbar flexion exercises include exercising on all fours, arching the back, or assuming the fetal position. Exercises that extend the spine should be avoided because they will likely initiate symptoms of spinal stenosis.

Bicycling is one aerobic exercise that a patient may tolerate because it is done with the spine in flexion. Improving abdominal muscle tone lifts the pelvis anteriorly and flexes the lumbar spine. Reduction of intra-abdominal fat is critical to achieving the objective. Thus, weight loss may be pivotal.

FOLLOW-UP AND REFERRAL

Follow-up with the patient at the primary care practice is variable, dependent on the severity of the patient's symptoms and what conservative management has been implemented. This can range from every few weeks to several months between visits.

The rate of progression is variable, but it is typically slow. Some patients may never develop any neurological deficits and tolerate the condition well. Pain and limited function, however, can become severe and lead to a secondary depression, which may necessitate referral to a pain management or mental health provider. Standing erect may become impossible due to exacerbation of symptoms and pain, and the patient may adopt a stooped posture for comfort. In significant disease, claudication may develop after walking only a few feet. CES develops in some patients, leading to loss of bowel and bladder function.

Spinal stenosis is the most common reason for surgery in people older than 65 years. Surgical consultation with a spine specialist should be considered when a patient is experiencing moderate to severe symptoms that persist despite 3 to 6 months of conservative measures or when the patient has symptoms of CES or myelopathy. A decompressive laminectomy opens the space within the spinal canal by removing all or a portion of the lamina. For those who have spinal stenosis accompanied by spondylolisthesis, decompression laminectomy and vertebral fusion are the procedures of choice. Implantation of interspinous spacers between the spinous processes is another option for surgical management of spinal stenosis without spondylolisthesis.

Patient Education: Lumbar Spinal Stenosis

The patient and family should be educated about potentially serious symptoms, such as changes in bowel and bladder function, change in neurological status, and gait disturbance. Symptoms of CES require urgent reporting and intervention. The patient should be informed about the side effects of NSAIDs. Weight loss may be helpful, and patients should be provided with dietary instructions and clear guidelines for activity and exercise. Because many of these patients are older adults, they may need a range of services arranged to accomplish these goals.

CAUDA EQUINA SYNDROME

CES is a rare but emergent surgical condition caused by compression and impaired function of the cauda equina portion of the spinal cord. The cauda equina consists of a bundle of nerve roots at the end of the spinal cord. The cauda equina extends from the level of the conus medullaris and provides innervation of the bladder, anus, perineum, and lower extremities.

CES has the potential for lasting neurological compromise and severe disability. Unfortunately, some patients are not identified early enough; they are not referred for emergency surgical intervention until it is too late to avoid or reverse neurological compromise. On average it takes 11 days for patients to receive treatment for CES after they have an onset of symptoms. Nearly one in five patients with CES will experience permanent negative outcomes, which can include sexual dysfunction and bowel or bladder dysfunction. It is essential for healthcare providers to quickly identify the signs and symptoms of CES and refer the patient for emergency management.

EPIDEMIOLOGY AND CAUSES

CES is rare, occurring in approximately 1% to 3% of those with a herniated lumbar disc. CES occurs most commonly with large central disc herniations at the

L4/5 level. People between 31 and 50 years of age have a greater incidence of CES. Risk factors for developing CES include obesity, female sex, a thickened ligamentum flavum (a ligament connecting laminae of neighboring vertebrae), and preexisting spinal stenosis. Although a large disc herniation is the most common cause of CES, it is essential to remember not all large disc herniations will cause CES. Aside from disc herniation, there are multiple etiologies for this syndrome (see Table 54.2).

PATHOPHYSIOLOGY

The cauda equina, Latin for "horse's tail," is a continuation of the spinal cord below the first lumbar vertebra in adults. The cauda equina consists of a bundle of spinal nerve roots that exit the conus medullaris and the tapered end of the spinal cord and continue down the lumbar spine, exiting at different lumbar and sacral levels through neuroforamina.

Innervation from the cauda equina is responsible for specific sensory and motor functions. Lower extremity limb movement and sensation are enabled by nerves of the cauda equina. Perineal, perianal, genital, bladder, and anal sphincter are all innervated by the cauda equina. CES involves a compression and injury to the nerve roots of the cauda equina within the spinal canal. Direct compression most often results from a large disc herniation. CES may also result from venous congestion or inflammation.

CES can be divided into four stages: suspected (CES-S), incomplete (CES-I), retention (CES-R), and complete (CES-C). CES-S is characterized by bilateral radicular pain in the lower extremities. There is an onset of neurogenic urinary symptoms with CES-I. This includes poor urinary stream, altered desire to void, or needing to strain to urinate. Fully developed neurogenic urinary retention is present with CES-R. These patients will have overflow incontinence as well as painless urinary retention. CES-C is present when a patient has an absence of perineal sensation and loss of sensation and tone of the bowel and bladder.

CLINICAL PRESENTATION

Cauda equina compression is characterized by bilateral lower extremity weakness and by anesthesia, or paresthesia, of the perineum and buttocks (saddle anesthesia). There may or may not be bowel or bladder incontinence or bladder retention. When there is a neurological deficit affecting the bowel or bladder, these changes may not be reversed with surgical decompression.

Subjective

The presenting symptoms may be acute onset or insidious. Early symptoms may prove to be somewhat subtle. The clinician should keep in mind that there may be existing pathology that may cloud the clinical picture by mimicking some CES symptoms. Nearly three-fourths of patients with CES have existing or chronic back pain. The patient may have underlying benign prostatic hypertrophy, leading to urinary symptoms. Ask the patient about acute changes in existing symptoms or new onset of back pain, weakness, sensory changes, or changes in bowel and bladder function. A majority of patients with chronic or preexisting symptoms, such as back pain, report an acute increase in symptoms over the previous day. Patients with CES often have worsening pain while lying in a supine position.

The clinician should attempt to accurately identify when the patient's symptoms began and how fast the symptoms are progressing. Time from onset of symptoms to surgical intervention is important. A greater time to surgery and a more rapid onset of symptoms lead to worse patient outcomes and slower recovery from CES.

The patient may complain of pain in both legs that may be more severe in one extremity. Unilateral pain is more common. Inquire about erectile dysfunction and any change in sensation the patient experienced with sitting or toileting. Some clinicians will ask about urinary incontinence and forget to ask about urinary retention. It is important to ask about retention as this is an earlier sign of CES than incontinence.

TABLE 54.2 Cauda Equina Syndrome Etiologies	
Etiology	**Pathology**
Degenerative disease	Disc herniation (L4/5; L5/S1) Lumbar spinal stenosis Spondylolisthesis Cysts Perineural cysts Facet joint cysts
Inflammatory	Acute and chronic ankylosing spondylitis
Traumatic	Spinal fracture Epidural hematoma Postprocedure Post–spinal manipulation
Infectious	Epidural abscess Tuberculosis (Pott's disease)
Malignant	Lymphoma Metastases Primary central nervous system malignancies (schwannoma, neurofibroma, etc.)
Vascular	Aortic dissection Arteriovenous malformation
Other space-occupying lesion(s)	Sarcoid

Objective

Patients suspected of having CES should have a thorough neurological examination including sensation, motor function, and reflexes. A key component of the examination is to assess for any abnormal neurological findings, as well as noting the pattern of the findings (e.g., radicular pattern vs generalized) and if the symptoms are unilateral or bilateral. Ambulation should be observed. The patient may have a stumbling gait from leg weakness. Quadriceps and/or hip extensor weakness may be observed as the patient has difficulty arising from a chair and uses the armrests or seat to push into standing position. The patient is unable to walk on heels and toes due to ankle dorsiflexor and plantar flexor weakness. Bilateral footdrop may be observed.

A sensory examination of the lumbosacral nerve roots should be performed to include at least light touch of lower extremities across dermatomes, as well as the perineal and perianal regions. A loss of strength and sensation frequently accompanies CES. Lower extremity strength and sensation are innervated by L2 to S3 spinal nerves. The S2 to S4 spinal nerves provide perianal and perineal sensation.

Deep tendon reflexes of the lower extremity are often diminished with CES. The Achilles reflex, innervated by S1 nerve, and the patellar reflex, innervated by L4, should be assessed. A patient who has hyperreflexia may have pathology affecting the spinal cord higher than the cauda equina. Anal wink reflex and bulbocavernosus reflex, both innervated by the S2 to S4 spinal nerves, may also be absent with CES. Although assessing rectal sphincter tone with a digital rectal examinations is a typical component of assessment for CES, more recently, the correlation between a loss of reflex and finding of CES on MRI has come into question.

Other tests to consider would include position sense, clonus, and Babinski's sign if the clinician is concerned about CNS or upper motor neuron pathology. It is essential for the clinician to remember that early symptoms and findings can be subtle and that not all of the examination findings described in this section need to be present for the patient to be diagnosed with CES.

DIAGNOSTIC REASONING

Diagnostic Tests

Although radiographs of the lumbar spine may provide some assessment of bony pathology such as arthritis or degeneration, the radiographs frequently are not necessary, and they bring little value in evaluating the patient with CES. Obtaining a stat MRI is the diagnostic test of choice as this will be best able to identify pathology causing CES (e.g., abscess, herniated disc, hematoma, or tumor). In patients who cannot tolerate MRI or in whom the test is contraindicated, CT myelogram is warranted.

If point-of-care ultrasound is readily available, scanning the bladder for postvoid residual urinary volume can provide evidence for CES. Urinary retention is a sign seen earlier in CES, and incontinence is seen as the syndrome progresses.

Differential Diagnoses

Differential diagnoses of CES are as follows:

- Guillain-Barré syndrome
- Herniated disc
- Metastatic disease
- Multiple sclerosis
- Pernicious anemia
- Tabes dorsalis
- Spinal cord tumor
- Hysteria and other psychiatric disorders

MANAGEMENT

If cauda equina compression is suspected or confirmed, an immediate consultation with a spine surgeon is necessary. The treatment for CES is emergent surgical lumbar decompression to halt neurological deterioration unless surgery is contraindicated for other medical reasons. Delaying surgical intervention, especially with rapidly progressing symptoms, increases the risk for greater negative outcome and varying degrees of permanent disability.

FOLLOW-UP AND REFERRAL

CES patients may have varying levels of postsurgical recovery, including ongoing chronic pain and residual neurological deficits. One in five patients may have physical or psychosocial issues after CES decompression. The need for intensive rehabilitation, learning self-catheterization, colostomy care, sexual dysfunction, depression, and loss of employment are all issues that the primary care provider should include as part of the office follow-up evaluation after discharge from surgery. Ongoing support for the patient with linkage to community resources and support groups assists in the long-term recovery process.

Patient Education: Cauda Equina Syndrome

The initial patient education is to explain CES and the sense of urgency for surgical intervention. Post–neurosurgical discharge, patient education should focus on providing any knowledge needed for self-care, ongoing health maintenance, giving information on community resources, and assuring that the social determinants of health are explored to address needs beyond physical health.

VERTEBRAL FRACTURE

Vertebral fractures commonly occur as a result of a high-energy injury. This may be from an MVC or a diving injury or due to a fall from a height. Fractures can also occur as a result of a relatively low-energy type of injury, typically in the presence of underlying pathology such as vertebral insufficiency due to osteoporosis, long-term steroid use, vertebral infection, or tumor. Stability of the vertebral fracture is based upon the extent and pattern of the fracture. The pattern of a fracture is often predictable, based upon the physical force applied to the spine during the injury. Vertebral fractures are classified by both the directional force of the injury and the pattern of the fracture.

EPIDEMIOLOGY AND CAUSES

Vertebral fractures can be caused by weakness of the bone due to underlying pathology or significant injury and trauma. Pathology that can increase risk or lead to fracture includes osteoporosis, neoplastic disease, infection, or other calcium or bone demineralization disease processes such as renal failure. Thoracic and lumbar vertebral fractures are frequently associated with osteoporosis.

Osteoporosis is a worldwide musculoskeletal and public health burden. The International Osteoporosis Foundation estimates that more than 200 million people worldwide are affected by this disease. In the United States, approximately 14 million men and women are diagnosed with osteoporosis. Osteoporosis affects nearly 30% of Caucasian postmenopausal females. Although many people consider osteoporosis a disease of older females, men can also develop osteoporosis. Hereditary factors, medications such as prolonged use of steroids, smoking, alcoholism, renal disease, other chronic wasting diseases, and lifestyle choices can cause or lead to an increased risk for osteoporosis (see Chapter 56 for more information).

Trauma and injuries constitute the second leading cause of all vertebral fractures and the leading cause of fractures of the cervical spine. Twenty-five percent of lumbar fractures occur after a fall from a height of greater than 6 feet, and 50% are due to an MVC. Approximately 11,000 spinal cord injuries occur each year in the United States. Approximately 1% to 2% of those with cervical fractures will have a spinal cord injury. The average age of spinal cord-injured patients is 32, and 80% are male. Two-thirds of cervical spine fractures occur between C3 and C7. Almost 60% of cervical fractures in people older than 60 years occur at the odontoid process of the C1 vertebra. One-half of the fractures that occur in the thoracolumbar spine arise between T11 and L1 with another 30% occurring between L2 and L5. Most lumbar fractures cause no neurological deficit and have a burst or compression pattern.

PATHOPHYSIOLOGY

For patients who experience a fracture after a trauma, the mechanism of injury and amount of force are key to the pattern and type of fracture that results. Compression injuries, distraction injuries, and displacement/dislocation injuries all have distinct and common patterns. A few classification systems for vertebral fractures exist, including the AO Spine Classification System, the Denis Classification system, and the Thoracolumbar Injury Classification and Severity Score (TLICS).

The anatomical theory published by Francis Denis (1983) describes the vertebrae and the attached ligaments that are involved during injury and divides the spinal column into three sections: anterior, middle, and posterior. The anterior column contains the anterior two-thirds of the vertebra and the anterior longitudinal ligament. The middle column is the posterior one-third of the vertebral body and the posterior longitudinal ligament. The posterior consists of the pedicles, ligamentum flavum, neural arch, facet joints, and interspinous ligaments. When fractures affect two contiguous columns or all three columns, these are considered unstable. Typically, if a fracture affects only one column, it is considered stable.

People with osteoporosis experience a decreased bone mineral density with a thinned cortex and decreased trabecula of the vertebra. Decreased density and strength of the vertebral body increase the risk for a compression fracture caused by relatively minor stress to the bone. Similarly, vertebral tumors, vertebral infection, or other calcium or bone demineralization disease processes such as renal failure can weaken the overall structure of the vertebra, allowing a fracture from a minor force.

CLINICAL PRESENTATION

Subjective

The primary presenting symptoms include point tenderness or generalized spinal discomfort. The pain may radiate from the neck to the shoulder or from the back to the hip. Numbness and tingling into the extremities can accompany spinal nerve irritation. Motor and sensory loss can accompany a spinal cord injury. The clinician should ask about symptoms that may indicate myelopathy or CES.

For the patient presenting with a potential spinal fracture, the clinician must understand how the neck or back pain began. Explore whether there is a traumatic injury, such as an MVC, or an insidious onset of pain that could occur with a fracture from osteoporosis or vertebral osteomyelitis. The mechanism of injury not only helps to guide needed imaging, but also gives some insight to the type of potential fracture pattern.

Some patients who present for their first evaluation after a traumatic injury may not experience neck or back pain. Some patients are distracted from noticing their neck or back pain by other overwhelming injuries. For those patients who have an insidious onset of spinal pain, the clinician must consider the potential for underlying pathology leading to a fracture. The clinician should ask about any constitutional symptoms (e.g., fever, unexplained weight loss, or change in appetite), as well as any red-flag symptoms (e.g., history of IV drug use).

Objective

Any patient with the potential for a spinal fracture requires a thorough neurovascular examination, including pulses; skin temperature; capillary refill; strength, sensation, and deep tendon reflexes; and inspection for edema or ecchymoses that may be present at the neck or back, as well as over the chest, abdomen, or pelvis. Lap-belt injuries will have contusions or ecchymosis over the anterior iliac spine. Hematoma and forward shift or "step off" of the spinous processes on palpation are an indication of an unstable fracture. Point tenderness over the vertebra may reveal a fracture. Percussion over a vertebral fracture can also elicit pain. If there is suspected CES, myelopathy, or spinal cord injury, evaluate for clonus, Babinski's reflex, bulbocavernosus reflex, rectal sphincter tone, and perineal sensation.

Many vertebral compression fractures may be found incidentally on other radiology examinations without indication or complaint of acute injury. An acute onset of vertebral compression fracture may occur from coughing, sneezing, or lifting. The fractures commonly occur between T8 and L4. Examination may be normal, or a patient may have kyphosis and midline spine tenderness to palpation. The location of the pain is specific to the level of injury and correlates well with radiology findings.

DIAGNOSTIC REASONING

Given the patient history, presenting symptoms, and physical examination, diagnostic considerations should include:

- Pott's disease
- Renal failure
- Spinal malignancy
- Osteomyelitis
- Hemangioma of vertebral body

Diagnostic Tests

The standard imaging study for those suspected of having a vertebral fracture includes the anterior/posterior (AP) and lateral views of the injured portion of the spine. An open-mouth odontoid view of the C1 to C2 vertebra is necessary to supplement the AP view of the cervical spine after a trauma with neck pain to evaluate for a C2 odontoid process fracture. The AP images are used to evaluate for fractures of the dens, the transverse processes, and the occipital condyles. Widening of the space between the pedicles may indicate a burst fracture of the vertebra body, whereas misalignment of the spinous processes can be indicative of a fractured or dislocated facet joint.

The lateral views of the spine are used to evaluate for fractures of the spinous process, vertebral body, and facet joints. Anterior soft tissue swelling of the cervical spine may be noted. Vertebral body misalignment on the lateral view may indicate instability, fracture, dislocation, and/or spondylolisthesis. Lateral flexion and extension views of the vertebrae may be necessary to evaluate for instability.

CT provides further diagnostic value when assessing a fracture pattern or stability and when a suspected fracture is not visible on plain films. CT provides optimal views of posterior vertebrae and the neural arch. Trauma centers frequently will obtain a CT of the spine initially for trauma patients with suspected neck or back injury and bypass the x-ray imaging. An MRI is indicated in situations when further soft tissue imaging (e.g., spinal cord or intervertebral disc) of the spine is necessary. Edema of soft tissue and the spinal cord and edema from fractures can be identified on MRI. An MRI or bone scan can be useful to visualize a stress fracture or hidden (occult) fracture that cannot be identified on plain x-rays.

Differential Diagnoses

Differential diagnoses include the following:

- Coccyx pain
- Degenerative disc disease
- Vertebral facet arthropathy
- Disc herniation
- Spondylolysis
- Spondylolisthesis
- Osteoporosis
- Hyperparathyroidism
- Musculoskeletal pain
- Visceral injury

MANAGEMENT

Although patients who experience major trauma will typically present to the emergency department (ED) for evaluation and management, the primary care clinician may certainly be expected to provide initial evaluation of a person with a suspected fracture. Patients who present to the ED will have immobilization and spinal precautions put in place until they are evaluated and cleared.

If the patient has an acute spinal fracture, they will be treated nonsurgical with the proper cervical collar, halo device, or thoraco-lumbosacral orthosis (TLSO) immobilization, based upon the fracture pattern, stability, and extent of the injury. A clinician must keep in mind that sometimes fractures may not be seen on the first evaluation but then show up on imaging 1 to 2 weeks after the injury. For patients who have no identified fracture on initial evaluation after a trauma and have an unremarkable neurological examination but continue to have neck or back pain, it may be necessary to provide immobilization (e.g., cervical collar) for a week or two and then reexamine and do further x-rays.

Although some clinicians choose to refer patients to a spinal specialist for care, it is not unusual for a primary care provider to evaluate and manage patients with vertebral insufficiency fractures but without neurological symptoms. Insufficiency fractures may be due to osteoporosis or long-term steroid use. Additionally, patients may fall at home and experience an injury with neck or back pain and a potential vertebral fracture. These patients may choose not to go to the emergency department but present initially to their primary care provider because the pain is not improving.

The goals for managing compression fractures of thoracic or lumbar vertebrae are pain relief and stabilization, maintaining function, preventing future fractures, and maintaining quality of life. A majority of patients with a vertebral compression fracture can be treated nonsurgically. Compression fractures can take many forms, more typically a wedge shape with most of the compression on the anterior vertebral body. Patients with a compression fracture with less than a 20-degree wedge shape and without disruption of the posterior elements of the vertebrae can be treated with bracing, using a Jewett extension brace or TLSO for 8 to 10 weeks. There is some growing controversy about the benefit of bracing and preventing further progression of the fracture. The patient should be instructed to avoid lifting more than 10 pounds, bending, and twisting.

Nasal calcitonin may be used for pain management after an acute vertebral compression fracture. This is usually initiated early after the fracture and often only used for 4 weeks. Oral pain medication may be used, depending on the degree of discomfort. NSAIDs should be avoided as they interfere with bone healing. A short course of opioids or tramadol may be warranted to assist with significant pain. If muscle spasm is present, a muscle relaxer can be utilized. Lidocaine patches applied topically to the neck or back may provide adjunctive pain relief.

Pain relief or pain tolerance assists in increased mobility and physical therapy with the goal to increase core strength. Vertebroplasty, a surgical procedure for compression fracture, has fallen out of favor due to lack of evidence to support the procedure. Another similar surgical procedure, kyphoplasty, has limited evidence but is indicated for patients who fail to improve with conservative management.

FOLLOW-UP AND REFERRAL

Any patient with a neurological deficit on examination should be referred to a spine specialist for further evaluation and management. Patients with significant potentially unstable fractures should be referred to a spine specialist for further evaluation and management. For conservative management, the patient should be seen within 1 week of the first visit to assess pain level, function, and neurological integrity. Physical therapy referral should be made as soon as pain is managed and fracture healing is progressing. The goal of physical therapy is to strengthen trunk flexion and extensor muscles. Prevention of other fractures is warranted. Prevention includes weight-bearing exercises and appropriate medication management including bisphosphonates, calcitonin, calcium and vitamin D, parathyroid hormone, denosumab, and/or teriparatide.

Patient Education: Vertebral Fracture

During recovery, patients should avoid bending, stooping, twisting, or lifting anything over 10 pounds. Walking is a beneficial activity. Additional patient education should include smoking cessation and avoidance of excessive alcohol. Weight-bearing and muscle-strengthening exercises should be encouraged when healing of the fracture is complete. A fall-risk assessment should be performed as part of a fall-prevention strategy.

REFERENCES

Cauda Equina Syndrome

Greenhalgh S, Finucane L, Mercer C, et al. (2018). Assessment and management of cauda equina syndrome. *Musculoskeletal science & practice, 37*, 69–74. https://doi.org/10.1016/j.msksp.2018.06.002

Long B, Koyfman A, Gottlieb M. (2020). Evaluation and management of cauda equina syndrome in the emergency department. *The American journal of emergency medicine, 38*(1), 143–148. https://doi.org/10.1016/j.ajem.2019.158402

Quaile A. (2019). Cauda equina syndrome-the questions. *International orthopaedics, 43*(4), 957–961. https://doi.org/10.1007/s00264-018-4208-0

Todd NV. (2017). Guidelines for cauda equina syndrome. Red flags and white flags. Systematic review and implications for triage. *British journal of neurosurgery, 31*(3), 336–339. https://doi.org/10.1080/02688697.2017.1297364

Cervical Muscle Strain

Cohen SP, Hooten WM. (2017). Advances in the diagnosis and management of neck pain. *BMJ (Clinical research ed.). 358*, j3221. https://doi.org/10.1136/bmj.j3221

DePasse JM, Durand W, Palumbo MA, et al. (2019). Sex- and sport-specific epidemiology of cervical spine injuries sustained during sporting activities. *World neurosurgery, 122*, e540–e545. https://doi.org/10.1016/j.wneu.2018.10.097

Martel JW, Potter SB. (2019). Evaluation and management of neck and back pain. *Seminars in neurology, 39*(1), 41–52. https://doi.org/10.1055/s-0038-1677044

Tanaka N, Atesok K, Nakanishi K, et al. (2018). Pathology and treatment of traumatic cervical spine syndrome: whiplash injury. *Advances in orthopedics, 2018*, 4765050. https://doi.org/10.1155/2018/4765050

Vijiaratnam N, Williams DR, Bertram KL. (2018). Neck pain: what if it is not musculoskeletal? *Australian journal of general practice, 47*(5), 279–282. https://doi.org/10.31128/afp-10-17-4358

Xu Y, Wang Y, Chen J. (2020). The comorbidity of mental and physical disorders with self-reported chronic back or neck pain: results from the China Mental Health Survey. *Journal of affective disorders, 260,* 334–341. https://doi.org/10.1016/j.jad.2019.08.089

Cervical Spondylosis

Battié MC, Joshi AB, Gibbons LE, ISSLS Degenerative Spinal Phenotypes Group (2019). Degenerative disc disease: what is in a name? *Spine, 44*(21), 1523–1529. https://doi.org/10.1097/BRS.0000000000003103

Cho SK, Safir S, Lombardi JM, et al. (2019). Cervical spine deformity: indications, considerations, and surgical outcomes. *The Journal of the American Academy of Orthopaedic Surgeons, 27*(12), e555–e567. https://doi.org/10.5435/JAAOS-D-17-00546

Kos N, Gradisnik L, Velnar T. (2019). A brief review of the degenerative intervertebral disc disease. *Medical archives, 73*(6), 421–424. https://doi.org/10.5455/medarh.2019.73.421-424

Sun Y, Muheremu A, Tian W. (2018). Atypical symptoms in patients with cervical spondylosis: comparison of the treatment effect of different surgical approaches. *Medicine 97*(20), e10731. https://doi.org/10.1097/MD.0000000000010731

Theodore N. (2020). Degenerative cervical spondylosis. *The New England journal of medicine, 383*(2), 159–168. https://doi.org/10.1056/NEJMra2003558

Weber C, Behbahani M, Baardsen R, et al. (2017). Patients' beliefs about diagnosis and treatment of cervical spondylosis with radiculopathy. *Acta neurochirurgica, 159*(12), 2379–2384. https://doi.org/10.1007/s00701-017-3356-0

Herniated Lumbar Disc (Herniated Nucleus Pulposus)

Anitua E, Padilla S. (2018). Biologic therapies to enhance intervertebral disc repair. *Regenerative medicine, 13*(1), 55–72. https://doi.org/10.2217/rme-2017-0111

Arts MP, Kuršumović A, Miller LE, et al. (2019). Comparison of treatments for lumbar disc herniation: systematic review with network meta-analysis. *Medicine, 98*(7), e14410. https://doi.org/10.1097/md.0000000000014410

Benzakour T, Igoumenou V, Mavrogenis AF, et al. (2019). Current concepts for lumbar disc herniation. *International orthopaedics, 43*(4), 841–851. https://doi.org/10.1007/s00264-018-4247-6

Chen BL, Guo JB, Zhang HW, et al. (2018). Surgical versus non-operative treatment for lumbar disc herniation: a systematic review and meta-analysis. *Clinical rehabilitation, 32*(2), 146–160. https://doi.org/10.1177/0269215517719952

Cunha C, Silva AJ, Pereira P, et al. (2018). The inflammatory response in the regression of lumbar disc herniation. *Arthritis research & therapy, 20*(1), 251. https://doi.org/10.1186/s13075-018-1743-4

Hareni N, Strömqvist F, Strömqvist B, et al. (2019). Predictors of satisfaction after lumbar disc herniation surgery in elderly. *BMC musculoskeletal disorders, 20*(1), 594. https://doi.org/10.1186/s12891-019-2975-4

Ilyas H, Savage J. (2018). Lumbar disk herniation and SPORT: a review of the literature. *Clinical spine surgery, 31*(9), 366–372. https://doi.org/10.1097/bsd.0000000000000696

Kim JH, van Rijn RM, van Tulder MW, et al. (2018). Diagnostic accuracy of diagnostic imaging for lumbar disc herniation in adults with low back pain or sciatica is unknown; a systematic review. *Chiropractic & manual therapies, 26,* 37. https://doi.org/10.1186/s12998-018-0207-x

Yousif S, Musa A, Ahmed A, et al. (2020). Correlation between findings in physical examination, magnetic resonance imaging, and nerve conduction studies in lumbosacral radiculopathy caused by lumbar intervertebral disc herniation. *Advances in orthopedics, 2020,* 9719813. https://doi.org/10.1155/2020/9719813

Low Back Pain

Becker BA, Childress MA. (2019). Nonspecific low back pain and return to work. *American family physician, 100*(11), 697–703.

Maher C, Underwood M, Buchbinder R. (2017). Non-specific low back pain. *Lancet, 389*(10070), 736–747. https://doi.org/10.1016/s0140-6736(16)30970-9

Park J, Krause-Parello CA, Barnes CM. (2020). A narrative review of movement-based mind-body interventions: effects of yoga, tai chi, and qigong for back pain patients. *Holistic nursing practice, 34*(1), 3–23. https://doi.org/10.1097/hnp.0000000000000360

do Carmo Silva Parreira P, Maher CG, Latimer J, et al. (2015). Can patients identify what triggers their back pain? Secondary analysis of a case-crossover study. *Pain, 156*(10), 1913–1919. https://doi.org/10.1097/j.pain.0000000000000252

Pfieffer ML. (2020). How to care for adults with low back pain in the primary care setting. *Nursing, 50*(2), 48–55. https://doi.org/10.1097/01.nurse.0000651624.64152.11

Popescu A, Lee H. (2020). Neck pain and lower back pain. *The Medical clinics of North America, 104*(2), 279–292. https://doi.org/10.1016/j.mcna.2019.11.003

Urits I, Burshtein A, Sharma M, et al. (2019). Low back pain, a comprehensive review: pathophysiology, diagnosis, and treatment. *Current pain and headache reports, 23*(3), 23. https://doi.org/10.1007/s11916-019-0757-1

Vlaeyen JWS, Maher CG, Wiech K, et al. (2018). Low back pain. Nature reviews. *Disease primers, 4*(1), 52. https://doi.org/10.1038/s41572-018-0052-1

Will JS, Bury DC, Miller JA. (2018). Mechanical low back pain. *American family physician, 98*(7), 421–428.

Lumbar Spinal Stenosis

Baker JF. (2020). Evaluation and treatment of tandem spinal stenosis. *The Journal of the American Academy of Orthopaedic Surgeons, 28*(6), 229–239. https://doi.org/10.5435/jaaos-d-18-00726

Deer T, Sayed D, Michels J., et al. (2019). A review of lumbar spinal stenosis with intermittent neurogenic claudication: disease and diagnosis. *Pain medicine, 20*(Suppl 2), S32–S44. https://doi.org/10.1093/pm/pnz161

Diwan S, Sayed D, Deer TR, et al. (2019). An algorithmic approach to treating lumbar spinal stenosis: an evidenced-based approach. *Pain medicine, 20*(Suppl 2), S23–S31. https://doi.org/10.1093/pm/pnz133

Lafian AM, Torralba KD. (2018). Lumbar spinal stenosis in older adults. *Rheumatic diseases clinics of North America, 44*(3), 501–512. https://pubmed.ncbi.nlm.nih.gov/30001789/

Oster BA, Kikanloo SR, Levine NL, et al. (2020). Systematic review of outcomes following 10-year mark of spine patient outcomes research trial (SPORT) for spinal stenosis. *Spine, 45*(12), 832–836. https://doi.org/10.1097/brs.0000000000003323

Patel EA, Perloff MD. (2018). Radicular pain syndromes: cervical, lumbar, and spinal stenosis. *Seminars in neurology, 38*(6), 634–639. https://doi.org/10.1055/s-0038-1673680

Vertebal Fractures

Browner BD, Jupiter JB, Krettek C, et al. (2020). *Skeletal trauma: basic science, management, and reconstruction.* Philadelphia PA: Elsevier.

Denis F. (1983). The three column spine and its significance in the classification of acute thoracolumbar spinal injuries. *Spine, 8*(8), 817–831. https://doi.org/10.1097/00007632-198311000-00003

Garfin SR, Eismont FJ, Bell GR, et al. (2018). *Rothman-Simeone: the spine e-book.* Elsevier Health Sciences.

Magnusson E, Spina N, Fernando ND. (2018). Classifications in brief: the thoracolumbar injury classification. *Clinical orthopaedics and related research, 476*(1), 160–166. https://doi.org/10.1007/s11999.0000000000000004

Rosenthal BD, Boody BS, Jenkins TJ, et al. (2018). Thoracolumbar burst fractures. *Clinical spine surgery, 31*(4), 143–151. https://doi.org/10.1097/bsd.0000000000000634

van Den Hauwe L, Sundgren PC, Flanders AE. (2020). Spinal trauma and spinal cord injury (SCI). In: J. Hodler et al, eds, *Diseases of the brain, head and neck, spine 2020–2023: Diagnostic imaging.* (pp. 231–240). Springer.

RESOURCES

Spine Universe: trusted source for quality spine health information
  https://www.spineuniverse.com/
Herniated Disk. OrthoInfo/American Academy of Orthopedic Surgeons
https://orthoinfo.aaos.org/en/diseases—conditions/herniated-disk/
Lumbar Spinal Stenosis. OrthoInfo/American Academy of Orthopedic Surgeons
  https://orthoinfo.aaos.org/en/diseases—conditions/lumbar-spinal-stenosis/
Neck Sprain. OrthoInfo/ American Academy of Orthopedic Surgeons
  https://orthoinfo.aaos.org/en/diseases—conditions/neck-sprain/
Spinal Stenosis. Cleveland Clinic
  https://my.clevelandclinic.org/health/diseases/17499-spinal-stenosis

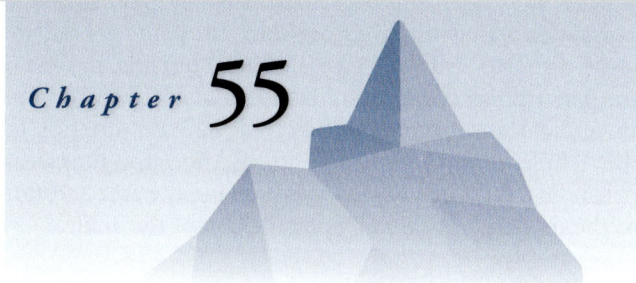

Chapter 55

Soft Tissue Disorders

Michael E. Zychowicz, DNP, ANP, ONP, FAAN, FAANP

Soft tissue disorders are extremely common and present frequently in primary care. These disorders are nonsystemic, focal, pathological syndromes involving periarticular tissues including muscles, tendons, ligaments, fasciae, aponeuroses, retinacula, bursae, and subcutaneous tissues. These disorders are classified as "nonarticular" disorders. Patients who present with a soft tissue disorder will frequently complain of regional pain such as "hip pain" or "elbow pain." This complaint often refers to pain in the general region of these joints, not in the joints themselves. Some may be a consequence of chronic, repetitive, low-grade trauma and overuse; many respond to conservative measures.

A general initial approach to these patients in the primary care setting is as follows:

- Exclude systemic disease.
- Eliminate aggravating factors.
- Explain the disorder.
- Provide pain relief on a short-term basis (e.g., medication, bracing, etc.).
- Educate about self-care and prognosis.
- Educate about prevention after this episode is resolved.

Underlying structural disorders are not uncommon even in healthy young adults and often contribute to pain syndromes. Body asymmetry is a common cause of many regional pain disorders.

BURSITIS

Bursitis, or inflammation of a bursa, is a common cause of painful musculoskeletal syndromes. Bursae are synovial sacs filled with synovial fluid, located between muscles, tendons, and bony prominences. Bursae cushion bony prominences from overlying muscles (deep bursae) or surface skin (superficial bursae); they may or may not communicate with the adjacent joint space. The bursa provides lubrication for movement of tendons over bones and can be affected by trauma, as in overuse, and by infection, inflammation, and neoplasms. The total number of bursae varies from person to person, but on average, this figure approaches 160. Some cases of bursitis may result from rheumatic disease and others from a pathological condition of adjoining tissues. It may be acute or chronic.

EPIDEMIOLOGY AND CAUSES

Bursitis is a common complaint, seen most often in patients who are skeletally mature. It is more common in males and tends to be more commonly associated with trauma (including overuse syndrome) in patients younger than 35 years. It is a common reason for visits to the primary care setting; the incidence is clearly related to increasing age. The incidence of bursitis of the lower extremities is increased by obesity. Bursitis commonly develops in the subdeltoid and subacromial bursa of the shoulder, the olecranon bursa of the elbow, the greater trochanteric bursa that is lateral to the hip, the ischial bursa, the prepatellar bursa of the knee, the pes anserine bursa that lies between the pes anserine tendons, and the retrocalcaneal bursa.

Trauma in the form of repetitive motion injury is a common cause of bursitis, as a result of constant friction between a bursa and musculoskeletal tissues surrounding it. Friction in turn causes irritation, edema, and inflammation. The end result is an engorged bursal sac with surrounding tissue that has become inflamed, tender, and painful. Movement around the bursa may result in increased pain and pressure. In turn, movement of the adjacent joint may be limited by the inflamed bursa. Aging connective tissues are at a higher risk for microtears with bursitis.

PATHOPHYSIOLOGY

Bursitis is an inflammatory process that may be acute or chronic. The exact etiology is often unknown. Bursitis may be caused by an infectious process, trauma (more common in patients younger than 35 years), repetitive movement disorders, pseudogout, gout, or neoplastic disease. Less often, it may be attributed to rheumatoid disease (especially with nodular or bilateral bursitis) or infection by *Mycobacterium tuberculosis* or *Candida* fungal infection. Far more commonly, however, septic bursitis is due to bacterial infection.

Up to 80% of septic bursitis cases are due to infection by *Staphylococcus aureus,* with 5% to 20% due to *Streptococcus* and other gram-positive skin flora, which are typically introduced via direct trauma that compromises the protective skin barrier. Immunocompromised conditions such as diabetes mellitus, HIV infection, chronic steroid use, or autoimmune conditions such as rheumatoid arthritis (RA) may all predispose the individual to septic bursitis, and causative trauma to the overlying skin surface may even be microscopic in nature.

Bursitis is essentially a soft tissue problem, rather than a joint problem such as arthritis, and often coexists with tendinitis or tenosynovitis. This overuse injury is characterized by repeated cycles of degeneration and regeneration with new collagen deposition. Synovial cells increase in thickness, and the normal bursal lining may be replaced by granulation tissue before eventual fibrosis. In turn, the bursa may become filled with transudative fluid with a high concentration of fibrin. At the conclusion of this inflammatory process, calcium deposition may occur proximal to the affected bursa.

CLINICAL PRESENTATION

Subjective

The presenting symptoms are usually pain and sometimes swelling over the known locations of bursal sacs, which may be accompanied by swelling and warmth over the involved bursa. When the subcutaneous bursal sacs (e.g., olecranon and prepatellar) are inflamed by systemic illnesses such as RA, gout, or infection, additional clues to diagnosis may include fever, chills, and arthralgias. The prepatellar and olecranon bursae frequently present with local redness, swelling, and warmth that must be distinguished from septic arthritis. Patients who develop subcutaneous bursitis may have a family history of articular problems. An occupational history may provide a clue to diagnosis. Some examples include "weaver's bottom" (ischial-gluteal bursitis), "miner's elbow" (olecranon bursitis), and "housemaid's knee" (prepatellar bursitis). Bursitis of a deep bursa is manifested by pain over the bursa with activity or direct pressure. The pain may radiate some distance, as in the case of gluteal bursitis, in which the patient may complain of pain in a sciatic distribution. In retrocalcaneal bursitis, there will be pain anterior to the Achilles tendon, just above its insertion into the calcaneus; the pain is aggravated by squeezing the area anterior to the tendon, as well as by dorsiflexion of the ankle.

Objective

Pain may be referred to other musculoskeletal structures contiguous to the bursa. Careful examination may be necessary to identify the precise source of the pain. Clinical signs and symptoms include induration, erythema, and effusion over the bursae. Gross distention of the bursal sac may be apparent. If there is significant limitation of range of motion (ROM) or pain on flexion, a coincident arthritis may be present. Bursitis may also develop from repeated microtrauma, leading to effusion and thickening of the bursal sac. As irritation and inflammation continue, the bursa is at risk for calcification and development of adhesions around the bursa, thereby limiting tendon movement.

DIAGNOSTIC REASONING

Diagnostic Tests

Laboratory findings will usually be normal with aseptic (noninfected) bursitis. Erythrocyte sedimentation rate and C-reactive protein may be elevated by gout, RA, or infection. In cases of gout, uric acid levels may be elevated; however, serum uric acid may be within normal range with a gouty flare-up. With infectious leukocytosis, the white blood cell (WBC) count may be elevated. Diagnosis of aseptic bursitis should be made, based on clinical examination and patient symptomatology.

Differential Diagnosis

When formulating a diagnosis, RA, gout, pseudogout, and septic arthritis must be ruled out. Frequently, aseptic bursitis can be a clinical diagnosis based upon history and physical findings. An x-ray image showing the involved joint or bursa, with or without calcified deposits, may be helpful to determine calcific tendonitis, calcification of the bursa, or degenerative joint disease. Aspiration and analysis of fluid from the affected bursa or possibly the underlying joint may be helpful to identify evidence of infection or gout. The fluid is cultured to assess the presence of bacterial infection. Elevated WBCs, low glucose, and elevated protein are characteristic of infection. An elevated red blood cell count is associated with trauma and bleeding into the bursa.

MANAGEMENT

Medical management and treatment of bursitis include avoidance of activities that can lead to irritation of the bursa and application of moist heat or ice to the affected area every 4 hours for 15 to 20 minutes. The use of moist heat versus ice is an individual preference. Immobilization of the affected area may help reduce pain and edema by providing support. Having the patient wear padding over the inflamed bursa can provide a layer of protection over body parts such as the elbow or knee. ROM exercises can be utilized if needed to prevent loss of mobility and to help maintain motion. Patients may use NSAIDs for symptom management.

If symptoms recur, an injection of a long-acting corticosteroid (triamcinolone 2 to 10 mg, hydrocortisone 25 to 37.5 mg, methylprednisolone 20 to 40 mg, or dexamethasone 4 to 16 mg, each mixed with an equal volume of lidocaine hydrochloride 1%) into the affected bursa is recommended, followed by application of ice for 10 to 20 minutes. Injections should not be repeated more than every 12 weeks. For fluid-filled bursae, aspiration of the fluid should be performed before injection. Additionally, if the clinician is suspicious for infection, a steroid should not be injected. Physical therapy through stretching and strengthening as well as modalities such as ultrasound may provide symptom relief. Failure of conservative therapy for 6 weeks should warrant orthopedic referral.

Patient Education: Bursitis

Patient education is an important part of recovery and prevention. Encouraging a patient to decrease certain activities may speed up recovery. Encourage preliminary stretching and warm-up exercises before activities to maintain flexibility and strength. If medications are part of the treatment regimen, reinforcement of proper administration and a discussion of their side effects are recommended.

TENDINITIS/TENOSYNOVITIS

Tendinitis is the inflammation of a tendon, which usually occurs at its point of insertion into bone or at the point of muscular origin. The term *tenosynovitis* refers to inflammation involving the tendon and the synovial sheaths surrounding the tendon. Common tendinitis/tenosynovitis syndromes include supraspinatus tendinitis, lateral epicondylitis or "tennis elbow," bicipital tendinitis, de Quervain's tenosynovitis (inflammation of the abductor pollicis longus [APL] and extensor pollicis longus and brevis tendons; discussed separately later in the chapter), "trigger finger" (volar flexor tenosynovitis; discussed separately later in the chapter), patellar tendinitis (patellar tendinosis or "basketball player's knee"), and Achilles tendinitis. Table 55.1 presents common sites for overuse injuries.

EPIDEMIOLOGY AND CAUSES

Overuse injuries frequently cause tendinitis, and they occur in both athletes and nonathletes of all ages. It is difficult to determine the true incidence because frequently overuse injuries are not brought to the attention of a health-care provider. Despite this, such injuries account for more than 50% of the injuries seen in a primary care setting, making them the most frequently encountered athletic injury. This problem occurs with a slightly increased frequency in males and is most likely related to sports or repetitive activity.

Athletes and manual laborers are especially prone to tendinitis because of repetitive use. Painful areas of a tendon are often labeled *tendinitis*, implying an inflammatory nature of the lesion. It is unclear, however, whether inflammation is truly present in all forms of the pathology. More chronic pathology tends to have a more

TABLE 55.1	Common Anatomical Sites: Overuse Syndrome
Anatomical Site	**Overuse Syndrome**
Shoulder	Rotator cuff tendinitis Thoracic outlet syndrome
Forearm	Lateral epicondylitis Medial epicondylitis Ulnar nerve entrapments
Hand and wrist	Carpal tunnel syndrome De Quervain's syndrome "Trigger finger"
Leg and foot	Chondromalacia patellae Iliotibial band syndrome Shin splints Achilles tendinitis Plantar fasciitis Stress fracture

degenerative component. Some sources advocate the use of the term *tendinosis* for this reason. *Tenosynovitis* may result from inflammatory arthropathies such as RA or gout but can be from overuse as well. Adults who overuse a joint with repeated motion are most likely to develop tendinitis. Some classifications are based on degree of function and whether there is a partial tear or complete rupture of the tendon.

The potential for repetitive use injury is enhanced by a wide variety of predisposing factors. Obesity and underlying anatomical imperfections aggravated by exercise or repeated motions have been identified as risk factors. In addition, poor cardiovascular or musculoskeletal conditioning, underlying cardiovascular disease, arthritis (osteoarthritis [OA] or RA), gout, and stress may all contribute to the development of overuse syndrome. In athletes, overtraining, running on uneven surfaces, poor equipment, inadequate footwear, and leg-length discrepancy may all contribute. In workers, unhealthy physical and emotional work environments are both thought to contribute. Repeatedly performing arm and hand movements with a very short repetitive cycle of less than 30 seconds during one's daily job is a risk factor. Repeatedly performing the same task in a short period of time in a factory can impose the same level of risk. Vibration, a cold environment, and the use of some specific hand tools also are considered risk factors.

Risk Factors: Overuse Syndrome

- Arthritis (OA and RA)
- Congenital defects
- Diabetes mellitus
- Ganglion cyst
- Gout
- Hobbies (knitting, musical instruments, electronic games)
- Hormonal factors (pregnancy, oral contraceptive use, menopause, thyroid disorders, hysterectomy with bilateral oophorectomy)
- Hypertension
- Impaired circulation
- Inflammation of tendons and tendon sheath
- Obesity
- Occupational activities (computer usage, cash registers)
- Paget's disease
- Raynaud's phenomenon
- Renal disease
- Sports (racquet sports, golf, softball, running)
- Underlying anatomical abnormalities

PATHOPHYSIOLOGY

Exact pathophysiological entities involved with tendinitis and tenosynovitis have not been clearly established. It is understood that tenosynovitis involves inflammation of the synovial-lined sheath around one or more tendons, whereas tendinitis involves inflammation of the tendinous tissue itself. Inflammation may be caused by repetitive microtrauma, which leads to repeated cycles of inflammation and tissue regeneration, characterized by fibroblast proliferation, collagen production, and resultant tissue contraction. Because flexor tendons typically run in tight fibro-osseous tunnels, thickening of the surrounding sheath caused by inflammatory changes may in turn limit movement and cause pain as the trapped tendon attempts to glide within the thickened, tight sheath. The parietal and visceral layers of the synovium that surround flexor tendons typically provide nutrition and stability to the tendons, and they also allow smooth movement of these connective tissues without extensive friction. Tenosynovitis may also be associated with an inflammatory or infectious process.

Tendinitis is usually associated with degenerative changes in the tendon. Calcium deposits may also be noted along the length of the tendon, known as *calcific tendinitis;* this is especially common in the shoulder joint and Achilles tendon. These tendons tend to stiffen without treatment. Loss of function often follows because they become progressively weaker and may eventually rupture.

CLINICAL PRESENTATION

Subjective

Patients typically complain of pain and swelling over a localized area of tendon. This may be in a region where the tendon passes through a fibro-osseous tunnel or at the point where a tendon attaches to the bone. Pain is usually worse with motion, especially motion that stretches the involved tendon. Patients who have significant tenosynovitis will describe squeaking, rubbing, crepitus, or sometimes a triggering or catching sensation. The pain associated with tendinitis can have a gradual or acute onset and can be associated with a repetitive-use activity or acute injury.

Objective

Tendinitis and tenosynovitis are typically clinical diagnoses. Early imaging is usually of minimal benefit, except in calcific tendinitis where calcium deposits in or around the tendon are seen on routine x-rays. A thorough history is essential, including all extracurricular activities as these may be the cause of the inflammation. The physical examination should include palpating any tender areas and ruling out any articular involvement. Swelling is usually minimal in tendinitis, but it may be pronounced in cases of infection or with inflammatory causes of tenosynovitis. Examination may reveal localized pain, swelling, and tenderness. The pain will worsen with certain motions that stretch the involved tendon or actively make the tendon work (stress the tendon) against resistance. Crepitus and sometimes triggering can be palpated if a significant tenosynovitis has developed. These signs vary, depending on the anatomical site of the inflammation:

- Tendinitis/tenosynovitis of finger flexors: possible fingertip numbness from median nerve compression may be present. Finger may physically get stuck in a flexed position (trigger finger). Crepitus and pain may be present with flexion and extension.
- Rotator cuff tendinitis: pain and tenderness are felt over the subacromial space with active motion of the shoulder including external rotation, forward flexion, and abduction. Pain can be triggered by overhead lifting. Lateral arm pain may be present. An "empty can" test is positive for pain and negative for weakness. In this test, the patient's affected arm is abducted to 90 degrees, in neutral rotation (the thumb is pointed toward the ground). The patient is instructed to turn their arm and hand forward as if emptying a can. The examiner places their fingers on the outstretched arm near the hand and applies downward pressure. This stresses the muscle and tendon of the most common inflamed rotator cuff tendons (supraspinatus).
- Lateral epicondylitis: pain over lateral epicondyle is worse with gripping or shaking hands. The patient may complain of stiffness at night and difficulty extending the arm in the morning.
- Achilles tendinitis: pain is felt at the posterior heel with pushing off while walking or running.
- Patellar tendinitis: pain is felt over the anterior aspect of the knee anteriorly with jumping or running.

If an inflammatory disease is present, associated redness, soft tissue swelling, and warmth may be present. Inflammatory processes of the tendon sheaths most commonly involve the dorsum of the hands, plantar surface of the feet, and ankle and may cause marked soft tissue swelling. The ROM of contiguous joints may be limited by pain.

DIAGNOSTIC REASONING

Diagnostic Tests

Plain films may be useful to rule out other potential causes of pain in affected areas, but they will not show tendinitis. An exception is calcific tendinitis, for which plain radiography can reveal calcium in a tendon, commonly the Achilles or rotator cuff tendons. Magnetic resonance imaging (MRI) is the diagnostic gold standard for tendinitis but should be reserved for patients who have failed conservative treatment or have weakness of the extremity. Generally, the diagnosis can almost always be made clinically without the need for imaging, including MRI.

Differential Diagnosis

Differential diagnoses to rule out include fracture, avulsion of the tendon, inflammatory arthritis, RA, and compartment syndrome. It is often not possible to differentiate tendinitis from bursitis, and because the two conditions are generally treated the same, it is clinically not necessary to do so. The pain in tendinitis is localized to the side of the joint where the tendon insertion is located. Infectious tenosynovitis occurs primarily in the hand. In addition, the tenderness and swelling are located along the synovial lines proximally instead of at the insertion site, and the pain is more marked, as are swelling and erythema. Erythrocyte sedimentation rate, C-reactive protein, and WBC count will likely be elevated in the case of infection.

Definitive diagnosis of tenosynovitis requires careful musculoskeletal examination, confirming the tendon source of the symptoms and excluding pathology from other contiguous musculoskeletal structures, including joints, bursae, and nerves. However, an inflammatory tenosynovitis of the dorsum of the hand or foot may require aspiration of synovial fluid, examination, and culture to confirm the diagnosis and determine whether an infectious process is present.

MANAGEMENT

Treatment depends on the stage of healing of the damaged tissue of the musculoskeletal system. There are three phases of healing: (1) inflammation, (2) proliferation of new collagen and ground substance, and (3) scar remodeling and maturation.

Initial management should include protection, rest, ice, compression, and elevation (PRICE). The injury should be protected and rehabilitated in parallel with the healing process. The injured tissue needs to be stressed to activate collagen remodeling and realignment but also protected from overstress, which will cause reinjury and incite a further inflammatory response. Taping and bracing can both be helpful in providing protection. Ice is useful for treating pain, hemorrhage, and edema. It induces vasoconstriction, which results in a decrease in local blood flow. Ice should be applied for 15 to 20 minutes; direct contact with the skin should be avoided to prevent cold injury. Treatment may be repeated every 1 to 2 hours in acute cases. In lowering the temperature, ice decreases metabolism and enzymatic function; furthermore, it slows the inflammatory process. It is useful during the first 48 hours in acute cases.

Compression in concert with cold therapy helps to reduce swelling. Elevation decreases edema by aiding lymphatic and venous return. In acute ankle sprains, for example, elevation has been shown to be one of the most effective methods of reducing swelling. The objective is to treat the initial symptoms with these techniques to prevent prolonged inflammation and avoid new tissue disruption. In addition, measures of relative rest are used to protect the tissue from further injury.

In the second stage of healing, the objective is to gradually introduce stress and apply modalities to increase collagen production, size, cross-linking, and alignment. The rate of collagen fiber formation is directly related to the functional state of the affected area. The collagen fibers reorient themselves in line with the tensile force applied to the tissue. In the third stage, the objective is to make the collagen as elastic as possible and decrease formation of scar tissue. Progressive stress is placed on tissue to promote an increase in collagen fibril size and to increase cross-linking in tissues. Flexibility training is needed to decrease cross-linking in the joint capsule. Home exercises or formal physical therapy can assist healing in stages 2 and 3.

Immobilization may be counterproductive, and absolute rest should be limited to 1 to 2 days at most until the inflammation response has settled or in severe, chronic cases of tendinitis, after active rest has failed. *Active rest* means that the injured area can be used, but it should be protected from significant stress, which may cause further damage. The frequency and intensity of an activity may be decreased or altered, for example, but all activity should not be completely eliminated. Physical therapy is a cornerstone of treatment and can aid in the development of an individualized plan for the patient. Ice plays an important role once exercise and activity are resumed. It should be applied at the end of every exercise session to help prevent recurrence of inflammation and swelling.

Heat is effective after 48 hours in the acute phase and in the chronic phase. After the acute phase of the healing process, heat is useful in improving blood flow, relieving muscle spasm, and decreasing tissue stiffness, allowing greater ease of deformation. A highly beneficial form of deep heat is ultrasound because the high-frequency waves render the tissues less stiff and more susceptible to remodeling by applied tensile forces. Ultrasound also increases local circulation.

NSAIDs can also help with tendinitis on two fronts. First, they decrease inflammation in the affected area; second, they help with palliative relief for the patient. NSAIDs are probably best prescribed at maximum dose for 10 to 14 days. If no benefit is noted in the first 3 days, it is unlikely further benefit will be gained. An alternate NSAID may be attempted. Although widely prescribed, they have not been shown to effectively shorten recovery time; they may be useful in their analgesic effect in supporting a patient's compliance with physical therapy.

Corticosteroids may be indicated in cases of chronic overuse syndromes. They should never be injected directly into a tendon because this can significantly increase the risk of tendon rupture. Tendon sheath injections, into the space between the tendon and the tendon sheath by contrast, are quite effective in treating tenosynovitis.

Activity generally needs to be decreased for 5 to 10 days after an injection. Intra-articular steroid injections can also be given when there is significant reactive synovitis with effusion. Providers should be taught proper injection technique before administering a joint or tendon sheath injection.

FOLLOW-UP AND REFERRAL

Soft tissue injuries cause considerable pain, discomfort, and potential dysfunction. A comprehensive team approach, structured in a Circle of Caring model, is necessary for these patients to avoid significant sequelae. As noted in the section on management, interventions need to be geared toward the stage of healing to be effective. The balance between rest and healing and the danger of erring in either direction can be great without thoughtful consideration by a team of providers, as well as maximum hearing of the patient's voice. Athletes may be overanxious and overdo activities; unhappy employees might have a psychogenic component to their pathology.

Referral to physical therapy is essential, as is referral to an orthopedic specialist if there is any question as to the nature of pathology. Treatment must be individualized, and the patient must be central to developing the plan of care. Patients requiring corticosteroid injections should be referred if the provider is not trained to deliver this injection. Occupational therapists can assist with fitting of splints or orthotic devices if necessary. Conservative management should be attempted for approximately 4 to 6 weeks. If the patient still has pain or dysfunction despite conservative treatment, orthopedic referral should be considered.

Patient Education: Tendinitis and Tenosynovitis

It is important that patients understand the nature of their injury and be involved in the plan of care. In the case of athletes, careful evaluation of training schedules and circumstances surrounding the injury is essential so that appropriate preventive measures can be put in place to support healing and avoid future injury. In the case of a work-related repetitive motion injury, evaluation of the workplace and nature of the work may be necessary.

For cases in which the patient's job is the source of repetitive strain injury, restrictions on work activity may be necessary. A careful and thorough occupational history can help make determinations about the contributing factors in the patient's job environment. A comprehensive ergonomic worksite evaluation may be conducted by a physical or occupational therapist in identifying specific problems. Ultimately, however, patients with severe forms of repetitive strain injury may need to change occupations.

HAND AND WRIST DISORDERS

CARPAL TUNNEL SYNDROME

Carpal tunnel syndrome (CTS) is the most common cause of peripheral nerve compression, affecting approximately 3% to 6% of adults. Pain and/or numbness affect some part of the median nerve distribution. Symptoms tend to affect the dominant hand, but more than one-half of patients experience bilateral symptoms. Females are three times more likely than males to be diagnosed with CTS.

EPIDEMIOLOGY AND CAUSES

CTS is most common in people aged 40 to 60 years and affects females significantly more frequently than males, most commonly middle-aged and pregnant females. Roughly 80% of patients are older than 40 years. Any condition that reduces the size or space of the carpal tunnel can cause compression of the medial nerve. Any movement that causes the wrist to repeatedly flex or extend out of the neutral position or that places pressure on the median nerve may contribute to the development of CTS. Direct compression may result from neoplasms, a misaligned fracture, or trauma to the carpal tunnel. The greatest risk is found in occupations that require repeated flexion or extension of the wrist, use of hand tools that require forceful gripping, or use of hand tools that vibrate. CTS has been reported to occur spontaneously, most often during conditions that affect hormone balance (e.g., pregnancy, menopause, myxedematous hypothyroidism, diabetes mellitus) or in patients with other underlying musculoskeletal disorders (e.g., gout, RA, acute injury, acromegaly). Although the mechanism is unclear, it is thought that the generalized fluid increase or deposition of matrix substances (e.g., myxedema, amyloidosis) in the body tissues causes impingement on the median nerve within the carpal tunnel. This is also likely to underlie the association of CTS with fluid overload in end-stage renal disease and chronic dialysis.

Past history of wrist trauma or Colles fracture, degenerative or inflammatory joint disease, ganglion cysts, obesity, fibromyalgia, and scleroderma are other risk factors for this disorder. There is no universal agreement that CTS is work related. Although no genetic mutations have been identified other than a rare chromosome 17 deletion that leads to an autosomal-dominant neuropathic disorder prone to pressure-related nerve palsies, CTS is well-known to occur in families and likely has a strong genetic component.

PATHOPHYSIOLOGY

The anatomy of the wrist extends from the distal radius and ulna to the carpometacarpal joint. The eight small carpal bones of the wrist, arranged in two rows, account for numerous articulations and enable the wrist to perform a wide ROM. The wrist is the second most mobile joint in the body, adding to the exceptional mobility of the hand. Radial ligaments and the triangular fibrocartilage complex work to maintain the stability of the carpal bones. The carpal tunnel is formed by the arrangement of the wrist bones and the inelastic flexor retinaculum ligament. Through this tunnel run the finger flexor tendons and the median nerve. Any source of inflammation or pressure within this canal can result in symptoms of CTS.

Patients with CTS are prone to developing increases in pressure within the carpal tunnel during wrist flexion and extension. In turn, this may lead to edema within the nerve tissue. These mechanisms may also result in venous congestion and stasis, compression of the median nerve, and resultant ischemia, leading to the pain and paresthesias associated with CTS.

CLINICAL PRESENTATION

Subjective

Typically, the patient will present with an aching sensation that radiates into the thenar area. A hallmark symptom is nighttime awakening with pain and numbness in the hand and fingers. Paresthesias and numbness in the median nerve distribution (thumb, second, third, and radial portion of the fourth digit) typically accompany the pain. In later disease, patients often report that they frequently drop objects and that they cannot open jars or twist off lids. Repetitive motions of the hand or stationary tasks with the wrist held flexed or extended for a period of time (such as when driving) worsen pain and numbness. Patients report that they must rub or shake the hand to get circulation back to normal. Persistent numbness, pain, and thenar atrophy can occur when the compression is severe and/or longstanding.

Objective

Examination of the patient with suspected CTS should include inspection of the wrist and hand for swelling, redness, nodules, deformity, and muscle atrophy. The thenar eminence, at the base of the thumb, is the best location to assess for atrophy. If the thenar eminence is atrophied or flattened, chronic CTS should be suspected. Palpation of the hand and wrist should be done to check for swelling, bogginess, or tenderness. Each distal interphalangeal (DIP), proximal interphalangeal (PIP), and metacarpophalangeal (MCP) joint should be palpated, as well as the joints of the carpal bones. Capillary refill time should be determined, and the radial and ulnar arteries should be assessed for patency. Allen's test, Phalen's test, and Tinel's test (see Advanced Assessment 53.10) should be performed to determine individual patency of both the radial and ulnar arteries, as well as irritation to the median nerve. In addition, the carpal compression test should be done. In this test, the examiner places the thumbs over the flexor retinaculum and applies even pressure over the area of the median nerve for 30 to 60 seconds. A positive test is indicated by the occurrence of pain, numbness, and tingling in the hand or first three digits. Finally, the patient should draw the pattern of numbness and tingling in their hand or indicate it on a preprinted picture of the hand and wrist.

The performance of sensory testing to aid in the diagnosis is generally of little clinical value. Many patients who do not have CTS have diminished ability to differentiate sharp and dull sensations on the fingers and therefore yield a high false-positive rate for this testing. Also remember that occupation and handedness may affect the muscular symmetry of the hands and wrists in the absence of a musculoskeletal condition.

DIAGNOSTIC REASONING

Diagnostic Tests

Radiographs are generally not performed for CTS; however, they may be warranted if the clinician is concerned about specific wrist pathology or if the patient has functional limitations in wrist movement. A useful diagnostic test is a median electromyogram/nerve conduction velocity study (EMG/NCV). By measuring the velocity of sensory conduction, nerve entrapment may be conclusively validated. Although the diagnosis of CTS is frequently a straightforward clinical diagnosis, if the clinical picture is unclear or if the patient is not improving with conservative management, the EMG/NCV can be an appropriate study. It is important to remember that this is an invasive test and that it can have a small percentage of false-negative and false-positive results.

Differential Diagnosis

The following is a list of differential diagnoses:

- Arthritis of the base of the thumb
- Cervical radiculopathy
- Diabetes mellitus with paresthesias
- Ganglion cyst within the carpal tunnel
- Median nerve compression at the elbow
- Wrist arthritis

MANAGEMENT

Conservative treatment is recommended for patients who present with acute symptoms. Nearly two-thirds of patients given conservative treatment will attain symptom relief. The goal of treatment is to prevent the sustained flexion of the wrist or compression of the carpal tunnel. This is best accomplished through use of a wrist splint that allows free movement of the fingers and the thumb while maintaining the wrist in the neutral position. Some providers recommend wearing the splint day and night, but others recommend nighttime only. Wearing the splint during the day can protect the wrist during work and daytime activities, whereas wearing the splint at night helps prevent prolonged wrist flexion that frequently occurs during sleep. People with carpal tunnel frequently complain of awakening from sleep often due to pain in their hands. Splinting is typically used for 3 months. If a patient continues to have symptoms after that, a surgical consultation is warranted.

Oral NSAIDs are another conservative measure that can be used in conjunction with splinting. These medications are effective in reducing the pain and edema of carpal tunnel.

Corticosteroid injections into the carpal tunnel space are performed by some providers and may provide relief and reduction in inflammation. This may be a short-term benefit for some patients because the anti-inflammatory effects of the steroid do not have an effect on the physical compression that can occur in the carpal tunnel space, regardless of inflammation, which can only be relieved with surgical release. There is also potential that the median nerve could sustain damage and scarring due to the injection.

The use of vitamin B_6 (pyridoxine) in CTS has been reported in the literature over the past several years to reduce symptoms. Although there are no conclusive studies on the utility of this vitamin in treating or preventing CTS, use of vitamin B_6 is becoming more prevalent. Care should be taken with dosing because larger doses may result in neuropathies. It is also important to determine whether the patient is on any other medications that may be affected by pyridoxine; for example, serum concentrations of phenytoin and phenobarbital may be decreased with pyridoxine.

Management of concurrent disease (e.g., hypothyroidism, diabetes mellitus) is an important aspect of the conservative treatment of CTS. Treatment that diminishes fluid retention, when used with other conservative methods, will produce better results in relieving the symptoms of CTS.

CTS that occurs during pregnancy usually resolves after pregnancy. Treatment consists of splinting and other nonoperative measures such as corticosteroid injections. CTS that is work related may respond to ergonomic modifications.

FOLLOW-UP AND REFERRAL

The presence of thenar atrophy or unremitting symptoms with conservative treatment warrants referral for surgical evaluation. In the absence of atrophy, conservative management should be attempted for 3 months before referral. Carpal tunnel release is one of the most commonly performed hand surgeries; it is usually done with local anesthesia on an outpatient basis. The surgery may be performed by a hand specialist, plastic surgeon, or neurosurgeon.

> ### Patient Education: Carpal Tunnel Syndrome
>
> Workers who are exposed to occupational risks for CTS should be educated on the causes and prevention of CTS. The work environment should be assessed for ergonomic risks to workers; often an ergonomic specialist is needed to perform these assessments. *Ergonomics* means fitting the job to the worker, as opposed to the worker accommodating to the workspace. Special attention should be paid to jobs with a known propensity to produce extreme or repeated flexion of the wrist. Ergonomic evaluations and recommendations include the following:
>
> - Evaluating the workstations of computer keyboard workers in regard to the height of the keyboard, chair, and monitor
> - Teaching lifting techniques and reviewing them annually
> - Rotating jobs for workers who perform repetitive tasks
> - Resting frequently or wearing specially designed hand wear; for example, workers who use vibrating tools should wear antivibration gloves or should be given frequent, short rest breaks
>
> Patients should be educated to consider risks outside of the workplace such as stress on the wrist during everyday activities like gardening and cleaning. Knitting, sewing, and playing musical instruments may irritate the carpal tunnel. Patients should be advised to avoid carrying heavy briefcases, packages, or purses with the hands. Bags with shoulder straps, backpacks, or bags with wheels should be recommended to patients with risk factors for CTS and those who do have it.

DE QUERVAIN'S TENOSYNOVITIS

EPIDEMIOLOGY AND CAUSES

De Quervain's tenosynovitis is a condition that affects the APL and the extensor pollicis brevis (EPB) tendons, as well as the tendon sheath enclosing those tendons. These traverse from the thumb, along the radial border of the wrist, to the forearm. De Quervain's tenosynovitis is characterized by pain at the base of the thumb or over the radial styloid on abduction and extension of the thumb and commonly occurs in patients who perform pinch-grip activities. This includes using hand tools with extreme pressure, carrying trays with a pinch grip, doing assembly work, and working on sewing/cutting activities. It is more common in middle-aged females and is often precipitated by repetitive use of the thumb. This condition is also common in pregnant females or those in the postpartum period.

PATHOPHYSIOLOGY

Within the wrist, there are six dorsal tunnels through which the extensor tendons pass. The first tunnel transports the APL and EPB tendons, which form the radial border of the anatomical snuffbox. The APL and EPB tendons are responsible for thumb flexion and extension and for establishing a grip. De Quervain's tenosynovitis occurs when the tendon sheath becomes inflamed. The tendon sheath becomes thickened and narrows, causing stenosis. This results in pain, impaired movement, and a possible triggering or locking when the tendons move within the sheath. Patients may have a sensation of crepitus as well. The alterations in hormones during pregnancy and in the postpartum period can contribute to the development of this condition during that time frame. Compounding the potentially hormonally induced tenosynovitis, new mothers may be aggravating the tendon while lifting and holding the baby.

CLINICAL PRESENTATION

Subjective

The history and physical examination should proceed in a similar fashion as described earlier for CTS. De Quervain's tenosynovitis presents with pain at the radial side of the wrist, usually with lifting. This pain is aggravated by attempts to move the thumb or make a fist. Patients may complain of pain while turning a key or a doorknob or while attempting to open a jar. Often the condition occurs as the result of lifting infants with the second metacarpal and the web between the thumb and the index finger under the baby's axillae. Chronic pain, loss of strength, and loss of thumb motion can occur. If there is a possible relationship to a patient's occupation or hobby, ask about the specifics of these activities.

Objective

Inspect the wrist for edema, erythema, or deformity. Palpation of the tendons along the radial border of the wrist may cause pain or discomfort. On palpation, the tendon sheath may feel thickened. Wrist and thumb ROM may produce pain. Allen's test, Phalen's maneuver, and Tinel's sign should be negative. The confirmation test for de Quervain's tenosynovitis is Finkelstein's test (see Advanced Assessment 53.10). This is performed by placing the thumb across the palm, and then covering the fingers over the thumb. While in this position, the wrist is deviated in the ulnar direction. If this causes pain, the Finkelstein test is positive for de Quervain's tenosynovitis.

DIAGNOSTIC REASONING

Diagnostic Tests

De Quervain's tenosynovitis is typically a fairly straightforward clinical diagnosis, and there is usually no need for additional diagnostic testing or imaging. Wrist x-ray studies are indicated if there is a history of trauma or other suspected causative pathology such as arthritis. Calcific tendonitis may be seen on radiographs.

Differential Diagnosis

The following is a list of differential diagnoses:

- CTS
- Intersection syndrome
- Radial neuritis
- Carpometacarpal joint arthrosis of the thumb
- Scaphoid fractures
- Wrist ganglion
- Arthritis of the thumb and/or wrist

MANAGEMENT

Noninvasive treatment includes rest, splinting, and NSAIDs. A 2-week course of NSAIDs, with the typical patient precautions, is usually helpful (see discussion about NSAIDs in Chapter 53). Splinting of the wrist and the thumb with a thumb spica splint can be used for 3 to 6 weeks. If conservative therapy fails to improve the patient's pain, a corticosteroid injection into the tendon sheath may be performed. A maximum of three steroid injections, separated by several weeks, can be performed, after which surgical intervention may be considered if the patient fails to improve.

FOLLOW-UP AND REFERRAL

Patients with unremitting symptoms after conservative treatment should be referred for orthopedic consultation and possible surgery. If steroid injection is warranted and the provider is not trained in this procedure, a referral to an orthopedic practice is reasonable. As noted, surgery is indicated if the patient fails to improve with steroid injections.

Patient Education: de Quervain's Tenosynovitis

Patients should be educated regarding the cause of de Quervain's tenosynovitis. Modifications to hand tools or the work environment may be necessary. For example, hand tools may be retrofitted with a larger grip surface, so that pressure is more evenly distributed over the palmar surface of the hand. Avoidance of the precipitating factor is often enough to permanently resolve early symptoms. The patient should also be educated about potential adverse events that can occur with the use of NSAIDs. If a steroid injection is to be performed, risks and benefits need to be discussed.

GANGLION CYST

A ganglion cyst arises from a tendon sheath or a joint capsule. It is filled with a thick, gel-like material that leaks from the joint or tendon sheath and forms a cystic mass. Ganglion cysts can be caused by strains, tears, contusions, or degeneration of the tendon sheath or joint capsule. They can also occur along with osteoarthritis. Due to this injury or degeneration, tears can develop in the sheath or capsule, allowing fluid to leak and lead to the development of a fluid-filled cystic mass. The connection between the capsule or sheath and the cyst is essentially a one-way valve allowing fluid to leak into the cyst but not out of it. The ganglion cyst can be asymptomatic with low fluid pressure; however, it can be painful when the cyst is significantly distended. The most common sites are at the base of a finger, on the dorsum of the wrist over the radiocarpal joint, and on the volar surface of the wrist near the flexor carpi radialis tendon. The ganglion cyst can be distinguished from a tumor by its soft consistency and transillumination. A conservative approach to a wrist ganglion cyst with wrist immobilization is appropriate. Treatment may include aspiration or surgical removal for a painful cyst that is not improving with immobilization. Diagnostic imaging is typically not necessary.

TRIGGER FINGER

Trigger finger is also known as *stenosing tenosynovitis of the flexor tendons* or *locked finger*. This problem can be painful and functionally limiting. Any digit can be affected, although it most commonly affects the ring or middle finger. Inflammation at the MCP joint pulley and/or inflammation of the tendon cause a size discrepancy between the tendon and the pulley. A pulley is a ligamentous strap that works to keep the flexor tendon close to the bone. A tendon may also have a nodule in the tendon, which can get stuck as the tendon slides back and forth under the pulley.

Because the tendon no longer slides freely through the pulley, there is a snapping or locking phenomenon. The digit remains flexed or extended until the tendon pops through the pulley, causing severe pain. Tenderness with palpation of the flexor tendon over the MCP joint is noted. Patients with CTS and de Quervain's stenosing tenosynovitis have a higher prevalence of trigger finger.

Trigger finger may be idiopathic and is more common in middle-aged females. RA, hypothyroidism, and diabetes have a higher association with trigger finger. Patients typically report pain and catching when they flex the affected finger and may describe the finger as locking in place. The patient may awaken with the finger locked in the palm, although the finger may gradually unlock during the day. Trigger finger present in a child can be due to a congenital or metabolic condition.

Physical examination reveals tenderness in the palm at the level of the distal palmar crease, usually overlying the MCP joint. A nodule on the flexor tendon, which moves when the patient flexes and extends the finger, may also be palpable. The finger may also lock when the patient flexes and extends the affected finger. This movement is almost always painful. Full flexion of the finger may not be possible.

Splinting, occupational therapy, and NSAIDs may be used initially. The most effective therapy for this problem is local anesthetic and corticosteroid injection into the tendon sheath, plus a modification of activities for about a month. A small number of patients require surgical release of the tendon if conservative therapy and steroid injection fail.

TENDON INJURIES OF THE HAND

Several finger deformities are caused by traumatic tendon ruptures or avulsions. The appearance of each type of deformity depends on the affected tendon:

- Jersey finger is caused by avulsion or rupture of the flexor digitorum profundus tendon and is characterized by the inability to actively flex the DIP joint (Fig. 55.1).
- Mallet finger is caused by rupture or avulsion of the extensor digitorum tendon and is characterized by inability to actively extend the DIP. The joint typically rests at 30 degrees of flexion (Fig. 55.2).
- Boutonnière deformity is caused by rupture of the central portion of the extensor tendon at its insertion into the middle phalanx. The finger is held partially flexed at the PIP joint and extended or hyperextended at the DIP joint. Flexion contracture of the PIP joint and extension contracture of the DIP joint are possible (Fig. 55.3). This injury is most commonly seen in patients with advanced RA (see Chapter 63).

Partial tendon injuries are treated with splinting and exercises to restore function to the tendons. Complete tears and avulsions of the flexor tendons often require surgical repair. For patients with a mallet finger, the DIP joint should be splinted in extension for 6 to 8 weeks. The PIP joint is left free. For boutonnière deformity, the PIP joint should be splinted in extension for 6 weeks, but

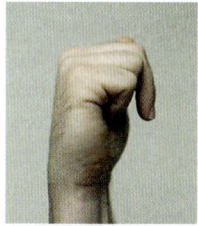

Figure 55.1 Jersey finger

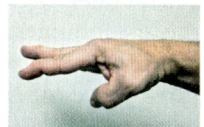

Figure 55.2 Mallet finger

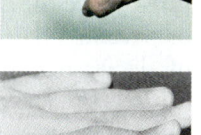

Figure 55.3 Boutonnière deformity

the DIP joint is left free. Active and passive ROM should be initiated if there is evidence of healing after splinting.

DUPUYTREN'S CONTRACTURE

Sometimes referred to as "Viking disease" or palmar fibromatosis, Dupuytren's contracture affects the palmar tissue between the skin and the distal palm and fingers, most often in the fourth and fifth fingers but also in the thumb–index finger web space. Visible, palpable fibrous bands, reminiscent of tendons, can extend from the palm to the PIP joint of Dupuytren-affected fingers.

It is a progressive condition that results in flexor contracture but does not affect the flexor tendons. As the contractures increase, patients have trouble grasping objects, pulling on gloves, and putting hands in pockets. Sensation in the affected fingers usually is normal. Dupuytren's contracture occurs most frequently in people aged 40 to 60 years and is a familial disorder, most commonly affecting males of northern European ancestry. It is dysfunctional and disfiguring but does not cause pain. Injections or surgery are the only therapeutic options. Patients should be referred to an orthopedic specialist for treatment.

SHOULDER DISORDERS

ADHESIVE CAPSULITIS

Adhesive capsulitis is defined as idiopathic loss of both active and passive ROM of the shoulder, often referred to as a *frozen shoulder*. There is no correlation between the affected arm and arm dominance. Additionally, approximately 50% of the patients will have both arms affected. Female patients aged 40 to 60 years are more likely to be affected. Type 1 diabetes has a high correlation with adhesive capsulitis, but other conditions also have a high degree of correlation, including Dupuytren's contracture, tumors, Parkinson's disease, herniated cervical disc, hypothyroidism, and stroke.

Adhesive capsulitis is characterized by contracture of the glenohumeral capsule. The natural history of this condition typically has the patient progress through three phases of the condition: a painful phase; a stiffness or *freezing* phase; and then a recovery or *thawing* phase of decreasing discomfort and increasing functionality. These phases are not distinct but have some overlap as the patient progresses though this disorder. Recovery may take anywhere from 6 months to 2 years. Some patients with adhesive capsulitis may continue to have long-term functional deficits and stiffness. Although adhesive capsulitis may result from conditions that cause pain and immobility, in patients without predisposing factors, the possibility of underlying organic disease, autoimmune disease, or neoplastic disease should be considered when night sweats, fever, unexplained weight loss, and/or malaise are also present. Cervical nerve compression should be considered for patients who also have radicular symptoms (pain, numbness, and tingling) in the upper extremity.

Disuse atrophy may be present at the shoulder girdle. Point tenderness on palpation is not typical and may be a sign of alternative pathology. Palpation usually results in nonspecific diffuse discomfort. Physical examination reveals a significant loss in both active and passive ROM with shoulder flexion, internal and external rotation, and abduction. Because patients can have substantial pain with motion, some clinicians may decide not to assess passive range of motion due to fear of causing the patient additional pain; however, it is essential to assess passive motion to secure the diagnosis. Pain may be present with motion and at the insertion of the deltoid, and diffuse tenderness about the shoulder is a typical finding. The patient's pain may have a sensation of radiation to the region of the biceps.

A clinician can make the diagnosis of adhesive capsulitis, based upon history and a physical examination. Anterior-posterior (AP) and axillary radiographs of the shoulder may be indicated to rule out underlying pathology such as arthritis, loose bodies, avascular necrosis, tendon calcification, pathological fracture, or tumor. Other studies, such as arthrography, computed tomography (CT), or MRI, are typically not indicated unless the clinician is suspicious for and needs to further investigate other potential shoulder pathology.

Differential diagnoses for adhesive capsulitis include chronic posterior shoulder dislocation, tumor, OA, post-traumatic stiffness, and rotator cuff tear. Adhesive capsulitis is differentiated from chronic posterior shoulder dislocation, tumor, and OA on radiograph. Post-traumatic shoulder stiffness will be associated with a history of trauma. Rotator cuff tear is differentiated due to the presence of normal passive ROM.

Treatment consists of the application of moist heat and use of analgesics (NSAIDs and nonnarcotic analgesics). Although NSAIDs are frequently recommended for patients with adhesive capsulitis—they do help with pain reduction—there is little evidence that they increase the speed of recovery from the condition. An intra-articular corticosteroid injection can potentially provide short-term pain relief and improvement in function.

Physical therapy is recommended to help improve function, along with gentle stretching exercises that can be performed at home. The patient should be advised that recovery time is often lengthy, and there is potential for chronic stiffness and residual pain. Patients with diabetes tend to be refractory to treatment. If improvement is not seen within 12 weeks with conservative treatment, the patient should be referred to an orthopedic specialist for consideration of an arthroscopic joint capsule release.

IMPINGEMENT SYNDROME

Impingement syndrome may result when the subacromial bursa and/or rotator cuff become inflamed because of injury, overuse, or compression in the subacromial space of the shoulder. It is the leading cause of shoulder pain. The four rotator cuff muscles (supraspinatus, infraspinatus, subscapularis, and teres minor) and tendons arise from the scapula and attach to the humerus, forming a cover (or cuff) over the humeral head. The rotator cuff muscles provide movement of the shoulder, including abduction, flexion, external rotation, and internal rotation. Additionally, the rotator cuff helps provide some stability for the glenohumeral joint.

Impingement syndrome is believed to be part of a continuum of rotator cuff pathology, including impingement and bursitis, partial tear of the rotator cuff, full-thickness tear, and rotator cuff arthropathy. Several etiological factors contribute to the development of impingement syndrome. Repeated impingement of the tendons from manual labor or overhead throwing activities can contribute to inflammation, irritation, and degradation of the anatomical structures in the subacromial space. A diminished microvasculature contributes to a diminished ability to heal injured tissue. As the supraspinatus degrades or degenerates, it is less able to hold the humeral head against the glenoid fossa. This allows the humeral head to move superiorly, causing a vicious cycle in which the subacromial space gets smaller and contributes to further degeneration of the supraspinatus.

Patients will describe a gradual, insidious onset of shoulder pain. This is typically located anterior and lateral at the affected shoulder. Patients will usually state the pain is worse with overhead motion. Some patients may

Academy of Orthopaedic Surgeons, 27(21), 794–805. https://doi.org/10.5435/JAAOS-D-18-00225

Rees HW. (2020). Management of osteoarthritis of the hip. The Journal of the American Academy of Orthopaedic Surgeons, 28(7), e288–e291. https://doi.org/10.5435/JAAOS-D-19-00416

Rivière C, Hardijzer A, Lazennec J-Y, et al. Spine-hip add understandings to the pathophysiology of femoro-acetabular impingement: a systematic review. Orthop Traumatol Surg Res. 2017; 103: 549–557.

Sanjaya A. (2020). Meralgia paresthetica: finding an effective cure. Postgraduate medicine, 132(1), 1–6. https://doi.org/10.1080/00325481.2019.1673582

Torres A, Fernández-Fairen M, Sueiro-Fernández J. (2018). Greater trochanteric pain syndrome and gluteus medius and minimus tendinosis: nonsurgical treatment. Pain management, 8(1), 45–55. https://doi.org/10.2217/pmt-2017-0033

Knee

Ardern CL, Ekås G, Grindem H, et al. (2018). 2018 International Olympic Committee consensus statement on prevention, diagnosis and management of paediatric anterior cruciate ligament (ACL) injuries. Knee surgery, sports traumatology, arthroscopy: official journal of the ESSKA, 26(4), 989–1010. https://doi.org/10.1007/s00167-018-4865-y

Bloom DA, Wolfert AJ, Michalowitz A, et al. (2020). ACL injuries aren't just for girls: the role of age in predicting pediatric ACL injury. Sports health, 12(6), 559–563. https://doi.org/10.1177/1941738120935429

Dingel A, Aoyama J, Ganley T, et al. (2019). Pediatric ACL tears: natural history. Journal of pediatric orthopedics, 39(Issue 6, Supplement 1 Suppl 1), S47–S49. https://doi.org/10.1097/BPO.0000000000001367

Filbay SR, Grindem H. (2019). Evidence-based recommendations for the management of anterior cruciate ligament (ACL) rupture. Best practice & research. Clinical rheumatology, 33(1), 33–47. https://doi.org/10.1016/j.berh.2019.01.018

Graham P. (2018). Meniscus tear. Orthopedic nursing, 37(4), 255–257. https://doi.org/10.1097/NOR.0000000000000476

Graham P. (2019). Tear of the anterior cruciate ligament. Orthopedic nursing, 38(1), 57–59. https://doi.org/10.1097/NOR.0000000000000536

Kramer DE, Miller PE, Berrahou IK, et al. (2020). Collateral ligament knee injuries in pediatric and adolescent athletes. Journal of pediatric orthopedics, 40(2), 71–77. https://doi.org/10.1097/BPO.0000000000001112

Lubowitz JH, Brand JC, Rossi MJ. (2020). Nonoperative management of degenerative meniscus tears is worth a try. Arthroscopy: the journal of arthroscopic & related surgery: official publication of the Arthroscopy Association of North America and the International Arthroscopy Association, 36(2), 327–328. https://doi.org/10.1016/j.arthro.2019.11.128

Moatshe G, Vap AR, Getgood A, et al. (2020). Medial-sided injuries in the multiple ligament knee injury. The journal of knee surgery, 33(5), 431–439. https://doi.org/10.1055/s-0039-3402768

Perkins CA, Willimon SC. (2020). Pediatric anterior cruciate ligament reconstruction. The Orthopedic clinics of North America, 51(1), 55–63. https://doi.org/10.1016/j.ocl.2019.08.009

Salzler MJ, Chang J, Richmond J. (2018). Management of anterior cruciate ligament injuries in adults aged >40 years. The Journal of the American Academy of Orthopaedic Surgeons, 26(16), 553–561. https://doi.org/10.5435/JAAOS-D-16-00730

Wolf, BR, Gulbrandsen TR. (2020). Degenerative meniscus tear in older athletes. Clinics in sports medicine, 39(1):197–209. https://doi.org/10.1016/j.csm.2019.08.005

Shoulder

Bechay J, Lawrence C, Namdari S. (2020). Calcific tendinopathy of the rotator cuff: a review of operative versus nonoperative management. The physician and sportsmedicine, 48(3), 241–246. https://doi.org/10.1080/00913847.2019.1710617

Chianca V, Albano D, Messina C, et al. (2018). Rotator cuff calcific tendinopathy: from diagnosis to treatment. Acta bio-medica: Atenei Parmensis, 89(1-S), 186–196. doi: 10.23750/abm.v89i1-S.7022

Cho CH, Bae KC, Kim DH. (2019). Treatment strategy for frozen shoulder. Clinics in orthopedic surgery, 11(3), 249–257. https://doi.org/10.4055/cios.2019.11.3.249

Dang A, Davies M. (2018). Rotator cuff disease: treatment options and considerations. Sports medicine and arthroscopy review, 26(3), 129–133. https://doi.org/10.1097/JSA.0000000000000207

Fields BKK, Skalski MR, Patel DB, et al. (2019). Adhesive capsulitis: review of imaging findings, pathophysiology, clinical presentation, and treatment options. Skeletal radiology, 48(8), 1171–1184. https://doi.org/10.1007/s00256-018-3139-6

Lawrence RL, Moutzouros V, Bey MJ. (2019). Asymptomatic rotator cuff tears. JBJS reviews, 7(6), e9. https://doi.org/10.2106/JBJS.RVW.18.00149

Micallef J, Pandya J, Low AK. (2019). Management of rotator cuff tears in the elderly population. Maturitas, 123, 9–14. https://doi.org/10.1016/j.maturitas.2019.01.016

Onks C, Silvis M, Loeffert J, et al. (2020). Conservative care or surgery for rotator cuff tears?. The Journal of family practice, 69(2), 66–72.

Redler LH, Dennis ER. (2019). Treatment of adhesive capsulitis of the shoulder. The Journal of the American Academy of Orthopaedic Surgeons, 27(12), e544–e554. https://doi.org/10.5435/JAAOS-D-17-00606

Stelter J, Malik S, Chiampas G. (2020). The emergent evaluation and treatment of shoulder, clavicle, and humerus injuries. Emergency medicine clinics of North America, 38(1), 103–124. https://doi.org/10.1016/j.emc.2019.09.006

Tendinopathy/Tenosynovitis

Cardoso TB, Pizzari T, Kinsella R, et al. (2019). Current trends in tendinopathy management. Best Practice & Research. Clinical Rheumatology, 33(1):122–140. https://doi.org/10.1016/j.berh.2019.02.001

Melton JK, Memarzadeh A, Dunbar WH, et al. Semimembranosus tenosynovitis: diagnosis and management of a commonly missed cause of posteromedial knee pain. Knee. 2017;24:305–309.

Patrick NC, Hammert WC. (2020). Hand and wrist tendinopathies. Clinics in sports medicine, 39(2):247–258. https://doi.org/10.1016/j.csm.2019.10.004

Wagner ER, Gottschalk MB. Tendinopathies of the forearm, wrist, and hand. Clinics in Plastic Surgery, 46(3):317–327. https://doi.org/10.1016/j.cps.2019.02.005

RESOURCES

American Academy of Orthopaedic Surgeons
https://www.aaos.org

American Academy of Physical Medicine and Rehabilitation
https://www.aapmr.org

American Academy of Physical Therapy
https://www.aaptnet.org

American Association of Clinical Endocrinology (AACE)
https://www.aace.com

American Association of Hip and Knee Surgeons
https://www.aahks.org

American Orthopedic Foot & Ankle Society
https://www.aofas.org

American Physical Therapy Association
https://www.apta.org

National Institute of Arthritis and Musculoskeletal and Skin Diseases
https://www.niams.nih.gov

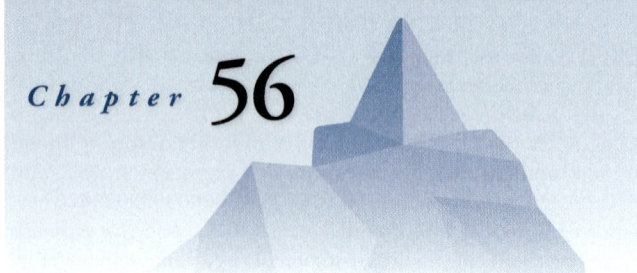

Chapter 56

Osteoarthritis and Osteoporosis

Margaret M. Harding, MSN, RN, AGPCNP-BC, RNFA, CPAN

Michael E. Zychowicz, DNP, ANP, ONP, FAAN, FAANP

OSTEOARTHRITIS

Osteoarthritis (OA), also known as *degenerative joint disease* (DJD) or "wear and tear" arthritis, is the most common articular disease in adults older than age 40. It is the most common form of arthritis and is a significant cause of functional impairment, chronic pain, and disability in the older population. OA is a gradual, progressive joint disease in which loss of articular cartilage and degeneration occur, leading to pain and often deformity.

OA affects both males and females of all races. In addition to advanced age, risk factors include genetics, female sex, joint injury, past trauma, obesity, and mechanical stress. OA that is not precipitated by an inciting event is classified as "primary" or idiopathic, resulting from advancing age, genetics, obesity, or overuse. In contrast, "secondary" OA develops at varying intervals as a result of preexisting joint abnormality, trauma, infection, osteonecrosis, or in the setting of inflammatory arthritis or metabolic disease. Other processes that could produce secondary OA include Paget's disease, osteopetrosis, osteochondritis dissecans, metabolic disorders (hemochromatosis, Wilson's disease), hemoglobinopathy, Ehlers-Danlos syndrome, and Marfan syndrome. Primary and secondary OA may coexist.

OA encompasses a group of subtypes with different etiological factors with a common response pattern in joint tissues, which is primarily noninflammatory and involves a combination of biomechanical stresses and biochemical changes in articular cartilage and synovial membrane. There is erosion and fibrillation of cartilage, with joint space narrowing and osteophyte formation. Principal sites for OA are the distal interphalangeal (DIP) joints, the proximal interphalangeal (PIP) joints, and the carpometacarpal (CMC) joint of the thumb in the hand; the first metatarsophalangeal or great toe joint; and the hips, knees, and cervical and lumbar spine. The ankle, wrist, shoulder, and elbow joints are at less risk of developing OA, unless the cause of the arthritis is traumatic or occupational.

Although both OA and rheumatoid arthritis (RA) affect the phalanges, they occur in different locations. RA usually presents as bilateral pain, swelling, and stiffness of the metacarpophalangeal and PIP joints with characteristic deformities and sparing the DIP joints. Generally, other systemic complaints will occur, and joints other than just those in the hand will be affected as well (see Chapter 63 for a full discussion of RA). OA affects the DIP joints (Heberden's nodes) and PIP joints (Bouchard's nodes) and presents with swelling, stiffness, pain, and deformity.

Apart from affecting physical health, OA may also have a negative effect on mental health. The Osteoarthritis Initiative (OAI) study demonstrated that those with lower limb OA had a greater likelihood of developing depressive symptoms, likely due to pain and immobility. OA has also been associated with greater odds of suicidal ideation.

EPIDEMIOLOGY AND CAUSES

OA is the most common joint disease worldwide, affecting 302 million people and causing disability in 43 million people. In the United States, it is estimated that 80% of the population older than 65 years has radiographic evidence of OA, although only about 48% have symptoms. With radiographic OA almost twice as common as symptomatic OA, it is important to note that radiographic changes do not necessarily prove OA as the cause of joint pain. OA also has a significant economic

MANAGEMENT

The principles of management of OA are to control pain and other symptoms, maximize functional independence and mobility, minimize disability, and preserve quality of life. Management choices can be categorized as nonpharmacological, pharmacological, complementary, alternative, and surgical. In general, treatment should begin with the safest and least invasive therapies before proceeding to more invasive therapies. All patients with OA should receive treatment from the first two categories. Surgical management (joint arthroplasty) for end-stage/severe OA of hip and knee has been shown to be cost-effective and improve quality of life.

Nonpharmacological Management

Self-Care Strategies

Initial management of OA includes educating the patient about the nature of the disease, delineating the role of the patient in self-management, and providing sources of information and support for the patient. The Arthritis Foundation is an excellent resource and offers information sheets, local support groups, and an arthritis self-help course that includes exercise, joint protection, and relaxation techniques, along with information on medications that are typically used to manage symptoms. Weight loss is often an important component of the plan of care.

The ACR and Arthritis Foundation guidelines strongly recommend that patients with OA participate in self-efficacy and self-management programs. The benefits of such programs are consistent across studies with minimal risk. These programs use a multidisciplinary group format to encourage goal-setting, problem-solving, and positive thinking. Additionally, education about the disease process of OA, medication effects and side effects, joint protection measures, and fitness and exercise are commonly included. Pain coping skills training (PCST) is another method of self-care that can be used in patients with OA. It is designed to help patients cope with pain by training them to self-regulate thoughts and behaviors. PCST is an effective method for improving pain, function, and psychological outcomes in patients with OA.

Physical Therapy

Nonpharmacological management strategies include physical therapy for muscle strengthening, particularly quadriceps strengthening for patients with knee OA. The physical therapist also evaluates mobility and the need for assistive devices such as canes or walkers to reduce load bearing on the arthritic joint. The physical therapist may recommend environmental modifications to maximize functional independence and safety. On an individual basis, physical therapists may also recommend other orthotic devices, such as shoe lifts, splints, or bracing, to improve biomechanics.

In addition to individual physical therapy, regular exercise is strongly recommended for all patients with OA. Whenever feasible, a supervised exercise program incorporating aerobic and resistive components should be instituted. Aquatic exercise programs are also excellent, particularly those that are tailored to the needs of arthritic patients. Exercise recommendations should focus on patient preferences and access to mitigate barriers to participation. In addition to regular aerobic exercise, the ACR and Arthritis Foundation guidelines conditionally recommend yoga in OA of the knee and strongly recommend tai chi in knee and/or hip OA.

Transcutaneous electrical nerve stimulation (TENS) therapy is sometimes used for arthritic pain, but studies to date have not established its effectiveness. The ACR and Arthritis Foundation guidelines strongly recommend against the use of TENS due to lack of supporting evidence.

Kinesiotaping is another method that is sometimes employed by physical therapists to support ROM of the joint to which it is applied. Quality of evidence is limited, but the ACR and Arthritis Foundation guidelines conditionally recommend kinesiotaping in patients with OA if the knee and/or first CMC joint.

Locally applied heat or cold may be used to decrease pain. Methods of thermal interventions vary greatly, including moist heat, electrically delivered heat, ultrasound, single-use hot and cold packs, and continuous circulating ice devices. The ACR and Arthritis Foundation guidelines conditionally recommend these types of interventions, as high-quality evidence is limited.

Occupational Therapy

Short-term occupational therapy to maximize ADLs and evaluate the need for adaptive devices is often overlooked, but it can be invaluable to the patient with arthritis. Devices such as a raised toilet seat, toilet side rails, elastic shoelaces, reachers, and various kitchen accessories can enhance functional capacity and independence.

Complementary Therapy

Acupuncture and massage are alternative therapies used for the management of OA and other musculoskeletal problems (see Complementary Therapies 56.1).

Pharmacological Management

The goal of pharmacological management of OA is pain control. The ACR and Arthritis Foundation have issued guidelines for pharmacological treatment of OA of the hand, hip, and knee. There are several different organizations that have published similar guidelines, including the American Academy of Orthopaedic Surgeons (AAOS) and the Osteoarthritis Research Society International (OARSI). A committee reviews the most current evidence and develops the guidelines. The voting on recommendations tends to differ slightly between organizations. The recommendations made by

> **Complementary Therapies 56.1: Osteoarthritis and Musculoskeletal Problems**
>
> **ACUPUNCTURE**
>
> Acupuncture has gained popularity as an option for many types of pain relief. Several systematic reviews have reported the efficacy of acupuncture in pain relief in patients with OA of the knee. Although acupuncture has been shown to be better than no treatment for pain, many studies show that it is not better than simulated, or placebo, acupuncture treatment in OA. Although there are few adverse effects when performed properly, complications such as infections and injuries can arise when acupuncture is not delivered properly. At this time, acupuncture is not widely recommended for the treatment of OA symptoms. The NIH National Center for Complementary and Integrative Health recommends that if patients choose to use acupuncture, they use only qualified and licensed professionals.
>
> **MASSAGE**
>
> Massage therapy was once taught as a core nursing skill but was long ago replaced by other interventions. In recent years, massage has gained popularity in Western culture. Massage therapy purports emotional and physiological benefits in a variety of conditions. In the treatment of OA, massage appears to be safe and offer short-term benefits. However, as with acupuncture, there are limitations in the available research. Massage is not widely recommended for the treatment of OA symptoms.
>
> **AROMATHERAPY**
>
> Like massage, aromatherapy is a nonpharmacological method that nurses and patients can directly and independently use to ease the symptoms of OA. Aromatherapy is a safe and supportive method, in which essential oils and aromatic herbs are used to decrease pain, fatigue, anxiety, and sleep disturbances. Several recent studies support the efficacy of aromatherapy in OA of the knee and hand. However, aromatherapy is not widely recommended, and there are no formal recommendations for or against its use in treatment of OA symptoms.

the ACR and Arthritis Foundation are summarized in Figure 56.1.

Acetaminophen

Acetaminophen (Tylenol) has long been considered a mainstay for pharmacological treatment of OA. However, the most recent OARSI guidelines do not recommend the use of acetaminophen in the treatment of OA, citing little to no efficacy and risk of hepatotoxicity. This may signal a shift away from the use of acetaminophen in individuals with OA.

NSAIDs

NSAIDs actually comprise several categories of pharmacological agents, all sharing comparable anti-inflammatory properties. Although each class acts in an individual manner, all inhibit the production of prostaglandins, which are inflammatory mediators. Cyclooxygenase (COX), or prostaglandin (PG) endoperoxide synthase, is the first enzyme in the PG synthesis pathway. This enzyme transforms arachidonic acid into other PG breakdown products. Two forms of COX are present: COX-1 is normally present in blood vessels, stomach, and kidneys and promotes the normal functioning of those systems, and COX-2 is generated in inflammatory settings by cytokines and inflammatory mediators. NSAIDs can be selective and nonselective COX inhibitors. All possess antipyretic, analgesic, and anti-inflammatory properties. Additionally, NSAIDs can be administered topically, orally, and intravenously.

Inhibition of COX-1 is largely responsible for the adverse effects associated with NSAID therapy, including gastrointestinal (GI) bleeding, ulcerogenic activity, fluid retention, and blockade of platelet aggregation. Patients taking NSAIDs are four to five times more likely to have GI bleeding than individuals who are not taking the drugs. The risk of bleeding is increased during the first month of treatment and with increased dosages of the NSAID; older age and polypharmacy are also risk factors. It was hoped that the use of the COX-2 inhibitors would be equally effective for pain while curbing GI side effects or platelets; however, subsequent data regarding the increased risk of vascular events such as myocardial infarction (MI) or transient ischemic attack (TIA)/stroke have resulted in withdrawal of several of these agents from the market. NSAIDs also interact with several other classes of medication and have the potential to cause nephrotoxicity.

The COX-2 inhibitor celecoxib (Celebrex) has been associated with increased risk of serious cardiovascular events, especially when used for long periods of time or in high-risk settings (such as after surgery). According to the U.S. Food and Drug Administration (FDA), patients who are at high risk of GI bleed have a history of intolerance to nonselective NSAIDs or are not doing well on nonselective NSAIDs may be appropriate candidates for COX-2 inhibitor therapy. However, individual patient risk for cardiovascular events and other risks commonly associated with NSAIDs should be considered.

There is considerable variability among patients in both effectiveness and tolerance of NSAIDs. If one particular drug proves ineffective or unacceptable, benefit may be obtained by changing to a drug of a different class. The doses of these drugs should be individualized.

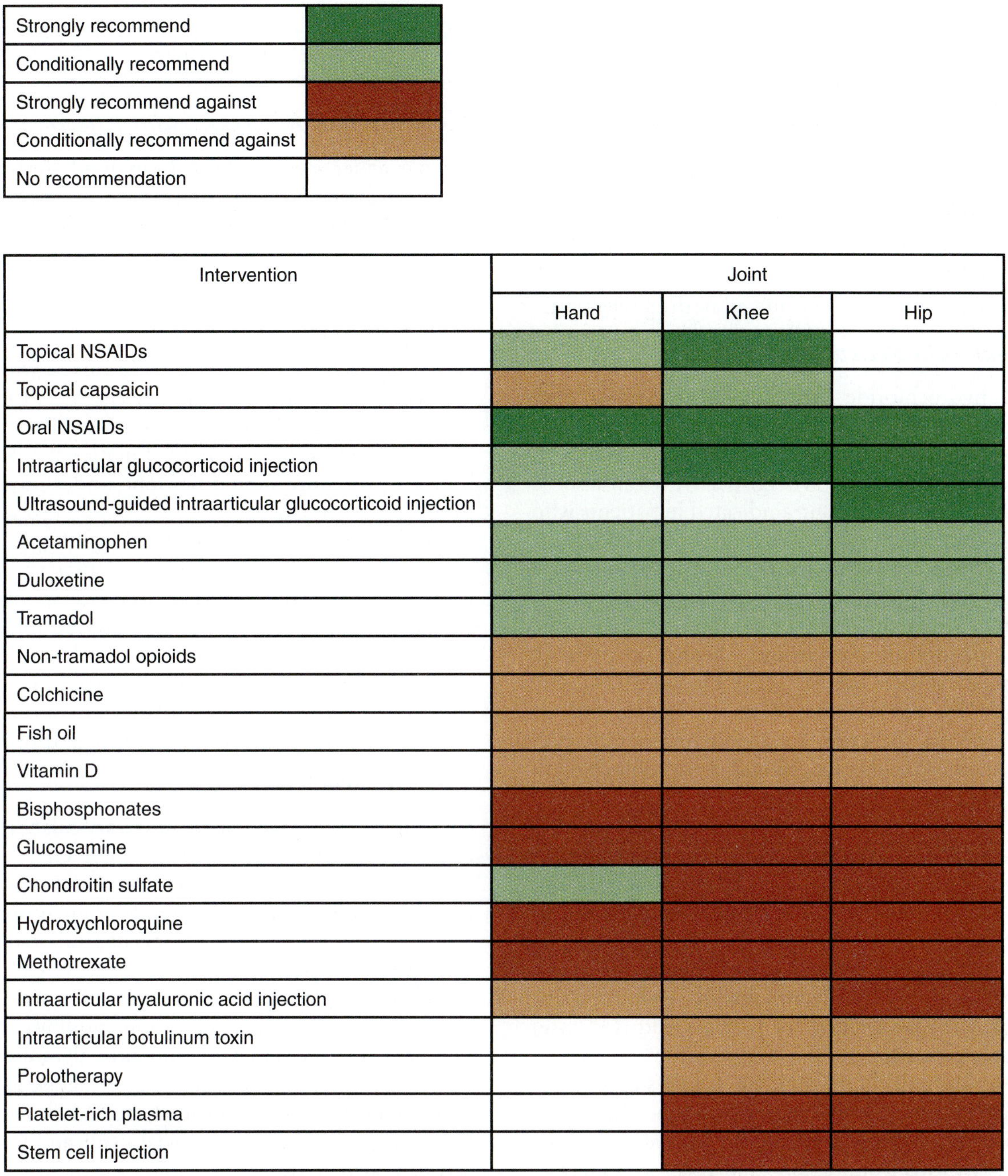

Strongly recommend	🟩
Conditionally recommend	🟢
Strongly recommend against	🟥
Conditionally recommend against	🟧
No recommendation	⬜

Intervention	Joint		
	Hand	Knee	Hip
Topical NSAIDs	Conditionally recommend	Strongly recommend	No recommendation
Topical capsaicin	Conditionally recommend against	Conditionally recommend	No recommendation
Oral NSAIDs	Strongly recommend	Strongly recommend	Strongly recommend
Intraarticular glucocorticoid injection	Conditionally recommend	Strongly recommend	Strongly recommend
Ultrasound-guided intraarticular glucocorticoid injection	No recommendation	No recommendation	Strongly recommend
Acetaminophen	Conditionally recommend	Conditionally recommend	Conditionally recommend
Duloxetine	Conditionally recommend	Conditionally recommend	Conditionally recommend
Tramadol	Conditionally recommend	Conditionally recommend	Conditionally recommend
Non-tramadol opioids	Conditionally recommend against	Conditionally recommend against	Conditionally recommend against
Colchicine	Conditionally recommend against	Conditionally recommend against	Conditionally recommend against
Fish oil	Conditionally recommend against	Conditionally recommend against	Conditionally recommend against
Vitamin D	Conditionally recommend against	Conditionally recommend against	Conditionally recommend against
Bisphosphonates	Strongly recommend against	Strongly recommend against	Strongly recommend against
Glucosamine	Strongly recommend against	Strongly recommend against	Strongly recommend against
Chondroitin sulfate	Conditionally recommend	Strongly recommend against	Strongly recommend against
Hydroxychloroquine	Strongly recommend against	Strongly recommend against	Strongly recommend against
Methotrexate	Strongly recommend against	Strongly recommend against	Strongly recommend against
Intraarticular hyaluronic acid injection	Conditionally recommend against	Conditionally recommend against	Strongly recommend against
Intraarticular botulinum toxin	No recommendation	Conditionally recommend against	Conditionally recommend against
Prolotherapy	No recommendation	Conditionally recommend against	Conditionally recommend against
Platelet-rich plasma	No recommendation	Strongly recommend against	Strongly recommend against
Stem cell injection	No recommendation	Strongly recommend against	Strongly recommend against

Figure 56.1 American College of Rheumatology and Arthritis Foundation Recommendations. *Adapted from Kolasinski SL, Neogi T, Hochberg MC, et al. 2019 American College of Rheumatology/Arthritis Foundation guideline for the management of osteoarthritis of the hand, hip, and knee. Arthritis Care Res. 2020;72(2):149–162.*

The addition of a proton pump inhibitor to NSAID therapy helps protect against gastroduodenal ulceration. In addition, meloxicam (Mobic) is a preferential inhibitor of COX-2 and appears to be well-tolerated with few drug-drug interactions.

Due to the risks associated with NSAID therapy, OARSI recommends topical NSAIDs over oral analgesics. Topical NSAID application to one joint results in substantially less systemic absorption than the recommended oral dose of the same drug, producing a more favorable balance of efficacy and transient side effects.

The American Academy of Family Practice Physicians has issued the following recommendations regarding oral NSAID use:

- Initiate therapy with acetaminophen, and if NSAIDs are needed, use the lowest dose for the shortest duration possible.
- Avoid NSAIDs in patients with preexisting renal disease, congestive heart failure, or cirrhosis.
- Avoid NSAIDs and aspirin in patients taking anticoagulants.

- Creatinine should be monitored in patients taking angiotensin-converting enzyme inhibitors or angiotensin receptor blockers who are prescribed NSAIDs on a regular basis.

Recommendations from other medical experts emphasize that conservative treatments such as physical therapy and exercise should be first-line management. If NSAIDs must be used, the topical route is preferred. In patients requiring oral NSAID therapy, medical history and risk factors should be carefully considered in drug selection.

Additional Pain Relievers

Tramadol hydrochloride (Ultram) is an opioid pain reliever that is indicated for moderate to moderately severe pain. It is available as a combination drug with acetaminophen that works synergistically; it can also be taken with NSAIDs. It is contraindicated in patients who use alcohol and who are taking hypnotics and should be used with caution in patients with the potential to abuse it. Caution also should be used in patients who are taking selective serotonin reuptake inhibitors (SSRIs) due to the risk of serotonin syndrome. There is no evidence that this medication is more effective than NSAIDs. Any prescription for opioids should be considered only if expected pain and function are anticipated to outweigh the risks to the patient and should be combined with nonpharmacological therapy.

There is no clear evidence that muscle relaxants or benzodiazepines are helpful adjuncts, although some clinicians continue to prescribe them if spasms of the paraspinous muscles are elicited on physical examination in the case of vertebral OA.

Other medications such as gabapentin (Neurontin), SSRIs, and tricyclic antidepressants have also proven effective in the management of patients with OA who have chronic pain.

Glucosamine and chondroitin are dietary supplements not regulated by the FDA. Glucosamine is one of the most widely used dietary supplements in the United States. The ACR and Arthritis Foundation guidelines strongly recommend against the use of glucosamine, citing a lack of efficacy and a large placebo effect. A single trial reported efficacy of chondroitin in hand OA; therefore, the ACR and Arthritis Foundation conditionally recommend the use of chondroitin in hand OA, but strongly recommend against its use in OA of the knee and/or hip.

Topical agents such as capsaicin (Zostrix) cream, applied three to four times daily to painful areas, either alone or in concert with oral pharmacotherapy, may be helpful. The patient should be cautioned to avoid rubbing the cream in the eyes and to wash hands carefully after using capsaicin to avoid irritation. The ACR and Arthritis Foundation guidelines conditionally recommend the use of topical capsaicin only in OA of the knee. Other topical agents, such as Bengay, Icy Hot, and similar preparations, are menthol-based and have a temporary local effect. Topical preparations also give the patient a sense of control over their own treatment (see Drugs Commonly Prescribed 56.1).

Corticosteroid Intra-Articular Injections

Intra-articular steroids have been used for some time in the treatment of OA of the knee. Several controlled studies document short-term efficacy of up to 4 weeks, although some patients report a response for up to 6 months after injection. There are multiple different types of injectable corticosteroid. Product selection is generally based on clinician preference and availability. A 1% lidocaine solution is usually mixed with the steroid before injection. Patients are instructed to rest the joint for a day and to limit physical activity for 48 to 72 hours after the injection. The hip may also be injected, but this procedure should be done under ultrasound or fluoroscopic guidance.

The use of intra-articular injections of corticosteroids should be judicious: No more than three to four injections should be done per year, and they should be used only in episodes of acute flares. If steroid injections are administered excessively, they can accelerate joint deterioration and increase the risk of avascular necrosis. The ACR and Arthritis Foundation strongly recommend the use of corticosteroid injections in knee and/or hip OA.

Viscosupplementation

Viscosupplementation with intra-articular hyaluronic acid is also used for treatment of knee OA. Hyaluronic acid is a naturally occurring component of synovial fluid; its purpose is to lubricate the joint for low-impact activities and potentially prevent mechanical joint damage during high-impact activities. In patients with OA, the viscosity and elasticity of synovial fluid are decreased; there may be a lower concentration and limited distribution of hyaluronic acid. Consequently, all of the rheological features of synovial fluid, such as shock absorption, lubrication, and protection are decreased, further increasing the risk of damage to synovial tissue and the articular cartilage surface.

Hyaluronan (Hyalgan), hylan G-F 20 (Synvisc), and hyaluronic acid (Orthovisc, a highly purified, high-molecular-weight form of hyaluronic acid) are intended to restore all of the protective functions found in normal synovial fluid. They are indicated for pain relief of knee OA that has failed to respond to conservative measures. Intra-articular injections of hyaluronic acid are marketed as medical devices, not medications, and may be used in conjunction with NSAIDs. Hyaluronic acid is injected once a week for 3 to 5 weeks depending on the preparation, and it may provide benefit for 6 months or longer. Adverse effects of hyaluronic acid injections include transient localized pain, burning, and swelling at the injection site.

Viscosupplementation remains a controversial treatment option. Although several studies have demonstrated dexamethasone suppression and other tests for hyperadrenocorticism, acid-base studies, serum or urine protein electrophoresis, and bone marrow examination or bone biopsy.

Differential Diagnosis

If a fracture has occurred, it is important to distinguish the underlying cause. Was it related to trauma, or was there an underlying pathological condition such as osteoporosis or neoplasm? Similarly, skeletal changes could result from a variety of underlying conditions, including a neoplasm, such as multiple myeloma or other neoplasias; osteomalacia; osteogenesis imperfecta tarda (type I); skeletal hyperparathyroidism (primary and secondary); and hyperthyroidism.

Screening for fracture risk involves appropriate history, physical examination, standard biochemical and hematological studies, and measurement of BMD. The clinical history should include inquiring about possible secondary causes of bone loss, such as social history, use of medications with potential adverse effects on bone health, and family history of osteoporosis. Approaches to BMD screening vary from country to country, in part due to cost and questions regarding the efficacy of a broad population screening policy.

MANAGEMENT

The goals for prevention and treatment of osteoporosis are to prevent fractures, stabilize or improve bone mass, maximize physical functioning, relieve symptoms of fractures and resulting skeletal deformity, and maximize psychosocial functioning and coping.

The ability to meet these goals is dependent on both the patient and the practitioner's dedication to work as a team, first in determining what therapeutic regimen will be most beneficial and acceptable to the patient. After this is the long-term commitment to continuing treatment, evaluating the therapeutic response, and assessing the need to redirect the management plan based on the response. An algorithm outlining prevention, detection, and management strategies for osteoporosis is presented in Figure 56.2.

In addition to the physical and functional limitations that can be quantified, practitioners must also address the human and emotional aspects of being diagnosed with osteoporosis. Although not often the direct cause of death and often identified as a "silent disease" until the patient sustains a fracture, for many individuals, a fracture can lead to a downward spiral in physical and mental health and well-being. There may be an abrupt descent into disease and disability. Osteoporosis can have a devastating effect on patients and their families, dramatically affecting functional status, leaving the patient feeling vulnerable, isolated, and uncertain of the future.

Lifestyle Management

For both prevention and treatment of osteoporosis, smoking cessation, moderation of alcohol use, weight-bearing exercise, and adequate calcium and vitamin D intake are advised. In addition, avoidance of falls by eliminating hazards in the home and gait training or other exercises that improve strength and agility through physical therapy are important considerations. Weight training and walking are effective interventions for prevention and treatment. An active lifestyle, including safe and appropriate exercise, should be actively encouraged by the provider. Interestingly, qualitative nursing research has shown that the current female-focused approach to osteoporosis prevention and treatment may influence how males with osteoporosis develop self-management strategies. Novel measures such as protective pads and inflatable devices worn around the outer thigh, which cover the trochanteric region of the hip, have been developed to prevent hip fractures in older adults. Patients with pain from osteoporotic fractures may find therapies such as massage, music, or acupuncture helpful.

Pharmacological Management

Calcium and Vitamin D

Optimal calcium and vitamin D intake vary according to age, sex, and other conditions (see Table 56.3). Adequate intake of calcium and vitamin D is necessary for the prevention of osteoporosis when consumed during childhood, adolescence, and early adulthood. An optimal diet for prevention and treatment of osteoporosis includes an adequate intake of calories (to avoid malnutrition), calcium, and vitamin D.

Those who reliably get adequate calcium from dietary intake alone do not need to take calcium supplements. Those with inadequate dietary intake should take supplemental elemental calcium in divided doses at mealtime, so that their total calcium intake reaches recommended levels. There is considerable controversy about the calcium supplements and the risk of cardiovascular disease; additionally, the evidence that ingestion of calcium supplementation truly prevents fractures is weak. The trend is to lessen emphasis on calcium supplementation and to encourage dietary intake.

Increased doses of vitamin D may be required if malabsorption or rapid metabolism of vitamin D is present due to concomitant anticonvulsant drug therapy or another condition. Most patients with osteoporosis require vitamin D supplementation because it is difficult to achieve goals with diet alone.

In general, the best source of calcium and vitamin D is from dietary sources. The National Osteoporosis Foundation offers a useful list of calcium-rich foods. Calcium and vitamin D are available in many forms, and patients may be confused about which type or brand is best. Product

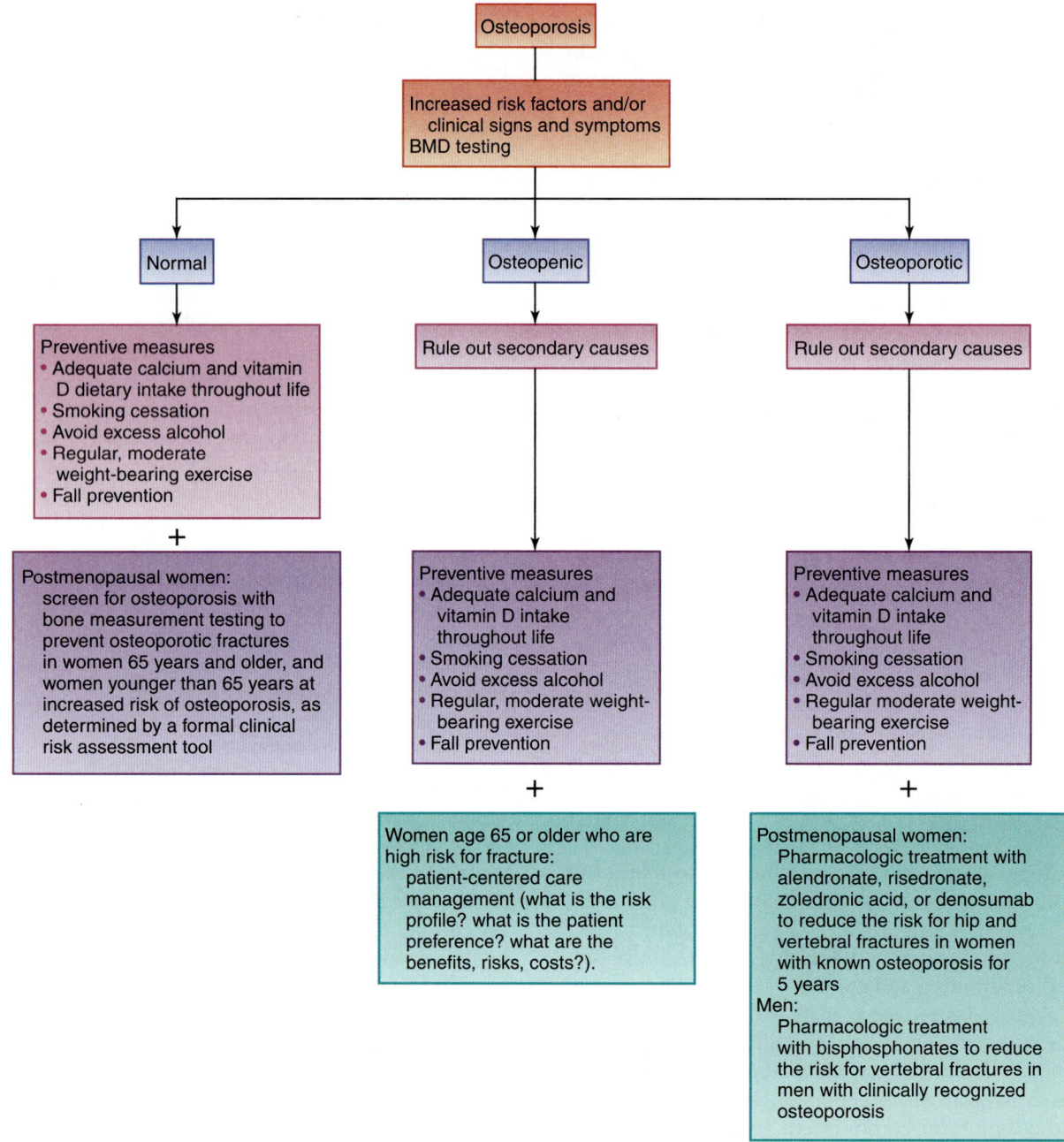

Figure 56.2 Prevention, detection, and management of osteoporosis.

selection generally depends on availability and affordability. The National Osteoporosis Foundation suggests that vitamin D_3 or cholecalciferol be used when available. Calcium carbonate is generally less expensive and more easily absorbed with meals. However, individuals with hypochlorhydria may absorb calcium citrate more efficiently, and it can be taken with or without food. As inadequate levels of vitamin D interfere with the body's absorption of calcium, adequate intake of both is essential.

Estrogen Therapy

Estrogen was the mainstay of treatment for osteoporosis for many years, until data from the Women's Health Initiative suggested that estrogen-progestin therapy reduced fracture risk at a cost of increased incidence of breast cancer, coronary heart disease (CHD), stroke, and venous thromboembolism, or in the case of unopposed estrogen, an increase in stroke and thromboembolism risk (but not CHD or breast cancer). As a result, the 2017 American College of Physicians treatment of low bone density or osteoporosis to prevent fractures in both sexes recommends against using menopausal estrogen or estrogen plus progesterone and raloxifene for treatment of osteoporosis in females.

Bisphosphonates

Bisphosphonates are the first-line pharmacological treatment for females with osteoporosis according to

TABLE 56.3 Recommended Daily Calcium Intake

Adult Females	Calcium (Daily)	Vitamin D_3 (Daily)
49 years and younger	1,000 mg	400–800 IU
50 years and older	1,200 mg	800–1,000 IU
Adult Males	**Calcium (Daily)**	**Vitamin D_3 (Daily)**
49 years and younger	1,000 mg	400–800 IU
50-70 years	1,000 mg	800–1,000 IU
71 years and older	1,200 mg	800–1,000 IU

Sources: Institute of Medicine (US) Committee to Review Dietary Reference Intakes for Vitamin D and Calcium; Ross AC, Taylor CL, Yaktine AL, et al. *Dietary Reference Intakes for Calcium and Vitamin D*. National Academies Press; 2011. https://www.ncbi.nlm.nih.gov/books/NBK56070/, doi: 10.17226/13050; National Osteoporosis Foundation. *Boning up on osteoporosis; 2018.* https://cdn.nof.org/wp-content/uploads/BoningUpBrochure_8.5x11.pdf.

TABLE 56.4 ACP Recommendations for Treatment of Low Bone Density or Osteoporosis to Prevent Fractures in Males and Females

Recommendation 1	Pharmacological treatment with alendronate, risedronate, zoledronic acid, or denosumab to reduce the risk for hip and vertebral fractures in females with osteoporosis
Recommendation 2	Clinicians treat osteoporotic females with pharmacological therapy for 5 years
Recommendation 3	Clinicians offer pharmacological treatment with bisphosphonates to reduce the risk for vertebral fractures in males who have clinically recognized osteoporosis
Recommendation 4	Recommends against bone density monitoring during the 5-year pharmacological treatment period for osteoporosis in females
Recommendation 5	Recommends against using estrogen plus progesterone therapy or raloxifene for the treatment of osteoporosis in females
Recommendation 6	Clinicians should make the decision to treat osteopenic females 65 years of age or older who are at a high risk for fracture based on patient preferences, fracture risk profile, and benefits, harms, and costs of medications

Adapted from The American College of Physician treatment of low bone density or osteoporosis to prevent fractures in men and women: a clinical practice guideline update from the American College of Physicians. *Ann Intern Med.* 2017;166:818–839. doi:10.73226/M15-1361.

the American College of Physicians. Specifically, their guidelines recommend that clinicians use pharmacological treatment with alendronate, risedronate, zoledronic acid, or denosumab to reduce the risk for hip and vertebral fractures in females who have known osteoporosis. Further, pharmacological therapy for 5 years with no bone density monitoring is recommended. Likewise, clinicians should offer pharmacological treatment with bisphosphonates to reduce the risk for vertebral fracture in males who have clinically recognized osteoporosis (see Table 56.4).

Bisphosphonates reduce the risk of fractures from osteoporosis by inhibiting bone resorption (see Drugs Commonly Prescribed 56.2). Alendronate sodium (Fosamax), a third generation bisphosphonate, binds to bone hydroxyapatite and specifically inhibits the activity of osteoclasts, thus reducing bone turnover. Treatment with alendronate sodium has been shown to increase BMD and reduce hip fracture risk by about 50% and other nonvertebral fractures by about 30%. Like other bisphosphonates, alendronate sodium has the potential to irritate upper GI mucosa. Alendronate sodium (Fosamax) and risedronate (Actonel) are available in weekly dosing and ibandronate (Boniva) is available in monthly dosing.

Risedronate (Actonel) prevents bone loss and reduces vertebral and nonvertebral fracture risk by about 40%. Similar effects have been noted in etidronate disodium (Didronel). Zoledronic acid (Reclast, Zometa) is an IV third generation bisphosphonate. A once-yearly dosage of zoledronic acid (Reclast) 5 mg IV has been noted to reduce the incidence of vertebral fracture risk by about 70% and hip and other nonvertebral fracture risk by about 35%. Adequate calcium and vitamin D must be maintained before, during, and after treatment. Zoledronic acid is approved for prevention and treatment of postmenopausal osteoporosis, glucocorticoid osteoporosis, osteoporosis in males, and treatment of Paget's disease.

Apart from the aforementioned GI side effects, adverse effects of bisphosphonates can be significant and include hypocalcemia, arthralgia and myalgia, rare ocular complications, atypical femur fractures, and osteonecrosis of the jaw. Contraindications to all bisphosphonate therapy include:

- History of hypersensitivity or allergic reaction to bisphosphonates
- History of atypical femur fracture or osteonecrosis of the jaw due to bisphosphonates
- History of hypocalcemia
- Chronic kidney disease with a glomerular filtration rate of less than 30 to 35 mL/min
- Esophageal disorders such as achalasia, esophageal stricture, esophageal varices, Barrett's esophagus
- Patient with an inability to stand or sit upright for at least 30 minutes
- History of bariatric surgery (Roux-en-Y gastric bypass)

The American College of Physicians advises providers offer bisphosphonates to males with clinically recognized

Drugs Commonly Prescribed 56.2: Osteoporosis

DRUG	PRESCRIBING CONSIDERATIONS
Bisphosphonates: therapy for 5 years	
Risedronate (Actonel) Available in daily, weekly, twice-monthly, and once-monthly dosage forms	• Swallow whole; take in the morning with a full glass of water before other food or drink; remain in upright position for at least 30 minutes. • Caution with other GI irritants such as aspirin
Alendronate (Fosamax) Also available with vitamin D; daily or once-weekly dosage	• Swallow whole; take in the morning with a full glass of water at least 30 minutes before other food or drink; remain in upright position for at least 30 minutes.
Ibandronate (Boniva) Available in oral daily or monthly preparations and IV preparation every 3-month dosing	• Swallow whole; take in the morning with full glass of water; remain upright and do not eat or drink for an additional 60 minutes; take on same day each month. • Caution with other GI irritants such as aspirin
Zoledronic acid (Reclast) IV preparation annual dosing	• Adequate hydration is important • Consider a drug holiday after three annual doses in moderate-risk patients or after six annual doses in higher-risk patients
Parathyroid Hormone	
Teriparatide (Forteo)	• Daily subcutaneous injection for up to 24 months • Stimulates bone formation • Contraindicated in hyperparathyroidism • Adverse reactions include dizziness, orthostatic hypotension, arthralgia, injection site reaction, secondary malignancy
Monoclonal Antibody	
Denosumab (Prolia)	• Subcutaneous injection every 6 months • Increases risk of serious infection • Drug holiday not recommended

osteoporosis. There is moderate-quality evidence that vertebral fractures in osteoporotic males were reduced by zoledronic acid.

Androgen Supplementation

Few studies have examined pharmacological therapy effectiveness in osteoporotic males. Preliminary data from one study showed an increase in BMD in males with idiopathic primary osteoporosis when treated with intramuscular testosterone over 6 months. Although no adverse cardiovascular events were found in the treatment group, studies of longer duration are indicated in this area to better estimate the risks versus benefits of testosterone supplementation in males.

Fluoride

Oral sodium fluoride has been used extensively in Europe for the treatment of osteoporosis and has been found to significantly increase vertebral bone density by increasing the number of osteoblasts. Large prospective studies have not shown a concurrent reduction in fractures, however, and until future research shows otherwise, it is believed the quality of bone produced by fluoride is more brittle than that formed by antiresorptive agents. Therefore, in the United States, sodium fluoride is currently not approved by the FDA for the prevention or treatment of osteoporosis.

FOLLOW-UP AND REFERRAL

Perhaps the most important part of managing the treatment of osteoporosis is improving adherence to treatment by individualizing the plan of care according to what is most effective in terms of increasing BMD and preventing fractures and what is most acceptable to the patient. There are currently no well-accepted guidelines for monitoring treatment of osteoporosis. Repeat BMD testing to monitor treatment response in osteoporotic patients should be limited to at least 2-year intervals. For patients with osteopenia or a normal baseline BMD, repeat measurement every 2 to 3 years is indicated to monitor for either stabilization or progression of the disease. Referral to an endocrinologist is warranted any time secondary causes of osteoporosis cannot be excluded or if the response to treatment is less than expected for the type of therapy instituted.

Patient Education: Osteoporosis

A number of informative patient education materials are available from a variety of sources, including pharmaceutical companies. Extensive, individualized education should be given to individuals when BMD results are available. This is particularly true for patients who are found to have osteoporosis and have an array of interventions available to them.

Reviewing potential hazards that may lead to falls and reinforcing the importance of maintaining agility are equally important in the ongoing care and management of patients who are at increased risk for fractures. Referral to a physical therapist and/or a home-care nursing evaluation is often of value in this area. Referral to local support groups, national osteoporosis education groups, and mental health counseling may also be of benefit for patients who seek further assistance in either learning about their condition or coping with their situation. Active exercise, such as weight training and/or walking, should be encouraged and supported.

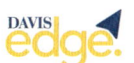 Go to Davis Edge for practice Q&A.

REFERENCES

Altman R, Alarcón G, Appelrouth D, et al. The American College of Rheumatology criteria for the classification and reporting of osteoarthritis of the hand. *Arthritis Rheum*. 1990;33(11): 1601–1610. https://doi.org/10.1002/art.1780331101

Altman R, Asch E, Bloch D, et al. Development of criteria for the classification and reporting of osteoarthritis. Classification of osteoarthritis of the knee. Diagnostic and Therapeutic Criteria Committee of the American Rheumatism Association. *Arthritis Rheum*. 1986;29(8):1039–1049. https://doi.org/10.1002/art.1780290816

American Academy of Orthopaedic Surgeons. (n.d.). Management of osteoarthritis of the hip: evidence-based clinical practice guidelines. https://aaos.org/globalassets/quality-and-practice-resources/osteoarthritis-of-the-hip/management-of-osteoarthritis-of-the-hip-7-31-19.pdf

American College of Rheumatology. (n.d.). Osteoarthritis. https://www.rheumatology.org/I-Am-A/Patient-Caregiver/Diseases-Conditions/Osteoarthritis

Bahr T, Allred K, Martinez D, et al. Effects of a massage-like essential oil application procedure using Copaiba and Deep Blue oils in individuals with hand arthritis. *Complement Ther Clin Pract*. 2018;33:170–176. https://doi.org/10.1016/j.ctcp.2018.10.004

Bannuru RR, Osani MC, Vaysbrot EE, et al. OARSI guidelines for the non-surgical management of knee, hip, and polyarticular osteoarthritis. *Osteoarthritis Cartilage*. 2019;27(11):1578–1589. https://doi.org/10.1016/j.joca.2019.06.011

Berenbaum F, Wallace IJ, Lieberman DE, et al. Modern-day environmental factors in the pathogenesis of osteoarthritis. *Nat Rev Rheumatol*. 2018;14(11):674–681. https://doi.org/10.1038/s41584-018-0073-x

Bortoluzzi A, Furini F, Scirè CA. Osteoarthritis and its management—epidemiology, nutritional aspects and environmental factors. *Autoimmun Rev*. 2018;17(11):1097–1104. https://doi.org/10.1016/j.autrev.2018.06.002

Choueiri M, Chevalier X, Eymard F. Intraarticular corticosteroids for hip osteoarthritis: a review. *Cartilage*. 2020;13(1 Suppl): 122S–131S. Advance online publication. https://doi.org/10.1177/1947603520951634

Donahue SW. Krogh's principle for musculoskeletal physiology and pathology. *J Musculoskelet Neuronal Interact*. 2018;18(3); 284–291.

Dowell D, Haegerich TM, Chou R.CDC guideline for prescribing opioids for chronic pain—United States, 2016. *MMWR Recomm Rep*. 2016;65(1):1-49. https://doi.org/10.15585/mmwr.rr6501e1

Efe Arslan D, Kutluturkan S. Effectiveness of aromatherapy in decreasing arthritis pain: a systematic review. *International Congress on Medicinal and Aromatic Plants*. 2017.

Efe Arslan D, Kutlutürkan S, Korkmaz M. The effect of aromatherapy massage on knee pain and functional status in participants with osteoarthritis. *Pain Manag Nurs*. 2019;20(1):62–69. https://doi.org/10.1016/j.pmn.2017.12.001

Fuggle NR, Cooper C, Oreffo R, et al. Alternative and complementary therapies in osteoarthritis and cartilage repair. *Aging Clin Exp Res*. 2020;32(4):547–560. https://doi.org/10.1007/s40520-020-01515-1

Henrotin Y, Raman R, Richette P, et al. Consensus statement on viscosupplementation with hyaluronic acid for the management of osteoarthritis. *Semin Arthritis Rheum*. 2015;45(2):140–149. https://doi.org/10.1016/j.semarthrit.2015.04.011

Ho KY, Cardosa MS, Chaiamnuay S, et al. Practice advisory on the appropriate use of NSAIDs in primary care. *J Pain Res*. 2020;13:1925–1939. https://doi.org/10.2147/JPR.S247781

Hsu H, Siwiec RM. Knee arthroplasty. In: StatPearls [Internet]. Treasure Island (FL): StatPearls Publishing; 2020, July 31. https://www.ncbi.nlm.nih.gov/books/NBK507914/

Hubertsson J, Turkiewicz A, Petersson IF, et al. Understanding occupation, sick leave, and disability pension due to knee and hip osteoarthritis from a sex perspective. *Arthritis Care Res*. 2017;69(2);226–233. https://doi.org/10.1002/acr.22909

Hunter DJ, Bierma-Zeinstra S. Osteoarthritis. *Lancet*. 2019; 393(10182):1745–1759. https://doi.org/10.1016/S0140-6736(19)30417-9

Kamaruzaman H, Kinghorn P, Oppong R. Cost-effectiveness of surgical interventions for the management of osteoarthritis: a systematic review of the literature. *BMC Musculoskelet Disord*. 2017;18(1):183. https://doi.org/10.1186/s12891-017-1540-2

Kolasinski SL, Neogi T, Hochberg MC, et al. 2019 American College of Rheumatology/Arthritis Foundation guideline for the management of osteoarthritis of the hand, hip, and knee. *Arthritis Care Res*. 2020;72(2):149–162. https://doi.org/10.1002/acr.24131

Krishnan Y, Grodzinsky AJ. Cartilage diseases. *Matrix Biol*. 2018; 71–72:51–69. https://doi.org/10.1016/j.matbio.2018.05.005

Le A, Enweze L, DeBaun MR, et al. Platelet-rich plasma. *Clin Sports Med*. 2019;38(1):17–44. https://doi.org/10.1016/j.csm.2018.08.001

Li J, Li YX, Luo LJ, et al. The effectiveness and safety of acupuncture for knee osteoarthritis: an overview of systematic reviews. *Medicine*. 2019;98(28):e16301. https://doi.org/10.1097/MD.0000000000016301

Mandl LA. Osteoarthritis year in review 2018: clinical. *Osteoarthritis Cartilage*. 2019;27(3):359–364. https://doi.org/10.1016/j.joca.2018.11.001

Marshall M, Watt FE, Vincent TL, et al. Hand osteoarthritis: clinical phenotypes, molecular mechanisms and disease management. *Nat Rev Rheumatol*. 2018;14(11):641–656. https://doi.org/10.1038/s41584-018-0095-4

McIntyre JA, Jones IA, Han B, et al. Intra-articular mesenchymal stem cell therapy for the human joint: a systematic review. *Am J Sports Med*. 2018;46(14):3550–3563. https://doi.org/10.1177/0363546517735844

Pehlivan S, Karadakovan A. Effects of aromatherapy massage on pain, functional state, and quality of life in an elderly individual with knee osteoarthritis. *Jpn J Nursing Sci*. 2019;16(4);450–458. https://doi.org/10.1111/jjns.12254

Perlman A, Fogerite SG, Glass O, et al. Efficacy and safety of massage for osteoarthritis of the knee: a randomized clinical trial. *J General Intern Med*. 2019;34(3):379–386. https://doi.org/10.1007/s11606-018-4763-5

Primorac D, Molnar V, Rod E, et al. Knee osteoarthritis: a review of pathogenesis and state-of-the-art non-operative therapeutic considerations. *Genes*. 2020;11(8):854. https://doi.org/10.3390/genes11080854

Rice SJ, Beier F, Young DA, et al. Interplay between genetics and epigenetics in osteoarthritis. *Nat Rev Rheumatol*. 2020;16(5):268–281. https://doi.org/10.1038/s41584-020-0407-3

Sen R, Hurley JA. Osteoarthritis. In: StatPearls [Internet]. Treasure Island (FL): StatPearls Publishing; 2022 Jan. https://www.ncbi.nlm.nih.gov/books/NBK482326/

Sharma L, Hochberg M, Nevitt M, et al. Knee tissue lesions and prediction of incident knee osteoarthritis over 7 years in a cohort of persons at higher risk. *Osteoarthritis Cartilage*. 2017;25(7):1068–1075. https://doi.org/10.1016/j.joca.2017.02.788

Varacallo M, Luo TD, Johanson NA. Total hip arthroplasty techniques. In: StatPearls [Internet]. Treasure Island (FL): StatPearls Publishing; 2020, July 8. https://www.ncbi.nlm.nih.gov/books/NBK507864/

Veronese N, Stubbs B, Solmi M, et al. Association between lower limb osteoarthritis and incidence of depressive symptoms: data from the osteoarthritis initiative. *Age Ageing*. 2017;46(3):470–476. https://doi.org/10.1093/ageing/afw216

Vina ER, Kwoh CK. Epidemiology of osteoarthritis: literature update. *Curr Opin Rheumatol*. 2018;30(2):160–167. https://doi.org/10.1097/BOR.0000000000000479

Wang L, Zhang L, Yang L, et al. Effectiveness of pain coping skills training on pain, physical function, and psychological outcomes in patients with osteoarthritis: a systemic review and meta-analysis. *Clin Rehabil*. 2021;35(3):342–355. Advance online publication. https://doi.org/10.1177/0269215520968251

Yazdany J, Schmajuk G, Robbins M, et al. Choosing wisely: the American College of Rheumatology's Top 5 list of things physicians and patients should question. *Arthritis Care Res*. 2013;65(3):329–339. https://doi.org/10.1002/acr.21930

Osteoporosis

Anthamatten A, Parish A. Clinical update on osteoporosis. *J Midwifery Womens Health*. 2019;64(3):265–275. https://doi.org/10.1111/jmwh.12954

Buckley L, Guyatt G, Fink HA, et al. 2017 American College of Rheumatology guideline for the prevention and treatment of glucocorticoid-induced osteoporosis. *Arthritis Care Res*. 2017;69(8):1095–1110. https://doi.org/10.1002/acr.23279

Colangelo L, Biamonte F, Pepe J, et al. Understanding and managing secondary osteoporosis. *Expert Rev Endocrinol Metab*. 2019;14(2):111–122. https://doi.org/10.1080/17446651.2019.1575727

Compton M, Ben Mortenson W, Sale J, et al. Men's perceptions of living with osteoporosis: a systematic review of qualitative studies. *Int J Orthop Trauma Nurs*. 2019;33:11–17. https://doi.org/10.1016/j.ijotn.2018.11.007

Eastell R, Rosen CJ, Black DM, et al. Pharmacological management of osteoporosis in postmenopausal women: an Endocrine Society Clinical Practice Guideline. *J Clin Endocrinol Metab*. 2019;104(5):1595–1622. https://doi.org/10.1210/jc.2019-00221

Ganesan K, Bansal P, Goyal A, et al. Bisphosphonate. In: StatPearls [Internet]. Treasure Island (FL): StatPearls Publishing; 2020. https://www.ncbi.nlm.nih.gov/books/NBK470248/

International Osteoporosis Foundation. (2020). About osteoporosis. https://www.osteoporosis.foundation/health-professionals/about-osteoporosis

National Osteoporosis Foundation. (2018). Boning up on osteoporosis. https://cdn.nof.org/wp-content/uploads/BoningUpBrochure_8.5x11.pdf

Porter JL, Varacallo M. Osteoporosis. In: StatPearls [Internet]. Treasure Island (FL): StatPearls Publishing; 2020. https://www.ncbi.nlm.nih.gov/books/NBK441901/

Qaseem A, Forciea MA, McLean RM, et al. Clinical Guidelines Committee of the American College of Physicians. Treatment of low bone density or osteoporosis to prevent fractures in men and women: a clinical practice guideline update from the American College of Physicians. *Ann Intern Med*. 2017;166(11):818–839. https://doi.org/10.7326/M15-1361

Troy KL, Mancuso ME, Butler TA, et al. Exercise early and often: effects of physical activity and exercise on women's bone health. *Int J Environ Res Public Health*. 2018;15(5):878. https://doi.org/10.3390/ijerph15050878

U.S. Department of Health and Human Services, National Institutes of Health Osteoporosis and Related Bone Diseases National Resource Center. (2018). Osteoporosis in men (NIH Publication No. 18-7885-E). https://www.bones.nih.gov/health-info/bone/osteoporosis/men

U.S. Preventive Services Task Force. Screening for osteoporosis to prevent fractures: US Preventive Services Task Force recommendation statement. *JAMA*. 2018;319(24):2521–2531. https://doi.org/10.1001/jama.2018.7498

Weaver CM, Gordon CM, Janz KF, et al. The National Osteoporosis Foundation's position statement on peak bone mass development and lifestyle factors: a systematic review and implementation recommendations. *Osteoporos Int*. 2016;27(4):1281–1386. https://doi.org/10.1007/s00198-015-3440-3

RESOURCES

American College of Rheumatology
https://www.rheumatology.org

Arthritis Foundation
https://www.arthritis.org

Calcium Fact Sheet for Health Professionals. National Institutes of Health Office of Dietary Supplements
https://ods.od.nih.gov/factsheets/Calcium-HealthProfessional

National Osteoporosis Foundation
https://www.nof.org

National Women's Health Resource Center (NWHRC)
https://www.healthywomen.org

Osteoporosis. American College of Obstetricians and Gynecologists
https://www.acog.org/Patients/FAQs/Osteoporosis

Osteoporosis. National Institute of Arthritis and Musculoskeletal Diseases
https://www.bones.nih.gov/health-info/bone/osteoporosis

Osteoporosis. OrthoInfo/American Academy of Orthopedic Surgeons
https://orthoinfo.aaos.org/en/diseases-conditions/osteoporosis

Osteoporosis and Arthritis: Two Common But Different Conditions. National Institute of Arthritis and Musculoskeletal Diseases
https://www.bones.nih.gov/health-info/bone/osteoporosis/conditions-behaviors/osteoporosis-arthritis#b

Osteoporosis Society of Canada
https://www.osteoporosis.ca

Section 11 ENDOCRINE AND METABOLIC PROBLEMS

SECTION EDITOR

Debera J. Thomas, PhD, RN, ANP/FNP

Chapter 57

Common Endocrine and Metabolic Complaints

Debera J. Thomas, PhD, RN, ANP/FNP
Brian Oscar Porter, MD, PhD, MPH, MBA

HYPOCALCEMIA

Hypocalcemia is defined as a calcium level of less than 8.5 mg/dL. In response to hypocalcemia, secretion of parathyroid hormone (PTH) increases, which leads to mobilization of calcium stores from bone and an increase in the absorption of calcium in the intestines. Neuromuscular signs and symptoms may occur in the presence of hypocalcemia because calcium is an important mediator in neuromuscular transmission and other intracellular biochemical activities.

Acute neuromuscular irritability occurs when the serum calcium drops abruptly by 2 to 3 mg/dL. Neuromuscular signs and symptoms include:

- Carpopedal spasm (Trousseau's sign) is a violent, painful contraction of the hands or feet. It is one of the neuromuscular signs indicating hypocalcemia and is a significant sign of tetany (hypocalcemia due to parathyroid dysfunction). It is often preceded by muscle cramps in the legs and feet. Carpal spasm consists of a flexed elbow and wrist, adducted thumb over the palm, flexed metacarpophalangeal joints, adduction of hyperextended fingers, and extended interphalangeal joints. The response is elicited by inflation of a blood pressure cuff to 20 mm Hg above the level of the systolic blood pressure. Inflation is maintained for 3 minutes to elicit the response, which is secondary to ulnar and median nerve ischemia.
- Chvostek's sign is another neuromuscular sign commonly associated with hypocalcemia. It is an abnormal unilateral spasm of the facial muscle when the facial nerve is tapped below the zygomatic arch anterior to the earlobe. In severe hypocalcemia, spontaneous spasms may also occur in the lower extremities and feet.

Other less specific symptoms of hypocalcemia include various neuropsychiatric disorders, including irritability, emotional instability, problems with memory, and psychosis. Complaints of paresthesias, fatigue, muscle cramps, or muscle weakness may be elicited on history. Gastrointestinal manifestations include dysphagia, nausea, vomiting, biliary colic, and abdominal pain or cramping. Patients may also complain of chronic constipation or diarrhea. Cardiovascular symptoms include hypotension, bradycardia, congestive heart failure (CHF), and dysrhythmias. Prolonged QT intervals may be seen on an electrocardiogram.

Chronic hypocalcemia may cause the skin to be coarse, dry, and scaly. Alopecia may present with thinning of the eyebrows and eyelashes. Nails are often rigid, brittle, and thin, with transverse grooves. Subcapsular cataracts, optic neuritis, intracranial calcification, papilledema, and parkinsonian-type movements may also be present in chronic hypocalcemia.

DIFFERENTIAL DIAGNOSIS

Patients exhibiting the discussed signs and symptoms should be immediately assessed for hypocalcemia, because it is critical to begin treatment in a timely fashion. Normal serum calcium values in adults range from 9 to 11 mg/dL. Immediate medical treatment is indicated in patients with marked hypocalcemia (less than 6.5 mg/dL). The etiology of hypocalcemia should be determined, and other conditions that present similarly should also be ruled out.

A focused history, clinical examination, and subsequent laboratory tests may determine the cause of hypocalcemia. In the absence of a clearly identifiable etiology such as a medication, chronic liver or renal disease, or an acute disease process, additional laboratory studies are needed. Further laboratory evaluation should begin with serum magnesium, serum phosphorus, and albumin levels. Depending on these findings, the clinician should initiate treatment if indicated. A serum PTH level will assist in the diagnosis of parathyroid disease. A direct measure of serum vitamin D levels is the 25-hydroxycholecalciferol (25-$[OH]D_3$) assay.

Patients exhibiting either Trousseau's sign or Chvostek's sign accompanied by respiratory distress (e.g., stridor, loud crowing noises, and cyanosis) require immediate referral for emergency care because the neuromuscular irritation produced by hypocalcemia may progress rapidly to laryngospasms, seizures, and dysrhythmias. In contrast, if serum calcium levels have declined gradually, symptoms are usually subtle.

PTH deficiency disease or inadvertent damage to the parathyroid glands during neck surgery may cause acute severe hypocalcemia. Acute transient hypocalcemia associated with significant intravascular fluid shifts may occur in burns, severe sepsis, pregnancy, extensive blood transfusions with citrated blood, acute pancreatitis, and acute renal failure.

Aggressive treatment of hypercalcemia with plicamycin (Mithracin), bisphosphonates, and calcitonin (Cibacalcin, Calcimar) may result in acute hypocalcemia. Other drugs that may produce hypocalcemia include radiographic contrast dyes that contain the calcium-chelating agent EDTA and the antiviral medication foscarnet (Foscavir).

Chronic hypocalcemia is usually caused by the absence of PTH, ineffective PTH function, vitamin D deficiency, chronic renal failure, hypomagnesemia, or hypoalbuminemia. Other potential causes of chronic hypocalcemia include alkalosis, malabsorption syndromes, chronic pancreatitis, laxative abuse, chronic liver failure, phosphate excess, and osteomalacia.

GYNECOMASTIA

Gynecomastia (GM) is the enlargement of glandular breast tissue in individuals assigned male at birth, resulting in increased breast size. True GM involves enlargement of the stromal and ductal tissues; it may present unilaterally and progress to bilateral symmetrical or asymmetrical enlargement. GM results from an imbalance of androgen and estrogen or an increase in prolactin. Growth hormones, estrogen, and corticosteroids stimulate ductal growth in the breasts. Progesterone and prolactin stimulate alveolar lobular growth of the breasts.

GM is estimated to affect 36% to 57% of the male population in the United States and is present in approximately 60% of males older than 50 years of age, due to a decrease in testosterone levels. Transient GM occurs in male neonates (65% to 90%) and at puberty (22% to 69%).

DIFFERENTIAL DIAGNOSIS

Asymptomatic GM may be an incidental finding on routine examination. It may also present as an acute unilateral (or bilateral), painful, tender mass beneath the areola or as a progressive, painless enlargement of breast tissue. The enlargement may be obvious by observation alone; however, less severe cases are noted only during palpation. Pain in the nipple or breast and tenderness often accompany GM, although GM lasting longer than 1 year is usually asymptomatic. Nipple discharge is rare, presenting in fewer than 5% of cases.

True GM must also be differentiated from pseudogynecomastia, which is fatty enlargement of the breast that often accompanies obesity in males. The patient is examined in a supine position while the examiner grasps breast tissue between the thumb and forefinger and gently moves the two digits toward the nipple. A firm or rubbery, mobile, disc-like mound of tissue at least 2 to 4 cm in diameter arising concentrically from beneath the nipple and areolar region confirms GM. The glandular enlargement of GM is usually resistive and ropy in texture. Severe cases present with more extensive enlargement.

Lack of a disc of tissue suggests the enlargement is the result of adipose tissue deposition (pseudogynecomastia). Mammography will distinguish between the two if the clinical examination is inconclusive. When GM is accompanied by other breast abnormalities, especially if they are unilateral, a mammogram is indicated to rule out a neoplasm. In addition, a disc that is greater than 4 cm in diameter should be evaluated via mammography.

When true GM has been established, the patient is evaluated for physiological (developmental) or pathological causes. Although physiological causes of GM are most common, pathological causes should always be ruled out with a thorough history and physical examination. The most common causes of GM are puberty (25%), idiopathic (25%), drug related (15%), cirrhosis or malnutrition (10%), and testicular failure (10%). Other

Pediatric/Adolescent Considerations:
Gynecomastia

GM associated with puberty has an age of onset of 12 to 14 years. The duration is approximately 6 months, followed by spontaneous regression. GM that presents before or after puberty and cannot be associated with physiological aging, a drug side effect, or chronic disease requires further investigation by an endocrinologist. Associated symptoms may assist in identifying the cause. Attention to any impact on body image, especially in adolescents, is important. A referral to an endocrinologist is also required for all cases in which GM appears before puberty, does not resolve within 2 years after puberty, occurs in the presence of abnormal serum levels of free testosterone and luteinizing hormone (LH), or when GM is accompanied by the abnormal presence or the absence of secondary sex characteristics, undermasculinization, or small asymmetrical testes.

causes include renal failure, thyroid disease, neoplasms (including testicular cancer), hyperprolactinemia, Klinefelter syndrome (XXY genotype), and gonadotropin deficiency. Decreased libido and impotence may accompany GM and may indicate the presence of chronic pulmonary, renal, or liver disease; testicular failure; or endocrine pathology. Idiopathic and pubertal GM should resolve spontaneously within 1 to 2 years and require no medication. The patient should be followed every 3 to 6 months, and the size of the disc should be measured until it has resolved.

Medications implicated in GM include highly active antiretroviral therapy for HIV infection, calcium channel blockers, tricyclic antidepressants, and selective serotonin reuptake inhibitors. Less common medication causes include amiodarone, human growth hormone, amphetamines, and diazepam.

Malignant breast tumors (which represent about 3% of all cases of GM) in males are typically unilateral, firm, and immobile; they grow rapidly and are often painful. Nipple retraction and discharge, skin dimpling, and axillary lymphadenopathy may also accompany breast neoplasms. Mammography and fine-needle biopsy are essential in confirming the diagnosis.

HIRSUTISM

Hirsutism is an increase in terminal hair growth on the face, chest, back, lower abdomen, pubic area, axillae, and inner thighs. It is typically considered an abnormal finding in females, as hair growth in these areas in males is often considered within the range of normal body hair distribution. In turn, hirsutism is present in approximately 5% of females. Almost 25% of these patients have terminal hair growth on the face, especially on the upper lip. Hirsutism is caused by increased secretion of androgens by the ovary or adrenal glands or an increased sensitivity to androgens. It is often accompanied by menstrual irregularities.

There are two major types of hair: vellus and terminal. Vellus hair is found over most of the body and is fine, soft, and unpigmented. During puberty, vellus hair often changes to terminal hair in the presence of increased androgens. Terminal hairs are characteristically dark, coarse, pigmented, and thicker compared with vellus hair. Terminal hairs are found on the scalp, eyebrows, and the axillary and pubic areas after puberty. They are found in lesser abundance on the extremities.

DIFFERENTIAL DIAGNOSIS

Androgen-dependent terminal hair growth may be caused by pathology in the adrenal glands or ovaries or by exogenous androgen administration. The characteristic increase in terminal hair growth occurs in areas most sensitive to androgenic activity: the upper lip, chin, chest, upper arms, upper abdomen, lower abdomen, thighs, and upper and lower back. The age, associated symptoms, and rapidity of onset are critical factors in differentiating potential causes of hirsutism, which helps guide the choice of treatment.

Although most (90%) cases of hirsutism are idiopathic or result from polycystic ovary syndrome (PCOS), more serious underlying disease entities must be ruled out. A targeted history with emphasis on when hirsutism was first recognized and how rapidly it has progressed, a detailed menstrual history, and a review of associated symptoms may provide some insight into the cause of hirsutism. When the cause of hirsutism is determined to be of adrenal or ovarian origin, the patient is referred to an endocrinologist for treatment.

The physical examination should focus on signs of adrenal disease and virilization that may further clarify possible causes. For example, accompanying signs of virilization, hoarseness of the voice, clitoromegaly, receding temporal hairline, acne, loss of body fat, and breast atrophy may be due to an ovarian or adrenal tumor. Markedly increased levels of plasma androgens often accompany this virilization.

Laboratory evaluation of hirsutism is indicated in female patients with menstrual irregularities, a history of sudden-onset or rapid progression of hirsutism, associated symptoms of ovarian or adrenal pathology, and moderate to severe clinical presentations. Evaluation of free and total testosterone, androstenedione, 17-hydroxyprogesterone, urine 17-hydroxycorticosteroids, thyroid-stimulating hormone, prolactin, LH, follicle-stimulating hormone (FSH), and dehydroepiandrosterone sulfate (DHEA-S) levels will provide insights into possible causes of hirsutism and the need for further evaluation. Slightly elevated levels of serum androgens (free testosterone) are found in 40% of females with idiopathic hirsutism, whereas LH and FSH levels are increased in 75% of cases of PCOS. Testosterone levels greater than 200 ng/dL (in females) and/or DHEA-S levels greater than 700 ng/dL indicate the need for an ovarian and adrenal work-up as these levels are rarely seen in idiopathic hirsutism or PCOS.

Idiopathic hirsutism in females is the result of excessive androgenic activity and begins during puberty, usually occurring in females 15 to 25 years of age without symptoms of virilization. There is a gradual development of the condition over 2 to 3 years, followed by a period of stability. It is usually mild and not accompanied by menstrual irregularities. There is a familial tendency toward hirsutism, and females of eastern European or Mediterranean descent are likely to have increased terminal hair growth. Obese females have increased androgen levels due to insulin-stimulated androgen production in ovarian theca cells. Thus, weight reduction may assist patients with this problem, because if the patient is obese, androgen production may be reduced with weight loss.

Hirsutism can also present in pregnancy, owing to the production of androgens by the placenta and corpus luteum. Postmenopausal patients experience an increase in androgen production, with 75% experiencing noticeable growth of facial hair.

Mild cases of hirsutism can be managed by cosmetic therapy, including physical hair removal, chemical depilatories, and bleaching. Electrolysis and laser therapy are more permanent solutions but are costly. Estrogen-dominant oral contraceptives are effective and will increase levels of sex hormone–binding globulin, which in turn, reduces free (nonprotein bound and, therefore, biologically active) testosterone levels. Progesterone-dominant contraceptives will increase clearance of testosterone. Medroxyprogesterone is also effective.

Hormonal therapy will stop further hair growth but will not reverse existing hair growth, which must be treated cosmetically. It may take 6 to 24 months to detect the results of hormonal treatment, which may need to be lifelong. Eflornithine 13.9% (Vaniqa) cream is U.S. Food and Drug Administration approved to reduce unwanted facial hair in biological and transgender women and has shown evidence of reducing hair growth on the upper lip, especially when combined with laser therapy.

INCREASED NECK SIZE

Along with an extensive muscular, vascular, and neurological network, the neck contains approximately 75 lymph nodes, the trachea, larynx, pharynx, submandibular and salivary glands, cervical vertebrae, and parathyroid and thyroid glands. Pathology in one of these structures or in an area that is drained by one of the many cervical lymph node chains may increase neck size.

A patient with increased neck size may present with complaints that shirt collars have become too tight. The patient should be evaluated immediately for difficulty swallowing or problems with breathing, as a rapid diagnostic work-up with a specialty referral is indicated in the presence of either of these red flag symptoms. Some patients may also complain of neck pain.

DIFFERENTIAL DIAGNOSIS

The most common cause of increased neck size is an enlarged thyroid gland, although increased neck size may be caused by a mass in any structure in the neck, including glands, lymph nodes, the larynx, or pharynx. Blockage of the salivary glands also produces neck enlargement, as can the development of cysts in the neck. Other potential causes include trauma and neoplasms.

A thorough history can assist in diagnosing the cause of increased neck size. For example, patients reporting a recent fall, automobile accident, or injury may have sustained cervical trauma, and a recent infection may have caused lymph node enlargement. The patient should be questioned about a history of thyroid problems or recent surgeries, allergies, sinus problems, and any complaints of headaches. Complaints of neck pain should be investigated, including if the pain is aggravated by range-of-motion movements, breathing, swallowing, or chewing. Symptoms of dysphagia, dyspnea, chest tenderness, cough, and hoarseness should be addressed. In addition, a patient with an increase in neck size may exhibit sleep apnea, which carries with it the risk of serious sequelae (see Chapter 29 for a full discussion).

The physical examination should assess whether the swelling (enlargement) of the neck is focal or diffuse. One or more focal masses may be enlarged lymph nodes related to Hodgkin disease, sarcoidosis, a thyroglossal cyst, thyroid adenoma, or other carcinoma. If the swelling is diffuse, venous distention due to CHF, Graves disease (autoimmune hyperthyroidism), subacute thyroiditis, superior vena cava syndrome, or subcutaneous emphysema (which is usually accompanied by subcutaneous crepitus) may be suspected. If the swelling is focal, it should be noted if the lesion is midline or lateral. Midline masses may indicate thyroglossal cysts or an adenoma of the thyroid; lateral masses are more likely related to a Virchow's node (a single lymph node in the left supraclavicular fossa that takes its supply from lymph vessels in the abdomen and may signify serious abdominal pathology if enlarged), Hodgkin lymphoma, bronchial cysts, a pharyngeal pouch, or a stone in a Wharton duct (submandibular salivary duct). Intermediate swelling suggests venous congestion of CHF, a bronchial cyst, a stone in a Wharton duct, or a neck aneurysm as possible etiologies.

A technique for detecting thyromegaly as the cause of neck swelling is to have the patient sit upright for examination and expose the neck down to the sternal notch while the examiner stands directly in front of the patient with the thyroid gland at the examiner's eye level. The patient should take several sips of water while the examiner observes for an enlarged thyroid gland. After visual examination, the thyroid is palpated anteriorly and posteriorly.

Thyroid nodules can be palpated in about 5% of the U.S. population. Females are more likely to have palpable thyroid nodules, and the frequency of nodules increases with age. Fewer than 10% of singular nodules are malignant, although thyroid-stimulating hormone and free thyroxine (T4) levels should be obtained on any patient with enlargement or any abnormality of the thyroid.

A single enlarged lymph node is unlikely to result in a significant increase in neck size, and a sudden complaint of lymph node enlargement suggests an infectious process. Patients who present with enlargement of a node over several months or multiple nodal involvement are more likely to have neoplastic disease. A hard, immobile mass is also suggestive of a neoplastic process. Laryngeal cancer also produces cervical lymphadenopathy and an increase in neck size, which may be accompanied by pain, dyspnea, dysphagia, hemoptysis, stridor, or hoarseness. In turn, a referral is indicated for biopsy of the nodes or neck mass in these situations.

POLYDIPSIA, POLYPHAGIA, AND POLYURIA

Polydipsia is defined as excessive thirst; it is associated with several endocrine diseases, psychiatric disorders, and the side effect profile of certain drugs. Polydipsia may accompany increased urine output (polyuria), which can be associated with excessive loss of water and salt.

Polyphagia refers to excessive eating before satiety. This symptom can present as a persistent or intermittent condition, resulting from various endocrinological and psychological disorders. Certain drugs are also known to cause polyphagia. Elevated thyroxine (T4) levels increase metabolism and thus the body's need for calories, often causing polyphagia.

Polyuria is a condition associated with increased urine production; it is defined as excretion of more than 3,000 mL (3 L) of urine per day. Any condition that increases hyperosmolar states will increase urination as a consequence of osmotic diuresis. The patient with polyuria is at risk for developing a fluid volume deficit that could result in hypovolemia.

DIFFERENTIAL DIAGNOSIS

Differential diagnoses for the patient with symptoms of polydipsia, polyphagia, and polyuria (also known as "The 3 P's") include diabetes mellitus (DM), diabetes insipidus, diuretic abuse, head trauma, and psychiatric disorders. See Figure 57.1 for other causes of these symptoms.

The patient should be asked about any history of head trauma, weight changes, thyroid disease, hypertension, and family history of DM. The patient should also be questioned about any history of psychiatric illness or changes in mental status, such as decreases in alertness or memory, as well as symptoms of fatigue. A detailed 48-hour history of fluid intake and output should be obtained, including the type of fluid intake over 48 hours, as well as the characteristics of urine output. As urine output is often difficult for patients to estimate, objective measurements may be needed, which can be challenging outside of a clinical or hospital setting.

The patient should be assessed for signs of dehydration and malnutrition, including measuring weight and vital

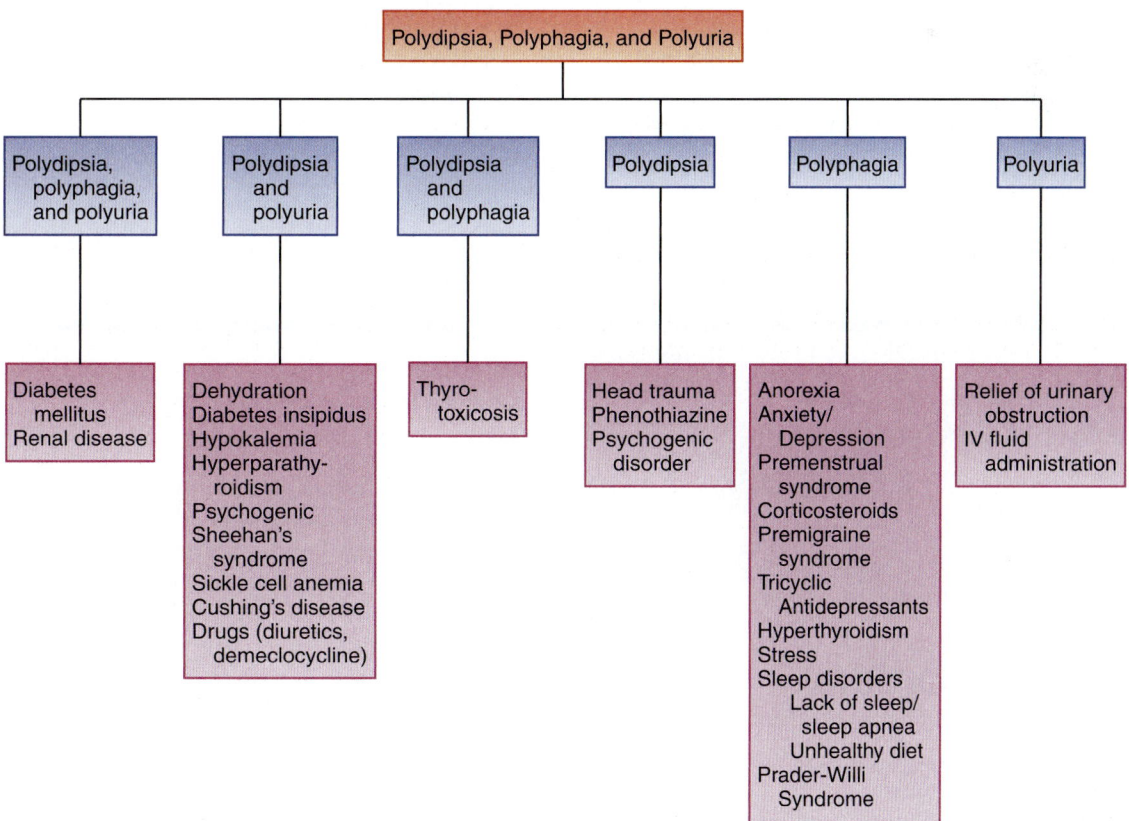

Figure 57.1 Diagnostic reasoning algorithm: Polydipsia, Polyphagia, and Polyuria

signs. Initial laboratory testing includes urinalysis, urine specific gravity, serum electrolytes, blood urea nitrogen, serum creatinine, complete blood count, fasting serum glucose, and glycosylated hemoglobin A1c (Hb A1c).

Polydipsia, polyphagia, and polyuria are the classic symptoms of DM. Thus, blood glucose levels should be evaluated in patients who experience these symptoms. An A1c equal to or greater than 6.5%, a fasting (after 8 hours of no caloric intake) blood glucose level equal to or greater than 126 mg/dL, a 2-hour postprandial plasma glucose level equal to or greater than 200 mg/dL after a 75-g oral glucose tolerance test, a random blood glucose level greater than 200 mg/dL in people with classic symptoms of hyperglycemia (e.g., polyuria, polydipsia, polyphagia, weight loss), or a hyperglycemic crisis confirms the diagnosis of DM. Additional symptoms of DM include weakness, fatigue, increased susceptibility to infections, and nocturia.

REFERENCES

Gynecomastia

Kanakis GA, Nordkap L, Bang AK, et al. EAA clinical practice guidelines—gynecomastia evaluation and management. *Andrology,* 2019;7(6):778–793.

Koch T, Bräuner EV, Busch AS, et al. Marked increase in incident gynecomastia: a 20-year national registry study, 1998–2017. *The Journal of Clinical Endocrinology & Metabolism,* 2020; 105(10):3134–3140.

Hirsutism

Matheson E, Bain J. Hirsutism in women. *American Family Physician,* 2019;100(3):168–175.

Schuler C, Rowe P, Stavropoulos A, et al. What are the most effective pharmacological treatments of hirsutism in women? *Evidence-Based Practice,* 2020;23(3):46–47.

Hypocalcemia

Falch C, Hornig J, Senne M, et al. Factors predicting hypocalcemia after total thyroidectomy—a retrospective cohort analysis. *International Journal of Surgery,* 2018;55:46–50.

Pepe J, Colangelo L, Biamonte F, et al. Diagnosis and management of hypocalcemia. *Endocrine,* 2020, 69:485–495.

Neck Enlargement

Bialek EJ, Jakubowski W. Mistakes in ultrasound diagnosis of superficial lymph nodes. *Journal of Ultrasonography,* 2017;17(68):59–65.

Yildirim Simsir I, Cetinkalp S, Kabalak T. Review of factors contributing to nodular goiter and thyroid carcinoma. *Med Princ Pract* 2020;29:1–5. doi: 10.1159/000503575

Polydipsia, Polyphagia, and Polyuria

Ahmadi L, Goldman MB. Primary polydipsia: update. *Best Practice & Research Clinical Endocrinology & Metabolism.* 2020:34(5): 101469

American Diabetes Association. Classification and diagnosis of diabetes. *Diabetes Care.* 2020;43(Suppl 1):S14–S31. https://doi.org/10.2337/dc20-S002

Refardt J. Diagnosis and differential diagnosis of diabetes insipidus: update. *Best Practice & Research Clinical Endocrinology & Metabolism.* 2020;34(5):101398.

RESOURCES

General

American Association of Clinical Endocrinologists
   https://www.aace.com

National Institute of Diabetes and Digestive and Kidney Diseases: Endocrine Diseases
   https://www.niddk.nih.gov/health-information/endocrine-diseases/

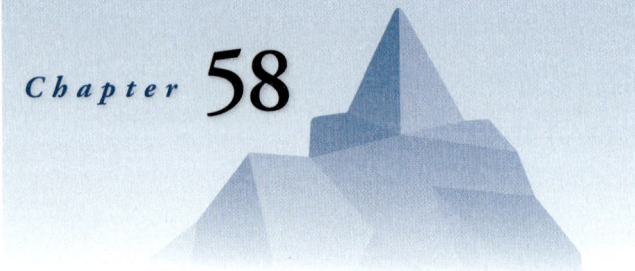

Chapter 58

Glandular Disorders

Debera J. Thomas, PhD, RN, ANP/FNP
Brian Oscar Porter, MD, PhD, MPH, MBA

HYPERTHYROIDISM

Hyperthyroidism, a common clinical condition, includes a heterogeneous group of conditions characterized by the excessive secretion and synthesis of one or both of the thyroid hormones thyroxine (T_4) and triiodothyronine (T_3). Although many clinicians use the terms interchangeably, *thyrotoxicosis* is a more general term that encompasses hyperthyroidism, as well as exogenous thyroid hormone intake and subacute thyroiditis, in which acute inflammation of the thyroid gland results in the rapid excretion (rather than overproduction) of stored thyroid hormones.

The clinical manifestations of hyperthyroidism result from the effects of excessive thyroid hormone on body tissues, resulting in alterations in growth, metabolism, and development. These manifestations are sometimes mistaken for signs of psychiatric illnesses. The long-term effects of inadequately treated overt hyperthyroidism are heart disease, osteoporosis (in postmenopausal females), mental illness, and infertility.

EPIDEMIOLOGY AND CAUSES

Hyperthyroidism occurs in about 1.2% of the U.S. population. It may occur at any age but peaks in persons 20 to 40 years of age. Only 10% to 15% of hyperthyroidism is diagnosed in older adults. The prevalence of hyperthyroidism is 2% in females older than 70 years of age and 4% in females 40 to 60 years of age, with an overall prevalence of 1% to 3%. Hyperthyroidism is much more common in females than in males (8:1).

Hyperthyroidism often occurs spontaneously from overproduction of thyroid hormones, but it can also result from the excessive intake of thyroid hormones. Graves' disease (more commonly called *Basedow disease* in Europe) is the most common cause of spontaneous hyperthyroidism in the United States. An autoimmune disorder characterized by autoreactive, agonistic antibodies to the thyroid-stimulating hormone (TSH; also called *thyrotropin*) receptor, Graves' disease accounts for 80% to 90% of hyperthyroid cases, peaking in young adults 20 to 40 years of age. It is also the most common form of hyperthyroidism that occurs during pregnancy.

Subacute thyroiditis accounts for 15% to 20% of thyrotoxicosis cases. Characterized by glandular inflammation and follicular cell destruction, it is thought to be of viral etiology, frequently occurring after an acute viral infection. More common in middle-aged adults between 40 and 50 years of age, subacute thyroiditis is more likely to develop in females than in males. Silent thyroiditis is a form of subacute thyroiditis in which the thyroid gland is moderately enlarged and nontender. It usually occurs in adults between 30 and 40 years of age and is also more common in females.

Toxic multinodular goiter (Plummer's disease) is as common as subacute thyroiditis, accounting for 15% to 20% of thyrotoxicosis cases. This type of goiter is more common in older adults and is a complication of chronic, inactive nodular goiter. This condition is more common in other parts of the world where dietary iodine deficiency is prevalent. A single, toxic thyroid adenoma is a less common cause of thyrotoxicosis, accounting for 3% to 5% of all cases.

The inappropriate use of thyroid replacement therapy or treatment errors may also produce symptoms of hyperthyroidism. Thyrotoxicosis factitia is a form of thyrotoxicosis in which a patient takes excessive amounts of either T_4 or T_3. This condition should be considered in a patient with access to hormone supplements or with psychiatric problems. An excess of dietary iodine may also precipitate symptoms of hyperthyroidism, as the exogenous iodine acts as a rich substrate for thyroid hormone overproduction.

A tumor of the pituitary gland causing hypersecretion of TSH is a rare cause of hyperthyroidism. Other uncommon causes of hyperthyroidism include metastatic follicular thyroid carcinoma, ingestion of iodine-containing drugs (e.g., certain expectorants, amiodarone, seaweed-containing health food supplements) or iodinated radiocontrast media, choriocarcinoma, or hydatidiform molar pregnancy producing high amounts of human chorionic gonadotropin that can weakly activate the receptor for TSH, struma ovarii (ectopic thyroid tissue) that is associated with dermoid tumors and ovarian teratomas, and testicular embryonal carcinoma (see Table 58.1).

	Disorder/Problem	Etiology/Comments
Common Causes	Graves' disease	Autoimmune disease
	Toxic nodular goiter	Unknown; development of nodules that progress from nontoxic to toxic over time
	Subacute thyroiditis	Thought to be caused by viral infection
	Thyrotoxicosis factitia	Excessive ingestion of exogenous thyroid hormones
	Jod-Basedow phenomenon	Large intake of dietary iodine or iodinated radiocontrast dye exposure in a person with thyroid disease
Rare Causes	Pituitary adenoma	Rare tumor of the pituitary gland
	Struma ovarii	Rare secretion of thyroid hormones by thyroid tissue located in ovarian dermoid tumors
	Metastatic thyroid cancer	Very rare cause
	High-dose amiodarone	Excessive dosage of iodine-containing amiodarone
	Pregnancy and trophoblastic tumors	Very high serum levels of human chorionic gonadotropin

TABLE 58.1 Hyperthyroidism: Common and Rare Causes

PATHOPHYSIOLOGY

All types of hyperthyroidism are a result of overproduction, overexposure (exogenous sources), and/or oversecretion of thyroid hormones, and the clinical manifestations of hyperthyroidism are a direct result of the effect of excessive thyroid hormones on essentially all organ systems and body tissues. Although thyroid hormones are required to regulate normal growth and development, excessive release of T_4 and T_3 from the thyroid into the circulation upregulates metabolism, leading to an increase in total body heat production, heart rate and contractility, and vasodilation. This explains the clinical manifestations of thyrotoxicosis, which include palpitations, diaphoresis, heat intolerance, and anxiety.

T_3 is normally 20 to 100 times more biologically active than T_4, which is converted into T_3 in peripheral tissues. Interestingly, however, the degree of symptomatology does not consistently correlate with the extent of thyroid hormone overproduction. In general, younger patients tend to have symptoms more reflective of sympathetic activation (e.g., tremors, anxiety, and hyperactivity), whereas older patients manifest more cardiovascular symptoms, including atrial fibrillation and dyspnea, as well as weight loss.

Graves' disease is an autoimmune disorder that results from aberrantly produced thyroid-stimulating immunoglobulins that activate TSH receptors in the thyroid gland, overriding the gland's normal regulatory mechanisms, thereby leading to thyroid hyperplasia (goiter) and increased synthesis of T_3. Thyroid hormone levels are typically highest with this form of thyrotoxicosis, and excessive thyroid hormone levels result in thyroid growth (hypertrophy), hypermetabolism, and sympathetic overactivity.

Graves' disease has a higher prevalence in people with human leukocyte antigen (HLA)-DRw3 and HLA-B89. It also strongly correlates with other autoimmune conditions including vitiligo, type 1 diabetes mellitus (DM), pernicious anemia, myasthenia gravis, and adrenal insufficiency. A diffusely enlarged goiter involving both thyroid lobes, hyperthyroid ophthalmopathy (e.g., periorbital edema, conjunctival edema and injection known as chemosis, proptosis, lid lag, and even diplopia), and excessive uptake of radioactive iodine with diagnostic imaging are all common characteristics. Circulating antithyroperoxidase (anti-TPO) antibodies are another common finding.

In contrast, subacute thyroiditis produces symptoms of thyrotoxicosis via the release of preformed thyroid hormones, in response to an inflammatory response after an acute viral infection. Thus, unlike other common causes of thyrotoxicosis, including toxic multinodular goiter and an isolated toxic adenoma that involve increased production and hypersecretion of thyroid hormones, subacute thyroiditis demonstrates a very low uptake of radioactive iodine on diagnostic testing. Subacute painful or granulomatous thyroiditis is associated with HLA-Bw35.

Toxic multinodular goiter typically arises in geographical areas where dietary iodine is deficient. As scattered portions of the thyroid gland increase in activity in an attempt to compensate for insufficient iodine, hormonal excess develops slowly over time. In fact, this condition may be asymptomatic at the time of diagnosis, especially in older individuals in whom the classic symptoms of hyperthyroidism may be blunted—a condition termed *apathetic hyperthyroidism*.

Nuclear scintigraphy demonstrates scattered areas of both increased and decreased iodine uptake, which reflect the increased thyroidal activity that manifests in the setting of adequate dietary iodine. In contrast, a single hyperfunctioning monoclonal follicular adenoma will show only one focus of increased uptake on a radioactive thyroid scan. Such nodules tend to be functional only once they reach at least 2.5 cm in size. As pituitary TSH production is suppressed by the adenoma, the remaining glandular tissue becomes hypofunctional and actually demonstrates decreased uptake on nuclear scintigraphy.

Autoregulation of the thyroid normally prevents thyrotoxicosis in the face of dietary iodine excess via a process known as the *Wolff-Chaikoff effect*, in which increased iodine transport to the thyroid triggers inhibition of the TPO enzyme, which is critical to the production of thyroid hormones. However, in the setting of a particularly concentrated iodine load (such as with iodinated radiocontrast media), patients with one or more autonomous thyroid nodules may lose this adaptive capability and be thrown into thyrotoxicosis (Jod-Basedow effect or Jod-Basedow syndrome).

CLINICAL PRESENTATION

The clinical presentation of hyperthyroidism depends on the duration and amount of excess thyroid hormone secretion. Signs and symptoms vary, depending on the cause and organ systems affected. Patients may be asymptomatic in the presence of mild elevations of thyroid hormones, and they are more likely to remain asymptomatic at increasing levels if the increased secretion is gradual.

Subjective

Because thyroid hormones affect most organ systems, a complete history and review of systems is indicated. Most patients with hyperthyroidism will complain of some combination of anxiety, nervousness, diaphoresis, fatigue, heat intolerance, palpitations, weight loss, and insomnia. In situations in which the thyroid tissue has become enlarged, the patient may report fullness or pressure in the neck. Additional complaints may include weakness, exercise intolerance, tremors, lower extremity edema, weight loss in the presence of an increased appetite, menstrual irregularities, frequent bowel movements or diarrhea, and exertional dyspnea.

Eye complaints include blurred vision, proptosis (downward displacement of the eyeball), photophobia, and double vision. Patients may also report that they are unable to concentrate and are extremely irritable and emotionally labile. Older patients may present with vague symptoms such as unexplained weight loss, apathy, worsening of angina, depression, a change in bowel habits, and weakness. A summary of potential signs and symptoms of hyperthyroidism is presented in Table 58.2.

TABLE 58.2 Hyperthyroidism: Clinical Presentation		
Body System	**Subjective Complaints**	**Objective Findings**
General	Fatigue Increased appetite Difficulty maintaining weight	Cognitive impairment Dementia Weight loss
Integumentary	Diaphoresis Heat intolerance	Warm, flushed, moist skin Onycholysis Hyperpigmentation Fine and silky hair Thinning hair Dermopathy of legs Pretibial myxedema Urticaria Pruritus Vitiligo
Gastrointestinal	Diarrhea Increased bowel movements Increased appetite	Increased liver function tests
Ophthalmological	Blurred vision Increased tearing Double vision Decreased visual acuity Photophobia Feelings of increased orbital pressure	Increased exophthalmos Lid lag Lid edema Corneal ulceration
Neurological	Hand tremors Confusion	Hyperactive reflexes Hand tremor
Cardiopulmonary	Palpitations Exertional dyspnea Breathlessness	Sinus tachycardia Elevated blood pressure Symptoms of congestive heart failure Dysrhythmias (atrial fibrillation) Increased respiratory rate
Genitourinary	Menstrual irregularities (decreased menstrual flow)	Gynecomastia
Head and neck	Pressure in neck Increased neck size	Enlarged thyroid gland
Psychosocial	Anxiety Nervousness Insomnia Irritability Restlessness	Emotional lability
Musculoskeletal	Weakness	Proximal muscle weakness Loss of muscle tone Muscle atrophy Osteoporosis (in postmenopausal females)
Laboratory findings	Not applicable	Normochromic normocytic anemia Hypercalcemia Potassium wasting Increased alkaline phosphatase

Patients should be questioned about current and prior endocrine diseases (in both the patient and family members), as well as a personal or family history of thyroid nodules, goiter, use of iodide-containing drugs, and thyroid neoplasms. Radiation to the head and neck increases the risk of thyroid cancer, which can rarely be associated with hyperthyroidism. A weight history should be obtained, including recent and long-term weight patterns. If the patient is currently taking thyroid hormone replacement medication, how the medication is being taken should be assessed. Patients should also be questioned about any recent viral infections or the possibility of pregnancy, as well as the use of other medications.

Objective

Signs of thyrotoxicosis are associated with the various forms of hyperthyroidism and range from overt manifestations in young adults with an acute onset to subtler presentations in older adults. Often, an older adult will present with signs and symptoms typically diagnosed as a failure to thrive.

The neck should be examined for visual enlargement of the thyroid and palpated for lymphadenopathy. The thyroid must be palpated thoroughly, noting any nodules or enlargement, both anteriorly and posteriorly. On physical examination, the thyroid may be enlarged, nodules may be palpable, and a bruit may be heard over the thyroid gland with the bell of a stethoscope. Whereas the goiter of Graves' disease is typically firm, the thyroid in toxic multinodular goiter may be softer, but with several palpable nodules. The neck should be moderately extended during the examination, and water should be provided to the patient to aid in swallowing. The thyroid gland normally moves with swallowing; however, a very large goiter or a large thyroid mass may prevent movement.

In subacute thyroiditis, the patient will present with firm and painful thyroid gland enlargement, fatigue, and possibly a low-grade fever. An enlarged painful thyroid is also consistent with degeneration or hemorrhage into a thyroid nodule, as well as either granulomatous or suppurative thyroiditis. In contrast, the thyroid gland is swollen but not usually tender in silent thyroiditis or subacute lymphocytic thyroiditis.

Cardiovascular manifestations include tachycardia (resting heart rate greater than 90 beats per minute), an irregular pulse, systolic murmurs, and a widening of the pulse pressure (the difference between the systolic and diastolic blood pressures). Although rare, an infiltrative dermopathy may be present in the lower extremities, which includes myxedema (deposition of glycosaminoglycan material in the dermis of the lower extremities, which causes nonpitting pretibial edema), erythema due to an inflammatory cell infiltrate, and skin thickening along the ankles and pretibial areas.

Visual acuity should be tested and lid lag assessed by instructing the patient to slowly gaze upward and downward. As the patient gazes downward, the upper lid will lag behind the eye movement. Lid lag can also be detected by the eyeball lagging behind the lower lid as the patient gazes upward. Hyperthyroid ophthalmopathy occurs in 40% of patients with Graves' disease and is rare in patients with subacute thyroiditis. The conjunctiva may be inflamed, and visual acuity may be affected. Exophthalmos, excessive lacrimation, lid retraction, and lid lag may be present.

The examiner should assess the skin and extremities for edema, general appearance, and signs of thinning hair. The skin may be moist and velvety to the touch, with increased pigmentation, spider angiomata, and vitiligo. Onycholysis (splitting and spooning of the nails) may also be present. Deep tendon reflexes may show a rapid relaxation of the reflexes, and the most predominant hyperactive reflex is usually the Achilles tendon reflex. The patient may have decreased strength in the extremities and fine tremors, especially of the hands when the arms are fully outstretched. Lymphadenopathy and splenomegaly may also be present.

Patients with longstanding hyperthyroidism may also have clubbing of the digits and signs of new bone growth in the hands, termed *thyroid acropachy*. Older adults with hyperthyroidism often appear apathetic. Physical examination may reveal atrial fibrillation (present in one-third of all older adults with hyperthyroidism), fine skin, brittle nails, and symptoms of congestive heart failure. However, the thyroid gland is often not enlarged in older adults.

Thyroid storm or crisis is a severe and sometimes fatal form of hyperthyroidism that requires immediate emergency medical care. Assessment, contributing factors, and treatments for thyroid storm are shown in Table 58.3.

DIAGNOSTIC REASONING

Diagnostic Tests

Initial Testing

Public health and medical organizations differ in their recommendations for routine screening of subclinical hyperthyroidism (SCHyper) in asymptomatic patients. In 2015, the U.S. Preventive Services Task Force (USPSTF) reviewed recommendations for thyroid hormone screening and reaffirmed that there is insufficient evidence for or against routine screening for thyroid disease in asymptomatic adults, which remains its current recommendation. If the patient is symptomatic or in a high-risk category, such as having a family history of thyroid disease or a previous history of thyroid disease or autoimmune disorders, screening is appropriate.

Levels of thyroid hormone often do not correlate reliably with the clinical presentation of hyperthyroidism. The initial screening tests for suspected hyperthyroidism are a serum TSH assay to detect suppressed thyrotropin

TABLE 58.5 Clinical Presentation: Hypothyroidism

Body System	Subjective Complaints	Objective Findings
General	Fatigue Lethargy Mild weight gain Cold intolerance Hypersomnia	Hypothermia Myxedema
Integumentary	Decreased sweating Hair loss	Dry, cool, rough skin Yellow skin (carotenemia) Alopecia Dry, coarse, thick hair
Gastrointestinal	Constipation Nausea	Hypoactive bowel sounds Enlarged tongue Ascites
Ophthalmological	Lid puffiness	Periorbital puffiness
Neurological	Memory deficits Personality changes	Hyporeflexia Bradykinesia Delayed relaxation of reflexes Slowing of mental processes
Cardiopulmonary	Inability to exercise	Bradycardia Cardiac enlargement Pleural effusion
Genitourinary	Menorrhagia Metrorrhagia	Decrease in fertility
Head and neck	Enlargement of the neck	Dull facial expression Facial pallor Facial swelling Enlarged tongue (late stage) Hoarseness
Psychosocial	Mild depression Decreased libido	Mild depression
Musculoskeletal	Ankle swelling Muscle weakness and cramping	Nonpitting edema

DIAGNOSTIC REASONING

Diagnostic Tests

Initial Testing

Although one in five females will develop an alteration in thyroid function in their lifetime, recently published clinical guidelines do not recommend routine screening of asymptomatic females before 50 years of age. Many clinicians, however, still use the age of 40 years as their criterion to begin screening. Although there are no universally accepted screening recommendations for hypothyroidism, the American Thyroid Association recommends baseline screening at age 35 years, with close attention to high-risk patients (e.g., pregnant patients, females older than 60 years, persons with other autoimmune diseases). The American Association of Clinical Endocrinologists recommends assessing TSH in females of childbearing age before pregnancy and in the first trimester of pregnancy. Females experiencing unexplained infertility should be screened for thyroid dysfunction, and postpartum patients with vague complaints may benefit from screening. In addition, congenital hypothyroidism is routinely screened for in neonates, as mandated in most states because failing to treat hypothyroidism promptly in this group may have serious sequelae (e.g., intellectual and developmental disabilities).

In 2015, the USPSTF reviewed its recommendations for thyroid screening and reaffirmed that there is insufficient evidence for or against routine screening for thyroid disease in adults without symptoms. In turn, the USPSTF does not recommend routine screening in adults without specific risk factors. However, all patients with an abnormal thyroid examination or prior history of any medically or surgically treated thyroid disease should be screened with a yearly serum TSH measurement while stable. In addition, patients with other autoimmune diseases such as type 1 DM or pernicious anemia, unexplained depression or other psychiatric diagnoses, cognitive dysfunction, prior external beam irradiation to the head and neck, previous radioablation of the thyroid, hypercholesterolemia, chronic amiodarone or lithium use, or a first-degree relative with autoimmune thyroid disease or other autoimmune disorders should be screened with TSH measurements.

The diagnosis of hypothyroidism is made by measuring serum TSH, and both TSH and FT_4 levels should be used to monitor treatment. When autoimmune thyroiditis is the suspected underlying cause of hypothyroidism, confirmation should be sought by performing antithyroid antibody titers—either for antimicrosomal (anti-TPO) antibodies or antithyroglobulin antibodies. The antimicrosomal antibody test is more sensitive and specific. If the TSH is low, inappropriately normal, or insufficiently elevated in the presence of low T_4 values, central hypothyroidism caused by hypothalamic or pituitary disease should be excluded before starting thyroid replacement therapy.

The sensitive thyrotropin assay is the most specific test for diagnosing primary hypothyroidism. A rise in TSH will precede any other abnormality of thyroid function as the first evidence of primary hypothyroidism. Hypothyroidism caused by primary thyroid failure can be confirmed by the concomitant finding of a decrease in serum FT_4. Patients in an early stage of hypothyroidism may present with an increase in serum TSH level together with a normal or low-normal serum FT_4 level.

By radioimmunoassay, primary hypothyroidism is associated with low FT_4 with an elevated TSH level. Values will differ depending on the laboratory method used. The normal range of ultrasensitive TSH is 0.4 to 4.0 mU/L. Older adults have a slightly higher normal range. TSH levels from 4.5 to 10 mU/L have varied treatment recommendations. Absent cardiovascular disease, there are no outcome data to suggest that treatment for levels between 2.5 and 4.5 mU/L is beneficial. An elevated TSH (up to 15 to 20 mU/L) may be temporarily observed in euthyroid patients with a systemic illness. In this situation, the TSH and T_4 should be repeated in 2 to 3 weeks for confirmation.

Patients with secondary or tertiary (central) hypothyroidism show a low, normal, or mildly elevated TSH level with low FT_4 and T_3 by radioimmunoassay. In subclinical hypothyroidism, these laboratory values show a mildly increased TSH level with a normal FT_4 concentration. Measurement of FT_4 is always preferred over total T_4, because of alterations in the protein-binding of thyroid hormone levels that can result in large fluctuations in total serum T_4 levels. The free thyroxine index (FTI), although not the test of choice, may be used in laboratories that do not have the capacity to measure FT_4. FTI uses a T_3 resin uptake test to calculate the percentage of hormone-binding sites available and multiplies this by the total T_4 level to give an estimation of the free T_4 level.

A high (1:400) antimicrosomal (anti-TPO) antibody titer is diagnostic for autoimmune thyroiditis. The degree of antibody elevation correlates directly with clinical hypothyroidism, although it is unclear whether the antibodies themselves are pathogenic because clinical disease may also be apparent with low or absent autoantibody titers, and when hypothyroidism is present for a long period of time, antibody titers typically fall. Antithyroglobulin antibody is also increased, but it is not as specific for Hashimoto's thyroiditis. If no antibodies are identified at the time of diagnosis, the condition is called *idiopathic hypothyroidism*, which is also considered a form of autoimmune thyroiditis. Antimicrosomal antibody titers and thyroid hormone (TSH and FT_4) levels should also be evaluated in patients with repeat miscarriages to screen for autoimmune hypothyroidism as a potential etiology.

Although the promotility GI agent metoclopramide (Reglan) can increase TSH levels in hypothyroidism, dopamine (Intropin), glucocorticoids, NSAIDs, and somatostatin (Sandostatin) can all decrease TSH levels. Other medications, such as phenytoin (Dilantin), amiodarone (Cordarone), and lithium carbonate, can also decrease thyroid hormone levels and function. Smoking (nicotine) also affects thyroid hormone levels and can both exacerbate hypothyroidism symptoms, as well as predispose to Graves' disease and hyperthyroidism. These medication and chemical exposures act via a number of mechanisms to affect thyroid function. A drug may bind with albumin and displace thyroid hormone off carrier proteins, or it may prevent albumin from binding with T_3 or T_4, thereby resulting in more active hormone in circulation. Other drugs may cause an upregulation of metabolic processing proteins (e.g., different cytochrome P450 oxidase isomers), which normally inactivate thyroid hormones; thus, their upregulation can lead to more rapid processing of thyroid hormones and, in turn, increase TSH levels.

Subsequent Testing

Once a diagnosis of hypothyroidism is confirmed, additional testing may be necessary to determine the effect of the disease on other body systems. Because the T_3 level is nonspecific and insensitive, it is not routinely used as an initial diagnostic tool. In the early stages of hypothyroidism, T_3 levels may be normal because of TSH-induced hyperstimulation. T_3 levels may not fall until late in the disease. Because the T_3 level correlates well with clinical status, the patient will not be as severely hypothyroid in clinical presentation until the T_3 falls to significantly low levels. In addition, the T_3 level may be below normal or elevated in patients with chronic disease.

Because anemia is a frequent complication of hypothyroidism, a CBC should be done. In addition, a serum chemistry profile should be done to assess for alterations in serum electrolytes, blood urea nitrogen, creatinine, serum osmolarity, and glucose, because glomerular filtration rate (renal function) may be decreased. A urinalysis should also be performed, with specific attention to the presence of protein (indicating possible renal impairment). Changes in blood chemistry may be an indication of deteriorating thyroid function leading to myxedema.

Patients with mild to moderate hypothyroidism have a tendency to develop hypertension (especially diastolic hypertension); therefore, blood pressure should be monitored. Interestingly, patients with longstanding or severe hypothyroidism tend to be normotensive or hypotensive. Depression of the uptake of LDL cholesterol by the liver in hypothyroid patients due to decreased LDL receptor expression (among other mechanisms) causes a decreased rate of cholesterol catabolism that leads to hypercholesterolemia. These patients tend to have elevated triglycerides and elevated LDL cholesterol. The combination of hypertension and hyperlipidemia increases the risk of atherosclerotic heart disease in hypothyroid patients. Thus, an annual lipid profile and an electrocardiogram (ECG) should be done. As the cardiac system continues to deteriorate, the ECG may show nonspecific ST and T-wave changes or low-voltage QRS complexes.

Unless there is reason to suspect a thyroid nodule or to confirm multinodular goiter, radioactive iodine scans and uptake are not usually necessary in hypothyroidism. As part of a complete examination of the patient with hypothyroidism, patients should have an annual chest x-ray examination to rule out cardiopulmonary complications, including cardiomegaly, congestive heart failure, and pleural effusion.

Ultrasound studies of the thyroid may be useful if a nodular thyroid is detected or if infiltrative disease is suspected (e.g., amyloidosis, sarcoidosis, tuberculosis). Fine-needle aspiration (FNA) is indicated for suspicious nodules, which may be found in patients with hypothyroidism, hyperthyroidism, or euthyroidism. In fact, 5% to 6% of isolated thyroid nodules are malignant, especially larger ones, and ultrasound may reveal suspicious findings for cancer such as irregular margins or microcalcifications.

Differential Diagnosis

Marked variations in TSH may occur in the setting of an acute illness or psychiatric disorder when the body's metabolic demands are altered. TSH levels normally peak in the evening and are at their lowest in the afternoon. Nonthyroidal illness is often associated with decreased TSH, T_3, and FT_4 levels without clinical hypothyroidism, with a reduction in the conversion of T_3 from T_4. In addition, usually the TSH level is normal or mildly increased during recovery from nonthyroidal illness.

In euthyroid hypothyroxinemia, the patient is euthyroid with a decreased T_4 level due to a decreased concentration of thyroid-binding globulin caused by nephrotic syndrome, exogenous testosterone exposure, or high-dose corticosteroids. Also, drugs that inhibit T_4 binding, such as phenytoin, phenobarbital, and salicylates, may decrease the total T_4 level.

MANAGEMENT

The goal of thyroid hormone replacement in primary hypothyroidism is to normalize, not suppress, the TSH, given the risks of overtreatment. Suppressed TSH, particularly in postmenopausal patients or individuals with levothyroxine overreplacement, causes decreased bone mineral density after several years, leading to osteoporosis. Hypothyroidism is typically treated medically (see Drugs Commonly Prescribed 58.2), though surgery may be indicated for particularly large, nonfunctional goiters that impair tracheoesophageal functioning. The goal of hormonal replacement in central hypothyroidism is to normalize the FT_4 because the TSH is not a reliable indicator of euthyroidism. The usual medication is levothyroxine (Levothroid, Levoxyl, Synthroid), a synthetic preparation of T_4, which has generally replaced desiccated bovine thyroid preparations, given their greater purity and consistency of dosing. Levothyroxine preparations are manufactured in numerous dosages, allowing for specific, precise titration to meet individual patient requirements.

According to the medical guidelines developed by the American Association of Clinical Endocrinologists, the usual dose of thyroxine is 1.6 µg/kg per day for full replacement. Otherwise healthy patients younger than 60 years may receive 50 to 100 µg daily as a full replacement dose. Patients who are older or have coronary artery disease should begin with one-half of the expected replacement dose or 25 to 50 µg/day orally, increasing the dose gradually by 25 µg/day once every 4 to 6 weeks. The TSH level should be measured every 4 to 8 weeks after initiating therapy and before each dosage increase. The common dosage is 75 to 150 µg/day. Dosing is best done in the morning to avoid nighttime insomnia. Many other medications and mineral supplements interfere with GI absorption of thyroid hormone replacements, including iron, calcium carbonate, aluminum hydroxide, sucralfate, and tube feedings. Thus, these medications require separation of dosing in time, whereas patients receiving continuous tube feedings require IV thyroxine dosing.

Replacement with T_3 preparations (liothyronine [Cytomel, Triostat]) is usually not indicated; however, anecdotal reports exist that indicated combination T_3/T_4 therapy may be helpful in patients who do not respond adequately to T_4 replacement alone. Although T_3 is better absorbed via the GI tract than T_4, the appropriate ratio of triiodothyronine preparations versus thyroxine in combination therapy has not been well established, and such treatment decisions require expert input from an endocrinologist.

Another treatment of historical importance that is still used today in some settings because of its relative lower cost is desiccated bovine thyroid (Armour Thyroid).

Drugs Commonly Prescribed 58.2: Hypothyroidism—Lifelong Pharmacological Treatment

DRUG	INDICATIONS	ADVERSE REACTIONS AND PRESCRIBING CONSIDERATIONS
Synthetic L-thyroxine T_4* (Levothroid, Levoxyl, Synthroid)	Patients with increased TSH level, usually three times the upper limit of normal Overt hypothyroidism Goal: administer enough thyroid supplement orally to result in normal free T_4 and TSH levels	Monitor effects of antihyperglycemics, oral anticoagulants, and potential sympathomimetics. Wait 4–5 hours after cholestyramine ingestion. Not to be prescribed for obesity. Increased sensitivity in myxedema and severe hypothyroidism. Start with the lowest dose and increase by 25 µg/day once every 3–6 weeks as needed, to no more than a maximum of 300 µg per day. Use with caution in patients with cardiovascular disease, diabetes mellitus, and adrenal insufficiency. Older adults require slightly lower initial doses.

*Synthetic T_3 supplements (e.g., Cytomel) are not recommended as a drug of choice.

Obtained from pooled thyroid extracts from cows, these preparations contain multiple foreign antigens, and the specific levels of active hormone are difficult to control. Some manufacturers standardize preparations based on bioassays, whereas others use iodine content as a surrogate measure of activity. T_3 and T_4 are both present, usually in a 1:4 ratio. Although some older patients who have been treated for many years with desiccated thyroid are wary of changing medications after decades of replacement therapy at stable doses, few clinicians in the United States will start new patients on these preparations. They should not be used for patients with underlying cardiac disease, given the varied concentrations of highly active T_3, which poses a greater risk of overreplacement and iatrogenic thyrotoxicosis.

Regardless of choice of replacement therapy, all patients should be monitored for signs of thyrotoxicity, especially angina pectoris and arrhythmias, because optimizing thyroid replacement dosing can be difficult and time-consuming. If significant adverse symptoms occur during levothyroxine replacement, the dose should be decreased and the patient should be referred to an endocrinologist for evaluation before reattempting replacement therapy at the original higher dose.

Concurrent severe illness or major surgery may alter dosing requirements in either direction in the hypothyroid patient. Pregnancy is also well known to increase replacement therapy requirements. Some clinicians suggest increasing replacement dosing by 30% on confirmation of pregnancy, with subsequent adjustments guided by TSH levels because untreated hypothyroidism in pregnancy is associated with preeclampsia, postpartum cardiac dysfunction, anemia, miscarriage, and low birth weight. The levothyroxine dose should be returned to the prepregnancy dose after delivery, and a serum TSH level should be obtained at 6 to 8 weeks postpartum.

Untreated hypothyroidism may progress steadily for 10 to 15 years before resulting in myxedema coma—a life-threatening state of multiorgan failure, characterized by progressive respiratory depression, decreased cardiac output, and fluid and electrolyte abnormalities (including hyponatremia)—or even death. Box 58.1 presents the assessment and management of patients with myxedema coma.

Treatment of Subclinical Hypothyroidism

Treatment for subclinical hypothyroidism has varied recommendations. The American Thyroid Association and the American Association of Clinical Endocrinologists recommend treating subclinical disease when antithyroid antibodies are present, when evidence of atherosclerotic cardiovascular disease exists, when heart failure exists, or if the patient is symptomatic at the respective TSH level.

Some patients with subclinical hypothyroidism feel better when treated with levothyroxine. Medication therapy has potentially dangerous adverse effects but may improve subtle abnormalities, prevent goitrous growth, and prevent the development of frank hypothyroidism. Therapy is advisable especially if thyroid autoantibodies are positive, because overt hypothyroidism frequently develops in these patients.

In young patients or patients with goiter and subclinical hypothyroidism, levothyroxine therapy should be considered. If the decision is made not to treat these patients, they should be evaluated at 6- to 12-month intervals for evidence of more severe clinical disease or biological loss of thyroid function as reflected in worsening laboratory indices. A lower dose (0.5 to 1.0 µg/kg) of levothyroxine may be given for the treatment of subclinical hypothyroidism. If the diagnosis of hypothyroidism is uncertain in a patient who is already on levothyroxine, the dose can be reduced by one-half, and FT_4 and TSH levels can be reassessed in 6 to 8 weeks. If the TSH level is increasing, the patient should resume the previous higher dose. If the TSH is normal, the patient should discontinue the levothyroxine, and the TSH level should be rechecked in 6 to 8 weeks for any increase.

Box 58.1 Assessment and Management of Myxedema Coma

Untreated hypothyroidism may progress steadily for 10 to 15 years before resulting in myxedema coma (a life-threatening condition characterized by progressive respiratory depression, decreased cardiac output, and fluid and electrolyte abnormalities) or death. Myxedema coma is a result of severe hypothyroidism, most commonly seen in older adult females, presenting with altered mental status (e.g., profound lethargy or coma), hypothermia, bradycardia, hypoventilation, hypoglycemia, and adrenal insufficiency. It is usually triggered by a precipitating factor such as noncompliance with levothyroxine therapy, ingestion of narcotics or analgesics, sepsis, cerebrovascular accident (stroke), myocardial infarction, trauma, or severe stress. The mortality rate can be greater than 50%, despite emergency medical intervention.

Assessment

The patient is usually pale with periorbital edema, dry skin, decreased body temperature, macroglossia, distant heart sounds, bradycardia, and delayed deep tendon reflexes. The patient may have hyponatremia, seizures, and hypotension, with secondary respiratory acidosis, hypoxia, and retention of CO_2. A clinical diagnosis is required, in addition to laboratory confirmation, as T_4 is usually low and TSH is high.

Management

Patients with myxedema coma need emergency medical intervention and should be treated by an endocrinologist in an intensive care setting. Provide ventilatory support if indicated, treat hypothermia, and administer levothyroxine (Synthroid, Levothroid) IV 300 to 500 µg over 15 minutes and then IV 100 µg every 24 hours to bring thyroxine concentrations back to normal levels quickly. Glucocorticoids should also be administered until coexistent adrenal insufficiency can be ruled out. Hydrocortisone hemisuccinate 100 mg IV bolus is initially given, followed by 50 mg IV every 12 hours or 25 mg IV every 6 hours until the plasma cortisol level is confirmed to be within normal limits. Administer IV hydration to correct hypotension, adding dextrose if hypoglycemia is present. Avoid overhydration because clearance of free water is impaired in these patients. Rule out and treat precipitating factors (e.g., if the patient has sepsis or another infection of bacterial origin, treat with antibiotics).

FOLLOW-UP AND REFERRAL

After therapy has been initiated with levothyroxine, the primary care practitioner should monitor the effect of therapy in 4 to 8 weeks by evaluating the TSH level to determine whether adjustment of the levothyroxine dose is necessary. The target TSH level is 0.3 to 2.4 mIU/L. Increasing the levothyroxine dose more often than at 6-week intervals may lead to thyroid hormone overreplacement. Once a stable dose of levothyroxine has been established, the TSH level in primary hypothyroidism or the FT_4 level in central hypothyroidism can be checked biannually or annually.

The patient should be examined annually for manifestations of thyrotoxicity (e.g., tachycardia, nervousness, or tremor) before increasing thyroid hormone replacement dosages. Laboratory values (FT_4 and TSH levels) within normal limits and a satisfactory clinical examination suggest that treatment is adequate. For maintenance treatment, the medication should be titrated to the lowest dose required to maintain euthyroidism, with a normal TSH level and a normal or slightly elevated T_4 concentration. Undetectable TSH levels suggest overtreatment, and the dose of thyroid hormone replacement should be decreased in these patients. TSH levels greater than 10 mIU/L indicate undertreatment, in which case the dose of hormone replacement medication should be increased.

Referral to an endocrinologist is necessary if the patient has cardiac disease, symptoms of myxedema, or central (secondary or tertiary) hypothyroidism. After starting hormone replacement therapy, if signs or symptoms of myxedema, chest pain, or thyrotoxicosis develop, an endocrinologist should be consulted. These patients are at a high risk for serious complications related to hypothyroidism or its treatment. Hypothyroid patients with severe illness or those who present with unusual or confusing laboratory findings should be referred to an endocrinologist. Referral to an endocrinologist is also indicated for patients younger than 18 years of age, those with evidence of pituitary disease, pregnant and postpartum patients, and patients taking lithium or amiodarone.

For asymptomatic patients with subclinical hypothyroidism who (after consultation) are not being treated with medication, a TSH should be performed yearly, along with a focused history and physical examination to monitor for disease progression that may require the initiation of therapy.

Patient Education: Hypothyroidism

During follow-up visits, emphasis should be placed on compliance with lifelong thyroid therapy (if indicated), reviewing the symptoms of hypothyroidism and hyperthyroidism, and stressing the importance of adherence to the follow-up schedule. Instructions should be simple and repeated frequently with written information in the patient's primary language. An older adult or patient with decreased cognition or depression with hypothyroidism may need additional emotional support, reinforcement, and follow-up teaching. Support in the home setting may be necessary until the symptoms of slowed mental processes and depression abate. Initially, a caregiver may be needed to remind the patient to take his or her daily dose of medication (see The Patient's Voice 58.1).

Patients should be encouraged to wear an extra layer of clothing if they have cold intolerance and should be warned not to

The Patient's Voice 58.1

HYPOTHROIDISM

I pretty much had a normal life. I was working in an administrative job, was in a bad relationship, and was perimenopausal. I would get home from work and it was a struggle to make dinner and clean up. I was exhausted all the time. I had trouble getting out of bed in the morning even after going to bed at 7 p.m.! On the weekends, I would sleep for 14 hours a night and still wake up tired. At meetings, where I had once been quick with suggestions, I couldn't seem to think straight and put two sentences together. I had trouble finding the right words and thought I was getting early Alzheimer's.

I was 50 years old, and I felt like 100! I was constipated and cold all the time and in a mental fog every day. I saw my primary care provider, and she told me I was probably depressed because of my life situation and being perimenopausal. Thus, I was prescribed an antidepressant. After taking it for more than a month, I was not feeling any better and saw a different provider. That provider did a bunch of tests, including a TSH level. The results were astonishing! My thyroid was almost entirely shut down. If someone had just done the test earlier, I could have been spared several years of total exhaustion.

---

use a heating pad, because patients with diminished cognition, deceased sensitivity, and slowed responses may be at risk for thermal burns. If psychomotor symptoms are present, the patient should be cautioned against operating dangerous machinery or driving a motor vehicle until the symptoms have resolved.

Patients who are at high risk for hypothyroidism (e.g., those who have had previous thyroid surgery, radioactive iodine treatment, a history of thyroiditis, and postpartum patients) should be taught the common symptoms of hypothyroidism (e.g., lethargy, fatigue, cold intolerance, constipation, weight gain, dry skin). The patient and family should be instructed that hypothyroidism is a chronic, sometimes progressive disease requiring monitoring every 6 to 12 months to confirm response to therapy. Patients and their families should be reassured that as treatment progresses, symptoms will resolve. Because heredity is implicated in hypothyroidism, patients with children should be instructed to advise their child's primary care practitioner of their diagnosis.

Practitioners are encouraged to write prescriptions for thyroid hormone replacement therapy that do not allow for substitution and use the same medication brand for the patient throughout treatment to maintain consistency of dosing. The same brand of thyroid preparation is recommended because the bioavailability, stability, and content of active thyroid hormone may vary with different formulations. Patients should be given the rationale for their choice treatment, potential adverse effect profile, and dosage of their medication. Emphasis should be on the realization that medication use is lifelong. The patient should understand that as the body ages or as there are changes in body weight (including loss in body mass from bulky surgical amputations), transitions from pregnant or nonpregnant states, or other significant changes in metabolic demand, the dosage of thyroid replacement medication may need to be adjusted.

The patient should be taught the signs of iatrogenic hyperthyroidism (thyrotoxicity) due to thyroid replacement overdosage (e.g., nervousness, palpitations, insomnia, tremor). It is important to explain that it will take 1 to 2 weeks for the medication to be effective. During this time, patients may experience an increase in urination and a decrease in periorbital puffiness.

The absorption of levothyroxine from the GI tract may be slowed by concurrent use of certain drugs, such as ferrous sulfate, sucralfate (Carafate), or antacids. The dose of thyroid hormone should be taken 2 hours before or 4 hours after ingestion of these medications. Because levothyroxine supplements may increase blood glucose levels, patients with DM should carefully monitor their blood sugar levels, as doses of insulin or oral hypoglycemic agents may need to be adjusted. Thyroid hormones may also affect the levels of phenytoin (Dilantin), lithium, tricyclic antidepressants, estrogen, digitalis, anticoagulants, and indomethacin (Indocin). The appropriate blood tests and screenings should be performed, and patients should be instructed on key adverse reactions of thyroid hormone replacement to report, should they occur.

Because of increased sensitivity to certain medications in hypothyroid patients, patients should be cautioned against the use of analgesics and sedatives. Even in small dosages, these medications can cause severe somnolence and respiratory depression. Infrequently, a patient treated for hypothyroidism with normal TSH levels may continue to feel fatigued but should be discouraged from increasing the dose of thyroid hormone without consultation with a clinician, which some patients may be tempted to do. Persistent fatigue warrants further investigation as to the underlying cause and should be discussed during a clinic visit. In cases where medication adherence may be a problem, weekly dosing can be established with the guidance of an endocrinologist because the half-life of T_4 is approximately 1 week.

Patients should be taught to follow a healthy diet, with an emphasis on low-fat, high-fiber foods. Some patients may need to follow a diet that promotes weight loss once medication has been started. Because many patients with hypothyroidism experience constipation, they should increase their intake of raw fruits and vegetables and bran or high-fiber cereals and breads, and add unprocessed bran (two tablespoons daily) to cereal or liquids. A bulk-forming laxative containing psyllium may also be taken on a daily basis. Increasing water intake to six to eight glasses a day is often beneficial in reducing constipation, as is increasing physical activity. A low-fat diet is recommended because there is a high incidence of atherosclerotic heart disease in patients with hypothyroidism.

Once therapy with levothyroxine is initiated, the patient should be able to resume all previous activities. Initially, rest periods with a gradual increase in exercise and activity, as tolerated, may be indicated. The patient must be instructed that if they develop any signs or symptoms of cardiac or respiratory difficulty, it is essential to seek immediate medical attention.

THYROID CANCER

Thyroid cancer is classified as differentiated (papillary and follicular) or undifferentiated (medullary and anaplastic) forms. Approximately 60% of thyroid cancers are papillary, 20% are follicular, and the remaining 20% of cases are medullary or anaplastic.

EPIDEMIOLOGY AND CAUSES

Thyroid cancer is the most common endocrine-related cancer. The incidence of thyroid cancer in the United States is low, with an approximate lifetime risk of 1.2%. The U.S. National Cancer Institute estimates 44,280 new cases of thyroid cancer diagnosed in 2021. This incidence increases with age and is more common in adults 20 to 54 years of age, but thyroid cancer can occur at any age and is three times more common in females than in males.

Most thyroid cancers are small and slow-growing. Nodules are often found on routine physical examinations, by the patient, or via imaging done for other purposes. Thyroid nodules found in persons younger than 20 years of age or in adults older than 60 years of age are more likely to be cancerous. Anaplastic tumors are the fastest-growing of all thyroid neoplasms; they are more common in older adults and are associated with a high mortality rate. Overall, thyroid cancer accounts for 0.4% of all cancer deaths per year.

The major risk factor for developing thyroid cancer is exposure to ionizing radiation. Several historical incidents resulting in high-dose radiation exposure have been linked to an increased incidence of papillary thyroid malignancies in children, including the atomic bombings of the Japanese cities of Hiroshima and Nagasaki during World War II, military testing of the atomic bomb near the Marshall Islands, and the nuclear power plant meltdown in the Russian city of Chernobyl.

Moreover, until the 1950s, radiation treatments were given to children as treatment for an enlarged thymus, enlarged tonsils, and acne. It is estimated that 1 to 2 million individuals were exposed to this risk factor. Studies have estimated that one-third of patients who received radiation therapy to the head and neck will develop a thyroid nodule, and one-third of those patients will later develop a thyroid malignancy. Thus, it may be advisable for patients who received head and neck irradiation as children to have a thyroid ultrasound for screening purposes.

Importantly, low-dose radiation exposure associated with routine radiographic imaging studies has not been shown to be tumorigenic. In addition, ^{131}I radioablation therapy for thyrotoxicosis and high-dose external beam radiotherapy have not been associated with papillary thyroid carcinoma, presumably because of the greater amount of cellular apoptosis associated with these doses of radiation.

There is also an increased incidence of follicular and anaplastic thyroid carcinoma in areas where iodine deficiency and goiter are more prevalent. Thyroid cancer is also more common in persons with autoimmune disease. Medullary carcinoma is an inherited form of family-based thyroid cancer, with 90% of those inheriting the autosomal dominant gene ultimately developing cancer. Metastatic cancer of the thyroid is less common, although renal cancer, breast cancer, lung cancer, and malignant melanoma can all metastasize to the thyroid gland.

PATHOPHYSIOLOGY

Thyroid carcinomas are relatively rare in the United States, but benign thyroid disease is significantly more common. An estimated 10% of the general adult population develops thyroid nodules; although the vast majority of these nodules represent benign disease, it is estimated that 5% to 6% of isolated nodules are malignant. Thus, distinguishing nonmalignant from malignant cases requires careful clinical evaluation. Thyroid cancers range from those that are well differentiated and slow-growing to those that are poorly differentiated and aggressive. As with other malignancies, poorly differentiated thyroid cancers have an unfavorable prognosis.

Cancers of the thyroid gland are typically classified into primary or secondary (metastatic) tumors. Primary tumors include papillary (80% of cases), follicular (10% of cases), medullary (5% to 10% of cases), and anaplastic (2% of cases) tumors, as well as sarcomas and rare cases of primary non-Hodgkin thyroid lymphomas (2% to 5% of cases), which should be considered in persons with a rapidly growing goiter. Hürthle cell carcinoma is another rare type of thyroid malignancy (2% to 3% of thyroid cancers) that is often considered a variant of follicular carcinoma. Consisting almost exclusively of Hürthle cells (also called *oxyphilic* or *oncocytic cells*) that contain abundant granular acidophilic cytoplasm, these malignancies are highly aggressive, metastasize in more than half of cases, and are difficult to follow because they do not respond to TSH or take up radioiodine.

Papillary, follicular, and anaplastic tumors arise from endodermally derived thyroxine and thyroglobulin-producing follicular epithelium, whereas medullary tumors arise from neuroendocrine-derived parafollicular or C cells. Thyroid lymphomas arise from intrathyroid lymph tissue and are strongly associated with chronic lymphocytic thyroiditis (autoimmune thyroiditis), whereas sarcomas are derived from the vascular and connective tissue interwoven throughout the thyroid gland.

As with all types of malignancies, thyroid cancer is believed to develop from a series of mutational events producing an immortalized cell that is genetically different from its source. This explains the strong association of thyroid cancer with radiation exposure, which increases the incidence of DNA mutations and leads to transformation of normal thyroid cells into malignant clones. Similarly, germline mutations in the *RET* proto-oncogene have been associated with the inherited cancer syndromes of multiple endocrine neoplasia (MEN) 2A, MEN 2B, familial adenomatous polyposis, and familial medullary thyroid carcinoma (FMTC) syndrome—all of which are associated with medullary thyroid carcinoma.

CLINICAL PRESENTATION

Subjective

The major symptom of thyroid cancer is a lump or nodule in the neck, which is usually painless. Patients may also complain of a tight or full feeling in the neck, difficulty breathing or swallowing, hoarseness, hemoptysis, and swollen lymph nodes. In particular, the new onset of hoarseness with hemoptysis is strongly suggestive of a malignant growth. Progressive dysphagia and shortness of breath may indicate invasiveness. Neck pain is usually a late symptom with thyroid cancer.

Objective

Differentiated thyroid carcinomas most commonly present as a thyroid mass or nodule. However, almost 10% of the adult U.S. population has a palpable thyroid nodule, making clinical examination of the thyroid an ineffective method of screening. Although malignant neoplasms of the thyroid are more likely to be fixed, nontender, firm, and irregular in shape, only a biopsy can rule in malignancy. The physical examination should also include evaluation of the tongue, oropharynx, and cervical spine for swelling, nodules, or tenderness, which may suggest extension of disease or alternative pathology.

DIAGNOSTIC REASONING

Although there are typical presentations of benign versus malignant nodules of the thyroid, many malignant lesions have an atypical presentation. Thus, a biopsy is the only reliable method of differentiating benign from malignant lesions, and patients should be referred for evaluation and probable biopsy upon palpation of a nodule. Fewer than 5% of nodules are malignant, and multiple nodules of the same consistency are more likely to be benign.

Diagnostic Tests

Initial Testing

High-resolution ultrasonography is beneficial in identifying thyroid nodules but is not reliable in differentiating benign from malignant lesions. Ultrasound is indicated when there is suspicion of multinodular disease or when the thyroid is difficult to evaluate clinically. RAIU testing is a means of determining functionality of a thyroid nodule; positive uptake portends a more favorable prognosis in thyroid cancer, owing to the ability to treat such tumors with high-dose radioactive iodine therapy.

Subsequent Testing

FNA biopsy is usually successful in differentiating benign from cancerous lesions of the thyroid gland and has 83% sensitivity and 92% specificity for thyroid cancer. Thus, FNA will not capture all cases of thyroid cancer and a repeat biopsy may be necessary. The sensitivity of FNA is increased if it is ultrasound-guided. Nondiagnostic FNA biopsies may require surgical lobectomy to confirm that the nodule is not, in fact, malignant. Psammoma bodies are found in 50% of papillary carcinomas; they are circular, laminated bodies found in the stroma of the tumor.

Thyroid function tests typically show levels within the normal range in the setting of thyroid cancer, unless the patient also has thyroiditis. Elevated serum calcitonin is a strong tumor marker of medullary thyroid carcinoma, but these cancers are somewhat rare overall, so this test is not usually used in the initial work-up. For the inherited cancer syndromes MEN 2A, MEN 2B, and FMTC, polymerase chain reaction assays are used to detect germline mutations in the *RET* oncogene.

Computed tomography (CT) and MRI are used when the tumor is large or recurrent or when there is suspected extrathyroidal extension of the tumor, but these imaging modalities are not helpful for evaluating a simple, isolated nodule. However, they can be used to assess for distant metastases and regional lymph node involvement. Spread to the lymph nodes is more common with papillary than follicular carcinomas, and if distant metastasis occurs, the lung and bone are the most common sites. Interestingly, lymph node metastases are not an important prognostic factor, but distant metastasis is associated with a nearly 70-fold increase in death.

Differential Diagnosis

Differential diagnoses of thyroid cancer include lymphocytic thyroiditis, multinodular goiter, a benign thyroid nodule, cystic nodules, and regional lymphadenopathy. Mass-related effects may be similar to those associated with laryngeal carcinoma or other forms of head and neck cancer (e.g., dysphagia or hoarseness due to recurrent laryngeal nerve involvement with vocal cord paralysis, hemoptysis due to local invasion through the trachea).

If medullary thyroid carcinoma is diagnosed, it is critical to take a thorough family history to assess whether this presentation occurs as a component of several inherited cancer syndromes, including MEN 2A or Sipple's syndrome (which may present with concurrent pheochromocytoma and hyperparathyroidism), MEN 2B (which may present with concurrent pheochromocytoma, a tall and slender Marfanoid body habitus, and ganglioneuromas), or FMTC syndrome.

MANAGEMENT

Initial Management

Any swelling suggestive of malignancy should be referred for evaluation of the mass. Early referral of patients with thyroid nodules to an endocrinologist for evaluation and treatment reduces costs, decreases patient hospital time, and increases the precision of the diagnosis. The prognosis is good for thyroid cancer that is found early, is less than 2 cm in diameter, is of a favorable histological type, and has not invaded locally or metastasized.

A surgeon and an oncologist (possibly a radiation or medical oncologist) will be necessary for determining the diagnosis and treatment plan, as thyroidectomy is the treatment of choice. The decision is based on the type of tumor, the size, and whether the tumor is compressing other structures. A surgeon with expertise in thyroid surgery should perform the procedure because of the potential to damage the laryngeal nerves and parathyroid glands. For small, noninvasive tumors, some surgeons prefer to perform a lobectomy as a more conservative approach. However, if there is local invasion by the tumor, there is a greater possibility of recurrence. Thus, radical neck surgery may be indicated for tumors with extensive local invasion.

Subsequent Management

After a total thyroidectomy, patients are often treated with radioactive iodine therapy to ablate any remnant thyroid tissue. Thyroid replacement therapy is initiated to suppress TSH to a goal of 0.1 mIU/L, and patients are monitored closely for response to therapy. Patients are subsequently followed every 6 to 12 months by an endocrinologist. A thorough neck examination, chest x-ray, and physical examination are performed to assess for evidence of thyrotoxicosis. Thyroglobulin levels may also be measured for well-differentiated carcinomas. The endocrinologist may perform a follow-up ^{131}I scan 6 to 12 months after a total thyroidectomy and may initiate further radioactive iodine ablation therapy if indicated. A follow-up ^{131}I scan is not useful in medullary cancer because medullary carcinoma does not take up the radioactive isotope.

Some forms of thyroid malignancy have unique treatments. In addition to thyroidectomy and postoperative radiation therapy, thyroid lymphomas may also require chemotherapy directed by a medical oncologist. Sarcomas are particularly aggressive and, after thyroidectomy, are poorly responsive to chemotherapy, thus carrying a poor prognosis.

The long-term prognosis of thyroid malignancy depends on tumor cell type, size of the primary growth, gender (males are twice as likely to die of thyroid cancer as females), age at diagnosis (death is more common in patients diagnosed at younger than 20 years or older than 40 years), and the extent of metastasis at the time of excision. Fortunately, papillary thyroid cancer is rarely fatal.

FOLLOW-UP AND REFERRAL

Follow-up is directed by the knowledge that no single diagnostic tool is sufficient to evaluate for recurrent disease. The follow-up of patients who have been treated for thyroid cancer includes periodic clinical examinations, serum thyroglobulin measurements, chest x-rays, and ultrasound examinations to assess for recurrence. The patient is followed closely during the first 3 to 4 years after surgery because recurrence is more likely within this time period. The patient with a total thyroidectomy will also require thyroid hormone replacement for life. Patients with medullary carcinoma should be offered *RET* (rearranged during transcription) proto-oncogene testing to assess for MEN2A or MEN2B. Provided the mutation is identified, all first-degree relatives should be offered *RET* mutational testing as well.

Patient Education: Thyroid Cancer

Patients with a family history of thyroid cancer should be advised to perform a "neck check" monthly. Patients with a history of goiter or irradiation should also perform this screening technique. The check is performed at home with a glass of water and a handheld mirror. The patient should be instructed to hold the mirror to visualize the area between the Adam's apple and clavicle. Then the head should be tilted backward, enough to adequately visualize the area without producing coughing or choking. As a sip of water is swallowed, the patient should observe the area for any bulging. The maneuver should be repeated several times. Any signs of bulging should be reported immediately. An instruction card on how to perform the *neck check* can be obtained through Thyroid Cancer Survivors' Association, Inc (ThyCa).

CUSHING'S SYNDROME

Cushing's syndrome includes myriad symptoms and physical features produced by persistent and inappropriate hypercortisolemia. The condition was named after Harvey Cushing, a physician who found pituitary adenomas in six of eight patients with symptoms of adrenocortical hyperfunctioning in 1932.

EPIDEMIOLOGY AND CAUSES

Cushing's syndrome can be caused by cortisol hypersecretion by the adrenal cortex due to cortical hypertrophy or to a tumor of the adrenal gland. However, the prolonged administration of large doses of exogenous glucocorticoid hormones will also cause this cluster of signs and symptoms and simulate dysfunctional adrenal overactivity. The term *Cushing's disease* refers to a specific form of Cushing's syndrome caused by excess secretion of adrenocorticotropic hormone (ACTH) from a pituitary adenoma, which results in overproduction of cortisol by the adrenal gland.

Cushing's syndrome may be classified mechanistically as ACTH-dependent or ACTH-independent hypercortisolemic states. The former mechanism results in adrenocortical hyperplasia and is most frequently (70% of cases) due to an ACTH-secreting pituitary adenoma (Cushing's disease), which occurs more commonly in females. These tumors are usually small (microadenomas) and may not be recognizable on pituitary imaging, with some patients demonstrating only hyperplasia of pituitary corticotrophs. Fewer than 10% of affected patients have a tumor greater than 10 mm in diameter. The tumors are present in the anterior pituitary and are not encapsulated. Spontaneous cases of Cushing's syndrome are rare, occurring in 2.6 persons per 1,000,000 patient years, and malignant pituitary tumors are particularly rare.

Nonpituitary tumors account for ectopic ACTH secretion in 10% to 15% of ACTH-dependent cases of Cushing's syndrome. In contrast, excessive administration of exogenous ACTH (as a therapeutic agent) and ectopic secretion of corticotropin-releasing hormone (CRH) by nonhypothalamic tumors each account for less than 1% of ACTH-hypersecretion cases.

The majority of ACTH-independent cases of Cushing's syndrome are due to iatrogenic administration of glucocorticoid hormones for therapeutic purposes. However, tumors of the adrenal cortex account for up to 20% of ACTH-independent cases, and both micronodular and macronodular dysplasia of the adrenal gland have been observed, although these etiologies are both quite rare, accounting for fewer than 1% of Cushing's syndrome cases.

PATHOPHYSIOLOGY

A basic knowledge of the hypothalamic-pituitary-adrenal neurohormonal axis is required to properly understand the pathophysiology of Cushing's syndrome. Ultimately regulated by the central nervous system, CRH is first produced by the hypothalamus and released into the hypophyseal portal circulation, where it stimulates the production of proopiomelanocortin (POMC) by corticotrophs in the anterior pituitary gland, from which ACTH (also called *corticotropin*) is derived as a cleavage product. ACTH then acts directly on the adrenal cortex to stimulate the production of cortisol and other adrenal hormones that act at peripheral tissue sites as intranuclear transcription factors for corticosteroid-responsive genes. Cortisol is then metabolized by the liver and kidneys, and its breakdown products are secreted in the urine as 17-hydroxycorticosteroids, 17-ketogenic steroids, and 17-ketosteroids.

A key regulatory mechanism of this neuroendocrine axis is the negative feedback exerted by each downstream product on its preceding hormone—namely, the inhibitory effects of ACTH on CRH secretion, as well as serum cortisol on the secretion of ACTH and CRH at the level of the pituitary and hypothalamus, respectively. In contrast, the pituitary gland is also likely subject to other forms of positive feedback from additional secretagogues. For example, pituitary corticotrophs have been shown to express receptors for growth hormone–releasing peptide (GHRP) and increase ACTH production in response to GHRP secretion.

The secretion of ACTH (and, subsequently, serum cortisol) is normally pulsatile in nature in terms of frequency, which remains constant in pattern. However, the extent of ACTH release with each pulse varies according to the body's circadian rhythms (i.e., sleep–wake cycles), which accounts for the variation in serum cortisol levels observed through serial measurements at different times of the day. Physical and emotional stressors that increase the body's metabolic demands also increase ACTH and cortisol secretion. In the normal diurnal sleep–wake cycle, levels are highest in the early morning on awakening and are lowest late in the evening and during the very early morning hours after midnight.

In patients with Cushing's disease, pituitary adenomas secrete excessive amounts of ACTH. The hypersecretion is random, episodic, and does not follow the usual circadian rhythm of physiological ACTH secretion in terms of amplitude and duration. ACTH stimulates the secretion of glucocorticoids, mineralocorticoids, and androgenic steroids from the adrenal cortex. As cortical hyperplasia increases, the adrenal glands secrete increasing amounts of cortisol in response to each incremental pulse of ACTH. Moreover, in the presence of an adenoma, the usual negative feedback mechanism of excessive glucocorticoid secretion does not suppress ACTH production to the same extent as in unaffected persons, possibly due to a defect in the glucocorticoid receptor in adenomatous corticotrophs. In turn, these patients present with hypercortisolemia and elevated levels of ACTH—particularly those with macroadenomas.

Importantly, however, in contrast to the ACTH-producing cells of relatively rarer ectopic nonpituitary adenomas that remain virtually unresponsive to negative feedback mechanisms, pituitary adenomatous corticotrophs appear to still retain a threshold level for cortisol-mediated negative feedback, albeit higher than in normal corticotrophs. This allows a high-dose dexamethasone suppression test (DST) to differentiate between pituitary and nonpituitary sources of ACTH hypersecretion. With ectopic nonpituitary ACTH secretion, both hypothalamic CRH secretion and pituitary ACTH secretion from normal corticotrophs are suppressed. A number of tumor types have been implicated with ectopic ACTH hypersecretion, most commonly small oat-cell carcinoma of the lung and carcinoid tumors of the thymus or pancreas, all of which arise from neuroendocrine cell precursors. Interestingly, most of these tumors secrete a greater proportion of POMC precursors than ACTH itself.

In patients with Cushing's syndrome, cortisol measurements taken at various times during a 24-hour period will demonstrate prolonged elevations of cortisol, even though some readings may be within the normal range. The normally tight regulatory relationship between ACTH and cortisol secretion is lost, with late evening cortisol levels being particularly high. This excessive production of cortisol over the entire 24-hour sleep–wake cycle results in the clinical signs and symptoms of Cushing's syndrome.

The most frequent cause of Cushing's syndrome, however, is prolonged administration of exogenous glucocorticoid hormones—an iatrogenic etiology that is ACTH independent. Thus, any medical problem requiring the prolonged use of corticosteroids predisposes the patient to develop this syndrome. Examples include autoimmune disorders, reactive airway disease, and COPD—all of which may involve long-term systemic corticosteroid use as maintenance therapy or for recurrent exacerbations. Rarely, megestrol acetate (Megace), which has intrinsic glucocorticoid activity, may also lead to Cushing's syndrome. Exogenous corticosteroid administration leads to suppression of CRH and ACTH excretion and corticosteroid production by native adrenal tissue. This results in bilateral adrenocortical atrophy and low salivary and urinary levels of 17-hydroxycorticosteroid and cortisol, unless cortisol itself is the steroid being administered.

Primary adrenocortical disease, including cortical tumors and both micronodular and macronodular hyperplasia, is much less common. Adrenal tumors may be benign adenomas or malignant carcinomas. Both types of tumors demonstrate altered expression of genes involved in apoptosis and telomeric function, which appears to underlie clonal immortalization. However, a number of significant differences exist between benign and malignant adrenal tumors. Adrenal adenomas produce cortisol from cholesterol backbones very efficiently, secreting relatively low levels of the cortisol precursors dehydroepiandrosterone (DHEA-S) and 17-ketosteroids. Benign adenomatous cells respond to beta-adrenergic agonists and multiple cytokines, including IL-1, gastric inhibitory peptide, vasopressin, and serotonin. In contrast, adrenal carcinomas are far less efficient at producing cortisol and secrete cortisol precursors at disproportionately higher concentrations. Adrenal carcinomas are still capable of leading to Cushing's syndrome, however, because of their size and secretory cell mass. They are also more likely than adrenal adenomas to produce elevated levels of the aldosterone precursor corticosterone and its hydroxy and deoxy variants. Adrenal carcinomas also produce high levels of vascular endothelial growth factor-A, insulin-like growth factor (IGF)-1, IGF-2, IGF-2 receptor, cell cyclins, cyclin-dependent kinase, and the chemokines IL-8 and epithelial neutrophil-activating protein-78. In contrast, levels of the antiangiogenic factor thrombospondin-1 are reduced.

With primary adrenocortical tumors, hypercortisolemia allows for negative feedback of both CRH and ACTH secretion. Thus, pituitary corticotrophs atrophy, as do the normal adrenal cells of the zona fasciculata and zona reticularis. In contrast, macronodular adrenal hyperplasia results in glands weighing 25 to 500 g or more, with multiple benign nodules greater than 5 mm in diameter and a hypertrophic (rather than atrophic) internodular cortex.

CLINICAL PRESENTATION

Subjective

The clinical presentation of Cushing's disease is usually gradual, developing over months or years. Signs and symptoms of Cushing's disease are those of hypercortisolism and androgen excess. The presentation of patients with Cushing's syndrome is similar. Common complaints include weight gain, back pain, headaches, skin changes, and muscle weakness. Females may complain of menstrual irregularities and hirsutism, and males often report decreased libido and impotence. Patients may also complain of emotional lability, increased appetite, increased irritability, anxiety, poor concentration and memory, and sleep disturbances.

Objective

Patients with Cushing's syndrome usually present with generalized or central obesity. In fact, obesity is the most common and often the first clinical manifestation of this disorder. Excessive accumulation of fat in the face leads to the typical "moon face" appearance. Facial plethora often accompanies the moon facies. The characteristic "buffalo hump" appearance is caused by excessive accumulation of fat in the supraclavicular and dorsocervical area of the upper back.

Most patients will have readily recognizable skin changes. There is atrophy of the epidermis and connective tissue, producing a thinning of the skin and easy bruising. Fungal infections of the skin, nails, and oral mucosa are common. Skin wounds heal slowly in the presence of excessive cortisol. Additional skin changes include hirsutism, acne, and striae (stretch marks). Striae are typically red to purple and are usually present on the abdomen but may be present on the hips, buttocks, thighs, breast, and axillae. Hyperpigmentation, commonly found in some types of Cushing's syndrome, is rare in patients with Cushing's disease.

Most patients have muscle weakness, which is more prominent proximally and in the lower extremities. The extremities are usually thin, with muscle wasting. Other manifestations include glaucoma and psychiatric symptoms. Less common clinical findings include renal calculi and edema. However, hypertension is often present on physical examination secondary to sodium and water retention.

DIAGNOSTIC REASONING

Diagnostic Tests

Initial Testing

Cushing's syndrome (and specifically Cushing's disease) is diagnosed via a combination of laboratory testing and radiographical examinations. The Endocrine Society (a large, multinational professional medical society focusing on endocrinology and metabolism) has released diagnostic guidelines recommending that one of four tests be used in the initial evaluation for Cushing's syndrome: urinary free cortisol (at least two measurements), late-night salivary cortisol (two measurements), a 1 mg overnight DST, or a longer low-dose (2 mg/day for 48 hours) DST as an alternative testing modality if the first three do not give conclusive results.

A urinary free cortisol 24-hour collection test requires the patient to collect urine for 24 hours, which is often not a practical expectation, unless the collection is done in an inpatient setting. The majority of patients with Cushing's syndrome will have an elevated urinary cortisol level; if it is at least fourfold the upper limit of normal, this result is considered diagnostic for Cushing's syndrome. However, mild Cushing's syndrome may still have normal levels; thus, normal urinary free cortisol levels (less than 50 μg/24 hours) do not rule out Cushing's syndrome entirely. If the test result is positive for Cushing's syndrome, the patient should be referred to an endocrinologist, who will conduct further testing to determine the cause and subtype of Cushing's syndrome.

If symptoms of Cushing's syndrome are present but tests do not confirm the diagnosis of hypercortisolism, a low-dose DST should be performed.

A nighttime (11 p.m.) salivary cortisol level is normally less than 4.2 nmol/L, and obtaining two samples within this range excludes the diagnosis of Cushing's syndrome. In contrast, levels twice this high are suggestive of Cushing's syndrome. Although this is a relatively easy test to perform (samples are stable at room temperature), it requires special sample collection tubes and a nighttime collection schedule. This test has a sensitivity of 93% to 100%.

The overnight DST assists in the confirmation of hypercortisolemia. In this test, the patient ingests 1 mg of dexamethasone (Decadron) orally at 11 p.m., and the plasma cortisol level is measured at 8 the next morning (when physiological cortisol levels are typically highest). A normal finding is a value less than 1.8 μg/dL, whereas an elevated morning cortisol level would indicate that the patient's endogenous cortisol secretion is insensitive to the negative feedback imparted by the exogenous dexamethasone dose. False-positive results may occur, however, in patients who are obese, depressed, or under extreme stress, given the elevated cortisol levels seen in these conditions. Medications that can also produce high cortisol levels include estrogens, antiseizure medications, and rifampin. Phenytoin (Dilantin), phenobarbital (Luminal), and primidone (Mysoline) accelerate the metabolism of dexamethasone and can also produce a false-positive DST.

Additional initial laboratory tests include a CBC, blood glucose level, and comprehensive metabolic panel. Hypercortisolemia impairs glucose tolerance because cortisol interferes with the transfer of insulin across the cell membrane; thus, it often produces hyperglycemia, hypokalemia, and leukocytosis (which may manifest as a granulocytosis in the setting of lymphopenia). Hypokalemic alkalosis is rare in Cushing's disease but is often seen in Cushing's syndrome.

Subsequent Testing

If urinary or salivary cortisol levels and an initial overnight DST do not provide conclusive results confirming Cushing's syndrome, a longer low-dose DST may be used. The low-dose DST involves administration of dexamethasone 0.5 mg PO every 6 hours for 48 hours, with urine collected on day 2 of the test. Urinary free cortisol greater than 20 μg/dL or a 17-hydroxycorticosteroid level greater than 4.5 μg/dL confirms the diagnosis of hypercortisolism. Many medications, including corticosteroids, phenothiazines, phenytoin, diuretics, quinidine, penicillin G, oral contraceptives, lithium, acetylsalicylic acid, and monoamine oxidase inhibitors, may affect the accuracy of these test results.

After testing to confirm a hypercortisolemic state, baseline plasma ACTH levels should be assessed. Levels are highest between 7 and 10 a.m. (8 to 80 pg/mL) and lowest just before bedtime (less than 10 pg/mL). Generally, levels less than 20 pg/mL indicate a possible adrenal tumor, whereas levels exceeding 20 pg/mL are indicative of a pituitary or ectopic ACTH-secreting tumor.

After completion of hormonal studies, radiological assessments are performed to localize the possible source of excess cortisol production. Most microadenomas of the pituitary gland are detected by imaging, and if the etiology of hypercortisolemia is determined to be the pituitary gland, an MRI assessment is indicated. An abdominal CT scan of the adrenal glands is done to detect adrenal tumors, although in Cushing's disease, the adrenal glands are also enlarged. A CT scan of the chest and abdomen is also beneficial in detecting possible sites of ectopic secretion. Because the lung is the most likely source of ectopic secretion, special attention to the chest is indicated.

Even if not evident from the initial laboratory and diagnostic testing for Cushing's syndrome, patients should be assessed during subsequent evaluation for sequelae such as hypokalemia, anemia, metabolic alkalosis, hyperglycemia, and hypercholesterolemia. In addition, osteoporosis is common in patients with prolonged elevated cortisol levels, and pathological fractures may be evident on radiographical examination. Thus, except for initial testing, the diagnosis of Cushing's syndrome and the differentiation as to its cause are best accomplished either by an endocrinologist or in collaboration with an endocrinologist.

Differential Diagnosis

Pregnancy, obesity, and excessive physical activity may produce elevated serum cortisol levels. Other conditions that may produce elevated cortisol levels are alcoholism, severe depression, obesity, hypertension, DM, glucocorticoid therapy, estrogen replacement therapy, and oral contraceptives. There are also various familial (genetic) predispositions to hypercortisolemia. Type 1 MEN 1 syndrome presents with pituitary corticotroph adenomas in 2% of cases, whereas Carney's syndrome is a rare autosomal dominant complex consisting of bilateral micronodular dysplasia, pigmented lentigines (liver spots), and blue nevi on the head and trunk, as well as multiple endocrine and nonendocrine neoplasms.

MANAGEMENT

The goals of treatment are to normalize the patient's cortisol level and treat the underlying cause of hypercortisolemia. The initial clinical management of patients with Cushing's syndrome should be handled by an endocrinologist. Despite successful treatment, some patients may relapse, so the patient must be evaluated for recurrence of hypercortisolemia.

Initial Management

Transsphenoidal pituitary microsurgery is the treatment of choice for a pituitary adenoma causing Cushing's disease. If surgery is unsuccessful, irradiation of the pituitary may be considered. Complications from surgery include transient diabetes insipidus, visual disturbances, cerebrospinal rhinorrhea, and meningitis. After microsurgery, 80% to 90% of patients will experience dramatic decreases in cortisol and may require exogenous glucocorticoid therapy for 6 to 36 months after surgery. For patients who fail to respond or who have a recurrence, treatment may include stereotactic pituitary radiosurgery (gamma knife) or laparoscopic bilateral adrenalectomy. Conventional pituitary irradiation therapy has a 23% cure rate. Failure rates with both types of treatment increase over time.

In younger patients who are not surgical candidates, mitotane (Lysodren) or alternatively ketoconazole (Nizoral) 200 mg every 6 hours can be used alone or in combination to reduce cortisol overproduction, as inhibitors of steroidogenesis. Older adults who are not surgical candidates may tolerate the use of ketoconazole; however, liver enzymes may be elevated with this treatment and need to be monitored.

Subsequent Management

After resection of a pituitary adenoma, corticotropins are suppressed, and temporary cortisone replacement therapy is indicated as directed by an endocrinologist for 9 to 12 months, but may be needed for as long as 36 months. The drugs of choice for adrenal replacement therapy are hydrocortisone (Cortef), prednisone (Deltasone), and fludrocortisone (Florinef). Dexamethasone (Decadron) is an alternative. The lowest dose effective in maintaining hormone levels is recommended. Complications of untreated or inadequately treated Cushing's disease are increased susceptibility to infections, nephrolithiasis, hypertension, and osteoporosis. Inadequate treatment may also lead to psychosis or uncontrolled DM. Medications for corticosteroid replacement are listed in Drugs Commonly Prescribed 58.3.

FOLLOW-UP AND REFERRAL

The follow-up for each patient depends on the selected therapy and is critical, because excessive corticosteroid treatment should be avoided as much as possible. The disorder is usually chronic and characterized by periods of cyclic exacerbation and rare remissions. Complications include osteoporosis, increased susceptibility to infection, hirsutism, and metastases of malignant tumors, depending on causality. Thus, the patient should be followed monthly for the first year and checked for signs of adrenal hypofunction, and then every 6 to 12 months.

Drugs Commonly Prescribed 58.3: Corticosteroid Replacement Therapy

DRUG	INDICATIONS	ADVERSE REACTIONS AND PRESCRIBING CONSIDERATIONS
Prednisone (Deltasone, Meticorten) oral	Adrenalectomy Pituitary resection	Glucocorticoid activity: moderate Mineralocorticoid activity: weak Use the lowest effective dose to prevent side effects such as diabetes mellitus, psychosis, osteoporosis, and infections.
Prednisolone (Delta-Cortef, Prelone)	Adrenalectomy Pituitary resection	Glucocorticoid activity: moderate Mineralocorticoid activity: weak Use the lowest effective dose to prevent side effects such as diabetes mellitus, psychosis, osteoporosis, and infections.
Methylprednisolone oral (Medrol), IM (Depo-Medrol), or IV (Solu-Medrol)	Adrenalectomy Pituitary resection	Glucocorticoid activity: moderate Mineralocorticoid activity: none Use the lowest effective dose to prevent side effects such as diabetes mellitus, psychosis, osteoporosis, and infections.
Hydrocortisone (Cortef, Hydrocortone) oral, IM, IV, topical, and ophthalmic	Adrenalectomy Pituitary resection	Glucocorticoid activity: high Mineralocorticoid activity: yes Use the lowest effective dose to prevent side effects such as diabetes mellitus, psychosis, osteoporosis, and infections.
Cortisone acetate (Cortone) oral and IM	Adrenalectomy Pituitary resection	Glucocorticoid activity: high Mineralocorticoid activity: yes Use the lowest effective dose to prevent side effects such as diabetes mellitus, psychosis, osteoporosis, and infections.
Dexamethasone (long-acting) oral, IM, and IV (Decadron)	Adrenalectomy Pituitary resection	Glucocorticoid activity: very high Mineralocorticoid activity: weak Use the lowest effective dose to prevent side effects such as diabetes mellitus, psychosis, osteoporosis, and infections.
Fludrocortisone (Florinef) oral	Adrenalectomy Pituitary resection	Glucocorticoid activity: none Mineralocorticoid activity: high Use the lowest effective dose to prevent side effects such as sodium and water retention, edema, hypertension, and hypokalemia.

An endocrinology referral is critical to establish a proper diagnosis and treatment plan, although ongoing management requires close coordination with the primary care practitioner. Referrals are suggested for surgical intervention for the following conditions associated with Cushing's syndrome:

1. *Primary hypersecretion of ACTH by the pituitary.* Transsphenoidal microsurgery is recommended and is often followed by radiation and sometimes by medication (e.g., adrenocortical inhibitors).
2. *Adrenocortical tumors.* Surgery is recommended, but the prognosis is poor. Replacement therapy is used but usually for only 3 to 12 months. The patient may need treatment with adrenocortical inhibitors if not treated with surgery, which should be managed by an endocrinologist.
3. *Ectopic ACTH production.* Surgery is recommended for removal of neoplastic tissue to manage symptoms, although surgical cure is unlikely. Sometimes a bilateral adrenalectomy is performed. Follow-up for these patients depends on the underlying cause and recommended treatment.

There is the potential for failure of any surgical intervention. Thus, the patient must be instructed to report any return of symptoms if they have been asymptomatic for a period after the surgery.

Patient Education: Cushing's Syndrome

The patient will need education to cope with lifelong symptomatology (e.g., information on the importance of early interventions for infections), strategies to manage overwhelming stress and emotional lability, use of potassium supplements, and maintenance of a high-protein diet.

Although patients with Cushing's syndrome will be managed initially by an endocrinologist, the primary care practitioner often manages other aspects of the patient's health; thus, the patient should understand that it is important to work collaboratively with the primary care practitioner to manage symptoms successfully.

Patients need a thorough understanding of their medications and the warning signs of undertreatment or overtreatment with cortisone. Cortisone preparations should be taken with food. Patients need to be told that they should consult with the primary care practitioner when initiating additional medications, both by prescription or over the counter. Patients on high doses of corticosteroids should wear a medical identification bracelet. Because these patients are prone to infections, they should be instructed on how to avoid common infections, both bacterial and fungal. Patients cannot rely on fever to indicate the seriousness of infection, given the anti-inflammatory effects of corticosteroids; therefore, they need to report any initial signs of infection promptly to the primary care practitioner.

Nutritional counseling may be indicated, including information on the avoidance of excessive sodium and on a well-balanced, low-fat diet. Many patients are obese, and the importance of weight loss must be addressed. In addition, patients should monitor their glucose levels at least weekly. During periods of stress or medication adjustment, glucose levels will need to be tested even more frequently (e.g., daily during periods of medication adjustment). If glucose levels are stable and within normal range, patients should continue testing glucose levels until at least 1 week after the final dose adjustment. Patients should resume daily glucose testing in times of stress or if any signs of infection are present. If the morning glucose level at any time is above normal, more frequent testing is indicated. The patient should be given a log to record the glucose test results and instructed to bring the log to each primary care visit.

Patients with Cushing's syndrome will need to have their blood pressure monitored weekly. As with glucose monitoring, the frequency of blood pressure monitoring will depend on their symptoms and coexisting cardiovascular disease. More frequent monitoring will be needed during times of stress. The patient should obtain a sphygmomanometer for home use and keep a log of their blood pressures so that the primary care practitioner can evaluate any patterns.

The patient should be instructed on fall prevention, and given the potential for osteoporosis with chronic corticosteroid treatment, the patient should avoid activities that are likely to cause falls. Simple environmental changes can be made in the home to increase safety, such as removing small rugs, placing rails around bathtubs and toilets, and using a shower chair.

Patients should also report any symptoms of GI upset (e.g., nausea, bloating, vomiting) and monitor themselves for signs of GI bleeding (e.g., vomiting blood, tarry stools, increasing fatigue).

Instructions on skin care are essential. Older adults with a history of long-term corticosteroid use are more prone to pressure ulcers, as their thin, easily traumatized skin must be protected. These individuals should avoid applying tape and adhesive bandages directly to their skin, and they should wear protective clothing for outdoor activities such as gardening.

ADRENAL INSUFFICIENCY

Abnormally low levels of cortisol secretion by the adrenal glands can result from inadequate stimulation of the adrenals by ACTH from the anterior pituitary or because the adrenals are unable to produce sufficient adrenocortical hormones. Addison's disease, also known as *primary adrenal insufficiency,* is relatively rare and results from a failure of the adrenal glands to produce hormones because of a problem in the gland, rather than a problem with the pituitary or ACTH production. Other types of adrenal insufficiency, or hypocortisolism, occur from secondary sources, such as a failure of the pituitary gland to produce adequate levels of the adrenal-stimulating hormone ACTH or the abrupt withdrawal of exogenously administered glucocorticoids, which previously suppressed endogenous adrenal hormone production.

EPIDEMIOLOGY AND CAUSES

Addison's disease is primarily caused by autoimmune destruction of the adrenal cortex in 80% of cases in the United States. Although it can occur at any age, Addison's disease most often occurs in persons 30 to 50 years of age. The prevalence of Addison's disease is 100 to 140 cases per 1,000,000 persons in the United States. Risk factors for Addison's disease include having a first- or second-degree relative with the disease.

Other causes of (secondary) adrenal insufficiency are chronic corticosteroid use followed by a physiologically stressful event, such as severe infection, trauma, or a surgical procedure, in which adrenal hormone levels are inadequate due to the iatrogenic suppression of endogenous hormone production. Tuberculosis infection is the most common infectious cause of adrenal insufficiency worldwide, whereas HIV is the most common infectious cause in the United States, resulting from the direct effects of infection on the adrenal glands themselves. Other causes include bilateral adrenal hemorrhage and infarction, tumors of the adrenal gland causing decreased function, antisteroidogenic drugs (e.g., ketoconazole [Nizoral], etomidate [Amidate]), sarcoidosis, hemochromatosis, amyloidosis, and congenital causes.

PATHOPHYSIOLOGY

Idiopathic Addison's disease is an autoimmune disorder that can occur at any age. Adrenal-specific autoantibodies are present in 50% to 70% of cases and are more likely to be present in younger patients and those with other autoimmune diseases. These autoantibodies are specific for cells of the adrenal cortex and for the enzyme(s) responsible for the production of cortisol and aldosterone. A combination of autoantibodies and cell-mediated immune responses is responsible for this disease. Frequently, idiopathic Addison's disease appears with other autoimmune diseases, which are collectively termed *autoimmune polyendocrine syndrome* (APS). Type 1 APS is an inherited autosomal recessive disease and, along with Addison's disease, includes hypoparathyroidism and mucocutaneous candidiasis. Type 2 APS is the more common type, with a constellation of disorders that includes Addison's disease, DM, celiac disease, immune thyroid disease, and hypogonadism.

Secondary hypocortisolism is usually a result of low ACTH levels and subsequent adrenal atrophy. The resulting hypocortisolism causes clinical manifestations similar to Addison's disease. However, in this type of hypocortisolism, there is no hyperpigmentation as typically seen in Addison's disease (as both ACTH and corresponding melanocortin levels are low), and the renin-angiotensin system functions normally, resulting in normal aldosterone and potassium levels.

CLINICAL PRESENTATION

Subjective

Clinical manifestations of Addison's disease include complaints of fatigue, weakness, lightheadedness, anorexia, weight loss, nausea, abdominal pain, and diarrhea.

Objective

On physical examination, patients typically demonstrate hypotension (particularly orthostatic hypotension), which is the result of both hypocortisolism and hypoaldosteronism. Patients with Addison's disease also typically exhibit hyperpigmentation due to elevated levels of ACTH, which is derived from the precursor protein POMC, which also gives rise to melanocyte-stimulating hormone. The decreased adrenal androgen secretion associated with Addison's disease also results in the loss of secondary sex characteristics (e.g., loss of pubic and axillary hair) in females, but because the adrenal glands are not a major source of androgens in males, they do not experience any loss of secondary sex characteristics.

In severe cases, when a patient has Addison's disease that is well managed but the patient subsequently experiences a physiological stressor of some kind (e.g., infection, surgery), the requirement for cortisol increases and the patient may experience an Addisonian crisis, manifesting as severe hypotension and vascular collapse.

DIAGNOSTIC REASONING

Diagnostic Tests

When Addison's disease or other forms of hypocortisolism are suspected, a plasma cortisol level should be obtained. A morning (8 a.m.) cortisol level of less than 3 µg/dL is consistent with Addison's disease, especially if accompanied by a plasma ACTH level greater than 200 pg/mL. The diagnosis is confirmed by a cosyntropin stimulation test, in which a synthetic form of ACTH is given intramuscularly (IM) and a serum cortisol level is obtained 45 minutes later. In Addison's disease, the exogenous ACTH dose does not result in a corresponding increase in cortisol secretion, demonstrating primary failure of the adrenal glands to respond to ACTH. Small, noncalcified adrenal glands on CT scan are indicative of autoimmune Addison's disease.

Patients with hypocortisolism are also prone to hypoglycemia, as adequate levels of cortisol are not available to counter the action of insulin in facilitating the transport of glucose across cell membranes. Thus, serum glucose levels tend to be low.

Differential Diagnosis

In any patient with unexplained hypotension, Addison's disease and other forms of hypocortisolism should be considered. Patients with Addison's disease generally have an elevated ACTH level, which is associated with hyperpigmentation of the skin. In contrast, patients with hypocortisolism that is a result of hypopituitarism resulting in a low ACTH level will have normal pigmentation. Other nonspecific clinical manifestations that may be associated with Addison's disease, but are also common in other conditions as well, include nausea, unintentional weight loss, weakness, and anorexia. Thus, hypocortisolism should be considered when other causes for these constitutional symptoms have been ruled out.

MANAGEMENT

Initial therapy for adrenal insufficiency consists of hydrocortisone 15 to 30 mg in two divided doses, with two-thirds of the dose given in the morning and one-third given in the early evening. Prednisone can be used if the patient does not respond well to hydrocortisone. The dose of prednisone is 2 to 4 mg in the morning and 1 to 2 mg in the evening. The doses of these replacement medications are then adjusted based on the patient's clinical response.

Stress hormone supplementation is necessary for patients who experience significant physiological stressors, such as serious infection, trauma, or surgery. In cases of severe stress, hydrocortisone is given IV or IM every 6 hours at a maximum dose of 50 mg. Oral medication at lower doses can be prescribed if the physiological stress is less severe and then reduced to normal when the stress subsides.

In addition to hydrocortisone (glucocorticoid), mineralocorticoids must be replaced, although not all patients require daily therapy. Fludrocortisone acetate (Florinef) is the drug of choice and has a potent sodium-retaining effect. The usual dosage is 0.05 to 0.3 mg PO daily, which should be determined in conjunction with an endocrinologist. Symptoms of fatigue, postural hypotension, hyponatremia, or hyperkalemia may indicate the need for a higher dose. Of note, in contrast to glucocorticoid requirements, increased mineralocorticoid supplementation is not required during times of increased physiological stress.

Some patients require androgen therapy along with the medications mentioned earlier. DHEA 25 to 50 mg PO daily has been shown to improve a patient's sense of well-being, increase muscle mass, and reverse bone loss. When prescribed DHEA, older females should be monitored for masculinizing effects.

FOLLOW-UP AND REFERRAL

Patients with adrenal insufficiency require chronic glucocorticoid and mineralocorticoid supplementation and are prone to Addisonian crises, due to the inability to mount an appropriate stress hormone response with endogenous cortisol. Determination of an appropriate replacement dose and regimen requires periodic assessment for signs of both underdosing (e.g., weakness, dizziness, and headaches on waking) and overdosing (e.g., Cushingoid physical features, as discussed in the previous section on Cushing's syndrome).

Once chronic maintenance dosing is established in conjunction with an endocrinologist, the primary care provider will be able to meet most of the patient's ongoing health-care needs but should also coordinate evaluation of the patient for iatrogenic complications of chronic corticosteroid use, including cataract formation (requiring annual ophthalmological examinations) and the development of osteopenia/osteoporosis (requiring periodic dual-energy x-ray absorptiometry scanning). Expert consultation with an endocrinologist should be sought if dose adjustments or a change in the class of hormone replacement therapy is indicated.

Patient Education: Adrenal Insufficiency

Patients with Addison's disease or other forms of adrenal insufficiency need to be well informed about their condition and the potential for an Addisonian crisis if the patient should develop a serious infection or experience other physiological stressors. Given the significant risk from systemic illness, patients should be instructed to see their health-care provider during times of illness. In these instances, additional corticosteroid (stress hormone) supplementation may be required, for example, a doubling or tripling of the dose of hormone replacement therapy in the setting of a significant illness, surgery, or dental procedure. This may require parenteral (e.g., IM, IV) dosing if oral supplementation is not possible (e.g., due to significant nausea, vomiting, or diarrhea). Thus, if possible, patients should be trained to self-administer IM injections and may be given a reserve prescription for parenteral hydrocortisone or similar agent to be used in these situations.

REFERENCES

Adrenal Insufficiency

Buonocore F, Ackermann JC. Primary adrenal insufficiency: new genetic causes and their long-term consequences. *Clin Endocrinol.* 2019;92:11–20.

Husebye ES, Pearce SH, Krone NP, et al. Adrenal insufficiency. *Lancet.* 2021;397(10274):613–629.

Martin-Grace J, Dineen R, Sherlock M, et al. Adrenal insufficiency: physiology, clinical presentation and diagnostic challenges. *Clin Chim Acta.* 2020;505:78–91.

Cushing's Syndrome

Braun LT, Reincke M. What is the role of medical therapy in adrenal-dependent Cushing's syndrome? *Best Pract Res Clin Endocrinol Metab.* 2020;34(3):101376. https://doi.org/10.1016/j.beem.2020.101376

Chaudhry HS, Singh G. Cushing syndrome. StatPearls, last updated December 25, 2020. Cushing Syndrome—StatPearls—NCBI Bookshelf. https://www.ncbi.nlm.nih.gov/books/NBK470218/. Accessed 5/17/2021.

Galm BP, Qiao N, Kilbanski A, et al. Accuracy of laboratory tests for the diagnosis of Cushing syndrome. *J Clin Endocrinol Metab.* 2020;105(6):2081–2094.

Nieman LK, Biller B, Findling JW, et al. Treatment of Cushing's syndrome: an Endocrine Society Clinical Practice Guideline. *J Clin Endocrinol Metab.* 2015;199(8):2807–2831.

Hyperthyroidism

Azizi F. Long-term treatment of hyperthyroidism with antithyroid drugs: 35 years of personal clinical experience. *Thyroid.* 2020;30(10):1451–1457. https://doi.org/10.1089/thy.2019.0814

Francis N, Francis T, Lazarus JH, et al. Current controversies in the management of Graves hyperthyroidism. *Exp Rev Endocrinol Metab.* 2020;15(3):159–169.

Gronich N, Lavi I, Rennert G, et al. Cancer risk after radioactive iodine treatment for hyperthyroidism: a cohort study. *Thyroid.* 2020;30(2):243–250.

Ross DS, Burch HB, Cooper DS, et al. 2016 American Thyroid Association guidelines for diagnosis and management of hyperthyroidism and other causes of thyrotoxicosis. *Thyroid.* 2016;26(10):1343–1421. http://online.liebertpub.com/doi/pdf/10.1089/thy.2016.0229. Accessed 5/17/2021.

Tsai K, Leung AM. Subclinical hyperthyroidism: a review of clinical literature. *Endocr Pract.* 2021;27(3):254–260.

Hypothyroidism

Bekkering GE, Agoritsas T, Lytvyn L, et al. Thyroid hormones treatment for subclinical hypothyroidism: a clinical practice guideline. *BMJ.* 2019;365:l2006. doi: https://doi.org/10.1136/bmj.l2006

Biondi B, Agoritsas T, Lytvyn L, et al. Subclinical hypothyroidism: a review. *JAMA.* 2019;322(2):153–160.

Grossman A, Weiss A, Koren-Morag N, et al. Subclinical thyroid disease and mortality in the elderly: a retrospective cohort study. *Am J Med.* 2016;129(4):423–430.

McAninch EA, Rajan KB, Miller CH, et al. Systemic thyroid hormone status during levothyroxine therapy in hypothyroidism: a systematic review and meta-analysis. *J Clin Endocrinol Metab.* 2018;103(12):4533–4542.

U.S. Preventive Services Task Force. Thyroid dysfunction: Screening. Final Recommendation Statement: Thyroid Dysfunction:

Screening | United States Preventive Services Taskforce; 2015. https://www.uspreventiveservicestaskforce.org/uspstf/document/RecommendationStatementFinal/thyroid-dysfunction-screening. Accessed 5/17/2021.

Thyroid Cancer

National Cancer Institute, Surveillance, Epidemiology, and End Results (SEER) Program. (2021). Cancer Stat Fact: Thyroid Cancer. https://seer.cancer.gov/statfacts/html/thyro.html.

Olson E, Wintheiser G, Wolfe KM, et al. Epidemiology of thyroid cancer: a review of the National Cancer Database, 2000–2013. *Cureus.* 2019;11(2):e4127. doi: 10.7759/cureus.4127

U.S. Preventive Services Task Force: Screening for thyroid cancer: recommendation statement. *Am Fam Physician.* 2018;98(6): 406B–407B.

RESOURCES

Adrenal Insufficiency/Cushing's Syndrome

National Adrenal Diseases Foundation (NADF)
http://www.nadf.us/

Hyperthyroidism/Hypothyroidism

American Thyroid Association
https://www.thyroid.org

Thyroid Cancer

American Cancer Society
http://www.cancer.org.

Chapter 59

Diabetes Mellitus

Debera J. Thomas, PhD, RN, ANP/FNP
Brian Oscar Porter, MD, PhD, MPH, MBA

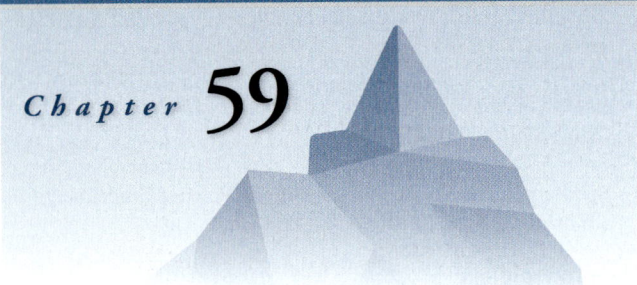

Diabetes mellitus (DM) is a syndrome of disordered carbohydrate, fat, and protein metabolism, resulting in hyperglycemia, that is caused by deficits in insulin secretion or insulin action or a combination of both. Impaired fasting glucose is a prediabetic state in which a person's fasting glucose is consistently elevated above the normal range but below the level of 126 mg/dL, which establishes a formal diagnosis of DM. Impaired glucose tolerance (IGT) describes a prediabetic state of hyperglycemia in which a 2-hour postglucose load glycemic level is 140 to 199 mg/dL. DM is the most common endocrine disorder, affecting 30.3 million people in the United States. Up to 7.2 million people may not be aware that they have DM. The National Diabetes Statistics Report for 2020 estimated that 10.5% of the population and 13% of the adult population in the United States have some form of DM.

There are four subtypes of DM, each with a distinct epidemiology and etiology: type 1 DM (T1DM), type 2 DM (T2DM), type 3c DM (T3cDM), and type 4 DM (gestational or pregnancy-related DM). The majority of patients with DM have T1DM or T2DM, with T3cDM being recognized with increased frequency. These three forms of DM are discussed in this chapter, as pregnancy-related DM is beyond the scope of this primary care text.

Tight control of blood glucose levels reduces the morbidity and mortality rates associated with DM, whereas the complications of inadequately treated DM include cardiovascular disease and peripheral vascular disease (PVD), decreased immune system functioning, renal failure, retinopathy, and nephropathy. Indeed, DM is the leading cause of both end-stage renal disease and acquired blindness in the United States.

DIABETES MELLITUS TYPE 1

T1DM is a metabolic disorder characterized by severe insulin deficiency resulting from pancreatic beta islet cell destruction, which produces hyperglycemia due to the altered metabolism of lipids, carbohydrates, and proteins. This chronic hyperglycemia results in damage to various body organs, especially the eyes, kidneys, nerves, heart, and both small and large blood vessels. Loss of vision, renal failure, loss of a lower extremity, and chronic foot ulcers due to peripheral neuropathy are common sequelae of long-term hyperglycemia. Such complications result in significant social, economic, and psychological demands on patients and their families.

EPIDEMIOLOGY AND CAUSES

T1DM occurs in approximately 1.25 million Americans, and it is estimated that 5 million Americans will have T1DM by 2050. T1DM was previously known as *insulin-dependent DM* or *juvenile-onset diabetes.* Although 60% of

The Iceberg of Diabetes Mellitus

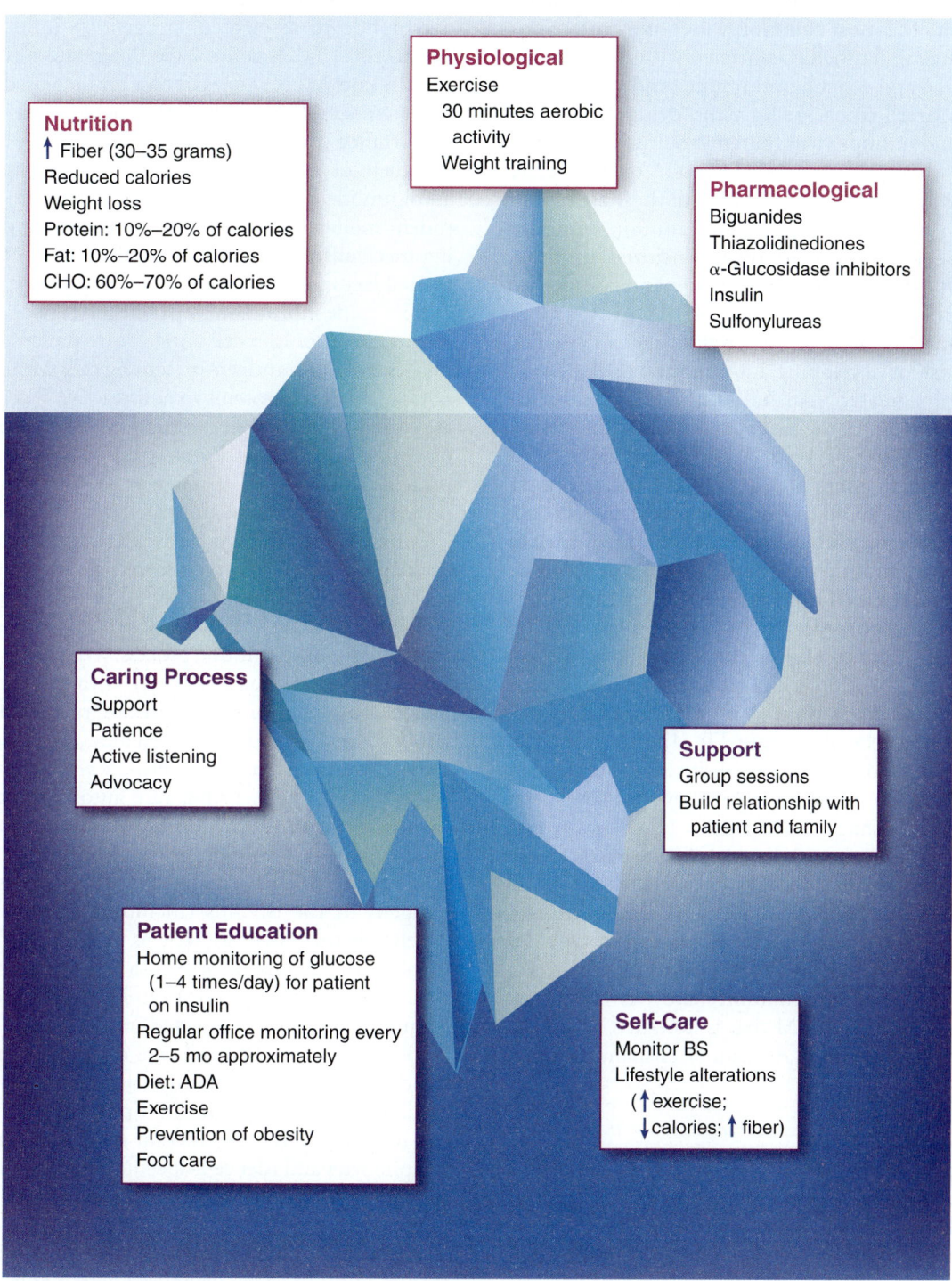

patients are younger than 18 years on first presentation, cases may occur at any age with a fairly abrupt onset. It is uncommon in children younger than 1 year and in adults older than 30 years. In nonpediatric patients, T1DM is sometimes known as *latent autoimmune diabetes of adults* (LADA). Although there is no sex predisposition, marked variations in sex predominance have been observed across ethnocultural groups, correlating with differential expressions of human leukocyte antigen (HLA) haplotypes. In turn, T1DM is 1.5 to two times more common in whites of European descent than in nonwhites.

T1DM has two forms—immune-mediated DM (type 1A) and idiopathic DM (type 1B). Immune-mediated DM accounts for 90% of cases and is generally referred to as T1DM. It is caused by autoimmune destruction of insulin-producing pancreatic beta islet cells. The triggering factor in the development of T1DM is thought to be an infection or toxic insult in people with a genetic predisposition. The most commonly identified infectious agents are congenital rubella (associated with the development of T1DM and other autoimmune syndromes up to 5 to 20 years later), coxsackie B4 virus, cytomegalovirus, adenovirus, and mumps virus (paramyxovirus). Although it is unclear whether direct viral infection of pancreatic beta islet cells plays a role, infections with these agents are believed to cause a cross-reactive autoimmune response against beta cell antigens. In turn, sensitized immune cells may release destructive cytotoxins and antibodies that contribute to the development of T1DM. Of note, immunization with viral or bacterial antigens does not increase the risk of developing autoimmune DM.

Birth weight greater than 4,000 g and higher-than-expected weight gain in the first year of life are associated with an increased risk of T1DM, but viral antigens and certain dietary influences appear to have the strongest impacts. Although food epitopes may not mimic beta cell antigens directly, proteins from other animal species may trigger autoimmune reactions, leading to T1DM. Epidemiological research from at least 10 countries implicated protein components of cow's milk (e.g., bovine serum albumin, beta-casein) as the most likely dietary triggers, but cross-sectional and prospective studies did not confirm these associations (with some work suggesting a protective effect of vitamin D). The introduction of gluten and rice-containing cereals into an infant's diet before 3 months or after 7 months of age has also been implicated in increasing T1DM risk.

Patients with immune-mediated DM are rarely obese and are prone to other autoimmune diseases such as Graves' disease, Hashimoto's thyroiditis, Addison's disease, vitiligo, and pernicious anemia. In contrast, idiopathic type 1B DM, which accounts for less than 10% of T1DM cases, shows no evidence of autoimmunity and has no known cause. It is a rare form of DM that is inherited and more common in people of Asian, African, or Hispanic origin.

PATHOPHYSIOLOGY

T1DM is characterized by a reduction or absence of functioning beta cells in the pancreatic islets of Langerhans. Genetic susceptibility has been mapped to the HLA region on chromosome 6p, with an increased risk associated with specific polymorphisms in several *HLA-DQ* and *HLA-DR* genes, preproinsulin (the primary protein product of the insulin gene), and PTPN22 (a tyrosine phosphatase involved in T-cell receptor signaling). Inheritance of T1DM appears to be polygenic, as expression of a particular HLA allele is insufficient by itself to lead to autoimmune beta cell destruction. However, there are rare forms of monogenic diabetes that account for 1% to 5% of all cases in young people (e.g., neonatal DM, maturity-onset diabetes of the young). Although other genes within the major histocompatability complex (MHC) loci and some non-MHC genes (e.g., cytotoxic T-lymphocyte–associated antigen 4) influence T1DM risk, class II HLA genes have the greatest effect. In fact, certain non-MHC genes confer an increased risk only in the presence of particular HLA haplotypes, showing the importance of polygenic interactions.

Much of our understanding of the pathogenesis of autoimmune DM stems from studies in diabetogenic rodent models. Animal studies demonstrate that a triggering mechanism, such as a viral infection or other environmental factor, can stimulate an inflammatory response and autoimmune infiltration of pancreatic beta cells—a process termed *insulitis*. Islet cell antigens are presented by macrophages and other antigen-presenting cells within the context of class II MHC proteins to autoreactive T cells that mediate subsequent beta cell destruction. Alterations in just one or two amino acid positions within certain class II MHC proteins can markedly increase or decrease their capacity to present autoantigens to autoreactive T cells, presumably by altering binding affinity. Molecular mimicry is often cited as the mechanism by which seemingly innocuous environmental (e.g., food-based epitopes) or infectious (e.g., viral) antigens that share homology with islet cell antigens initiate a destructive autoimmune process.

T1DM is clearly associated with an increased incidence of other autoimmune disorders, including thyroid, adrenal, and gonadal insufficiency. The coexistence of these conditions has been termed *polyglandular autoimmune disease type 2*. Other rare autoimmune syndromes involving insulitis include autoimmune polyendocrine syndrome type 1, which results from a mutation in the *AIRE* gene, which normally allows for expression of autoantigens in the thymus (including insulin) to mediate T-cell self-tolerance, as well as IPEX syndrome, which involves mutations in *foxp3*—a master control gene for regulatory T cells—that lead to DM and potentially fatal fulminant enteritis in affected infants.

Both Th1 and Th2 cells are capable of inducing beta cell destruction, underscoring the importance of both cell-mediated and humoral immune processes in the pathogenesis of T1DM. The presence of functional autoreactive B lymphocytes and islet cell–specific autoantibodies has been shown to both increase the incidence and shorten the time to progression of T1DM. Islet cell–specific antibodies may be identified in 70% to 80% of individuals with prediabetes and in those newly diagnosed with T1DM. Antibodies specific for insulin are usually detected first, followed by antibodies against the islet cell enzyme glutamic acid decarboxylase (GAD), which shares homology with the proteins of certain viruses implicated in the development of T1DM such as coxsackie B4 virus, and later antibodies specific for insulinoma-associated protein 2 (IA-2), a tyrosine phosphatase. Development of at least two of these three types of autoantibodies (anti-insulin, anti-GAD, anti-IA-2) is strongly predictive of progression to type 1A

DM in genetically predisposed individuals. However, it is unclear if these autoantibodies are pathogenic or simply formed as a consequence of immunological upregulation, as they are not essential for the pathogenesis of T1DM.

Genetic predisposition alone does not fully account for disease pathogenesis, however. Identical (monozygotic) twin studies reveal only a 30% lifetime risk of developing T1DM in twin siblings of probands, compared with a 5% risk in nonidentical siblings. Twin studies also demonstrate that autoantibodies against beta islet cells may be present for years in the sibling of a proband before autoimmune diabetes develops. Thus, destruction of a significant amount of beta cell mass may take months to years before resulting in a lack of insulin. The inflammatory cytokine milieu plays an important role in diabetic pathogenesis, and some patients with T1DM may have a reversible component to their disease if the autoinflammatory process can be stopped early enough and an adequate number of beta cells salvaged (e.g., insulin-like growth factor–1 has a role in preserving beta cell function).

Progressive beta cell destruction remains the hallmark of T1DM, with hyperglycemia typically developing once 80% to 90% of a patient's beta cells have been destroyed. This hyperglycemia leads to both microvascular and macrovascular complications, which underlie long-term diabetic damage. Vascular endothelial dysfunction and inflammation result in fibrosis and intimal thickening in blood vessels, leading to progressive narrowing of the vascular lumen. The resultant decreased blood flow through the microvasculature leads to tissue ischemia throughout the body and functional impairment of multiple end organs. Several clinical trials have demonstrated that careful glycemic control reduces the development and delays the progression of microvascular manifestations of DM, including nephropathy and retinopathy.

CLINICAL PRESENTATION

Subjective

Although the symptom manifestations of T1DM vary, the majority of patients seek medical attention due to symptoms related to hyperglycemia, with the initial diagnosis in children often being made when patients present in frank diabetic ketoacidosis (DKA). The classic symptoms of T1DM are polyuria (increased urination); polydipsia (increased fluid intake due to excessive thirst); nocturnal enuresis; polyphagia with paradoxical weight loss (due to reduced glucose metabolism, despite increased consumption); visual changes (especially blurred vision); and eventual fatigue, weakness, and anorexia. Polyuria results from osmotic diuresis secondary to sustained hyperglycemia; this loss of glucose, free water, and electrolytes in the urine induces a hyperosmolar state, which causes excessive thirst and compensatory polydipsia. Blurred vision results from the lens and retina being exposed to hyperosmolar fluids. A decreased plasma volume resulting from significant fluid losses may cause dizziness and fatigue, and weakness results from the catabolism of muscle proteins and potassium loss.

Because hyperglycemia worsens humoral immunity and leukocyte function, patients with DM may present with repeated or complicated infections, decreased wound healing, and/or infections that are uncommon in the general public, such as serious staphylococcal and *Klebsiella pneumoniae* infections, malignant (necrotizing) otitis externa due to *Pseudomonas aeruginosa,* or rhinocerebral mucormycosis, which occurs almost exclusively in patients with DM. Pathogens are able to multiply rapidly because the increased glucose in bodily fluids acts as an energy source. If a patient complains of nausea, abdominal pain, or genitourinary discomfort, urinary tract infection must be ruled out because individuals with DM are more likely to experience serious complications of pyelonephritis, such as renal papillary necrosis and emphysematous (necrotizing) pyelonephritis, or progression to gram-negative bacterial sepsis. Female patients may also present with complaints of vaginal pruritus or burning caused by vulvovaginitis.

Objective

Signs of dehydration such as poor skin turgor and dry mucous membranes may be present. Weight loss despite a normal or increased appetite may be noted, as water, glycogen, and triglyceride stores are depleted and as glucose cannot be metabolized for its nutritional value due to insulinemia. A reduction in muscle mass may be seen, as muscle proteins are broken down to generate amino acids used by the liver for gluconeogenesis, resulting in the formation of ketone bodies. Thus, ketoacidosis is usually present and may be mild to severe.

Signs of severe ketosis known as DKA include extreme fatigue, abnormal cramping, and alterations in breathing pattern. In addition, a telltale sign of ketosis is halitosis (malodorous breath), which smells like a combination of nail polish remover (acetone) and rotting fruit (ketones). In contrast, hyperosmolar hyperglycemic state (HHS) is a serious form of nonketotic acidosis resulting from prolonged hyperglycemia that is less common than DKA but has a higher mortality rate. HHS is seen most frequently in adults who have a restriction in fluid intake for some reason, such as a concurrent illness, impaired physical function, or reduced cognition.

The physical examination should include a funduscopic examination because longstanding DM predisposes patients to diabetic retinopathy as a result of retinal ischemia. Five stages of retinopathy are evident on physical examination: (1) dilation of retinal venules and retinal capillary microaneurysms; (2) increased vascular permeability; (3) retinal ischemia due to vascular occlusion; (4) angiogenesis (proliferation of new retinal surface blood vessels); and (5) retinal hemorrhage with fibrovascular proliferation and contraction, which may lead to retinal detachment. Such findings are discernible on funduscopic examination and require expert evaluation by an ophthalmological specialist.

Patients with poorly controlled DM can present with various skin complications, such as chronic pyogenic infections or necrobiosis lipoidica diabeticorum, which consists of well-demarcated granulomatous plaques with a shiny yellow surface that occur on the anterior surfaces of the legs or dorsal aspect of the ankles. The physical examination must include a comprehensive foot evaluation because patients can present with paresthesias related to dysfunction of peripheral sensory nerves, which can decrease sensitivity to extremity trauma. The typical stocking-glove distribution of anesthesia classically leads to unrecognized foot ulcers or burns on the hands from cooking or smoking. Thus, diabetic foot ulcers result from a combination of factors, including decreased circulation, infection, decreased immune response, and peripheral neuropathy. Moreover, neurological complications may also impact the third (oculomotor), fourth (trochlear), or (abducens) cranial nerves, resulting in deviations in gaze of the affected eye.

DIAGNOSTIC REASONING

Diagnostic Tests

The American Diabetes Association (ADA) does not recommend screening for T1DM in apparently healthy individuals who have no risk factors for this disorder. However, if suspected, point-of-care testing can be accomplished by using a portable blood glucose monitor to determine capillary blood glucose level as a random plasma glucose measurement taken without regard to the timing of a patient's last meal. If elevated, the patient's urine should be tested for ketones, and additional plasma glucose testing should be initiated.

Initial Testing

Current guidelines for the diagnosis of DM include any one of the following:

- Glycosylated hemoglobin (A1c) of 6.5% or higher
- Symptoms of diabetes (e.g., polyuria, polydipsia, weight loss) plus a random plasma glucose level of 200 mg/dL or higher
- Fasting plasma glucose level of 126 mg/dL or higher (after 8 hours of no caloric intake)
- Two-hour plasma glucose level of 200 mg/dL or higher during an oral glucose tolerance test (OGTT) with a 75-g glucose load

The first three criteria should be confirmed by repeat testing (preferably with the same test) without delay, except in the setting of unequivocal hyperglycemia with acute metabolic decompensation.

Patients with borderline glucose intolerance at risk for developing T1DM or those with suspected LADA can be tested for antibodies against GAD, insulin, tyrosine phosphatases (e.g., IA-2), or zinc transporters (e.g., ZnT8), as these autoantibodies help differentiate LADA from T2DM. If two or more of these antibody classes are positive in the setting of diagnostic hyperglycemia, then the diagnosis of T1DM is confirmed. However, such antibodies are not a diagnostic requirement for T1DM.

Another test to assess beta cell function and insulin production in a patient with T1DM is C-peptide level. Proinsulin is cleaved into insulin and C-peptide, the latter being biologically inactive. Therefore, C-peptide levels are found in amounts equal to endogenous insulin. However, exogenous insulin preparations do not include C-peptide. Thus, a patient with residual pancreatic beta cell function will have decreased but nonetheless detectable levels of C-peptide, whereas if no insulin is being produced, the levels of C-peptide will be negligible (normal fasting level = 0.51 to 2.72 ng/mL [0.17 to 0.90 mmol/L]).

The International Expert Committee on Diabetes recommends that an A1c of 6.5% or greater can be used to diagnose DM with a repeat level obtained for confirmation. Confirmatory testing is not needed if a patient has the clinical symptoms of DM or if the random plasma glucose level is greater than 200 mg/dL. Of note, this test cannot be used for diagnosis in the setting of pregnancy, hemoglobinopathy, or other situations with abnormal rates of erythrocyte turnover.

Subsequent Testing

A1c determination gives valuable insight into the mean plasma glucose concentration over the preceding 2 to 3 months and is helpful in documenting the degree of glycemic control at the time of diagnosis and as part of continuing care. The risk of developing complications of T1DM, such as retinopathy, nephropathy, and neuropathy, are significantly reduced when A1c levels are maintained below 7%, which is recommended as a treatment goal by the ADA. The A1c level roughly correlates to mean plasma glucose concentration as follows: 6% = glucose of 135 mg/dL; 7% = 170 mg/dL; 8% = 205 mg/dL; 9% = 240 mg/dL; 10% = 275 mg/dL; 11% = 310 mg/dL; 12% = 345 mg/dL. A1c testing should be done at least twice a year in patients with good glycemic control and quarterly in patients whose therapy has changed or in patients who have not yet achieved their glycemic goals.

Additional laboratory tests that are appropriate to the evaluation of the patient's general medical condition and cardiovascular risk status should be performed. These include a fasting lipid profile (total cholesterol, high-density lipoprotein [HDL], low-density lipoprotein [LDL], and triglyceride levels), urinalysis, microalbuminuria, thyroid function tests (thyroid-stimulating hormone, free T4), liver enzymes (aspartate aminotransferase, alanine aminotransferase [ALT], gamma glutamyl-transferase), and blood urea nitrogen and serum creatinine if proteinuria is present. Urine cultures may be obtained if indicated by symptom complaints or urinalysis results.

A 12-lead electrocardiogram (ECG) should be done on adults at the time of diagnosis, and screening for other autoimmune diseases (e.g., vitamin B_{12} deficiency, celiac disease, hypothyroidism, hyperthyroidism) should be considered as well.

Differential Diagnosis

With the classic symptoms of DM confirmed by blood plasma glucose testing, a diagnosis of DM can be made; however, other potential causes of hyperglycemia should be considered. Hyperglycemia and glucosuria are present in patients with Cushing's disease, pheochromocytoma, and acromegaly. Extreme stress or trauma, such as that seen in extensive burns, may produce transient hyperglycemia. Renal tubular disease may produce glycosuria without concurrent hyperglycemia. Several pharmacological agents can cause hyperglycemia, including glucocorticoids, furosemide (Lasix), thiazide diuretics, sympathomimetic agents, estrogen-containing products, beta blockers, and nicotinic acid.

Nonimmune secondary causes of hyperglycemia may mimic either T1DM or T2DM, depending on whether the mechanism is destruction of beta islet cells with subsequent insulin deficiency or peripheral insulin resistance in which the body produces insulin that is utilized inefficiently by the peripheral tissues. Nonimmune mechanisms of beta cell destruction that produce a T1DM-like state include hemochromatosis, cystic fibrosis, and pancreatitis.

MANAGEMENT

T1DM is a chronic illness that requires ongoing health care and patient education to prevent acute and chronic complications. The complexity and lifelong management regimens necessitate that the patient and clinician work as a team to develop and implement the treatment plan. The ADA recommends a team approach to care, including the primary care provider, an endocrinologist for periodic evaluation, a certified diabetes educator, a dietitian, the patient, and the patient's family/support people. To achieve successful implementation of the treatment plan, it is essential that the plan fit with the patient's lifestyle to the greatest extent possible. This is where a diabetes educator is of greatest assistance. Children with T1DM will also need school personnel involved in the treatment team.

A comprehensive treatment program requires exogenous insulin, frequent self-monitoring of blood glucose (SMBG), medical nutrition therapy, regular exercise, continuing education in the prevention and treatment of diabetic complications (e.g., cardiovascular disease [CVD]), and the periodic reassessment of treatment goals. As with any chronic illness, a diagnosis of DM requires incorporation of the diagnosis and subsequent management strategy into the patient's lifestyle. Often, it may take a traumatic event or "turning point" in a patient's management to break the complacency of a treatment plan to one that focuses on lifestyle changes. The principles of assessment and management of T1DM are summarized in Table 59.1.

TABLE 59.1 Outpatient Assessment and Management of the Patient With T1DM

Assessment	Laboratory Monitoring	General Health Maintenance
Every visit: • Symptoms of hypoglycemia and hyperglycemia • Results of SMBG • Any self-adjustments based on SMBG or symptoms • Problems with adherence • Symptoms of complications of chronic hyperglycemia • Any other medical illnesses • Medications (prescription and over the counter) • Height and weight • Blood pressure • Cardiovascular assessment • Thyroid examination • Ophthalmic examination (with an annual dilated retinal eye examination) • Peripheral vascular assessment • Feet and skin assessment • Neurological assessment • Oral examination	A1c every 3 months during the first year of initiation of insulin therapy and during periods of insulin dosage adjustment In patients who have met treatment goals, measure A1c twice a year, if stable. Initially upon diagnosis and annually, if stable: • Lipid profile • Urinalysis • Serum creatinine Microalbuminuria screening annually: • Method 1: Spot UACR (can be performed in clinic; first morning void is preferred because of diurnal variation in albumin excretion; greater than 30 mcg albumin/mg creatinine indicates microalbuminuria) • Method 2: 24-hour urine collection	Immunizations and prophylaxis: • Pneumococcal vaccine • Influenza vaccine annually • Cardioprotective aspirin in patients older than 40 years Patient education: • Smoking cessation, if applicable

Abbreviations: A1c, glycosylated hemoglobin; SMBG, self-monitoring of blood glucose; UACR, urinary albumin-to-creatinine ratio.

Of note, although type 1A DM is essentially insulin dependent, the need for insulin replacement therapy in patients with type 1B DM is variable. Clinical trials are currently evaluating prevention strategies to delay the onset of clinical disease in type 1B DM, and the ADA is hopeful that effective preventive therapies will eventually be found.

Initial Management

Insulin Therapy

The initial goal of treatment for T1DM is to normalize the blood glucose level. This is best accomplished by intensive insulin regimens to achieve the following goals: plasma glucose levels of 80 to 130 mg/dL before meals, peak postprandial (1 to 2 hours after the beginning of a meal) glucose levels of less than 180 mg/dL, and an A1c below 7% for adults with T1DM. The patient with new-onset T1DM often presents in hyperglycemic crisis and requires hospitalization. These patients should be managed by or in close collaboration with an endocrinologist and a comprehensive health-care team. When patients present in acute hyperglycemia, it is essential not only to treat the hyperglycemia but also to determine its underlying cause (e.g., medication nonadherence, dietary indiscretions, or underlying infection, which is the most common cause of DKA, the inpatient treatment of which is detailed in Table 59.2).

The Diabetes Control and Complications Trial conclusively demonstrated that in patients with T1DM, the risk of development or progression of retinopathy, nephropathy, and neuropathy is reduced by 50% to 75% with intensive insulin regimens, compared with conventional treatment regimens. Individual treatment goals should take into account the patient's capacity to understand and carry out the treatment, the risk for severe hypoglycemia, and any other factors that increase risk or decrease

TABLE 59.2 Diabetic Ketoacidosis		
Overview	*Clinical Presentation*	*Management*
Diabetic ketoacidosis (DKA) is an acute life-threatening decompensation of glucose metabolism seen in DM (most commonly in T1DM) that requires immediate medical attention. Cardinal features: • Hyperglycemia—blood glucose level greater than 359 mg/dL • Ketonemia—plasma ketone level greater than 5 mmol/L • Acidosis—plasma bicarbonate level less than 9 mEq/L Causes: • Lack of insulin • Stress (physical or emotional), even with continued insulin therapy Pathophysiology: • As insulin levels decrease, the concentration of glucagon rises, which increases glucose levels. • Epinephrine inhibits glucose transport in peripheral tissues, thereby stimulating the production of glucose from noncarbohydrate substrates in the liver. • Free fatty acids from adipose stores are oxidized in the liver for energy, causing release of ketones and resultant acidosis.	Initial signs of DKA: • Anorexia • Increased thirst • Nausea/vomiting • Halitosis (malodorous breath), which smells like nail polish remover (acetone) and rotting fruit (ketones) • Abdominal cramping • Increased urine formation • Fatigue Later signs: • Kussmaul respiration • Signs of dehydration (usual fluid deficit of 3–5 L) • Oliguria • Altered consciousness Left untreated: • Coma • Vascular collapse • Renal shutdown • Blood glucose increases from 300–800 mg/dL Diagnostic tests: • Serum glucose • Sodium potassium • Phosphate • Bicarbonate • Beta-hydroxybutyrate • Osmolality • pH • Calculated anion gap	Goals: • Correct hyperglycemia • Correct dehydration • Normalize electrolytes (replenish deficiencies) • Correct acidosis First line of treatment is insulin: • Continuous-dose insulin infusion: 0.1–0.2 U/kg/hr Correcting dehydration and electrolyte imbalances: • Rapid IV infusion of normal saline (0.9% NaCl) or Ringer's lactate: 1–2 L • Potassium replacement 3–4 hours after initiation of insulin and fluid therapy • Phosphorus replacement • Magnesium replacement • Bicarbonate therapy if pH is 7.0 or below After recovery, causes of DKA should be explored. Patients should be taught about increased insulin needs during periods of illness and stress.

Abbreviation: DM, diabetes mellitus.

benefit. Tight glycemic control increases the chance of hypoglycemic episodes and may not be appropriate for many older patients, patients with coronary artery disease (CAD) who may be prone to hypoglycemia, or those with diabetic neuropathy who may lack the early neurological (adrenergic) warning signs of hypoglycemia.

The initiation of insulin therapy in newly diagnosed T1DM patients should be managed by or in close collaboration with an endocrinologist. The majority of insulin used today is made chemically identical to human insulin by recombinant DNA technology or by chemical modification of pork insulin; however, beef and pork insulin preparations are still available. Insulin is available in rapid-, short-, intermediate-, and long-acting forms. The optimal dosage is highly individualized and can depend on the site and depth of injections, skin temperature (related to subcutaneous and superficial blood circulation in the skin), and exercise. Human insulin is preferred for patients newly beginning insulin therapy, pregnant patients, and people with allergies.

In the United States, insulin is available in concentrations of 100 or 500 U/mL, but highly concentrated preparations are used only in rare cases of insulin resistance, when a patient requires large doses. The 2021 ADA Standards of Medical Care in Diabetes state that the majority of patients with T1DM should be treated with multiple daily injections of prandial insulin and daily basal insulin or with a continuous subcutaneous insulin infusion pump. Both strategies require diligent and frequent blood glucose monitoring by the patient and should be selected on the basis of what is most appropriate for the patient's current or future lifestyle choices, given the severe consequences of therapeutic nonadherence. Commercially mixed neutral protamine Hagedorn (NPH) and regular insulin preparations are also available to reduce the number of injections needed, or the patient can custom mix a personalized insulin preparation. Both insulin dosage and timing should be individualized for the patient according to specific health needs and lifestyle choices (see Drugs Commonly Prescribed 59.1).

Some patients may experience early morning hyperglycemia due to complete absorption of the evening insulin dose before the early morning hours (termed the dawn phenomenon), particularly if an intermediate-acting form of insulin is used, such as NPH (isophane insulin), which has a peak effect at 6 to 10 hours after

Drugs Commonly Prescribed 59.1: Diabetes Mellitus Type 1 Insulin Regimens

SINGLE-DOSE THERAPY

Single Injection

- Intermediate- or long-acting insulin with or without regular insulin in the morning *or* intermediate- or long-acting insulin at bedtime
- Recommend at a minimum SMBG in the morning and at bedtime

CONVENTIONAL SPLIT-DOSE THERAPY

Two Injections

- Mixture of NPH and regular insulin in the morning and evening
- Recommend at a minimum SMBG before each dosing and at bedtime

INTENSIVE INSULIN THERAPY

Three Injections

- NPH and regular insulin in the morning; regular insulin at dinner; NPH insulin at bedtime
- Monitor for increased risk of hypoglycemic episodes

Four Injections

- Regular or lispro insulin before meals and long-acting insulin to maintain basal insulin levels
- Monitor for increased risk of hypoglycemic episodes

TYPES OF INSULIN	SPECIES	ONSET, PEAK, AND DURATION*	ROUTE
Insulin Glulisine			
Apidra	Recombinant DNA (usually used in combination with longer-acting insulins)	<5 min, 1–2 hr, 2–3 hr	SC
Insulin Aspart			
Novolog	Recombinant DNA (usually used in combination with longer-acting insulins)	<10 min, 1–3 hr, 3–5 hr	SC
Insulin Lispro			
Humalog	Recombinant DNA (usually used in combination with longer-acting insulins)	<15 min, 1–2 hr, 3–4 hr	SC

Continued

Drugs Commonly Prescribed 59.1: Diabetes Mellitus Type 1 Insulin Regimens—cont'd

TYPES OF INSULIN	SPECIES	ONSET, PEAK, AND DURATION*	ROUTE
Regular Insulin			
Humulin R	Human	30–60 min, 2–6 hr, 6–8 hr	SC, IM, IV
Iletin II Regular	Pork	30–60 min, 2–6 hr, 6–8 hr	SC, IM, IV
Novolin R	Human	30–60 min, 2–6 hr, 6–8 hr	SC, IM, IV
Purified Pork Regular	Pork	30–60 min, 2–6 hr, 6–8 hr	SC, IM, IV
Velosulin	Human	30–60 min, 2–4 hr, 6–8 hr	SC, IM, IV
Insulin Isophane Suspension (NPH)			
Humulin N	Human	1–1.5 hr, 4–12 hr, 18–24 hr	SC
Iletin II NPH	Pork	1–1.5 hr, 4–12 hr, 18–24 hr	SC
Novolin N	Human	1–1.5 hr, 4–12 hr, 18–24 hr	SC
Purified Pork NPH	Pork	1–1.5 hr, 4–12 hr, 18–24 hr	SC
Insulin Isophane Suspension (NPH)/Regular Insulin			
Humulin 70/30	Human	30–60 min, 2–12 hr, 24 hr	SC
Humulin 50/50	Human	30–60 min, 3–5 hr, 24 hr	SC
Novolin 70/30	Human	30–60 min, 2–12 hr, 24 hr	SC
Insulin Glargine			
Lantus	Insulin analog	Slowly absorbed with gradual onset, peakless, lasting up to 24 hr	SC
Insulin Detemir			
Levemir	Insulin analog	Slowly absorbed with gradual onset, relative constant concentration with peak at 6–10 hr, lasting up to 24 hr	SC

Abbreviations: IM, intramuscular; NPH, neutral protamine Hagedorn; SC, subcutaneous; SMBG, self-monitoring of blood glucose.
*General guidance, affected by multiple factors.

subcutaneous injection and a duration of action of 10 to 16 hours. In addition, humans have an increased insulin requirement in the morning because of early morning secretion of growth hormone and cortisol. Thus, increasing the nighttime insulin dose to address early morning hyperglycemia may lead to late evening hypoglycemia in the absence of an adequate insulin effect in the early morning hours. Therefore, if NPH is used, the evening dose should be given later. Alternatively, it may be more efficient to prevent early morning hyperglycemia by switching the regimen from NPH to a longer-acting form of insulin, such as glargine (Lantus) or detemir (Levemir).

Self-Monitoring of Blood Glucose Levels

SMBG is the testing of capillary blood to determine blood glucose level. Typically, plasma venous glucose measurements are within 15% of the results of whole blood capillary test results. SMBG is recommended for patients with T1DM to evaluate the effectiveness of the insulin regimen, medical nutrition therapy, and exercise. Used properly, it is the most practical mechanism to maintain glucose levels as close to normal as possible and to prevent the most common complication of DM therapy—hypoglycemia.

The frequency and timing of blood glucose monitoring are dependent on the needs and goals of the individual patient. Optimal SMBG for patients with T1DM occurs three to four times a day—before each meal and before bedtime, but with intensive control, blood glucose checks could be up to 10 times a day, as postprandial assessment is added. Common barriers to frequent SMBG in patients with T1DM include cost (e.g., test strips, multiple glucometers), inconvenience, and discomfort produced by the finger pricks. The benefit versus cost ratio must be thoroughly explored with each patient, as a treatment plan is developed and individualized goals are established. Table 59.3 presents the goals of glucose management for patients without symptoms of hypoglycemia.

Continuous Glucose Monitoring

Continuous glucose monitoring (CGM) utilizes a device that measures interstitial glucose concentration and can be utilized with intensive insulin therapy. This measurement correlates with SMBG. Such devices have been studied in adults older than 25 years of age and found to reduce the amount of time T1DM patients experience hyperglycemic and hypoglycemic episodes. The measurement of CGM must be calibrated with SMBG, however, and SMBG should be used to make acute treatment decisions. Patients who have limited awareness of hypoglycemic episodes or experience them frequently may also benefit from CGM.

There are many different types of blood glucose meters, and one should be selected that best fits the needs and resources of the patient. Many glucometers have the ability to download records into personal computers or smartphones, which allows clinicians to readily review the data. This can provide helpful information regarding trends in SMBG. The patient should, nevertheless, be instructed to keep a log of results along with insulin doses so that adjustments can be made to the treatment plan. There are more than 1,100 smartphone apps available to help manage DM. The proper function of the glucometer, as well as the patient's SMBG testing technique, should be assessed for accuracy at each visit while the patient's ideal dose is being adjusted and then annually once the patient's regimen is stabilized.

Management of Hypoglycemia

Hypoglycemia is a common occurrence in patients with T1DM and occurs for a variety of reasons: excessive exogenous insulin, missed meals or inadequate food intake, excessive exercise, alcohol ingestion, drug interactions, or decreases in liver or kidney function. Signs and symptoms include diaphoresis, tachycardia, hunger, shakiness, altered mentation (ranging from an inability to concentrate to frank coma), slurred speech, and seizures. The signs and symptoms exhibited by the patient are highly individual and can vary from mild to severe. In 2017, the International Hypoglycemia Study Group of the ADA Standards of Medical Care in Diabetes classified a plasma glucose level of less than 54 mg/dL as serious, clinically significant hypoglycemia. A blood glucose level of 70 mg/dL is considered a threshold level that requires intervention.

The goal of treatment is to normalize the plasma glucose level promptly. If the patient is conscious and able to swallow, this is best accomplished by the prompt ingestion of glucose or carbohydrate-containing food with a high glycemic index for rapid absorption. Pure glucose is the treatment of choice according to the ADA, but any carbohydrate that can increase the blood glucose level can be given. Food with significant fat content may delay the glycemic response. Examples of appropriate foods to rapidly raise blood sugar include one-half cup of any fruit juice (with no additional sugar added), 6 ounces of regular soda (not diet or sugarless), 1 cup of milk, or glucose tablets. Candy (other than chocolate) can be used in dire situations but is not recommended when other sources of sugar are available. Blood glucose should be checked 15 minutes after treatment, and additional carbohydrates should be given if the blood glucose remains less than 70 mg/dL. For severe hypoglycemia in a patient who is unconscious or unable to swallow, 1 mg of glucagon can be given subcutaneously to mobilize hepatic glucose stores. An alternative treatment in the inpatient setting is to administer 50 mL of a 50% dextrose solution intravenously.

Nocturnal hypoglycemia can occur if the predinner, intermediate-acting insulin dose is too high or if the patient skips dinner or eats an inadequate amount of food. The patient may not awaken with symptoms but on arising may note an increased fasting glucose level. This is due to a compensatory mechanism in the liver, which responds by mobilizing glucose from hepatic glycogen stores in response to sustained hypoglycemia. After the hypoglycemia has been resolved, the possible causes should be reviewed with the patient and preventive measures discussed. The Somogyi effect, for example, is a unique combination in which a diabetic patient develops hypoglycemia during the night with rebound hyperglycemia in the morning. Although several studies have failed to confirm the validity of this pathological process, many clinicians still feel the Somogyi effect exists and is most commonly observed in children with T1DM.

Diet

Once the patient has been educated in insulin therapy, SMBG, and the treatment of hypoglycemia, subsequent management includes education in meal planning and dietary practices. Meal planning or medical nutritional therapy is one of the most challenging aspects of diabetes management because achievement of treatment goals may require substantial lifestyle changes related to food intake. The goals of nutritional therapy are to maintain normal blood glucose levels, prevent hypoglycemia, maintain normal serum lipid levels, attain or maintain a reasonable body weight, and promote healthy eating

TABLE 59.3 Goals of Glucose Management*	
Time	Goal
Before meals	80–120 mg/dL
Postprandial	Less than 180 mg/dL
Bedtime	100–140 mg/dL

*Goals are for glucose management without symptoms of hypoglycemia.

practices. There is no evidence that establishes the ideal percentages of macronutrients for people with DM. The meal plan should be based on the patient's food choices; exercise habits; medical history; current and goal weight; and lifestyle, cultural, ethnic, and financial factors.

Most patients will benefit from a referral to a certified diabetes educator for a group program or individual counseling. Thus, referral to a dietitian for an initial consultation should be ordered for all diabetic patients at a minimum.

The first step of a nutritional consultation is the initial assessment of the patient's nutritional status, including a detailed diet history. Recommendations for dietary changes should not be made until the patient's current eating patterns are determined. Individuals on insulin should eat at consistent times that are synchronized with their insulin administration. Most patients with T1DM are lean, so weight loss is generally not a major factor in meal planning. The following formulas can be used to determine the total number of kilocalories needed to maintain current weight:

- For males: 66 + 13.7 (weight in kg) + 5 (height in cm) − 6.8 (age)
- For females: 65 + 9.6 (weight in kg) + 1.7 (height in cm) − 4.7 (age)

Multiply the result by 1.2 for a fairly active person and by up to 1.5 for an ill person, given increased caloric requirements.

A nutritionally balanced meal plan is important for the patient with T1DM, taking into account the higher prevalence of atherosclerosis typically seen in patients with DM. The ADA acknowledges that no single dietary plan is appropriate for all patients and that each patient needs an individualized eating plan. The current recommendation is for each patient to receive medical nutrition therapy provided by a registered dietitian knowledgeable in diabetes management. The goals of the eating plan are to maintain a healthy body weight, support glycemic control, facilitate blood pressure and lipid goals, and delay or prevent the complications of DM. Examples of nutrient dense, high-quality eating plans for DM are the Mediterranean Diet, the Dietary Approaches to Stop Hypertension (DASH) diet, and plant-based diets.

Nutritive sweeteners (such as fructose, dextrose, and maltose) and sugar alcohols (such as sorbitol, mannitol, and xylitol) have not demonstrated a significant advantage over sucrose in improving overall diabetes control, and sugar alcohols in excessive amounts may have a laxative effect. The caloric and carbohydrate content of all these sweeteners should be taken into account in the meal plan. Nonnutritive sweeteners such as saccharin, aspartame, acesulfame potassium, sucralose, and the Latin American herb stevia are noncaloric and do not affect the blood glucose level. The majority of patients with T1DM can safely use them. It is unclear, however, whether nonnutritive sweeteners and the products that contain them (e.g., sugarless diet sodas) provide any advantage over nutritive sweeteners, in terms of weight management.

Although soluble fiber can inhibit the absorption of glucose from the small intestine, the amount of fiber contained in most foods will not have a significant effect on blood glucose levels. Fiber recommendations for individuals with DM, therefore, are the same as for the general population (20 to 35 g/day).

Vitamin and mineral supplements are not generally recommended for people whose dietary intake is adequate. For example, chromium replacements have no known benefit except for the patient who may be chromium deficient as a result of long-term parenteral nutrition. In addition, magnesium and sodium replacements should be given only if medically warranted.

The same recommendations for the general population concerning alcohol ingestion are appropriate for the patient with T1DM. Alcohol consumption in some patients can increase hypoglycemia with insulin or insulin secretagogues; patients with DM should be made aware of this and instructed to drink alcohol cautiously. Additionally, calories from alcohol should be included as part of the total caloric intake. Heavily sweetened alcoholic drinks should be avoided, and alcohol intake should be considered as part of the meal plan.

Physical Activity

According to the ADA standards, all patients should undergo a careful evaluation of their medical history and assessment for cardiovascular risk factors (e.g., hypertension, hyperlipidemia, family history) before being provided assistance in developing a regular program of physical activity. A physical activity program should be individualized to take into account the patient's activity interests, lifestyle, physical condition, and motivation. The recommendations by the ADA include 150 minutes or more of moderate to vigorous aerobic activity per week. The activity should be spread over at least 3 days per week, with no more than 2 consecutive days with no activity. In addition, resistance training and flexibility training should each be done 2 to 3 times per week. All adults with DM should decrease the amount of time spent in sedentary activity. The patient should be instructed to interrupt prolonged sitting every 30 minutes with some type of physical activity.

Because the metabolic adjustments that maintain blood glucose levels during physical activity in a nondiabetic individual are impaired in patients with T1DM, physical activity can exacerbate hyperglycemia if the patient with DM has too little insulin available. Conversely, if there is too much insulin present, hypoglycemia may occur. Thus, the patient with DM must use the following general guidelines regarding physical activity to regulate the glycemic response:

- Check blood glucose before, every 30 to 60 minutes during, and after physical activity.

- Avoid physical activity if fasting glucose is more than 250 mg/dL and ketosis is present or if the glucose level is more than 300 mg/dL, regardless of whether ketosis is present.
- Consume additional carbohydrates if the glucose level is less than 100 mg/dL and as needed to avoid hypoglycemia.
- Identify when changes in insulin dose or food intake are necessary.

Urine Ketone Testing

Urine ketone testing is recommended for patients with T1DM when the patient experiences documented hyperglycemia or stressful events that can lead to hyperglycemia. For instance, during an acute illness, particularly if the patient is nauseated and vomiting, urine ketones can be monitored, especially if the patient is prone to ketosis, with documented ketotic episodes in the past. Because pregnancy places stress on the diabetic patient, it may also be recommended that pregnant patients perform periodic ketone assessments. Ketonuria can reflect dehydration and the need for increased fluid intake, as well as increased insulin requirements.

FOLLOW-UP AND REFERRAL

Continuity of care is essential in the management of T1DM, and patients typically benefit from a long-term relationship with their primary care practitioner. Long-term surveillance for potential complications of DM demands almost as much daily attention by the patient and office time of the primary care practitioner as does the daily insulin regimen needed to manage the disease effectively.

The frequency of follow-up visits depends on the degree to which blood glucose levels are controlled, changes in insulin therapy, and the presence and severity of complications or other medical conditions. If the patient uses SMBG effectively, telemedicine or phone consultations instead of clinic visits may be possible. Once glycemic levels are effectively regulated (e.g., A1c consistently below 7%) and insulin regimens are stabilized, patients with diabetes should be seen at least quarterly. These visits should include a discussion of SMBG results; adjustments to therapy made by the patient; symptoms of DM and its complications; problems with adherence to the treatment plan; changes in lifestyle behaviors; any modifications to the patient's medications; and the frequency, causes, and severity of hyperglycemia or hypoglycemia.

The U.S. National Institutes of Health has created a multicenter program called the type 1 Diabetes TrialNet, which is an international research network that accepts referrals of relatives of patients with T1DM for screening with islet cell antibody measurements. It offers treatment with various agents that are being investigated as potentially preventing the development of the disease.

The potential for the development of long-term complications of DM affecting almost every major organ system necessitates regular follow-up of all diabetic patients. For example, diabetic retinopathy remains the leading cause of new-onset blindness among adults 20 to 74 years of age, and at 20 years postdiagnosis of T1DM, nearly all patients have some degree of retinopathy. In addition, growth impairment, an increased susceptibility to infection, and autonomic neuropathy may occur, resulting in gastrointestinal (GI), genitourinary, and cardiovascular symptoms, including sexual dysfunction. Indeed, people with DM have an increased incidence of atherosclerotic heart disease, PVD, and cerebrovascular disease. The development of the life-threatening sequelae of hyperglycemia, DKA (more common in T1DM), and HHS (more common in T2DM) may first be detected by the primary care practitioner at unscheduled sick visits; however, these conditions call for immediate referral to an emergency department (see Table 59.2 and the section on T2DM for more information on these serious complications).

If any of these complications are detected or suspected, referral to a specialist to guide management may be indicated. Key follow-up and management principles with respect to the diabetic patient are as follows:

- *Retinopathy:* The ADA recommends that adults with T1DM should be seen by an ophthalmologist or optometrist and have a dilated comprehensive eye examination within the first 5 years of diagnosis. If there is no retinopathy at the first evaluation, an eye examination should be done every 2 years. If retinopathy is detected, a full eye examination should be done by an ophthalmologist or optometrist at least annually to assess for appropriate intervention.
- *Hyperlipidemia:* Adults with T1DM should be tested annually for lipid disorders with a complete fasting lipid profile, given the increased risk in these individuals for CAD.
- *Nephropathy:* The ADA recommends assessing urinary albumin to monitor for developing nephropathy at least once a year in patients with T1DM. Screening with a spot urinary albumin-to-creatinine ratio (UACR) and an estimated glomerular filtration rate (eGFR) should be done after a disease duration of 5 years or sooner if the patient has hypertension. Persistent albuminuria (greater than 30 mg/g of creatinine) is the earliest stage of diabetic nephropathy, and overt nephropathy with albuminuria equal to or greater than 300 mg/g creatinine will develop over a period of 10 to 15 years in approximately 80% of patients with microalbuminuria, many of whom will also present with hypertension.

Transient elevations of albumin excretion occur with acute febrile illnesses, marked hypertension, short-term hyperglycemia, exercise, urinary tract infections, and heart failure. Angiotensin-converting enzyme inhibitors (ACEIs) have been found to postpone the progression of microalbuminuria and, ultimately, nephropathy. Thus, they are suggested as part of the initial therapy for diabetic patients with nephropathy. Their use is contraindicated in pregnant patients, however, and they should be used with caution in females of childbearing age. ACEIs may also exacerbate hyperkalemia in patients with advanced renal insufficiency or hyporeninemic hypoaldosteronism. Older adults with advanced renal disease and patients with renal artery stenosis may experience a decline in renal function with ACEIs. If a patient does not tolerate the use of ACEIs, angiotensin receptor blockers (ARBs) can be used. Some studies suggest these agents can be used together in diabetic patients with nephropathy because they act by different, albeit related, mechanisms.

- *Hypertension:* In a patient with T1DM, hypertension is often a manifestation of nephropathy. Control of hypertension has been demonstrated to reduce the rate of progression of nephropathy and to reduce the complications of CVD. ADA guidelines recommend that the goal for blood pressure control in nonpregnant adults is to maintain the systolic blood pressure at less than 140 mm Hg and the diastolic blood pressure at less than 90 mm Hg. Even lower systolic and diastolic blood pressure should be targeted in patients who are at high risk of CVD. The goal for patients with isolated systolic hypertension is also less than 140 mm Hg. Patients at high risk for CVD may target a lower goal of 130/80 mm Hg, if this can be achieved without significant side effects. Studies have shown that the closer patients with DM approach the target blood pressure, the less likely they are to develop cardiac sequelae. Initial treatment for diabetic patients with hypertension should include lifestyle management and, if medication is required, an ACEI or ARB should be started, unless contraindicated. Patients with signs of congestive heart failure and an abnormal ejection fraction should be immediately referred for a cardiology consult.
- *Macrovascular disease:* Patients with DM are at risk for developing macrovascular complications including stroke, PVD, CAD, and other forms of CVD. Evidence of uncontrolled angina, carotid bruits, and ECG abnormalities may require advanced intervention. Daily intake of aspirin has been shown to reduce cardiovascular events in patients with DM. Patients with disabling claudication or nonhealing ulcers require a vascular consultation for their PVD. All patients with DM should be screened for these diseases, because symptoms may not be present until late in the course of the disease.
- *Neuropathy:* One-half of the patients with hyperglycemia extending over 15 years will develop some degree of neuropathy. Foot ulcers and related problems resulting from decreased peripheral sensation in diabetic patients with significant neuropathy are a major cause of morbidity in DM, with potentially life-threatening consequences if such infections spread systemically. Peripheral neuropathy may result in pain, loss of sensation, and muscle weakness. The feet and ankles are affected most often, but many patients also complain of pain in the knees and upper extremities. Severe pain from neuropathy can lead to sleep and mood disturbances. A thorough initial foot examination followed by annual follow-up foot examinations are indicated in asymptomatic patients. A 10-g Semmes-Weinstein monofilament should be used to assess sensation at least annually. Abnormal findings indicate the need for a thorough vascular, neurological, musculoskeletal, and soft tissue evaluation.

   Many patients take several medications to control the pain or discomfort of neuropathy. Nonopioid analgesics, calcium channel blockers, narcotic analgesics, tricyclic antidepressants, antiarrhythmics, and local anesthetics are frequently prescribed. Pregabalin (Lyrica) and duloxetine (Cymbalta) have received U.S. Food and Drug Administration (FDA) approval for the treatment of neuropathic pain in DM. The opioid tapentadol (Nucynta, Palexia, Tapal) has also received FDA approval, but the evidence is weaker related to its effectiveness in diabetic neuropathy. Tricyclic antidepressants are commonly prescribed for painful neuropathies, as are gabapentin (Neurontin), venlafaxine (Effexor), carbamazepine (Tegretol), tramadol (Ultram), and topical capsaicin. Patients with chronic pain syndromes may benefit from a referral to a chronic pain clinic.

   Patients with neuropathy require professional nail and callus care because most ulcers begin at the site of a callus. Supportive athletic shoes are recommended for all patients for walking. Extra-depth shoes and custom-molded shoe inserts are indicated for patients who are at high risk for foot ulcers. Patients at high risk include those with neuropathy; those with structural deformities of the feet, skin, or nails; and those with a history of previous ulcers. Charcot foot disorders occur in 9% of patients with neuropathy, leading to bony destruction, joint subluxation, and bony remodeling of the foot. Patients with abnormal findings on radiological examination should be referred to an orthopedist for further evaluation.
- *Pregnancy:* Of the 10% of all pregnancies that are complicated by DM, 0.2% to 0.5% are in patients with T1DM. There is an increased risk for pregnancy-related complications in these patients, including preeclampsia, preterm delivery, intrauterine fetal demise, and cardiac and renal malformations. These patients should undergo preconception counseling and then frequent follow-up to stress the importance of extremely tight glucose control.
- *Diabetes distress:* This distinct psychological disorder related to DM is very common. The constant demands of medication dosing, monitoring of blood glucose,

food tracking, and increased attention to physical activity have an adverse psychological impact on up to 45% of patients. Annual screening for this disorder should be done with a validated measurement tool, such as the Diabetes Distress Scale for Adults with Type 1 Diabetes. If the patient screens positive for this condition, they should be referred to a mental health professional. In some cases, the demands of glycemic control on the patient's lifestyle can lead to depression, and patients should be evaluated for depression by the primary care practitioner after the initial diagnosis of DM and then annually.

- *Other:* Autonomic involvement can affect GI, cardiovascular, and genitourinary function. Sexual dysfunction, particularly erectile dysfunction, occurs frequently in older patients.

Patient Education: T1DM

A key focus in the education of patients with T1DM is insulin self-injection and the appropriate use of insulin syringes and autoinjectors. Insulin administration involves the use of subcutaneous syringes marked in insulin units. Regulations governing the purchase of syringes vary greatly from state to state. Syringes should be recapped by the patient, using a one-handed technique, and they should be discarded according to state requirements. Patients with visual or dexterity difficulties may benefit from prefilled syringes. Prefilled insulin syringes may be stored in a vertical position in the refrigerator for up to 30 days with the needle pointing upward.

Alternatives to syringes include jet injectors and penlike autoinjector devices. Jet injectors are useful for patients who have needle phobias, but they are expensive. Penlike devices hold insulin cartridges and are useful if the patient is visually or neurologically impaired, as they help increase the accuracy of insulin administration. Unlike older insulins, newer varieties of insulin do not require constant refrigeration, which makes them more convenient for patients. Another alternative insulin delivery device is the implanted insulin pump, which is a small device that is worn externally. Continuous subcutaneous insulin is delivered from the pump via tubing attached to the pump reservoir. Use of the insulin pump requires oversight by skilled professionals, the careful selection of patients, frequent blood glucose monitoring, and comprehensive patient education.

Insulin should be injected at room temperature, but insulin storage bottles not in use should be refrigerated. Insulin should be injected into the subcutaneous tissue of the upper arm or anterior or lateral aspects of the thigh, the buttocks, or the abdomen. Rotation of the site within one area is recommended rather than rotating to a different site with each injection.

Education in foot care should also be reviewed at each visit. Patients at high risk for foot ulcer development should be encouraged to follow through with periodic professional foot care and daily foot hygiene. Patients at low risk should be encouraged to continue good hygiene, wear properly fitting footwear, avoid trauma to the feet, stop smoking if applicable, and immediately report any blisters, macerated skin, or hemorrhaging into a callus, as well as to limit weight-bearing on the affected extremity.

Patients should understand that any illness maximizes stress, and this is especially true for individuals with DM. When acutely ill, all patients must continue to take their insulin and increase blood glucose monitoring to every 2 hours. Supplemental dosages of regular insulin may be needed to control blood glucose levels. If the patient's blood sugar is higher than 240 mg/dL, the urine should be checked for ketones every 4 hours. A caloric intake of 50 g of carbohydrates every 4 hours should be maintained. A variety of clear fluids, including some with glucose, should be encouraged, as well as gelatin, ice pops, regular soda, soup, and toast, if tolerated. Patients should be encouraged to maintain an oral fluid intake of 6 to 9 oz/hr to avoid dehydration. If the illness is accompanied by vomiting or diarrhea for more than 2 hours, a fever of 101°F (38.3°C) or higher, or blood glucose of 240 mg/dL or higher and if ketones continue to appear in the urine despite additional insulin, the patient should be instructed to seek medical attention immediately, given the risk of developing DKA.

DIABETES MELLITUS TYPE 2

T2DM is characterized by the abnormal secretion of insulin, resistance to the action of insulin in the target tissues, and/or an inadequate response at the level of the insulin receptor. T2DM reduces life expectancy because of complications that are affected by the duration of DM, the degree of blood glucose control, and other cardiovascular risk factors such as smoking and hypertension.

EPIDEMIOLOGY AND CAUSES

According to the U.S. Centers for Disease Control and Prevention (CDC), the prevalence of T2DM in the United States is 9.4%. Approximately 90% to 95% of all Americans diagnosed with DM have T2DM. Approximately 28 million American adults have T2DM, but nearly 24% of individuals are unaware that they have the disorder. The disease is often asymptomatic in its early stages; as a result, individuals can remain undiagnosed for many years. However, chronic hyperglycemia is associated with long-term damage and dysfunction of various organs, including the kidneys, liver, eyes, nerves, heart, and blood vessels. In turn, T2DM is the seventh leading cause of death in the United States, as it contributes to many other diseases of major organ systems, such as cardiovascular, cerebrovascular, and kidney disorders. The comorbidities associated with T2DM are extensive and are reflected in the per capita health-care costs of people with DM in the United States, which are five times higher than those without DM.

T2DM has a stronger genetic association than T1DM. First-degree relatives of patients with T2DM have a five-to 10-fold higher lifetime risk of developing DM than age-matched control subjects with no family history. Moreover, nearly 40% of patients have at least one affected parent with the disease, and monozygotic twin studies have demonstrated between 60% and 90% concordance.

Risk Factors: T2DM

Family history (first-degree relative)
Body mass index greater than 25 kg/m² (lower for Asian Americans)
Older than 45 years
Impaired fasting glucose or A1c greater than 5.7%
History of gestational diabetes
Hypertension (greater than 140/90 mm Hg or on antihypertensive therapy)
Hyperlipidemia (HDL less than 35 mg/dL, triglycerides greater than 250 mg/dL)
Females with polycystic ovarian syndrome
Race/ethnicity
- African American
- Latino
- Native American
- Asian American
- Pacific Islander

The overall prevalence of T2DM is increasing in the U.S. general population, as well as among certain ethnic minority groups. A disproportionate number of African Americans, Latinos, Native Americans, Asian Americans, and Pacific Islanders have T2DM, compared with the general population. Native Americans and Alaskan Natives have the highest prevalence of diagnosed T2DM. Along with genetic differences, additional factors that may underlie this disparity in disease prevalence include socioeconomic factors, differential health-care practices, unequal access to health-care resources, and ethnocultural influences in diet and activity level.

Unlike T1DM, the incidence of T2DM increases with age, reaching 25% in individuals aged 65 years and older. However, it is important to note that this form of DM may be diagnosed at any age. Rates of newly diagnosed cases of T2DM among children are on the rise, reflecting the marked increase in childhood obesity over the past several decades. Indeed, the CDC estimates that the prevalence of T2DM in children and adolescents will quadruple over the next 40 years.

Several pharmacological agents are associated with iatrogenic hyperglycemia and the eventual development of overt DM. These include glucocorticoids; hormonal therapies such as oral contraceptives; the immunosuppressants tacrolimus and cyclosporine; nicotinic acid (niacin); antiretroviral protease inhibitors used for HIV (which also cause central fat redistribution known as *lipodystrophy syndrome*); several atypical antipsychotic agents including clozapine (Clozaril) and olanzapine (Zyprexa); and certain antihypertensives including beta blockers, calcium channel blockers, clonidine (Catapres), and thiazide diuretics. In contrast, both ACEIs and ARBs appear to improve insulin sensitivity and reduce the development of T2DM in hypertensive nondiabetic patients.

PATHOPHYSIOLOGY

T2DM is associated with two physiological abnormalities: insulin resistance and impaired insulin secretion by the beta islet cells of the pancreas. Initially, as insulin resistance increases, insulin levels begin to rise but the glucose level remains normal, resulting in a state of hyperinsulinemia. Insulin resistance worsens in conjunction with hyperinsulinemia, eventually resulting in the development of fasting hyperglycemia, because hepatic gluconeogenesis increases due to glucagon being produced by pancreatic alpha cells in response to the hyperinsulinemia. As hyperglycemia is ultimately toxic to pancreatic beta cells, over time this results in relative hypoinsulinemia, which ultimately necessitates exogenous insulin in cases of advanced T2DM.

Unlike the pathophysiology in T1DM, there is no autoimmune destruction of pancreatic beta cells in T2DM. Rather, there is a decline in beta cell function, with impaired insulin secretion in response to a glycemic load, which results in elevated plasma glucose levels. This first manifests as postprandial elevated glucose levels, and because insulin also supports the transport of amino acids and fatty acids, alterations in lipid and protein levels may be seen. Thus, multiple metabolic processes are affected.

The sequence of worsening insulin resistance preceding impaired insulin secretion has been observed in prospective studies, although other studies have indicated these two pathophysiological mechanisms are independent risk factors for the development of T2DM and occur in concert, rather than sequentially. Although insufficient to cause DM alone, insulin resistance appears to be the strongest predictor of T2DM development, an observation that is reinforced by the importance of insulin resistance as a component of metabolic syndrome (see Chapter 35).

Insulin resistance is primarily thought to be caused by toxicity due to elevated levels of free fatty acids and pro-inflammatory cytokines that are associated with acquired traits, such as aging and obesity, in which these substances are produced by adipose tissue. Obesity is characterized by low-grade systemic inflammation, which has been linked to beta cell dysfunction. For example, adipocyte-derived tumor necrosis factor-α has been positively correlated with increasing insulin resistance, as has the adipocyte-derived hormone resistin. In contrast, the adipocyte-derived hormone adiponectin appears to be negatively correlated with insulin resistance.

Obesity is a major modifiable risk factor for T2DM, affecting up to 90% of individuals with the disease.

Physical exercise with a corresponding weight loss of just 5% to 10% of total body weight can prevent or delay the development of T2DM in obese individuals, generating marked improvement in insulin resistance. Patients who are not obese but who have a disproportionate percentage of body weight distributed in the visceral area rather than at the hips are also at greater risk of developing T2DM.

The interaction of genetic and environmental factors may be responsible for producing epigenetic changes that underlie the heterogeneity of T2DM. More than 40 single nucleotide polymorphisms have been identified that increase the risk of developing T2DM. Genetic variants have been identified that affect incretin hormones (which normally decrease glucose levels), beta cell function, and key protein regulators of glucose metabolism. The intestinal microbiome may also play a role in determining the risk of developing T2DM, as the gut flora impacts nutrient absorption. Studies demonstrate the ability to improve insulin sensitivity by altering the gut biome.

Elevated plasma glucose levels may be tolerated for many years by the patient with DM who, in turn, may not seek treatment until significant complications result. Eventually, insulin secretion will become insufficient to compensate for insulin resistance. Moreover, hyperinsulinemia and hyperglycemia increase lipid synthesis, raising serum levels of fatty acids, triglycerides (greater than 150 mg/dL), and LDL cholesterol, while lowering HDL cholesterol. This increase in lipids is also toxic to beta cells and is referred to as *lipotoxicity*.

Overall, the pathogenesis of T2DM has been labeled the "ominous octet," consisting of eight distinct factors: (1) beta cell failure; (2) insulin resistance in muscle cells; (3) insulin resistance in liver cells; (4) adipocyte resistance to the antilipolytic effect of insulin, which results in increased plasma free fatty acids; (5) decreased incretin; (6) increased glucagon secretion and enhanced hepatic sensitivity to glucagon; (7) enhanced renal glucose reabsorption; and (8) resistance of the central nervous system to the anorectic effect of insulin, which results in appetite dysregulation and weight gain.

GI tissues contribute to this pathophysiology through the actions of the incretins glucagon-like peptide-1 (GLP1) and gastric inhibitory polypeptide (GIP). These two hormones play a significant role in glucose absorption. In T2DM, GLP1 is deficient, and there is resistance to the GIP effect on the stimulation of insulin secretion. GLP1 normally inhibits glucagon secretion postprandially. Pancreatic alpha cells stimulate glucagon secretion and are normally responsive to beta cell function. In T2DM, this communication becomes dysfunctional, and alpha cells begin to hypersecrete glucagon.

The kidneys are designed to filter glucose through the sodium-glucose transport 2 (SGLT2) transporter system. A small amount of glucose is also filtered through the related SGLT1 transporter located in the descending proximal tubule of the renal nephron. The kidneys reabsorb even more glucose in hyperglycemic states. Eventually, this hyperglycemia leads to renal microvascular damage and eventually diabetic kidney disease.

CLINICAL PRESENTATION

Because the onset of T2DM may occur years before a diagnosis is made, individuals who are asymptomatic tend to be diagnosed during a routine physical examination or during treatment for another condition.

Subjective

Because the onset of T2DM is usually insidious, only a minority of patients are initially symptomatic. A patient may present with pruritus, fatigue, neuropathic complaints such as numbness and tingling, or blurred vision. The symptoms of T1DM and T2DM are essentially the same due to hyperglycemia (see the previous section on T1DM for a complete discussion), although the severe ketoacidosis that may occur in T1DM is rare in patients with T2DM. Thus, some patients present with increased urination, nocturia, thirst, or polydipsia. In many cases, T2DM initially presents as an infection, such as vaginitis (candidiasis) in females, balanitis (especially in older males), or a skin infection. Cardiovascular symptoms such as angina may also prompt a heretofore undiagnosed patient with T2DM to seek health care.

Objective

There may be no dramatic change in objective findings with T2DM, although the typical patient is often obese, with a history of dyslipidemia, hypertension, and CAD. Abnormal healing and an increased occurrence of infection, especially yeast infection, may also be present.

In severe cases, patients may present with HHS, in which profound dehydration results from prolonged hyperglycemia (see Table 59.4). Formerly known as *hyperosmolar hyperglycemic nonketotic coma,* HHS is associated with a high mortality rate and is typically seen in older diabetic adults who have developed an infection, such as pneumonia or other illness. Patients with undiagnosed DM may develop this condition due to prolonged hyperglycemia in the absence of treatment. Other risk factors for developing HHS in the diabetic patients include peritoneal dialysis; hemodialysis; tube feedings with high-protein formulas; and the use of mannitol, phenytoin, corticosteroids, immunosuppressive agents, and diuretics. Symptoms of HHS are dramatic, including severe hyperglycemia (greater than 600 mg/dL), plasma or serum hyperosmolality (more than 340 mOsm), and profound dehydration. Although classically thought of as a nonketotic condition, ketosis may or may not be present in HHS, and neurological symptoms range from a clouded sensorium to frank coma. HHS requires immediate referral for acute care management.

TABLE 59.4 Hyperosmolar Hyperglycemic Syndrome

Overview	Clinical Presentation	Management
Hyperosmolar hyperglycemic syndrome (HHS) characterized by: • Severe hyperglycemia—blood sugar greater than 600 mg/dL • No ketosis • Hyperosmolality • Dehydration • High mortality rate Occurs in: • Older patients with DM who develop infection or other illness • Undiagnosed patients with DM • Patients with DM diagnosed after a prolonged period of hyperglycemia Precipitating factors: • Peritoneal dialysis • Hemodialysis • Tube feeding with high-protein formulas • Mannitol infusion • Phenytoin (Dilantin) • Corticosteroids • Immunosuppressive agents • Diuretics • Surgery • Myocardial infarction • Sepsis • Renal insufficiency • Congestive heart failure	Insidious onset with subtle initial symptoms; history may indicate decreased fluid intake Patients may present with: • Polyuria • Polydipsia • Weakness • No ketoacidosis • Lethargy and confusion that develop when serum osmolality is greater than 310 mOsm/kg • Coma Laboratory tests: • Severe hyperglycemia—blood glucose greater than 600 mg/dL • Initial serum sodium decreased • Serum sodium that increases as dehydration progresses • Serum osmolality greater than 400 mOsm/kg	Goals: • Correct dehydration • Normalize electrolytes (replenish deficiencies) Correct dehydration and electrolyte imbalances: • Rapid infusion of hypotonic saline (0.45% NaCl). • In cases of hypovolemia, use normal saline (0.9% NaCl). • Fluid needs may be 4–6 L over 8–10 hours. • Correct serum sodium with the following equation, given dilutional effect of hyperglycemia: corrected sodium = measured sodium + (0.8 × every 50 mg/dL increment of plasma glucose above 100 mg/dL) • Once blood glucose is less than 250 mg/dL, fluid replacement should be with 5% dextrose in 0.45% saline solution or normal (0.9%) saline. • Endpoint of fluid therapy is to return urine output to ≥50 mL/hr. • Less potassium replacement is typically needed than in diabetic ketoacidosis.

Abbreviations: DM, diabetes mellitus.

DIAGNOSTIC REASONING

Diagnostic Tests

Because early detection and prompt treatment may reduce the complications of T2DM, screening for DM as part of routine medical care is appropriate under certain circumstances. Screening for prediabetes and DM should be considered in all individuals who are overweight or obese, regardless of age, and for all adults aged 45 years and older. Testing should be repeated at a minimum of 3-year intervals, with several laboratory approaches capable of diagnosing T2DM, as described in the following section.

Initial Testing

Immediate testing for hyperglycemia in the clinical setting can be accomplished by using a portable monitor to assess capillary blood glucose level. This test is referred to as a *random capillary blood glucose measurement* and may be taken without regard to timing of the patient's last meal. It is important to note that certain drugs can produce hyperglycemia, including glucocorticoids, furosemide (Lasix), thiazide diuretics, phenytoin (Dilantin), estrogen-containing products, beta blockers, and nicotinic acid. A result of 200 mg/dL or greater should be followed up by screening for elevated blood glucose, using a whole blood sample. If the random plasma glucose level is elevated, additional blood glucose testing should be done.

There are four laboratory-based criteria to confirm DM:

1. Glycosylated hemoglobin (A1c) level greater than or equal to 6.5%*
2. Random plasma glucose level of 200 mg/dL in the presence of classic symptoms of hyperglycemia or a hyperglycemic crisis*
3. Fasting plasma glucose level of 126 mg/dL or higher on two occasions (*fasting* is defined as no caloric intake for at least 8 hours)
4. Two-hour postload plasma glucose level of 200 mg/dL or higher during an OGTT, after consumption of a glucose load containing the equivalent of 75 g of anhydrous glucose dissolved in water (an OGTT is also used to screen for diabetes during pregnancy)

*In the absence of unequivocal hyperglycemia, results should be confirmed by repeat testing on a new blood sample without delay, preferably using the same type of test.

Subsequent Testing

An A1c determination gives valuable insight into the mean glycemic level over the preceding 2 to 3 months and is helpful in documenting the degree of glycemic control at the time of diagnosis and as part of continuing care. An A1c value of less than 7% indicates strong control; however, a value of less than 6.5% has been shown to significantly decrease the occurrence of complications, provided this can be achieved without hypoglycemia or other adverse effects.

Additional laboratory tests that are appropriate to the evaluation of the patient's general medical condition should be performed at the time of diagnosis and at least annually thereafter. These include a fasting lipid profile, serum creatinine, eGFR, liver function tests, and spot urinary UACR. A C-peptide measurement (reflecting endogenous insulin production) may be ordered if the diagnosis between T1DM and T2DM is unclear. In T2DM, the C-peptide level is normal or elevated, but it is decreased in T1DM, given the lack of insulin production.

Specific evaluations should be performed to assess for end-organ damage at diagnosis and annually thereafter. These include, but are not limited to, body mass index assessment, blood pressure measurement including orthostatic blood pressure (especially in older adults), funduscopic eye examination, thyroid palpation, full skin examination to evaluate for acanthosis nigricans, and a comprehensive foot examination to assess for diabetic ulcers.

Differential Diagnosis

Differential diagnoses for T2DM include prediabetes (glucose intolerance), gestational diabetes (new-onset DM developing at any stage of pregnancy), Cushing's syndrome, pheochromocytoma, and drug-induced hyperglycemia. In addition, a patient who fails to respond to metformin (Glucophage) or other antihyperglycemic agents should be evaluated for the possibility of T1DM. Although T1DM occurs infrequently in older adults, it should be considered in patients with other autoimmune disorders, patients without a family history of T2DM, or patients of normal weight.

Increasing evidence points to linkages among CAD, hyperlipidemia, obesity, and T2DM; thus, such comorbidities must be ruled out in all diabetic patients. A prediabetic state of glucose intolerance has also been associated with hypertension, obesity, and hyperlipidemia as a collection of comorbidities known as *metabolic syndrome*, which is a strong predictor of eventual development of DM and CVD (see Chapter 35 for further information on metabolic syndrome).

MANAGEMENT

T2DM is a chronic, complex illness that requires ongoing health care and education to prevent acute and chronic complications. Interventions should include treatments directed at both risk reduction and glycemic control. Lifestyle management is an important part of treatment and comprises nutrition therapy, activity prescriptions for exercise, decreased prolonged sitting, and, in older adults, training in balance and flexibility. Lifestyle management should also focus on mental health, sleep, and smoking cessation.

Preventing or delaying complications is accomplished by active screening and frequent clinical assessments, as well as the use of medications. Obesity management has become a high-level target in the treatment of patients with T2DM, including the possible use of medications and surgery for the treatment of obesity. The pharmacological approach to antihyperglycemic treatment changes rapidly as new medications and drug classes are approved and older medications are combined with newer agents.

Although the primary care practitioner's focus is often on glycemic control and risk reduction, the patient's focus is typically on the need to fit these treatment interventions into an acceptable lifestyle and ensure they are minimally disruptive. Research has identified that dietary modifications, the need for frequent blood glucose monitoring, and subsequent follow-up with health-care providers place a financial and psychological burden on patients and their families/support people.

Lifestyle Management

Lifestyle management encompasses nutritional education including the treatment of obesity, physical activity, adequate sleep and sleep hygiene practices, the evaluation of psychosocial status and stress reduction, and smoking cessation if applicable.

The 2021 ADA Standards of Medical Care recommend that every patient receive diabetes self-management education (DSME) and diabetes self-management support (DSMS) at the time of diagnosis. Patients should be evaluated for the need for specialty referrals annually and with the onset of any new complication or transition in care. Comprehensive diabetes treatment programs are designed to be person centered and to provide patients with the information to empower them to self-treat and become the leader in their own DM management. Studies of patients who complete DSME demonstrate lower A1c values, lower weight, and improved quality of life. Unfortunately, in contrast to newly diagnosed (mostly pediatric) patients with T1DM, not many patients with T2DM receive formal DSME and DSMS.

Nutritional Therapy

Meal planning or nutritional therapy is one of the most fundamental and challenging components of DM management. The goal of nutritional therapy is to achieve and maintain body weight goals, blood glucose and lipid levels, and blood pressure goals, and to delay or prevent the complications of DM. Most patients with T2DM are obese or overweight; therefore, weight loss is generally a significant factor in meal planning. Although hypocaloric diets and weight loss usually improve blood glucose control, traditional dietary strategies have not proven to be particularly effective in achieving long-term weight loss.

As research continues to explore why weight loss and weight maintenance are so difficult, the emphasis of dietary counseling should be on the consumption of nutrient-dense foods in appropriate portion sizes to control serum glucose levels and promote healthy eating practices. The meal plan should be based on the patient's food preferences, activity level, medical history, and both current and target weights, as well as lifestyle, cultural, ethnic, and financial factors. Ideally, a registered dietitian or certified diabetes educator should be consulted to assist patients. It is important for the clinician to be nonjudgmental and to help patients enjoy their healthy food choices.

If weight loss is indicated, a moderate caloric restriction of 500 to 750 calories less than the patient's average daily intake, as calculated from a detailed food history (which can be tracked with a food diary), can be instituted. A hypocaloric diet, independent of weight loss, is associated with increased insulin sensitivity and the improvement of blood glucose levels. Moderate weight loss, irrespective of the patient's starting weight, has significant benefits, especially in decreasing morbidity and mortality rates. In fact, weight loss is a primary intervention because it improves the serum lipid profile, reduces blood pressure, decreases insulin resistance, and ameliorates glucose intolerance.

Individuals on most oral glucose-lowering agents and/or insulin therapy should eat at consistent times that are synchronized with their medication administration. A nutritionally balanced meal plan is important for the patient with T2DM and should take into account the higher prevalence of atherosclerosis in patients with DM. Specific diets for patients with DM are no longer recommended by the ADA; instead, the ADA recommends that macronutrient distribution within the diet is individualized for each patient, with total calorie and metabolic needs used as guides (see Table 59.5 for nutritional information on different classes of macronutrients).

Physical Activity

Physical activity is an integral component of the management of T2DM. Activity-based interventions include increasing general movement through activities of daily living and decreasing sedentary behavior. Exercise is a specific type of physical activity, and the recommendation is 150 minutes per week of moderate to intensive physical effort. The exercise should occur at least 3 days per week, with no more than 2 consecutive days without exercise.

TABLE 59.5 Macronutrient Information

Macronutrient	Recommend	Avoid
Carbohydrates	Whole grains Vegetables (fresh preferred) Fruits (fresh preferred) Legumes Emphasis on high-fiber content	Refined (simple) sugars Refined flour Sugar-sweetened beverages Minimize foods with added sugar
Protein	Daily intake: 1–1.5 g/kg Daily intake with chronic kidney disease: 0.8 g/kg	Do not use protein-containing foods to treat nocturnal hypoglycemia; unclear whether protein-containing bedtime snacks prevent nocturnal hypoglycemia
Fats	Monounsaturated fats Foods rich in long chain omega-3 fatty acids Daily intake: 25%–30% of total calories	Trans fatty acids

In addition, decreasing sedentary behavior is critical, and not sitting for more than 30 minutes at a time is recommended. Older adults should have flexibility and balance training two to three times per week. Also, studies have demonstrated that older adults have improved A1c control if resistance training is added 2 days per week to their exercise routine.

Before beginning an exercise program, patients should be screened for the presence of macrovascular and/or microvascular complications of DM that may be worsened by exercise. These include CAD, PVD, retinopathy, nephropathy, and peripheral or autonomic neuropathy. The patient with T2DM can perform all levels of exercise, as long as glycemic control is adequate and there is no evidence of DM complications. If there are complications, consultation with the appropriate specialists should be completed before starting an exercise program. If the patient is taking particular oral antidiabetic agents (e.g., sulfonylureas) or is on insulin therapy, exercise can lead to hypoglycemia. Thus, patients initiating an exercise regimen should be aware of the signs and symptoms of hypoglycemia and be prepared to treat such an event. Any exercise prescription should be individualized to take into account the patient's level of interest in physical activity, lifestyle practices, physical condition, financial situation, and motivation.

Psychosocial Issues

Appropriately addressing psychosocial issues is included in ADA treatment guidelines. The ADA suggests screening patients for depression, diabetes distress, anxiety, eating disorders, and impaired cognitive function at least annually. For patients to provide their own self-care, they need to have emotional well-being. DM is a risk factor for depression and anxiety. Thus, screening and appropriate referrals to mental health providers are important for the overall care and support of diabetic patients and their families.

Monitoring Blood Glucose Levels

The optimal monitoring of blood glucose levels in patients with T2DM has not been clearly established. SMBG is useful for guiding the effectiveness and safety of treatment with antihyperglycemic medications or insulin, especially in patients who have not consistently achieved blood glucose treatment goals. These patients should be instructed to keep a log of their results for periodic review by the primary care practitioner.

CGM may play a role for patients who have difficulty achieving glycemic control or who are using an intensive insulin regimen. Patients who are unaware of their hypoglycemic episodes may also benefit from CGM, given the life-threatening risk of hypoglycemia and the need for immediate intervention. Both types of blood glucose monitoring can assist patients and their healthcare providers in understanding the patient's individual response to treatment. Continuous monitoring requires more intensive education than SMBG, however.

Pharmacological Therapy

Pharmacological therapy for T2DM is required when lifestyle management does not result in adequate blood glucose control. Drug therapy should always be considered an adjunctive therapy to lifestyle management, as the latter is typically initiated first. However, for particular patients with significant disease, the American Association of Clinical Endocrinologists (AACE) and American College of Endocrinology agree with the ADA Standards of Medical Care that pharmacotherapy can be initiated at the time of diagnosis simultaneously with lifestyle management.

Selecting a medication for glycemic control involves analyzing the risks and benefits of the agent according to patient age, comorbidities, and hypoglycemia risk. Basic recommendations from professional organizations differ with regard to initiating pharmacological therapy. The AACE recommends that patients with recent-onset T2DM or mild hyperglycemia (A1c less than 7.5%) start with lifestyle treatment and monotherapy. The ADA and AACE recommend metformin (Glucophage) if there are no contraindications, such as renal disease or abnormal creatinine clearance, acute myocardial infarction, or septicemia. The AACE recommends adding a second agent to lifestyle treatment and metformin if the A1c is more than 7.5% at the time of diagnosis or after 3 months of metformin monotherapy without achievement of the patient's blood glucose goals. In contrast, the ADA does not recommend dual-agent pharmacotherapy until the A1c is 9% or greater. This differs from AACE guidelines, which recommend starting insulin if the patient's A1c is 9% or higher at the time of presentation and if the patient is symptomatic. The ADA, on the other hand, recommends starting insulin when the A1c is 10% or greater with symptoms.

Current therapy for T2DM includes drugs that alter insulin action, stimulate insulin secretion, affect the absorption of glucose, mimic the effects of incretin, act as an insulin secretagogue, or suppress postprandial glucagon release. Insulin itself is also a treatment for T2DM. Both AACE and ADA guidelines list (in no selected order) sulfonylureas, thiazolidinediones, dipeptidyl peptidase-4 inhibitors (DPP4-Is), SGLT2 inhibitors, GLP1 analogues, and insulin as therapeutic choices.

Metformin (Glucophage) is a biguanide that works by suppressing excessive hepatic glucose production and by increasing glucose utilization in peripheral tissues. Metformin reduces fasting and postprandial hyperglycemia and reduces hepatic gluconeogenesis. It may also improve glucose levels by reducing intestinal glucose absorption. Metformin does not stimulate endogenous insulin secretion, but it can provide cardiovascular protection and contribute to weight loss.

Metformin can be used as a monotherapy unless the patient has contraindications or intolerance. Although metformin is the first-line medication recommended by the ADA and the AACE for T2DM, it should be used only in patients with adequate renal function and should not be used in patients with an eGFR less than 45 mL/min/1.73 m^2. Metformin also has a boxed warning in its FDA-approved prescribing information for lactic acidosis, although this side effect is very rare. Patients at risk for developing lactic acidosis include those with liver impairment, alcohol abuse, and cardiopulmonary insufficiency. Metformin should be discontinued 24 to 48 hours before diagnostic or surgical procedures due to the risk of decreased kidney function, and its administration should not be resumed for at least 6 hours after these procedures or until the patient is adequately hydrated.

Initial dosing is 500 mg once a day with breakfast or dinner for 1 week and then twice daily with breakfast and dinner. The dosage should be titrated up to a maximum dose of 2,000 mg. Several weeks of therapy may be needed to achieve maximum effects of the given dose. Common adverse reactions include diarrhea, nausea, anorexia, and abdominal discomfort, which usually resolve with a gradual increase of dosage. Metformin has been shown to cause decreased vitamin B$_{12}$ absorption, and patients on long-term metformin therapy should undergo periodic testing for B_{12} deficiency, especially if the patient complains of peripheral neuropathy. At the maximum dose, the monthly cost of metformin in the United States is approximately $4 on many generic formularies. Metformin is currently found in 20 combination formulations with other medications (see Drugs Commonly Prescribed 59.2).

Sulfonylureas work by stimulating pancreatic insulin secretion; thus, pancreatic beta cells must still be producing insulin in order for sulfonylureas to be effective, as they do not reduce insulin resistance. The advantages of second generation sulfonylureas over older first generation agents include their improved safety profile, shorter half-life, and relatively greater effects on reducing A1c, with an approximate 1.5% average absolute decrease. However, these agents carry a higher risk of hypoglycemia and weight gain than other medications. In addition, patients with severe insulin resistance may

Drugs Commonly Prescribed 59.2: Noninsulin Agents for Diabetes Mellitus Type 2

DRUG CLASS AND EXAMPLES	INDICATION	ADVERSE REACTIONS AND PRESCRIBING CONSIDERATIONS
Biguanides		
• Metformin (Glucophage)	Monotherapy; may be used as an adjunct to diet in T2DM or with a sulfonylurea or insulin therapy	Monitor for hypoglycemia, especially in older adults. Adverse reactions include GI disturbances and metallic taste. Rare cases of lactic acidosis. Contraindicated in renal disease; renal function should be assessed before starting.
First Generation Sulfonylureas *(no longer recommended, given newer agents)*		
• Chlorpropamide (Diabinese) • Tolbutamide (Orinase)	For use as an adjunct to diet and exercise in T2DM (largely replaced by second generation sulfonylureas)	Adverse reactions include hypoglycemia with high doses or, in fasting patients, weight gain, headache, GI upset, skin rashes, severe anemia, and hypersensitivity. Increased risk of cardiovascular mortality Contraindicated for patients with impaired liver or kidney function, given the increased risk of hypoglycemia; not for use in T1DM or DKA Worse safety profile than second generation sulfonylureas, so no longer recommended
Second Generation Sulfonylureas		
• Glimepiride (Amaryl; sometimes considered as third generation) • Glipizide (Glucotrol) • Glyburide (Diaßeta, Micronase)	For use as an adjunct to diet and exercise in T2DM	Same as for first generation sulfonylureas, but with relatively improved safety profile compared with older agents Increased potency by weight compared with first generation drugs
Alpha-Glucosidase Inhibitors		
• Acarbose (Precose) • Miglitol (Glyset)	For use as an adjunct to diet and exercise in T2DM; used as monotherapy or added to insulin, metformin, or a sulfonylurea	Adverse reactions include flatulence, diarrhea, and abdominal pain (advise patient to take with first bite of main meal, starting with a low dose and gradually increasing). Contraindicated in DKA and in patients with inflammatory bowel disease, colonic ulceration, intestinal obstruction, and chronic intestinal diseases impacting digestion. Do not use if serum creatinine is greater than 2 mg/dL. Use glucose (tablets, gel), not fructose (such as in fruit juices), to treat hypoglycemia, as the metabolism of complex carbohydrates will be inhibited.

Drugs Commonly Prescribed 59.2: Noninsulin Agents for Diabetes Mellitus Type 2—cont'd

DRUG CLASS AND EXAMPLES	INDICATION	ADVERSE REACTIONS AND PRESCRIBING CONSIDERATIONS
Thiazolidinediones		
• Pioglitazone (Actos) • Rosiglitazone (Avandia)	For use as an adjunct to diet and exercise in T2DM; used as monotherapy to reduce insulin resistance or added to metformin; not for use with T1DM or DKA	Adverse reactions include exacerbation of congestive heart failure, swelling of legs, fluid retention, weight gain, upper respiratory tract infection, and hypersensitivity. Increased risk of bladder tumors reported Do not give to patients with liver disease or if ALT is greater than 2.5 × upper limit of normal; monitor transaminases at baseline every 2 months for first 12 months and then periodically; discontinue if levels increase or jaundice occurs. Contraindicated in New York Heart Association class III or IV heart failure May cause resumption of ovulation in an anovulatory patient (and thus may result in unintended pregnancy)
Dipeptidyl Peptidase-4 Inhibitors		
• Alogliptin (Nesina) • Linagliptin (Tradjenta) • Saxagliptin (Onglyza) • Sitagliptin (Januvia)	Can be used as monotherapy as incretin mimetic, but usually used as an add-on drug for T2DM; available in combination with metformin, thiazolidinediones, and SGLT2 inhibitors	Adverse reactions include Stevens-Johnson syndrome, nasopharyngitis, diarrhea, abdominal pain, pancreatitis, joint pain, and renal failure. May cause hypoglycemia when used with sulfonylureas
Glucagon-like Peptide-1 Analogues		
• Albiglutide (Tanzeum) • Dulaglutide (Trulicity) • Exenatide (Byetta, Bydureon) • Liraglutide (Victoza) • Lixisenatide (Adlyxin)	Can be used as monotherapy as incretin mimetic, but usually used as an add-on drug for T2DM; available in combination with insulin	Adverse reactions include severe pancreatitis, nausea, dyspepsia, injection site reactions, and arthralgias. Do not use with gastroparesis and use with caution in patients with renal impairment. Contraindicated for patients with a family history of multiple endocrine neoplasia type 2 or medullary thyroid carcinoma, given an increased risk of thyroid C-cell tumors
Sodium-Glucose Transport-2 Inhibitors		
• Canagliflozin (Invokana) • Dapagliflozin (Farxiga) • Empagliflozin (Jardiance)	Can be used as monotherapy, but usually used as an add-on drug for T2DM	Adverse reactions include acute renal failure, ketoacidosis, hypotension, urinary and/or genital fungal infections, and nausea. Contraindicated in patients with congestive heart failure, nephrotoxicity, or volume depletion
Meglitinides (Glinides)		
• Mitiglinide (Glufast) • Nateglinide (Starlix) • Repaglinide (Prandin)	For use as an adjunct to diet and exercise in T2DM; used as monotherapy as an insulin secretagogue or can be added to a thiazolidinedione; not for use with T1DM or DKA	Adverse reactions include weight gain, GI complaints, hypoglycemia, cardiovascular events, and hypersensitivity. Contraindicated in patients taking gemfibrozil

Abbreviations: DKA, diabetic ketoacidosis; DM, diabetes mellitus; GI, gastrointestinal.

respond better to treatment with metformin or thiazolidinediones than with sulfonylureas.

Therapy with sulfonylureas should be initiated at the lowest possible dose and usually begins with a once-daily dose before breakfast. The dosage can be increased every 2 weeks until the desired response is achieved, the maximum dosage is reached, or side effects preclude further increases. Common adverse reactions are mild GI upset, weight gain, and skin rashes. Serious effects include hypoglycemia and severe anemias. Sulfonylureas are metabolized in the liver, and their use should be avoided in people with significant hepatic dysfunction. Sulfonylureas are not recommended for use during the third trimester of pregnancy or for females who are planning a pregnancy.

Numerous drugs can interfere with the metabolism of sulfonylureas and can alter their effects. NSAIDs, azole antifungal drugs, salicylates, sulfonamides, warfarin (Coumadin), monoamine oxidase inhibitors, quinolones, and beta blockers can all potentiate the effects of sulfonylureas and lead to hypoglycemia. In contrast, thiazide diuretics, corticosteroids, phenothiazines, oral contraceptives, nicotinic acid, sympathomimetics, calcium channel blocking drugs, and isoniazid (INH) can reduce the effects of sulfonylureas and result in loss of glycemic control.

Acarbose (Precose) and miglitol (Glyset) are alpha-glucosidase inhibitors that slow the breakdown of complex carbohydrates into monosaccharides. This effect occurs on the brush border of the small intestine, thus reducing postprandial blood glucose levels. The recommended initial dosage of acarbose is 50 mg/day, which should be slowly titrated up to the maintenance dosage of 50 to 100 mg three times daily with meals. Miglitol also delays absorption of carbohydrates, thereby lowering the postprandial glucose level. Therapy is initiated with the lowest effective oral dosage of 25 three times daily, eventually increasing to the maintenance dose of 50 mg three times daily. Both drugs have similar common adverse effects—flatulence and diarrhea—which are thought to be caused by the osmotic effect of undigested carbohydrates in the distal bowel. Contraindications to alpha-glucosidase inhibitors include any chronic intestinal disease that could be worsened by increased bowel gas formation.

The thiazolidinediones pioglitazone (Actos) and rosiglitazone (Avandia) work by sensitizing peripheral tissues to insulin by activating the nuclear glitazone receptor (also known as *peroxisome proliferator-activated receptor-γ*), which lowers serum glucose levels without increasing pancreatic insulin secretion. The thiazolidinediones can decrease A1c from 0.5% to 1.4%, with a low risk of hypoglycemia. They can be used either alone or in combination with other antihyperglycemic medications, including insulin. Thiazolidinediones should be used cautiously in patients at risk for fractures. Common side effects include significant weight gain, upper respiratory tract infection, edema, fluid retention, anemia, and hypoglycemia. These medications carry a boxed warning for congestive heart failure in their prescribing information. In addition, due to possible liver damage, hepatic enzyme levels should be monitored before their initiation and during treatment.

There are two categories of incretin mimetics: DPP4-Is and GLP1 analogues. DPP4-Is prolong and enhance the activity of incretins, which suppresses glucagon secretion and modestly reduces A1c by 0.5% to 0.8%. Although medications from this class can be used as monotherapy, they are more likely to be used as add-on therapy to metformin. Common adverse effects include nasopharyngitis, abdominal pain, and hypoglycemia when used with sulfonylureas. Severe adverse effects include pancreatitis, Stevens-Johnson syndrome, and renal failure. In 2015, the FDA issued a warning for this medication class because it can cause severe joint pain. DPP4-Is are given once daily and are available in combination with metformin, thiazolidinediones, and SGLT2 inhibitors.

GLP1 analogues enhance insulin secretion in a glucose-dependent manner in response to food intake. GLP1 analogues also improve insulin sensitivity, increase beta cell mass, and decrease glucagon secretion. GLP1 analogues affect satiety and hunger by decreasing the hedonic value (appeal) of food, prolonging the time food remains in the stomach, and decreasing the patient's motivation to eat. GLP1 analogues are injected with daily or weekly dosing and must be slowly increased over time from initial dosing. The 2016 LEADER trial demonstrated a reduced risk of mortality from cardiovascular causes with these medications, and the 2017 CSALE trial demonstrated a delayed onset of DM for patients with prediabetes taking these medications. Common side effects include GI distress (e.g., nausea, vomiting, and diarrhea), headache, fatigue, and pancreatitis. There is also a boxed warning in their prescribing information for an increased risk of thyroid C-cell tumors with these medications due to studies in rodents; they are contraindicated in patients with medullary thyroid carcinoma and multiple endocrine neoplasia type 2. A modest reduction in A1c of 0.5% to 0.8% can be expected with their use.

SGLT2 inhibitors block the activity of SGLT proteins in the renal proximal tubule, thereby reducing glucose reuptake and increasing the secretion of glucose in the urine. The medication is given once daily. Patients often lose weight due to the loss of sugar through the kidney. The 2015 EMPA-REG OUTCOME study demonstrated a reduced rate of cardiovascular events and a slowed progression of kidney disease with this class of antidiabetic medication. Common adverse effects include mycotic urinary and genital infections. Severe adverse reactions include renal failure, ketoacidosis, and pancreatitis. SGLT2 inhibitors are contraindicated in patients with congestive heart failure, nephrotoxicity, and volume depletion.

Meglitinides (or glinides) are insulin secretagogues that act similarly to sulfonylureas but with a more pronounced effect in reducing A1c and with a lower risk of hypoglycemia than sulfonylureas. Side effects include weight gain and GI complaints, and they are not intended for patients with T1DM or DKA. Dosing is multiple times a day before meals. Certain drugs such as gemfibrozil (contraindicated with meglitinides) and azole antifungals can markedly increase the level of these drugs and increase their risk of hypoglycemia.

There are several other medications that are infrequently used for T2DM. Bromocriptine is a dopamine agonist and increases insulin sensitivity at the level of the dopamine receptor. Common side effects include nausea and orthostatic hypotension. Colesevelam is a bile acid sequestrant that binds bile acid in the intestinal tract, increasing hepatic glucose production and incretin levels. Hypoglycemia is rare with this agent, although LDL levels often decrease; other side effects include constipation and decreased absorption of other medications.

Individual treatment goals should take into account the patient's capacity to understand and carry out the management plan, the risk of severe hypoglycemia, and any other factors that increase risk or decrease benefit of selected treatments. When lifestyle management plus antidiabetic agents fails to control blood glucose levels or if the patient's A1c at diagnosis is high, the addition of insulin is recommended. Relatively large doses of insulin may be required for T2DM patients, given their degree of insulin resistance, in comparison to patients with T1DM. The 2021 Standards of Medical Care in Diabetes published by the ADA recommends starting at 0.1 to 0.2 U/kg/day of basal insulin (approximately 10 U), increasing the dosage by 10% to 15% or 2 to 4 U once or twice a week, as guided by fasting blood glucose levels. The normal target fasting blood glucose level is less than 140 mg/dL. Metformin and thiazolidinediones can be used with insulin therapy, as they facilitate lower doses of insulin in maintaining glycemic control. However, sulfonylureas should be discontinued if insulin is started, given the significant risk of hypoglycemia when these drugs are combined with exogenous insulin. A description of the properties of long-acting basal insulin formulations can be found in the previous section on T1DM (see Drugs Commonly Prescribed 59.1).

Because several types of oral antidiabetic agents can be used as monotherapy, in combination with one another, or with insulin therapy, treatment decisions in T2DM can be complex. The following is a synopsis of treatment recommendations in T2DM. Each patient's treatment plan will require individualization that is dependent on the starting A1c value at the time of pharmacotherapy initiation and specific lifestyle issues or comorbidities:

- Immediately upon diagnosis of T2DM, begin lifestyle management with medically assisted obesity treatment.
- If glycemic goals are still not met 3 months after initiating therapy, begin single-agent or dual-agent therapy with oral antidiabetic agents, depending on whether A1c is less than (single-agent) or greater than (dual-agent) 7.5%, respectively.
- If glycemic goals are not met in 3 months, initiate triple-agent therapy.
- If after 3 additional months (or at the time of diagnosis) A1c is 9% or higher and the patient is symptomatic, add insulin therapy.

The ADA Standards of Medical Care differ slightly from these guidelines. Dual-agent therapy is not started at diagnosis unless A1c is greater than or equal to 9%, and insulin therapy is not initiated until A1c is greater than or equal to 10% and the patient is symptomatic.

Monitoring for Hypoglycemia

Hypoglycemia (defined as a plasma glucose less than 54 mg/dL, although the glucose alert value is typically set at less than 70 mg/dL) may occur in patients with T2DM for a variety of reasons: excessive exogenous insulin, excessive dosing of oral antidiabetic agents, missed meals or inadequate food intake, excessive exercise, alcohol ingestion, drug interactions, and a decrease in liver or kidney function. When using two oral antidiabetic agents, the potential for hypoglycemic episodes is increased, and the patient and family members/support people should be aware of this. Signs and symptoms of hypoglycemia include diaphoresis, tachycardia, hunger, shakiness, altered mentation (ranging from an inability to concentrate to coma), slurred speech, and seizure. The signs and symptoms exhibited by the patient are highly individualized and can vary from mild to severe. If the patient becomes acutely ill for any reason, blood glucose levels will need closer monitoring, given the body's increased metabolic demands. Parenteral insulin may be necessary in this situation, if oral agents cannot be tolerated due to nausea, vomiting, or impaired oral intake.

FOLLOW-UP AND REFERRAL

Because T2DM is a chronic disease, continuing care is essential, and the goal of treatment is to prevent or slow the development of diabetic complications. The frequency of patient visits depends on the degree to which blood glucose levels are controlled, changes in antihyperglycemic therapy, and the presence and degree of complications or other medical conditions. If the patient is performing SMBG, telephone consultations may be possible instead of clinic visits. Once glycemic levels are adequately regulated, the patient should be seen at least quarterly. These visits should include a discussion of the results of SMBG, symptoms of hypoglycemia and other illnesses, patient adjustments to therapy and changes in lifestyle due to disease management, problems with adherence to the treatment plan and medications, as well as the frequency, causes, and severity of hyperglycemia or hypoglycemia if the patient is on insulin therapy and/or antidiabetic agents.

On initial diagnosis, the patient should be referred to a dietitian and a certified diabetes educator. Effective dietary modification as directed by a qualified nutritionist may also be a key factor in preventing the development of T2DM in a prediabetic patient. A1c determination should be performed at least twice a year in patients with adequate glycemic control and quarterly in patients whose therapy has changed or who are not meeting glycemic goals. Patients should also undergo annual examinations of the feet and eyes (including fundoscopy), the latter of which requires referral to a qualified ophthalmologist or optometrist.

If any of the following complications are detected or suspected, referral to a specialist to guide management may be indicated. Key follow-up and management principles with respect to the diabetic patient are as follows:

- *Retinopathy:* T2DM is the leading cause of acquired blindness in adults aged 20 to 74 years, and up to 25% of newly diagnosed patients may present with retinopathy at the time of diagnosis. Comprehensive visual eye examinations and dilated retinal examinations should be performed at the time of diagnosis by an ophthalmologist or optometrist who is knowledgeable and experienced in the management of diabetic retinopathy. If the examination is normal, follow-up examinations can be conducted every 2 years, but if there is any concern for abnormalities, then the examinations should be done annually. Optimizing blood pressure and lipid levels can reduce the risk or slow the progression of retinopathy.
- *Hyperlipidemia:* Adults with T2DM should be tested at diagnosis for lipid disorders and every 5 years thereafter if the initial lipid panel is normal. The AACE recommends an annual fasting lipid profile, including serum cholesterol, triglycerides, HDL, and calculated LDL cholesterol measurements. Some patients can achieve recommended lipid goals with lifestyle management (i.e., modifications to diet and physical activity), but the majority will need pharmacological therapy. The purpose of hyperlipidemia treatment is to reduce cardiovascular events. ADA guidelines suggest that the emphasis in clinical management be based on risk profiles using the American College of Cardiology (ACC) Atherosclerotic Cardiovascular Disease (ASCVD) risk calculator. Aggressive therapy is indicated because it has been shown to lower the risk of CAD. The LDL level should be less than 100 mg/dL in a patient with no overt CVD and less than 70 mg/dL with overt CVD. In patients with an extreme risk of CVD, the LDL level should be less than 55 mg/dL. The use of statins (HMG CoA-reductase inhibitors) as antihyperlipidemic therapy is indicated in these patients, with nutritional treatment (dietary modification) initiated as first-line management. Moderate- to high-intensity dosing is based on patient age and cardiovascular risk level.
- *Diabetic kidney disease:* A routine spot UACR (normal less than 30 mg/g albumin/mg creatinine) and eGFR should be performed annually on all patients with DM. Screening for the patient with T2DM should begin at the time of diagnosis because it is not known how long the patient has had DM before the formal diagnosis. The ADA recommends screening for diabetic kidney disease at the time of DM diagnosis, followed by annual screening. Albuminuria is found more often in patients with DM and hypertension. Thus, in addition to maintaining normal serum glucose levels, controlling BP is the most effective method to slow or reduce the risk of diabetic kidney disease. ACEIs or ARBs are the recommended treatment for patients with DM and hypertension, abnormally high UACR, or a lower-than-normal eGFR.
- *Hypertension:* In a patient with T2DM, hypertension is often part of a syndrome that includes glucose intolerance, insulin resistance, obesity, dyslipidemia, and CAD. It is present in one-third of patients diagnosed with T2DM, and control of hypertension has been shown to reduce the rate of progression of nephropathy and reduce the complications of CVD. Systolic blood pressure should be less than 140 mm Hg and diastolic blood pressure below 90 mm Hg. A lower blood pressure goal of 130/80 mm Hg may be appropriate for patients at high risk for cardiovascular events but only if this can be achieved without significant risk or burden to the patient. Treatment can be with ACEIs, ARBs, thiazide-like diuretics, or dihydropyridine calcium channel blockers.
- *Macrovascular disease:* Patients with DM are at risk for developing macrovascular complications including stroke, PVD, and CAD. All diabetic patients should be screened for these diseases, because symptoms may not be present until late in the course of the disease process. Evidence of uncontrolled angina, carotid bruits, or ECG abnormalities may require advanced intervention and referral to a cardiologist. Patients with disabling claudication or nonhealing ulcers require a vascular consultation for their PVD. T2DM is the leading cause of nontraumatic lower extremity amputation due to PVD and peripheral neuropathy. Problems involving the feet may require care by a podiatrist, orthopedic surgeon, vascular surgeon, or rehabilitation specialist. Daily aspirin is recommended for cardiac prophylaxis in patients with a 10-year risk of CVD greater than 10% at a dose of 81 to 165 mg/day. Given the increased risk of bleeding due to its antiplatelet effects, aspirin is not recommended in low-risk patients with a 10-year CVD risk of less than 5%.
- *Neuropathy:* All patients should be screened for neuropathic symptoms at the time of diagnosis and then at least annually. Peripheral neuropathy may result in pain, loss of sensation, and muscle weakness. Its incidence increases

over time in patients with T2DM, and it is more prevalent in patients with low serum insulin concentrations and poor glycemic control. Autonomic involvement can affect GI, cardiovascular, and genitourinary functions. Patients with significant urinary symptoms or impotence should be referred to a urologist.

- *Pregnancy:* To reduce the risk of fetal malformation and maternal and fetal complications, every pregnancy in a woman with T2DM should be planned in advance. Insulin is the first-line medication for the treatment of diabetes in pregnancy. No long-term pregnancy studies of oral diabetic agents have been conducted. A pregnant patient with T2DM requires tight blood glucose control and should be monitored closely by a multidisciplinary team, including an obstetrician or certified nurse midwife. Maintaining A1c at less than 6.0% during pregnancy is recommended to prevent adverse fetal outcomes, although this goal increases the risk of hypoglycemia.

Patient Education: T2DM

Successful diabetes management involves a team effort to achieve mutually agreed-upon treatment goals. To achieve these goals, it is crucial that the patient, family, and significant others be educated in all aspects of the treatment plan. The following list is a synopsis of the salient topics for patient education in T2DM:

- *Introduction:* Definition and causes of T2DM; function of the pancreas in insulin production
- *Regulation of blood glucose:* Role of food, physical activity, and insulin in glucose utilization; signs and symptoms, causes, treatment, and prevention of hyperglycemia and hypoglycemia; guidance on when to contact the primary care practitioner
- *Blood glucose monitoring and urine testing:* How to perform SMBG and how often to test; recording and reporting blood glucose results; urine ketone testing
- *Medication and insulin administration:* Actions and adverse reactions of antidiabetic agents; actions and types of insulin, including effects on blood glucose; storage of medication supplies; drawing, mixing, and injecting insulin and GLP1 analogues; injection site selection and rotation; needle disposal
- *Meal planning:* Types of macronutrients (carbohydrates, proteins, fats); dietary practices, including timing of meals, portion control, use of sweeteners, dining out, consumption of alcohol, and dietary modification during acute illness
- *Physical activity:* Benefits of exercise; types of activity best suited to the patient; effects on blood glucose; planning and measuring exercise effort, including snack intake
- *Prevention of long-term complications:* Importance of blood glucose control; periodic eye examinations and regular foot care; prevention of infection; early detection of the signs and symptoms of complications

DIABETES MELLITUS TYPE 3C

Although T1DM and T2DM are well-known forms of DM, T3cDM is less so, being due to diseases or conditions specifically affecting the exocrine pancreas that also affect nutrient digestion. Both the ADA and the World Health Organization classify pancreatogenic diabetes as T3cDM.

EPIDEMIOLOGY AND CAUSES

T3cDM refers to glycemic dysregulation resulting from a lack of available insulin due to diseases of the exocrine pancreas that also impact nutrient digestion, including pancreatitis, pancreatectomy, trauma, neoplasia, cystic fibrosis, hemochromatosis, and fibrocalculous pancreatopathy. T3cDM occurs in an estimated 5% to 10% of the population in Western countries and is mostly a result of chronic pancreatitis. Because many patients with T3cDM are misclassified initially due to a lack of understanding of the disease process, the actual prevalence of T3cDM is unknown.

PATHOPHYSIOLOGY

The pathophysiology in T3cDM differs from other types of DM. Because there is a complex interplay of nutrient digestion, absorption, and utilization, damage to the pancreas disrupts this process. There is inflammation of the pancreatic beta islet cells, which causes destruction of these cells and impairs insulin production. However, this differs from the pathophysiology of T1DM because in T3cDM, there is also a loss of glucagon and pancreatic polypeptide (PP) from the pancreatic islets, in addition to the loss of insulin specifically from the beta cells. Moreover, because of the disruption in nutrient digestion, absorption, and utilization, there is a concomitant impairment of incretin secretion and, therefore, a diminished release of insulin from the remaining pancreatic beta cells. In addition to low circulating levels of insulin, there is a compensatory increase in peripheral insulin sensitivity but a decrease in insulin sensitivity in the liver as well as unsuppressed hepatic glucose production, resulting in hyperglycemia. There is also a reduction in PP secretion associated with persistent hepatic glucose production, which further decreases insulin sensitivity in the liver. In turn, this collection of processes causes T3cDM to be erratic in nature with wide swings in blood glucose levels from hyperglycemia to hypoglycemia, making T3cDM particularly difficult to control.

CLINICAL PRESENTATION

Subjective

There are few data demonstrating differences in clinical presentation between T1DM, T2DM, and T3cDM. The latter has been characterized as "brittle diabetes" because of the unsuppressed hepatic glucose production and exaggerated peripheral sensitivity to insulin that results in reports of severe hyperglycemia, punctuated by episodes of significant hypoglycemia. However, in common practice, the term "brittle diabetic" has been used to refer to any patient who presents with this pattern of widely erratic blood sugars, regardless of diabetic etiology.

Objective

Close monitoring of blood sugars reveals hypoglycemia to be common in T3cDM, which may be severe due to the deficiency in compensatory glucagon secretion, poor dietary intake, impaired food digestion, and decreased insulin sensitivity in the liver that, over time, reduces the availability of hepatic glycogen stores to compensate for hypoglycemia. In contrast to T1DM, ketoacidosis is rare. In contrast to T2DM, patients with T3cDM are rarely overweight or obese. However, in the presence of chronic pancreatitis, patients with T3cDM may be overweight or obese, while also having notable muscle wasting. Indeed, these patients are usually undernourished, with deficiencies in fat-soluble vitamins (e.g., vitamins A, D, E, and K) due to pancreatic exocrine insufficiency.

DIAGNOSTIC REASONING

There is no specific test to determine T3cDM, but rather the diagnosis is made on the basis of a history of pancreatic issues (e.g., pancreatitis, pancreatic trauma, cystic fibrosis, etc.) and elevated blood sugars.

Diagnostic Tests

The initial diagnosis of T3cDM includes fasting blood glucose levels and A1c, which should be repeated annually for patients with pancreatitis. Proposed diagnostic guidelines for T3cDM include both major and minor criteria.

The major diagnostic criteria for T3cDM must all be present and include the following:

- Pancreatic exocrine insufficiency
- Pathological pancreatic imaging (e.g., computed tomography, magnetic resonance imaging, ultrasound, endoscopy)
- Absence of T1DM-associated autoimmune antibodies

Minor criteria include the following:

- Impaired PP secretion
- Impaired incretin secretion
- Absence of excessive insulin resistance
- Impaired pancreatic beta cell function
- Low serum levels of fat-soluble vitamins

Differential Diagnosis

The diagnosis of T3cDM is often missed. Although T1DM may be distinguished on the basis of its autoimmune etiology, patients with T3cDM are often misclassified as having T2DM, especially if T3cDM is due to chronic pancreatitis, in which case overweight and obesity are more common. Thus, the diagnosis is complicated not only by similar clinical presentations related to the long-term complications of hyperglycemia, but also by the fact that people with T2DM are at a higher risk for developing pancreatitis, resulting in a degree of overlap between these different diabetic etiologies.

MANAGEMENT

There are currently no specific guidelines to manage T3cDM separately from other forms of DM. The goal of management is to prevent retinopathy, neuropathy, nephropathy, and other microangiopathic complications, which occur at the same rate as for other forms of DM. Management centers around glycemic control, lifestyle modifications, and appropriate nutrition.

Glycemic Control

The ADA does not address T3cDM glycemic control specifically. The guidelines for T1DM and T2DM of an A1c less than 7% should be followed for T3cDM as well to minimize the risk of chronic complications. However, because of the increased risk for hypoglycemia in "brittle diabetes," a slightly higher-than-normal blood glucose level may improve quality of life in T3cDM and avoid this potentially life-threatening complication.

Because the pathophysiology of T3cDM differs from other forms of DM, treatment is based on the underlying cause and resultant pathology. For example, for patients with T3cDM related to chronic pancreatitis who exhibit only mild hyperglycemia (A1c less than 8%), oral hypoglycemic agents may be the treatment of choice. Metformin (Glucophage) may be considered when concomitant insulin resistance is present; however, it is often not well tolerated because of adverse GI effects and weight loss. Sulfonylureas and meglitinides are not generally used because of an increased risk of tumors observed in laboratory animals and the risk for hypoglycemia. However, patients with chronic pancreatitis and T3cDM benefit from incretin-based antidiabetic therapy, including GLP1 analogues (semaglutide [Ozempic]; dulaglutide [Trulicity]) and DPP4-Is (sitagliptin [Januvia]; saxagliptin [Onglyza]; linagliptin [Tradjenta]).

Because most patients with T3cDM have an insulin deficiency, treatment with insulin is the preferred therapy, particularly in patients with cystic fibrosis. Insulin therapy is also used for chronically or acutely ill patients, hospitalized patients, or severely malnourished patients with T3cDM. In the case of the malnourished patient, the anabolic effect of insulin is beneficial. For patients with advanced T3cDM, multidose insulin treatment is used, and guidelines for T1DM should be followed. Because patients with T3cDM are prone to hypoglycemic episodes, all insulin regimens should be monitored closely.

Lifestyle Modifications

Because the majority of patients with T3cDM have a history of chronic pancreatitis, attempts should be made to reduce toxic and modifiable contributors to pancreatic dysfunction. These include abstaining from alcohol and smoking cessation. Abstaining from alcohol is particularly important because alcohol inhibits hepatic glucose production and can cause hypoglycemia if the patient is on insulin therapy. Patients should also be instructed in the same physical activity guidelines as for all patients with DM, of at least 150 minutes of moderate physical activity per week.

Appropriate Nutrition

The goal of nutrition therapy is to prevent and/or treat malnutrition, control the symptoms of steatorrhea (diarrhea with fat malabsorption), and minimize meal-induced hyperglycemia, particularly in T3cDM patients with chronic pancreatitis. A diet high in soluble fiber and low in fat is recommended. In patients with pancreatic exocrine insufficiency, oral pancreatic enzyme replacement (e.g., pancrelipase [Creon, Pancreaze, Zenpep, Ultresa, Viokace, Pertzye]) is important for fat digestion and nutrient absorption, particularly the absorption of fat-soluble vitamins. For patients with cystic fibrosis and T3cDM, a well-balanced diet with no specific restrictions on calories, fat, or carbohydrates is indicated.

FOLLOW-UP AND REFERRAL

T3cDM patients with chronic pancreatitis or DM from a pancreatic origin should be referred to an endocrinologist/diabetologist for treatment. Follow-up by the primary care provider should be tailored to each individual patient and their specific etiology of T3cDM.

Patient Education: T3cDM

Patients with T3cDM require education about the nature of their disease and its specific connection to pancreatic dysfunction, which forms the basis for understanding ways to minimize episodes of hyper- and hypoglycemia. As with other forms of DM, patients should be educated as to the long-term complications of T3cDM, including target organ damage due to chronic hyperglycemia, as well as the life-threatening nature of acute hypoglycemic episodes, which are more common in this type of DM. Given the propensity of these patients to experience "brittle diabetes," patients with T3cDM and their families should be taught to convey this to health-care providers, particularly in situations in which they require emergency care. Given the high rate of chronic pancreatitis in these patients, the importance of abstinence from alcohol and smoking cessation should be emphasized at all clinical visits.

HYPOGLYCEMIA

Hypoglycemia is a clinical syndrome of subnormal plasma glucose concentration that may affect infants through older adults, although the primary etiology of the disorder differs markedly among various age-groups. Adult hypoglycemia is characterized by blood glucose levels of less than 55 mg/dL, whereas neonatal hypoglycemia is defined as a level below 30 mg/dL in the first 24 hours of life. There is no universal agreement about hypoglycemia thresholds, however, with some research supporting a level of less than 50 mg/dL for males, 45 mg/dL for females, and 40 mg/dL for infants and children. Regardless, clinical hypoglycemia occurs when the blood glucose level is low enough to cause signs or symptoms.

EPIDEMIOLOGY AND CAUSES

Classic hypoglycemia denotes a low plasma glucose level in the setting of insulin-dependent DM. Inconsistent subcutaneous absorption of insulin, decreased food intake, missed meals, increased insulin secretion during exercise, physical and emotional stress, and antidiabetic medications such as sulfonylureas can all produce hypoglycemia in patients with DM. However, hypoglycemia occurs more commonly with insulin-treated T1DM and T3cDM.

Hypoglycemia with DM is the most commonly occurring endocrine emergency; however, it is not common in patients without DM. Hypoglycemia as a separate disease entity is most common in older adults and is more prevalent in females overall. About 1% of the nondiabetic population is affected. Although endocrine disorders are the most frequent cause of hypoglycemia, bariatric surgery, insulinomas, non–islet cell neoplasms, liver disease, pregnancy, certain medications, and alcohol consumption are also causes. Hypoglycemia in neonates is a unique phenomenon, largely related to the immature developmental stage of the neonatal endocrine system.

There are three types of hypoglycemia—fasting, reactive, and induced—the causes of which are summarized in Table 59.6. Fasting hypoglycemia is a low blood sugar level more than 5 hours after eating; it can be subacute or chronic, and blood glucose will not return to normal levels without glucose ingestion or administration.

TABLE 59.6 Causes of Hypoglycemia

Type of Hypoglycemia	Causes
Fasting hypoglycemia	Renal failure (decreases urinary excretion of insulin) Hepatic disease Insulinomas Pancreatic tumors Autoimmune disease Hypopituitarism Extrapancreatic tumors Ethanol intake Septicemia
Reactive hypoglycemia	Postgastrectomy Gastric bypass surgery Hereditary fructose intolerance Congenital enzyme deficiency Pancreatic beta cell dysfunction Meals high in carbohydrates Exercise Pregnancy
Drug-induced hypoglycemia	Exogenous insulin Sulfonylureas Propranolol (Inderal) Salicylates Quinidine Pentamidine (Pentam) Disopyramide (Norpace)

The possible causes of fasting hypoglycemia include pancreatic beta cell tumors, extrapancreatic tumors, hypopituitarism, myxedema, glycogen storage diseases, medications, ethanol-induced hypoglycemia, severe malnutrition, septicemia, pregnancy, and renal failure, which results in decreased insulin clearance from the body. In adrenocortical insufficiency, there is a decreased production of cortisol that is required for gluconeogenesis, thus leading to hypoglycemia. Liver diseases including hepatitis, cirrhosis, hepatomas, and hepatic congestion interfere with the uptake and release of glycogen from the liver and can ultimately lead to hypoglycemia.

The list of drugs that can cause fasting hypoglycemia is lengthy: insulin, sulfonylureas, fluoroquinolones, propranolol (Inderal), salicylates, quinidine, pentamidine (Pentam, NebuPent), warfarin (Coumadin), sulfonamides, tricyclic antidepressants, disopyramide (Norpace), didanosine (Videx), chlorpromazine (Thorazine), isoniazid (INH), selective serotonin reuptake inhibitors, clofibrate (Atromid), thiazide diuretics, lithium (Lithobid), and ACEIs. Poisoning with organophosphates and carbamate-based pesticides also results in hypoglycemia. The illegal sexual-enhancement drug methylenedioxymethamphetamine ([MDMA] Ecstasy) has also been associated with severe hypoglycemia.

Reactive or postprandial hypoglycemia is less common than fasting hypoglycemia and is most often acute in nature. Reactive hypoglycemia usually produces symptoms 2 to 4 hours after a carbohydrate-rich meal, and symptoms in these patients rarely occur in a fasting state. Within 5 to 6 hours after a meal, the blood glucose level will return to normal. Reactive hypoglycemia may also be caused by GI surgery or any other GI tract disorder that affects carbohydrate absorption, congenital deficiency of any of the enzymes necessary for carbohydrate metabolism, and late insulin release caused by beta cell dysfunction. Postprandial hypoglycemia is an early manifestation of T2DM and has also been seen with extreme exertion in untrained, physically unfit people, as well as in patients with sepsis or heart failure. Idiopathic or functional postprandial hypoglycemia also exists that cannot be ascribed to any discrete cause.

Induced hypoglycemia is the most common form of hypoglycemia. Medications and alcohol are the most frequent causes of induced hypoglycemia, which may be factitious or self-induced by the excessive intake of sulfonylureas or insulin. The timing of these types of hypoglycemic events is unrelated to food intake. If this type of hypoglycemia is suspected in patients with known access to these drugs (e.g., health-care workers, caregivers of diabetic patients), serum and urine sulfonylurea levels should be obtained. In addition, a very low or nonexistent serum C-peptide level confirms that insulin is being injected exogenously, rather than being produced endogenously.

Lifestyle patterns may contribute to hypoglycemia in nondiabetic patients as well. The excessive consumption of simple sugars, an excessively refined and processed diet, excessive exercise, stress, irregular eating patterns, or missing meals can all cause abnormal fluctuations in blood sugar levels. Nutrient deficiencies, food allergies, and poor digestion also contribute to hypoglycemia, and cigarette smoking and high caffeine intake can produce instability in blood glucose levels as well.

PATHOPHYSIOLOGY

To understand the clinical and biochemical phenomenon of hypoglycemia, it is important to grasp the mechanics behind the body's careful maintenance of euglycemic plasma glucose levels between 80 and 90 mg/dL. After a carbohydrate-containing meal in which glucose is absorbed from the gut into the bloodstream, plasma glucose levels transiently increase to 120 to 140 mg/dL. Glucose subsequently enters pancreatic beta cells via the glucose transporter 1 (GLUT1) and GLUT2 cell membrane transporters, where the enzyme glucokinase phosphorylates it to glucose-6-phosphate. This acts as a glucose sensor and triggers the passive entry of calcium into beta cells, causing insulin secretion. Insulin lowers plasma glucose levels by decreasing hepatic glycogenolysis (glycogen breakdown) and gluconeogenesis (*de novo* glucose synthesis), driving glucose uptake by skeletal, muscle, and adipose tissue via the translocation of intracellular GLUT molecules to the cell membrane surface and decreasing both proteolysis and lipolysis, which reduces the number of gluconeogenic precursors. In turn, under physiological circumstances, plasma glucose concentration typically returns to normal levels within several hours after a carbohydrate-containing meal.

As part of the body's homeostatic mechanisms, hypoglycemia is sensed by central nervous system receptors in the hypothalamus, as well as peripheral receptors that act via afferent nerves, to trigger an appropriate hormonal response to restore euglycemia. The body counters glucose levels below 80 mg/dL by decreasing pancreatic insulin production and eventually secreting several counterregulatory hormones once blood glucose levels fall to below 70 mg/dL. These include glucagon from pancreatic alpha cells that acts directly on the liver and epinephrine from the adrenal medulla that acts similarly to glucagon via hepatic beta-adrenergic receptors, mediating the autonomic (i.e., sympathetic, adrenergic) symptoms of hypoglycemia (e.g., diaphoresis, tachycardia, anxiety) while inhibiting insulin secretion via alpha-2-adrenergic receptors. If the hypoglycemia becomes severe (less than 60 mg/dL) or persists for several hours, additional counterregulatory hormones are mobilized, including cortisol from the adrenal cortex and growth hormone from the pituitary gland.

Counterregulatory hormones increase hepatic glucose production via a number of mechanisms, including glycogen breakdown into individual glucose monomers and, once intrahepatic glycogen stores are depleted, *de novo* glucose synthesis (gluconeogenesis) from amino acids, pyruvate, glycerol, and free fatty acid precursors. The body also metabolically shifts away from glucose utilization toward alternate sources of fuel to maintain euglycemia, such as proteins and ketone bodies converted from fats. Increased lipolysis is reflected in increased plasma free fatty acids, and increased protein breakdown is reflected in higher concentrations of the amino acids alanine and glutamine.

The brain uses glucose almost exclusively as its fuel source; however, it is not capable of synthesizing or storing it. Thus, the brain is particularly sensitive to dramatic changes in blood glucose concentration. Hypoglycemia, in which plasma glucose falls below 60 mg/dL, prevents the brain from receiving an adequate supply of blood glucose, thereby impairing function. In adults, cognitive dysfunction can be detected in otherwise normal individuals at plasma glucose levels between 50 and 55 mg/dL; older males are particularly prone to this type of neurological impairment. At levels between 45 and 50 mg/dL, lethargy and obtundation follow, with coma occurring at levels below 30 mg/dL, followed by convulsions below 20 mg/dL and eventually death. Severe hypoglycemia has also been associated with cardiovascular dysfunction. Even in infants and children, otherwise asymptomatic hypoglycemia has been associated with neurocognitive impairment.

The histological structure of the pancreas is specifically designed to prevent these events, however. Within the pancreas, each islet of Langerhans consists of several hundred cells, including a core of insulin-producing beta cells surrounded by glucagon-secreting alpha cells and an outer layer of somatostatin-producing delta cells and PP cells, which make pancreatic polypeptide. As arterial blood enters the islet core, the beta cells are the first to encounter plasma glucose concentrations. Thus, the function of alpha cells is determined largely by the normal activity of beta cells. For example, insulin directly inhibits glucagon secretion by pancreatic alpha cells.

In adults, reactive hypoglycemia occurs when these counterregulatory responses fail after the person consumes a carbohydrate load, causing blood glucose to fall 2 to 5 hours after eating. Patients with decreased glucagon and epinephrine responses to low blood glucose levels have up to a 25-fold greater risk of experiencing hypoglycemia, particularly during sleep, as sleep itself decreases counterregulatory hormonal responses.

Unfortunately, an initial hypoglycemic episode appears to contribute to a vicious cycle of hypoglycemia, as recurrent hypoglycemia has been associated with autonomic failure and a delay in onset of the early warning signs associated with subsequent hypoglycemic episodes. This may relate to an increased production of cortisol, which decreases glucagon and epinephrine responses, as well as an upregulation of glucose transport in the brain, which renders the central nervous system less sensitive in producing neuroglycopenic symptoms.

CLINICAL PRESENTATION

The clinical presentation of hypoglycemia, especially subjective symptoms, varies, depending on the physical status of the person. For example, older adults with neuropathy may lack awareness of hypoglycemic symptoms unless they are severe. In addition, with accidental exposures to hypoglycemic agents, symptoms are often neither recognized nor associated with hypoglycemia.

Subjective

Symptoms of hypoglycemia may be present when blood glucose levels fall below 60 mg/dL, and brain function is often impaired when glycemic levels fall below 50 mg/dL. Moreover, some patients exhibit symptoms with abnormal fluctuations of glucose and insulin. Symptoms vary from very mild to severe and are classified as adrenergic or neuroglycopenic. Adrenergic symptoms include sweating, tremulousness, dizziness, confusion, anxiety, and palpitations. Neuroglycopenic symptoms include headaches, fatigue, weakness, drowsiness, syncope, diplopia, blurred vision, and personality changes. Seizures and coma are severe presentations. The medical history should focus on eating habits, mealtimes, exercise habits, alcohol intake, any history of liver or renal disease, and any family history of endocrine disorders, including DM and hypoglycemia.

Hypoglycemic symptoms are often relieved with the ingestion of carbohydrates. The neurological manifestations of hemiparesis, convulsions, confusion, and coma are more common in patients with DM.

Objective

Objective findings that accompany hypoglycemia include tachycardia with or without premature ventricular contractions, diaphoresis, hypothermia or hyperthermia, coma, seizures, tremors, positive Babinski's sign, aphasia, and hemiparesis. A physical examination with special attention to objective signs of endocrinological disease is indicated initially. Assessment for an enlarged liver and neurological signs of chronic alcohol abuse should also be performed to evaluate for this key cause of hypoglycemia. In patients unable to provide an adequate medical history, the skin should be examined for needle marks, which may reflect possible insulin injections.

DIAGNOSTIC REASONING

Diagnostic Tests

Blood glucose levels are used to diagnose hypoglycemia, which is suspected if a random glucose level is between 45 and 60 mg/dL or if an overnight fasting glucose level is less than 60 mg/dL. Hypoglycemia is considered present if the blood glucose level is 45 mg/dL or less. Evaluation of the etiology, when not attributed to the treatment of DM, requires subsequent laboratory testing.

Initial Testing

Initial testing for suspected hypoglycemia includes measurement of the blood glucose level. Chronic hypoglycemia may be evident by measuring a low A1c level; however, the most informative time to obtain a blood glucose level is when the patient is experiencing acute symptoms. If hypoglycemia and symptoms occur concurrently and if both are relieved with eating, the diagnosis of postprandial hypoglycemia is confirmed. Of note, finger-stick monitors are not highly accurate at extremes of high or low glucose concentrations. Thus, they are helpful in detecting high and low blood glucose levels in general, but the specific numerical result may not accurately reflect the true blood glucose concentration. It is also important to recognize that whole blood glucose levels are 10% to 15% lower than serum glucose levels, because red blood cells consume glucose.

More than one-third of normal patients have hypoglycemia with or without symptoms during a short-term 4-hour fasting test. Thus, as an alternative, a 5-hour OGTT may be done, using a 100-g glucose load, by taking hourly glucose and insulin measurements. Hypoglycemia is typically diagnosed if the patient experiences a decrease in blood glucose concentration of greater than 100 mg/dL per hour or a blood glucose level of less than 50 mg/dL at any point during the test. However, overinterpretation of this test may lead to an overdiagnosis of hypoglycemia. In turn, some experts caution the use of the OGTT as a diagnostic test for hypoglycemia, requiring that low blood glucose levels be accompanied by clinical signs and symptoms of hypoglycemia, which must ameliorate upon subsequent glucose ingestion in order to diagnose hypoglycemia. These three criteria are known as Whipple's triad (i.e., low blood glucose, accompanying signs and symptoms, resolution upon glucose ingestion).

In turn, for a definitive diagnosis of hypoglycemia, the patient should have (1) documented occurrences of low blood glucose levels, (2) symptoms that occur when the blood glucose level is low, (3) evidence that symptoms are relieved by sugar or other carbohydrate-containing foods, and (4) identification of the particular type of hypoglycemia. The most reliable method of diagnosing hypoglycemia is a supervised 72-hour fasting plasma glucose test. During this test, the patient is allowed calorie- and caffeine-free fluids, while fasting at least overnight and for up to 72 hours to detect whether symptoms develop in the presence of hypoglycemia. Before and after the fast, baseline measurements of serum glucose, insulin, proinsulin, and C-peptide concentration are obtained. Urine is tested for ketones throughout the test, and capillary glucose measurements are taken every 6 hours. The test is terminated when symptoms of hypoglycemia appear, and a blood glucose level is measured immediately. A positive test result is considered to be a blood glucose level of less than 55 mg/dL in males and less than 45 mg/dL in females. If after 72 hours of fasting and light exercise, hypoglycemia (less than 60 mg/dL) is not demonstrated, the test is negative. This test is performed in a hospital setting under close observation, as either glucagon or glucose must be administered after the symptomatic blood draw to reverse hypoglycemic manifestations.

Subsequent Testing

The following laboratory tests assist in the diagnostic reasoning during a hypoglycemic episode: plasma insulin level, insulin antibodies, plasma and urine sulfonylurea levels, and C-peptide concentration. Other tests include a blood urea nitrogen, serum creatinine, blood alcohol level, and liver function tests. Fasting insulin levels range from <17 µU/mL of 42–243 pmol/L. An abnormally elevated insulin level in the absence of blood glucose variation is suggestive of an insulinoma, exogenous insulin administration, insulin resistance syndrome, or reactive hypoglycemia in developing DM. Elevated insulin levels in response to glucose fluctuations suggest functional or reactive hypoglycemia. To rule out endocrinological pathology if suspected, cortisol and adrenocorticotropic hormone levels are obtained. The first morning urinary void can be tested for ketones, as a lack of ketone bodies implies a defect in the fatty acid oxidation pathway.

C-peptide analysis is done via radioimmunoassay and provides an index of beta cell function; normal values range from 0.9 to 4.2 ng/mL. A low C-peptide level with an elevated insulin level confirms exogenous insulin administration. In contrast, C-peptide levels are elevated with insulinomas. To differentiate the effects of an insulinoma from factitious hypoglycemia, the ratio of insulin to C-peptide is determined. If the insulin to C-peptide ratio is equal to or less than 1, the hypoglycemia is a result of endogenous insulin secretion; if it is greater than 1, then exogenous insulin administration is confirmed.

Differential Diagnosis

Differential diagnoses that share many of the same signs and symptoms of hypoglycemia include generalized anxiety disorder, panic attacks, hyperventilation, pheochromocytoma, drug or alcohol intoxication, transient ischemic attack, cerebrovascular accident, and psychosis. Causes of reactive hypoglycemia include meals high in refined carbohydrates, because certain nutrients such as fructose and galactose can cause a burst of insulin secretion. Certain drugs (e.g., sulfonylureas, salicylates) can cause excess glucose utilization or deficient glucose production, resulting in hypoglycemia. Oral diabetic medications are especially prone to causing reactive hypoglycemia when used in combination therapy, especially with concurrent insulin treatment. Insulinomas (adenomas of the islets of Langerhans), although rare, should be considered in an otherwise healthy adult who is found to have fasting hypoglycemia.

MANAGEMENT

The goal of the management of hypoglycemia is to normalize blood glucose levels and treat the underlying cause of the hypoglycemia. As acute severe hypoglycemia may be life-threatening, treatment to increase low glycemic levels must occur immediately and should be administered locally wherever the hypoglycemia is first detected (e.g., in the home), in the field by emergency medical services first responders, in an emergency department, or in an urgent care setting. After stabilization, the patient with identifiable pathology is typically referred to an endocrinologist for further evaluation and treatment. In cases of functional and idiopathic hypoglycemia, the management plan may be developed by the primary care practitioner in consultation with an endocrinologist.

Initial Management

The treatment of acute hypoglycemia for alert patients who can ingest by mouth is 6 to 12 ounces of orange juice or other fruit juice without additional sugar. One cup (8 oz) of milk can be substituted if juice is unavailable. Glucose tablets or gel, if available, can also be used as rapidly absorbed glucose sources. In acute care settings, glucose is provided emergently as standardized IV bolus preparations of dextrose diluted to various concentrations in water (e.g., D25% or D50%), as opposed to standardized hypotonic saline solutions with lower amounts of dextrose that are used primarily for maintenance glucose requirements (e.g., D5% 0.45% NaCl). The blood glucose level should be monitored closely after IV bolus administration of dextrose and then periodically while the patient is on a dextrose-containing continuous IV drip. Glucagon hydrochloride (0.03 to 0.1 mg/kg per dose: 1 to 2 mg in adults; 1 mg in children older than 5 years or weighing more than 20 kg; 0.5 mg in children younger than 5 years or weighing less than 20 kg) may be given intramuscularly (IM), subcutaneously (SC), or IV if the patient is unresponsive. Doses may be repeated as needed every few hours in adults and even more frequently in children (up to every 20 to 30 minutes initially).

Hypoglycemia is a medical emergency because of the seriousness of potential sequelae (e.g., seizures, coma, cardiovascular dysfunction, death). Thus, even if euglycemia is readily restored, patients must be evaluated for potential hospital admission for inpatient care and close observation if there is any concern for the recurrence of hypoglycemia. Patients requiring hospital admission include those with hypoglycemia without an obvious cause or with severe or persistent neurological deficits.

Subsequent Management

The long-term management of hypoglycemia includes treatment of its underlying causes and dietary modifications as needed. If hypoglycemia is a result of pancreatic or extrapancreatic tumors, surgical excision is recommended. Although the treatment of choice for insulinoma is surgical resection, there is only an 85% success rate with an experienced surgeon. If the tumor is small, it may not be found on an exploratory laparotomy. When surgery is unsuccessful, an endocrinologist may initiate diazoxide (Hyperstat, Proglycem) 3 to 8 mg/kg per day orally in divided doses three times daily or 200 mg every 4 hours in adults to reduce insulin secretion. If hypoglycemia is caused by rapid gastric emptying after a gastrectomy, an anticholinergic drug may provide relief by delaying gastric emptying and decreasing intestinal motility.

In patients with inoperable pancreatic tumors or in whom resection has been unsuccessful, small frequent feedings (every 2 to 3 hours) that are high in carbohydrates may be effective in preventing acute hypoglycemic episodes. In patients with renal failure, frequent small high-carbohydrate meals may prevent hypoglycemic episodes. Similarly, in patients with pseudohypoglycemia or idiopathic hypoglycemia, in which a cause cannot be identified, treatment consists primarily of dietary modifications. A high-protein, low-carbohydrate diet divided into six small meals per day often relieves symptoms. Caffeine, refined sugars, and alcohol should be restricted. If food allergies are suspected, allergy testing may be indicated to identify offending foods to avoid. If a medication is suspected as a causative factor, alternative agents must be considered.

SMBG is the cornerstone of long-term self-management of hypoglycemia. Patients may need to monitor blood glucose levels frequently during the initiation of lifestyle changes or dietary modifications to evaluate success. Monitoring glucose levels during exercise, eating at regularly scheduled intervals, understanding the importance of SMBG for self-diagnosis, and early detection may prevent severe hypoglycemic reactions.

FOLLOW-UP AND REFERRAL

Patients with a history of hypoglycemic events require frequent follow-up and evaluation, as determined on an individual basis. More frequent SMBG may be indicated, especially from 12 to 24 hours after a hypoglycemic event. At each visit, the patient's record of cumulative hypoglycemic events should be reviewed for patterns or clues as to triggering factors, such as postprandial associations. Patients who continue to experience hypoglycemic episodes despite intervention should be referred to an endocrinologist.

Patient Education: Hypoglycemia

The importance of dietary modifications must be stressed. Nondiabetic patients with reactive, functional, or fasting hypoglycemia should eat five or six small meals daily to steady the release of glucose into the blood. These meals should be balanced with carbohydrates, protein, and some fat. Patients who experience symptoms after a meal that is high in refined sugar but not after a nonsugary meal should restrict refined sugars in the diet. Patients who cannot eat small meals throughout the day should be encouraged to carry raw seeds and nuts mixed with dried fruits for periodic snacking.

Patients with DM who experience hypoglycemia should be instructed to maintain their glycemic goals, report all episodes of hypoglycemia, and monitor blood glucose levels at bedtime and before, during, and after exercise to assist in glycemic management. Alcohol, cigarette smoking, and caffeine should be avoided in these patients.

REFERENCES

Diabetes Mellitus Type 1

American Diabetes Association. Standards of medical care in diabetes—2021 Abridged for Primary Care Providers. *Clinical Diabetes*. 2021;39(1):14–43.

Centers for Disease Control and Prevention: Diabetes. Incidence of Newly Diagnosed Diabetes | Diabetes | CDC. https://www.cdc.gov/diabetes/data/statistics-report/newly-diagnosed-diabetes.html. Accessed 05/25/2021.

Centers for Disease Control and Prevention. (2020). National Diabetes Statistics Report. https://www.cdc.gov/diabetes/library/features/diabetes-stat-report.html. Accessed 5/25/2021.

Dhatariya KK, Vallanki P. Treatment of diabetic ketoacidosis (DKA)/hyperglycemic hyperosmolar state (HHS): novel advances in management of hyperglycemic crisis (UK versus USA). *Curr Diab Rep*. 2017;17(5):33.

DiMeglio LA, Evans-Molina C, Oram RA. Type 1 diabetes. *The Lancet*. 2018;391(10138):2449–2462.

Eizirik DL, Pasquali L, Cnop M. Pancreatic β-cells in type 1 and type 2 diabetes mellitus: different pathways to failure. *Nature Reviews Endocrinology*. 2020;16, 349–362. https://doi.org/10.1038/s41574-020-0355-7

Foster NC, Beck RW, Miller KM, et al. State of type 1 diabetes management and outcomes from the T1D Exchange in 2016–2018. *Diabetes Technology & Therapeutics*. 2019;21(2):66–72.

Funnell MM, Piatt GA. Incorporating diabetes self-management education into your practice: when, what and how. *J Nurse Pract*. 2017;13(7):466–474.

Mobasseri M, Shirmohammadi M, Amiri T, et al. Prevalence and incidence of type 1 diabetes in the world: a systematic review and meta-analysis. *Health Promotion Perspectives*. 2020;10(2):98–115.

Rawshani A, Rawshani A, Sattar N, et al. Relative prognostic importance and optimal levels of risk factors for mortality and cardiovascular outcomes in type 1 diabetes mellitus. *Circulation*. 2019;139(16):1900–1912.

Diabetes Mellitus Type 2

Arnott C, Li Q, Kang A, et al. Sodium-glucose cotransporter 2 inhibition for prevention of cardiovascular events in patients with type 2 diabetes mellitus: a systematic review and meta-analysis. *Journal of the American Heart Association*. 2020;9(3). https://doi.org/10.1161/JAHA.119.014908

Galicia-Garcia U, Benito-Vicente A, Jebari S, et al. Pathophysiology of type 2 diabetes mellitus. *International Journal of Molecular Sciences*. 2020;21(17):6275. https://doi.org/10.3390/ijms21176275

Garber A, Handelsman Y, Grunberger G, et al. Consensus statement by the American Association of Clinical Endocrinology and American College of Endocrinology on the comprehensive type 2 diabetes management algorithm. *Endocr Pract*. 2021;26(1):107–139.

Gomes MB, Rathmann W, Charbonnel B, et al. Treatment of type 2 diabetes mellitus worldwide: baseline patient characteristics in the global DISCOVER study. *Diabetes Research and Clinical Practice*. 2019;151:20–32.

Halim M, Halim A. The effects of inflammation, aging and oxidative stress on the pathogenesis of diabetes mellitus (type 2 diabetes). *Diabetes & Metabolic Syndrome: Clinical Research & Reviews*. 2019;13(2):1165–1172.

Kriska AM, Rockette-Wagner B, Edelstein SL, et al. The impact of physical activity on the prevention of type 2 diabetes: evidence and lessons learned from the Diabetes Prevention Program, a long-standing clinical trial incorporating subjective and objective activity measures. *Diabetes Care*. 2021;44(1):43–49.

Malone JI, Hansen BC. Does obesity cause type 2 diabetes mellitus (T2DM)? Or is it the opposite? *Pediatric Diabetes*. 2019;20:5–9. https://doi.org/10.1111/pedi.12787

Scheen AJ. Sodium-glucose cotransporter type 2 inhibitors for the treatment of type 2 diabetes mellitus. *Nature Reviews Endocrinology*. 2020;16:556–577.

Sikalidis AK, Maykish A. The gut microbiome and type 2 diabetes mellitus: discussion a complex relationship. *Biomedicines*. 2020;8(1):8. https://doi.org/10.3390/biomedicines8010008

Vesa CM, Popa L, Popa AR, et al. Current data regarding the relationship between type 2 diabetes mellitus and cardiovascular risk factors. *Diagnostics*. 2020;10:314. https://doi.org/10.3390/diagnostics10050314

Diabetes Mellitus Type 3c

Johnston PC, Thompson J, Mckee A, et al. Diabetes and chronic pancreatitis: considerations in the holistic management of an often neglected disease. *Journal of Diabetes Research.* 2019;(article ID 2487804). https://doi.org/10.1155/2019/2487804

Kaminski BA, Goldsweig BK, Sidhaye A, et al. Cystic fibrosis related diabetes: nutrition and growth considerations. *Journal of Cystic Fibrosis.* 2019;18(S2):S32–S37.

Petrov MS, Basina M. Diagnosis of endocrine disease: diagnosing and classifying diabetes in disease of the exocrine pancreas. *European Journal of Endocrinology.* 2021;184(4):R151–R163.

Richardson A, Park WG. Acute pancreatitis and diabetes mellitus: a review. *Korean Journal of Internal Medicine.* 2021;36(1):15–24.

Wynne K, Devereaux B, Dornhorst A. Diabetes of the exocrine pancreas. *Journal of Gastroenterology and Hepatology.* 2018; 34(2):346–354.

Hypoglycemia

Johnson-Rabbett B, Seaquist ER. Hypoglycemia in diabetes: the dark side of diabetes treatment. A patient-centered review. *Journal of Diabetes.* 2019;11:711–718.

Ratner RE. Hypoglycemia: new definitions and regulatory implications. *Diabetes Technology & Therapeutics.* 2018;20(S2): 50–53.

Salehi M, Vella A, McLauglin T, et al. Hypoglycemia after gastric bypass surgery: current concepts and controversies. *Journal of Clinical Endocrinology & Metabolism.* 2018;103(8):2815–2826.

RESOURCES

General

Academy of Nutrition and Dietetics
https://www.eatright.org

Diabetes Mellitus Type 1/Type 2/Type 3c

American College of Cardiology/American Heart Association: Atherosclerotic Cardiovascular Disease Risk Calculator
http://tools.acc.org/ASCVD-Risk-Estimator-Plus/#!/calculate/estimate/

American Diabetes Association
https://www.diabetes.org

Association of Diabetes Care & Education Specialists
https://www.diabeteseducator.org

Behavioral Diabetes Institute: Diabetes Distress Scale
http://behavioraldiabetes.org/scales-and-measures/#1448434304201-ce67e63c-8e90

Indian Health Service: Division of Diabetes Treatment and Prevention
https://www.ihs.gov/MedicalPrograms/Diabetes

JDRF (Juvenile Diabetes Research Foundation)
http://www.jdrf.org/about/fact-sheets/type-1-diabetes-facts/

National Eye Institute: Diabetic Retinopathy
https://www.nei.nih.gov/learn-about-eye-health/eye-conditions-and-diseases/diabetic-retinopathy

National Institute of Diabetes and Digestive and Kidney Diseases: Diabetes
https://www.niddk.nih.gov/health-information/diabetes

U.S. Centers for Disease Control and Prevention: National Diabetes Statistics Report
https://www.cdc.gov/diabetes/pdfs/data/statistics/national-diabetes-statistics-report.pdf

Hypoglycemia

National Institute of Diabetes and Digestive and Kidney Diseases: Hypoglycemia
https://www.niddk.nih.gov/health-information/diabetes/overview/preventing-problems/low-blood-glucose-hypoglycemia

---

Chapter 60

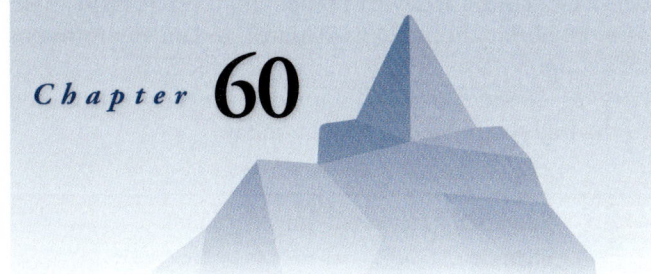

Metabolic Disorders

Debera J. Thomas, PhD, RN, ANP/FNP
Brian Oscar Porter, MD, PhD, MPH, MBA

OBESITY

Obesity, defined as an excess amount of adipose tissue (body fat), is a chronic endocrinological and metabolic disease that is multifactorial and neurobehavioral in nature. The World Health Organization classifies obesity as one of the world's most neglected public health problems, which is at epidemic proportions worldwide. The increase in body fat promotes adipose tissue dysfunction that results in significant adverse metabolic, biomechanical, and psychosocial health consequences. It is associated with multiple comorbidities, including an increased risk of cancer, cardiovascular disease, disability, type 2 diabetes mellitus (T2DM), gallbladder disease, hypertension, osteoarthritis, obstructive sleep apnea, cerebrovascular accident (stroke), and susceptibility to infection (including more severe SARS-CoV-2 infection resulting in COVID-19 disease).

EPIDEMIOLOGY AND CAUSES

The American Medical Association classified obesity as a disease in 2013. The U.S. Centers for Disease Control and Prevention (CDC) bases its classifications of overweight and obesity on body mass index (BMI). Although not an entirely accurate reflection of increased body fat, the BMI provides a "ballpark" figure from which to estimate obesity (Table 60.1).

Published clinical guidelines on the identification, evaluation, and treatment of overweight and obesity cite the complex etiology of overeating that makes this chronic illness poorly understood and often intractable to medical management. The two major types of obesity are central (apple-shaped) and lower body (pear-shaped) obesity. Patients with central obesity have excessive body fat in the abdomen and flank areas and are at a greater risk for T2DM, coronary artery disease (CAD), stroke, and early death, compared with those with lower body obesity who have excessive adipose tissue in the buttocks and thighs.

Being overweight and obesity are epidemic in the United States today, and rates are increasing across the globe. Obesity has tripled worldwide since 1975. In the United States, obesity affects 42.4% of adults, with more than one-third being overweight with a BMI between 25 and 29.9 kg/m². Thus, overall, 70.2% of American adults are overweight or obese: 73.7% of males and 66.9% of females. Moreover, the World Health Organization reports that 38 million children younger than 5 years were overweight or obese in 2019. African Americans are more likely to be obese than European Americans, and the incidence of obesity is higher in those of lower socioeconomic status, regardless of race.

The health-care costs of obesity in the United States are estimated to be $147 to $210 billion annually. Job absenteeism as a result of obesity and its related comorbidities costs about $4.3 billion each year. Moreover, Americans spend more than $64 billion a year on diets, weight-loss supplements, and low-calorie food products in an attempt to treat obesity. In fact, obesity kills more people than being underweight. In addition, the psychological costs and effects of obesity, which are difficult to quantify, include stigmatization, discrimination, and social isolation.

The causes of obesity are complex and research is rapidly examining causal mechanisms, complications, and treatment. Predisposing factors include genotype and gene-environment interactions. Obesity is generally polygenic and often associated with other phenotypes, including endocrinological disorders and intellectual disability. Some of these associated endocrinological disorders are T2DM and hypothyroidism, whereas associated intellectual disorders include Down's syndrome and Prader-Willi syndrome. Rarer single-gene defects that can result in obesity include mutations in the melanocortin-4 receptor, leptin, or leptin receptor genes, which affect the leptin and melanocortin pathways that control appetite and regulate energy homeostasis, either directly or indirectly.

Cushing's syndrome, Cushing's disease, polycystic ovary syndrome, growth hormone deficiency, hypothyroidism, and hypothalamic injury are metabolic abnormalities that also contribute to obesity (see Chapter 58). There are also complex cultural and environmental risk factors that contribute to obesity such as geographical location, family structure, low socioeconomic status, high intake of low-nutrient but energy-dense foods, low levels of physical activity, disrupted sleep cycles, medication side effects, increased stress, neurological dysfunction (e.g., central nervous system trauma, hypothalamic inflammation, leptin resistance), viral infections, and alterations in the gut microbiome. In fact, an energy-dense diet combined with a sedentary lifestyle is the main cause of obesity in the United States, and an environment that supports a sedentary lifestyle and facilitates access to fatty, processed foods and refined sugars has contributed to the high incidence of obesity today.

TABLE 60.1 Calculating Body Mass Index and Classifying Obesity

Calculating Body Mass Index

The most recent formula for calculating body mass index (BMI) was developed by a panel convened by the National Heart, Lung, and Blood Institute and the National Institute of Diabetes and Digestive and Kidney Diseases of the National Institutes of Health. The equation for BMI is weight (kg) divided by height (m) squared (kg/m²).

Classifying Obesity

Classification	BMI
Overweight	25–29.9 kg/m²
Obesity Class 1	30–34.9 kg/m²
Class 2	35–39.9 kg/m²
Class 3 (severe, extreme)	>40 kg/m²

Pediatric/Adolescent Considerations: Obesity

Specific factors have also been identified that uniquely affect children's propensity for obesity. For example, during gestation, unhealthy maternal nutrition, particularly in pregnant women who are overweight or obese, may increase nutrient transfer through the placenta into the fetal circulation that cause alterations in fetal gene expression that may increase the child's predisposition to being overweight or obese. As a postpregnancy example, early exposure to antibiotics in childhood has also been shown to be a risk factor in the development of overweight and obesity later in life, although the mechanism is unclear.

PATHOPHYSIOLOGY

Obesity affects almost every body system and is associated with an increased risk of multiple comorbid diseases (Box 60.1). The health risks associated with obesity are directly correlated with its severity and include metabolic and structural effects on the body, as well as the psychosocial disability that results from the social stigma attached to obesity. Mortality risk increases as complications of obesity develop, approaching 50% when a patient's weight is 30% to 40% greater their ideal body weight. Obesity is associated with an increased risk of colon, rectal, and prostate cancer in males, and uterine, gallbladder, biliary tract, breast, and ovarian cancer in females. Patients who are obese also have increased surgical and obstetrical risks. A reduction in body weight of 5% to 20% significantly decreases these comorbid risk factors in obese individuals.

Obesity is a complex, multifactorial disease that involves interactions among lifestyle, behavioral, genetic, and environmental factors. An increase in weight, and ultimately obesity, results when one's intake of calories persistently exceeds energy expenditures. The control of appetite and the mechanisms that govern food intake are complex and incompletely understood. Neurologically, the hypothalamus controls certain aspects of appetite and appears to have a role in an individual's food preferences. Other important central nervous system sites contributing to weight control include the solitary tract of the hindbrain, the arcuate and paraventricular nuclei, and the amygdala. Mediated by an array of neurotransmitters including norepinephrine, dynorphin, hypocretin, serotonin, neuropeptide Y, and ghrelin, both the central and peripheral nervous systems produce and integrate a complex array of neural inputs that regulate appetite, energy metabolism, and body fat mass.

> **Box 60.1   Consequences of Obesity**
>
> - Coronary heart disease/congestive heart failure
> - Hypertension
> - Dyslipidemia/hyperlipidemia
> - Type 2 diabetes mellitus/insulin resistance
> - Metabolic syndrome
> - Sleep apnea
> - Restrictive lung disease
> - Asthma
> - Varicose veins and venous insufficiency
> - Gout/hyperuricemia
> - Osteoarthritis
> - Reflux esophagitis
> - Gallbladder disease
> - Thromboembolic disease
> - Cancers: Endometrial, breast, prostate, colon
> - Depression
> - Low self-esteem

When properly regulated, the body is known to have neuroendocrinological homeostatic feedback control mechanisms involving both the peripheral and central nervous systems, which seek to maintain adequate nutrient intake and an ideal body weight. Examples include glycemic levels (hypoglycemia is a trigger to eat), serum leptin concentrations, glucocorticoids that act as appetite stimulants, sympathomimetic hormones that act as appetite suppressants, and the peptide ghrelin—a ligand for the growth hormone secretagogue receptor that increases appetite (ghrelin levels increase in anticipation of a meal and in response to diet-induced weight loss).

Differences in fat-free body mass also correlate strongly with the variable energy expenditure seen across different individuals, contributing to counterbalancing mechanisms. In particular, weight gain is associated with increased metabolic demands and energy expenditure that retard further weight gain, whereas weight loss is associated with reductions in energy expenditure that counter further weight loss. Thus, a formerly obese individual who loses weight will experience a relative decrease in energy expenditure compared with a nonobese individual and will thus require 15% fewer calories to maintain their reduced weight. In turn, failing to reduce one's caloric intake appropriately may result in progressive weight gain after a period of weight loss in a formerly obese individual (i.e., part of the basis for the inefficacy of "yo-yo dieting").

Adipocytes, the cellular basis of obesity, secrete hormones and cytokines known as adipokines, which underlie the neuroendocrinological regulatory mechanisms that contribute to obesity if dysregulated. These include leptin (which inhibits hunger), adiponectin (which is insulin-sensitizing, anti-inflammatory, and antiatherogenic), resistin (which causes insulin resistance and is a feedback regulator for adipogenesis), apelin (which regulates blood sugar), visfatin (which mimics insulin and comes from visceral fat), vaspin (which is insulin-sensitizing and anti-inflammatory), and retinol-binding protein 4 (which promotes insulin resistance and fat deposition). Adipokines also include regulators of lipoprotein metabolism (e.g., lipoprotein lipase, lipotransin, apolipoprotein E, cholesterol ester transfer protein) and inflammatory cytokines (e.g., prostaglandins, tumor necrosis factor-α [TNF-α], various interleukins [ILs], plasminogen activator inhibitor 1, monocyte chemoattractant protein 1).

Expressed by adipose, intestinal, and placental cells, the leptin gene in particular has been the subject of much controversy in human obesity research. Serum leptin concentrations strongly correlate with body fat content, and leptin-deficient mice demonstrate insulin resistance, hyperinsulinemia, and hyperphagia. Leptin has been shown to reduce levels of neuropeptide Y, a potent stimulus for food intake produced in the brain's arcuate nucleus. Human obesity due to leptin deficiency has been identified in two consanguineous families, as has obesity due to leptin receptor deficiency. However, leptin overexpression has not been shown to reduce appetite or weight, and most obese patients express normal levels of this protein, albeit with decreased sensitivity to leptin. Thus, decreased leptin levels appear to signal that fat stores are insufficient for growth and reproduction; however, the hormone itself is not a negative regulator of appetite or weight gain.

There is a well-documented genetic predisposition for the development of obesity. Twin studies have revealed strong correlations in obesity prevalence between siblings raised together by the same set of parents, as well as apart in separate households. In addition, the BMIs of adoptees correlate closer with those of their biological parents rather than their adoptive parents, also suggesting genetic predispositions. Moreover, obesity is a presenting feature of at least 24 genetic syndromes that display a wide range of heritability patterns. These syndromes are relatively rare, but the most common are Prader-Willi syndrome, a neurodegenerative disorder resulting from genetic abnormalities in the long arm of chromosome 15q11 to 13, and the autosomal recessive Bardet-Biedl syndrome, which involves concurrent hypogenitalism, intellectual disability, and renal abnormalities.

On a molecular level, the bulk of our understanding of the pathophysiology and genetics of obesity stems from preclinical animal models—particularly that of the obese mouse, for which a number of genetically altered strains are available. Through genetically engineered knockout mice that lack one or more target genes, as well as transgenic models that overexpress either a functional or nonfunctional version of a target gene, researchers have identified several single gene defects that result in obesity. Some of these genetic findings have been further generalized to humans.

There is recent evidence that alterations in the gut microbiome are linked to obesity. Research is ongoing, but evidence obtained thus far shows a parallel between the obesity pandemic and the increase in antibiotic use and the development of microbial resistance. Antibiotic use, diet, and bariatric surgery alter the gut microbiome, which in turn alters energy metabolism and body habitus. The gut microbiome is likely a factor in the complex interplay of genetics, environment, and gut permeability in the development of obesity and other chronic diseases.

CLINICAL PRESENTATION

Subjective

Patients often present to their health-care provider with some or all of the following symptoms as a result of obesity: fatigue, decreased energy, weakness, joint pain, shortness of breath, increased daytime sleepiness, and depression. Most will seek help for another medical condition or present with one or more of the aforementioned complaints. A comprehensive history includes probing for a weight history and attempts at weight loss, as patients often report several attempts with repeated ("yo-yo") dieting with poor long-term success. A family history of obesity and cultural food preferences must be assessed, and the amount of control the patient maintains in food purchasing and preparation should also be considered. The patient should be questioned about any periods of rapid weight gain and environmental or psychosocial changes in lifestyle or behavior during these periods. Self-induced weight gain may be a protective defense mechanism in psychologically disturbing or physically threatening situations, such as with sexual abuse in adolescents or young adults. Thus, specific questions to assess current or past eating disorders are essential. A history of physical activity should also be obtained, with special emphasis on the relationship of any weight-gain or weight-loss periods to physical activity.

Objective

A complete physical examination should be done, with a focus not only on body weight, but also on signs of possible secondary causes (e.g., Cushing's syndrome, thyroid disease) and complications (e.g., diabetes mellitus, peripheral vascular disease) of obesity. The diagnosis of obesity is based on a BMI of 30 kg/m² or greater (Table 60.1). However, in extremely muscular individuals, BMI is not an accurate gauge of obesity; in such cases, a body fat analysis will yield more accurate information about body composition. In children, obesity is diagnosed as a BMI in the 95th percentile or higher on age- and gender-specific CDC-generated pediatric growth charts.

Historically, ideal body weight has been calculated by comparing actual body weight to population tables from the Metropolitan Life Insurance Company. Weights for the original and updated tables were calculated based on data from middle-class, mostly white Americans seeking insurance; as Americans grew heavier, the weights in the tables increased. Measurements of weight and height are used to calculate the BMI for the precise classification of obesity. BMI remains the measurement most frequently used in research and clinical practice to assess overweight and obesity because it is easily calculated without laboratory equipment. In clinical studies, BMI correlates with measurements of body fat percentage taken with underwater displacement weighing, but this measure is not as reliable in older adults.

Two methods can be used to assess for central obesity, which is the type of obesity most associated with significant complications. The first is to measure waist circumference, with values greater than 40 inches in men and more than 35 inches in women indicating central obesity. The second method is to calculate a waist-to-hip ratio using the following formula:

$$\text{Waist-to-hip ratio} = \frac{\text{Waist measurement at the smallest part}}{\text{Hip measurement at largest circumference}}$$

A ratio of greater than 1.0 in males and more than 0.85 for females indicates central obesity.

DIAGNOSTIC REASONING

A complete history and physical examination with anthropometric measurements are essential elements of the initial assessment. A past medical history and complete medication profile are also critical, especially regarding the intake of corticosteroids or appetite stimulants, as well as past use of appetite suppressants, laxative, diuretics, or herbal supplements as evidence of past weight-loss attempts.

Diagnostic Tests

Initial assessment of the obese patient should include the following laboratory tests: thyroid-stimulating hormone (TSH), fasting glucose, glycosylated hemoglobin A1c, fasting lipid profile, liver function tests (serum transaminases), alkaline phosphatase, total bilirubin, serum electrolytes, creatinine, blood urea nitrogen, uric acid, vitamin D level, and general laboratory tests, including a complete blood count, urinalysis, and urinary microalbumin. An electrocardiogram should also be obtained to assess cardiac health.

Also included in initial testing may be an evaluation of body composition (body fat percentage) using calipers or bioelectrical impedance. Both are inexpensive assessment methods; however, calipers are not as accurate in patients with a high BMI, whereas the impedance-based measurement is hydration dependent and can give less accurate measurements in dehydrated or edematous states. Dual-energy x-ray absorptiometry (DXA) is accurate but relatively expensive, and DXA machines may not accommodate very obese patients.

Differential Diagnosis

The diagnosis of obesity is usually straightforward, although underlying causes may not always be evident. Thus, the differential diagnosis of obesity is geared toward determining the underlying etiology. Secondary causes of obesity, such as Cushing's syndrome, hypothalamic injury, and hypothyroidism, must be ruled out before initiating a treatment plan with the patient. For example, edematous states and water balance must be considered, as acute or chronic fluid retention should be distinguished from increased adiposity. Although the vast majority of obesity cases are due to nonnutritive dietary choices and sedentary lifestyle behaviors, certain medical conditions such as hypothyroidism can be ruled out with simple laboratory tests (e.g., TSH, free thyroxine). In general, an extensive laboratory work-up is not necessary. Rare syndromes may also be associated with severe or morbid obesity, such as Pickwickian syndrome that consists of hypersomnia, congestive heart failure, and hypertension in an obese patient.

Patients should also be evaluated for other risk factors associated with obesity—especially those implicated in CAD, such as hyperlipidemia and insulin resistance associated with T2DM. *Metabolic syndrome* is defined as a constellation of risk factors including hypertension, hyperlipidemia, insulin resistance, and overweight/obesity that significantly increases an individual's risk of cardiovascular disease and diabetes mellitus (see Chapter 35 for more information on metabolic syndrome). The American Diabetes Association has published a statement with multiple professional societies addressing metabolic syndrome, and the Endocrine Society has a practice guideline stressing the importance of recognizing these at-risk patients.

MANAGEMENT

Whether weight gain is related to exogenous or endogenous factors is an important determination in developing a comprehensive treatment plan, as many secondary causes of obesity may be treatable. For example, with obesity caused by hypothyroidism, treating the thyroid issues may solve the weight-gain problem. Ultimately, the clinical management of obesity requires the balancing of energy intake versus expenditure. Current clinical evidence suggests that successful treatment must include a combination of diet, physical activity, and behavioral interventions, as multidisciplinary approaches to weight loss have a higher success rate. Continued close contact with a health-care provider is more important for long-term success than any particular diet program. Given the chronic nature of obesity, the patient must learn long-term weight management skills. Cognitive therapy in conjunction with education is effective in increasing self-esteem, improving depression, and decreasing patients' dissatisfaction with their bodies.

The management plan should focus on reducing comorbidity and visceral obesity, not solely on improving cosmetic outcomes. Dietary instructions are essentially the same for the obese individual as they are for a healthy nonobese person. The National Heart, Lung, and Blood Institute of the National Institutes of Health (NIH) recommends following a heart-healthy eating plan with an emphasis on portion control that includes abundant fruits and vegetables, whole grains, low-fat protein sources, and small amounts of whole foods containing high levels of monounsaturated and polyunsaturated fats, such as nuts and seeds. A management plan that is realistic, can fit into the patient's lifestyle, and includes gradual changes in diet and activity is more likely to be successful than extreme or fad dieting.

Cultural and socioeconomic factors affect not only the prevalence of obesity but also attitudes as to acceptable weight and its implications. For example, some cultures view being overweight as a sign of good health and prosperity. In many Western cultures, obesity is seen more as a cosmetic problem and an issue of willpower, rather than as a major health problem. Thus, patient counseling should stress the health benefits of weight loss, such as reductions in blood pressure, serum triglycerides, and blood glucose levels (especially in patients with T2DM who may experience decreased A1c levels as a consequence of weight loss), as well as an increase in the level of cardioprotective high-density lipoprotein cholesterol. In addition, identifying reasons for overeating may benefit patients in managing their dietary behaviors. Being tired, anxious, socially isolated, and angry are all major triggers for overeating, as denoted by the HALT acronym, which stands for Hungry, Angry, Lonely, and Tired. Depression is also a key comorbidity that must be addressed if present.

Weight management should be directed toward an initial goal of decreasing the patient's weight by 5% to 10% over 6 months, which has been shown to improve the risk factor profile associated with obesity. Subsequent goals are set after achieving this initial weight-loss goal. Treatment guidelines include measuring BMI at each patient encounter, and if a patient has a BMI of 25 kg/m² or more or a waist circumference greater than 35 inches in females or greater than 40 inches males, care should be taken to assess for comorbidities and cardiovascular risk factors. All patients, regardless of their BMI, should be counseled about healthy lifestyle behaviors, including healthy dietary and physical activity habits. Weight-loss goals and treatment plans should be made in consultation with the patient to devise a program that is practical and feasible. If on repeated visits the patient has failed to lose weight, the provider should explore barriers to behavioral change and alternative approaches with the patient.

Dietary Management

Before dietary modifications are initiated, a 3- to 7-day diet history should be evaluated. The patient should keep a diary, recording all oral intake, including water and drinks. It is often beneficial to have the patient record daily activities along with food intake. Clues as to lifestyle patterns and behavioral eating patterns can be assessed more adequately with both sets of data. Ideally, a more plant-based eating plan with whole (nonprocessed) foods should be suggested. There is an abundance of research to indicate that this type of eating plan can reduce weight, blood pressure, blood sugar, and other complications of obesity. The overall goal of weight loss depends on a calorie deficit in which caloric expenditure exceeds caloric intake. A daily caloric deficit of 500 to 750 calories has been shown to be effective in achieving weight loss, regardless of the manipulation of macronutrients (fats, carbohydrates, and protein). Thus, the goal is to create a caloric deficit following a healthy eating plan. Besides calorie restriction, dietary recommendations must consider minimum recommended daily nutrient requirements, the patient's food preferences, and the patient's lifestyle.

Physical Activity

Physical activity is a significant part of a weight loss and maintenance program. It is especially beneficial in the long-term management of weight loss, lowering blood pressure, increasing muscle mass, increasing insulin sensitivity, improving the lipid profile, and improving glucose metabolism. Unless specific contraindications exist, physical activity should be prescribed for all patients. The NIH recommendation for physical activity for everyone is 150 minutes of moderate-intensity aerobic physical activity per week. Moderately intense physical exertion is equal to a brisk walk of 3 to 4 miles per hour. Patients are more likely to continue low-intensity physical activity than high-intensity physical activity. A 20-minute walk is usually acceptable to most patients as a starting point. Including resistance exercises in the physical activity prescription will also help maintain lean body mass.

Younger patients with obesity may begin an aerobic exercise program if physical examination results are within normal levels. Older, sedentary patients should begin with walking programs. Exercise tolerance testing may be indicated for older adults and adults at risk for CAD before beginning a physical activity program.

Behavioral Modification

Behavioral modification is essential for initial weight loss and weight maintenance. Unless the patient can identify eating patterns and lifestyle patterns that have contributed to weight gain and change those within their control, long-term weight management will not be achieved. Effective control over eating behaviors includes cognitive strategies for portion control and healthy food selections. The need to identify impulsive and binge eating is also important. Behavioral management is enhanced by avoiding high-risk environments or altering the environment to reduce triggers to overeating.

Stress has a significant effect on eating behavior. During times of stress, the patient may find it impossible to implement behavior modification techniques. Relaxation techniques can assist in managing stress. These relaxation techniques must also be practiced frequently in times of low stress, so they can be effectively used in times of excessive stress.

Pharmacological Management

Pharmacological therapy for obesity has been available for decades, although the medications currently approved by the U.S. Food and Drug Administration (FDA) for use in overweight and obesity all have notable side effect profiles. Medications approved by the FDA for weight loss include orlistat (Xenical, Alli), phentermine plus topiramate extended-release (Qsymia), naltrexone-bupropion (Contrave), and liraglutide (Saxenda). The selective serotonin antagonist lorcaserin (Belviq), previously approved for chronic weight management, was voluntarily removed from the market in 2020 due to an increased risk of cancer and is no longer available.

Orlistat functions by blocking the absorption of fat in the gastrointestinal (GI) tract. Orlistat 60 mg is available as an over-the-counter formulation (Alli) and is taken with each fat-containing meal to inhibit gastric and pancreatic lipases, thereby reducing fat absorption. It is also available by prescription at a dose of 120 mg (Xenical). Demonstrated results are a weight loss of 2 to 4 kg maintained for 2 years. Adverse effects of orlistat at either dose include diarrhea, gas, and abdominal cramping. Some studies suggest it may also inhibit the absorption of fat-soluble vitamins.

Phentermine-topiramate (Qsymia) suppresses appetite and increases feelings of satiety. Phentermine-topiramate has four dose formulations to allow for titration when starting and stopping the drug. The usual dose for weight loss is 7.5 mg/46 mg or 15 mg/92 mg. It should be taken each morning to suppress the appetite (phentermine component) and increase satiety, decrease food appeal, and increase metabolic rate (topiramate component). In studies, patients lost approximately 8% of their starting body weight using this combination medication. Side effects include dry mouth, paresthesias, constipation, insomnia, changes in taste sensation, and seizures if abruptly discontinued.

Naltrexone-bupropion (Contrave) works by targeting the hypothalamic melanocortin system and the mesolimbic reward system to affect weight loss, but the exact mechanism of action is not fully characterized. Naltrexone-bupropion is supplied in tablets that contain 8 mg of naltrexone and 90 mg of bupropion. One tablet should be taken during week 1 and then increased by one tablet per day each week subsequently to reach a maintenance dose of 2 tablets twice a day at week 4. Side effects include constipation, dry mouth, headache, diarrhea, hypertension, insomnia, liver damage, tachycardia, and nausea and vomiting.

Liraglutide 3 mg (Saxenda) is an injectable glucagon-like peptide 1 (GLP-1) analog that causes weight loss by slowing gastric emptying and suppressing food intake; it is also approved at a lower dose (Victoza) to treat T2DM. The starting injection dose of liraglutide (Saxenda) is 0.6 mg daily for the first week. The dose is increased by 0.6 mg daily per week until the full dose of 3.0 mg is achieved by week 5. Side effects include nausea, diarrhea, constipation, abdominal pain, headache, and tachycardia. Liraglutide may also cause medullary thyroid carcinoma in rodents and has been associated with postmarketing cases of pancreatitis.

Surgical Intervention

Surgical intervention for obesity should be reserved for those patients who have a BMI over 40 kg/m^2 or over 35 kg/m^2 with comorbid conditions. Surgery is usually not considered until the obese patient has failed more conventional weight-loss methods. The rate of bariatric surgery is increasing in the United States today. The most common surgical procedure is the Roux-en-Y gastric bypass (RYGB), which may be performed laparoscopically. Gastric banding is another option, but the weight-loss results are less dramatic than with RYGB. However, short-term complications of gastric banding are fewer than with RYGB. A third surgical option that is gaining in popularity is a sleeve gastrectomy. In this procedure, about 75% of the stomach is removed but the rest of the GI tract is left intact. Weight loss is less than with RYGB but greater than with gastric banding, with a lower complication rate than RYGB.

Some studies have shown that weight-loss surgery can produce up to a 50% loss of initial body weight. Complications may occur in up to 40% of patients after surgery and include peritonitis, abdominal wall hernia, dumping syndrome, infection, acute cholecystitis, hypoglycemia, pyloric outlet obstruction, chronic diarrhea, nausea, and vomiting. Patients should be counseled regarding these potential complications of surgical interventions. They should also be informed of the possibility of regaining much of the lost weight if lifestyle changes are not also undertaken and sustained.

Additional Clinical Considerations

The increasing number of obese and morbidly obese patients brings a challenge to primary care practitioners. Although caring for patients who are obese certainly includes treating the obesity, many of these patients also have diseases and illnesses that first bring them to the provider's office. The National Institute of Diabetes and Digestive and Kidney Diseases Weight-Control Information Network offers suggestions for health-care providers in the care of these individuals separate from the need to treat the underlying obesity. Health-care providers and clinic staff need to receive education related to respect for patients, the need for size-appropriate equipment in the clinic, and providing the same level of care for obese patients as nonobese patients. Box 60.2 provides details to guide providers in creating an accessible and comfortable clinic environment for obese patients, including medical equipment that can accurately assess patients who are obese and ways to reduce patient fears about their weight.

FOLLOW-UP AND REFERRAL

Most patients on weight-loss programs require close follow-up. The severity of the problem and the nature of the interventions should govern how frequently the primary care practitioner sees the patient, though patients are more successful in maintaining weight loss with frequent follow-up visits. Many patients will benefit

> **Box 60.2 Provider's Guide to Caring for Obese Patients**
>
> Create an accessible and comfortable clinic environment:
>
> - Provide sturdy, armless chairs and high, firm sofas in waiting rooms.
> - Provide sturdy, wide examination tables that are bolted to the floor to prevent tipping.
> - Provide a sturdy stool or step with handles to help patients get on the examination table.
> - Provide extra-large examination gowns.
> - Install a split lavatory seat and provide a specimen collector with a handle.
>
> Use medical equipment that can accurately assess patients who are obese:
>
> - Use large adult blood pressure cuffs or thigh cuffs on patients with an upper-arm circumference greater than 34 cm.
> - Have extralong phlebotomy needles, tourniquets, and large vaginal speculae available.
> - Have a weight scale with adequate capacity (greater than 350 pounds) for obese patients.
>
> Reduce patient fears about weight assessment:
>
> - Weigh patients only when medically appropriate.
> - Weigh patients in a private area.
> - Record weight without comments.
> - Ask patients if they wish to discuss their weight or health.
> - Avoid using the term *obesity* when discussing weight-related health issues. Patients may be more comfortable with phrases such as "difficulties with weight" or "being overweight" (patients may be asked what terms they prefer when discussing their weight).

from frequent clinician visits that provide medical guidance, goal-setting, and emotional support throughout the weight-loss process. In addition, the importance of clinical follow-up once weight-loss goals have been achieved should be emphasized, because recurrent weight gain after periods of significant weight loss is common. The patient should be seen for a weigh-in, blood pressure measurement, and discussion of progress at least monthly, but once a week is often most beneficial until the patient has developed habituated lifestyle changes.

Specialty referrals are driven by the identification of underlying causes of overweight and obesity, such as endocrinological causes that may be reversible or genetic etiologies that may require further counseling for patients and their families (if heritable). In addition, patients may benefit from a referral to a dietitian who specializes in weight loss. A surgical referral may be indicated for morbidly obese patients if nonsurgical interventions have proven unsuccessful. In addition, referrals to comprehensive weight-loss programs at specialized weight-loss centers have become increasingly popular, although such programs are often not covered by health insurance plans or other third-party payers, and thus may prove costly for the patient. Referrals to weight-loss support groups may be beneficial regardless of the type of weight-loss interventions selected.

In addition, given the critical role that maladaptive psychosocial coping mechanisms play in driving the behavior of many obese patients, referrals to mental health professionals specializing in weight-loss assessment and counseling are typically indicated. For example, weight-loss surgery will typically not be attempted unless a thorough psychological evaluation of the patient and his or her social support network has been completed and the patient's psychological status is deemed capable of supporting the postsurgical practices needed to maintain weight loss.

Patient Education: Obesity

Patient education includes instruction on how to maintain a balance between caloric intake and energy expenditure. Physical activity, a healthy diet that includes more fruits and vegetables, and lifestyle changes should be emphasized. Many patients are unaware of techniques to reduce fat in their diet by cooking methods alone, including, for example, the use of nonstick cookware that obviates the need to use fat or grease in the pan. Other suggestions are to bake, broil, or braise foods, rather than to fry them with oil or solid animal and dairy fats such as lard, shortening, margarine, or butter. In addition, many obese persons skip breakfast and, as a consequence, eat more in the late afternoon and evening, which is unhelpful.

Obese patients must be guided to set realistic weight-loss goals and educated about the importance of combining therapeutic approaches (e.g., dietary changes plus increased physical activity, even if pharmaceutical or surgical approaches are utilized). Sustaining weight loss requires behavioral changes, and patients should plan out their weight-loss strategy in writing. The plan should include dietary modifications, a physical activity routine, and behavioral strategies. A calendar should be developed outlining this intervention schedule. If lapses in the plan are experienced, the patient should explore the reasons for the lapse. In turn, the primary care provider should review the plan and schedule of interventions at each visit.

Adequate social support is a key element to successful weight loss. Patients who feel "sabotaged" or undermined by family members who do not support the same type of effective weight-loss behaviors as the patient (especially home-based dietary practices) will need to explore methods for support outside of the family. Patients typically benefit from weight-loss support groups, and the primary care provider can use online resources to find a support group in the patient's geographical area. Finding a walking partner and initiating a walking program immediately after work before returning home are strategies that can be suggested.

GOUT

Gout is a metabolic disease that produces an inflammatory crystal-induced arthritis. Gout was characterized as far back in history as the time of Hippocrates. It has been referred to as "the disease of kings" because of its prevalence in the wealthy, who were able to afford the traditionally expensive, purine-rich foods that typically trigger this disorder. Once a disabling chronic disease, modern medical diagnostics and treatment modalities have decreased its disabling effects.

EPIDEMIOLOGY AND CAUSES

Persons from the United States, the Pacific Islands, and countries with abundant lifestyles have an increased incidence of gout. In the United States, gout affects 8.3 million adults. It rarely occurs in children, premenopausal females, or males younger than 30 years of age. Seventy percent of people with gout are males, with a peak incidence between 40 and 50 years of age. The increased incidence of gout in older adults has been associated with an increased use of diuretics. Twenty percent of patients who present with gout have a family history of the disease. Gout is also more prevalent in African American males, possibly because of the increased prevalence of hypertension in this group.

Hyperuricemia (i.e., uric acid levels exceeding 7 mg/dL in males and 6 mg/dL in females) occurs in 5% to 10% of the U.S. population. Most of these adults, however, are asymptomatic. One in five persons with hyperuricemia will develop urate deposits in a joint, soft tissue, or cartilage. Patients with gout may experience an acute attack with rapid fluctuations of serum urate levels. Surgery, dehydration, binge alcohol consumption, emotional stress, infections, diuretics, and uricosuric drugs can all cause rapid fluctuations in serum urate levels.

Causes of primary gout include idiopathic inborn errors of purine metabolism, decreased renal clearance of uric acid, and specific enzymatic defects such as those resulting in Lesch-Nyhan syndrome and glycogen storage disease. Secondary causes of gout include other disease processes and medications, such as thiazide diuretics, that result in an overproduction or underexcretion of uric acid. Predisposing risk factors for the development of gout are listed next.

Risk Factors: Gout

Primary Risk Factors

- Decreased renal clearance of uric acid
- Enzyme defects (Lesch-Nyhan syndrome, glycogen storage diseases)

Secondary Risk Factors

- Excessive (daily) intake of purine-rich foods
- Obesity
- Starvation
- Dehydration
- Alcohol abuse
- Medications: thiazide diuretics, ethambutol, nicotinic acid, pyrazinamide, low-dose salicylates, cyclosporine
- Paget's disease
- Chronic hemolytic anemia
- Psoriasis
- Cytotoxic drugs
- Sarcoma and other carcinomas
- Chronic renal disease
- Hypothyroidism
- Lead poisoning
- Hyperparathyroidism
- Diabetes insipidus
- Diabetic ketoacidosis

PATHOPHYSIOLOGY

Overproduction and/or underexcretion of uric acid with tissue deposition of monosodium urate crystals is the metabolic disorder underlying gout. Most individuals (90%) with gout have inappropriate underexcretion of uric acid. At the time of puberty, serum uric acid levels are known to increase in males; however, most (90% to 95%) males remain asymptomatic throughout life. In addition, estrogen is believed to be protective from hyperuricemia in females.

Gout is a direct result of hyperuricemia (high serum uric acid) and the increased saturation of urate in the plasma and other body fluids. Supersaturation of body fluids results in a precipitation of monosodium urate crystals out of body fluids and into the joints, soft tissues, and cartilage. This leads to the symptoms and clinical findings of gout, as the deposition and crystallization of urate in the joints triggers an inflammatory response. Thus, the arthritis produced by gout is characterized by recurrent, painful attacks of monoarticular joint inflammation caused by the phagocytosis of urate crystals, which deposit in joints, soft tissues, and cartilage.

Several mechanisms may trigger an acute attack of gout, the most common being trauma or surgery. Gout attacks may also be paradoxically triggered by prophylactic or uricosuric agents, which are known to lower serum uric acid levels. Acute attacks are also more likely to occur at lower serum uric acid levels in persons with alcoholism due to decreased urinary excretion. There is also an increased incidence of hypothyroidism in persons with crystal aspirates in synovial fluid.

Gouty arthritis may extend to several joints and is classified into four stages based on timing and clinical presentation (Table 60.2): asymptomatic, acute phase, intercritical, and chronic tophaceous. For unclear reasons, gouty arthritis has a predilection for the first metatarsophalangeal joint (the great toe)—a condition known

TABLE 60.2 Stages of Gout

Stage	Subjective Findings	Objective Findings	Diagnostic Findings
I. Asymptomatic	None	None	Microtophaceous deposits of urate in joints and bursae
II. Acute phase (inflammatory phase)	Extremely painful monoarticular or polyarticular attack Pruritus and desquamation of the skin surrounding affected joints as the inflammation subsides	Affected joints are red, warm, and swollen Early acute attack subsides within a few days, but may last up to 2 weeks, as inflammation gradually subsides 10% of patients experience only one acute attack during their lifetime	Elevated WBC count Elevated temperature Elevated serum uric acid or normouricemia
III. Intercritical (interval between acute attacks)	None; patient is asymptomatic	Duration of intervals between attacks decreases as the disease progresses If a second acute attack occurs, it usually presents within the first year after the initial attack	Microtophaceous deposits of urate in joints and bursae serum urate levels should be less than 6 mg/dL if adequately treated
IV. Chronic tophaceous (results from recurrent attacks with multiple sites of urate deposits [tophi] in articular and periarticular tissue)	May restrict movement of affected joints Chronic pain, stiffness, decreased joint function, joint derangement, and secondary joint degeneration affecting the upper and lower extremities	More than 50% of patients progress to this stage within 20 years of their initial attack if not properly managed Occasionally, tophus ulceration and erosion with chalk-textured drainage observed Uric acid kidney stones in 5% to 10% of patients	Tophi

as *podagra*. This may result from the relative coolness of this peripheral joint that allows for greater crystal deposition, the constant microtrauma to which this joint is subjected, and the differential affect that weight-bearing alternating with recumbency has on the resorption of joint fluid and intra-articular urate.

In general, urate crystallization is more likely to occur at lower temperatures. Noninflamed synovial fluid in the knee is significantly cooler (90 to 91°F [32.2 to 32.78°C]) than core body temperature. Thus, although a serum uric acid concentration of 7 mg/dL appears to be the threshold level above which gout is more likely to develop, crystallization may be more likely to occur at lower urate concentrations intra-articularly. In addition, hyperuricemia alone is insufficient to lead to crystallization. As part of the inflammatory process, urate-specific immunoglobulin (Ig) molecules coat monosodium urate crystals in gouty synovial fluid, likely serving as a promoter of nucleation for more urate crystal formation.

As gout progresses, crystals are deposited into multiple body tissues. In severe cases with repeated attacks, monosodium urate monohydrate crystals form into a nodular deposit known as a *tophus*, surrounded by granulomatous inflammation consisting of monocytes and giant cells. In addition to the skin and joints, tophaceous swellings may be found in a number of body tissues, including the heart valves, kidneys, and larynx, capable of leading to significant pathology. Microtophi, consisting of collections of urate crystals surrounded only by a thin fibrocytic ring, may also be present in gouty synovial fluid. Some research has suggested that these microtophi release their urate crystals into the joint fluid after the initiation of synovial inflammation in the early stages of a gout attack.

Urate crystals induce intra-articular inflammation via a number of mechanisms. Synovial lining cells, monocytes, and endothelial cells have all been shown to phagocytose urate crystals in vitro and subsequently increase their production of inflammatory mediators via transcriptional upregulation and mRNA stabilization, including IL-1, IL-6, IL-8, and TNF-α. Blockade of IL-8 and TNF-α activity has been further shown to counter urate-induced inflammation.

Neutrophilic migration into affected joints and their subsequent phagocytosis of urate crystals appears to play a central role in the pathogenesis of gouty arthritis. Neutrophils undergo an oxidative burst during this process, releasing lysosomal enzymes, superoxide anions, leukotriene B4, and IL-1, among other inflammatory mediators. Indeed, the complexities of neutrophilic chemotaxis and function within gouty joints have been a central focus of gout research. Studies have indicated tyrosine kinases, phospholipases, adhesion molecules such as E-selectin, and several chemotactic factors play key roles in neutrophilic recruitment and activation by urate crystals. This explains the efficacy of colchicine in treating acute attacks, because it inhibits neutrophil tyrosine kinase activity in response to both gout and pseudogout crystals, as well as downregulates the activity of adhesion molecules on both neutrophils and endothelial cells.

A number of proteins interact with urate crystals to increase their proinflammatory properties. For example, Igs bound to urate crystals lead to a greater release of lysosomal and superoxide enzymes by neutrophils. The complement and kinin systems have also been implicated in urate crystal pathology, but they are not requisite for acute gouty inflammation. Although acute attacks of gout typically resolve spontaneously within several weeks, if left untreated or if inadequately treated, gout leads to chronic arthritis and bony erosions within 5 to 10 years, resulting in joint deformities and ultimately restricting function.

The self-limited nature of an acute gout attack involves several mechanisms. Neutrophil mediators have been shown to cleave Ig molecules from urate crystals to reduce their inflammatory nature. The inflammatory properties of tophaceous urate crystals are also reduced after protease treatment in vitro. Lipoproteins (specifically apolipoprotein B) reduce the inflammatory potential of urate crystals after binding, indicating that they may be involved in the self-limited resolution of acute attacks. In addition to the deactivation and death of inflammatory cells and the inactivation of secreted proinflammatory mediators, leukocytes, monocytes, and macrophages have been shown in vitro to alter their cytokine transcriptional activity over time. In turn, they secrete several anti-inflammatory cytokines on resolution of an acute gout attack, including IL-1 receptor antagonist, transforming growth factor-β, and peroxisome-proliferator-activated receptor-γ.

CLINICAL PRESENTATION

Subjective

A thorough evaluation of the onset, characteristics, and potentiating causes of gouty joint pain should be completed on initial evaluation. The patient presents during an acute attack with pain, tenderness, erythema, and swelling of the affected joints. The usual presentation is monoarticular, and the joint most frequently affected is the first metatarsophalangeal joint of the great (big) toe; however, the midfoot, knees, fingers, wrists, and elbows may also be affected. The typical presentation is excruciating pain that awakens the patient at night. Patients often describe the pain as throbbing, crushing, and pulsating. The pain is not relieved by rest or positional changes and prevents weight-bearing on the affected limb. Often the patient cannot tolerate anything coming into contact with the affected joint—even bed clothing touching the limb can be extremely painful.

The patient's past medical history, including any joint or musculoskeletal trauma, should be reviewed, along with any family history of gout. The patient may also report an episode of recent trauma to the affected joint, a recent alcohol binge, or an eating binge of gout-triggering foods before the acute attack. Patients may report a recent operation or severe illness, especially one producing a shift in fluid balance. Because gout is more prevalent in patients with hypertension, obesity, and hyperlipidemia, questioning should focus on these contributing factors. In addition, a medication history, specific for recently increased intake of aspirin or cyclosporine, should also be obtained.

Objective

Although a typical patient with gout initially presents with monoarticular joint complaints, a complete bilateral examination of all joints should be performed. Bilateral joints should be assessed for symmetry in appearance and range of motion. Asymmetrical presentation of joint inflammation, redness, tenderness, and limitations in range of motion are typical of gout. On physical examination, the affected area is warm or hot to the touch. The patient will complain of pain on palpation, and range of motion will be limited. Skin overlying the affected area is often red and taut. Several days after an acute attack, desquamation of skin over the affected joints may be evident.

The manifestation of podagra is experienced by approximately 90% of patients with gout. Subsequent attacks may progress to include several joints (polyarticular disease). Other joints that are frequently affected include the instep of the ankle, the heels, knees, wrists, fingers, and elbows. Peripheral joints are more likely to be involved because central joints are warmer and less conducive to crystal formation. In polyarticular episodes or those involving a large joint, the patient may have an elevated temperature, tachycardia, anorexia, malaise, headache, and/or chills.

Patients who have progressed to the chronic tophaceous stage of gout will have palpable tophi, which are nodular deposits of monosodium urate monohydrate crystals that initiate the inflammatory process. Most tophi are firm and movable, whereas the overlying skin is thin and red. Tophi are most likely to develop on the pinnae of the ears, olecranon tips, and the distal interphalangeal joints of the hands and feet. Extensive tissue deposits of urate may also occur on the helices and antihelices of the ears, the eyelids, the sclerae, and the corneas.

DIAGNOSTIC REASONING

Diagnostic Tests

The clinical presentation and medical history findings are often sufficient to diagnose gout. Serum uric acid levels and radiographic imaging may provide supportive evidence; however, a definitive diagnosis is only made with identification of sodium urate crystals in the aspirated fluid from affected joints.

Initial Testing

Initial testing for gout includes a serum uric acid level. Most patients will have an elevated serum urate level in the absence of elevated blood urea nitrogen, as serum urate is greater than 7.5 mg/dL in up to 95% of persons with gout. However, some studies have suggested that serum urate levels may be normal in up to 15% of patients at the time of an acute gout attack. Thus, elevated serum urate levels are not diagnostic of gout in the absence of characteristic joint signs and symptoms, and the clinician should look for other supportive laboratory findings. The erythrocyte sedimentation rate and white blood cell (WBC) count may also be elevated during an acute attack. The WBC count is typically greater than 10,000 cells/µL, but values up to 100,000 cells/µL may occasionally be observed.

The classic radiographic findings of gout are tophi, normal mineralization of bone, joint space preservation without narrowing, an asymmetrical polyarticular distribution, an overhanging cortical edge, and punched-out erosions of bone. However, radiographs of affected joints may show no changes in early stages of disease. The only radiographic evidence of gout in its early stages may be asymmetrical soft tissue swelling. With recurrent attacks and progressive disease, however, radiolucent urate tophi and punched-out appearing areas become apparent in bone. Tophi appear as cloud-like increases in density, which may show signs of calcification. Urate crystals may also be seen in subcutaneous tissue, cartilage, joints, and other tissues. Uric acid kidney stones will also be present in 5% to 10% of patients. In the very late stages of gout, demineralization and loss of articular structures may be apparent on radiographic examination. Most changes are asymmetrical and occur predominantly in the feet, ankles, and knees. Patients with severe disease often have involvement of the hands and elbows as well.

Subsequent Testing

The definitive test to confirm the diagnosis of acute gout is microscopic observation of urate crystals in aspirated joint fluid. The synovial fluid will be turbid during an acute attack, and needle-shaped uric acid crystals are identified as strongly negatively birefringent when examined by compensated polariscopic examination of wet smears of aspirated joint fluid. This means that when examined with a polarizing filter and red compensator filter, uric acid crystals appear yellow when aligned in parallel to the slow axis of the red compensator and blue when aligned perpendicularly to the direction of polarization. Of note, patients who present with gout and comorbid symptoms of abdominal pain, peripheral neuropathy, and proteinuria should be assessed for lead exposure, as hyperuricemia has been associated with acute exposure to high lead levels.

Differential Diagnosis

Differential diagnoses for gout include other arthritides and infectious musculoskeletal and skin conditions, including septic arthritis, rheumatoid arthritis, psoriatic arthritis, bursitis, fracture, cellulitis, acute joint trauma, pseudogout (i.e., joint inflammation due to calcium pyrophosphate crystal deposition), and reactive arthritis (a postinfectious form of inflammatory arthritis associated with GI and genitourinary infections).

Septic arthritis should be considered when a patient presents with joint pain, swelling, and erythema. Septic arthritis occasionally coexists with gout and should also be strongly considered when a patient does not respond to initial management for gout, given the need for antibiotics. Septic arthritis more commonly occurs in larger joints. Gram stains and cultures of synovial fluid are positive for bacteria in septic arthritis, and patients often present with fever and chills. Radiographic examination often reveals joint-space narrowing and erosions within 1 to 2 weeks of the onset of septic arthritis.

A rheumatoid factor titer may help rule out rheumatoid arthritis, as either rheumatoid factor or antibodies against citrullinated cyclic peptides are more likely to be positive in rheumatoid arthritis than in gout. Clinically, rheumatoid arthritis may resemble gout, but it typically has a symmetrical joint presentation of clinical signs, symptoms, and radiographic findings. Joint-space narrowing is also typical of rheumatoid joint disease but not gout. Psoriatic arthritis, a seronegative (i.e., rheumatoid factor-negative) peripheral spondyloarthritis, may resemble gout in its early stages; however, the initial joints affected are frequently in the hands, feet, and sacroiliac and spinal joints. Fusiform soft tissue swelling is typical of psoriatic arthritis, and early joint-space narrowing also commonly differentiates it from gout.

Pseudogout is an inflammatory joint pathology that presents with many similar characteristics as gout. However, polarized microscopic examination of joint fluid aspirates reveals rhomboid-shaped calcium pyrophosphate dihydrate crystals that are weakly positively birefringent, rather than the strongly negatively birefringent needle-shaped uric acid crystals associated with gout. Thus, the calcium pyrophosphate crystals of pseudogout appear blue when aligned in parallel to the slow axis of the red compensator and yellow when aligned perpendicularly to the axis of polarization. Pseudogout usually presents at a later age, and the symptoms are characteristically less acute and less severe than gout. Pseudogout is polyarticular in approximately 75% of patients and typically affects the knees and larger joints. Pseudogout is associated with hyperthyroidism and hypothyroidism, hypomagnesemia, amyloidosis, hypercalcemia, hypophosphatemia, and hemosiderosis.

The development of an inflamed joint in a young patient after a GI (e.g., *Campylobacter, Salmonella,*

Section 12: HEMATOLOGICAL AND IMMUNOLOGICAL PROBLEMS

SECTION EDITOR

Brian Oscar Porter, MD, PhD, MPH, MBA

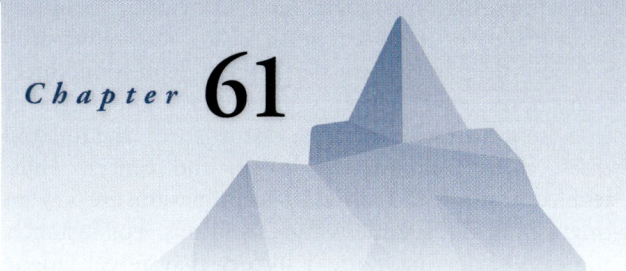

Chapter 61

Common Hematological and Immunological Complaints

Monica Giovannini, MD
Jill E. Winland-Brown, EdD, APRN, FNP-BC, FAANP
Brian Oscar Porter, MD, PhD, MPH, MBA

BRUISING

A bruise (ecchymosis) is an integumentary manifestation of extravasated blood. Discoloration of the skin is attributed to a local interstitial pool of erythrocytes, which causes a light- to dark-blue skin color associated with red pigment. The bruise sets off a local inflammatory event that includes macrophage invasion and histamine release, which may be associated with edema. Macrophages engulf red blood cells (RBCs) to clear the area of extravasated blood.

Macrophages that contain the RBCs excrete hemosiderin and hematoidin. Hemosiderin is brown, and hematoidin is yellow. The release of these molecules from macrophages accounts for the characteristic color changes of bruises during their resolution. In general, the initial redness of a bruise transitions into a blue or purple hue in 1 to 2 days and may even darken to black several days later. After this, a color change to green occurs approximately 1 week after the initial onset of the bruise, and then the bruise acquires a yellowish-brown appearance, which gradually fades over time. Hematomas (larger bruises resulting from collections of blood that pool under the skin) require more time to resolve than smaller bruises.

Bruising may result from blunt trauma or occur spontaneously in the absence of trauma. Thrombocytopenia (platelet counts less than 50,000 cells/mL) predisposes an individual to bruise formation with minor trauma, given the integral role of platelets in the formation of blood clots.

Spontaneous bruising may be seen with platelet counts less than 30,000 cells/mL, particularly on the arms and legs. Hematological cancers, such as (but not limited to) leukemia and myeloma, can induce bruising or bleeding because of the production of abnormal malignant cells in the blood and bone marrow and the consequent drop in the number of normal blood cells like platelets. Spontaneous bruising may also be associated with the chronic use of corticosteroid or anticoagulant therapies. Corticosteroids weaken vascular walls, making them prone to release erythrocytes. Anticoagulants, when their levels exceed the therapeutic range, can permit microvascular ruptures to spill blood into interstitial spaces. Cancer treatments can also predispose to bruising, due to their propensity to cause thrombocytopenia.

One of the most common forms of anticoagulant therapy consists of warfarin (Coumadin) in oral dosages that are intended to keep the international normalized ratio (INR) between 2.0 and 3.0 for most disease-related prophylaxis, such as the prevention of valvular thrombi formation in atrial fibrillation. Although dosing guidelines must be individualized for each patient, initial dosing of warfarin is typically 2 to 5 mg per day for 3 days, followed by measurement of prothrombin time (PT) and INR. This initial loading dose starts the process of anticoagulation. Dosages thereafter range from 2 to 7.5 mg daily, although dosages can be higher than 10 mg if the INR dictates. Excessive dosing of warfarin or other anticoagulants may lead to easy bruising as one of the most obvious clinical signs of overdose. If the INR is above the therapeutic target, the clinician should consider withholding 1 or more days of anticoagulant therapy and possibly starting reversal therapy with vitamin K if active bleeding is present. PT and INR should be reevaluated within 3 to 5 days of the dosage adjustment, and treatment should be restarted at a lower dose after a hiatus of therapy.

DIFFERENTIAL DIAGNOSIS

Unexplained or suspicious bruising may be the primary care practitioner's first clue to an underlying medical condition or physically dangerous circumstances in a patient's life. A thorough history and physical examination by the clinician should focus on the etiology of the bruising and distinguish between extrinsic versus intrinsic causes. The differential diagnoses of the causes of bruising include chronic use of corticosteroid and anticoagulant therapies, thrombocytopenia, hemolytic anemia, nutritional deficiencies (e.g., inadequate dietary vitamin K), domestic violence, self-inflicted injury or other blunt trauma, and hypersensitivity vasculitis. Hematological cancers also always need to be considered in the differential diagnosis of bruising. Some cancer treatments, such as chemotherapy and targeted therapies, can increase the risk of bleeding and bruising, primarily due to medication-induced thrombocytopenia.

FATIGUE

Fatigue presents as a complaint of tiredness that cannot be explained on the basis of exercise or other activity. It may be either acute or chronic, associated with a disease or independent of other pathophysiology.

Acute fatigue is most often associated with viral or bacterial infections and may serve as a harbinger of impending symptoms such as fever. Determining the etiology of chronic fatigue that may last for months is far more complex. A patient seeking relief from chronic fatigue may see their clinician many times before the cause can be identified. The patient usually cannot explain the cause of chronic fatigue without the clinician asking appropriate assessment questions.

The clinical history of fatigue offers insights into the nature of the cause. Patient reports of fatigue that increases over the course of the day and abates after rest suggests an underlying medical condition that may account for the fatigue. For example, fatigue may reflect hematological abnormalities associated with other disease conditions, such as chronic anemia that results in decreased oxygen-carrying capacity, which makes the patient less tolerant of physical exertion and may contribute to persistent fatigue.

Functional fatigue is more typically characterized by fatigue on awakening that may improve after exercise. The close associations of depression and anxiety with fatigue make for a difficult task in distinguishing functional causes of fatigue from the fatigue itself. Depression has been cited as one of the most common comorbidities underlying complaints of fatigue in the primary care setting. Mental health disorders, in general, are more likely to be found in patients reporting significant fatigue to primary care practitioners, whereas underlying serious somatic disorders may be found in only a small percentage of these patients. Nonetheless, the strong association between fatigue and hematological abnormalities, in particular, should raise suspicion for easily ruled-out physical conditions, such as anemia, as contributing factors.

Cancer-related fatigue is one of the most common side effects of cancer and its treatments. It is often described as "paralyzing." Usually, it comes on suddenly, does not result from activity or exertion, and is not relieved by rest or sleep. It may not end—even when treatment is complete. Fatigue can have a profoundly negative impact on a person's ability to function and quality of life.

DIFFERENTIAL DIAGNOSIS

Fatigue carries an extensive differential diagnosis, as it seldom presents without additional comorbidities. Acute fatigue is perhaps the simplest type to diagnose and treat. For example, acute fatigue typically appears in a clinical history that is positive for viral or bacterial exposure, combined with examination findings of fever and other systemic abnormalities. Chronic fatigue has many causes, including chronic anxiety or stress reactions, lack of restorative sleep due to poor sleep hygiene or sleep apnea, depression, infectious mononucleosis, hepatitis, tuberculosis, anemia, heart disease, lung disease, electrolyte disturbances, rheumatoid diseases, chronic fatigue syndrome, and cancer. Thus, a detailed history and physical examination are key to distinguishing these underlying conditions. For instance, in the case of anemia, patient history may reveal fatigue that worsens with exertion, and physical examination may demonstrate conjunctival pallor and pale nailbeds, gingivae, or tongue, along with sinus tachycardia.

FEVER

Fever is defined as a temperature elevation above a patient's normal baseline, which may result from any pathology and is often multifactorial. On average, most individuals maintain a body temperature close to 98.6°F (37°C), which may normally fluctuate by ±0.9°F (±0.5°C) throughout the day. Physical exertion can elevate body temperature temporarily, followed by a return to baseline after the activity ends. A persistent elevation in temperature clearly reflects an underlying pathology, however.

Fever may be either acute or chronic. If acute, body temperature tends to be greater than 101.3°F (38.5°C). Acute fever is associated with upper respiratory infections that are either bacterial or viral in etiology, drug reactions, gastroenteritis, or urinary tract infections. Physiologically, fever is associated with the release of inflammatory immune mediators (e.g., interleukin-6, tumor necrosis factor–α), which act as pyrogens, presumably to create an environment within the body that is not conducive to microbial growth and replication. The ability of the body to elevate its temperature in the event of infection diminishes with advancing age due to a weakening of the immune system as one gets older. Therefore, acute fever in an older adult might not be as elevated compared with that in a younger patient. Quite often, the older patient may not even mount a febrile response; therefore, other symptoms may be more commonly indicative of an infection, such as malaise, fatigue, decreased appetite, decreased mentation, delirium, or confusion.

Chronic fevers tend to be low-grade temperature elevations. Temperatures rise to 100.4°F (38°C), for example, in cases of infectious hepatitis, infectious mononucleosis (especially in the third and fourth weeks after the onset of symptoms), sinusitis, dental abscess, prostatitis, and tuberculosis (TB). Cancer patients will often have a fever as a presenting symptom, which is usually a sign that the cancer has spread or that it is in an advanced stage. Fever is rarely an early symptom of cancer, but it may be if a person has a blood cancer, such as leukemia or lymphoma. Neutropenic fever occurs in patients with infection and underlying neutropenia, and fever may often be the first and sometimes only sign of infection in these patients. Cancer treatments can also induce fever; for example, fever is a cardinal symptom of cytokine release syndrome after chimeric antigen receptor (CAR)-T-cell therapy or cytolytic chemotherapy used to treat a number of hematological cancers.

The origin of a fever may not be apparent from the patient's history, physical examination, or laboratory testing. If the cause is not evident after a thorough workup, a persistent fever should be classified as a fever of unknown origin (FUO). Specifically, FUO is defined as a fever of greater than 101.3°F (38.5°C) that occurs on at least three occasions over a 3-week period in an ambulatory patient. A hospitalized patient is diagnosed with FUO if the unexplained fever persists for 1 week, despite a standard diagnostic evaluation.

DIFFERENTIAL DIAGNOSIS

The differential diagnosis of fever is extremely broad, with FUO alone having several hundred potential causes. Thus, the primary care practitioner should approach diagnostic decision making for fever with several large etiological categories in mind, including infection, malignancy, noninfectious inflammatory diseases (e.g., rheumatological disorders), drug or environmental exposures, thromboembolic disease, and even factitious causes.

The magnitude of fever elevation may guide the clinician in differentiating its cause. Fevers can vary widely, however, based on the patient's age, history of pathogenic exposure, and many other factors. Fevers less than 101.3°F (38.5°C) are characteristic of infectious hepatitis, some acute viral infections, and TB. Fevers between 101.3°F (38.5°C) and 104°F (40°C) are associated with urinary tract infections and some acute viral syndromes. Fevers in excess of 104°F (40°C) tend to be associated with pancreatitis, pyelonephritis, and intracranial pathology (e.g., bacterial meningitis).

Correlated with history and physical examination findings, differential temperature elevations determine the type of laboratory testing of blood or other bodily fluids to be ordered. In the absence of definitive test results, knowledge of different fever categories may help guide the clinician in evaluating a more focused differential diagnosis. For example, a middle-aged female patient with a 3-day fever of 102.2°F (39°C) who presents with a nonproductive cough, chills, inspiratory chest discomfort, and clear lungs that are dull to percussion at the bases raises the suspicion for a pulmonary consolidative process (e.g., pneumonia) that should prompt the clinician to order a chest x-ray and complete blood count to assess for pulmonary infection. However, the clinician may decide not to order blood cultures for this patient, as there are focal symptoms to explain the fever and localize its source, and the fever is not high enough to suggest systemic infection, for which blood cultures would be indicated.

Medications and environmental toxins may also cause fever. When this etiology is suspected, the history should focus on exposure to drugs (including both prescribed medications and illicit drugs) and industrial chemicals, including pesticides and herbicides used in animal husbandry and agriculture. Fevers of environmental origin tend to follow an indolent course, often demonstrating peaks and troughs. Physical signs may also be absent, thus adding to the insidious nature of their presentation.

LYMPHADENOPATHY

The term *lymphadenopathy* is used in clinical practice to designate any abnormality of lymph nodes and, in particular, enlarged lymph nodes. *Lymphadenitis* is a term that suggests inflammation as the cause of the lymph node enlargement, which may be associated regionally or systemically. If the inflammation is regional, the lymph nodes that are proximal to a site of infection will show enlargement. If the disease process is systemic, lymph nodes in three or more sites dispersed across the body may become enlarged. An example of regional lymph node enlargement is cervical lymphadenopathy associated with infectious pharyngitis. An example of systemic lymphadenopathy is HIV infection, in which there may be lymphadenopathy in three or more extrainguinal lymphatic chains. Lymphadenopathy can also be a sign of cancer spread; cancers that originate in the lymph nodes are called *lymphomas*.

Lymphadenopathy follows the course of the underlying disease. Thus, lymph nodes may be acutely or chronically enlarged, depending on actual disease pathology, the natural history of the condition, as well as the duration of disease. Acute infection often leaves the regional lymph nodes proximate to the site of infection tender to the touch, whereas chronically enlarged nodes, such as in HIV infection or cancer, may be nontender.

DIFFERENTIAL DIAGNOSIS

The differential diagnosis of lymphadenopathy depends on the location of nodal involvement, patient characteristics, and associated findings. Neck masses, for example, involve a differential that is based on nodal abnormalities manifesting in specific locations of the neck (e.g., anterior lymphadenopathy being associated with streptococcal pharyngitis, posterior lymphadenopathy being associated with viral pharyngitis), the age of the patient, and associated comorbidities or risk factors such as tobacco use. The clinician should distinguish between slow growth in nodes versus rapid or acute onset of lymphadenopathy. An acute onset is more characteristic of inflammation or acute infection, whereas slow-growing nodes in the neck suggest neoplasm, such as lymphoma. However, there are exceptions. For example, a young patient with no history of tobacco or ethanol use may present with slow-growing cervical lymphadenopathy, but the likelihood of neoplasm is minimal in a patient of this age and with this history. In contrast, a patient older than 70 years with even a remote history of tobacco use is likely to be diagnosed with lymphoma if presenting with slow-growing neck lymphadenopathy. Thus, the patient's age is an important consideration in the differential diagnosis of lymphadenopathy, and cancers, either solid or hematological, should always be considered in this context. In turn, persistent slow-growth enlargement is a reason to consider lymph node aspiration and cytological evaluation.

HIV-associated lymphadenopathy presents challenges to the differential diagnosis. The average HIV-infected patient is younger than 50 years, has a history of alcohol and/or tobacco use, and may also test positive for other sexually transmitted infections that can cause nodal abnormalities. Lymphadenopathy in these patients can affect the neck, axillae, inguinal region, breasts, and thorax. Reactive lymphadenopathy is characteristic of early and middle stages of the disease and is often attributable to the HIV infection itself. Later manifestations contributing to lymphadenopathy in advanced stages of HIV disease include lymphoma, human papillomavirus–associated cancers, or concurrent infection with cytomegalovirus, toxoplasmosis, or *Mycobacterium avium* complex.

REFERENCES

Bruising

Harrison L, Nash M, Fitzmaurice D, et al. Investigating easy bruising in an adult. *BMJ*. 2017;356:j251. doi: https://doi.org/10.1136/bmj.j251

Neutze D, Roque J. Clinical evaluation of bleeding and bruising in primary care. *Am Fam Physician*. 2016;93(4):279–286.

Fatigue

Hulme K, Safari R, Thomas S, et al. (2018) Fatigue interventions in long term, physical health conditions: A scoping review of systematic reviews. PLOS ONE 13(10): e0203367. https://doi.org/10.1371/journal.pone.0203367

Stadje R, Dornieden K, Baum E, et al. The differential diagnosis of tiredness: A systematic review. *BMC Fam Pract*. 2016;17:147.

Fever

Wright W, Auwaerter P. Fever and fever of unknown origin: Review, recent advances, and lingering dogma. *Open Forum Infectious Diseases*, Volume 7, Issue 5, May 2020. https://doi.org/10.1093/ofid/ofaa132

Lymphadenopathy

DeVita VT, Lawrence TS, Rosenberg SA. (2018). DeVita, Hellman, and Rosenberg's Cancer: Principles and Practice of Oncology, 11th Edition. United States: Wolters Kluwer Health.

Gaddey H, Riege A. Unexplained lymphadenopathy: Evaluation and differential diagnosis. Am Fam Physician. 2016 Dec 1;94(11): 896-903.

RESOURCES

American Cancer Society
https://www.cancer.org/
American Society of Hematology
http://www.hematology.org/patients/

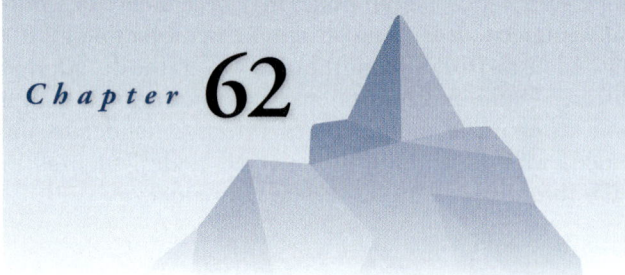

Chapter 62

Hematological Disorders

Monica Giovannini, MD

Jill E. Winland-Brown, EdD, APRN, FNP-BC, FAANP

Brian Oscar Porter, MD, PhD, MPH, MBA

ANEMIA

Evaluation of anemia is extremely common in clinical practice and is one of the most common laboratory abnormalities encountered in the primary care setting. *Anemia* can mean any one of several problems that involve suboptimal red blood cell (RBC) numbers or functions. The diagnosis suggests low hemoglobin, low hematocrit (Hct), and/or a low number of RBCs. All of these problems involve a reduced amount of oxygen circulating in the body, because RBCs carry oxygen to tissues and other cells. The World Health Organization (WHO) identifies anemia as a hemoglobin of less than 13 g/dL (less than 42% Hct) in males and less than 12 g/dL (less than 36% Hct) in females. Slightly higher normal ranges of hemoglobin and Hct values are considered standard in developed versus underdeveloped regions of the world.

The evaluation of anemia may be uncomplicated, unless the patient has comorbidities that can impact the evaluation of anemia, including the interpretation of laboratory results. Past medical history, family history, concurrent medical problems, and predisposing risk factors for anemia are important to consider in the evaluation of all forms of anemia and other hematological disorders. It is important to determine whether the anemia is due to decreased RBC production, maturation defects of RBC precursors, destruction (hemolysis) of RBCs in the peripheral blood, or acute blood loss.

MICROCYTIC ANEMIA

Microcytic anemia is a category of anemia based on the small size (*micro-*) of RBCs (*-cytic*). It has been linked to nutritional deficiencies, particularly a deficiency in dietary intake or gastrointestinal (GI) uptake of iron. The small size of RBCs is identified via the mean corpuscular volume (MCV). Microcytosis, therefore, refers to an MCV value of less than 80 fL.

EPIDEMIOLOGY AND CAUSES

Microcytic anemia related to iron deficiency is one of the most common anemias throughout the world. The incidence is high among females of childbearing age, with up to one-third of pregnant females developing anemia in the third trimester. Worldwide, the ratio of incidence between females and males is 4:1, but in the United States, 20% of adult females are affected by the condition, compared with 3% of adult males. These statistics have remained constant for the past decade. The main causes of microcytic anemia include (1) inadequate oral intake or GI uptake of dietary iron, (2) anemia of chronic disease (ACD), (3) thalassemia, and (4) sideroblastic anemia.

The incidence of iron-deficiency anemia has been estimated to be 1:2.0 to 2.5 among pregnant females and 1:6 in people older than 75 years of age. Iron-deficiency anemia is often the easiest type of anemia to correct, unless it is caused by a GI malignancy. In turn, iron deficiency is straightforward to identify and remains the most common cause of microcytic anemia. Most adults in the United States ingest and absorb an adequate amount of iron in their diets to avoid anemia. It is estimated that the average dietary intake of iron in the United States is 10 to 15 mg per day, of which not more than 10% is absorbed in the stomach, duodenum, and jejunum. The average healthy adult, therefore, absorbs approximately 1 to 2 mg of iron per day. In addition, the same adult loses an amount of iron equal to that ingested and absorbed, thereby maintaining homeostasis.

ACD, unlike iron-deficiency anemia, presents a more complex diagnostic picture because of the many and varied causes of inflammatory disorders in chronic disease, which include rheumatoid arthritis, malignancies, and serious infections. Given its complex diagnostic picture, ACD must always be considered in the differential for microcytic anemia; the precise incidence and prevalence of ACD are unknown.

The thalassemias constitute a group of inherited diseases of alpha- or beta-globin chains. Microcytic anemia is caused by hemolysis that results from the suboptimal synthesis of alpha- or beta-globin chains, known as alpha- or beta-thalassemia, respectively. Beta-thalassemia is associated with descendants of individuals who originated in areas around the Mediterranean Sea. Alpha-thalassemia is far more widespread, occurring in individuals with ancestry from the Asian continent, including China and Southeast Asia. A high prevalence of alpha-thalassemia has also been noted among people living along the western coast of Africa.

Sideroblastic anemia results from a disorder of heme synthesis, resulting in abnormal hemoglobin and disordered RBC function. It may be caused by chronic alcoholism or lead poisoning or may be a stage in the evolution of a generalized bone marrow disorder that may progress to acute leukemia.

PATHOPHYSIOLOGY

Normal Hemoglobin Formation

The predominant normal adult hemoglobin (hemoglobin A; hemoglobin A_1; $\alpha_2\beta_2$) consists of one pair of alpha-globin chains and one pair of beta-globin chains, accounting for 90% to 95% of total adult hemoglobin. Each of these globin chains is linked to an individual heme group, which consists of a protoporphyrin IX molecule bound to a ferrous (Fe^{2+}) reduced iron ion. It is this heme unit that reversibly binds oxygen, allowing for transport of oxygen by the hemoglobin tetramer to the bodily tissues.

Several other forms of hemoglobin are formed during human development. At least three distinct forms of hemoglobin consisting of different combinations of zeta (ζ), epsilon (ε), gamma (γ), and alpha (α) chains present themselves throughout embryonic development in the following order: hemoglobin Gower I ($\zeta_2\varepsilon_2$), hemoglobin Portland ($\zeta_2\gamma_2$), and hemoglobin Gower II ($\alpha_2\varepsilon_2$). In contrast, the predominant normal hemoglobin form in infancy is hemoglobin F or fetal hemoglobin (approximately 80%), which has two gamma-globin chains substituted for the beta-chains ($\alpha_2\gamma_2$). Hemoglobin F has a stronger affinity for oxygen than hemoglobin A does, allowing for oxygen transport across the placenta from the mother to the developing fetus. As a newborn ages, this form of hemoglobin slowly clears from the circulation, accounting for less than 1% of hemoglobin by 6 months of age, with a corresponding increase in hemoglobin A. Finally, an additional form of adult hemoglobin, hemoglobin A_2, also exists, which is present in far smaller amounts than hemoglobin A (about 2% to 5% of total adult hemoglobin). With a slightly higher oxygen affinity than hemoglobin A, hemoglobin A_2 has two delta (δ)-globin chains substituted for the beta-globin chains ($\alpha_2\delta_2$).

Iron-Deficiency Anemia

Because the reduced ferrous (Fe^{2+}) ion is a critical component of the heme moiety in hemoglobin, sufficient iron stores are critical for adequate erythropoiesis in the bone marrow. In low-iron states, the production of hemoglobin is severely reduced, resulting in marked microcytosis. Iron deficiency remains the most common cause of microcytic anemia in the United States. Because most adults receive enough iron in their diets to prevent microcytosis (other than strict vegan vegetarians, who consume no animal-based products of any kind), the clinician's attention should turn to malabsorption or occult loss of blood as the primary causes of iron-deficiency anemia.

The majority of iron uptake occurs in the duodenum and upper jejunum. Thus, malabsorption of iron is linked to underlying GI problems such as celiac sprue; surgical resections involving the stomach, duodenum, or jejunum; inflammatory bowel disease such as Crohn's disease; rapid GI motility; gastroenteritis; and selected drugs such as the histamine receptor 2 (H_2) antagonist cimetidine (Tagamet). Decreased levels of iron can also occur as the result of molecular bonds between plasma iron stores and certain drugs. These bonds develop during the distribution phase of pharmacokinetics, sequestering iron ions and decreasing its plasma pool available for integration into heme molecules. For example, sulfonamide drugs such as sulfamethoxazole-trimethoprim (cotrimoxazole, Bactrim, Septra) can cause decreased plasma levels of iron.

Iron deficiency resulting from acute or chronic (occult) blood loss with inadequate iron intake to compensate is perhaps the most prevalent cause of microcytic anemia. A net loss of blood depletes iron stores and impairs the bone marrow's ability to synthesize new RBCs, due to progressively decreased heme synthesis. Thus, RBCs are decreased not only in number but also in size, producing a characteristic microcytic anemia. Common sites of bleeding (which may be either painless or painful) include the GI tract (e.g., upper GI tract lesions such as peptic ulcers or gastritis; lower GI tract lesions such as colon cancer, ulcerative colitis, Crohn's disease, diverticulosis, and ruptured hemorrhoids) and the genitourinary tract (e.g., heavy endometrial bleeding known as *menorrhagia*, hematuria from bladder cancer). In fact, microcytic anemia may be the first laboratory finding that initiates a line of investigation identifying underlying malignancy. For example, heme-positive stools or melena are strong indications for colonoscopic cancer screening in patients older than 50 years or younger individuals with a strong family history.

Anemia of Chronic Disease

ACD may cause microcytic or normocytic anemia. ACD as a cause of microcytic anemia results from mechanisms that involve inflammation, infection, and/or underlying malignancy. Inflammation may lead to occult and progressive blood loss, because microvascular eruptions may result from histamine release and immune complexes that physically invade the involved region. When these eruptions occur in the GI tract, occult blood escapes through the intestines. Thus, of particular concern is the relationship of occult blood in the stool to GI malignancy. Alternatively, chronic use of NSAIDs such as ibuprofen (Motrin, Advil) and aspirin for chronic pain conditions (e.g., routine management of rheumatoid arthritis and osteoarthritis) must also be considered as a cause of occult blood loss. Blood loss results from erosion of the protective mucosal lining of the stomach due to decreased production of prostaglandin formed by the enzymes cyclooxygenase-1 and cyclooxygenase-2—the molecular targets inhibited by NSAIDs.

ACD has also been referred to as *anemia of inflammation*. Although multiple pathophysiological processes may contribute, in general, the inflammatory processes mediated by cytokines such as interleukin (IL)-6 lead to increased iron sequestration (iron loading) by macrophages and heightened ferritin synthesis, which consequently decrease serum iron levels. In turn, less iron is available for formation of the heme moiety of hemoglobin, thereby leading to resultant anemia.

Thalassemia

The pathology of thalassemia is related either to depletion or mutation in the genes that code for the subunits of the protein component of adult hemoglobin—the alpha- and beta-globin chains. Alpha-thalassemia is caused by gene depletion that leads to a reduction of alpha-globin chain synthesis. Because two copies of the alpha-globin chain gene are inherited from each parent on chromosome 16, mutations or deletions may exist in one or more of these four gene copies, producing distinct clinical manifestations. Mutations or deletions in all four genes result in *alpha (O)–thalassemia* or *alpha-thalassemia major*. No hemoglobin A, A_2, or F can form in this disorder, which is incompatible with extrauterine life. Rather, there is an excess of Bart's hemoglobin, which consists of gamma chain tetramers (γ_4). Bart's hemoglobin has an oxygen affinity at least 10-fold greater than that of hemoglobin A and thus cannot effectively release oxygen to fetal tissues. This causes severe anemia with resultant congestive heart failure, widespread capillary leak, and anasarca known as *hydrops fetalis* (i.e., widespread edema of all fetal tissues), typically resulting in fetal demise by the third trimester of pregnancy.

Mutations in three of the four alpha genes result in hemoglobin H disease, characterized by the widespread formation of hemoglobin H, which consists of a tetramer of four beta-globin chains (β_4). This results in moderate to severe lifelong hemolytic anemia, which typically requires repeated blood transfusions. Having mutations in only two of the four alpha genes is called *alpha-thalassemia minor* or *alpha-thalassemia-1 trait*. This results in a mild anemia with only minor clinical manifestations. Having a mutation in only one of the four alpha-globin genes is a silent carrier state called *alpha-thalassemia minima* or *alpha-thalassemia-2 trait* and can be diagnosed only through DNA analysis because it has no clinical manifestations.

In contrast, only one gene for the beta-globin chain is inherited from each parent. Mutation or deletion of one of these genes results in beta-thalassemia minor or beta-thalassemia trait, characterized by a mild anemia that is typically asymptomatic. Deletions or severe mutations in both beta-globin genes result in beta-thalassemia major (Cooley's anemia), characterized by a severe, transfusion-dependent, lifelong anemia with skeletal abnormalities due to bone marrow expansion in the body's attempt to increase hematopoiesis. An intermediate form of the disorder known as *beta-thalassemia intermedia* also exists; in this form, a patient inherits two mutated, albeit expressed, beta-globin genes, each with a different type of mutation (a compound heterozygote), a situation that results in varied levels of expression or functionality. Clinical manifestations may be worsened by acute illness or infection that impairs erythropoiesis and exacerbates the anemia.

Sideroblastic Anemia

Sideroblastosis and its resulting microcytic anemia are caused by a host of molecular defects that affect the biosynthesis of the heme moiety of hemoglobin. Heme is normally formed first by the creation of 5-aminolevulinic acid (ALA) from glycine and succinyl-coenzyme A by the erythroid isoform of the mitochondrial enzyme ALA synthase, which requires vitamin B_6 (pyridoxine) as a cofactor. Although the underlying genetic defects in many forms of hereditary sideroblastic anemia have not been characterized, known mutations occur most commonly in the genes for the erythroid form of ALA synthase (located on the X chromosome); the mitochondrial transporter ABC7; pyridoxal 5-phosphate (resulting in a reversible form of the disease that is responsive to pyridoxine therapy); ferrochelatase, the copper-dependent enzyme cytochrome oxidase; and pseudouridine synthase–1.

In most forms of sideroblastic anemia, elemental iron is typically delivered appropriately to erythrocyte precursors. However, underlying enzymatic mutations prevent or reduce the ability of heme to incorporate into protoporphyrin IX. A reduced number of RBCs form from ring sideroblast precursors (a diagnostic hallmark) found in the bone marrow, because peripheral reticulocytosis is markedly diminished. Despite an increase in the RBC growth factor erythropoietin, anemia results from the destruction of abnormal erythroid precursors in the bone marrow via apoptosis and intramedullary hemolysis.

Sideroblastic mutations result in excessive iron deposition in the mitochondria of affected erythrocytes (erythropoietic hemochromatosis), which, nonetheless, are hypochromic and microcytic because this form of mitochondrial ferritin cannot be utilized for cytoplasmic maturation in the developing erythrocyte. Intestinal iron absorption is actually increased in sideroblastic anemia, owing to ineffective erythropoiesis, as is also observed in the thalassemias. Thus, iron overload occurs not only in erythroid cells but throughout the body, similarly to genetic (familial) hemochromatosis, with predictable end-organ damage due to iron deposition (e.g., cirrhosis [liver], cardiomyopathy [heart], and endocrine defects [pancreas and adrenal glands]).

Acquired forms of sideroblastic anemia also exist. The most common causes include chronic alcoholism, which results in a multifactorial pathogenesis including many of the hypoproliferative mechanisms previously cited; iatrogenic associations with the antituberculous drug isoniazid and the antibiotic chloramphenicol; zinc toxicity, in which zinc ions preferentially bind to protoporphyrin in place of iron; and copper deficiency, which leads to decreased intestinal absorption of iron and diminished reduction of iron ions from the ferric (3+) state to the bioavailable ferrous (2+) form as a result of reduced cytochrome oxidase activity. Lead poisoning is also often cited as an acquired cause of sideroblastic anemia because lead inhibits ALA synthase. However, with lead toxicity, true ring sideroblasts are typically not seen in the bone marrow, owing to the inhibitory effect of lead on the enzyme ferrochelatase, which prevents the integration of ferrous ions into heme. Idiopathically acquired sideroblastic anemia may also occur when a single erythroid progenitor cell develops a mutation affecting the heme synthesis pathway but also confers a survival advantage. As clonal proliferation of this precursor cell ensues, the bone marrow is largely replaced by cells of this single sideroblastic lineage, which is prone to apoptosis, a situation that results in a myelodysplastic anemia.

CLINICAL PRESENTATION

Subjective

Overall, patients with microcytic anemia present with subjective findings of tachycardia, fatigue, shortness of breath, dyspnea on exertion, palpitations, listlessness, poor concentration, anorexia, and dizziness or lightheadedness.

Because similar subjective findings are also associated with many diagnoses other than microcytic anemia, the history of patient complaints is unlikely to be conclusive.

Objective

As the patient's hemoglobin drops below 10 g/dL (approximately 30% Hct), many patients present with a facial mask of fatigue, sallow-colored skin, pale mucous membranes, tachycardia, and tachypnea at rest. It is possible also to note a prolonged blanching response in the nailbeds (more than 3 seconds), although many patients never present with this sign. Severe iron-deficiency anemia can also cause progressive skin and mucosal changes, such as brittle nails, cheilosis (reddened appearance of the lips, with fissures formed at the angles of the mouth), and a smooth appearance to the tongue. In addition, pica is considered an objective finding associated with severe iron deficiency. *Pica* is identified as an eating disorder of craving for food substitutes, such as clay, dirt, ice chips, or cotton.

DIAGNOSTIC REASONING

Diagnostic Tests

Knowing when to screen for anemia is key. Screening is recommended in pregnant female patients and in children at 1 year of age when metabolic demands are extremely high and the patient appears otherwise healthy. Adult males and postmenopausal females should not be routinely screened for anemia unless the clinical picture suggests it is the possible cause of symptomatology, such as fatigue, generalized weakness, shortness of breath with exertion, pallor, dizziness, fainting, headaches, chest pain, or evidence of GI bleeding (either occult or gross bleeding).

Initial diagnostic testing is focused on obtaining a complete blood count (CBC), including RBC count and RBC indices (e.g., MCV, mean corpuscular hemoglobin [MCH], and mean corpuscular hemoglobin concentration [MCHC]). A low RBC count, hemoglobin level, and/or Hct identify anemia (see Table 62.1). As a rule of thumb, Hct is three times the value of the hemoglobin. For example, a hemoglobin value of 13 g/dL suggests an estimated Hct of 39%.

Iron-deficiency Anemia

The diagnostic tests for iron-deficiency anemia are relatively simple to perform and are readily available to the primary care practitioner. Serum ferritin is a reliable test of low-iron stores, provided the patient does not have advanced liver disease. A serum ferritin value of less than 30 mg/L is considered pathological. As the ferritin level falls, the total iron-binding capacity (TIBC) rises above the normal range. If the drop in ferritin level and rise in TIBC continue without intervention, the serum iron level will eventually fall (to less than 30 mg/L), as will transferrin

TABLE 62.1 Classification of Anemia

Anemia	Examples of Causes	Mean Corpuscular Volume (fL)	Mean Corpuscular Hemoglobin (pg/cell)	Mean Corpuscular Hemoglobin Concentration (%)
Microcytic, hypochromic	Iron deficiency, lead poisoning, thalassemia, rheumatoid arthritis	50–80	12–25	25–30
Microcytic, normochromic	Renal disease, infection, liver disease, malignancies	Less than 80	20–25	27
Normocytic, normochromic	Sepsis, hemorrhage, hemolysis, drug-induced aplastic anemia (e.g., chloramphenicol), radiation, hereditary spherocytosis	82–92	25–30	32–36
Macrocytic, normochromic	Vitamin B_{12} and folic acid deficiency, antimetabolite drugs (e.g., hydroxyurea, methotrexate), pernicious anemia	95–150	30–50	32–36

INDICATIONS FOR HEMOGLOBIN ELECTROPHORESIS

- Suspected thalassemia, especially in individuals with positive family history for the disorder
- Differentiation among the types of thalassemia
- Evaluation of a positive sickle cell anemia screening test (e.g., Sickledex) to differentiate sickle cell trait (20%–40% Hgb S) from sickle cell disease (greater than 70% Hgb S)
- Diagnosis of hemoglobin C disease or combined hemoglobin C/sickle cell anemia (hemoglobin SC disease)
- Identification of the numerous types of abnormal hemoglobin, most of which do not produce clinical disease

TABLE 62.1 Classification of Anemia—cont'd		
Hemoglobin Electrophoresis	Normal Percentage of Hemoglobin (%)	Comments
Hgb A_1 (adults) Infants	Greater than 95 10–30	Low: Alpha- and beta-thalassemia major and minor
Hgb A_2 (adults) Cord blood Birth–6 months Older than 6 months	2–5 0–1.8 0–3.5 1.5–3.5	Elevated: Beta-thalassemia major and minor up to 9%
Hgb F (adults) Neonates 1 month 2 months 3 months 6 months–1 year	Less than 10 70–80 70 50 25 3	Elevated: Thalassemia major and minor (after 6 months) Elevated: Beta-thalassemia minor up to 9%
Hgb C	Absent	Usually asymptomatic but can cause red blood cells to sickle due to osmotic fragility; occurs in 2%–3% of individuals of African descent
Hgb D	Absent	Rarely occurs alone but worsens disease when in combination with sickle cell anemia or thalassemia
Hgb E	Absent	Rarely occurs alone but worsens disease when in combination with sickle cell anemia or thalassemia
Hgb H	Absent	Unstable tetramer of beta-hemoglobin chains; 30% of hemoglobin in severe alpha-thalassemia with three of four mutated alpha genes (hemoglobin H disease)
Hgb M	Absent	Any of several mutated forms of hemoglobin that cannot be reduced to an oxygen-carrying state, resulting in congenital methemoglobinemia
Hgb S	Absent	Elevated in sickle cell anemia: Less than 40% in sickle cell trait; 85%–95% in sickle cell disease Most common beta-hemoglobin chain variant: If both beta-chain genes are affected, then sickle cell anemia (0.25% of African Americans). If only one gene affected, then sickle cell trait (8%–10% of African Americans)

Abbreviation: Hgb, hemoglobin.

saturation (to less than 15%). In addition, secondary testing should focus on the RBC morphology indices from the CBC. Findings such as anisocytosis (variable RBC size), poikilocytosis (variable RBC shape), and hypochromasia (pale-colored RBCs) may be seen when severely iron-deficient samples are microscopically evaluated.

Anemia of Chronic Disease

Diagnostic tests for ACD focus on distinguishing ACD from iron-deficiency anemia. Unlike iron-deficiency anemia, ACD presents with a low serum iron level, along with a low TIBC. Ferritin levels, however, are often normal or elevated, given the iron sequestration associated with chronic inflammation. Similarly, the serum transferrin level is either normal or increased in patients with ACD. Finally, the clinician should expect transferrin saturation to be low, as it is in iron-deficiency anemia.

Thalassemia

The diagnosis of both alpha- and beta-thalassemia requires a CBC and hemoglobin electrophoresis to identify the type and amount of each hemoglobin chain. The CBC is essential to determine the diagnosis of microcytic anemia, as the hemoglobin and MCV are low for each type of thalassemia. In alpha-thalassemia trait, the hemoglobin electrophoresis reveals no increase in hemoglobin A_2 or hemoglobin F. In addition, no hemoglobin H is present. Plasma iron parameters are normal. The level of anemia in alpha-thalassemia is modest, as evidenced by an Hct between 27% and 40%.

Beta-thalassemia minor patients have modest anemia. Unlike those with alpha-thalassemia trait, hemoglobin electrophoresis in these patients reveals elevated hemoglobin A_2 and, in some cases, elevated hemoglobin F (given the reduction in β-chains available for hemoglobin formation). Neither type of hemoglobin will typically be elevated to greater than 9%, however.

Patients with beta-thalassemia major present very differently from patients with other forms of thalassemia, as the degree of anemia is severe. If left untreated, Hct levels fall to less than 10%. Electrophoresis reveals little to no hemoglobin A, with variable amounts of hemoglobin A_2 present. The clinician should expect hemoglobin F to be the primary hemoglobin detectable in these patients. As with all of the thalassemias, findings in patients with beta-thalassemia will include abnormal RBC morphology, such as poikilocytosis and anisocytosis.

Sideroblastic Anemia

A diagnosis of sideroblastic anemia is confirmed by a Prussian blue stain of a bone marrow aspirate. The Prussian blue stain reveals ringed sideroblasts, which have iron deposits located in the mitochondria surrounding the RBC nucleus, forming a visible ring. In addition, erythroid hyperplasia is present in the aspirate from patients with sideroblastic anemia. A high level of serum iron and a high transferrin saturation should accompany these findings. Without a stain of the bone marrow aspirate, the laboratory profile could mimic iron-deficiency anemia, with a moderately low Hct of 20% to 30% and a low MCV.

Differential Diagnosis

The differential diagnosis as to the type of microcytic anemia depends on blood-work results. Microcytic anemia is typically distinguished as to its four predominant etiologies, as discussed earlier: iron-deficiency anemia, ACD, thalassemia, and sideroblastic anemia. The ultimate goal of the diagnostic evaluation is to identify the underlying cause of the microcytic anemia, such as GI malignancy, iron malabsorption, blood loss, menorrhagia, and so forth. For example, iron-deficiency anemia in a patient older than 50 years should be ruled out as due to GI malignancy with a screening colonoscopy done as soon as possible.

MANAGEMENT

The management of microcytic anemia focuses on treating and eradicating the cause of the anemia. If amelioration of the cause is not possible, symptomatic care is indicated. The severity of the anemia will direct the intervention. For example, the decision to transfuse a patient with RBCs is a major clinical step that may be indicated if the Hct is 27% or less. This decision requires a thoughtful analysis of the overall clinical setting and hemodynamic status of the patient, however, which may not be severely compromised, even at low hemoglobin levels. For instance, transfusing patients with volume-sensitive comorbidities, such as congestive heart failure, calls for great caution, given the risks of fluid overload and high output cardiac failure. In addition, the risk of iron overload after repeated RBC transfusions must be carefully considered. Therefore, more conservative treatments are initiated in nonemergent settings.

Iron-deficiency Anemia

Iron-deficiency anemia is first treated with an increase in dietary iron and thereafter with supplemental iron. Foods rich in iron should be recommended, such as animal proteins; legumes; and dark-green leafy vegetables, such as spinach. Diet alone may be sufficient in treating iron deficiency if the patient is either young or middle-aged or the cause of the anemia is short-lived. However, as the patient ages (particularly beyond the age of 65 years) and if the cause of the anemia is chronic, iron deficiency must be treated with either supplemental oral or parenteral iron.

Supplemental oral iron is best given as ferrous sulfate 325 mg three times daily; 10 to 20 mg will be absorbed from the total daily regimen if the serum iron level is moderately low. In more severe cases, however, the level of absorption will increase. The clinician should recheck the RBC indices and iron values in 2 to 4 weeks after starting the regimen to ascertain the effectiveness of the oral regimen. The patient's adherence to the regimen could be complicated by the requirement that iron supplements be taken on an empty stomach to achieve maximal absorption. Some individuals have GI intolerance to oral iron, and some may develop constipation on oral iron. Both of these can lead to difficulty for the patient in adhering to the regimen.

If no measured improvements in anemia (e.g., Hct elevated by one-half of baseline), MCV, and iron stores appear after 1 month of therapy, the clinician should confirm adequate adherence to the iron regimen along with the underlying cause of the iron deficiency. The patient should continue to take supplemental iron for 3 to 6 months after normal levels in the blood and serum indices have been restored. Within 1 to 2 weeks, there should be an increase in hemoglobin (reticulocytes begin to increase within 3 to 4 days). Thereafter, the clinician should recheck laboratory values as indicated by the clinical assessment.

It is uncommon that the patient will not respond to oral iron, unless the patient is on hemodialysis (with low erythropoietin levels); there is severe recurrent blood loss, such as with GI or uterine hemorrhage; or a malabsorption syndrome is present. However, if the patient does not respond to supplemental iron and none of the confounding factors mentioned plays a role, the clinician should doubt the initial diagnosis of iron-deficiency anemia. In particular, ACD should be suspected as the cause, or the clinician should reconsider whether the rate of GI or uterine blood loss might exceed stem-cell deployment from the bone marrow.

Given the risk of anaphylaxis, supplemental parenteral iron is indicated only when there is documented failure of therapy with oral iron supplements. The clinician should calculate the daily dose by subtracting the patient's measured MCV from the normal lower range value (which varies by age and gender). This value is considered the total number of milligrams of iron to add according to the MCV. In addition, the clinician must add 1,000 mg to the delivered dose to cover the storage of iron in the body. Overall, the daily dosage of supplemental parenteral iron is approximately 1,300 to 2,000 mg (1.3 to 2 g) of iron. The preferred parenteral route of administration is IV. However, because anaphylaxis is possible with IV iron, the initial dose should be delivered slowly over 4 to 6 hours to minimize adverse effects; some practitioners advocate giving just 50 mg over the first hour as a trial.

Anemia of Chronic Disease

Treatment of ACD is focused on treating the underlying cause (i.e., the precipitating illness). Because these patients are less likely to respond to oral iron supplementation, parenteral iron is recommended. Red blood cell transfusions may become necessary for symptomatic treatment if Hct falls to 27% to 30%. In most cases of ACD, however, Hct will stay above 30%. ACD due to chronic renal failure, HIV infection, and cancer chemotherapy (not anemia related to the cancer itself) might require treatment with drugs that stimulate erythropoiesis given subcutaneously, such as erythropoietin alfa or darbepoetin alfa. The dosage varies according to patient tolerance and hematological requirements. The U.S. Food and Drug Administration recommends the lowest possible dose necessary to eliminate the need for transfusions, so as to prevent dangerously high increases in hemoglobin.

To protect against a potentially dangerous rise in hemoglobin, it is recommended that hemoglobin be checked twice weekly for 2 to 6 weeks after an increase in dose of these erythropoietic agents. Administration should be held for a hemoglobin that exceeds 12 g/dL or rises more than 1 g/dL in any 2-week period. Erythropoietin alfa (Epogen, Procrit) is given three times weekly and then adjusted in dose according to therapeutic response. Darbepoetin alfa (Aranesp) may initially be given weekly and then adjusted in frequency to every 2 weeks. These medications can be administered IV in the hospital or clinical setting. In addition, patients can learn to self-inject these medications subcutaneously, just as diabetic patients learn to self-inject insulin.

Thalassemia

Thalassemia often requires no treatment other than vigilance by the clinician concerning hematological markers. If a clinician diagnoses microcytosis with mild anemia, the patient should not be subjected to further checks for iron deficiency if there is a distinct thalassemic etiology. Thus, clinical vigilance may be all that is required for microcytosis with mild anemia.

Patients with severe anemia, however, such as that associated with beta-thalassemia major and hemoglobin H disease, require regular transfusion with packed RBCs. In addition, these patients require folate supplementation and possibly oral iron chelation therapy to prevent hemosiderosis (focal iron deposition) and hemochromatosis (systemic iron overload) resulting from multiple transfusions. Hemosiderosis of chronic standing may also require referral for a splenectomy, given the high concentration of iron-laden splenic macrophages.

Sideroblastic Anemia

There are few options for the treatment of sideroblastosis. Depending on the severity of anemia, RBC transfusions may be required, with the attendant risks discussed earlier. Large doses (200 mg/day) of vitamin B_6 (pyridoxine, e.g., Beesix) have benefited some patients. Erythropoietin alfa has proven to be of little aid in supporting these patients.

FOLLOW-UP AND REFERRAL

In general, the plan of referral for microcytic anemia should be to isolate the cause of the anemia, initiate treatment in the primary care setting, and involve specialty care referral only as needed. The primary care practitioner, therefore, has the responsibility to perform all screening tests and to determine the underlying cause.

Iron-deficiency Anemia

Mild iron-deficiency anemia necessitates follow-up every 4 to 6 months. There should be no need to retest iron stores after the first follow-up visit after the initial diagnosis, unless indicated by patient complaints or physical examination findings. Thus, typical follow-up testing may consist only of serial CBCs, and referral to a specialist is almost never required unless iron-deficiency anemia is complicated by concurrent diagnoses, including other causes of microcytic anemia, such as GI malignancy or other type of occult blood loss. Such patients may require upper and/or lower endoscopy or other type of work-up to exclude serious pathology. Similarly, anyone 50 years or older with heme-positive stools or evidence of iron-deficiency anemia should be referred for a colonoscopy, unless the risks of colonoscopy outweigh the potential benefits of catching a GI cancer early—such as in much older patients with an increased risk of intestinal perforation with colonoscopy that could prove fatal. Along these lines, iron-deficiency anemia secondary to menorrhagia would necessitate appropriate gynecological referral if procedural interventions, such as uterine ablation or hysterectomy, are indicated.

Anemia of Chronic Disease

ACD follow-up can be more complicated than the follow-up of iron-deficiency anemia. If patients require erythropoietin injections, they should be maintained on a 30-day follow-up schedule once the hemoglobin level is acceptable and has stabilized, to continue for approximately 6 months after initiating therapy. In most cases, only a CBC will be required to determine the effectiveness of therapy. It is exceptional for patients with ACD to require transfusions. Based on initial evaluation, the clinician should refer patients with ACD to gastroenterologists, hepatologists, oncologists, rheumatologists, hematologists, or other specialists depending on the suspected underlying pathology. For example, if the clinician were to detect occult blood in the stool of a patient with microcytic anemia and the history did not reveal a likely cause, referral to a gastroenterologist would be warranted.

Thalassemia

Patients diagnosed with one of the thalassemias may or may not require referral to a hematologist. Although patients with more aggressive thalassemia (such as beta-thalassemia major or hemoglobin H disease) must be referred promptly to a hematologist who will be entrusted with managing the plan of care, patients with alpha- or beta-thalassemia minor may be managed by the primary care practitioner after initial diagnosis. In these patients, it may only be necessary to monitor serial CBCs every 3 to 4 months. More frequent observation and intervention are required, however, for the other types of thalassemia, which require transfusion therapy, and the plan of care established by the hematologist will dictate the follow-up schedule.

Sideroblastic Anemia

Because sideroblastosis is diagnosed by examination of a bone marrow aspirate, early referral to a hematologist is required for suspected sideroblastic anemia. The hematologist may also perform tests to determine lead exposure and resultant damage from lead toxicity, a common etiology of sideroblastic anemia. Follow-up evaluation will become the responsibility of the primary care practitioner, however, and CBCs in these patients should be monitored every 2 to 3 months.

Patient Education: Microcytic Anemia

Education should focus on self-care and primary care management of the underlying cause of microcytic anemia. Self-care teaching encompasses topics such as adherence to the medication regimen, dietary changes, level of activity, self-monitoring for signs and symptoms of anemia, and adjustment to the requirements of new health-related practices. For example, patients with iron-deficiency anemia must be educated to perform the following self-care behaviors: (1) take ferrous sulfate (supplemental iron) on an empty stomach or at most with a small snack; (2) eat foods that are rich in iron, vitamin C, and B-complex vitamins, which are all necessary for proper RBC development; (3) remain as active as possible, and if fatigued, rest before resuming activity; (4) self-monitor for fatigue, shortness of breath, pale-colored stools (before initiating supplemental iron), and palpitations or tachycardia, which may all be associated with decreased oxygen-carrying capacity due to anemia; and (5) share information about iron deficiency so that friends and/or family can assist in lifestyle adjustments that new health-related behaviors will require.

Additional patient education focuses on primary care management. Patients need to understand the importance of timely clinical laboratory evaluations, return follow-up visits, recognizing signs and symptoms of recurrent anemia that should be reported to the clinician, and proper techniques for administering or receiving drugs that must be delivered via a parenteral route, such as erythropoietin or IV iron supplements. The need to remain vigilant for the signs of potential iron overload in patients with severe anemia who are receiving chronic blood transfusions is key, including monitoring for the signs of liver dysfunction, such as nausea, loss of appetite, weight loss, yellowing of the skin, and swelling of the lower legs.

NORMOCYTIC ANEMIA

Normocytic anemia is defined as an anemia associated with normally sized RBCs (MCV = 81 to 99 fL), although normal ranges vary with age. Many forms of normocytic anemia have normally shaped RBCs as well, although some conditions are recognized by characteristically abnormal morphological findings on a peripheral blood smear. Most commonly, this type of anemia results from chronic disease states that lead to a hypoproliferative anemia. However, acute blood loss, hemolysis, volume overload, and some drugs that induce aplastic anemia (e.g., chloramphenicol) are other important etiologies of normocytic anemia.

EPIDEMIOLOGY AND CAUSES

Normocytic anemias cover a broad range of diseases and conditions, each with its own epidemiology and prevalence rate. Thus, normocytic anemia is also an important form of ACD. In turn, it is possible to estimate the incidence of normocytic ACD by recognizing that at least half of all patients with an underlying chronic disease will develop normocytic anemia over the course of their illness, whereas some will develop microcytic ACD as discussed previously.

PATHOPHYSIOLOGY

One mechanism by which normocytic ACD develops is the reduction of the erythrocyte life cycle, presumably through increased phagocytosis by macrophages, which results in the increased clearance of erythrocytes from the circulation. It is not known how or why this happens because there appear to be no intrinsic defects in the erythrocytes. ACD can also be considered a hypoproliferative anemia because of bone marrow suppression (myelosuppression) resulting from the direct effects of inflammatory cytokines. Animal studies have shown that certain inflammatory cytokines such as tumor necrosis factor–α, interferon (IFN)-β, and IFN-γ may underlie this hypoproliferative mechanism in normocytic ACD.

The combination of a reduced erythrocyte lifespan and impaired stem cell production (hypoproliferation) associated with chronic illness typically results in a normocytic, normochromic anemia. Any condition that creates inflammation can therefore cause normocytic ACD. These include but are not limited to chronic infection, chronic inflammatory disorders, autoimmune activation, malignancy (with or without bone marrow invasion), cardiac disease, diabetes mellitus, endocrine disorders (e.g., hypothyroidism, hypoadrenalism, hypopituitarism, hypogonadism), acute renal insufficiency (due to the accumulation of uremic metabolites that decrease RBC lifespan), and chronic renal insufficiency (due to impaired erythropoietin synthesis by the kidneys). Severe trauma, surgery, or major acute disease states such as sepsis and myocardial infarction may also result in normocytic anemia, possibly due to the significant tissue damage and inflammatory responses associated with these events.

Iron metabolism also plays a critical role in the pathogenesis of normocytic ACD. The human body does not have a defined pathway to excrete excess iron. Thus, it is essential to life that the absorption of dietary iron be regulated efficiently. Decreased dietary ingestion or decreased absorption can lead to iron deficiency, whereas excess ingestion or absorption can result in iron overload. This regulation is mediated by the iron-regulatory hormone hepcidin, which binds to the iron export protein ferroportin and induces its internalization and degradation, thus limiting the amount of iron released into the blood.

The major factors that are implicated in hepcidin regulation include tissue iron stores, transferrin saturation, hypoxia, inflammation, and erythropoiesis. Upregulated by the proinflammatory cytokines IL-6 and IL-1 and by the bacterial superantigen lipopolysaccharide, hepcidin has been shown in animal models to directly inhibit iron absorption by the gut, resulting in decreased plasma iron levels. It is known that the erythropoietic demand reduces hepcidin levels in order to increase iron availability for the production of RBCs; however, the molecular details of this mechanism are still being elucidated. Moreover, patients with ACD are less capable of adequate erythropoietin upregulation in response to their anemic state, compared with patients with non-iron-sequestering anemia (e.g., iron-deficiency anemia). Although absolute erythropoietin levels may be increased in ACD, compared with nonanemic normal values, the bone marrow in ACD demonstrates a decreased erythropoietic response to this growth factor.

Aplastic anemia also results in a hypoproliferative normocytic anemia. This may be a primary condition affecting only the erythroid lineage or it may encompass more than one cell line (e.g., white blood cells [WBCs] or platelets), which would indicate a hypoproliferative defect in an earlier common progenitor cell that gives rise to more than one bone marrow lineage. Aplastic anemia may also be secondarily associated with certain types of viral infections in high-risk individuals, such as parvovirus B19 infection in patients with sickle cell disease or hereditary spherocytosis. A failure of erythropoietin production by the kidneys, as is also observed in chronic renal insufficiency, will similarly result in reduced RBC production and decreased reticulocytosis.

Normocytic anemia may also be caused by a relative increase in plasma volume, such as that which occurs in pregnancy or iatrogenic parenteral overhydration. This results in a dilutional drop in plasma hemoglobin, which may be physiological, as in pregnancy, or which may be reversible via pharmacological diuresis, as in the case of fluid overload.

Increased blood loss, such as from acute bleeding or hemolysis, is another major cause of normocytic anemia. As bleeding progresses and the marrow undergoes reticulocytosis, MCV may be transiently increased due to the relatively larger size of reticulocytes. However, once plasma and bone marrow iron stores are exhausted, hemoglobin production decreases, and this anemia transitions to a normocytic state and then eventually into a microcytic anemia characteristic of iron-deficiency anemia, as discussed previously in this chapter.

If hemolysis occurs intravascularly, fragmented RBCs termed *schistocytes* are seen on peripheral blood smear. This type of anemia is most commonly associated with hemolytic uremic syndrome (HUS), thrombotic thrombocytopenic purpura (TTP), disseminated intravascular coagulation (DIC), or heart valve abnormalities that cause mechanical RBC shearing. Hemolysis may also occur extravascularly with clearance of RBCs by the reticuloendothelial system. This is characterized by rounded RBCs termed *spherocytes* on peripheral blood smear and occurs most commonly due to splenic removal of RBCs, as seen in hypersplenism or autoimmune hemolytic anemia (AIHA).

Immune-mediated hemolysis typically occurs when RBC-specific antibodies coat erythrocytes, rendering them prone to splenic removal or direct hemolysis by antibody-mediated complement fixation. RBC-specific antibodies may form as a consequence of antibody upregulation from viral infections such as mononucleosis, malignancies (especially chronic lymphocytic leukemia), or autoimmune disorders such as systemic lupus erythematosus. When these antibodies are primarily of the immunoglobulin (Ig)G class, they are known as *warm agglutinins* because they result in RBC aggregation (agglutination) at warmer temperatures, due to the binding of two RBCs at a time (one to each of the IgG molecule's two antigen-binding sites). In contrast, IgM RBC-specific antibodies, such as those associated with *Mycoplasma* infection, are called *cold agglutinins* because they are capable of causing RBC aggregation at relatively lower temperatures by virtue of their greater number of antigen-binding and complement fixation sites that results from their tendency to cluster in pentamers (i.e., aggregates of 5 IgM molecules with a total of 10 antigen-specific binding sites).

Extravascular hemolysis may also result from a host of intrinsic RBC membrane defects, such as mutations in the membrane protein spectrin that cause hereditary spherocytosis. In addition, mutations in certain cytoplasmic enzymes render RBCs more prone to hemolysis. A prime example involves disorders of glucose-6-phosphate dehydrogenase (G-6-PD), an enzyme critical to the production of glutathione, a powerful reducing agent and the RBC's main protective mechanism against highly oxidizing compounds such as naphthalene (the active chemical agent found in mothballs) and certain drugs such as trimethoprim-sulfamethoxazole (Bactrim), primaquine, and dapsone.

CLINICAL PRESENTATION

Subjective

A patient's clinical presentation will depend on the severity of the anemia. Because normocytic anemia rarely presents with moderate to severe anemia of less than 30% Hct, many patients with this diagnosis do not report subjective findings. On closer questioning, however, they might note malaise or fatigue.

Objective

The objective findings of normocytic anemia are the same as for microcytic anemia, as discussed previously in this chapter.

DIAGNOSTIC REASONING

Diagnostic Tests

Initial testing begins with a CBC. The clinician should expect the finding of anemia unaccompanied by an alteration in RBC indices (MCV, MCH, MCHC) to establish the diagnosis of normocytic normochromic anemia, such as that associated with acute blood loss, sepsis, underlying malignancy, mechanical shearing of RBCs from prosthetic heart valves, aplastic anemia, or normocytic ACD.

Subsequent testing includes an absolute reticulocyte count (normal range for adults is 0.5% to 2.5% of the total RBC count), reticulocytes being the less mature stage of RBCs. They acquire their name from their fine cytoplasmic network of ribosomal RNA used for hemoglobin synthesis, which is called a *reticulum;* this network appears when stained with certain cellular dyes such as new methylene blue. The reticulum is lost as the RBC matures but is prominent in these less mature cells, which are larger than their mature RBC counterparts. Thus, the reticulocyte count is always higher than normal in any proliferative condition (e.g., proliferative normocytic anemia). Although overall MCV may be elevated due to this abundance of immature reticulocytes in some forms of anemia, MCV may paradoxically be normal in a true microcytic anemia with a significant reticulocytosis, because the average (mean) RBC size may appear normal in the face of both smaller mature RBCs and larger reticulocytes. Thus, the clinician must keep in mind that size descriptions such as normocytic and microcytic typically refer to the RBC itself, whereas MCV is an average size assessment of the overall erythroid cell lineage.

Proliferative microcytic anemia may be difficult to diagnose solely from laboratory testing. If the patient has a recent (but not acute) history of trauma, a diagnosis of proliferative microcytic anemia secondary to hemorrhage should be considered. However, when hemorrhage is not part of the clinical picture, attention should turn to evaluating the patient for hemolysis as a potential etiology. Testing for hemolysis requires a peripheral smear, as RBC morphology is useful in determining the cause of the hemolysis. Possible morphological changes in RBC appearance include spherocytes, sickle cells, and schistocytes. Spherocytes are erythrocytes shaped like rounded spheres or globes, which are abnormal shapes for an erythrocyte. Sickle cells assume the shape of a quarter moon or the curved metal blade of a sickle cutting tool, from which these erythrocytes take their name. Schistocytes, on the other hand, are classically described as "fragmented" and appear on microscopy as many varied shapes.

Further genetic testing may be required if these abnormal RBC morphologies are detected on a peripheral smear. The presence of spherocytes necessitates obtaining a Coombs' test to detect anti-RBC antibodies, because a positive Coombs' test suggests hemolysis due to AIHA, whereas a negative test may suggest hereditary spherocytosis. The presence of sickle cells on a smear implies a sickle cell anemia diagnosis or one of its variants, such as sickle beta-thalassemia or sickle C disease. Schistocytes require the clinician to order tests for prothrombin time (PT) and partial thromboplastin time (PTT), because elevated PT and PTT values may reflect disseminated intravascular coagulation (DIC) if there is also thrombocytopenia, given that platelet consumption from widespread thrombi and microthrombi is characteristic of this disorder. This results in bleeding and/or oozing, which may be refractory to treatment and ultimately prove fatal. Normal PT and PTT values in the presence of schistocytes suggest any one of several diagnoses, including severe hypertension, HUS or TTP, heart valve abnormalities (such as mitral valve stenosis), vasculitis, or hemolysis with concurrent elevated liver enzymes and low platelets (HELLP) syndrome. HELLP syndrome is typically associated with pregnancy, especially later-term pregnancies, and delivery of the baby is the primary intervention.

Although a peripheral blood smear typically reveals morphological changes in RBCs in the patient with hemolysis, RBC shape may be normal in some forms of hemolysis, such as with G-6-PD deficiency. A low level of G-6-PD in the absence of morphological changes in the peripheral blood smear of a patient with normocytic anemia strongly implicates the lack of this enzyme as the cause for the hemolysis. However, G-6-PD levels measured during an acute attack of hemolytic anemia may appear paradoxically elevated in patients with underlying G-6-PD deficiency because of the relatively higher concentration of G-6-PD found in reticulocytes, which are upregulated during acute hemolysis as the bone marrow attempts to compensate for blood loss due to hemolyzed RBCs. Thus, serum levels are often normal during acute hemolytic attacks, and the diagnosis of G-6-PD deficiency must be confirmed by redrawing G-6-PD levels several weeks after the acute anemia has resolved.

Should the G-6-PD level be within normal limits in a patient who reports voiding dark-red urine in the morning, then it is necessary to consider conducting the Ham acidified serum lysis test, as dark-red urine raises suspicion of paroxysmal nocturnal hemoglobinuria (PNH). The traditional Ham acidified serum lysis test may provide a definitive diagnosis, although state-of-the-art diagnostic testing typically involves flow cytometric analysis, which directly evaluates RBCs for reduced or absent levels of the cell surface molecules CD55 and CD59 that result from the genetic defects underlying PNH.

In patients diagnosed with a hypoproliferative normocytic anemia with a normal MCV and low reticulocyte count, attention should turn to the WBC and platelet counts. If both are low, the clinician should suspect pancytopenia affecting all the major bone marrow lineages. If the WBC and thrombocyte counts are high, however, then either ACD or renal disease is the likely cause of the normocytic anemia. Subsequent evaluation should therefore involve renal function studies (e.g., blood urea nitrogen and creatinine) and a careful review of the patient's medical history to guide further evaluation. Assessing endogenous erythropoietin levels is an important part of this work-up as well.

Differential Diagnosis

The differential for normocytic anemia includes mixed anemias of other classifications. Differentiation should be made between three major causative mechanisms: *deficiency* of various factors needed for normal RBC development (e.g., iron, vitamin B_{12}, folic acid, pyridoxine [vitamin B_6]); *central* RBC production abnormalities—caused by impaired bone marrow function (e.g., ACD, anemia of older adults, malignant blood disorders); and *peripheral* disorders of RBC loss (e.g., bleeding, hemolysis). Mixed anemias may appear normocytic because the MCV is within normal range, even though iron-deficient RBCs may be small and vitamin B_{12}- or folate-deficient RBCs are megaloblastic. Moreover, because ACD is part of the differential for microcytic anemia as well as normocytic anemia, the clinician must distinguish between the RBC indices of these two forms of ACD, in addition to focusing on the underlying chronic pathology.

MANAGEMENT

The management of normocytic anemia focuses on the cause of the disorder. In the initial phase of management, treatment should be symptomatic, alleviating the common downstream effects of anemia. Subsequent management consists of correcting, stabilizing, or preventing the underlying cause of the normocytic anemia (e.g., ACD, AIHA, heart valve abnormalities, vasculitis, severe hypertension, HELLP syndrome, DIC).

Apart from appropriately treating the underlying disease pathology, management of ACD may sometimes consist of only watchful waiting; however, if the patient's Hct drops below 30%, the clinician may consider using recombinant human erythropoietin (rhEPO) or darbepoetin. Dosing with rhEPO or darbepoetin for ACD is highly individualized and is dependent on the underlying causative disease pathology. In general, treatment should be targeted to increase hemoglobin to 10 to 12 g/dL, but not by more than 1 g/dL in a 2-week period.

Starting doses of rhEPO range from 50 to 150 U/kg subcutaneously (SC) three times per week (or 50 to 200 mcg every 2 weeks for darbepoetin), depending on the underlying pathology, and should only be initiated after carefully reviewing dosing guidelines in the specific product labeling. For the first 3 weeks of therapy, the clinician should check Hct twice weekly until the dosage level is stabilized. An interval of 2 to 6 weeks may pass before the Hct undergoes an appreciable elevation. These agents should ideally be used with oral iron supplementation if the patient is able to tolerate it. If there is no response after 6 weeks, the clinician should confirm compliance with iron therapy. If noncompliance with iron therapy is noted, the patient should restart iron supplementation if possible. If there is no response after 6 weeks, the patient may receive a trial of IV iron supplementation.

Endogenous erythropoietin levels do not aid in determining the starting dose of exogenous erythropoietin alfa therapy. Moreover, the clinician may increase the dosage and frequency of administration until the Hct rises to an appropriate level. As the dosage level rises, however, it is possible that polycythemia (i.e., Hct greater than 60% to 65%) may develop as a side effect of exogenous erythropoietin usage. Thus, if hemoglobin rises to 12 or 13 g/dL or the patient becomes frankly polycythemic, the drug should be discontinued. Within a week of discontinuing therapy, the Hct should start to decline. Otherwise, in rare cases, it may be necessary to phlebotomize the patient, removing enough volume to cause a drop in Hct.

After the clinician achieves and maintains a normal Hct, the dosage level may be reduced and/or the frequency of administration changed. Thus, the management of dosing of exogenous RBC growth factors such as erythropoietin alfa (Epogen, Procrit) or darbepoetin-alfa (Aranesp) requires expert consultation with a hematologist or other appropriate specialist, given the significant risks of overdosage associated with polycythemia, including thrombosis, stroke, and myocardial infarction. As a result, RBC growth factors are rarely used to treat anemia outside of chronic kidney disease.

First-line treatment of AIHA consists of oral or IV corticosteroid therapy, such as prednisone 1 to 2 mg/kg per day in divided doses. Thus, an adult who weighs 70 kg would receive between 70 and 140 mg of prednisone in two or three divided doses each day. After an initial response is documented, the prednisone dose is decreased to 20 to 30 mg/day within several weeks, followed by a slow taper over several months to prevent recurrence. As for other patients on chronic corticosteroid therapy, supplementation with calcium, vitamin D, and folic acid may be initiated, along with bisphosphonate therapy, as prophylaxis against osteoporosis. If transfusion is required for severe anemia, the clinician should be aware that the risk of transfusion reaction is very high because of crossmatching difficulties for these patients, given their Coombs' test positivity. The clinician should expect that transfused cells will survive no better than the patient's own erythrocytes if the underlying AIHA is left untreated.

Surgical consultation is required for possible splenectomy, should prednisone become ineffective or too toxic from chronic administration. In emergency situations, short-term hemolytic control in 1 to 3 weeks may be achieved with IV immune globulin (500 mg/kg per day for 1 to 4 days). In addition, off-label use of rituximab (Rituxan), an anti-CD20 B-cell-depleting monoclonal antibody therapy, has been used as second-line therapy for AIHA.

Heart valve abnormalities resulting in hemolysis require an individualized plan of care developed with referral to an interventional cardiologist, which may include surgical correction of the abnormality. Many patients with heart valve abnormalities will have already started taking warfarin sodium (Coumadin) to prevent thromboembolic complications. They should not stop taking anticoagulant therapy unless their platelet counts fall along with the Hct or active bleeding is present. However, anticoagulation should be stopped in the face of a rapidly falling hemoglobin, even in the setting of a normal platelet count.

Treatment of vasculitis as an etiology of hemolysis consists of high-dose prednisone, which it may be necessary to raise to 60 mg daily. The clinician should slowly taper the corticosteroid dose as the manifestations of vasculitis resolve, fever declines, and other symptoms abate. Additional immunosuppressive therapy may be required to augment the prednisone. Cyclophosphamide (Cytoxan) in a dose range of 1 to 2 mg/kg per day may be added to the prednisone regimen. These drugs should be taken either along with or after a meal to avoid GI upset. If the dosage of cyclophosphamide exceeds 100 mg, the clinician can anticipate that only 75% of the dose will be absorbed via the GI tract. Therefore, for doses that exceed 100 mg, the dose should be split. Weekly or biweekly monitoring of the patient's CBC, liver and renal function tests, and uric acid level monitoring are necessary, given the potential toxicities of these agents.

Severe hypertension (greater than 180 mm Hg systolic and 110 mm Hg diastolic) can be treated with one antihypertensive agent or a combination of agents. If hemolysis secondary to severe hypertension presents in a patient who is known to the clinician, drug therapy should be adjusted according to the history of treatment for the individual patient (see the section on management of hypertension in Chapter 35).

HELLP syndrome typically occurs during the third trimester of pregnancy. Because of its late onset in pregnancy, delivery of the infant is the treatment of choice. Most hematological indices return to baseline within 2 to 3 days after delivery; however, thrombocytopenia may persist for a week or more.

DIC requires treatment with heparin and platelet transfusions (replacement therapy). Platelet transfusion thresholds run as low as 20,000/mcL to minimize the risk of spontaneous bleeding, 50,000/mcL in the setting of active bleeding, or higher in the anticipation of invasive procedures. Platelet transfusions, however, are often futile because of severe consumptive coagulopathy that quickly extracts platelets from the circulation.

Although the role of heparin is controversial in the treatment of DIC, especially before or after surgery, heparin is mandated if thrombus is diagnosed in DIC. In addition, fresh frozen plasma is an important therapy in DIC. It is often used empirically, rather than waiting for tests that specifically confirm deficits in certain clotting factors. Before symptoms are present, anticoagulation in the form of low molecular weight heparin (LMWH) such as enoxaparin (Lovenox) is an accepted therapy for patients at risk of postoperative deep vein thrombosis, provided renal function is normal (because LMWH is renally cleared). There are also recombinant versions of certain human clotting factors such as factor VIII that are available for use in significant bleeding disorders.

Because patients who require heparin therapy for DIC need around-the-clock nursing care, they require hospitalization and typically intensive care, where they can receive 500 to 750 U/hr of heparin, according to established weight-based dosing nomograms. Platelet transfusions should be used to maintain the thrombocyte count. In addition, cryoprecipitate should be given to raise the fibrinogen level to 150 mg/dL or more.

Prevention of hemolysis in G-6-PD deficiency by avoiding hemolytic triggers is preferred to treating the hemolysis once an attack has initiated; however, the primary care clinician must understand both prevention and treatment strategies for hemolysis resulting from G-6-PD deficiency. The avoidance of oxidant drugs, such as dapsone (Avlosulfon), quinidine (Quinaglute Duratabs), and sulfonamide drugs (e.g., sulfamethoxazole/trimethoprim), as well as environmental triggers such as naphthalene (moth balls), is critical to prevent hemolysis in patients who are G-6-PD-deficient. Treatment for acute hemolytic attacks consists of discontinuing all oxidant drugs, increasing oral and/or IV fluids, and administering RBC transfusions as indicated by the Hct level. Screening for G-6-PD deficiency among patients who may require one or more oxidant drugs has become standard in the management of patients with HIV/AIDS (e.g., sulfamethoxazole/trimethoprim prophylaxis or treatment for *Pneumocystis jirovecii* pneumonia) and patients who are susceptible to urinary tract infections (UTIs) and may require frequent antibiotic treatment, such as older females.

FOLLOW-UP AND REFERRAL

If normocytic anemia is not accompanied by an abnormal reticulocyte count or abnormal erythrocyte morphology, then follow-up every 6 months is sufficient for most patients, and no referral is required for these patients. Follow-up should consist of a history and physical examination, along with a CBC and reticulocyte count. The patient's records should be constructed so that these values are readily retrievable to allow long-term monitoring.

If the peripheral smear is positive for spherocytes, sickle cells, or schistocytes, the primary care practitioner should refer the patient to a hematologist for further diagnostic evaluation and management. The hematologist will create a plan of care, which the primary care practitioner can comanage. Routine follow-up with the hematologist should occur every 3 to 6 months, depending on the severity and chronicity of the underlying pathological mechanism of the anemia, such as hemolysis.

If the reticulocyte count is low and the clinician discovers low WBC and platelet counts as well, the patient is diagnosed with pancytopenia, and referral to a hematologist is indicated. If the evaluation of a bone marrow aspirate suggests the need for treatment, the hematologist will determine the plan of care. Normal or high WBC and platelet counts rule out pancytopenia, which suggests the need for referrals to specialists who can diagnose and treat the underlying cause of the normocytic anemia. These referrals may include gastroenterologists, hepatologists, rheumatologists, infectious disease specialists, nephrologists, or cardiologists.

Patient Education: Normocytic Anemia

Education for patients should follow the pattern outlined in the section on microcytic anemia, addressing self-care regimens and primary care management. Self-care of normocytic anemia is similar to that for other anemias. Patients should be instructed to remain as active as possible, and, if they become fatigued, to rest. In addition, the patient must remain vigilant for the signs and symptoms of a declining Hct—malaise, fatigue, shortness of breath, tachycardia, and palpitations. Individualized patient education should also address the underlying cause of normocytic anemia. For example, if a deficiency in G-6-PD is diagnosed, the patient should be made aware of this and of all the potential oxidant drugs and chemical exposures that could trigger hemolysis and should be avoided.

Because of the chronicity of several of these causes, patients must be instructed at every visit to adhere to their treatment regimens and follow-up plan, including pertinent laboratory testing. For example, patients with sickle cell disease require frequent follow-up, infectious disease prophylaxis, and assistance from their families/support person(s) during sickle crises. Establishing a plan for the management of sickle cell crises is an important preparatory step in anticipation of an event and is discussed in greater detail later in this chapter in the section on sickle cell anemia.

MACROCYTIC ANEMIA

Macrocytic anemia (or megaloblastic anemia) is defined as anemia with an MCV equal to or greater than 100 fL. These anemic states are typically normochromic and may be normoblastic or megaloblastic with large erythroid precursors. Macrocytic anemia results most commonly from defects in DNA metabolism or changes in RBC membrane structure.

EPIDEMIOLOGY AND CAUSES

The prevalence of macrocytic anemia is greatest among people of northern European and Caucasian descent. Incidence increases past 60 years of age, but it has been observed in all age-groups. Overall, both sexes are equally affected by macrocytic anemia, although certain forms show a gender predisposition, particularly as related to autoimmune phenomena that are more common in females.

Macrocytic anemia has four general categories of causes: (1) vitamin B_{12} deficiency, (2) folate deficiency, (3) antimetabolite drugs such as methotrexate, and (4) miscellaneous etiologies. The most common cause of megaloblastic anemia is a hereditary autoimmune disorder called *pernicious anemia,* which results from a deficiency of vitamin B_{12}, a critical component of the RBC maturation pathway and effective erythropoiesis. In contrast to other forms of macrocytic anemia, pernicious anemia affects females more than males at a rate of 5:1, with peak onset occurring in midlife, often after age 40 years.

PATHOPHYSIOLOGY

Vitamin B_{12} Deficiency

Pernicious anemia is a macrocytic anemia caused by a hereditary autoimmune disorder in which destructive antibodies are directed against intrinsic factor, a 45 kDa protein produced by gastric parietal cells that binds to dietary vitamin B_{12} (cobalamin) during the digestion and absorption of nutrients, which is critical to DNA synthesis and RBC maturation. Under normal conditions, dietary vitamin B_{12} is cleaved from carrier proteins in the acidic environment of the stomach by the protease pepsin. It is then rapidly bound by cobalamin-binding factors known as *R-proteins,* which are found in gastric secretions and the saliva. As these complexes are not absorbable, they pass out of the stomach and into the duodenum. However, the alkaline environment produced by pancreatic proteases in the duodenum allows for the release of vitamin B_{12} from R-factor and its subsequent rapid, high-affinity binding to intrinsic factor. This newly formed vitamin B_{12}–intrinsic factor complex then binds to specific receptors for this complex (e.g., cubilin) in the ileum, where absorption into ileal enterocytes is mediated primarily by transcobalamin II (complexes bound to transcobalamin I and transcobalamin III are metabolically inert).

Vitamin B_{12} is essential to the maturation of erythrocytes via the conversion of homocysteine into methionine and the demethylation of tetrahydrofolate. Demethylated tetrahydrofolate is a key component in the conversion of deoxyuridate to thymidylate and in purine synthesis involved in DNA metabolism. Anti-intrinsic factor antibodies are present in up to three-fourths of all patients with pernicious anemia and act either by blocking the binding of vitamin B_{12} to intrinsic factor or by blocking the binding of the cobalamin-intrinsic factor complex to ileal enterocyte receptors. In addition, autoantibodies produced against gastric parietal cells and pathogenic CD4+ T cells act in concert to destroy gastric parietal cells, producing a morphological change in the stomach lining known as *atrophic gastritis.*

A subsequent decrease in gastric acid production compounds vitamin B_{12} deficiency, as cobalamin cannot be freed from its carrier proteins in the less acidic stomach environment, thereby preventing its subsequent binding to intrinsic factor in the duodenum. Prolonged use of medications that counter gastric acid production such as histamine-2 blockers (e.g., ranitidine, famotidine, cimetidine) and proton pump inhibitors (e.g., esomeprazole, omeprazole, pantoprazole) have a similar effect. The widely used diabetic drug metformin (Glucophage) also decreases vitamin B_{12} absorption in up to one-third of patients taking this medication.

Thus, insufficient levels of vitamin B_{12} cause erythrocytes to expand in size compared with normal RBCs, thereby producing a characteristic megaloblastic anemia. In turn, pernicious anemia is characterized by a macrocytic anemia, a low serum level of vitamin B_{12}, atrophic gastritis, achlorhydria secondary to gastric atrophy, and a greater probability of other autoimmune diseases, such as hypothyroidism and vitiligo.

Normally, the complex of vitamin B_{12} and intrinsic factor is absorbed through the terminal ileum and then travels to the liver where it is stored. Studies have estimated that the liver may store up to 5,000 mcg/day of vitamin B_{12}. Because the body requires no more than 10 mcg/day, liver stores of vitamin B_{12} typically last for several years before anemia ensues. Therefore, megaloblastic anemia is insidious in onset. In patients with HIV disease and liver dysfunction, both the depletion of liver stores of vitamin B_{12} and the destruction of storage sites within the liver have been identified as underlying causes of megaloblastic anemia.

Dietary deficiency of vitamin B_{12} in the typical American diet is rare because of its rich supply of animal proteins. However, because meats and dairy products are the only dietary source of vitamin B_{12}, vegetarians and particularly vegans (who completely avoid all meat and dairy products) may consume inadequate amounts of vitamin B_{12}. Other reasons for poor absorption include a number of mechanical causes, such as those associated with surgical GI resections (e.g., partial or total gastrectomy, resections of the terminal jejunum or proximal ileum) and Crohn's disease, which can destroy sections of the small intestine where absorption of vitamin B_{12} would otherwise occur.

Folic Acid Deficiency

Folic acid is a critical nutrient that acts in concert with vitamin B_{12} to further nuclear maturation in erythrocytes. Folate deficiency leads to decreased levels of tetrahydrofolate, an important building block of DNA. As with vitamin B_{12} deficiency, abnormal erythroid precursors deficient in folate are prone to intramedullary hemolysis within the bone marrow, leading to a characteristic macrocytic anemia clinically indistinguishable from that of vitamin B_{12} deficiency. Animal models have also demonstrated that RBC precursors in folate deficiency are more prone to apoptosis (programmed cell death), although human studies are less definitive. However, in contrast to vitamin B_{12} deficiency, folic acid deficiency does not produce neurological sequelae.

Macrocytic anemia due to folate deficiency presents with a low serum folate level and a normal level of vitamin B_{12}. It is almost always related to inadequate dietary intake, although folic acid is found in citrus fruits, dark-green leafy vegetables, and animal proteins. Adequate dietary intake is 50 to 100 mcg/day, except in pregnant patients who need 800 mcg/day to prevent neural tube defects during fetal development. Even in developed countries such as the United States, pregnant patients may not consume adequate amounts of folate in their diets, with folic acid deficiency increasing in incidence in multigravid patients and with multigestational pregnancies.

Less common causes of folic acid deficiency are impaired metabolism and storage of folate. The liver typically stores enough folic acid as N^5-methyltetrahydrofolic acid (approximately 5,000 mcg) to serve the body's needs for several months, given the body's use of 50 to 100 mcg/day, as long as hemolysis and increased erythrocyte production are not issues, as in sickle cell anemia. There are many causes of impaired folate metabolism and hepatic storage, including chronic alcohol use, which results in decreased enterohepatic cycling, and drugs such as phenytoin (Dilantin), sulfamethoxazole/trimethoprim (Bactrim), methotrexate (Trexall, Rheumatrex), and oral contraceptives, which contribute to folic acid deficiency via a variety of mechanisms.

Impaired absorption of folic acid is another cause of folic acid deficiency. Tropical sprue, surgical removal of part of the GI tract, inflammatory bowel diseases such as Crohn's disease and ulcerative colitis, and some intestinal parasitic infections are the primary causes of impaired folic acid absorption. Unlike vitamin B_{12}, however, folic acid can be absorbed along the entire GI tract.

Antimetabolite Drugs

Any chemical that serves as a potential inhibitor of DNA or RNA synthesis is a potential cause of macrocytic anemia. Drugs such as hydroxyurea (an inhibitor of ribonucleotide reductase), the antiviral zidovudine, and the chemotherapies methotrexate, azathioprine, and 6-mercaptopurine can all cause macrocytosis, with methotrexate being best known for leading to anemia. Methotrexate interrupts purine metabolism in the liver by competitively preventing molecular binding of folic acid with dihydrofolate reductase, an enzyme required for the storage of folic acid. Thus, less folic acid can be stored, thereby leading to a reduction in serum folate levels and subsequent macrocytic anemia.

Miscellaneous Etiologies

Various unrelated causes of macrocytic anemia include thiamine (vitamin B_1) or pyridoxine (vitamin B_6) deficiencies and Lesch-Nyhan syndrome. Macrocytic anemia may also be caused by chronic alcoholism (i.e., ingestion of at least 80 g of alcohol per day) via mechanisms other than folate deficiency, such as changes in RBC membranes caused by the alcohol breakdown product acetaldehyde. In addition, liver disease may lead to macrocytic anemia, possibly via increased lipid deposition in RBC membranes and myelodysplasia, which causes a normoblastic (albeit macrocytic) anemia.

PRESENTATION

Subjective

Patients with macrocytic anemia may present with complaints of stomatitis, glossitis, nausea, anorexia, diarrhea, peripheral neuropathies, and malaise if they have pernicious anemia. Macrocytic anemia due to other causes will present similarly. Patients may also have complaints consistent with peripheral neuropathy (e.g., numbness or tingling of the hands and feet, decreased reflexes, positive Babinski sign [upward plantar flexion]), which typically do not occur in folate deficiency, but are part of the symptom constellation associated with chronic vitamin B_{12} deficiency.

Objective

The clinician may note any of the following findings on physical examination with macrocytic anemia: pale or icteric mucosa, a dry and cracked oropharynx, a thickened and smooth-surfaced tongue, tachycardia, a systolic ejection murmur, tachypnea, and diffuse abdominal tenderness without organomegaly. Long standing vitamin B_{12} deficiency may also result in a variety of neurological signs and pathological manifestations, including peripheral neuropathy in a glove-and-stocking distribution on the distal extremities, increased or decreased deep tendon reflexes, impaired positional sense, diminished vibratory sensation in the lower extremities, a positive Romberg sign, a variable Babinski sign, and pronounced irritability or other mental status changes, including frank dementia in severe cases. Of the megaloblastic anemias, neurological signs related to myelin defects in the dorsal and lateral spinal columns present only in vitamin B_{12} deficiency and not with isolated folic acid deficiency.

DIAGNOSTIC REASONING

Diagnostic Tests

Initial testing involves confirmation of megaloblastic macrocytic anemia on a peripheral blood smear. Expected findings include anemia and an elevated MCV (greater than 100 fL). MCHC is typically within normal limits, as megaloblastic anemia is usually normochromic. It is important to note that the pathological processes that underlie macrocytic anemia may occur simultaneously with causes of microcytic or normocytic anemia, such as iron deficiency and thalassemia (microcytic) or ACD (normocytic). In these mixed anemias, MCV may actually be within a normal range, and the RBC indices are difficult to predict and interpret, typically requiring referral to a hematologist.

Reticulocytes may be either low or normal in number, depending on the cause of the anemia. If the cause of macrocytosis is a deficiency in vitamin B_{12}, then the serum vitamin B_{12} level should be less than 0.1 mcg/mL, and hypersegmented neutrophils will be present on the peripheral blood smear. Macro-ovalocytes will also be evident. In the case of folic acid deficiency, the serum folate level will typically be less than 3 ng/mL, although levels may vary in patients with chronic deficiency. Homocysteine and methylmalonic acid levels can distinguish between these two etiologies, with both values being elevated in vitamin B_{12} deficiency, whereas only homocysteine levels are elevated in folic acid deficiency. Common to both etiologies is a high serum iron level and findings consistent with mild hemolysis, including low haptoglobin, elevated lactate dehydrogenase (LDH), and mildly increased unconjugated bilirubin.

The Schilling test is rarely performed today but was classically used to diagnose GI malabsorption as a common etiology of vitamin B_{12} deficiency. The Schilling test uses orally administered radiolabeled vitamin B_{12} to measure the ability of the small intestine to absorb vitamin B_{12}, which is subsequently secreted in the urine. It involves a two-stage 24-hour urine collection that needs to be done before any radioactive diagnostic scans are performed, as the material used in these scans may confound measurements of the radiolabeled vitamin B_{12}.

When diagnosing iatrogenic etiologies of macrocytic anemia, it is important to recognize that blood levels of specific drugs such as the antimetabolite methotrexate may vary according to individual laboratory standards. Additional tests may be indicated to assess for changes in liver function that may also be impaired by drugs, as reflected in elevations of hepatic transaminases (alanine aminotransferase [ALT] and aspartate aminotransferase [AST]), bilirubin, and LDH. Urobilinogen may also be detected in the urinalysis.

Differential Diagnosis

The differential diagnoses for macrocytic anemia include all of the causes identified in this section: vitamin B_{12} deficiency, folate deficiency, antimetabolite drugs, and miscellaneous causes. In addition, the differential diagnosis includes anemia of chronic liver disease and myelodysplasia.

A thorough patient history often leads the clinician to the cause of the anemia even when diagnostic laboratory results might be equivocal. For example, if the patient is pregnant, then the clinician should suspect folate deficiency over vitamin B_{12} deficiency. In addition, megaloblastic anemia due to vitamin B_{12} or folate deficiency is also often characterized by thrombocytopenia and neutropenia due to defects in megakaryocyte and myeloid precursors. This same pancytopenia is also commonly seen in the various types of myelodysplasia.

MANAGEMENT

A general management approach to the patient with macrocytic anemia should address the cause of the anemia, as well as downstream effects of the anemia itself. Thus, the goal is to correct or ameliorate the underlying cause while addressing clinically significant sequelae of the anemia. For example, it might be appropriate to deliver supplemental vitamin B_{12} or folate while providing RBC transfusions as needed. However, transfusion is rarely indicated for macrocytic anemia, other than in severe cases. These patients are often older and unable to handle large volume transfusions, given the risk of fluid overload.

If the cause of vitamin B_{12} deficiency anemia is not pernicious anemia or malabsorption, then the clinician may use the following guideline for oral supplementation: prescribe up to 1,000 mcg/day of oral cobalamin until normal serum levels of vitamin B_{12} are achieved (usually in 6 to 12 weeks after the initiation of therapy). High doses such as these may even be effective in some cases of pernicious anemia, despite the lack of intrinsic factor, given the presence of an additional, albeit less efficient, GI absorption pathway that functions independently of intrinsic factor and does not require absorption through the terminal ileum. Daily oral therapy, however, requires a high degree of patient commitment and compliance.

In most cases of pernicious anemia, especially if neurological symptoms are present, more aggressive therapy is warranted. In these cases, the preferred route of administration is parenteral with 1,000 mcg of vitamin B_{12} given intramuscularly once daily for the first 7 days and then weekly for 1 month, followed by once monthly administration for life. Lower parenteral doses of 100 mcg have been advocated, although toxicity related to vitamin B_{12} overtreatment is not typically observed, as excess vitamin B_{12} is excreted in the urine. After depleted stores are replaced, patients may transition to oral, sublingual, or nasal preparations of vitamin B_{12} for ease of administration; however, serum levels of vitamin B_{12} and methylmalonic acid should still be followed periodically to ensure compliance with these medication regimens.

For folic acid deficiency, the clinician should prescribe 1 mg/day of supplemental folic acid, and the effects of therapy should be reassessed after 2 to 3 months. It is critical to understand that treatment of folic acid deficiency will reverse many of the hematological defects shared with vitamin B_{12} deficiency; however, the neurological manifestations of cobalamin deficiency will progress and may be devastating if treated inappropriately with folic acid supplementation alone. Thus, it is important to rule out vitamin B_{12} deficiency before starting a folate replacement regimen, and if empiric therapy must be started before testing is available, patients should be treated with both folic acid and vitamin B_{12} supplementation until each deficiency is ruled out. Patients suspected of having either condition who do not respond with a significant reticulocytosis after 1 week of therapy should be evaluated further for a mixed anemic process, which may have been originally masked by megaloblastic manifestations. Note that even one nutritious and well-balanced meal eaten occasionally can normalize folate levels in a person with true deficiency.

If the cause of the macrocytic anemia is an antimetabolite drug or other iatrogenic drug toxicity, the patient should discontinue all suspected drugs. Laboratory tests for elevated drug levels should be ordered, and liver transaminases (AST, ALT) should be monitored for evidence of liver dysfunction, as well as coagulation times (PT/INR and PTT) as indications of hepatic synthetic function. For patients with macrocytic anemia from miscellaneous causes, the individual etiologies and underlying disorders must be addressed.

It is also important to evaluate serum potassium levels in profoundly anemic patients once they start treatment, as increased erythropoiesis will markedly increase potassium utilization. As a result, as the anemia corrects, these patients may become significantly hypokalemic, requiring oral potassium repletion.

FOLLOW-UP AND REFERRAL

Follow-up of the patient with vitamin B_{12} deficiency involves assessing the severity of the anemia. Serial CBCs and monitoring of vitamin B_{12} levels are required on a monthly basis after starting oral cobalamin therapy. If parenteral therapy is initiated, more frequent testing is required (e.g., every 2 weeks). Additional testing includes liver function tests; if these reveal elevated transaminase levels before cobalamin replacement is started, then their course should be evaluated every 2 to 4 weeks. If liver enzyme levels rise after the start of therapy, more frequent testing might be required, as well as additional diagnostic testing for evolving hepatotoxicity.

Referral for vitamin B_{12} deficiency is often not required unless the diagnosis is pernicious anemia or the patient suffers from a particularly difficult-to-diagnose mixed anemic process. A hematologist and gastroenterologist should be consulted in the event of pernicious anemia, as these patients are at greater risk for gastric cancer, carcinoid tumors, and colorectal carcinoma. Thus, stool should be monitored periodically for occult blood as a trigger for colonoscopy. In addition, the hyperhomocysteinemia that accompanies vitamin B_{12} or folic acid deficiency is a risk factor for atherosclerosis and venous thromboembolism and should be addressed as an independent risk factor.

Follow-up of the patient with folic acid deficiency consists of a CBC and serum folate level drawn 2 to 3 months after starting therapy. The problem should be corrected by this point if the patient has adhered to the daily regimen of folic acid replacement. No referrals are indicated unless the anemia does not resolve.

Patient Education: Macrocytic Anemia

Patients need to learn how to enrich their diets with folic acid and vitamin B_{12}. Increasing dark-green leafy vegetables in one or two meals eaten daily can support supplements and other therapies. In addition, patients should be educated about the basic signs and symptoms of macrocytic anemia so that they can self-monitor the effectiveness of therapy and possible recurrence of the anemia.

SICKLE CELL ANEMIA

Sickle cell anemia is an autosomal recessive disorder. The disease is caused by a point mutation in the DNA sequence of the gene for the beta-hemoglobin chain (termed the *hemoglobin S gene*), resulting in a marked hemoglobinopathy in which intracellular hemoglobin molecules form abnormal polymers that cause gross sickling of RBCs under hypoxic conditions. It is therefore diagnosed by the detection of sickled (scythe-shaped) cells on peripheral blood smear, a positive family history, recurrent painful episodes of vaso-occlusive pain, and a pattern demonstrating mutated hemoglobin S on a hemoglobin gel electrophoresis profile.

EPIDEMIOLOGY AND CAUSES

Sickle cell anemia and sickle cell trait are inherited conditions that occur most commonly in people of West African descent. The disease has also been identified in people of European or Middle Eastern ancestry, although these cases are extremely rare. The disease is not prevalent among people of Asian or Pacific Islander descent.

Initial symptoms appear within the first year of life for those born with sickle cell anemia. Given the perinatal manifestations and associated comorbidities, prenatal screening is now available for at-risk patients, consisting of DNA analysis from fetal cells. The procedure should be offered to these patients as part of their prenatal counseling. If both the father and mother have sickle cell trait and each carries one copy of the mutated hemoglobin S gene, their offspring have a one-in-four chance of developing true homozygous sickle cell anemia. In more than 40 states, newborns undergo universal neonatal screening for hemoglobinopathies, including hemoglobin protein electrophoresis screening for sickle cell disease, the thalassemias, and other variant hemoglobinopathies.

Autosomal recessive genes for hemoglobin S are distributed equally between the sexes. Individuals who are homozygous for the hemoglobin S gene will develop sickle cell anemia and experience recurrent sickle cell crises throughout their lives. In addition, overall life expectancy is typically reduced to between 40 and 50 years of age. Those who are heterozygous for the hemoglobin S gene are said to carry the sickle cell trait, which is asymptomatic because hemoglobin A accounts for more than half of their hemoglobin. Approximately 8% to 10% of people of West African descent in the United States carry the sickle cell trait, whereas one in 400 African Americans suffers from actual sickle cell anemia. Sickle cell disease also affects individuals of other ethnicities, but at much lower rates, with approximately 100,000 Americans in total affected by the disease, the vast majority of which are of African descent.

PATHOPHYSIOLOGY

The cause of sickle cell anemia is a point mutation in the genetic sequence of the beta-chain hemoglobin gene, which results in the replacement of glutamic acid by valine at the N-terminal amino acid position 6 of this protein chain. The substitution of valine leads to the production of hemoglobin S, which is poorly soluble and prone to rigid polymerization when in its deoxygenated state. This typically occurs under conditions of physiological stress (such as physical overexertion), muscle tissue ischemia (causing lactic acidosis), dehydration, infection, or exposure to cold environmental temperatures. However, the majority of acute sickling events have no identifiable cause.

Polymerized deoxyhemoglobin S takes on a ropelike form, aligning itself with other polymerized strands and transforming erythrocytes into a rigid, sickled, crescent-like shape. In turn, these sickled erythrocytes regularly become lodged in the microvasculature of various organs and bodily tissues, causing small but highly symptomatic infarcts throughout the body. Sickled cells adhere rigidly to the inner membranes lining small blood vessels, inducing intimal hyperplasia that contributes to the obstruction of free blood flow in the smaller capillaries, as well as RBC hemolysis due to adherence to the inner vessel wall. In turn, RBCs in patients with sickle cell disease have an average lifespan of 17 days, versus the normal length of 100 days.

Sickled cells become lodged in the microvasculature as small thrombi. Once the thrombi are situated against the vascular membrane, they attract plasma proteins, leukocytes, and platelets, creating an occlusion to blood flow. This inflammatory process escalates, as ischemia to the surrounding tissue unfolds. Ischemic injury and infarcts cause pain as perimeter tissue is increasingly starved for oxygen and other nutrients. The rate of sickling increases as tissues become more hypoxic and acidotic. Erythrocytes, with or without hemoglobin S, that are lodged in and around the microthrombi lose intracellular water, which results either in hemolysis occurring before RBC sickling or in escalated sickle cell formation and plasma hyperviscosity. As hypoxia and acidosis increase, more erythrocytes begin to sickle, and nearly all the sickled cells in the area of the thrombus will eventually hemolyze.

The body attempts to compensate for this resultant anemia (which is typically normocytic, unless also associated with iron deficiency or a form of thalassemia) with expansion and upregulation of the bone marrow, which has several pathological implications. Chronically elevated WBC counts result in the production of inflammatory cytokines, which further complicates vaso-occlusive crises. The additional blood cell production and vascular flow may also lead to cardiomegaly and eventually high-output congestive heart failure. This results in greater metabolic and caloric requirements as the affected individual ages, leading to stunted growth and lower-than-average adult weight if the condition is poorly controlled and nutritional requirements are not met with dietary supplements.

Anemia is also worsened by impaired production of the RBC growth factor erythropoietin (which is normally produced in the kidney), due to progressive renal disease from microinfarction of the vasa recta capillaries in the renal medulla. Hemolysis results in hyperbilirubinemia, which predisposes to the development of pigmented cholelithiasis (gallstones). In turn, cholecystectomy is the most common surgical procedure in patients with sickle cell anemia.

The formation of microthrombi occurs in many parts of the body but is especially prone to occur in the chest, vertebrae, and long bones of the legs. In pediatric patients, swelling, tenderness, and inflammation of the hands and feet (especially the fingers and toes, termed *dactylitis*), known as hand–foot syndrome, is a common manifestation before age 2 years. Leg ulcers are also common, typically affecting the skin over the lateral and medial malleoli; these leg ulcers are subject to infection by *Staphylococcus aureus, Pseudomonas, Streptococcus* species, or *Bacteroides.*

Bone manifestations also occur. As ischemia progresses due to vaso-occlusion, the affected bone eventually infarcts and becomes susceptible to osteomyelitis by *Salmonella* species and, less commonly, *S aureus.* Severely debilitating noninfectious aseptic necrosis of the hip or shoulder joints may also occur due to vaso-occlusion of the arterial supply to the femoral or humeral heads, resulting in eventual loss of the entire joint.

Organs including the heart, liver, penis, and kidney also tend to be affected by vaso-occlusive crises, particularly during childhood and adolescence. Priapism (painful and sustained penile erection often lasting several hours) is an emergent condition requiring inpatient treatment with hydration, transfusion, and in some cases surgical intervention to release engorged blood, as ischemia of the penis can lead to tissue necrosis. Retinopathy and its associated complications caused by microvascular ischemia increase in prevalence with age as well; associated complications include proliferative retinopathy and retinal hemorrhage and detachment, as well as retinal artery occlusion. Such changes may begin in childhood, and, in turn, many patients with sickle cell anemia become blind before age 40 years.

Splenic sequestration results when large numbers of sickled erythrocytes become lodged in an engorged, functional spleen during early childhood, resulting in severe anemia and potentially fatal hypovolemic shock, with a mortality rate of 10% to 15%. Because this condition tends to be recurrent, splenectomy is often performed after the first episode. Later in adult life, vaso-occlusive episodes in the spleen lead to autoinfarction, with replacement of the splenic parenchyma by fibrotic tissue, resulting in functional asplenia. Although this precludes the occurrence of splenic sequestration syndrome, splenic autoinfarction results in increased susceptibility to infection by encapsulated organisms, such as *Streptococcus pneumoniae* and *Haemophilus influenzae*.

In addition to splenic sequestration, severe anemia may also result from aplastic crises, in which patients experience extreme suppression of bone marrow erythropoiesis. This is often a postinfectious phenomenon that may follow infection with Epstein-Barr virus, *S. pneumoniae, Salmonella,* and especially parvovirus B19, seen classically in pediatric patients, which directly infects erythroid progenitors. The bone marrow is also susceptible to infarction, which may further exacerbate the chronic anemia.

Sickle cell disease patients are at risk for other life-threatening conditions, as well. In acute chest syndrome, bilateral pulmonary infiltrates occur with fever and significant pleuritic chest pain, resulting in a "splinting" pattern of respiration with shallow breaths of suboptimal volume and leading to progressive atelectasis and hypoxia. This condition may be triggered by vaso-occlusion, pulmonic infection, *in situ* thrombus formation with pulmonary infarction, or pulmonary emboli associated with bone marrow infarction (including fat emboli). Respiratory failure can occur if the condition is not treated aggressively with IV hydration, RBC transfusion, pain management to relieve respiratory splinting, supplemental oxygen, and antibiotics for documented infection (e.g., community-acquired pneumonia or less commonly bacteremia).

Another serious complication of sickle cell disease is the tendency for cerebrovascular accidents (e.g., strokes, transient ischemic attacks). In fact, a significant percentage of these patients will experience strokes before reaching adulthood, some repeatedly—with the first episode most commonly occurring between 2 and 8 years of age. Myocardial infarction may also occur in the presence or absence of documented coronary artery disease, believed to be due either to vaso-occlusion of the coronary vasculature or to severe hypoxemia resulting from the reduced oxygen-carrying capacity of the blood.

CLINICAL PRESENTATION

Subjective

Subjective findings are associated with the severity of the anemia and manifest predominantly with pain. Although pain is evident only when there is a crisis, the subjective findings of anemia may be apparent without a concurrent sickle cell crisis. Thus, apart from these crises, the subjective findings of sickle cell anemia are similar to those of other types of chronic anemia.

The cardinal subjective symptom of a sickle cell crisis is pain. Pain appears suddenly in the back, chest, abdomen, or extremities, which patients typically characterize as excruciating. It may last for several hours or several days and is unrelieved by rest or change in body position. Massaging the site is of little value in relieving pain. Other subjective findings may include nausea, anorexia, light-headedness, significant anxiety or feelings of panic, heart palpitations, and shortness of breath.

Personality traits characteristic of patients who have lived with a chronic debilitating disease may also be present, including depression, anxiety, negative thinking, catastrophizing, delayed psychological maturation, learned helplessness, and addiction disorders involving alcohol or opioid use as a means of self-medicating. Given the ethnic predominance of sickle cell disease in patients of African descent, health-care providers should be self-aware of their own inherent biases that may influence their assessment or treatment of these patients, compared with patients with other types of chronic or recurrent debilitating medical conditions who may also develop socially maladaptive behaviors as coping mechanisms.

Objective

The patient may present with a low-grade fever (less than 101.3°F [38.5°C]) during and preceding a sickle cell crisis. Additional signs may include point tenderness and guarding at the sites of pain, pinpoint pupils, an inability to follow commands, photophobia, tachycardia and a systolic heart murmur, tachypnea, diminished respiratory excursion, hepatomegaly, a nonpalpable spleen (due to infarction and fibrosis), and pretibial leg ulcers affecting the skin and underlying tissue.

Outside of a sickle cell crisis, the clinician may note characteristic physical findings resulting from chronic bone marrow expansion including a lengthened tower-shaped skull, frontal bossing of the forehead, and fish-mouth deformities of the vertebrae. During the objective examination, the clinician may note chronic effects of hemolysis, such as jaundice or a sallow color to the skin. Patients may appear older than their stated age.

DIAGNOSTIC REASONING

Diagnostic Tests

Initial testing involves a CBC and a peripheral blood smear. It should be clear, however, that adults with sickle cell disease do not present *de novo*. They are typically diagnosed soon after birth and learn to cope with sickle cell crises even as they face delayed physical and psychological maturation. Postnatal infant screening in the United States, therefore, typically includes a hemoglobin electrophoresis to detect sickle cell disease and the various thalassemias, as well as a CBC and peripheral blood smear, although the specific panel of postnatal screening tests differs by state.

Sickled cells will constitute 5% to 10% of the peripheral blood smear in most patients. The elevated reticulocyte count (greater than 10% of the total erythrocyte count) is characteristically accompanied by the presence of Howell-Jolly bodies, which are small remnants of nuclear material from hemolyzed erythrocytes that reflect hyposplenia from autoinfarction, as well as target cells, which are erythrocytes with a deeply stained core surrounded by a lighter-stained margin that resembles a target with a bull's eye. The clinician should also expect the WBC count to be elevated to 12,000 cells/mcL or greater, especially during and soon after a sickle cell crisis.

Further testing may include an indirect bilirubin level, which will be elevated after a sickle cell crisis due to hemolysis. Conversely, haptoglobin, a glycoprotein that binds free hemoglobin released from hemolyzed erythrocytes, will be significantly decreased, as it cannot be replaced quickly enough after a severe hemolytic episode.

Differential Diagnosis

The differential diagnosis for sickle cell anemia includes anemia resulting from other causes, sickle thalassemia (a combination of the hemoglobin S and one of the various thalassemia mutations), hemoglobin C disease (a glutamic acid to lysine mutation in the sixth position residue of the beta-hemoglobin chain), nonspecific abdominal pain, urinary tract infection (UTI), poisoning, and diabetes mellitus. Each of these mimics some or all of the subjective and objective findings elicited from the history and physical examination in sickle cell anemia patients.

Sickle cell anemia is differentiated from sickle thal-assemia by the MCV, which will be low if there is any combination of sickle cell anemia and beta-thalassemia (a microcytic anemia) or normal if only sickle cell anemia is present. Sickle beta-thalassemia is typically milder than homozygous sickle cell disease but nonetheless a significantly morbid condition. If there is no production of protein from the other beta-hemoglobin gene (known as *sickle beta thal^0*), these patients will be the most symptomatic, as all of their hemoglobin will be of the S form. Alternatively, reduced but detectable protein production from the other beta-chain gene (*sickle beta thal$^+$*) results in a milder condition, as some functional hemoglobin A remains present.

A combination of sickle cell anemia with alpha-thalassemia may have a slower rate of sickling due to a reduced MCHC in the erythrocytes resulting from the concurrent alpha-thalassemia. Therefore, sickle cell crises in these patients are typically less damaging and possibly less painful than those in patients without this sickle/thalassemia combination.

Hemoglobin C disorders are differentiated by a milder course of anemia than sickle cell anemia. Indeed, some patients with hemoglobin C disorders may live their lives without any crises caused by the disorder. The underlying pathology is differentiated from sickle cell anemia by the substitution of lysine instead of valine at amino acid position 6 of the beta-hemoglobin chain. Morphological differentiation between these disorders comes with a peripheral blood smear, which reveals rectangular crystals of hemoglobin C in erythrocytes. With heterozygous sickle cell/hemoglobin C disease (sickle C disease or SC disease), adult patients may still be prone to splenic sequestration crises, as their spleens typically do not auto-infarct and fibrose. There are also rarer forms of doubly heterozygous hemoglobinopathies in which hemoglobin S is combined with hemoglobins A, G, or O.

Nonspecific abdominal pain that mimics sickle cell anemia will have none of the characteristic laboratory markers of sickle cell anemia, other than possibly an elevated WBC count or a low Hct. Sickle cell anemia in crisis usually also manifests with extra-abdominal pain. In addition, sickle cell anemia patients experience UTIs more frequently than other individuals. A UTI can present with excruciating abdominal pain and referred pain to the back and chest. The WBC count is typically elevated, and there could be a low-grade fever with either frank or microscopic blood present in the urine. Thus, the distinguishing features between isolated cases of UTI and those associated with sickle cell anemia are the history and laboratory markers reflective of sickle cell anemia itself.

Poisoning with certain agents may present with hypoxemia and acidosis, similar to a sickle cell crisis. For example, the ingestion of strong alkalines, such as those contained in household cleaning compounds, causes nausea, vomiting, acute abdominal pain, and dyspnea. The patient history and a CBC should aid in the rapid and almost certain differentiation of poisoning from sickle cell anemia. Diabetes mellitus is also in the differential for sickle cell anemia because of the similarities in blood chemistries in these conditions, including renal and hepatic function tests and an acidic blood pH, as well as urinalysis results and physical examination findings.

Again, as is the case with the other differential diagnoses, the history, CBC, and peripheral blood smear should readily differentiate these etiologies, even in an emergent situation.

MANAGEMENT

Initial Management

Folic acid supplementation of 1 mg/day by mouth is indicated, along with a diet that is rich in the B complex vitamins and vitamin C. Significant rehydration is needed as a part of management and is key to reversing sickle cell crises. It aids in keeping the blood pH normal, thereby preventing acidosis and the sequela of RBC sickling. Hydroxyurea, a chemotherapeutic agent, is a common treatment to increase hemoglobin F levels, an infant hemoglobin form with a higher affinity for oxygen than hemoglobin A or S, which results in less hypoxemia and less sickling of RBCs. In turn, this reduces the frequency of painful sickle cell crises.

Although packed RBC transfusions may be indicated in sickle cell anemia treatment to decrease the fraction of hemoglobin S prone to polymerization, especially in children, transfusions are less commonly used in adults and must always be weighed against the risks of infection (especially with hepatitis C), transfusion reactions, and iron overload. Anemia with a hemoglobin of less than 7 g/dL has been associated with a greater risk of stroke, severe vaso-occlusive episodes, acute chest syndrome, and death in children. Chronic transfusions, however, lead to iron overload and iatrogenic hemochromatosis, which can destroy solid organs such as the liver and adrenal glands. Exchange transfusion may be used when the clinical manifestations of sickle cell anemia (e.g., acute chest syndrome, priapism) are severe and refractory to initial treatment to decrease hemoglobin S to less than 50% of total hemoglobin.

If osteomyelitis is confirmed with magnetic resonance imaging (MRI), which is the diagnostic imaging test of choice, then antibiotic therapy is required. *Salmonella* predominates in osteomyelitis in sickle cell patients over *S. aureus,* which is seen more commonly in non–sickle cell patients. Dactylitis requires urgent treatment, as does aseptic necrosis of the hip and priapism.

Subsequent Management

The management of sickle cell crises often requires hospitalization. General goals include symptomatic control of pain with opioid-type drugs; IV rehydration; oxygen supplementation to reestablish normal or near-normal oxygen saturation and to prevent or control acidosis; and vigilance against possible damage to vital organs such as the heart, liver, lungs, and kidneys. Parents, other family members, or support person(s) should also be taught how to assess for splenic size so that they can recognize the early signs of splenic sequestration syndrome in affected individuals.

Given the increased risk of infection by encapsulated organisms (e.g., *S. pneumoniae, H. influenzae*) in sickle cell anemia patients, prophylactic penicillin should be used in children 2 months to 5 years of age and lifelong in children and adults who have had a splenectomy secondary to splenic sequestration crises. In addition, patients should receive all age-appropriate immunizations according to current vaccine guidelines, including both protein-conjugate (13-valent Prevnar in infants 2 months and older, children, and adults) and polysaccharide (23-valent Pneumovax in children 2 years and older and adults) antipneumococcal vaccines, *H. influenzae* type b (Hib) vaccine, influenza (trivalent inactivated injected but not attenuated intranasal) vaccine, and meningococcal vaccine.

Given the chronicity of sickle cell anemia and the propensity for recurrent sickle cell crises, there is a phenomenon of learned helplessness, narcotic addiction, and drug-seeking behavior that may develop in some sickle cell disease patients who are afflicted with chronic pain. These are critical conditions that must be considered when developing a treatment plan for the management of sickle cell anemia, because they can significantly affect the patient's capacity for effective self-care.

Crizanlizumab (Adakveo) is a monoclonal antibody therapy specific for P-selectin, a cell-surface molecule expressed on vascular endothelial cells that has been associated with vaso-occlusive sickle cell crises. This biological agent was recently approved to reduce the frequency of vaso-occlusive crises in sickle cell anemia patients aged 16 years and older.

Currently, the only cure for sickle cell disease and its variant hemoglobinopathies previously discussed is transplantation of hematopoietic stem cells from a human leukocyte antigen–identical related donor, which is the major factor limiting its use, given the paucity of matched donors. However, the ethical challenge of balancing transplant-related morbidity and mortality, which includes strokes and seizures in the early years, has led to changes in transplant protocols in the United States, with the avoidance of total body irradiation in preparing the patient's bone marrow to receive transplanted stem cells, as well as the use of less toxic conditioning regimens (such as cyclophosphamide, busulfan, and T-cell depletion using antithymocyte globulin or the anti-CD52 monoclonal antibody alemtuzumab [Campath]). A combination of methotrexate and cyclosporine or cyclosporine and prednisone is used for prophylaxis against graft-versus-host disease. The success rate with these techniques is now at least 93%, with a graft rejection rate of 5% to 7%. Gene therapy trials aimed at increasing beta-hemoglobin or fetal hemoglobin levels to increase the oxygen-carrying capacity of a patient's blood are also ongoing to further advance the treatment options for sickle cell disease.

FOLLOW-UP AND REFERRAL

Follow-up visits for patients with sickle cell anemia should occur every 3 months during periods of stability when patients have not been in crisis for a period of 6 months or more; however, the frequency and duration of crises may increase the required frequency of follow-up examinations with appropriate laboratory evaluations. Routine clinical markers to be assessed at follow-up include a CBC, fasting blood sugar, serum electrolyte panel, renal and liver function studies, and urinalysis. Annual or biannual 12-lead electrocardiograms are also necessary to screen for cardiac pathology.

Every patient with sickle cell anemia should be evaluated at least twice per year by a hematologist. In addition, retinal examinations should be performed by an ophthalmologist on an annual basis. Retinal photographs may be required once retinopathies have been diagnosed. The need for other referrals becomes evident as complications arise or organ function decreases, which may include cardiologists, gastroenterologists, nephrologists, orthopedic surgeons (for aseptic joint necrosis), and general surgeons (for splenectomy).

Patient Education: Sickle Cell Anemia

Education for patients with sickle cell disease should focus on the patient's maturation and personality development, within the context of living with this chronic disease.

Self-care behaviors that may prevent sickle cell crises should be reinforced regularly. These include adequate hydration, folic acid supplementation, avoidance of situations that tax the patient's physical and emotional stamina, and adequate sleep and rest as part of everyday activities. Additional self-care actions include participation in peer support groups; pregnancy prevention (unless the patient is prepared for the possibility of additional sickle cell crises during pregnancy and lactation); prenatal counseling and testing of the fetus for DNA evidence of sickle cell disease; and avoidance of alcohol and adrenergic dietary elements, such as caffeine, which can cause diuresis and dehydrate the body, thereby triggering a sickle cell crisis.

Coping may also involve the patient's own spiritual or self-care practices, which may provide a unique contribution to the course of adaptation to any disease.

Because sickle cell disease is a lifelong condition, problems unique to children and adolescents with chronic disease are abundant. There is an important transition period in which the specialty care of these patients typically transitions from a pediatric to an internal medicine setting. Peer support groups can be particularly helpful for these patients.

POLYCYTHEMIA

Polycythemia involves an increase in erythrocyte number or concentration, which results in an increase in blood viscosity. The disorder may be either relative or absolute. An Hct greater than 51% in females and 54% in males is characteristic of the condition. The term *polycythemia* is somewhat misleading, as it literally means too many blood cells (*poly* = "many"; *cythemia* = "blood cells"), rather than too many erythrocytes, in particular. Nevertheless, the name is only associated with an increase in erythrocytes.

EPIDEMIOLOGY AND CAUSES

The incidence of polycythemia increases with age. It is more prevalent in males older than 70 years compared with females of similar age by a ratio of 2:1. Overall, the incidence is 1.9:100,000 people. These statistics have remained stable for the past 60 years, according to multiple retrospective analyses. The incidence and prevalence of polycythemia increase among people who reside at high altitudes, given the body's compensation for the relatively lower environmental oxygen tension through the upregulation of erythropoiesis.

Causes of relative polycythemia include decreased fluid intake, increased fluid loss from the body, and extravasation (redistribution) of vascular fluid into the tissues. Absolute polycythemia, on the other hand, may be caused by either primary or secondary mechanisms. Primary polycythemia involves the proliferation of stem cells independent of erythropoietin and is termed *polycythemia vera*. In contrast, causes of secondary absolute polycythemia include Cushing's syndrome, erythropoietin-secreting tumors, and chronic hypoxia, such as that associated with carboxyhemoglobinemia and residence at high altitudes.

PATHOPHYSIOLOGY

Relative Polycythemia

Relative polycythemia is a condition in which there is a decrease in plasma volume while the total number of circulating erythrocytes remains constant. The underlying pathology is almost always dehydration, which may be either acute or chronic. Acute dehydration is associated with vomiting, burns, crush-type injuries, and fevers, whereas chronic dehydration is an outcome of long-term use of diuretics, such as furosemide. Another chronic cause of dehydration is decreased oral fluid intake, a condition frequently encountered in older adults. Cigarette smoking, though also an important cause of absolute polycythemia, is known to decrease plasma volume. Interestingly, this reduction reverses on cessation of smoking (with a reduction in Hct of 4 or more percentage points in just a matter of days). Terms such as *pseudo-* or *spurious polycythemia, stress erythrocytosis,* and *Gaisböck's disease* have all been used to label chronic states in which plasma volume is reduced, but Hct and hemoglobin are elevated.

distinguish the type of leukemia as either acute or chronic. Further classification of leukemia specifies the stage of development and type of WBC (immunophenotype) that are involved in the malignant transformation (see Table 62.2). The involved leukocytes proliferate and occupy space previously filled by nonmalignant cell lines. Thus, one significant outcome of the malignancy is the suppression of nonmalignant blood cells.

EPIDEMIOLOGY AND CAUSES

The incidence of leukemias varies according to childhood and adult age-groups. Overall, there is a slight predominance of male cases to female cases. Acute lymphoblastic (lymphocytic) leukemia (ALL) is the predominant form in children between 2 and 15 years of age, with a higher prevalence among children younger than 5 years of age. Other types of leukemia more commonly strike adults. Acute

TABLE 62.2 Types of Leukemia and General Treatment Considerations

	Age at Onset	Combination Chemotherapy	Treatment—Other*
Acute Leukemia			
Acute myelogenous leukemia (AML)	All adults, but more prominent at greater than 40 years	Daunorubicin (Cerubidine) OR idarubicin (Idamycin) OR mitoxantrone (Novantrone) PLUS cytarabine (Ara-C) Targeted therapy CD33+ patients: gemtuzumab ozogamicin (Mylotarg) in combination with daunorubicin (Cerubidine) and cytarabine (Ara-C) FLT3-mutated patients: Combination of daunorubicin (Cerubidine), cytarabine (Ara-C), and midostaurin (Rydapt) IDH1-mutated patients: ivosidenib (Tibsovo) IDH2-mutated patients: enasidenib (Idhifa) Older patients: venetoclax (Venclexta)-based combination as low- or nonintensive induction option	Autologous or allogeneic bone marrow transplantation (BMT) for high-risk patients in first remission
Acute lymphoblastic leukemia (ALL)	2–15 years, rarely in adults	*Induction:* Four-drug regimen of daunorubicin (Cerubidine), vincristine (Oncovin), prednisone (Deltasone), and asparaginase (DVP L-asp) *Consolidation:* daunorubicin (Cerubidine) cytarabine (Ara-C) *Maintenance:* Four-drug regimen as explained earlier Other treatment pillars: imatinib (Gleevec), dasatinib (Sprycel), rituximab (Rituxan), antibody-drug conjugates like inotuzumab ozogamicin (Besponsa), and the chimeric antigen receptor-T-cell immunotherapy tisagenlecleucel (Kymriah)	Central nervous system involvement: intrathecal methotrexate (Trexall) and cranial irradiation Allogeneic BMT in high-risk patients in first remission

Continued

TABLE 62.2 Types of Leukemia and General Treatment Considerations—cont'd			
	Age at Onset	Combination Chemotherapy	Treatment—Other*
Chronic Leukemia			
Chronic myelogenous leukemia (CML)	All patients, but more prominent in people older than 60 years of age Median age 42 years	First-line treatment with tyrosine kinase inhibitors like imatinib (Gleevec), bosutinib (Bosulif), dasatinib (Sprycel), or nilotinib (Tasigna)	Allogeneic BMT in chronic phase (greater success in younger patients)
Chronic lymphocytic leukemia (CLL)	Greater than 60 years of age	Preferred first-line treatment: ibrutinib (Imbruvica) Alternative options: venetoclax (Venclexta) and rituximab (Rituxan)-based combinations, obinutuzumab (Gazyva), duvelisib (Copiktra), and idelalisib (Zydelig) Chemoimmunotherapy: cladribine (Mavenclad) OR fludarabine (Fludara) OR chlorambucil (Leukeran) PLUS cyclophosphamide (Cytoxan) used in combination with rituximab (Rituxan) or alemtuzumab (Campath, Lemtrada)	Allogeneic BMT

*For all leukemias, the need for erythropoietin (Epogen, Procrit), darbepoetin (Aranesp), and/or pegfilgrastim (Neulasta) to treat specific cytopenias must be assessed.

myelogenous (myelocytic/myeloid) leukemia (AML) may be seen in adults of all ages, but its incidence increases after 40 years of age. Chronic lymphocytic leukemia (CLL) is more prevalent among adults older than 60 years of age; however, it may appear in people of any age. CLL is the most common leukemia in Western (developed) countries, with a median age of onset of 70 years. Chronic myelogenous (myelocytic/myeloid) leukemia (CML) strikes middle-aged people, with a median age of onset of 42 years.

The etiology of leukemia is complex and not fully understood. Researchers have linked leukemia to environmental toxins such as chemical solvents, petroleum products, and insecticides, as well as heredity factors, although familial leukemias are rare. It is unclear whether the incidence of leukemia is higher among adult identical twins compared with other adults with affected nontwin siblings; however, CLL in particular appears to have a familial predisposition.

The complications of mutagenic pharmacotherapies used to treat lymphoma, rheumatoid arthritis, or to maintain immunosuppression post-transplantation have provided insight into disease etiology. For example, alkylating agents such as melphalan (Alkeran) and cisplatin (Platinol) have been associated with a 5% to 10% increased incidence of leukemia among patients who have been receiving them for an extended period of time.

Likewise, prolonged exposure to high doses of ionizing radiation is also associated with the later development of leukemia. In cases of prolonged toxin and radiation exposure, a latency period of up to 20 years may pass before a leukemia diagnosis develops. Shorter latency periods are seen after exposure to chemotherapeutic agents that inhibit the DNA-splicing enzyme topoisomerase II, such as etoposide (VePesid), doxorubicin (Adriamycin), and mitoxantrone (Novantrone).

PATHOPHYSIOLOGY

There are two staging and classification systems for leukemia. The French-American-British (FAB) classification system, which was first described in 1976, is based on morphology and cytochemical features of the leukemic cells. It is still in use today, despite the emergence of cytogenetics and immunophenotyping as important markers in the diagnosis and prognosis of leukemia. A newer, more commonly used classification system was generated by the WHO, which incorporates morphological features, cytochemistry, immunophenotyping, cytogenetics and clinical features.

The 2016 revision to the WHO classification of tumors of the hematopoietic and lymphoid tissues reflects numerous advances in the identification of biomarkers associated with some myeloid neoplasms, lymphoid neoplasms, and AML. These have been derived in large part from gene expression analysis and next-generation sequencing. This update enables the implementation of improved diagnostic criteria, as well as genetic factors of prognostic significance to guide therapy, for the disease entities present in the previous WHO classification.

For example, AML now has several subcategories, one of which is AML with recurrent genetic abnormalities. Within this subcategory alone, there are now eleven types of AML:

- AML with t(8;21)(q22;q22.1); RUNX1-RUNX1T1
- AML with inv(16)(p13.1q22) or t(16;16)(p13.1;q22); CBFB-MYH11
- Acute promyelocytic leukemia (APL) with PML-RARA
- AML with t(9;11)(p21.3;q23.3); KMT2A-MLLT3
- AML with t(6;9)(p23;q34.1); DEK-NUP214
- AML with inv(3)(q21.3q26.2) or t(3;3)(q21.3;q26.2); GATA2, MECOM
- AML (megakaryoblastic) with t(1;22)(p13.3;q13.3); RBM15-MKL1
- Provisional entity: AML with BCR-ABL1
- AML with mutated NPM1
- AML with biallelic mutations of CEBPA
- Provisional entity: AML with mutated RUNX1

Thus, the full complexity of the revised WHO classification system is beyond the scope of this text. However, an overview of the FAB classification system of myeloid and lymphocytic leukemias in both acute and chronic forms is illustrative of the genetic mutations and prognostic factors that underlie the wide variety of leukemias and help to explain their underlying pathophysiology.

Acute Nonlymphocytic Leukemia

By far, the largest number of adults with acute leukemia (as high as 80%) suffer from acute nonlymphocytic leukemia (ANLL), which mainly presents after 40 years of age and increases in incidence with each year thereafter. It originates in the malignant transformation of a single stem cell or a few select cells. At least 85% of all cases have been associated with defined clonal karyotypic abnormalities in all cells of the progenitor line.

ANLL is a category that includes the leukemias also known as AML and acute granulocytic leukemia (AGL), although some classification systems have eliminated the ANLL and AGL nomenclature altogether, in favor of a more comprehensive classification system that categorizes all acute leukemias of nonlymphocytic origin as forms of AML. In the FAB system, ANLL is divided into eight distinct morphological classes (M0 to M7), with classes M3 to M5 further subdivided into two subclasses each. Each of these subtypes is characterized by one or more cytogenetic abnormalities that can be used to predict prognosis and guide treatment, as they can determine responsiveness to specific chemotherapies. Some of these same genetic abnormalities are incorporated into the revised 2016 WHO classification system. For example, acute promyelocytic leukemia (AML class M3) is associated with a translocation between chromosomes 15 and 17 that juxtaposes the promyelocytic leukemia (PML) and retinoic acid receptor-alpha (RARA) genes, repressing the latter and preventing retinoic acid–induced differentiation of promyelocytes. Nonetheless, this mutation portends a favorable prognosis, as promyelocytic M3 cells are particularly sensitive to therapy with all-trans retinoic acid.

Genetic abnormalities that carry a particularly poor prognosis in ANLL include mutations resulting in monosomy (an entire chromosomal deletion) of chromosomes 5 or 7 or trisomy of chromosome 8. The former monosomies are particularly associated with AML resulting from previous chemotherapy with alkylating agents or exposure to ionizing radiation. In contrast, AML associated with past exposure to topoisomerase II inhibiting agents is often associated with mutations in chromosome 11.

Acute myeloblastic leukemia (AML class M2) and acute myelomonocytic leukemia (AML class M4) have both been associated with a balanced translocation between chromosomes 8 and 21, which juxtaposes the transcription factor genes *AML1* and *ETO,* leading to dysregulated transcription of genes directly involved in myeloid cell division (e.g., granulocyte-monocyte colony-stimulating factor, IL-3, and the antiapoptotic gene *BCL-2*). AML class M4 has also been associated with inversions or translocations in chromosome 16, creating a fusion of the genes *CBFB* and *MYH11,* which leads to repressed transcription of genes involved in myelocytic differentiation. Acute monoblastic leukemia (AML class M5) is associated with rearrangements of chromosome 11, whereas mutations in chromosome 3 appear to confer thrombocytosis in the setting of AML.

Acute Lymphoblastic Leukemia

ALL can appear among people of all ages but is clearly a disease predominantly of early childhood, as noted previously. B-cell lymphoblasts or, in far fewer cases, T-cell lymphoblasts increase in number after a single hematopoietic stem cell undergoes transformation (immortalization). Interestingly, the cytogenetics of ALL in children differs from those in adults. For instance, the Philadelphia chromosome (a balanced translocation between chromosomes 9 and 22 that juxtaposes and activates the *BCR* and *ABL* oncogenes) is seen in only 5% of childhood cases, but this is the most common abnormality in adult ALL and is found in up to 40% of cases. In contrast, hyperdiploidy (in which greater than 50 chromosomes are found in malignant clones) is seen in up to 30% of childhood cases but in no more than 5% of affected adults.

In contrast to CML (see next section), the presence of the Philadelphia chromosome is a poor prognostic indicator in ALL, contributing to dysregulated activation of the *RAS* intracellular signaling pathway that leads to uncontrolled cell division. These patients often have additional karyotypic abnormalities such as monosomy of chromosome 7. Studies have shown that ALL patients with the Philadelphia chromosome may be divided into two subsets that are distinguished by differing translocation breakpoints along the BCR gene—one in which this karyotypic abnormality appears restricted to a B lineage lymphoblastic cell clone and another in which the Philadelphia chromosome is further identified in myelogenous cell lines as well, indicating these patients may have an indolent form of CML that underwent a B lineage lymphoblastic crisis at the time of diagnosis.

As with AML, different forms of ALL have been distinguished on the basis of morphology, with certain cytogenetic profiles correlating with each presentation. For instance, ALL of L3-type B-cell origin often shares a translocation of chromosomes 8 and 14 that is also seen in B-cell-derived Burkitt's lymphoma, suggesting that these cancers are varied manifestations of the same underlying malignant transformation event. Pre–B-cell ALL has been associated with translocations between chromosomes 1 and 19, which lead to a fusion protein between the highly active transcription factors *E2A* and *PBX1*, with subsequent immortalization of this early B-cell progenitor that portends a particularly poor prognosis. Infantile ALL has been associated in up to 80% of cases with translocations involving the mixed lineage leukemia (MLL) gene at chromosome 11q23, which is thought to regulate a number of downstream genes involved in lymphocyte differentiation, thereby resulting in extremely poor outcomes. A poor prognosis is also seen in ALL associated with translocations between chromosomes 4 and 11, a mutation that is commonly seen in AML class M5.

A translocation between chromosomes 12 and 21 that produces a fusion protein between the transcription factors *TEL* and *AML1* is the most common mutation seen in childhood ALL. Fortunately, this translocation confers a favorable prognosis in ALL, as does the presence of hyperdiploidy (with 50 to 60 chromosomes) with occasional structural abnormalities such as partial chromosomal duplications and translocations. Multiple copies of chromosome 21 and the X chromosome are the most common findings in hyperdiploidy, but several other duplications have been noted as well (e.g., chromosomes 4, 6, 10, and 14). The high prevalence of these karyotypic abnormalities in childhood ALL underlies the generally favorable outcomes associated with this form of leukemia in children.

T-cell ALL is a less common entity that typically strikes young males. Related to T-cell lymphomas, these patients may present with particularly high WBC counts, invasion of malignant cells into the CNS via the cerebrospinal fluid, and the presence of a mediastinal tumor. Well over half of these cancers are characterized by mutations in genes coding for the various protein components of the T-cell receptor—alpha, beta, gamma, or delta subunits. The T-cell receptor is a heterodimeric protein composed of either alpha–beta or gamma–delta subunit pairs expressed on the surface of the T cell, which allow for the recognition of specific antigens. Mutations commonly occur in chromosome 14, which encodes the alpha and delta receptor subunits, or chromosome 7, which encodes the genes for the beta and gamma chains. Translocations at these sites typically juxtapose these genes with various transcription factors that lead to dysregulated expression of the receptor subunit and proliferation of the T-cell clone. Mutations in these same chromosomes that do not involve these receptor subunits, as well as in others such as chromosomes 6 and 11, have also been identified in T-cell ALL. Interestingly, prognosis does not appear tied to these particular cytogenetics, and outcomes are generally favorable in both adults and children with T-cell ALL.

Chronic Myelogenous Leukemia

CML (chronic myelocytic leukemia, chronic myeloid leukemia) is most commonly associated with the development of the Philadelphia chromosome in a hematopoietic stem cell that commits to the myeloid lineage. Although differentiation is typically unaffected, the leukemic stem cell is self-renewing and produces a tremendous number of daughter cells, with the same leukemic clone dominating up to 90% of the bone marrow at the time of diagnosis. In this mutation, breaks occur in the DNA, resulting in an equivalent exchange of genetic material between chromosomes 9 and 22. Oncogene activation occurs, as the reciprocal translocation [t(9;22)(q34;q11)] juxtaposes the *BCR* and c-*ABL* genes, creating a BCR–ABL fusion protein that confers a proliferative advantage to the leukemic clone, even in the absence of cellular growth factors.

The functions of the native BCR and ABL proteins are not fully elucidated, and neither gene alone is capable of malignant transformation; however, the fusion protein is oncogenic, giving rise to malignant clones through upregulated tyrosine kinase (phosphorylation) activity within a number of intracellular signaling pathways contributing to cell division (e.g., RAS, c-Myc, and JAK/STAT molecular pathways). This explains the effectiveness of treatment with the tyrosine kinase inhibitor imatinib (Gleevec). Depending on the site of the chromosomal breaks, various types of the BCR-ABL fusion protein may be formed. In turn, cells transformed by these different species of fusion protein appear to respond differentially to specific therapies.

Although IL-3 and G-CSF mRNA transcripts are both upregulated in leukemic cell clones, the precise role of cytokines in the dysregulated growth of these cells remains unclear. As with other forms of leukemia, leukemic cell clones in CML appear to arise from a self-renewing pool of mutated leukemic stem cells, which are typically less mature than the differentiated granulocytic leukemic clones themselves. In fact, the Philadelphia chromosome has been identified in a number of cell lineages in CML, including granulocyte, macrophage, erythrocyte, megakaryocyte (platelet), and B-lymphocyte precursor cells, indicating that the mutation first occurs in an early, noncommitted, multilineage hematopoietic stem cell.

The creation of the Philadelphia chromosome may predate the onset of disease symptoms by many years—a pattern suggesting that the disease progresses through a latent or asymptomatic phase before becoming active. For example, the karyotypic abnormality may first arise in the third decade of life, with symptom onset as much as 10 to 20 years later. In fact, normal bone marrow function is characteristic of the disease trajectory in the early years after development of the Philadelphia chromosome. The pool of leukemic stem cells may not be expanded in number; however, leukemic daughter cells undergo clonal expansion and eventually crowd out normal bone marrow components. In addition, cell surface adhesion factors (e.g., beta-1 integrin) are downregulated, eliminating adhesion-dependent growth inhibition in which normal cells are triggered to stop proliferating after coming into contact with one another.

As with any chronic leukemia, a dreaded complication of CML is degeneration into a leukemic blast crisis, in which leukemic progenitor cells develop self-renewing properties as they undergo further mutations resulting in clonal proliferation of either myeloid or lymphoid (almost exclusively B lineage) blasts, given the widespread presence of the Philadelphia chromosome in multiple lineages. Most commonly, the additional mutations described include trisomies of chromosomes 8 or 19, duplications of the Philadelphia chromosome itself, or mutations in the *p53* tumor suppressor gene on chromosome 17.

These blast cells may express many of the same proteins as hematopoietic stem cells, such as the transcription factor beta-catenin. Both leukemic stem cells and their progeny appear more resistant to apoptosis than wild-type (nonmutated) cells, but the significance of this to the pathogenesis of CML is not fully known, as the lifespan of leukemic cell clones is not significantly greater than that of wild-type granulocytes and does not appear to account for their increase in number.

Finally, CML may also occur in the absence of the Philadelphia chromosome mutation, which is known as *atypical CML*. Up to 15% of CML patients may suffer from this condition, although some hematologist-oncologist specialists have chosen to classify these patients as having a distinct myeloproliferative disease, rather than true CML. For reasons that are poorly understood, these patients have a worse prognosis with a poorer response to therapy and shorter survival times.

Chronic Lymphocytic Leukemia

CLL is a chronic lymphoproliferative disorder typically associated with increased numbers of small B lymphocytes and is clinically indistinguishable from small lymphocytic B-cell lymphoma. After malignant transformation occurs in a B-cell precursor, thus forming an immortal cell line, this clonal abnormality is passed on to slowly replicating progeny that are functionally incompetent.

The genetics of the malignant alteration in CLL are not as well established as they are for CML. Malignant B-cell clones are known to be frozen in a state of differentiation somewhere between the pre-B and mature B-cell phases, with rates of proliferation and cell death varying widely among different individuals. These cells express very low levels of surface immunoglobulin, with various B lineage–specific cell surface proteins (e.g., CD19, CD20, CD21), as well as CD5, which is primarily considered a T-cell marker. Variant forms exist that do not adhere to these criteria, although some hematologist-oncologists feel that a proliferation of non–CD5-expressing B cells represents a leukemic phase of non-Hodgkin lymphoma, rather than true CLL.

The relative percentages of both T cells and natural killer cells are reduced in CLL, although absolute numbers of T lymphocytes may be increased, given the tremendous expansion of lymphocytes. Moreover, some CLL patients demonstrate unusual forms of T cells with low levels of surface CD4 and CD8 proteins. Such nonclassical T cells are also found in other autoimmune diseases. In addition, although hypogammaglobulinemia is common in patients with CLL, immunoglobulin receptors on leukemic cells may demonstrate autoimmune specificity, which may explain the increased frequency of AIHA, idiopathic thrombocytopenic purpura, and pure-red blood cell aplasia in people with CLL. Because of patients' lack of protective antibodies, infection by gram-negative or encapsulated organisms is the most frequent cause of morbidity and mortality in people with CLL.

Cytogenetic analysis of CLL cell clones has revealed chromosomal abnormalities in up to 70% of cases. The most frequent karyotypic abnormalities include trisomy of chromosome 12, partial deletions in chromosome 13 that affect the tumor suppressor retinoblastoma (*Rb*) gene, and partial deletions in chromosomes 11 and 17 that are associated with a particularly poor prognosis and shorter survival. The *p53* tumor suppressor gene located on chromosome 17 is often affected, either by deletion or expression of a mutated nonfunctional protein, with both conditions leading to unregulated cellular proliferation. The overexpression of survival factors has also been identified in B lineage CLL, including the antiapoptotic molecules BCL-2 and inducible nitric oxide synthetase.

CLINICAL PRESENTATION

Subjective

Patients with acute leukemia commonly report bone and joint pain, as well as fevers, chills, palpitations, shortness of breath, and symptoms of infection. Patients may also have gingival bleeding associated with gingival hyperplasia. Complaints of skin eruptions, easy bruising, or prolonged bleeding from simple wounds form a significant part of the subjective history.

Patients with chronic leukemia report fatigue, night sweats, and low-grade fevers. Although there is no clear differentiation in subjective findings between CML and CLL, CML may present with the symptoms of leukostasis associated with very high WBC counts (greater than 500,000 cells/mcL). The syndrome of leukostasis is characterized by blurred vision, respiratory distress, and occasionally priapism (prolonged and painful penile erections that last for several hours). Nausea and vomiting may be associated with organomegaly in both types of chronic leukemia. Bone and joint pain are typically limited to the myeloproliferative stages of CML.

Objective

The clinician will often note a high fever in patients with acute leukemia. Tachycardia and tachypnea are related findings. Patients appear pale due to anemia and manifest skin eruptions related to impaired platelet function, such as petechiae and purpura. Confusion due to hypoxemia and fever may be revealed using standardized evaluation tools such as the Folstein Mini-Mental State Examination.

In chronic leukemia patients, heart and lung sounds are typically within normal limits except during states of infection, in which the lungs may produce adventitious sounds. Splenomegaly may be evident and variably associated with hepatomegaly and/or lymph node enlargement. Temperature may not be elevated in chronic leukemia, as is often observed in acute leukemia, unless the disease has progressed or there is a concurrent infection. In addition, the patient's skin may appear pale in chronic leukemia due to accompanying anemia, while few, if any, skin eruptions are evident.

DIAGNOSTIC REASONING

Diagnostic Tests

Initial testing for suspected acute leukemia includes a CBC with peripheral blood smear and platelet count. The WBC count may be significantly elevated (more than 300,000 cells/mcL). Granulocytes (polysegmented and banded forms) are typically diminished in number, as are platelets (often less than 50,000/mcL). An Hct of less than 30% is a common finding, especially if the WBC count is markedly elevated. The peripheral smear reveals a blastocystosis of greater than 25% in almost all cases.

Initial tests for suspected chronic leukemia are the same as for acute leukemia: CBC, peripheral blood smear, and platelet count. The WBC count should be elevated in CML and CLL, but typically more so in CML (elevations of more than 100,000 cells/mcL are common). Lymphocytosis, however, differentiates CLL from CML. Lymphocytes occupy as much as 90% of the peripheral blood smear in CLL, whereas the peripheral smear of CML is characterized by a left-shifted myeloid series, with mature forms of myeloid cells predominating. Platelets may also be elevated in CML and are rarely diminished.

Once leukemia is suspected in the primary care setting, referral to a hematologist-oncologist should be initiated to conduct further specialized testing, such as a bone marrow aspirate and morphological, immunophenotypic, and cytogenetic studies to determine the specific type of leukemia and guide treatment based on prognostic factors in the updated 2016 WHO classification system. Results should parallel the peripheral blood smear, thus confirming the initial diagnosis with greater accuracy in quantitative and qualitative indices.

For example, in acute leukemia, the bone marrow aspirate reveals hypercellular components, which are dominated by blasts. At least 30% of bone marrow cells must be blasts to diagnose acute leukemia. Auer bodies are rod-shaped structures, present in the cytoplasm of myeloblasts, myelocytes, and monoblasts in leukemic patients; they predominate within myeloblasts in the bone marrow aspirates of patients with AML. Serum chemistry profiles are critical for secondary testing in acute leukemia patients because of rapid cell turnover in the WBC population, which liberates intracellular uric acid and leads to significant increases in serum uric acid concentration.

In CML, bone marrow evaluation typically reveals the presence of the Philadelphia chromosome, along with a left-shifted myelopoiesis. Blasts occupy less than 5% of the aspirated sample. Subsequent testing of CML also includes measuring leukocyte alkaline phosphatase, which is usually low, thus reflecting the abnormal function of neutrophils. Additional testing includes measuring vitamin B_{12} and serum chemistries. Vitamin B_{12} is typically elevated, as is uric acid.

In CLL, bone marrow biopsy results confirm the initial peripheral blood smear findings, as small, mature lymphocytes dominate the field. Monoclonal surface immunoglobulin on the malignant lymphocytes aids in distinguishing these small cells from their normal counterparts. Another secondary test, immunoelectrophoresis, further supports the diagnosis of CLL in about half of patients, as the profile from the electrophoresis demonstrates hypogamma globulinemia. A particularly recognizable variant of CLL on microscopy is hairy cell leukemia (HCL). This rare and slow-growing form of leukemia is named for the characteristic "hairy" appearance of its abnormal B cells, due to radial cytoplasmic projections from the cell surface that look like strands of hair. These malignant B cells are generated in the bone marrow and can crowd out other cell lines, resulting in pancytopenia on the peripheral blood smear.

Molecular methods of cytogenetic analysis (e.g., fluorescent *in situ* hybridization, Southern blot, reverse transcriptase–polymerase chain reaction) to identify the Philadelphia chromosome and other karyotypic abnormalities are critical for predicting the prognosis and determining the most effective treatment plan for each type of leukemia. These analyses have revolutionized leukemia treatment by facilitating the use of individualized, directed therapy, and they form the basis of the revised 2016 WHO classification system for these blood cancers.

Differential Diagnosis

Acute Leukemia

The left-shifted (immature) bone marrow aspirates of acute leukemia must be distinguished from left-shifted aspirates associated with recent exposure to toxic chemicals and radiation. The clinician should expect that the full recovery period after certain toxic exposures will be at least 6 weeks and may extend to 12 weeks. If exposure to toxins and not monoclonal malignant transformation was the cause of the cellular left-shift, then subsequent testing should reveal maturing cell lines. It is also important to rule out false-positive left-shifted aspirates by repeating bone marrow sampling several days after the initial procedure, although some patients may not want to be subjected to this invasive procedure again so soon, unless the results will influence imminent treatment decisions.

Acute leukemias must be distinguished from their chronic counterparts and from similar myeloproliferative disorders, such as polycythemia. ALL may also resemble other lymphoproliferative diseases, such as lymphoma and mononucleosis. Therefore, a skilled pathologist is required to differentiate these lymphoproliferative conditions, given their differences in prognosis and treatment plans.

Chronic Leukemia

The Philadelphia chromosome of CML distinguishes this disease from myeloproliferative responses to infection, systemic inflammation, and other malignancies. Clinical wisdom will also help the practitioner to distinguish the leukocytosis of CML from other reactive immunological states. CML will likely present with more than 50,000 cells/mcL, but reactive states will not mount as great an immune response. In addition, CML differs from other myeloproliferative diseases, as the erythrocyte count, RBC indices, and Hct are generally normal in CML.

Microscopic evaluation of a bone marrow aspirate differentiates CLL from other lymphocytic disorders, such as viral infections, based on the findings described earlier. In addition, unlike in CLL, viral infections will present with flu-like symptoms, which include fever, chills, myalgias, and arthralgias. Thus, CLL is perhaps the easiest among the leukemias to distinguish.

Box 62.1 Anemia and Cancer

Anemia is one of the most frequently reported problems in patients with cancer and is associated with worsening of cognitive function, performance status, activity level, overall energy, and survival. Anemia may develop either before or after the onset of cancer therapy, either due to the underlying disease (especially with blood cancers like leukemia) or as a consequence of treatment. Patients with normal Hgb concentration before medical treatment often receive only postsurgical adjuvant therapy to address microscopic tumor burden; however, those with preceding cancer-related anemia (CRA) often undergo chemotherapy for clinically detectable tumors. Thus, in the former patients, anemia is typically considered a side effect of cancer treatment, whereas for the latter patients, CRA may result from the chronic inflammation associated with advanced cancer.

Multiple lines of evidence implicate inflammatory mediators in the pathophysiology of CRA, as proinflammatory cytokines reduce the proliferation of erythroid progenitor cells, erythropoietin production, and erythrocyte survival. This chronic inflammatory state is further evidenced by elevated plasma C-reactive protein levels induced by increased IL-6, along with weight loss, hypoalbuminemia, and erythropoietin-resistant anemia. IL-6 also increases the synthesis and activity of hepcidin, which is involved in iron homeostasis by inhibiting duodenal iron absorption and iron release from macrophages. Thus, increased hepcidin activity appears directly correlated to the development of ACD or, more specifically, anemia of chronic inflammation. Other mechanisms of inflammation-associated anemia include the cytokine-induced production of reactive oxygen species that may inhibit erythropoiesis, as well as worsened nutritional status associated with chronic inflammation.

Management

In cancer patients, all potentially contributing factors leading to anemia should be considered, especially before initiating treatment that may worsen anemia, such as chemotherapy or radiation. Although erythropoiesis-stimulating agents (ESAs) are not appropriate in most patients with nonchemotherapy–associated CRA, other than in certain myelodysplastic syndromes, these agents may be given to patients with chemotherapy-associated anemia if Hgb has fallen to less than 10 g/dL and in whom cancer treatment is not intended to be curative. Even though RBC transfusion may be an option for these patents, ESAs are given to increase Hgb to the lowest concentration above which transfusions are not needed. In addition, iron supplementation may be used to improve Hgb response to ESAs and reduce the need for RBC transfusions in these patients, regardless of whether iron deficiency is apparent. Considering the complexity and multifactorial pathogenesis of CRA, close monitoring by the treating oncologist/hematologist is paramount to follow up and adjust the treatment regimen in such patients.

Sources: Bohlius J, Bohlke K, Castelli R, et al. Management of cancer-associated anemia with erythropoiesis-stimulating agents: ASCO/ASH clinical practice guideline update. *Blood Adv.* 2019;3(8):1197–1210. doi:10.1182/bloodadvances.2018030387

MANAGEMENT

The probability of successful treatment and subsequent cure for acute leukemia decreases with advancing age. In addition, a cure for acute leukemia is less probable if the patient is diagnosed late in the disease trajectory, after several physiological systems have become involved. In general, treatment begins with combination chemotherapy to induce remission (i.e., an induction phase), and this stage of treatment is followed by the consolidation phase (a stage of chemotherapy) and then a prolonged maintenance phase. Unlike the acute leukemias, chronic leukemias usually follow an indolent course, which means that myelosuppressive chemotherapy may not be initiated until symptoms necessitate intervention. Symptoms, therefore, are managed as they appear.

Acute Leukemia

Treatment options for AML are customized, based on several factors, such as patient age (either older or younger than 60 years), cytogenetic risk, the presence of FLT3/IDH1/IDH2 mutations, a history of prior myelodysplastic syndrome, and whether the AML is treatment induced. AML patients typically receive combination chemotherapy (see Table 62.2). The oncologist will set the dose ranges for at least two drugs—daunorubicin (Cerubidine), idarubicin (Idamycin), or mitoxantrone (Novantrone) plus cytarabine (Ara-C). $CD33^+$ patients may also receive gemtuzumab ozogamicin (Mylotarg) in combination with daunorubicin and cytarabine. FLT3-mutated patients may be candidates for a combination of daunorubicin, cytarabine, and midostaurin (Rydapt), and the kinase inhibitor gilteritinib (Xospata) is a subsequent treatment option for these patients. Other kinase inhibitors include ivosidenib (Tibsovo), which is an option for IDH1-mutated patients, and enasidenib (Idhifa), which can be used in IDH2-mutated patients. Combination therapy with the BCL-2 inhibitor venetoclax (Venclexta) is used in older patients as a low- to nonintensive induction option.

The primary care practitioner should monitor hepatic function throughout the course of combination therapy, which may run in 3- to 6-day cycles every 3 to 4 weeks for a total of 3 to 6 months, depending on successful remission and patient tolerance. Combination therapy produces bone marrow aplasia, which abates 2 weeks after the conclusion of therapy. Aplastic patients, therefore, require supportive antibiotic prophylaxis, vigorous stoma care due to severe denuding of mucosal surfaces, and possible RBC transfusions. The primary care practitioner's role is to comanage the adverse effects of chemotherapy and monitor serum chemistries, including liver function tests. In addition, follow-up bone marrow aspirate and biopsy are common practice 2 to 3 weeks after the initiation of induction therapy.

Of note, acute promyelocytic leukemia is cured more often than other types of AML and is usually treated with all-trans retinoic acid in combination with other therapies like arsenic trioxide. The targeted immunotherapy gemtuzumab ozogamicin (Mylotarg) or chemotherapy is an alternative option. In case of an incomplete response to such therapies, hematopoietic cell transplantation should be considered.

Adult patients with ALL may enter remission with initial management (albeit not as quickly or as easily as children with ALL) without the aplastic disorders associated with the initial treatment of AML. Combination four-drug chemotherapy is the mainstay for the initial management of ALL, including daunorubicin (Cerubidine), vincristine (Oncovin), prednisone (Deltasone), and asparaginase (collectively called DVP L-asp), whereas other combinations are under investigation. Additional treatment pillars include targeted therapies like the tyrosine kinase inhibitors imatinib (Gleevec) and dasatinib (Sprycel), monoclonal antibodies like rituximab (Rituxan) directed against $CD20^+$ ALL cells, antibody-drug conjugates like inotuzumab ozogamicin (Besponsa) directed against $CD22^+$ ALL cells, stem cell transplantation, and chimeric antigen receptor (CAR)-T-cell immunotherapy. CAR-T-cell therapy, also called *adoptive cell transfer,* is a relatively new form of immunotherapy in which a sample of a patient's T cells is collected from the blood and then modified to produce special cell-surface structures called *chimeric antigen receptors,* which enhance their cancer-fighting ability upon reinfusion. The CAR-T therapy tisagenlecleucel (Kymriah) targets the B-cell surface receptor CD19 to treat B-cell ALL; other CAR-T therapies have been developed to treat specific types of B-cell lymphomas.

Comanagement of ALL with the oncologist is the same as for patients with AML. Glucose intolerance may develop due to prednisone therapy, particularly in patients suffering from diabetes mellitus at baseline. Thus, the primary care practitioner is responsible for making adjustments to any antidiabetic agents during chemotherapy.

After remission has been achieved for the patient with acute leukemia, a consolidation course of treatment is begun. Consolidation cycles differ for the acute leukemias, depending on type (see Table 62.2). AML patients receive one complete chemotherapy consolidation cycle. Alternatively, they may receive a bone marrow transplantation to consolidate the gains of earlier therapy. Transplantation may be autologous (an individual's own marrow saved before treatment), allogeneic (marrow donated by another individual), or syngeneic (marrow donated by an identical twin). Therapeutic Procedure 62.1 presents information that should be provided to the patient who will be undergoing bone marrow transplantation. Patients with ALL, on the other hand, face different challenges during the consolidation phase of management. They must receive CNS

Type 1: IgE-mediated Immediate Hypersensitivity Response

In the first step of initial exposure to an allergen, the immune system must recognize that the allergen is foreign. IgE is a class of antibody present in relatively low concentration in the circulation. As with all immunoglobulins, IgE molecules are antigen specific in their variable arms, allowing for binding of more than one IgE molecule to a single circulating antigenic molecule. However, the constant portion of the IgE molecule (Fc) allows it to bind to the surface of cells specifically expressing high-affinity receptors for the IgE molecule (FcɛRI). IgE molecules are bound to tissue-derived mast cells located primarily in the skin, respiratory system, and gastrointestinal (GI) tract, where external environmental allergens are most likely to contact or invade the body. In addition, allergen-specific IgE molecules are bound to circulating basophils.

Antibody cross-linking is the process by which two or more cell surface-bound IgE molecules bind a common antigen, thereby triggering intracellular signaling and degranulation of the immune cell, with the release of cytokine mediators. Such responses do not typically occur on initial exposure to an allergen. On first exposure, specific IgE molecules are formed via class-switching of monoclonal antibodies produced by preexisting antigen-specific B cells from the IgG or IgM classes to IgE, based on the constant Fc portion of cell surface antibody molecules. Once secreted by the B cell, these IgE molecules then bind to mast cells and basophils. On reexposure (when the same allergen binds to cell-bound antigen-specific IgE), a cascade of cellular events occurs, resulting in intracellular calcium shifts that facilitate cyclic nucleotide signaling molecules to trigger degranulation of the immune cell.

Degranulation results in the excretion of preformed inflammatory mediators from the immune cell, including histamine, heparin, tryptase, other proteolytic enzymes, thromboxane, arachidonic acid, prostaglandins, superoxides, and several eosinophilic and neutrophilic chemotactic factors. In addition, the synthesis of newly formed inflammatory mediators, including leukotrienes and certain cytokines, is also triggered.

These inflammatory mediators cause venules, capillaries, and arterioles to dilate and become hyperpermeable. The mucous membranes are triggered to increase mucus secretion and the walls of hollow visceral structures to spasm as a result of smooth muscle contraction. Dehydration may result from the relative shift of fluid that follows intravascular proteins out of the vasculature and into the extravascular space, thus potentially lowering blood pressure. Hypotension may also be aggravated by environmental factors, such as relative heat and humidity.

IgE activation and cellular excretion of inflammatory mediators may take place within seconds to minutes after antigenic exposure. Whereas the effects of initially released inflammatory mediators may last for 30 minutes or less, repeated allergenic exposure can prolong the inflammatory cycle for hours. A prolonged and intractable inflammatory cycle produces the clinical picture of atopic hypersensitivity diseases characterized by type 1 allergic responses, such as allergic rhinitis and allergic asthma, which are heavily dependent on inflammatory cells, including mast cells, eosinophils, and Th2 cells.

A second category of type 1 allergic reaction is anaphylaxis. Unlike atopic diseases, which are typically characterized by localized effects in the skin or respiratory tract, anaphylaxis produces systemic effects. All of the inflammatory processes of hypersensitivity become exaggerated, leading to life-threatening hypotension, bronchospasm, laryngospasm, angioedema, smooth muscle and visceral organ contractions, and raised inflammatory skin eruptions (generalized urticaria or hives). Anaphylaxis may follow exposure in susceptible individuals to well-known allergens, such as insect venom (bee or wasp stings) or certain drugs such as penicillin. However, these responses are not limited to individuals with a history of atopic disease and may occur unexpectedly in any individual. Therefore, a history of atopy does not predict anaphylaxis. If left untreated, anaphylaxis is typically fatal. Therapeutic Procedure 63.1 describes a seven-step treatment algorithm for anaphylaxis.

Therapeutic Procedure 63.1: Seven-step Treatment for Anaphylaxis

- Step 1: Administer aqueous epinephrine 1:1,000 dilution 0.3–0.5 mg (0.3–0.5 mL) intramuscularly into the upper lateral thigh, in a supine position with the head below heart level, if possible.
- Step 2: Repeat epinephrine every 5–15 minutes as required by the clinical presentation. If hypotensive, position the patient supine with feet elevated.
- Step 3: Support bronchodilation if patient is without laryngospasm by administering albuterol 3 mL (2.5 mg) inhalation via nebulizer.
- Step 4: If patient is in laryngospasm or pulmonary arrest, perform emergency endotracheal intubation and provide respiratory support.
- Step 5: Start IV fluids using normal saline or Ringer's lactate solution to maintain systolic blood pressure greater than 90 mm Hg. The rate of flow should be determined by the blood pressure reading but typically may be bolused.
- Step 6: If the patient is conscious and without laryngospasm, administer diphenhydramine (Benadryl) 25–50 mg to relieve cutaneous symptoms. H_2 blockers may also be added (particularly if GI symptoms are present) but have not been shown to be as effective as H_1 blockers.
- Step 7: Transfer the patient to an acute-care emergency center for continued support and observation. Add corticosteroids (IV or PO) to prevent late-phase anaphylactic reactions, which may be as severe as early phase reactions.

See Patient Education: Allergic Reactions regarding teaching about injectable epinephrine (e.g., EpiPen, Auvi-Q).

Type 2: Antibody-mediated Cellular Cytotoxicity Response

Type 2 antibody-mediated cellular cytotoxicity responses introduce an immune mechanism different from type 1 immediate hypersensitivity responses. Type 2 responses involve the activation of antigen-specific IgM and IgG molecules. These humoral immune molecules bind to foreign antigens and activate serum immune complement. This leads to destruction of any cell to which an allergen-antibody complex is bound; thus, a type 2 immune response is cytotoxic. Examples of such type 2 responses include neonatal Rh (Rhesus blood group factor)-incompatibility hemolytic disease and immune-mediated hemolytic anemia. In addition, when these antibodies bind to foreign antigens such as microbial cell surface proteins, the invading microbes become prone to phagocytosis and destruction by host immune cells—a process known as *opsonization*.

Type 3: Antibody–allergen Immune Complex Response

The third category of immune responses also requires IgM and IgG activation, as is characteristic of a type 2 immune response. However, type 3 responses denote a free-standing immune complex that is formed between these immunoglobulins and the allergen. These complexes become deposited into the various tissues of the body, activating serum complement that in turn triggers multiple inflammatory mediators. These reactions tend to be systemic, as immune complexes affect multiple organs and tissue types throughout the body. The reaction is not immediate, and, in fact, may occur up to 2 to 3 weeks after antigenic exposure. Hypersensitivity-type pneumonitis secondary to an inhaled allergen and serum sickness are two examples of type 3 immune responses. Delayed drug reactions are also classic examples of type 3 responses, and the most common offenders are the antiepileptic drugs phenytoin, phenobarbital, and carbamazepine, as well as various antibiotics.

Type 4: Delayed-type Cellular Hypersensitivity Response

The fourth category of immune responses is defined as a cell-mediated delayed-type immune response that is unlike the three previous categories, which are all mediated by humoral factors (antibody dependent). The other three categories directly involve few, if any, T lymphocytes. However, type 4 reactions are T cell–dependent and usually begin in the skin, where large numbers of T cells are found. Antigen contacting the skin is endocytosed (taken up) by antigen-presenting cells, which process and relocate small antigenic peptides to the cell surface, coupled to antigen-presenting proteins known as *major histocompatibility complex* (MHC) molecules.

Antigen-specific T cell receptors recognize and bind to these antigenic peptide–MHC complexes, which leads to a series of inflammatory reactions including cellular lysis of the antigen-presenting cell and cytokine production. Because of this delay in cellular lysis, which may occur up to 2 to 3 days after antigenic exposure, skin eruptions do not appear immediately. Contact dermatitis (e.g., poison ivy, chemical irritations, nickel metallic allergies) is the classic example of a type 4 immune response, typically referred to as delayed-type hypersensitivity. In addition, the positive wheal-and-flare response to *Mycobacterium tuberculosis* (TB) purified protein derivative (PPD) used in TB screening is also a type 4 immune response, which is why the tuberculin skin test (TST) is read 48 to 72 hours after it is administered.

CLINICAL PRESENTATION

Subjective

Patients with classic atopic disease report fatigue and/or malaise, irritability, itchy and watery eyes, sneezing, rhinorrhea, nasal congestion, coughing without sputum production (unless a secondary bacterial infection accompanies the allergy), pruritus, and, in more severe cases, wheezing. Two elements are common to subjective complaints associated with allergies. First, an exposure to an allergen precedes the onset of symptoms. Thus, allergic rhinitis can be distinguished from perennial rhinitis because environmental seasonal allergen exposure precedes the former. Second, patients typically attempt to control their symptoms with self-care. For example, their subjective picture usually includes self-medication and may be somewhat controlled with over-the-counter (OTC) agents. A history of subjective allergic symptoms, therefore, requires accompanying inquiry concerning the use of OTC antihistamines and decongestants.

Objective

The sinuses may be tender to percussion if nasal congestion has predisposed a patient to sinusitis (due to impeded mucous drainage); otherwise, the sinuses are typically nontender in uncomplicated allergic rhinitis. The conjunctivae and mucous membranes in general will be injected. Nasal turbinates are erythematous. Cervical nodes may feel small and hard ("shotty"), with few greater than 1 cm in size. Postauricular nodes and thoracic nodes are less commonly involved. Tympanic membranes may appear dull to light but will be otherwise unremarkable.

Tachycardia typically accompanies OTC decongestant use, but fever does not contribute to the tachycardia, as it is almost always absent from allergic reactions. Drowsiness is also typical with OTC antihistamine use (especially with first generation H_1-blocking agents with greater central nervous system [CNS] penetration). Lungs will be clear after several deep breaths and coughs, unless allergic asthma results in wheezing. Except in patients with anaphylaxis or allergenic invasion of the GI tract, the abdominal examination will be unremarkable. In these exceptional cases, profound abdominal tenderness may inhibit deep palpation.

Skin eruptions will depend on the type of allergic reaction and may include urticaria (type 1 response), fissures, circumscribed papules, bullae, and petechiae. The clinician should expect no singular picture of skin eruptions that corresponds with the allergenic source; however, there are associations in skin presentation and history that may lend themselves to diagnostic conclusions. For example, a history of exposure to poison ivy and multiple circumscribed papules in the anatomical place of exposure provides an association that is diagnostic of delayed-type hypersensitivity to a specific exposure. Poison ivy, poison oak, and poison sumac all produce contact dermatitis caused by the oily irritant substance urushiol, which is contained in the leaves of these plants, leading to a delayed, cell-mediated (type 4) immune response.

If the patient's sensorium is affected, an objective mental status examination may reveal diminished problem-solving ability, impairment in recent recall, and unfocused attention. These signs are particularly evident in older adults.

DIAGNOSTIC REASONING

Diagnostic Tests

Initial evaluation begins with the clinical history. The clinician should ask the patient to describe any changes in diet, skin-care products, or activities involving environmental exposures that preceded the onset of allergic symptoms. Suspicions raised by the history will often be confirmed or at least supported by subsequent diagnostic testing. Thus, particularly with regard to the evaluation of environmental exposures, a detailed history informed by the clinical presentation should largely drive diagnostic allergy testing.

Type 1 Response

Some clinicians recommend initial testing with skin tests by allergists to diagnose the response to specific allergens. Skin tests involve first pricking the epidermis with a small amount of a liquid extract of each allergen of interest. Later, to test suspicious allergens that initially result as negative on prick testing, small amounts of these extracts can be injected into the intradermal layers of the skin, which is believed to be a more sensitive form of skin testing than prick testing. (Patch testing, in which small amounts of emulsions of potential allergens are applied directly to the skin and left in place for 24 to 48 hours, is generally performed to diagnose contact dermatitis and other manifestations of type 4 hypersensitivity reactions.) Skin prick testing is the first stage of allergen testing because of the very slight but potentially fatal risk that the applied allergen could cause a serious systemic allergic response (anaphylaxis). Thus, for every negative prick test, an intradermal injection may be placed as a more sensitive, albeit potentially higher risk, method of allergen testing.

The selection of antigens to be tested follows a pattern of reasoning based on the question: What are the most likely culprits? The exact composition of skin-test panels is determined by regional and patient-specific determinants. An allergist will expose the patient to small amounts of regional and suspected environmental allergens in skin test panels by prick or injection. If the test is positive, a wheal should appear in 15 to 20 minutes. The reliability and sensitivity of skin testing make it the preferred test for initial diagnosis. Skin tests are done with both positive (histamine) and negative (inert substances, such as saline) controls, and results must be judged against these controls as some individuals are sensitive to any kind of scratching or pricking of the skin, just by nature of the insult to the skin, and not due to hypersensitivity to the antigen.

The rate of false-positive responses in allergen skin testing is high. Testing should not be done indiscriminately or overinterpreted. In fact, many environmental and food allergens may test positive in up to half of the general population who otherwise demonstrate no other manifestations of hypersensitivity to these antigens. In turn, skin tests are far more useful in ruling out (i.e., excluding, rather than confirming) specific antigenic hypersensitivities, when reactions are negative.

Alternatives to allergen skin testing include in vitro serum-based testing methods, such as the radioallergosorbent test (RAST), the enzyme-linked immunosorbent assay (ELISA), and the fluorescent antibody staining technique (FAST). These serum tests reduce the risk of hypersensitivity-type reactions from allergens as seen in skin testing because they only measure antigen-specific IgE levels in the blood, rather than assess for functional

---

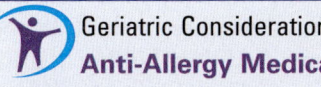

Geriatric Considerations: Anti-Allergy Medications

Older adults and others who practice polypharmacy with combination OTC agents may have a diminished mental status. Thus, it may be difficult to distinguish between the sedative effects of anti-allergy medications (in particular, antihistaminic agents) versus the effect of a chronic atopic condition that is affecting the patient's sleep–wake cycle, such as severe allergic rhinitis or nighttime asthma.

The risk of sedation may require dose reduction or a limited drug trial. Second generation antihistamines are typically less sedating than first generation agents. At prescribed doses, second generation agents dry secretions without causing excessive drowsiness in most patients and can be dosed once daily.

hypersensitivity responses. Thus, skin tests are typically more sensitive than serum RAST tests in detecting true hypersensitivity responses because more atopic individuals will be positive on skin tests than will have elevated antigen-specific IgE serum levels. RAST tests are usually considered more specific than allergen skin testing, as nonatopic individuals are unlikely to have high allergen-specific IgE levels, which must be balanced with their relatively decreased level of diagnostic sensitivity.

Consideration of sensitivity and specificity of allergy testing is particularly important for food challenge testing, which often uses skin prick testing as an initial screen to rule out specific food allergies, given its high sensitivity. Some clinicians also complement skin testing with RAST testing because although some food allergies may be type 3 immune complex responses, others are type 1 anaphylactic food allergy reactions that are IgE mediated and clinically severe. Definitive testing for such reactions may take place via blinded food challenges in an office setting by an allergy specialist (with ready access to endotracheal intubation supplies and injectable epinephrine) in the presence of physicians or other persons qualified to treat anaphylactic reactions. Set amounts of food are given to persons suspected of food allergy (typically children) in progressively increasing amounts, and individuals are subsequently monitored for several hours for any reaction. This is a highly specific test and is thus very effective in ruling out food allergies. Obviously, however, this testing method carries a risk of anaphylaxis. Thus, RAST testing may be done instead of an observed food challenge to avoid needlessly subjecting individuals with high food-specific IgE levels to intentional exposure with the corresponding food trigger.

The most common form of asthma is an allergen-driven atopic disease characterized by type 1 immune responses to environmental allergens, although it is distinct from systemic anaphylaxis. Atopic airway hyperreactivity may also be triggered by environmental irritants, such as tobacco smoke, which is not a true allergen. Thus, these individuals do not express tobacco-specific IgE levels, although smoke and other environmental pollutants may trigger an asthma attack. Reactive airway disease (bronchial hyperresponsiveness), therefore, may be either allergic or nonallergic in origin. As asthma is largely an atopic, allergen-driven disease, sputum from an asthmatic patient may reveal eosinophils after staining with methylene blue dye; sputum from atopic individuals typically demonstrates higher levels of eosinophils than in the nonatopic population.

Type 2 Response

Rh testing of blood during pregnancy is the initial test to determine prospective Rh incompatibility. In infants with suspected immune-mediated hemolytic anemia, an elevated indirect bilirubin level indicates hemolysis. Red blood cell (RBC) hemolysis is further associated with decreased serum haptoglobin levels. Autoimmune hemolytic anemia is also associated with a positive Coombs test, which detects RBC-specific antibodies in the blood.

Type 3 Response

Initial tests are employed to detect complement activation, as an underlying step in immune-complex reactions. A complement-based ELISA will give specific evidence of complement activation and consumption of complement proteins. For example, the ELISA might show lower levels of C_3 and/or C_4, which are two complement factors that may be diminished if an allergic inflammatory reaction has activated the complement system. Similarly, the CH50 test, which is a measure of overall complement protein levels, will also be low in this setting. Skin manifestations in type 3 immune responses may be biopsied and stained for immune complex deposition, which is a hallmark of such reactions.

Type 4 Response

Skin testing is the initial test of preference for cell-mediated hypersensitivity. Allergens are either injected intradermally or applied topically onto patches of skin. Results are then read 48 to 72 hours after application to assess for a delayed-type hypersensitivity reaction. Positive responses consist of induration (for injected allergens) and erythema and papules (for topically applied allergy skin patch testing).

Antigen-specific serum IgE levels may aid in distinguishing allergic from nonallergic immune responses. For example, classic type 1 hypersensitivity reactions are IgE-mediated, whereas cell-mediated type 4 responses are not. Although both type 2 and type 3 responses are antibody mediated, the IgE immunoglobulin class is not typically involved in those reactions. An elevated peripheral eosinophil count may also provide secondary confirmation of recent IgE-mediated atopic disease.

Differential Diagnosis

Clinical history is the mainstay of differentiating allergic disease. Allergies are triggered by exposure to environmental antigens. The history, therefore, must support allergenic exposure proximal to the onset of symptoms and may often reveal partial or temporary relief of symptoms from OTC allergy remedies, as well as possible familial allergic patterns. Additional differentiation of classic allergic disease from other types of immune responses comes from skin test results, antigen-specific IgE levels, and other diagnostic tests aimed at identifying antibody-mediated immune responses.

Alternatively, irritants that enter the body but do not initiate classical immune-mediated hypersensitivity responses include nonallergic sources, such as air pollutants and tobacco smoke. In addition, some research has suggested that susceptible asthmatic patients may experience worsening of symptoms associated with barometric changes in the atmosphere, although it is unclear whether this weather-related phenomenon may actually be due to increases in airborne pollen levels associated with atmospheric pressure changes.

MANAGEMENT

Allergy management requires both symptomatic relief and prevention of exposure to specific allergens. After the initial diagnosis and treatment of acute symptoms, priority should be given to identifying and avoiding triggering allergens, whether with respect to respiratory symptoms (asthma, allergic rhinitis), cutaneous manifestations (urticaria), ocular allergies, or systemic allergic reactions (anaphylaxis). (Atopic dermatitis, another core atopic disorder, is covered in detail in Chapter 16.) For both allergic rhinitis and asthma patients, long-term immunomodulatory therapy with allergy vaccines (i.e., allergen immunotherapy) offers both effective prophylaxis and attenuation of future atopic symptoms.

Initial Management

The patient must become vigilant in avoiding further allergenic exposure. After clinical history, skin testing, and antigen-specific IgE levels have identified likely triggering allergens, avoidance behaviors should be initiated. For example, individuals diagnosed with hypersensitivity to penicillin must avoid not only penicillin but also cephalosporins, given the likelihood of cross reactivity. However, although penicillin remains one of the most common triggers of antibiotic hypersensitivity, penicillin allergy is typically overdiagnosed based on often unreliable self-reporting. Thus, a detailed patient history should focus on whether an anaphylactic reaction to penicillin truly occurred, as research involving confirmatory skin testing and antibiotic challenge has consistently demonstrated that most patients who report penicillin allergies do not have true penicillin hypersensitivity reactions or contraindicating anaphylaxis. Moreover, when use of a specific antibiotic class is deemed essential in an allergic patient, desensitization to penicillin or other antibiotics can be performed in a controlled clinical environment with the capacity to treat anaphylaxis and other forms of hypersensitivity (e.g., intensive care or step-down unit).

Many other preventive behavioral interventions can be recommended to the allergic patient. Bee venom reactions can be avoided in venom-allergic patients by not disturbing beehives or wasp nests. Dust mite–allergic patients may use specially designed mattress and pillow covers that seal in dust mites and their allergenic fecal matter, avoid dust-collecting ceiling fans, remove carpets from bedrooms to limit dust mite exposure during sleeping hours, and regularly wash plush toys and any other potential dust reservoirs in hot water. Patients with pollen allergies should keep windows closed in favor of using air conditioning in both the home and car, as well as bathe soon after outdoor exposure to pollen, which can adhere to clothes and hair. Air conditioning filters should be changed regularly, although high-efficiency particulate air (HEPA) filters and chemical agents purported to reduce the concentration of aeroallergens have not been shown to be consistently effective.

Subsequent Management

Subsequent management consists of ongoing symptom control and immunotherapy. Although some of these treatments are available only by prescription, OTC formulations are commonly used for most respiratory, ocular, and cutaneous allergic manifestations (see Drugs Commonly Prescribed 63.1). There are many classes of drugs that have demonstrated efficacy for symptom management in allergic disease; for example, sympathomimetics (used as decongestants), antihistamines (both oral and topical), corticosteroids (topical, inhaled, or systemic), cromolyn, and theophylline. Newer generation antihistamines have been designed to have less anticholinergic effects and CNS penetration; therefore, they cause less tachycardia and sedation than first generation agents.

Drugs Commonly Prescribed 63.1: Over-the-Counter (OTC) Drugs for Allergic Reactions

DRUG	INDICATION/FORMULATION	CONSIDERATIONS
Oral first generation H$_1$ antihistamines	First-line therapy: allergy, hay fever, initial-onset urticaria (with or without angioedema)	Sedating; anticholinergic side effects
Diphenhydramine (Benadryl)	As above; common cold (for mucosal drying effect)	As above; may be used in pregnancy and lactating women
Chlorpheniramine (Chlor-Trimeton)	As above; common cold (for mucosal drying effect)	Sedating; anticholinergic side effects; also has sympathomimetic effects
Oral second generation H$_1$ antihistamines	First-line therapy: allergy (seasonal or perennial allergens), hay fever, ocular allergies, pruritus; once-daily dosing	Minimally or nonsedating at recommended doses

Continued

Drugs Commonly Prescribed 63.1: Over-the-Counter (OTC) Drugs for Allergic Reactions—cont'd

DRUG	INDICATION/FORMULATION	CONSIDERATIONS
Cetirizine (Zyrtec)	As above	As above; may be used in pregnancy and lactating women
Levocetirizine (Xyzal)	As above	Minimally or nonsedating at recommended doses
Loratadine (Claritin)	As above	As above; may be used in pregnancy and lactating women
Desloratadine (Clarinex)	As above	Minimally or nonsedating at recommended doses
Fexofenadine (Allegra)	As above; chronic idiopathic urticaria	Minimally or nonsedating at recommended doses
Oral H_2-receptor antagonists	May be useful for mild allergic reactions, especially with gastrointestinal manifestations	May have mood-altering and significant anticholinergic effects in older patients
Cimetidine (Tagamet)	As above	As above
Ranitidine (Zantac)	As above	As above
Intranasal corticosteroids	Chronic (seasonal or perennial) nasal and ocular allergic symptoms; persistent symptoms despite antihistamines; may be used once or twice daily (titratable)	Continuous use needed to prevent symptoms, because it is ineffective if used sporadically; side effects associated with chronic use (mucosal thinning, epistaxis, possible systemic corticosteroid effects in children with overuse)
Fluticasone propionate (Flonase)	As above	As above
Fluticasone furoate (Flonase Sensimist)	As above	As above
Mometasone furoate (Nasonex)	As above	As above
Oral sympathomimetics (α-receptor agonists)	Hay fever; nasal and ocular allergy symptoms including congestion, ocular pruritus, and watery ocular discharge; common cold (for mucosal decongestion and drying effect)	May increase heart rate and cause palpitations
Chlorpheniramine (Chlor-Trimeton)	As above	As above
Pseudoephedrine (Sudafed)	As above; breathing problems related to congestion, including for bronchitis	As above
Intranasal sympathomimetics (α-receptor agonists)	Nasal decongestion and mucosal drying	May induce tachyphylaxis (rebound nasal congestion after withdrawal from chronic use) known as *rhinitis medicamentosa*
Oxymetazoline (Afrin)	As above; short-term use only (not recommended for use more than several times a day or continuously for more than 3 days)	As above
Inhaled sympathomimetics (α-receptor agonists)	Bronchodilation; inhalational mist	May increase heart rate and cause palpitations
Epinephrine (Primatene Mist)	Reformulated to be chlorofluorocarbon (CFC)-free	As above

Of note, in addition to future allergen avoidance, the most severe form of allergic disease, anaphylaxis, requires emergent treatment (e.g., epinephrine, IV fluids) for immediate life-threatening manifestations caused by preformed inflammatory mediators, as well as prophylactic treatment (e.g., corticosteroids) for delayed, late-phase manifestations caused by de novo (newly formed) immune mediators, as described in Therapeutic Procedure 63.1. Because late-phase anaphylactic reactions may occur up to 24 hours after allergen exposure and can prove fatal, prophylactic corticosteroids should be given, although they are ineffective in treating acute symptoms, given their slow onset of action.

Symptom Control

Many OTC oral and topical agents are sympathomimetic (alpha-receptor agonist) in activity. Common examples of oral drugs in this class include pseudoephedrine (Sudafed), chlorpheniramine (Chlor-Trimeton), and intranasal oxymetazoline (Afrin) spray, which is also widely used on an as-needed basis. In addition, epinephrine is available OTC as an inhalational sympathomimetic therapy (Primatene Mist). Of note, the sale of the chlorofluorocarbon (CFC)–containing formulations of inhaled epinephrine was prohibited by the U.S. Food and Drug Administration (FDA) in 2012, given environmental concerns over the effect of CFC on ozone levels; in turn, inhaled formulations are now CFC free.

Sympathomimetic agents may display both alpha-adrenergic and beta-adrenergic properties. They vasoconstrict engorged mucosa (an alpha-adrenergic property) and dilate the bronchioles by relaxing smooth muscle (a beta-adrenergic property). Therefore, these medications support antihistamines in drying secretions while opening the airways of the nasopharynx and bronchial tree. In addition, however, they also typically increase heart rate and may lead to palpitations (a beta-adrenergic effect). Because of their low molecular weight and solubility, sympathomimetics may cross the blood–brain barrier, resulting in irritability, anxiety, and addiction potential, particularly when combined with other psychoactive substances such as ethanol. In addition, topical intranasal agents such as oxymetazoline are known to induce tachyphylaxis (i.e., a decreased response to the drug after frequent use over a relatively short period of time), resulting in rebound nasal congestion on withdrawal after chronic use (rhinitis medicamentosa).

The abuse potential of OTC sympathomimetics remains high for many reasons. They are available for purchase and consumption without professional supervision, are relatively inexpensive, provide rapid symptomatic relief, and are heavily marketed. In addition, sympathomimetic formulations may be readily manipulated to form highly addictive illicit drug substances, such as methamphetamine (which resulted in increasing restrictions on the OTC availability of some of these drugs, such as pseudoephedrine). In addition, regular use of short- and long-acting beta-adrenergic inhalants, such as albuterol (Proventil) and salmeterol (Serevent, Advair), may increase disease-related morbidity in asthmatic patients, including both exacerbations and asthma-related deaths.

Another class of agents widely used for allergic reactions and chronic atopic disease are the antihistamines. With both first and second generation agents now available OTC, antihistamines are widely used in allergic disease for their ability to block H_1-histamine receptors, thereby reducing the effects of histamine released early in the inflammatory cascade. The blockade of H_1-receptor sites also contributes to the therapeutic effect of drying secretions. Adverse effects include overdryness and sedation. The risk of sedation, particularly in older adults and children, may require dose reduction or a limited drug trial. Newer generation antihistamines such as desloratadine (Clarinex), fexofenadine (Allegra), and cetirizine (Zyrtec) are typically less sedating than first generation agents (e.g., diphenhydramine [Benadryl], hydroxyzine [Atarax]). At prescribed doses, second generation agents dry secretions without causing excessive drowsiness in most patients and can be dosed once daily. They are also not associated with untoward cardiac events (e.g., QTc prolongation, fatal arrhythmias), which have been observed with other long-acting second generation antihistamines now withdrawn from the market (e.g., astemizole [Hismanal], terfenadine [Seldane]), particularly when used in combination with macrolide antibiotics or azole antifungals. Anticholinergic agents such as intranasal ipratropium (Atrovent) are also effective at drying secretions.

H_2-receptor antagonists such as cimetidine (Tagamet) may also be useful in managing mild allergic reactions, although they are primarily used to decrease the production of stomach acid for GI symptoms. In some cases when allergy patients have failed to improve after receiving epinephrine and diphenhydramine, they have responded to cimetidine. However, H_2 blockers are known to cross the blood–brain barrier and may have mood-altering and significant anticholinergic effects, particularly in older patients.

Corticosteroids form a third group of drugs used in symptom control. Given their long onset of action (several hours), they have little role in the acute treatment of symptoms. However, they may prevent the recurrence of symptoms in patients with mild allergic reactions, such as urticaria. They also constitute part of the long-term treatment regimen of life-threatening allergic reactions, such as the manifestations of systemic anaphylaxis, including severe laryngeal edema, bronchospasm, and hypotension. For most hypersensitivity reactions, a dosage of 1 to 2 mg/kg per day of prednisone for 4 or 5 days is usually sufficient to prevent recurrent or late-onset symptoms. Short-term pulse dosing such as this does not require tapering. However, the clinician should consider tapering the regimen if the patient has received corticosteroid therapy in the recent past or if there are plans to continue therapy for more than several weeks. When given as short-term therapy, prednisone and other corticosteroids typically have benign adverse effect profiles. However, prolonged use of systemic corticosteroids has several implications, including the development of Cushingoid syndrome, adrenal insufficiency, and hyperglycemia.

Inhaled corticosteroids such as fluticasone propionate (Flovent) are used as standard prophylactic controller medications in allergic asthma (see Chapter 31). Intranasal corticosteroids such as mometasone furoate (Nasonex) are extremely effective for long-term control of both nasopharyngeal and ocular allergic rhinitis symptoms (see Chapter 24). Because corticosteroids are immunosuppressive anti-inflammatory agents, they effectively downregulate the allergic immune responses characteristic of atopic disease.

Immunotherapy

Allergen immunotherapy (allergy vaccine) offers the patient long-term control of atopic disease. Given the small, albeit well-documented, risk of anaphylaxis or other hypersensitivity reactions associated with allergen immunotherapy, its use is usually limited in scope to patients with intractable allergic rhinitis or asthma whose disease fails to be controlled with symptom management or for whom consistent allergen avoidance is not possible. Immunotherapy regimens should be prescribed and administered by a qualified specialist with expert knowledge in allergic diseases, as the first step is the proper identification of key allergens, which are the patient's most troublesome environmental triggers. Depending on the number of allergens identified, these extracts are combined into one or more allergy vaccine admixtures, taking into account both cross reactivity of individual allergens and the reduced stability of certain allergen extracts (e.g., plant pollens, animal dander) in combination with others, given the presence of proteolytic enzymes in many fungal and insect (e.g., dust mite, wasp, or bee venom) extracts.

Injections of commercially prepared extracts of these allergens are given subcutaneously in 0.5 mL allotments of diluent that progress from minimal dilutional strength to higher concentrations. The weekly injections continue, increasing in concentration until symptoms are controlled and/or the maximum concentration of allergen extract is achieved, at which time the frequency of injections may be decreased to once monthly. Immunotherapy may require more than 12 months of treatments before maximal effects are observed. There are also "rush immunotherapy" protocols that are being evaluated, which are shorter-course regimens that escalate a patient to maximal allergen extract concentrations more quickly than traditional regimens, although this raises the concern for an increased risk of anaphylaxis.

Current guidelines recommend continuing allergen immunotherapy for 3 to 5 years, after which many individuals experience lasting suppression of allergic hypersensitivity, allowing for the tapering and eventual cessation of extract injections. However, many patients experience a recurrence of allergic symptoms when they attempt to stop or even taper the frequency of maintenance immunotherapy. Thus, although not generally recommended, some patients may continue immunotherapy for life.

Injection allergen immunotherapy has been used therapeutically for well over a century. However, a more recent development is sublingual allergen immunotherapy formulations, in which liquid extract is administered in drops under the tongue for systemic absorption. The concept behind these regimens is the same as traditional subcutaneous and intradermal injection immunotherapy, although the convenience of this dosing route is self-evident, particularly given the potential for self-administration in nonclinical settings. Although sublingual immunotherapy has gained acceptance in Europe, its use is not as widespread in the United States, and evaluations of its safety and efficacy are ongoing.

Other forms of biological immunotherapy exist for allergic diseases. For extremely refractory cases of atopy, such as severe allergic asthma with atopic dermatitis, the anti-IgE monoclonal antibody omalizumab (Xolair) may be effective. Xolair is approved by the FDA for moderate to severe persistent asthma in persons 12 years and older. This therapy acts by binding circulating IgE and preventing its interaction with cell surface molecules on blood cells that mediate allergic hypersensitivity responses, including mast cells, basophils, and eosinophils, thereby preventing initiation of the allergic cascade.

Nursing Situation: Immunotherapy

A 55-year-old woman has severe and persistent allergic rhinitis refractory to both OTC and prescription controller medications. Her primary triggering allergens are dust mites, ragweed pollen, egg, and *Aspergillus*. Food-based allergen immunotherapy is not considered an acceptable therapeutic strategy, given the relatively higher risk of anaphylaxis to food antigens. Thus, she completely avoids egg in her diet. To avoid dust mite exposure, she has removed all carpeting from her bedroom and replaced her curtains with window blinds. However, she cannot relocate from her home in the midwestern United States, where ragweed pollen levels are elevated between July and October. Her husband cleans the bathroom tiles and kitchen cabinets where *Aspergillus* might grow.

For the past 3 months, she has seen her primary care practitioner on six occasions. Her medication regimen includes a prescribed inhaled intranasal corticosteroid and both long- and short-acting antihistamines. Despite treatment, her symptoms keep her awake at night, and recently she has started to wheeze, requiring use of an albuterol metered-dose inhaler (MDI). Her primary care practitioner referred her to an allergist, who identified her specific allergens and recommended allergen immunotherapy on the basis of the severity and recurrence of her symptoms, as well as her refractoriness to other medications. Because of the risk of anaphylaxis associated with allergen immunotherapy, the risk–benefit ratio of this approach is discussed extensively with the patient before she initiates an immunotherapy regimen. The patient undergoes allergen skin testing, and the results confirm allergic sensitivity to ragweed, dust mites, egg, and *Aspergillus*. The patient initiates weekly injections of an individual prepared allergy admixture at the lowest dilution. She continues this therapy and notes that after 3 months, she is able to control her symptoms with the inhaled intranasal corticosteroid and no longer needs the albuterol inhaler. The allergist recommends continuation of the immunotherapy for at least 1 year, after which the patient's condition and treatment regimen will be reassessed.

FOLLOW-UP AND REFERRAL

Follow-up of the patient with an allergic reaction is directly dependent on the severity and chronicity of the atopy and may consist of both regular visits and increased consultations during seasonal allergy periods, depending on symptoms. An allergist should be consulted if the patient's symptoms cannot be controlled. The allergist is responsible for ordering and evaluating skin tests and for prescribing, administering, and evaluating the effectiveness of immunotherapy. Follow-up tests include a complete blood count (CBC) to evaluate for leukocytosis and eosinophilia, as well as fasting blood sugar tests to assess for hyperglycemia if the patient requires systemic corticosteroids.

Patient Education: Allergic Reactions

Depending on the clinical manifestations, the patient must know what foods or other environmental allergens to avoid. The patient and clinician should decide together how to identify and control exposure to triggering allergens that may have been unknown by the patient before the diagnosis. For example, few patients know the places that dust mites hide or understand how to eradicate *Aspergillus* with simple household chemicals.

Patients with significant respiratory symptoms may need to learn how to use nasal inhalants for significant rhinitis symptoms or MDIs for bronchial/pulmonary symptoms. Initial use under the clinician's supervision can provide both the patient and clinician with reassurance that the drug will be delivered correctly. For patients with asthma, the use of spacers for MDIs should be taught and encouraged as a means of maximizing medication delivery (see Chapter 31). The patient should learn which drugs may be taken together without significant risk of interaction and which should be administered alone or with food to facilitate absorption. The narrow therapeutic index of some drugs, such as theophylline used for asthma treatment, requires vigilance on the part of the patient to report early symptoms of drug toxicity.

Patients with a history of anaphylaxis must have epinephrine available at all times for emergencies, should they encounter offending allergens. The immediate use of epinephrine after any exposure to a known anaphylactic triggering agent is crucial. The clinician should prescribe self-administered intramuscular epinephrine (e.g., EpiPen, Auvi-Q) and have the patient demonstrate an understanding of the injectable device before leaving the clinic. The patient should be instructed that whenever a dose is self-administered, emergency department care should be sought in case the reaction worsens or recurs, requiring more advanced therapy such as IV epinephrine or crystalloid infusion. Given the life-threatening nature of anaphylaxis, susceptible individuals with a history of systemic hypersensitivity reactions to environmental triggers must always have access to a readily available source of epinephrine.

Many patients will take OTC agents to help with allergy symptoms and should be taught to read and interpret drug labels correctly to check for ingredients that might cause tachycardia, drowsiness, or other adverse effects. Given safety concerns with several adrenergic agents when used in combination with other drugs, patients should be cautioned to be alert for any OTC formulations containing ephedrine, phenylephrine, phenylpropanolamine, or pseudoephedrine.

RHEUMATOID ARTHRITIS

Rheumatoid arthritis (RA) is a chronic, progressive, systemic inflammatory disease that primarily affects the synovial joints, although it may affect many organ systems. Joints are destroyed over a long course of disease remissions and exacerbations. Structural deformities, which create physical as well as emotional trauma for the patient, are common as the disease progresses. *Healthy People 2030* has four objectives related to this chronic debilitating condition: (1) reduce the proportion of adults with arthritis whose arthritis limits their activities, (2) reduce the proportion of adults with arthritis whose arthritis limits their work, (3) increase the proportion of adults with arthritis who get counseling for physical activity, and (4) reduce the proportion of adults with arthritis who have moderate or severe joint pain.

EPIDEMIOLOGY AND CAUSES

RA is one of the most common connective tissue diseases in the United States and one of the most destructive to the joints. Females with the disease outnumber males at a ratio of 2.5 to 3.1:1, with a worldwide incidence of approximately 3 in 10,000 persons. Prevalence increases with age, with a peak of cases occurring between the ages of 40 and 60 years, after an onset of disease between 20 and 40 years of age. RA has been observed across all racial and ethnic groups, and familial patterns have been observed, with first-degree relatives of affected patients having approximately a two- to three-fold higher risk of developing the disease. An association between RA and the human leukocyte antigen (HLA) system, a series of linked genes on the chromosome 6, has been observed. Although genetic risk factors have been identified, the cause of the disease is unknown. Other potential etiological factors that have been implicated include infection, autoimmune responses, environmental triggers, and hormonal influences.

PATHOPHYSIOLOGY

RA causes joint destruction through many immunopathogenic mechanisms. Proteolytic enzymes (proteases) digest the tissue components of affected joints. This is speculated to occur due to local antigens that evoke the inflammatory cascade in the joint space. These antigens may be autoimmune targets (e.g., type II collagen found only in articular cartilage and the vitreous of the eye, glycoprotein-39 found in cartilage, cyclic citrullinated peptides [CCPs] including citrullinated fibrin, and glucose-6-phosphate isomerase), which activate self-reactive T cells that initiate the inflammatory cascade.

T cells comprise nearly half the immune cells in an inflamed rheumatoid joint and are characterized by an activated T helper phenotype based on the cell surface expression of HLA-DR (MHC class II) antigens, CD27, CD4, as well as the costimulatory molecules CD28 and CD40. Interestingly, some evidence indicates that it may not be the antigens themselves that trigger self-reactive T cells, but rather genetic mutations that alter specific amino acids within MHC class II antigen-presenting molecules (such as HLA-DRβ1) found on antigen-presenting cells. Other work has implicated superantigen interactions, in which several different T-cell clones are activated independently of their association with MHC class II molecules.

Cells of the synovial (joint) lining including joint endothelium, T cells, and fibroblast-like cells proliferate, producing cytokines (e.g., IL-1, IL-6, IL-8, IL-15, IL-18, IFN-γ), neuropeptides such as substance P, and chemotactic factors that induce expression of cell adhesion molecules (e.g., intercellular adhesion molecule [ICAM]-1, vascular cell adhesion molecule [VCAM]-1, P-selectin, E-selectin). This leads to increased recruitment of an array of immune cells into the affected joint, including mast cells that produce histamine, tryptase, leukotrienes, cytokines, and chymase; multinucleated cells and macrophages, which are the main source of potentially toxic nitric oxide and destructive matrix metalloproteinases (MMPs) (e.g., collagenase [MMP-1], stromelysin [MMP-3], macrophage elastase [MMP-12]); and self-reactive plasma cells capable of producing autoantibodies (e.g., rheumatoid factor [RF]). Synovial fibroblasts further produce MMP-13, which has great specificity for type II collagen and is primarily responsible for soft tissue destruction in the affected joint.

Particularly noteworthy in the pathogenesis of RA is the production of RF—polyclonal antibodies typically of the IgM class that have specificity for the constant FC region of IgG. RF forms large immune complexes capable of activating complement proteins that are cytolytic and chemotactic. The plasma cell genes that encode RF undergo somatic mutations that increase their affinity for IgG, a process known as *affinity maturation*. Although RF is not pathognomonic of RA (as it may also be present in scleroderma, systemic lupus erythematosus [SLE], and even some viral infections) and may be absent in up to 25% of RA cases, the presence of these antibodies in the peripheral circulation correlates with invasive disease of greater severity.

Another type of autoantibody found in the blood of RA patients, anti-CCP antibodies (ACPAs), primarily directed against the connective tissue protein filaggrin, are considered more specific for RA than RF and are now widely used in the diagnosis of early RA. In addition, antimutated citrullinated vimentin (anti-MCV) antibodies have been shown to be more specific than ACPAs in patients with early RA.

Tumor necrosis factor-alpha (TNF-α) is one of the main cytokines that triggers the proliferative rheumatoid synovium, which explains the efficacy of anti–TNF-α immunotherapies in treating RA. However, in addition to TNF-α, a wide array of cytokines has been implicated in the pathophysiology of the rheumatoid joint, including granulocyte-macrophage colony-stimulating factor, IL-2, IL-6, IL-13, IL-17, and transforming growth factor-beta (TGF-β). Moreover, cells of the synovial lining undergo transformation into a rapidly proliferating state (although incapable of true metastasis) in which several types of transcription factors (NF-κB, Fos, Jun, Raf, Myc) and intracellular kinases (e.g., mitogen-activated protein kinase) are upregulated.

As these various inflammatory pathways manifest over time, joints are progressively destroyed by an invasive rheumatoid pannus. The rheumatoid pannus consists of granulated vascular tissue extending from the vascular bed into the joint space. Acting similarly to a destructive malignancy, the pannus is characterized by increased angiogenesis (new blood vessel formation), which is mediated by the upregulation of several angiogenic cytokines and growth factors, including hypoxia-inducible factor-1, vascular endothelial growth factor (VEGF), heparin-binding growth factors, macrophage angiogenic factor, epithelial neutrophil activating peptide-78, TNF-α, prostaglandin E_1 (PGE_1), PGE_2, and IL-8. Despite this increased vascularity, circulation is often inadequate for the exaggerated level of cellular proliferation in the rheumatoid synovium. In addition, the increased intra-articular pressure within the affected joint resulting from cellular proliferation, fibrin and clotting factor deposition, and fluid accumulation may compress articular vessels, resulting in progressive joint ischemia and more tissue destruction.

Mutations and overexpression of certain cell cycle regulatory proteins such as the *p53* tumor suppressor gene have been identified in cells of the rheumatoid synovium, which may render them less susceptible to apoptosis (programmed cell death). Proteolytic enzymes (e.g., MMP, glycosidases) released by cells in the pannus destroy the connective tissue matrix, including glycosaminoglycans, fibronectin, proteoglycans such as chondroitin sulfate, and collagen, and eventually subchondral bony structures. In addition, certain components of the rheumatoid pannus, such as regulatory T cells and bone marrow stromal cells, induce differentiation and proliferation of bone osteoclasts, which leads to further joint destruction. However, the pannus remains responsive to antiproliferative immunosuppressant treatments.

Within the synovial fluid, an inflammatory response also ensues but with a notably different distribution of immune cells. Polymorphonuclear neutrophils are the most prominent cellular infiltrate, numbering upward of one billion in severely inflamed joints. These cells secrete a host of proteolytic enzymes into the joint fluid (e.g., myeloperoxidase, collagenase and other MMPs, elastase, and lysozyme), as well as inflammatory cytokines (e.g., prostaglandins, IL-1β), and chemotactic factors (e.g., leukotriene B4, platelet-activating factor). Because accumulation of joint fluid distends the joint capsule and contributes greatly to articular pains, aspiration of this exudative fluid may provide immediate relief.

The immunopathology of RA is widespread and extends beyond the joint synovium. Constitutional signs and symptoms including fever, anorexia, weight loss, and fatigue may be prominent during acute flares, reflecting the systemic nature of the disease, which may involve layers of the heart muscle, cardiac valves, pulmonary visceral pleura, the spleen, larynx, dura mater, and sclera (extra-articular manifestations). Other organ manifestations of RA may include pericardial effusions, cardiac dysfunction (including myocardial infarction), and rarely pericarditis. Lung manifestations may include pleural effusion, pleuritis, interstitial fibrosis, and bronchiolitis obliterans with organizing pneumonia. Hematological findings are not uncommon and may include anemia of chronic disease or thrombocytosis. RA associated with both splenomegaly and neutropenia is termed *Felty's syndrome*. Ocular manifestations include keratoconjunctivitis associated with dry eye syndrome (sicca), as well as episcleritis, uveitis, and nodular scleritis, which can lead to blindness.

Rheumatoid nodules are another common extra-articular manifestation of RA. These nodules typically appear on the elbows but may be found on any extensor surface of the body that is subject to repeated mechanical stress, pressure, or irritation. Found in up to 25% of RA patients, these initially microscopic nodules are subcutaneous and may form into larger granulomas, characterized by a central section of fibrinoid necrosis that is surrounded by a palisade of radially arranged, elongated connective tissue cells enveloped by chronic granulation tissue.

CLINICAL PRESENTATION

Subjective

In the early stages of the disease, the RA patient may complain of malaise, diffuse arthritis, weight loss, anorexia, and low-grade fever. In addition, the patient may complain of neuropathic pain in the extremities, ocular pain, and chest pain on deep inspiration. Joint swelling and immobility on rising, which abate or diminish throughout the day, characterize early rheumatoid disease. The patient typically awakens with joint pain and stiffness but reports that it improves as the day progresses. As the disease progresses over time, recurrent pain and swelling in both small and large peripheral joints may result in diminished activity and worsening pain and immobility.

Objective

Key physical findings of RA are peripheral symmetric polyarthritis and morning stiffness, which typically last longer than 1 hour. The clinician may note that certain joints are affected more than others, such as the proximal interphalangeal (PIP) and metacarpophalangeal (MCP) joints in the hands and wrists, as well as the knees. The toes and ankles also tend to be affected. The clinician should expect the affected joints to be tender (painful to pressure), edematous, and partially immobile. Unlike radiographic x-ray, advanced magnetic resonance imaging (MRI) has shown promise as an imaging modality capable of detecting early joint manifestations with increased sensitivity compared with x-ray studies.

As the disease progresses, affected joints will appear more deformed and rigid, with diminished range of motion. Characteristic findings of advanced disease include Boutonnière deformity of affected fingers, in which the PIP joint is in a nonreducible state of flexion with hyperextension of the distal interphalangeal (DIP) joint, as well as the associated swan neck deformity, in which the PIP joint is hyperextended and the DIP joint is in a constant state of flexion. The most severe form of structural joint damage in the hands is known as *arthritis mutilans,* which is characterized by extensive bone resorption, complete loss of the joint space, shortening and malpositioning of the fingers, and almost complete loss of function.

Physical examination may also reveal additional significant findings associated with extra-articular organ manifestations of the disease. A cardiac rub associated with pericarditis may be detected. A pulmonary friction rub or diminished respiratory excursion may suggest inflammation of the visceral pleura, as well as involvement of the bony structures of the ribs and sternum. Dry crackles may reflect an interstitial pulmonary process in advanced chronic disease. A finding of injected sclera suggests scleritis. Loss of sensation, especially in the lower extremities, indicates peripheral neuropathy, and ecchymotic lesions may appear on the arms and legs. Rheumatoid nodules are commonly observed over the olecranon process or other extensor surfaces of the limbs and may be tender.

DIAGNOSTIC REASONING

Diagnostic Tests

The preferred initial test for diagnosis of RA is measurement of peripherally circulating RF. The test result provides both qualitative and quantitative information that is useful in correlating with physical markers of RA. For example, a positive RF titer of greater than 1:150 indicates a poorer prognosis and is often accompanied by findings of severe disease, such as rheumatoid nodules. It is necessary to interpret both the presence of RF (qualitative) with the dilutional titer (quantitative) because RF may be present in other diseases and its incidence increases with age. A more specific test than RF is to check for circulating ACPAs in the peripheral blood. These autoantibodies are more specific for RA and may be detected earlier in the disease process.

Initial testing should also include an erythrocyte sedimentation rate (ESR), which will be elevated if the disease is active. C-reactive protein (CRP) is an acute-phase reactant, which, like ESR, is reflective of a heightened inflammatory state. Thus, CRP may be evaluated in addition to or in place of ESR as an indicator of systemic inflammation. Other tests include a CBC to rule out anemia as a potential cause of fatigue and to evaluate for an associated leukocytosis or, alternatively, neutropenia. A platelet count (showing normal or high values) will become more elevated as joints become more inflamed. In addition, joint fluid analysis may aid in distinguishing RA from other causes of joint inflammation, such as infection. Aspirates from rheumatoid joints will show between 2,000 and 50,000 white blood cells (WBCs) per μL, with a pronounced neutrophil component.

Subsequent laboratory tests may be used as markers of disease progression. For example, ESR and CRP act as markers of inflammation, which may be helpful in tracking the course of disease and response to therapy. Quantitative antinuclear antibodies (ANAs) may also help in differentiating RA from SLE, because lower titers suggest rheumatoid disease. If the diagnosis is in doubt, a comprehensive autoantibody panel may be done to help distinguish RA from other autoimmune connective tissue disorders, such as Sjögren's syndrome (SS), although interpretation of such panels typically requires expert rheumatological knowledge.

Radiographic x-ray changes become evident after the disease has run its course for 6 months or more; radiographs will reveal bone erosions in the joints of the hands and feet. Plain films may show bone erosions in up to 30% of patients within 1 year of diagnosis and in up to 90% of cases after the first 2 years. MRI has gained wider acceptance in recent years as a more sensitive (albeit more expensive) detection method for joint changes in early disease.

Differential Diagnosis

In general, an array of connective tissue diseases must be considered in the differential diagnosis of RA. These include osteoarthritis, gout, chronic Lyme disease, SLE, infection by human parvovirus B19, polymyalgia rheumatica, SS, sarcoidosis, and various neoplasms. Osteoarthritis almost never affects the wrists and the MCP joints. Osteoarthritis is classically known for affecting the DIP joints with Heberden's nodes (hard, bony swellings) in the fingers. In contrast, the distal joints are less commonly affected in RA, and there are typically no Heberden's nodes in the hands. Within the thumb, the carpophalangeal joint is typically affected in osteoarthritis, whereas the interphalangeal joint is more often affected in RA.

A diagnosis of gout is confirmed by the finding of urate crystals in synovial aspirate. For crystalline arthritides, gout crystals are negatively birefringent, whereas pseudogout has positively birefringent calcium pyrophosphate crystals. Chronic Lyme disease usually involves only a single joint. A characteristic expanding bull's-eye rash (erythema migrans) is typical, and positive serological markers against the causative agent (*Borrelia burgdorferi*) distinguish Lyme disease from RA.

Infection with human parvovirus B19 may also manifest with joint pain. Serological evidence of antiparvovirus B19 IgM antibody and a characteristic rash with an erythematous "slapped cheek" appearance distinguish this infection from RA. When considering acute viral polyarthritis, other causative infections include hepatitis C and rubella (rubeola virus), which may be distinguished from RA via specific immunoassays and organism-specific antibody titers. Apart from infections, some neoplasms can mimic rheumatoid disease, but RF is typically negative or quantitatively low in this setting.

SLE arthritic changes are almost never deforming and erosive changes are absent on radiographs. Patients with polymyalgia rheumatica are usually negative for RF or have low titers. In addition, this disease usually affects persons older than 50 years of age. Whereas qualitative RF positivity increases with age and may be nonspecifically present in older adults, patients with polymyalgia rheumatica may report myalgias but not distinctive arthralgias or arthritis.

A more challenging disease to distinguish from RA is psoriatic arthritis (PsA), because joint manifestations may not occur concurrently with cutaneous psoriatic findings in these patients. However, as a predominantly seronegative form of inflammatory arthritis, RF is usually not detected in PsA. If psoriatic lesions are not present at the time of evaluation, a family history of psoriasis and joint manifestations in one or more relatives usually supports this diagnosis. Another form of seronegative (RF-negative) spondyloarthritis, ankylosing spondylitis (AS), may also present with peripheral arthritis; however, the predominant feature of this condition is axial (spinal) stiffness due to arthritis and dysfunctional bony changes in the vertebral joints, which is not typically seen in RA. The distinguishing features of PsA, AS, and the other common forms of spondyloarthritis are summarized in Table 63.1.

MANAGEMENT

The management of RA progresses from conservative interventions to aggressive symptom management. Although the disease is debilitating over time, clinicians also recognize the potential adverse effects of immunosuppressive and anti-inflammatory therapies, including increased infection risk and hepatotoxicity.

The overall goals of management are to reduce pain and inflammation and preserve joint function. It is possible to achieve these goals in early management without pharmacological agents. This section on management, therefore, includes nonpharmacological interventions as therapy for RA, particularly early in the disease process.

Initial Management

Early disease symptoms can be managed by one or a combination of the following: physical and occupational therapies, heat and cold applications, exercise, rest, assistive devices, splints, meditation, chiropractic adjustments, and weight loss. Physical and occupational therapists are educated to identify strategies that promote function and prevent immobility. Their special skills in motivating patients to remain active should not be underestimated in early disease management. Often patients attend therapy sessions and derive accompanying educational and emotional benefits from associating with other patients diagnosed with RA.

Heat and cold applications provide analgesia and relaxation to muscles and connective tissue. It is usually necessary to try both heat and cold therapy with individual patients because some patients respond better to one rather than the other. Application in anticipation of exercise may enhance joint mobility during exercise. Particularly helpful to some patients is to remain seated in warm water for 10 to 30 minutes.

Exercise reduces pain and inflammation only if the affected joints are not stressed during an inflammatory period. Outside of an inflammatory event, the joints may undergo judicious stress through an increase in resistance exercises to promote strength and endurance. Thus, isometric exercises (in which the joint angle and muscle length are held constant) should be prescribed for inflamed joints, and isotonic exercises (in which muscle length is shortened with contractions against a constant load) should be done at other times. Patients may also benefit from low-resistance aerobic exercise at the shallow end of a swimming pool.

Rest reduces pain and inflammation by controlling joint movement. However, one must distinguish between systemic rest and resting of the joints. Systemic rest signifies a prescribed period of relaxation that may involve sleep. Patients with mild inflammation may benefit from systemic rest in the prone position for 1 to 2 hours per day; the rest period may extend to 2-hour periods three or four times daily during waking hours, as necessitated by severe inflammation. Like systemic rest, resting of the joints should be done in a prone position to avoid hip contractures; however, the duration of rest is much shorter than with systemic rest, usually lasting only 20 to 40 minutes. In either case, the patient should prepare a method for awakening to avoid excessive systemic rest, as excessive rest may signal depression or other underlying disease.

Assistive devices include equipment that the patient requires to complete activities of daily living. Canes or crutches can relieve stress on affected weight-bearing joints during periods of acute inflammation. Once the inflammation subsides, the patient may walk without such devices. When the clinician or physical therapist recommends using a cane or crutches, it is important to the patient's self-esteem and inner hope to explain that these may be needed only temporarily. Other assistive devices for the home include bars for gripping the inside of a shower or bathtub or beside the toilet, a raised toilet seat, retrieval–extension devices for picking up items from the floor or at a distance, and an electronic chair lift to help the patient manage stairs.

Splints reduce pain, promote function, and stabilize involved joints. The hands and wrists are the preferred regions for splints, which are usually applied at night. Splints of the hips and knees are usually not preferred over lying prone. The position of optimal function should be considered when applying the splint. Moreover, the material of the splint should be lightweight, nonabrasive, and durable enough to withstand frequent applications. Because self-application is preferred, the splint should be structured so that the patient can apply it without assistance.

Meditation may be helpful in relieving depression and anxiety associated with chronic disease and disability. In addition, it promotes self-care practices and self-efficacy. Meditation may follow traditional spiritual paths, whereby patients learn from teachers in traditional religious communities. Alternatively, meditation may involve guiding the attention using restful music, images, spiritual charms, and breath work. Patients with RA should meditate in a prone position to prevent postmeditation joint stiffness and pain.

TABLE 63.1 Distinguishing Features of Spondyloarthritides

The spondyloarthritides encompass a group of inflammatory arthritides with distinct disease mechanisms that differ in both pathophysiology and clinical presentation from rheumatoid arthritis (RA). Unlike RA, these disorders are termed seronegative arthritides, because of the typical absence of rheumatoid factor (RF). The group of spondyloarthritides comprises both axial and peripheral spondyloarthritis (SpA), which together occur in 0.3% to 1.9% of the population, similar to the prevalence reported for RA. Axial SpA refers to conditions that display disease manifestations with predominantly axial (spinal) involvement, e.g., ankylosing spondylitis (AS) and nonradiographic axial spondyloarthritis (nr-axSpA). Peripheral SpA features include arthritis, enthesitis, and dactylitis, with psoriatic arthritis (PsA) being the most prevalent entity. Similar patterns of inflammatory arthritis may be seen after distal infection (e.g., sexually transmitted *Chlamydia* infection or *Salmonella, Shigella, Yersinia,* or *Campylobacter* gastrointestinal infection) as reactive arthritis or associated with inflammatory bowel disease (e.g., Crohn's disease, ulcerative colitis) as enteropathic arthritis, with other forms classified as undifferentiated inflammatory arthritis.

Classification	Epidemiology	Diagnosis	Clinical Presentation	Pathophysiology	Management	Prognosis
Spondyloarthritis Patients who are classified as having axial or peripheral SpA by Assessment of the Spondyloarthritis International Society (**ASAS**) criteria, including PsA by Classification Criteria for the Study of Psoriatic Arthritis (**CASPAR**) criteria	Prevalence 0.3%–1.9%	Systemic inflammatory disorders characterized by musculoskeletal manifestations (sacroiliitis, enthesitis, peripheral arthritis, reactive arthritis) associated with nonmusculoskeletal features (mucocutaneous, ocular, gastrointestinal, cardiovascular)	Chronic systemic inflammatory rheumatic disorders with skeletal involvement and inflammation at tendon and ligament bone insertion sites (enthesitis) Extra-articular manifestations are common, and some patients present associations with psoriasis or inflammatory bowel disease	Seronegative: RF negative and anti-cyclic citrullinated peptide (anti-CCP) antibody-negative arthritides Evidence for a central role of immune dysregulation and involvement of proinflammatory cytokines (e.g., TNF-α, IL-17, IL-23) in disease pathogenesis	Nonpharmacological treatment of patients with SpA consists of physical exercise, with adequate patient education Initial symptomatic response to NSAIDs and analgesics as first-line treatment for pain and stiffness Glucocorticoids administered as local injections or low-dose systemic glucocorticoids Conventional disease-modifying antirheumatic drugs (cDMARDs), such as methotrexate and sulfasalazine Biological DMARDs that neutralize proinflammatory cytokines (e.g., inhibitors of TNF-α, IL-17, IL-23) Immunomodulatory drugs (e.g., Janus kinase [JAK] inhibitors)	Long-term disability and negative socioeconomic impact are common in patients suffering from SpA Longer disease duration, reduced physical functioning, and physically demanding daily activities are risk factors for work disability and lower quality of life

Subcategory:					
Axial Spondyloarthritis	Full spectrum of disease is estimated to be as prevalent as RA	Predominance of spinal inflammatory arthritis of the central bony axis	Chronic inflammatory lower back pain, stiffness, and limitation of spinal mobility. Acute anterior uveitis occurs in up to 40% of patients as a comorbidity	Strong genetic predisposition associated with human leukocyte antigen (HLA)-B27	Same treatments are effective across full spectrum of disease (regardless of nonradiographic or radiographic disease manifestations)	Survival may be reduced compared with general population, but has improved with current standard of care, as mortality risk correlates with disease activity; cardiovascular disease is the most common cause of death
Non-radiographic Axial Spondyloarthritis (nr-axSpA)	Prevalence estimated to be equal to AS	Diagnosis of nr-axSpA requires a combination of clinical, laboratory, and imaging parameters: inflammatory back pain in the absence of sacroiliitis on x-ray, but with MRI evidence of spinal structural damage or elevated inflammatory markers (e.g., C-reactive protein [CRP]) in the presence of HLA-B27	Back pain lasting 3 months or longer, which worsens with rest. Equal male:female ratio of 1:1, with onset before the age of 45 years. Active inflammation showing subchondral bone edema on MRI distinguishes nr-axSpA from mechanical back pain	HLA-B27 plays a role in disease pathogenesis; overlap of susceptibility loci with inflammatory bowel disease loci have been reported. Altered intestinal microbiota could also play an important pathogenic role	Similar effectiveness of biological DMARDs (e.g., inhibitors of TNF-α, IL-17) in nr-axSpA and AS patients	Rates of progression from nr-axSpA to AS are between 5% and 30% over 2 to 30 years; thus, not all patients with nr-axSpA progress to AS

Continued

TABLE 63.1 Distinguishing Features of Spondyloarthritides—cont'd

Classification	Epidemiology	Diagnosis	Clinical Presentation	Pathophysiology	Management	Prognosis
Ankylosing Spondylitis (AS)	Prevalence: 0.1%–1.4% Incidence: 7.2 per 100,000 adults	1984 modified New York Criteria for the classification of AS: sacroiliitis or spondylitis noted on x-ray	Chronic inflammatory disease affecting the spine, entheses, and occasionally peripheral joints Male-female ratio 2–3:1 Hip involvement predictive of severe disease; disability and deformities usually occur within first 10 years of disease	HLA-B27 believed to be directly involved in disease pathogenesis Arthritogenic Peptide Hypothesis proposes that different HLA-B27 subtypes have the ability to present peptides to cross-reacting cytotoxic T cells; inflammation ensues at fibrocartilaginous sites, such as the sacroiliac joints and peripheral sites adjacent to entheses	Patient education and physical therapy, especially early in the diagnosis Symptomatic response to NSAIDs and analgesics as first-line treatment for pain and stiffness to facilitate physical therapy Oral DMARDs (e.g., sulfasalazine and methotrexate) have some efficacy on peripheral but not axial joint manifestations Biological DMARDs that neutralize proinflammatory cytokines (e.g., inhibitors of TNF-α, IL-17) suppress symptoms and reduce disability	Early diagnosis and screening in primary care setting is important for starting physical therapy early Treatment with NSAIDs and biological DMARDs can delay or prevent surgical interventions (e.g., hip replacement, spinal surgery) and can even achieve remission in a substantial group of patients with AS
Subcategory: Peripheral Spondyloarthritis *Psoriatic Arthritis (PsA)*	Prevalence: 0.3%–1% Incidence: 3.6 to 9.8 per 100,000 adults	Chronic inflammatory arthritis associated with psoriasis or psoriatic nail disease Multiple subtypes: peripheral arthritis with distal interphalangeal joint involvement; oligoarticular arthritis; symmetric polyarthritis; arthritis mutilans	Multidomain disease characterized by inflammatory arthritis, often associated with psoriasis and psoriatic nail disease Equally affecting males and females, with onset in patients age 50 years or older Radiographic structural damage reveals joint erosions and joint space narrowing, as well as proliferative new bone formation Typical clinical features include distal interphalangeal joint swelling and tenderness, dactylitis, and enthesitis, often associated with plaque psoriasis	Heritable disease mediated by multiple genes with low-risk effect (e.g., IL12B, IL23R, HLA-Cw6) Etiology unknown, although an association with HIV infection has been suggested Systemic inflammation with increased erythrocyte sedimentation rate (ESR) and/or CRP that positively correlate with disease activity Positivity for autoantibodies (e.g., RF, anti-CCP, antinuclear antibody [ANA]) found in up to 10% of patients	Moderate efficacy of cDMARDs (e.g., methotrexate, sulfasalazine, leflunomide) for peripheral arthritis inadequately controlled by NSAIDs and glucocorticoids Strong efficacy and safety with biological DMARDs (e.g., inhibitors of TNF-α, IL-17, IL-12 and/or IL-23) for treatment of peripheral arthritis, psoriasis, enthesitis, dactylitis, and inhibition of structural damage) Immunomodulatory small molecule inhibitors of Janus kinase (JAK) administered orally	Patient education, physical therapy, and occupational therapy associated with conventional treatments can improve quality of life and prevent irreversible joint damage and the need for surgical joint replacement

The role of chiropractic adjustment remains controversial among traditional Western medicine practitioners; however, its benefits to the patient with RA must be considered. Chiropractors can relieve pressure on unaffected joints that compensates for decreased weight-bearing or activity in the affected joints. Although adjustments may require repeated manipulations and therapeutic benefits may be short-lived, other benefits include an increased sense of well-being and improved quality of life.

Weight loss reduces pressure on weight-bearing joints in the lower extremities and enhances activity. Alternatively, overeating may be a sign of depression. Thus, weight gain must be addressed in an overall plan of encouraging weight reduction (if applicable) to achieve ideal body weight.

Subsequent Management

Drug therapies include analgesics, NSAIDs, corticosteroids, nonbiologic and biological disease-modifying antirheumatic drugs (DMARDs), and older therapies as described in the following sections.

Analgesics

Analgesics such as acetaminophen (Tylenol) or capsaicin cream, gel, lotion, or roll-on may be effective, even though they have no anti-inflammatory effects. Although aspirin has been the mainstay of therapy for RA, acetaminophen may be helpful for mild pain. Of note, opioid analgesics have also been used for more significant pain, although these agents are addictive and are not disease modifying in RA. Given the public health risks associated with the overuse of prescription opioids, reliance on narcotic analgesics as primary RA therapy is strongly discouraged and presents a significant danger for the patient.

NSAIDs

Subsequent management begins with a consideration of cyclooxygenase (COX) inhibitors, which include aspirin and other NSAIDs. Drugs of this class may not need to be used daily during the early stages of disease; rather, the patient can take them only for pain that is unrelieved by nonpharmacological means. Patients may be individually more responsive to one type of NSAID than another, and trial courses are sometimes required to determine the most effective agent, although simultaneous use of multiple NSAIDs is discouraged. Different NSAIDs may also differ in their side-effect profiles (e.g., sulindac 150 mg by mouth [PO] twice daily, conferring fewer GI side effects than other NSAIDs). However, the adverse effects of NSAIDs as a class are well documented, including renal toxicity, GI side effects, platelet inhibition, and idiosyncratic hypersensitivity reactions. Thus, they should not be used indiscriminately.

Extra-strength (1,000 mg) aspirin can be used up to three to four times per day if baseline liver function studies, platelet count, renal function studies, and hemoglobin level are within normal limits. Caution must be exercised when prescribing 4 g of aspirin per day to persons older than 65 years of age, however, as their hepatic and renal function may be impaired by age. Dose reductions are warranted if adverse effects ensue or laboratory markers dictate. Aspirin should always be taken with 8 ounces of water or milk to avoid pill erosion or ulceration of the gastric mucosa. Enteric-coated aspirin is preferred to prevent gastric erosion. Concurrent anticoagulant therapy is a relative contraindication to aspirin and other NSAID use. Patients on anticoagulant therapy should avoid these medications or, if benefits of these medications are thought to outweigh their risks, lower doses may be used.

If adverse effects of aspirin occur or if its therapeutic efficacy diminishes, other NSAIDs may be used. With chronic use, individual drugs of the same NSAID class can lose their effectiveness in a specific patient. However, many different NSAIDs are available, and clinicians may recommend a different NSAID in these cases.

The primary adverse effect of NSAIDs is GI discomfort. Their inhibition of gastric PGE (a natural stomach protectant) predisposes the gastric mucosa to erosion. Most NSAIDs can be taken with an H_2 blocker such as cimetidine (Tagamet) to reduce dyspepsia; however, H_2 blockers do not reduce hemorrhage or mucosal erosions. Proton pump inhibitors such as omeprazole (Prilosec) OTC or esomeprazole magnesium (Nexium) suppress gastric acid secretion and may be preferred to H_2 blockers for GI prophylaxis with NSAID use.

Minimal elevations in serum transaminase levels are to be expected at daily doses of 2,400 mg ibuprofen (Motrin, Advil) for adults younger than 65 years of age; the maximum dose may be as high as 3,200 mg/day if no adverse effects are apparent, but prolonged use of such doses may confer significant renal, hepatic, or GI toxicity, as well as iatrogenic hypertension. Should transaminase levels exceed two times the upper limit of normal, a dose reduction is indicated, along with laboratory evaluation for infectious causes of elevated liver enzymes, such as screening for hepatitis B and C.

Toxicity from prolonged NSAID use may result in renal impairment and present with acute renal failure requiring emergent care, as patients are prone to overuse NSAIDs, given their OTC availability and highly marketed nature. Thus, renal toxicity is as important a consideration as gastritis and ulcer formation. A rise in serum creatinine or blood urea nitrogen after starting NSAID therapy is an indication for further testing and initiating a possible dose reduction or cessation. Should renal failure develop, it is usually reversible after withdrawing the agent, given the proper supportive care.

Corticosteroids

Corticosteroids (up to 7.5 mg prednisone daily by mouth or injected intra-articularly, such as triamcinolone) may be helpful in RA. However, side effects of prolonged corticosteroid use include adrenal insufficiency, hyperglycemia, osteoporosis, increased infection risk, and skin discoloration, which explains why maximal daily therapy is not recommended for more than 6 months. In addition, calcium, vitamin D, and bisphosphonates are indicated with prolonged corticosteroid use to mitigate bone demineralization. (The adverse effect profile of corticosteroids is thoroughly covered in the atopic dermatitis section of Chapter 16.)

Disease-modifying Antirheumatic Drugs

DMARDs include immunosuppressants and immunomodulators of various types, many of which have been used for decades. However, the newest class of DMARDs are biological immunotherapeutic agents, including anticytokine immunotherapies (TNF-α inhibitors, IL-1 inhibitors, IL-6 inhibitors) and anti–B-cell and anti–T-cell agents (see Drugs Commonly Prescribed 63.2). Active disease should be treated early with DMARDs within 3 months of disease onset and even more aggressively in severe disease. Because anti–TNF-α therapy inhibits cell-mediated immunity, a potential side effect of this therapy is reactivation of latent (dormant) TB infection. TB screening should be instituted in all patients before starting biological immunosuppressive agents.

Combination therapy with DMARDs is more effective than monotherapy, and several different combinations have been tested. There is strong evidence for the greater efficacy of the combination of three DMARDs—methotrexate,

Drugs Commonly Prescribed 63.2: Disease-modifying Antirheumatic Drugs (DMARDs)

DRUG	ADVERSE REACTIONS AND PRESCRIBING CONSIDERATIONS
Aminoquinolines	
Hydroxychloroquine (Plaquenil)	May cause irreversible retinopathy, alopecia, blood dyscrasias, and QT interval prolongation.
Immunosuppressants	
Cyclosporine (Neoral)	Indicated only in patients who have not responded to methotrexate. Should not be used in pregnancy unless benefits outweigh potential risks to the fetus. Monitor renal and hepatic function. Reduce dose if hypertension occurs.
Pyrimidine Synthesis Inhibitors	
Leflunomide (Arava)	Monitor liver function. May cause GI upset, leukopenia, and thrombocytopenia.
Salicylate Sulfonamides	
Sulfasalazine (Azulfidine)	Monitor liver function. May cause nausea, dyspepsia, abdominal pain, vomiting, leukopenia, thrombocytopenia, and urine or skin discoloration.
Folic Acid Antagonists	
Methotrexate (Rheumatrex)	Monitor liver function. May cause blood dyscrasias (risk of cytopenia can be reduced with folic acid supplements), GI upset, hepatotoxicity, opportunistic infections, and fatal skin reactions.
Tumor Necrosis Factor (TNF)-α Blockers	
Caution with all TNF-α blockers for reactivation of TB and hepatitis B, predisposition to serious infection, development of lupus-like syndrome, development of selective cytopenias and pancytopenias, worsening of demyelinating syndromes, worsening of heart failure, increased malignancy rates, and cautious use in patients at risk for hepatic injury or with elevated liver function enzymes.	
Adalimumab (Humira)	May be used with or without methotrexate in moderate to severe RA.
Etanercept (Enbrel)	May be used with or without methotrexate in moderate to severe RA.
Infliximab (Remicade)	Should be used in combination with methotrexate for moderate to severe RA.
Certolizumab pegol (Cimzia)	May be used with or without methotrexate in moderate to severe RA.
Golimumab (Simponi)	Should be used in combination with methotrexate for moderate to severe RA.
Interleukin-1 Receptor Antagonists	
Anakinra (Kineret)	May cause predisposition to infections, headache, nausea, vomiting, diarrhea, stomach pain, and neutropenia.

Drugs Commonly Prescribed 63.2: Disease-modifying Antirheumatic Drugs (DMARDs)—cont'd

DRUG	ADVERSE REACTIONS AND PRESCRIBING CONSIDERATIONS
Interleukin-6 Receptor Antagonists	
Tocilizumab (Actemra)	May be used with or without methotrexate in patients with an inadequate response to one or more DMARDs, including TNF-α blockers. May predispose to infections, hyperlipidemia, GI perforation in at-risk patients.
Sarilumab (Kevzara)	May be used with or without methotrexate in patients with an inadequate response to one or more DMARDs, including TNF-α blockers. May predispose to infections, hyperlipidemia, and GI perforation in at-risk patients.
Anti–B-Cell Agents	
Rituximab (Rituxan)	Indicated for use with methotrexate in patients who do not respond to TNF-α blockers. Stop hypertension medications during treatment. May cause angioedema, abdominal pain or black tarry stools, and blood dyscrasias.
Anti–T-Cell Agents	
Abatacept (Orencia)	May be used as monotherapy or with other DMARDs, other than TNF-α blockers. May predispose to infections, headache, or respiratory adverse events in COPD patients.
Janus Kinase (JAK) Inhibitors	
May predispose to infections, hepatic enzyme elevations, neutropenia, anemia, and GI perforation in at-risk patients. Do not use in combination with TNF-α blockers or potent immunosuppressants such as azathioprine, cyclosporine, or other JAK inhibitors.	
Tofacitinib (Xeljanz)	May be used as monotherapy or with other DMARDs (other than indicated above) for moderate to severe RA.
Baricitinib (Olumiant)	May be used as monotherapy or with other DMARDs (other than indicated above) for moderate to severe RA.
Upadacitinib (Rinvoq)	May be used as monotherapy or with other DMARDs (other than indicated above) for moderate to severe RA.

sulfasalazine, and hydroxychloroquine—versus methotrexate monotherapy or dual therapy with only sulfasalazine and hydroxychloroquine. There is also strong evidence for adding a TNF-α blocking agent to methotrexate therapy in patients with moderately or highly active disease after 3 months of methotrexate monotherapy.

Although the anti–TNF-α agents are considered first-line biological DMARDs, other biological agents have been approved for use in RA patients with an inadequate therapeutic response or intolerance to anti–TNF-α agents (e.g., abatacept, rituximab, tocilizumab, sarilumab), as well as the small molecule oral Janus tyrosine kinase (JAK) inhibitors tofacitinib. It is not recommended, however, that immunosuppressive biological agents with different mechanisms of action be used in combination, given the risk of serious infection. Thus, therapies should be crafted based on the patient's tolerance of side effects and the presence of comorbid conditions.

Older Therapies

Other DMARDs are possible options in the event of treatment failure with aspirin and other NSAIDs, but these are used less often now, given their low therapeutic index (i.e., higher toxicity risk) and the development of newer biological agents, as discussed previously. These include azathioprine (Imuran), gold sodium thiomalate (Myochrysine), antimalarials, penicillamine (Depen), sulfasalazine (Azulfidine), and minocycline hydrochloride (Minocin). Hydroxychloroquine (Plaquenil) is an antimalarial usually used in milder disease, compared with sulfasalazine, which is used more often in moderate disease. Most of the COX-2 inhibitors, which were a mainstay of therapy in the past, are no longer marketed because of their cardiovascular risks. Celecoxib (Celebrex) is one of the last remaining COX-2 inhibitors.

Methotrexate (Rheumatrex) is an older agent that is also used in many common chemotherapeutic regimens for the treatment of cancer, as an inhibitor of tetrahydrofolate reductase, which prevents DNA and RNA synthesis and, therefore, cellular proliferation. In contrast to many other older DMARDs, methotrexate remains highly effective in RA, including when used in low-dose regimens early in the disease process. It may be administered in adults younger than 65 years of age at an initial weekly dose of 7.5 mg PO. The dosage may be doubled during the second week if tolerance and therapeutic aims necessitate, although its full therapeutic effect may take 4 to 6 weeks to manifest. The maximum dosage of methotrexate in RA is typically 25 mg per week.

The potential toxic effects of methotrexate include interstitial pneumonitis, hepatic cirrhosis, and teratogenicity. It is therefore not used in women who may become pregnant or in patients with chronic liver disease or elevated hepatic function enzymes. Combined use of methotrexate with NSAIDs, sulfonamides (e.g., trimethoprim-sulfamethoxazole [TMP-SMX]) or sulfonylureas such as glipizide [Glucotrol]) increases the chance of hepatotoxicity, so concurrent use of these drugs is discouraged. Increased risk of hepatotoxicity is also seen with diabetes mellitus, obesity, and renal disease. Chronic methotrexate use can also lead to cytopenias, which may be prevented through the use of folic acid supplementation. Thus, the decision to initiate methotrexate therapy must be weighed against its potential risks and the availability and appropriateness of alternative therapeutic options.

FOLLOW-UP AND REFERRAL

The follow-up of patients with RA requires routine clinical laboratory evaluation and episodic adjustments in therapeutic interventions. Routine clinical laboratory evaluation is performed every 90 days and includes CBC, platelet count, serum liver and renal function studies, and fasting blood sugar. Most of the adverse effects of drugs used in the management of RA can be monitored with this routine panel. If methotrexate is used, a serum albumin level should be added to the routine panel of tests to monitor hepatic synthetic function.

The CRP blood test is a nonspecific method for evaluating the severity and course of the inflammatory process in RA. CRP is normally less than 0.8 mg/dL and is typically elevated in RA before treatment. Failure to decrease the CRP level after initiating treatment may thus indicate a lack of efficacy of the therapeutic agent or the presence of an underlying infection or tissue necrosis; therefore, CRP should be monitored to determine the effectiveness of therapy.

After scheduled laboratory evaluations, each visit to the clinician should address the interim clinical history since the last visit. Attention should focus on the efficacy of relief measures and the onset, duration, and frequency of pain and swelling of the joints. Standardized and validated disease activity assessment tools may be completed by the clinician at each visit to assess how well treatment interventions have achieved the targeted goals of low disease activity and complete disease remission, commonly known as "treating to target."

The primary care practitioner should refer the patient to a rheumatologist if initial management (including aspirin or NSAID therapy) fails. The rheumatologist is responsible for initiating therapies such as methotrexate and other DMARDs, including newer biological agents. Comanagement may mean that the rheumatologist will evaluate the patient twice each year once stable or more frequently, as signs and symptoms necessitate. In particular, specialist input is typically required to effectively treat to target.

Patient Education: Rheumatoid Arthritis

Patient education focuses on the goals of therapy, which are reduction of pain, control of inflammation, and preservation of function. Many of the key patient education topics were covered under the earlier section on Initial Management. In addition, education should address the therapeutic and adverse effects of all drugs used. Because RA is a chronic disease, education should also encompass the emotional, social, and spiritual sequelae of living with recurrent bouts of pain and disability.

The goals of therapy are best realized by promoting self-care. Education concerning self-care should include caregivers who must share common therapeutic goals for the patient before they can support the patient's self-care practices. To help keep the patient from sinking into a cycle of seeking secondary gains from the "sick" role, the caregiver should support normal social role behaviors by encouraging self-care. The caregiver, therefore, becomes integral to achieving the therapeutic goals of therapy, which should be reviewed at each visit. This is an ideal context to employ the Circle of Caring model involving all medical modalities, nursing modalities, complementary therapies, and the patient's family.

CHRONIC FATIGUE SYNDROME AND FIBROMYALGIA SYNDROME

Chronic fatigue syndrome (CFS), also known as *myalgic encephalomyelitis* (ME), remains poorly understood, despite abundant attention in the scientific literature and lay press. Although an Institute of Medicine report recommended this condition be renamed *systemic exertion intolerance disease*, the lack of agreement as to its cause, laboratory markers, and clinical course may explain why the syndrome is not discussed in some medical texts. There appears to be significant overlap between CFS and fibromyalgia syndrome (FMS), another controversial chronic pain syndrome. Most patients with CFS meet criteria for FMS, and at least 70% of patients with FMS meet criteria for CFS. Moreover, both disorders have been widely recognized in persons with comorbid psychiatric illness, because nearly two-thirds of CFS patients and one-third of FMS patients meet criteria for depression or anxiety disorders. Many clinicians have criticized the historical and physical diagnostic criteria for both conditions as having a strong potential for overlap with somatization disorders.

EPIDEMIOLOGY AND CAUSES

Without a generally accepted working definition of CFS, it is difficult to systematically ascertain its epidemiology. Chronic fatigue is an initial complaint in up to 25% of patients in ambulatory care settings, and it is estimated that approximately 10% of these individuals meet diagnostic criteria for CFS. This syndrome has been hypothesized to be autoimmune or infectious in etiology; however, the causes for CFS have yet to be determined. Importantly, it is a diagnosis of exclusion, with the incidence ranging from 4 to 8.6 cases per 100,000 adults. In terms of prevalence, in 2015, the National Academies of Sciences, Engineering, and Medicine estimated that 2.5 million Americans suffer from CFS. Numerous books in the popular press have advanced the belief that females are affected twice as often as males, and the same references tend to agree that younger females are affected by CFS more often than older females.

More epidemiological data for FMS than CFS exist in the medical literature. An estimated 11 million people in the United States have FMS, 80% to 90% of whom are female. The prevalence of FMS has been estimated to be 0.5% for males and 3.4% for females, with some studies claiming an increased prevalence in females compared with males of up to 10:1. Prevalence is higher in older patients, at more than 7% for females aged 60 to 79 years.

These numbers are reflected in the clinical effect of FMS, as up to 20% of all patient visits to rheumatology practices are for FMS. It is now considered the most common cause of generalized musculoskeletal pain in females aged 20 to 55 years. FMS may occur with greater frequency in patients with disorders characterized by systemic inflammation, including RA, SLE, and hepatitis C infection. However, an underlying inflammatory etiology to FMS is unclear, because relatives of patients with fibromyalgia are seven times more likely than relatives of patients with RA to have FMS. In addition, several studies have shown that up to 50% of patients with FMS have a history of sexual and/or physical abuse, suggesting the importance of psychological factors in the development of FMS.

PATHOPHYSIOLOGY

Despite extensive investigation, the pathophysiologies of CFS and FMS are unclear. It has been hypothesized that both syndromes may be disorders of muscle energy metabolism, inflammatory or immunopathological diseases of muscle, generalized disorders of pain perception, neuronally mediated hypotension, neuroendocrine disturbances, dysregulated serotonin secretion, sleep disturbances, or a sequela of sexual abuse or domestic violence. Although depression and anxiety disorders demonstrate great overlap with both CFS and FMS, it is controversial as to whether these conditions occur concurrently, whether CFS and FMS lead to psychiatric sequelae, or whether these chronic conditions are somatic manifestations of underlying mood disorders. Patients commonly experience accusations of malingering (intentionally fabricating symptoms for secondary gain).

Extensive work has explored a potential infectious etiology for CFS, focusing on Epstein-Barr virus (EBV), retroviruses, and human herpesvirus-6 (HHV-6) as causative agents. However, there has been difficulty in reproducing positive results across different laboratories. Moreover, no consistent serological profile has been identified that distinguishes patients with CFS from control groups across multiple studies.

Several studies, however, have demonstrated qualitative and quantitative differences in immune function between patients with CFS and controls, including reduced numbers of natural killer cells with depressed function, reduced levels of immunoglobulin and immune complexes, and increased numbers of cell surface adhesion molecules, among others. However, the differences are of questionable clinical significance and have been inconsistent and even conflicting among different studies.

Studies that have examined neuroendocrine differences between affected patients and controls have produced similarly inconclusive results. Although some evidence points to diminished secretion of adrenocorticotropic hormone and reduced serum cortisol levels, these findings are not specific for CFS and have also been observed in FMS, as well as in healthy subjects with altered sleep patterns related to overnight work shifts.

Studies attempting to clarify the etiology of FMS have also not been definitive. For many years, FMS was considered a disorder of muscle metabolism, possibly related to chronic hypoxia of muscular tissue. However, studies of lactate levels, muscle force studies, and postexertional pain have demonstrated a marked similarity between patients with FMS and sedentary controls. Thus, the most current theories suggest that patients with FMS have disproportionate perceptions of pain, exacerbated by muscle inactivity and deconditioning. In fact, lower pain perception thresholds have been documented in first-degree relatives of patients with FMS.

Although no studies have been conclusive, altered pain perception is more likely to be a central rather than peripheral nociceptor (pain receptor) phenomenon. This is supported by observations in FMS patients of altered patterns of sleep and mood, decreased blood flow to pain centers in the brain, and alterations in serotonin secretions and functioning of the hypothalamic-pituitary-adrenal neuroendocrine axis. In addition, autonomic dysregulation of heart rate and systemic blood pressure has also been implicated on the basis of tilt-table testing for orthostatic hypotension; again, however, these findings have not been consistently reproduced. An inflammatory component to the myalgias of FMS has also not been consistently demonstrated, which likely explains the lack of efficacy of NSAID and corticosteroid therapies in this condition.

CLINICAL PRESENTATION

Subjective

The symptomatic presentation of CFS and FMS may overlap considerably. Patients may report postexercise malaise, fatigue, polyarthralgia, headaches, impaired memory and concentration, depressed mood, cognitive disturbances, sore throat, myalgias, and restless and disordered sleep which is not restorative for the patient. Often, the patient will also report having consulted one or more specialists concerning these vague symptoms.

CFS may also severely affect a person's ability to conduct activities of daily living, including occupational, educational, social, or personal activities, for at least 6 months. Patients typically have profound fatigue, which may be accompanied by cognitive dysfunction, sleep abnormalities, and generalized pain that may be exacerbated by physical exertion.

Objective

The onset of CFS is sudden and may be preceded by a mononucleosis-like illness or by significant GI findings. This same type of preceding event may also herald the onset of FMS. The patient will appear tired and the skin may be pale. Cervical lymph nodes, if enlarged, will be shotty and nontender. Otherwise, the examination may be unremarkable. Despite complaints of impaired memory and concentration, the results of objective mental status assessments may vary with reference to recent recall and problem-solving abilities.

For a diagnosis of FMS to be made, the patient must have widespread muscular pain that has been present for at least 3 months. The pain should be present in at least 11 of 18 tender points on digital palpation with an applied pressure of 4 kg/cm (enough force to whiten the examiner's nailbed). The 18 tender points are bilateral sites at nine key locations (see Table 63.2). Pain at these sites should be significantly greater than at control sites, which are not expected to be tender, such as the patient's thumbnail or midforearm.

DIAGNOSTIC REASONING

Diagnostic Tests

CFS tends to affect active, highly functional adults. The physical examination for CFS is typically normal. Advanced imaging tests such as computed tomography (CT) and MRI are not indicated in the absence of significant physical findings. In addition, virus-specific serologies against EBV or Lyme disease are also not recommended without a strong suspicion from history or physical examination findings, because any positive result is likely to be falsely positive in the setting of low suspicion.

Laboratory testing for FMS should include the same screening tests as for CFS, as well as muscle enzymes (e.g., creatine kinase, aldolase). ANA testing is typically not helpful unless an autoimmune disorder such as SLE is strongly suspected, as it may generate a false-positive result that incorrectly labels these patients as having lupus.

TABLE 63.2 Diagnostic Criteria for Fibromyalgia*	
History Criteria	Pain is considered widespread when ALL of the following are present: • Pain in the left side of the body • Pain in the right side of the body • Pain above the waist • Pain below the waist • Axial skeletal pain (cervical spine, anterior chest, thoracic spine, or lower back)
Pain Criteria	Pain exists in at least 11 of 18 tender points on digital palpation (at a force of at least 4 kg/cm): • Occiput: bilateral, at the suboccipital muscle insertions • Low cervical: bilateral, at the anterior aspects of the intertransverse spaces at C5–C7 • Trapezius: bilateral, at the midpoint of the upper border • Supraspinatus: bilateral, at the origins above the scapular spine near the medial border • Second rib: bilateral, at the second costochondral junctions, just lateral to the junctions on upper surfaces • Lateral epicondyle: bilateral, 2 cm distal to the epicondyles • Gluteal: bilateral, in upper quadrants of the buttocks in anterior fold of muscle • Greater trochanter: bilateral, posterior to the trochanteric prominence • Knee: bilateral, at the medial fat pad proximal to the joint line For a tender point to be "positive," the patient must state that the palpation was painful. A statement of "tender" is not considered "painful."

*Patient must have a history of widespread pain (present for at least 3 months) in specific anatomic areas and must exhibit this pain during an examination of tender points.
Source: Running AF, Berndt AE: *Management guidelines for nurse practitioners working in family practice*. Philadelphia, PA: FA Davis; 2003:586.

Differential Diagnosis

There is a wide differential diagnosis for both CFS and FMS. Many diagnoses can be ruled out with the laboratory studies mentioned in the preceding text. The differential diagnoses includes rheumatic diseases, such as SLE, RA, and polymyalgia rheumatica; endocrinological diseases, such as thyroid and parathyroid disease; metabolic myopathies; neuropathies; infectious diseases, such as Lyme disease and EBV-related mononucleosis; mood disorders and psychiatric illnesses, including depression, anxiety disorders, personality disorders, and psychosis; malingering; and other conditions such as irritable bowel syndrome, cancer, and parkinsonism.

Myofascial pain syndrome involves a more limited number of tender muscular trigger points than FMS, as well as involuntary constrictions of muscular fascia (fibrous connective tissue that surrounds muscles). This condition has been considered either a separate clinical entity or a regional variant of FMS. The multiglandular connective tissue disorder known as *Sjögren's syndrome* (SS) should also be considered in the differential diagnosis, as many CFS patients present with anhidrosis that mirrors the dry mouth and dry eye manifestations (sicca symptoms) commonly seen in SS.

MANAGEMENT

The management of CFS and FMS remains controversial. A supportive approach to the patient–clinician relationship is critical for effective treatment, as this reinforces that CFS or FMS is a genuine diagnosis and, thus, avoids the debate between psychological and "organic" etiologies. Ultimately, the goal of therapy is to enable the patient to have the best quality of life possible within the limitations of chronic disability related to fatigue and/or pain.

The two therapies that have been shown to be beneficial in terms of symptom relief and increased function (albeit not curative) are cognitive-behavioral therapy, which changes beliefs and behaviors that are barriers to recovery, and graded exercise. In contrast, increased bedrest should not be encouraged.

The following pharmacotherapies have been tried with little consistent success: galantamine (Reminyl), a drug used to treat Alzheimer's disease; IV immune globulin (IVIG); acyclovir (Zovirax); and selective serotonin reuptake inhibitors (SSRIs), such as citalopram (Celexa), fluoxetine (Prozac), and paroxetine (Paxil). Corticosteroids have shown some benefit in uncontrolled studies but increase the risk of adrenal suppression; moreover, controlled and blinded studies have not confirmed their benefit.

The long-term prognosis of CFS is better than the short-term prognosis, as treatment may be a lifelong process. However, certain factors have been cited as predicting a poor prognosis: (1) having more than eight medically unexplained physical symptoms, other than ones associated with CFS diagnostic criteria (e.g., functional impairment for at least 6 months with profound fatigue, postexertional malaise, unrefreshing sleep), (2) a lifetime history of dysthymia, (3) chronic fatigue lasting for more than 1.5 years, (4) having less than 16 years of formal education, and (5) an age greater than 38 years at the onset of disease.

For FMS, acetaminophen (Tylenol) 650 mg four times daily and tramadol (Ultram) 75 mg four times daily as combination therapy may be helpful analgesics, but there is little to no evidence that NSAID or corticosteroid therapy is beneficial. Tramadol is a synthetic opioid that carries some abuse potential, but it is generally considered of less risk than oxycodone, hydrocodone, or morphine. Amitriptyline (Elavil) 75 mg daily in divided doses remains one of the medications most frequently prescribed for FMS. Although it helps some patients, studies have shown that after 3 months, it has no greater effect than placebo. Additionally, this and other tricyclic antidepressants have anticholinergic side effects.

A similar transient therapeutic effect has also been seen with cyclobenzaprine (Flexeril), which appears effective for the first 3 months, initially taken at 5 mg three times daily and then increasing to 10 mg three times daily. The adage of "start low and go slow" applies to this medication as well. Desipramine (Norpramin) is an alternative tricyclic agent with fewer side effects and may work in patients who respond to amitriptyline but cannot tolerate it. Of all the SSRIs, fluoxetine has been most promising when taken in doses from 20 to 80 mg daily. Dual norepinephrine and serotonin reuptake inhibitors, such as duloxetine (Cymbalta) 40 to 60 mg daily, have shown some benefit as well. Although management guidelines are not well established, tramadol should probably be added only after psychotropic medications are tried first. In addition, low-dose clonazepam (Klonopin) 0.5 mg at bedtime may be helpful, and research is ongoing on the use of antiseizure medications. Pregabalin (Lyrica) was approved for FMS in 2007; it may be started at 75 mg twice daily and increased to a maintenance dose of 150 to 225 mg twice daily. Pregabalin may cause dizziness or somnolence, however, and has the potential to cause severe allergic reactions.

An ongoing low-impact aerobic (cardiovascular) exercise program (e.g., walking, swimming, biking, water aerobics) with cognitive-behavioral therapy, hypnotherapy, or electromyogram biofeedback therapy may be a useful adjunct in certain patients, because these therapies have been shown in limited trials to increase quality of life (albeit not affecting symptom severity). Chiropractic and massage therapies are only weakly supported. Trials with ultraviolet (UV) light (especially blue-spectrum light) exposure have shown mixed results. Vitamin supplementation also has received mixed results in small studies.

FOLLOW-UP AND REFERRAL

Follow-up for CFS and FMS should occur according to the symptoms reported. Typically, patients are referred to rheumatologists initially to assist in confirming the diagnosis by ruling out autoimmune syndromes. Referral to regional specialists who study and treat CFS and FMS may be required. Psychiatric referral could be necessary if mood disorders are apparent or mental status test results warrant. Because many patients with CFS or FMS have been treated for affective psychiatric disorders in the past, they may already know what psychological manifestations should trigger professional assistance.

Patient Education: Chronic Fatigue Syndrome and Fibromyalgia Syndrome

For both CFS and FMS, management relies on helping the patient cope with a chronic condition by learning methods to deal with long-term symptoms. While validating its effect on the patient's life, clinicians should stress that the patient does not have a fatal disease. Although symptomatic, it may be relatively benign in terms of the risk of complications, and the patient can live a normal and productive life. Living with the uncertainty of the diagnosis and the chronicity of symptoms are continuing challenges for both the patient and clinician. This is illustrated in The Patient's Voice 63.1.

As no definitive evidence supports standardized treatments for these conditions, patients may use alternative therapeutic means which they believe could assist them with pain relief, such as chiropractic, therapeutic touch, guided imagery, or hypnosis therapy, provided the risks of these therapies are understood, including practical considerations such as cost and time commitment. Pain is highly subjective, and any treatment may help relieve pain in these conditions if the patient believes it to be helpful.

Patients should understand that physical and emotional stress can worsen their symptoms. Patient education has been shown in unblinded studies to improve FMS symptoms and quality of life and is, thus, a critical component of treatment. The Circle of Caring model is tested in cases in which a patient is frustrated and experiences daily pain. It is especially trying when a patient outwardly appears to be fine physically but is mentally suffering. In turn, patients with CFS and FMS may require multiple resources, with all those involved with the patient focusing on finding what works best for each individual patient. Evidence-Based Nursing Practice 63.1 explores the associations between adolescent fatigue and distress and parental fatigue and distress, as well as family functioning, including both mothers and fathers.

SJÖGREN'S SYNDROME

SS is a chronic inflammatory autoimmune disorder caused by exocrine gland dysfunction. It presents as dryness in all areas of the body where there are exocrine glands associated with mucous membranes (sicca syndrome), most notably the salivary and lacrimal glands. However, SS has the potential to affect a wide array of organ systems including the skin, lung, kidney, and heart. In addition, the hematopoietic system may be affected with a propensity for lymphoma.

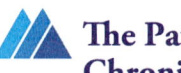

The Patient's Voice 63.1: Chronic Fatigue Syndrome

I have been chronically tired for years. It started out that I would drive the kids to school in my nightgown, and then I'd go back to bed. I had given up my job the year before. Thank goodness we could afford it. My husband thought that I was depressed, so I went to doctor after doctor and tried all sorts of antidepressant medications with no relief. One doctor suggested that I needed to see a psychiatrist because the antidepressants were not working, and he said I was obviously depressed. I knew "deep down" that I wasn't depressed, but I also knew that something wasn't right. I knew I had to do something when I overheard one of my kids on the phone telling his friend not to come over because his mom was just "having another lazy day in her PJs."

That same week, I heard an ad on the radio inviting participants for a study on chronic fatigue syndrome. I had heard about the syndrome vaguely and thought it was just a "catch-all term" for tiredness. I didn't really think it was a medical condition. I called the phone number given for the study and after answering just a few questions over the phone, I felt 200% better! There actually is a medical name for the condition that I know I have. Now, I know I'm not crazy or just lazy. I can't wait to participate in the study. Even if it doesn't help me, I'll feel better knowing that what I have is "real."

EPIDEMIOLOGY AND CAUSES

SS has a worldwide distribution with an annual incidence of 4 in 100,000 people; 70% of these cases may be primary, whereas the other cases are associated with comorbid conditions (these were traditionally considered secondary cases of SS in the past, although more recently this nomenclature has fallen out of favor due to the subjective nature of this designation). Nonetheless, because SS often accompanies underlying rheumatic diseases (e.g., RA, SLE, systemic sclerosis), investigations evaluating the etiological links among these conditions are ongoing.

Accurate estimates of disease prevalence are complicated by a lack of agreement as to the defining diagnostic criteria of the disease. However, it is generally agreed that SS affects females nine times more often than males, and the typical age range for disease onset is 40 to 60 years. The cause of SS has not been fully characterized, although it is generally considered to be autoimmune in nature, as biopsy of impacted exocrine glands reveals an

> ### Evidence-Based Nursing Practice 63.1
>
> #### CHRONIC FATIGUE SYNDROME
>
> Loades, ME, Lievesley, K, Rimes, K, et al. (2019). Does fatigue and distress in a clinical cohort of adolescents with chronic fatigue syndrome correlate with fatigue and distress in their parents? *Child Care Health Dev*. 2019;45:129-137.
>
> **Objectives:** Previous studies have found that parents of children with chronic fatigue syndrome (CFS) are more fatigued, and mothers are more distressed than healthy controls. Managing the disabling symptoms of CFS can result in disruption and burden for the family. Most research has focused on mothers. This study sought to further explore the associations between adolescent fatigue and distress and parental fatigue and distress, as well as family functioning, including both mothers and fathers.
>
> **Design:** Cross-sectional study of a clinical cohort of consecutive attenders at a specialist chronic fatigue unit.
>
> **Methods:** Questionnaires were completed by adolescents (N = 115, age 11–18) with a confirmed diagnosis of CFS and their mothers (N = 100) and fathers (N = 65).
>
> **Results:** Maternal fatigue was significantly correlated with maternal distress, but not with adolescent fatigue, depression, anxiety, or functioning. This pattern held true for paternal fatigue. Maternal and paternal anxiety and depression were significantly correlated with family functioning. Paternal and maternal distress were correlated with each other. Mothers and fathers tended to have a consistent view of family functioning. Family functioning, specifically being overwhelmed by difficulties and scoring lower on strengths and adaptability, was positively associated with adolescent depression. Unexpectedly, higher levels of adolescent fatigue and poorer physical functioning were associated with better family functioning as rated by the mother.
>
> **Conclusions:** Parents of adolescents with fatigue scored near to or within normative range for nonclinical samples on distress, fatigue, and family functioning. Parental distress may contribute to or result from poorer family functioning. Family functioning, particularly building strengths and adaptability, may be clinically important in CFS, as well as attending to parental (particularly paternal) distress in families where adolescents are low in mood.

inflammatory lymphocytic cellular infiltrate that results in glandular dysfunction.

PATHOPHYSIOLOGY

As an autoimmune disorder, lymphocytic infiltration in all affected organs is the pathophysiological hallmark of SS. Pooling of lymphocytes and plasma cells in the lacrimal glands causes the characteristic dry eye conjunctivitis of the syndrome called *keratoconjunctivitis sicca*, whereas parotid enlargement and diminished salivary excretions result from a similar infiltrate within the salivary glands along with hyperplasia of the ductal epithelium, which produce the characteristic dry mouth (xerostomia) of SS.

At least three-quarters of these infiltrating cells are T lymphocytes, primarily of the $CD4^+$ T helper subset, with classical $TCR\alpha\beta$ receptors and expressing a memory cell phenotype including LFA-1 surface adhesion molecules. About 10% of the infiltrating cells are B lymphocytes and plasma cells that produce significant amounts of oligoclonal immunoglobulin. The adjacent glandular epithelium expresses high levels of class II MHC (HLA-DR) and costimulatory molecules such as B7, suggesting antigenic T-cell stimulation is central to the pathogenesis of SS. However, it is unclear whether these stimulatory antigens are autoantigens and/or specific viral antigens.

Evidence for a genetic predisposition to SS is supported by studies that recognize a familial propensity for specific HLA-DR3, HLA-DR5, and HLA-DRB3 alleles in affected patients and their relatives. Primary SS has also been linked to genetic polymorphisms in regulatory DNA sequences of the IL-10 gene, a cytokine that influences cell-mediated immunity. However, IFN-γ and IL-2 appear to be the primary immunomodulatory cytokines in SS. Produced by ductal epithelium, IFN-γ upregulates the expression of HLA-DR molecules on epithelial antigen-presenting cells and potentiates T-lymphocyte cellular cytotoxicity. Cytolytic destruction of exocrine gland tissue does not appear to explain the full pathology of SS, however, as decreased saliva and tear production do not correlate well with the degree of histological damage on glandular biopsies.

The importance of autoantibodies in the pathophysiology of SS has long been emphasized. Autoantibodies specific for acetylcholine receptors in salivary glands have been suggested to impair the secretion of saliva in histologically normal glands. Far more common, however, are autoantibodies to specific nucleoproteins associated with RNA, including anti-Ro (SSA) antibodies seen in up to 90% of SS cases and anti-La (SSB) antibodies seen in up to half of cases. Although the pathogenetic role of these autoantibodies is unclear, the same antibodies can be found in a variety of other autoimmune disorders, including neonatal lupus, in which they mediate complete heart block after crossing the placenta from mother to child. Anti–α-fodrin antibodies may be even more sensitive and specific for SS than anti-Ro or anti-La antibodies, but their pathological significance is not fully established.

Infection by various viruses, including EBV, retroviruses such as human T-cell lymphotropic virus (HTLV-1), hepatitis C virus, and coxsackievirus, has been suggested as an underlying cause of primary SS. In vitro studies and preclinical animal models have demonstrated that infection with these viruses is capable of leading to lymphocytic infiltrates of the salivary and lacrimal glands, recreating many of the same symptoms as in SS. Although viral particles are typically not present in high numbers, viral infection has been suggested to break tolerance to autoantigens and lead to SS via autoimmune activation. The relationship between SS and viral infection is not entirely clear, however, because much of the etiological evidence is indirect and does not predominate for any single virus.

Disorders of estrogen have also been indirectly implicated because primary SS is seen predominantly in females. Postmenopausal females taking estrogen therapy have a higher incidence of ocular dryness compared with controls. This evidence remains circumstantial, however.

CLINICAL PRESENTATION
Subjective

A patient may complain of dryness of the eyes and the feeling that a particulate is in them. Keratoconjunctivitis sicca is dryness of the cornea caused by a deficiency of tear secretion in which the corneal surface appears dull and rough and the eye feels gritty and irritated. The patient may also complain of dryness of the mouth caused by cessation of normal salivary secretions. In addition, the patient may complain of loss of taste and smell, recurrent dental caries, dysphagia, vaginismus, and rectal bleeding. Associated complaints can include RA-like signs and symptoms of joint swelling, pain, and malaise, as well as low-grade fever. Fatigue is another important aspect of the presentation, due to disrupted sleep patterns from mucosal dryness or accompanying systemic symptoms such as arthralgias and myalgias.

Objective

The patient may appear chronically ill, particularly if RA-like joint symptoms precede SS. The patient's breath may smell fetid because of dental caries and mucosal dryness, and the mucosal beds of the nose and throat will be pale and may reveal small fissures. The tongue can be beefy red because of dryness. Similar findings are associated with the vagina and anus.

Many other systemic, albeit rare, manifestations of SS may be present: a macular, papular, vesicular, or purpuric skin rash; arthralgias and myalgias; cardiopulmonary manifestations such as pericarditis or pulmonary hypertension from lymphocytic interstitial pneumonitis; pulmonary emboli due to circulating antiphospholipid/anticardiolipin antibodies; interstitial nephritis leading to renal tubular acidosis or glomerulonephritis (similar to that seen in SLE); gastroesophageal reflux disease (GERD); hypothyroidism due to autoimmune thyroiditis; neurological sequelae including peripheral (mononeuritis multiplex or symmetric neuropathies) and autonomic neuropathies, CNS manifestations mimicking multiple sclerosis, transverse myelitis, optic neuritis, and ischemic strokes that may be due to vasculitis or thrombosis, which result in demyelination.

DIAGNOSTIC REASONING
Diagnostic Tests

SS is diagnosed via clinical and laboratory findings, rather than identification of a single causative agent. Clinical diagnosis of SS includes six defining criteria:

1. Inadequate tear production (evaluated using the Schirmer test with filter paper to blot tears on the lateral third of the lower eyelid [less than 5 mm of wetting in 5 minutes is abnormal] or using artificial replacement tears more than 3 times daily)
2. Signs of corneal epithelial damage from dry eye using Rose-Bengal or fluorescein staining and slit-lamp examination
3. Decreased saliva production
4. Lymphocytic infiltration of labial salivary gland tissue on histopathology after biopsy—the closest test to a gold standard for diagnosis (greater than 50 immune cells surrounding an intact glandular lobule)
5. Impaired salivary gland function by objective testing via radionuclide technetium scanning (quantitative salivary gland scintigraphy demonstrating poor uptake), parotid sialography with parotid gland cannulation and injection of oil-based contrast material, or spontaneous saliva production of less than or equal to 1.5 mL/15 min
6. Autoantibodies including anti-Ro (SSA) and/or anti-La (SSB)

Initial laboratory tests include a CBC, RF, ANA, and γ-globulin profile. The CBC may reveal anemia of chronic disease that is typically mild, leukopenia, and/or eosinophilia caused by autoimmune factors and not by external antigens. RF is positive in three-fourths of samples. ANA is typically elevated, as are γ-globulin levels.

Electrophoresis studies are required to determine whether SS is present alone or in combination with other rheumatoid disease. SS alone typically manifests more specific autoantibodies—anti-Ro and anti-La—whereas SS and rheumatoid disease together may reveal antibodies against exocrine ducts and RA-associated nuclear antigens.

Differential Diagnosis

Because patients with SS have a higher prevalence of hypothyroidism, this should be screened for via a thorough history and thyroid-stimulating hormone (TSH) and free T_4 levels. Further laboratory work-up includes a basic metabolic panel with hepatic function tests (liver transaminases), RF (to assess for RA), and ANA (to assess for SLE). HIV and hepatitis C testing may also be indicated. Presence of sarcoidosis could be checked with a chest x-ray examination to evaluate for hilar lymphadenopathy or interstitial lung disease. An MRI or ultrasound and biopsy should be done if there is unilateral salivary gland enlargement to rule out malignancy or specific glandular pathology, such as acute bacterial sialadenitis. Bilateral salivary gland swelling may be due to acute viral infection (e.g., mumps, coxsackievirus, echovirus, or EBV) or chronic infection with HIV or hepatitis C; granulomatous diseases such as sarcoidosis, amyloidosis, or TB; malnutrition; alcoholism; and eating disorders such as bulimia or anorexia with purging features.

Additional differential diagnoses for SS include other autoimmune disorders that may exist concurrently, such as SLE, scleroderma (systemic sclerosis), or RA. In fact, RF may be positive in up to 75% of SS cases. It is also critical to distinguish SS from patients with FMS or depression who may have significant anticholinergic toxicities from psychiatric medications, which can lead to dry eyes and especially dry mouth. Dry eyes may also result from impaired blinking due to muscular or neurological disorders, vitamin A deficiency leading to mucin deficiency (xerophthalmia), conjunctivitis, infiltration of the lacrimal glands (from sarcoidosis, lymphoma, or amyloidosis), or blepharitis from meibomian gland dysfunction. Dry mouth can also result from sialadenitis from obstructing salivary gland stones, chronic viral infections (e.g., hepatitis C, HIV), or iatrogenic anticholinergic drug effects. In fact, the following conditions are exclusion criteria for the diagnosis of SS: previous head/neck irradiation or preexisting lymphoma, comorbid infection with hepatitis C or HIV with AIDS, sarcoidosis, graft versus host disease, or recent use of anticholinergic medications. Symptoms of mucosal dryness are also common in liver disease and depression, which should also be considered as part of the differential.

MANAGEMENT

The management of this syndrome consists primarily of symptom-directed supportive care, although research into immunomodulatory therapies is ongoing. To address the primary manifestations of dry eyes and dry mouth, saline eye drops can relieve lacrimal dryness, and hard candies and gum may be used to stimulate salivation but should be sugar free to avoid worsening dental caries. Dried fruits that contain malic acid may also be helpful in stimulating salivation. In extreme cases of salivary dryness, the patient should be encouraged to apply an artificial salivary gel or use a mouth spray. Fluids can also keep the mouth lubricated as long as they do not contain caffeine (a diuretic) or ethanol (as used in mouthwash), which can be drying. Special toothpastes and toothbrushes designed for a dry mouth are also available. Quarterly dental evaluations, along with vigorous flossing and regular brushing, may prevent dental caries. Dry lips may be treated with petroleum jelly (Vaseline), dry skin with moisturizing lotions, and vaginal dryness with intravaginal lubricant gel.

Artificial tears and salivary gels containing hypromellose (0.3%) or methylcellulose (0.3%) may be used every 2 to 4 hours if needed, although these preparations can be irritating to certain individuals. Pilocarpine (Salagen) 5 mg PO three to four times daily and cevimeline (Evoxac) 30 to 60 mg PO three times daily are specific cholinergic (muscarinic) agonists (parasympathomimetics) for stimulating aqueous secretions. These drugs are contraindicated in persons with narrow-angle glaucoma or iritis because of their mydriatic effects. Cevimeline should not be used if a patient has asthma, because it can worsen respiratory secretions.

Acetylcysteine can be used as a mucolytic if thick mucus fibers coat the eye, but it may be unacceptable to some patients because of its characteristic "rotten egg smell" due to its sulfur content. Spreading agents such as polyethylene glycol and dextran-70 0.1% eye drops are also available for dry eyes. Topical cyclosporine 0.05% 1 gtt every 12 hours is approved by the FDA to increase tear production, presumably by decreasing T-cell infiltration within the conjunctivae. If these treatments prove ineffective, the patient may undergo punctal occlusion, in which collagen plugs are placed by an ophthalmologist into the lacrimal puncta on the inferior eyelid so that tears (artificial or natural) cannot drain into the nasolacrimal duct.

The following are rarer systemic manifestations of SS, along with specific treatments:

- Macular, papular, vesicular, or purpuric skin rashes may require biopsy and treatment as a form of vasculitis.
- Arthralgias and myalgias may respond to NSAIDs or hydroxychloroquine.
- Inflammatory cardiopulmonary manifestations such as pericarditis or pulmonary hypertension from lymphocytic interstitial pneumonitis may require treatment with corticosteroids (prednisone) or other immunosuppressants (e.g., azathioprine, chlorambucil, cyclophosphamide).
- Interstitial nephritis leading to renal tubular acidosis or glomerulonephritis (similar to that of SLE) may require corticosteroid or immunosuppressant therapy (e.g., cyclophosphamide, mycophenolate).
- Rare neurological sequelae, such as peripheral mononeuritis multiplex or symmetrical neuropathies and autonomic dysfunction (confirmed by tilt-table tests), may require mineralocorticoid therapy.
- Neuropathies and CNS manifestations mimicking multiple sclerosis, transverse myelitis, optic neuritis, or ischemic strokes may be due to vasculitis, thrombosis, or demyelination and require treatment with immunosuppressants.

Most recently, treatment guidelines from the Sjögren's Syndrome Foundation have put forth the anti-CD20 monoclonal antibody therapy rituximab (Rituxan) for patients with systemic symptoms severe enough to require biological therapy. However, this therapy is not approved by the FDA for SS. Multiple biological therapies are currently in development for this significant area of unmet medical need, including inhibitors of B cell proliferation and activation.

FOLLOW-UP AND REFERRAL

Follow-up of SS consists of ongoing evaluation to assess the effectiveness of symptom management and the need for alterations in treatment. If SS presents as an isolated condition, follow-up evaluations may occur as infrequently as twice per year. However, more frequent evaluations are necessitated by the presence of concurrent disease. Referrals may not be necessary except when this syndrome accompanies other diseases. The primary care provider should consult with a rheumatologist initially to differentiate the disease from other rheumatic conditions and to confirm the diagnosis.

During follow-up examinations, it is important to monitor for dental caries and oral candidiasis predisposed by dry mouth, which can lead to severe oral pain and requires antifungal therapy. It is also important to screen for infectious conjunctivitis predisposed by dry eye and complications from nasal dryness and laryngotracheal reflux, which can stimulate vagal responses and mimic symptoms of allergy and recurrent sinusitis, including repeated throat clearing and postnasal drip-like symptoms. This type of reflux may be treated with proton pump inhibitors (similar to GERD), with referral to an ear, nose, and throat specialist if needed.

Patient Education: Sjögren's Syndrome

The patient with SS should learn that mucosal dryness can be controlled with conservative interventions. Regular application of artificial lubricants locally can prevent the soreness and untoward effects of dry mucosae. The patient should be encouraged to wear sunglasses to protect the eyes from strong light, wind, and dust, as well as to avoid low-humidity environments that exacerbate dryness. If the patient has sore lesions in the mouth, tobacco, alcohol, and both spicy and salty foods should be avoided. OTC medications that decrease pharyngeal secretions, such as antihistamines, antidepressants, anticholinergics, and atropine derivatives, should be avoided. Patients should be warned that they are at greater risk for complications from surgeries requiring general anesthesia and intubation, given their increased risk for thick, inspissated mucus and atelectasis.

SYSTEMIC LUPUS ERYTHEMATOSUS

SLE is an inflammatory autoimmune disease that affects many organ systems. Spontaneous remissions and exacerbations characterize the clinical picture. SLE can be mild, moderate, or aggressive to life-threatening in presentation.

EPIDEMIOLOGY AND CAUSES

The prevalence of SLE is 40 to 50 cases per 100,000 people and is associated with age, gender, race, and underlying genetics. Nearly 85% of patients with SLE are female, most often in their third or fourth decade of life. However, 15% of cases present after the age of 55 years. Juvenile cases are not uncommon, however, with 20% of diagnosed patients being younger than 16 years. In children, the female to male ratio is 3:1, and in adults, it is 10 to 15:1. Epidemiological studies have identified sex hormones as potential causative factors for SLE, because the onset of the disease in females typically occurs before menopause. Estrogen has been shown to stimulate T cells, B cells, and macrophages, as well as increase the expression of cytokines, endothelial cell adhesion molecules, and antigen-presenting MHC molecules. SLE flares have also been associated with hyperprolactinemia.

In contrast, androgenic hormones such as testosterone tend to be immunosuppressive, which may also contribute to the gender specificity of SLE. Although males with lupus typically experience less photosensitivity than females, they are often considered to have more severe disease manifestations, with a greater incidence of serositis and a higher 1-year mortality rate, although they tend to present at an older age of onset.

Persons of African descent are four times more likely to develop the disease compared with European descent. SLE also disproportionately affects patients of Asian ancestry, and some studies show higher rates of disease in Hispanic patients compared with the general population. Several lines of evidence have demonstrated a genetic component to SLE, such as a high concordance rate between monozygotic twins, a propensity for specific HLA-DR class II MHC genes in affected individuals, and positive gene linkage studies in affected siblings. Poor prognostic factors include concurrent hypertension, male gender, developing active disease at a young age, low socioeconomic status, and being of African descent.

Trends related to ethnic background (i.e., higher disease rates in people of color) have been observed with many chronic diseases and are multifactorial in nature. They must not be attributed solely to genetic differences between races, as worse outcomes in SLE are also associated with the presence of prothrombotic antiphospholipid antibodies (e.g., lupus anticoagulant, anticardiolipin, anti–beta 2-glycoprotein) and highly active inflammatory disease, both of which may be addressed through individualized treatment plans to decrease the risk of morbidity.

Although not causative of SLE, several triggering factors for acute exacerbations have been identified. These include exposure to UVB and UVA light rays, which is believed to cause increased cytokine and cell adhesion molecule expression; certain infections (e.g., EBV, *Mycobacteria*, trypanosomiasis) that may stimulate cross-reacting autoantibodies; emotional stress, which has been tied to mild disease flares; pregnancy and postpartum hormonal fluctuations; and surgery, which may increase the formation of autoantibody-containing immune complexes via the release of intracellular antigens into the circulation from tissue trauma. Exposure to cigarette smoke or silica dust also increases the risk of developing SLE, which implicates inflammatory lung pathology.

PATHOPHYSIOLOGY

The pathophysiology of SLE is best understood by a review of the diagnostic criteria. The diagnosis of SLE is made after 4 or more of the following 11 criteria are met in the absence of medications or other disorders known to induce these effects, as defined by the American College of Rheumatology (ACR):

- Arthritis—nonerosive and usually involving two or more joints
- Photosensitivity—often triggering skin rashes, exposure to the sun's UVB rays may be a triggering event for SLE exacerbations
- Oral (or nasal) ulcers—typically painless
- Malar rash—bilateral butterfly formation across the cheeks and nasal bridge
- Discoid rash—raised red patches, sometimes with denuded central areas
- Serositis (inflammation) of the pleura or pericardia
- Renal disease (any one of three indicators): more than 0.5 g/day proteinuria, 3+ or more proteinuria (as detected by dipstick), or cellular casts
- Hematological disorders (any one of four indicators): hemolytic anemia, leukopenia (less than 4,000 WBCs/µL), lymphopenia (less than 1,500 lymphocytes/µL), thrombocytopenia (less than 100,000 platelets/µL)
- Neurological disease (e.g., seizures, psychoses) not otherwise explained by iatrogenic or metabolic causes
- Positive ANA antibodies
- Immunological abnormalities (any one of four indicators): positive antiphospholipid antibodies such as anticardiolipin or lupus anticoagulant, antibody to double-stranded native DNA (anti-dsDNA), anti-Smith (anti-Sm) antibody, false-positive serological test for syphilis (Venereal Disease Research Laboratory [VDRL] or rapid plasma reagin [RPR] tests)

SLE is, at its core, a condition of disordered immunity in which mechanisms that normally prevent immune cell activation by autoantigens are eliminated. Many factors have been identified that contribute to this autoimmune activation; for example, an inhibition of suppressor T cells that normally downregulate immune responses, an increase in $CD4^+$ T helper cells, increased cytokine production (e.g., IFN-α, IL-4, IL-6, IL-10, IL-17), polyclonal B-cell activation, and dysregulated intracellular signaling (particularly pathways involving cytosolic calcium). These changes contribute to a significant production of autoantibodies that are considered a hallmark of the disease. Mouse models of SLE have demonstrated dysregulated apoptosis in which nuclear antigens (e.g., DNA, ribonucleoprotein, histones) are exposed on the cell surface that are capable of recognition by autoreactive lymphocytes. In turn, autoantibodies often appear in the serum years before the actual onset of SLE symptoms.

Autoantibodies are also formed against cell surface antigens, including antibodies specific for RBCs and WBCs, platelets, and neuronal and renal cells. These antibodies mediate cellular destruction via complement activation, antibody-dependent cellular cytotoxicity, and opsonization. Although not seen universally, autoantibody-derived immune complexes are believed to underlie the pathology of most of clinical manifestations of SLE. Histochemical staining has identified immune complex deposition along the basement membrane in nephritic kidneys, at the dermal–epidermal junction in skin lesions, within the choroid plexus, as well as in the pleural cavity and pericardium—all major sites of SLE pathology. The biochemical nature of both the autoantigen and autoantibody (e.g., size, charge, binding affinity, rate of phagocytic clearance, ability to be neutralized by complement proteins) determines where these complexes form and the extent of tissue damage after their deposition.

One of the organ systems most severely affected by immune complex deposition is the renal system. In addition to the deposition of circulating immune complexes along the glomerular basement membrane, autoreactive IgG_1 and IgG_3 anti-DNA antibodies also bind directly to autoantigens in the basement membranes, serving as a nidus for complement activation. These chemotactic complement proteins then attract leukocytes and mononuclear cells that phagocytose the immune complexes, releasing cytokines and clotting factors that lead to fibrinoid necrosis, ongoing inflammation, renal scarring, and kidney dysfunction, known collectively as *lupus nephritis*. Diffuse proliferative glomerulonephritis is the most common histological form of lupus nephritis, which results from this inflammation. In contrast, lupus membranous nephropathy is not associated with inflammation; rather, in this setting, immune complex activation is separated physically from circulating immune cells by the glomerular basement membrane, resulting in epithelial injury and proteinuria without active inflammation.

A subset of individuals with SLE is also prone to developing antiphospholipid antibodies, including antibodies against the β_2-glycoprotein I complex and cardiolipin, as well as the lupus anticoagulant. These individuals have more severe disease, related primarily to an increased thrombogenic state, which predisposes to both venous and arterial thromboembolism, resulting in a greater incidence of deep venous thrombosis, pulmonary embolism, cerebrovascular accidents (strokes and transient ischemic attacks), and recurrent first-trimester miscarriages due to placental infarcts. Normally, β_2-glycoprotein has an anticoagulant effect, which is abrogated by these antiphospholipid antibodies.

One of the most characteristic physical findings of SLE is a bilateral malar rash, often called a "butterfly rash" due to its characteristic shape and location across the nose and cheekbones. This and other SLE skin rashes are exacerbated by sun exposure, largely due to UV damage to DNA in skin keratinocytes and alterations in membrane phospholipid metabolism. Thus, anti-DNA, anti-RNA, anti-Ro, anti-La, and antiphospholipid autoantibodies form that mediate keratinocyte destruction and local skin inflammation.

CLINICAL PRESENTATION

Subjective

The patient may complain of malaise, fever, anorexia, and unplanned weight loss. The patient may also complain of blurred vision and conjunctival swelling. Sleeplessness and depression are also common complaints. Joints may be reported to be swollen and painful by history, but this may not be evident on examination. Shortness of breath and painful inspiration may be present if lung pathology exists. Vague abdominal pain and/or abdominal cramping may also be part of the history.

Objective

Integumentary findings may include the following:

- A characteristic "butterfly" rash, as well as other photosensitive rashes, are common.
- Alopecia and scalp exanthema are typical findings.
- Splinter hemorrhages, periungual erythema, and fingertip lesions may be observed on the fingers and toes.
- Lymphadenopathy in several regions of the body indicates systemic disease.
- Discoid lupus presents with scarring and highly inflammatory (even ulcerating) skin lesions, but often does not present with the familiar autoantibodies of SLE, such as ANA, anti-dsDNA, and anti-Sm antibodies.
- Raynaud's phenomenon, a vascular condition, may be seen in up to 40% of patients as whitish-blue skin color changes in response to cold temperatures, which then change to red on rewarming, often predating other symptoms.

Musculoskeletal findings may include the following:

- Musculoskeletal joint pains (asymmetrical, nondeforming, migratory arthritis—often in the hands and fingers) occur in 90% of cases and are often the presenting complaint.
- Swollen joints may not follow a particular pattern, as in other rheumatic diseases; joint inflammation is typically nonerosive on radiographs.

Neurological findings may include the following:

- Cognitive thought processes may be impaired. Therefore, the clinician should carefully listen to the patient's explanations in response to questioning to establish lapses in logic; however, these deficits are often not evident in mental functioning assessments commonly used in primary care settings, such as the Folstein Mini-Mental State Examination.
- Evidence of peripheral paresthesias and diminished deep tendon reflexes may be present.

CNS and psychiatric manifestations of SLE are quite varied and may require aggressive immunosuppressive treatment. These may include cognitive defects, delirium, depression, mania, anxiety, psychosis (which may also result iatrogenically from corticosteroid use), headache, aseptic meningitis, and various neuropathies. Ischemic CNS damage from a thromboembolic cerebrovascular accident may underlie these symptoms as well.

Cardiopulmonary findings may include the following:

- A systolic murmur may be present.
- Distended jugular veins suggest right-sided cardiac failure, which may be seen with pulmonary hypertension or interstitial lung disease.
- Lung inflammation may lead to pleuritis with a pleural friction rub, lung effusions, pneumonitis, interstitial lung disease, alveolar hemorrhage, or eventually pulmonary hypertension.

The cardiovascular system may also manifest with pericarditis or a verrucous form of nonbacterial endocarditis known as *Libman-Sacks endocarditis*. This is associated with antiphospholipid antibodies and can produce emboli due to valvular insufficiency and turbulent blood flow. There is also a well-documented phenomenon of transmission of anti-Ro and anti-La anti–single-stranded DNA antibodies from a mother with SLE to the developing fetus, which can result in potentially fatal third-degree heart block in newborns. This is known as *neonatal lupus,* which is not a manifestation of primary lupus in the fetus, however, and is different from pediatric manifestations of SLE.

GI findings may include the following:

- Painless oral and nasal ulcers may be seen.
- Right upper abdominal quadrant tenderness may accompany the finding of hepatomegaly; hepatitis is a common finding.
- Right lower quadrant tenderness suggests right colon enlargement, which may be caused by intestinal vasculitis.

Of note, GI manifestations often relate to SLE treatments, rather than to the disease itself, such as gastritis and peptic ulcers resulting from chronic NSAID and corticosteroid use. However, SLE-related vasculitis can lead to inflammation of the pancreas, large intestine, and serosal layers of the peritoneum, as well as to esophagitis and GERD. In addition, both hepatomegaly and splenomegaly may be detected, along with lymphadenopathy.

Kidney involvement may be clinically apparent in up to one-half of all SLE patients and is the primary reason for lupus-related hospitalization. Renal biopsy may reveal several histological subtypes of lupus nephritis. Class I is normal. Class II is pure mesangial and carries with it a good prognosis. Class III is segmental and focal proliferative lupus nephritis and usually responds to corticosteroids. Class IV is diffuse proliferative lupus nephritis, which is typically considered to carry the worst prognosis, presenting with hypertension and leading to end-stage renal disease (ESRD) or death in up to 50% of cases. Class V is membranous nephritis with a variable presentation that worsens as complement levels decrease due to immune complex formation and organ deposition. Class VI is advanced sclerosing lupus nephritis, which nearly always leads to ESRD, given the irreversibility of renal fibrosis.

DIAGNOSTIC REASONING

Diagnostic Tests

Initial testing should include a CBC with platelet count, basic metabolic panel (serum electrolytes and kidney function tests), serum albumin (which will be reduced in nephropathy), ANA, urinalysis, and screening tests for anti-dsDNA antibodies (highly specific, with 75% to 95% sensitivity), antiphospholipid antibodies, and anti-Sm antibodies (highly specific, but with only 25% sensitivity). ANA results are likely to be elevated in more than 90% of cases; however, this finding is not specific for SLE, as numerous other inflammatory diseases are also associated with elevated ANA. Other common autoantibodies include those against single-stranded DNA and nucleoprotein, including antiribonucleoprotein antibodies as seen in scleroderma (systemic sclerosis) and both anti-Ro (SSA) and anti-La (SSB) antibodies as seen in SS. Increasing levels of autoantibodies and decreasing levels or activity of serum complement components (e.g., CH50, C3, C4) correlate with SLE disease activity.

The CBC may reveal either anemia or leukopenia or both. If the patient is leukopenic, the differential count may reveal lymphocytopenia. One-third of patients with SLE will be thrombocytopenic. Elevated ESR and CRP levels are nonspecific markers of active inflammation in SLE, and proteinuria is also a possible finding on urinalysis in nephrotic or nephritic patients, with hematuria seen in the latter.

All test results should be interpreted in conjunction with clinical presentation (history and physical examination) to evaluate for worsening of the disease state and should not be overinterpreted or under interpreted in isolation. These initial laboratory tests, along with characteristic clinical manifestations, should be sufficient to confirm a diagnosis of SLE. Of note, as reflected in the SLE diagnostic criteria, the RPR test for syphilis may be falsely positive due to anticardiolipin antibodies or other SLE-related phenomena.

Pertinent imaging tests should be guided by the patient's clinical presentation, such as chest radiography for pulmonary symptoms, renal ultrasound in the face of kidney failure, and plain films for arthritic joints. If indicated in the setting of pulmonary findings, pulmonary function tests often have a restrictive pattern, given inflammation and scarring in the lungs. More invasive procedures such as renal biopsy are indicated when histology is needed to determine prognosis and guide therapy. Electrocardiography and echocardiography are indicated to evaluate for pericarditis and other cardiac pathology, and specific tests such as ventilation–perfusion scans or high-resolution spiral CT scans of the lungs may be needed to evaluate for pulmonary emboli in prothrombotic patients. As with other thrombotic phenomena, a negative D-dimer test may effectively rule out thrombosis; however, the nonspecific nature of this test in inflammatory conditions typically decreases its diagnostic utility in SLE.

As with SS, keratoconjunctivitis sicca may be present, as can pathognomonic (albeit rare) cotton wool retinal exudates from retinal vasculitis. Scleritis and anterior uveitis may also occur but are both uncommon. Mild to moderate cytopenias may affect all three major cell lines (i.e., leukopenia, anemia, thrombocytopenia), with thrombocytopenia leading to easy bruising and purpura. Rarely, severe autoimmune hemolytic anemia can also result.

In contrast, thrombophilia may occur, increasing the risk of thrombosis, including deep vein thrombosis and arterial blood clots, especially if antiphospholipid antibodies or lupus anticoagulant are present (the latter being paradoxically named, as it increases the risk of thrombosis). This prothrombotic state is the cause of recurrent miscarriages (abortions) seen in SLE patients early in pregnancy, usually in the first trimester. Thus, such an obstetric history should always make the clinician think of antiphospholipid syndrome and SLE as potential underlying diagnoses.

Classification Criteria for SLE

In addition to their utility in diagnosis, classification criteria are essential for the identification of relatively homogeneous groups of SLE patients for inclusion in research studies and clinical trials. The 1982 revised ACR SLE classification criteria and their 1997 revisions have been used worldwide. Since then, additional specific manifestations were described, certain clinical symptoms have become better understood, and immunological tests for diagnostic work-ups entered into routine clinical practice. An increased understanding of organ system involvement also led to questions about whether some of the independently counted criteria were in fact manifestations of the same disease phenomenon. In turn, new SLE classification criteria were recently developed with support from both the ACR and the European League Against Rheumatism (EULAR), including over 200 SLE experts from multiple medical disciplines and over 4,000 SLE patients. These new classification criteria use rigorous methodology and have excellent sensitivity and specificity (see Fig. 63.1).

Differential Diagnosis

The differential diagnosis for SLE includes vasculitis, RA, scleroderma, SS, juvenile idiopathic arthritis (particularly the systemic form), chronic active hepatitis, drug reactions, drug-induced lupus, and polyarteritis. The diagnostic criteria described in the section on Pathophysiology of SLE and in Figure 63.1 should aid in distinguishing SLE from these other diseases. Hypothyroidism also needs to be ruled out as a cause of fatigue via a TSH and free T_4 level. Drug-induced lupus has a milder presentation and is associated predominantly with procainamide, hydralazine, and minocycline, as well as the anti–TNF-α biological immunomodulators.

MANAGEMENT

The principal goal of therapy in SLE is symptom control, as current treatment is not curative. Many patients require little or no intervention. Mild joint pain may be managed with nonpharmacological interventions, as described in the section on RA. Emotional support and referral to SLE support groups are both helpful in establishing control over some symptoms. Dietary modifications should consider the specific clinical presentation. For example, active inflammatory states may require higher-calorie diets if weight loss is a concern; in contrast, corticosteroid-induced surges in appetite may call for lower-calorie diets. Corticosteroid- or NSAID-induced hypertension and hyperlipidemia (or that accompanying lupus nephritis) may call for low-salt and low-fat/low-cholesterol diets, respectively. Likewise, a lack of sun exposure because of photosensitivity may require vitamin D and calcium supplements to prevent bone loss, especially given chronic corticosteroid use. If conservative management fails, however, the patient may require antimalarials, corticosteroids, immunosuppressants, or immunomodulatory biological agents.

Constitutional symptoms are often the most troubling for patients. Fatigue is the most common symptom and tends to be the most debilitating. It can happen even in the absence of signs of active inflammation. Fatigue may be multifactorial, but if due predominantly to SLE, it tends to respond to treatment with hydroxychloroquine, corticosteroids, or dehydroepiandrosterone. In addition to weight loss associated with hyperinflammatory states, weight gain may also occur due to generalized edema (anasarca) resulting from hypoalbuminemia in nephrotic syndrome or fluid retention and increased appetite associated with glucocorticoid use. If fever is present, it is important to deduce whether it is due to the SLE itself, infection (more likely if fever is episodic and occurs while the patient is on active corticosteroids or immunosuppressive therapies), or a drug reaction that may also present with a morbilliform rash and be prolonged, without an antipyretic response to NSAIDs or acetaminophen.

NSAIDs are effective for mild musculoskeletal symptoms and mild serositis (inflammation of serosal layers, such as the pleura or pericardia). COX-1 inhibitors are used most frequently, as several COX-2 inhibitors have been withdrawn from the market due to serious cardiovascular health risks. In turn, the remaining COX-2 inhibitors (e.g., celecoxib) should be used with caution.

Entry criterion
Antinuclear antibodies (ANA) at a titer of ≥1:80 on HEp-2 cells or an equivalent positive test (ever)

↓

If absent, do not classify as SLE
If present, apply additive criteria

↓

Additive criteria
Do not count a criterion if there is a more likely explanation than SLE.
Occurrence of a criterion on at least one occasion is sufficient.
SLE classification requires at least one clinical criterion and ≥10 points.
Criteria need not occur simultaneously.
Within each domain, only the highest weighted criterion is counted toward the total score§.

Clinical domains and criteria	Weight	Immunology domains and criteria	Weight
Constitutional		**Antiphospholipid antibodies**	
Fever	2	Anti-cardiolipin antibodies OR	
Hematologic		Anti-β2GP1 antibodies OR	
Leukopenia	3	Lupus anticoagulant	2
Thrombocytopenia	4	**Complement proteins**	
Autoimmune hemolysis	4	Low C3 OR low C4	3
Neuropsychiatric		Low C3 AND low C4	4
Delirium	2	**SLE-specific antibodies**	
Psychosis	3	Anti-dsDNA antibody* OR	
Seizure	5	Anti-Smith antibody	6
Mucocutaneous			
Nonscarring alopecia	2		
Oral ulcers	2		
Subacute cutaneous OR discoid lupus	4		
Acute cutaneous lupus	6		
Serosal			
Pleural or pericardial effusion	5		
Acute pericarditis	6		
Musculoskeletal			
Joint involvement	6		
Renal			
Proteinuria >0.5g/24h	4		
Renal biopsy Class II or V lupus nephritis	8		
Renal biopsy Class III or IV lupus nephritis	10		
Total score:			

↓

Classify as Systemic Lupus Erythematosus with a score of 10 or more if entry criterion fulfilled.

Figure 63.1 The 2019 EULAR Classification Criteria for Systemic Lupus Erythematosus (*Source: Aringer M, et al. 2019 European League Against Rheumatism/American College of Rheumatology classification criteria for systemic lupus erythematosus. Ann Rheum Dis. 2019;7:1151-1159.*)

Cutaneous manifestations of lupus, including discoid lupus, respond well to antimalarials such as hydroxychloroquine (Plaquenil), which are also second-line agents for joint pains and myalgias. Antimalarials are also effective in treating serosal inflammation (pleuritis and pericarditis) and constitutional symptoms including fatigue and fever. Given their association with the long-term reduction of multiple SLE-related complications, their use is recommended in nearly all SLE patients. However, these agents are not without side effects and require appropriate monitoring, including for potential ocular toxicity and QT prolongation.

When multiple organ systems are involved or manifestations within a given organ system are moderate to severe, glucocorticoids may be given alone or in combination with another immunosuppressant. Prednisone and other glucocorticoids are effective at treating and preventing relapses if started as soon as a marked rise in anti-dsDNA antibodies is observed in the setting of clinical disease manifestations. Many SLE patients can be maintained on low doses of corticosteroids. However, although these medications are often considered a mainstay of SLE treatment, the clinician must be aware of the important side effects of systemic (IV or PO) corticosteroids, which include avascular necrosis (i.e., a reduction in blood supply to a major joint such as the knee or hip that results in joint necrosis), osteopenia and osteoporosis with bone fractures or vertebral collapse, growth inhibition in children, glaucoma and cataracts, hyperglycemia and diabetes mellitus, hypertension, weight gain, early atherosclerosis that can lead to long-term coronary artery disease and cardiac damage, and cognitive dysfunction and behavioral changes, which may be associated with both short-term and chronic use of corticosteroids. Thus, although corticosteroid therapy is associated with a delayed onset of organ damage after diagnosis, the side effects and health risks of corticosteroids are well documented and may cause significant morbidity in SLE patients. Many lupus specialists strive to decrease corticosteroid use whenever possible by use of steroid-sparing agents.

One of the newest drugs approved by the FDA for SLE treatment is the biological immunomodulatory agent belimumab (Benlysta), a monoclonal antibody therapy that binds the soluble B-cell growth factor B-lymphocyte stimulator (BLyS), thereby preventing signaling through its cognate B-cell surface receptor. As BLyS is known to support autoreactive B cells in SLE, belimumab effectively inhibits the production of autoantibodies capable of mediating organ damage and inflammation. Although not a curative therapy for SLE and not indicated to treat acute flares, belimumab has been shown to decrease disease activity, reduce symptom flare rates, and improve symptoms in autoantibody-positive lupus patients, as well as lead to reductions in corticosteroid controller therapy.

Persistent evidence of SLE-related organ damage or symptomatic flares in the face of NSAID or antimalarial therapy may signal the need for more aggressive immunosuppressive therapy, such as higher-dose glucocorticoid pulse therapy or the addition of other immunosuppressants such as mycophenolate mofetil (CellCept) or enteric-coated mycophenolate sodium (Myfortic), azathioprine (Imuran), methotrexate, and cyclophosphamide (Cytoxan). However, the severity of organ damage does not always correlate with the severity of inflammation. For instance, kidney dysfunction may relate to irreversible scarring from past kidney inflammation that has since resolved and, in turn, may not be effectively treated with immunosuppressants. This is an important distinction for the clinician to make because worsening or ongoing inflammation may be treated with corticosteroids or immunosuppressants, whereas treating noninflammatory organ damage with this same regimen just increases the risks of side effects and iatrogenic complications due to immunosuppression, without improving the underlying organ damage.

For example, class IV lupus nephritis patients typically require a remission induction and maintenance regimen with high-dose corticosteroids and immunosuppressants such as azathioprine (Imuran), mycophenolate mofetil (CellCept), or cyclophosphamide (Cytoxan). In contrast, one-third of class V lupus nephritis patients need no treatment other than for other SLE symptoms, one-third require low to moderate dose corticosteroids, and one-third need high-dose corticosteroids. Class VI lupus nephritis, on the other hand, is characterized by advanced fibrosis and no longer responds to immunosuppressive treatment, requiring instead dialysis and eventual kidney transplantation. Importantly, effective therapy for lupus nephritis should aim for at least partial remission of kidney disease, with a reduction of proteinuria to 0.5 to 0.7 g/24 hr and a normal or near-normal glomerular filtration rate after 12 months of therapy. Apart from class VI patients with advanced disease, complete renal remission is achievable in about 40% of lupus nephritis patients, although some patients may require a longer treatment duration of 12 to 24 months.

An important concept in SLE management is to treat to target, in which standardized disease activity assessment tools are used to monitor signs and symptoms and guide adjustments to the patient's treatment regimen. In turn, treatment in SLE should aim at remission (defined as a Systemic Lupus Erythematosus Disease Activity Index [SLEDAI] score = 0 and no corticosteroid use, in the presence of hydroxychloroquine) or low disease activity (SLEDAI of 4 or less, prednisone use of 7.5 mg/day or less, and immunosuppressives in stable doses, in the presence of hydroxychloroquine). The prevention of lupus disease flares is an additional important milestone of SLE treatment.

Disease progression in the face of potent immunosuppressants, such as cyclophosphamide, portends a particularly poor prognosis in SLE. Several immunomodulatory treatments are being explored for such refractory cases, including immune system ablation with high-dose chemotherapy, with or without stem cell transplantation. In addition, although not approved by the FDA to treat lupus, the anti–B-cell (anti-CD20) monoclonal antibody immunotherapy rituximab (Rituxan) is often used in refractory SLE patients, given its familiar side-effect profile and relatively long record of clinical use in other indications.

Five-year survival in SLE has greatly improved in recent decades, given the therapeutic advances discussed in this section, and is currently greater than 90%. However, the course of SLE tends to be relapsing and remitting, characterized by recurrent flares with intermittent periods of quiescence, sometimes resulting in prolonged periods of remission lasting several years. CNS and renal involvement, especially diffuse proliferative nephritis or advanced sclerosing nephritis, portend the worst prognosis. Indeed, most SLE inpatients are admitted to inpatient care for renal complications, whereas patients with isolated cutaneous and joint/muscle manifestations have the best prognosis. Short-term risk of death is also often due to infection related to immunosuppression by multiple classes of SLE medications, in addition to organ involvement associated with active inflammation in the heart, kidney, or CNS.

FOLLOW-UP AND REFERRAL

Follow-up of SLE patients is critical to track the course of the disease, which is highly variable. SLE patients who require only nonpharmacological management should still be seen at least twice per year to assess for disease progression. Patients requiring medication are typically seen at least every 3 months after stabilization on an optimal controller regimen. Before consultation with a rheumatologist, patients should receive laboratory evaluation in the primary care setting including a CBC, urinalysis (to check for proteinuria), CRP, and ANA to follow the course of the disease.

In addition, SLE patients have a greater risk of lymphoma. A greater risk of breast cancer, abnormal Pap smears, and squamous cell skin cancer has also been suggested. Thus, appropriate cancer screening in the primary care setting is critical.

Referral to a rheumatologist is indicated if antimalarials, corticosteroids, immunosuppressants, or biological immunomodulators are to be prescribed.

Patient Education: Systemic Lupus Erythematosus

Newly diagnosed patients should receive referrals to information hotlines for SLE and an array of patient advocacy groups, given the potential life-changing effect of this disease. These organizations provide patients with access to materials that support symptom control and facilitate social supports. In addition, patients should learn their individualized trajectory of disease progression and prognosis, depending on their clinical manifestations.

Patients should learn that rest is essential during disease exacerbations (lupus flares). The need for increased oral fluids and appropriate dosing of NSAIDs during such flares are also essential parts of the educational plan. Patients should understand the need for professional intervention when their temperature escalates beyond 101.5°F (38.5°C), because fevers can signal the onset of an opportunistic infection or a lupus flare, for which the primary care practitioner should be consulted immediately.

Immunizations have not been shown to induce SLE flares and should not be avoided, except for live attenuated vaccines in immunocompromised patients. If possible, sulfonamide antibiotics (e.g., TMP-SMX [Bactrim]) and tetracyclines should be avoided, because they may lead to adverse effects in SLE patients, including exacerbation of photosensitivity. Females should be encouraged to avoid pregnancy until the disease is in remission for at least 6 months, given the high miscarriage risk due to thromboembolic complications. In addition, birth control pills may exacerbate disease manifestations, although low-dose estrogen pills appear to be better tolerated. Corticosteroids, NSAIDs, and hydroxychloroquine are usually used to treat pregnant women, whereas other immunosuppressants such as methotrexate and cyclophosphamide are contraindicated in pregnancy due to their potential teratogenic effects.

REFERENCES

Allergic Reactions

Ansotegui IJ, Melioli G, Canonica GW, et al. IgE allergy diagnostics and other relevant tests in allergy, a World Allergy Organization position paper. *World Allergy Organ J.* 2020;13(2):100080. https://www.sciencedirect.com/science/article/pii/S1939455119312360?via%3Dihub. Accessed March 2, 2021.

Lieberman P, Nicklas RA, Randolph C, et al. Anaphylaxis—a practice parameter update 2015. *Ann Allergy Asthma Immunol.* 2015;115:341–384.

Schrijvers R, Gilissen L, Chiriac AM, et al. Pathogenesis and diagnosis of delayed-type drug hypersensitivity reactions, from bedside to bench and back. *Clin Transl Allergy.* 2015;5:31.

Chronic Fatigue Syndrome and Fibromyalgia Syndrome

Bush M. Chronic fatigue syndrome. *Nurs Manage.* Oct. 2020;51(10):24-28.

Ganiats T. Redefining the chronic fatigue syndrome. *Ann Intern Med.* 2015;162:653-654.

Institute of Medicine. *Beyond myalgic encephalomyelitis/chronic fatigue syndrome: Redefining an illness.* Washington, DC: The National Academies of Sciences, Engineering, and Medicine. http://www.nationalacademies.org/hmd/Reports/2015/ME-CFS.aspx. Published February 10, 2015.

Kia S, Choy E. Update on treatment guideline in fibromyalgia syndrome with focus on pharmacology. *Biomedicines.* 2017;5(20):1-24.

Okifuji A, Gao J, Bokat C, et al. Management of fibromyalgia syndrome in 2016. *Pain Manage.* 2016;6(4):383-400.

Rheumatoid Arthritis

Mian A, Ibrahim F, Scott D. A systematic review of guidelines for managing rheumatoid arthritis. *BMC Rheumatol.* 2019;3(42):1-13.

Smolen J, Landewé R, Bijlsma J, et al. EULAR recommendations for the management of rheumatoid arthritis with synthetic and biological disease-modifying antirheumatic drugs: 2016 update. *Ann Rheum Dis.* 2017;76(6):960–977.

Sjögren's Syndrome

Jonsson R, Brokstad K, Jonsson M, et al. Current concepts on Sjögren's syndrome – classification criteria and biomarkers. *Eur J Oral Sci.* 2018;126(Suppl. 1):37-48.

Sjögren's Syndrome Foundation. Clinical practice guidelines: Systemic manifestations in Sjögren's patients. https://www.sjogrens.org/home/research-programs/clinical-practice-guidelines. Published 2017. Accessed November 13, 2017.

Stefanski A, Tomiak C, Pleyer U, et al. The diagnosis and treatment of Sjögren's syndrome. *Dtsch Arztebl Int.* 2017;114:354–361.

Systemic Lupus Erythematosus

Aringer M, Costenbader K, Daikh D, et al. 2019 European League Against Rheumatism/American College of Rheumatology classification criteria for systemic lupus erythematosus. *Ann Rheum Dis.* 2019;78:1151–1159.

Hui-Yuen J, Li XQ, Askanase AD. Belimumab in systemic lupus erythematosus: a perspective review. *Ther Adv Musculoskel Dis.* 2015;7(4):115–121.

Lam N, C, Ghetu MV, Bieniek ML. Systemic lupus erythematosus: primary care approach to diagnosis and management. *Am Fam Physician.* 2016;94(4):284–294.

RESOURCES

Allergic Reactions

National Institute of Allergy and Infectious Diseases (National Institutes of Health)
http://www.niaid.nih.gov

Chronic Fatigue Syndrome and Fibromyalgia Syndrome

American Fibromyalgia Syndrome Association, Inc.
http://www.afsafund.org

National Fibromyalgia Association
http://www.fmaware.org

Solve M.E./CFS Initiative
http://solvecfs.org

Rheumatoid Arthritis

American College of Rheumatology
http://www.rheumatology.org

Arthritis Foundation
http://www.arthritis.org

Sjögren's Syndrome

Sjögren's Foundation
http://www.sjogrens.org

Systemic Lupus Erythematosus

Autoimmune Related Disease Association
http://www.aarda.org

Lupus Foundation of America
http://www.lupus.org

Lupus Research Alliance
http://www.lupusresearch.org

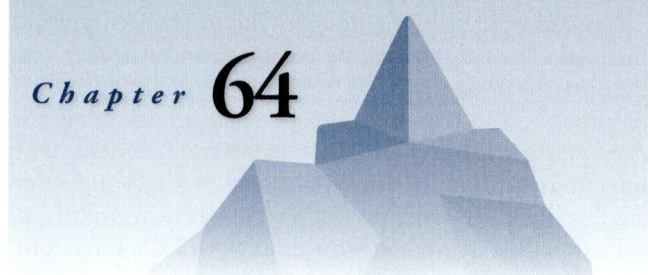

Chapter 64

Infectious Disorders

Virginia Sheikh, MD, MHS
Jill E. Winland-Brown, EdD, APRN, FNP-BC, FAANP
Brian Oscar Porter, MD, PhD, MPH, MBA

INFECTIOUS MONONUCLEOSIS

Infectious mononucleosis, formerly called "glandular fever," is a viral syndrome characterized by prolonged malaise and fatigue, fever, sore throat, and tender cervical lymphadenopathy. The majority (90%) of infectious mononucleosis cases are caused by infection with Epstein-Barr virus (EBV). Cytomegalovirus (CMV) is a less common viral cause.

EPIDEMIOLOGY AND CAUSES

Both EBV and CMV infections are widespread; up to 95% of adults are seropositive for EBV exposure, and 59% of individuals aged 6 years or older are seropositive for CMV exposure. Both EBV and CMV are members of the Herpesviridae family of viruses and cause lifelong, usually asymptomatic infection. Humans are the major reservoir for latent EBV infection, which typically spreads through intimate contact with asymptomatic viral shedders. Humans, along with monkeys, are the major reservoir for CMV infection, which can be transmitted to others by direct contact with urine or saliva (especially from babies and young children), through sexual contact, and via breast milk.

Symptomatic cases of infectious mononucleosis are most common in teenagers and young adults, for whom the most important mode of transmission is kissing. Preadolescent children, especially those who live in crowded conditions, are commonly infected with EBV and CMV through saliva, although they are typically asymptomatic. The incidence of infectious mononucleosis is equal among genders, economic classes, and educational levels, although the incidence of clinical infection is up to 30 times higher in whites than blacks. There is no seasonal variation in rates of infectious mononucleosis cases.

PATHOPHYSIOLOGY

EBV is most commonly spread through saliva. Once inside the oral cavity, the virus initially infects and replicates in oropharyngeal epithelial cells. Infectious virions then infect B cells, which migrate and disseminate the infection widely throughout the lymphoreticular system, which includes the lymph nodes, spleen, and liver. At the time of infectious mononucleosis symptom onset, high levels of EBV can be detected in the blood. The immune response to EBV viremia includes an atypical peripheral lymphocytosis, which is characterized by a large number of activated CD8+ T cells and natural killer cells. These cells are key to preventing the acute lysis of virally infected cells (i.e., the lytic phase of infection) and establishing nonlytic, subclinical lifelong infection. CMV is transmitted through close contact with body fluids (saliva, urine, and stool), blood or tissue exposure, sexual exposure, or perinatal exposure.

Although the majority of individuals with chronic EBV and/or CMV infection remain asymptomatic throughout their lifetimes, both viruses have the potential to cause serious disease. For example, many cases of Hodgkin and non-Hodgkin lymphoma are associated with EBV. Babies born to patients who experienced infectious mononucleosis caused by CMV during pregnancy are at risk of congenital CMV infection, which can cause serious complications, including preterm birth, seizures, and central nervous system (CNS) impairment. CMV reactivation causes significant disease in severely immunosuppressed patients, such as those with HIV/AIDS and bone marrow transplant recipients.

CLINICAL PRESENTATION

Subjective

Patients with infectious mononucleosis typically present with complaints of fever, sore throat, adenopathy, and fatigue. Gastrointestinal (GI) manifestations including nausea, vomiting, and anorexia may also be present, as may hepatosplenomegaly, headache, and, occasionally, a morbilliform viral exanthem (rash). Patients may also report neuropathies, headache, photophobia, dysphagia, sore throat, diffuse chest pain, dyspnea, cough, nausea, myalgia, and arthralgia. They usually cannot identify a known contact with EBV infection before the onset of symptoms.

Objective

Children and teenagers with mononucleosis may present with fevers as high as 39°C (greater than 102.5°F). Almost all patients with infectious mononucleosis will have tender, cervical lymphadenopathy, although this finding is not specific. Posterior cervical, axillary, and inguinal adenopathy are more specific findings. Nuchal stiffness associated with painful lymph nodes may be present, although it is not as rigid as in meningitis. The pharynx is typically infected. The tonsils may be enlarged, and tonsillar exudate may be present. Splenomegaly is present in up to 60% of patients. The liver may also be enlarged and tender to deep palpation, but jaundice is uncommon. Patients with infectious mononucleosis as a result of CMV infection are less likely to develop lymphadenopathy, tonsillitis, or splenomegaly, compared with those with EBV infection.

Patients with infectious mononucleosis may present with a fine, maculopapular rash (viral exanthem). More commonly, patients with infectious mononucleosis who have been treated with antibiotics (especially amoxicillin or ampicillin), either due to a misdiagnosis or concurrent bacterial infection, may develop a pruritic, morbilliform rash that can be mistaken for antibiotic allergy.

DIAGNOSTIC REASONING

The symptoms of mononucleosis are seen in many diseases; therefore, laboratory findings play an important role in the differential diagnosis. Although limited diagnostic

Pediatric/Adolescent Considerations: Infectious Mononucleosis

Infectious mononucleosis is common in teens, who may be experiencing a range of new physical, cognitive, and emotional challenges as they cope with the symptoms and clinical manifestations of infectious mononucleosis. In turn, adolescents may be reticent to express relevant health concerns, especially those pertaining to sexual, behavioral, and mental health. They may also feel less comfortable undergoing physical examinations and more anxious when subjected to medical testing. Thus, clinicians should recognize that adolescents may need additional assurance of confidentiality and require more time to feel comfortable communicating their concerns and questions.

testing may establish the diagnosis in straightforward cases, additional testing may be required for certain presenting symptoms that are less specific (e.g., pharyngitis) and in more complex situations.

Diagnostic Tests

Often the diagnosis of infectious mononucleosis can be made with clinical symptoms and with results from a complete blood count (CBC), serum chemistries, and a heterophile antibody test (Monospot). The CBC usually shows at least 50% lymphocytes, including 10% "atypical" lymphocytes. Mild thrombocytopenia and neutropenia are frequent transient findings. Liver enzyme levels, particularly serum transaminase levels, are mildly or moderately elevated in about 90% of patients.

The Monospot test detects heterophile antibodies, which are circulating immunoglobulin (Ig)M antibodies that target red blood cell antigens. Heterophile antibodies are present in 80% to 90% of patients with acute infectious mononucleosis, although they are not specific and may take several weeks to become positive. The Monospot test is less sensitive in younger patients (75% sensitivity in children aged 24 to 28 months and 25% in children aged 10 to 24 months); therefore, EBV-specific serologies should be checked in children. In fact, further testing of EBV-specific serum IgM antibodies may prove useful in adult patients as well, if the diagnosis based on initial testing is questionable. Anti-EBNA (EBV nuclear antigen) and anti-VCA (viral capsid antigen) are two specific anti-EBV serology tests that are widely available, although they are also less sensitive in younger patients (60% sensitivity in infants but up to 100% sensitivity in young adults). False-positive results for EBV have been noted in HIV-infected individuals but are considered rare.

For patients with infectious mononucleosis with negative Monospot test results, serological testing for CMV should be considered, especially in patients who are immunocompromised or pregnant. The U.S. Centers for Disease Control and Prevention (CDC) recommends measurement of IgG, commonly via an enzyme-linked immunosorbent assay (ELISA) in paired samples taken 1 to 3 months apart after initial presentation. Evidence of seroconversion (i.e., first sample IgG negative and second sample IgG positive) establishes the diagnosis of acute CMV infection.

Differential Diagnosis

Although infectious mononucleosis due to EBV or CMV is relatively common, the differential diagnosis for the common presenting symptoms of fever, pharyngitis, and lymphadenopathy is broad. Glandular variant infectious mononucleosis, in which lymphadenopathy is out of proportion to the pharyngitis, differs from systemic variant mononucleosis that presents with fever and fatigue and typically has mild or absent lymphadenopathy and pharyngitis.

Other conditions that can mimic the clinical presentation of infectious mononucleosis include streptococcal infection, peritonsillar abscess, and acute HIV. Throat culture and/or rapid antigen detection testing should be performed routinely in these cases to rule out group A streptococcal disease (i.e., strep throat). Peritonsillar abscess should be suspected in patients who present with severe unilateral sore throat, drooling, muffled voice, or trismus (lockjaw). For cases in which acute HIV is a possibility, a fourth generation combined antigen/antibody immunoassay should be ordered to detect recent HIV infection (refer to the section on HIV for more information on acute HIV infection and HIV testing).

Acute toxoplasmosis, caused by infection with the parasite *Toxoplasma gondii*, can also cause fever and cervical adenopathy in immunocompetent individuals. Acute infection with *T. gondii*, which is uncommon, can typically be excluded via serological testing, as the absence of anti-*Toxoplasma* IgM and IgG antibodies essentially excludes this diagnosis. Acute leukemia may also present with fever, fatigue, and lymphadenopathy, and certain medications such as isoniazid, phenytoin, or carbamazepine can also induce a mononucleosis-like illness.

Table 64.1 presents a comparison of the signs and symptoms of different forms of infectious mononucleosis and other EBV-related conditions. These include oral hairy leukoplakia, which is caused by EBV infection in an immunocompromised host (such as with AIDS), and Duncan's disease, which is a rare X-linked lymphoproliferative disorder with a dysfunction immune response to

TABLE 64.1 Signs and Symptoms of Infectious Mononucleosis and Other Epstein-Barr Virus-related Conditions				
	EBV-related Infectious Mononucleosis	CMV-related Infectious Mononucleosis	Oral Hairy Leukoplakia	Duncan's Disease (X-Linked Lymphoproliferative Disorder)
Malaise	+	+	+/−	+
Lymphadenopathy	+	+/−	+	+
Fever	+	+	+/−	+/−
Splenomegaly	+ (50% of cases)	+/−	+/−	+
Pharyngeal exudate	+	−	−	−

Abbreviations: + present; − absent; CMV, cytomegalovirus; EBV, Epstein-Barr virus.

EBV infection characterized by widespread lymphocyte proliferation that is nonetheless ineffective at clearing the infection.

MANAGEMENT

The mainstay of management of infectious mononucleosis is supportive care. No effective antiviral medications are available for the treatment of infectious mononucleosis caused by EBV infection. Infectious mononucleosis caused by CMV is usually self-limiting, and therefore, antiviral therapy is not typically indicated. NSAIDs or acetaminophen (in the absence of significant liver injury) can help minimize fever and discomfort. Adequate hydration and nutrition should be emphasized. Supportive measures such as gargling with warm salt water and throat lozenges may alleviate throat pain. Although strict bedrest is not required, adequate rest to support recovery is recommended.

FOLLOW-UP AND REFERRAL

Because patients with infectious mononucleosis are at risk of serious sequelae including splenic rupture, airway compromise, bone marrow suppression, and neurological complications, patients should be followed regularly until symptom resolution. Repeat laboratory testing may also be necessary if significant abnormalities were present at the time of initial diagnosis, such as elevations in liver-associated enzymes. The primary care practitioner should provide the patient with a full clinical picture of the disease, including its prolonged course of recovery, so that the patient may play an active role in self-assessment during the follow-up period.

Although severe complications are unlikely, prompt referral may be necessary. Splenic rupture is a rare (2 in 1,000) but potentially fatal complication of infectious mononucleosis. Patients with splenic rupture may experience abdominal pain and/or progressive anemia due to internal bleeding. Patients with these symptoms should be referred for surgical consultation on an urgent or emergent basis, depending on the acuity of symptoms. Patients with infectious mononucleosis who complain of difficulty breathing should be evaluated for airway obstruction, caused by cervical lymphadenopathy or mucosal swelling. The initiation of corticosteroid therapy and emergent consultation with an otolaryngologist are warranted in these cases.

Other uncommon but serious sequelae may develop and require ongoing monitoring and/or referral to a specialist. Rare hematological complications can include hemolytic or aplastic anemia, thrombocytopenia, thrombotic thrombocytopenic purpura, hemolytic uremic syndrome, or disseminated intravascular coagulation. Cardiovascular complications include myocarditis. Renal and genitourinary complications include glomerulonephritis or genital ulceration, and GI complications include pancreatitis. Neurological complications include Guillain-Barré syndrome, facial nerve palsy, meningoencephalitis, aseptic meningitis, transverse myelitis, or optic neuritis. Any patient with encephalitis will require an immediate neurological consultation.

Patient Education: Infectious Mononucleosis

Young, school-aged patients must be warned of the dangers of contact sports and rough-housing for at least 4 weeks after the onset of symptoms because splenic rupture predominantly occurs within 3 weeks of symptom onset and may also occur in the absence of frank splenomegaly (50% of splenic rupture cases). In addition, up to one-half of all splenic rupture cases may occur without any preceding trauma, and the risk of rupture does not correlate with symptom severity or abnormal laboratory results. A good rule of thumb is that the patient's energy level must be at baseline before the resumption of strenuous or risky physical activity, and this must not occur before 4 weeks. However, strict bedrest is not required during this entire period and will be driven largely by the patient's energy level.

Patients must learn that their recurrent fevers will typically disappear long before they feel recovered. Fevers will typically subside after 10 to 14 days, although energy levels will not rebound to baseline until 1 to 3 months postinfection. Therefore, teenagers and young adults who typically manage busy schedules and active lives will need to accept that they require rest for a prolonged recovery period that will last weeks, rather than days.

Other elements to consider in patient education include providing information about prescribed drugs, such as appropriate doses and adverse effects. The primary care practitioner should also caution patients to avoid alcohol and cigarette use because they aggravate coughing and nausea. Alcohol should be avoided for a minimum of 3 months after liver function tests return to normal. In addition, patient education should include age-appropriate counseling regarding sexual practices and the risk of sexually transmitted infections (STIs), other than EBV-associated infectious mononucleosis, that may affect future fertility (e.g., pelvic inflammatory disease) or even be life-threatening (e.g., HIV).

LYME DISEASE

Lyme disease is a multisystem inflammatory disease caused by *Borrelia burgdorferi*, a tick-borne spirochete (bacterium). Most of the early signs and symptoms are nonspecific including fever, chills, headache, fatigue, myalgia, arthralgia, and lymphadenopathy. Some patients, however, develop erythema migrans ("bull's eye" rash), which is classically associated with Lyme disease. Later manifestations of Lyme disease may include meningitis, arthritis, facial palsy, arrhythmias, nerve pain, and short-term memory loss.

EPIDEMIOLOGY AND CAUSES

The CDC estimates that approximately 300,000 people get Lyme disease in the United States every year. Only about 10% of these cases are reported to the CDC, however, which relies on a passive reporting system.

Although Lyme disease is named for a town in Connecticut (Old Lyme), where it was isolated among residents in the 1970s, it is prevalent in much of the northeastern and mid-Atlantic United States. The states with the highest incidence of Lyme disease in 2018 included Connecticut, Delaware, Maine, Maryland, Massachusetts, Minnesota, New Hampshire, New Jersey, New York, Pennsylvania, Rhode Island, Vermont, Virginia, West Virginia, and Wisconsin. Up to one-half of the ticks found in these states may be infected with the spirochete. In Europe and Asia, other species of *Borrelia* cause disease with somewhat different clinical manifestations. The diagnosis of Lyme disease, which can be challenging, as described later in this section, causes some difficulty in collecting reliable incidence data.

Lyme disease affects individuals with exposure to *B. burgdorferi* via a tick bite, without regard to race, gender, or other demographic traits. *B. burgdorferi* is transmitted to humans primarily through the bite of the *Ixodes scapularis* (black-legged or deer) tick, which is common throughout wooded areas in the eastern part of the United States. The tick survives on blood meals from mammals, birds, reptiles, and amphibians at each stage of its life, and it is through these blood meals that the tick is infected with *B. burgdorferi*.

Most human infections occur in the late spring, summer, and early fall and are a result of tick nymph bites. The tick eggs hatch in springtime and develop into larvae over the following summer. The tick larvae acquire spirochetes on taking their first blood meal from infected mice, birds, or other small mammals. The larvae eventually detach from their hosts to molt and emerge the following spring as infected nymphs. Nymph ticks are very small (less than 2 mm), and, therefore, humans are less likely to see or remove nymphs after a bite. Nymphs detach and molt into adults in the early fall.

Adult ticks survive throughout fall and winter, feeding exclusively on large mammals (primarily white-tailed deer) before laying eggs in the spring. Although infected adult ticks are also able to transmit the infection, adult ticks are larger, and therefore more likely to be recognized and removed by humans. Thus, the tick life cycle and the ability to identify bites from larger adult ticks help to explain the seasonal preference for Lyme disease being spread by nymphs in the summer months, rather than in the winter.

PATHOPHYSIOLOGY

After the bite of an infected tick, the likelihood of *B. burgdorferi* infection depends on the duration of tick exposure. The infected tick must feed for at least 24 to 48 hours before it transmits the spirochete to the host. After infection, spirochetes are believed to bind fibronectin and epithelial cell–derived proteoglycans (e.g., heparin, dermatan sulfate) in the extracellular matrix via glycosaminoglycan receptors. This initiates a mild local inflammatory response that causes cutaneous erythema at sites of spirochetal invasion and centrifugal (outward) spread from the original tick bite, resulting in the bull's eye–appearing rash termed *erythema migrans*. Subsequent spirochetemia and tissue-specific binding may cause neurological sequelae, vasculopathy, and cardiac conduction defects in certain individuals. Arthritis is thought to be due to joint inflammation from localized exposure to spirochetal antigens, such as outer surface protein A (OspA) or the heat shock protein groEL.

B. burgdorferi has been shown to exert immunomodulatory influences on host cells, including decreasing major histocompatibility complex (MHC) class II antigen-presenting molecules on Langerhans cells isolated from late-phase cutaneous skin lesions, while upregulating the class II MHC molecules human leukocyte antigen (HLA)-DR1, HLA-DR2, and HLA-DR4 on synovial endothelial cells in arthritic joints. The role of cytokines in this disease has not been fully elucidated, but several studies have demonstrated increased levels of macrophage-derived tumor necrosis factor-alpha, interleukin (IL)-1, and IL-6 in the blood, synovial fluid, and cerebrospinal fluid (CSF) of affected persons.

In addition, an autoimmune pathology has also been implicated in late disease manifestations. Most notably, the predominant T-cell receptor found on activated T lymphocytes after infection is specific for an epitope of OspA presented within certain class II MHC molecules that are upregulated in affected patients. Moreover, this OspA epitope has been shown to be cross-reactive with the leukocyte adhesion molecule human lymphocyte function-associated antigen-1 (LFA-1), which is highly expressed on T lymphocytes. Studies of transgenic mice tolerant to OspA suggest that cross reactivity of this protein does not fully explain these autoimmune phenomena.

Some evidence suggests the importance of a *Borrelia*-specific superantigen. In addition, IgM antibodies against the spirochete protein flagellin are cross-reactive with human axonal proteins and myelin, which has been suggested to mediate the neurological sequelae of Lyme disease. Several other types of autoantibodies have been identified in the CSF of Lyme disease patients. However, it is not known whether these antibodies play a role in the actual pathogenesis of the disease or are simply a benign secondary consequence of infection.

CLINICAL PRESENTATION

Subjective

Early in the course of the disease, the patient typically complains of a flu-like illness, including fever, chills, and myalgia. The patient may also report a rash that grew in size. Importantly, most patients with Lyme disease do not recall a tick bite.

Later in the course of the disease, malaise, fatigue, headache, neck pain and stiffness, and generalized pain may constitute presenting symptoms. Left untreated, the disease may progress to include arthritis of one or more joints. Late in the disease trajectory, the patient may complain of memory loss, cognitive disturbances, mood changes, and peripheral neuropathy in addition to arthritis.

Objective

In early localized disease, occurring 3 to 30 days after exposure, 70% to 80% of Lyme disease presentations include an erythema migrans rash. Erythema migrans is typically located on parts of the body where the tick selectively feeds, such as the axilla, groin, and waistline. The bull's eye–appearing rash grows in size, as it spreads from the site of the tick bite. This classic rash is occasionally pruritic and/or burning, may develop central clearing, and is typically greater than 5 cm in size. The presence of this rash is essentially diagnostic of Lyme disease and should prompt treatment in the appropriate clinical and epidemiological setting, without the need for serological confirmation.

In early disseminated disease, which occurs days to 10 months after infection and often in the absence of erythema migrans, infected patients may present with systemic manifestations including carditis (less than 10% of cases) and neurological manifestations (10% of cases) such as lymphocytic meningitis, cranial nerve (CN) palsies (especially of CN VII), and radiculoneuritis. This neurological triad is known as *Bannwarth syndrome* and is more common in European cases of Lyme disease than in the United States.

Objective findings later in the disease include regional or organ-specific physical abnormalities. In late disease, which may be months to years after exposure, symptoms are characterized by intermittent arthritis (50% of cases, which respond to oral antibiotic therapy) and arthralgias (20%), with 10% of patients having monoarthritis of the knee. Very late in the disease trajectory, musculoskeletal findings predominate. In particular, joints become edematous and are associated with tenderness to touch. Gait disturbances may also occur in association with encephalopathy.

Patients may have neurological manifestations known as *tertiary neuroborreliosis,* including encephalopathy, neurocognitive impairment, and peripheral neuropathy.

Objective findings may include nuchal rigidity, sensorimotor disturbances, and paresthesias. A mental status examination may be positive for impaired problem resolution. Cardiac findings include dysrhythmias, a prolonged P-R interval, and rarely third-degree heart block. Skin eruptions resembling the erythema migrans rash of early infection may recur later in the disease course, as well.

DIAGNOSTIC REASONING

Diagnostic Tests

The presence of one or more skin lesions compatible with an erythema migrans rash in a Lyme-endemic area should prompt a clinical diagnosis of Lyme disease, without the need for laboratory testing. Because erythema migrans typically occurs in the first 1 to 2 weeks after *B. burgdorferi* infection before many patients develop antispirochetal antibodies, serological testing is only 40% sensitive in this setting. Furthermore, prompt treatment triggered by erythema migrans may inhibit the subsequent development of antispirochetal antibodies. Therefore, laboratory testing at a later time is not recommended either in this setting. If the patient has one or more skin lesions that are suggestive of but atypical for erythema migrans, antibody testing of acute and convalescent sera is recommended.

For patients who present with extracutaneous symptoms concerning for Lyme disease such as arthritis, carditis, or facial palsy, laboratory testing is necessary to make a Lyme disease diagnosis. Currently, the CDC recommends a two-step process for testing blood for antibodies to *B. burgdorferi*. The first step is an enzyme immunoassay (EIA) and the second step, performed only if the EIA is positive, is a confirmatory Western blot assay. Often, laboratories will offer "reflex" testing that automatically proceeds with Western blot testing of positive EIA samples.

Serological testing performed within the first few weeks of symptoms (and presumably *B. burgdorferi* infection) should assay IgM antibodies, whereas serological testing performed later in infection should assess IgG antibodies, which develop approximately 1 month after initial exposure. IgM levels can remain elevated for more than a year, so they cannot be used to make a diagnosis of active disease. Repeated serological testing 4 to 6 weeks after exposure (during the convalescent period) may be appropriate if early serological testing is negative.

A Western blot is considered positive if two of three of the following IgM bands are positive (OspC/24, 39, and 4) or if five of the following IgG bands are positive (18, 23, 28, 30, 39, 41, 45, 58, 66, and 96). False-positive Western blot results are relatively common in uninfected individuals; therefore, the CDC does not recommend performing Western blot testing unless the screening EIA result is positive. In addition, Lyme disease serological testing should only be performed if findings clearly suggest this disease, rather than with only nonspecific chronic complaints. Testing results should be measured against CDC testing standards because results may vary significantly between individual laboratories. When used appropriately, Lyme disease serological testing is highly sensitive and specific for the diagnosis of Lyme disease.

For a number of reasons, the following tests for Lyme detection are not widely accepted and are considered experimental, rather than confirmatory or diagnostic: variable surface antigen ELISA, polymerase chain reaction (PCR), urinary antigen testing, T-cell proliferative responses, and immune complex disruption. Thus, providers should not use these tests to confirm a diagnosis of Lyme disease.

For patients who present with symptoms suggestive of infection of the CNS (e.g., neuroborreliosis), lumbar puncture should be performed. Analysis of the CSF typically reveals modest pleocytosis (up to several hundred white blood cells [WBCs]) and moderately elevated protein. CSF glucose is typically normal. CSF should be sent for antibodies against *B. burgdorferi*, and positive results are highly specific for the diagnosis of Lyme meningitis. Negative results do not, however, rule out the diagnosis. Testing for other etiological causes of the patient's symptoms, such as herpes simplex virus, West Nile virus, and syphilis, should also be performed on the CSF fluid.

Because Lyme arthritis is a late manifestation of *B. burgdorferi* infection, IgG antibodies to *Borrelia* are almost always strongly positive. Therefore, the two-step serological testing of the blood described earlier may be adequate to establish the diagnosis of Lyme arthritis in the appropriate clinical setting. Arthrocentesis may be appropriate to rule out other causes of arthritis. Synovial fluid analysis in Lyme disease typically reveals characteristics consistent with an inflammatory arthritis, in which WBCs are elevated with a neutrophilic predominance. *B. burgdorferi* rarely grows in culture. PCR testing of *B. burgdorferi* may be useful in seropositive patients for whom more definitive information is required for clinical decision making.

Differential Diagnosis

For patients who present with a viral-like illness and skin lesions within 1 month of a tick bite, human granulocytic anaplasmosis (HGA), babesiosis, and southern tick–associated rash illness (STARI) should be considered as alternative or comorbid diagnoses. Both HGA and babesiosis are transmitted by *Ixodes* ticks. HGA is caused by *Anaplasma phagocytophilum* and may present with a high fever and severe constitutional complaints, elevated liver enzymes, and leukopenia and/or thrombocytopenia. Babesiosis is caused by infection with the parasite *Babesia microti* and can present with fatigue, high fever, headache, and myalgia. STARI is associated with *Amblyomma americanum* (lone star tick) bites and can present with a similar erythema migrans–like rash, low-grade fever, and lymphadenopathy. Although the cause of STARI is not known, these patients appear to respond to the same treatment used for Lyme disease (e.g., doxycycline). Thus, although STARI presents similarly, Lyme disease remains more common than STARI in Lyme-endemic areas; therefore, patients in these areas with erythema migrans lesions should be presumed to have Lyme disease.

Differential diagnoses for Lyme disease also include viral syndromes, Rocky Mountain spotted fever, and relapsing fever. It is important not to confuse Lyme disease with fibromyalgia syndrome (FMS) or chronic fatigue syndrome (CFS or myalgic encephalomyelitis), which are not inflammatory disorders and have never been shown to be clearly infectious in etiology. Although FMS may develop after the onset of Lyme disease, it is important not to simply accept a diagnosis of "chronic Lyme disease" made previously by another clinician, because there is little evidence that this condition actually exists, as opposed to late manifestations of Lyme disease, which are considered genuine aspects of the disease process.

MANAGEMENT

The goal of management for the infected patient is to minimize the manifestations of the disease at the time of diagnosis, although protective measures to prevent primary infection are a key component of any comprehensive management program to benefit others. Patients living in Lyme-endemic areas should be advised to avoid tick bites by use of both protective clothing and tick repellents. After outdoor activities, patients should check for ticks daily and remove attached ticks promptly.

For children 8 years of age and older and nonpregnant adult patients with attached ticks, the Infectious Disease Society of America (IDSA) suggests that clinicians offer a single dose of doxycycline 200 mg when *all* the following circumstances are met: (1) the attached tick can be identified as an *I. scapularis* nymph or adult tick that has been attached for 36 hours or longer based on the degree of engorgement and exposure, (2) prophylaxis can be started within 72 hours of the time the tick was removed, (3) ecological information indicates the local rate of infection is 20% or greater, and (4) doxycycline is not contraindicated.

Approximately 90% of early localized Lyme disease responds to antibiotic therapy. The duration of treatment depends on the extent of involvement. Regimens for early localized disease should last for 10 to 14 days, whereas 30 days of therapy are required for cardiac, neurological, and arthritic manifestations. IDSA recommends doxycycline (Vibramycin) 100 mg twice daily for the initial management of erythema migrans. (Doxycycline is also effective against the tick-borne bacterial infection ehrlichiosis.) All tetracyclines, including doxycycline, are not recommended for children younger than 8 years of age or in pregnant females, given the risk of tooth discoloration. In children older than 8 years of age, the dosage is 2 mg/kg.

Alternative antibiotic agents include amoxicillin (Amoxil), cefuroxime (Ceftin), and erythromycin (E-Mycin). Cefuroxime is typically more expensive than doxycycline or amoxicillin. The amoxicillin dose is 500 mg three times daily (50 mg/kg per day divided every 8 hours with the same maximum dose in children). The cefuroxime dose is 500 mg twice daily in adults and up to 30 mg/kg per day divided twice daily with the same maximum dose in children. Macrolides such as erythromycin are not as effective in Lyme disease as doxycycline, amoxicillin, or cefuroxime and should be used only for patients intolerant to these other first- and second-line antibiotic choices. First generation cephalosporins, such as cephalexin (Keflex), should not be used because these antibiotics are not active against *Borrelia*.

Up to 15% of patients may display worsening of symptoms with rigors, fever, or hypotension in the first 24 hours of antibiotic therapy due to an increase in acute inflammatory cytokines associated with bacterial death. This phenomenon is referred to as the *Jarisch-Herxheimer reaction* and is well-documented in tick- and louse-borne relapsing fever conditions. Thus, clinicians should inform patients that this reaction may occur.

Early disseminated disease with mostly musculoskeletal manifestations should be treated with these same oral antibiotic agents for 2 to 3 weeks, as long as meningitis or third-degree heart block is not noted. First- and second-degree heart block and isolated facial nerve palsy can be treated with 3 weeks of oral antibiotics. If neurological sequelae (other than isolated facial nerve palsy) or third-degree heart block are noted, IV antibiotic therapy should be started with ceftriaxone (Rocephin) 2 g daily or cefotaxime (Claforan) 2 g three times daily for 2 to 4 weeks. Specifically, a lumbar puncture should be done to analyze the CSF for anti-*Borrelia* antibodies or inflammatory cells (WBCs), because neurological manifestations may be subclinical. If subclinical meningitis is suspected with elevated WBCs in the CSF, IV antibiotic therapy is required. Third-degree heart block should be treated with IV ceftriaxone or cefotaxime, and prednisone (Deltasone) 40 to 60 mg/day in divided doses may be added if patients do not respond within 4 days, although this approach has not been validated in randomized trials.

Late Lyme disease is treated with amoxicillin or doxycycline for at least 4 weeks if arthritis is the primary manifestation. If patients fail one or two courses of oral antibiotic therapy or if late disease presents with neurological sequelae (or if a lumbar puncture shows subclinical meningitis with WBC or autoantibodies), IV antibiotic therapy with ceftriaxone or cefotaxime for 4 weeks should be given.

All IV antibiotic therapy may be completed on an outpatient basis if the patient has reliable IV access (e.g., a peripherally inserted central catheter or a central venous catheter, as opposed to a peripheral IV line) and a stable social situation. In addition, at least the first IV dose should be given in a monitored setting to evaluate for drug hypersensitivity. Weekly CBCs should be done to monitor for leukopenia, which may be seen with ceftriaxone and cefotaxime. Ceftriaxone may cause biliary sludging, which can be monitored with weekly hepatic panels to evaluate for hyperbilirubinemia. If this occurs, the patient should be switched to cefotaxime. GI side effects, including the development of *Clostridium difficile* colitis, may also occur. Doxycycline causes photosensitivity, and amoxicillin and cefuroxime can cause drug rashes.

Combination antibiotic therapy, an oral course of antibiotics after IV courses, pulse antibiotic therapy with weekly IV treatments, and extended IV antibiotic regimens lasting beyond 2 to 4 weeks have never been validated for Lyme disease through randomized clinical trials and should be avoided, as these are only likely to increase drug toxicity with no value-added benefit. There is also no evidence that pharmacological treatment of asymptomatic seropositivity, found on routine screening for instance, provides any benefit. These patients should be thoroughly evaluated, however, to determine whether an asymptomatic phase is actually latent infection that will eventually manifest as late disease, because such individuals typically do not progress through early disease manifestations.

Symptoms may persist after appropriate antibiotic treatment, as some Lyme disease symptoms such as headache, fatigue, and malaise commonly take months or years to resolve after treatment. In other cases, persistent symptoms may be attributable to another, inadequately treated tick-borne pathogen, such as the *Ehrlichia* species. Continued infection with *B. burgdorferi* after appropriate Lyme treatment should only be suspected if Lyme-specific symptoms worsen after treatment or if new Lyme-specific signs or symptoms develop.

FOLLOW-UP AND REFERRAL

Follow-up for symptomatic presentations of Lyme disease, before the actual diagnosis is confirmed, may require weekly clinic visits. Thus, antibiotic therapy may be started after initial laboratory testing if Lyme disease is highly suspected, and then stopped later if the diagnosis is not confirmed on follow-up.

The rash of erythema migrans usually begins to resolve after the fifth dose of oral antibiotics, whereas fibromyalgic and CFS-like symptoms (e.g., headache, weakness, fatigue, arthralgias) may persist for years after infection. Actual FMS is also recognized as a postinfectious complication of Lyme disease.

Referral to a specialist may not be required if the diagnosis is straightforward. However, if the diagnosis is unclear, rather than overtreating with antibiotic therapy, a referral to an infectious disease specialist is indicated for further evaluation and treatment recommendations. Neurological, cardiac, and other serious organ-specific manifestations may necessitate appropriate specialist referrals, should these manifestations persist despite appropriate primary care management.

Patient Education: Lyme Disease

People should be encouraged to avoid foliage (where ticks may reside), especially at the ankle level, along wooded paths and to walk in the center of the path to avoid low-lying brush. Hikers should wear clothing that can prevent ticks from attaching to the skin. When planning an activity in the woods, individuals should wear long pants and boots, and pant cuffs should be tucked inside the boot lip. Shirt collars should be closed. Tick repellent should be applied to any exposed skin and the scalp. After removing clothing, the patient should inspect the axillae, groin, and waistband areas, in particular, for evidence of attached ticks or bites.

If infection has already occurred, the patient needs to understand the course of the disease and that an initial worsening of symptoms early in treatment or a recurrence of symptoms after initial treatment might occur. Moreover, patients who are seropositive are not necessarily immune from reinfection. Reinfection is possible with *Borrelia* of a different strain if the patient remains exposed to high-risk environments.

HIV INFECTION

More than one million people in the United States are living with HIV infection, and about 15% of them are unaware of their infection. Although patients may experience a flu-like illness with acute HIV infection, many patients are asymptomatic for years, despite having high levels of HIV in the blood and other bodily fluids, such as semen. HIV infects the key immune cells, CD4+ T cells, leading to the death of most of these infected cells. Over a period of months, years, or decades, HIV kills more CD4+ T cells than the body can produce, and the patient's CD4+ T cell count begins to decline. When the CD4+ T cell count drops below 200/μL, the patient becomes particularly susceptible to opportunistic infections (OIs) and is considered to have AIDS. Table 64.2 presents the CDC HIV classification system for adults and adolescents.

This section of the chapter covers screening, pre-exposure prophylaxis (PrEP), and postexposure prophylaxis (PEP) for HIV. In addition, the section discusses the diagnosis and management of HIV infection in the acute setting and before the progression to AIDS. Refer to the section on AIDS for the diagnosis and management of AIDS and OIs.

EPIDEMIOLOGY AND CAUSES

At the end of 2019, the World Health Organization estimated 38 million people were living with HIV worldwide, but only 68% of adults and 53% of children living with HIV globally were receiving antiretroviral therapy (ART). That same year, 1.7 million people were newly infected with HIV, and 690,000 people died from AIDS. Although HIV has affected all regions of the world, over two-thirds of new HIV infections occur in Africa.

Today, HIV infection in the United States affects people of any sexual orientation, gender, race, and ethnicity. According to the CDC, men who have sex with men (MSM) still account for the majority (69%) of new infections, but nearly a quarter (24%) of new infections occurs in individuals who are heterosexual. In 2018, transgender people accounted for 2% of newly diagnosed HIV infections. Although a quarter (25%) of newly infected individuals are white/European American, black/African American (42%) and Hispanic/Latino (27%) people are disproportionately affected, relative to the demographic distribution of the U.S. population at large. Additionally, in 2018 the highest rates of

TABLE 64.2 U.S. Centers for Disease Control and Prevention HIV Classification System for Adults and Adolescents

This system emphasizes the importance of CD4+ T lymphocyte testing in the clinical management of HIV-infected persons. The system is based on three ranges of CD4+ T cell counts and three clinical categories, giving a matrix of nine exclusive categories.

Criteria for HIV Infection
Persons aged 13 years or older with repeatedly (two or more) reactive screening tests (ELISA and HIV-specific antibodies identified by a supplemental test such as the Western blot). Other specific methods of diagnosis of HIV-1 include virus isolation, antigen detection, and detection of HIV genetic material by PCR or branched DNA assay.

AIDS-defining Conditions
The term *AIDS-defining illness* refers to any of a list of infections, diseases, or conditions that, when occurring in an HIV-infected person, leads to a diagnosis of AIDS, the most advanced stage of HIV infection. AIDS is also diagnosed if an HIV-infected person has a CD4+ T cell count less than 200 cells/μL, regardless of whether that person has an AIDS-defining condition. Twenty-six conditions were identified and classified as AIDS-defining conditions in 1993 by the CDC.

Continued

TABLE 64.2 U.S. Centers for Disease Control and Prevention HIV Classification System for Adults and Adolescents—cont'd		
Clinical Category	CD4+ T Cell Count*	Clinical Manifestations
A1	≥500 cells/μL	Category A consists of one or more of the following conditions in a person with documented HIV infection. Conditions listed in Categories B and C must not have occurred. • Asymptomatic HIV infection • Persistent generalized lymphadenopathy (noted in two or more extrainguinal sites, at least 1 cm in diameter for ≥3 months) • Acute (primary) HIV infection with accompanying illness or history of acute HIV infection
A2	200–499 cells/μL	See A1
A3	<200 cells/μL	See A1
B1	≥500 cells/μL	Symptomatic HIV infection (but not A or C conditions) Examples include but not limited to: • Bacillary angiomatosis • Candidiasis, vulvovaginal: Persistent >1 month, poorly responsive to treatment • Candidiasis, oropharyngeal • Cervical dysplasia, severe, or carcinoma in situ • Constitutional symptoms such as fever or diarrhea >1 month (The previous examples must be attributed to HIV infection or have a clinical course or management complicated by HIV.)
B2	200–499 cells/μL	See B1
B3	<200 cells/μL	See B1
C1	≥500 cells/μL	Category C includes the following clinical conditions; for classification purposes, once a category C condition has occurred, the person will remain classified as category C: • Bacterial pneumonia, recurrent (≥2 episodes in 1 year) • Candidiasis: esophageal, tracheal, bronchi, or lungs • Cervical cancer, invasive • Coccidioidomycosis, disseminated or extrapulmonary • Cryptococcosis, extrapulmonary • Cryptosporidiosis, chronic intestinal >1 month • Cytomegalovirus (CMV) disease, other than in liver, spleen, or lymph nodes (e.g., CMV retinitis) • Encephalopathy, HIV-related • Herpes simplex with mucocutaneous ulcer >1 month, bronchitis, pneumonia, or esophagitis • Histoplasmosis, disseminated or extrapulmonary • Isosporiasis, chronic intestinal >1 month • Kaposi's sarcoma • Lymphoma: Burkitt's, immunoblastic, or primary central nervous system • *Mycobacterium avium* complex or *M. kansasii,* disseminated or extrapulmonary • *M. tuberculosis,* pulmonary or extrapulmonary • *Mycobacterium,* other species, disseminated or extrapulmonary • *Pneumocystis jiroveci* pneumonia • Progressive multifocal leukoencephalopathy • *Salmonella* bacteremia, recurrent • *Toxoplasma gondii* (brain) • Wasting syndrome due to HIV (involuntary weight loss >10% of baseline body weight) with either chronic diarrhea (≥2 loose stools per day for ≥1 month) or chronic weakness and fever ≥1 month
C2	200–499 cells/μL	See C1
C3	<200 cells/μL	See C1

*There is diurnal variation in CD4+ counts, averaging slightly higher in the afternoon, in HIV-positive persons. Blood for sequential CD4+ counts should be drawn at the same time each day.
Source: Selik R, Mokotoff ED, Branson B, et al. Revised surveillance case definition for HIV infection—United States, 2014. *MMWR Recomm Rep.* 2014;63(RR03):1-10.

HIV infection were among people aged 25 to 29 years (32.6 cases/100,000 people), followed by people aged 20 to 24 years (27.9 cases/100,000 people). Although the number of new HIV diagnoses has declined among females in recent years, females made up 19% of new HIV diagnoses in the United States in 2018.

The opioid crisis has led to increased numbers of people who inject drugs (PWID), and PWID now account for about 1 in 15 people newly diagnosed with HIV in the United States. Importantly, many of these people live in nonurban areas where HIV-related health and social services may be more limited.

There are two strains of HIV: HIV-1 and HIV-2. HIV-1 is the predominant strain of HIV worldwide and in the United States. HIV-1 has been genetically divided into subtype Groups M, N, and O. Group M has been further subdivided into subclasses known as *clades,* designated A through J. In the United States, nearly all HIV infections are caused by HIV-1 clade B. HIV-2, found most commonly in West Africa, is associated with slower disease progression and appears less readily transmissible. HIV-2 infection should be considered in patients who were born in Africa, have traveled in Africa, or have had sexual contact or shared needles with someone from Africa. Co-infection with both strains of HIV may occur. As is discussed under Diagnostic Tests, the CDC now recommends screening for HIV using an antigen/antibody combination immunoassay, most of which detect both HIV-1 and HIV-2.

HIV is acquired through sexual intercourse, exposure to infected blood or tissue, perinatal transmission, or breastfeeding. HIV cannot be transmitted by casual contact (e.g., handshakes, closed or open-mouth kissing, hugs). HIV is considered an STI because both HIV and infected $CD4^+$ T cells may be present in semen and vaginal secretions. During vaginal or anal sex, friction can cause minute tears to these highly vascular mucous membranes. These tears can allow systemic exposure to HIV-infected bodily fluids during penetrative intercourse, particularly on ejaculation. The use of latex condoms can help prevent the exchange of secretions.

Anyone who has had unprotected sex (without a condom or other adequate form of barrier protection) is considered potentially at risk for HIV infection. The risk of HIV transmission from a single episode of unprotected receptive vaginal intercourse with a known HIV-positive sexual partner is estimated to be between 0.08% and 0.2%, and the infection risk associated with a similar episode of receptive anal intercourse is 0.1% to 0.3%. The risk of HIV transmission from oral sex (mouth to genital or mouth to anal contact) is difficult to determine because most people who practice oral sex also practice other forms of sex during the same encounter. Oral to vaginal (cunnilingus), oral to anal (anilingus), and receptive oral to penile (fellatio) sex carry little risk of HIV transmission. The highest risk of HIV transmission from oral sex is to a person performing fellatio on an HIV-infected individual who ejaculates. Factors that increase the risk of HIV transmission from oral sex include oral or genital ulcers or cuts, bleeding gums, and concurrent STIs.

HIV can also be transmitted through the sharing of needles, syringes, or other or drug injection equipment (e.g., cookers) with an HIV-infected person; therefore, PWID are a high-risk group for HIV infection, as well as hepatitis B and C infection. The use of a new sterile needle and syringe for every injection can substantially reduce the risk of acquiring and transmitting these viruses. These sterile supplies are often available through pharmacies without a prescription or through syringe services or needle exchange programs.

Before blood banks began universal testing for HIV, people who had blood transfusions were at high risk for HIV infection (e.g., individuals with hemophilia), given the presence of contaminated blood products in the blood banking system. Routine testing of all blood products for HIV-1 and HIV-2 has now virtually eliminated this route of transmission in the United States and other developed nations with universal blood testing standards. However, given the potential of an HIV-positive individual to donate blood during the asymptomatic and undetectable window period before seroconversion with the presence of HIV-specific antibodies has occurred, transmission rates as low as 1 in 1,000,000 to 1 in 2,000,000 transfusion procedures are typically cited during informed consent procedures for transfused blood products.

HIV can be transmitted from mother to newborn perinatally and with breastfeeding. In 2018, perinatal transmission accounted for 65 new HIV diagnoses in the United States. In turn, maternal-to-child transmission of HIV has become increasingly rare in the United States in the context of current CDC guidelines that recommend the following:

- Routine prenatal and perinatal HIV screening
- Prompt initiation of ART with the goal of providing full HIV viral load suppression (i.e., plasma HIV RNA less than 200 copies/mL) for pregnant individuals throughout pregnancy and delivery
- Elective cesarean delivery for HIV-infected mothers to avoid birth canal exposure when full HIV viral suppression is not achieved
- Preemptive antiretroviral (ARV) treatment of the newborn
- Because HIV is present in the breast milk of mothers living with HIV and can be a mode of HIV transmission, the CDC recommends that mothers living with HIV should not breastfeed their infants, provided they have ready access to clean water and infant formula.

PATHOPHYSIOLOGY

HIV infection begins with transfer of the virus from one host to another. In the case of sexual transmission, infectious virus is exposed to mucocutaneous tissue, such as in the genital tract or anus. Dendritic cells called *Langerhans cells* found within the mucosal epithelium are believed to be the earliest targets of HIV infection. After these cells are infected with HIV, they bind to CD4+ T cells and subsequently migrate to draining lymph nodes via regional lymphatic channels. Within these lymph nodes, HIV further infects follicular dendritic cells capable of presenting virus to circulating CD4+ T cells. HIV, both as free virus and in CD4+ T cells, then enters the bloodstream and disseminates via lymphatic tissues throughout the body. These events are responsible for the fever, malaise, and lymphadenopathy associated with acute HIV infection.

Initial HIV infection of a human CD4+ T cell requires several steps. First, the gp120 molecule of HIV attaches to the CD4 receptor. This interaction causes a conformational change in gp120 that allows for additional interaction with the coreceptors CXCR4 or CCR5. X4-tropic viruses bind to CXCR4 coreceptors, and R5-tropic viruses bind to CCR5 coreceptors. Engagement of one of these two coreceptors promotes membrane fusion and internalization of the HIV virion and its components. Humans cells that lack the CCR5 receptor cannot be infected by R5-tropic viruses, and the drug maraviroc (Selzentry), which blocks the human CCR5 receptor, is an effective antiviral drug in patients infected with R5-tropic virus. Maraviroc is not effective, however, in the treatment of patients infected with an X4-tropic virus or dual-tropic viruses.

Once HIV infects the CD4+ T cell, HIV begins its replication activities by converting its RNA genetic material into complementary DNA strands, using the RNA-dependent DNA polymerase enzyme reverse transcriptase (RT)—the hallmark of retroviruses. Because mammalian cells do not express RT, this enzyme was the first retrovirus-specific therapeutic target for HIV medications in the form of nucleoside (and nucleotide) RT inhibitors (NRTIs), as well as the nonnucleoside RT inhibitors (NNRTIs). These agents either serve as competitive chain terminators of elongating viral DNA strands (NRTIs) or interfere with the DNA template-primer activity of RT (NNRTIs). Importantly, RT lacks the histone repair enzymes characteristic of mammalian DNA polymerases. This results in a high rate of uncorrected mutations during each cycle of viral DNA replication. In turn, this leads to the rapid development of resistance by HIV to most ARV agents, particularly if used suboptimally as monotherapy or, alternatively, as combination therapy with a high degree of patient nonadherence.

After a complementary DNA strand is generated off the viral RNA template, viral DNA then becomes double-stranded and is incorporated into the host cell genome by viral integrase. This new DNA acts as a blueprint for viral replication, directing the infected host cell to make new viral particles of HIV. Integrase inhibitor ARVs, such as raltegravir (Isentress) and dolutegravir (Tivicay), inhibit the genomic integration step in the viral replication process.

In addition to genomic replication, a large portion of viral DNA is transcribed and subsequently translated into a large polyprotein, which must then be activated by the HIV protease enzyme. This enzyme acts like "chemical scissors" and catalyzes the cleavage of these polyproteins into mature structural proteins and enzymes. This process results in formation of a large number of infectious viral particles, which bud from the host cell and seek out new cells to infect. The HIV protease enzyme is the target of one of the most potent classes of ARV agents—the protease inhibitors (PIs).

CLINICAL PRESENTATION

Subjective

Most patients with HIV infection are minimally symptomatic or asymptomatic for years after initial infection, so routine HIV screening should be part of regular health maintenance for all healthy adults. Providers should discuss risk behaviors with their patients and annually test patients at high risk of HIV. In addition, patients who present with STIs should also be tested for HIV. The Focus on History: Evaluating Risk of HIV Infection provides a template for the discussion of HIV risk factors, and the section on HIV management further details specific risk factors that should prompt annual testing.

Focus on History: Evaluating Risk of HIV Infection

Sexual history and STIs

- Describe your sexual relationships.
- Describe your sexual orientation.
- Describe your sexual practices. Have you ever had anal sex?
- Have you ever had an STI?
- Have you ever had a vaginal discharge or other problem (for females)? Penile discharge or other problem (for males)?
- Have any of your sexual partners been tested for STIs?
- Do you practice safer sex, such as using condoms or other forms of barrier protection?
- What form of birth control do you use, if any?
- Have any of your sexual partners been told that they were HIV positive or had AIDS?
- Would you expect any of your sexual partners to have been exposed to an STI or HIV? Why or why not?

Substance abuse

- Have you ever injected drugs (legal or illegal [street])?
- Have you ever shared needles, such as for injections, piercings, or tattoos?
- Have you ever used (in any form) illegal or street drugs?
- Do you drink alcohol? If so, how much?

Transfusion history

- Did you receive any blood or blood products between 1977 and 1985?

- Are you or any of your sexual partners a hemophiliac?
- Have you ever received any donor sperm during artificial insemination?

Infection history

- Have you or any of your sexual partners ever had any form of hepatitis?
- Have you or anyone close to you been diagnosed with tuberculosis (TB)? If so, what is (or was) the treatment?
- Have you ever had a positive test for TB?
- Have you ever taken medications for TB?

Occupational history

- Do you work in the health-care field? In a long-term residential facility? In a jail or prison?
- Are you exposed to blood or other body fluids while on the job?
- Have you ever had a needle-stick injury?

After acute HIV infection, approximately 8% of patients experience flu-like symptoms such as fever, sore throat, myalgia, headache, cervical lymphadenopathy, and night sweats. Although the differential diagnosis for this constellation of symptoms is very broad, providers should keep this diagnosis in mind, because early HIV treatment leads to better health outcomes for patients and decreased risk of HIV transmission to their sexual partners. The symptoms associated with acute HIV infection may be the only symptoms the patient has before developing AIDS years later, so recognition of the infection during this phase may prevent subsequent morbidity and mortality and prevent transmission of HIV to the patient's sexual partners.

In the years that follow initial HIV infection, as the disease slowly progresses, HIV-infected patients may become more vulnerable to outbreaks of common infections. For example, they may experience herpes zoster (i.e., shingles or reactivation of varicella zoster virus) or unusually aggressive or frequent outbreaks of herpes labialis. Patients may also present with oral candidiasis (thrush). Although these infections also occur in individuals without HIV infection (e.g., in patients prescribed corticosteroids) and are not considered AIDS-defining illnesses, providers should consider testing for HIV in this setting.

Objective

Many patients with HIV infection will have no objective signs of infection. However, the following physical or laboratory signs should prompt consideration of HIV testing:

- Persistent generalized lymphadenopathy: This is a relatively common feature in early HIV infection, when the patient is often asymptomatic. During the assessment, the clinician must be alert for enlarged lymph nodes involving two noncontiguous sites, other than inguinal nodes. The clinician should measure and record the size of nodes if palpable, although significant nonpalpable lymphadenopathy may also be evident on imaging examinations.
- Localized *Candida* infections: Thrush is a common finding in HIV infection. In the context of HIV, the presence of thrush indicates advanced immunosuppression, with a high probability of a serious or OI within 3 years. The clinician should carefully assess the oral cavity, using a high-quality flashlight and look for the presence of white plaques (thrush), dark purplish lesions (possibly Kaposi's sarcoma), or a whitish hair-like growth on the tongue (oral hairy leukoplakia caused by EBV, seen in advanced states of immunosuppression). If white plaque is found, the clinician should attempt to lightly scrape off a portion with a tongue blade. If thrush is present, the plaque may bleed as it is scraped off. The presence of oral candidiasis should prompt consideration of potential *Candida* esophagitis, a late complication of HIV infection that is typically associated with odynophagia and thrush. *Candida* vaginitis in female patients with HIV infection is more likely to be recurrent or refractory to therapy than in other females.
- STIs: They increase the likelihood of HIV transmission or acquisition. The clinician should do a thorough examination of the rectal and genital area, inspecting for perianal and genital herpes simplex lesions, genital warts, as well as penile or vaginal discharge reflective of gonorrhea or other STI.
- Weight loss: The clinician should document the patient's height and weight at the time of the examination and record the patient's description of weight loss (i.e., amount lost over what period of time) because this is a common presenting sign in patients with undiagnosed HIV infection and may herald progressive immunosuppression.
- Cytopenias: Anemia, leukopenia, and/or thrombocytopenia often complicate HIV infection. The clinician should check the CBC with leukocyte differential, in addition to specific T lymphocyte subset (CD4+ and CD8+) counts to assess the level of HIV-associated immunosuppression.

DIAGNOSTIC REASONING

HIV testing should be part of routine care for individuals aged 15 to 65 years. Patients with risk factors for HIV infection should be tested annually.

Diagnostic Tests

Before 2014, routine screening for HIV was performed using a two-tiered algorithm, which utilized an ELISA followed by a confirmatory Western blot test if the initial ELISA was positive. Both of these tests rely on the presence of host antibodies to HIV. This approach was sensitive and specific overall but was not as sensitive at diagnosing acute HIV infection, given the lag in seroconversion with detectable anti-HIV antibodies. In 2013, the CDC updated its guidelines for the diagnosis of HIV to recommend the use of a U.S. Food and Drug Administration (FDA)-approved HIV-1/2 antigen/antibody combination immunoassay (sometimes referred to as a *fourth generation HIV immunoassay*) for the initial screening of HIV.

Unlike previous serological tests used to screen for HIV that relied solely on an individual's antibody response to HIV infection, the HIV-1/2 antigen/antibody combination immunoassay detects an HIV antigen (p24) in addition to IgM and IgG antibodies to HIV-1 and HIV-2. Detection of the p24 antigen, which is present in the blood earlier than HIV antibodies, allows for earlier detection of HIV, effectively shortening the "window period" between HIV infection and a positive HIV test result. For specimens that are positive by the HIV-1/2 antigen/antibody combination immunoassay, HIV infection is then confirmed with an additional immunoassay to distinguish between HIV-1 and HIV-2 antibodies or, if the differentiating assay is inconclusive, nucleic acid amplification testing (NAT), which is often referred to as HIV viral load testing.

Using the new algorithm utilizing an antigen/antibody combination immunoassay, determining viral load via NAT is only needed in certain circumstances to establish the diagnosis of HIV. First, as described previously, NAT testing of HIV-1 is used when the HIV-1/HIV-2 antibody distinguishing assay is inconclusive. Second, NAT testing is used for screening of blood donors. Third, the diagnosis of neonatal HIV infection in infants born to HIV-infected mothers is made using NAT because maternal antibodies are present in the infants' blood for the first 6 to 12 months of life and may lead to a false-positive result with respect to the infant. Lastly, NAT testing may be considered when acute HIV is suspected, although HIV-1 RNA is present in the blood only 1 or 2 days before the rise in p24 antigen, which is detected in the HIV-1/2 antigen/antibody immunoassay. Of note, detectable HIV RNA at low levels may represent false-positive results in some cases.

Several rapid HIV serological tests are now available for use in high-throughput clinical settings (such as emergency departments or labor and delivery units) or in the home. Numerous portable, rapid HIV tests are commercially available, and two types of home-based HIV tests are currently approved in the United States:

- There is currently one FDA-approved rapid self-test (OraQuick) that can be done entirely at home and provides results in 20 minutes.
- Mail-in self-tests include a collection kit that is then sent into a laboratory, with results provided to the patient by a health-care provider.

Every state and territory of the United States, as well as the District of Columbia, requires that laboratories report positive HIV test results to the public health authority serving the patient's geographic area. However, primary care practitioners should become familiar with the specific reporting requirements of their state and local health departments, as specific guidance may differ.

Differential Diagnosis

The signs and symptoms of acute HIV infection are very similar to those seen in other common infections and systemic conditions, such as infectious mononucleosis (due to EBV or CMV infection, as described earlier in this chapter), toxoplasmosis, rubella, viral hepatitis, and drug reactions. The symptoms and signs seen in chronic HIV, before the onset of AIDS, are commonly observed in other immunosuppressed patients, such as those on chemotherapy, radiation therapy, or long-term corticosteroid treatment. Certain cancers can also cause a decrease in the $CD4^+$ T cell count. Cytopenias including lymphopenia may be due to a primary or infiltrative bone marrow disorder and may require a diagnostic bone marrow biopsy if an HIV test is negative.

There is also a well-documented condition, idiopathic CD4 lymphocytopenia (ICL), that was first noted around the same time HIV infection was characterized. In ICL, patients present with the same laboratory profile as HIV-infected patients (i.e., low $CD4^+$ T cell counts), but with no direct evidence of HIV infection, as no virus is detectable in the blood of ICL patients even using the most sensitive assays. In turn, this condition is not attributed to HIV nor to any other infectious agent as yet identified, although patients may suffer from the same OIs and AIDS-defining illnesses as seen with advanced HIV infection.

MANAGEMENT

This section addresses screening for HIV in at-risk patients, PrEP, PEP, and the management of HIV in infected patients who have not yet developed AIDS.

Screening

Approximately 166,000 people in the United States are living with HIV but are unaware of their infected status. Most of these individuals are likely asymptomatic. Testing is the first step toward earlier HIV treatment, as results from the START study demonstrated that earlier treatment of HIV offered patients clear health benefits. Thus, the CDC recommends that everyone between the ages of 13 and 64 years get tested for HIV at least once, unless the patient actively declines (opt-out screening). Although many states previously required written consent before HIV testing, most states have eliminated this requirement because it was a barrier to early diagnosis. In turn, primary care practitioners should inform themselves of individualized state laws regarding HIV testing.

It is important not to neglect certain demographic segments of the population, with regard to HIV testing. For example, pregnant females should also be tested for HIV. In addition, although older adults may be at lower risk overall of acquiring HIV infection than younger adults, older people and their health-care providers are less likely to discuss sexual or drug use behaviors, and HIV testing is often neglected in this population. However, over half of the people diagnosed with HIV in 2018 were aged 50 years and older.

Risk Factors: Special Considerations for Individuals With Higher Risk for HIV

The following groups of people are at higher risk of HIV infection and should be offered HIV testing at least once a year:

- MSM
- Individuals who have had sex (anal or vaginal) with a partner with HIV
- Individuals with more than one sexual partner since their last HIV test
- Individuals who injected drugs and shared needles, syringes, or other drug injection equipment with others
- Individuals who exchanged sex for drugs or money
- Individuals who were diagnosed with or treated for another STI
- Individuals who were diagnosed or treated for viral hepatitis or TB
- Individuals who have had sex with someone who falls into one or more of the previous categories or someone whose sexual history is not known by the individual

Sexually active MSM may benefit from more frequent testing, such as every 3 to 6 months.

Pre-exposure Prophylaxis

Recent clinical trials have demonstrated that certain populations at high risk for HIV can reduce their likelihood of acquiring the infection by taking certain antiviral drugs daily as PrEP in combination with condoms and other safer sex measures. PrEP reduces the risk of acquiring HIV from sex by approximately 99% when taken as prescribed. Less information is known about the effectiveness of PrEP among PWID. The U.S. Public Health Service provides comprehensive guidelines for PrEP (https://www.cdc.gov/hiv/guidelines/preventing.html) and recommends consideration of PrEP for all HIV-negative individuals who are at substantial risk of acquiring HIV infection. Risk groups include HIV-uninfected individuals for whom one of the following is true:

- Male or female in an ongoing relationship with an HIV-infected partner
- MSM who have anal sex without a condom and are not in a mutually monogamous relationship with a HIV-uninfected male or has been diagnosed with an STI in the past 6 months
- MSM who has been diagnosed with an STI in the past 6 months
- Heterosexual male or female who does not regularly use condoms during sex with partners of unknown HIV status or who are at substantial risk of HIV infection
- Individual who has injected illicit drugs in the past 6 months and shared injection equipment or has been in drug treatment for injection drug use in the past 6 months

Candidates for PrEP must be willing to adhere to PrEP daily and follow up with a provider every 3 months for repeat HIV testing and other follow-up assessments. Before the initiation of PrEP, the following laboratory tests should be performed: HIV testing immediately before PrEP initiation to confirm negativity, hepatitis B virus (HBV) serology, hepatitis C virus (HCV) serology, and serum chemistry for estimation of renal function. Two drug combinations are approved by the FDA for PrEP for at-risk adults and adolescents weighing at least 35 kg: emtricitabine 200 mg/tenofovir disoproxil fumarate 300 mg (Truvada) and emtricitabine 200 mg/tenofovir alafenamide 25 mg (Descovy). Because tenofovir disoproxil fumarate treatment is associated with renal toxicity, individuals with creatinine clearance lower than 60 mL/min should not be offered PrEP with a regimen containing this drug.

As the same population who would benefit from PrEP is also at high risk of HBV infection, all individuals who are susceptible (i.e., uninfected and nonimmune to HBV) should be vaccinated against HBV. For individuals who are HBV-infected, both components of Truvada and Descovy are active against HBV, therefore, individuals with HBV who stop either PrEP medication are at risk for a flare of HBV infection, which is characterized by elevations in hepatic enzymes. Thus, liver function tests should be monitored in these patients.

Postexposure Prophylaxis

PEP should be considered after an HIV-uninfected individual has a recent (less than 72 hours) exposure that carries a substantial risk of HIV infection. Substantial risks include percutaneous contact or exposure of mucosal surfaces (e.g., vagina, eye, or nonintact skin) with blood, semen, vaginal secretions, rectal secretions, breast milk, or any bodily fluid contaminated with blood from a known HIV-infected source.

PEP should be provided only for infrequent exposures. Individuals who engage in high-risk behaviors may be offered PEP, but PEP should be followed by PrEP, as described in the preceding section. Nonoccupational HIV exposures might include sexual assault or a nonoccupational needlestick. The most common cause of occupational exposure to HIV is a needlestick injury in a health-care setting. Although the risk of acquiring HIV through a single occupational or nonoccupational exposure is low (e.g., approximately 0.3% for an occupational needlestick from an HIV-positive patient versus 0.08% for receptive penile-vaginal intercourse), exposed individuals may experience significant anxiety. The Patient's Voice 64.1 presents one health-care worker's perspective when faced with such a situation.

PEP should be initiated within 72 hours of exposure and is unlikely to be effective if started later. The following laboratory tests should be performed on presentation: HIV antibody/antigen testing, HBV serology (hepatitis B surface antigen [HBsAg], hepatitis B surface antibody [HBsAb], and hepatitis B core antibody [HBcAb]), HCV serology, serum creatinine, alanine transaminase (ALT), and aspartate aminotransferase (AST). For those who have been sexually exposed, testing for syphilis, gonorrhea, chlamydia, and pregnancy should be performed. If the individual who is the source of the exposure is available, the following tests should be performed on the source: HIV antibody/antigen testing for those with unknown HIV status or HIV viral load and HIV genotypic testing for those with known HIV infection, HBV serology (HBsAg, HBsAb, and HBcAb), and HCV serology.

In 2016, the CDC published updated guidance for nonoccupational PEP and recommended that all PEP regimens should include a 28-day course of a three-drug ARV regimen. For adults and adolescents aged 13 years and older with creatinine clearance of 60 mL/min or greater, the CDC recommends emtricitabine 200 mg/tenofovir 300 mg (Truvada) once daily and either raltegravir (Isentress) 400 mg twice daily or dolutegravir (Tivicay) 50 mg once daily. The recommended alternative regimen is a four-drug combination of emtricitabine 200 mg/tenofovir 300 mg once daily, darunavir (Prezista) 800 mg once daily, and ritonavir (Norvir) 100 mg once daily.

The most recent updates to the recommendations for occupational PEP were published in 2013. All recommended regimens contain three or more ARV drugs. The preferred PEP regimen is raltegravir 400 mg twice daily with emtricitabine 200 mg/tenofovir 300 mg once daily. Most clinicians, however, would likely consider dolutegravir 50 mg once daily with emtricitabine 200 mg/tenofovir 300 mg once daily. Of note, data from an observational surveillance study of birth outcomes among pregnant females receiving HIV treatment in Botswana suggested that dolutegravir exposure at the time of conception, but not later in pregnancy, may be associated with a small increase of neural tube defects in infants born to these patients. Before prescribing dolutegravir or another integrase strand transfer inhibitor (INSTI) to an individual of childbearing potential, clinicians should refer to CDC guidelines (https://www.cdc.gov/hiv/risk/pep/index.html) for updated information on this topic. In addition, the CDC maintains a 24-hour, 7-day per week National Clinicians' Postexposure Prophylaxis Hotline (PEPline: 1-888-448-4911) for health-care professionals managing occupational exposures to HIV and hepatitis B and C viruses.

Immediate expert consultation may be appropriate before the initiation of PEP. The CDC guidance provides recommended regimens for children younger than 13 years of age. However, a pediatric HIV expert may be better equipped to manage the dosing, administration challenges, side effects, and counseling in this population. Expert consultation is also indicated when the exposed individual is pregnant. When the source individual is infected with an HIV strain with known resistance mutations, consultation with an HIV expert is advised. Of note, abacavir sulfate (Ziagen) should not be included in any PEP regimen because the rapid initiation of PEP does not allow sufficient time to perform HLA-B*5701 testing, and patients with the HLA-B*5701 allele are at high risk of abacavir hypersensitivity syndrome, which can lead to death.

Health-care providers prescribing PEP should educate patients regarding the potential risks of each of the components of their PEP regimen and provide counseling on ways to prevent transmission of HIV. Because many exposed individuals feel considerable stress at the time of exposure, providers should consider scheduling an early follow-up visit (3 to 7 days after initiation of PEP) and be prepared to reiterate some of the initial counseling discussion. Providers should also assess patients' needs for mental health and other services

Four to 6 weeks after the HIV exposure, HIV antigen/antibody testing should be repeated, along with other tests based on the PEP regimen selected, such as serum creatinine, ALT, and AST. Exposed individuals whose HIV testing is negative should undergo repeat testing again at 3 months and 6 months postexposure. For exposed

The Patient's Voice 64.1: Occupational Exposure and HIV Infection

I am furious! I've been a nurse for 20 years and have always been proud of my skills and techniques. I have been stuck by needles, but only a few times during my career . . . usually when a patient suddenly moved, not through negligence on my part. I thought nothing of it until last month when I went to my doctor because I was feeling so tired and run down. He asked if I had been tested for HIV, and I said no. Just to appease him, I had the test done, and it was positive.

The only thing I can relate it to is a needlestick that occurred when I was working in home health several years ago. I didn't even think anything of it at the time, and I didn't even fill out an incident report. I don't have any recourse now since I can't prove I was infected "on the job." Now, I hear about the needleless syringes and all the safeguards in place. If I had them back then, I probably wouldn't be in the situation I am now. I am so angry! What do I do now?

individuals with positive HIV testing, HIV treatment should be continued. The management of acute and early HIV infection is discussed next.

Treatment for Acute HIV and Early HIV Infection (before AIDS)

All patients with HIV should be treated with ART, regardless of CD4+ T cell count, as soon as possible after diagnosis. Although there is no cure at this time for HIV infection, numerous effective combinations of ART are available, and early HIV treatment provides patients with health benefits. With early detection and early initiation of treatment, HIV infection can be managed as a chronic but controllable infectious disease. Additionally, prompt treatment has potential public health benefits because maintenance of HIV RNA (viral load) at less than 200 copies/mL with ART prevents sexual transmission of HIV to sexual partners.

The key goals of ART are to durably suppress HIV viral load and improve the patient's immune system, thereby preventing AIDS-related complications, such as OIs and death. Principles of management for early HIV infection include (1) initial disclosure of HIV status, (2) initiation of multidrug therapy to suppress the virus, and (3) monitoring of viral activity to determine any need to modify or revise drug therapy.

Initial Disclosure

Disclosure of HIV test results is a critical event in the clinician–patient relationship. Disclosure counseling sets the tone and foundation for the patient's acceptance, knowledge base, and attitudes about their HIV infection (see The Iceberg of Living with HIV). Disclosure of HIV test results is typically a stressful period for the patient, who may experience significant denial toward a positive test result. Some guidelines and concepts for disclosure counseling are summarized here, although certain testing strategies, such as mail-in HIV self-tests, may not allow for all of the following:

- Disclosure counseling should be done face to face. In planning the disclosure of the patient's HIV status, the clinician should assess the degree to which the patient or parent/guardian is prepared to receive the results. The clinician should also assess the patient's social, demographic, cultural, and psychological characteristics, which may relate to coping with a positive HIV test. During the disclosure session, the provider should discuss the natural history of HIV infection, the potential effects of HIV infection on physical and mental health, the role of health maintenance practices, the availability of treatment, and the need to practice HIV transmission prevention behaviors.
- The disclosure counseling process is an opportunity to provide immediate interventions and involve the patient in ongoing medical, mental health, social, and family support networks. Immediate interventions may include the following: assessing the patient for the risk of inflicting violence to self or others, ensuring the patient will receive a thorough medical evaluation for staging and initial care; informing the patient of the ongoing availability of services, scheduling the patient's next appointment, addressing prevention of further HIV transmission, assessing the availability of an immediate support person and other care providers, providing local and national resources for information on HIV infection, and making appropriate referrals for any ongoing services that cannot be provided on-site.
- The provider must reassure the newly diagnosed patient that medical advances have led to the availability of numerous ARV drugs, which have led to prolonged survival and improved quality of life for HIV-infected patients. In fact, some recent studies have suggested that with early and attentive medical care, optimized medication adherence, and healthy lifestyle habits, HIV-infected people may experience nearly the same life expectancy as noninfected individuals in the United States. Many newly diagnosed patients and their family members think that HIV is a "death sentence," so learning the facts about the effectiveness of modern HIV treatments can provide patients with great relief.
- Clinicians should assist patients in understanding the advantages and disadvantages of disclosing their HIV status to others by providing counseling, factual information regarding legal aspects of disclosure, opportunities for patient education and dialogue, and referrals as needed.
- The patient should be strongly advised and encouraged to disclose their HIV status to significant others, particularly sexual and needle-sharing partners. Some local and state health departments will conduct partner notification without disclosing the name of the HIV-positive person, informing partners that they have been exposed to a sexually transmitted disease and that HIV testing is advised. Some patients prefer to have a provider present at the time of disclosure to significant others.
- The prevention of HIV transmission must be discussed at the time of the initial diagnosis of HIV infection. The patient's blood and semen become infectious to others shortly after the patient is initially infected, so risky sexual behaviors need to be addressed immediately. The patient should also be advised against donating blood, plasma, tissue, body organs, sperm, or eggs.
- The patient must also understand that the virus mutates within each host; therefore, the HIV-infected person remains at risk of acquiring a slightly different HIV strain from another HIV-infected individual—a phenomenon known as *superinfection*. The existence in a patient of a second viral strain with a different mutation profile can complicate the selection of an appropriate ARV regimen, increase the likelihood of infectious complications, and hasten the progression of disease. Patients from West Africa are also at risk of co-infection with strains of both HIV-1 and HIV-2.

The Iceberg of Living with HIV

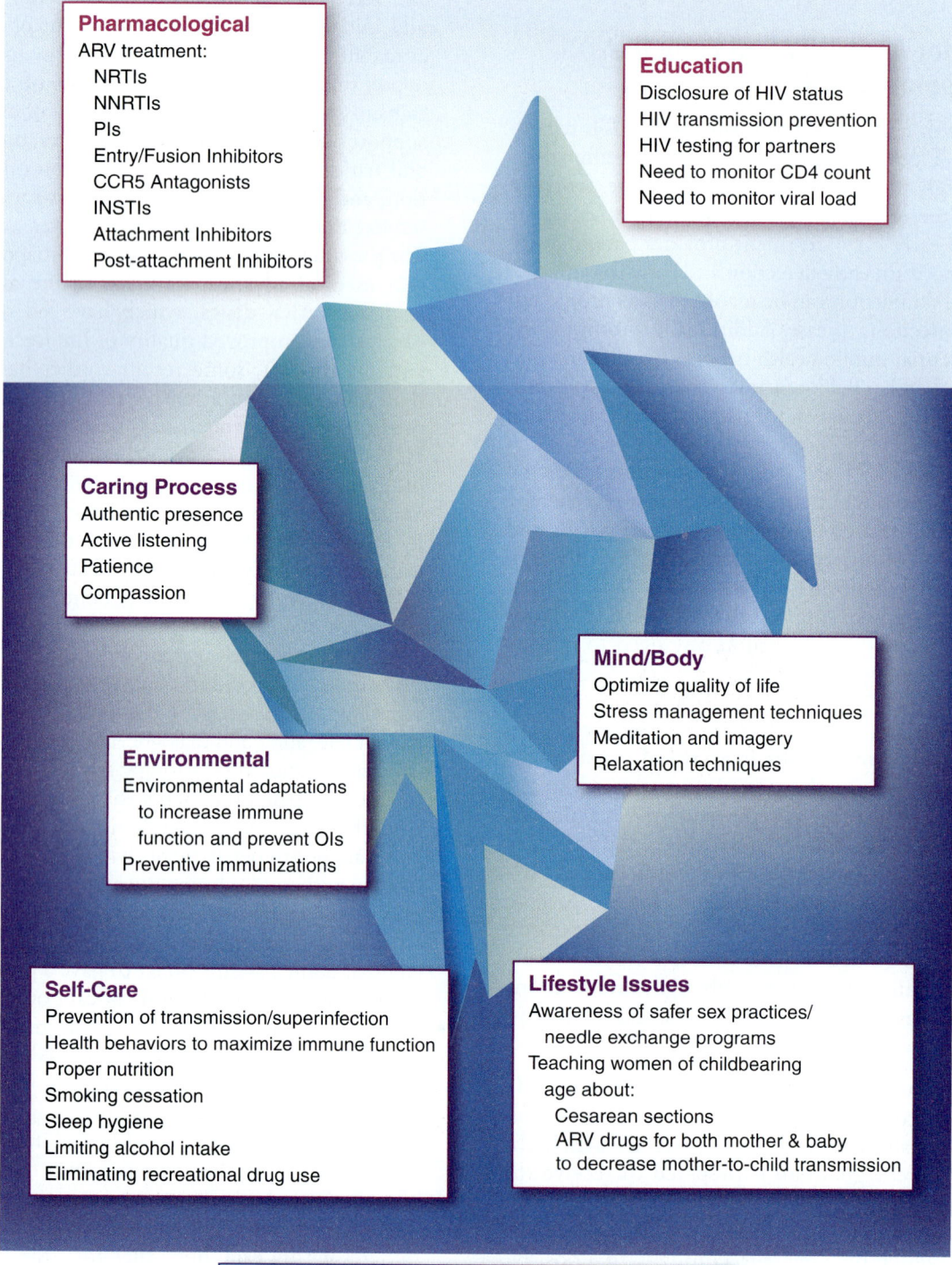

Pharmacological
ARV treatment:
- NRTIs
- NNRTIs
- PIs
- Entry/Fusion Inhibitors
- CCR5 Antagonists
- INSTIs
- Attachment Inhibitors
- Post-attachment Inhibitors

Education
- Disclosure of HIV status
- HIV transmission prevention
- HIV testing for partners
- Need to monitor CD4 count
- Need to monitor viral load

Caring Process
- Authentic presence
- Active listening
- Patience
- Compassion

Mind/Body
- Optimize quality of life
- Stress management techniques
- Meditation and imagery
- Relaxation techniques

Environmental
- Environmental adaptations to increase immune function and prevent OIs
- Preventive immunizations

Self-Care
- Prevention of transmission/superinfection
- Health behaviors to maximize immune function
- Proper nutrition
- Smoking cessation
- Sleep hygiene
- Limiting alcohol intake
- Eliminating recreational drug use

Lifestyle Issues
- Awareness of safer sex practices/needle exchange programs
- Teaching women of childbearing age about:
  - Cesarean sections
  - ARV drugs for both mother & baby to decrease mother-to-child transmission

Legend
- ARV = antiretroviral
- NRTIs = nucleoside reverse transcriptase inhibitors
- NNRTIs = non-nucleoside reverse transcriptase inhibitors
- PIs = protease inhibitors
- INSTIs = integrase strand transfer inhibitors
- OIs = opportunistic infections

If the results of the two tests are similar, a stable baseline is established and used to monitor the effects of drug therapy. The viral load should be repeated 4 to 6 weeks after the initiation of drug therapy or after any alteration in an ARV regimen is made. The initiation of ARV therapy should correspond with a decrease in viral load, typically by a factor of 10 after 2 to 4 weeks. Effective ART will often suppress viral load fully after 8 to 12 weeks of therapy.

Thus, if viral load is about the same or higher than the baseline level after initiating treatment, changes in the drug regimen or counseling regarding adherence are likely needed. It should be noted that reestablishment of complete suppression of the virus to below the detection limit of established viral load assays (e.g., HIV RNA less than 20, 40, or 50 copies/mL, depending on the assay) should remain the primary goal of ARV therapy. Once adequate viral suppression has been achieved, a viral load test should be repeated every 3 to 6 months to confirm chronic viral suppression.

$CD4^+$ T cell count is typically followed with similar frequency to assess for adequate immune reconstitution after initiating ART, although cellular immune reconstitution typically lags behind decreases in viral load, with an expected increase in $CD4^+$ T cells of 100 to 150 cells/mL annually in adequately treated patients. Immunological nonresponders who fail to undergo adequate cellular immune reconstitution on ART, despite viral load suppression, remain at increased risk for OIs and may require alterations in their ARV regimen, as directed by an HIV specialist.

FOLLOW-UP AND REFERRAL

Follow-up for a patient infected with HIV will be required for the rest of the patient's life. In general, a primary care practitioner should refer the patient to an HIV specialist to help establish a treatment plan. Often, HIV specialists are trained in infectious diseases; however, many primary care providers, nurse practitioners, and physician assistants are experienced and well-trained in the care of HIV-infected patients. Stable patients with suppressed viral loads and adequate $CD4^+$ T cell counts may be seen every 6 months for ongoing monitoring, provided medication adherence and social stability are apparent. However, the clinician caring for HIV-infected patients must always be vigilant for the need for rapid evaluation if patients develop intercurrent complaints that could signal breakthrough viral replication or other forms of disease progression.

For patients with $CD4^+$ T cell counts less than 200 cells/μL (see the following section on AIDS), prophylactic medications against common opportunistic diseases, including pneumocystis pneumonia (PCP) may be necessary. In addition, concurrent chronic viral infections, such as hepatitis B or hepatitis C, require specialty referral to an appropriate clinical specialist (such as a hepatologist) because these infections are typically more aggressive with a worse prognosis in the HIV-infected patient. Patients with HIV/HCV co-infection should be evaluated for HCV therapy and potential drug interactions should be considered when selecting an ART regimen.

Recent studies have demonstrated that, in the era of effective ART, HIV-infected patients are at high risk of morbidity and mortality from non-AIDS conditions, such as cardiovascular disease, diabetes mellitus, or liver disease. The prevention and treatment of many of these chronic diseases that are also seen in the general population are now a large focus of HIV management. In turn, healthy lifestyle choices should be encouraged, such as maintaining a healthy diet with regular exercise, whereas tobacco, alcohol, and drug use should be discouraged.

Health maintenance of the HIV-infected patient also requires close attention to preventive immunizations, which may include pneumococcal vaccine (23-valent polysaccharide vaccine; Pneumovax) that may be readministered after 5 years, annual influenza vaccination, tetanus toxoid boosters every 10 years, human papillomavirus (HPV) vaccine, COVID-19 vaccine, and vaccination for both hepatitis A (two vaccinations spaced 6 months apart) and hepatitis B (three vaccinations spaced 1 and 6 months apart). Importantly, attenuated live virus vaccines including measles, mumps, rubella (MMR), oral polio virus (OPV), bacillus Calmette-Guérin anti-TB vaccine (BCG), intranasal influenza vaccine, and those for varicella (chickenpox) and yellow fever are contraindicated in HIV-infected patients with advanced disease and significant immunosuppression. However, the MMR and varicella vaccines may be given early in the course of disease to nonimmunosuppressed HIV-infected individuals.

Patient Education: HIV Infection

HIV infection is a chronic lifelong disease. Education may facilitate self-care activities that can decrease the risk of superinfection with other HIV strains, hepatitis viruses, and opportunistic pathogens. HIV-infected patients require extensive personalized education for their specific medical conditions and therapeutic ART regimens, including specific drug contraindications and interaction warnings. It is also critical to provide adequate support to facilitate adherence to what may be a demanding ART regimen.

Likewise, the patient will need continual reinforcement and education on the need to attain and maintain effective HIV transmission prevention behaviors, such as safer sex practices (e.g., barrier protection, a single exclusive sexual partner) to decrease the potential of transmitting HIV to others or acquiring new HIV strains. A wide variety of patient education materials are available from pharmaceutical companies, AIDS support organizations, and government and health-care agencies (see Resources at the end of this chapter). Educational programs for clinicians are also available through the Association of Nurses in AIDS Care (ANAC) at 1-800-260-6780.

AIDS

A person with HIV is classified as having progressed from HIV infection to AIDS if the CD4+ T cell count falls below 200 cells/μL or if the patient develops an OI or other AIDS-defining illness.

EPIDEMIOLOGY AND CAUSES

The CDC estimates that approximately 1.2 million people aged 13 years and older were living with HIV in the United States at the end of 2018, including an estimated 160,000 people who have not been diagnosed. Despite the availability of sensitive and specific HIV testing and numerous effective ART options, more than 15,000 adults and adolescents with HIV died in 2018. Worldwide, nearly 700,000 people died from AIDS-related illnesses in 2019.

PATHOPHYSIOLOGY

HIV is recognized for its lengthy latency period after acute infection, in which infected persons remain relatively asymptomatic in the absence of ART, despite persistent low-level viremia and progressive CD4+ T cell destruction (with a loss of approximately 40 to 80 CD4+ T cells/μL per year in untreated patients). Over a period of months or years, however, the replication activity of the virus supersedes the capacity for CD4+ T-cell regeneration, except in rare cases. In turn, as the CD4+ T cell count declines, patients become increasingly susceptible to OIs and malignancies.

The natural history of HIV infection can vary significantly from one patient to another. Thus, it is impossible to predict precisely when HIV will progress to AIDS in a person infected with HIV without treatment. Studies conducted in the 1980s to the mid-1990s, before the widespread availability of effective ART, indicated the usual survival time after the diagnosis of AIDS was just 3 years. It is clear, however, that effective ART has dramatically improved the survival and quality of life for many HIV-infected persons, including those with AIDS.

CLINICAL PRESENTATION

Subjective

Patients with AIDS may present with a variety of viral, bacterial, fungal, and/or protozoal OIs. Common viral infections include CMV, herpes simplex virus, varicella zoster virus, and progressive multifocal leukoencephalopathy (PML, which is caused by infection with the John Cunningham or JC virus). Common bacterial infections include *Mycobacterium avium* complex (MAC, which is caused by *M. avium* and *Mycobacterium intracellulare*) and TB. Common fungal infections include candidiasis, PCP, histoplasmosis (*Histoplasma capsulatum*), and cryptococcosis (*Cryptococcus neoformans*). Common protozoal infections include cryptosporidiosis, which causes chronic diarrhea, and cerebral toxoplasmosis (*T. gondii* infection of the CNS), which can be life-threatening. Other potential problems include malignancies, such as Hodgkin's and non-Hodgkin's lymphoma, and AIDS wasting syndrome.

In assessing the patient with AIDS, it is important to realize these patients may have more than one, and sometimes several, active OIs. Therefore, a careful history, thorough review of systems, physical examination, and frequent follow-up assessments are extremely important. Advanced Assessment 64.1 provides a framework for the evaluation of an HIV-infected patient with advanced disease.

Advanced Assessment 64.1: HIV-positive Individual

HISTORY	
Present Illness	When were you diagnosed with HIV? Why did you take the HIV test? Why did you come to the doctor today? How are you feeling physically? How are you feeling emotionally?
Past Medical History	Have you been to a health-care provider for HIV care? Do you know what your viral load is? What your CD4+ T cell count is? When were these tests last done? Have you had any opportunistic infections, such as PCP or thrush? Were you ever hospitalized for these infections? What is your past medical history? Surgical history? Have you ever had a heart problem or a history of high cholesterol? Are you using any nontraditional (alternative or complementary) therapies? If so, please explain.

Advanced Assessment 64.1: HIV-positive Individual—cont'd

Social History	What is your living situation (e.g., home life, support system [friends, relatives], financial situation, emotional situation, occupational situation, sexual relationships)? What do you know about HIV infection? Are you sexually active? Do you know how to prevent the spread of HIV from one person to another? If so, do you use those methods?
Medication History	What HIV drugs have you taken in the past? How long were you on them? How long have you been off them (if applicable)? Have you been taking any medications for prophylaxis? Do you take them all of the time or just some of the time? What other medications are you taking (prescription drugs, over-the-counter drugs, herbal remedies)?
Nutritional History	Tell me about your usual diet. Do you eat raw eggs or raw fish? How do you cook your meat? Do you take any appetite enhancers? Do you take any nutritional supplements?
Travel History	Do you travel often? If so, where? Have you traveled or lived in other states or out of the country? If so, when, where, and for how long?

PHYSICAL EXAMINATION

General Condition and Mental Status	Fatigue Change in activities of daily living Level of consciousness Difficulty remembering Confusion Change in mental status or mood
Neurological System	Headaches and associated signs and symptoms Cranial nerve examination Neurological examination
Respiratory System	Shortness of breath or dyspnea and associated signs and symptoms Cough and associated signs and symptoms Hiccups Lung sounds Respiratory rate, rhythm, and characteristics; use of accessory muscles
Cardiovascular System	Heart sounds Pulse rate, rhythm, and characteristics
Hematological and Lymphatic System	Swollen, enlarged, or tender glands Fever
Gastrointestinal System and Nutrition	Sores or white spots in the mouth or on the lips; dental assessment Problems eating or swallowing Nutritional intake Nausea/vomiting Change in weight or appetite Change in bowel habits (diarrhea, constipation) Anorectal symptoms, lesions, masses, or warts
Integumentary System (Dermatological)	Active rash or evidence of previous rashes (e.g., herpes zoster) Kaposi's sarcoma
Genitourinary System	Abnormal Papanicolaou test (Pap smear) Condylomata acuminata (genital warts) Signs or symptoms of other STIs (e.g., discharge, dysuria, pruritus, rash)

Abbreviation: STI, sexually transmitted infection.

The patient may complain of visual problems, such as a loss of central or peripheral vision, blurred vision, loss of visual acuity, eye pain, photophobia, or the development of "floaters." Such complaints should raise suspicion for CMV retinitis or fungal endophthalmitis (ocular histoplasmosis).

Neurological symptoms or alterations in mental status, including headaches, confusion, mood swings, personality changes, dizziness, neck stiffness, fever, lethargy, malaise, nausea, vomiting, photophobia (intolerance of light due to resulting eye pain), neurological deficits, hemiparesis, ataxia, CN palsies, or seizures, may be the result of herpes encephalopathy, PML, cryptococcal meningitis, or cerebral toxoplasmosis.

GI problems such as diarrhea and abdominal pain may be present concurrently with unintentional weight loss, fever, chills, or night sweats, as a result of CMV enterocolitis, viral gastroenteritis, pancreatitis, AIDS wasting syndrome, MAC, *Salmonella* or other enteric bacterial infection, cryptosporidiosis, giardiasis, isosporiasis, or histoplasmosis. Dermatological problems may develop, such as stinging or burning papules or bumpy rashes in a linear or clustered pattern, which may be indicative of herpes simplex or HPV infection, particularly if located in the anogenital region. Other painless lesions, such as the purplish plaques of Kaposi's sarcoma, may go unnoticed in areas poorly visible to the patient (e.g., the back).

The patient may also complain of pulmonary symptoms, such as shortness of breath or a persistent cough. These symptoms may be accompanied by fever, chills, night sweats, weight loss, purulent or blood-tinged sputum, or chest pain, which may be indicative of PCP, bacterial pneumonia, or active TB. The clinician should determine the onset of pulmonary symptoms, because PCP and TB are usually insidious in presentation, with worsening of symptoms over days to weeks, whereas pulmonary toxoplasmosis progresses more rapidly. In addition, nonspecific complaints of fatigue, weakness, and fever with anemia and leukopenia could signify disseminated MAC with bone marrow involvement.

Objective

A complete physical examination is indicated for the patient with AIDS because an array of OIs and malignancies may affect literally any organ system. Some of the most common physical presentations of AIDS are described in this section by organ system.

For example, with CMV retinitis, retinal changes are seen on ophthalmoscopic examination. With toxoplasmosis encephalitis (the most common presentation of *Toxoplasma* infection), the clinician should check for an altered level of consciousness, impaired cognition, and any stroke-like symptoms. Of note, the physical examination findings of cryptococcal meningitis are typically not as striking as the fulminant meningitic symptoms of bacterial meningitis.

Oropharyngeal examination may reveal erythematous mucosal ulcers, which should raise suspicion for herpes simplex or CMV, or if patchy white lesions are present, candidiasis or EBV-associated oral hairy leukoplakia, which is typically limited to the tongue, gingivae, and/or buccal mucosa.

A wide variety of skin lesions may present with AIDS. Herpes simplex lesions are initially papulovesicular (fluid-filled), painful, and pruritic; these clustered lesions become progressively erythematous and ulcerated, eventually crusting over before healing. The lesions of shingles are exquisitely painful papules and vesicles, which present with a burning sensation and are distributed over a well-demarcated region of the skin known as a dermatome, corresponding to the cutaneous area innervated by a single spinal nerve. Genital warts associated with HPV infection (condylomata acuminata) appear as raised, flesh-colored papules, with or without stalks, in isolation or in clusters. Cutaneous Kaposi's sarcoma presents with one or more raised, dark-colored lesions that may occur anywhere on the body, whereas cutaneous cryptococcosis usually presents as a single ulcerated nodule at the site of infection. Papular pruritic eruption (PPE) of HIV is a highly pruritic rash that presents as widespread papular to nodular skin lesions; as a diagnosis of exclusion, the etiology of PPE is unclear but has been suggested to be due to a dysregulated immune response to arthropod bites because it often improves after initiating ART. Eosinophilic folliculitis is an overlapping diagnosis with PPE in which a skin biopsy will confirm perifollicular eosinophilic infiltration that has been suggested to be of autoimmune etiology.

Findings on pulmonary examination may be nonspecific in the setting of a wide variety of infectious processes, such as PCP, TB, or community-acquired pneumonia. Therefore, physical examination findings should be considered within the context of a careful medical history detailing the patient's clinical presentation and timing of symptom onset, along with appropriate diagnostic imaging and laboratory studies. Advanced Assessment 64.1 presents additional physical examination information to be gathered from the HIV-positive patient.

DIAGNOSTIC REASONING

Diagnostic Tests

Table 64.4 includes some of the diagnostic tests a healthcare provider should consider in evaluating an HIV-infected patient with AIDS, including $CD4^+$ T cell count and HIV viral load, as well as additional laboratory tests and how to interpret them, as guided by the patient's presenting signs and symptoms.

For patients with suspected TB or PCP, the clinician should order a purified protein derivative (PPD) or interferon-gamma release assay (IGRA), chest x-ray, and sputum examination for acid-fast bacilli (AFB) smear, AFB culture,

TABLE 64.4 Diagnostic Tests for the HIV-infected Patient With AIDS

Test	Interpreting the Results
CD4+ T cell count	<200 cells/µL or <14%: Prophylaxis for *Pneumocystis jiroveci* pneumonia (PCP) <100 cells/µL or <14%: Prophylaxis for toxoplasmosis (often the same as PCP prophylaxis) <50 cells/µL or <14%: Prophylaxis for *Mycobacterium avium* complex (MAC) CD4+ T cell counts may also help narrow or broaden the differential diagnosis of a presenting complaint because some opportunistic infections are rare at higher CD4+ T cell counts.
HIV viral load	An increase in viral load while on ART indicates poor adherence, poor absorption, and/or emergence of drug-resistant mutations.
HIV genotypic resistance testing	If a change in regimen is required, viral resistance testing will guide the choice of components in the next ART regimen. Viral amplification for resistance testing may not always be possible for patients who have HIV RNA levels <500 to 1,000 copies/mL.
Tropism testing (if considering treatment with CCR5 antagonist)	Patients who are infected with X4-tropic or dual-tropic viruses should not be treated with a CCR5 antagonist. In contrast, R5-tropic viruses are susceptible to a CCR5 antagonist. Tropism can change over time in the same individual; therefore, this test may need to be repeated if significant time has elapsed since the last test.
HLA-B*5701 testing (if considering treatment with abacavir)	Abacavir and abacavir-containing regimens should not be prescribed in patients who are positive for HLA-B*5701 or in whom testing has not been performed, given the increased risk of abacavir hypersensitivity.
Hepatitis A, B, and C serologies	HBV co-infection is an important factor to consider in selecting an ART regimen and, subsequently, in withdrawing or changing ARV components. Several ARV drugs (e.g., emtricitabine, lamivudine, tenofovir disoproxil fumarate, and tenofovir alafenamide) have activity against HBV, and HBV-infected patients are at risk for an HBV flare after withdrawal of these ARV drugs.
Complete blood count with differential	Anemia is common; may be related to HIV disease, underlying infection, or medication (particularly zidovudine [AZT]). Bone marrow biopsy may be done to check for fungi, *M. avium* or tuberculosis, cytomegalovirus, parvovirus, or malignancy. Thrombocytopenia is often seen. In early infection, idiopathic thrombocytopenic purpura may be seen; in later infection, thrombocytopenia may occur due to bone marrow suppression. Thrombocytopenia may also be seen with Kaposi's sarcoma. Leukopenia is common; WBC counts less than 2,000 cells/µL are common and, in isolation, are not cause for alarm. If using medications that cause neutropenia, may need to prescribe colony-stimulating factors such as filgrastim (Neupogen).
Basic serum chemistries	Renal function may be impaired because of HIV nephropathy, ARV drugs, dehydration, volume depletion from diarrhea, or wasting. Electrolytes may need repletion due to diarrhea or malnutrition. Low phosphorus may indicate Fanconi syndrome with renal tubular dysfunction, due to tenofovir-containing regimens.
Liver-associated chemistries	Liver-associated enzymes (e.g., AST, ALT, alkaline phosphatase) may be elevated as a result of HBV or HCV co-infection, medications, alcohol abuse, or nonalcoholic fatty liver disease, which is common in HIV-infected patients. Elevations in bilirubin may indicate disseminated MAC infection. Bilirubin may also become elevated after starting certain ARV drugs (e.g., atazanavir). Elevated lactate dehydrogenase may be nonspecific or related to PCP, lymphoma, hemolysis, muscle wasting, or may be caused by HIV or AZT. Low albumin levels may indicate malnutrition.
Interferon-gamma release assay or purified protein derivative tuberculin skin test (TST)	A positive interferon-gamma assay result or TST induration of 5 mm or more is considered a positive reaction (no reaction may be due to anergy); evaluate for signs/symptoms of active tuberculosis with physical examination and chest x-ray.
Urinalysis	Patients infected with HIV are at risk of renal disease both from HIV and from some ARV drugs (e.g., tenofovir).

Abbreviations: ALT, alanine transaminase; ART, antiretroviral therapy; ARV, antiretroviral; AST, aspartate aminotransferase; HBV, hepatitis B virus; HCV, hepatitis C virus; WBC, white blood cell.

and at least one nucleic acid amplification (NAA) test for TB screening, if available. The clinician should be aware that both PPD and IGRA tests rely on the patient's immune response to detect latent infection with TB; therefore, both tests are less reliable in the context of severe immunosuppression. Repeat AFB smears are still recommended to diagnosis active TB, but NAA tests are additionally recommended because they are more sensitive, offer a more timely diagnosis, and are becoming more widely available. For establishing TB drug susceptibility, AFB cultures have been used traditionally, but commercial NAA tests and line probe assays (LPAs) are now available that can provide rapid information about TB susceptibility. Using bronchoalveolar lavage or an induced sputum sample, the diagnosis of PCP can be made using a PCR test to detect PCP-specific nucleic acids, a direct fluorescent antibody test to visualize the causative organisms, or special microscopic staining techniques, including a Giemsa stain, a Wright stain, or a Diff-Quik preparation that incorporates both eosinophilic and basophilic counterstains.

For patients with neurological symptoms, a referring physician should order a computed tomography scan or magnetic resonance imaging of the brain to check for the presence of ring-enhancing lesions, which could be associated with *T. gondii* or CNS lymphoma, or nonenhancing areas of white matter (demyelination), which could indicate PML. A lumbar puncture may be indicated.

If diarrhea is present, with or without other GI symptoms, the clinician should send stool cultures for infectious organisms, including examination for protozoal forms, ova, and parasites. Viral infections such as CMV colitis may require colonoscopic biopsy of the GI mucosa for a definitive diagnosis.

Differential Diagnosis

The differential diagnoses for AIDS-associated illnesses are extensive, particularly with regard to pulmonary, neurological, and GI manifestations, and are geared toward identifying underlying disease processes and infections. In the pulmonary differential, the clinician should consider TB, PCP, MAC, histoplasmosis, or other bacterial, viral, fungal, or protozoal infections of the pulmonary system, as well as internal Kaposi's sarcoma affecting the lungs. Regarding the neurological system, the clinician should consider CNS lymphoma or other malignancy, in addition to the cerebral infections discussed earlier of toxoplasmosis and PML. In the GI system, CMV must be considered, as well as protozoal infections (e.g., cryptosporidiosis, isosporiasis, giardiasis) and malabsorption syndromes. Pancytopenia should raise suspicion of disseminated MAC infection in the bone marrow.

Although the identification of HIV in the setting of CD4+ T cell lymphopenia of less than 200 cells/μL is diagnostic of AIDS, the same clinical and hematological laboratory presentation in the absence of a history and currently detectable HIV infection may be consistent with the rare condition known as *idiopathic CD4 lymphocytopenia* or ICL. With mild to severe clinical presentations possible, ICL may manifest with pure CD4+ T cell lymphopenia or dual lymphopenia of both CD4+ and CD8+ T cells.

MANAGEMENT

The overall focus of HIV management is to help the patient maintain HIV viral suppression, thereby improving immune function and preventing AIDS-defining illnesses and improving quality of life. Providing support for ART adherence is essential to that goal.

However, OIs still affect a substantial number of HIV patients, even in resource-abundant settings, given factors such as therapeutic nonadherence, barriers to health-care accessibility, and comorbid medical conditions that interfere with effective HIV treatment. Thus, correctly identifying the causative organism of a presenting OI is crucial to initiating appropriate treatment in a timely fashion. Because CD4+ T cell count serves as the major clinical indicator of immunocompetence in HIV-infected individuals, when the CD4+ T cell count falls below 200 cells/μL, an HIV-positive patient becomes increasingly prone to OIs. PCP prophylaxis is required for CD4+ T cell counts of less than 200 cells/μL, and *T. gondii* prophylaxis is needed for counts of less than 100 cells/μL. For patients who are not receiving ART or who remain viremic on ART without a fully suppressive regimen, MAC prophylaxis is recommended for CD4+ T cell counts of less than 50 cells/μL.

Candidiasis

The diagnosis of oral candidiasis can generally be made clinically without laboratory testing. Oral candidiasis can be treated with fluconazole 100 mg/day for 1 to 2 weeks. Esophagitis can be treated similarly, except with a 3-week course of antifungal medication.

Chronic Diarrhea

Patients with AIDS are at risk for many OIs associated with diarrhea. The diagnostic work-up of such a presentation should include stool analysis for ova and parasites (cryptosporidiosis, isosporiasis, giardiasis, strongyloides), stool culture for enteric bacterial infection, and testing for *C. difficile*. For diarrhea that persists in the absence of a diagnosis, CMV colitis (discussed subsequently) should be considered. Colonoscopy with biopsy may be necessary to identify an etiology.

Cytomegalovirus

CMV viremia is common in HIV-infected patients and should not be treated in the absence of end-organ disease, which may include colitis, pneumonitis, or sight-threatening retinitis. The diagnosis of CMV end-organ disease generally requires a tissue biopsy or, in the case of eye disease, ophthalmological consultation. Ganciclovir (Cytovene) may be given at 5 mg/kg IV every 12 hours for 14 days or foscarnet (Foscavir) 90 mg/kg IV every 12 hours for 14 days. The dose of either drug should be reduced in patients with renal failure. Valganciclovir (Valcyte) is an oral formulation of the drug ganciclovir and is now used frequently when a patient's disease is managed in the outpatient setting. Valganciclovir is used at 900 mg by mouth (PO) every 12 hours for induction therapy and 900 mg PO once daily for maintenance therapy. In addition, cidofovir (Vistide) 5 mg/kg IV may be given with probenecid (Benemid) for 1 week, then reduced to every 2 weeks. Cidofovir should not be used in patients with renal insufficiency. Also, a combination of foscarnet/ganciclovir or intravitreal injections or implants of ganciclovir (which treat only the affected area) may be tried. For maintenance, ganciclovir 5 mg/kg IV daily or foscarnet 90 to 120 mg/kg IV daily may be given.

Cryptococcosis

For acute treatment of *C. neoformans* infection, amphotericin B deoxycholate (Fungizone) 0.7 to 1.0 mg/kg IV daily for 14 days with or without 5-flucytosine (Ancobon) 100 mg/kg PO divided four times daily and then followed by fluconazole (Diflucan) 400 mg daily or itraconazole (Sporanox) 200 mg PO twice daily for 8 weeks is used. In milder cases, fluconazole 400 to 800 mg daily for 8 to 12 weeks may be used, although inadequate treatment may lead to antifungal resistance. CNS infection (cryptococcal meningitis) should be treated with an initial period of IV induction therapy. Serum cryptococcal antigen titers should be followed, as well as CSF titers if applicable, to evaluate the response to therapy. Secondary antifungal prophylaxis with fluconazole 200 mg PO daily is typically continued for life or until the CD4+ T cell count is greater than 200 cells/μL for at least 6 months.

Cryptosporidiosis

There is no effective treatment for *Cryptosporidium* infection other than immune reconstitution with continued ART. In severe cases, nitazoxanide (Alinia) 500 to 1,000 mg PO twice daily given with food for 14 days may help to clear the infection.

Herpes Simplex

For treatment of acute herpes simplex virus manifestations, the clinician should prescribe acyclovir (Zovirax) 200 to 400 mg PO three times daily for 7 to 10 days, famciclovir (Famvir) 250 mg PO three times daily, or valacyclovir (Valtrex) 1 g PO twice daily for 7 to 10 days. For suppressive treatment, acyclovir 400 mg PO twice daily for 3 to 7 days per week should be given. Foscarnet (Foscavir) 40 mg/kg IV every 8 hours for 10 days can be used for acyclovir-resistant herpes simplex.

Herpes Zoster

Herpes zoster (varicella zoster virus, shingles) should be treated with acyclovir (Zovirax) 800 mg PO five times daily for 7 to 10 days or famciclovir (Famvir) 500 mg PO three times daily for 7 days plus topical silver sulfadiazine for skin lesions. In severe cases, the patient may require IV acyclovir (10 mg/kg per dose) every 8 hours. Valacyclovir (Valtrex), a prodrug of acyclovir, may also be used at 1 g PO every 8 hours for 7 days; although more expensive than acyclovir, its simplified dosing regimen may result in greater adherence.

Histoplasmosis

Primary prophylaxis with itraconazole (Sporanox) 200 mg PO daily is indicated for patients with CD4+ T cell counts less than 150 cells/μL who live in endemic areas. Disseminated *Histoplasma capsulatum* infection is treated with a 2-week induction period of liposomal amphotericin B (Ambisome) 3 mg/kg IV daily (5 mg/kg for meningitis), followed by itraconazole 200 mg PO three times daily for 3 days and then twice daily for at least 1 year. Secondary prophylaxis with itraconazole 200 mg PO daily, initiated after resolution of initial histoplasmosis infection, is often continued for life.

Kaposi's Sarcoma (Human Herpesvirus-8)

Although Kaposi's sarcoma has been associated with underlying human herpesvirus-8 infection, herpes-specific antiviral therapies are not utilized in current treatment regimens. Rather, cutaneous Kaposi's sarcoma typically improves on ART, as HIV viral load is suppressed and immune status improves. However, disseminated disease may require more aggressive treatment, particularly if any internal organs are affected. Local treatment consists of cryotherapy, excision, intralesional vinblastine (Velban), or radiation. Systemic chemotherapy for more severe disease may include vinblastine, vincristine (Oncovin), doxorubicin (Adriamycin), liposomal doxorubicin (Doxil), liposomal daunorubicin (DaunoXome), bleomycin (Blenoxane), or paclitaxel (Taxol). For more severe cases requiring chemotherapy, treatment is typically guided by a qualified oncology specialist.

Mycobacterium avium Complex

For acute treatment, at least two drugs should be used for initial therapy: clarithromycin (Biaxin) 500 mg PO twice daily plus ethambutol (Myambutol) 15 mg/kg PO per day OR azithromycin (Zithromax) 500 to 600 mg PO daily plus ethambutol 15 mg/kg PO per day. The duration of treatment is at least 12 months and should not be discontinued unless signs and symptoms of MAC have resolved and CD4+ T cell count is greater than 100 cells/μL in response to ART.

Mycobacterium tuberculosis

Most public health departments manage or comanage the treatment of active TB infection. Several ARV drugs are contraindicated or require dosage adjustments when coadministered with TB medications capable of affecting the cytochrome p450 enzymatic pathway, such as rifampin and rifapentine. Thus, it is critical to review current guidelines for each HIV drug the patient is prescribed, using a frequently updated resource such as the DHHS *Guidelines for the Use of Antiretroviral Agents in Adults and Adolescents Living with HIV*. This document is available at https://clinicalinfo.hiv.gov/en/guidelines/adult-and-adolescent-arv, the official Web site sponsored by the National Institutes of Health, which posts regularly updated treatment and prevention guidelines for HIV infection.

Patients with latent TB infection (LTBI) diagnosed by a positive tuberculin skin test greater than or equal to 5 mm or a positive IGRA in the absence of active pulmonary disease (i.e., negative radiological imaging and absence of clinical signs and symptoms) should be offered treatment to prevent active disease. The CDC recommends one of the following regimens for LTBI:

- Isoniazid (INH, Nydrazid) daily or twice weekly for 6 to 9 months
- Isoniazid plus rifapentine (Priftin) once weekly for 12 weeks
- Rifampin (Rifadin) daily for 4 months.

For active infection with drug-susceptible TB, the CDC recommends a 6- to 9-month course of treatment that is based on four key drugs: isoniazid, rifampin, pyrazinamide (Zinamide), and ethambutol (Myambutol). ARV regimens should be modified to avoid potentially dangerous drug interactions between certain agents, such as rifampin and PIs/NNRTIs. Rifabutin (Mycobutin) may be used as an alternative to rifampin, given its improved drug interaction profile. Patients on pyrazinamide should undergo regular serum uric acid monitoring, whereas ethambutol use requires periodic visual acuity and red-green color perception testing, given its risk of ocular toxicity. Pyrazinamide and ethambutol may be discontinued after 2 months to minimize toxicity, if supported by TB susceptibility testing. Thus, it is critical to send sputum AFB cultures as soon as possible. Combination treatment for active TB infection should be continued for at least 6 months after conversion to AFB-negative sputum cultures.

Oral Hairy Leukoplakia (Epstein-Barr Virus Infection)

These common oral lesions found mainly on the tongue typically improve after the initiation of effective ART and do not require EBV-specific antiviral therapy.

Pneumocystis jiroveci Pneumonia

There are several options for prophylaxis of PCP at CD4+ T cell counts of less than 200 cells/μL. The first is trimethoprim-sulfamethoxazole (TMP/SMX, Bactrim, Septra), one double-strength (DS) tablet daily or three times per week. Prophylaxis may be better tolerated when begun with small doses leading to incremental increases, such as TMP/SMX suspension 1 mL PO daily for 3 days, then 2 mL PO daily for 3 days, then 5 mL PO daily for 3 days, then 10 mL PO daily for 3 days, then 20 mL PO daily for 3 days, and then 1 DS TMP/SMX tablet daily.

Between 10% and 40% of all patients on this oral course will develop an allergic reaction with fever and a pruritic morbilliform rash and will have to stop treatment. However, this reaction is typically not IgE-mediated, nor is it considered an immediate hypersensitivity reaction. It may be mediated by an allergic reaction to the sulfa moiety, particularly in individuals of the slow acetylation phenotype who metabolize sulfonamides at slower rates. Given the effectiveness of TMP/SMX for PCP prophylaxis, rechallenge with TMP/SMX may be attempted at a later date.

Dapsone (Avlosulfon) 100 mg PO daily, inhaled nebulized pentamidine (NebuPent) 300 mg every month, or atovaquone (Mepron) 1500 mg PO daily can also be used for PCP prophylaxis, although these regimens are not as effective as TMP/SMX prophylaxis. PCP prophylaxis may be stopped if CD4+ T cell counts increase above 200 cells/μL for more than 3 months.

For the treatment of mild to moderate PCP, the clinician may prescribe TMP/SMX at 15 mg TMP/kg total daily dose, divided three times daily PO or IV. A typical adult dose is 2 DS tablets of TMP/SMX PO every 8 hours. Other treatments include pentamidine 4 mg/kg daily IV; dapsone 100 mg daily (check glucose-6-phosphate dehydrogenase level before dosing, given the risk of anemia) plus TMP (Primsol) 15 mg/kg total daily dose, divided three times daily; clindamycin (Cleocin) 600 mg PO or IV three times daily plus primaquine 30 mg daily; atovaquone 750 mg PO twice daily with meals plus pyrimethamine (Fansidar) 50 to 75 mg PO daily; or trimetrexate (Neutrexin) plus dapsone plus leucovorin (folinic acid; Wellcovorin), with continuation of therapy for 3 weeks before switching to maintenance therapy.

Patients with acute PCP who develop respiratory distress will require hospitalization. If patients develop hypoxia, as documented on a room air arterial blood gas with a PaO_2 of less than 70 mm Hg or an arterial-alveolar O_2 gradient of greater than 35 mm Hg, patients should also be started on corticosteroids (prednisone [Deltasone] 40 mg PO 2 times daily for 5 days, then 40 mg PO daily for 5 days, then 20 mg PO daily for 11 days—all doses given 30 minutes before TMP/SMX dosing) to reduce pulmonary inflammation associated with PCP.

Progressive Multifocal Leukoencephalopathy

There is no treatment for PML, a progressively deteriorating disease caused by JC virus infection of the CNS, except reversal of immunosuppression. Therefore, patients who are suspected of having PML should be started on ART as soon as possible. Some patients stabilize or improve on ART; however, advanced or progressively deteriorating cases of PML should prompt the clinician to discuss the goals of care with the patient, family, or significant others, as PML is often fatal.

Toxoplasmosis

Prophylaxis against *T. gondii* at CD4+ T cell counts of less than 100 cells/μL, is TMP/SMX (Bactrim, Septra) 1 DS tablet PO daily or three times per week or dapsone (Avlosulfon) 50 mg PO daily plus pyrimethamine (Daraprim) 50 mg PO every week with folinic acid (Wellcovorin) 25 mg PO per week. Prophylaxis may be stopped if CD4+ T cell counts increase above 200 cells/μL for more than 3 months.

For acute treatment, pyrimethamine 75 to 100 mg PO daily plus folinic acid 10 to 20 mg PO daily plus either sulfadiazine (Neotrizine) 1 to 1.5 g PO four times daily or clindamycin (Cleocin) 600 to 900 mg PO four times daily for 6 to 8 weeks is used. Maintenance suppressive therapy is pyrimethamine 25 to 50 mg PO daily plus either sulfadiazine 1 g PO twice daily or clindamycin 300 to 450 mg PO four times daily.

FOLLOW-UP AND REFERRAL

Clinical and immunological status, medication adherence, and the availability of social supports all influence how often the patient with AIDS will need follow-up appointments. Follow-up visits should be more frequent at the time of initiation of ART or any new medications to assess for response to therapy and drug tolerance, as a CD4+ T cell count should be obtained every 3 to 6 months. HIV viral load should be determined when initiating or switching ARV regimens, and a follow-up viral load must be done 2 to 8 weeks later to determine effectiveness of the medication regimen. Specifically, HIV viral load should fall by at least a factor of 10 after 2 weeks of ART. Resistance testing should be considered if a therapeutic response is not noted with ART or HIV viral rebound occurs despite adequate medication adherence. In stable patients, HIV viral load may be checked every 6 months. The goal of ART should be complete viral suppression to below the limit of detection on standardized commercial HIV viral load assays.

Specialty referrals are unique to each patient and are guided by HIV-related complications, such as OIs and malignancies, which develop in the immunosuppressed individual. For example, in addition to periodic visits to an infectious disease or HIV specialist, a referral should be made to an ophthalmologist whenever the patient complains of visual problems, whereas unresolved diarrhea or GI problems may require referral to a gastroenterologist. Similarly, an oncology referral may be necessary for patients with Kaposi's sarcoma or if there is a suspicion of malignancy.

Patient Education: AIDS

Patient education is an ongoing process and does not end with counseling after the initial diagnosis. Patient-centered education should include an ongoing review of health maintenance and HIV transmission prevention behaviors because sexual abstinence should not be assumed for any patient, regardless of HIV status. Patient education is particularly important regarding the early detection of visual problems. Other healthful behaviors, such as smoking cessation and limiting alcohol intake, should be discussed within the larger context of HIV infection, given the increased morbidity and mortality risk imparted by these behaviors.

The clinician should also work with the patient to convey the risks of drug interactions, given the complicated nature of ARV metabolism and both prophylactic and treatment regimens for OIs. Because blood levels of ARV medications may be increased or decreased by several other common medications, the patient must understand the need to discuss any other concurrent medications. In addition, a thorough understanding of self-care practices to avoid OIs is critical.

Because over the past decade, an increasing number of females have become affected by AIDS, the need for female patients to use effective contraception and infection prevention methods has taken on a new urgency. Female patients with HIV should have regular age-based cervical cancer screening. If abnormalities are present, they tend to be more severe and progress more rapidly in HIV-infected patients.

All patients should be encouraged to complete advance directives early in the course of HIV infection. If the clinician broaches this topic at a later stage of the disease (i.e., after a patient has developed AIDS), the patient may mistakenly assume that the clinician has additional information regarding their prognosis of which the patient is unaware. Thus, lines of communication need to be kept open between the clinician, the patient, significant others, and family members, depending of the extent of diagnosis disclosure by the patient.

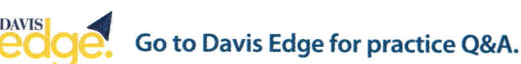

Go to Davis Edge for practice Q&A.

REFERENCES

HIV Infection/AIDS

American College of Obstetricians and Gynecologists' Committee on Practice Bulletins–Gynecology. Practice Bulletin No. 167: Gynecologic Care for Women and Adolescents With Human

Immunodeficiency Virus. *Obstet Gynecol.* 2016 Oct;128(4):e89-e110. doi: 10.1097/AOG.0000000000001707.

Bavinton BR, Pinto AN, Phanuphak N, et al. Viral suppression and HIV transmission in serodiscordant male couples: an international, prospective, observational, cohort study. *Lancet HIV.* 2018;5(8):e438-e447.

Calabrese SK, Mayer KH. Providers should discuss U = U with all patients living with HIV. *Lancet HIV.* 2019;6(4):e211-e213.

Centers for Disease Control and Prevention. Updated guidelines for antiretroviral postexposure prophylaxis after sexual, injection drug use, or other nonoccupational exposure to HIV—United States, 2016. *MMWR Morb Mortal Wkly Rep.* 2016;65:458.

Cohen MS, Chen YQ, McCauley M, et al. Antiretroviral therapy for the prevention of HIV-1 transmission. *N Engl J Med.* 2016;375(9):830-839.

Insight Start Study Group, Lundgren JD, Babiker AG, et al. Initiation of antiretroviral therapy in early asymptomatic HIV infection. *N Engl J Med.* 2015;373:795-807.

Lifson AR, Grund B, Gardner EM, et al. Improved quality of life with immediate versus deferred initiation of antiretroviral therapy in early asymptomatic HIV infection. *AIDS.* 2017;31:953-963.

Panel on Opportunistic Infections in Adults and Adolescents with HIV. Guidelines for the prevention and treatment of OIs in adults and adolescents with HIV: Recommendations from the Centers for Disease Control and Prevention, the National Institutes of Health, and the HIV Medicine Association of the Infectious Diseases Society of America. Available at https://clinicalinfo.hiv.gov/en/guidelines/adult-and-adolescent-opportunistic-infection. Accessed May 18, 2021.

Phillips, JC, Hidayat J, Clark K, et al. A review of the state of HIV nursing science with sexual orientation, gender identity/expression peoples. *J Assoc Nurses AIDS Care.* May-June 2021;32(3): 225-252. https://journals.lww.com/janac/Fulltext/2021/06000/A_Review_of_the_State_of_HIV_Nursing_Science_With.2.aspx. Accessed May 25, 2021.

Rodger AJ, Cambiano V, Bruun T, et al. Risk of HIV transmission through condomless sex in serodifferent gay couples with the HIV-positive partner taking suppressive antiretroviral therapy (PARTNER): final results of a multicentre, prospective, observational study. *Lancet.* 2019;393(10189):2428-2438.

Rodger AJ, Cambiano V, Bruun T, et al. Sexual activity without condoms and risk of HIV transmission in serodifferent couples when the HIV-positive partner is using suppressive antiretroviral therapy. *JAMA.* 2016;316(2):171-181.

Infectious Mononucleosis

Bartlett A, Williams R, Hilton M. Splenic rupture in infectious mononucleosis: a systematic review of published case reports. *Injury.* 2016;47:531-538.

De Paor M, O'Brien K, Fahey T, et al. Antiviral agents for infectious mononucleosis (glandular fever). *Cochrane Database Syst Rev.* 2016;12:CD011487.

Ebell MH, Call M, Shinholser J, et al. Does this patient have infectious mononucleosis?: the rational clinical examination systematic review. *JAMA.* 2016;315:1502-1509.

Yager JE, Magaret AS, Kuntz SR, et al. Valganciclovir for the suppression of Epstein-Barr virus replication. *J Infect Dis.* 2017;216: 198-202.

Lyme Disease

Berende A, ter Hofstede HJ, Vos FJ, et al. Randomized trial of longer-term therapy for symptoms attributed to Lyme disease. *N Engl J Med.* 2016;374:1209-1220.

Butler T. The Jarisch-Herxheimer Reaction after antibiotic treatment of spirochetal infections: a review of recent cases and our understanding of pathogenesis. *Am J Trop Med Hyg.* 2017;96:46-52.

Cadavid D, Auwaerter PG, Rumbaugh J, et al. Antibiotics for the neurological complications of Lyme disease. *Cochrane Database Syst Rev.* 2016;12:CD006978.

Chaaya G, Jaller-Char JJ, Ali SK. Beyond the bull's eye: recognizing Lyme disease. *J Fam Pract.* 2016;65:373-379.

Cutler SJ, Rudenko N, Golovchenko M, et al. Diagnosing *Borreliosis*. *Vector Borne Zoonotic Dis.* 2017;17:2-11.

Eisen L, Dolan MC. Evidence for personal protective measures to reduce human contact with blacklegged ticks and for environmentally based control methods to suppress host-seeking blacklegged ticks and reduce infection with Lyme disease spirochetes in tick vectors and rodent reservoirs. *J Med Entomol.* 2016 Sep 1;53(5): 1063-1092. doi: 10.1093/jme/tjw103.

Lantos P, Rumbaugh J, Bockenstedt L, et al. Clinical Practice Guidelines by the Infectious Diseases Society of America (IDSA), American Academy of Neurology (AAN), and American College of Rheumatology (ACR): 2020 Guidelines for the Prevention, Diagnosis and Treatment of Lyme Disease. *Clin Infect Dis,* 2021;72(1):e1-e48. https://doi.org/10.1093/cid/ciaa1215.

Sanchez E, Vannier E, Wormser GP, et al. Diagnosis, treatment, and prevention of Lyme disease, human granulocytic anaplasmosis, and babesiosis: a review. *JAMA.* 2016;315:1767-1777.

Theel ES. The past, present, and (possible) future of serologic testing for Lyme disease. *J Clin Microbiol.* 2016;54:1191-1196.

Waddell LA, Greig J, Mascarenhas M, et al. The accuracy of diagnostic tests for Lyme disease in humans, a systematic review and meta-analysis of North American research. *PLoS One.* 2016;11:e0168613.

RESOURCES

HIV Infection/AIDS

Centers for Disease Control and Prevention: National Prevention Information Network
https://npin.cdc.gov

Health Options and Positive Energy (H.O.P.E.) Foundation
https://www.hopedc.org

U.S. Department of Health and Human Services, National Institutes of Health: HIVinfo
https://hivinfo.nih.gov

Infectious Mononucleosis

Centers for Disease Control and Prevention: Epstein-Barr Virus Information
https://www.cdc.gov/epstein-barr/about-mono.html

Lyme Disease

American Lyme Disease Foundation
https://www.aldf.com

Section 13: PSYCHOSOCIAL PROBLEMS

SECTION EDITOR

Karen Jennings Mathis, PhD, APRN-CNP, PMHNP-BC, FAED

Chapter 65

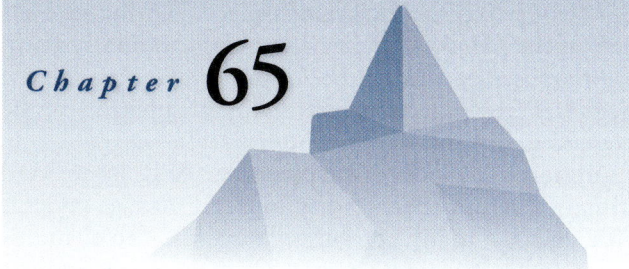

Common Psychological Complaints

Jamison Lord, DNP, APRN, PMHNP-BC
Rachele Lipsky, PhD, APRN, PMHNP
Katerina Melino, MS, PMHNP
Lynne M. Dunphy, PhD, APRN-CNP, PMHNP-BC, FAED

OVERVIEW

In the past decade, there has been a substantial increase in the number of people living with serious mental illness and substance use disorders who receive mental health care from primary care and emergency department services. This increase is typically related to the long wait times for initial evaluation by mental health providers and the nationwide shortage of these specialists, particularly in rural communities. Unfortunately, the outbreak of the novel coronavirus in 2019 (COVID-19) plunged the nation into a mental health crisis as the daily deaths, isolation, and fear generated widespread psychological trauma. The wave of mental health issues surged, including depression, anxiety, substance use, post-traumatic stress disorder, and suicide. Approximately 20% of people with COVID-19 developed mental health problems within 3 months of the diagnosis. In addition, healthcare workers reported feeling overwhelmed and suffered from serious levels of stress contributing to exhaustion, frustration, anxiety, and burnout.

Nearly one-half of Americans report that the coronavirus crisis has harmed their mental health, according to a Kaiser Family Foundation poll. As the COVID-19 pandemic hit an underfunded and understaffed mental health system, it worsened fragmentation and difficulty accessing care, leaving the nation overwhelmed. Despite trillions of dollars distributed by the U.S. Congress for emergency funding, only a small fraction was allocated for mental health. Community behavioral health centers, treating the most at-risk populations, struggled to stay open, and many closed. People are turning to emergency departments for care, overwhelming the system. Confounding the situation is that people in mental health crises consistently struggle to obtain approval from insurance companies, and even with insurance, many people are unable to find therapists and psychiatrists willing to accept their insurance. Primary care facilities and providers play a key role by identifying mental health challenges and providing initial treatment options for mental health.

The chronic debilitating nature of serious mental health disorders places a heavy emotional and financial burden on individuals, families, communities, and society. Mental health disorders top the list of the costliest conditions in the United States. A market intelligence survey reported that the national expenditure on mental health services totaled $225.1 billion in 2019 and accounted for 5.5% of all health spending. Spending increased by 52.1% from 2009 to 2019 in the United States, and this number is expected to be surpassed in 2022 with the COVID-19 pandemic and Americans reporting worsening mental health.

The National Alliance of Mental Health (NAMI, 2020) reports one in five Americans experiences a mental health disorder annually. Currently, 19.86% of American adults (nearly 50 million) are experiencing a psychiatric disorder. These statistics are also on the rise for youth in America, which has been exacerbated by the pandemic. Suicide and suicidal ideation are on the upswing, with the U.S. Centers for Disease Control and Prevention (CDC, 2022) reporting that an estimated 12.2 million American adults seriously thought about killing themselves in 2020 and that suicide is the second leading cause of death for people aged 10 to 14 years and aged 25 to 34 years. Despite the prevalence of significant mental health problems in young Americans, up to 60% are not receiving any mental health care.

According to the CDC, 45,979 individuals died by suicide in the United States in 2020, which is higher than the number of deaths from breast cancer and prostate cancer added together, 3.5 times the number of deaths from HIV, and 2.5 times the number of deaths from homicides. Furthermore, U.S. veterans are 1.5 times more likely to die by suicide than nonveterans, with approximately 17 suicides a day, according to the 2019 National Veteran Suicide Prevention Annual Report (U.S. Department of Veterans Affairs,

2020). Overall, the suicide rate in the U.S. increased by 35% from 1999 to 2018 and declined in 2019 and 2020.

Increased suicide rates are linked to major disasters: COVID-19, political unrest, difficulties in race relations, financial instability, job loss, and weather (increased temperatures) have all contributed significantly to suicidal ideation and attempts. Indeed, inequalities that exist in the United States create additional stressors, leading to mental health problems. The needs of underserved and marginalized populations, including black, Indigenous, and people of color (BIPOC); new immigrants; people living in poverty; LGBTQ+; and older adults, require special attention. In fact, poverty can lead to poor physical and mental health. Emotional costs of the pandemic are much higher for the poor and vulnerable, compared to others, heightening deep preexisting inequities in well-being in the United States and globally. Increases in unemployment and lack of income during the pandemic compound this issue. Many have turned to unhealthy coping behaviors, expanding the need for mental health services.

Racism undermines mental health and creates a sense of mistrust in psychiatric services. BIPOC populations are less likely, for instance, than whites to utilize psychiatric services and typically receive a lower quality when they do obtain mental health care. Subsequently, there is an unmet need for mental health care among individuals who identify as BIPOC.

Another subset of individuals who are especially susceptible to social isolation, loneliness, and social vulnerability consists of older adults. Family care providers are in a unique position to identify mental health problems, initiate services for this vulnerable population, and help to decrease this treatment gap.

A mental health disorder affects the patient's functional capacity, family relationships, and economic stability. It often leads to the development of comorbid chronic diseases and premature mortality, as well as daily suffering for the individual and family. A shorter life expectancy, varying by 10 to 20 years, has been reported for patients with mental health disorders. Most of this early mortality is attributed to acute and chronic comorbid medical conditions such as heart, pulmonary, and infectious diseases.

Psychological health and physical health influence each other greatly and are best approached in an integrated manner. Signs and symptoms of mental health disorders exist on a continuum and affect patients, families, and society, each in a unique way. What determines the burden of illness is the severity of symptoms, their duration, and the level of functional impairment (see Table 65.1 for screening tools for psychological disorders). The *Diagnostic and Statistical Manual of Mental Disorders, Fifth Edition, Text Revision (DSM-5-TR)* notes the relevance and significance of cultural factors and their influence on the expression and management of mental illness. The Cultural Formulation Interview in the *DSM-5-TR* (2022, pp 864–867) provides a mechanism for assessing the impact of culture on an individual's clinical presentation, prognosis, and treatment course. For individuals and families for whom English is not their first language, it is crucial that a bicultural, appropriately trained interpreter be provided for all interviews, ideally, one with specialized expertise and training in interpreting mental health issues.

Primary care clinicians should be familiar with the *DSM-5-TR* (see Advanced Assessment 65.1 for an overview of the *DSM-5-TR* diagnostic classification system). For purposes of this textbook, the primary psychiatric diagnoses are discussed; various clinical subtypes can be referenced directly from the *DSM-5-TR*.

Advanced practice registered nurses (APRNs) are ideal primary care providers to diagnose and manage patients with mental health problems that are often multidimensional. Psychiatric mental health nurse practitioners (PMHNPs), psychiatric mental health (PMH) clinical nurse specialists, family nurse practitioners, and adult-gerontology nurse practitioners have training and the ability to treat mental health issues. Psychiatric disorders are often comorbid and combined with physiological issues. Primary care has become a major source of mental health treatment. Patients, especially in rural areas, are more likely to seek mental health care from their primary care provider than a PMH specialist. Patients may present to primary care with a constellation of signs and symptoms that have medical and psychological underpinnings. Primary care providers should consider both mental health problems and social determinants of mental health when evaluating every patient. Ensuring mental health access for vulnerable patients, such as older adults, people from BIPOC communities, individuals with severe mental illness, immigrants, and the homeless, is critical, especially during a national crisis like COVID-19, which presents additional barriers. Moreover, providers should consider the intersectionality of these identities and the impact on clinical presentation, treatment options, and access to mental health care. Mounting evidence indicates early recognition and treatment of mental health issues prevent complications, improve quality of life, and reduce health care costs.

Primary care provides an opportunity for patients to benefit from continuity and a person-centered care approach, like the Circle of Caring model, to detect and treat mental health issues. Models of integrated and collaborative care are effective and lead to better outcomes for patients with mental health problems. Patient-centered medical homes (PCMH) have assumed prominence in our health-care delivery system, providing continuity of care over time, as well as access to an entire health-care team. PCMH-based care has been found to be superior to standard primary care in chronic disease management (John et al, 2020). The collaborative method is based on Wagner's Chronic Care Model and emphasizes behavioral change via a team approach utilizing high-level expertise for illness management and strong community linkages. Patients score higher on scales for quality of life and social

TABLE 65.1 Screening Tools

Mental Health Criterion	Resource	Screening Tool	Links
General Overview of Tools	Wisconsin Department of Public Instruction	Behavioral Health Screening Tools: Ten Free Assessment Tools	https://dpi.wi.gov/sspw/mental-health/mental/behavioral-health-screening/behavioral-health-screening/tools#cds
	American Psychiatric Association	Assessment Measures for Baseline and to Monitor Treatment Progress Includes Adult and Child/Adolescent Tools	https://www.psychiatry.org/psychiatrists/practice/dsm/educational-resources/assessment-measures#Disorder
	Medicare Preventive Services	Screening ICD-10 codes, Overview of Coverage for Depression, Alcohol Misuse, Other Medical Screenings	https://www.cms.gov/Medicare/Prevention/PrevntionGenInfo/medicare-preventive-services/MPS-QuickReferenceChart-1.html
	Health Measures Northwestern University/NIH Grant	PROMIS Tools	https://www.healthmeasures.net/explore-measurement-systems/promis
	World Health Organization	World Health Organization Disability Assessment Schedule (WHODAS 2.0)	https://www.who.int/classifications/icf/whodasii/en/
Anxiety Disorders	National HIV Curriculum	Generalized anxiety disorder 7-item scale (GAD-7)	https://www.hiv.uw.edu/page/mental-health-screening/gad-7
	Adult attention-deficit/hyperactivity disorder (ADHD) Toolkit Assessment Tools	Hamilton Anxiety Rating Scale	https://dcf.psychiatry.ufl.edu/files/2011/05/HAMILTON-ANXIETY.pdf
Depressive Disorders	University of Michigan	Patient Health Questionnaire (PHQ)	https://www.med.umich.edu/1info/FHP/practiceguides/depress/phq-9.pdf
	Ohio State University	Mood Disorder Questionnaire (MDQ)	https://www.ohsu.edu/sites/default/files/2019-06/cms-quality-bipolar_disorder_mdq_screener.pdf
Bipolar Disorders	American Psychiatric Association	Young Mania Rating Scale	https://dcf.psychiatry.ufl.edu/files/2011/05/Young-Mania-Rating-Scale-Measure-with-background.pdf
Suicide	SAMHSA	SAFE-T	https://store.samhsa.gov/product/SAFE-T-Pocket-Card-Suicide-Assessment-Five-Step-Evaluation-and-Triage-for-Clinicians/sma09-4432
	Health Resources & Services Administration (HRSA)	Columbia Suicide Severity Rating Scale (C-SSRS)	https://suicidepreventionlifeline.org/wp-content/uploads/2016/09/Suicide-Risk-Assessment-C-SSRS-Lifeline-Version-2014.pdf
Substance Use Disorder	SAMHSA	SBIRT: Screening, Brief Intervention, and Referral for Treatment	https://www.samhsa.gov/sbirt
	SAMHSA	Examples of Screening and Assessment Tools for SUD (AUDIT-C), CAGE	https://ncsacw.samhsa.gov/files/SAFERR_AppendixD.pdf
	National Institute on Alcohol Abuse and Alcoholism (NIAA)	Alcohol Screening and Brief Intervention for Youth Guide: A Practitioner's Guide	https://www.niaaa.nih.gov/alcohols-effects-health/professional-education-materials/alcohol-screening-and-brief-intervention-youth-practitioners-guide
	NIAA	TWEAK	https://pubs.niaaa.nih.gov/publications/AssessingAlcohol/InstrumentPDFs/74_TWEAK.pdf

> **⊕ Advanced Assessment 65.1: The *Diagnostic and Statistical Manual of Mental Disorders, Fifth Edition, Text Revision (DSM-5-TR)***
>
> The *DSM-5-TR* is a descriptive manual of mental health disorders authored by the American Psychiatric Association. It provides the diagnostic criteria for each mental health disorder, which enables clinicians to diagnose, communicate about, and treat people with various mental health disorders. Using the *DSM-5-TR* enhances agreement among clinicians.
>
> Precise *DSM-5-TR* criteria have been defined for each diagnosis with the addition and reorganization of some previously identified conditions. This manual is divided into three sections: Section I contains user information, Section II contains the diagnostic criteria, and Section III addresses cultural aspects and conditions that need further research, including emerging measurement tools.
>
> Effective October 2015, the *International Classification of Diseases*, 10th Edition, Clinical Modifications (*ICD-10-CM*), Classification of Mental and Behavioral Disorders was published, which correlates to the *DSM-5-TR*. The use of *ICD-10-CM* codes for psychiatric disorders in the *DSM-5-TR* has been mandated by the Health Care Financing Administration for purposes of reimbursement. Both the *DSM-5-TR* and *ICD-10-CM* codes are used for diagnosis, and the *DSM-5-TR* guides the provider to the applicable *ICD-10-CM* codes that are used for billing.
>
> ### Nonaxial System
>
> The first category combines the psychiatric disorder with known medical conditions; category two identifies the applicable environmental and psychosocial stressors; and category three provides a global assessment of functioning. In previous editions, a companion resource for primary care was developed. There are no plans to provide such a companion because one of the goals of the *DSM-5-TR* revision was to reorganize the text to incorporate clinical decision making for the disciplines of psychiatry and primary care, where many individuals seek and receive mental health care. Accurate identification and treatment have the potential to improve morbidity and mortality from mental health disorders.
>
> ### Using *DSM-5-TR* Symptom Criteria
>
> Specific symptom criteria are listed and defined for *DSM-5-TR* disorders including symptom type, number, intensity, and duration. To meet the symptom criteria for a disorder, the patient must have experienced the minimal number of specified symptoms for a defined period of time, and the symptoms experienced should be sufficient to cause distress or impair psychosocial functioning. Persons who have fewer symptoms of less duration or less intensity may have an atypical form of the disorder, or their condition may be described as subclinical. The term *subclinical* does *not* imply that treatment is unnecessary. Atypical symptoms and subclinical symptoms can cause significant distress.
>
> ### Using *DSM-5-TR* Distress Criteria
>
> Patients with symptoms typically report subjective distress. However, a patient's distress may also be observed by others or assessed by the practitioner. There are no absolute measures of symptom-induced distress: Symptoms that are highly distressing to one person may be only mildly distressing to another. The experience of distress should not be confused with the way a person expresses their distress. It is possible for a highly distressed person who is suffering a great deal to have trouble expressing their distress, whereas others may be able to describe their distress in painful detail. Whether or not a distressed person is expressive should not overly influence the assessment. Often, simple verbal statements of symptom-related discomfort and suffering are sufficient.

role function, as well as for management of specific illnesses in practices using chronic care collaborative models compared with other care approaches. The collaborative model is ideal for APRNs to optimize the use of their clinical and relationship skills to improve patient outcomes.

This chapter presents the most common psychosocial concerns the primary care provider is likely to encounter in practice. It gives a general overview of each complaint and a discussion of the potential differential diagnoses to consider. These specific diagnoses are presented in detail within this section.

ANXIETY DISORDERS

Anxiety disorders are the most common psychiatric disorders in the United States with up to 31% of adults and adolescents experiencing an anxiety disorder in their lifetime (National Institute of Mental Health, 2020). Anxiety disorders most commonly present in individuals aged 20 to 45 years and are more frequently seen in females. Anxiety is an unpleasant state of physical and psychological arousal that interferes with effective psychosocial functioning. Occasional, mild anxiety is a normal fact of life and can be positive; however, severe or chronic anxiety can become debilitating. Although anxiety disorders were once thought to be of minor clinical significance, it is now clear that they are serious mental illnesses, responsible for substantial morbidity and potentially mortality.

Anxiety symptoms are typically manifested in several dimensions: affective, cognitive, behavioral, and somatic. Anxiety can be an experience of dread, foreboding, or panic, often accompanied by autonomic hyperactivity—primarily sympathetic—manifested as bodily symptoms. The patient may attempt to counter the affective component of anxiety by cognitive thoughts that seek to make sense of or minimize the discomfort. Additional affective symptoms of anxiety are apprehension, fear, irritability, intolerance, frustration, and overreaction or hypersensitivity to personal feelings of shame. Behaviors such as avoidance, distractibility, and restlessness reflect the anxiety or may evolve in response to it. Behavioral symptoms of anxiety may include apathy, compulsions, rigidity, overreactions, preoccupation, and repetitive actions such as hair pulling or nail biting. Somatic symptoms of anxiety range in intensity from a loss of appetite, dry mouth, and fatigue to diarrhea, sweating, chest pain, hyperventilation, vomiting, and paresthesias. People with anxiety may experience the full range of anxiety symptoms or may have only one or two symptoms. The classification of anxiety disorders is largely based on clinical presentation and is discussed in depth in Chapter 70.

DIFFERENTIAL DIAGNOSIS

Anxiety symptoms are present in a variety of disorders (see Differential Diagnosis 65.1):

- *Specific phobia disorders,* such as agoraphobia, social phobias, and assorted specific phobias
- *Anxiety disorders,* such as panic disorder, generalized anxiety disorder, and other anxiety disorders (see Chapter 70)
- *Obsessive-compulsive and related disorders,* both specified and unspecified (see Chapter 71)
- *Trauma- and stressor-related* disorders, such as prolonged grief disorder, post-traumatic stress disorder and adjustment disorders (see Chapter 70)
- *Dissociative disorders,* such as dissociative identity disorder
- *Somatic symptom and related disorders,* such as conversion disorder and factitious disorder
- *Body dysmorphic disorder* (see Chapter 71)
- *Nonpsychotic mental disorders,* such as depersonalization-derealization syndrome

The extreme variability of anxiety presentations in primary care makes anxiety disorders the most seen mental health issue. Primary care providers must differentiate between patients with a relatively mild and transient anxiety state, often externally situated, and patients with a pervasive and more debilitating anxiety disorder. Screening questions may include the following: *Are you a constant worrier, unnecessarily anxious all the time about a lot of different things? How long have you felt like this? Does this interfere with your day-to-day functioning?* A diagnosis of generalized anxiety disorder is reserved for those patients who experience extensive, pervasive, and disabling anxiety that lasts for more than 6 months. These criteria are necessary to avoid overdiagnosis of the "worried well."

The age of the patient is important in considering the differential diagnoses. For example, older adult patients are more likely to have an underlying physiological

> ### Differential Diagnosis 65.1: Anxiety Disorders
>
> - Realistic worries
> - Generalized anxiety disorder: Excessive worry and anxiety about various events or activities.
> - Adjustment disorders (usually transient): The emotional or behavioral symptoms are in response to an identifiable stressor.
> - Panic disorder: The specific worry is focused on the symptoms of panic.
> - Social anxiety disorder (social phobia): The concern is related to social situations.
> - Obsessive-compulsive disorder: The worry becomes focused on a specific object or activity.
> - Separation anxiety disorder: The fear is about being away from parents and caregivers.
> - Somatic symptoms disorder: The worry is focused on physiological symptoms.
> - Body dysmorphic disorder: The concern is focused on a perceived defect in physical appearance.
> - Post-traumatic stress disorder and acute stress disorder: The worry is focused on reminders of a traumatic event.
> - Anxiety disorder due to another medical condition (for example, hyperthyroidism)
> - Psychotic disorders: The worries are not reality tested (delusions).
> - Substance/medication-induced anxiety disorder: The anxiety is caused by substance/medication intoxication (stimulants, caffeine) or substance/medication withdrawal (alcohol, alprazolam, fluoxetine).

Source: Adapted from American Psychiatric Association. (2022). Anxiety disorders. *Diagnostic and statistical manual of mental disorders, fifth edition, text revision (DSM-5-TR),* pp 215-261.

component, such as a vascular dementia, that must be ruled out. Undiagnosed arrhythmias, metabolic conditions, and drug reactions may also manifest as anxiety. Many medical conditions involving stimulation of the sympathetic nervous system may produce anxiety symptoms, complicating the diagnosis. Anxiety caused by a medical disorder may be intermittent, such as anxiety associated with transient cardiac arrhythmias or abrupt changes in blood glucose levels. In all cases, potential physical explanations for anxiety symptoms should be evaluated first. Patients with constant anxiety may warrant an electrocardiogram (ECG), a drug screen, and a thyroid profile, especially if there is accompanying weight loss.

Some psychiatric disorders, such as mood disorders, psychotic disorders, dementias, and substance use or substance-induced disorders, may present with anxiety as a prominent part of their constellation of symptomatology. For example, an average of 67% of patients with a depressive disorder have anxiety symptoms, about 33% have panic attacks, and about 40% of patients with an anxiety disorder and about 33% of patients with panic disorder also have depressive symptoms. The complexity of these disorders can pose considerable diagnostic and treatment challenges for the primary care clinician. Referral for psychiatric evaluation may be needed to establish a correct diagnosis and offer treatment guidance.

DEPRESSED MOOD

Depressive disorders are commonly seen in primary care settings. People use the term "depression" to describe a wide variety of negative emotional experiences, ranging broadly from sadness to disinterest in pleasurable activities to self-hate. Those who are experiencing a depressed mood may describe feeling hopeless, discouraged, sad, or "down in the dumps."

Major depressive disorder (MDD) is the most common depressive disorder. The overall 12-month percentage prevalence of MDD in the United States is 7%, with 18- to 29-year-olds experiencing a prevalence three times higher than individuals who are 60 years and older. Beginning in early adolescence, females experience depression at a twofold higher rate than males (APA, 2022). However, MDD can occur in any age-group and sex. That is why it is important to screen for MDD universally in every patient. The U.S. Preventive Services Task Force (USPSTF) recommends "screening for depression in the general adult population, with an emphasis on pregnant and postpartum women." Chapter 69 discusses screening tools for depression. The most common characteristics of MDD are sadness and apathy, but other symptoms of depression can be easily remembered by the mnemonic SIGECAPS (Table 65.2).

Depressive disorders can commonly present in primary care as fatigue, loss of appetite, general aches and pains, digestive problems, abdominal pain, menstrual symptoms, severe headaches, sexual dysfunction, and changes in sleep patterns. Sex can also influence the presentation of depression. Male patients are more likely to report substance use disorders, risk-taking, and poor impulse control, whereas female patients are more likely to report depressed mood, appetite disturbance, weight change, and sleep disturbances. Although sex may influence the clinical presentation of depression, it should not influence how a clinician conducts an assessment.

The presentation of depressive symptoms is often marked with cultural variations, yet even within cultural expressions, a person's unique responses can be observed, based on the patient's individualized perception of the disorder. Some patients may focus less on personal experiences and more on physical aches and pains. Ethnic and cultural norms concerning privacy, embarrassment, and disclosure will have an impact on the patient's presentation and willingness to discuss symptoms.

No description of depression, whether as a symptom or as a disorder, is complete without addressing the psychological pain and suffering it can generate. The pain of depression can become so severe that some people are willing to go to any length, even contemplating or attempting suicide, to obtain even a moment of relief. Those who are at an increased risk for death by suicide have one or more of the following characteristics: male, living alone, being single, feelings of hopelessness, early life adversity, availability of lethal methods, sleep disturbance, social disconnectedness, and previous instances of suicidal ideation or attempts. Thoughts of death or suicide exist at times throughout a major depressive episode, and they should be assessed by asking the question: "Are you thinking of harming yourself or committing suicide?" A referral to a mental health specialist should be considered if the depression is severe, especially if suicidal ideation is present (see Chapter 69 for information about acute suicide risk).

DIFFERENTIAL DIAGNOSIS

Depressive disorders, such as MDD, belong to a broad category of psychiatric disorders known as *mood (affective) disorders*, which include bipolar disorder. Chapter 69 has an informative, in-depth discussion of these mental health disorders. The clinician needs to be aware that depression can be heterogeneous in presentation; it may, for example, contain a seasonal component, or it may be triggered by external stressors and be more responsive to context, such as grief (see "Grief" later in this chapter). Moreover, in some patients, depressive preoccupations can become delusional convictions (see Differential Diagnosis 65.2).

The clinician should rule out organic causes such as anemia; neurological disorders such as Parkinson's disease; sleep apnea; infectious diseases such as HIV, syphilis, or Lyme disease; endocrine disorders such as hypothyroidism; myocardial infarction; cancer; and vitamin deficiencies such as B_{12} and folate. To rule out organic causes, the following tests should be considered: drug screen, chemistry panel, serum cortisol and cortisol suppression test, thyroid panel, follicle-stimulating hormone (FSH),

TABLE 65.2 Mnemonic for Depression Symptoms—SIGECAPS
S: Sleep disturbances (increased or depressed sleep)
I: Interest deficit (anhedonia)
G: Guilt (hopelessness, worthlessness, regret)
E: Energy deficit
C: Concentration deficit
A: Appetite changes (increased or decreased appetite)
P: Psychomotor retardation or agitation
S: Suicidal ideation and/or behaviors

> **Differential Diagnosis 65.2: Types of Depression**
>
> - **Bereavement** (see "Grief" in this chapter).
> - **Sadness:** Periods of sadness are inherent of the human experience.
> - **Major depressive disorder:** At least one major depressive episode, and one symptom must be depressed mood or loss of interest or pleasure.
> - **Depressive disorder due to another medical condition:** Consider in older patients
> - **Substance/medication-induced mood disorder:** Most common in younger patients
> - **Bipolar disorders:** Recurrent or previous symptoms of hypomania or hypermania, such as racing thoughts, impulsivity, spending sprees, and/or not needing sleep
> - **Persistent depressive disorder (dysthymia):** Depressive symptoms are milder than those of major depressive disorder but may persist for years.
> - **Schizoaffective disorder:** Delusions and hallucinations occur during periods with no mood symptoms.
> - **Premenstrual dysphoric disorder:** Depressed mood can be seen during the premenstrual phase of the cycle and remit around the onset of menses or shortly after.
> - **Adjustment disorder with depressed mood:** A depressive episode that occurs in response to a psychosocial stressor. The full criteria for major depressive disorder are not met.
> - **Depressive disorders with psychotic features:**
>   Mood congruent: Delusions and/or hallucinations are present during the major depressive episode, and the content is consistent with depressive themes of guilt, disease, death, nihilism, deserved punishment, or personal inadequacy.
>   Mood incongruent: Delusions and/or hallucinations are present during the major depressive episode, and the content is **NOT** consistent with depressive themes of guilt, disease, death, nihilism, deserved punishment, or personal inadequacy.
> - **Major depressive disorder with a seasonal pattern:** Recurring major depressive episodes, but the onset of major depressive episodes is temporal and occurs at a particular time of the year
> - **Depressive disorders with peripartum onset:** Major depressive episode occurs during pregnancy or in the 4 weeks after delivery.
> - **Depressive disorders with anxious distress:** At least two of the following symptoms occur during a major depressive episode or persistent depressive disorder: keyed up or tense, unusually restless, difficulty concentrating because of worry, fear that something awful may happen, and/or feeling that the individual might lose control of self.
> - **Depressive disorders with atypical features:** Experiencing mood reactivity during a major depressive episode or persistent depressive disorder with at least two of the following symptoms: significant weight gain or increase in appetite, hypersomnia, leaden paralysis, long-standing pattern of interpersonal rejection sensitivity resulting in significant social/occupational impairment
> - **Depressive disorders with melancholic features:** Major depressive episode where the person experiences either the loss of pleasure in all, or almost all, activities or the lack of reactivity to usually pleasurable stimuli (does not feel much better, even temporarily, when something good happens) with three (or more of the following): distinct quality of depressed mood (i.e., the depressed mood is experienced as distinctly different from the kind of feeling experienced after the death of a loved one), depression regularly worse in the morning, early morning awakening (at least 2 hours before usual time of awakening), marked psychomotor retardation or agitation, significant anorexia or weight loss, and/or excessive or inappropriate guilt
> - **Depressive disorders with mixed features:** At least three of the following manic/hypomanic symptoms are present nearly every day during the majority of days of a major depressive episode: elevated, expansive mood; inflated self-esteem or grandiosity; more talkative; racing thoughts; increase in energy or goal-directed activity.
>
> Source: Adapted from American Psychiatric Association. (2022). Depressive disorders. *Diagnostic and statistical manual of mental disorders, fifth edition, text revision (DSM-5-TR)*, pp 177-214.

rapid plasma reagin (RPR), B_{12} and folate levels, and a complete blood count.

GRIEF

Grief, mourning, and *bereavement* are terms that define a universal human response to loss, and their distinct and diverse manifestations tell us a great deal about the nature of what it means to be human. From a dry clinical perspective, *grief* refers to the emotional process of reacting to the loss of a loved one, mourning is the public display of grief, and bereavement is the time period after having experienced grief and mourned that loss. A better understanding of these phenomena, however, is achieved outside of the clinical realm.

The COVID-19 pandemic has vividly underscored how important these various manifestations of grief and mourning are to the human experience. It has done so through the deprivation of these elemental experiences from those who have been forced to remain isolated from their dying loved ones and deprived of the ability to comfort and to ultimately say goodbye to those parents and grandparents who have played such an important role in their lives.

Typically, while we think of the loss of a spouse, a child, a sibling, or a parent, as most associated with this concept—and these losses are undoubtedly the prime manifestation of the experience—grief may also be triggered by the loss of a variety of things of value to an individual: loss of a pet, a home, social status, occupation and/or job, imprisonment, or loss of a homeland. The universal importance of grief is highlighted by its omnipresence in the continuum of our lives.

Grieving is both an emotional and a physiological response that can lead to an increased risk of mortality and morbidity. One prime example of this can be seen in loving couples who have been together for decades, and when one dies, the other soon passes away because the sense of loss has taken away the will to live. Here we can vividly see how grief punctuates life's meaning for so many people.

From the more clinical perspective, experiencing acute grief often leads to a disruption of biological rhythms. It is well-documented that grief is accompanied by impaired immune function, specifically decreased lymphocyte proliferation and impaired functioning of natural killer cells, although it is not known how clinically significant these changes are. Manifestations of grief are also curated through a cultural context, an individual's personality, previous life experiences, the significance of the loss, past psychological history, the relationship with the deceased, existing family and social networks, other life events, resources, educational level, and general state of health. In other words, it is a complex phenomenon that must be broken down by the multiple variables that impact its significance.

Each person grieves in a manner that is meaningful for them. Grief can be understood as a unique individual journey along a well-marked psychological path that's given expression through individuation. The way a person grieves, and, consequently, the amount of time a person needs to move from agony to acceptance is heavily influenced by personal, social, cultural, religious, and spiritual norms.

Lifestyle is also a factor to be considered. As we have seen in the discussion on the impact of the pandemic, individuals who live in social isolation find it more difficult to grieve a loss without close significant others who can offer mutual comfort and assistance. Grieving for a loss alone can drain psychosocial resources needed for day-to-day functioning.

Equally difficult modern problems are the overvaluation of immediacy and the loss of human interdependence. Living with technology has increased our cultural expectations for speed, while loosening direct personal interaction that creates the conditions for properly mourning loss. Human experiences that require time may appear suspect in this context. Busy employers, families, and friends may support grieving, if (in their perceptions) it does not take too long—the implication being that personal grief should not take too much time or demand too many valuable social resources. After a year has passed, family and friends may begin to ask why the grieving person is not "over" their loss yet.

With normal grief, there is consistent progress toward acceptance, although daily functioning can be very difficult at times. Normal grief appears to occur in up to 85% of people after they have experienced a loss. There are a few common theories of grieving. Regardless of the theoretical lens used to understand the grieving process, common emotional reactions to normal grief may include the following: disbelief, shock, emotional numbness, and/or denial, especially if the loss of a loved one comes unexpectedly. Additionally, emotional distress may be exhibited; it tends to focus on separation from the person who died.

Grief can be anticipatory, absent, or delayed; excessively intense and prolonged emotions; complicated grief associated with suicidal ideation; or frank psychosis. The risk factors for a more complicated grief reaction include (1) sudden and/or violent death; (2) social isolation; (3) individuals who believe that they are in some way responsible for the death (real or imagined); (4) individuals with a history of traumatic losses; and (5) individuals who had an intensely ambivalent or dependent relationship with the deceased. In some instances, reduced or absent grief may be an appropriate reaction.

Grief can also be collective in nature. *Collective grief* refers to when a group of people (community, village, society, nation, etc.) all experience loss or trauma. This can occur in events such as natural disasters, terrorism, mass shootings, war, pandemics, structural racism, and genocide. An example of this can be seen in the trauma experiences and re-experienced from violence inflicted on BIPOC communities in the United States and internationally.

Another example is the impact of the COVID-19 pandemic. Globally, people have experienced the loss of loved ones; lack of social connectedness such as physical touch, standing next to people, and shaking people's hands; changes to daily routines; loss of work; loss of participating in sports or other leisure activities; and loss of social and spiritual gatherings. We are still learning how the forceful elimination of the grieving process, a phenomenon that was emblematic of the Nazi extermination of European Jewish populations, impacts individuals both interpersonally and genetically. Where grieving had to be repressed during the Nazi extermination of European Jewish populations, long-term damage has been found to impair people's ability to love and function normally.

DIFFERENTIAL DIAGNOSIS

Cultural, ethnic, religious, and social beliefs; community and family traditions; and personal characteristics determine how and when a person, a couple, or a family will mourn a loss. For some people, grieving is a well-defined, highly satisfying ritual. For others, particularly those who have never suffered a major loss before, grief can be confusing and disturbing. In terms of mental health and well-being, the process of mourning should allow the person to experience pain but achieve acceptance.

Grief and depression share many characteristics, and it can sometimes be difficult to evaluate when the scope of normal grieving has slipped into a pathological realm. It is important to distinguish the grieving process from a major depressive episode and prolonged grief disorder. The *DSM-5-TR* points out several features that help define each process. Specifically, in distinguishing between grief and a major depressive episode, providers should consider that the mood disturbance in depression is typically pervasive and unrelenting: one's thoughts are not linked to specific preoccupations or thoughts, and there is an inability to anticipate happiness or pleasure. In prolonged grief disorder, individuals have a maladaptive grief reaction that continues to be severe and impairing after at least one year (six months for children and adolescents) since the death of the person close to the bereaved person. However, when one is experiencing adaptive grief, fluctuations of mood are common; the pain of grief may also be accompanied by humor and positive emotions, and self-esteem is usually preserved.

Early detection of grief and preventive interventions can alleviate suffering and lead to earlier and more effective treatment. This includes normalizing grief. In the case of terminal illness, early and ongoing bereavement assessment and a collaborative process are essential components of a preventive approach to bereavement care. Interventions include bereavement education and counseling that assist in facilitating communication with the dying person. There is strong evidence that involvement and caregiving benefit survivors.

Primary care clinicians can assist individuals by doing the following:

- Validating pain and distress related to loss
- Providing appropriate pharmacological therapy
- Making bereaved patients aware of the many supportive therapies available and having ready a list of referrals

Utilizing the Circle of Caring model, community services that focus on grief—especially traumatic grief (miscarriage, death of a child at birth, death from violence or war)—church resources, family support, and other support services to deal with special issues, for example, single parenting, may be beneficial. Appropriate medical therapy should be given as indicated. For example, a brief course of a short-acting sedative may be appropriate during acute grief to induce sleep or to help manage the funeral and burial, especially when supportive interventions have not succeeded. The use of drugs such as tranquilizers or alcohol, which numb emotions, should be discouraged. Antidepressant therapy may be considered for patients with particularly prolonged or complex grief reactions, especially for those who have depression alongside complicated grief.

Specific counseling sessions for the bereaved may be extremely valuable and may assist in the prevention of pathological mourning or depressive reactions. These sessions with trained counselors/therapists can assist the grieving person to recognize and express angry or ambivalent feelings toward a deceased person. Group counseling, as well as self-help groups, can be important adjunctive therapies.

The goals for treating grief include facilitating mourning and helping the patient find new activities and relationships to alleviate the loss. Studies have found that effective treatment of depressive syndromes, even as early as 6 to 8 weeks after the death of a loved one, reduces suffering and facilitates the work of grief. The notion that medications or psychotherapy impedes the process of grief is unsubstantiated and may at times serve to prolong suffering and disability. Obviously, elements of psychosis clearly indicate a need for more aggressive treatment: some patients may even become suicidal and should be referred for psychiatric care for further assessment and treatment.

What we ultimately need to understand, however, is that the mental health of the individual and the mental health of the larger social structure are inextricably intertwined. As healers, primary care practitioners need to be aware of the need to not only treat individuals but to work collectively to address underlying social conditions that create a fertile climate for individual dysfunction.

SUBSTANCE USE DISORDER

The primary care provider should assess, educate, treat, and refer patients for substance-related disorders. All agents in the substance use disorder (SUD) category can cause tolerance, habituation, and physical dependence. Types of SUD that are frequently encountered in primary care settings include nicotine, alcohol, cannabis, hallucinogen, inhalant, opioid, sedative, hypnotic, anxiolytic, and stimulant use disorders. Many times, a combination of disorders is present. Sedatives, hypnotics, and anxiolytics may be prescribed for a variety of reasons on a short-term basis by providers, and they can lead to dependence and subsequent abuse, causing the individual to seek the substance illegally. Using substances such as stimulants to enhance cognitive function or athletic performance has the potential for misuse. Caffeine is unique in that it is not classified as an SUD agent, but symptom criteria for intoxication and withdrawal are provided in the *DSM-5-TR*. The *DSM-5-TR* also includes gambling. There has been lobbying for inclusion of diagnoses for additional behavioral addictions, such as internet shopping and internet gaming, but evidence is currently lacking.

The science of addiction has grown over the past 20 years, and evidence demonstrates a common neurophysiological basis to addictive behaviors. Addiction changes the brain and how it works. The brain experience pleasure from many things the person enjoys doing. The way the brain signals pleasure is through the release of the neurotransmitter dopamine into the nucleus accumbens, the brain's pleasure center. This is generally a good thing; it ensures that people will seek out things needed for survival. Drugs of misuse also cause the release of dopamine in the nucleus accumbens, and in some cases these drugs cause much more dopamine release than natural nondrug rewards. Drugs of misuse provide a shortcut to the brain's reward system by flooding the nucleus accumbens with dopamine. These drugs can release up to 10 times more dopamine than natural rewards with higher velocity and efficiency. Eventually, the drug becomes less rewarding, and the craving for the substance dominates. The brain adapts to the effects of the drug, referred to as *tolerance*, and because of these brain adaptations, dopamine has less impact. People who develop an addiction find the substance does not provide as much pleasure as it once did, and a larger dose is needed to experience similar effects. There is a distinction between liking and wanting the drug; over time, the liking decreases, and the wanting increases. Individuals with an SUD continue to seek and use the substance, despite the negative consequences. These disorders are considered chronic and relapsing because, despite significant negative consequences, the behaviors continue.

Pharmacological agents have been introduced to target certain areas of the brain, based on research. Targeted treatments, often referred to as *medication-assisted treatments* (MATs), for tobacco, alcohol, and opioids are now available. There has been resistance to MATs by members of the recovery community, especially those dedicated to the model of abstinence from all substances and recovery through interpersonal support, spiritual growth, and the shared self-help community. However, many areas in the United States are in the grip of a multifactorial epidemic of opioid addiction, with significant numbers of deaths from overdoses. The reality of this epidemic, combined with increasing biological knowledge and superior pharmacological products, has led to an increasing acceptance by the recovery community. The Substance Abuse and Mental Health Services Administration (SAMHSA, 2021) recommends the use of medication in combination with therapy to provide a holistic patient approach to the treatment of SUDs. Medications used in MAT are approved by the U.S. Food and Drug Administration (FDA). MAT programs are clinically driven and tailored to meet the individual's needs. Research shows a combination of medication and therapy can successfully treat these disorders and assist in sustaining recovery.

DIFFERENTIAL DIAGNOSIS

Some individuals can use substances recreationally without impairment or distress. SUDs are recognized when a person's use of a substance affects the ability to function (employment, academic performance, interpersonal relationships). The hallmarks of SUDs are tolerance (the person needs more and more of the substance for the same effect), withdrawal (stopping brings on painful physical and/or psychological symptoms), and compulsive use. The person no longer just enjoys the substance; they *need* it (see Differential Diagnosis 65.3). Screening questions that may uncover a substance abuse problem include the following: *Has anyone ever suggested that you have an alcohol or drug problem?* and *Have you ever gotten into trouble because of alcohol or drugs?*

Chapter 67 discusses SUDs in greater depth and includes a section dedicated to opioid use disorder.

> **Differential Diagnosis 65.3: Substance Use Disorders**
>
> - Recreational use: Substance use—even heavy substance use—that does not cause clinically significant impairment or distress
> - Substance intoxication: A set of symptoms and behaviors that occurs shortly after taking the substance. Each substance tends to have a pattern of intoxication, but for this diagnosis to be applied, there must be evidence of clinically significant distress or behavioral impairment to distinguish it from recreational use.
> - Substance withdrawal: Signs and symptoms that occur when an individual attempts to stop using a substance. A screening question might be the following: *Do you ever get troubling symptoms when you try to stop drinking or using a drug?*
> - Substance-induced mental disorders: Substance misuse can amplify many psychiatric disorders and needs to be considered in many instances of altered mental status and function.
>
> Source: Adapted from American Psychiatric Association. (2022). Substance-related and addictive disorders. *Diagnostic and statistical manual of mental disorders*, fifth edition, text revision (DSM-5-TR), pp 543-665.

INTIMATE PARTNER VIOLENCE

Intimate partner violence (IPV) is defined as a pattern of assaultive and coercive behaviors that may include inflicted physical injury, psychological abuse, sexual assault, progressive social isolation, stalking, deprivation, intimidation, and threats perpetrated by a current or former partner. The aim of such behavior is control by one partner over the other. IPV may be experienced by people of all gender identities and sexual orientations and may occur in any community regardless of ethnicity, religion, socioeconomic level, level of education, employment, or age.

The 2015 U.S. National Intimate Partner and Sexual Violence Survey reported that one in four females and one in 10 males in the United States are physically, sexually, or emotionally abused by their partners over the course of their lifetime and experience IPV-related effects. These numbers may be artificially low, as victims of IPV fear potential escalation of violence and/or increase in safety risks. More than one type of violence may occur in any given family; for example, in one study, up to 70% of females who experienced abuse reported that the perpetrator also abused their children.

Between 2013 and 2018, the World Health Organization (WHO), the USPSTF, and Cochrane Reviews released identification and treatment recommendations for IPV. All guidelines encourage clinicians to be alert to physical and behavioral signs of abuse. Risk for IPV increases during times of psychosocial stress, such as financial difficulties or loss of employment. In 2020, the National Domestic Violence Hotline warned of a growing number of crisis calls spurred by the COVID-19 pandemic. Pregnancy is also a high-risk time for IPV perpetration. Although alcohol/substance abuse and a history of childhood abuse are correlates of perpetrating IPV, they do not cause or explain IPV.

DIFFERENTIAL DIAGNOSIS

It is difficult to know when to include violence in the differential diagnosis. Routine screening for IPV is recommended by the USPSTF for all females of childbearing age at initial visits and periodically. Presenting symptoms or behaviors in a primary care setting that may signal abuse in any patient include the exacerbation or poor control of chronic illness, sleep disturbances, chronic pain, or frequent unexplained appointment changes. Behavioral red flags are (1) a patient who is reluctant to speak in front of their partner or gives evasive answers and (2) an overly protective or controlling partner. Any patient presenting with multiple complaints or whose symptoms are not consistent with their history should be assessed for violence and reassessed as indicated (see Box 65.1). Exposure to IPV is frequently linked with mental health issues such as depression, anxiety, suicide attempts, and/or substance misuse. Problems or injuries during pregnancy should raise the level of suspicion, as should delays in seeking medical care.

ASSESSMENT

The first goal of assessment is to determine whether an individual is a target of violence. The second goal is to evaluate the level of danger. The patient must be seen alone. The partner, children, and family members should be asked to leave the room. If an interpreter is needed, a professional interpreter of the same sex as the patient should be used, rather than a family member. If the partner refuses to leave, the clinician should avoid confrontation and instead strategize a way to get the patient alone later. Requesting a urinalysis or chest x-ray examination is often an effective approach.

Safety and confidentiality are of utmost importance to establish before asking questions about IPV. The clinician should always preface IPV questioning with an appropriate and nonthreatening explanation such as, "I ask all my patients these questions because these problems affect many people's health." Avoid using stigmatizing words such as *domestic violence* or *abuse*. In some instances, a patient may disclose a past experience with violence that may provide useful information in providing appropriate care. It is crucial to use a trauma-informed approach to patient assessment for IPV (see Box 65.2).

Box 65.1 Advanced Practice Nursing Interventions for Intimate Partner Violence

Prevention:
- Teach conflict resolution skills.
- Create a safety plan to remove the individual(s) from the violent situation.
- Inquire about the abuse. Questions to ask include the following:
    1. Has the physical violence increased in frequency/severity over the past year?
    2. Have you ever been choked?
    3. Has a weapon or threat with a weapon been used?
    4. Have you been threatened with death, or do you believe the individual could kill you?
    5. Is there a gun in the house?
    6. Have you ever been forced to have sex when you did not wish to?
    7. For women, have you ever been abused while you were pregnant?
    8. Is alcohol or substance abuse a factor? How often is the alcohol or substance used?
    9. Have your daily activities been controlled?
    10. Is the individual violent and constantly jealous of you?
- Provide community resources.
- Provide counseling and other therapy as indicated (e.g., crisis intervention, post-traumatic stress disorder therapy, physical rehabilitation).
- Document findings and interventions.

Source: Adapted from Jezierski, M. (1994). Abuse of women by male partners: Basic knowledge for emergency nurses. *Journal of Emergency Nursing;20*(5): 361–368. https://pubmed.ncbi.nlm.nih.gov/7823432/

Use of a validated assessment instrument should be considered. The following instruments demonstrate sensitivity and specificity for identifying IPV: Hurt, Insult, Threaten, Scream (HITS); Ongoing Abuse Screen/Ongoing Violence Assessment Tool (OAS/OVAT); Slapped, Threatened, and Throw (STaT); Humiliation, Afraid, Rape, Kick (HARK); Modified Childhood Trauma Questionnaire–Short Form (CTQ-SF); and Woman Abuse Screen Tool (WAST). Patients may disclose emotional abuse before they are comfortable disclosing physical abuse, even if both are occurring. A key component of the abuse experience is intrusion; many patients who are in an abusive relationship may perceive questioning as intrusive. Again, sensitivity is crucial.

FOLLOW-UP AND REFERRAL

Any evidence of IPV requires full compliance with local reporting and referral laws. Local and state agencies for victims have established protocols and systems for providing services that include emergency housing, health care, foster care, and displacement counseling. Despite the significant

> **Box 65.2 Practical Framework for Communication With Patients Who May Be Experiencing IPV or Any Traumatic Event**
>
> Kimberg's (2016) practical framework, called the "4 C's," are principles for providers working with patients who may be experiencing IPV or any traumatic event.
>
> 1) Calm (notice how you feel when you are with a patient, taking deep and grounding breaths along with a patient)
> 2) Contain (limit trauma history data gathering to essentials to ensure emotional and physiological safety)
> 3) Care (share support when patients disclose trauma; normalize and destigmatize trauma responses, symptoms, and coping behaviors)
> 4) Cope (emphasize coping and relationships that build resilience)
>
> Source: Kimberg L. (2016). Trauma and trauma-informed care. In: TE King, MB Wheeler (Eds.). Medical management of vulnerable and underserved patients: Principles, practice, and populations (2nd ed.). McGraw-Hill.

incidence of IPV, there is still a shortage of referral services for violent offenders. Individuals who are violent and are motivated to stop their violent behaviors may benefit from community support groups. Local crisis services and police hotlines should be contacted to protect victims of IPV. Victims of IPV should have the phone numbers and addresses for local emergency services, legal advocacy programs, and support groups, or at least be informed regarding how to obtain this information. Due to historical emphasis on IPV in heterosexual relationships perpetrated by males against females, males and/or victims in non-heterosexual relationships may have fewer available resources and may perceive law enforcement as being less helpful.

Clinicians should consider referral for mental health evaluation for associated psychiatric problems. Those living with any form of abuse may have associated MDD, panic disorder, post-traumatic stress disorder, suicidal ideation, and SUD. A patient who may decline referrals for IPV services may accept a referral to obtain help with their mental health problems.

Clinicians may also want to consider participating in preventive services by working with local and state coalitions against domestic violence, child abuse, and older adult abuse. The work environment should have clear policies and procedures defining abuse-reporting procedures. This is important in every office, because primary care clinicians are often the "first stop" for victims of IPV.

REFERENCES

General

Alang SM. (2019). Mental health care among blacks in America: Confronting racism and constructing solutions. *Health Services Research*, 54(2), 346–355. https://doi.org/10.1111/1475-6773.13115

American Psychiatric Association. (2022). *Diagnostic and statistical manual of mental disorders, text revision* (5th ed). American Psychiatric Association.

American Psychological Association. (2022, March 11). *Stress in America: Covid second anniversary.* Retrieved April 11, 2022, from https://www.apa.org/news/press/releases/stress/2022/march-2022-survival-mode?utm_source=twitter&utm_medium=social&utm_campaign=apa-stress&utm_content=sia-mar2022-unhealthy-behaviors#health

Centers for Disease Control and Prevention. (2022, April 6). *Facts about suicide.* Retrieved April 11, 2022, from https://www.cdc.gov/suicide/facts/index.html

Egede LE, Ruggiero KJ, Frueh BC. (2020). Ensuring mental health access for vulnerable populations in COVID era. *Journal of Psychiatric Research*, 129, 147-148. https://doi.org/10.1016/j.jpsychires.2020.07.011

Freedman A, Nicolle J. (2020). Social isolation and loneliness: The new geriatric giants: Approach for primary care. *Canadian Family Physician*, 66(3), 176–182. https://cfp.ca/content/66/3/176

John JR, Jani H, Peters K, et al. (2020). The effectiveness of Patient-Centered Medical Home-Based Models of care versus standard primary care in chronic disease management: A systematic review and meta-analysis of randomized and non-randomized controlled trials. *International Journal of Environmental Research and Public Health*, 17(18), 6886. doi: 10.3390/ijerph17186886.

National Alliance of Mental Illness. (2020, December). *Mental health by the numbers.* Retrieved January 10, 2020, from https://www.nami.org/mhstats

Open Minds. (2020, May 6). *The U.S. mental health market: $225.1 billion in spending in 2019: An Open Minds market intelligence report.* https://openminds.com/intelligence-report/the-u-s-mental-health-market-225-1-billion-in-spending-in-2019-an-open-minds-market-intelligence-report/

Panchal N, Kamal R, Orgera K, et al. (2020, August 21). *The implications of COVID-19 for mental health and substance use.* Kaiser Family Foundation. https://www.kff.org/coronavirus-covid-19/issue-brief/the-implications-of-covid-19-for-mental-health-and-substance-use/

Renahy E, Mitchell C, Molnar A, et al. (2018). Connections between unemployment insurance, poverty, and health: A systematic review. *European journal of public health*, 28(2), 269–275. https://doi.org/10.1093/eurpub/ckx235

Sadock BJ, Sadock VA, Ruiz, P. (2015). *Kaplan and Sadock's synopsis of psychiatry* (11th ed.). Wolters Kluwer.

Substance Abuse and Mental Health Services Administration. (2014). *Projections of national expenditures for treatment of mental and substance use disorders, 2010–2020.* https://store.samhsa.gov/sites/default/files/d7/priv/sma14-4883.pdf

Taquet M, Lucaino S, Geddes JR, et al. (2020, November 9). Bidirectional associations between COVID-19 and psychiatric disorder: Retrospective cohort studies of 62354 COVID-19 cases in the USA. *Lancet Psychiatry.* https://www.thelancet.com/action/showPdf?pii=S2215-0366%2820%2930462-4

U.S. Department of Veterans Affairs. (2019, September 20). *VA releases 2019 national veteran suicide prevention report.* https://www.va.gov/opa/pressrel/pressrelease.cfm?id=5317

Anxiety

Anxiety and Depression Association of America (n.d.). *Facts and statistics.* https://adaa.org/about-adaa/press-room/facts-statistics

Balon R, Starcevic V. (2020). Role of benzodiazepines in anxiety disorders. *Advances in Experimental Medicine and Biology, 1191*, 367–388. https://doi.org/10.1007/978-981-32-9705-0_20

Balsamo M, Cataldi F, Carlucci L, et al. (2018). Assessment of anxiety in older adults: a review of self-report measures. *Clinical interventions in aging, 13*, 573–593. https://doi.org/10.2147/CIA.S114100

Bandelow B, Michaelis S, Wedekind D. (2017). Treatment of anxiety disorders. Dialogues in clinical neuroscience, 19(2), 93–107. https://doi.org/10.31887/DCNS.2017.19.2/bbandelow

Brahmbhatt A, Richardson L, Prajapati S. (2020). Identifying and managing anxiety disorders in primary care. *The Journal for Nurse Practitioners, 16*(10). https://doi.org/10.1016/j.nurpra.2020.10.019

Edmund SJ, Sheppard KG. (2018). The challenge of generalized anxiety disorder in primary care. *The Nurse Practitioner, 43*(4), 14-18. doi:10.1097/01.NPR.0000531075.19182.0b

Kuru E, Safak Y, Özdemir İ, et al. (2018). Cognitive distortions in patients with social anxiety disorder: Comparison of a clinical group and healthy controls. *The European Journal of Psychiatry, 32*(2), 97-104. https://psycnet.apa.org/record/2019-05099-006

Kwak YT, Yang Y, Koo MS. (2017). Anxiety in dementia. *Dementia and neurocognitive disorders, 16*(2), 33–39. https://doi.org/10.12779/dnd.2017.16.2.33

Love AS, Love R. (2019). Anxiety disorders in primary care settings. *The Nursing Clinics of North America, 54*(4), 473–493. https://doi.org/10.1016/j.cnur.2019.07.002

Metzler DH, Mahoney D, Freedy JR. (2016). Anxiety disorders in primary care. *Primary Care, 43*(2), 245-261. doi:10.1016/j.pop.2016.02.002

National Institute of Mental Health. (n.d.). *Any anxiety disorder.* https://www.nimh.nih.gov/health/statistics/any-anxiety-disorder.shtml

Pappa S, Ntella V, Giannakas T, et al. (2020). Prevalence of depression, anxiety, and insomnia among healthcare workers during the COVID-19 pandemic: A systematic review and meta-analysis. *Brain, Behavior, and Immunity, 88*, 901–907. https://doi.org/10.1016/j.bbi.2020.05.026

Salcedo B. (2018, January 19). The comorbidity of anxiety and depression. National Alliance on Mental Illness. https://www.nami.org/Blogs/NAMI-Blog/January-2018/The-Comorbidity-of-Anxiety-and-Depression

Thibaut F. (2017). Anxiety disorders: a review of current literature. *Dialogues in clinical neuroscience, 19*(2), 87–88. https://doi.org/10.31887/DCNS.2017.19.2/fthibaut

Depression

Cavanagh A, Wilson CJ, Kavanagh DJ, et al. (2017). Differences in the expression of symptoms in men versus women with depression: A systematic review and meta-analysis. *Harvard Review of Psychiatry, 25*(1), 29–38. https://doi.org/10.1097/HRP.0000000000000128

Chand SP, Arif H. (2020). Depression. In: *StatPearls*. StatPearls Publishing.

Eliacin J, Coffing JM, Matthias MS, et al. (2018). The relationship between race, patient activation, and working alliance: Implications for patient engagement in mental health care. *Administration and Policy in Mental Health, 45*(1), 186–192. https://doi.org/10.1007/s10488-016-0779-5

Ferenchick EK, Ramanuj P, Pincus HA. (2019). Depression in primary care: Part 1- screening and diagnosis. *British Medical Journal (Clinical research ed.), 365*, l794. https://doi.org/10.1136/bmj.l794

Jackson JL, Machen JL. (2020). From the Editors' Desk: The Importance of screening for depression in primary care. *Journal of General Internal Medicine, 35*, 1–2.

Maki PM, Kornstein SG, Joffe H, et al. (2019). Guidelines for the evaluation and treatment of perimenopausal depression: Summary and recommendations. *Journal of Women's Health, 28*(2), 117-134. doi:10.1089/jwh.2018.27099.mensocrec

Maurer DM, Raymond TJ, Davis BN. (2018). Depression: Screening and diagnosis. *American Family Physician, 98*(8), 508-515. https://pubmed.ncbi.nlm.nih.gov/30277728/

Nelson B, Kaminsky DB. (2020, September 4). COVID-19's crushing mental health toll on health care workers. *Cancer Cytopathology, 128*(9), 597-598. https://doi.org/10.1002/cncy.22347

Park LT, Zarate Ca Jr. (2019). Depression in the primary care setting. *The New England Journal of Medicine, 380*(6), 559–568. https://doi.org/10.1056/NEJMcp1712493

Siu AL, US Preventive Services Task Force (USPSTF), Bibbins-Domingo K, et al. (2016). Screening for depression in adults: U.S. Preventive Services Task Force recommendation treatment. *JAMA, 315*(4), 380–387. https://doi.org/10.1001/jama.2015.18392

Stahl SM. (2013). *Stahl's essential psychopharmacology: Neuroscientific basis and practical applications* (4th ed.). Cambridge University Press.

Grief

Farber T, Eagle G, Smith C. (2018). Catastrophic grief and associated defenses in elderly child holocaust survivors. *Psycho-analytic Psychotherapy in South Africa, 26*(2), 49 83. https://journals.co.za/content/journal/10520/EJC-14f2fbe76f

Gesi C, Carmassi C, Cerveri G, et al. (2020). Complicated Grief: What to Expect After the Coronavirus Pandemic. *Frontiers in Psychiatry, 11*, 489. https://doi.org/10.3389/fpsyt.2020.00489

Hopf D, Eckstein M, Aguilar-Raab C, et al. (2020). Neuroendocrine mechanisms of grief and bereavement: A systematic review and implications for future interventions. *Journal of Neuroendocrinology, 32*(8), e12887. https://doi.org/10.1111/jne.12887

Kübler-Ross E. (1965). *On death and dying.* Basic Books.

McKee KY, Kelly A. (2020). Management of Grief, Depression, and Suicidal Thoughts in Serious Illness. *The Medical Clinics of North America, 104*(3), 503–524. https://doi.org/10.1016/j.mcna.2020.01.003

Mughal S, Azhar Y, Siddiqui WJ. (2020). *Grief reaction.* In: *StatPearls*. StatPearls Publishing. https://www.ncbi.nlm.nih.gov/books/NBK507832/

Nakajima S. (2018). Complicated grief: Recent developments in diagnostic criteria and treatment. *Philosophical Transactions of the Royal Society of London. Series B, Biological Sciences, 373*(1754), 20170273. https://doi.org/10.1098/rstb.2017.0273

Näppä U, Lundgren AB, Axelsson B. (2016). The effect of bereavement groups on grief, anxiety, and depression—A controlled, prospective intervention study. *BMC Palliative Care*, 15: 58e1–e8. https://doi.org/10.1186/s12904-016-0129-0

National Cancer Institute. (2020, December 3). *Grief, bereavement, and coping with loss (PDQ®)–Health professional version.* https://www.cancer.gov/about-cancer/advanced-cancer/caregivers/planning/bereavement-hp-pdq

Intimate Partner Violence

Centers for Disease Control and Prevention (2020, October 9). *Intimate partner violence.* https://www.cdc.gov/violenceprevention/intimatepartnerviolence/index.html

Feltner C, Wallace I, Berkman N, et al. (2018). Screening for intimate partner violence, elder abuse, and abuse of vulnerable adults. Evidence report and systematic review for the US Preventive

Services Task Force. *JAMA, 320*(16):1688–1701. doi:10.1001/jama.2018.13212

Godin M. (2020, March 18). As cities around the world go on lockdown, victims of domestic violence look for a way out. *Time.* https://time.com/5803887/coronavirus-domestic-violence-victims/

Kimberg L. (2016). Trauma and trauma-informed care. In: TE King, MB Wheeler (Eds.). *Medical management of vulnerable and underserved patients: Principles, practice, and populations* (2nd ed.). McGraw-Hill. https://accessmedicine.mhmedical.com/content.aspx?bookid=1768&sectionid=119151819

Machtinger EL, Davis KB, Kimberg LS, et al. (2019). From treatment to healing: Inquiry and response to recent and past trauma in adult health care. *Women's Health Issues, 29*(2), 97–102. https://doi.org/10.1016/j.whi.2018.11.003

Reddy KS. (2016). Global burden of disease study 2015 provides GPS for global health 2030. *Lancet, 388*(10053),1447–1449. doi: 10.1016/S0140-6736(16)31743-3. PMID: 27733278.

Swailes AL, Lehman EB, McCall-Hosenfeld JS. (2017). Intimate partner violence discussions in the healthcare setting: A cross-sectional study. *Preventive Medicine Reports, 8*, 215–220. https://doi.org/10.1016/j.pmedr.2017.10.017

Substance Use Disorders

Substance Abuse and Mental Health Services Administration. (2021, January 4). *Medication-assisted treatment (MAT).* https://www.samhsa.gov/medication-assisted-treatment

Volkow ND, Michaelides M, Baler R. (2019). The neuroscience of drug reward and addiction. *Physiological Reviews, 99*(4), 2115–2140. https://doi.org/10.1152/physrev.00014.2018

RESOURCES

General

National Institute of Health. (2017, July 10). *Psychiatric genomics in the era of team science symposium.*
https://videocast.nih.gov/Summary.asp?File=23388&bhcp=1

National Institute of Mental Health. (2018, January). *Statistics.*
https://www.nimh.nih.gov/health/statistics/index.shtml

Anxiety

Brain & Behavior Research Foundation. (2020). *Advice for parents of children with anxiety disorders.*
https://www.bbrfoundation.org/blog/advice-parents-children-anxiety-disorders

National Alliance on Mental Illness. (2017, December). *Anxiety disorders.*
https://www.nami.org/Learn-More/Mental-Health-Conditions/Anxiety-Disorders/Overview

National Institute of Mental Health. (2016). *Generalized anxiety disorder: When worry gets out of control.*
https://www.nimh.nih.gov/health/publications/generalized-anxiety-disorder-gad/index.shtml

National Institute of Mental Health. (2016). *Panic disorder: When fear overwhelms.*
https://www.nimh.nih.gov/health/publications/panic-disorder-when-fear-overwhelms/index.shtml

National Institute of Mental Health. *Social anxiety disorder: More than just shyness.*
https://www.nimh.nih.gov/health/publications/social-anxiety-disorder-more-than-just-shyness/index.shtml

Depression

Department of Veterans Affairs and Department of Defense. (2016). *VA/DoD clinical practice guideline for the management of major depressive disorder. Department of Veterans Affairs and Department of Defense.*
https://www.healthquality.va.gov/guidelines/MH/mdd/MDDCPGClinicianSummaryFINAL1.pdf

Department of Veterans Affairs and Department of Defense. (2016, April). *VA/DoD pocket card.*
https://www.healthquality.va.gov/guidelines/MH/mdd/MDDCPGPocketcardFINAL1.pdf

National Institute of Mental Health. (2018, February). *Depression.*
https://www.nimh.nih.gov/health/topics/depression/index.shtml#part_145398

National Institute of Mental Health. (2016). *Depression basics.*
https://www.nimh.nih.gov/health/publications/depression/index.shtml

National Institute of Mental Health. (2020). *Depression in women: 5 things you should know.*
https://www.nimh.nih.gov/health/publications/depression-in-women/index.shtml

National Institute of Mental Health. *Men and depression.*
https://www.nimh.nih.gov/health/publications/men-and-depression/index.shtml

National Institute of Mental Health. *Older adults and depression.*
https://www.nimh.nih.gov/health/publications/older-adults-and-depression/index.shtml

National Institute of Mental Health. *Teen depression: more than just moodiness.*
https://www.nimh.nih.gov/health/publications/teen-depression/index.shtml

U.S. Preventive Services Task Force. (2020, August 27). *Screening for depression, anxiety, and suicide risk in adults, including pregnant and postpartum persons.*
https://www.uspreventiveservicestaskforce.org/uspstf/draft-update-summary/screening-depression-anxiety-suicide-risk-adults

U.S. Preventive Services Task Force. (2020, August 6). *Screening for depression and suicide risk in children and adolescents.*
https://www.uspreventiveservicestaskforce.org/uspstf/document/final-research-plan/screening-depression-anxiety-suicide-risk-children-adolescents

Grief

Aging With Dignity. (2021).
https://agingwithdignity.org/

American Cancer Society. (2021). *Grief and bereavement.*
https://www.cancer.org/treatment/end-of-life-care/grief-and-loss/grieving-process.html

American Hospice Foundation.
https://americanhospice.org/

American Psychological Association. (2021). *Grief: Coping with the loss of your loved one.*
http://www.apa.org/helpcenter/grief.aspx

Elizabeth Kübler-Ross Foundation. (2021).
http://www.ekrfoundation.org/

Grief.com. *Five stages of grief.*
https://grief.com/the-five-stages-of-grief/

Mayo Clinic. (2016, October 19). *What is grief?*
https://www.mayoclinic.org/patient-visitor-guide/support-groups/what-is-grief

National Hospice and Palliative Care Organization. (2020). https://www.nhpco.org/

National Hospice and Palliative Care Organization. (2020). *Grief and loss.* https://www.nhpco.org/about-nhpco/patients-and-caregivers/the-grief-experience/types-of-grief-and-loss/

Intimate Partner Violence (IPV)

American Family Physicians. *Intimate partner violence.* https://www.aafp.org/afp/2016/1015/p646.html

Centers for Disease Control and Prevention. *Violence Prevention.* https://www.cdc.gov/violenceprevention

IPV Health Partners. *Health care centers are key to violence prevention.* http://ipvhealthpartners.org/

Mayo Clinic. (2020, February 8). *Adult health (violence against men).* https://www.mayoclinic.org/healthy-lifestyle/adult-health/in-depth/domestic-violence-against-men/art-20045149?p=1

Mayo Clinic. (2020, February 25). *Adult health (violence against women).* https://www.mayoclinic.org/healthy-lifestyle/adult-health/in-depth/domestic-violence/art-20048397?p=1

National domestic violence hotline. *Here for you.* https://www.thehotline.org/

National Institute on Aging (NIH). (2020, July 29). *Elder abuse.* https://www.nia.nih.gov/health/elder-abuse#caregiver

National Institute of Justice. (2016, September 30). *Evaluating what works for victims and offenders: The domestic violence homicide prevention demonstration initiative.* https://www.nij.gov/topics/crime/intimate-partner-violence/Pages/evaluation-of-domestic-violence-homicide-prevention-demonstration-initiative.aspx

National Institute of Justice (2017, April 3). *Family context is an important element in the development of teen dating violence and should be considered in prevention and intervention.* https://www.nij.gov/topics/crime/intimate-partner-violence/teen-dating-violence/Pages/family-context-in-development-of-teen-dating-violence.aspx

National Institute of Justice. (2017, October 12). *Risks in adolescence that lead to intimate partner violence in young adulthood.* https://www.nij.gov/topics/crime/intimate-partner-violence/Pages/risks-in-adolescence-that-lead-to-intimate-partner-violence-in-young-adulthood.aspx

National Sexual Violence Resource Center (NSVRC). https://www.nsvrc.org/

National Sexual Violence Resource Center. (2017, April 25). *Talking points: National Intimate Partner and Sexual Violence Survey (NISVS) 2010-2012 state report – sexual violent data and prevention implications.* https://www.nsvrc.org/sites/default/files/nsvrc_publications_talking-points-nisvs_state_report_0.pdf

Recovery Research Institute. (2020). *The brain in recovery.* https://www.recoveryanswers.org/recovery-101/brain-in-recovery/

Substance Abuse and Mental Health Service Administration. (2020). *Intimate partner violence. and child abuse considerations during COVID-19.* https://www.samhsa.gov/sites/default/files/social-distancing-domestic-violence.pdf

U.S. Department of Health & Human Services. *Child welfare information gateway.* https://www.childwelfare.gov/

United States Department of Justice Archives. (2018, November 5). *Protecting students from sexual assault.* https://www.justice.gov/archives/ovw/protecting-students-sexual-assault

---

Chapter 66

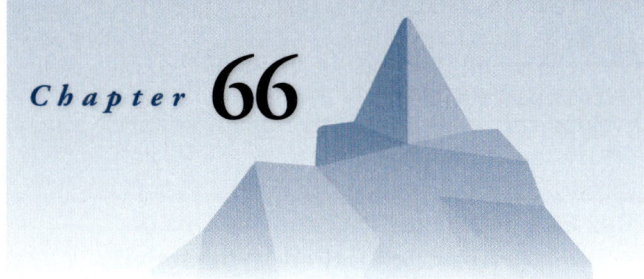

Neurodevelopmental Disorders

Elizabeth Hutson, PhD, APRN-CNP, PMHNP-BC

Karen Jennings Mathis, PhD, APRN-CNP, PMHNP-BC, FAED

A major change from the *Diagnosis and Statistical Manual of Mental Disorders IV (DSM-IV)* to the *DSM-5-TR* was relabeling of the chapter "Diagnosis usually first made in infancy, childhood, or adolescence." The new chapter, called "Neurodevelopmental Disorders," was meant to signify the advances in research on the developing brain. These disorders are commonly still diagnosed in infancy, childhood, or adolescence, but it is important for the primary care clinician to be keenly aware of how these disorders can present across the life span. In this chapter, we will discuss four neurodevelopmental disorders, attention deficit-hyperactivity disorder, autism spectrum disorder, intellectual disability, and tic disorders, and how these disorders can be evaluated and managed, not only during the developmental period but across the life span. Diagnostic terms and labels often change, but many of the disorders discussed in this chapter can be thought of as differences in typical versus atypical development.

ATTENTION DEFICIT-HYPERACTIVITY DISORDER

Attention deficit-hyperactivity disorder (ADHD) is one of the most common neuropsychiatric disorders and manifests with persistent patterns of hyperactivity/impulsivity and/or inattention. Though previously thought of as a disorder of childhood, studies have consistently shown that this disorder continues into adulthood. Many individuals diagnosed with ADHD in childhood and adolescence continue to manifest significant impairment in occupational, academic, and social functioning into adulthood. Additionally, there is recognition that some individuals will present for diagnosis and treatment of ADHD for the first time in adulthood, although the symptoms must start before age 12 years, according to the *DSM-5-TR*. The symptoms of ADHD affect academic, occupational, behavioral, cognitive, emotional, and social functioning in individuals across the life span. Emotional dysregulation in individuals with ADHD is common, and in some instances, this can lead to comorbid conditions.

EPIDEMIOLOGY AND CAUSES

The reported prevalence of ADHD ranges from 0.1% to 10.2% in children and up to 2.5% in adults. In children, the male-to-female ratio is 2:1, and this skewed ratio of males-to-females continues into adulthood. There is debate as to whether differences among the sexes have to do with differences in referrals and presenting symptoms. Females tend to present with more symptoms of inattention, which can be harder to observe, compared to a more hyperactive presentation in males. Prevalence is also influenced by cultural variations in behavioral norms and expectations of youth in different social contexts, differences in interpretations of youth's behaviors, parental demand for diagnosis of behaviors, and clinician bias. In fact, underdetection may result from mislabeling of ADHD symptoms as oppositional or disruptive in historically marginalized racial and ethnic groups, leading to overdiagnosis of disruptive disorders.

The *DSM-5* made significant changes to the diagnostic criteria of ADHD. Although there is no specific age of onset, the symptoms must have been present before age 12. The rationale behind this change was to note that it was challenging for adults presenting with ADHD symptoms to remember symptoms prior to age 7, as previously required by the *DSM-IV*. The *DSM-5-TR* also includes specific adult examples of the required diagnostic criteria, which makes it easier for primary care providers to ask questions related to impairments in functioning for adult patients (e.g., forgetful about paying bills and keeping appointments, difficulty sustaining attention in lengthy reading and conversations).

In ADHD, comorbidities are the rule, not the exception. There appears to be a dose–response relationship between ADHD and comorbidity: the higher the number of ADHD symptoms, the greater the comorbidities (see Box 66.1). To date, no single etiology for ADHD has been identified. Data from biological, environmental, and psychosocial research suggest several *possible* risk factors or causes for the disorder. There is no strong scientific evidence that food additives, colorings, preservatives, or sugar contributes to ADHD, although some literature argues that certain subsets of populations, especially children, may benefit from some forms of dietary controls.

Risk Factors: Attention Deficit-Hyperactivity Disorder

- Very low birth weight
- Prenatal tobacco exposure
- Prenatal toxin exposure
- Genetic factors
- Child abuse
- Lead exposure

There is a strong genetic component to ADHD. Children with parents or siblings with ADHD have two to eight times increased risk, with heritability estimated at 74% based on pooled data from twin studies. Results of behavioral genetic investigations using family, twin, and adoption studies converge with those of molecular genetic studies in showing that genes influence susceptibility to ADHD. Despite these correlations, genome-wide association studies have not found any specific genetic variant to be significantly related to ADHD. To date, there is no genetic testing for a patient who presents with symptoms of ADHD.

PATHOPHYSIOLOGY

Imbalances among the levels of norepinephrine, dopamine, and epinephrine appear to be involved in the development of ADHD, suggesting a complex genetic

Box 66.1 Psychiatric Comorbidities of Attention Deficit-Hyperactivity Disorder

- Oppositional defiant disorder/conduct disorder
- Social phobia
- Substance-use disorders
- Bipolar disorder
- Major depressive disorder
- Post-traumatic stress disorder
- Generalized anxiety disorder
- Obsessive-compulsive disorder

Source: Leahy LG. (2018). Diagnosis and treatment of ADHD in children vs adults: What nurses should know. *Archives of psychiatric nursing*, 32(6), 890–895. https://doi.org/10.1016/j.apnu.2018.06.013

mechanism through which the disorder is caused by the combined actions of several genes interacting with environmental risk factors. In structural imaging examinations of the brains of children with and without ADHD, several differences emerge as well. For example, studies have found a delay in cortical maturation of both cortical thickness and surface area in children with ADHD, but these delays tend to normalize with long-term stimulant medication treatment. Research indicates that those with ADHD demonstrate impaired executive functioning and/or difficulties with response inhibition on neuropsychological testing, confirming neuroimaging studies that demonstrate structural and functional abnormalities in prefrontal structures and basal ganglia. The noradrenergic system is involved in the modulation of higher cortical functions, and animal models suggest that there is an imbalance in norepinephrine and dopamine systems in the prefrontal cortex that would account for the decrease in inhibitory dopamine activity and increase in norepinephrine activity.

CLINICAL PRESENTATION

Parents may be the first to note excessive motor activity (hyperactivity) during the toddler years. The disorder is not usually diagnosed during this time, however, because that is the normative developmental stage. By preschool, children with ADHD may have difficulty participating in sedentary activities, such as sitting still while listening to a story. Parents may describe the child as "always on the go," and the child may appear to constantly run, jump, and not sit still. There may also be excessive talking and interrupting of others. For children who have more of an inattentive presentation, parents and teachers may describe the child as "always daydreaming," and the child may appear to be constantly needing redirection to focus and pay attention.

ADHD is most often diagnosed during the childhood years (especially during elementary school) when the child's decreased attention span affects classroom work and academic performance. The school-aged child with ADHD will usually have difficulty remaining seated, be unable to complete assignments and turn them in, and talk out of turn. Hyperactivity behaviors may include constantly tapping their hands, frequent fidgeting, shaking of their feet or legs, getting up repeatedly during meals, and talking excessively. Inattentive behaviors may include constantly not paying careful attention to assignments, frequent forgetfulness, misplacing possessions, frequent daydreaming or spacing out, and difficulty following instructions.

In childhood and adolescence, many of the same symptoms continue, and the symptoms of impulsivity can lead to risky and dangerous behaviors. Disruptive behaviors and poor social skills can make bonding with peers difficult and may lead to self-esteem issues, depressive and anxiety symptoms, and substance and tobacco abuse.

As individuals age, the symptoms of hyperactivity tend to abate while the symptoms of inattention remain. Adults may describe difficulties with focusing and prioritizing, leading to challenges in work and social relationships. Restlessness may lead to difficulty participating in sedentary activities and to avoiding occupations, such as desk jobs, that provide limited opportunity for spontaneous movement. Adults with ADHD often complain of boredom and frustration with job and life routines. Consequently, adults with ADHD may have challenges in occupational performance and social relationships.

Symptoms are often present and visible during the assessment of ADHD in the primary care office, although inattention may be less obvious if the assessment is structured and the individual answers questions appropriately. Lack of symptoms displayed during a short primary care office visit does not preclude the diagnosis of ADHD. Individuals with ADHD may not be able to report their own symptoms accurately (1) due to age if they are a child or (2) due to challenges in recall of childhood if they are an adult; therefore, information should be gathered from parents or guardians as well as significant others and supplemented by reports from teachers/professors. Additional questions related to family history of ADHD should be conducted. Adult patients may need to question their parents regarding ADHD behaviors that were evident from childhood. Key areas for questioning relate to complaints of boredom, disorganization or frustration in work, and a tendency for impulsive, impatient, and restless behavior.

Generally, diagnostic tests are not indicated, but serum lead, ferritin, and/or thyroid levels may be considered. An electroencephalogram (EEG), diagnostic imaging, and genetic testing may be indicated for those patients who present with anomalies or soft neurological signs.

DIAGNOSTIC REASONING

Screening for psychosocial issues has become more common as providers become increasingly aware that many children exhibit emotional and behavioral problems. Utilizing a tool at regular well-child visits may help to identify this chronic condition, particularly in children with academic and behavioral issues. For adults, assessment should include prior history of ADHD, previous school performance, history of mental health diagnoses, substance abuse, and current or past medication use. When there are concerns for ADHD, various screening tools can be used (see Box 66.2).

Symptoms

The diagnosis of ADHD is based on *DSM-5-TR* criteria; please refer to the *DSM-5-TR* for complete diagnostic criteria. Symptoms must have been present for at least 6 months prior to age 12, although the diagnosis can be

Box 66.2 ADHD Rating Scales

Commonly used

- The National Institute for Children's Health Quality (NICHQ) Vanderbilt Assessment Scale (forms for teachers and parents)
- The Swanson, Nolan and Pelham Questionnaire (SNAP IV)
- Connors-3 (forms for teachers and parents)
- Adult ADHD self-report scale (ASRS)
- Achenbach Child Behavior Checklist (CBCL)

Computerized ADHD testing

- The Test of Variables of Attention (TOVA)
- Conners Continuous Performance Test

Differential Diagnosis 66.1: Attention Deficit-Hyperactivity Disorder

- Normal, age-appropriate behaviors
- Medical conditions
  - Thyroid disease
  - Lead toxicity
  - Iron deficiency
  - Fetal alcohol syndrome
- Genetic conditions
  - Fragile X syndrome
  - Turner syndrome
  - Neurofibromatosis type 1
  - Prader-Willi syndrome
  - Williams syndrome
- Psychiatric conditions
  - Learning disabilities
  - Autism spectrum disorder
  - Tic disorders
  - Conduct disorder
  - Oppositional defiant disorder
  - Major depressive disorder
  - Generalized anxiety disorder
  - Substance use disorder
- Drug-seeking behaviors

made at any age. Importantly, symptoms must be present across at least two settings (e.g., home, school, work, social interactions), as symptoms in only one setting may indicate an environmental etiology and subsequent intervention. Categories of symptoms include:

- Inattention: Difficulty focusing or sustaining attention, forgetfulness, or difficulty following instructions
- Hyperactivity: Excessive motor activity and difficulty sitting still or in quiet activities
- Impulsivity: Interrupting others, not thinking before acting or speaking

Diagnosis of ADHD occurs after a careful assessment including an interview with the individual and their guardian if available. The interview should focus on the onset of symptoms, clinical course, and current symptomology. Although neuropsychological testing may be helpful, it is not required for the diagnosis of ADHD.

Differential Diagnosis

Various medical, psychological, and genetic conditions need to be assessed (see Differential Diagnosis 66.1). It is important for the clinician to be able to distinguish symptoms of ADHD from developmentally age-appropriate behaviors in children and adolescents and from other neurological concerns in adults. In addition, because many psychiatric conditions are associated with inattention, it is important to rule out other disorders such as depressive and anxiety disorders.

MANAGEMENT

A comprehensive plan needs to address the chronic nature of ADHD, treatment options (pharmacological and nonpharmacological), and community and school resources. Reappraisal of the plan with medication reassessment needs to be done periodically and appropriate changes made.

Pharmacological Management

Pharmacotherapy in preschool-age children warrants precaution, given their young age, and behavioral interventions are the first line of treatment. However, stimulants are approved for this age group if the symptoms are severe or nonresponsive to behavioral treatment, and nonstimulants can be considered as well. For older children, adolescents, and adults, pharmacotherapy should be considered when symptoms cause clinically significant impairment at home, school, and/or work. There is strong evidence for the stimulant medications, given their robust efficacy (with response rates of 75% to 80%), and they are considered the first-line pharmacological treatment for ADHD in these populations.

The two stimulant classes are methylphenidate-based and amphetamine-based agents, with both immediate-release and sustained-release formulations available. The advantages of once-daily dosing include compliance, convenience, and confidentiality. Management includes beginning a stimulant at a low dose and titrating upward until symptoms are controlled (generally every 1 to 3 weeks) or side effects prohibit further titration. There is no advantage to either a methylphenidate-based or amphetamine-based class. It is not necessary to begin with a short-acting agent before using a sustained-release agent, although this can be useful in dose titration, particularly with younger children. If the maximum dosage does not control the symptoms, switching to another stimulant class is indicated. If the chosen stimulant does not provide adequate symptom control later in the day, augmenting with an alpha-agonist (guanfacine or clonidine) can be effective. If children cannot swallow pills, consider chewable or liquid options; in addition, some long-acting preparations are available in capsules that can be opened and sprinkled. Medication diversion or abuse, especially to improve academic performance, is a consideration when prescribing for patients with ADHD. Stimulants may increase levels of seizure drugs, selective serotonin reuptake inhibitors, tricyclics, and warfarin (see Drugs Commonly Prescribed 66.1).

Drugs Commonly Prescribed 66.1: Attention Deficit-Hyperactivity Disorder (ADHD) Medications

MEDICATION	INDICATION	ADVERSE REACTIONS AND PRESCRIBING CONSIDERATIONS
Methylphenidate (MPH) Derivatives†		
Adhansia XR‡ Aptensio XR‡ Concerta‡ Cotempla XR Daytrana Focalin‡, Focalin XR‡ Jornay PM‡ Metadate CD, Metadate ER‡ Methylin Chewable, Methylin ER‡ QuilliChew ER‡ Quillivant‡ Ritalin‡, Ritalin LA	ADHD, narcolepsy	• Side effects: Insomnia, weight loss, tics, tachycardia, elevated blood pressure, irritability • Age 6 years and older • **Black-box warning:** Abuse and dependence
Amphetamine Derivatives†		
Adderall‡, Adderall XR‡ Adzenys ER‡, Adzenys XR-ODT‡ Desoxyn‡ Dexedrine Dyanavel XR Vyvanse‡ Evekeo‡, Evekeo ODT Mydayis‡ ProCentra Zenzedi	ADHD, narcolepsy	• Side effects: Insomnia, weight loss, tics, tachycardia, elevated BP, irritability • Stop slowly, not suddenly • Age 3 years and older (mixed amphetamine salts) • Extended release: Age 6 years and older • **Black-box warning:** Abuse and dependence
Selective Norepinephrine Reuptake Inhibitors		
Atomoxetine (Strattera)‡	ADHD	• Side effects: Gastrointestinal upset; weight loss; mood swings, sedation, headaches • Once daily in a.m. (can split dose or give all at night if daytime sedation) • **Black-box warning:** Suicide ideation
Alpha-Agonists		
Clonidine (Catapres, Kapvay) Guanfacine (Tenex, Intuniv)	ADHD, Tourette's disorder	• More effective in treatment of impulsivity/hyperactivity than inattention • Must be tapered on discontinuation • Beneficial in comorbid Tourette's disorder and tics • Side effects: Sedation, dizziness, hypotension • Helpful in treatment of stimulant-induced insomnia • Advantages of guanfacine over clonidine: Less sedation and longer duration of action

Continued

Drugs Commonly Prescribed 66.1: Attention Deficit-Hyperactivity Disorder (ADHD) Medications—cont'd

MEDICATION	INDICATION	ADVERSE REACTIONS AND PRESCRIBING CONSIDERATIONS
Tricyclic Antidepressants*		
Imipramine (Tofranil)* Desipramine (Norpramin)*	ADHD, depression	• ECG recommended at baseline and with dose increases • Monitoring blood levels is useful in guiding dosing • **Black-box warning:** Suicide ideation • Anticholinergic effect • Limited use due to risk of sudden death; use only if other agents not effective
Dopamine/Norepinephrine Reuptake Inhibitor		
Bupropion (Wellbutrin)*	ADHD, depression	• Side effects: Insomnia, decreased appetite • Seizure risk
Antinarcoleptic		
Modafinil*	ADHD, narcolepsy	• Insomnia • Headache • Decrease in appetite • Stevens-Johnson syndrome

Abbreviations: ECG, electroencephalogram; FDA, Food and Drug Administration.
*Off-label use.
†C-II controlled substance; available in short- and extended-release formulations; monitor growth parameters (height, weight), blood pressure, and pulse; do not use in severe cardiac disease or with family history of sudden cardiac death at young age; use caution in administration with history of drug or alcohol dependence; doses of stimulants should advance slowly every several days until appropriate response is obtained; stimulants may increase levels of seizure drugs, selective serotonin reuptake inhibitors, tricyclics, and warfarin.
‡Approved by the U.S. FDA for adults with ADHD.

Common side effects of stimulants include weight loss, appetite suppression, abdominal pain, insomnia, and headache. The practitioner needs to be aware of the common side effects and have strategies to offset them, including dose reduction, changing medication, and prescribing adjunctive medications. Tics are not an absolute contraindication to stimulant use, and more research is finding no association between tics and stimulant use (Cohen et al., 2015). Congenital heart disease including hypertrophic cardiomyopathy or significant cardiac-related symptoms should prompt cardiac evaluation, including an electrocardiogram, before initiating pharmacological therapy. The practitioner should closely monitor patients with ADHD and an eating disorder because two common side effects of stimulants are weight loss and appetite suppression.

Atomoxetine (Strattera) is a selective norepinephrine reuptake inhibitor (SNRI), which is used if stimulant drugs are not tolerated or contraindicated (active substance abuse, tics, comorbid anxiety, or mood lability). Atomoxetine has an effect both on ADHD and on comorbid anxiety. Atomoxetine affects weight and sleep less than stimulants, and unlike stimulants (the effects of which are often seen soon after initiation), the full clinical effect of atomoxetine may take up to 6 weeks. Although stimulants can be stopped on weekends or school holidays if side effects warrant this and symptoms can be managed in the home, atomoxetine must be taken daily without "drug holidays."

Nonpharmacological Management

Behavioral interventions can be quite useful for all patients, particularly with younger children. Behavioral techniques include parental training, classroom management techniques, and peer interventions. Evidence-based group parent training programs and early educational programs are recommended as the initial step for preschool-age children, although these can be conducted in conjunction with medications in older patients. Referral for early intervention services or to a behavioral specialist may be useful. For adolescents and adults, study and organizational skills training including time management, study strategies, and empowerment to minimize distractions may increase functioning.

FOLLOW-UP AND REFERRAL

Follow-up for patients diagnosed with ADHD includes gathering information from the patient, parents, and teachers regarding symptom progression, often on standardized rating scales. The focus of follow-up visits includes physical parameters (height, weight, cardiac evaluation including blood pressure and pulse), assessment of behavioral progress (utilizing an ADHD scale helps to objectively identify and track behavioral changes from the parent and teacher), monitoring of medication compliance and side effects, and continued education and referral to support services if indicated. It is often useful to set specific parameters for tracking progress, such as grades, homework completion, or frequency of calls home from school. If appetite is significantly affected such that the patient is falling on their growth chart, reevaluation of the treatment plan is necessary (including considering decreasing the dose, drug holidays, increasing caloric intake at the start and end of the day, or switching to a nonstimulant).

Children with ADHD are at increased risk for abuse, bullying, depression, and social isolation and should be monitored. Parents will need regular support and advice and may need referral for family therapy to cope with the added demands. Parents, teachers, and advisors should encourage career choices that allow autonomy and mobility. Adolescence offers new challenges, and the practitioner needs to address these issues both with the adolescent and the family. Increased independence, decision making, and risk-taking behaviors need to be addressed. In addition, discussion about the continued need for and the benefit of medication may ensue. In general, if the patient has been symptom free for longer than 1 year with no adjustment in medication dosage despite increases in weight and height, consideration about remission should occur. Summer vacation or a prolonged vacation may be a good time to trial a drug holiday.

Nursing Situation: Attention Deficit-Hyperactivity Disorder

Brianna, a 7-year-old child, presents to her primary care provider after her teacher met with her mother for parent-teacher conferences. During this conference, behavioral concerns in school were noted. Her teacher reported that Brianna often gets up out of her seat and moves around. She leaves the classroom so often her teacher started putting a badge on her to say where she is going and where she needs to be. The teacher also noted some spurts of anger at school when she has difficulty waiting her turn, but no physical aggression. The teacher sent in a NICHQ Vanderbilt Assessment Scale, and Brianna scored 5 out of 9 for inattentive symptoms of ADHD, 8 out of 9 for hyperactive symptoms of ADHD, 3 out of 9 for oppositional/conduct behaviors, and 0 out of 6 for depressive/anxiety symptoms.

Mom reports at home Brianna is constantly in motion and is very hard to interrupt. During the COVID-19 pandemic, when Mom was helping Brianna with online schooling, Mom reports having a very difficult time helping her to get her schoolwork done. Brianna would rush through her work and make careless mistakes. Her mom denied seeing depressive symptoms in Brianna but did endorse that she is very emotional and moody. She becomes upset easily and has a hard time controlling her emotions.

Brianna has a history of ADHD and oppositional defiant disorder (ODD), and in the past had been linked with psychiatry outpatient services at the local children's hospital. Brianna was started on a stimulant medication when she was in preschool for behavioral issues and ADHD. Mom reports Brianna first took dextroamphetamine/amphetamine (Adderall XR) 5 mg, which was helpful. Then medication was switched to methylphenidate (Concerta) 18 mg. Mom is unsure why; the change made her behaviors worse. Mom reports Brianna has been off medication for the past year, and Mom would like her to start medication again.

In an interview with Brianna, she sheepishly reports that she gets into trouble at school "a lot" and wishes she could control her behaviors. She appeared fidgety and got into many of the items in the examination room during the assessment.

The diagnoses of ADHD and ODD were continued, and Brianna was restarted on dextroamphetamine/amphetamine (Adderall XR) 5 mg and titrated up to 10 mg with benefit. Brianna was referred to behavior therapy, where she worked on self-control and building her self-esteem to improve impulsiveness and reduce emotional dysregulation. Mom also participated in parent training where the concepts of positive reinforcement and consistent discipline were discussed with other parents in a group setting. Mom also found the group setting with other parents of children with ADHD and ODD to be supportive.

Many children with ADHD suffer from self-esteem issues related to getting into trouble often in school and at home. Many parents of children with ADHD find parenting more difficult than anticipated and could use extra support in managing difficult behaviors. The combination of medication plus behavioral therapies and parent training for children with ADHD often leads to the best long-term outcomes.

Monitoring for diversion of controlled substances is essential. If there are concerns regarding this, use of atomoxetine, extended-release guanfacine, or extended-release clonidine should be considered. In some situations, treatment with a stimulant agent that possesses a smaller risk for abuse could be used. High school and college students are at high risk for nonmedical use of prescription stimulants as a study aid, particularly during examination time. Providers should be cautious when making a first-time diagnosis of ADHD in a college student, and retrospective history is extremely important, including speaking with previous providers and family, if possible.

Patient Education: Attention Deficit-Hyperactivity Disorder

Adherence to the treatment plan improves when the patient and family understand the chronic nature of ADHD and its potential effects on school, social life, and occupational functioning.

Continued education about medications and management of side effects may improve adherence. Utilization of various community support groups may also help families and adults deal with developmental challenges. There are many interventions that parents, family members, and teachers can do in addition to administering medication (Box 66.3). Parents should be educated regarding realistic expectations and should be made aware of support groups for themselves, as well as child advocate groups.

AUTISM SPECTRUM DISORDER

Autism spectrum disorder (ASD) is a neurodevelopmental disorder with two core categories of symptoms, delays/deficits in social interaction and restricted or repetitive behaviors. A major change from the *DSM-IV* to *DSM-5* was labeling the diagnostic category autism spectrum disorders, encompassing the former diagnoses of pervasive developmental disorder not otherwise specified (PDD NOS), autistic disorder, Asperger syndrome, child disintegrative disorder, and Rett syndrome. The rationale for using one umbrella term was to show how the symptoms lie on a spectrum. ASD has been frequently thought of as a diagnosis associated with childhood, but as individuals age and more individuals are diagnosed later in life, the adult primary care provider needs to be aware of the assessment and treatment of ASD across the life span. Additionally, ASD is associated with an increased prevalence of medication complications, such as seizures, gastrointestinal (GI) distress, and sleep disorders, which often present first to primary care.

EPIDEMIOLOGY

The prevalence of ASD is thought to be between 1% and 2% of the U.S. population, with similar estimates in youth and adults. Recent increases in the incidence of ASD may reflect a true increase in cases, increased awareness of the diagnosis, or the broadening of the criteria in *DSM-5* (Myers et al, 2018). ASD is more common in males than females (3:1), and females are more likely to experience intellectual disability compared to males. Prevalence appears to be lower among historically marginalized racial and ethnic groups compared to non-Hispanic white children, which may be the result of misdiagnosis, delayed diagnosis, or underdiagnosis. Severity of ASD is often increased with impairment in language or cognition, comorbid mental illness, or comorbid epilepsy. ASD can present with or without intellectual disability or language impairment and may be associated with some genetic disorders.

PATHOPHYSIOLOGY

The underlying etiology of ASD remains under investigation, although there is an apparent role for genetics, given the elevated rate of diagnosis in siblings (up to 10 times higher than the general population) and the high concordance rate in monozygotic twins. Approximately 15% of cases of ASD are associated with a known genetic mutation. Repeated epidemiological studies have demonstrated no association between the MMR (measles, mumps, and rubella) vaccine and subsequent development of ASD, despite an initial faulty study that suggested otherwise. Environmental factors may contribute to ASD, including closer spacing of pregnancies, advanced parental age, premature birth, low birth weight, and fetal exposure to certain drugs or teratogens like valproic acid.

CLINICAL PRESENTATION

The *DSM-5-TR* includes two core categories of symptoms of ASD, of which individuals must meet a certain number of criteria. The first category includes delays/deficits in social interaction, which can manifest as deficits in social-emotional reciprocity; deficits in nonverbal communication; and deficits in developing, maintaining, and understanding relationships. The second category is restricted, repetitive patterns of behavior, interests, or

---

Box 66.3 Patient Education: Attention Deficit-Hyperactivity Disorder (ADHD)

Teach parents to do the following:

- Have the child do one task at a time.
- Use "time-out" periods for bad behavior.
- Make eye contact each time they are making a request.
- Reinforce good behavior or tasks the child does well with rewards and attention.
- Use behavior therapy, such as token systems.
- Stop unacceptable behavior before it escalates.
- Make use of parent support and advocacy groups.
- Deal with negative feelings and unrealistic expectations.
- Incorporate family therapy, anger-management training, and social training.
- Coordinate homework with teachers.
- Work closely with teachers for consistent behavioral plan.

Teach teachers to do the following:

- Make sure the child has a second set of books at home.
- Make work sessions short.
- Help the child deal constructively with negative feelings.
- Provide immediate consequences for bad behavior.
- Reinforce good behavior.
- Coordinate homework with parents.
- Work closely with parents for a consistent behavioral plan.

activities, which can manifest as stereotyped or repetitive behaviors; insistence on sameness; adherence to routines; highly restricted, fixated interests; and hyper- or hypoactivity to sensory input.

Symptoms of ASD usually appear during the second year of life but can be noted earlier or later, depending on the severity of deficits. ASD is not a degenerative disorder, and the individual will continue to develop throughout life, although at an altered pace compared with peers. Many patients with ASD will struggle socially throughout their lives, although those who are less impaired intellectually and behaviorally can lead independent lives. About 70% of individuals with ASD may have one comorbid mental disorder, and 40% may have two or more comorbid mental disorders. There are frequent co-occurring psychiatric disorders including specific phobias, obsessive-compulsive disorders (OCD), and ADHD. In addition, up to 25% of individuals with ASD will have EEG abnormalities or seizure activity.

Individuals with ASD can present with a variety of symptoms. A complete developmental history can provide context for the diagnosis, and this can be important to complete in both pediatric and adult populations.

Focus on History: Autism Spectrum Disorder

- Were there any difficulties with the pregnancy or in utero exposures?
- Were there any difficulties at delivery (e.g., preterm, low birth weight, need for emergent caesarian section)?
- Did the individual experience any illness as an infant or toddler?
- At what age did the individual reach developmental milestones (e.g., walking, talking, toileting)?
- Did the individual develop normally and then experience a regression?
- How did the individual interact with the caregiver when they were a child or currently?
- Does the individual maintain eye contact, point at desired objects, seek out the caregiver?
- Does the individual show empathy if someone appears hurt?
- How does the individual engage socially?
- Does the child engage in pretend play?

Clinical Presentation of ASD in Children

Children with ASD have difficulty with imaginary play or sharing, which may be appropriate to their age level. These children may present in primary care with the chief complaint of "sameness," such as self-restricted diet, and/or self-restricted activities such as lining up cars or watching the fan or toilet spin for hours at a time. Some may spin or twirl, and some may have repetitive movements such as hand flapping. They are inflexible about routine and become distressed over small changes, and parents may complain about their activities of daily living such as lack of or difficulty with showering, dressing, or eating. Although there are not exact percentages, most children with ASD have difficulty sleeping and may function with less sleep.

Clinical Presentation of ASD in Adolescents

As mentioned, individuals with ASD continue with developmental maturation but at an altered pace. Therefore, school-age and adolescent individuals with ASD have increased communication and intellectual abilities. Similar to children, they may experience distress with changes in routine. Repetitive behaviors may appear as self-stimulating behaviors, such as posturing, chewing or mouthing objects, staring at lights or rotating objects, or rearranging objects. Less often, these behaviors can become self-injurious in the form of head banging and biting. School-age individuals with ASD may be at an increased risk for learning difficulties, such as specific learning disorders or nonverbal learning disabilities. Challenges in the classroom may occur, such as difficulties with emotional regulation and behavioral disturbances, due to difficulties with social communication (see Box 66.4).

Clinical Presentation of ASD in Adults

Adults with ASD may have difficulty starting or continuing back-and-forth conversations with others. They may display difficulties with eye contact and difficulties interpreting nonverbal communication. Similar to children, adults with ASD may experience distress with changes in

Box 66.4	Common Presentations of ASD Across the Life Span
Preschool	Lack of interest in others, absent or delayed speech and communication, resistance to change, stereotyped movements, picky eating, selective interests
Childhood	Increase in social and communication skills, problems dealing with change and transitions, self-stimulation behaviors (self-injury, head banging)
Adolescence	Can have large developmental gains, but may have emotional and behavioral challenges related to communication deficits (tantrums, self-injury, aggression)
Adulthood	Difficulty understanding social cues and sarcasm, rigid adherence to rules, follows specific routines, may be more prone to anxiety and depression

routines or expectations and have highly fixated interests. It is becoming more common for adults to present later in life for the diagnosis and treatment of ASD, although their symptoms began during the early developmental period. This may reflect the individual's difficulty obtaining or sustaining employment, difficulty in their social life, or their difficulty integrating into the community as an adult.

Primary care clinicians should pay attention to age-appropriate development. Individuals with ASD may present with sensory issues and may be hyper- or hypoactive to pain, temperature, textures, certain smells, and specific sounds. Some nonverbal and individuals with severe ASD have self-harming behavior such as banging their head on the wall, scratching or biting themselves, and/or displaying aggression toward others. Physical examinations, including providing immunizations and obtaining a blood pressure or blood work, may prove difficult in some patients. Using clear, direct statements about what you are about to do will help to prepare individuals with ASD. It is also important to ask caregivers for self-soothing techniques that the individual has found helpful that can be used during the examination.

DIAGNOSTIC REASONING

To diagnose a patient with ASD, there must be persistent deficits in social communication and interaction and restrictive, repetitive patterns in behavior, interests, and activities. When children or adults with ASD are evaluated, the clinician may observe a lack of emotional back-and-forth conversation, deficiencies in verbal and nonverbal communication, and deficiencies in understanding the interpersonal relationship. ASD may not have been diagnosed earlier in childhood, depending on the level of disability, verbal skills, English as second language, cultural beliefs, and social demands on the child. Mild ASD is at times not diagnosed until during or after high school when social demands increase during early adulthood and compensatory behaviors or actions no longer suffice. Although the diagnosis can be made later in life, the symptoms must have been present during the early developmental period on retrospect.

All young children should be screened for the presence of ASD features as part of routine developmental assessment. In addition, several tools are available that can be used to screen for ASD in primary care or mental health settings (see Box 66.5 for examples); some are rated by the clinician, others by the caregivers.

If there are significant concerns on screening, the child should undergo a comprehensive diagnostic evaluation, often accomplished through a referral to a developmental specialist (e.g., in developmental pediatrics or mental health). This assessment would ideally occur in a multidisciplinary team and include medical, developmental, psychological, and mental health assessments.

Box 66.5 Selected Screening Tools for Autism Spectrum Disorder

Infant and toddler screening tools

- Infant Toddler Checklist (ITC) (In Communication and Symbolic Behavior Scale [CSBS] Developmental Profile)
- The Modified Checklist for Autism in Toddlers (M-CHAT)
- Ages and Stages Questionnaire (ASQ)

Adolescent and Adult Screening Tools

- Autism-Spectrum Quotient (AQ)
- Social Responsiveness Scale (SRS)

A frequently used assessment tool is the ADOS (Autism Diagnostic Observation Schedule), which is administered by trained clinicians. Diagnoses should specify whether impairments in intellect or language are present. A comprehensive medical evaluation for organic causes of ASD should be completed (see Box 66.6).

Differential Diagnosis

Differential diagnoses for ASD must be ruled out. Many medical conditions mimic or cause ASD (see Differential Diagnosis 66.2).

MANAGEMENT

ASD requires individualized treatment and referral, as no two patients with ASD are alike. History obtained from parents/caregivers and observation of the individual patient are critical.

Pharmacological Management

There is no pharmacological intervention for ASD. Psychotropic medications should be considered when there is comorbid mental illness or if there are specific

---

Box 66.6 Medical Evaluation of Suspected Autism Spectrum Disorder

- Complete physical examination
- Motor assessment
- Hearing assessment
- Vision assessment
- Sensory assessment
- Genetic testing (chromosomal microarray, whole-exome sequencing)
- Fragile X testing

Source: Hyman SL, Levy SE, Myers SM, et al. Identification, evaluation, and management of children with autism spectrum disorder. *Pediatrics*. 2020;145:e20193447.

Differential Diagnosis 66.2: Autism Spectrum Disorder

- Deafness
- Tic or movement disorder
- Attention deficit-hyperactivity disorder
- Selective mutism
- Social (pragmatic) communication disorder
- Language disorder
- Speech sound disorder
- Childhood-onset fluency disorder (stuttering)
- Stereotypic movement disorder
- Developmental coordination disorder or motor skill deficits
- Intellectual disability
- Schizophrenia
- Reactive attachment disorder
- Obsessive-compulsive disorder
- Fragile X syndrome
- Rett syndrome (when developmental regression is noted)
- Landau-Kleffner syndrome
- Tuberous sclerosis

problematic target symptoms to address, such as severe irritability or aggression, sleep disturbances, or hyperactivity. Two agents have been approved by the U.S. Food and Drug Administration for the treatment of irritability (often manifesting as severe tantrums or aggression): risperidone and aripiprazole. Other medications have off-label uses for various target symptoms (see Drugs Commonly Prescribed 66.2). Medications should be considered if behavioral interventions were ineffective or if symptoms are severe. Because of the communication difficulties of some patients with ASD, response to medication may be judged by caregivers.

Nonpharmacological Management

Educational and behavioral interventions have been shown to be effective for ASD and are first-line treatment options. Young children should be referred for early intervention services. The most frequently used behavioral intervention is applied behavioral analysis (ABA), in which functional analyses are undertaken when maladaptive behaviors occur so that behavioral techniques can be identified to promote the desired behavior.

Assessment of the level and ability of the individual's communication is critical. For individuals with minimal or absent verbal communication skills, forms of augmentative communication should be used, such as sign language, pictures, or communication boards. This augmented communication can be used for adults later in life, even when they were not introduced during childhood. Individuals with fluent speech may lose the ability to speak when particularly stressed, something that can happen in the primary care setting.

In addition, caregivers should be encouraged to speak with the school to discuss academic accommodations that may be beneficial, and they could consider requesting an evaluation for an individualized education program (IEP). Because individuals with ASD benefit most from structure and predictability, designing the school or workday to minimize disruptions can be beneficial. Consider the need to involve physical, occupational, and speech therapy. Finally, referral to a social skills program can help the patient develop and practice social pragmatic skills across the life span.

FOLLOW-UP AND REFERRAL

Because ASD is chronic and lifelong, the primary care provider plays an important role in developing and maintaining a long-term relationship with the patient and family/caregivers. Additionally, the needs of the patient and support people will change over time and as the individual develops. If the primary care clinician is a pediatric provider, plans around transition of care to an adult provider are crucial. As these patients approach adulthood, planning around vocational training and the ability to live independently become highlighted. The primary care provider should refer the patient to a multidisciplinary team for initial diagnostic assessment and support in management, and the provider should work in conjunction with this specialist team.

Patient Education: Autism Spectrum Disorders

Families and caregivers should be encouraged to access local and national resources for ASD, engage in support groups, link with other families, access medical and mental health care, and maintain close lines of communication with the school system. Some schools are overwhelmed and underfunded; consequently, some children are classified incorrectly and receive inappropriate interventions. Some caregivers are not aware of their rights when schools refuse to do special education evaluations, especially when the signs and symptoms of autism are not severe. Parents should request IEP assessments in writing, and by law the school needs to provide the assessment within a specified amount of time. There are laws and advocacy groups that can assist families with this process, and parents and clinicians should become familiar with educational advocates in the area. Parents can be referred to the Autism Speaks Website for further guidance on their rights, https://www.autismspeaks.org/.

INTELLECTUAL DISABILITY

Intellectual disability (ID), replacing the outdated term *mental retardation*, is present when there are deficits in intellectual and adaptive functioning. Determining the

Drugs Commonly Prescribed 66.2: Medications Used in the Treatment of Autism Spectrum Disorder

MEDICATION	INDICATION	ADVERSE REACTIONS AND PRESCRIBING CONSIDERATIONS
Second Generation Antipsychotics (SGAs)		
Risperidone (FDA approved)	Autism-associated irritability (including aggression, temper tantrums, self-injurious behavior, and quickly changing moods), bipolar disorder, disruptive behavior disorders, ADHD, Tourette's disorder, schizophrenia, delirium	• EPS (e.g., akathisia, dystonia, etc.) • Drowsiness • Parkinsonian-like syndrome (common in children) • Increase in LFTs • Metabolic syndrome • Hyperprolactinemia, gynecomastia • Galactorrhea • Cardiovascular effect including prolongation of the QTc interval
Aripiprazole (FDA approved)	Autism-associated irritability (including aggression, temper tantrums, self-injurious behavior, and quickly changing moods), bipolar disorder, disruptive behavior disorders, ADHD, Tourette's disorder, schizophrenia, delirium	• EPS (particularly akathisia) • Drooling • Drowsiness • Parkinsonian-like syndrome (common in children) • Metabolic syndrome • Cardiovascular effect
Olanzapine	Bipolar disorder (including acute mania), schizophrenia, acute agitation, anorexia nervosa, Tourette's disorder	• EPS • Cardiovascular effect • Drowsiness • Weight gain • Metabolic syndrome
Alpha-Agonists		
Clonidine	ADHD (particularly hyperactivity/impulsivity), disruptive behavior disorders, tic disorder, Tourette's disorder, hypertension, insomnia, anxiety	• Hypotension • Bradycardia • Drowsiness • Rebound hypertension • Epistaxis
Guanfacine	ADHD (particularly hyperactivity/impulsivity), tic disorder, Tourette's disorder, hypertension	• Hypotension • Bradycardia • Drowsiness • Increase in serum ALT • Skin rash
Melatonin		
Melatonin	Initial insomnia (difficulty falling asleep)	(Rare) headache, confusion, and fragmented sleep

Abbreviations: ADHD, attention deficit-hyperactivity disorder; ALT, alanine aminotransferase; ASD, autism spectrum disorder; CNS, central nervous system; EPS, extrapyramidal symptoms; FDA, Food and Drug Administration; LFTs, liver function tests; NMS, neuroleptic malignant syndrome; ODD, oppositional defiant disorder; SGAs, second generation antipsychotics.

presence of ID is important as it assists in the determination of the level of support that an individual requires. ID onset must be during the developmental period and has a range of severity. The severity of ID is specified in the *DSM-5-TR* and is based on adaptive functioning in three domains: conceptual, social, and practical. The conceptual domain encompasses language, reading, writing, and reasoning skills; social domain encompasses empathy, communication skills, and friendships; and the practical domain encompasses self-management in personal care, money, and jobs. The most common conditions associated with ID are Down syndrome, fragile X syndrome, and fetal alcohol syndrome.

EPIDEMIOLOGY AND CAUSES

The prevalence of ID is estimated to be 1% of the general population, with a significant proportion being males. The predominance of males being diagnosed with ID is thought to be related to the many X-linked genetic disorders that can cause ID. Individuals with ID are living longer than in the past, and most are living in the community rather than in institutional settings. Individuals with Down syndrome live, on average, twice as long as they did 25 years ago. Thus, the adult and family primary care clinician will be providing health care for increasing numbers of patients with ID. Prevalence rates vary for the differing severity levels of ID, with the estimated prevalence of severe ID being six in 1,000. Challenging behaviors are present in up to 10% of individuals with ID. ID is a diagnosis in and of itself, although it can be associated with many underlying conditions that need to be assessed for and treated appropriately. Comorbidity with medical, psychiatric, and neurodevelopmental conditions is common. In addition to treatment of the underlying cause of the ID, supports often need to be put in place in school, home, and the community to address the differences in learning and adaptability that these individuals have.

PATHOPHYSIOLOGY

Intellectual disability describes a syndrome rather than a discrete diagnostic entity. As such, there is no unifying pathophysiological mechanism to explain the intellectual deficits observed in patients. ID can be the result of in utero insults (including genetic, toxic/metabolic, environmental, and structural malformations), perinatal/delivery complications, or postnatal illness (including ischemia, infection, traumatic brain injury, or toxic/metabolic exposures) that impede normal neurological development, and subsequently, intellect. As ID can be associated with underlying medical causes, a comprehensive medical evaluation needs to be undertaken as part of the diagnostic process (see Box 66.7). Clinical evaluation and testing can determine as many as 70% of cases of ID. Primary care providers should consider referral to a medical geneticist and work closely with the geneticist in making the diagnosis.

CLINICAL PRESENTATION

The clinical presentation of ID varies across the severity spectrum. Many individuals with a more severe presentation will have delays in their motor, social, and language milestones, and these delays can be identified within the first 2 years of life. Milder levels of severity may not be identified until the school-age years. Patients with ID will present with varying deficits in cognitive and adaptive functioning, depending on the severity of the disability. See Table 66.1 for clinical features in the conceptual, social, and practical domains that appear with increasing severity of ID.

DIAGNOSTIC REASONING

There are two major diagnostic and classification systems for ID in the United States, the *DSM-5-TR* and the *American Association on Intellectual and Developmental Disabilities (AAIDD)*. The *DSM-5-TR* bases the diagnosis on severity, whereas the AAIDD bases the diagnosis on supports based on severity. Please see the *DSM-5-TR* criteria in the next section.

The diagnostic process includes diagnosing the ID and the underlying medical etiology, if one exists. To assess for the criteria, neuropsychological testing of cognition (in the form of intelligence quotient [IQ]) and adaptive functioning must be undertaken by a trained psychologist. Intellectual testing is often undertaken, using standardized, structured assessments (e.g., Wechsler Intelligence Scale for Children) to assess IQ. It is important to note that there are many challenges with using a standardized, norm-referenced test for individuals with ID, especially those affected on severe and profound levels.

Adaptive functioning is also often assessed, using standardized instruments, including the Vineland Adaptive Behavior Scale. Per *DSM-5-TR* criteria, intellectual deficits can be in the domains of problem-solving, planning, abstract thinking, judgment, academic learning, and learning from experience. Adaptive functioning deficits manifest in the activities of daily life, such as communication, school/occupational participation, and independent living.

Symptoms

The diagnosis of ID is based on *DSM-5-TR* criteria; please refer to the *DSM-5-TR* for complete diagnostic criteria. Although patients can present at any age, onset

---

Box 66.7 Evaluation for Medical Etiology of Intellectual Disability

- Complete medical history, including a family history spanning three generations
- Complete physical examination, including assessment for dysmorphic features and a neurological examination
- Lead poisoning
- Genetics referral for consideration of:
  - Chromosomal microarray
  - Karyotype
  - Screening for inborn errors of metabolism
  - Testing for X-linked genetic disorders in boys, particularly fragile X syndrome
  - Testing for *MECP2* gene mutation in females to rule out Rett syndrome
- Neuroimaging

Source: Huang J, Zhu T, Qu Y, et al. Prenatal, perinatal and neonatal risk factors for intellectual disability: A systemic review and meta-analysis. *PLoS One.* 2016;11:e0153655.

TABLE 66.1 Severity Levels for Intellectual Disability

Severity	Conceptual Domain	Social Domain	Practical Domain
Mild	• Difficulties learning academic skills • Impaired abstract thinking, executive functioning, or short-term memory	• Immature in social interactions and judgment • Concrete use of language and communication	• Functions well in personal care • Needs support in independent ADLs • Can excel in jobs that do not require conceptual skills
Moderate	• Language and academic skills markedly lagging behind peers • Ongoing support needed into adulthood to manage day-to-day tasks	• Spoken language simpler than peers' • May misperceive social cues • Limited decision-making abilities	• With support, can manage ADLs and household tasks by adulthood • Considerable support required in employment
Severe	• Little understanding of written language or numbers • Limited attainment of conceptual skills	• Speech that consists of single words or phrases • Understands simple language and gestures	• Support required for all ADLs • Cannot make responsible decisions regarding well-being
Profound	• Can use objects in a goal-directed way • Little understanding of conceptual processes • Motor or sensory impairments possibly present	• Very limited understanding of symbolic communication • Mostly uses nonverbal communication and gestures	• Dependent on others for all aspects of daily care and recreational activities

Abbreviation: ADLs, activities of daily living.
Source: Patel DR, Apple R, Kanungo S, et al. Intellectual disability: definitions, evaluation and principles of treatment. *Pediatr Med.* 2018;1:11.

of symptoms must be during the developmental period. Common symptoms include:

- Intellectual deficits, such as reasoning, problem-solving, planning, and abstract thinking, based on clinical assessment and testing
- Deficits in adaptive functioning occurring across multiple environments that limit the patient's ability to successfully perform their activities of daily living

Differential Diagnosis

In addition to diagnosis of the ID itself, a diagnostic assessment for underlying etiologies must be undertaken. Some children will present with characteristic physical features (e.g., Down syndrome) or behavioral features (e.g., Lesch-Nyhan syndrome) of the underlying cause. Discerning if children had a period of normal development prior to onset of symptoms will also help narrow the differential diagnosis (see Differential Diagnosis 66.3). Assessment of comorbid mental illness should be undertaken as well (see Box 66.8).

> **Differential Diagnosis 66.3: Intellectual Disability**
>
> - Down syndrome
> - Fragile X syndrome
> - Fetal alcohol syndrome
> - Autism spectrum disorder
> - Duchenne muscular dystrophy
> - Lesch-Nyhan syndrome
> - Rett syndrome
> - Inborn errors of metabolism
> - Structural brain malformations
> - Maternal disease during the prenatal period
> - Encephalopathy
> - Hypoxic ischemic brain injury
> - Traumatic brain injury
> - Infections (e.g., meningitis, encephalitis)
> - Seizure disorders
> - Toxic metabolic syndromes
> - Cerebral palsy

MANAGEMENT

Pharmacological Management

There are no medications indicated for the treatment of ID. Treatment should be directed at any underlying or comorbid medical or psychiatric conditions. Challenging or dangerous behavior that is not responsive to behavioral or psychosocial interventions can be managed in a way similar to that described earlier for ASD. Off-label use of alpha-agonists (such as guanfacine and clonidine) or atypical antipsychotics (such as risperidone and aripiprazole) can be useful in managing challenging behaviors but should often be reserved for use only if there is a comorbid mental illness that would indicate use of these agents, given the risk of side effects.

meta-analysis of resting-state functional connectivity. *Psychological medicine*, *49*(15), 2475–2485. https://doi.org/10.1017/S003329171900237X

Gomez R, Corr PJ. (2014). ADHD and personality: a meta-analytic review. *Clinical psychology review*, *34*(5), 376–388. https://doi.org/10.1016/j.cpr.2014.05.002

Gossé LK, Bell SW, Hosseini SMH. (2021). Functional near-infrared spectroscopy in developmental psychiatry: a review of attention deficit hyperactivity disorder. *European archives of psychiatry and clinical neuroscience*, 10.1007/s00406-021-01288-2. Advance online publication. https://doi.org/10.1007/s00406-021-01288-2

Graziano PA, Garcia A. (2016). Attention-deficit hyperactivity disorder and children's emotion dysregulation: A meta-analysis. *Clinical psychology review*, *46*, 106–123. https://doi.org/10.1016/j.cpr.2016.04.011

Harrison AG, Nay S, Armstrong IT. Diagnostic accuracy of the Conners' adult ADHD Rating Scale in a postsecondary population. *J Atten Disord*. 2016. https://doi.org/10.1177%2F1087054715625299.

Hart H, Radua J, Nakao T, et al. Meta-analysis of functional magnetic resonance imaging studies of inhibition and attention in attention-deficit/hyperactivity disorder: Exploring task specific, stimulant medication, and age effects. *JAMA Psychiatry*. 2013; 70:185–198.

Hauser TU, Iannaccone R, Ball J, et al. Role of the medial prefrontal cortex in impaired decision making in juvenile attention-deficit/hyperactivity disorder. *JAMA Psychiatry*. 2014; 71:1165–1173.

Huang H, Huang H, Spottswood M, et al. (2020). Approach to Evaluating and Managing Adult Attention-Deficit/Hyperactivity Disorder in Primary Care. *Harvard review of psychiatry*, *28*(2), 100–106. https://doi.org/10.1097/HRP.0000000000000248

Katzman MA, Bilkey TS, Chokka PR, et al. Adult ADHD and comorbid disorders: clinical implications of a dimensional approach. *BMC Psychiatry* 17, 302 (2017). https://doi.org/10.1186/s12888-017-1463-3

Kim JH, Kim JY, Lee J, et al. (2020). Environmental risk factors, protective factors, and peripheral biomarkers for ADHD: an umbrella review. *The Lancet. Psychiatry*, *7*(11), 955–970. https://doi.org/10.1016/S2215-0366(20)30312-6

Klein M, Walters RK, Demontis D, et al. (2019). Genetic Markers of ADHD-Related Variations in Intracranial Volume. *The American journal of psychiatry*, *176*(3), 228–238. https://doi.org/10.1176/appi.ajp.2018.18020149

Leahy LG. (2018). Diagnosis and treatment of ADHD in children vs adults: What nurses should know. *Archives of psychiatric nursing*, *32*(6), 890–895. https://www.doi.org/10.1016/j.apnu.2018.06.013

McCarthy H, Skokauskas N, Frodl T. Identifying a consistent pattern of neural function in attention deficit hyperactivity disorder: A meta-analysis. *Psychol Med*. 2014; 44:869–880.

Mechler K, Banaschewski T, Hohmann S, et al. (2021). Evidence-based pharmacological treatment options for ADHD in children and adolescents. *Pharmacology & therapeutics*, 107940. Advance online publication. https://doi.org/10.1016/j.pharmthera.2021.107940

Moriyama TS, Polanczyk GV, Terzi FS, et al. Psychopharmacology and psychotherapy for the treatment of adults with ADHD—a systematic review of available meta-analyses. *CNS Spectr*. 2013; 18:296–306.

MTA Cooperative Group. Moderators and mediators of treatment response for children with attention-deficit/hyperactivity disorder: The Multimodal Treatment Study of children with attention-deficit/hyperactivity disorder. *Arch Gen Psychiatry*. 1999;56(12):1088–1096. https://www.researchgate.net/publication/236585378_Moderators_and_mediators_of_treatment_response_for_children_with_Attention-Deficit_Hyperactivity_Disorder. Accessed February 19, 2018.

Musser ED, Raiker JS Jr. (2019). Attention-deficit/hyperactivity disorder: An integrated developmental psychopathology and Research Domain Criteria (RDoC) approach. *Comprehensive psychiatry*, *90*, 65–72. https://doi.org/10.1016/j.comppsych.2018.12.016

Nimmo-Smith V, Merwood A, Hank D, et al. (2020). Non-pharmacological interventions for adult ADHD: a systematic review. *Psychological medicine*, *50*(4), 529–541. https://doi.org/10.1017/S0033291720000069

Pelsser LM, Frankena K, Toorman J, et al. (2017). Diet and ADHD, Reviewing the Evidence: A Systematic Review of Meta-Analyses of Double-Blind Placebo-Controlled Trials Evaluating the Efficacy of Diet Interventions on the Behavior of Children with ADHD. *PloS One*, *12*(1), e0169277. https://doi.org/10.1371/journal.pone.0169277

Pollak Y, Dekkers TJ, Shoham R, et al. (2019). Risk-Taking Behavior in Attention Deficit/Hyperactivity Disorder (ADHD): a Review of Potential Underlying Mechanisms and of Interventions. *Current psychiatry reports*, *21*(5), 33. https://doi.org/10.1007/s11920-019-1019-y

Rigler T, Manor I, Kalansky A, et al. New *DSM-5* criteria for ADHD—Does it matter? *Compr Psychiatry*. 2016;68:56–59.

Ross MM, Arria AM, Brown JP, et al. College students' perceived benefit-to-risk tradeoffs for nonmedical use of prescription stimulants: Implications for intervention designs. *Addict Behav*. 2018;79:45–51

Shaw P, Malek M, Watson B, et al. Development of cortical surface area and gyrification in attention-deficit/hyperactivity disorder. *Biol Psychiatry*. 2012; 72(3): 191-197.

Shaw P, Sudre G. (2021). Adolescent Attention-Deficit/Hyperactivity Disorder: Understanding Teenage Symptom Trajectories. *Biological psychiatry*, *89*(2), 152–161. https://doi.org/10.1016/j.biopsych.2020.06.004

Spencer TJ, Brown A, Seidman LJ, et al. Effect of psychostimulants on brain structure and function in ADHD: A qualitative literature review of magnetic resonance imaging-based neuroimaging studies. *J Clin Psychiatry*. 2013;74:902–917.

Storebø OJ, Elmose Andersen M, Skoog M, et al. (2019). Social skills training for attention deficit hyperactivity disorder (ADHD) in children aged 5 to 18 years. *The Cochrane database of systematic reviews*, *6*(6), CD008223. https://doi.org/10.1002/14651858.CD008223.pub3

Thomas R, Sanders S, Doust J, et al. Prevalence of attention-deficit/hyperactivity disorder: a systematic review and meta-analysis. *Pediatrics*. 2015 Apr;135(4):994-100.

Ustun B, Adler LA, Rudin C, et al. The World Health Organization adult attention-deficit/hyperactivity disorder self-report screening scale for *DSM-5*. *JAMA Psychiatry*. 2017;74:520–526.

van der Burg D, Crunelle CL, Matthys F, et al. (2019). Diagnosis and treatment of patients with comorbid substance use disorder and adult attention-deficit and hyperactivity disorder: a review of recent publications. *Current opinion in psychiatry*, *32*(4), 300–306. https://doi.org/10.1097/YCO.0000000000000513

Wilens TE, Kaminski TA. (2019). Prescription Stimulants: From Cognitive Enhancement to Misuse. *Pediatric clinics of North America*, *66*(6), 1109–1120. https://doi.org/10.1016/j.pcl.2019.08.006

Wolraich ML, Hagan JF, Allan C, et al. Subcommittee on Children and Adolescents with Attention-Deficit/Hyperactive Disorder. Clinical Practice Guideline for the Diagnosis, Evaluation, and Treatment of Attention-Deficit/Hyperactivity Disorder in Children and Adolescents. *Pediatrics*. 2019;144(4):e20192528 - March 01, 2020.

Yadav SK, Bhat AA, Hashem S, et al. (2021). Genetic variations influence brain changes in patients with attention-deficit hyperactivity disorder. *Translational psychiatry*, 11(1), 349. https://doi.org/10.1038/s41398-021-01473-w

Ziegler S, Pedersen ML, Mowinckel AM, et al. (2016). Modelling ADHD: A review of ADHD theories through their predictions for computational models of decision-making and reinforcement learning. *Neuroscience and biobehavioral reviews*, 71, 633–656. https://doi.org/10.1016/j.neubiorev.2016.09.002

Autism Spectrum Disorder

American Psychiatric Association. *Diagnostic and statistical manual of mental disorders*. 5th ed. Arlington, VA: American Psychiatric Association; 2013.

Antshel KM, Polacek C, McMahon M, et al. Comorbid ADHD and anxiety affect social skills group intervention treatment efficacy in children with autism spectrum disorders. *J Dev Behav Pediatr*. 2011;32:439–446.

Bearss K, Johnson C, Smith T, et al. Effect of parent training vs parent education on behavioral problems in children with autism spectrum disorder: A randomized clinical trial. *JAMA*. 2015;313:1524.

Cândido RCF, Menezes de Padua CA, Golder S, et al. (2021). Immediate-release methylphenidate for attention deficit hyperactivity disorder (ADHD) in adults. *The Cochrane database of systematic reviews*, 1(1), CD013011. https://doi.org/10.1002/14651858.CD013011.pub2

Ching H, Pringsheim T. Aripiprazole for autism spectrum disorders (ASD). *Cochrane Database Syst Rev*. 2012;(5):CD009043.

Dellapiazza F, Vernhet C, Blanc N, et al. (2018). Links between sensory processing, adaptive behaviours, and attention in children with autism spectrum disorder: A systematic review. *Psychiatry research*, 270, 78–88. https://doi.org/10.1016/j.psychres.2018.09.023

Estes A, Munson J, Rogers SJ, et al. Long-term outcomes of early intervention in 6-year-old children with autism spectrum disorder. *J Am Acad Child Adolesc Psychiatry*. 2015;54:580–587.

Farmer C, Thurm A, Grant P. Pharmacotherapy for the core symptoms in autistic disorder: current status of the research. *Drugs*. 2013;73:303–314.

Goel R, Hong JS, Findling RL, et al. (2018). An update on pharmacotherapy of autism spectrum disorder in children and adolescents. *International review of psychiatry (Abingdon, England)*, 30(1), 78–95. https://doi.org/10.1080/09540261.2018.1458706

Gringras P, Nir T, Breddy J, et al. Efficacy and safety of pediatric prolonged-release melatonin for insomnia in children with autism spectrum disorder. *J Am Acad Child Adolesc Psychiatry*. 2017;56:948–957.

Guénolé F, Godbout R, Nicolas A, et al. Melatonin for disordered sleep in individuals with autism spectrum disorders: Systematic review and discussion. *Sleep Med Rev*. 2011;15:379–387.

Händel MN, Rohde JF, Rimestad ML, et al. (2021). Efficacy and Safety of Polyunsaturated Fatty Acids Supplementation in the Treatment of Attention Deficit Hyperactivity Disorder (ADHD) in Children and Adolescents: A Systematic Review and Meta-Analysis of Clinical Trials. *Nutrients*, 13(4), 1226. https://doi.org/10.3390/nu13041226

Harfterkamp M, van de Loo-Neus G, Minderaa RB, et al. A randomized double-blind study of atomoxetine versus placebo for attention-deficit/hyperactivity disorder symptoms in children with autism spectrum disorder. *J Am Acad Child Adolesc Psychiatry*. 2012;51:733–741.

Hazlett HC, Gu H, Munsell BC, et al. Early brain development in infants at high risk for autism spectrum disorder. *Nature*. 2017;542:348–351.

Huffman LC, Sutcliffe TL, Tanner IS, et al. Management of symptoms in children with autism spectrum disorders: A comprehensive review of pharmacologic and complementary-alternative medicine treatments. *J Dev Behav Pediatr*. 2011;32:56–68.

Hyman SL, Levy SE, Myers SM, Council on Children With Disabilities, Section on Developmental and Behavioral Pediatrics. Identification, evaluation, and management of children with autism spectrum disorder. *Pediatrics*. 2020;145:e20193447.

Kasari C, Kaiser A, Goods K, et al. Communication interventions for minimally verbal children with autism: A sequential multiple assignment randomized trial. *J Am Acad Child Adolesc Psychiatry*. 2014;53:635–646.

Kasari C, Lawton K, Shih W, et al. Caregiver-mediated intervention for low-resourced preschoolers with autism: An RCT. *Pediatrics*. 2014;134:e72–e79.

Kasari C, Rotheram-Fuller E, Locke J, et al. Making the connection: Randomized controlled trial of social skills at school for children with autism spectrum disorders. *J Child Psychol Psychiatry*. 2012;53:431–439.

Landa RJ, Gross AL, Stuart EA, et al. Developmental trajectories in children with and without autism spectrum disorders: The first 3 years. *Child Dev*. 2013;84:429–442.

Landa RJ, Holman KC, O'Neill AH, Stuart EA. Intervention targeting development of socially synchronous engagement in toddlers with autism spectrum disorder: A randomized controlled trial. *J Child Psychol Psychiatry*. 2011;52:13–21.

Maenner MJ, Shaw KA, Baio J, et al. Prevalence of Autism Spectrum Disorder Among Children Aged 8 Years—Autism and Developmental Disabilities Monitoring Network, 11 Sites, United States, 2016 [published correction appears in MMWR Morb Mortal Wkly Rep. 2020 Apr 24;69(16):503]. *MMWR Surveill Summ*. 2020;69(4):1-12. Published 2020 Mar 27. doi:10.15585/mmwr.ss6904a1

McElhanon BO, McCracken C, Karpen S, et al. Gastrointestinal symptoms in autism spectrum disorder: A meta-analysis. *Pediatrics*. 2014;133:872–883.

McGuire K, Fung LK, Hagopian L, et al. Irritability and problem behavior in autism spectrum disorder: A practice pathway for pediatric primary care. *Pediatrics*. 2016;137(suppl 2):S136–S148.

Miller M, Iosif AM, Hill M, et al. Response to name in infants developing autism spectrum disorder: A prospective study. *J Pediatr*. 2017;183:141–146.

Myers SM, Voigt RG, Colligan RC, et al. Autism spectrum disorder: Incidence and time trends over two decades in a population-based birth cohort. *J Autism Dev Disord*. 2019;49:1455–1474. https://doi.org/10.1007/s10803-018-3834-0

Oono IP, Honey EJ, McConachie H. Parent-mediated early intervention for young children with autism spectrum disorders (ASD). *Cochrane Database Syst Rev*. 2013;(4):CD009774.

Orefice L. L. (2020). Peripheral Somatosensory Neuron Dysfunction: Emerging Roles in Autism Spectrum Disorders. *Neuroscience*, 445, 120–129. https://doi.org/10.1016/j.neuroscience.2020.01.039

Ozonoff S, Iosif AM, Young GS, et al. Onset patterns in autism: Correspondence between home video and parent report. *J Am Acad Child Adolesc Psychiatry*. 2011;50:796–806.

Pacia C, Holloway J, Gunning C, et al. (2021). A Systematic Review of Family-Mediated Social Communication Interventions for Young Children with Autism. *Review journal of autism and developmental disorders*, 1–27. Advance online publication. https://doi.org/10.1007/s40489-021-00249-8

Pearson DA, Santos CW, Aman MG, et al. Effects of extended release methylphenidate treatment on ratings of attention-deficit/hyperactivity disorder (ADHD) and associated behavior in children with autism spectrum disorders and ADHD symptoms. *J Child Adolesc Psychopharmacol.* 2013;23:337–351.

Pickles A, Le Couteur A, Leadbitter K, et al. Parent-mediated social communication therapy for young children with autism (PACT): Long-term follow-up of a randomised controlled trial. *Lancet.* 2016;388:2501–2509.

Reichow B, Steiner AM, Volkmar F. Social skills groups for people aged 6 to 21 with autism spectrum disorders (ASD). *Cochrane Database Syst Rev.* 2013;8(2):266–315.

Robberecht H, Verlaet AAJ, Breynaert A, et al. (2020). Magnesium, Iron, Zinc, Copper and Selenium Status in Attention-Deficit/Hyperactivity Disorder (ADHD). *Molecules (Basel, Switzerland), 25*(19), 4440. https://doi.org/10.3390/molecules25194440

Saint-Georges C, Mahdhaoui A, Chetouani M, et al. Do parents recognize autistic deviant behavior long before diagnosis? Taking into account interaction using computational methods. *PLoS One.* 2011;6(7):e22393.

Scahill L, McCracken JT, King BH, et al. Extended-release guanfacine for hyperactivity in children with autism spectrum disorder. *Am J Psychiatry.* 2015;172:1197–1206.

Section on Complementary and Integrative Medicine; Council on Children With Disabilities; American Academy of Pediatrics, Zimmer M, Desch L. Sensory integration therapies for children with developmental and behavioral disorders. *Pediatrics.* 2012;129(6):1186–1189.

Siemann JK, Veenstra-VanderWeele J, Wallace MT. (2020). Approaches to Understanding Multisensory Dysfunction in Autism Spectrum Disorder. *Autism research.* 13(9):1430–1449. https://doi.org/10.1002/aur.2315

Solomon R, Van Egeren LA, Mahoney G, et al. PLAY Project Home Consultation intervention program for young children with autism spectrum disorders: A randomized controlled trial. *J Dev Behav Pediatr.* 2014;35:475–485.

Storebø OJ, Ramstad E, Krogh HB, et al. Methylphenidate for children and adolescents with attention deficit hyperactivity disorder (ADHD). *Cochrane Database Syst Rev.* 2015;(11):CD009885.

Thurm A, Manwaring SS, Luckenbaugh DA, et al. Patterns of skill attainment and loss in young children with autism. *Dev Psychopathol.* 2017;26:212–222.

Volkmar F, Siegel M, Woodbury-Smith M, et al. Practice parameter for the assessment and treatment of children and adolescents with autism spectrum disorder. *J Am Acad Child Adolesc Psychiatry.* 2014;53:237–257.

Wang X, Zhao J, Huang S, et al. (2021). Cognitive Behavioral Therapy for Autism Spectrum Disorders: A Systematic Review. *Pediatrics, 147*(5), e2020049880. https://doi.org/10.1542/peds.2020-049880

Warren Z, Veenstra-VanderWeele J, Stone W, et al. Therapies for children with autism spectrum disorders. Rockville, MD: Agency for Healthcare Research and Quality; 2011.

Weitlauf AS, Sathe N, McPheeters ML, et al. Interventions targeting sensory challenges in autism spectrum disorder: A systematic review. *Pediatrics.* 2017;139.

World Health Organization. The ICD-10 classification of mental and behavioural disorders. Clinical descriptions and diagnostic guidelines. https://apps.who.int/iris/handle/10665/37958. Accessed April 27, 2022.

Yates K, Le Couteur A. (2016). Diagnosing autism/autism spectrum disorders. *Paediatrics and Child Health. 26*(12), 513–518. https://doi.org/10.1016/j.paed.2016.08.004

Intellectual Disabilities

Abrahamson EE, Head E, Lott IT, et al. (2019). Neuropathological correlates of amyloid PET imaging in Down syndrome. *Developmental neurobiology, 79*(7), 750–766. https://doi.org/10.1002/dneu.22713

Anderson LL, Larson SA, MapelLentz S, et al. (2019). A Systematic Review of U.S. Studies on the Prevalence of Intellectual or Developmental Disabilities Since 2000. *Intellectual and developmental disabilities, 57*(5), 421–438. https://doi.org/10.1352/1934-9556-57.5.421

Benevides TW, Shore SM, Andresen ML, et al. (2020). Interventions to address health outcomes among autistic adults: A systematic review. *Autism: the international journal of research and practice, 24*(6), 1345–1359. https://doi.org/10.1177/1362361320913664

CDC response to Advisory Committee on Childhood Lead Poisoning Prevention Recommendations. Low level lead exposure harms children: A renewed call of primary prevention. https://www.cdc.gov/nceh/lead/acclpp/cdc_response_lead_exposure_recs.pdf. Accessed April 27, 2022.

Cipriani G, Danti S, Carlesi C., et al. (2018). Aging With Down Syndrome: The Dual Diagnosis: Alzheimer's Disease and Down Syndrome. *American journal of Alzheimer's disease and other dementias, 33*(4), 253–262. https://doi.org/10.1177/1533317518761093

Glover G, Bernard S, Branford D, et al. Use of medication for challenging behaviour in people with intellectual disability. *Br J Psychiatry.* 2014;205:6–7.

Hoffman-Zacharska D, Kmieć T, Poznański J, et al. Mutations in the PLP1 gene residue p. Gly198 as the molecular basis of Pelizeaus-Merzbacher phenotype. *Brain Dev.* 2013;35:877–885.

Hoffman-Zacharska D, Mierzewska H, Szczepanik E, et al. The spectrum of PLP1 gene mutations in patients with the classical form of the Pelizeaus-Merzbacher disease. *Med Wieku Rozwoj.* 2013;17:293–300.

Huang J, Zhu T, Qu Y, et al. Prenatal, perinatal and neonatal risk factors for intellectual disability: A systemic review and meta-analysis. *PLoS One.* 2016;11(4):e0153655.

Jarjour IT. Neurodevelopmental outcome after extreme prematurity: A review of the literature. *Pediatr Neurol.* 2015;52:143–152.

Jensen KM, Bulova PD. Managing the care of adults with Down's syndrome. *BMJ.* 2014;349:g5596.

McCarron M, Lombard-Vance R, Murphy E, et al. (2019). Effect of deinstitutionalisation on quality of life for adults with intellectual disabilities: a systematic review. *BMJ open, 9*(4), e025735. https://doi.org/10.1136/bmjopen-2018-025735

McCarron M, McCallion P, Coppus A, et al. (2018). Supporting advanced dementia in people with Down syndrome and other intellectual disability: consensus statement of the International Summit on Intellectual Disability and Dementia. *Journal of intellectual disability research: JIDR, 62*(7), 617–624. https://doi.org/10.1111/jir.12500

McCormick F, Marsh L, Taggart L, et al. (2020). Experiences of adults with intellectual disabilities accessing acute hospital services: A systematic review of the international evidence. *Health & social care in the community,* 10.1111/hsc.13253. Advance online publication. https://doi.org/10.1111/hsc.13253

McQuire C, Hassiotis A, Harrison B, et al. (2015). Pharmacological interventions for challenging behaviour in children with intellectual disabilities: a systematic review and meta-analysis. *BMC psychiatry, 15,* 303. https://doi.org/10.1186/s12888-015-0688-2

Moeschler JB, Shevell M, Committee on Genetics. Comprehensive evaluation of the child with intellectual disability or global developmental delays. *Pediatrics.* 2014;134(3):e903–e918.

Moran JA, Rafi MS, Keller SM, et al. The National Task Group on Intellectual Disabilities and Dementia Practices consensus recommendations for the evaluation and management of dementia in adults with intellectual disabilities. *Mayo Clin Proc.* 2013;88: 831–840.

Nevala N, Pehkonen I, Teittinen A, et al. (2019). The Effectiveness of Rehabilitation Interventions on the Employment and Functioning of People with Intellectual Disabilities: A Systematic Review. *Journal of occupational rehabilitation*, 29(4), 773–802. https://doi.org/10.1007/s10926-019-09837-2

Patel DR, Apple R, Kanungo S, et al. Intellectual disability: definitions, evaluation and principles of treatment. *Pediatr Med.* 2018;1:11.

Scott Schwoerer J, Laffin J, Haun J, et al. MECP2 duplication: Possible cause of severe phenotype in females. *Am J Med Genet A.* 2014;164A:1029–1034.

Toth K, de Lacy N, King BH. Intellectual Disability. In: M Dulcan Editor (Eds.) Dulcan's textbook of child and adolescent psychiatry. American Psychiatric Association Publishing. 2016.

van de Kamp JM, Betsalel OT, Mercimek-Mahmutoglu S, et al. Phenotype and genotype in 101 males with X-linked creatine transporter deficiency. *J Med Genet.* 2013;50:463–472.

Tic Disorder

Albanese A, Bhatia K, Bressman SB, et al. Phenomenology and classification of dystonia: a consensus update. *Mov Disord.* 2013;28:863–873.

Albanese A, Jankovic J. Distinguishing clinical features of hyperkinetic disorders. In: Albanese A, Jankovic J, eds. *Hyperkinetic movement disorders.* Oxford: Wiley-Blackwell; 2012:3.

Baizabal-Carvallo JF, Jankovic J. Movement disorders in autoimmune diseases. *Mov Disord.* 2012;27:935–946.

Baizabal-Carvallo JF, Stocco A, Muscal E, et al. The spectrum of movement disorders in children with anti-NMDA receptor encephalitis. *Mov Disord.* 2013;28:543–547.

Cavanna AE, Ganos C, Hartmann A, et al. (2020). The cognitive neuropsychiatry of Tourette syndrome. *Cognitive neuropsychiatry*, 25(4), 254–268. https://doi.org/10.1080/13546805.2020.1760812

Cohen SC, Mulqueen JM, Ferracioli-Oda E, et al. Meta-Analysis: Risk of Tics Associated With Psychostimulant Use in Randomized, Placebo-Controlled Trials. *J Am Acad Child Adolesc Psychiatry.* 2015 Sep;54(9):728-36.

Conte G, Valente F, Fiorello F, et al. (2020). Rage attacks in Tourette Syndrome and Chronic Tic Disorder: a systematic review. *Neuroscience and biobehavioral reviews*, 119, 21–36. https://doi.org/10.1016/j.neubiorev.2020.09.019

Deng H, Gao K, Jankovic J. The genetics of Tourette syndrome. *Nat Rev Neurol.* 2012;8:203–213.

Hacohen Y, Dlamini N, Hedderly T, et al. N-methyl-D-aspartate receptor antibody-associated movement disorder without encephalopathy. *Dev Med Child Neurol.* 2015;56:190.

Hirschtritt ME, Lee PC, Pauls DL, et al, Tourette Syndrome Association International Consortium for Genetics. Lifetime prevalence, age of risk, and genetic relationships of comorbid psychiatric disorders in Tourette syndrome. *JAMA Psychiatry.* 2015 Apr;72(4):325-33.

Jankovic J. Medical treatment of dystonia. *Mov Disord.* 2013;28: 1001–1012.

Knight T, Steeves T, Day L, et al. Prevalence of tic disorders: a systematic review and meta-analysis. *Pediatr Neurol.* 2012 Aug; 47(2):77-90.

Mohammad SS, Fung VS, Grattan-Smith P, et al. Movement disorders in children with anti-NMDAR encephalitis and other autoimmune encephalopathies. *Mov Disord.* 2014;29:1539–1542.

Pauls DL, Fernandez TV, Mathews CA, et al. The inheritance of Tourette Disorder: A review. *J Obsessive Compuls Relat Disord.* 2014;3:380–385.

Scharf JM, Yu D, Mathews CA, et al. Genome-wide association study of Tourette's syndrome. *Mol Psychiatry.* 2013 Jun;18(6):721-8.

Singer HS, Mink JW, Gilbert DL, et al. *Movement disorders in childhood.* 2nd ed. Philadelphia, PA: Butterworth-Heinemann (Elsevier); 2015.

van Egmond ME, Kuiper A, Eggink H, et al. Dystonia in children and adolescents: A systematic review and a new diagnostic algorithm. *J Neurol Neurosurg Psychiatry.* 2015;86:774–781.

Yang C, Cheng X, Zhang Q, et al. (2020). Interventions for tic disorders: An updated overview of systematic reviews and meta analyses. *Psychiatry research*, 287, 112905. https://doi.org/10.1016/j.psychres.2020.112905

RESOURCES

Attention Deficit-Hyperactivity Disorder

Attention Deficit Hyperactivity Disorders: Diagnosis and Treatment in Children and Adolescents
https://effectivehealthcare.ahrq.gov/products/adhd-update/systematic-review-2018

AHRQ, Attention Deficit-Hyperactivity Disorder Information Page. National Institute of Neurological Disorders and Stroke
https://www.ninds.nih.gov/Disorders/All-Disorders/Attention-Deficit-Hyperactivity-Disorder-Information-Page

Attention-Deficit Hyperactivity Disorder: Overview, Symptoms, Causes, Diagnosis, Treatment, and Resources. American Academy of Family Physicians
https://familydoctor.org/condition/attention-deficit-hyperactivity-disorder-adhd/?adfree=true

Bright Futures: What to Expect & When to Seek Help
https://www.brightfutures.org/tools/index.html

Children and Adults with Attention-Deficit/Hyperactivity Disorder (CHADD)
https://chadd.org/

College Students with ADHD. American Academy of Child and Adolescent Psychiatry
https://www.aacap.org/AACAP/Families_and_Youth/Facts_for_Families/FFF-Guide/College-Students-with-ADHD-111.aspx

Autism Spectrum Disorder

AASPIRE Healthcare Toolkit: Primary Care Resources for Adults on the Autism Spectrum and their Primary Care Providers
https://autismandhealth.org/

Autism. Healthy Children.org.
https://www.healthychildren.org/English/health-issues/conditions/Autism/Pages/default.aspx

Autism Resource Center. American Academy of Child and Adolescent Psychiatry
http://www.aacap.org/AACAP/Families_and_Youth/Resource_Centers/Autism_Resource_Center/Home

Autism Society
http://www.autism-society.org/

Autism Speaks
https://www.autismspeaks.org/

Intellectual Disability

American Association on Intellectual and Developmental Disabilities
https://www.aaidd.org/

Children with Intellectual Disabilities. American Academy of Pediatrics and Healthy Children.Org
https://www.healthychildren.org/English/health-issues/conditions/developmental-disabilities/Pages/Intellectual-Disability.aspx

Fact Sheet on Intellectual Disability. Center for Parent Information & Resources
http://www.parentcenterhub.org/intellectual/

Individuals with Disabilities Education Act
https://sites.ed.gov/idea/

Intellectual Disabilities: Facts for Families Guide. American Academy of Child & Adolescent Psychiatry
https://www.aacap.org/AACAP/Families_and_Youth/Facts_for_Families/FFF-Guide/Children-with-an-Intellectual-Disability-023.aspx

Intellectual Disabilities. National Institute of Child Health and Human Development
https://www.nichd.nih.gov/health/topics/idds/conditioninfo/Pages/default.aspx

Tic Disorder

Tourette Association of America
http://www.tourette.org

Chapter 67

Substance-Related and Addictive Disorders

Jamie Lord, DNP, APRN, PMHNP-BC

Sean Convoy, DNP, PMHNP-BC

Karen Jennings Mathis, PhD, APRN-CNP, PMHNP-BC, FAED

Substance-use disorders (SUDs) affect millions of adolescents and adults in the United States, contributing heavily to the burden of morbidity and mortality. In 2020, related to the COVID-19 pandemic, the Centers for Disease Control and Prevention (CDC) data demonstrate significant increases in SUDs. There were approximately 20.3 million people in 2018, aged 12 and older, with an SUD related to alcohol or illicit drug in the past year, including 14.8 million individuals with alcohol-use disorder (AUD) and 8.1 million people with illicit drug-use disorder.

The *Diagnostic and Statistical Manual of Mental Disorders, 5th edition, Text Revision* (*DSM-5-TR*) defines an SUD as chronic, relapsing, compulsive use of a drug, varying from mild to severe. Additionally, the criteria for SUD consist of cravings for the substance, inability to decrease or stop use despite desire, taking more of the substance or for longer periods, neglecting other areas in life due to use, continuation of the substance despite consequences, and using the substance when it is unsafe. Denial and rationalization develop and promote continuation of the substance without regard to unexpected or dangerous consequences. The substance use creates a cluster of cognitive, behavioral, and physiological symptoms for the individual. These conditions have a dramatic effect on the lives of individuals, their families and partners, and society.

Types of SUDs that are frequently encountered in primary care settings include nicotine (covered in Chapter 33), alcohol, cannabis, hallucinogen, inhalant, opioid, sedative-hypnotic, anxiolytic, and stimulant-use disorders. Many times, a combination of disorders is present. Most individuals struggling with SUD do not receive treatment until the advanced stages of the disease, despite the existence of effective, evidence-based treatments. SUDs are psychiatric disorders requiring treatment, with primary prevention being an effective strategy to thwart their development. Primary care clinicians are in an ideal position to screen for alcohol and illicit substance-use problems because these conditions develop slowly, with the individual often initially presenting for medical concerns. It is critical that primary care providers recognize individuals at risk, tailor interventions, and provide education and referrals to prevent the development of an SUD. Accurate terminology for SUDs is detailed in Box 67.1. Risk factors for SUD include a history of trauma, chronic health problems, environmental factors, family history, social determinants, grief, and loss.

It is essential to introduce the potential for dual diagnosis, sometimes referred to as *co-occurring* or *comorbid conditions*. A dual diagnosis condition is defined as the active presence of both an SUD and another psychiatric disorder. Comorbidities are common in persons with SUD. The most common comorbidities are depressive disorders, bipolar disorders, anxiety disorders, antisocial personality disorder, borderline personality disorder, attention deficit-hyperactivity disorder, and schizophrenia.

> **Box 67.1 Terminology**
>
> **Intoxication:** A transient condition of altered consciousness and behavior with recent use of a substance. This process is considered reversible; as the effect of the substance wears off, a return to baseline generally occurs. Several symptoms of intoxication include impaired judgment and alertness along with psychomotor and behavioral changes.
>
> **Substance withdrawal:** Functional impairment related to the cessation or reduction of a substance; demonstrated in physiological, cognitive, and behavioral symptoms.
>
> **Substance use:** Sporadic or intermittent utilization of alcohol or drugs with no adverse consequences.
>
> **Substance abuse:** Utilization of drugs or alcohol that causes the individual some type of adverse consequence.
>
> **Substance dependence:** Involves physiological and/or psychological components.
>
> **Physical dependence:** The physiological effects of withdrawal from rapid dose reduction, abrupt cessation of the drug, or administration of an antagonist drug.
>
> **Psychological or behavioral dependence:** Pathological use patterns and substance-seeking activities; a subjective need for the substance.
>
> **Substance-use disorder:** A chronic illness characterized by impaired control, social impairment, and use despite significant consequences, tolerance, and withdrawal.
>
> **Tolerance:** The diminished response to a drug when a person uses a drug for a long time.

Source: Barnett AI, Hall W, Carter A. Substance use terminology. *JAMA*. 2017;317(7):769-770. https://doi.org/10.1001/jama.2016.20475

Pediatric/Adolescent Considerations: Substance-use Disorder

Substance use among teenagers is a growing concern. The most used substances are alcohol, marijuana, and tobacco. The CDC reports almost 67% of adolescents have tried alcohol by 12th grade, 50% have used marijuana, and 20% have used prescription medications without a prescription. In fact, 10% of all alcohol consumed in the United States is among individuals aged 12 to 20 years.

The risk of substance use among adolescents is significant. Risk factors include but are not limited to family history of substance use, parental substance use, family rejection of sexual orientation or gender identity, peers who use illicit substances or engage in delinquent behaviors, lack of school connectedness, childhood sexual abuse, and mental health issues. Moreover, substance use affects adolescents' growth and development, especially brain development. The brain is not fully developed until approximately age 25 years. Substance use overloads the brain with dopamine, which causes the reward system to send too many pleasurable feelings. As a result, the brain releases less dopamine in an attempt to balance the levels and damages neuronal connections, reducing the ability to experience pleasure. Substance use increases with other risky behaviors like unprotected sex and unsafe driving. Use of substances contributes to the formation of adult health issues such as high blood pressure, heart disease, and sleep problems. The earlier adolescents start using substances, the greater is their chances of continuing to use substances with an increase in dependency.

The advanced practice nurse is in an excellent position to talk to adolescent patients and support systems about avoiding and reducing substance use. Protective factors for high-risk substance use include parent or family engagement and support, parental disapproval of substance use, parental monitoring, and school connectedness. The following guide by the CDC provides information to implement screening for adolescent substance use and brief counseling in practice: https://www.cdc.gov/ncbddd/fasd/alcohol-screening.html.

Substance use is a risk factor for both fatal and nonfatal overdoses, suicide attempts, and death by suicide. Compared with the general population, individuals with alcohol dependence and persons who use illicit drugs have a 10- to 14-fold greater risk of death by suicide. The frequency of suicide among individuals in this group is second only to that among individuals with major depressive disorder. Many individuals with AUD or alcohol dependency may have an underlying depressive disorder, which increases the risk of death by suicide. The National Institute on Drug Abuse (2020) reported comorbidity of SUD and mental health issues is triggered by overlapping factors such as genetic and epigenetic vulnerabilities, issues with similar areas of the brain, and environmental influences such as early exposure to stress or trauma.

EPIDEMIOLOGY AND CAUSES

In the United States, among people aged 12 years and older, the percentage with an SUD within the past year remained stable between 2015 and 2019. In 2019, an estimated 20.4 million individuals aged 12 years and older met criteria for SUD and more than 70,000 Americans died from drug-involved overdose. However, only 4.2 million people received any substance-use treatment and 2.6 million received substance-use treatment at a specialty facility in the past year.

Unfortunately, there was an acceleration of overdose deaths during the COVID-19 pandemic such that more than 100,000 deaths occurred in the United States in the 12 months ending in April 2021. In the following sections, we provide information about the three most used substances: alcohol, cannabis, and opioids.

Alcohol

An estimated 14.1 million adults in the United States aged 18 years and older (5.6% of the age group) met criteria for AUD in 2019. This includes 8.9 million men (7.3 % in the age group) and 5.2 million women (4% in the age group). An additional 414,000 adolescents (ages 12 to 17) were diagnosed with AUD in 2019 (1.7% in the age group). Currently, AUD contributes to approximately 95,000 deaths a year and 31% of all traffic fatalities. The economic cost related to AUD is estimated to be $250 billion a year.

Females are affected by alcohol differently than males. Recommendations for daily alcohol use limits are lower for females than for males because females have less body water and slower alcohol metabolism. Studies demonstrate a positive association between trauma, negative life events, chronic stress, and vulnerability in developing AUD. Unfortunately, females have more exposure to high-impact trauma (e.g., sexual abuse) than males, increasing the risk of alcohol initiation and maintenance. Among heavy drinkers, females develop problems with alcohol at an accelerated rate and are at greater risk for heart muscle damage, brain damage, and cirrhosis than males. Females who are heavy drinkers also have an increased risk of miscarriage.

Risk factors for AUD include but are not limited to other psychiatric disorders, family history of AUD, and early age of alcohol use. The younger the age at drinking onset, the greater the chance that an individual will develop an AUD at some point in their life. Research suggests that the risk of AUD in adulthood *decreases* by 14% for each additional year of age drinking onset is delayed. Moreover, it is estimated that one in five adults in the United States lived with an individual with AUD during childhood. Unfortunately, children around adults with AUD are at increased risk for childhood abuse and developing AUD in adulthood.

Cannabis

Cannabis is the second most used psychotropic drug in the United States, after alcohol. An estimated 43.5 million Americans, aged 12 or older in 2018, used cannabis in the past year, corresponding to 15.9% of the population. The largest increase in use was among adolescents 12 years and older. One in 10 people who use cannabis will become dependent. When the individual starts before the age of 18 years, the rate of dependency escalates to 1 in 6. Cannabis is rapidly becoming more widely available in the United States, with at least 18 states legalizing recreational use and more for medicinal purposes. In the United States, cannabis remains an illegal substance under federal law.

Opioids

An estimated 1.7 million people in the United States suffer from opioid-use disorder (OUD) involving prescription opioid pain relievers and 652,000 suffer from a heroin-use disorder. Up to 29% of people prescribed opioids for chronic pain misuse the medication with 8% to 12% developing OUD. Stricter prescribing regulations and cost of opiates triggered an estimated 4% to 6% of patients to transition to heroin and fentanyl use. Up to 80% of individuals who use heroin first misused prescription opioids. The current national opioid health crisis in the United States involves an increase in opioid-related overdoses; neonatal abstinence syndrome; and the spread of infectious diseases like HIV, hepatitis B and C, tuberculosis, and serious bacterial infections related to intravenous opioid use. Additionally, the economic burden of opioid misuse is an estimated $78.5 billion per year, including medical care, lost productivity, addiction treatment, and criminal justice involvement. Social issues related to opioid use involve justice issues, interference with education and employment, loss of social functioning, and significant family/significant other distress.

Unfortunately, the COVID-19 pandemic has negatively affected the opioid crisis because stakeholders are focused on COVID-19; there is a lack of treatment infrastructure; and people have lost their jobs, are isolated from their supports, and are struggling with depression and anxiety—all risk factors for recurrence, lapses, and increased opioid use (Box 67.2).

Risks factors include other substance use disorders, externalizing traits (such as novelty-seeking and impulsivity), genetics, and various peer, family, and environmental factors. Pregnant females with OUD are more likely to seek prenatal care late in pregnancy, miss appointments, experience poor weight gain, or exhibit signs of withdrawal or intoxication. Prescription opioid misuse has become a leading cause of unintentional injury and death among adolescents and young adults. A study conducted with 7,374 high school seniors found that 12.9% of participants used opioids recreationally and 80% of these nonmedical uses originated from previous prescriptions. Misuse of opioids by adolescents aged 12 to 17 years in 2018 comprised 2.8% of the population with a 1% use of heroin. Opioid misuse in adolescents is strongly associated with later heroin use. Although unhealthy substance use by older adults is often overlooked, misuse of prescribed medications by older adults needs to be recognized as a serious public health concern.

There is a significant increase in unintentional opioid poisoning among adolescents. One in 13 high school seniors reported use in the past year of nonprescription opioids. Despite these increases in use, only a small percentage, less than 10%, receive treatment. The Academy of Pediatrics endorsed a policy recommending pediatricians offer medication-assisted treatment (MAT) for adolescents with OUD along with therapy (individual and family) as an integral part of treatment. Amid a shortage of treatment options for adolescents in many settings, primary care practices can provide effective care even without extensive resources to meet the needs of this population.

Box 67.2 The COVID-19 Pandemic and SUD

What happens when an epidemic meets a pandemic? The COVID-19 pandemic has caused an increase in opioid-related deaths. In the United States, by the fifth month into the pandemic, there was a record upsurge in opioid-related deaths with more than 40 states reporting up to a 50% increase. When stay-at-home orders began in many states to mitigate the spread of virus transmission, alcohol consumption increased significantly. The Nielsen ratings reported a 54% increase in national sales of alcohol for the week ending on March 21, 2020, compared with the year before; online sales increased by 262%. The World Health Organization sent a warning that alcohol use during the pandemic may potentially exacerbate health concerns and risk-taking behaviors. Individuals affected by SUDs are also higher risk for COVID-19 infection and related mortality.

Social and economic changes caused by the pandemic, along with the traditional difficulties regarding treatment access and adherence intensified. The economic recession caused isolation, unemployment, boredom, and emotional distress, triggering relapses and increases in use. Transportation to treatment facilities was already a barrier to many and amplified with public transportation being limited related to COVID-19 restrictions. Medicare responded by relaxing coverage to allow telemedicine implementation in the treatment of OUD. Telemedicine for mental health problems including SUDs took a more central role during the crisis, showing its feasibility and minimizing the risk of virus transmission while providing continuity of care. Telemedicine offers the promise of increased adherence to treatment, because several logistical barriers associated with physical attendance at treatment services are removed. Telemedicine made care more accessible and person-centered than before the pandemic, especially to rural populations.

Even if patients did not have computer access, most had phone capabilities to initiate or continue treatment. The stigma of being seen at a treatment facility was also removed with telemedicine. Research demonstrates telemedicine shows favorable results for reduction of alcohol use, depressive symptoms, and cost with increases in quality of life, patient satisfaction, and accessibility.

SAMHSA responded to the COVID-19 public health emergency by permitting stable patients in an outpatient treatment practice to receive 28 days of take-home doses of medications for OUD. Patients who are less stable could receive up to 14 days of medications, if the provider felt that the patient could manage this level of responsibility. Although such a response decreased the amount of travel to the clinics and less risk for exposure to the virus, the access to more medication may have been an impetus for misuse and diversion for some patients.

Support groups also moved to a virtual platform, which assisted some individuals in recovery. Other patients missed the social connections of in-person meetings. The lapse of support facilitated many relapses as their support system and coping skills diminished. Conversely, financial restrictions and reduced availability and higher prices of illicit drugs during the lockdowns have been well documented and may have reduced alcohol and drug use for some individuals.

Person-centered care was implemented during COVID-19 to best meet the needs of the patient. Patient preferences for fewer in-person visits and testing, easier access to receive treatment, and fewer prescribing restrictions are likely to have improved the quality of care. Despite the many challenges created by the COVID-19 pandemic, a unique opportunity emerged to update SUD treatment services.

Geriatric Considerations: Substance-use Disorders

Due to the physiological changes of aging and increased chronic medical disease, older adults are particularly vulnerable to overdose, especially when using other prescribed medications.

Older adults are at an increased risk of OUD and adverse effects. This growing population presents several challenges with ranges of complex mental and physical health disorders along with multiple medication use. Polypharmacy is common, with a risk for poor health outcomes, hospitalization, and mortality. Adverse drug reactions and drug interactions increase the risk of harm for this vulnerable population. Focus needs to be placed on universal screening of older adults for substance use and prescription drug misuse, to help minimize the use of opioids, sedatives, and tranquilizers. As primary care providers, you must be aware of the need to deprescribe potentially inappropriate medications for older adults who are at high risk for adverse events from prescription drug misuse. Patient education is necessary to inform patients of the risks of overdose from concurrent use of opioids and alcohol. Understanding prescription opioid misuse among older adults can inform providers of unique risks and the development of focused interventions.

PATHOPHYSIOLOGY

SUDs have diverse pathophysiological and symptomatic variation. This section will emphasize the unifying genetics and pathophysiology associated with SUDs, followed by a broader exploration into epigenetics, which informs a stress diathesis that summarizes the relative risk for developing an SUD.

Much progress has been made in identifying and weighing genomic vulnerability associated with SUD through the seminal work of the genome-wide association studies (GWAS), which illuminate the effect of genome sequencing and identified single nucleotide polymorphisms (SNPs). An SNP represents a single letter change in the genetic code between people. Although there are some recognized single-gene (or Mendelian) disorders (e.g., cystic fibrosis, sickle cell, fragile X syndrome, Huntington's disease), there are no recognized single-gene psychiatric or substance-related disorders. Our developing understanding of psychiatric disorders suggests that multiple SNPs interact with environmental variables during critical periods of development, which best explains the underlying pathophysiology. For example, a recent study has implicated varied SNPs (e.g., glucokinase regulatory protein or *GCKR*, Klotho beta or *KLB*, Alcohol Dehydrogenase 1B or *ADH1B*, Alcohol Dehydrogenase 1C or *ADH1C*, and Solute Carrier Family 39 Member 8 or *SLC39A8*) as being associated with an increased risk for developing AUD. Another example is in recent research that recognized SNPs of the butyrylcholinesterase gene (BCHE) as influencing how drugs like cocaine are metabolized in the body.

It is recognized that neurodevelopment persists through young adulthood. This evidence provides necessary context into the epigenetics that take place between our SNPs and environment, which informs our neurodevelopment. Evidence suggests that substance use during adolescence can facilitate both acute and chronic alterations in neuropsychiatric development and function, which may result in neuropsychiatric pathophysiology. Based on this genomic premise, an impulsive-compulsive disorder construct hypothetically links a host of different psychiatric disorders including SUDs, with dysregulation of varied neural circuits and neurotransmitter systems. The current understanding of impulsivity (an inability to resist the urge to initiate an action) implicates dysregulation among several different neural circuits involving the anterior cingulate cortex, ventromedial prefrontal cortex, ventral striatum, and thalamus. Likewise, the developing understanding of compulsivity (the inability to resist the urge to stop an action) implicates other neural circuits connecting the orbitofrontal cortex, dorsal striatum, and thalamus.

Stahl provides a user-friendly illustration of a stress diathesis model—a suspension bridge. The main and suspender cables, deck, tower, and anchors of the bridge are analogous to a person's genomic constitution. The number of SNPs in one's genomic makeup speaks to the relative degree of integrity of the "suspension bridge." The more SNPs associated with a particular condition the greater the person's vulnerability is to that condition. Cars and trucks on the suspension bridge are analogous to stressors. The greater the number, the heavier the weight, and the longer the time spent on the bridge in relation to the bridge's structural integrity defines stress diathesis. The metaphor's larger message is clear: The confluence of genomic vulnerability in dynamic interaction with neurodevelopment and stress exposure provides insight into why certain people manifest symptoms above a clinical threshold at a particular time.

Let's apply this knowledge in the form of an exemplar to crystallize the concepts (see the following Nursing Situation).

Nursing Situation: Substance-use Disorder and Genomic Profile

Karen is a 43-year-old executive with a remote history of extensive childhood trauma with biparental SUD history who presents to her primary care provider with complaints of increased work-related stress associated with recent changes in her organization's corporate structure. The primary care provider evaluating Karen performs a comprehensive evaluation to include the administration of a Patient Health Questionnaire-9 (PHQ-9) and an Alcohol Use Disorder Identification Test (AUDIT) screening tool, which yielded scores of 15 and 16, respectively. In this situation, the PCP was able to evaluate Karen's genomic profile subsequently identifying SNP variations in *ADH1B*, *ADH2C*, and *SLC39A8*. Given the presenting information, it could be reasonable to conclude that on birth, Karen's genomic profile brought with it an increased risk for AUD. Subsequent exposure to trauma during childhood, early socialization to alcohol, and current occupational stress provide necessary context for her neurodevelopment and the subsequent stress diathesis that informs her clinical presentation.

As it relates to this specific exemplar, current evidence suggests that heritability estimates for AUD range from 50% to 60% for both females and males. As the evidence that informs genomic vulnerability evolves, the primary care provider is challenged to resist the fatalistic notion that suggests we are merely subservient to our genetics. Primary care providers need to understand the underlying and still-developing pathophysiology of SUDs, and not become overwhelmed by it. Primary care providers are challenged to shift their locus of control away from that which they are not able to control (e.g., genomic vulnerability, adverse childhood events, established psychopathology) to that which they can meaningfully influence (e.g., establishing a therapeutic relationship, delivering evidence-based care, and embracing continuing education).

CLINICAL PRESENTATION

Persons of all ages, races, religions, and every socioeconomic status are susceptible to SUDs. Moreover, SUDs among older adults are among the fastest-growing health concerns in the United States and expected to expand and intensify. SUDs are common among patients in primary care settings making this an excellent venue for identification and treatment. The clinical presentation of a person with substance intoxication, misuse, or withdrawal varies depending on the substance used.

Integration of SUDs and primary care services is a major goal for health-care reforms to improve quality of care. Primary care providers report a low level of preparedness, however, in identifying and assisting patients with SUDs. An effective approach to identifying, treating, and managing SUDs is Screening, Brief Intervention, and

Referral to Treatment (SBIRT). SBIRT is a model used to identify and address risky substance use, including motivational interviewing and specific strategies to promote behavior change. SBIRT is flexible and easy to apply, allowing primary care providers opportunities for early intervention for at-risk substance users before more severe consequences occur. The integration of motivational interviewing techniques by the provider is critical to elicit change within the individual in a nonconfrontational style during the screening, counseling, and treatment planning stages to improve patient outcomes. SBIRT interventions include brief treatment for those with less severe SUDs and referrals to specialized treatment programs for those with more severe clinical presentation (see Table 65.1, Screening Tools). The Treatment Improvement Protocol (TIP) expert panel recommends providers use medical terminology (positive urine drug screen vs. dirty urine) and first-person language (a person with an SUD, not an addict or user), see Table 67.1. Selectively choose words decreasing bias and discrimination to promote treatment, retention, and recovery.

Alcohol

Alcohol consumption is extremely variable, as are its effects on the health and well-being of an individual. The National Institute of Alcohol Abuse and Alcoholism (NIAAA, 2019) defines *low-risk drinking* for males younger than 65 as no more than two drinks per day and no more than 14 drinks per week. Females and males aged 65 and older low-risk drinking is defined as no more than one drink per day and no more than seven drinks per week. *At-risk drinking* is defined as consuming volumes higher than these guidelines. *Binge drinking,* defined as drinking five or more alcoholic beverages in a 2-hour period for males and four or more alcoholic beverages in a 2-hour period for females, often results in acute intoxication and is the proximate cause of many alcohol-related deaths. *Heavy drinking* is defined as five or more days of binge drinking in a 30-day period with an increase in physical, psychological, or social harm. Any alcohol consumption for individuals younger than age 21 years is illegal in the United States and problematic. One drink is defined as a can or bottle of beer, a glass of wine or a wine cooler, a shot of liquor, or a mixed drink with liquor.

Consumption of alcohol exceeding the liver's rate of metabolism will result in elevations in blood alcohol concentration (BAC) and various levels of intoxication:

- BAC of 0.05: mild sedation, slowed reaction time, inhibitions lowered
- BAC of 0.1: slurred speech, reaction time, judgment and coordination impaired
- BAC of 0.2: stupor, disorientation, loss of muscle control, blackouts (memory loss)
- BAC of 0.3: loss of consciousness, irregular breathing, tachycardia, loss of bladder control
- BAC of 0.4+: coma, cardiac or respiratory difficulty, death

AUD typically has a slow, progressive course and many people seek treatment only after complications arise after long-term use. AUD is correlated with numerous health consequences that affect multiple organ systems. Health consequences related to excessive alcohol use include the following:

- Cardiovascular: hypertension, arrhythmias, dyslipidemia, cardiomyopathy, and stroke
- Gastrointestinal: dyspepsia progressing to gastritis, peptic ulcers, alcoholic hepatitis, fatty liver, cirrhosis, pancreatitis, portal hypertension, and esophageal varices
- Neuropsychiatric: peripheral neuropathy, memory impairment, suicidality, cortical atrophy, and dementia
- Neoplastic: increased risk of cancer, particularly oral, pharyngeal, laryngeal, esophageal, and possibly breast and colon cancer
- Safety issues: motor vehicle accidents, falls, burns, episodes of violence, and high-risk sexual behaviors

In primary care, screening tools such as the CAGE and AUDIT may be used to help detect possible problematic use, and ongoing assessment and monitoring may identify signs of AUD before severe consequences occur. Assessment should include family history (genetic risk, attitudes about alcohol and substance use), legal problems (arrest for driving under the influence [DUI]), work issues (job loss, poor work performance), and relationship issues (marital strain, divorce, poor relationship with children). Furthermore, the Adverse Childhood Events Scale (ACES) should be performed to identify vulnerable patient's risk for AUD.

Abrupt cessation of alcohol consumption in dependent persons can result in a range of symptoms from mild (characterized by symptoms such as irritability, tremulousness, and insomnia) to severe (characterized by withdrawal seizures, delirium tremens [disorientation, diaphoresis, visual hallucinations, tachycardia, hypertension, and agitation] and possibly death). Alcohol withdrawal is considered a medical emergency and is best evaluated in a setting equipped to manage symptoms.

Caffeine

Caffeine can be found in numerous dietary sources, supplements, and prescribed medications. Average U.S. daily consumption of caffeine over the last decade remains stable at around 400 mg/day. Dietary guidelines vary by both gender and age. At elevated doses (more than 1,000 mg/day), caffeine can induce arrhythmia, psychomotor agitation, and anxiety. Lethal doses of caffeine at blood concentration levels can range between 800 and 1,200 µg/mL. Conversely, there is evidence to suggest that responsible use of caffeine can be associated with improvements in physical performance, mood, and prevention of several chronic medical conditions.

TABLE 67.1 National Institute of Drug Abuse: Words Matter—Terms to Avoid When Talking About Addiction

Instead of...	Use...	Because...
• Addict • User • Substance or drug abuser • Junkie • Alcoholic • Drunk • Former addict • Reformed addict	• Person with substance use disorder • Person with opioid-use disorder (OUD) or person with opioid addiction [when substance in use is opioids] • Patient • Person with alcohol use disorder • Person who misuses alcohol/engages in unhealthy/hazardous alcohol use • Person in recovery or long-term recovery • Person who previously used drugs	• Person-first language. • The change shows that a person "has" a problem, rather than "is" the problem. • The terms avoid eliciting negative associations, punitive attitudes, and individual blame.
• Habit	• Substance-use disorder • Drug addiction	• Inaccurately implies that a person is choosing to use substances or can choose to stop. • "Habit" may undermine the seriousness of the disease.
• Abuse	**For illicit drugs:** • Use **For prescription medications:** • Misuse • Used other than prescribed	• The term "abuse" was found to have a high association with negative judgments and punishment. • Legitimate use of prescription medications is limited to their use as prescribed by the person to whom they are prescribed. Consumption outside these parameters is misuse.
• Opioid substitution replacement therapy	• Opioid agonist therapy • Medication treatment for OUD • Pharmacotherapy	• It is a misconception that medications merely "substitute" one drug or "one addiction" for another.
• Clean	**For toxicology screen results:** • Testing negative **For nontoxicology purposes:** • Being in remission or recovery • Abstinent from drugs • Not drinking or taking drugs • Not currently or actively using drugs	• Use clinically accurate, nonstigmatizing terminology the same way it would be used for other medical conditions. • Set an example with your own language when treating patients who might use stigmatizing slang. • Use of such terms may evoke negative and punitive implicit cognitions.
• Dirty	**For toxicology screen results:** • Testing positive **For nontoxicology purposes:** • Person who uses drugs	• Use clinically accurate, nonstigmatizing terminology the same way it would be used for other medical conditions. • May decrease patients' sense of hope and self-efficacy for change.
• Addicted baby	• Baby born to mother who used drugs while pregnant • Baby with signs of withdrawal from prenatal drug exposure • Baby with neonatal opioid withdrawal/neonatal abstinence syndrome • Newborn exposed to substances	• Babies cannot be born with addiction because addiction is a behavioral disorder—they are simply born manifesting a withdrawal syndrome. • Use clinically accurate, nonstigmatizing terminology the same way it would be used for other medical conditions.

Source: National Institute on Drug Abuse. (2021, November 29). Words matter: Terms to use and avoid when talking about addiction. https://nida.nih.gov/nidamed-medical-health-professionals/health-professions-education/words-matter-terms-to-use-avoid-when-talking-about-addiction

Cannabis

The potency of THC in cannabis has increased from 0.5% in the 1970s to over 15% in 2020, producing higher levels of dependency. Drug-related emergency department visits involving cannabis (either alone or in combination) have increased over time, corresponding to the increase in the potency of the drug. High doses of cannabis are associated with a variety of physiological symptoms from red eyes, mild increases in heart rate, orthostatic hypotension, polyphagia, and dry mouth. Memory impairment appears to be the most significant long-term effect of cannabis use. Heavy daily users of cannabis experience significant physical and psychological withdrawal symptoms and cravings. Withdrawal symptoms include irritability, insomnia, decrease in appetite, restlessness, cravings, nausea, and abdominal pain. Cannabis withdrawal symptoms peak the first week of stopping use and can last up to 2 weeks with mood issues and physical discomforts. Research demonstrates the cannabinoid receptors in the brain return to normal after 2 days without cannabis and regain regular functioning within 4 weeks after stopping use. The psychological symptoms of withdrawal are typically the most difficult for the individual with cravings lingering.

Numerous health risks are associated with the inhalation of cannabis. Circulatory changes include variability of blood pressure, arrhythmias, and cerebellar infarction. Immune system dysfunction and fertility issues, including erratic ovulation and reduced sperm count, have been reported. The most significant changes are in mood and cognition including exacerbations of panic attacks, anxiety, and depression. Other behavior changes may include a lack of desire to participate in activities; persistent cognitive and memory impairment, especially if misuse began in adolescence; and psychotic symptoms. In fact, in genetically predisposed adolescents, exposure to cannabis has been associated with an onset of psychosis and worsening of schizophrenia. Furthermore, cannabis affects the developing adolescent brain, not considered fully developed until age 25 years. The long-term effects include impairment of cognition, memory, and learning functions along with neuronal connections in the brain. Declines in IQ scores related to cannabis use have been documented, especially in adolescents and young adults.

Hallucinogens

Several chemical agents (e.g., d-lysergic acid diethylamide or LSD, 4-phosphoryloxy-N, N-dimethyltryptamine or psilocybin, mescaline or peyote, dimethyltryptamine or DMT, ayahuasca or hoasca, phencyclidine or PCP, ketamine or Ketalar, dextromethorphan or DXM, and *Salvia divinorum* or diviner's sage) potentially fit into this diagnostic category. LSD is known to elevate vital signs, generate dizziness, anorexia, diaphoresis, paresthesias, weakness, tremors, impulsiveness, and marked mood lability. Psilocybin has been known to generate feelings of profound relaxation, paranoia, panic-like reactions, and introspective/spiritual experiences. Peyote has been known to generate hyperthermia, tachycardia, ataxia, diaphoresis, and gooseflesh. DMT has been known to generate tachycardia and foment agitation and hallucinatory effects defined by radical alternations in environments and spatial distortions. Hoasca has been known to elevate blood pressure, induce vomiting, and alter states of awareness and perceptual experience. PCP has been known to generate hypoesthesia, dysarthria, ataxia, nystagmus, auditory hallucinations, mood and affect dysregulation, paranoia, aggression, and the subjective experience of strength and invulnerability. Ketamine has been known to generate hypotension, nausea, vomiting, anorexia, hyperopia, oneirophrenia, drowsiness and hallucinations. DMX has been known to generate nausea, vomiting, constipation, dizziness, sedation, cognitive impairment, and anxiety. Lastly, salvia has been known to induce hallucinations, mood and affect instability, depersonalization, emotional incontinence, cognitive impairment, intensified sensory experiences, and out-of-body experiences. These agents can potentially produce a host of reactions ranging from dissociation to stupor to death. Given these agents' common hallucinatory effects, primary care providers may anticipate a presentation with a co-occurring fall, injury, or accident.

Primary care providers should be aware of a relatively new phenomenon referred to as *microdosing*, which is taking small fractions of what would otherwise be considered a recreational dose of a hallucinogen. Microdosing LSD and psilocybin-containing mushrooms is most common. Early research suggests that microdosing might influence mood, cognition, energy, and creativity.

Inhalants

Several chemical agents across numerous agent classifications potentially fit into this category including glues and adhesives (e.g., ethyl acetate, hexane, toluene, methyl chloride, benzene, and chloroform), aerosols (e.g., butane, fluorocarbons, chlorofluorocarbons, dimethyl ether, and ethyl chloride), alkyl nitrites, anesthetics (e.g., nitrous oxide, halothane, enflurane, isoflurane), cleaning agents (e.g., tetrachloroethylene, xylene, petroleum distillates, acetone, methanol), and solvents and gases (e.g., acetone, bromochlorodifluoromethane, esters, isoparaffins). Street names for these agents include laughing gas, poppers, snappers, and whippets. These substances can produce neurocognitive problems, as well as pulmonary and cardiac issues. Inhalants have been associated with sudden death related to cardiac arrhythmias but also through respiratory depression and aspiration. Dependent on the specific chemical agent, acute inhalant intoxication can generate a wide array of symptoms ranging from dizziness, ataxia, dysarthria, euphoria, lethargy, hyporeflexia, cognitive impairment, tremors, hyperopia, nystagmus, and myasthenia. Alternatively, chronic exposure to this classification of chemical agents promotes cognitive, learning, memory, attention, impulse control, judgment, and reasoning problems, as well as other neurological, hepatic, and renal impairment.

Opioids

Opioids decrease the perception of pain with side effects of drowsiness, mental confusion, nausea, constipation, and euphoria. High doses depress respirations and increase the incidence of death. The symptoms of opioid withdrawal affect people differently based on the severity and duration of use in combination with the health and genetic disposition of the individual. The typical symptoms, however, begin approximately 24 hours after the last opioid use. Early symptoms include muscles aches, restlessness, anxiety, tearing of the eyes, runny nose, excessive sweating, inability to sleep, and frequent yawning. Later symptoms are more intense with diarrhea, abdominal cramping, piloerection, nausea, vomiting, dilated pupils, rapid heart rate, and high blood pressure. Many patients report symptoms comparable to influenza. Although these issues are unpleasant and painful, they are not life-threatening and usually begin to improve within 72 hours. However, vomiting and diarrhea may result in dehydration and hypernatremia, which can lead to death. A significant decrease in acute symptoms occurs within 1 week. Some patients, however, may experience a protracted abstinence involving a negative emotional state characterized by a loss of motivation, heightened stress reactivity, inability to identify and describe emotions, chronic irritability, malaise, dysphoria, and sleep disorders.

The key for primary care providers is to identify opiate misuse to assist with the treatment process. The Opioid Risk Tool is a popular, validated screening instrument commonly used in primary care practice to predict risk of developing an OUD. This tool assumes there are predisposing factors related to the patient's history and experiences. The benefit of this tool is the brevity (five questions) and accessibility, as it is available as a phone app. Other assessment tools include Current Opioid Misuse Measure, Patient Medication Questionnaire, and Screener and Opioid Assessment for Patients with Pain—Revised. These tools rely on self-reporting, are dependent on patients answering questions honestly, and should not be used in isolation. A combination of a typical clinical examination with a urine drug screen when indicated and a validated risk assessment tool improves the ability to detect opioid misuse.

Sedative-Hypnotics and Anxiolytics

This classification group combines three different drug classes: barbiturates (e.g., methohexital, pentobarbital, secobarbital, amobarbital, butalbital, phenobarbital, and primidone), benzodiazepine hypnotics (e.g., alprazolam, oxazepam, temazepam, lorazepam, diazepam, and clonazepam), and nonbenzodiazepine hypnotics (e.g., zalepion, zolpidem, zopiclone, buspirone, clomethiazole, promethazine, diphenhydramine, and melatonin). These substances generally operate as central nervous system (CNS) depressants and can cause various neurological deficits in memory, cognition, coordination, and respiratory depression. Given the epidemic of polypharmacy that affects patients in the primary care setting, providers should be aware of the synergistic risks between these drugs and other CNS depressants like alcohol, opioids, and muscle relaxants. Suspicions of misuse and diversion can be seen with repeated attempts by a patient (or significant other) to attain additional supplies earlier than the dosage plan requires and larger doses of these medications over time.

Physiological withdrawal from both the barbiturate and benzodiazepine classes of drugs should be considered a potential medical emergency. The primary care provider is encouraged to seek a referral and consultation with a psychiatrist or psychiatric mental health nurse practitioner because an unsupervised outpatient taper is rife with risk. In fact, the safest course of action is hospitalization for a medically supervised taper guided by evidence-based tools like the Clinical Institute Withdrawal Assessment Scale – Benzodiazepine (CIWA-B).

Stimulants

Cocaine intoxication is characterized by subjective experiences of euphoria, elation, grandiosity, and the perception of improved task performance. Intoxication can also produce agitation, irritability, impaired judgment, impulsive sexual behavior, aggression, hyperactivity, and mania. Cocaine withdrawal is characterized by subjective experiences of cognitive impairment, impaired concentration, fatigue, restlessness, sexual impairment, anhedonia, impaired sleep, chills, tremors, muscle aches, and nerve pain. Chronic cocaine use has been associated with increased risks for varied psychiatric (e.g., depressive, anxiety, bipolar, and thought) and general medical (e.g., olfactory impairment, epistaxis, asthma, increased risk for HIV and hepatitis) conditions.

Amphetamines are associated with violent, bizarre behavior at a time when mellow "highs" were more socially acceptable. Methamphetamine (e.g., speed, meth, chalk, ice, and crystal) is a synthetic form of amphetamine. Users describe a methamphetamine high as feeling "amped" (amplified) or "tweaked." Methamphetamine is a potent, easy-to-make, inexpensive stimulant, which can deliver an extreme amphetamine high that can last for hours. Intoxication includes elation, increased self-esteem, increased physical endurance, insensitivity to fatigue, and feelings of being invulnerable. Several side effects of methamphetamine use are hyperthermia, dehydration, a significant anxiety, insomnia, mood disturbances, and violent behavior, as well as psychosis. These symptoms can persist even after the behavior of use has stopped. Additional physical signs and symptoms include dermatological changes such as sores and dental issues, including tooth decay and tooth loss. Chronic users experience acute episodes of euphoria and dysphoria that can mimic bipolar disorder. Other medical issues that can occur with stimulant use include nasal septum perforation, and respiratory and cardiovascular issues such as chest pain, myocardial infarction, arrhythmias, and stroke.

DIAGNOSTIC REASONING

The *DSM-5-TR* divides the substance-related and addictive disorders category into two subcategories (substance-related and non–substance-related disorders). The substance-related disorder section is stratified by SUD (e.g., those pathological behaviors associated with substance-seeking activities) and substance-induced disorders (e.g., intoxication, withdrawal, and mental disorders caused by a medication or a substance) and includes nine specific substance classifications (e.g., Alcohol-Related; Caffeine-Related; Cannabis-Related; Hallucinogen-Related; Inhalant-Related; Opioid-Related; Sedative-, Hypnotic-, or Anxiolytic-Related; Stimulant-Related; and Tobacco-Related), whereas the non–substance-related disorder section exclusively houses gambling disorder.

Each condition within the substance-related and addictive disorders category is defined by a specific set of diagnostic criteria reflecting varying degrees of symptomatic intensity, symptomatic duration, and associated functional impairment. Almost every condition within this disorder category is defined by the transdiagnostic phenomena of cravings, tolerance, withdrawal, and functional impairment. The SUDs are further stratified by clinical specifiers (e.g., mild, moderate, and severe) with an increased number of diagnostic criteria met being associated with a higher specifier category.

Differential Diagnosis

Much like in other fields of medicine, differential diagnosis is both an art and a science. Each substance-related and substance-induced disorder brings with it a unique set of symptoms that can mimic a whole host of other medical and psychiatric symptoms and conditions. A key tactic to successfully navigating differential diagnostic challenges in this area is associated with extensive case research, laboratory testing, and context. For example, the symptoms associated with physiological withdrawal from alcohol and benzodiazepines are near identical. Likewise, those who use synthetic cathinones (e.g., bath salts) can experience symptoms of psychosis. Consequently, the only way to differentially parse out the diagnosis between a substance/medication-induced psychotic disorder and stimulant intoxication with perceptual disturbances is by conducting a detailed history, collateral research, and laboratory testing.

According to the U.S. Department of Justice, the pipeline of new psychoactive substances (NPS) entering the country are steadily on the rise. This reality suggests that primary care providers will encounter patients using NPS for which we do not yet have formal testing. This reality makes an already opaque process muddier. In situations like this and absent available testing, primary care providers will have to double down on detailed history and collateral research to parse out the differential diagnosis.

It is also essential for the clinician to depict any dual diagnoses present in the individual to properly treat each disorder. Dual diagnosis presentations are significantly more challenging to diagnose and treat, and are commonly and regrettably mutually reinforcing. The primary care provider is encouraged to take great care to distinguish between the psychiatric symptoms of depression, anxiety, and trauma and the physiological expressions of commonly associated substance intoxication or withdrawal.

MANAGEMENT

Primary care practitioners are often the first health-care professionals to observe the health and psychosocial effect of SUDs. Primary care is an excellent opportunity to address substance-related issues, provide education and information, and offer therapeutic intervention or referral. The NIAAA recommends screening as part of routine evaluations, in response to medical conditions related to or affected by alcohol use, and before prescribing medications that may interact with alcohol. For information on screening tools, please refer to Table 65.1.

Primary care providers have the advantage of an established relationship with their patients, allowing them to recognize substance misuse and initiate the first steps toward intervention. SBIRT is recommended and involves screening every patient at least annually for alcohol and drug use with a structured screening tool to assess and document symptoms. Brief counseling is offered to all patients with positive scores. If indicated, the primary care clinician will provide referrals to counseling and specialists along with treatment options based on the preferences of the patient. The final step of the SBIRT process is the emphasis on follow-up with monitoring and support. The goal of this approach is to promote early engagement and retention of patients with SUDs or problematic use. Many patients may initially decline voluntary referral or express ambivalence, but the primary care provider's encouragement and support may help the patient to eventually be more willing to pursue treatment options. There is considerable evidence indicating that factors such as the strength of the therapeutic alliance and the structure provided by regular clinical contact have a powerful effect on engagement and result in positive patient outcomes. Once the disorder is identified, it is important for the clinician to utilize motivational interviewing skills to empower the individual to make a change.

Most patients require a variety of interventions in the promotion of treatment for SUDs. The following strategies are recommended:

- Use motivational interviewing (see Chapter 87) and emphasize the common elements of effective interventions including improving self-efficacy for change, promoting a therapeutic relationship, strengthening coping skills, changing reinforcement contingencies for recovery, and enhancing social support for recovery.
- Reiterate to the patient that the most consistent predictors of successful outcome are retention in formal treatment and/or active involvement with community support for recovery.
- Discuss strategies demonstrated to be effective to promote active involvement in available mutual help programs (e.g., Alcoholics Anonymous [AA], Narcotics Anonymous [NA]).
- Coordinate addiction-focused psychosocial interventions with evidence-based intervention(s) for other biopsychosocial problems to address identified concurrent problems consistent with patient priorities.
- Provide intervention in the least restrictive setting necessary to promote access to care, safety, and effectiveness.
- Attempt to reengage the patient in treatment if the patient stops participating or relapses. If the patient remains unwilling to engage in any addiction-focused care, maintain motivational interviewing style of interactions. Emphasize that options remain available in the future and determine whether treatment for medical and psychiatric problems can be effectively and safely provided while looking for windows of opportunity to engage the patient in addiction treatment. Even when patients refuse referral or are unable to participate in specialized addiction treatment, many are accepting of general medical or mental health care.
- Identify underlying mental and physical health conditions and provide treatment for the comorbidities.

Treatment programs tend to be multidisciplinary and often include a specific set of procedures. Broadly, programs may focus on controlling acute withdrawal (detoxification), long-term behavioral change, and/or may provide treatment for a few days or a few months. Most treatment centers incorporate individual psychotherapy, AA or other 12-step principles, and therapeutic community principles. Multimodal approaches are utilized with shared decision making between the patient and provider about the recommended approach that might work best for this person. Publicly and privately funded treatment programs for drug dependence are categorized as methadone maintenance (mostly outpatient), outpatient drug-free programs, therapeutic communities, or short-term inpatient programs.

MAT is available for nicotine, alcohol, and opioid disorders. Nicotine agents are listed in Chapter 33 (see Drugs Commonly Prescribed 33.1). Pharmacological options for maintenance of alcohol abstinence include disulfiram (Antabuse), oral and extended-release injectable naltrexone (Revia), and acamprosate (Campral). Naltrexone is the primary drug choice unless co-occurring opioid use is present. Treatment options for opioid disorders encompass detoxification (managed opiate withdrawal), behavioral strategies, and pharmacological intervention. Long-term maintenance of abstinence can be achieved by methadone, buprenorphine, and naltrexone. Methadone can only be prescribed by a Substance Abuse and Mental Health Services Administration (SAMHSA)-certified opioid treatment programs. In fact, nurse practitioners and physician assistants can prescribe medications for the treatment of OUD through the 2016 Comprehensive Addictions and Recovery Act (CARA). This involves free training via SAMHSA to complete the federal waiver online to prescribe buprenorphine for OUD. This initiative along with the Drug Addiction Treatment Act of 2000 that allows physicians to offer office-based opioid treatment (OBOT) decreased the gap by providing more treatment services to patients with OUD. See Box 67.3 for an example of a medication initiation checklist.

SAMHSA highly recommends the integration of nonpharmacological interventions with MAT for improved patient outcomes. Nonpharmacological interventions include but are not limited to cognitive behavioral therapy (CBT), the community reinforcement approach (CRA), motivational enhancement therapy (MET), and/or 12-step programs (AA). Increasingly, the recovery

---

Box 67.3 Medication Initiation Checklist for Treatment of Severe Opioid Use Disorder

- Review of confidentiality
- Opioid use disorder assessment and diagnosis with use of appropriate screening tools
- Assessment of other substance-use disorders, including tobacco-use disorder
- Discussion of treatment options
- Laboratory tests: Complete blood cell count, liver function tests, HIV, syphilis, hepatitis panel (hepatitis A and C antibodies, hepatitis B surface antibody and surface antigen), gonorrhea/chlamydia culture, urine pregnancy test
- Vaccination: Hepatitis A, hepatitis B. Confirm hepatitis A and B virus immunity before vaccinating
- Sign release to obtain information about previous treatment

If medication therapy is indicated, before medication initiation:

- Sign the treatment agreement and consent form
- Assess for co-occurring mental health disorders
- Refer to behavioral health (or offer within program)
- Discuss safe medication storage planning
- Review urine drug testing expectations and visit frequency

community has embraced integrated and individualized approaches. The first goal of treatment should be the restoration of the physical, psychological, and social well-being of the person and family/significant others. Approaches include specific procedures or techniques such as MAT along with individual therapy, family therapy, group therapy, relapse prevention, pharmacotherapy, and treatment programs. Significant damage often occurs to the patient's support system. The family/significant others may have additional codependent and enabling issues to address with the need for treatment. *Codependence* refers to an unhealthy relationship or interactions between family or loved ones and the person with substance use. Related concepts of enabling and denial may characterize the support system of patients who misuse substances.

FOLLOW-UP AND REFERRAL

In addition to primary care, patients being treated for SUDs will need access to several information and support resources, which should include education services, treatment programs, and support groups. It is unlikely that any single program or support group will be sufficient, so patients are encouraged to make repeated contact with several different types of programs and groups. Follow-up includes monitoring self-reported use, adherence, laboratory markers, response to treatment, and adverse effects. Education about SUD consequences and treatments should be ongoing with encouragement to abstain from nonprescribed opioids and other substances. Emphasizing the connection with community supports (e.g., mutual help groups) and initiation of lifestyle changes to support recovery are vital elements. There must be shared decision making with the patient and support persons and a variety of approaches tried, monitored, and evaluated. Accentuating the fact that SUD is a chronic, potentially recurring, and progressive disease is key to promote necessary lifelong treatment for the patient.

Nursing Situation: Patient–treatment Planning in MAT From SAMHSA, Treatment Improvement Protocol for MAT in the Treatment of Opiate-use Disorder

The patient is a 30-year-old Hispanic mother of two children who has been divorced for 3 years. She dropped out of high school at age 15 when she became pregnant. As a single mother receiving Temporary Assistance for Needy Families (TANF), she first began using heroin intranasally at age 17 and began injecting 1 year later.

The patient was born in Puerto Rico, and her family came to the mainland United States when she was 10 years old. She is the youngest of five children. Her father was an unemployed painter and alcoholic who physically abused her mother. He died in Puerto Rico from cirrhosis. The patient's relationship with her mother always has been strained. Her mother has had numerous relationships that the patient resented. The patient stated that, as the youngest child, she feels that she never received enough attention or love from her mother. To support her lifestyle, which includes alcohol, cocaine, and heroin use, the patient earned money through prostitution, which led to selling drugs, theft, and other criminal activities.

The patient married after giving birth to her second child. She has an arrest history and a pending case for selling cocaine. After a divorce, the patient lived with her mother. An anonymous call was made to Child Protective Services (CPS) reporting her chronic drug use and criminal history. As a result, her children were placed in foster care. After the patient's arrest and the removal of her children, the patient's mother asked her to move out of the house; she then lived with whomever she could. The patient has enrolled in an opioid treatment program (OTP), motivated by her desire to regain custody of her children. She considers cessation of her cocaine habit secondary to cessation of her heroin use. She initially stated that she wanted to change her life, including having her own permanent housing and stopping commercial sex work. Although stabilized on methadone, she continued to use cocaine on a regular basis during her first 6 months in treatment. While in the program, she tested positive for HIV. She was assessed as having severe depression with suicidal ideation and escalation of cocaine use. Although attempts have been made to motivate the patient to stop cocaine use, these attempts have been unsuccessful.

Patient's Treatment Plan Might Include the Following Short- and Long-Term Goals:

Short-Term Goals

1. Address imminent danger of suicide by developing a service plan in conjunction with mental health provider
   - Objective: To rule out suicide; to treat patient's depression and assess need for medication
   - Action: Have patient sign a consent form for a psychiatric evaluation and communication between provider and OTP staff; set up appointment with psychiatric mental health nurse practitioner or psychiatrist; set up appointment for psychotherapy with a mental health provider; obtain evaluation, diagnosis, and treatment recommendations from the psychiatric mental health nurse practitioner or psychiatrist and the mental health provider
   - Target date: Immediately for suicidal ideation; within 1 month for ongoing mental health needs
   - Responsible persons: Patient, psychiatric mental health nurse practitioner or psychiatrist, mental health provider, caseworker (possibly)
   - Measurable outcome: Patient is stable and no longer at high risk for suicide; medication needs are assessed
   - Long-term goal: Stable mental health status with ongoing treatment plan
2. Obtain housing for patient, with long-term goal of stable permanent housing
   - Objective: To refer to a shelter
   - Action: Make appointment to apply for housing assistance program

- Target date: Immediately
- Responsible persons: Patient, mental health provider, caseworker (possibly), housing staff
- Measurable outcome: Copy of lease, patient self-report, or both
- Long-term goal: Access to stable housing

3. Obtain HIV counseling
   - Objective: To provide support and education about HIV status
   - Action: Provide education, resources, and counseling about safer sexual practices and spread of HIV
   - Target date: 4 to 6 months
   - Responsible persons: Medical staff, mental health provider, and patient
   - Measurable outcome: Patient has obtained and integrated accurate information; myths are dispelled; patient reports readiness to explore treatment options
   - Long-term goal: Initiation of antiretroviral treatment

4. Address cocaine use
   - Objective: To educate the patient on the psychological and physiological effects of cocaine use; to develop a recovery intervention
   - Action: Assess level of use and readiness for change; develop plan with patient to address use (e.g., motivational groups, Cocaine Anonymous, skills-building interventions, drug testing)
   - Target date: 2 to 4 months
   - Responsible persons: Patient, mental health provider, group leader, and medical staff members
   - Measurable outcome: Patient decreases cocaine use based on self-report, observable behavior, drug testing, and adherence to counseling plan

Long-Term Goals

1. Manage or eliminate depression
   - Objective: To stabilize depression; to increase self-esteem and motivation to work on treatment goals
   - Action: Provide regular psychiatric and psychotherapy treatments on site or by referral; communicate with providers
   - Target date: 6 months
   - Responsible persons: Patient, mental health provider, and psychiatric mental health nurse practitioner or psychiatrist
   - Measurable outcomes: Patient regularly attends to psychiatric treatment plan, adherence to medication regimen if prescribed, elimination of or reduction in depression (as assessed by patient report, depression assessment tools, observed behaviors)

2. Regain custody of children once in stable housing situation
   - Objective: To reconcile the patient with her family; to maintain a stable living situation
   - Action: Assist patient in obtaining public assistance to ensure stable, safe, appropriate environment for children; access legal assistance for custody issues; obtain permission to communicate with CPS; assist patient in remaining abstinent from substance use
   - Target date: 1 year
   - Responsible persons: Patient, mental health provider, caseworkers (possibly), internal or external social services worker, and lawyer
   - Measurable outcomes: Patient self-report, family and CPS agency reports, rent receipts, progress toward obtaining custody of children

3. Continue HIV medical care
   - Objective: To obtain ongoing HIV education and treatment
   - Action: Provide access and communication with HIV and primary care providers; provide referral to support group meetings for individuals who are HIV positive
   - Target date: Ongoing
   - Responsible persons: Patient, health-care providers, mental health provider, caseworker (possibly), group counselor or facilitator
   - Measurable outcomes: Patient self-report, health-care providers' report, laboratory reports, and group leader reports about adherence to health-care needs

Referral to a specialist should be made immediately when the patient's behavior represents a danger to self or others. SUDs, particularly AUD, is a factor in motor vehicle accidents, family violence, and suicide. It can also be beneficial for patients to have at least one appointment with a specialist to develop a comprehensive assessment of the patient's substance use and misuse. This assessment for the patient is a critical source of information that can reduce her ambivalence toward making needed changes in substance-related behaviors. Seeing a specialist may also be motivational because one of the most common reasons for not trying to make required changes in behavior is the patient's unspoken fears of failure.

Patient Education: Substance-use Disorder

Individuals who have developed psychological and physical needs for a substance often have formed strong attachments to their substance-use lifestyle and substance-based relationships. It is critical for the primary care clinician to consider these connections to effectively address a patient's SUD. A person can become strongly attached to the people, places, and community that make up their substance-use lifestyle. These relationships range from friendships among coworkers in designated smoking areas to football parties and alternative lifestyles. Many people find it more difficult to relinquish these attachments than the substance used. The fear of losing these valued relationships is frequently used to rationalize continued substance use.

Personal losses may increase or decrease the motivation to significantly change substance-use behaviors. Years of substance use can result in the loss of all non–substance-based relationships, significant loss of self-esteem, financial losses, and loss of physical and mental health. These personal losses can have a devastating psychological effect on the individual and family/significant others. The person may become overwhelmed and develop feelings of hopelessness that may manifest as ambivalence about making needed changes in substance-use behaviors. Providers should remember to be aware of these confounding variables for the individual suffering from SUDs.

Clinicians should educate patients and their support persons regarding the effects of alcohol and drugs and provide information on substance use and treatment options. This includes information regarding the danger of exposure to HIV, hepatitis, and other infections. Additionally, education about cannabis use for parents and children should focus on the threat cannabis poses to the developing adolescent brain and multiple physical and mental issues. Primary care providers should teach the patient's support persons about the dynamics that may continue to enable substance misuse because quite often support persons are unaware. Primary care clinicians can provide the patient's support persons with specific feedback and discuss strategies to decrease any enabling or codependency behaviors. Twelve-step programs should not only be encouraged for the individual with SUD, like AA or NA, but their support system as well, available as Al-Anon in the community. Treating the individual and their support system is imperative to the recovery process.

Based on the high risk of overdose, prevention education with a naloxone prescription for safety should be incorporated. The prevention of infections is another important facet of education with the teaching of the importance of sterilizing injection equipment and acquisition of new needles. Communication by the provider of the importance of follow-up appointments and referrals is pertinent to promote recovery.

REFERENCES

Afuseh E, Pike CA, Oruche UM. Individualized approach to primary prevention of substance use disorder: age-related risks. *Subst Abuse Treat Prev Policy*. 2020;15(1):58. https://doi.org/10.1186/s13011-020-00300-7

American Psychiatric Association. *Diagnostic and Statistical Manual of Mental Disorders: Diagnostic and Statistical Manual of Mental Disorders*. 5th ed. American Psychiatric Association; 2013.

American Psychological Association. *Publication Manual of the American Psychological Association*. 7th ed. American Psychological Association; 2019.

Anderson T, Petranker R, Christopher A, et al. Psychedelic microdosing benefits and challenges: an empirical codebook. *Harm Reduct J*. 2019;16(1):43. https://doi:10.1186/s12954-019-0308-4

Andrade C. Risk of major congenital malformations associated with the use of methylphenidate or amphetamines in pregnancy. *J Clin Psychiatry*. 2018;79(1):18f12108. https://doi:10.4088/JCP.18f12108

Barnett AI, Hall W, Carter A. Substance use terminology. *JAMA*. 2017;317(7):769-770. https://doi.org/10.1001/jama.2016.20475

Beheshti D. Adverse health effects of abuse-deterrent opioids: Evidence from the reformulation of OxyContin. *Health Econ*. 2019;28(12):1449-1461. https://doi.org/10.1002/hec.3944

Brook K, Bennett J, Desai SP. The chemical history of morphine: an 8000-year journey, from resin to de-novo synthesis. *J Anesth Hist*. 2017;3(2):50-55. https://doi.org/10.1016/j.janh.2017.02.001

Brott NR, Cascella M. Opioid, risk tool. In: *StatPearls*. StatPearls Publishing; 2020. https://www.ncbi.nlm.nih.gov/books/NBK553147/

Carney BL, Hadland SE, Bagley SM. Medication treatment of adolescent opioid use disorder in primary care. *Pediatr Rev*. 2018;39(1):43-45. https://doi: 10.1542/pir.2017-0153.

Carvalho AF, Heilig M, Perez A, et al. Alcohol use disorders. *Lancet*. 2019;394(10200):781-792. https://doi.org/10.1016/S0140-6736(19)31775-1

Centers for Disease Control and Prevention. CDC guideline for prescribing opioids for chronic pain; 2019, August 28. https://www.cdc.gov/drugoverdose/pdf/Guidelines_At-A-Glance-508.pdf

Centers for Disease Control and Prevention. Data overview. The drug overdose epidemic: behind the numbers; 2020, December 7. https://www.cdc.gov/drugoverdose/data/index.html

Centers for Disease Control and Prevention. Reported law enforcement encounters testing positive for fentanyl increase across US; 2019, August 24. https://www.cdc.gov/drugoverdose/data/fentanyl-le-reports.html

Centers for Disease Control and Prevention. Drug overdose deaths in the U.S. top 100,000 annually; 2022, April 27. https://www.cdc.gov/nchs/pressroom/nchs_press_releases/2021/20211117.htm

Centers for Disease Control and Prevention. CDC WONDER; 2020, March 3. https://wonder.cdc.gov/

Cohen K, Weizman A, Weinstein A. Positive and negative effects of cannabis and cannabinoids on health. *Clin Pharmacol Ther*. 2019;105(5):1139-1147. https://doi.org/10.1002/cpt.1381

Deak JD, Miller AP, Gizer IR. Genetics of alcohol use disorder: a review. *Curr Opin Psychol*. 2019 Jun;27:56-61. doi: 10.1016/j.copsyc.2018.07.012

Department of Veteran Affairs. VA/DoD clinical practice guideline for the management of substance use disorders; 2015. https://www.healthquality.va.gov/guidelines/MH/sud/VADoDSUDCPGRevised22216.pdf

DISA Global Solutions. Map of cannabis legality by state; 2020, November 4. https://disa.com/map-of-marijuana-legality-by-state

Dowell D, Haegerich TM, Chou R. CDC guideline for prescribing opioids for chronic pain–United States, 2016. *JAMA*. 315(15): 1624-1645. https://www.doi.com/10.1001/jama.2016.1464

Ducharme J, Moore S. Opioid use disorder assessment tools and drug screening. *Missouri Med*. 2019;116(4):318-324. https://www.ncbi.nlm.nih.gov/pmc/articles/PMC6699803/

Edelman EJ, Oldfield BJ, Tetrault JM. Office-based addiction treatment in primary care: approaches that work. *Med Clin North Am*. 2018;102(4):635-652. https://doi.org/10.1016/j.mcna.2018.02.007

ElSohly MA, Mehmedic Z, Foster S, et al. Changes in cannabis potency over the last 2 decades (1995-2014): analysis of current data in the United States. *Biol Psychiatry*. 2016;79(7):613-619. https://doi.org/10.1016/j.biopsych.2016.01.004

Esang M, Ahmed S. A closer look at substance use and suicide. *Am J Psychiatry Residents J*. 2018;6:6-8. https://psychiatryonline.org/doi/pdf/10.1176/appi.ajp-rj.2018.130603

Farzam K, Faizy RM, Saadabadi A. Stimulants. In: *StatPearls*. StatPearls Publishing; 2020, November 27. https://www.ncbi.nlm.nih.gov/books/NBK539896/

Galanter M, Kleber HD, Brady KT. *The American Psychiatric Association Textbook of Substance Abuse Treatment: DSM-V Edition*. American Psychiatric Publishing; 2015.

Guina J, Merrill B. Benzodiazepines I: upping the care on downers: the evidence of risks, benefit, and alternatives. *J Clin Med.* 2018;7(2):17. https://doi.org/10.3390/jcm7020017

Guinle MI, Sinha R. The roles of stress, trauma, and negative affect in alcohol misuse and alcohol use disorder in women. *Alcohol Res.* 2020;40(2):05. https://www.arcr.niaaa.nih.gov/arcr402/article05.pdf

Hamilton I, Kaufman G. Approaches to managing older people using opiates and their risk of dependence. *Nurs Older People.* 2019;31(3):40-48. https://doi.org/10.7748/nop.2019.e1100

Han BH, Sherman SE, Palamar JJ. Prescription opioid misuse among middle-aged and older adults in the United States, 2015-2016. *Prev Med.* 2019;121:94-98. https://doi.org/10.1016/j.ypmed.2019.02.018

Holmes AJ, Hollinshead MO, Roffman JL, et al. Individual differences in cognitive control circuit anatomy link sensation seeking, impulsivity, and substance use. *J Neurosci.* 2016;36(14):4038-4049. https://doi:10.1523/JNEUROSCI.3206-15.2016

Howard MO, Bowen SE, Garland EL, et al. Inhalant use and inhalant use disorders in the United States. *Addict Sci Clin Pract.* 2011;6(1):18-31. https://www.ncbi.nlm.nih.gov/pubmed/22003419

Jodra P, Lago-Rodriguez A, Sanchez-Oliver AJ, et al. Effects of caffeine supplementation on physical performance and mood dimensions in elite and trained-recreational athletes. *J Int Soc Sports Nutr.* 2020;17(1):2. https://pubmed.ncbi.nlm.nih.gov/31900166/

Johns Hopkins University and Medicine. Coronavirus resource center; 2022, April 27. https://coronavirus.jhu.edu/

Johnson BA. *Addiction Medicine: Science and Practice.* 2nd ed. Elsevier; 2020.

Kahn SA, Bierman TV, Larson KJ, et al. Killing brain cells and skin cells simultaneously with inhalant abuse: pearls from the national burn repository. *J Burn Care Res.* 2019;40(3):347-348. https://pubmed.ncbi.nlm.nih.gov/30806464/

Korownyk C, Perry D, Ton J, et al. Managing opioid use disorder in primary care: PEER simplified guideline. *Can Fam Physician.* 2019;65(5):321-330. https://www.ncbi.nlm.nih.gov/pmc/articles/PMC6516701/

Kuhn C, Swartzwelder S, Wilson W. *Buzzed: The Straight Facts About the Most Used and Abused Drugs From Alcohol to Ecstasy.* 5th ed. Norton, 2019.

Lee RD, Chen J. Adverse childhood experiences, mental health, and excessive alcohol use: Examination of race/ethnicity and sex differences. *Child Abuse Negl.* 2017;69:40-48. https://doi.org/10.1016/j.chiabu.2017.04.004

Lee RSC, Hoppenbrouwers S, Franken I. A systematic meta-review of impulsivity and compulsivity in addictive behaviors. *Neuropsychol Rev.* 2019;29(1):14-26. https://link.springer.com/article/10.1007/s11065-019-09402-x

López-Pelayo H, Aubin HJ, Drummond C, et al. "The post-COVID era": challenges in the treatment of substance use disorder (SUD) after the pandemic. *BMC Med.* 2020;18(1):241. https://doi.org/10.1186/s12916-020-01693-9

Ludwig IA, Clifford MN, Lean ME, et al. Coffee: biochemistry and potential impact on health. *Food Funct.* 2014;5(8):1695-1717. https://doi:10.1039/c4fo00042k

Madras BK. The President's commission on combating drug addiction and the opioid crisis: origins and recommendations. *Clin Pharmacol Ther.* 2018;103(6):943-945. https://doi.org/10.1002/cpt.1050

Maldonado JR. Novel algorithms for the prophylaxis and management of alcohol withdrawal syndromes-beyond benzodiazepines. *Crit Care Clin.* 2017;33(3):559-599. https://pubmed.ncbi.nlm.nih.gov/28601135/

Martin CE, Terplan M, Krans EE. Pain, opioids, and pregnancy: historical context and medical management. *Clin Perinatol.* 2019;46(4):833–847. https://doi.org/10.1016/j.clp.2019.08.013

McGuire S. Institute of Medicine. 2014. Caffeine in food and dietary supplements: examining safety—workshop summary. Washington, DC: The National Academies Press. *Adv Nutri.* 2019;5(5):585-586. https://academic.oup.com/advances/article/5/5/585/4565775

Mecca MC, Thomas JM, Niehoff KM, et al. Assessing an interprofessional polypharmacy and deprescribing educational intervention for primary care post-graduate trainees: a quantitative and qualitative evaluation. *J Gen Intern Med.* 2019;34(7):1220-1227. https://link.springer.com/article/10.1007%2Fs11606-019-04932-9

Moore DJ. A nurse practitioner's perspective on prescribing suboxone for opioid use disorder. *J Addict Nurs.* 2018;29(3):226-229. https://doi.org/10.1097/JAN.0000000000000242

Mostofsky E, Chahal HS, Mukamal KJ, et al. Alcohol and immediate risk of cardiovascular events: a systematic review and dose-response meta-analysis. *Circulation.* 2018;133(10):979-987. https://pubmed.ncbi.nlm.nih.gov/26936862/

Munir S, Habib R, Awan S, et al. Biochemical analysis and association of butyrylcholinesterase SNPs rs3495 and rs1803274 with substance abuse disorder. *J Mol Neurosci.* 2019;67(3):445-455. https://link.springer.com/article/10.1007/s12031-018-1251-7

Murray A, Traylor J. Caffeine toxicity. In: *StatPearls.* StatPearls Publishing; 2020. https://pubmed.ncbi.nlm.nih.gov/30422505/

National Council for Behavioral Health. Implementing care for alcohol and other drug use in medical settings: An extension of SBIRT; 2018, February. https://www.thenationalcouncil.org/wp-content/uploads/2018/03/021518_NCBH_ASPTReport-FINAL.pdf?daf=375ateTbd56

National Institute on Alcohol Abuse and Alcoholism. Drinking levels defined; 2020. https://www.niaaa.nih.gov/alcohol-health/overview-alcohol-consumption/moderate-binge-drinking

National Institute of Drug Abuse. Genetics and epigenetics of addiction drugfacts; 2019, August 5. https://www.drugabuse.gov/publications/drugfacts/genetics-epigenetics-addiction

National Institute of Drug Abuse. Hallucinogens and dissociative drugs research report. How do hallucinogens (LSD, psilocybin, peyote, DMT, and Ayahuasca) affect the brain and body?; 2020, June 2. https://www.drugabuse.gov/publications/research-reports/hallucinogens-dissociative-drugs/how-do-hallucinogens-lsd-psilocybin-peyote-dmt-ayahuasca-affect-brain-body

National Institute of Drug Abuse. Inhalants drugfacts; 2020, April 16. https://www.drugabuse.gov/publications/drugfacts/inhalants

National Institute on Drug Abuse. Opioid overdose crisis; 2020, May 27. https://www.drugabuse.gov/drug-topics/opioids/opioid-overdose-crisis

National Institute on Drug Abuse. Research Report Revised April 2020 Common Comorbidities with Substance Use Disorders Research Report; 2020, April. https://www.drugabuse.gov/download/1155/common-comorbidities-substance-use-disorders-research-report.pdf?v=5d6a5983e0e9353d46d01767fb20354b

National Institute on Drug Abuse. Word Matter-Terms to Avoid When Talking About Addiction; 2020, October 28. https://www.drugabuse.gov/nidamed-medical-health-professionals/health-professions-education/words-matter-terms-to-use-avoid-when-talking-about-addiction

Nestler EJ, Lüscher C. The molecular basis of drug addiction: linking epigenetic to synaptic and circuit mechanisms. *Neuron.* 2019 Apr 3;102(1):48-59. doi: 10.1016/j.neuron.2019.01.016

Nieber K. The impact of coffee on health. *Planta Med.* 2017;83(16):1256-1263. https://pubmed.ncbi.nlm.nih.gov/28675917/

Nuckols TK, Anderson L, Popescu I, et al. Opioid prescribing: a systematic review and critical appraisal of guidelines for chronic pain. *Ann Intern Med*. 2014;160(1):38-47. https://doi.org/10.7326/0003-4819-160-1-201401070-00732

Nyatanga B. COVID-19 pandemic: changing the way we live and die. *Br J Commun Nurs*. 2020;25(5):254. https://doi.org/10.12968/bjcn.2020.25.5.254

Ogbonna CI, Lembke A. Tapering patients off of benzodiazepines. *Am Fam Physician*. 2017;96(9):606-610. https://www.ncbi.nlm.nih.gov/pubmed/29094883

O'Grady MA, Kapoor S, Kwon N, et al. Substance use screening and brief intervention: evaluation of patient and implementation differences between primary care and emergency department settings. *J Eval Clin Pract*. 2019;25(3):441-447. doi: 10.1111/jep.13060

Ona G, Bouso JC. Potential safety, benefits, and influence of the placebo effect in microdosing psychedelic drugs: a systematic review. *Neurosci Biobehav Rev*. 2020;119:194-203. https://pubmed.ncbi.nlm.nih.gov/33031815/

Ornell F, Moura HF, Scherer JN, et al. The COVID-19 pandemic and its impact on substance use: Implications for prevention and treatment. *Psychiatry Res*. 2020;289:113096. https://www.ncbi.nlm.nih.gov/pmc/articles/PMC7219362/

Osilla KC, Watkins KE, D'Amico EJ, et al. Effects of motivational interviewing fidelity on substance use treatment engagement in primary care. *J Subst Abuse Treat*. 2018;87:64-69. https://doi.org/10.1016/j.jsat.2018.01.014

Pace CA, Uebelacker LA. Addressing unhealthy substance use in primary care. *Med Clin North Am*. 2018;102(4):567-586. https://doi.org/10.1016/j.mcna.2018.02.004

Piano MR. Alcohol's effects on the cardiovascular system. *Alcohol Res*. 2017;38(2):219-241. https://www.ncbi.nlm.nih.gov/pmc/articles/PMC5513687/

Pollard MS, Tucker JS, Green HD Jr. Changes in adult alcohol use and consequences during the COVID-19 pandemic in the US. *JAMA Ntw Open*. 2020;3(9):e2022942. https://doi.org/10.1001/jamanetworkopen.2020.22942

Rahimi-Movaghar A, Gholami J, Amato L, et al. Pharmacological therapies for management of opium withdrawal. *Cochrane Database Syst Rev*. 2018;6(6):CD007522. https://www.cochranelibrary.com/cdsr/doi/10.1002/14651858.CD007522.pub2/full

Reyes CM, Cornelis MC. Caffeine in the diet: Country-level consumption and guidelines. *Nutrients*. 2018;10(11). https://www.mdpi.com/2072-6643/10/11/1772

Richmond-Rakerd LS, Slutske WS, Lynskey MT, et al. Age at first use and later substance use disorder: shared genetic and environmental pathways for nicotine, alcohol, and cannabis. *J Abnorm Psychol*. 2016;125(7):946-959. https://www.ncbi.nlm.nih.gov/pmc/articles/PMC5061603/

Rizk AH, Simonsen SE, Roberts L, et al. Maternity care for pregnant women with opioid use disorder: a review. *J Midwifery Womens Health*. 2019;64(5):532-544. https://doi.org/10.1111/jmwh.13019

Russell C, Rueda S, Room R, et al. Routes of administration for cannabis use—basic prevalence and related health outcomes: a scoping review and synthesis. *Int J Drug Policy*. 2018;52:87-96. https://doi.org/10.1016/j.drugpo.2017.11.008

Saitz R, Daaleman TP. Now is the time to address substance use disorders in primary care. *Ann Fam Med*. 2017;15(4):306-308. https://doi.org/10.1370/afm.2111

Sajadi-Ernazarova KR, Anderson J, Dhakal A, et al. Caffeine withdrawal. In: *StatPearls*. StatPearls Publishing; 2020, November 10. https://www.ncbi.nlm.nih.gov/books/NBK430790/

Salmond S, Allread V. A population health approach to America's opioid epidemic. *Ortho Nurs*. 2019;38(2):95-108. https://doi.org/10.1097/NOR.0000000000000521

Sanchez-Roige S, Fontanillas P, Elson SL, et al. Genome-wide association study of alcohol use disorder identification test (AUDIT) scores in 20 328 research participants of European ancestry. *Addict Biol*. 2019;24(1):121-131. https://onlinelibrary.wiley.com/doi/abs/10.1111/adb.12574

Skolnick P. The opioid epidemic: Crisis and solutions. *Ann Rev Pharmacol Toxicol*. 2018;58:143-159. https://www.annualreviews.org/doi/abs/10.1146/annurev-pharmtox-010617-052534

Stahl SM. *Stahl's Essential Psychopharmacology: Neuroscientific Basis and Practical Application*. 4th ed. Cambridge University Press; 2013.

Stoicea N, Costa A, Periel L, et al. Current perspectives on the opioid crisis in the US healthcare system: a comprehensive literature review. *Medicine*. 2019;98(20):e15425. https://doi.org/10.1097/MD.0000000000015425

Substance Abuse and Mental Health Services Administration. 2015 National Survey on Drug Use and Health: Methodological Summary and Definitions; 2016, September. https://www.samhsa.gov/data/sites/default/files/NSDUH-MethodSummDefsHTML-2015/NSDUH-MethodSummDefsHTML-2015/NSDUH-MethodSummDefs-2015.htm

Substance Abuse and Mental Health Services Administration. Co-occurring disorders and other health conditions; 2020, August 19. https://www.samhsa.gov/medication-assisted-treatment/medications-counseling-related-conditions/co-occurring-disorders

Substance Abuse and Mental Health Services Administration. Key substance use and mental health indicators in the United States: results from the 2019 National Survey on Drug Use and Health; 2020. https://store.samhsa.gov/sites/default/files/SAMHSA_Digital_Download/PEP20-07-01-001-PDF.pdf

Substance Abuse and Mental Health Services Administration. Substance use disorder treatment for people with co-occurring disorders: Updated 2020; 2020. https://store.samhsa.gov/sites/default/files/SAMHSA_Digital_Download/PEP20-02-01-004_Final_508.pdf

Substance Abuse and Mental Health Services Administration. The DAWN Report: Benzodiazepines in Combination With Opioid Pain Relievers or Alcohol: Greater Risk of More Serious ED Visit Outcomes; 2014, December 18. https://www.samhsa.gov/data/sites/default/files/DAWN-SR192-BenzoCombos-2014/DAWN-SR192-BenzoCombos-2014.pdf

Thorpe HHA, Hamidullah S, Jenkins BW, et al. Adolescent neurodevelopment and substance use: Receptor expression and behavioral consequences. *Pharmacol Ther*. 2020;206:107431. https://pubmed.ncbi.nlm.nih.gov/31706976/

U.S. Department of Justice. 2019 Drug Enforcement Administration: National Drug Threat Assessment; 2019, December. https://www.dea.gov/sites/default/files/2020-01/2019-NDTA-final-01-14-2020_Low_Web-DIR-007-20_2019.pdf

U.S. Food and Drug Administration. FDA and cannabis: research and drug approval process; 2020, October 1. https://www.fda.gov/news-events/public-health-focus/fda-and-cannabis-research-and-drug-approval-process

U.S. National Library of Medicine. What are single nucleotide polymorphisms (SNPs)?; 2020, September 18. https://ghr.nlm.nih.gov/primer/genomicresearch/snp

van den Heuvel OA, van Wingen G, Soriano-Mas C, et al. Brain circuitry of compulsivity. *Eur. Neuropsychopharmacol*. 2016;26(5):810-827. https://pubmed.ncbi.nlm.nih.gov/26711687/

Wang S. Historical review: opiate addiction and opioid receptors. *Cell Transplant.* 2019;28(3):233-238. https://doi.org/10.1177/0963689718811060

Welsch L, Bailly J, Darcq E, et al. The negative affect of protracted opioid abstinence: progress and perspectives from rodent models. *Biol Psychiatry.* 2020;87(1):54-63. https://doi.org/10.1016/j.biopsych.2019.07.027

Wilming C, Alford M, Klaus L. Gabapentin use in acute alcohol withdrawal management. *Fed Pract.* 2018;35(3):40-46. https://www.ncbi.nlm.nih.gov/pmc/articles/PMC6368058/

Wilson J, Freeman TP, Mackie CJ. Effects of increasing cannabis potency on adolescent health. *Lancet Child Adolesc Health.* 2019;3(2):121-128. https://doi.org/10.1016/S2352-4642(18)30342-0

Wood AM, Kaptoge S, Butterworth AS, et al. Risk thresholds for alcohol consumption: combined analysis of individual-participant data for 599 912 current drinkers in 83 prospective studies. *Lancet.* 2018;391(10129):1513-1523. https://www.thelancet.com/action/showPdf?pii=S0140-6736%2818%2930134-Xhttps://doi.org/10.1016/S0140-6736(18)30134-X

Yarnelle S, Luming L, MacGrory B, et al. Substance use disorders in later life: a review and synthesis of the literature of an emerging public health concern. *Am J Geriatr Psychiatry.* 2020;28(2):226-236. https://pubmed.ncbi.nlm.nih.gov/31340887/

Zehra A, Burns J, Liu CK, et al. Cannabis addiction and the brain: a review. *Focus.* 2019;17(2):169-182. https://doi.org/10.1176/appi.focus.17204

Zhu S, Noviello CM, Teng J, et al. Structure of a human synaptic $GABA_A$ receptor. *Nature.* 2018;559(7712):67-72. https://doi.org/10.1038/s41586-018-0255-3

RESOURCES

General

Alcoholics Anonymous
   http://www.aa.org/

Narcotics Anonymous
   http://www.na.org/

National Institute on Alcohol Abuse and Alcoholism (NIAAA)
   http://pubs.niaaa.nih.gov/publications/Treatment/treatment.htm http://rethinkingdrinking.niaaa.nih.gov

National Institute on Drug Abuse
   https://www.drugabuse.gov/sites/default/files/Commonly-Used-Drugs-Charts_final_June_2020_optimized.pdf

Substance Abuse and Mental Health Services Administration (SAMHSA)
   https://www.samhsa.gov/disorders/substance-use

Alcohol

American Psychological Association
   http://www.apa.org/helpcenter/alcohol-disorders.aspx

National Institute on Alcohol Abuse and Alcoholism
   https://www.niaaa.nih.gov/

Substance Abuse and Mental Health Services Administration
   https://www.samhsa.gov/atod/alcohol

Anxiolytic, Hypnotic, and Sedative Drugs

Drug Enforcement Administration
   https://www.deadiversion.usdoj.gov/drug_chem_info/benzo.pdf

Harvard Medical School
   https://www.health.harvard.edu/a_to_z/sedative-hypnotic-or-anxiolytic-drug-use-disorder-a-to-z

Cannabis

Substance Abuse and Mental Health Services Administration
   https://www.samhsa.gov/marijuana

Hallucinogens

National Institute on Drug Abuse
   https://www.drugabuse.gov/publications/drugfacts/hallucinogens
   https://www.drugabuse.gov/publications/research-reports/hallucinogens-dissociative-drugs/what-are-dissociative-drugs

Opioids

American Academy of Family Physicians
   https://familydoctor.org/condition/opioid-addiction/

Centers for Disease Control and Prevention
   https://www.cdc.gov/drugoverdose

National Institute on Drug Abuse
   https://www.drugabuse.gov/publications/principles-substance-abuse-prevention-early-childhood/index
   https://www.drugabuse.gov/publications/effective-treatments-opioid-addiction/effective-treatments-opioid-addiction

Stimulants

National Institute on Drug Abuse
   https://www.drugabuse.gov/publications/research-reports/cocaine/how-does-cocaine-produce-its-effects
   https://www.drugabuse.gov/publications/drugfacts/cocaine
   https://www.drugabuse.gov/publications/drugfacts/prescription-stimulants
   https://www.drugabuse.gov/publications/drugfacts/mdma-ecstasymolly
   https://www.drugabuse.gov/publications/drugs-brains-behavior-science-addiction/preface

Substance Abuse and Mental Health Services Administration
   https://store.samhsa.gov/product/Treatment-of-Stimulant-Use-Disorder/PEP20-06-01-001

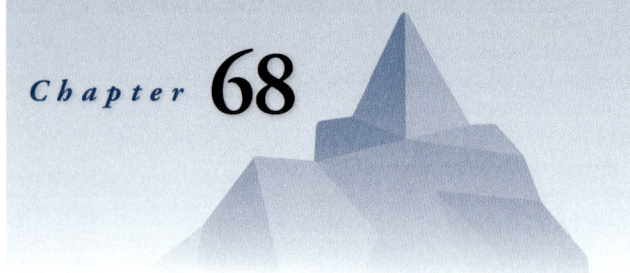

Chapter 68

Schizophrenia Spectrum and Other Psychotic Disorders

Amanda Ling, MS, RN, PMHNP

Kara Birch, DNP, PMHNP, FNP

Karen Jennings Mathis, PhD, APRN-CNP, PMHNP-BC, FAED

Psychotic disorders are disturbances of thought content and/or process that signal a departure from reality, often accompanied by a combination of hallucinations and delusions, disorganized thinking (recognized in speech), disorganized or abnormal motor behavior (including catatonia), and negative symptoms (including apathy and diminished expression). A person with psychosis may exhibit difficulties with communication, insight, behavior, and relationships. Psychosis may be the direct result of substance use or medication effects, such as illicit drugs or prescribed steroids. It may also be confused with delirium, which most often signals a medical rather than psychiatric cause. Psychotic disorders often coexist with other psychiatric and medical disorders, requiring a team approach to patient care. Psychotic disorders can be classified into several categories, as outlined in Table 68.1. Although most of the presented information will focus on schizophrenia, it is applicable to schizophrenia spectrum and other psychotic disorders. Schizophrenia is ranked by the World Health Organization as one of the top 15 illnesses contributing to the global burden of disease. Though less prevalent than substance-use disorders or depression, schizophrenia is among the most disabling mental illnesses with immense personal and societal costs. For example, reviews of U.S. public health insurance claims found annual health-care expenses for someone with schizophrenia averaged between $11,000 and $22,000 (Chapel et al, 2017). The total economic burden of schizophrenia annually including health care and lost productivity is estimated at $155 billion in the U.S. (Cloutier et al, 2016).

People with schizophrenia often experience symptoms such as hearing internally generated voices not heard by others or believing that other people are reading their minds, controlling their thoughts, or plotting to harm them. These symptoms may leave them fearful, withdrawn, and hesitant to trust providers, which makes it difficult for individuals to engage in treatment, and/or adhere to treatment recommendations. Because symptoms may be severe or disruptive, a diagnosis of schizophrenia can have serious implications for patients and

TABLE 68.1 Psychotic Disorders	
Psychotic Disorder	**Description**
Schizophrenia	Onset: Acute or insidious. Symptoms present for at least 6 months with at least two or more positive or negative symptoms present for at least 1 month. Social, employment, or self-care impairment.
Bipolar I disorder, manic, severe, with psychosis	Onset: Variable. Signs and symptoms must be present for 1 week or if hospitalization is required. Psychotic signs and symptoms present only during mood disorder. Social and employment impairment during episode.
Bipolar I disorder, mixed episode, with psychosis	Onset: Variable. Signs and symptoms must be present for 1 week or if hospitalization is required. Meets criteria for depression and mania. Positive signs and symptoms only with mood symptoms. Social and employment impairment during episode.
Major depression, severe, with psychotic features	Onset: Variable. Lasts 2+ weeks. Positive signs and symptoms occur only during mood episode. Impairment during episode (includes postpartum).
Schizoaffective disorder	Presence of psychosis independent and concurrent with major mood symptoms.
Brief psychotic disorder	Onset: Acute. Full expression within 2 weeks and complete remission in 1 to 3 months, lasts at least 1 day but less than 1 month. May have an acute stressor.
Schizophreniform	Usually acute onset of symptoms. Criteria of schizophrenia are met, but for fewer than 6 months.
Delusional disorder	Criteria for schizophrenia are not met. Onset subtle, nonbizarre delusions, symptoms last more than 1 month. Impairment usually less severe.

Sources: American Psychiatric Association. *Diagnostic and Statistical Manual of Mental Disorders, Text Revision.* 5th ed. Arlington, VA; American Psychiatric Association; 2022. Mojtabai R, Fochtmann LJ, Bromet EJ. Other psychotic disorders. In: Sadock BJ, et al, eds. *Kaplan and Sadock's Comprehensive Textbook of Psychiatry*. Philadelphia, PA: Lippincott Williams & Wilkins; 2017.

families. Schizophrenia is a serious psychological disorder that is also highly treatable. Although there is no cure for schizophrenia, combined treatment with antipsychotic medications and psychosocial therapies can significantly improve symptoms, functioning, and quality of life.

EPIDEMIOLOGY AND CAUSES

The number of people meeting criteria for schizophrenia at any given time is about 1 in 4,000. Currently, about 20 million people worldwide and about 1.1 million people in the United States are diagnosed with schizophrenia (Charlson et al, 2018). The risk of developing the illness over one's lifetime averages 0.7%, with minor variations related to race and ethnicity, immigration status, and socioeconomic and geographical factors. Males are up to 1.4 times more likely to develop schizophrenia than females, although some studies have found no difference in prevalence. Age of onset is typically during adolescence or early 20s; however, females tend to present in their late 20s to mid-30s. Childhood and late-life onset (older than 45 years) is rare.

Early symptoms can be subtle and occur long before a definitive diagnosis is made, making close evaluation for early intervention critical. The prevalence of schizophrenia in adolescents is low, and although rare, it can occur in childhood before age 13. Early onset tends to point to a poor prognosis; however, early intervention and early use of medications lead to better medical outcomes for the patient. Recent research increasingly shows that the disease process of schizophrenia gradually and significantly damages the brain, and that earlier treatments (medications and other therapies) seem to result in less damage over time. The earlier someone with schizophrenia is diagnosed and stabilized on treatment, the better the long-term prognosis for their illness.

There is a higher incidence of co-occurring disorders in those with schizophrenia such as depressive disorders; anxiety disorders (specifically social anxiety); post-traumatic stress disorder (PTSD); obsessive-compulsive disorders; and alcohol, tobacco, and substance use. Additionally, there are higher rates of metabolic and neurological problems. The rate of suicide is higher in those with schizophrenia compared with the general population. Among adolescents diagnosed with schizophrenia, 20% to 40% will attempt suicide, and 5% to 10% of all people with schizophrenia die by suicide. The risk for suicide is highest within several years of initial diagnosis and during or shortly after hospitalization. Comorbid personality disorders are more common in individuals with schizophrenia and can also convey higher risk for suicide and violence (Hor and Taylor, 2010; Popovic et al, 2014).

The disease course is variable, with some patients exhibiting only mild symptoms, whereas others follow a chronic course resulting in functional impairment, including social deficits and an inability to maintain independent housing and gainful employment. Poor engagement in health maintenance initiatives such as cancer screenings, exercise, nutrition, tobacco cessation, and identification of other comorbid chronic medical diseases plays a role in poor outcomes. Overall, among those diagnosed with schizophrenia, one-third recover, one-third wax and wane, and one-third have a chronic course and slow deterioration.

Identified but poorly understood risk factors for schizophrenia include immigration, living in an urban area, adverse childhood events, obstetrical complications, late-winter/early spring birth (perhaps related to exposure to influenza virus during neural development), prenatal maternal stress, and advanced paternal age (thought to be related to increased risk of de novo mutations). Leading theories suggest that schizophrenia is a result of genetic predisposition combined with environmental exposures and/or stresses during pregnancy or childhood that contribute to, or trigger, the disorder.

PATHOPHYSIOLOGY

Though current practice approaches schizophrenia as a single diagnosis, variations in pathophysiology have led some researchers to suspect schizophrenia may be a syndrome comprising multiple diseases presenting with similar signs and symptoms. Twin studies and prevalence among close family members support some genetic, heritable basis. For monozygotic twins sharing 100% of their DNA, if one twin meets criteria for schizophrenia, the other also meets criteria about 50% of the time. Several genes have been identified as contributing to risk, but no single gene is strongly associated with development of schizophrenia. Environmental factors must also play a role, otherwise

Pediatric/Adolescent Considerations:
Schizophrenia Spectrum Disorders

Primary care providers should consider schizophrenia spectrum disorders as differential diagnoses for youth with changes in social or academic behavior. These changes occur gradually, and individuals who later develop psychosis may exhibit signs of cognitive decline, more difficulty socializing, and blunted facial expressions as adolescents. Other risk factors include first-degree relatives with bipolar or schizophrenia spectrum diagnoses, legal involvement or hospitalizations for other mental health diagnoses, and cannabis use, which may precipitate psychosis in individuals who already have genetic vulnerabilities. None of these features are diagnostic, but providers should maintain a low threshold for referral to specialty psychiatric evaluation. Hallucinations, particularly auditory hallucinations of voice, are more commonly experienced in earlier-onset psychosis. However, the presence of psychosis in youth combined with a lack of family history, cognitive changes, or substance use should prompt a thorough neurological and medical work-up.

monozygotic twins would meet criteria near 100% of the time. Many individuals with schizophrenia have differences in brain anatomy, including a smaller prefrontal cortex and hippocampal region; however, the effect of these differences on the disease is still being studied. Several neurotransmitter systems are involved in the pathology of schizophrenia, including dopamine, glutamate, gamma aminobutyric acid (GABA), and acetylcholine, and represent the current best targets for pharmacological interventions. One of the oldest and best supported theories suggests that hyperdopaminergic activity causes most positive symptoms based on the observation that dopamine receptor blockade is the primary mechanism of antipsychotic drugs.

It is safe to say that various genetic and environmental factors combine to cause schizophrenia, although the mechanisms are poorly differentiated. Indeed, a complex interplay of factors may result in eventual diagnosis. For instance, someone born with predisposing genes and brain structure may experience childhood trauma and developmental delays that encourage distrusting and paranoid thought patterns. In early adulthood, neurodevelopmental factors, substance use, or stress may then sensitize the dopamine system with cascading effects causing an initial psychotic episode (Sadock et al, 2017).

CLINICAL PRESENTATION

The onset of schizophrenia may be abrupt or insidious. The illness begins for many individuals in adolescence and shows a slow and gradual development of clinical symptoms, with the first frank episode usually presenting between 15 and 25 years of age in males and 25 and 35 years of age in females. Rare later presentations beyond 40 years of age can also occur and tend to be in females. Depressive symptoms occur in approximately half of cases and should not habitually be diagnosed as schizoaffective disorder (discussed later in this chapter). Schizophrenia presents with four symptom clusters that are used to describe the disorder, and each has implications for therapeutic treatment. Positive symptoms, negative symptoms, cognitive impairments, and affective disturbances comprise these clusters.

Positive symptoms are the "active" qualities that are abnormal and are synonymous with psychosis. Positive symptoms include delusions, hallucinations, disorganized thinking (speech), and grossly disorganized or abnormal behavior (catatonia). Delusions are the hallmark of positive symptoms, occurring in more than half of patients. Delusions are fixed beliefs that are not amenable to change despite conflicting evidence. They can include persecutory, referential, somatic, religious, or grandiose themes. Hallucinations are sensory impressions without basis in reality. They can be vivid and clear to the individual experiencing them and may occur in any sensory modality such as auditory, visual, somatic, olfactory, or gustatory, with auditory followed by visual hallucinations most common. Auditory hallucinations are distinct from the individual's own thoughts and are the most common type of hallucination. They must occur in the context of a clear sensorium. Disorganization is seen in behavior and/or thinking. Disorganized thinking is typically inferred from speech and must substantially impair effective communications. Commonly observed forms of abnormal speech include the following:

- Tangentiality—getting off topic without answering questions appropriately
- Circumstantiality—will answer question in markedly roundabout manner
- Derailment—switching topics without a logic sequence
- Neologisms—creation of new, idiosyncratic words
- Word salad—words are placed together without any sensible meaning

Grossly disorganized or abnormal motor behavior (including catatonia) may occur with schizophrenia with problems noted in goal-directed activities and activities of daily living.

Negative symptoms are diminished or there are a lack of normal characteristics—diminished emotional expression and avolition. Diminished emotional expression encompasses reductions in expression of the face; eye contact; intonation of speech; and movements of the hands, head, and face, which contribute to emotion of speech. Avolition is a decline in motivated, self-initiated, purposeful activities. This encompasses loss of affective responsiveness; verbal expression; and communication, personal and social motivation, and enjoyment. Primary negative symptoms can be resistant to treatment and closely related to functional outcome. Secondary negative symptoms may be rooted in other manifestations such as depression of the illness or treatment including sedating antipsychotics.

Cognitive impairments in schizophrenia often are seen early in life and correlate with everyday functional outcomes such as the ability to keep a job or live independently. Cognitive impairments include difficulties with memory, attention, psychomotor speed, and executive function. Cognitive impairments, along with negative symptoms, are the most common contributors to disability in schizophrenia.

Affective disturbances, which are difficulties with mood and affect, are seen with schizophrenia. Depression and anxiety can be detected before, during, or after a psychotic episode, and providers must be alert for risk of suicide, particularly at the initiation of treatment, immediately after an acute psychotic crisis, and throughout outpatient encounters (see Box 68.1).

DIAGNOSTIC REASONING

Symptoms

The Diagnostic and Statistical Manual of Mental Disorders, Fifth Edition, Text Revision (*DSM-5-TR*) provides detailed symptom criteria for schizophrenia. Two or more positive

Box 68.1 Symptom Clusters of Schizophrenia

Positive Symptoms—Exaggeration of Normal Processes

- Hallucinations: Perception of a sensory process in the absence of an external source; can be auditory (most common), visual, somatic, olfactory, or gustatory, alone or in combination.
- Delusions: Fixed false belief; classified as bizarre delusion—clearly implausible; or nonbizarre delusions—although not true, is understandable with possibility of being true. Categorized as grandiose, paranoid, nihilistic, and erotomanic.
- Disorganization: Affective or cognitive chaos; manifested in speech and behavior as loose or illogical thoughts lacking connectivity.
- Movement disorders: Grossly disorganized or abnormal motor behavior including catatonia.

Negative Symptoms—Absence or Diminution of Normal Processes

- Flat or blunted affect
- Alogia: Poverty of speech
- Asociality/anhedonia: Lack of pleasure in acts that are normally pleasurable; failure to engage with peers socially
- Apathy: Lack of self-motivation, poor grooming and hygiene, anergy

Cognitive Impairments

- Poor executive functioning, concrete thoughts, diminished processing speed
- Difficulty focusing, maintaining attention
- Verbal and visual learning and memory deficits
- Poor verbal comprehension
- Impaired social cognition

Affective Disturbances

- Blunted or flat affect, loss of affective reactivity, odd affect
- Poor self-esteem
- Depression and anxiety
- Increased risk of suicide

Source: Adapted from American Psychiatric Association. *Diagnostic and Statistical Manual of Mental Disorders, Text Revision.* 5th ed. Arlington, VA; American Psychiatric Association; 2022.

---

or negative symptoms must be present, with one of the positive symptoms being delusions, hallucinations, or disorganized speech. Dysfunction in one or more areas such as interpersonal relations, work or education, or self-care also must be present. Associated features include inappropriate affect, anhedonia, dysphoric mood, abnormal psychomotor activity, cognitive dysfunction, confusion, lack of insight, and depersonalization. Abnormal neurological findings may show a broad range of dysfunction including slow reaction time, poor coordination, abnormalities in eye tracking, and impaired sensory gating.

Schizoaffective disorder appears to be one-third as common as schizophrenia with an estimated prevalence of 0.3% and requires an uninterrupted period of illness during which the criteria for schizophrenia and a major mood disorder are met. There must also be a period of 2 weeks or longer during which there are psychotic symptoms in complete absence of mood symptoms. The incidence is higher in females than in males. Age of onset is typically early adulthood, although it may occur in adolescence to adulthood. Social dysfunction and exclusion of autism spectrum disorder or other communication disorders of childhood onset required for schizophrenia do not have to be met. Occupational function and social functioning are often impaired but need not be defining criteria for diagnosis, in contrast to schizophrenia. There may be restricted social contact, anosognosia (poor insight), and difficulties with self-care; however, negative symptoms may be less severe and less persistent. Alcohol and substance abuse can be associated with schizoaffective disorder. Individuals may go on to a diagnosis of schizophrenia, major depressive disorder, or bipolar disorder. As with schizophrenia, schizoaffective disorder carries a 10% lifetime risk of suicide, and suicide lethality must be always assessed (see the *DSM-5-TR* for complete diagnostic criteria).

Table 68.1 briefly identifies the schizophrenia spectrum and other psychotic disorders for consideration.

Differential Diagnosis

Initial presentation may occur in the primary care setting. The role of the primary care provider is to identify and refer any suspected or new cases of schizophrenia for urgent psychiatric evaluation. In some settings, especially in rural settings, this may be difficult because of a paucity of mental health services and psychiatric providers. The primary care provider is responsible for evaluating the patient's current risk to self and others. Any person presenting with psychosis for the initial or "first break" should be fully evaluated for underlying medical conditions. Consideration of substance use should be one of the primary differentials, and toxicology testing should be performed. Alcohol, opioids, cocaine, amphetamines, MDMA-receptor antagonists (ecstasy), and hallucinogens are some of the most common offenders. In addition, it is not only consumption of these agents, but also withdrawal from them, that may precipitate symptoms. Commonly prescribed medications such as anticholinergic agents, phenytoin, steroids, H_2 blockers (cimetidine), and anxiolytics may produce similar symptoms. Other differentials to consider include delirium, in which the onset of symptoms can occur rapidly and are accompanied by confusion, and in which visual hallucinations are more common, versus schizophrenia, in which the sensorium remains clear, symptoms occur over a longer time period, and auditory hallucinations occur more frequently. For individuals with acute, later-onset psychotic conditions, medical illnesses such as hepatic encephalopathy, hyponatremia, hypoglycemia, hypoxia, intracranial bleed, infection, and meningitis/encephalitis should be considered. A complete history and physical examination with attention to neurological and mental status examination are essential. Laboratory evaluation should include complete blood count (CBC) with differential, electrolytes, renal function, liver profile, thyroid function, drug and alcohol toxicology, and pregnancy. Attention should be paid to potential infectious disease processes with screening for syphilis, HIV, and hepatitis C. It may be determined that further testing for heavy metals, electroencephalogram, or brain imaging with magnetic resonance imaging or computed tomography is warranted. Diagnosis of schizophrenia spectrum and other psychotic disorder is appropriate only after other possible causes for symptoms have been ruled out.

MANAGEMENT

Depending on the individual long-term course, schizophrenia can be a chronic illness that influences many aspects of everyday life for patients and their families (see The Patient's Voice 68.1). Treatment goals should include reducing or eliminating symptoms, maximizing quality of life, improving function, and promoting and maintaining recovery within the context of an early intervention model of care. Treatment involves a multidisciplinary approach: assertive outreach and education for patients who may be hesitant to engage, family involvement and interventions, psychological therapy and interventions, vocational and educational interventions, and antipsychotic medication and monitoring (American Psychiatric Association, 2020).

Pharmacotherapy with antipsychotic medications is the mainstay of treatment for schizophrenia and should be prescribed in the context of a person-centered treatment plan (McDonagh et al, 2017; American Psychiatric Association, 2020). Early treatment is important and improves long-term outcomes. Pharmacological intervention is quite effective in addressing the positive symptoms of schizophrenia but less successful for negative and cognitive symptoms. The negative and cognitive symptoms are best addressed in a more multifaceted approach, including cognitive behavioral therapy (CBT) and cognitive remediation therapy in combination with psychiatric rehabilitation approaches. Strategies to prevent relapse and encourage medication adherence are essential. The first step may be working with patients to determine whether lack of adherence is intentional or unintentional. Intentional nonadherence may stem from negative attitudes toward medication, believing the medication is unnecessary, distressing side effects, or poor therapeutic alliance. Reasons for unintentional nonadherence may include substance use, lack of family or social support, and poor cognitive or social functioning needed to access and organize medications (Velligan et al, 2017). Social support plays a crucial role in minimizing the social disability associated with schizophrenia. The Circle of Caring (see Chapter 1) is essential in helping the patient navigate the complex system of primary care and mental health services, as well as providing education for patients and significant others to access available community resources. Understanding the lived experience of the patient, family, and community of those living with schizophrenia, as well as their definition of wellness and recovery, helps foster insight and adherence to the treatment plan. Of critical importance is the establishment of the therapeutic alliance, providing a supportive environment, maintaining continuity of provider when possible, and developing a trusting relationship where the patient is an active participant in their care. Recovery includes wellness and provision of primary care. Management of comorbid conditions is central to that effort.

Targets of Treatment

The goals of therapy include management of symptoms; evaluation of community issues such as housing, employment, homelessness, justice issues, and victimization; and assessment of co-occurring illnesses such as PTSD, substance abuse, and depression (McDonagh et al, 2017). In addition, it is essential to provide education to patients and their families and significant others to enhance understanding of the disorder, shared decision making, and adherence with the treatment plan (American Psychiatric Association, 2020).

Pharmacological Management

Antipsychotic medications can be divided into two categories: (1) conventional first generation antipsychotics (FGAs) or "typical" and (2) second generation "atypical" antipsychotic (SGA) medications. Conventional FGAs vary in affinity for D2 receptor antagonism with higher affinity, leading to increased efficacy but increased extrapyramidal symptoms (EPS). SGAs are equally as effective

> **The Patient's Voice 68.1: Schizophrenia**
>
> The first voice I heard was friendly, and I didn't make much of it. He sounded male and would comment on my day: "she's going outside" as I walked out the door, or "she should wash her hair" in the evening. The voices multiplied, and eventually I told a friend, who said I needed to see a doctor. She told other people and got my teachers involved, but the more people who told me I needed help, the less I wanted it. I didn't want to be sick and was convinced that if I ignored the evidence, it would go away. Instead, it got worse. I became confused and scared as my reality fragmented. Things were so busy and noisy inside my head that I had a hard time understanding what was happening in the world around me, and honestly, I didn't much care.

as FGAs in the treatment of positive symptoms, but SGAs are generally considered first line in first episodes of psychosis due to their reduced risk of motor side effects. Although SGAs are less likely to cause motor side effects, they have commonly been associated with weight gain and metabolic disturbances such as elevated blood glucose and lipids, type 2 diabetes mellitus, and cardiovascular disease (see Table 68.2). In addition, a greater response to medication is often seen when it is started early in the course of the disease. Initiation of early and effective doses of antipsychotic medication is important because it may influence the effect on the patient and family, as well as decrease the risk of injury to self or others (see Drugs Commonly Prescribed 68.1 and 68.2).

TABLE 68.2 Comparison of the First Generation Antipsychotics and Risk of Side Effects

High Potency	Low Potency	Shared Side Effects
High risk of extrapyramidal effects	Lower risk of extrapyramidal effects	Moderate risk of weight gain
Moderate risk of sedation	High risk of sedation	Low risk of metabolic effects
Low risk of orthostatic hypotension and tachycardia	High risk of orthostatic hypotension and tachycardia	High risk of sexual dysfunction
Low risk of anticholinergic and antiadrenergic effects	High risk of anticholinergic and antiadrenergic effects	Seizures (rare)
Higher risk of neuroleptic malignant syndrome	Lower risk of neuroleptic malignant syndrome	Allergic and dermatological effects

Drugs Commonly Prescribed 68.1: Typical Antipsychotics

DRUG	INDICATION	ADVERSE REACTIONS AND PRESCRIBING CONSIDERATIONS
High Potency		
Perphenazine* (Trilafon)	Psychosis Severe behavioral disturbances due to cognitive impairment Nausea/vomiting	• Risk for neuroleptic malignant syndrome • Monitor: AIMS, CBC, LFTs, annual eye examination, renal function, serum prolactin, weight, waist circumference, BP, FPG, and lipids, photosensitivity • Administration 2×/day
Fluphenazine (Prolixin)*+	Psychosis	• Monitor: AIMS, CBC, LFTs, annual eye examination, serum prolactin, skin exanthemas, weight, waist circumference, BP, FPG, and lipids • Administration 2×/day
Haloperidol (Haldol)*+	Acute psychosis Schizophrenia ADHD Tourette's disorder	• EPS, hyperprolactinemia, sedation, weight gain • QT prolongation risk: continuous cardiac monitoring recommended in IV administration • Monitor: AIMS, CBC, LFTs, serum prolactin, urinalysis, weight, waist circumference, BP, FPG, and lipids
Medium Potency		
Loxapine (Loxitane)*	Bipolar disorder Schizophrenia	• Photosensitivity, seizures • Monitor: CBC, ophthalmological examination, TFTs, urinalysis, weight, waist circumference, BP, FPG, and lipids
Low Potency		
Chlorpromazine (Thorazine)*	Acute intermittent porphyria Acute psychosis Nausea/vomiting Tetanus Schizophrenia Hiccups	• Photosensitivity, sulfite sensitivity, QT interval prolongation, orthostatic hypotension • Monitor: AIMS assessment, CBC, ophthalmological examination, prolactin, weight, waist circumference, BP, FPG, and lipids

*Black box warning: dementia.
+Also available as long-acting depot injection to be given biweekly (fluphenazine) or monthly (haloperidol).
Abbreviations: ADHD, attention deficit-hyperactivity disorder; AIMS, Abnormal Involuntary Movement Scale; BP, blood pressure; CBC, complete blood count; EPS, extrapyramidal symptoms; FPG, fasting plasma glucose; LFTs, liver function tests; TFTs, thyroid function tests.

Drugs Commonly Prescribed 68.2: Atypical Antipsychotics

DRUG	INDICATION	ADVERSE REACTIONS AND PRESCRIBING CONSIDERATIONS
Asenapine (Saphris)	Bipolar disorder Schizophrenia	• Sublingual (avoid eating/drinking for at least 10 mins after administration), transdermal patch • Somnolence, dizziness, EPS, anticholinergic, prolonged QT interval+, oral hypoesthesia postsublingual administration that normally dissipates, application site irritation with transdermal, metabolic effects • Monitor: weight gain,++ increased lipids,++ FPG,++ waist circumference, BP, CBC with differential, LFTs, QT interval, and AIMS
Brexpiprazole (Rexulti)	Schizophrenia Adjunct to antidepressant in major depressive disorder	• EPS, dizziness, drowsiness, metabolic effects, prolonged QT interval+ • Monitor: weight gain,+ increased lipids,++ FPG,+ waist circumference, BP, CBC with differential, LFTs, and AIMS
Clozapine (Clozaril)*	Schizophrenia Schizoaffective disorder	• Agranulocytosis, lowered seizure threshold,† rare myocarditis • Anticholinergic effects, EPS, postural hypotension, prolong QT interval,++ sedation, metabolic effects • Monitor: weight gain,+++ increased lipids,+++ FPG,+++ waist circumference, BP, CBC with differential, LFTs, and AIMS
Olanzapine (Zyprexa)*ᴵ	Bipolar depression Bipolar disorder Depression Mania Schizophrenia	• Anticholinergic effects, dizziness/hypotension, sedation, EPS, metabolic effects, prolactinemia, prolonged QT intervalᴵ+ • Monitor: weight gain,+++ increased lipids,+++ FPG,+++ waist circumference, AIMS assessment, LFTs, prolactinemia,++ neurological function
Quetiapine (Seroquel)*	Bipolar depression Bipolar disorder Depression Mania Schizophrenia	• Anticholinergic effects, postural hypotension, somnolence, prolonged QT interval++ • Monitor: weight gain,++ FPG,++ increased lipids,+++ AIMS, waist circumference, LFTs, neurological function, BP
Risperidone (Risperdal)*ᴵ	Autism Bipolar disorder Mania Schizophrenia	• Anxiety, agitation, hypotension, sedation, metabolic side effects, prolonged QT interval,++ EPS • Monitor: weight gain,++ hyperlipidemia,+ FPG,++ hyperprolactinemia,++ AIMS, waist circumference, LFTs, BP, neurological function, lipid profile
Aripiprazole (Abilify)*ᴵ	Autism Bipolar disorder Depression Mania Schizophrenia	• EPS, metabolic side effects, prolactin elevation • Monitor: AIMS, weight gain,+ FPG,+ BP LFTs, neurological function, hyperlipidemia,+ FPG +
Ziprasidone (Geodon)*	Bipolar disorder Mania Schizophrenia	• More likely to prolong QT interval, recommended baseline and monitoring • EPS, less often metabolic side effects, prolactin elevation • Monitor: ECG, AIMS, body weight, FPG,+ BP, LFTs, neurological function, lipid profile, QT interval,+++ prolactinemia++
Paliperidone (Invega)*ᴵ	Schizoaffective disorder Schizophrenia	• May prolong QT interval, EPS, tachycardia, metabolic side effects, prolactinemia • Monitor: AIMS, ECG, weight gain,++ FPG,+ BP, lipid profile, LFTs, neurological function
Iloperidone (Fanapt)*	Schizophrenia	• Anticholinergic,+ dizziness, tachycardia, orthostatic hypotension,+ sedation, metabolic side effects, prolonged QT interval,++ EPS+ • Monitor: AIMS, ECG, weight gain,++ FPG,++ BP, prolactinemia++
Lurasidone (Latuda)	Bipolar depression Schizophrenia	• EPS, nausea, drowsiness, insomnia, metabolic side effects • Monitor AIMS, ECG, weight gain,+ FPG,++ BP, hyperlipidemia,++ LFTs

Drugs Commonly Prescribed 68.2: Atypical Antipsychotics—cont'd

DRUG	INDICATION	ADVERSE REACTIONS AND PRESCRIBING CONSIDERATIONS
Cariprazine (Vraylar)	Bipolar disorder Schizophrenia	• EPS, nausea, headache, insomnia, metabolic side effects • Monitor AIMS, ECG, weight gain,++ FPG,+ BP, hyperlipidemia,+ LFTs

*Black box warning: dementia.
†Doses greater than 600 mg.
+Mild
++Moderate
+++High risk.
ⁱMedications available in long-acting injectable form ranging from 2- to 12-week dosing interval requirement depending on drug pharmacology.
Abbreviations: AIMS, Abnormal Involuntary Movement Scale; BP, blood pressure; CBC, complete blood count; ECG, electrocardiogram; EPS, extrapyramidal symptoms; FPG, fasting plasma glucose; LFT, liver function test.

Because medication-naive patients are more sensitive to the psychotropic effects of medications (they respond to lower doses and may show heightened sensitivity to side effects), initiation at the lower end of the standard dose is recommended. Response rates are variable; slow titration of antipsychotic medication is recommended to help reduce the risk of intolerable side effects that may affect long-term adherence, although more rapid dose escalation is sometimes required. Patients who experience a first episode are typically more responsive to treatment than those who have experienced multiple episodes of illness; remission is achieved within 3 to 4 months for 70% of patients, and 83% have a stable remission by 1 year. Unfortunately, some individuals will not seek treatment because of paranoid symptoms or impaired thinking process.

The Clinical Antipsychotic Trials of Intervention Effectiveness project (CATIE) sponsored by the National Institute of Mental Health looked at the various antipsychotic medications, comparing a number of the newer drugs with the conventional antipsychotic perphenazine. The newer "atypical" drugs were not superior to perphenazine, a "typical" antipsychotic, although olanzapine had the highest rate of "persistence" (i.e., was switched less often because of side effects or lack of efficacy). Given the magnitude of the problem of nonadherence with antipsychotic medications, depot medications are particularly important for patients who have difficulty with adherence. Injectable formulations are given intramuscularly ranging from biweekly to 12-week intervals and may aid patients with adherence. Adjunctive medications help with controlling side effects and assisting with comorbid illnesses such as anxiety and depression.

EPS are potentially troubling side effects of antipsychotics and include Parkinson-like symptoms, akathisia (an inability to sit still), and dystonia (involuntary muscle contraction). Antipsychotic dose reduction, cessation, or switching to an SGA if on an FGA may be required and anticholinergics may be prescribed to reduce symptoms. Any dystonia involving the airway requires medication cessation and may require acute stabilization. Tardive dyskinesia (TD) is involuntary choreoathetoid movements that may also require dose reduction, cessation, or switching to an SGA. Treatment with benzodiazepines, botulinum toxin injections, valbenazine, or tetrabenazine is considered to improve TD symptoms, but symptoms may become persistent or disabling. Patient education is essential in discussing EPS to identify and treat these symptoms and to ensure adherence to the pharmacological regimen (see Table 68.3).

It is important to consider that dose adjustment, reduction, or medication changes may be required in various situations. FGAs largely undergo hepatic metabolism, which may require dose reduction in hepatic impairment and many antipsychotics may interact with other drugs that affect CYP metabolism. Patients with sexual dysfunction or abnormal lactation will require evaluation of prolactin, with elevation being more common with certain medications such as risperidone and paliperidone. Antipsychotics have varying cardiac risks including prolonged QT interval. Risks versus benefits must be considered carefully in those with a cardiac history. Baseline electrocardiogram (ECG) and monitoring recommendations should be considered in collaboration with cardiology and psychiatry services, and it is important to avoid medications with more pronounced cardiac risks such as ziprasidone.

Geriatric Considerations: Antipsychotic Medications

Antipsychotic medications should be used cautiously in older patients. These medications remain appropriate for treating psychosis and severe agitation; however, providers should titrate slowly and use the lowest effective dose. All antipsychotics are included in the American Geriatric Association Beers Criteria with particular concern for sedation, falls, and orthostatic hypotension. SGAs are safer for older patients but carry a Food and Drug Administration (FDA) black box warning for death and cerebrovascular events in patients with dementia. These patients require individualized treatment planning and careful monitoring for side effects, neurological changes, and medication interactions. Nonpharmacological options should be used whenever possible to reduce distress and agitation, and antipsychotics should be discontinued if they are not providing clear benefit.

TABLE 68.3 Extrapyramidal Symptoms, Description, and Treatment

Movement Disorder/Timing	Description	Treatment
Akathisia Occurs a few days to a few weeks after initiation of medication	Restlessness Subjective: Unable to sit still, unable to remain calm Objective: Pacing, foot-tapping, shifting weight from foot to foot	Discontinue medication Benzodiazepines: lorazepam, diazepam, alprazolam Beta blockers such as propranolol
Dystonia May occur after a single dose of medication to several days later	Involuntary muscle contractions affecting the head and neck (hoarseness, laryngeal spasms, oculogyric crisis, torticollis) May involve the torso and extremities (opisthotonos)	Anticholinergics Antiparkinsonian medication
Pseudoparkinsonism May occur after a single dose, but typically seen a few weeks later as the dosage is increased	Slow pill-rolling tremor of hands, cogwheel rigidity, shuffling gait, mask-like face, loss of arm swing, and bradyphrenia After prolonged use, "rabbit syndrome": tremor of lips characterized by constant chewing motion	Anticholinergics
Tardive Dyskinesia More often late-appearing manifestation, months to years	Involuntary rapid movements of the face (lip smacking, grimacing, facial distortions), torso, and extremities 6% irreversible	Prevention and screening tools for movement disorders every 3–6 months Anticholinergic agents Antiparkinsonian agents Removal of agent

Antipsychotics have varying incidence of metabolic side effects including weight gain and metabolic changes such as elevated glucose, hyperlipidemia, and hypertension, with medications such as olanzapine and clozapine being higher risk and medications such as aripiprazole and ziprasidone showing less metabolic side effects. These side effects necessitate screening, ongoing monitoring, clinical management and risk/benefit evaluation, and discussion with the patient and psychiatric provider. Primary care providers can play a pivotal role in managing metabolic conditions for patients who feel the risk of uncontrolled psychiatric symptoms necessitates ongoing medications that may affect their physical health. Frequent monitoring is recommended for all patients receiving antipsychotics including baseline and sequential measurement of body mass index (BMI); waist circumference; blood pressure; fasting glucose; and fasting lipid profile at baseline, 1 month, 3 months, and annually. Pregnancy testing at baseline and routinely in females of childbearing age is recommended.

Patients with schizophrenia are more likely than the general population to die of chronic obstructive pulmonary disease (COPD); influenza; pneumonia; diabetes; and cardiovascular disease; and to develop lung, breast, and gastrointestinal cancers, making the clinician's role in identification and management of comorbidities and side effects crucial. Ongoing education that builds on previous medical encounters is essential to assist the patient and family with methods to reduce the increased risk of cardiac- and pulmonary-related events. The clinician can also aid in harm reduction and education around dietary, nicotine, and controlled substance use that may contribute to poor health outcomes. Ensuring routine dental, eye, and age-appropriate screening examinations are conducted to prevent delays in treatment or problem identification is important. Strong patient and clinician alliance can be of support to patients with schizophrenia. Clinicians can play a role in helping patients with adherence to pharmacological and nonpharmacological therapies with the goal of sustained remission of symptoms. It is recommended that patients continue on the lowest effective dose of antipsychotic medications to prevent recurrence of symptoms. There is a risk of relapse with medication cessation and varying recommendations for length of time before considering a trial cessation of medications. Person-centered engagement in discussion of the risks/benefits and treatment decisions is essential and, if the patient desires, they may find benefit from inclusion of their support system in the education and decision-making processes. Treatment of coexisting behavioral health conditions such as depression, substance use, or anxiety may also benefit patients with schizophrenia. Antidepressants may improve overall functioning.

Most antipsychotics show some improvement in symptoms in 2 to 4 weeks of treatment; however, improvement may slowly continue over many months. Patients who do not show improvement or have intolerable side effects may require switching to a different antipsychotic medication. For those with treatment-resistant schizophrenia or persistent suicidal behavior, clozapine has been shown to be efficacious. It can be challenging, however, for patients to adhere to the mandatory regular neutrophil monitoring (weekly for the first 6 months, every 2 weeks for the second 6 months, and then every 4 weeks after 1 year) that is required due to a rare but dangerous risk of agranulocytosis. Clozapine also requires a slow taper to initiate, which must be restarted if the medication dose is missed for 72 hours. Myocarditis is also a potential adverse reaction to clozapine and patients presenting with fatigue, tachypnea, chest pain, fever, and/or dyspnea need emergent evaluation with an ECG, white blood cell count, and serum troponin levels. If myocarditis is diagnosed, clozapine must be stopped, and when abruptly discontinued, may require anticholinergic replacement therapy to prevent anticholinergic rebound.

Nonpharmacological Management

For patients with persistent positive symptoms, CBT has been found helpful in the reduction of both symptoms and relapse rates while improving function and quality of life. Specific CBT strategies developed for individuals with psychosis (CPTp) can improve insight and help patients develop more personal, realistic, and adaptive explanations for their positive symptoms (American Psychiatric Association, 2020). Patients who have experienced a high incidence of relapse may benefit from an assertive community treatment (ACT) team approach. The ACT approach forgoes the constraints of timed clinic appointments, and instead team members meet patients at their home or at shelters or community locations and spend more time on individualized support. This multidisciplinary team-based approach is evidence based and provides culturally sensitive services for people with severe and persistent mental illnesses who have not benefited from traditional outpatient care and who also have a significant history of relapse or hospitalization. A hallmark of ACT is to develop a positive, trusting relationship with each patient to improve their compliance with mental health treatment and focus on mental health and recovery.

ACT services have a strong emphasis on recovery principles individualized to meet the patient's needs, and patient participation can be either voluntary or court mandated. Services may include case management, medication management, vocational counseling and placement, family counseling and psychoeducation, and wellness management education. The team approach typically includes a psychiatric prescriber, nurse, counselor, case manager, and peer support. The original ACT model included a medical provider, but this is no longer an integral part of the model.

FOLLOW-UP AND REFERRAL

Treatment of schizophrenia requires integrated care and close communication among primary care, specialty care, patients, and families. Families' support and encouragement are crucial for patients who may be hesitant to accept treatment, especially early in the disease course. Patients who present a danger to themselves or others and those who are unable to care for basic personal needs must be hospitalized, but all patients with schizophrenia should receive specialty psychiatric assessment or consult after initial presentation and during acute episodes that do not respond to straightforward medication adjustments.

Primary care settings are important in recognizing early symptoms for referral and treatment, supporting early aggressive treatments through patient education and trusting relationships with family, and long-term management and monitoring. The course of illness of schizophrenia is variable and often chronic, with symptoms, cognitive deficits, and medical health issues combining to create high levels of disability. Patients with schizophrenia have an average life span shorter by 20 years compared with population norms, which is due to suicide and medical comorbidities that lead to diabetes and cardiovascular disease. Typically, 15% of patients have a good outcome, 30% have an intermediate outcome, and 55% have a poor outcome.

Long-term primary care follow-up requires assessing for changes in symptoms or suicidality and managing medical comorbidities and medication side effects. Supporting a patient in developing a healthy lifestyle and reducing substance use through tobacco cessation and harm-reduction methods improves prognosis and reduces medical morbidity and mortality. Poor prognosis is suggested by a gradual onset of symptoms, earlier onset, disorganized thoughts and behavior, and comorbid substance use.

Patient Education: Schizophrenia

Because schizophrenia is best viewed as a chronic and potentially lifelong illness, looking at a variety of strategies to optimize functional status and quality of life is important. Patients and families should have an opportunity to learn about the diagnosis and risks and benefits of different treatment options. The Circle of Caring model, encompassing the concepts of authentic presence, advocacy, knowing, commitment, and patience, is the essence of humanistic, quality medical care for all populations, but is critically important for those living with schizophrenia and other serious mental illnesses. This model must be fostered in staff training and incorporated into the culture of the health-care setting to reduce the negative effects of stigma.

Individuals living with schizophrenia regularly face public stigma, as represented by negative stereotypes and discrimination enacted by others, as well as internalized stigma, in which individuals become aware of these negative stereotypes and apply these beliefs to themselves. Stigmatization reduces schizophrenia to a set of negative attitudes and fears and may have negative effects on patients' willingness to engage with treatment and the clinical course of the disease. Labels and social disapproval influence health-care access, damage self-esteem and self-efficacy, and increase depressive symptoms. Increased likelihood of the misuse of alcohol and drugs may be related to the prejudice and discrimination related to schizophrenia.

There is some evidence that practicing active coping strategies and sharing stories with peers may reduce stigma and facilitate attendance at primary care. Peers are individuals who have the unique lived experience of being mental health consumers themselves. Services delivered by trained peers have been shown to diminish feelings of isolation and improve coping skills that support recovery. Peer support services can also include assistance with housing and benefits advisement, employment and career counseling, justice issues, advocacy, and independent living skills.

Social centers, sometimes called "clubhouses," can be found in most U.S. states. These provide a voluntary semi-structured program where patients can meet in a safe environment to share conversation and participate in activities with others having similar concerns. Groups run by the Hearing Voices Network can also support individuals who feel isolated or stigmatized by their experiences.

Social skill training improves social adjustment and coping skills. Supportive individual and group psychotherapy along with medications can reduce relapses and enhance occupational and vocational functioning. Employment may destigmatize a person coping with both psychiatric disability and a criminal record, and paid employment may aid in community integration. Family education helps improve communication between the patient and mental health services and subsequently helps reduce relapse rates and improve family functioning. Social centers aim to address isolation experienced by most patients. Community resources such as the National Alliance on Mental Illness are invaluable sources of support for patients and families.

REFERENCES

American Diabetes Association, American Psychiatric Association, American Association of Clinical Endocrinologists, North American Association for the Study of Obesity. Consensus development conference on antipsychotic drugs and obesity and diabetes. *Diabetes Care.* 2004;27:596-601.

American Psychiatric Association. *Practice Guideline for the Treatment of Patients with Schizophrenia.* 3rd ed. American Psychiatric Association; 2020. https://psychiatryonline.org/doi/book/10.1176/appi.books.9780890424841

American Psychiatric Association. *Practice Guideline on the Use of Antipsychotics to Treat Agitation or Psychosis in Patients with Dementia.* American Psychiatric Association; 2016. https://psychiatryonline.org/doi/book/10.1176/appi.books.9780890426807

Barbui C, Girlanda F, Ay E, et al. Implementation of treatment guidelines for specialist mental health care. *Cochrane Database Syst Rev.* 2014;1:CD009780.

Bartels SJ, DiMilia PR, Fortuna KL, et al. Integrated care for older adults with serious mental illness and medical comorbidity: evidence-based models and future research directions. *Psychiatr Clin North Am.* 2018;41(1):153-164.

Belbasis L, Köhler CA, Stefanis N, et al. Risk factors and peripheral biomarkers for schizophrenia spectrum disorders: an umbrella review of meta-analyses. *Acta Psychiatr Scand.* 2018 Feb;137(2):88-97.

Bora E, Murray RM. Meta-analysis of cognitive deficits in ultra-high risk to psychosis and first-episode psychosis: do the cognitive deficits progress over, or after, the onset of psychosis? *Schizophr Bull.* 2014;40:744.

Bowie CR, Bell MD, Fiszdon JM, et al. Cognitive remediation for schizophrenia: An expert working group white paper on core techniques. *Schizophr Res.* 2020 Jan;215:49-53.

Cella M, Price T, Corboy H, et al. Cognitive remediation for inpatients with psychosis: a systematic review and meta-analysis. *Psychol Med.* 2020 May;50(7):1062-1076.

Ceraso A, Lin JJ, Schneider-Thoma J, et al. Maintenance treatment with antipsychotic drugs for schizophrenia. *Cochrane Database Syst Rev.* 2020 Aug 11;8:CD008016.

Cernea S, Dima L, Correll CU, et al. Pharmacological management of glucose dysregulation in patients treated with second-generation antipsychotics. *Drugs.* 2020 Nov;80(17):1763-1781.

Chapel JM, Ritchey MD, Zhang D, et al. Prevalence and medical costs of chronic diseases among adult medicaid beneficiaries. *Am J Prevent Med.* 2017;53(6):S143-S154. https://doi.org/10.1016/j.amepre.2017.07.019

Charlson FJ, Ferrari AJ, Santomauro DF, et al. Global epidemiology and burden of schizophrenia: findings from the Global Burden of Disease Study 2016. *Schizophr Bull.* 2018;44(6):1195-1203. https://doi.org/10.1093/schbul/sby058

Chien WT, Yip AL. Current approaches to treatments for schizophrenia spectrum disorders, part I: an overview and medical treatments. *Neuropsychiatr Dis Treat.* 2013;9:1311-1132.

Clemmensen L, Vernal DL, Steinhausen HC. A systematic review of the long-term effects of early onset schizophrenia. *BMC Psychiatry.* 2012;12:150.

Cloutier M, Sanon Aigbogun M, Guerin A, et al. The economic burden of schizophrenia in the United States in 2013. *J Clin Psychiatry.* 2016;77(06):764-771. doi: 10.4088/JCP.15m10278

Cunningham KC, Lucksted A. Social cognition, internalized stigma, and recovery orientation among adults with serious mental illness. *Psychiatr Rehab J.* 2017;40(4):409-411.

Davies C, Segre G, Estradé A, et al. Prenatal and perinatal risk and protective factors for psychosis: a systematic review and meta-analysis. *Lancet Psychiatry.* 2020;7(5):399-410.

De Sousa A, Shah B, Shrivastava A. Suicide and schizophrenia: an interplay of factors. *Curr Psychiatry Rep.* 2020 Oct 8;22(12):65.

Debbané M, Eliez S, Badoud D, et al. Developing psychosis and its risk states through the lens of schizotypy. *Schizophr Bull.* 2015;41(suppl 2):S396.

Drapalski AL, Lucksted A, Perrin PB, et al. A model of internalized stigma and its effects on people with mental illness. *Psychiatr Serv.* 2013;64:264.

Fantini G, Tibaldi G, Rucci P, et al. Quality of care indicators for schizophrenia: Determinants of observed variations among Italian Departments of Mental Health. Results from the ETAS DSM study. *Epidemiol Psychiatr Sci.* 2016:1-15.

Francey SM, Jovev M, Phassouliotis C, et al. Does co-occurring borderline personality disorder influence acute phase treatment for first-episode psychosis? *Early Intev Psychiatry.* 2018;12(6):1166-1172. https://doi.org/10.1111/eip.12435

Glick ID, Correll CU, Altamura AC, et al. Mid-term and long-term efficacy and effectiveness of antipsychotic medications for schizophrenia: a data-driven, personalized clinical approach. *J Clin Psychiatry.* 2011 Dec;72(12):1616-1627.

Habtewold TD, Rodijk LH, Liemburg EJ, et al. A systematic review and narrative synthesis of data-driven studies in schizophrenia symptoms and cognitive deficits. *Transl Psychiatry.* 2020 Jul 21;10(1):244.

Haddock G, Eisner E, Boone C, et al. An investigation of the implementation of NICE-recommended CBT interventions for people with schizophrenia. *J Ment Health.* 2014;23(4):162-165.

Harrison RNS, Gaughran F, Murray RM, et al. Development of multivariable models to predict change in Body Mass Index within a clinical trial population of psychotic individuals. *Sci Rep.* 2017;7(1):14738.

Hasan A, von Keller R, Friemel CM, et al. Cannabis use and psychosis: a review of reviews. *Eur Arch Psychiatry Clin Neurosci.* 2020 Jun;270(4):403-412.

Henssler J, Brandt L, Müller M, et al. Migration and schizophrenia: meta-analysis and explanatory framework. *Eur Arch Psychiatry Clin Neurosci.* 2020 Apr;270(3):325-335.

Hor, K., Taylor, M. (2010). Suicide and schizophrenia: A systematic review of rates and risk factors. *Journal of Psychopharmacology,* 24(4 Suppl), 81–90. https://doi-org.uri.idm.oclc.org/10.1177/1359786810385490

Kane JM, Robinson DG, Schooler NR, et al. Comprehensive versus usual community care for first-episode psychosis: 2-year outcomes from the NIMH RAISE early treatment program. *Am J Psychiatry.* 2016;173:362.

Kuepper R, van Os J, Lieb R, et al. Continued cannabis use and risk of incidence and persistence of psychotic symptoms: 10 year follow-up cohort study. *BMJ.* 2011;342:d738.

Leaune E, Dealberto M, Luck D, et al. Ethnic minority position and migrant status as risk factors for psychotic symptoms in the general population: a meta-analysis. *Psychol Med.* 2019;49(4):545-558.

Lipner E, Murphy SK, Ellman LM. Prenatal maternal stress and the cascade of risk to schizophrenia spectrum disorders in offspring. *Curr Psychiatry Rep.* 2019 Sep 14;21(10):99. doi: 10.1007/s11920-019-1085-1.

Lundström S, Jormfeldt H, Hedman Ahlström B, et al. Mental health nurses' experience of physical health care and health promotion initiatives for people with severe mental illness. *Int J Ment Health Nurs.* 2020 Apr;29(2):244-253.

Lynskey MT, Strang, J. The global burden of drug use and mental disorders. *Lancet.* 2013;382(9904):1540-1542.

McDonagh MS, Dana T, Selph S, et al. Treatments for schizophrenia in adults: a systematic review (Comparative Effectiveness Review No. 198; prepared by the Pacific Northwest Evidence-based Practice Center under Contract No. 290-2015-00009-I). AHRQ Publication No. 17(18)-EHC031-EF. Rockville, MD: Agency for Healthcare Research and Quality; 2017. https://effectivehealthcare.ahrq.gov/products/schizophrenia-adult/research-2017.

Mitchell AJ, Vancampfort D, De Herdt A, et al. Is the prevalence of metabolic syndrome and metabolic abnormalities increased in early schizophrenia? A comparative meta-analysis of first episode, untreated and treated patients. *Schizophr Bull.* 2013 Mar;39(2):295-305.

Moore EA, Green MJ, Carr VJ. Comorbid personality traits in schizophrenia: prevalence and clinical characteristics. *J Psychiatr Res.* 2012;46(3):353-359. https://doi.org/10.1016/j.jpsychires.2011.11.012

Moore TA. Schizophrenia treatment guidelines in the United States. *Clin Schizophr Relat Psychoses.* 2011;5:40-49.

Moreno-Küstner B, Martín C, Pastor L. Prevalence of psychotic disorders and its association with methodological issues. A systematic review and meta-analyses. *PLoS One,* 2018;13(4):e0195687. https://doi.org/10.1371/journal.pone.0195687

Morriss R, Vinjamuri I, Faizal MA, et al. Training to recognise the early signs of recurrence in schizophrenia. *Cochrane Database Syst Rev.* 2013;(2):CD005147.

Murray RM, Bhavsar V, Tripoli G, et al. 30 years on: how the neurodevelopmental hypothesis of schizophrenia morphed into the developmental risk factor model of psychosis. *Schizophr Bull.* 2017 Oct 21;43(6):1190-1196.

National Institute of Health. *CATIE: Schizophrenia trial.* Published 2021, February. https://www.clinicaltrials.gov/ct2/show/NCT00014001

National Institute for Health and Clinical Excellence. *Psychosis and schizophrenia in adults: prevention and treatment.* https://www.nice.org.uk/guidance/cg178. Published March 2014.

Pillinger T, Beck K, Gobjila C, et al. Impaired glucose homeostasis in first-episode schizophrenia: a systematic review and meta-analysis. *JAMA Psychiatry.* 2017;74:261.

Popovic D, Benabarre A, Crespo JM, et al. Risk factors for suicide in schizophrenia: systematic review and clinical recommendations. *Acta Psychiatr Scand.* 2014;130(6):418-426. https://doi.org/10.1111/acps.12332

Rosen C, Grossman LS, Harrow M, et al. Diagnostic and prognostic significance of Schneiderian first-rank symptoms: a 20-year longitudinal study of schizophrenia and bipolar disorder. *Compr Psychiatry.* 2011;52:126.

Sadock BJ, Kaplan, VA, Ruiz P. *Kaplan and Sadock's Comprehensive Textbook of Psychiatry.* 10th ed. Lippincott Williams & Wilkins; 2017.

Selten JP, van der Ven E, Rutten BP, et al. The social defeat hypothesis of schizophrenia: an update. *Schizophr Bull.* 2013 Nov;39(6):1180-1186.

Somaiya M, Grover S, Avasthi A, et al. Changes in cost of treating schizophrenia: comparison of two studies done a decade apart. *Psychiatry Res.* 2014;215:547.

Sommer IE, Tiihonen J, van Mourik A, et al. The clinical course of schizophrenia in women and men—a nationwide cohort study. *NPJ Schizophr.* 2020;6(1):1-7. https://doi.org/10.1038/s41537-020-0102-z

Stentebjerg-Olesen M, Pagsberg AK, Fink-Jensen A, et al. Clinical characteristics and predictors of outcome of schizophrenia-spectrum psychosis in children and adolescents: a systematic review. *J Child Adol Psychopharmacol.* 2016;26(5):410-427.

Strauss GP, Horan WP, Kirkpatrick B, et al. Deconstructing negative symptoms of schizophrenia: Avolition-apathy and diminished expression clusters predict clinical presentation and functional outcome. *J Psychiatr Res.* 2013;47:783.

Suijkerbuijk YB, Schaafsma FG, van Mechelen JC, et al. Interventions for obtaining and maintaining employment in adults with severe mental illness, a network meta-analysis. *Cochrane Database Syst Rev.* 2017 Sep 12;9(9):CD011867.

Tandon, R, Nasrallah, HA, Keshavan MS. Schizophrenia, "just the facts" 5. Treatment and prevention. Past, present, and future. *Schizophr Res.* 2010;122(1-3):1-23.

Thornicroft G, Bakolis I, Evans-Lacko S, et al. Key lessons learned from the INDIGO global network on mental health related stigma and discrimination. *World Psychiatry.* 2019 Jun;18(2):229-230.

Vaucher J, Keating BJ, Lasserre AM, et al. Cannabis use and risk of schizophrenia: a Mendelian randomization study. *Mol Psychiatry.* 2018 May;23(5):1287-1292.

Velligan DI, Sajatovic M, Hatch A, et al. Why do psychiatric patients stop antipsychotic medication? A systematic review of reasons for nonadherence to medication in patients with serious mental illness. *Patient Prefer Adherence.* 2017;11:449.

Ward PB, Firth J, Rosenbaum S, et al. Lifestyle interventions to reduce premature mortality in schizophrenia. *Lancet Psychiatry.* 2017;4(7):e14.

Werbeloff N, Levine SZ, Rabinowitz J. Elaboration on the association between immigration and schizophrenia: A population-based national study disaggregating annual trends, country of origin and sex over 15 years. *Soc Psychiatry Psychiatr Epidemiol.* 2012;47:303.

WFSBP Task Force on Treatment Guidelines for Schizophrenia. World Federation of Societies of Biological Psychiatry (WFSBP) guidelines for biological treatment of schizophrenia—a short version for primary care. *Int J Psychiatry Clin Pract.* 2017;21(2):82-90.

Wood L, Byrne R, Varese F, et al. Psychosocial interventions for internalised stigma in people with a schizophrenia-spectrum diagnosis: a systematic narrative synthesis and meta-analysis. *Schizophr Res.* 2016;176(2-3):291-303.

World Health Organization. Schizophrenia, schizotypal and delusional disorders. *International Statistical Classification of Disease and Related Health Problems.* 10th revision. http://apps.who.int/classifications/icd10/browse/2015/en#/F20-F29. Published 2015.

Wykes T, Huddy V, Cellard C, et al. A meta-analysis of cognitive remediation for schizophrenia: methodology and effect sizes. *Am J Psychiatry.* 2011 May;168(5):472-485.

Zhao S, Sampson S, Xia J, et al. Psychoeducation (brief) for people with serious mental illness. *Cochrane Database Syst Rev.* 2015;(4):CD010823.

Zhuo C, Tao R, Jiang R, et al. Cancer mortality in patients with schizophrenia: systematic review and meta-analysis. *Br J Psychiatry.* 2017;211(1):7-13.

RESOURCES

Advice for Parents of Children With Behavioral and Psychiatric Disorders. Brain and Behavior Research Foundation
https://www.bbrfoundation.org/blog/advice-parents-children-behavioral-and-psychiatric-disorders

Clubhouse International
https://clubhouse-intl.org/

Delusional Disorder. Harvard Health Publishing
https://www.health.harvard.edu/a_to_z/delusional-disorder-a-to-z

Delusional Disorder Health Library. Cleveland Clinic
https://my.clevelandclinic.org/health/diseases/9599-delusional-disorder

Delusional Infestation: Overview and Recommendations. DynaMed Plus
http://www.dynamed.com/topics/dmp~AN~T114682/Delusional-infestation#Overview-and-Recommendations

Expert Q & A: Schizophrenia. American Psychiatric Association
https://www.psychiatry.org/patients-families/schizophrenia/expert-q-and-a

Fact Sheet: Early Warning Signs of Psychosis. National Institute of Mental Health
https://www.nimh.nih.gov/health/topics/schizophrenia/raise/fact-sheet-early-warning-signs-of-psychosis

Fact Sheet: First Episode Psychosis. National Institute of Mental Health
https://www.nimh.nih.gov/health/topics/schizophrenia/raise/fact-sheet-first-episode-psychosis#:~:text=FACTS%20ABOUT%20PSYCHOSIS&text=Psychosis%20often%20begins%20when%20a,some%20time%20in%20their%20lives

Guidelines and Measures. Agency for Healthcare Research and Quality.
https://www.guideline.gov/summaries/summary/48381?

Hearing Voices Network.
https://www.hearing-voices.org/

Patient Story: Schizophrenia. American Psychiatric Association.
https://www.psychiatry.org/patients-families/schizophrenia/patient-story

Schizophrenia. Medline Plus Patient Information
https://medlineplus.gov/schizophrenia.html

Schizophrenia. National Alliance on Mental Illness.
https://www.nami.org/Learn-More/Mental-Health-Conditions/Schizophrenia

Schizophrenia. National Institute of Mental Health
https://www.nimh.nih.gov/health/topics/schizophrenia/index.shtml

Publications about Schizophrenia. National Institute of Mental Health
https://www.nimh.nih.gov/health/publications/schizophrenia-listing

Schizophrenia. National Alliance on Mental Illness
https://www.nami.org/Learn-More/Mental-Health-Conditions/Schizophrenia/Discuss

Schizophrenia: Overview and Recommendations. DynaMed Plus
http://www.dynamed.com/topics/dmp~AN~T115234#Overview-and-Recommendations

Schizophrenia: Overview Treatment. DynaMed Plus
http://www.dynamed.com/topics/dmp~AN~T115234#Treatment

Schizotypal Personality Disorder. Mayo Clinic.
https://www.mayoclinic.org/diseases-conditions/schizotypal-personality-disorder/symptoms-causes/syc-20353919

Schizophrenia Statistics. National Institute of Mental Health
https://www.nimh.nih.gov/health/statistics/prevalence/schizophrenia.shtml

Schizotypal Personality Disorder. Medline Plus Health Information
https://medlineplus.gov/ency/article/001525.htm

Schizotypal Personality Disorder. Targeting the D1 Dopamine Receptor to Improve Working Memory in Schizotypal Personality Disorder. Brain and Behavior Research Foundation.
https://www.bbrfoundation.org/content/targeting-d1-dopamine-receptor-improve-working-memory-schizotypal-personality-disorder

Chapter 69

Mood Disorders

Michaela K. Hogan, DNP, APRN, PMHNP-BC
Ashley Love, DNP, PMHNP-BC
Rene Love, PhD, DNP, PMHNP-BC, FNAP, FAANP
Karen Jennings Mathis, PhD, APRN-CNP, PMHNP-BC, FAED

OVERVIEW

Depression is a common disorder with more than 254 million people suffering globally. Worldwide, depression is a leading cause of disability and an overall contributor to the global burden of diseases. In the United States, 4.7% of adults aged 18 and older have regular feelings of depression with 9.3% of physician office visits documenting depression on the medical record. The following sections include major depressive, dysthymic, and bipolar disorders. Major depressive disorder (MDD) is the primary diagnosis in this category. Sequelae from mental illness contribute to the almost 800,000 people worldwide who die by suicide. Suicide is the second leading cause of death in 10- to 14-year-olds and 25- to 34-year-olds. In 2020, over 45,000 people died by suicide in the United States, making suicide among the top 9 leading causes of death in 10- to 64-year-olds. Therefore, in this chapter, acute suicide risk will be discussed in detail.

MAJOR DEPRESSIVE DISORDER

Depression is a common condition seen in primary care settings. People use the term *depression* to describe a wide variety of negative emotional states, ranging from sadness to loss of interest or pleasure in activities to irritability to self-hate. The hallmarks of MDD, however, are sadness and anhedonia (loss of pleasure). In most cases, the sadness and anhedonia associated with MDD can be distinguished from ordinary changes in mood.

Individual variations in the clinical presentation of depression can be great, sometimes making the condition difficult to recognize. In primary care settings, patients often present with ambiguous symptoms of unexplained fatigue, changes in appetite, and changes in sleep patterns; only when questioned will they admit to feelings of "sadness." Others will complain of moderate to significant feelings of apathy. Additional presentations include complaints of irritability, anger, anxiety, or hyperactivity. Many people with depression are unaware of the level of functional impairment resulting from their illness. Slowed thinking and emotional numbness—two significant symptoms of depression—can contribute to a lack of awareness of depression. Sex and culture can impact presentation, but neither should influence assessment of depression. Depression causes great psychological pain, prompting many people with depression to consider any solution that they think may bring relief. Patients may have difficulty describing their pain and may make vague references to "hurting" or "feeling bad." Thoughts of death or suicide are not uncommon (see Evidence-Based Nursing Practice 69.1).

MDD is characterized by substantial negative changes in mood, thinking, and behavior. A person who is severely depressed will have intense feelings of sadness, irritability, or apathy. These feelings may persist and are unrelieved by situational changes; for example, whether at home, school, work, or in recreational situations, the mood of the person with depression will vary little, without significant improvement.

Negative changes in thinking associated with depression are common. Depressed thinking can be described as global, distorted, and circular. Rather than dealing with today, the person with depression may instead focus

---

 Evidence-Based Nursing Practice 69.1
Depression

DEPRESSION

Beck CT. Teetering on the edge: A substantive theory of postpartum depression. *Nurs Res*. 1993;42(1):42–48.

This classic study used a qualitative approach to develop a theory regarding women's perceptions of postpartum depression. Drawing a sample of 12 from a postpartum support group, the researcher conducted in-depth interviews with the women about their experiences of postpartum depression. What emerged was a rich description of the nature of postpartum depression and how these women managed their depression. "Teetering on the edge" was the hallmark metaphor that the researcher extracted to describe the process that the participants confronted during their depression. They felt "between" sane and insane, and the researcher identified several stages: "Encountering the terror" described the unpredictable nature of feelings that overwhelmed them, anxiety and panic attacks, obsessions, and loss of concentration. In the next stage, called "the dying of self," the women experienced isolation, withdrawal, and feelings of dissociation and depersonalization. Most had suicidal ideation. In the next stage, "struggling to survive," they began to grapple with their feelings. They searched out support groups, used prayer and faith to manage the depression, and began, hesitantly, and with some steps forward and some steps backward, to recover.

on past events or think about a bleak future. The balance between positive and negative thoughts about self, life, and the future becomes distorted. Negative views can seem more valid than positive views. Global negative thinking can take on a ruminative or circular pattern, so that the person's negative thinking seems to always depart from and arrive at the same painful conclusions.

MDD interferes with decision making and concentration. The smallest decision, such as whether to make a phone call, becomes difficult. The person with depression may become alarmed by their inability to make choices or concentrate. Although others may recognize negative changes in the patient's thinking, it can develop without warning to the patient. The negative thinking may include thoughts of death and suicide. Some clinicians attempt to make a clear distinction between passive thoughts of death and active thoughts of suicide, but both patterns are alarming.

The individual with depression may begin behaving uncharacteristically. For this reason, significant others may become aware of the depression before the patient. Depression-related behavioral changes range from changes in grooming and interpersonal interactions to substance abuse, irritability, aggression, and social withdrawal.

Cultural variations in the presentation of depression are also individualized. Based on how traditional or nontraditional the individual's attitudes and behaviors are, patients may focus less on personal experiences and more on physical aches and pains. Ethnic and cultural norms concerning privacy, embarrassment, and disclosure will also have an impact on the patient's presentation.

EPIDEMIOLOGY AND CAUSES

It is estimated that 8.4% of adults in the United States will experience MDD in their lifetime. The prevalence of MDD is higher in adult females (10.5%), individuals aged 18 to 25 years (17%), and adults reporting ancestry of two or more races (15.9%). It is estimated that 17% of adolescents aged 12 to 17 years will experience MDD. The prevalence is higher in adolescent females (25.2%) and adolescents reporting ancestry of two or more races (29.9%). In certain segments of the older adult population, usually those who are sicker and/or in pain, the prevalence of depression can be higher. Some studies document prevalence as high as 40% in nursing home patients and as high as 30% in community-dwelling older adults with chronic medical conditions. Older adults have many risk factors for depression because of the frequent losses experienced in this age group.

The economic burden of serious mental health problems in the United States equals $210.5 billion lost earnings per year. Within the United States, depression is the leading cause of disability among people aged 15 to 44 years. Depression ranks among the top three workplace issues, along with family crises and stress.

There is a higher incidence of depression in females (21%) than in males (13%). Researchers have studied this phenomenon for decades, yet there does not appear to be a single, universal explanation for females' greater susceptibility to depression. Depression may also occur during the peripartum period. Peripartum depression (PPD) usually occurs within 1 to 3 weeks after childbirth, but PPD can occur during pregnancy or up to 4 weeks after delivery. About 9% of females will develop PPD. One-half of all episodes begin before delivery. Risk factors for PPD include a history of depression before, during, or after pregnancy; a current history of depression; unplanned pregnancy; preterm birth; giving birth to a child with a medical condition or birth defect; lack of social, economic, and personal support; and concurrent stressful life events.

In general, once a person experiences one major depressive episode, the possibility of another episode is high, which makes treatment challenging. Individuals who suffer from an initial major depressive episode have a 40% to 60% chance of recurrence. This number increases to 60% to 70% with two recurrences and then to 90% with three episodes. The recurrence usually happens within the first 3 years after the initial episode and then 1 to 1.5 years after future episodes. In the absence of systematic screening, usual care by primary care providers fails to detect the disorder in between 30% and 50% of patients with depression. This makes it imperative that primary care practitioners use evidence-based screening tools and inquire sensitively about depression (see "The 15-Minute Hour: Practical Psychotherapy for Primary Care," Chapter 87).

Risk Factors: MDD

Age

- Peak age: Mid- to late adolescence to the early 40s

Sex

- Female

Family History

- Strong family history of depression, suicide or suicide attempts, alcohol abuse, or other substance abuse

History

- Adverse childhood events (ACEs)

Current Medical Condition

- Current chronic disease (especially multiple diseases)
- Chronic pain
- Insomnia

Life Events That Affect Mood

- Stress
- Social determinants of health such as unemployment, poor education, food and housing instability, limited access to health care
- Recent traumatic event
- Retirement

Depression is also an independent risk factor for increased morbidity and mortality from cardiac disease. In patients with coexisting atrial fibrillation and congestive heart failure, even with optimal treatment, a higher rate of depressive symptoms correlates with increased cardiovascular mortality. Even before the coronavirus 2019 (COVID-19) pandemic, the World Health Organization (WHO) reported depression as the leading cause of disability worldwide, which is a major contributor to the overall global burden of disease. A systematic review showed that depression increased by 27.6% in 2020 due to the effects of COVID-19 (COVID-19 Mental Disorders Collaborators, 2021). In fact, daily COVID-19 infection rates and reductions in human motility were associated with increased prevalence of MDD, and females and young age groups were more affected than males and older age groups.

PATHOPHYSIOLOGY

Although there are still many unknowns about the pathophysiology of depression, until recently, neurochemical deficits had been the focus of attention in depression. Yet chemical imbalances do not capture the complexity of the disorder. More recently, the focus has begun to shift to neural circuits and neurobehavioral systems. This means that monoamine transmitters are one part of a bigger system.

Several areas of the brain within the limbic system are affected by depression. Activity in the amygdala has been shown to be higher in a person who is depressed. The amygdala is associated with emotions that affect mood regulation and dysregulation. The hippocampus has a role in processing long-term memory and recollection. Some research has shown the hippocampus to be smaller in people with depression, and it becomes smaller still as more episodes of depression occur. It may also suppress the production of new nerve cells in this area of the brain. Other key areas in the limbic system are the prefrontal cortex and the anterior cingulate. The prefrontal cortex houses the representations of goals and appropriate responses to obtain these goals. The anterior cingulate serves as the point of integration of attentional and emotional inputs.

There are many neurotransmitters identified as having a role in depression. Serotonin is the most discussed as playing a role in regulating sleep, appetite, and mood. People with depression have reduced serotonin transmission. A functional polymorphism in the serotonin transporter gene (*5-HTT*) may interact with stressful life events to markedly increase the risk for depression and suicide, especially when the stressors are encountered early in life. Norepinephrine, which increases heart rate, blood pressure, and blood sugar in the body, may be seen in low levels in depression. Dopamine is another neurotransmitter that is essential in movement and reward-driven behaviors. Low levels of dopamine will be demonstrated through feelings of boredom and apathy, loss of satisfaction, and chronic fatigue. A correlation between the hypersecretion of cortisol and depression is one of the oldest observations in biological psychiatry. Neurovegetative signs and symptoms of depression may correlate with various neuroendocrine abnormalities.

More recently, the focus has expanded toward network and circuit models to describe how the limbic system and beyond can interact to affect mood. Some of the findings indicate volume reductions in the thalamus, basal ganglia, hippocampus, prefrontal cortex, and orbitofrontal cortex, and possibly the amygdala and anterior cingulate cortex. It is not clear what contributes to the changes in volume. Continued studies have supported a network of brain areas altered in depression. As brain imaging continues to improve, better understanding of how the different regions interact will be better understood. Alterations in sleep, appetite, and sexual behavior, as well as biological changes in endocrine, immunological, and chronobiological measures in patients with depression, all suggest dysregulation of the hypothalamus. The stooped posture of patients with depression, motor slowness, and minor cognitive impairments are similar to the signs of disorder of the basal ganglia, such as those found in Parkinson's disease and other subcortical dementias.

Approximately 5% to 10% of all patients with depression have a coexisting thyroid disorder. A subset of patients with depression may have an unrecognized autoimmune disorder that affects the thyroid gland. Some patients with depression benefit from liothyronine. A thyroid-stimulating hormone (TSH) level should be obtained on all patients with depression. The pathophysiology of PPD has included etiological theories of decreased maternal estrogen, as well as abnormalities in maternal neurotransmitters.

Genetic factors are strongly implicated in the development of depressive disorders, although it is impossible to rule out psychosocial factors, as well as other nongenetic factors. Adoption studies have provided data supporting a genetic basis for the inheritance of mood disorders. For MDD, the concordance rate in monozygotic twins is about 50%, arguing strongly for a genetic disposition.

Stressful life events commonly precede first episodes of mood disorders. Some speculate that the stress accompanying the first episode results in long-lasting changes in neurocircuitry. Thus, the person is at high risk for subsequent mood episodes unrelated to an external stressor. The external psychosocial factor most often associated with the onset of a major depressive episode is the loss of a spouse or a parent if it occurs before age 11. Another risk factor is unemployment: people out of work are three times more likely to report symptoms of an episode of MDD than those who are employed. However, what may seem to be a relatively mild stressor from an outside perspective may be devastating to the person because of whatever personal meaning they assign to the event.

CLINICAL PRESENTATION

A comprehensive assessment extends beyond the presence or absence of sadness or anhedonia, although these symptoms may be reported by the patient, observed and reported by significant others, or observed by the practitioner. Two quick questions, recommended by the U.S. Preventive Services Task Force, that provide a preliminary screen for depression are:

- Have you felt down or hopeless over the past few weeks?
- Have you had little interest in doing things over the past few weeks?

These questions are from the screening questionnaire called the Patient Health Questionnaire-2 (PHQ-2). A positive response to one or both questions in this screen indicates possible MDD, but the test has a high false-positive rate. Thus, confirmatory testing should be conducted with a validated screening instrument and a clinical interview.

The clinical diagnosis of MDD can be assisted by the Patient Health Questionnaire-9 (PHQ-9). Its sensitivity (85%) and specificity (84%) make it an excellent tool to utilize in primary care. Consisting of a checklist of nine symptoms, the PHQ-9 provides an effective supplement to the two-question screen. The patient is asked to indicate the frequency with which depressive symptoms have occurred over the preceding 2 weeks. It can be filled out quickly either in the waiting room or examination room before a primary care visit. The PHQ-9 may also be used to track the progress of treatment at each follow-up visit. A similar measure of symptom severity, the self-rated Quick Inventory of Depressive Symptomatology (QIDS-SR) with 16 items, can be used for the same purpose and has the additional benefit of including symptom severity; thus it may provide a sensitive measure of change with treatment. Both of these instruments are free to the provider.

Other scales frequently employed include the Geriatric Depression Scale (GDS), a widely used and validated screening tool for use in older adults. The Edinburgh Postnatal Depression (EPSD) scale is one of the most used screening tools for PPD.

Some patients with MDD may, as a result of the disorder, find it difficult to list their symptoms. In this case, direct observations, yes-or-no questions, or a referral to a specialist may be substituted. When yes-or-no assessment questions are used, all yes responses should be explored. Extremely depressed patients may not tolerate assessment in any form that requires effort on their part. They can become irritable and impatient with the practitioner for asking questions that, to them, seem "unnecessary." This situation can sometimes be improved by indicating that the purpose of asking questions is to better understand the patient's situation.

Programs aimed at enhancing public awareness of depression have been impactful. As such, more patients are likely to seek professional health care from their primary care provider for MDD because of having assessed their symptoms via surveys published in popular magazines, online, or in local newspapers. Primary care practitioners can help determine symptom intensity, duration, and impact on functioning. It is also valuable to ask patients to identify which symptoms they consider treatment priorities.

DIAGNOSTIC REASONING

Symptoms

The Diagnostic and Statistical Manual of Mental Disorders, Fifth Edition, Text Revision (*DSM-5-TR*), symptom criteria for a major depressive episode require five (or more) symptoms to be present during the same 2-week period and represent a change from previous functioning. The symptoms must be present nearly every day. At least one of the symptoms is either (1) depressed mood or (2) anhedonia, meaning loss of interest or pleasure. See the *DSM-5-TR* for complete diagnostic criteria for MDD.

In terms of mental disorders, depression can be a feature of many disorders listed in the *DSM-5-TR*. Depression has a high comorbidity with anxiety disorders, as well as alcohol-use disorders, eating disorders, schizophrenia, schizophreniform disorder, and somatic symptom disorders. Bereaved patients also need careful assessment. In patients with comorbid anxiety and depression, the symptom profile may be balanced, or either symptom can predominate. In addition, some patients with so-called mixed anxiety and depression may demonstrate symptoms of both disorders but may not meet the full diagnostic criteria for either. Any patient who has symptoms of either depression or anxiety should be evaluated for current symptoms of both disorders.

Differential Diagnosis

Consensus recommendations from a panel of experts representing psychiatry, primary care, pharmacy, and managed care state that every patient suspected of having unipolar depression should be evaluated for bipolar disorder, using a quick screening tool before, being treated with antidepressants to prevent a switch into mania. It is also necessary to rule out other medical conditions and substance use. The patient's depressive symptoms must be assessed for severity, duration, and recurrence to differentiate among the depressive disorders. One consideration is persistent depressive disorder or dysthymia, which is distinguished by a protracted time course.

All patients must also be carefully evaluated for underlying medical conditions. Many medical and neurological disorders and pharmacological substances can produce symptoms of depression. Careful medical history and physical examination should be done on all patients, including a neurological examination and routine blood work and urinalysis. The history needs to include the patient's personal as well as family history of depression and suicide. Tests for thyroid and adrenal function should be included because disorders of these endocrine systems can mimic depression. Cardiac drugs, antihypertensive agents, sedatives, hypnotics, antipsychotics, antiepileptics, antiparkinsonian drugs, analgesics, antibacterials, steroids, and antineoplastics have all been associated with depressive symptomatology. A careful medication review, including over-the-counter (OTC) drugs and herbal agents, as well as evaluation of alcohol and substance use, is imperative. The most common neurological disorders that may manifest depressive symptoms are Parkinson's disease (50% to 75% of patients have depressive symptoms that do not correlate with physical disability), dementing illnesses (including Alzheimer-type), epilepsy, cerebrovascular disease, and tumors. The interictal changes associated with temporal lobe epilepsy can mimic a depressive disorder, especially if the epileptic focus is on the right side. There is increasing evidence of linkages between depression and cardiovascular disease, not limited to sequelae but actually preceding the event. In brain tumors, depression is more common in cases of anterior lobe tumor as opposed to posterior lobe lesions, and both respond to antidepressants. The "pseudodementia" of MDD can be differentiated from dementia with regard to onset (sudden in the case of pseudodementia) and its co-occurrence with low mood. Patients with MDD will sometimes not answer questions, whereas those with dementia may confabulate. Patients with depression may be encouraged into remembering during an interview; those with primary dementia cannot. It is important to differentiate postpartum "blues" from PPD as presenting symptoms are similar. Symptoms of postpartum blues are less severe and transient in nature, although their presence increases the risk of PPD. The main distinguishing features of PPD are the longer duration of symptoms and the severity of symptoms with features of hopelessness and worthlessness.

MANAGEMENT

Remission of symptoms should be the standard for successful treatment of depression. *Remission* is defined as a virtual absence of depressive symptoms or a PHQ-9 score of less than five. Alternatively, *response* is defined as a substantial reduction in symptoms. On the PHQ-9, it is at least a 50% decrease in the score. In clinical trials, less than one-half of patients experience complete remission of depressive symptoms with an initial course of antidepressant therapy across 4 to 6 weeks. Remission is important, though, because incomplete relief of symptoms may increase the risk of relapse and further impairment. The mainstays of treatment are the use of antidepressants and/or psychotherapy. For mild to moderate depression, either medication or psychotherapy is recommended; if the depression is more severe, evidence-based guidelines support the simultaneous use of both. If a patient expresses suicidal intent or plan or has a history of suicidal attempt, referral to a specialty provider is recommended. For patients from differing ethnic groups or cultures, discussion of acceptable treatments should form the basis of therapeutic management. Guidelines for the treatment of depression can be found in multiple places. A list of these resources can be found in Box 69.1.

Pharmacological Management

Pharmacological therapy in patients with MDD may require several trials to find the right medication. Agents that are effective in front-line treatment of MDD are selective serotonin reuptake inhibitors (SSRIs); serotonin-norepinephrine reuptake inhibitors (SNRIs); tricyclic antidepressants (TCAs); and bupropion (Wellbutrin), which is a norepinephrine dopamine reuptake inhibitor, among others (Michigan Quality Improvement Consortium, 2016).

Antidepressant medications can be prescribed, based on their half-life, neurotransmitter or receptor activity, side-effect profile, and/or clinical efficacy. The half-life for newer antidepressant medications ranges from hours to several days. Neurotransmitter or receptor activity accounts for differences in medication effects, including sedation, activation, and anxiolytic (antianxiety) activity. In general, antidepressant medications with significant norepinephrine effects (e.g., bupropion) tend to be activating.

Box 69.1 Clinical Practice Guidelines for Treatment of Depression

- American Psychological Association Clinical Practice Guidelines for the Treatment of Depression Across Three Age Cohorts
- The Institute for Clinical Systems Improvement Health Care Guideline for Depression, in Primary Care
- Michigan Quality Improvement Guidelines for Depression
- The American Academy of Pediatrics Guidelines for Adolescent Depression in Primary Care Part 1
- The American Academy of Pediatrics Guidelines for Adolescent Depression in Primary Care Part 2
- American College of Physicians Clinical Guideline for Nonpharmacologic versus Pharmacologic Treatment of Adult Patients with Major Depressive Disorder
- National Institute for Health and Care Excellence Guidelines for Depression in Children and Young People
- National Institute for Health and Care Excellence Guidelines for Depression in Adults
- The National Center of Excellence in Youth Mental Health

Important common side-effect risks with serotonin-specific antidepressants include decreased sexual desire, decreased sexual response, headache, stomach upset, sedation, fatigue, or nervousness. For some patients, dramatic decreases in adverse effects can be obtained by adjusting the time of day the medication is taken. Patients who are bothered by adverse effects when they take an antidepressant in the morning may experience milder side effects if they take the same medication with dinner or at bedtime. Starting with a low dose and increasing it slowly (start low, go slow) may be necessary when it is clear that a patient seems to benefit from an antidepressant but cannot tolerate medication side effects during the early stages of treatment. Absolute medication dose limitations have been defined for patients with seizure disorders, renal disease, and liver disease. Some antidepressants, such as bupropion, are contraindicated for people with bulimia, and some drugs, such as paroxetine (Paxil), fluoxetine (Prozac), and fluvoxamine (Luvox), have significant liver cytochrome (CYP) P450 interaction effects. In older adults, antidepressants should be started at lower doses and titrated slowly. For some pregnant women, antidepressants are a safer option than untreated depression. For breastfeeding mothers, sertraline (Zoloft) and paroxetine have demonstrated undetectable serum levels in infants with no short-term effects, although further research is needed on the long-term effects. TCAs are not less effective than newer antidepressant medications, but they can produce more side effects and have greater lethality in overdose.

If the patient has seen some benefit from the medication but not remission of the depression, after 4 to 6 weeks, it is important to maximize the dosage before switching to a new medication. Switching between SSRIs and SNRIs can be done by prescribing the new drug at an equivalent dosage. Switching from an SSRI to a TCA or an SNRI can be accomplished through cross-tapering, where the SSRI is gradually reduced over a 1- to 2-week period as the new drug is introduced and gradually increased to therapeutic levels. Cross-tapering is also recommended for mirtazapine (Remeron). Because paroxetine possesses the most distressing discontinuation symptoms, one approach may be to switch to fluoxetine and then slowly taper. Discontinuation symptoms are generally not a problem for bupropion because it does not possess strong serotonergic properties. It is recommended to taper bupropion over a 1-week period while initiating the new drug at full dosage. Paroxetine, fluvoxamine, and fluoxetine are metabolized by the liver and could potentially increase the blood level of bupropion and the risk of seizures, especially at high doses of bupropion. Refer to specific prescribing considerations and patient information regarding monoamine oxidase inhibitors. The most important aspect is to warn patients about abrupt cessation and formulate a plan to discontinue by tapering over a 2- to 3-week period.

Providers are advised to identify all supplements or medications the patient is currently taking before starting an antidepressant medication, particularly if the patient has not taken a psychotropic medication previously. This list should include all compounds—prescribed and self-administered. Many people take OTC products—vitamins, minerals, herbal remedies—that they may not consider "medications." The high number of such products available makes this information vital. Patient use of megadose vitamin and mineral supplements, weight-loss or weight-gain products, and nutritional supplements should also be noted. At present, the standard of practice regarding the use of prescribed and herbal compounds is that the two treatments should not be used simultaneously. For example, there is no compelling evidence for the efficacy of St. John's wort in either mild or moderate depression; neither is the herb recommended in cases of more serious MDD. St. John's wort, however, when taken with an antidepressant, can precipitate serotonin syndrome. It also induces the hepatic metabolism of many drugs. For information on specific drugs for MDD, see Drugs Commonly Prescribed 69.1.

Pharmacogenetic testing for pharmacokinetics and pharmacodynamic assays, based on individual genetic variations, may be considered after at least one failed medication. The results can inform the provider about how the individual's genes can affect the metabolization or response to medications such as antidepressants. When pharmacogenetic testing is utilized, it can reduce time lost to efficacy and may speed recovery through introduction to more targeted medication based on the patient's genetic structure.

Lastly, each patient should be given information to ensure that they understand the potential benefits of taking medication, the specific medication being prescribed, possible adverse effects and how to handle them, and what to do in an emergency. When possible, this information should be made available in writing. Effective patient education makes it possible for patients to participate in their care and decreases the risks of having a patient agree to take medications without being fully informed of the medication's risks and benefits.

Nonpharmacological Management

Both interpersonal and cognitive behavioral therapy (CBT) have been shown to be effective for the treatment of depression, and there is evidence that the combination of psychotherapy and pharmacotherapy may be more effective than either alone. Patients with MDD need hope and reassurance. Both are particularly important with patients who may have lived with untreated depression. Informing a person that their disorder is MDD and that the disorder can be treated sets the stage for patients to define goals for improvement and begin to combat the demoralization that can develop after months of untreated depression. False reassurances and unrealistic expectations must be avoided, however.

Drugs Commonly Prescribed 69.1: Major Depressive Disorder

DRUG	INDICATION	ADVERSE REACTIONS AND PRESCRIBING CONSIDERATIONS
Selective Serotonin Reuptake Inhibitors (SSRIs)		
All SSRIs		Common to most SSRIs: • Response rates: 60%–70% • Remission rates: 20%–35% • Safest class of antidepressants in overdose • Avoid sudden discontinuation due to possible withdrawal syndrome. • Do not prescribe with MAOIs due to risk of serotonin syndrome. • Agitation, dizziness, headache, drowsiness (dose in evening), insomnia (dose in morning), nausea/vomiting (self-limiting 1–3 weeks), and xerostomia • SIADH, risk is highest in older adults • Serotonin syndrome (caution with "triptans") • SSRI-induced mania in BD patients • If anxiety/panic disorder develops or patient has a history of these disorders, start low and adjust dose slowly. • Increased risk of suicidal behavior in children, adolescents, and young adults • Absent or slight weight gain except for paroxetine • Sexual dysfunction in 30%–40%, resolving after medication is discontinued • Wait 2 weeks after discontinuing an SSRI to start an MAOI (wait 5 weeks after fluoxetine is discontinued). • Wait 2 weeks after discontinuing an MAOI to start an SSRI.
citalopram (Celexa)*	Depression SAD† Panic disorder,† PTSD†/OCD† Hot flashes*,† PMDD†	• Tolerability similar to sertraline • Minimal CYP P450 effects • Causes dose-dependent QT interval prolongation, which can cause torsades de pointes, ventricular tachycardia, and sudden death • Monitor weight
escitalopram (Lexapro)*	Depression Generalized anxiety disorder Depression in children aged 12–17 years	• Minimal CYP P450 effects • Insomnia increases 50% with each 20-mg dose. • Monitor weight.
fluoxetine (Prozac)*	Bulimia Depression OCD Panic disorder PMDD Depression and OCD in children	• Less severe discontinuation syndrome due to long half-life • Nausea (20%), headache, GI complaints (10%), anxiety, nervousness, insomnia, drowsiness, fatigue, dizziness, tremor • Strong inhibition of CYP 2D6 can lead to drug–drug interactions. • Monitoring parameters: weight and growth rate • Must wait 5 weeks after discontinuing before initiating MAOI
fluvoxamine (Luvox)*	OCD Social anxiety disorder	• More side effects than other SSRIs • Inhibition of CYP 1A2 and 3A4 results in high potential for drug–drug interactions. • Monitor growth rate and weight.
paroxetine (Paxil)*	Depression GAD Hot flashes Menopause OCD Panic PTSD PMDD SAD	• Most severe discontinuation syndrome • Causes the most weight gain of the SSRIs • Nausea/vomiting (25%), xerostomia, sedation, insomnia, tremor • Strong inhibition of CYP 2D6 can lead to drug–drug interactions. • Exposure to paroxetine in the first trimester has been associated with an increased risk of cardiac birth defects.

Continued

Drugs Commonly Prescribed 69.1: Major Depressive Disorder—cont'd

DRUG	INDICATION	ADVERSE REACTIONS AND PRESCRIBING CONSIDERATIONS
sertraline (Zoloft)*	Depression OCD Panic PTSD PMDD SAD	• Nausea, vomiting, diarrhea, drowsiness, headache • Monitor weight. • Considered the safest for pregnancy and nursing
fluoxetine/ olanzapine (Symbyax)	Bipolar depression Treatment-resistant depression (treatment failure with two separate antidepressants)	• Remission rate: 25.5% • Side effects—see individual medications
Serotonin-Norepinephrine Reuptake Inhibitors (SNRIs)		
All SNRIs		Common to most SNRIs: • Response rates: 60%–70% • Remission rates: up to 50% • Safety in overdose is intermediate, between SSRIs and TCAs. • Avoid sudden discontinuation • Do not prescribe with MAOIs • Agitation, weakness, dizziness, headache, drowsiness, insomnia, nausea/vomiting (self-limiting 1–3 weeks), and xerostomia • Increased risk of suicidal behavior in children, adolescents, and young adults • SIADH, risk is highest in older adults • Serotonin syndrome (caution with "triptans") • SNRI-induced mania in BD • If anxiety/panic disorder develops or if the patient has a history of these disorders, start low and adjust dose slowly. • Contraindicated in uncontrolled closed-angle glaucoma • Sexual dysfunction, resolving in days after medication discontinuation • Monitor blood pressure for diastolic hypertension. • Wait 2 weeks after discontinuing an SNRI to start an MAOI. • Wait 2 weeks after discontinuing an MAOI to start SNRI.
desvenlafaxine (Pristiq)*	Depression	• Dose adjustment required with renal impairment
levomilnacipran (Fetzima)*	Depression	• May cause tachycardia • May cause hypertension • May cause ejaculatory dysfunction
duloxetine (Cymbalta)*	Depression Diabetic neuropathy Fibromyalgia GAD Musculoskeletal pain Osteoarthritis	• Do not use with hepatic impairment or seizure disorder • May cause rare hepatotoxicity, monitor LFTs periodically • May cause orthostatic hypotension • May cause hypertension
venlafaxine (Effexor)*	Depression GAD Panic disorder SAD	• Monitor blood pressure due to risk of hypertension. • Insomnia, nervousness

Drugs Commonly Prescribed 69.1: Major Depressive Disorder—cont'd

DRUG	INDICATION	ADVERSE REACTIONS AND PRESCRIBING CONSIDERATIONS
Tetracyclic Antidepressants		
All tetracyclic antidepressants		Common to most tetracyclic antidepressants: • Increased risk of suicidal behavior in children, adolescents, and young adults
mirtazapine (Remeron)*	Depression	• Response and remission rates: 53%–63% • Somnolence (high incidence) and weight gain • May cause dizziness, increased cholesterol levels, and orthostatic hypotension. • Can cause rare agranulocytosis • Monitor glucose, lipids • Weight gain
Serotonin Modulators		
Serotonin Modulators		Common to most serotonin modulators: • Increased risk of suicidal behavior in children, adolescents, and young adults
vortioxetine (Trintellix)*	Depression	• Withdrawal symptoms if abrupt D/C • May cause hyponatremia • May cause angle-closure glaucoma • May cause increased chance of bleeding
vilazodone (Viibryd)*	Depression	• May cause trouble sleeping • Withdrawal symptoms if abrupt D/C • May cause hyponatremia • May cause angle-closure glaucoma • May cause increased chance of bleeding
trazodone (Desyrel)*	Depression Insomnia	• Rarely used as an antidepressant; often prescribed at low doses for insomnia in depressed patients • Do not give after myocardial infarction • Potentiates alcohol, other CNS depressants; sedative effect
Norepinephrine-Dopamine Reuptake Inhibitor (NDRIs)		
bupropion (Wellbutrin, Zyban)*	Depression Smoking cessation SAD ADHD	• Response rate: 52%–70% • May cause weight loss • Fewer sexual side effects • Avoid use in patients with seizure disorders, history of eating disorders, or history of alcohol dependence/withdrawal due to increased risk of seizures • Increased risk of suicidal behavior in children, adolescents, and young adults
Tricyclic Antidepressants (TCAs)		
All TCAs	In addition to major indications, may be used in conjunction with mood stabilizers and antipsychotics to treat concomitant depression	Common to most TCAs: • Response rates: 43%–70% • Remission rates: 25%–60% • High lethality with overdose • Analgesic, anticholinergic, and antimuscarinic actions; high side-effect burden • Avoid in patients with narrow-angle glaucoma or prostatic hypertrophy • Risk of cardiotoxicity, QTc prolongation • Wait 2 weeks to start after discontinuation of fluoxetine, MAOIs • Do not use with history of seizures, glaucoma, urinary retention • Increased risk of suicidal behavior in children, adolescents, and young adults • Drug levels helpful to monitor for some agents • Monitor ECG and blood pressure. • Treat constipation with fiber and exercise.

Continued

Drugs Commonly Prescribed 69.1: Major Depressive Disorder—cont'd

DRUG	INDICATION	ADVERSE REACTIONS AND PRESCRIBING CONSIDERATIONS
amitriptyline (Elavil)*	Depression	• Monitor BP, HR, ECG, serum concentrations.

amoxapine (Asendin)*	Depression	• Moderate sedation
		  • Monitor orthostatic blood pressure.
		  • May cause tardive dyskinesia and neuromuscular symptoms
		• Monitor ECG.

clomipramine (Anafranil)*	OCD	• Strong anticholinergic effect, sedation, orthostatic hypotension • Monitor BP, ECG, and liver transaminases if hepatic disease
desipramine (Norpramin)*	Depression	• Less sedating • Monitor ECG and serum concentrations.
doxepin (Sinequan)*	Anxiety Atopic dermatitis Depression Eczema Insomnia Lichen simplex	• Strong sedation and orthostatic hypotension • Monitor ECG.
imipramine (Tofranil)*	Depression Enuresis	• Moderate sedation and hypotension • Monitor ECG and serum concentrations.
nortriptyline (Pamelor)*	Depression	• Monitor ECG and serum concentrations.
protriptyline (Vivactil)*	Depression	• Strong anticholinergic effects • Can be activating • Monitor ECG
trimipramine (Surmontil)*	Depression	• Strong sedation effect; monitor orthostatic blood pressure • Monitor ECG.
Monoamine Oxidase Inhibitors (MAOIs)		
All MAOIs		Common to most MAOIs: • Increased risk of suicidal behavior in children, adolescents, and young adults
isocarboxazid (Marplan)*	Depression	• 60%–70% remission rates; may be better in atypical depression • Requires dietary (tyramine) restrictions: Aged, smoked, or fermented meat; aged cheeses; tap/unpasteurized beers; sauerkraut; soy/tofu • Avoid dextromethorphan, other serotoninergic compounds. • Potential for hypertensive crisis • Potential for serotonin syndrome • Because of the potential for serious adverse effects and drug interactions and the necessity of dietary restrictions, MAOIs (e.g., phenelzine, tranylcypromine) generally are not used as initial therapy for MDD. • Monitor liver transaminases and for orthostatic hypotension
tranylcypromine (Parnate)	Depression	• Monitor liver transaminases and blood pressure.
phenelzine (Nardil)*	Depression	• Monitor liver transaminases and blood pressure.

*Black-box warning: children, suicide ideation.
†Not approved by the U.S. Food and Drug Administration for this indication.

Abbreviations: CNS, central nervous system; Cr, creatinine; ECG, electrocardiogram; GAD, generalized anxiety disorder; GI, gastrointestinal; LFTs, liver function tests; MAOI, monoamine oxidase inhibitor; OCD, obsessive-compulsive disorder; PMDD, premenstrual dysphoric disorder; PTSD, post-traumatic stress disorder; SAD, social anxiety disorder; SIADH, syndrome of inappropriate antidiuretic hormone secretion; SNRI, selective norepinephrine reuptake inhibitor; SSRI, selective serotonin reuptake inhibitor; TCA, tricyclic antidepressant; TSH, thyroid-stimulating hormone.

The support needs of patients with depression can be significant. It is unlikely that, in a primary care setting, practitioners will be able to meet all of their patients' needs. For this reason, new sources of support should be identified. Friends, relatives, and spouses or partners are important potential sources of information, comfort, and assistance. Professional-led support groups and peer self-help groups are also highly effective. Additional wrap-around services including case management and coordination of care can be offered in a mental health clinic.

Support is an important resource for patients with depression, but patients who are anxious or irritable may require a great deal of practitioner patience. Patients who are anxious and/or irritable can be indecisive, critical, demanding, and appear uncooperative or uninterested. Every effort must be made to avoid getting into a power struggle or challenging patients who are upset. In the long run, reassuring acceptance is easier and more effective.

Establishing a routine and focusing on increasing activities and behaviors may be a constructive approach. Massage, relaxation therapies, exercise, good nutrition, and a variety of forms of self-care should also be initiated and supported.

For some patients, the only important outcome of treatment for MDD is symptom relief. Normalized sleep, appetite, mood, energy, and concentration should, however, be viewed as minimal patient outcomes. If the patient's risk for future episodes of depression is to be significantly lowered, additional outcomes need to be addressed. Improved patient depression awareness is important. Patients treated for depression should, as a stated outcome of treatment, increase their understanding of the illness and improve their abilities to cope with depression. The most important outcome is that the patient will immediately seek help should symptoms of depression return. Depressive episodes that persist for months despite an adequate course of therapy, relapse despite ongoing treatment, or are characterized by extremely high symptom levels, including inability to function or thoughts of suicide, require referral and specialized care, sometimes in an inpatient setting.

> **Pediatric/Adolescent Considerations**
>
> For children and adolescents, classic symptoms of depression include irritability, fatigue, insomnia or sleeping more, and decline in academic performance. Specific screening tools for the pediatric population include the Pediatric Symptom Checklist (PSC-17) and the Columbia Suicide Severity Rating Scale–Pediatric (C-SSRS-Pediatric). When treating children and adolescents with pharmacological interventions, always start with a low dose and increase slowly. There is a Black Box warning on antidepressants, based on increased risk of suicidal thoughts and behaviors among children and adolescents, and thus, it is imperative to assess for safety as you initiate and monitor pharmacological treatments.

> **Geriatric Considerations**
>
> Classic symptoms of depression in older patients are a depressive mood; anhedonia; excessive feelings of guilt; and vegetative, cognitive, and somatic symptoms. A specific screening tool for older adults is the Geriatric Depression Scale-15 (GDS). Once again, start low and go slowly when using pharmacological interventions. Due to co-occurring medical conditions in older adults, drug–drug interactions need to be considered. The American Geriatrics Society's Beers Criteria for Potentially Inappropriate Medication Use in Older Adults can assist in guiding the provider and patient away from harmful medications, and it improves effectiveness and safety for prescription practices in the older adult population.

FOLLOW-UP AND REFERRAL

Follow-up during treatment of depression is absolutely necessary to ensure adherence to therapy. The provider should discuss medication compliance with the patient to ensure that the patient is taking the medications as prescribed. Treatment outcome should be assessed regularly, using formal diagnostic assessment tools. Target symptoms are used to evaluate the effectiveness of medication during early stages of treatment and until full symptom remission is obtained. In moderate to severe depression, follow-up is determined by the severity of the initial PHQ-9.

A reasonable criterion for extending the initial treatment is to assess whether the patient is experiencing a 50% or greater reduction in baseline symptom severity at 6 weeks of the therapeutic dose. If the patient's symptoms are reduced by 50% or more, but the patient is not yet at remission, and if medication has been well tolerated, continue to prescribe and continue to raise the dosage. In the acute phase of treatment and recovery, the patient should be seen or contacted every 1 to 2 weeks within the first month of therapy and at least once in the succeeding 4 to 8 weeks. For patients who can be treated effectively with antidepressant medication, satisfactory symptom relief often is achieved within 4 to 6 weeks. Many patients begin to feel better in 2 to 3 weeks. The duration of medication treatment for uncomplicated MDD is at a minimum 6 to 12 months at the treatment dose (Michigan Quality Improvement Consortium, 2016). A longer treatment period is recommended for patients with complicated or multiple disorders or patients who have a history of one or more years of untreated depression. In these instances, treatment duration should extend from 15 months to an indefinite time. When the patient reports target symptom relief or when the assessment indicates symptom remission has been achieved, the practitioner and patient develop a treatment and discontinuation plan. Short half-life antidepressants are discontinued gradually over a period of 2 to 3 weeks. People who experience significant discontinuation symptoms may report flu-like symptoms that last a few days. Consultation with a specialist should be considered if the patient has failed two medications after adequate trials and dosing. Consultation can also be sought if discontinuation symptoms appear to be significant or persistent.

Suicide Assessment

If a patient is having thoughts of suicide, it is important to assess if the patient has a plan. If they have a plan, the next question is to determine whether they have the means to complete the plan. There should also be an assessment of family or personal history of suicide attempts. Lastly, the provider needs to determine whether the person has the intention to follow through on the plan. If the patient answers yes to any of these questions, an emergency referral is needed. If a patient has thoughts of suicide but has no plan or intent, a referral to a specialist is recommended.

Patient Education: Major Depressive Disorder

It is important for the provider to educate the patient and their support people to report signs of increased agitation, irritability, and suicidal thoughts and/or behaviors. Emergency phone numbers (such as crisis services) and tertiary care sites need to be given to the patient and their support people should such symptoms emerge. Some patients may experience an increase in suicidal thoughts or urges during the first few weeks of treatment. Danger signs and symptoms include the following:

- Hallucinations or delusions
- Severe adverse effects from antidepressant medications (e.g., severe urinary retention, fluctuation in blood pressure, seizures, cardiac complications)
- Suicidal thoughts
- Extreme self-care deficits (e.g., not able to care for basic needs)

The person and their support people should understand that depression generates feelings of helplessness, powerlessness, and pessimism; major decisions should be delayed. The practitioner should reassure the patient that current feelings will change. All side effects of drugs should be clearly understood, and the provider should stress the importance of taking medication daily as ordered for maximum effect. The clinician should advise the patient and their support people that drugs to offset adverse effects are available or that medication can be changed. Patients should be encouraged to maintain a schedule of activities and keep their regularly scheduled visits with their primary care clinician.

The Substance Abuse and Mental Health Services Administration's (SAMHSA) National Helpline is a confidential, free 24-hour, 365-day service in English and Spanish for individuals and family members facing mental and/or substance use disorders. The National Suicide Prevention Lifeline is available 24 hours, 365 days a year with information in English and Spanish. The number links to a national network of local crisis centers that will provide free and confidential emotional support to people in suicidal crisis or emotional distress. (See Resources in this chapter for more information.)

BIPOLAR AND RELATED DISORDERS

Bipolar disorder (BD) is characterized by episodes of mania, hypomania, and major depression. Mania is characterized by excessive excitement, elation, delusions of grandeur, distractibility, restlessness, agitation, flight of ideas, frenzied movement, decreased sleep, and poor judgment. The spectrum of bipolar disorders includes (1) bipolar I (BD I), the essential feature of which is mania accompanied most often with major depressive and hypomanic episodes; (2) bipolar II (BD II), characterized by at least one hypomanic episode (a persistent period of excitement or hyperactivity with a moderate change in behavior) and at least one major depressive episode; (3) cyclothymic disorder, characterized by alternating cycles of hypomania and depressive episodes of lesser severity than those of manic or MDD; (4) substance-/medication-induced bipolar disorder; and (5) bipolar and related disorders due to another medical condition.

More than 90% of patients who have at least one manic episode will develop recurrent mood episodes. Manic episodes immediately precede depressive episodes in 60% of patients. During interepisode periods, one-half of patients may experience subsyndromal symptoms, such as cognitive impairment and impulsivity; the length of these intervals tends to decrease progressively across multiple recurrences.

BD is commonly seen in the primary care setting. Patients with BD report having received treatment for their mental illness in primary care settings as frequently as specialty settings. It is estimated that patients diagnosed with BD make up about 4% of a primary care provider's total patient caseload. Up to 10% of all patients seen in primary care will be diagnosed with BD at some point in their lifetime. Emerging data from a variety of sources have confirmed a typical delay between symptom onset and diagnosis, ranging from 5 to 10 years, with patients being evaluated by an average of four health-care providers before the correct diagnosis is given. In the primary care setting, BD is frequently mistaken for other conditions, most commonly MDD, which occurs at a rate of around 15%. Clinicians must be able to distinguish between depressive episodes occurring in the context of unipolar depression versus depressive episodes occurring in bipolar disorders because misdiagnosis can lead to harmful patient care outcomes, including the emergence of mania with antidepressant monotherapy. Additionally, inappropriate pharmacological treatment for BD is associated with increases in morbidity and mortality and suicide. The three major categories—BD I, BD II, and cyclothymic disorder—are discussed here.

EPIDEMIOLOGY AND CAUSES

BD is the sixth leading cause of disability worldwide in patients aged 15 to 55 years. The direct and indirect costs of BD I in 2015 alone exceeded $202 billion in the United States. The greater proportion of these costs overall is due to bipolar depression; however, manic or mixed (mood episodes presenting with concurrent symptoms of opposite polarity) symptoms result in higher direct costs from inpatient hospitalization and treatment expenses. The financial burden of this disorder eclipses that of diabetes, and the impact on occupational function from BD is more extensive than MDD. Patients with BD are more likely to be unemployed, based on the severity of their depressive episodes and symptoms, rather than their manic ones. Two-thirds of patients with BD are substantially adversely affected by their illness, but the negative impact of BD goes beyond its morbidity rate. The rates of suicide in BD are 10 to 30 times higher than in the general population with up to 60% attempting suicide at least once in their lifetime. Attempts can occur during the manic, hypomanic, depressed, or mixed phases of BD but are most likely to occur in depressed or mixed states.

BD I has a lifetime prevalence of 1% to 3%; however, when the entire spectrum of bipolar disorder is included, the prevalence approaches 7% to 10%. Males and females are equally affected, although BD II is more common in females. The mean age of onset of BD I is 22 years, and for BD II, 20 years. It can occur in early childhood, adolescence, or as late as 60 to 70 years of age; however, 50% of initial onsets of BD symptoms occur before age 25 years. New onset of mania after age 50 years is rare and should prompt consideration of a medical condition, such as neurological disease, thyroid dysfunction, or substance abuse or withdrawal.

PATHOPHYSIOLOGY

The exact pathophysiology of BD is unknown. Greater understanding of the complex gene–environment interactions for these disorders is likely to emerge in the future and holds promise for attaining a clearer understanding of affective illnesses. However, from the current research and clinical findings, BD is thought to be a combination of biological, psychological, and social factors.

The pathogenesis of BD involves several aspects of genetics including candidate genes, gene expression, and epigenetics. There has been no single candidate gene identified in BD. Genetic susceptibility therefore is thought to be based on the interactions of many genes versus a singular gene with a large effect. Several genes implicated in recent genome-wide association studies (GWAS) have also been identified including *CACNA1C*, which plays a role in calcium channel coding and channel gating. Other biological pathways thought to be involved in expression of BD are signaling by corticotropin-releasing hormone, endothelin-1, glutamate, cardiac hypertrophy, cardiac b-adrenergic, and phospholipase C.

Genetic expression and epigenetics have both been demonstrated in postmortem tissues of patients with BD. Two studies of ribonucleic acid sequencing, one of postmortem tissue from the dorsolateral prefrontal cortex and the other of postmortem tissue from the anterior cingulate gyrus, both found downregulated genes associated with neuroplasticity and neurotransmitter and hormone receptor targets of psychotropic drugs. Other research has indicated that epigenetic changes in genetic expression are seen via methylation changes of glutamic acid decarboxylase in patients with BD. In monozygotic twins, concordance rates approach up to 70%, indicating that BD is highly heritable, although its expression is also influenced by environmental factors. If one parent has BD, the risk of their offspring developing BD increases by 20%. The exact mechanism by which these epigenetic changes occur is unclear, but it may involve early life stressors, chronic stress, and/or environmental factors such as toxins and air pollutants.

Neurobiological changes have been found in both brain structure and function of patients with BD, but it is unclear whether these changes are etiological causes, sequelae, neither, or both. Neuroimaging studies have shown decreased neuronal connections in the prefrontal cortex, limbic structures (especially the amygdala), and among gray matter volumes. Thus, one of the proposed models of the functional neuroanatomy of BD I theorizes that early developmental changes modulating emotional behavior become disrupted, leading to reduced connectivity among prefrontal networks and limbic structures. Inflammatory markers such as C-reactive protein, interleukin-4, and tumor necrosis factor-(have been elevated in patients with BD, compared with healthy controls, which seems to suggest that BD is also associated with immune system dysregulation.

Current evidence regarding risk of prenatal and perinatal factors as independent risk factors for development of BD in offspring has been inconsistent. There is some evidence of maternal *Toxoplasma gondii* infections leading to higher rates of BD, but further research is needed before conclusions can be made. Early life traumas and childhood maltreatment are well-studied environmental risk factors for development of BD later in life. Patients with BD are four times more likely to have experienced emotional abuse than their peers. Childhood maltreatment is also associated with earlier onset of diagnosis and poorer clinical outcomes including more severe and frequent mood episodes.

CLINICAL PRESENTATION

Presenting symptoms of BD manifest as manic, hypomanic, mixed, or depressive episodes; however, significant subsyndromal symptoms are commonly present between mood episodes. For a mixed episode, the symptom presentation must meet the full diagnostic criteria for a manic/hypomanic episode or depressive episode and have at least three symptoms present from the opposite polarity to make the diagnosis. For a clinical diagnosis, a patient must have the following symptoms:

- Bipolar disorder I: Patients with BD I have had at least one episode of mania. A major depressive episode is not required for diagnosis.
- Bipolar disorder II: BD II is characterized by a history of both depression and hypomania.
- Cyclothymic disorder: Cyclothymia involves 2 years of symptoms of hypomania and depression that do not meet the full criteria for either mood episode.

A mnemonic for bipolar disorder is presented in Box 69.2 with a more detailed comparison of these disorders in Table 69.1. Complete diagnostic criteria can be found in the *DSM-5-TR*.

> **Box 69.2 DIGFAST Mnemonic for Bipolar Disorder**
>
> The following mnemonic, DIGFAST, is useful for identifying BD:
>
> - Distractibility
> - Insomnia (decreased need for sleep)
> - Grandiosity (inflated self-esteem)
> - Flight of ideas (racing thoughts, negative for rumination)
> - Activities (increased, goal directed)
> - Speech (pressured, increased talkativeness)
> - Thoughtlessness (pleasure-seeking activities that show poor judgment such as spending sprees, sexual indiscretions, reckless driving, arguments if irritable)

TABLE 69.1 Comparison of Bipolar Disorders

Bipolar Disorders	Key Characteristics
Bipolar I Disorder	Presence of one or more manic episodes lasting at least 1 week, most of or nearly every day with inflated, irritable, or expansive mood and increased energy or activity. During this time, three (if inflated/expansive mood) or four (if irritable mood only) of the following symptoms must also be present and must demonstrate a significant change from usual behavior and cause marked impairment in overall functioning: 1. Pressured speech or more talkative and social than normal 2. Increased distractibility 3. Decreased need for sleep (i.e., feels rested after only 2 to 3 hours of sleep) 4. Increased self-esteem and/or grandiose thinking 5. Racing thoughts and/or flight of ideas 6. Increased psychomotor agitation or goal-directed activity (i.e., starting more projects than normal) 7. Impulsivity regarding activities that have high risk of negative consequences (i.e., gambling, speeding, spending money they do not have, sexual indiscretions, etc.) Note: If mania emerges during antidepressant treatment and persists beyond the effect of the antidepressant treatment, it warrants a bipolar I diagnosis. Note: Major depressive episodes are not required for bipolar I disorder diagnosis. Hypomanic episodes commonly occur but do not constitute a diagnosis of bipolar I disorder.
Bipolar II Disorder	Presence of one or more hypomanic episodes lasting at least 4 days, most of or nearly every day, with inflated, irritable, or expansive mood and increased energy or activity. During this time, three (if inflated/expansive mood) or four (if irritable mood only) of the following symptoms must also be present and must demonstrate a significant change from usual behavior: 1. Pressured speech or more talkative and social than normal 2. Increased distractibility 3. Decreased need for sleep (i.e., feels rested after 3 hours of sleep) 4. Increased self-esteem and/or grandiose thinking 5. Racing thoughts and/or flight of ideas 6. Increased psychomotor agitation or goal-directed activity (i.e., starting more projects than normal) 7. Impulsivity regarding activities that have high risk of negative consequences (i.e., gambling, speeding, spending money they do not have, sexual indiscretions, etc.) Note: Symptoms are not severe enough to cause marked impairment in functioning and do not include the presence of psychosis and/or the need for hospitalization.
Cyclothymic Disorder	Presence of hypomanic and depressive symptoms that do not meet full criteria of hypomanic episode or depressive episode. They must occur at least over 2 consecutive years, and patients may not have symptom-free periods for more than 2 months.

The majority of patients with BD initially present with depressive symptoms, making it more difficult to accurately diagnose in the clinical setting. Almost 90% of all people with BD experience depression, which is the most difficult phase of BD to treat. It is estimated that depressed mood occurs at least two-thirds of time spent unwell, even with treatment and can last an average of 5.2 months. In older adult populations, BD may present with more significant cognitive decline and functional disturbances than in younger adults with the same condition.

An initial manic episode may be related to an adverse life event or stressor; however, subsequent episodes may occur without an identifiable trigger. Known stressors or triggers for manic and hypomanic episodes include seasonal changes, particularly in the spring and summer months; excessive light exposure; or hormonal changes in females that occur during menstrual cycles. Manic episodes usually last 3 to 6 months if untreated, and the symptoms typically escalate rapidly over a period of days. Patients presenting in a manic or hypomanic state frequently exhibit symptoms of anxiety and agitation. If present, these symptoms are a predictor of poorer outcomes including longer times to remission and increased severity of manic symptoms. In up to 30% of patients presenting with mania, depressive symptoms are also present. Clinicians should be aware that these patients are at higher risk of suicide. Older adult patients may manifest irritability rather than an elated mood. Psychotic symptoms are present in at least one-half of manic episodes. Psychotic depression should raise an index of suspicion that the patient may have underlying BD.

DIAGNOSTIC REASONING

A complete physical examination is needed, as well as neurological assessment, to exclude other etiologies of mood symptoms or psychosis. The patient's mental status should be assessed, including general appearance, attitude, behaviors, mood, affect, speech, thought processes and content, concentration, and memory. Focus the physical and neurological examination (e.g., cranial nerves, reflexes, muscle tone, gait) on identifying or excluding a medical cause of the patient's symptoms. Comorbidity, and the possibility of precipitating factors such as thyroid disorder, head injuries, or substance abuse, should also be considered.

Diagnostic testing includes a complete blood count (CBC) with differential, platelet count, comprehensive blood chemistry panel, free thyroxine (T4), thyroid-stimulating hormone (TSH), rapid plasma reagin (RPR), HIV antibody test, urinalysis, urine toxicology screen, and pregnancy test. In the setting of HIV/AIDS, hepatitis C, and other infectious causes, new-onset mood or bipolar-like symptoms require further studies to exclude identifiable causes of mood changes. Consider conducting a Mini-Mental State Examination to assess cognition. Refer to a neurologist or infectious disease specialist to assist with diagnosis if indicated. Brain magnetic resonance imaging or computed tomography scans may be helpful if clinical findings suggest an underlying central nervous system (CNS) disorder.

Information to be obtained includes patient's childhood history, family history and family life, school performance, substance abuse history, medical history, and current and/or past symptoms of mania and depression. For a variety of reasons, patients often leave out these episodes when reviewing their medical history, and clinicians may fail to query or recognize previous hypomanic or manic symptoms. Some patients even identify periods of normal mood as depressed compared with mania. Therefore, if possible, a patient's self-report as well as collateral information from family members can assist in assessment and diagnosis of BD.

Clinicians should inquire about chronic or recurrent nonspecific physical symptoms (e.g., fatigue, headache, or gastrointestinal distress) and about depressive or manic feelings and behaviors. Clinicians should also assess the severity, frequency, and longitudinal course of depressive and manic episodes and determine whether the symptoms meet the specific diagnostic criteria for bipolar or another psychiatric disorder. Medical disorders that may coexist or appear similar to BD should be considered, including thyroid dysfunction, vasculitis, chronic infection, malignancies, and metabolic disorders. Clinical and laboratory findings may help to exclude these causes. Family history, particularly of first-degree relatives, should be reviewed. Recent medications, including hormonal contraceptives, and treatment during prior episodes should be noted, especially any temporal association between drugs and symptoms; many drugs can induce or exacerbate manic or depressive symptoms. Levodopa and corticosteroids are the most common causes of drug-induced mania; these agents can also cause depressive symptoms.

In over 50% of patients with BP, a comorbid substance use disorder is present at some point during their lifetime. Patients with BD often self-medicate with drugs and alcohol to relieve anxiety, insomnia, agitation, and excessive fatigue. The risk of BD diagnosis increases four times in those with comorbid alcohol use disorder and up to five times more in illicit substance users. Drugs, alcohol, and some medications may also contribute to these symptoms and are an important potential differential diagnosis, discussed later in this chapter.

Patients with BD appear especially sensitive to sleep deprivation, which may occur in conjunction with stressors such as bereavement, childbirth, vacation, longer work hours, and shift changes. They may experience periods of decreased need for sleep while manic. Disrupted sleep can also precipitate manic episodes. Specific details about sleep–wake periods, including daytime naps, mealtimes, social activities, hobbies and other areas of interest, interpersonal attitudes, and ability to work and perform household tasks are helpful. Patients should be asked about a typical day and about deterioration in the baseline level of functioning at work or school or in personal relationships.

Patients with mania or depression usually do not report characteristic psychological descriptors (e.g., elation, grandiosity, inflated self-esteem, racing thoughts, irritability, or agitation), so activities may provide diagnostic clues. For example, grandiose thinking may manifest as reckless gambling, spending sprees, or sexual promiscuity. Conversely, increased productivity, enhanced perceptual ability, altered view on interpersonal relationships, and fluctuating symptoms without substantial negative social or occupational consequences suggest hypomania.

Routine screening for depression is advised in primary care settings, but attention should also focus on screening for past episodes of hypomania or mania. The Mood Disorder Questionnaire (MDQ) is a validated screening tool for BD, which lessens the likelihood of underdiagnosis or missed diagnosis. Use of the MDQ can identify 70% of people with BD while eliminating the diagnosis for 90% of persons without it. More recently, there has been some question about whether the MDQ underdiagnoses BD II because of the requirement for moderate to severe impairment of functioning, as many patients feel that during a hypomanic episode they function better. Another instrument, the Bipolar Spectrum Diagnostic Scale, is better for ruling out the diagnosis of BD than for giving a positive diagnosis. If a patient scores positive for BD on this scale, further clinical evaluation is necessary to make the diagnosis. Other diagnostic screening instruments can be found in Table 69.2.

Assessment for suicide risk is essential. Clinicians should inquire openly about suicide ideation and intentions, and about extent of plans or preparations for, prior attempts at, family history of, and recent exposure to suicide. This is essential both at presentation and during subsequent mood episodes because the lifetime risk for suicide in patients with BD is up to 15%. Most suicide attempts are associated with depressive episodes or during depressive features of mixed episodes.

Differential Diagnosis

General Considerations for All Bipolar Disorders

Among those patients who have not experienced psychotic symptoms or classic recurrent episodes of MDD,

TABLE 69.2 Available Online Psychometric Scales for Bipolar Disorders					
Scale	Description	Length of Time/ Number of Items	Administration	Psychometric Properties	Obtainable
Structured Clinical Interview for DSM Disorders, DSM-5-TR (SCID-5-SV)	Interviewing tool to assist in diagnosis of bipolar disorders	30–120 minutes	Administered by clinician	Sensitivity greater than 90%; specificity greater than 97%, reliability greater than 90%	Purchased from: https://appi.org/Products/Interviewing/Structured-Clinical-Interview-for-DSM-5-Disorders?sku = 62461
Mood Disorder Questionnaire (MDQ)	Screening tool for bipolar disorders	17 items	Self-administered; parent version for children and adolescents ages 5–18 years	Sensitivity 58%; specificity 93% in primary care settings in adult populations	Free: http://www.sadag.org/images/pdf/mdq.pdf
Bipolar Spectrum Diagnostic Scale (BSDS)	Measurement of bipolar symptoms over time	20 items (19 within paragraph format)	Self-administered	Specificity 90%, responses psychometrically equivalent between older and younger adults	Free: https://static1.squarespace.com/static/5a0df2b3692ebe9b1a7973e0/t/5c7847c8e4966b2709f6f94d/1551386569187/Bipolar+Spectrum+Diagnostic+Scale+%28BSDS%29..pdf
Young Mania Rating Scale (YMRS)	Assessment of manic symptoms over previous 48 hours	11 items	Patient subjected report and clinician observed; parent version for children and adolescents ages 5–18	Sensitivity 93%; specificity 96%; area Under the Receiver Operating Curve (AUROC) value of 0.66	Free: https://dcf.psychiatry.ufl.edu/files/2011/05/Young-Mania-Rating-Scale-Measure-with-background.pdf

TABLE 69.2 Available Online Psychometric Scales for Bipolar Disorders—cont'd					
Scale	Description	Length of Time/ Number of Items	Administration	Psychometric Properties	Obtainable
Hypomania Checklist 32 (HCL-32)	Assist in identification of hypomanic symptoms in patients with MDD	32 items	Self-administered	Sensitivity 80% in distinguishing between major depressive disorder and bipolar disorders; higher accuracy in identification of bipolar II disorders versus MDQ	Free: http://www.oacbdd.org/clientuploads/Docs/2010/Spring%20Handouts/Session%20220b.pdf
Altman Self-Rating Mania Scale (ASRM)	Assessment of presence and severity of manic or hypomanic symptoms over past week	Five items	Self-administered	Sensitivity 85.5%; specify 87.3%	Free: https://psychology-tools.com/test/altman-self-rating-mania-scale
Kiddie Schedule for Affective Disorders and Schizophrenia for School-Age Children-Present and Lifetime Version (K-SADS-PL)	Semistructured interview to measure current and past symptoms of mood, anxiety, psychotic, and disruptive behaviors in children and adolescents ages 6–18 years	45–75 minutes to administer	Self-report from parent and child	Reliability range 93%–100%	Free with stipulations: https://www.pediatricbipolar.pitt.edu/resources/instruments

two diagnoses that are sometimes confused with BD are substance abuse and cluster B personality disorders, and there may be comorbidities with these entities. Cluster B personality disorders describe individuals who often present as erratic, emotional, and/or dramatic and include borderline, antisocial, histrionic, and narcissistic personality disorders. However, in substance abuse, euphoria/dysphoria is temporally related to drug intoxication and withdrawal state. In cluster B personality disorders, "mood swings" last from minutes to hours to days, not weeks to months, and are typically closely associated with interpersonal disruptions or alliances.

Bipolar I Disorder

The differential diagnoses to consider are MDD, other BD, schizophrenia, anxiety disorders, attention deficit-hyperactivity disorder, personality disorders, and substance use. See Table 69.3 for further information on differential diagnoses. It is essential to obtain a full psychiatric history, and with the patient's consent, to interview family and friends to corroborate information and help establish the diagnosis of BD. Patients with mania often lack insight into their symptoms and do not report them. They feel euphoric during a manic episode and value their productivity during an episode of hypomania. Family members and friends may be able to report historical clues, personal factors, and suicidal ideation that may be associated with increased suicide risk and point to a diagnosis of BD. To help differentiate between bipolar and unipolar depression, as part of the history, ask about the onset, frequency, and duration of symptoms, as well as about distractibility, seasonality, and other characteristics of a depressed patient's high and low moods (see Box 69.3).

Bipolar II Disorder

The differential diagnoses for BD II are the same as for BD I. However, because of some patients' reluctance to view hypomania as a pathological state, it can be difficult to distinguish from other forms of recurrent depression. It is essential to inquire about suicide, because most suicide attempts are associated with depressive or mixed episodes.

Cyclothymic Disorder

Differentiating the milder, subsyndromal form of BD can be challenging, especially in determining the length of previous episodes. In addition, borderline personality

TABLE 69.3 Differential Diagnoses for Bipolar Disorders

Disorder	Clinical Features	Distinguishing Features
Generalized Anxiety Disorder	Presentation can be similar to hypomania but with more significance on generalized worries and stress.	Inability to control excessive and pervasive worry about one's life. Constantly feeling overwhelmed. Although a person with anxiety may have difficulty sleeping, they feel tired during the day unlike a manic patient who has energy despite lack of sleep. Although thoughts may race in both disorders, speech is not usually pressured in a person with anxiety. People with anxiety symptoms may exhibit constricted body language versus expansive body language, which is noted when a person is manic. People with generalized anxiety disorder often have co-occurring somatic symptoms.
Post-Traumatic Stress Disorder	Patient has a history of significant trauma but no history of manic or hypomanic episodes.	The symptoms are related to a traumatic life event. Symptoms may include intrusive memories about the event, and attempts are made to avoid stimuli associated with the event. Patient may experience negative alterations in cognition and mood associated with trauma and alterations in arousal and reactivity associated with the trauma. If sleep is affected, it is usually disrupted with nightmares, not because of a decreased need for sleep.
Substance Use Disorder/Acute Intoxication	Symptoms typically occur in setting of intoxication or withdrawal.	Symptoms occur within the context of substances. A diagnosis of bipolar disorder should be made during a period of time when the person is not actively using mood-altering substances.
Borderline Personality Disorder	Mood swings last minutes to hours with mood symptoms typically triggered by external stimuli (such as perceived failure or abandonment), chronically unstable and intense interpersonal relationships, and self-reported feelings of emptiness.	Extreme emotions are reactions to situations, and duration may be minutes to hours versus days to weeks. Responses are often related to fears of abandonment. Symptoms are characterized by unstable relationships, self-harm behavior, and feelings of emptiness along with a self-image that is unclear.
Psychotic Disorder	Psychotic symptoms occur without presence of mania or depression.	Psychotic symptoms include one or more of the five domains (delusions, hallucinations, disorganized thinking, grossly disorganized or abnormal motor behavior, and negative symptoms). They occur outside the context of mood.
Attention Deficit–Hyperactivity Disorder	Symptoms are persistent and not episodic with onset typically presenting in early childhood. Patient can have difficulty falling asleep but does not have decreased need for sleep.	Symptoms typically start before age 12 years. Primary features surround inattention and hyperactive-impulsive behavior. Outbursts and meltdowns are related to poor distress tolerance and not mood.

disorder and substance-induced mood disorders need to be considered.

MANAGEMENT

Pharmacological Management

The ideal treatment goals for patients with BD include complete remission of current symptoms, mood stabilization, prevention of future affective episodes, and return to premorbid function. Mainstays of therapy are mood-stabilizing medications. Pharmacotherapy is used to achieve symptom remission and improve function in patients with BD. Mood stabilizers, second generation antipsychotics, first generation antipsychotics, and adjunctive anxiolytics and antidepressants are used to treat BD. Factors in determining which medication will most likely result in treatment remission depend on the diagnosis—BD I or BD II, manic versus depressed, acute or maintenance, rapid cycling versus nonrapid cycling, and whether psychotic symptoms exist. Attempts should be made to use the lowest possible dose to minimize side effects, particularly with first generation agents. For a complete list of FDA-approved pharmacological agents used in BD, see Drugs Commonly Prescribed 69.2.

Box 69.3 Distinguishing Between Bipolar and Unipolar Depressive Episodes

- Ask all depressed patients about history of mania and hypomania.
- Ask about family history of bipolar disorder— "loaded" family history is a clue to bipolarity in "unipolar" patients.
- Involve family member and/or significant other in screening process.
- Administer a screening instrument for bipolar disorder, such as the Mood Disorder Questionnaire.
- Early age at onset (younger than 25 years) is another clue for bipolarity.
- Psychotic features are another clinical clue for bipolarity in the seemingly unipolar patient, as is a seasonal pattern.
- Adverse and/or inadequate antidepressant response such as treatment-emergent hypomania or agitation, erratic or uneven antidepressant responses, multiple antidepressant failures, or "treatment-resistant depression."

Sources: Hirschfeld RM, Vornik LA. Recognition and diagnosis of bipolar disorder. *J Clin Psychiatry*. 2004;65(suppl 15):5–9; Lohano K, Loganathan M, Roberts RJ, et al. When to suspect bipolar disorder. *J Fam Pract*. 2010;59(12):682–688.

Considerations before initiating therapy include the patient's age, because older patients may be more sensitive to side effects of antipsychotic medications and anticonvulsants. It is essential to prescribe the lowest possible dose and monitor for side effects, unless in acute manic, psychotic, and/or depressive situations where more urgent titration may be needed. In these more acute stages of the illness, urgent titrations typically occur in an inpatient psychiatric setting. The possibility of pregnancy should always be considered in females of childbearing age before initiating psychotropic medications. Knowledge of past treatment history, effectiveness, tolerability, failures, and side-effect profiles allows the practitioner to provide individualized, person-centered care. It is likely there will be a need to change treatment modalities over time. Several weeks are required to assess the effects of a new treatment.

Collaboration with a psychiatrist will aid the clinician in selecting appropriate drug therapy to treat acute manic episodes in patients with BD. Treatment options for patients with BD I with hypomania, mania, or mixed episodes should begin with mood stabilizers or atypical

Drugs Commonly Prescribed 69.2: Bipolar Disorder

DRUG	INDICATION	ADVERSE REACTIONS AND PRESCRIBING CONSIDERATIONS
Adults		
Mood stabilizer		Risk for nausea, insomnia, somnolence, jitteriness, diarrhea, sexual dysfunction, drug reaction with eosinophilia and systemic symptoms (DRESS) Monitor: Propranolol 20–30 mg two to three times per day may reduce tremor if side effect
Valproate	Acute manic or mixed episodes, bipolar depression, maintenance treatment of bipolar disorder	Risk for headache, drowsiness, nausea/vomiting, increased appetite/weight gain, alopecia Considerations: Can cause major congenital malformations; not recommended for use in hepatic disease; trough concentrations should be drawn within 3 to 4 days of dosage adjustments or initiation and should be drawn before next dosage. Therapeutic range for mania 50–125 mcg/mL; multivitamin with zinc and selenium may reduce alopecia; do not use in patients with pancreatitis, serious liver disease, urea cycle disorder
Lamotrigine	Bipolar disorder maintenance, acute bipolar major depression	Risk for nausea/vomiting, drowsiness, *serious skin rash/reactions (Steven-Johnson's syndrome)* Monitor: Discontinue medication *immediately* if skin rash occurs and do not resume; if lamotrigine has been withheld for more than five half-lives (most patients more than 6 days) must restart according to initial dosage titration schedule; for patients taking medications that have interactions with lamotrigine, dosage adjustments are required; one of the more weight neutral options; oral contraceptives may decrease efficacy; dosage adjustments for moderate to severe hepatic impairment

Continued

Drugs Commonly Prescribed 69.2: Bipolar Disorder—cont'd

DRUG	INDICATION	ADVERSE REACTIONS AND PRESCRIBING CONSIDERATIONS
Lithium	Acute manic or mixed episodes, maintenance treatment for patients with a history of mania, acute hypomania, acute bipolar depression	Risk for weight gain, ataxia, tremor, memory problems, polyuria, polydipsia, diarrhea, nausea, acne, alopecia, leukocytosis, thyroid goiters, cardiac arrhythmias, hypotension, sedation Monitor: Trough levels (12 hours after last dosage) should be every 1 to 2 weeks until desired concentration is achieved and then every 2–3 months for the first 6 months and then repeat every 6–12 months; symptoms of lithium toxicity are life threatening and include tremor, ataxia, diarrhea, vomiting, sedation, muscular weakness, confusion; avoid use in renal impairment where creatinine clearance (CrCl) is less than 30 mL/minute; should be tapered off over 3-month period if used as long-term maintenance
Carbamazepine	Acute manic or mixed episodes, bipolar depression, bipolar maintenance	Risk for sedation, dizziness, confusion, unsteadiness, headache, nausea, vomiting, diarrhea, blurred vision, leukopenia, rash, *serious skin reactions (including toxic epidermal necrolysis and Stevens-Johnson syndrome)* Monitor: Discontinue medication *immediately* if skin rash occurs and do not resume; use with caution in hepatic and/or cardiac impairment; dosage adjustment recommended for renal impairment; can reduce effectiveness of oral birth control
Oxcarbazepine	Bipolar disorder	Risk for sedation, dizziness, headache, ataxia, nystagmus, abnormal gait, confusion, nausea, vomiting, diplopia, vertigo, abnormal vision, rash, hyponatremia Monitor: Can reduce effectiveness of oral birth control; monitoring of sodium may be required; dosage adjustments recommended for renal impairment; use with caution in hepatic impairment; same mechanism of action as carbamazepine but with fewer side effects
Second Generation Antipsychotics		Risk for akathisia, tardive dyskinesia, extrapyramidal side effects, metabolic side effects, neuroleptic malignant syndrome; increased risk of death in older adult patients with dementia-related psychosis; risk of dysphagia (use with caution in patients at risk of aspiration pneumonia) Benztropine or trihexyphenidyl for motor side effects
Quetiapine	Acute manic episodes, mixed episodes (use ER), mixed episodes (use IR), acute hypomania, **bipolar depression monotherapy**, bipolar depression adjunct with antimanic therapy, **maintenance treatment adjunct to antimanic therapy**, maintenance treatment monotherapy	Risk for increased blood pressure, increased cholesterol, weight gain, increased appetite, drowsiness, dizziness, agitation, headache Monitor: Dosage adjustment required in hepatic impairment; rare but serious side effect, drug reaction with eosinophilia and systemic symptoms (DRESS), can occur
Lurasidone	**Bipolar depression, acute.** Bipolar depression maintenance	Risk for increased triglycerides, increased cholesterol, nausea, drowsiness, extrapyramidal reactions, akathisia, insomnia Monitor: Must take with at least 350 calories; dosage adjustments recommended for hepatic and/or renal impairment; one of the more weight-neutral options
Aripiprazole	Acute manic episodes, mixed episodes, bipolar maintenance, bipolar depression	Risk for sedation, dizziness, insomnia, akathisia, activation, nausea, vomiting, orthostatic hypotension, constipation, headache Monitor: One of the more weight-neutral options; rare but serious side effect, drug reaction with eosinophilia and systemic symptoms (DRESS), can occur

Drugs Commonly Prescribed 69.2: Bipolar Disorder—cont'd

DRUG	INDICATION	ADVERSE REACTIONS AND PRESCRIBING CONSIDERATIONS
Cariprazine	Acute manic episodes, mixed episodes, bipolar depression	Risk for akathisia, restlessness, sedation, gastrointestinal distress, extrapyramidal symptoms Monitor for side effects for several weeks after starting due to long half-life; not recommended in severe hepatic or renal impairment; one of the more weight-neutral options
Olanzapine	Acute manic episodes, mixed episodes, maintenance, bipolar depression	Risk for dizziness, sedation, dry mouth, constipation, dyspepsia, weight gain, increased risk of diabetes and dyslipidemia, orthostatic hypotension, tachycardia, increased prolactin, extrapyramidal reactions Monitor: Dosage adjustment recommended in hepatic impairment; use with caution in cardiac impairment; increased risk of stroke in older adults; rare but serious side effect, drug reaction with eosinophilia and systemic symptoms (DRESS), can occur
Risperidone	Acute manic episodes, mixed episodes, maintenance, bipolar depression	Risk for sedation, weight gain, increased prolactin, dizziness, hypotension, increased risk of diabetes and dyslipidemia, extrapyramidal reactions, nausea, constipation, tachycardia Monitor: Use with caution in patients predisposed to hypotension; dosage adjustment required for renal and hepatic impairment; use with caution in cardiac impairment
Children and Adolescents		
Mood stabilizer		Risk for nausea, insomnia, somnolence, jitteriness, diarrhea, sexual dysfunction Monitor: Antidepressants increase the risk of suicidal thinking and behavior in children, adolescents, and young adults (18–24 years of age) with major depressive disorder (MDD) and other psychiatric disorders
Lithium	Bipolar disorder	Risk for weight gain, ataxia, tremor, memory problems, polyuria, polydipsia, diarrhea, nausea, acne, alopecia, leukocytosis, thyroid goiters, cardiac arrhythmias, hypotension, sedation. *Side effects are typically more pronounced in pediatric/adolescent populations.* Monitor: Trough levels (12 hours after last dosage) should be every 1–2 weeks until desired concentration is achieved and then every 2–3 months for the first 6 months and then repeat every 6–12 months; symptoms of lithium toxicity are life-threatening and include tremor, ataxia, diarrhea, vomiting, sedation, muscular weakness, confusion; avoid use in renal impairment where Crcl is less than 30 mL/minute; should be tapered off over 3-month period if used as long-term maintenance; rare but serious side effect, drug reaction with eosinophilia and systemic symptoms (DRESS), can occur
Second Generation Antipsychotics		
Quetiapine	Bipolar disorder, mania or mixed episodes	Risk for increased blood pressure, increased cholesterol, weight gain, increased appetite, drowsiness, dizziness, agitation, headache Monitor: Dosage adjustment required in hepatic impairment; rare but serious side effect, drug reaction with eosinophilia and systemic symptoms (DRESS), can occur
Lurasidone	Bipolar depression	Risk for increased triglycerides, increased cholesterol, nausea, drowsiness, extrapyramidal reactions, akathisia, insomnia Monitor: Must take with at least 350 calories; dosage adjustments recommended for hepatic and/or renal impairment; one of the more weight-neutral options

Continued

Drugs Commonly Prescribed 69.2: Bipolar Disorder—cont'd

DRUG	INDICATION	ADVERSE REACTIONS AND PRESCRIBING CONSIDERATIONS
Aripiprazole	Acute manic episodes, mixed	Risk for sedation, dizziness, insomnia, akathisia, activation, nausea, vomiting, orthostatic hypotension, constipation, headache Monitor: One of the more weight-neutral options; side effects more pronounced in pediatric/adolescent populations; rare but serious side effect, drug reaction with eosinophilia and systemic symptoms (DRESS), can occur
Olanzapine	Acute manic episodes, mixed episodes	Risk for increased prolactin, weight gain, increased appetite, akathisia, drowsiness, headache, extrapyramidal reaction, tremor Monitor: May need more monitoring than adults; use with caution with hepatic impairment; long-term metabolic risks and side effects—monitor closely; rare but serious side effect, drug reaction with eosinophilia and systemic symptoms (DRESS), can occur
Risperidone	Acute manic episodes, mixed episodes	Risk for sedation, weight gain, increased prolactin, dizziness, hypotension, increased risk of diabetes and dyslipidemia, extrapyramidal reactions, nausea, constipation, tachycardia

Note: Bold for FDA approved.

antipsychotic agents. Lithium is a typical first-line therapy in manic, hypomanic, and/or depressed states. Valproic acid (Depakote) is another option but should not be used in pregnant patients and should be avoided in patients with liver disease. Carbamazepine (Tegretol) or oxcarbazepine (Trileptal) may also be used. If there is no response or a partial response in acute manic episodes, combination therapy such as lithium plus valproic acid, lithium plus an atypical antipsychotic, or an atypical antipsychotic plus valproic acid may be considered. If still not effective, clozapine (Clozaril) may be added, or electroconvulsive therapy (ECT) may be introduced in treatment-resistant cases.

It is important that lithium be prescribed at a therapeutic dose. Valproic acid is usually preferred, however, due to its ease of administration. Carbamazepine, another anticonvulsant agent, is an alternative. Combinations of these agents may be used if patients do not respond to a single agent. If the patient does not respond fully, atypical antipsychotics may be added to one or more mood stabilizers. Long-acting benzodiazepines, such as clonazepam (Klonopin) and lorazepam (Ativan), may be used for rapid treatment of manic symptoms and to calm and sedate patients until acute mania or hypomania has subsided and the mood stabilizer has taken effect. In the case of psychotic symptoms, antipsychotics may be added. ECT may be used for patients with severe BD with drug treatment–resistant mania, psychotic depression, and/or catatonia.

Episodes of depression pose particular challenges. There are fewer approved treatments for bipolar depression. Typical first-line medications for depression include lurasidone (Latuda) and quetiapine (Seroquel). If these are ineffective, valproic acid as an adjunct or alone is a second-line option. Lithium can also be used alone or as adjunct with quetiapine, lurasidone, or valproate. Overall, antidepressant medications do not control depression as effectively in bipolar as in unipolar depression, and they may trigger mania. A newer combination of olanzapine (Zyprexa) and fluoxetine is another choice (Silva et al., 2013). If depression persists 2 to 4 weeks after optimization of the mood stabilizer, it is recommended that either lamotrigine (Lamictal), anticonvulsant, mood stabilizer, or an atypical antipsychotic be added. Antidepressants may be effective against depression but can precipitate mania. They should not be given to a patient with BD without a mood stabilizer, and even then, they are reserved for extremely ill patients after other options have failed. Bupropion is often the first antidepressant started because it is considered the least likely to induce mania. Any patient developing symptoms of hypomania while taking an antidepressant should stop taking it; in addition, patients should be slowly tapered off any antidepressants after a period of sustained remission. Patients with psychotic symptoms, such as delusions or hallucinations, will require treatment with antipsychotic medications.

Lithium remains the gold standard for treatment of BD and has been shown to be uniquely effective in decreasing suicidal behavior. Lithium appears to be most effective early in the course of the illness for classic manic symptoms in patients in whom depression immediately follows mania and in patients with a strong family history of BD. However, lithium also has a number of potential adverse effects, including life-threatening neurotoxicity that can occur at serum levels higher than 2 mEq/L. Lithium levels should be obtained twice weekly until the patient's clinical status and levels are stable, at which time the levels may be obtained every 1 to 3 months. Serum trough lithium levels are drawn 8 to 12 hours after the last dose. Adverse drug interactions can occur when lithium is prescribed with thiazide diuretics, NSAIDs, angiotensin-converting enzyme inhibitors, and COX-2 inhibitors. Additional potential adverse effects include nausea, diarrhea, tremor, polyuria, polydipsia, and weight gain. Lithium may exacerbate psoriasis and acne, cause hypothyroidism (5% to 35%), and in 20% of patients (usually after 15 or more years of treatment) lead to renal insufficiency. Lithium has also been associated with a rare birth defect called Ebstein's anomaly, a congenital heart defect in which the opening of the tricuspid valve is displaced toward the apex of the right ventricle of the heart. Lithium takes several weeks to become effective. Owing to potential adverse effects, lithium therapy should be preceded by an evaluation of renal, cardiac, and thyroid function, as well as a pregnancy test. Many patients do not stay on lithium. Some regret the loss of the exhilaration that occurs during a manic episode; some patients are concerned about weight gain or tremor. In one study, 50% of patients acknowledged some degree of medication nonadherence in the previous 2 years, and 32% reported only partial adherence in the preceding month.

Anticonvulsant medications are effective for the treatment and/or maintenance of mania and/or BD. These agents have become alternative treatments for patients who need a mood-stabilizing agent but who do not fare well with lithium; these medications also may be used in combination with lithium. Divalproex/valproic acid is considered a first-line pharmacological treatment for acute mania, mixed episodes, rapid cycling, and maintenance treatment. There is some evidence of antidepressant effect as well. Divalproex appears to be most effective for rapid cycling and mixed episodes in patients who have had more than three manic episodes and in patients with comorbid alcohol abuse. Valproic acid is comparable to lithium in efficacy and generally better tolerated. The most frequently observed side effects are nausea, vomiting, weight gain, tremor, dizziness, and sedation. Serious adverse effects include hepatotoxicity, pancreatitis, thrombocytopenia, and teratogenicity. Serum valproate levels, liver function tests, and CBCs should be monitored closely during treatment with valproic acid.

Valproic acid is a cytochrome 450 enzyme inhibitor and may engender metabolic interactions with other drugs. Valproic acid can induce menstrual irregularities and cause polycystic ovary syndrome (PCOS), affecting 2% to 7% of female patients in their reproductive years. PCOS is characterized by chronic anovulation and hyperandrogenism. Valproic acid is teratogenic and can cause neural tube defects in 1% to 4% of neonates. Valproic acid is also associated with congenital malformations, including spina bifida, atrial septal defect, cleft palate, hypospadias, polydactyly, and craniosynostosis. Troubling reports of lower intelligence quotient (IQ) in children exposed in utero to valproate have been published. As a result, many authorities recommend avoiding valproic acid altogether in females of childbearing age.

Carbamazepine is approved for the treatment of bipolar mania and mixed episodes. Therapeutic serum levels for BD have not been established; usually concentrations used for seizure disorders (4 to 12 mcg/mL) are applied. Serum levels as well as CBC, platelets, and liver function must all be monitored as potential side effects, which include agranulocytosis, aplastic anemia, hepatic failure, Stevens-Johnson syndrome, and pancreatitis. Carbamazepine reduces levels of other drugs, such as oral contraceptives and dihydropyridine calcium-channel blockers. Carbamazepine is contraindicated during pregnancy or lactation. It is associated with congenital malformations, including spina bifida, craniofacial defects, fingernail hypoplasia, and developmental delays.

Lamotrigine received approval as maintenance therapy for BD in 2003. This medication's antidepressant effects are stronger than its antimanic properties, and it usually is not used as monotherapy for patients with BD I. The most significant adverse effect is rash (about 5% risk), which, in some cases, can be Stevens-Johnson syndrome or toxic epidermal necrolysis, both of which can be fatal.

Typical antipsychotic agents such as haloperidol (Haldol) have been frequently used to treat acute bipolar mania. These agents work well in reducing symptoms such as paranoia, hallucinations, delusions, and thought disturbances. However, they are usually not used for the longer term or preventive management of BD and carry the risk of extrapyramidal symptoms (EPS), such as akathisia, dystonia (e.g., torticollis), parkinsonism, and tardive dyskinesia, as well as depression.

Newer second generation, or atypical, antipsychotics have a lower propensity to induce EPS, but have been linked to weight gain and metabolic syndrome. Both classes of drugs block dopaminergic transmission, but the newer drugs also block serotonin receptors. These are standard agents for schizophrenia, but most are now approved for use as monotherapy in mania and depression or for maintenance with and without mood stabilizers. Examples of medications used in BD mood stabilization include aripiprazole (Abilify), olanzapine, risperidone (Risperdal), quetiapine, and lurasidone. See Chapter 68 for further discussion of typical and atypical antipsychotics.

Maintenance drug therapy should be based on the patient's response to initial treatment and in conjunction with a psychiatrist. Patients at high risk for recurrence should consider lifelong therapy, generally with mood stabilizers. Lithium and valproic acid are first-line agents used in maintenance therapy, alone and in combination. Although there are some differences in side effects, the dropout rates are similar, and both agents demonstrate equal effectiveness. Carbamazepine may be used as an alternative.

Adjunctive drug therapy should be considered for comorbid disorders. For example, if a patient with BD is compliant with medication yet has a concurrent anxiety or substance use disorder, an antidepressant may be used with either a mood stabilizer or an antipsychotic. If a patient is persistently anxious, most psychiatrists will assess for a mixed state, occult substance abuse, or a medical condition. In summary, management options are based on the patient's primary symptoms of mania, depression, or mixed states (see Table 69.1).

Nonpharmacological Management

Psychotherapy, although not as effective as monotherapy, can significantly enhance treatment response and prevent relapse. Interpersonal, family-focused, cognitive behavioral, dialectical behavioral, supportive, and psychoeducational approaches increase illness awareness, improve collaboration with health-care professionals and supportive family and friends, and may assist in lifestyle regulation. There is good evidence that CBT protects against relapse, results in better treatment response, and helps support greater maintenance of treatment gains. Dialectical behavioral therapy (DBT) is another modality that has been shown to improve well-being, decrease emotional reactivity, increase mindfulness and distress tolerance, and benefit psychosocial functioning. Common themes among these therapy modalities include psychoeducation about the disease, identification of prodromal syndromes, problem-solving strategies to reduce and cope with stress, and plans for treatment adherence and interventions.

It is important to note that BD not only affects the patient but also the patient's family and friends. Ways in which BD can affect others in the patient's sphere include:

- Changes in family roles
- Coping with emotional distress, such as grief, worry, and guilt
- Coping with the patient's unusual and/or dangerous behaviors
- Increased financial stressors as a result of excessive spending or reduced income
- Strained relationships
- Difficulty with relationships outside the family
- Increased risk of health problems as a result of stress

Resources should be provided to the patient's support people such as support groups (i.e., National Alliance on Mental Illness), case management (through their insurance and/or local behavioral health organizations), individual therapists, and psychoeducation.

Psychoeducation is a key component and foundation of psychotherapy for management of BD. Meta-analysis has shown that patient education combined with drug treatment helps to improve adherence. It is aimed at providing comprehensive information about BD and treatment and is an important resource for patients, families, and support people. The goals of psychoeducation are to increase knowledge and acceptance of the disorder, to address denial and nonadherence to the treatment plan, and to provide information on self-management strategies including stress reduction, healthy lifestyle changes, and ways to identify early signs of recurrence.

The onset of manic and depressive episodes is often associated with psychosocial stress. Patients should be encouraged to pace their activities at work and to maintain a regular schedule. A change in sleep patterns often heralds the onset of a manic or depressive episode. Insomnia may be a precipitant or a prodromal warning sign. Maintenance of regular sleep habits helps prevent escalation of mood symptoms into a full-blown episode. Educate patients with BD and their support people about the risks of stress, substance abuse, irregular and inconsistent sleep patterns, meals, and other daily habits.

Patients with BD may have difficulty discussing unusual events or thoughts and often have poor insight regarding symptoms or the need for treatment. They respond best to proactive, collaborative, and individualized treatment, as exemplified in the Circle of Caring model. Developing a therapeutic alliance is imperative, because BD is chronic and needs long-term management. Establishing a trusting relationship with the patient, their family and support people, and other medical and behavioral health providers gives patients the opportunity to experience continuity of care, to attend to health maintenance and any chronic medical problems, and to maintain a collaborative connection with their behavioral health providers and support systems.

Current Considerations: Coronavirus Disease 2019 (COVID-19)

Since the first COVID-19 case was reported in the United States, millions of Americans have been infected, and hundreds of thousands have died. Many states imposed stay-at-home orders and limits on social gatherings to combat the disease and slow the spread. Although these measures were needed to protect public health and safety, they came with dire psychological consequences. Research has shown an increase in depression, feelings of helplessness, anger, anxiety, and alienation. It remains unclear how COVID-19 specifically impacted patients with BD. In general, providing ways to reduce stress for patients with BD can be helpful. All options should be person-centered and include a treatment plan tailored to the patient's needs, given their personal life and environment. Additionally, more frequent follow-up appointments may be required to ensure compliance with the treatment plan and stabilization of symptoms.

FOLLOW-UP AND REFERRAL

Education is a key component to effective adherence to therapy and support systems. Open discussion of all treatment options, side effects, and their management is critical and is a hallmark of person-centered care. It is essential to monitor and manage symptoms over time, including triggers and early warning signs. Personal monitoring and better symptom recognition are desirable goals. The prevalence of nonadherence with mood stabilizers ranges from 18% to 52%. Reasons include denial of diagnosis, unwillingness to take medication long-term, perceived improvement in health, and adverse side effects of medications. Patient adherence to the medication regimen can make a difference in patient outcomes. In one 18-month study, 81% of partially adherent patients required hospitalization versus just 9% of adherent patients. Primary care providers may improve patient medication adherence by asking patients to reflect on what life would be like without their medication, possible consequences of medication nonadherence, and things that may interfere with medication adherence such as social rhythms and/or stigmas around the illness. Patients may ask if they will need to continue taking the same medication for life. The specific medications prescribed may change as new agents are introduced and as the individual's treatment needs are reassessed. What will remain constant is the need to monitor the patient with BD over their lifetime as risk of relapse after one affective episode is over 85% within a 5-year period.

The practitioner can help the patient and family/support people develop realistic treatment goals by actively listening and being responsive to patient needs and by regularly addressing mixed feelings about adherence to treatment. Patients with BD struggle with a variety of interpersonal and/or occupational issues. As stabilization management and supervision are lessened after an acute affective episode, patient attendance at follow-ups may decrease. During this postacute period, intensive collaboration with the patient and support people can be invaluable for establishing the framework for long-term interactions that build on the therapeutic Circle of Caring; however, collaboration with support people is pertinent throughout the course of the illness.

Involvement of family and/or friends is critical to successful follow-up because progression of BD may be difficult to validate via self-report. Sensitivity to early warning signs of potential mood destabilization is important. Many patients do not try to achieve treatment goals. Symptoms of illness often preclude sound judgment, and patient unwillingness to tolerate medication side effects is one of the causes of apparent nonadherence.

Regularly reviewing with the patient "quality of life" versus "effects of treatment" and emphasizing the improved prognosis associated with maintenance therapy may improve medication compliance. CBT, family therapy, or interpersonal therapy should all target self-monitoring, treatment adherence, communication skills, and coping strategies to complement pharmacotherapy.

If a patient presents with early manifestations of relapse, promptly assess the clinical scenario and review the drug regimen. It is essential to investigate possible medication nonadherence, drug–drug interactions, and substance use and to obtain a drug level before initiating a change in the current regimen. If the cause of relapse is unclear or if the symptoms fail to respond to standard treatment, a psychiatrist should be consulted. Periodically, the patient should be reevaluated for known or new medical conditions or medication use that may complicate management; at every encounter, they should also be assessed for suicide risk.

The primary care provider should obtain a consultation with a psychiatrist or psychiatric mental health nurse practitioner (PMHNP) if BD is suspected once medical etiologies have been excluded. Accurate diagnosis can be complicated because other psychiatric disorders may appear similar. Consultation will provide clinicians with a more accurate diagnosis, as well as assistance with managing pharmacological regimens and acute crises should it be necessary. Consider referral to an integrated treatment provider for dual-diagnosed patients with substance and/or alcohol dependence. Hospitalization is necessary for patients with BD who may be a danger to themselves or others or who are unable to care for their needs. Patients with mood disorders, particularly mania, are often unwilling to enter a hospital voluntarily and may require involuntary commitment.

A supportive primary care provider can help monitor the patient's overall status, as well as encourage adherence to the medication regimen. The clinician can also provide referral for specific psychosocial interventions for patients with BD. Along with a PMHNP or a psychiatrist, a behavioral health specialist may aid recovery by relieving depression, delaying episodes, and improving function and treatment adherence.

Patient Education: Bipolar and Related Disorders

Educate the patient and support people about the nature of bipolar illness and about the importance of medication compliance, regular visits for clinical and laboratory monitoring, and contacting their health-care provider before stopping or starting any medication (prescribed or OTC). Patients should avoid complementary therapies such as St. John's wort, because they may interfere with some psychotropics or precipitate mania. Educating the patient and support people about potential side effects of all medications is important, as is informing them of the many options available to minimize or eliminate side effects. Patients and support people need to understand the importance of maintaining adequate blood levels of medication in prevention of relapse and of contacting the health-care provider in the event of unpleasant side effects rather than stopping the medication.

At follow-up visits, the practitioner can counsel the patient and support people about coping with stressors that may precipitate manic or depressive episodes, about maintaining a consistent lifestyle, about signs of relapse, and about medication adherence. Written patient instructions can reinforce the following recommendations:

- Limit "everyday" stimulants such as coffee, alcohol, and OTC medications that contain these substances because they can trigger mood episodes.
- Maintain regular sleep patterns.
- Avoid taking unnecessary or illegal drugs because they can trigger mood episodes; they can also prevent the benefits or increase the adverse side effects of necessary medications.
- Try to maintain a regular work schedule. If necessary, take time off rather than "tough it out" if mood symptoms hinder your ability to work.

As patients learn more about the stress their illness places on support people and family members, it may help them reduce both their own stress and the disruption that it can cause. Patients may develop such insights by learning more about bipolar illness and by joining a bipolar support group or a mental health organization for laypeople. Patients and support people should be instructed to watch for early signs of relapse, including changes in sleep patterns, grooming habits, energy or sexual interest; concentration problems; mood instability; or changes in self-esteem. Most patients experience a change in sleep patterns early in the development of an episode of mania or depression. Even small amounts of stimulants may interfere with sleep patterns or mood and possibly trigger a relapse. Insomnia may be either a precipitant or a warning sign. Early recognition of these signals, promptly followed by contacting the primary care provider, can help prevent relapse. Maintenance of regular sleep patterns, sometimes via judicious medication use, can prevent escalation of early symptoms into full episodes.

Patients with BD tend to minimize their limitations and vulnerabilities and may decide to discontinue treatment. There should be an individual action plan for coping and seeking assistance whenever the patient or support people suspect the patient is experiencing early manifestations of relapse. Knowledge of assigned roles in the patient's action plan may be an important resource when the patient is tempted to stop therapy. They should feel free to contact their psychiatrist, counselor, or primary care provider for advice whenever necessary, especially in light of self-destructive, aggressive behavior or any changes in daily routine that cause concern.

SUICIDE

Suicide is the result of wide-ranging disease states, disrupting biological, psychological, and social processes. In recent years, suicide has become an intensifying national public health crisis. In 2020, more than 45,000 Americans completed suicide, making it among the top 9 leading causes of death in the country. Since 1999, the suicide rate has increased each year in the United States (except in 2019 and 2020, rates declined), which results in an estimated $70 billion annually in lifetime medical and work-loss related costs. Suicide leaves a devastating legacy. Survivors are confronted with myriad distressing emotions and thoughts, which often continue to affect loved ones, family, children, friends, clinicians, and society long after the event.

Several terms are associated with suicidal behavior. *Completed suicide* refers to self-inflicted death. *Attempted suicide* describes potentially lethal acts that did not result in death. *Aborted suicide* indicates potentially suicidal behavior that was stopped before the action was completed. *Suicidal ideation* denotes thoughts of causing one's own demise. It can be accompanied by planning, intent, rehearsals, and obtaining the means for suicide. *Parasuicidal behavior* describes patients who injure themselves in nonlethal, occasional attention-seeking gestures, such as superficial cuts on wrists, but who do not wish to die. The behavior is a risk factor for suicide.

Each person and their life circumstances are unique. Unfortunately, there is no way to predict suicide. However, risk for suicide can be assessed through analysis of risk factors, suicidal intent, and protective factors. If there is a shared personal characteristic, it is likely to be a profound sense of hopelessness, in the sense that the individual perceives there is no future or that the future they envision is somehow unattainable. Suicidal patients may be angry, sad, or confused. They may be quite honest about their suicidal plans or refuse to disclose their hidden thoughts and feelings.

Suicidal thoughts and feelings commonly are associated with mood disorders, principally MDD and BD, although they also occur in other psychiatric disorders. People who are overwhelmed by severe psychosocial problems and/or medical illnesses may also experience suicidal thoughts. Approximately 54% of individuals completing suicide have no known mental health condition.

Suicidal ideation can have acute onset, meaning that for a period of time, the person is at risk for acting on thoughts of suicide. Chronic suicidal thoughts are also not uncommon. In this case, the person never feels completely free of thoughts of taking their life. Impulsive suicidal behavior is the most difficult to assess because this type of behavior is likely to occur without warning. Patients who are troubled by thoughts of suicide but are clear about their determination not to act on their suicidal thoughts may be appropriate candidates for primary care management. Any suggestion of impulsive behavior, chronic suicidal thoughts, or evidence of acute suicidal ideation with intent, plan, and/or means is an indicator for emergent evaluation by a specialist.

In the month before completing suicide, nearly one-half of patients visit their primary care provider, but only 20% see a mental health professional. Females and older patients are more likely to seek care before suicide, compared with males and younger patients. Most antidepressant prescriptions (~ 80%) in the United States are written by generalists, such as internists, pediatricians, and family physicians. Taken together, it is clear that primary care clinicians provide the most depression treatment in the United States and are also the group most likely to see patients at risk of suicide in the month preceding their death. Therefore, they may have the greatest opportunity to intervene (see The Patient's Voice 69.1.)

EPIDEMIOLOGY AND CAUSES

Suicide is among the top 9 leading causes of death in the United States and the second leading cause of death among adolescents, aged 10 to 14 years, and young adults, aged 25 to 34 years. Every 11 minutes, another life is lost to suicide. Every day, 132 Americans take their own lives, and more than 3,300 attempt suicide. For every victim of homicide in the United States, there are two deaths from suicide, and there are now three times as many deaths due to suicide than HIV/AIDS. More than one-half of all suicides occur in adult males aged 25 to 65 years. Although females are three times more likely to attempt suicide, a risk that increases directly with age, males are more likely to complete suicide. Males are almost four times more likely to die from suicide than females because they may use more lethal means, such as firearms. Sadly, many who make suicide attempts never seek professional care after the attempt. About 10% of all people who attempt suicide eventually die by suicide.

Divorced, separated, single, and widowed people of both sexes have a higher incidence of suicide. Adolescents and young adults (aged 10 to 34 years) as well as older adults (65 years and older) are at elevated risk, especially Native Americans and Caucasian males. Suicide is lowest in non-white females, including Hispanics and Asian/Pacific Islanders.

In terms of methods, the most lethal means are firearms, suffocation, and poisoning (overdose). In 2019, firearms accounted for about 50% of suicide deaths. Suffocation/hanging was the second leading method of completed suicide at 28.5% of suicide deaths.

Special at-risk occupations include physicians (especially female physicians and psychiatrists), musicians, dentists, law enforcement officers, firefighters, lawyers, and insurance agents. A number of CNS diseases increase the risk of suicide, specifically epilepsy, multiple sclerosis, head injury, cardiovascular disease, Huntington's disease, and AIDS. All of these diseases are associated with mood disorders. Loss of mobility, disfigurement, and intractable pain are also associated with an increased risk of suicide. Certain drugs such as reserpine (Serpasil), isotretinoin, montelukast, corticosteroids, antihypertensive agents, statins, anticonvulsants, and some antineoplastic agents can produce depression that may lead to suicide. Exposure to traumatic or life-threatening events may also increase risk for mental illness and suicide. When surveyed, twice as many Americans reported suicidal ideation in June 2020 than in the previous year, a statistic that has been attributed to the COVID-19 pandemic. During this time, 40% of adults reported significant symptoms of mood and anxiety disorders.

Suicide in Veterans

Among U.S. veterans, the rate of suicide is rising, too. On average, 17.6 veterans die by suicide each day. Veterans account for 13.7% of all suicide deaths but constitute only 7% of the adult population. Risk for suicide is 1.5 times higher in veterans, compared with civilians. In male veterans, suicide rates are highest in the younger and older years, whereas in female veterans, suicide rates are highest in the younger years.

Suicide in Older Adults

In 2019, older adults comprised 16.5% of the U.S. population but accounted for 19.3% of suicide deaths. Suicide rates are highest among older non-Hispanic white males, rising in this population to more than 47.8 suicides per 100,000 people annually. Although older females account for 20% of suicide deaths among those 65 and older, this number is expected to rise as the population of older females increases.

Older age has been associated with more determined and planned self-destructive acts and with fewer warnings of suicidal intent. The most common mechanisms for suicide are firearms, hanging, poisoning, and falls from heights. Among those who attempt suicide, older people are the most likely to die. In the general population, the ratio of attempted to completed suicides is estimated to be 25:1; in contrast, there are approximately four attempts for each completed suicide in older adults.

Several factors contribute to suicide in later life. Depression is the most closely associated and modifiable mental health risk factor. Poor physical health and functional impairment also contribute to suicide in older adults. Specific illnesses or conditions associated with suicide include congestive heart failure, chronic obstructive lung disease, seizure disorders, arthritis, urinary incontinence, liver disease, moderate to severe pain, visual impairment, neurological disorders, malignancy, and poor sleep quality. Serious physical illness in any organ category is an independent risk factor for suicide in older adults, and treatment for multiple illnesses is strongly

> **The Patient's Voice 69.1**
>
> **SUICIDE**
>
> The pain of the suicidal is private and inexpressible, leaving family members, friends, and colleagues to deal with an almost unfathomable kind of loss, as well as guilt. Suicide carries in its aftermath a level of confusion and devastation that is, for the most part, beyond description.
>
> Kay Redfield Jamison

related to higher risk of suicide. Serious physical illness and high overall burden of illness seem to be stronger risk factors for suicide in males than in females. In addition to physical illness, the perception of poor health can contribute to suicidal behavior. Socially, disruption of ties, resulting in loneliness and loss of a confidant, are also significantly and independently associated with risk for suicide in later life.

Suicide in LGBTQ+ Populations

The LGBTQ+ community in the United States experiences a wide array of health disparities, including increased risk for depression, anxiety, and suicidal behaviors. Although sampling methods have been debated, most recent estimates suggest 20% of LGBTQ+ adults have attempted suicide in contrast to approximately 11% of the general population. Increased suicidal risk among LGBTQ+ youth is also well established, with approximately 8% of adolescent suicide attempts attributed to LGBTQ+ status. Additional research is needed to identify specific risk factors and interventions for this vulnerable population.

PATHOPHYSIOLOGY

Although exact pathophysiological mechanisms are unknown, recent research has been informed by the stress-diathesis model, which posits health outcomes are the results of both genes and life events. A family history of suicide increases the risk of attempted suicide and of completed suicide in most diagnostic groups, likely due to both genetic and environmental factors. Genetic factors lowering the threshold for suicidal behavior may be decreased ability to control impulsive behavior. Hypothalamic–pituitary–adrenal axis (HPA axis) genetic vulnerabilities have also been identified, suggesting some individuals may have genetic loading for not only mood disorders but also increased susceptibility to ACEs. These factors have been strongly correlated with suicidal ideation and completion. As such, environmental stress, in the presence of a psychiatric disorder, can be a potentiating mechanism that triggers impulsive behavior in the direction of suicide.

CLINICAL PRESENTATION

Primary care clinicians must assess a patient's risk for suicide during clinical examination. Suicidal behavior is multidimensional, with complex factors contributing to the overall risk of a future suicide attempt. Factors typically elicited include psychiatric symptoms such as depression, mania, psychosis, substance use, trauma, anxiety, personality pathology, sleep quality, and pain. When suicidal ideation is assessed, further detail should be obtained by asking about plan, intent, and availability of means, such as firearms or medications. Other factors contributing to suicidality include recent or severe psychological and social stressors. Asking about suicidal ideation does not trigger suicide or increase the risk of suicide but could save a life.

DIAGNOSTIC REASONING

Acute risk factors may include severe anxiety, rumination, insomnia, depression with psychotic features, and alcohol or other substance use. A prior suicide attempt is the most important risk factor for suicide. As such, suicide screening tools often focus on previous attempts or intent to complete suicide, with various supportive items such as demographic information, level of social support, and coexisting mental health disorders. The Modified SAD PERSONS Scale has an administration time of 1 to 2 minutes, and the authors suggest using this as a rapid screening tool for nonpsychiatrists to obtain the objective information necessary to make an initial assessment of suicidality. The Columbia-Suicide Severity Rating Scale (C-SSRS) and the SAMHSA Suicide Assessment Five-Step Evaluation and Triage (SAFE-T) are both effective tools for assessing suicide risk in clinical settings. SAFE-T pocket guides and mobile app are available to guide clinicians through the following five steps: (1) identifying risk factors; (2) identifying protective factors; (3) conducting a suicide inquiry; (4) determining risk level and interventions; (5) documenting a treatment plan. C-SSRS has been validated for use with adolescents and adults in a variety of settings by researchers, clinicians, and nonclinicians alike. The C-SSRS for primary care clinicians provides a decision-making algorithm, based on assessment data that help determine suicide risk level and needed interventions. For adolescents and young adults aged 10 to 24 years, the Ask Suicide-Screening Questions (ASQ) Toolkit is a free resource for medical settings that can help clinicians identify youth at risk for suicide. The ASQ is a set of four screening questions that takes 20 seconds to administer.

Risk Factors: Acute Suicide Risk

The mnemonic "SAD PERSONAS" may be used to evaluate a person's suicide risk. Consider risk factors within the context of the clinical presentation.

- S = Sex
- A = Age
- D = Depression
- P = Previous attempt
- E = Ethanol abuse
- R = Rational thinking loss
- S = Social support loss
- O = Organized plan

- N = No spouse
- A = Availability of lethal means
- S = Sickness

Hopelessness about the future, helplessness, and lack of future orientation are "red flags" for possible suicidal intent, as well as suicidal thoughts, especially if accompanied by a plan and intent. Giving away personal possessions, quitting a job, and an appearance of peace may all signal that the person has made the decision to complete suicide. Patients who are suicidal may state their intentions, but many will find it hard to volunteer this information unless asked. The impulsive patient will often appear to be so and will give information that shows a great deal of recent poor judgment. The determined patient may refuse to answer questions or may give information freely, thinking that their plan cannot be deterred. Confused patients are more likely to seem unable to protect themselves from harm. Confused patients include people with auditory hallucinations instructing them to complete suicide and patients who are under the influence of drugs and alcohol. Suicidal patients may also express anger and rage and have hidden thoughts or fantasies of homicide, as though taking their own life might be equivalent to taking the object of their anger's life.

MANAGEMENT

Suicide prevention is carried out at two levels—individual and community. Individual prevention includes risk assessment, intervention (e.g., medications, counseling, hospitalization), and referral to a specialist. Community prevention is based on the crisis model of 24-hour community hotline services and walk-in crisis counseling services. Crisis counseling services should include a crisis response team that is dispatched immediately to schools or locations where assistance may be needed. These response teams can intervene to reduce the risk of suicide pacts among peers or "copycat" suicides. Reducing access to lethal means (e.g., firearms) was effective in reducing the risk of suicide, especially among military service members and veterans.

Community Prevention

In 2001, the Surgeon General organized the National Strategy for Suicide Prevention, under the auspices of the National Institutes of Health, which proposes public health methods to address suicide. The public health approach to suicide prevention represents a rational and organized way to marshal prevention efforts and ensure they are effective. Only within the past few decades has a public health approach to suicide prevention emerged with a better understanding of the biological and psychosocial factors contributing to suicidal behaviors. Its five basic steps are:

1. Clearly define the problem.
2. Identify risk and protective factors.
3. Develop and test interventions.
4. Implement interventions.
5. Evaluate effectiveness.

Individual Prevention

Careful assessment of suicide risk factors, consultation with other practitioners and specialists, and planning are the hallmarks of effective suicide risk management. The assessment should cover the patient's personal history and pay special attention to recent stressful life events and changes in mental status. Reports of losses, humiliations, demoralizing experiences, substance use and abuse, and relationship problems should be explored. People who have been abusing drugs and/or alcohol can suddenly become highly motivated to end their lives due to various factors, including loss of control over their use, legal problems, financial issues, homelessness, and/or loss of social supports. Even a person who is recovering from substance abuse and has stopped using the substance can be at high risk for suicide when faced with the painful consequences of substance abuse, including withdrawal or severe drug cravings.

All suicidal statements should be considered *seriously*. One of the most valuable assessment tools for practitioners is the willingness to question a patient directly about their suicide risk.

Two general questions are:

- "How long can you go on the way you are?"
- "Are you feeling so bad that sometimes you wish you could go to bed and not wake up?"

Examples of more specific questions are:

- "Have you thought about hurting yourself or ending your life?"
- "Do you have a plan for suicide?"
- "Have you assembled what you need?"
- "Do you have a location picked out?"
- "What has stopped you so far?"

Suicide plans are assessed on their specificity, availability, and lethality (SAL). The more specific and detailed the plan and the more available and lethal the method, the higher the risk of suicide.

Once it is determined that the patient is suicidal, the level of risk will determine the direction of the intervention. A major decision to be made is whether the patient needs to be hospitalized. The absence of a strong social support system, history of impulsive behavior, an intention to die, a suicidal plan of action, hopelessness, helplessness, lack of future orientation, and the availability of means such as weapons are indications for hospitalization. If hospitalization is deemed necessary but the patient has no way of getting there or if they refuse to go, it will be necessary to call 911 (or other local emergency services) to escort the patient involuntarily to the hospital. The primary goal of the intervention is to maintain the patient's safety. Therefore, the following considerations are important:

- Reduce or eliminate imminent danger.
- Never leave a patient alone who is actively suicidal.
- Involve family members or support people who care so that they can stay with the patient until the crisis has passed.

The best predictor of suicide risk is a history of a previous suicide attempt. All people with suicide gestures, attempts, and/or threats should be thoroughly screened for suicide risk factors and referred to a specialist for a full mental status examination, as well as psychiatric consultation and treatment. It is important to diagnose and treat any underlying psychiatric and/or substance abuse disorders. The clinician and the patient's family or support people should ensure the patient's safety by the least restrictive method, starting with removing potentially lethal objects, such as firearms, and providing close supervision. Some patients at acute high risk will require inpatient hospitalization for constant supervision and ongoing treatment.

Crisis management may also include the development of a safety plan that mobilizes resources for the patient during periods of suicidal ideation not requiring hospitalization (see Table 69.4). Safety plans do not replace the need for a higher level of care—inpatient hospitalization—when acute suicide risk is moderate to high. Primary care safety plans for low-risk patients may include warning signs, coping strategies, social support, clinical support, crisis-line contact information, and restriction of access to lethal means. Safety plans do not replace clinical judgment, referral to a mental health specialist, or a higher level of care.

In rare cases, a no-suicide contract can be initiated; however, a mental health professional should be the person to implement such an intervention. In the case of an angry or manipulative patient, this is usually not advisable. If a patient who is considered seriously suicidal cannot make the commitment to abide by a no-suicide contract, immediate hospitalization is necessary. A no-suicide contract is not a guarantee that a suicide will not happen, nor is it a substitute for clinical judgment. In fact, research does not support the use of no-harm contracts as a method for preventing suicide nor for protecting clinicians from malpractice litigation in the event of a patient suicide.

After acute risk for suicide is assessed and managed, it is essential to implement an ongoing program of help. This should involve the following:

- Treatment of the presenting symptoms, including specialist referrals
- Referral for individual or group therapy
- Referral for support groups and community programs
- Continual assessment and monitoring for safety

Appropriate documentation is critical. Follow agency guidelines for documenting situations involving suicide risk. Records should include statements made by the patient, the decision-making process followed, potential ramifications of no treatment, what has been shared with the patient and the family/support people, and the consultation process. To avoid malpractice litigation, practitioners need to perform and document a complete assessment addressing both the risk and the precautions taken and follow evidence-based guidelines. A standard of care exists for assessment of suicide risk but not for the prediction of suicide. Complete and accurate documentation is key.

FOLLOW-UP AND REFERRAL

Safety plans for patients who are not acutely suicidal include a follow-up appointment within 24 hours of assessment and a follow-up telephone call for missed appointments. Patients and involved family and support people should be given the local 24-hour crisis telephone number and information regarding access to emergency services. Practitioners must take responsibility to ask

TABLE 69.4 Primary Care Mental Health Crisis Safety Plan	
1. Recognize warning signs.	List thoughts, images, moods, behaviors that indicate a crisis may be developing.
2. Utilize internal coping strategies.	List things the person can do to soothe their emotions without contacting another person (e.g., relaxation techniques, physical activity).
3. Engage with people and social settings that provide distraction.	List names and contact information for people and places that can provide distraction without necessarily being informed of the suicidal crisis.
4. Contact people who can help.	List names and contact information for family and friends with whom the person is comfortable discussing their suicidal thoughts.
5. Contact professionals and/or agencies who can help.	List names and contact information for clinicians, urgent care services, emergency departments, and suicide hotlines.
6. Restrict access to lethal means.	Work with the patient and family members to restrict access to lethal means.

From: Dueweke AR, Bridges AJ. (2018). Suicide interventions in primary care: A selective review of the evidence. *Families, Systems, & Health, 36*(3), 289-302. http://dx.doi.org/10.1037/fsh0000349

patients about weapons and pill stashes and then take steps to have these items located and removed for safekeeping. If medications are prescribed, the amount should not exceed a 1-week supply, and the prescription should not have refills. Patients who are at risk should be referred to a mental health professional or seen at least weekly, and social support systems must be mobilized. Be aware that caring for a patient contemplating suicide can be clinically challenging, and it involves litigation risk.

Patient Education: Suicide

Education for the patient and family/support people includes providing suicide crisis hotline numbers to the patient and/or family members and support people. Patients should be instructed to avoid alcohol. Encourage the patient to seek adequate treatment for uncomfortable symptoms of physical illness, possibly including a prescription for analgesics to reduce pain. The patient should be informed that options often appear narrowed when a person is feeling depressed and suicidal. Alternative ways of thinking should be explored with the patient. Focus on building hope, especially for the future. Teach the patient to use specific, more constructive outlets for anger rather than self-destructive ones. Encourage patients to reach out for support and to reach out immediately when feeling the urge to harm themselves. Mobilize a social support system for the patient and educate support people regarding suicidal risk and danger signs. Educate the patient and family/support people that as the patient's mood "lifts" in response to antidepressant treatment, there can be an increased risk of suicide related to increased energy. At these times, patients must be monitored closely.

In the event a patient does complete suicide, the clinician should prepare the family and support people for a complex grief reaction that may follow. Suicide is particularly tragic because of the fallout that the death bequeaths to survivors. *Postvention* refers to an intervention strategy that attempts to minimize the impact of a patient's suicide and ensure that survivors of suicide have adequate services and support available to them. Postvention by the clinician includes the following:

- Educating family members and support people about suicide
- Allowing family members and support people to share their grief, including any burdens or other factors that they may feel (e.g., guilt, shame, anger, inability to do anything, situation out of their control)
- Encouraging family members and support people to attend support groups, such as Survivors of Suicide (SOS), which are available in most communities

The typical SOS group is sponsored by a mental health or social services agency and is facilitated by mental health professionals, survivor peers, or a combination of both. Referrals to such groups following a completed suicide are essential. Clinicians may also require support after a patient suicide.

REFERENCES

Bipolar Disorder

Agnew-Blais J, Danese A. (2016). Childhood maltreatment and unfavourable clinical outcomes in bipolar disorder: a systematic review and meta-analysis. Lancet Psychiatry, 3, p. 342–349.

Akula N, Barb J, Jiang X, et al. (2014). RNA-sequencing of the brain transcriptome implicates dysregulation of neuroplasticity, circadian rhythms and GTPase binding in bipolar disorder. Molecular Psychiatry, (19)11, p. 1179-1185.

Altman EG, Hedeker D, Peterson JL, et al. (1997). The Altman self-rating mania scale. Biologic Psychiatry, 42(10), p. 948-955.

Amann B, Gomar JJ, Ortiz-Gil J, et al. (2012). Executive dysfunction and memory impairment in schizoaffective disorder: A comparison with bipolar disorder, schizophrenia and healthy controls. Psychol Med., 42 (10), p. 2127-2135.

American Psychiatric Association. (2002). Practice guidelines for the treatment of patients with bipolar disorder. 2nd ed. https://psychiatryonline.org/pb/assets/raw/sitewide/practice_guidelines/guidelines/bipolar.pdf.

Baldessarini RJ, Tondo L, Visioli C. (2014). First-episode types in bipolar disorder: Predictive associations with later illness. Acta Psychiatr Scand., 129, p.383.

Bellani M, Hatch JP, Nicoletti MA, et al. (2012). Does anxiety increase impulsivity in patients with bipolar disorder or major depressive disorder? J Psychiatr Res., 46 (5), p. 616-621.

Brenner C, Shyn S. (2014). Diagnosis and management of bipolar disorder in primary care. A DSM-5 update. Medical Clinics of North America, 98, p. 1025-1048

Brooks SK, Webster RK, Smith LE, et al. (2020). The psychological impact of quarantine and how to reduce it: Rapid review of the evidence. Lancet, 395(10227), p. 912-920.

Burton CZ, Ryan KA, Kamali M, et al. (2017). Psychosis in bipolar disorder: Does it represent a more "severe" illness? Bipolar Disord, 20 (1), p. 18-26.

Calver L, Drinkwater V, Gupta R, et al. (2015). Droperidol v. haloperidol for sedation of aggressive behaviour in acute mental health: randomised controlled trial. Br J Psychiatry, 206 (3), p. 223-228.

Castle DJ. (2014). Bipolar mixed states: Still mixed up?, Current Opinion Psychiatry, 27, p. 540-549.

Cerimele JM, Goldberg SB, Miller CJ, et al. (2019). Systematic review of symptom assessment measures for use in measurement-based care of bipolar disorders. Psychiatric Services, 70, p. 396-408.

Cerimele JM, Kern JS. (2017). Bipolar disorder in primary care: Integrated care experiences. Journal of Lifelong Learning in Psychiatry, 15(3), p. 244-248. 10.1176/appi.focus.20170005

Chou YH, Lin CL, Wang SJ, et al. (2013). Aggression in bipolar II disorder and its relation to the serotonin transporter. J Affect Disord., 147 (3), p. 59-63.

Cloutier M, Greene M, Guerin A, et al. (2018). The economic burden of bipolar I disorder in the United States in 2015. Journal of Affective Disorders, 226, p. 45-51.

Coghill DR, Fazel S, Geddes JR, et al. (2016). Evidence-based guidelines for treating bipolar disorder: Revised third edition recommendations from the British Association for Psychopharmacology. J Psychopharmacol., 30(6), p.495–553.

Coryell W, Leon AC, Turvey C, et al. (2001). The significant of psychotic features in manic episodes: A report from NIMH collaborative study. Journal of Affective Disorders, 67, p. 79-88.

COVID-19 Mental Disorders Collaborators (2021). Global prevalence and burden of depressive and anxiety disorders in 204 countries and territories in 2020 due to the COVID-19 pandemic. *Lancet*,

398(10312), 1700–1712. https://doi.org/10.1016/S0140-6736(21)02143-7

Craddock N, Sklar P. (2013). Genetics of bipolar disorder. Lancet, 381, p.654–1662.Cusi, A.M., Macqueen, G.M., & McKinnon, M.C. (2012). Patients with bipolar disorder show impaired performance on complex tests of social cognition. Psychiatry Res., 200, p.258.

Daveney J, Panagioti M, Waheed W, et al. (2019). Unrecognized bipolar disorder in patients with depression managed in primary care: A systematic review and meta-analysis. General Hospital Psychiatry, 58, p. 71-76.

Dennehy EB, Marangell LB, Allen MH, et al. (2011). Suicide and suicide attempts in the Systematic Treatment Enhancement Program for Bipolar Disorder (STEP-BD). J Affect Disord., 133 (3), p. 423-427.

Depp CA, Mausbach BT, Harmell AL, et al. (2012). Meta-analysis of the association between cognitive abilities and everyday functioning in bipolar disorder. Bipolar Disord., 14 (3), p. 217-226.

Desmarais SL, Van Dorn RA, Johnson KL, et al. (2014). Community violence perpetration and victimization among adults with mental illnesses. Am J Public Health., 104 (12), p. 2342-2349.

Eisner L, Eddie D, Harley R, et al. (2017). Dialectical behaviour therapy group skills training for bipolar disorder. Behavioral Therapy, 48 (4), p. 557-566.

Feske U, Frank E, Mallinger AG, et al. (2000). Anxiety as a correlate of response to the acute treatment of bipolar I disorder. The American Journal of Psychiatry, 157(6), p. 956-962.

Fornaro M, De Prisco M, Billeci M, et al. (2021). Implications of the COVID-19 pandemic for people with bipolar disorders: A scoping review. *Journal of affective disorders, 295,* 740–751. https://doi-org.uri.idm.oclc.org/10.1016/j.jad.2021.08.091

Forte A, Baldessarini RJ, Tondo L, et al. (2015). Long-term morbidity in bipolar-I, bipolar-II, and unipolar major depressive disorders. Journal of Affective Disorders, 178, p.71-80.

Friborg O, Martinsen EW, Martinussen M, et al. (2014). Comorbidity of personality disorders in mood disorders: a meta-analytic review of 122 studies from 1988 to 2010. J Affect Disord., p. 152–154.

Geddes JR, Miklowitz DJ. (2013). Treatment of bipolar disorder. *Lancet, 381*(9878), 1672–1682. https://doi.org/10.1016/S0140-6736(13)60857-0

González-Pinto A, Galán J, Martin-Carrasco M, et al. (2012). Anxiety as a marker of severity in acute mania. Acta Psychiatrica Scandinavica, 126, p. 351-356.

González-Pinto A, Gonzalez C, Enjuto S, et al. (2004). Psychoeducation and cognitive-behavioral therapy in bipolar disorder: An update. Acta Psychiatr Scand., 109 (2), p. 83–90.

Goodwin GM, Haddad PM, Ferrier IN, et al. (2016). Evidence-based guidelines for treating bipolar disorder: Revised third edition recommendations from the British Association for Psychopharmacology. *Journal of Psychopharmacology, 30*(6), 495–553. https://doi.org/10.1177/0269881116636545

Grande I, Berk M, Birmaher B, Vieta E. (2016). Bipolar disorder. *Lancet, 387*(10027), 1561–1572. https://doi.org/10.1016/S0140-6736(15)00241-X

Harford TC, Yi HY, Grant BF. (2013). Other- and self-directed forms of violence and their relationships to DSM-IV substance use and other psychiatric disorders in a national survey of adults. Compr Psychiatry, 54, p.731.

Hirschfeld RM, et al. (2000). Development and validation of a screening instrument for bipolar spectrum disorder: The Mood Disorder Questionnaire. Am J Psychiatry, 157, p.1873.

Hirschfeld RM, Calabrese JR, Weissman MM, et al. (2003). Screening for bipolar disorder in the community. J Clin Psychiatry, 64 (1), p. 53–59.

Hirschfeld RM, Cass AR, Holt DC, et al. (2005). Screening for bipolar disorder in patients treated for depression in a family medicine clinic. Journal of American Board of Family Practice, 18(4), p. 233.

Hunt GE, Malhi GS, Cleary M, et al. (2016). Comorbidity of bipolar and substance use disorder in national surveys of general populations, 1990-2015: Systematic review and meta-analysis. Journal of Affective Disorders (206), p. 321-330.

Jamison KR. (1995). An unquiet mind. New York, NY: Vintage Books.

Jentink J, Loane MA, Dolk H, et al. (2010). Valproic acid monotherapy in pregnancy and major congenital malformations. N Engl J Med., 362 (23), p. 2185–2193.

Johnson MW, Fields SA, Bluett E. (2020). Bipolar disorder: Managing the peaks and valleys. The International Journal of Psychiatry in Medicine. https://doi.org/10.1177/0091217420952573

Judd LL, Akiskal HS, Schettler PJ, et al. (2002). The long-term natural history of the weekly symptomatic status of bipolar I disorder. Archives of General Psychiatry, 59(6), p. 530-537.

Kahn D, et al. Treatment of bipolar disorders: A guide for patients and families. Postgrad Med Rep. 2004;209–116.

Kato T. (2015). Searching for the molecular basis of bipolar disorder. American Journal of Psychiatry, (11)172, p. 1057

Kaufman J, Birmaher B, Brent D, et al. (1997). Schedule for affective disorders and schizophrenia for school-age children-present and lifetime version (K-SADS-PL): Initial reliability and validity data. Journal of American Academy Child Adolescent Psychiatry, 36(7), p. 980-988.

Kaye NS. (2005). Is your depressed patient bipolar? J Am Board Fam Pract., 18 (4), p. 271–281.

Kendall T, Morriss R, Mayo-Wilson E. et al. (2014). Assessment and management of bipolar disorder: Summary of updated NICE guidance. BMJ, 349, p. g5673.

Kessler RC, Berglund P, Demler O, et al. (2005). Lifetime prevalence and age-of-onset distributions of DSM-IV disorders in the national comorbidity survey replication. Archives of General Psychiatry, (62), p. 593-602.

King DB, Sixsmith A, Yaghoubi Shahir H, et al. (2016). Developing an ecological momentary sampling tool to measure movement patterns and psychiatric symptom variability. Gerontechnology, 14, p. 105–109.

Lewandowski KE, Cohen BM, Ongur D. (2010). Evolution of neuropsychological dysfunction during the course of schizophrenia and bipolar disorder. Psychol Med., 41, p. 225.

Management of Bipolar Disorder Working Group. (2010). VA/DoD clinical practice guideline for management of bipolar disorder in adults. Washington, DC: Department of Veterans Affairs, Department of Defense.

McCraw S, Parker G, Fletcher K, et al. (2013). Self-reported creativity in bipolar disorder: Prevalence, types and associated outcomes in mania versus hypomania. J Affect Disord., 151, p. 831.

McDermid J, Sareen J, El-Gabalawy R, et al. (2015). Co-morbidity of bipolar disorder and borderline personality disorder: Findings from the National Epidemiologic Survey on Alcohol and Related Conditions. Compr Psychiatry, 58, p. 18-28.

McIntyre RS, Soczynska JK, Cha DS, et al. (2015). The prevalence and illness characteristics of DSM-5-defined "mixed feature specifier" in adults with major depressive disorder and bipolar disorder:

Results from the International Mood Disorders Collaborative Project. J Affect Disord., 172, p. 259-264

Merikangas KR, Jin R, He JP, et al. (2011). Prevalence and correlates of bipolar spectrum disorder in the world mental health survey initiative. Arch Gen Psychiatry, 68(3), p. 241-251.

Messer T, Lammers G, Muller-Siecheneder F, et al. (2017). Substance abuse in patients with bipolar disorder: A systematic review and meta-analysis. Psychiatry Research, 253, p. 338-350.

Miklowitz DJ, George EL, Richards JA, et al. (2003). A randomized study of family-focused psychoeducation and pharmacotherapy in the outpatient management of bipolar disorder. Arch Gen Psychiatry, 60(9), p. 904-912.

Miller S, Dell'Osso B, Ketter TA. (2014). The prevalence and burden of bipolar depression. Journal of Affective Disorders, (169)1, p. 3-11.

Mohammadi Z, Pourshahbaz A, Poshtmashhadi M. (2018). Psychometric properties of the Young Mania Rating Scale as a mania severity measure in patients with bipolar I disorder. Practice in Clinical Psychology, 6(3), p. 175-182.

National Institute for Health and Care Excellence (NICE). (2014). Antenatal and postnatal mental health: clinical management and service guidance (NICE clinical guideline 192). http://www.nice.org.uk/guidance/cg192. Accessed May 16, 2016.

National Institute for Health and Care Excellence (NICE). (2014). Bipolar disorder: Assessment and management. https://www.nice.org.uk/guidance/cg185. Accessed February 26, 2021.

Nurnberger JI Jr, Koller DL, Jung J, et al. (2014) Identification of pathways for bipolar disorder: a meta-analysis. JAMA, 71 (6), p. 657-664.

Osorio FL, Loureiro SR, Hallak JEC, et al. (2019). Clinical validity and intrarater and test-retest reliability of the Structured Clinical Interview for DSM-5-Clinician Version (SCID-5-CV). Psychiatry and Clinical Neurosciences, 73(12), p. 754-760.

Ostergaard SD, Bertelsen A, Nielsen J, et al. (2013). The association between psychotic mania, psychotic depression and mixed affective episodes among 14,529 patients with bipolar disorder. J Affect Disord., 147(1-3), p.44-50.

Palmier-Claus JE, Berry K, Bucci S, et al. (2016). Relationship between childhood adversity and bipolar affective disorder: systematic review and meta-analysis. British Journal of Psychiatry, 209, p. 454–459.

Phillips ML, Swartz HA. (2014). A critical appraisal of neuroimaging studies of bipolar disorder: Toward a new conceptualization of underlying neural circuity and a road map for future research. The American Journal of Psychiatry, 171, p. 829-843.

Post R. (2016). Treatment of bipolar depression. Psychiatric Clinics of North America, 6(39), p. 11-33.

Post RM, Denicoff KD, Leverich GS, et al. (2003). Morbidity in 258 bipolar outpatients followed for 1 year with daily prospective ratings on the NIMH life chart method. Journal of Clinical Psychiatry, 64, p. 680-690.

Regier DA, Farmer ME, Rae DS, et al. (1990). Comorbidity of mental disorders with alcohol and other drug abuse. Results from the Epidemiologic Catchment Area (ECA) Study. JAMA, 264(19), p. 2511-2518.

Reinares M, Bonnín CDM, Hidalgo-Mazzei D, et al. (2015). Making sense of DSM-5 mania with depressive features. Australian and New Zealand Journal of Psychiatry, 49(6), p. 540-549.

Rihmer Z, Gonda X, Döme P. (2017). The assessment and management of suicide risk in bipolar disorder. The Treatment of Bipolar Disorder: Integrative Clinical Strategies and Future Directions.

Rowland TA, Marwaha S. (2018). Epidemiology and risk factors for bipolar disorder. Therapeutic Advances in Psychopharmacology, (9)8, p. 251-269.

Ruzicka WB, Subburaju S, Benes FM. (2015). Circuit- and diagnosis-specific DNA methylation changes at y-aminobutryic acid-related genes in postmortem human hippocampus in schizophrenia and bipolar disorder. JAMA, (6)72, p. 541-551.

Sachs G. (1998). Approach to the patient with elevated, expansive, or irritable mood. In: Stern TA, Herman JB, Slavin PL, eds. The MGH guide to psychiatry in primary care. New York, NY: McGraw-Hill.

Samamé C. (2013). Social cognition throughout the three phases of bipolar disorder: A state-of-the-art overview. Psychiatry Res., 210, p.1275.

Samamé C, Martino DJ, Strejilevich SA. (2014). Longitudinal course of cognitive deficits in bipolar disorder: a meta-analytic study. J Affect Disord., 164, p. 130.

Santos JL, Aparicio A, Bagney A, et al. (2014). A five-year follow-up study of neurocognitive functioning in bipolar disorder. Bipolar Disord., 16, p.722.

Simon GE, Ludman EJ, Unützer J, et al. (2008). Severity of mood symptoms and work productivity in people treated for bipolar disorder. Bipolar Disorder, 10(6), p. 718-725.

Stahl SM, Grady MM. (2017). Stahl's essential psychopharmacology: The prescriber's guide (6th ed.). Cambridge, UK; New York: Cambridge University Press.

Stefana A, Youngstrom E, Chen J, et al. (2020). The covid-19 pandemic is a crisis and opportunity for bipolar disorder. Clinical Care, 22(6), p. 641-643.

Subramaniam M, Abdin E, Vaingankar JA, et al. (2013). Prevalence, correlates, comorbidity and severity of bipolar disorder: Results from the Singapore Mental Health Study. J Affect Disord., 146, p. 189.

Sylvia LG, Dupuy JM, Ostacher MJ, et al. (2012). Sleep disturbance in euthymic bipolar patients. J Psychopharmacol., 26(8), p. 1108-1112.

Ten Have M, de Graaf R, van Weeghel J, et al. (2014). The association between common mental disorders and violence: To what extent is it influenced by prior victimization, negative life events and low levels of social support? Psychol Med., 44, p.1485.

Tondo L, Vázquez GH, Baldessarini RJ. (2017). Depression and mania in bipolar disorder. Currently Neuropharmacology, 15, p. 353-358.

Valiengo LCL, Stella F, Forlenza OV. (2016) Mood disorders in the elderly: prevalence, functional impact, and management challenges. Neuropsychiatric Disease and Treatment, 12, p. 2105-2114.

Weissman MM, Bland RC, Canino GJ, et al. (1996). Cross-national epidemiology of major depression and bipolar disorder. JAMA, 276(4), p. 293-299.

Work Group on Psychiatric Evaluation, American Psychiatric Association Steering Committee on Practice Guidelines. (2006). Psychiatric evaluation of adults. Second edition. American Psychiatric Association. Am J Psychiatry, 163(3).

Yatham LN, Kennedy SH, Parikh SV, et al. (2013). Canadian Network for Mood and Anxiety Treatments (CANMAT) and International Society for Bipolar Disorders (ISBD) collaborative update of CANMAT guidelines for the management of patients with bipolar disorder: update 2013. Bipolar Disord., 15, p.1-44.

Yatham LN, Kennedy SH, Parikh SV, et al. (2018). Canadian Network for Mood and Anxiety Treatments (CANMAT) and International Society for Bipolar Disorders (ISBD) 2018 guidelines for the management of patients with bipolar disorder. Bipolar Disord., 20(2), p. 97–170.

Youngstrom E, Meyers O, Demeter C, et al. (2005). Comparing diagnostic checklists for pediatric bipolar disorder in academic and community mental health settings, Bipolar Disorder, 7(6), p. 507-517.

Major Depressive Disorder

American Academy of Pediatrics (2018). Guidelines for Adolescent Depression in Primary Care (GLAD-PC): Part I. Practice Preparation, Identification, Assessment, and Initial Management. https://pediatrics.aappublications.org/content/pediatrics/141/3/e20174081.full.pdf

American Academy of Pediatrics. (2018). Guidelines for Adolescent Depression in Primary Care (GLAD_PC): Part II. Treatment and Ongoing Management. https://pediatrics.aappublications.org/content/pediatrics/early/2018/02/22/peds.2017-4082.full.pdf

American Psychiatric Association. (2013). *Diagnostic and statistical manual of mental disorders* (5th ed.). Washington, DC: American Psychiatric Publishing

American Psychological Association (2019). Clinical Practice Guidelines for the Treatment of Depression Across Three Age Cohorts. https://www.apa.org/depression-guideline/guideline.pdf

Arroll B, Goodyear-Smith F, Crengle S, et al. (2010). Validation of PHQ-2 and PHQ-9 to screen for major depression in the primary care population. *The Annals of Family Medicine, 8*(4), 348-353.

Beck AT, et al. *Cognitive therapy of depression.* New York, NY: Guilford Press; 1979.

Beck CT. (1993). Teetering on the edge: a substantive theory of postpartum depression. *Nurs Res,* 42(1), 42–8.

Centers for Disease Control (2016). National Ambulatory Medical Care Survey: 2016 National Summary Table. https://www.cdc.gov/nchs/data/ahcd/namcs_summary/2016_namcs_web_tables.pdf

Centers for Disease Control and Prevention (CDC) (2018). WISQARS Leading Causes of Death Reports (https://www.cdc.gov/injury/wisqars/index.html)

D'Ath P, Katona P, Mullan E, et al. (1994). Screening, detection and management of depression in elderly primary care attenders. I: The acceptability and performance of the 15 item Geriatric Depression Scale (GDS15) and the development of short versions. *Family practice,* 11(3), 260-266.

Eberhard-Gran M, Eskild A, Tambs K, et al. (2001). Review of validation studies of the Edinburgh Postnatal Depression Scale. *Acta Psychiatrica Scandinavica,* 104(4), 243-249.

Ettman CK, Abdalla SM, Cohen GH, et al. (2020). Prevalence of depression symptoms in US adults before and during the COVID-19 pandemic. *JAMA network open,* 3(9), e2019686-e2019686.

Falana S, Carrington JM. (2019), Postpartum Depression: Are you Listening? *Nursing Clinics of North America.* 54 (4), 561-567

Fick DM, Semla TP, Steinman M. (2019). American Geriatrics Society 2019 updated AGS Beers Criteria® for potentially inappropriate medication use in older adults. *Journal of the American Geriatrics Society,* 67(4), 674-694.

Jellinek MS, Murphy M. Pediatric symptom checklist. Massachusetts General Hospital. https://www.massgeneral.org/psychiatry/treatments-and-services/pediatric-symptom-checklist

Kroenke K, Spitzer RL, Williams JB. (2001). The PHQ-9: validity of a brief depression severity measure. *Journal of general internal medicine,* 16(9), 606-613.

McCoy KT, Costa CB, Pancione K, et al. (2019). Anticipating Changes for Depression Management in Primary Care. *Nursing Clinics of North America,* 54(4), 457-471

Michigan Quality Improvement Consortium Guideline (2020). Primary Care Diagnosis and Management of Adults with Depression. http://www.mqic.org/pdf/mqic_primary_care_diagnosis_and_management_of_adults_with_depression_cpg.pdf (2020).

National Center for Health Statistics (2020). Early Release of Selected Estimates Based on Data From the 2019 National Health Interview Survey. https://www.cdc.gov/nchs/data/nhis/earlyrelease/EarlyRelease202009-508.pdf

National Centre of Excellence in Youth Mental Health (2017). Treating depression in young people: Guidance, resources, and tools for assessment and management. https://www.orygen.org.au/Training/Resources/Depression/Clinical-practice-points/Treating-depression-in-yp/orygen_Clinical_practice_guide_depression_in_young?ext=.

National Institute for Health and Care Excellence (2009. Updated 2018). Depression in adults: recognition and management. https://www.nice.org.uk/guidance/cg90

National Institute for Health and Care Excellence. (2019). Depression in children and young people: identification and management. https://www.nice.org.uk/guidance/ng134/resources/depression-in-children-and-young-people-identification-and-management-pdf-66141719350981

National Institute of Mental Health (2019). Major Depression. Data courtesy of 2017 National Survey on Drug Use and Health from SAMHSA. https://www.nimh.nih.gov/health/statistics/major-depression.shtml

National Networks of Depression Centers (2020). Get the facts. https://nndc.org/facts/?gclid=EAIaIQobChMIubv3sP3j7AIVjeDICh3b_wCQEAAYASAAEgLx7PD_BwE

Nuggerud-Galeas S, Sáez-Benito Suescun L, Berenguer Torrijo N, et al. (2020). Analysis of depressive episodes, their recurrence and pharmacologic treatment in primary care patients: A retrospective descriptive study. *Plos one,* 15(5), e0233454.

Posner K, Brown GK, Stanley B, et al. (2011). The Columbia–Suicide Severity Rating Scale: initial validity and internal consistency findings from three multisite studies with adolescents and adults. *American journal of psychiatry,* 168(12), 1266-1277.

Qaseem A, Barry MJ, Kansagara D. (2016). Nonpharmacologic versus pharmacologic treatment of adult patients with major depressive disorder: a clinical practice guideline from the American College of Physicians. *Annals of internal medicine,* 164(5), 350-359.

Rush AJ, Trivedi MH, Ibrahim HM, et al. (2003). The 16-Item Quick Inventory of Depressive Symptomatology (QIDS), clinician rating (QIDS-C), and self-report (QIDS-SR): a psychometric evaluation in patients with chronic major depression. *Biological psychiatry,* 54(5), 573-583.

Saddock BJ, Saddock VA, Ruiz P. (2015). Kaplan & Saddock's Synopsis of psychiatry: behavioral sciences, clinical psychiatry. Eleventh Edition. Wolters Kluwer

Silva MT, Zimmermann IR, Galvao TF, et al. (2013). Olanzapine plus fluoxetine for bipolar disorder: a systematic review and meta-analysis. *Journal of affective disorders,* 146(3), 310–318. https://doi.org/10.1016/j.jad.2012.11.001

Spellman T, Liston C. (2020). Toward circuit mechanisms of pathophysiology in depression. *American Journal of Psychiatry,* 177(5), 381-390.

Trangle M, Gursky J, Haight R, et al. (2016). Institute for Clinical Systems Improvement. Adult Depression in Primary Care. https://www.icsi.org/wp-content/uploads/2021/11/Depr.pdf

World Health Organization (2020). Depression. Accessed at who.int/news-room/fact-sheets/detail/depression

Suicide

Arias SA, Zhang Z, Hillerns C, et al. (2014). Using structured telephone follow-up assessments to improve suicide-related adverse event detection. *Suicide and Life-Threatening Behavior, 44*(5), 537-547.

Bachmann S. Epidemiology of Suicide and the Psychiatric Perspective. Int J Environ Res Public Health. 2018 Jul 6;15(7):1425. doi: 10.3390/ijerph15071425. PMID: 29986446; PMCID: PMC6068947.

Ballard ED, Patel AB, Ward M, et al. (2015). Future disposition and suicidal ideation: Mediation by depressive symptom clusters. *Journal of affective disorders, 170*, 1-6.

Beck AT, Steer RA, Beck JS, et al. (1993). Hopelessness, depression, suicidal ideation, and clinical diagnosis of depression. *Suicide and Life-Threatening Behavior, 23*(2), 139-145.

Brådvik L. (2018). Suicide Risk and Mental Disorders. *International journal of environmental research and public health, 15*(9), 2028. doi: 10.3390/ijerph15092028

Campbell WH. (2004) Pearls: Revised "SAD PERSONS" helps assess suicide risk. *Current Psychiatry*, 3 (3):102-102.

Centers for Disease Control and Prevention. (2020, February 20). *Fatal Injury Reports, National, Regional and State, 1981-2018.* Web-based Injury Statistics Query and Reporting System. https://webappa.cdc.gov/sasweb/ncipc/mortrate.html

Centers for Disease Control and Prevention. (2022, February 25). *Suicide Prevention.* CDC Injury Center, Violence Prevention. https://www.cdc.gov/ViolencePrevention/suicide/index.html

Centers for Disease Control and Prevention. (2018, June 7). *Suicide Rising Across the US.* CDC Vital Signs. https://www.cdc.gov/vitalsigns/suicide/index.html

Conwell, Y., Van Orden, K., & Caine, E. D. (2011). Suicide in older adults. *Psychiatric Clinics, 34*(2), 451-468.

Czeisler MÉ, Lane RI, Petrosky E, et al. Mental Health, Substance Use, and Suicidal Ideation During the COVID-19 Pandemic — United States, June 24–30, 2020. MMWR Morb Mortal Wkly Rep 2020;69:1049–1057. DOI: https://www.cdc.gov/mmwr/volumes/69/wr/mm6932a1.htm

Drapeau CW, McIntosh JL. *U.S.A. suicide: 2019 official final data.* Washington, DC: American Association of Suicidology; December 23, 2020. https://suicidology.org/wp-content/uploads/2021/01/2019datapgsv2b.pdf.

Dueweke AR, Bridges AJ. (2018). Suicide interventions in primary care: A selective review of the evidence. *Families, Systems, & Health, 36*(3), 289-302. http://dx.doi.org/10.1037/fsh0000349

Eaton DK, et al. Youth risk behavior surveillance—United States, 2007. *MMWR Surveill Summ.* 2008;57:SS-4.

Esang M, Ahmed S. (2018). A closer look at substance use and suicide. *American Journal of Psychiatry Residents' Journal.*

Fässberg MM, Cheung G, Canetto SS, et al. (2016). A systematic review of physical illness, functional disability, and suicidal behaviour among older adults. *Aging & mental health, 20*(2), 166–194.

Fässberg MM, Orden KAv, Duberstein P, et al. (2012). A systematic review of social factors and suicidal behavior in older adulthood. *International journal of environmental research and public health, 9*(3), 722-745.

Gaynes BN, West SL, Ford CA, et al. (2004). Screening for suicide risk in adults: a summary of the evidence for the US Preventive Services Task Force. *Annals of internal medicine, 140*(10), 822-835.

Gipson PY, Agarwala P, Opperman KJ, et al. (2015). Columbia-suicide severity rating scale: predictive validity with adolescent psychiatric emergency patients. *Pediatric emergency care, 31*(2), 88–94. https://doi.org/10.1097/PEC.0000000000000225

Haas AP, Eliason M, Mays VM, et al. (2011). Suicide and suicide risk in lesbian, gay, bisexual, and transgender populations: Review and recommendations. Journal of Homosexuality, 58(1), 10–51.

Holkup P. *Evidence-based protocol: Elderly suicide – Secondary prevention.* University of Iowa Gerontological Nursing Interventions Research Center; 2002. https://www.healio.com/nursing/journals/jgn/2003-6-29-6/%7Bdeca3678-aca1-4059-9ce0-8c179682dd48%7D/evidence-based-protocol-elderly-suicide---secondary-prevention.

Horowitz LM, Bridge JA, Teach J, et al. (2012). Ask Suicide-Screening Questions (ASQ): a brief instrument for the pediatric emergency department. *Archives of pediatrics & adolescent medicine, 166*(12), 1170-1176.

Horowitz LM, Snyder DJ, Boudreaux ED, et al. (2020). Validation of the Ask Suicide-Screening Questions (ASQ) for adult medical inpatients: a brief tool for all ages. *Psychosomatics,* 61(6):713–722.

Hottes TS, Bogaert L, Rhodes AE, et al. (2016). Lifetime Prevalence of Suicide Attempts Among Sexual Minority Adults by Study Sampling Strategies: A Systematic Review and Meta-Analysis. *American journal of public health, 106*(5), e1–e12. https://doi.org/10.2105/AJPH.2016.303088

Juruena MF, Bocharova M, Agustini B, et al. (2018). Atypical depression and non-atypical depression: Is HPA axis function a biomarker? A systematic review. *Journal of affective disorders, 233*, 45–67. https://doi.org/10.1016/j.jad.2017.09.052

Lewis LM. (2007). No-harm contracts: A review of what we know. *Suicide and Life-Threatening Behavior, 37*(1), 50-57.

Li J, Yoshikawa A, Meltzer HY. (2017). Replication of rs300774, a genetic biomarker near ACP1, associated with suicide attempts in patients with schizophrenia: Relation to brain cholesterol biosynthesis. Journal of Psychiatric Research, 94, 54-61.

Mercier A, Auger-Aubin I, Lebeau JP, et al. (2014). Why do general practitioners prescribe antidepressants to their patients? A pilot study. *BioPsychoSocial medicine, 8*, 17. https://doi.org/10.1186/1751-0759-8-17

Miranda-Mendizábal A, Castellví P, Parés-Badell O, et al. (2017). Sexual orientation and suicidal behaviour in adolescents and young adults: systematic review and meta-analysis. *The British journal of psychiatry : the journal of mental science, 211*(2), 77–87. https://doi.org/10.1192/bjp.bp.116.196345

Mitchell J, Trangle M, Degnan B, et al. Institute for Clinical Systems Improvement. Adult Depression in Primary Care. Updated September 2013. https://www.bcbsnm.com/pdf/cpg_depression.pdf

Murri MB, Prestia D, Mondelli V, et al. (2016). The HPA axis in bipolar disorder: systematic review and meta-analysis. *Psychoneuroendocrinology, 63*, 327-342.

National Guideline Clearinghouse (NGC). Guideline summary: Final recommendation statement. Depression in adults: Screening. Rockville, MD: Agency for Healthcare Research and Quality; January 26, 2016. https://www.uspreventiveservicestaskforce.org/Page/Document/RecommendationStatementFinal/depression-in-adults-screening1. Accessed November 14, 2020.

National Institute of Mental Health. (September 2020). *Suicide by Method.* Mental Health Information: Suicide. https://www.nimh.nih.gov/health/statistics/suicide.shtml#part_154971

Normann C, Buttenschøn HN. (2020). Gene-environment interactions between HPA-axis genes and childhood maltreatment in depression: a systematic review. *Acta neuropsychiatrica*, 1–11. Advance online publication. https://doi.org/10.1017/neu.2020.1

Office of the Surgeon General (US), & National Action Alliance for Suicide Prevention (US). (2012). *2012 National Strategy for Suicide Prevention: Goals and Objectives for Action: A Report of the U.S. Surgeon General and of the National Action Alliance for Suicide Prevention.* US Department of Health & Human Services (US).

https://www.surgeongeneral.gov/library/reports/national-strategy-suicide-prevention/index.html

Patterson WM, Dohn HH, Bird J, et al. (April 1983). Evaluation of suicidal patients: the SAD PERSONS scale. *Psychosomatics*. 24 (4): 343–5, 348–9.

Posner K, Brown GK, Stanley B, et al. (2011). The Columbia-Suicide Severity Rating Scale: initial validity and internal consistency findings from three multisite studies with adolescents and adults. *The American journal of psychiatry*, 168(12), 1266–1277. https://doi.org/10.1176/appi.ajp.2011.10111704

Substance Abuse and Mental Health Services Administration. (September 2009). *SAFE-T Pocket Card: Suicide Assessment Five-Step Evaluation and Triage for Clinicians*. https://store.samhsa.gov/product/SAFE-T-Pocket-Card-Suicide-Assessment-Five-Step-Evaluation-and-Triage-for-Clinicians/sma09-4432

Turvey CL, Conwell Y, Jones MP, et al. (2002). Risk factors for late-life suicide: a prospective, community-based study. *The American journal of geriatric psychiatry*, 10(4), 398–406.

U.S. Department of Veterans Affairs, Office of Mental Health and Suicide Prevention. 2020 National Veteran Suicide Prevention Annual Report. 2020. Retrieved November 14, 2020 from https://www.mentalhealth.va.gov/docs/data-sheets/2020/2020-National-Veteran-Suicide-Prevention-Annual-Report-11-2020-508.pdf

U.S. Preventive Services Task Force. (2013, December 18). *Suicide Risk in Adolescents, Adults and Older Adults: Screening*. https://www.uspreventiveservicestaskforce.org/uspstf/recommendation/suicide-risk-in-adolescents-adults-and-older-adults-screening

RESOURCES

Edinburgh Postnatal Depression Scale
http://perinatology.com/calculators/Edinburgh%20Depression%20Scale.htm

National Suicide Prevention Lifeline
https://suicidepreventionlifeline.org/
1-800-273-8255

Substance Abuse and Mental Health Services Administration
https://findtreatment.samhsa.gov/
National Helpline: 1-800-662-435

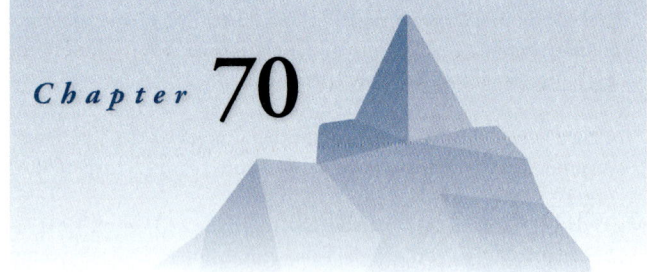

Chapter 70

Anxiety Disorders and Post-Traumatic Stress Disorder

Kara Birch, DNP, PMHNP, FNP

Katelyn Brady, MSN, PMHNP-BC

Amanda Ling, RN, PMHNP

Karen Jennings Mathis, PhD, APRN-CNP, PMHNP-BC, FAED

ANXIETY DISORDERS

Anxiety disorders are frequently encountered in primary care and one of the most common psychological disorders in the United States, with 31% of adults and adolescents experiencing an anxiety disorder in their lifetime. Anxiety may be broad, specific to certain thoughts or situations, with or without identifiable triggers, or a result of a prior negative experience. Anxiety is most often accompanied by an overestimation of the level of threat and an activated sympathetic nervous system response. Anxiety disorders differ from typical stress, fear, or worry due to their persistent nature and disruption to functioning. Early identification and evidence-based treatment are important in reducing disability and suffering, as approximately 56% of adults with an anxiety disorder may display moderate to serious impairment.

The American Psychiatric Association's *Diagnostic and Statistical Manual of Mental Disorders, Fifth Edition, Text Revision* (*DSM-5-TR*) differentiates anxiety disorders from trauma- and stressor-related disorders, which are connected to a distressing event(s) and classifies anxiety disorders into the following categories with associated approximate 12-month prevalence rates (see Box 70.1).

Additional classifications of anxiety secondary to substance use or withdrawal, medications, or other medical conditions should be thoroughly assessed and considered as ongoing potential differential diagnoses. Screening for comorbidities is prudent, with a high prevalence of depressive and trauma-related disorders in patients that present with anxiety symptoms. The *DSM-5-TR* has an anxious distress specifier that may be appropriate for those patients with depressive disorders who do not meet full criteria for an anxiety disorder. A detailed initial psychiatric assessment including review of symptoms, medical and psychological history, medications, and laboratory testing as indicated should be completed.

Vulnerability

Anxiety disorders appear to have multifactorial influences including genetic, environmental, psychological, and developmental. There is no single gene identified as

Box 70.1 Categories of Anxiety Disorders

Anxiety Disorder	12-Month Prevalence
Specific phobia	In adults: 8%–12%
Social anxiety disorder	In adults: 7%
Panic disorder	In adults: 2%–3% In adolescents: 2%–3%
Generalized anxiety disorder	In adults: 2.9% In adolescents: 0.9%
Agoraphobia	In adults: 1%–1.7% In adolescents: 1%–1.7%
Separation anxiety disorder	In adults: 0.9%–1.9% In adolescents: 1.6% In children: 4%

Source: American Psychiatric Association. (2022). *Diagnostic and statistical manual of mental disorders, text revision* (5th ed.). Washington, DC: American Psychiatric Association.

causing anxiety symptoms, but patients have an increased risk of anxiety disorder if they have a first-degree relative with an anxiety disorder. Changes in the hypothalamic-pituitary-adrenal (HPA) axis and the fear response areas of the brain, such as the amygdala, are believed to play a role in anxiety disorders. Epigenetic factors such as alterations in DNA methylation may lie at the intersection of genetics and environment. Exposure to childhood trauma can affect children during critical developmental periods, and its effects in health and behavioral outcomes have been well documented in the Adverse Childhood Experience (ACE) study. Individuals with a history of trauma or significant life stressors—recent, childhood, or adolescent—can be more vulnerable to anxiety disorders.

Screening

The first step in improving outcomes for those suffering from anxiety disorders is identification of symptoms. Screening for depression and anxiety in primary care can be done via a variety of available questionnaires, many of which are brief and available online for free in multiple languages. Providers must consider that some patients may need assistance due to limited literacy or English proficiency and clinic support staff often can provide aid. Common screening tools include the Beck Anxiety Inventory, the Hamilton Anxiety Rating Scale, the Generalized Anxiety Disorder-7 (GAD-7) Scale, and the Zung Self-Rating Anxiety Scale. The Panic Disorder Severity Scale screens for panic disorder. The Patient Health Questionnaire (PHQ-9) for depression, the GAD-7 for anxiety, and the PHQ-15 for somatic symptoms are often given together as the Patient Health Questionnaire—Somatic, Anxiety, and Depressive Symptoms Screener (PHQ-SADS), which is prudent given the frequency of comorbidities in anxiety disorders. In children and adolescents, common screening tools include the Youth Anxiety Measure for *DSM-5-TR* (YAM-5), the Screen for Child Anxiety-Related Emotional Disorders (SCARED), and the Pediatric Anxiety Rating Scale (PARS). The Fear Survey Schedule for Children is a tool used to detect the presence and severity of specific fears including phobias.

Numerous epidemiological and survey studies have demonstrated high rates of comorbid psychiatric conditions in children and adults with anxiety disorders. Therefore, assessment for anxiety, depression, or other psychiatric disorders is essential because, left untreated, they can significantly disrupt an individual's life. Moreover, because of familial correlations, consider screening children of parents with anxiety disorders, as well as parents of children with anxiety disorders.

Treatment Overview

Treatment for an anxiety disorder should be collaborative and nonjudgmental, building a therapeutic alliance with the patient. For most anxiety disorders, first-line treatment options include psychotherapy such as cognitive behavioral therapy (CBT), medications such as serotonin reuptake inhibitors (SRIs), or both. Individual and program-based therapy modalities, including telehealth, have been shown to be beneficial for individuals with difficulty leaving the home, with scheduling challenges, or in areas with limited access. In considering treatment options, the patent's unique risk factors, costs, preferences, previous treatment experiences, comorbidities, and severity of symptoms must be carefully considered (see Box 70.2).

GENERALIZED ANXIETY DISORDER

GAD is characterized by persistent (at least 6 months), excessive, and difficult to control anxiety and worry over multiple concerns that lead to impairment in functioning. Persons with GAD may experience a range of upsetting physical and cognitive symptoms such as restlessness, difficulty concentrating, insomnia, fatigue, and muscle tension. In primary care settings, patients with GAD often have somatic complaints, and medical illnesses should be ruled out because of their co-occurrence and similar symptoms.

EPIDEMIOLOGY AND CAUSES

GAD may occur across the life span, with a 12-month prevalence of about 3% among adults and lifetime prevalence of about 5.7%. Risk factors include lower socioeconomic status, comorbid physical or psychiatric disorders,

> **Box 70.2 Psychopharmacogenetic Testing**
>
> "Precision medicine" or "personalized medicine" is a care approach that seeks to tailor treatment to the individual with the utilization of genetic testing as it relates to pharmacokinetics and pharmacodynamics for psychiatric medication to predict potential side effects and accelerate effective treatment. Most drugs are prescribed in a "one-size-fits-all" fashion and are expected to work the same for every patient; however, genetics can affect medication efficacy. Pharmacogenomics uses information about a person's genetic makeup to help clinicians select the best drug and doses that will have the best efficacy for the person. The same concept is used when addressing mental disorders, and it is referred to as *psychopharmacogenetics*. This approach to care is extremely helpful because patients living with mental illness often undergo multiple trials of medications while experiencing negative side effects resulting in lower adherence to treatment before arriving at the right medication. Differences in each person's genes affect how their bodies respond to medications.
>
> Understanding individual's genetic uniqueness can help clinicians make more meaningful medication decisions. For example, a person's genes can affect blood levels of a drug (pharmacokinetic) by causing a medication to metabolize too slow, too fast, or normally, thus having an effect on how much drug reaches the brain to target a specific symptom. In this case, it may be as simple as increasing or decreasing the recommended medication dosage to reach the target outcome based on psychopharmacogenetic test results. On the other hand, if a patient is taking the correct dosage and reaches a therapeutic blood level but symptoms have not improved, this may be due to the lack of receptor binding (pharmacodynamics). This gene–drug interaction problem can be solved by learning the patient's specific phenotyping and selecting the best medication to target the correct sequence. Genetic test results can provide guidance on potential gene–drug interactions, side effects, and drug metabolization speeds and thus determine which medications may work best for the patient.
>
> Some genetic tests are covered by health insurance, but most are not. Patients sign consent for this type of test and should pay attention to how these test results can be used, which may include clinical decision making, billing and office operation, and quality improvement evaluation. Providers are reminded that test results are only part of the assessment. The use of psychopharmacogenetics has shown some early signs of clinical validity, as well as utilization and health cost savings, compared with patients receiving standard care.
>
> Psychopharmocogenetics can be a powerful tool if used appropriately and in combination with a detailed clinical assessment, laboratory results, and patient education. Patients seem to appreciate that a test is available that can increase reliability and validate the provider's clinical decision. This may lead to greater patient optimism that medications will work, increasing adherence to the medication regimen and follow-up care. When patients and clinicians understand that pharmacogenetics is just one piece of the overall assessment, the additional information obtained from this type of testing may lead to faster symptom improvement.

adverse or traumatic experiences, being female, and a genetic heritability rate of about 30%. In primary care, the prevalence of GAD increases to about 7% to 8% and often presents with somatic symptoms. GAD is often chronic and recurrent with up to half of patients who recover having a recurrence and about 42% of patients experiencing anxiety symptoms after several years. Coping with anxiety through substance use is common and requires screening as well as harm reduction psychoeducation if indicated. The increased occurrence of negative cardiovascular health outcomes, other comorbid psychiatric disorders, and impairment in function makes appropriate psychological and pharmacological interventions and monitoring important in improving outcomes.

PATHOPHYSIOLOGY

GAD symptomatology can be independent from external stimuli and appear to have a complex process, with functional magnetic resonance imaging (MRI) showing variability in limbic and prefrontal cortex changes in the brain. There is evidence for the role of changes in neuromodulation secondary to developmental trauma affecting anxiety symptoms, and treatment is thought to play a role in enhancing neuroplasticity. Three major neurotransmitters associated with anxiety are norepinephrine, serotonin, and gamma-aminobutyric acid (GABA). Changes in neurotransmission of GABA inhibitory and glutamate excitatory processes have been associated with GAD and are ongoing targets for pharmacological research. Monoamine availability has been shown to be reduced by proinflammatory cytokines and there is evidence to suggest that inflammatory markers are increased in GAD. Although GAD is more common in those with comorbid inflammatory conditions, larger-scale psychiatric neuroinflammatory research studies are needed to elucidate the causes or effects of inflammation.

CLINICAL PRESENTATION

Primary symptoms of GAD are excessive worry or anxiety often presenting with restlessness, fatigue, difficulty concentrating, irritability, muscle tension, and sleep disturbance. Shakiness, restlessness, headaches, and pain syndromes are common manifestations of motor tension. Autonomic hyperactivity is commonly manifested by excessive sweating, various gastrointestinal symptoms (increased acidity, nausea, and epigastric pain), palpitations, concentration problems, tachycardia, and shortness of breath. Irritability and a quick-to-startle response are typical of cognitive vigilance. Patients may be talkative about their excess worry or they may appear distracted and quietly ruminative. In primary care, patients with GAD often seek help for their somatic symptoms. The distinction between GAD and normal anxiety is emphasized by the specification that the symptoms of GAD must cause significant impairment or distress.

Several theories involving a propensity toward negative cognitions, an intolerance of uncertainty, an inability to manage distressing emotions, and the use of worry as an ineffective coping mechanism have been developed to better understand the thought processes involved in GAD. Worrying may be a way to avoid negative reactions to one's own internal experiences or emotional distress, and patients may be hard on themselves about their worry, thereby creating more negative cognitions. Excessive worrying may be a means to solve a problem or prevent a negative outcome and tends to be reinforced when positive outcomes occur.

DIAGNOSTIC REASONING

Symptoms

The main diagnostic criteria for GAD are excessive anxiety and worry predominating for at least 6 months. The intensity, duration, or frequency of the anxiety and worry are out of proportion to the actual likelihood or effect of the feared event. The anxiety is excessive and persistently interferes with functioning in one or more aspects of the patient's life.

Differential Diagnosis

Many physiological symptoms included in the *DSM-5-TR* criteria for GAD, such as fatigue, impaired concentration, and sleep disturbance, overlap with symptoms of medical, psychiatric, or substance-use diagnoses. Differential diagnoses should include medical illnesses that may cause anxiety such as heart disease and hyperthyroidism (Box 70.3). Typically, a medical work-up is necessary, including standard blood chemistry, electrocardiogram, and thyroid function tests. Caffeine intoxication; substance use; and sedative, anxiolytic, and hypnotic withdrawal should also be ruled out. A comprehensive list of medications, both prescribed and over the counter including herbal and homeopathic agents, must be reviewed. Additionally, an environmental/occupational assessment should be completed to determine potential inhalation of volatile gases—such as gasoline, paint, insecticides, carbon monoxide, and carbon dioxide—which are causes of anxiety symptoms.

Other psychiatric disorders to rule out include panic disorder, phobias, depressive and obsessive-compulsive disorders, and substance-use disorders. In patients with both depressive and anxiety disorders, the symptomatic profile may be balanced or either depressive or anxiety symptoms can predominate. Identification and treatment of depressive disorders can lead to improved outcomes and quicker recovery. Finally, a thorough suicide and homicide risk assessment must be completed with all patients.

Box 70.3 Physiological Causes of Anxiety

- *Cancers:* carcinoid syndrome, pancreatic cancer, lung cancer, pheochromocytoma
- *Cardiac:* mitral valve prolapse, arrhythmia, congestive heart failure, ischemic heart disease
- *Pulmonary:* asthma, chronic obstructive pulmonary disease, sleep apnea, pulmonary embolism, hypercapnia, hypoxia
- *Neurological:* Ménière's disease, cerebrovascular accident (stroke), transient ischemic attack, multiple sclerosis, encephalopathy, subdural hematoma
- *Hematological:* anemia
- *Metabolic:* thyroid disease, hyperparathyroidism, Cushing's syndrome, Addison's disease, hypoglycemia, hyperglycemia, hyponatremia, hypokalemia
- *Nutritional:* Folate deficiency, vitamin B_{12} deficiency, iron deficiency

Medications and Medication Side Effects

Significant anxiety can develop as an adverse effect of prescribed or over-the-counter (OTC) medications. Medications commonly associated with drug-induced anxiety include:

- *Prescription drugs:* aminophylline, digitalis, dopamine, epinephrine, levodopa, lidocaine, neuroleptics, NSAIDs, steroids, SSRIs, theophylline, sympathomimetics, thyroid preparations
- *OTC drugs:* certain decongestants containing ephedrine and pseudoephedrine, caffeine, certain cough syrups, salicylates (in large doses), nicotine, monosodium glutamate, phenylpropanolamine
- *Herbal preparations:* ephedrine, ginseng, yohimbine
- *Illicit drugs:* amphetamines, marijuana, cocaine, ecstasy, methamphetamine, hallucinogenics
- *Others:* alcohol, caffeine, organic solvents

MANAGEMENT

Education and Self-Care Management

Planning care for the patient with GAD begins with psychoeducation and a positive therapeutic alliance. The person with GAD may have little understanding of GAD symptoms, prognosis, or management. Early intervention may include education and treatment planning involving GAD symptom recognition (physiological symptoms, maladaptive thought patterns), decrease in intake of stimulants, enhanced physical activity, improved sleep hygiene, self-directed relaxation, mindfulness, and CBT therapies. Patients who develop routine methods of preventing acute anxiety and promoting relaxation may be more successful than patients who attempt to cope with their GAD on an as-needed basis. Patient functioning in various areas of their life should be well defined, and clear goals of improvement should be developed for each area affected by GAD.

Pharmacological Management

SRIs and serotonin norepinephrine reuptake inhibitors (SNRIs) are first-line medications for the treatment of GAD and can be helpful for patients with coexisting depressive disorders (see Drugs Commonly Prescribed 70.1). Slow titration to a therapeutic dose may reduce the likelihood or severity of side effects, including medication-induced anxiety for serotonergic agents. Patient education about initial side effects that often improve after several weeks, along with the delayed mechanism of action for improved anxiety, may improve adherence. Pharmacological treatment should be continued for approximately 1 year after remission of symptoms. If no response is noted with the first medication at maximum dosage, consider changing to another SRI or SNRI. When first-line medications are not fully effective and insomnia is a significant concern, second-line medications with sedating effects such as mirtazapine, pregabalin, and tricyclic antidepressants (TCAs; amitriptyline, imipramine) can be considered. Nonpharmacological interventions should be strongly encouraged to augment pharmacological treatment.

Short-acting medications should be considered to augment initial pharmacological treatments before serotonergic medications become effective or if symptoms remain. Options include benzodiazepines, which are

Drugs Commonly Prescribed 70.1: Antianxiety Agents

DRUG	INDICATION	ADVERSE REACTIONS AND PRESCRIBING CONSIDERATIONS
Short-Acting Non-Benzodiazepines		
Hydroxyzine (Vistaril, Atarax)	Anxiety, insomnia	• Antihistamine with anticholinergic properties • Sedating, beneficial for sleep but may require lower dose for daytime anxiety • Along with benzodiazepines, identified in Beers Criteria as potential risk for falls, confusion in older patients • Can increase risk for prolonged QTC interval in patients with other risk factors
Gabapentin (Neurontin)	Anxiety, neuropathic pain, alcohol withdrawal	• Highly adjustable depending on patient needs and tolerance to side effects such as drowsiness, dizziness • Some abuse potential • Increased risk for CNS depression, particularly patients taking concurrent opioids or risk factors such as COPD
Propranolol (Inderal)	Social anxiety, performance anxiety	• Especially helpful in anxiety with strong somatic or "fight or flight" component • Monitor for dizziness, hypotension
Benzodiazepines: Half-Life <12 Hours		
Alprazolam* (Xanax)	Anxiety, GAD, panic disorder	• Sedation, memory deficits, ataxia, narrow-angle glaucoma; association with falls and injury in older adults • Caution with depressed patients and substance abuse, impaired hepatic or renal function • Most contraindicated in obstructive sleep apnea • Metabolized by CYP450 3A4; check drug–gene interactions • Withdrawal symptoms with abrupt discontinuation • The onset of withdrawal symptoms is usually seen on the first day without drug and lasts 5–7 days—slow taper • Use lowest and shortest possible effective dose and time; risk of dependence for treatment longer than 12 weeks. • Avoid valerian, St. John's wort, kava kava, gotu kola • Potential severe allergic reactions (anaphylaxis, angioedema) and complex sleep-related behaviors, which may include sleep-driving, cooking, and eating food while asleep, and making phone calls while asleep

Drugs Commonly Prescribed 70.1: Antianxiety Agents—cont'd

DRUG	INDICATION	ADVERSE REACTIONS AND PRESCRIBING CONSIDERATIONS
Oxazepam* (Serax)	Anxiety and alcohol withdrawal	• See above
Temazepam* (Restoril)	Insomnia, short-term	• See above • Administer 30 minutes before bedtime • Lack of active metabolites; excellent option for older adults
Triazolam* (Halcion)	Insomnia, short-term	• Not a drug of first choice for older patients because of the higher incidence of CNS adverse reactions in this population
Benzodiazepines: Intermediate Half-life (12–24 hours)		
Alprazolam XR* (Xanax XR)	GAD, panic disorder, anxiety with depression	• Extended-release tablet: Should be taken once daily in the morning; do not crush, break, or chew • Onset 1 hour and duration 12 hours
Estazolam* (Prosom)	Insomnia short-term	• No active metabolites
Lorazepam* (Ativan)	Amnesia induction Anxiety sedation induction Status epilepticus	• Available in liquid and injectable formulation • Contraindicated if patient has angle-closure glaucoma
Benzodiazepines: Long Elimination Half-Life (>24 hours)		
Chlordiazepoxide* (Librium)	Anxiety, alcohol withdrawal	• The onset of withdrawal symptoms is usually seen after 5 days, with a duration of 10–14 days
Clonazepam* (Klonopin)	Absence seizures Lennox-Gastaut syndrome Myoclonic seizures Panic disorder	• Less sedating than other anxiolytics; onset of full anxiolytic effect can take 3–6 weeks; less dependence • Risk of suicidal ideation when used for seizures; monitor CBC, LFTs
Clorazepate* (Tranxene)	Anxiety, alcohol withdrawal, partial seizures (adjunctive)	• Increased risk of suicidal ideation when used for seizures • Long-acting metabolites; do not use in older adults • Monitor CBC, LFTs
Diazepam* (Valium)	Amnesia induction, anxiety, drug-induced seizures, alcohol withdrawal, muscle spasms, partial seizures, sedation induction Status epilepticus, tetanus, tonic-clonic seizures	• Monitor CBC, LFTs • Only benzodiazepine with a rectal administration formulation
Maintenance Medications		
Buspirone (Buspar)	Anxiety, GAD	• Low risk of cognitive or motor impairment, may cause dopamine-related movement disorders (restlessness) • Avoid St. John's wort, valerian, gotu kola, kava kava • May take 2–3 weeks to see full effect, little potential for abuse, needs continuous use, does not potentiate the effects of alcohol
Serotonin Reuptake Inhibitors (SRIs)		See Drugs Commonly Prescribed 69.1
Serotonin-Norepinephrine Reuptake Inhibitors (SNRIs)		See Drugs Commonly Prescribed 69.1

*All benzodiazepines are Schedule IV controlled substances with risk for building tolerance and dependence and are subject to increased state and federal regulations. All benzodiazepines are associated with potential anterograde amnesia, CNS depression, and paradoxical reactions.

Abbreviations: CBC, complete blood count; CNS, central nervous system; COPD, chronic obstructive pulmonary disease; GAD, generalized anxiety disorder; LFTs, liver function tests.

highly effective but can contribute to long-term risks, or the nonbenzodiazepines hydroxyzine (Vistaril), gabapentin (Neurontin), or propranolol (Inderal). Benzodiazepines can be helpful in the acute management of GAD; however, these medications should be avoided or limited for patients with a history of substance-use disorder. Moreover, benzodiazepines may exacerbate depressive symptoms.

Frequent monitoring and appropriate titration of medication to a therapeutic dose are important aspects of initial pharmacological treatment. The goal of medication treatment for GAD should be to reduce or relieve symptoms, which will enable effective self-care and engagement in nonpharmacological treatments and promote satisfactory levels of functioning.

Nonpharmacological Management

Nonpharmacological management is considered a first-line option that has similar efficacy to pharmacological therapy and may enhance the benefits of pharmacological interventions. Patient preference, costs, accessibility, and risks and benefits must be considered in determining treatment choices for patients with GAD. CBT (see Box 70.4) has been shown to be effective in improving anxiety symptoms comparably to SRIs. However, lack of head-to-head studies limits direct comparisons of CBT and pharmacological interventions. Mindfulness and acceptance-based therapy modalities have also shown to improve anxiety symptoms. Other treatment options include nonpharmacological approaches aimed at finding meaning and social connection and addressing structural inequities. The latter is based on theories that structural societal issues contribute to the current rates of anxiety and depression, and noninvasive brain stimulation via transcranial magnetic stimulation (TMS) or transcranial direct current stimulation (tDCS) may be of benefit.

Geriatric Considerations: Anxiety Disorders

In geriatric patients, it is important to consider other potential age- and medical-related needs, including but not limited to

- Addressing potential sensory-related limitations that may impair assessment
- Minimizing polypharmacy, addressing potential drug–drug interactions, and emphasizing deprescribing when appropriate
- Utilizing psychotherapy treatment and social support resources to avoid social isolation
- Considering the American Geriatric Society's Beers Criteria and potential for increased risk of medication side effects; medications are often required to treat anxiety symptoms, but judicious use and close monitoring are critical
- Addressing comorbidities that may contribute to physiological anxiety symptoms
- Having an awareness that anxiety may present with somatic complaints, while ensuring there is no medical etiology for complaints
- Screening and monitoring for neurocognitive disorders and delirium, which can present with anxiety symptoms

Box 70.4 Cognitive-Behavioral Strategies

Assumptions

- Alterations in content of underlying cognitive processes alter affective states and behavioral problems (i.e., thinking alters feeling and doing).
- Correction of these faulty constructs ("stinking thinking") can lead to clinical improvement.
- A person's appraisal/perception of situations is reflected in their cognitions (both thoughts and visuals).
- Through therapy, patients become aware of these faulty constructs and learn to alter them.

Processes

- Identify and alter cognitive distortions that maintain symptoms
- Time limited, usually 15–25 weeks, once weekly
- Collaborative empiricism
- Structured and directive
- Assigned readings
- Homework and behavioral techniques
- Desensitization in some patients
- Identification of irrational beliefs and automatic thoughts
- Identification of attitudes and assumptions underlying negative thoughts

Source: Buland R, Verduin ML, Ruiz P. *Kaplan & Sadock's Synopsis of Psychiatry*. 12th ed. Wolters Kluwer Health; 2022.

FOLLOW-UP AND REFERRAL

Monthly or bimonthly follow-up appointments may be needed until the patient with GAD has established alternative resources for support and assistance. A person-centered follow-up plan should include patient goals, supports, treatment interventions, and crisis resources. Staff check-ins via phone or electronically to ensure patients have access to their medications and supports may reduce return visits with limited change in clinical presentation. Referrals to support groups may be helpful.

Ongoing follow-up should include an evaluation of symptoms using a standardized screening tool, assessment of side effects from pharmacological interventions, and risk assessment for harm toward self or others. Referral to a specialist should be considered in patients with multiple comorbidities, severe symptoms, or if no improvement is noted within 8 weeks from initiation of treatment.

Patient Education: Generalized Anxiety Disorder

Education about symptoms, treatments, and course of illness should be addressed with the patient and, if appropriate, their support system. Discussion about potential side effects of pharmacological interventions that often dissipate, and the delayed onset of symptom relief, may help to prepare patients to manage their expectations. Setting the expectation that although therapy may provide lifelong coping mechanisms, it will take time and ongoing engagement to be effective. Written instructions including information about medication recommendations, coping strategies, and crisis contact information may help patients better understand the treatment plan and supports if they are feeling overwhelmed.

The provider may want to suggest complementary methods of anxiety management such as relaxation techniques, guided imagery, music therapy, physical activity, yoga, and acupuncture (see Complementary Therapies 70.1). Additionally, physical activity has consistently been shown to have a positive effect on anxiety, and changes in dietary intake may be helpful, such as reducing activating substances like sugar or caffeine. Consistent self-care can significantly improve anxiety symptoms. At the same time, providers must remember that patients with poorly controlled anxiety symptoms—no matter how motivated—are less likely to learn and engage in self-care because they struggle with learning and retaining new information. Primary care settings now have access to comprehensive patient education programs and team-based approaches in which the primary care nurse practitioner can play a pivotal role. Giving patients time to practice newly adopted self-care skills, such as mindfulness-based stress reduction programs and meditation, may assist patients to cope with ongoing symptoms.

Complementary Therapies 70.1: Relaxation Therapy Techniques

This breathing technique will help you relax, as well as provide increased energy, health, and concentration. Try using this technique for at least 15 minutes each day on an empty stomach. Do not stand up suddenly after performing these exercises because they can lower blood pressure, making you dizzy.

Step 1: Sit in a comfortable chair and in a quiet location to minimize distractions.
Step 2: Close your eyes.
Step 3: Begin by taking a slow, deep breath in through your nose and breathe out through your mouth slowly and deeply, like blowing out a candle.
Step 4: Breathe in slowly for a count of four, hold for a count of seven, and breathe out for a count of eight. Repeat this several times.
Step 5: The following techniques may also help you relax while doing the breathing exercise:
   a. Visualize a favorite, peaceful setting, such as a beach, forest, desert, or meadow.
   b. Play peaceful music in the background.
   c. Begin at your feet and repeat to yourself that your feet are warm and heavy. Once you have achieved that, move up to your legs, your torso, and then your arms and hands. The sensation of heaviness and warmth should spread throughout your entire body.
   d. Repeat a favorite phrase, or mantra, with each breath.
   e. Tighten different muscles while inhaling and relax them while exhaling (start with your feet and move systematically up your body).

Utilization of Technology for Meditation

There are many free downloadable applications for phones and portable devices that walk a person step by step through how to meditate. See the following:

- Calm: https://www.calm.com/
- Headspace: https://www.headspace.com/
- Simple Habit: https://www.simplehabit.com/

PANIC DISORDER

Panic disorder, like other anxiety disorders, overlaps in presentation with and has shown increased prevalence with many comorbid medical conditions, including asthma, sleep apnea, migraines, irritable bowel syndrome, cardiovascular illnesses, and diabetes. Thus, a comprehensive assessment and understanding of the condition is necessary. Patients with panic disorder experience recurrent unexpected episodes of panic with psychological and physical symptoms such as palpitations, shortness of breath, nausea, or dizziness. Panic disorder is specified by a cycle of anticipatory anxiety or avoidance that are related directly to panic symptoms. A panic episode may last from minutes to an hour, and the secondary distress that follows a panic episode may be prolonged. To the patient, panic symptoms feel life-threatening, and primary care providers must carry out due diligence to rule out underlying medical conditions.

EPIDEMIOLOGY AND CAUSES

The 12-month prevalence of panic disorder is estimated at 2% to 3% with lifetime prevalence of 4.7%. About three-fourths of patients with panic disorder report moderate to serious impairment. Panic disorder typically begins in late adolescence to young adulthood and affects females approximately twice as often as males. Patients with pulmonary, depressive, trauma, substance use, and other anxiety disorders more often develop panic disorder. Panic disorders are more common in those with a first-degree relative with an anxiety disorder.

Pediatric/Adolescent Considerations: Panic Disorder

In adolescent patients with anxiety or panic disorder, it is important to consider the following:

- Worry may be developmentally appropriate such as concerns over peer groups or school performance, and adolescents may find support through increased social support or therapy
- Anxiety disorder may present with somatic complaints or oppositional types of behavior that patients may have difficulty expressing
- Assess symptoms and functioning across varying settings including school, home, and social activities to determine whether there is a specific fear, potential relational challenge, or traumatic experience (e.g., bullying on a sports team, fighting at home)
- Providing the adolescent with normalization, privacy, and independence in the interview as much as possible (e.g., normalizing drug experimentation and assessing without parents present if possible)

Several studies have suggested that patients with panic disorder are at high risk for suicidal ideation and attempts. Comorbidity with major depressive disorder can increase the rate of suicide attempts. Research has also shown that patients with panic disorder typically experience greater distress about life events than those without panic disorder, and that in the months before the onset of panic episodes, individuals reported a higher incidence of stressful life events. Indeed, what was primarily a mild feeling of anxiety suddenly becomes an overwhelming feeling of apprehension and dread, replete with somatic symptoms.

PATHOPHYSIOLOGY

Structural brain-imaging studies, such as MRI, have demonstrated pathological involvement in the temporal lobes, particularly the hippocampus, in patients with panic disorder. Some studies use specific panic-inducing substances (such as caffeine, lactate, or yohimbine) to assess effects of panic on cerebral blood flow. Anxiety disorders and panic attacks are specifically associated with cerebral vasoconstriction. This in turn may cause central nervous system symptoms such as dizziness and peripheral nervous system symptoms (hyperventilation and hypercapnia).

Genetic predisposition to panic disorders, especially in those with agoraphobia, has been established. The *DSM-5-TR* now allows for panic disorder and agoraphobia to be diagnosed irrespective of each other, meaning that both diagnoses can be given to a patient if they meet criteria for each disorder.

First-degree relatives of those with panic disorder have a fourfold to eightfold higher risk for the development of the disorder than first-degree relatives of other psychiatric patients. Twin studies have demonstrated a higher concordance for panic disorder in monozygotic twins than in dizygotic twins. No data indicating association between a specific chromosomal location or mode of transmission and panic disorder exist.

CLINICAL PRESENTATION

As with anxiety disorders, certain at-risk patients should be considered for panic disorder, including those with a family history of panic and/or anxiety disorders and patients with another psychiatric disorder, such as major depression, bipolar disorder, or substance-use disorder. Due to the physical nature of panic symptoms, patients may present only with physical complaints and astute clinicians must rule out comorbid medical conditions while assessing for underlying psychiatric symptoms. Patients with panic disorder often develop anticipatory anxiety, frequently worrying over when their next panic attack will occur and can feel overwhelmed by the loss of control with physiological symptoms arising even from a state of calm. Frequency and severity of panic attacks vary, and unlike panic attacks secondary to trauma or phobia, in panic disorder, panic attacks are not expected and may occur in any setting. Although panic disorder may develop without any obvious causative events, it can occur after a period of intense stress such as loss, threat of a loss, or physical illness.

After having several panic attacks, up to 80% of patients begin to fear the next attack. This anticipatory anxiety may be more disabling than the panic attacks themselves and patients may develop ways to ensure that they have support or are able to escape when panic attacks occur. Patients may become agoraphobic, culminating in increasingly circumscribed lives with approximately 30% to 50% of individuals with agoraphobia also being diagnosed with panic disorder.

DIAGNOSTIC REASONING

Symptoms

Panic disorder can be distinguished from other anxiety disorders based on the patient's history of repeated unexpected panic attacks. The patient should be asked to describe the panic attacks in detail, noting onset, frequency, duration, coping or avoidance methods, and precipitating events. Panic disorder is diagnosed in patients with recurrent, intense, unexpected, short episodes of panic with psychological and physical symptoms of anxiety that peak within minutes and include four or more of the following: sweating, trembling or shaking, feeling short of breath, feelings of choking, chest pain or discomfort, nausea or abdominal distress, feeling dizzy/unsteady/lightheaded/faint, chills or heat, paresthesia, feelings of unreality or being detached from oneself, fear of losing control, going "crazy," or dying (American Psychiatric Association, 2022). Patients with panic disorder should be assessed for avoidance and behavioral change secondary to panic symptoms.

Agoraphobia is a separate diagnostic criterion in the *DSM-5-TR* and is characterized by overwhelming symptoms of anxiety when leaving home on at last two occasions. Symptoms include rapid heartbeat, chest pain, difficulty breathing, weakness, faintness, sweating, and a feeling of impending doom or fear of dying. Individuals with agoraphobia must also demonstrate avoidance behaviors, such as reluctance or refusal to leave home. See the *DSM-5-TR* for complete diagnostic criteria for agoraphobia.

Differential Diagnosis

For evaluating for panic symptoms, the Panic Disorder Severity Scale (Shear, 1997) is a seven-question self-administered measure. Panic symptoms may occur in other psychiatric disorders that do not meet the criteria for panic disorder. Appropriate diagnosis will then structure appropriate treatment and follow-up. The array of medical or other psychiatric conditions that may mimic symptoms/signs of panic disorder should be considered, especially with the onset of any anxiety disorder. Clinicians should take into account cultural considerations and concepts of distress when assessing for panic disorder. The *DSM-5-TR* has integrated cultural sensitivity tools to reflect cross-cultural presentations of mental disorders and notes cultural variation in expression of panic such as headache, tinnitus, and sobbing.

A comprehensive physical examination should be performed to rule out organic causes for the patient's symptoms. If the history suggests that organic disease is unlikely, the physical examination should focus primarily on the organ system of most concern (e.g., the heart in a patient with chest pain). Laboratory tests to rule out physical causality should be considered. Medical conditions may accompany, contribute to, or cause panic symptoms, such as pheochromocytoma, hyperthyroidism, seizure disorder, and cardiac arrhythmias or acute myocardial infarction. Panic attacks can also be the result of the use of or withdrawal from therapeutic or recreational drugs including theophylline, steroids, cocaine, amphetamines, and caffeine. Drug withdrawal symptoms are typically associated with drugs such as alcohol, barbiturates, and benzodiazepines. The differential diagnosis of panic disorder is complicated by a high rate of comorbidity with other psychiatric conditions including alcohol- and benzodiazepine-use disorders, which patients may initially use in an attempt alleviate panic symptoms.

MANAGEMENT

Pharmacological Management

SRIs, SNRIs, TCAs, and benzodiazepines are effective in the management of panic disorder. Generally, due to low side-effect profile, low cost, and efficacy, SRIs are initially utilized (see Table 69.1). Patients with panic disorder are often very sensitive to the pharmacological effects of various medications and may benefit from slow titration and frequent encouragement and education around likelihood of early side effects and delayed anxiolytic effect. When initiating pharmacological therapy, the practitioner may consider starting the drug at half of the recommended dose and gradually increasing the dose over several days. This strategy allows patients to slowly acclimate to the effects of medication. It is important to monitor and increase the dose until remission of symptoms or maximum recommended therapeutic dose is achieved. If the response to the initial SRI is inadequate or side effects intolerable, the clinician may consider changing to another SRI, or switching to an SNRI such as venlafaxine, or augmentation. Augmentation with short-acting medication may be appropriate, particularly when titrating upward on an SRI or SNRI. If benzodiazepines are used, longer-acting formulations are preferred for more consistent and extended coverage. When shorter-acting benzodiazepines are used "as needed," the risk is increased for greater tolerance and possible misuse or dependence. Once the primary maintenance medication becomes effective, the benzodiazepine augmentation should slowly taper down and be discontinued. After panic attacks have ceased, patients should be maintained on medications for a minimum of 6 months.

Nonpharmacological Management

CBT (see Box 70.4) is a first-line treatment for panic disorder, and useful adjuncts are self-help CBT-based books and self-help programs. Patients who receive CBT have shown periods of remission and longer-term benefits. CBT is also useful to facilitate the gradual withdrawal from benzodiazepines, which are often used for immediate symptom relief in panic disorder. CBT is aimed at altering the unproductive and dysfunctional thinking that helps generate and maintain anxiety. Patients with panic disorder learn to address cognitive distortions that arise in panic attacks such as "I am going to die." CBT is effective in treating maladaptive behaviors associated with anxiety through a range of treatments including breathing techniques, education, continuous panic monitoring, development of anxiety management skills, cognitive restructuring, and in vivo exposure. Additionally, sources recommend brief, highly focused behavioral and cognitive psychotherapeutic techniques for panic disorder. Acceptance and Commitment Therapy, or ACT, has shown to benefit patients with panic disorder and smaller studies have shown improvement with psychoanalytic therapy focused on panic symptoms. Hypnosis and alternative therapies (yoga, meditation, acupuncture) are sometimes useful tools for patients as part of combined therapies but lack rigorous clinical evidence compared with CBT, ACT, and psychoanalytic therapy.

FOLLOW-UP AND REFERRAL

Patients with mild to moderate panic disorder may be managed in primary care settings once a plan of care has been established and implemented. However, referral and coordination with psychiatric providers may be necessary for patients with moderate to severe symptoms who are willing to engage in therapeutic treatments. Generally, pharmacological follow-up is scheduled every 1 to 2 weeks when initiating therapy, and then every 2 to 4 weeks until therapeutic dosage is achieved. Appointments can be spaced further apart as the dosage is stabilized and symptoms reduced (see Box 70.5). As with any serious psychological condition, referral to specialist consultation or to hospital care should be made as appropriate. This includes *mandatory* inquiry about suicidal and homicidal history, ideation, or intent. The practitioner should consider referring the patient to a psychiatric provider, if the patient fails to respond after 6 to 8 weeks of standard treatment or experiences worsening or severe symptoms. Similarly, patients should be referred to an appropriate medical specialist if an underlying organic disorder is suspected. The practitioner should assess the patient's response to treatment and symptom intensity and reinforce patient education at every visit, as well as review strategies to manage panic attacks. The ongoing therapeutic alliance with the primary care clinician is crucial for long-term successful treatment.

Patient Education: Panic Disorder

Nonjudgmental, person-centered education about the symptoms, course, and multiple management options for panic disorder should be provided. Patients should be encouraged to actively participate in treatment planning and be curious self-observers including enhancing their own self-efficacy of identifying and managing symptoms. Moreover, patients and their support persons should be aware of potential benefits and adverse effects of drugs prescribed and engagement in therapy, relaxation techniques, deep breathing, and complementary strategies to reduce panic symptoms. Other approaches shown to be effective in treating panic disorder include physical exercise and healthy nutrition.

PHOBIAS

Phobias are intense fears of specific things or situations that are further specified into categories including natural environment, blood-injection-injury, animal, or situational. The phobia causes severe anxiety and avoidance, is disproportionate to the situation, and the patient may or may not have insight into the irrationality of the fear.

EPIDEMIOLOGY AND CAUSES

With both 1-year prevalence and lifetime prevalence being up to 12%, phobias are not uncommon in the primary care setting. Due to the ability to avoid specific phobias, such as elevators or dogs, some patients may not suffer from symptoms that significantly impair their day-to-day functioning. Unfortunately, about half of patients with phobias experience moderate to serious impairment from symptoms and may benefit from astute primary care assessment, management, and referral.

PATHOPHYSIOLOGY

Like other anxiety disorders, overactivation of the fear response to neutral stimuli is thought to lead to sympathetic hyperarousal and hypervigilance. In phobias, this has been largely explored and managed through the concepts of behavioral conditioning and learning. A once-neutral stimulus becomes feared secondary to a negative experience that evokes a significant emotional and physiological response, such as developing a fear of water after witnessing a near-drowning. The actual phobic stimuli may be secondary in certain situations such as a patient who develops their first panic attack at the grocery store. The grocery store may become associated with panic attacks leading to a phobia, even though the panic attack could occur elsewhere. It is important to realize the limitations in our understanding of phobias and to not expect patients to have a clear negative experience linked to their phobia.

Box 70.5 Advanced Practice Nursing Interventions for Panic Disorder

Management
- Goal: full remission, elimination of panic attacks, anxiety, phobias, and disability; restoration of well-being.
- Institute treatment with low-dose selective serotonin reuptake inhibitors (SSRIs); increase dose as tolerated to target dose.
- Monitor closely for adverse effects.
- Continue treatment for 12 to 24 months; phase out treatment slowly (over 4 to 6 months).
- Refer to an anxiety disorder specialist if response is not satisfactory or if comorbid conditions are present.

Patient and Family Education
- Teach the patient and family about panic disorder.
- Advise patient not to abruptly stop medication.

Source: Adapted from American Psychiatric Association. *Practice Guideline for the Treatment of Patients With Panic Disorder.* Retrieved from https://psychiatryonline.org/pb/assets/raw/sitewide/practice_guidelines/guidelines/panicdisorder.pdf. Updated January 2009.

Phobias are more likely to develop in individuals with family members with phobias, although there is variation in the specific types, and genetic and neurological research explores the complexities of these disorders. Evidence suggests that patients with phobias experience overactivation of certain brain areas including the amygdala, fusiform gyrus, insula, anterior cingulate cortex, and dorsomedial prefrontal cortex. Research continues to explore these areas of the brain and their complex connections with new approaches showing that administration of glucocorticoids or CBT may reduce amygdala activation and phobia symptom severity.

CLINICAL PRESENTATION

Patients with phobias may not be easily identified in primary care unless they are specifically screened for the phobia that is interfering with their day-to-day life (fear of driving a car), or it is related to their health-care treatment (fear of needles). Phobias are often seen in the presence of comorbid anxiety, depressive, or substance-use disorders. Thus, providers should ask patients with other mood symptoms directly about phobias. Remember that phobias may develop from a direct or witnessed negative experience, but the cause may be unknown and often begins in childhood.

DIAGNOSTIC REASONING

Symptoms

The criteria for a specific phobia include marked disproportionate fear or anxiety to a specific object or situation. Exposure to the phobic stimulus results in significant anxiety or fear, leads to avoidance of the stimulus, and persistently causes clinically significant distress. In more severe symptoms, the thought or mention of the phobia may provoke the fear response. Like many anxiety disorders, sympathetic arousal is common in phobias, but some patients experience a subsequent vasovagal response, which is often seen in patients with phobia of blood draws.

Differential Diagnosis

When considering a differential diagnosis for phobias, clinicians should assess for thoughts, feelings, and situations that trigger the anxiety or fear response. For example, patients that have triggers related to others' evaluation of them in situations may require further assessment for a social anxiety disorder, whereas those with phobias regarding specific food or eating patterns may require further assessment for an eating disorder. Obsessive, trauma, psychotic, and panic attack symptoms should be ruled out, and depressive and anxiety disorders should be screened for in patients with phobias.

MANAGEMENT

Pharmacological

Psychotherapy is first-line treatment for phobias, but pharmacological treatment may be needed for additional support. Acute severe phobias that are not encountered often, such as flying, are often managed with a limited course of benzodiazepines, but risks must be considered particularly if repeated exposure will be required. Any underlying anxiety disorder should be appropriately managed with medications such as SRIs.

Nonpharmacological

Exposure therapy is the most common and well-studied treatment for phobias, particularly CBT with exposure, which incorporates changing cognitions surrounding the phobia. Engaging a patient in treatment may be supported by a therapeutic alliance and assurance that the patient is in control of the level of distress or exposure they are willing to tolerate. Patients may demonstrate more success in exposure therapy treatment if they have high internal motivation and self-efficacy. Emerging research has shown that sleep or administration of D-cycloserine, a glutamatergic n-methyl-D-aspartate (NMDA) receptor partial agonist, after therapeutic intervention may improve outcomes, but additional research is needed.

FOLLOW-UP AND REFERRAL

Referral to a therapist with experience in the management of phobias is key, particularly for patients with debilitating symptoms. Patients with mild symptoms may be able to forgo follow-up, referral, or treatment. Patients with phobias should be educated that reengagement in treatment is always a future option and should be encouraged to report worsening or additional symptoms.

> **Patient Education: Phobias**
>
> Normalizing the feelings of fear, shame, embarrassment, or distress that the patient might experience in a nonjudgmental way is important. Discussions about level of impairment or distress and treatment options should be an integral component of care. As always, information about the risks, benefits, and alternatives to pharmacotherapy and psychotherapy should be provided.

POST-TRAUMATIC STRESS DISORDER

Post-traumatic stress disorder (PTSD) is a psychiatric illness that develops after a person witnesses, participates in, or experiences direct exposure to actual or threatened trauma, such as death, threatened death, serious injury, war, natural disasters, assault, and environmental and social experiences. Repeated or extreme exposure to aversive details of the trauma, usually in the course of professional duties for military personnel, police officers, medics, and other first responders, may lead to the development of PTSD. This exposure can be repeated or a one-time event. Reactions to this experience often include fear and a sense of helplessness; reliving the event repeatedly; and avoidance of events, people, or places that may trigger memories of the trauma.

Symptoms fall into four categories, intrusion, avoidance, alterations in cognition and mood, and alterations in arousal and reactivity, and may present differently in each individual. People with PTSD often continue to reexperience the trauma through flashbacks, intrusive thoughts, or nightmares, and will make an effort to avoid reminders of the traumatic event. They may report feeling "numb" and disengaged, or present with hyperarousal and increased reactivity that can manifest as reckless or destructive behaviors. Comorbid psychiatric disorders including major depression and anxiety, cognitive difficulties, and substance use are also common.

PTSD symptoms must be severe enough to persist and/or develop more than 30 days after the initial exposure. These manifestations must be disabling and significantly affect critical areas in the person's life such as interpersonal relationships and occupational roles. In the *DSM-5-TR, acute stress disorder* is separated from PTSD and refers to the development of trauma-related symptoms in the immediate aftermath of the exposure that persist for a minimum of 3 days, up to 30 days.

Nursing Situation: Post-traumatic Stress Disorder

Jennifer, a 45-year-old nurse and married woman with two children, presented to the Veteran's Administration Medical Center (VAMC). She lived in a rural community and served a total of 24 years in the military (13 years active duty in the U.S. Army and 11 years in the U.S. Army Reserves). She was deployed for 7 months during the Gulf War and for 19 months to Kuwait and Iraq. The deployment to Kuwait and Iraq was extended several times, and her support system was affected when various individuals of the medical team were reassigned to different locations. Jennifer denied any previous psychiatric history but reported a one-time sexual assault at age 20 for which she never received treatment.

During her Operation Iraqi Freedom deployment, she was at Abu Ghraib prison for 4 months and experienced mortar attacks, multiple casualties, prolonged working hours, and exposure to horrific injuries and death. She became adept at dissociating herself from these conditions until her 14th month of deployment. At that time, she lost interest in activities she normally enjoyed and became isolated from colleagues; her communication with family members also decreased. After redeployment, she began to have panic attacks, and she had intrusive symptoms and nightmares. Sensory experiences such as hearing helicopters, seeing blood, or smelling seared meat would provoke intrusive symptoms. She became increasingly isolated and alienated.

Jennifer's recovery encompassed the three stages of PTSD recovery. Providing a safe environment is a prerequisite to begin the process. During empowerment, the survivor can choose to speak about the experience, to remember, and to mourn. Narrative reconstruction and reconnection allow the survivor to reprocess the traumatic events into a tolerable form. And third, reconnection allows the individual to confront the traumatic past, accept the personal changes, and to reengage with the world and actively recreate a future.

Jennifer sought treatment at a VAMC outpatient psychiatric clinic 3 months after redeployment with the initial diagnoses of major depression and panic attacks. Her initial treatment included an SSRI and trazodone for sleep. On her third appointment, after utilizing a validated tool for PTSD, she was diagnosed with mild-moderate PTSD. As her medications began to improve her symptoms, she began to verbalize the traumatic experiences she had witnessed and could then reframe those experiences. Unfortunately, her psychiatrist retired after four sessions, and Jennifer was referred to group therapy, which she was unable to do. She sought care at a community health provider for the next year and continued the medications. Jennifer continued to heal through family support, retiring from the military, and receiving new career training.

Many veterans receive treatment outside of the VA system, and it is important for advanced practice registered nurses (APRNs) to be aware of the evidence-based pharmacological and nonpharmacological treatments for PTSD.

Source: Adapted from Feczer D, Bjorklund, P. Forever changed: posttraumatic stress disorder in female military veterans, a case report. *Perspect Pscyhiatr Care.* 2009;45(4):278–291.

EPIDEMIOLOGY AND CAUSES

PTSD affects approximately 4.5% of U.S. adults every year, and lifetime prevalence estimates range from 6.1% to 8.3%. Females are more than twice as likely to develop PTSD compared with males, 11% and 5.4%, respectively. Females are more likely to develop PTSD as a result of sexual assault, abuse, or rape either as a child or adult, whereas males are more likely develop PTSD resulting from physical assault; disaster; combat; or witnessing death, injury, and other forms of extreme violence. Rates of PTSD are higher among veterans and individuals whose jobs increase the risk of traumatic exposure (e.g., first responders, police officers, firefighters, emergency medical personnel). PTSD is more likely to occur in persons who are single, divorced, widowed, socially withdrawn, lower education, of lower socioeconomic status, and exposure to prior trauma. Moreover, blacks, Indigenous people, and Latinos are disproportionately affected and have higher rates of PTSD than non-Latino whites. Exposure to racial and ethnic discrimination has been associated with a more chronic course of PTSD among African American and Latinx adults.

Psychosocial factors that increase risk for PTSD after trauma exposure in both males and females include preexisting behavioral health problems, family history of mental illness, additional life stressors, adverse childhood experiences, and lack of social support after the traumatic incident. Age, race, socioeconomic status, sexual identity, and educational level are all contributing factors to development of PTSD. Psychiatric comorbidities include anxiety disorders, substance-use disorders, and mood disorders, with up to 70% of individuals with PTSD reporting at least one concurrent psychiatric condition.

Risk Factors: Post-traumatic Stress Disorder

- Childhood trauma (physical, emotional, sexual, neglect)
- Sexual assault, abuse, or rape
- Experiencing a dangerous event or physical injury
- Combat exposure
- Surviving a fire, flood, hurricane, or other natural disaster
- Witnessing another person being badly injured or killed
- History of mental illness or substance abuse
- Refugees resettled in Western countries

Multiple factors influence prognosis for patients with PTSD, including acuity, psychiatric comorbidities, personality, support resources, treatment adherence, and patients' ability and desire to learn new coping strategies. An adaptive person who develops acute PTSD after exposure to a traumatic event has a better chance for full recovery, especially if they have social supports. If left untreated, about 30% of patients with PTSD experience full recovery, about 40% of patients will experience mild symptoms, about 20% of patients will experience moderate symptoms, and about 10% of patients will experience severe or worsening symptoms. Thus, the development of PTSD varies with degree of exposure, type of traumatic event, and severity of precipitating event.

PATHOPHYSIOLOGY

Although much of the pathophysiology of PTSD is unclear, there is a growing body of research to suggest that biological processes may contribute to the development of PTSD. In magnetic imaging studies, patients with PTSD were found to have decreased volume of the hippocampus, left amygdala, and anterior cingulate cortex compared with matched controls. There also appears to be dysregulation of the HPA axis and the balance between excitatory and inhibitory brain neurocircuitry, as well as the adrenergic mechanisms that modulate the fight, flight, or freeze response. Patients with PTSD appear to have much greater variation in their levels of adrenocorticoids compared with those without PTSD, with recent studies showing decreased salivary cortisol variability in persons engaged in prolonged exposure therapy. Genetics and family history may also contribute to an individual's susceptibility to developing PTSD.

Personal predisposition may enhance the likelihood of symptom development after a traumatic event, and individuals who develop PTSD may have a personal or family history of mood or anxiety disorders, which is a risk factor. Patients with existing serious mental disorders are at risk for victimization and, at times, assault, and may be more likely to develop PTSD compared with others.

CLINICAL PRESENTATION

Principal clinical features of PTSD include persistent reexperiencing of the event, often in the form of flashbacks; avoidance behaviors such as staying away from places, events, or objects that are reminders of the trauma, and even avoiding thoughts and feelings related to the event; arousal and reactivity symptoms such as sleep disturbances or feeling "on edge"; and cognitive and mood symptoms. Symptoms may initially resolve within a short period of time, and then recur at intermittent intervals in response to a significant stressor, whereas other symptoms may be chronic and never fully remit after the precipitating event. Typically, a combination of the severity of the trauma, the patient's risk factors, and a variety of post-traumatic factors all must coalesce for the person to develop PTSD. Patients should also be screened for suicide and psychiatric comorbidities such as anxiety, depressive, and substance-use disorders.

PTSD symptoms may not be obvious in a routine office visit. A short screening tool such as the Primary Care PTSD Screen for *DSM-5-TR* (PC-PTSD-5), the Short Post-Traumatic Stress Disorder Rating Interview, or Trauma Screening Questionnaire (TSQ) can help quickly assess PTSD-related symptoms and provide an objective dimension to the clinical assessment to track patient outcome over time. In addition to a thorough assessment of trauma-related symptoms, the practitioner must determine the patient's level of insight and functional status to help establish person-centered treatment goals.

DIAGNOSTIC REASONING

Symptoms

To meet *DSM-5-TR* criteria for PTSD, the following symptoms must have persisted for more than 1 month and must have caused clinically significant distress in social, occupational, or other areas of functioning:

- At least one reexperiencing symptom, such as intrusive thoughts, nightmares about the event, flashbacks about the event, emotional distress after exposure to traumatic reminders, and physical reactivity after exposure to traumatic reminders. This experience can manifest itself as a nightmare; a flashback; or simply sudden, vivid memories that are accompanied by painful emotions or images related to the trauma.

- At least one avoidance symptom, such as staying away from any situation or activity that might revive memories of the trauma. This symptom can severely impair the patient's relationships with others because close emotional ties with family, friends, and colleagues may be included among the situations that the patient intentionally avoids.
- At least two cognition and mood symptoms, such as trouble remembering key features of the traumatic event, negative thoughts about oneself and the world, distorted feelings like guilt or blame, or loss of interest in enjoyable activities. These symptoms can lead the patient to feel detached from friends and family members.
- At least two arousal and reactivity symptoms, such as being easily startled, such as hypervigilance and hyperarousal. As a result of being hypersensitive or on edge, patients may experience episodes of unprovoked anger, jumpiness, and seem to be "on guard" most of the time. Patients may behave as though they are facing constant threats of danger or further trauma. They can become hyperreactive to unexpected sounds or encounters. Problems with concentrating or remembering current information are common, and terrifying nightmares can lead to severe insomnia. See the *DSM-5-TR* for the complete diagnostic criteria for PTSD.

Differential Diagnosis

Psychiatric differential diagnoses for PTSD symptoms are relatively broad and include mood or anxiety disorders, which can also be comorbidities. A thorough psychiatric history and assessment can aid in identifying other behavioral health conditions. Clinicians should rule out organic causes of physical symptom presentations and complete a full mental status and physical examination. Furthermore, a complete medication review should occur to rule out any side effects, and substance use or withdrawal should be assessed. If the thorough history assessment suggests that organic disease is unlikely, the physical examination should be comprehensive to document ways that the disorder may physiologically affect the patient. Laboratory tests to rule out physical causality should be considered.

MANAGEMENT

Pharmacological Management

Although trauma-focused psychotherapy is recommended as a first-line treatment for PTSD, pharmacological interventions can be used to help regulate biological responses, along with co-occurring psychiatric diagnoses, and may benefit psychological and social symptoms as well. Significant evidence indicates that SSRIs and the SNRI venlafaxine (Effexor) are efficacious in the treatment of trauma-related symptoms. Indeed, these medications have been shown to improve core PTSD clusters (intrusion, avoidance, negative alterations in cognition and mood, and alterations in arousal and reactivity), although symptoms may improve at varying rates during pharmacotherapy.

Prazosin is recommended for treatment of PTSD-associated nightmares and has been found to improve the quality of sleep for combat-related PTSD. Trazodone is also an effective medication for insomnia, and for some patients, TCAs such as imipramine may be effective. Anxiolytic medications can be used for acute or short-term symptom management. Buspirone (Buspar) may reduce intrusive symptoms for some patients and is a relatively safe anxiolytic.

Nonpharmacological Management

The Department of Veterans Affairs, Department of Defense Clinical Practice Guidelines for the Management of Post-traumatic Stress Disorder (2017) recommends *trauma-focused psychotherapy,* defined as therapy that uses cognitive, emotional, or behavioral techniques to facilitate processing a traumatic experience and in which the trauma focus is a central component of the therapeutic process, over other nonpharmacological or pharmacological treatments. The trauma-focused psychotherapies with the strongest evidence from clinical trials are prolonged exposure (PE), cognitive processing therapy (CPT), and eye movement desensitization and reprocessing (EMDR). These treatments have been tested in numerous clinical trials, in patients with complex presentations and comorbidities, compared with active control conditions, have long-term follow-up, and have been validated. PE is based in emotional processing theory, which posits that PTSD symptoms arise from cognitive and behavioral avoidance of trauma-related thoughts, reminders, activities, and situations. PE helps the patient interrupt and reverse this process by blocking cognitive and behavioral avoidance, introducing corrective information, and facilitating organization and processing of the trauma memory and associated thoughts and beliefs. PE was developed originally for females with sexual assault trauma and is an effective first-line treatment with sustained benefit over time. One technique of PE, called "imaginal exposure" has the patient imagine and describe the trauma and associated emotions, and has been proven effective in reducing PTSD symptom severity. In vivo exposure uses systematic desensitization to triggers of trauma. With desensitization, the patient is exposed to their trauma "trigger" in a controlled environment. Improvement is achieved by gradually increasing the time of exposure to the trigger until the patient no longer reacts with panic.

Other protocols that have sufficient evidence to recommend use are specific CBTs for PTSD, brief eclectic psychotherapy (BEP), narrative exposure therapy (NET), and written narrative exposure. Stress inoculation therapy (SIT) may be considered a "toolbox" for managing anxiety and focuses on correcting the patient's intrusive symptoms by teaching relaxation techniques, such as breathing exercises, that can be used to help self-manage intrusive symptoms when they occur. Individual-, manualized-, and non-trauma-focused therapies such as present-centered therapy (PCT) and interpersonal psychotherapy (IPT) are also suggested as alternatives to trauma-focused psychotherapy. Another intervention for PTSD is psychodynamic psychotherapy, although there is insufficient evidence to recommend for or against. This method focuses on helping the patient to examine personal values and how the experience of the traumatic event violated them. The goal is to resolve the conscious and unconscious mental conflicts that were created by the trauma. Patient work on strengthening their self-esteem as a way of increasing the ability to cope with the trauma.

Manualized group therapy or peer-counseling groups are also effective interventions for PTSD, although there is insufficient evidence to recommend using one type of group therapy over any other. The group dynamic can help encourage members to share similar traumas and symptoms safely, and through participation in these groups individuals with PTSD can gain benefits such as group support and decreased isolation. Patients may also find it easier to learn new coping techniques from other group members with similar lived experience. Relaxation therapy and other forms of complementary therapies are also helpful for persons with PTSD. Massage, positive imagery, meditation, and yoga have all been shown to be beneficial adjuncts to treatment.

FOLLOW-UP AND REFERRAL

If a patient with PTSD is not fully recovering from a traumatic experience and is experiencing suicidal ideation or other psychiatric comorbidities, then they should be referred to a psychiatric specialist. Symptoms of PTSD can be very disturbing, and some patients will require more time and support than is available in primary care settings. Pharmacological management may also require specialized management, especially if an SSRI has been tried and the patient's symptoms prove refractory to treatment. Recovery from trauma is a slow process, and patients may stop and start treatment for several months or even years. When this is the case, their relationship with their primary care practitioner may be a stabilizing force and the patient can be encouraged to engage in treatment or support at any time.

Patient Education: Post-traumatic Stress Disorder

It is important that the patients with PTSD and their support systems have a good understanding of the disorder, the chronic nature of PTSD, treatment options, and the potential benefits and adverse effects of any pharmacological intervention. Normalizing nonpharmacological interventions and their need for repeated specialty visits can help set the stage for patients with PTSD to understand that engaging in improving symptoms may take time. Regular physical activity, good nutritional practices, and other self-care interventions may help improve symptoms. Disease progression could lead to suicidal ideation and/or violence, and patients and their support persons should be informed about the danger signs, local crisis support services, and the need for close follow-up and possible intervention.

REFERENCES

Generalized Anxiety Disorder

American Geriatrics Society Expert Panel. American geriatrics society 2019 updated AGS Beers Criteria for potentially inappropriate medication use in older adults. *J Am Geriatr Soc.* 2019;67(4): 674-694. DOI: https://doi.org/10.1111/jgs.15767

American Psychiatric Association. (2022). Diagnostic and statistical manual of mental disorders, text revision (5th ed.). Washington, DC: American Psychiatric Association.

American Psychiatric Association. *Practice Guideline for the Treatment of Patients with Panic Disorder.* 2nd ed. Washington, DC: American Psychiatric Association; 2009.

Andrews G, Bell C, Boyce P, Gale C, Lampe L, Marwat O, Rapee R, Wilkins G. Royal Australian and New Zealand College of Psychiatrists clinical practice guidelines for the treatment of panic disorder, social anxiety disorder and generalised anxiety disorder. *Aust N Z J Psychiatry.* 2018;52(12):1109-1172. https://doi.org/10.1177/0004867418799453

Aylett E, Small N, Bower P. Exercise in the treatment of clinical anxiety in general practice – a systematic review and meta-analysis. *BMC Health Serv Res.* 2018;18(1):559. https://doi.org/10.1186/s12913-018-3313-5

Baker SL, et al. The Liebowitz Social Anxiety Scale as a self-report instrument: a preliminary psychometric analysis. *Behav Res Ther.* 2002;40:701-715.

Benitez J, Jablonski MR, Allen JD, Winner JG. The clinical validity and utility of combinatorial pharmacogenomics: enhancing patient outcomes. *Appl Transl Genom.* 2015;5:47-49.

Brenes GA, Danhauer SC, Lyles MF, et al. Telephone-delivered cognitive behavioral therapy and telephone-delivered nondirective supportive therapy for rural older adults with generalized anxiety disorder: a randomized clinical trial. *JAMA Psychiatry.* 2015;72:1012-1020.

Brown TA, Barlow DH. *Anxiety and Related Disorders Interview Schedule for DSM-5 (ADIS-5). Disorders Interview Schedule for DSM-5: Lifetime Version (ADIS-5L), Clinician's Manual.* Oxford University Press; 2014.

Carpenter JK, Andrews LA, Witcraft SM, Powers MB, Smits JAJ, Hofmann SG. Cognitive behavioral therapy for anxiety and related disorders: a meta-analysis of randomized placebo-controlled trials. *Depress Anxiety*. 2018;35(6):502-514. https://doi.org/10.1002/da.22728

Centers for Disease Control and Prevention. (n.d.). *About the CDC-Kaiser ACE Study*. https://www.cdc.gov/violenceprevention/aces/about.html?CDC_AA_refVal=https%3A%2F%2Fwww.cdc.gov%2Fviolenceprevention%2Facestudy%2Fabout.html

Cirillo P, Gold AK, Nardi AE, Ornelas AC, Nierenberg AA, Camprodon J, Kinrys G. Transcranial magnetic stimulation in anxiety and trauma-related disorders: a systematic review and meta-analysis. *Brain Behav*. 2019;9(6), e01284. https://doi.org/10.1002/brb3.1284

Connolly SD, Suarez L, Sylvester C. Assessment and treatment of anxiety disorders in children and adolescents. *Curr Psychiatry Rep*. 2011 Apr;13(2):99-110. doi: 10.1007/s11920-010-0173-z. PMID: 21225481.

Costello H, Gould RL, Abrol E, Howard R. Systematic review and meta-analysis of the association between peripheral inflammatory cytokines and generalised anxiety disorder. *BMJ Open*. 2019;9(7):e027925. https://doi.org/10.1136/bmjopen-2018-027925

Dear BF, Titov N, Sunderland M, et al. Psychometric comparison of the Generalized Anxiety Disorder Scale—7 and the Penn State Worry Questionnaire for measuring response during treatment of generalised anxiety disorder. *Cogn Behav Ther*. 2011;40:216-227.

Gloster AT, Sonntag R, Hoyer J, et al. Treating treatment-resistant patients with panic disorder and agoraphobia using psychotherapy: a randomized controlled switching trial. *Psychother Psychosom*. 2015;84:100-109.

Grant BF, Goldstein RB, Saha TD, et al. Epidemiology of *DSM-5* alcohol use disorder: results from the National Epidemiologic Survey on Alcohol and Related Conditions III. *JAMA Psychiatry*. 2015;72:757-766.

Hall J, Kellett S, Berrios R, et al. Efficacy of cognitive behavioral therapy for generalized anxiety disorder in older adults: systematic review, meta-analysis, and meta-regression. *Am J Geriatr Psychiatry*. 2016;24:1063-1073.

Hunt TKA, Slack KS, Berger LM. Adverse childhood experiences and behavioral problems in middle childhood. *Child Abuse Negl*. 2017;67:391-402.

Kimmel R, Roy-Byrne PP, Cowley DS. Pharmacological treatments for panic disorder, generalized anxiety disorder, specific phobia and social anxiety disorder. In: Nathan PE, Gorman JM, eds. *A Guide to Treatments That Work*. 4th ed. New York, NY: Oxford University Press; 2015:337-353.

Kladnitski N, Smith J, Uppal S, James MA, Allen AR, Andrews G, Newby JM. Transdiagnostic internet-delivered CBT and mindfulness-based treatment for depression and anxiety: a randomised controlled trial. *Internet Interv*. 2020;20:100310. https://doi.org/https://doi.org/10.1016/j.invent.2020.100310

Klahn AL, Klinkenberg IA, Lueken U, et al. Commonalities and differences in the neural substrates of threat predictability in panic disorder and specific phobia. *Neuroimage Clin*. 2017;14:530-537.

Locke, A, Kirst, N, Schultz, CG. Diagnosis and management of generalized anxiety disorder and panic disorder in adults. *Am Fam Physician*. 2015;91(9):617-624.

Metzler M, Merrick MT, Klevens J, et al. Adverse childhood experiences and life opportunities: shifting the narrative. *Child Youth Serv Rev*. 2017;72:141-149.

Meuret AE, Kroll J, Ritz T. Panic disorder comorbidity with medical conditions and treatment implications. *Ann. Rev. Clin. Psychol*. 2017;13(1):209-240. https://doi.org/10.1146/annurev-clinpsy-021815-093044

Milrod B, Chambless DL, Gallop R, et al. Psychotherapies for panic disorder: a tale of two sites. *J Clin Psychiatry*. 2016;77(7):927-935.

Möller H-J, Bandelow B, Volz H-P, Barnikol UB, Seifritz E, Kasper S. The relevance of "mixed anxiety and depression" as a diagnostic category in clinical practice. *Eur Arch Psychiatry Clin Neurosci*. 2016;266(8):725-736.

National Institute of Mental Health. Any anxiety disorder. https://www.nimh.nih.gov/health/statistics/any-anxiety-disorder.shtml. Published 2017. Accessed November 3, 2020.

National Institute of Mental Health. Generalized anxiety disorder. https://www.nimh.nih.gov/health/statistics/generalized-anxiety-disorder.shtml. Published 2017. Accessed November 3, 2020.

National Institute of Mental Health. Panic disorder. https://www.nimh.nih.gov/health/statistics/panic-disorder.shtml. Published 2017. Accessed November 3, 2020.

Sagliano L, Atripaldi D, De Vita D, D'Olimpio F, Trojano L. Non-invasive brain stimulation in generalized anxiety disorder: a systematic review. *Prog Neuropsychopharmacol. Biol. Psychiatry*. 2019;93:31-38. https://doi.org/https://doi.org/10.1016/j.pnpbp.2019.03.002

Schiele MA, Domschke K. Epigenetics at the crossroads between genes, environment and resilience in anxiety disorders. *Genes Brain Behav*. 2018;17(3):e12423. https://doi.org/https://doi.org/10.1111/gbb.12423

Shear MK, Brown TA, Barlow DH, Money R, Sholomskas DE, Woods SW, Gorman JM, Papp LA. Multicenter collaborative Panic Disorder Severity Scale. *Am J Psychiatry*. 1997;154.1571-1575.

Singh SK, Gorey KM. Relative effectiveness of mindfulness and cognitive behavioral interventions for anxiety disorders: meta-analytic review. *Soc Work Ment Health*. 2018;16(2):238-251. https://doi.org/10.1080/15332985.2017.1373266

Smitherman TA, Kolivas ED, Bailey JR. Panic disorder and migraine: comorbidity, mechanisms, and clinical implications. *Headache*. 2013;53:23-45.

Stahl S. *Essential Psychopharmacology: The Prescriber's Guide*. 5th ed. New York, NY: Cambridge University/Stahl Press; 2014.

Stein MB, Sareen J. Clinical Practice. Generalized anxiety disorder. *N Engl J Med*. 2015;373(21):2059-2068.

Strawn JR, Geracioti L, Rajdev N, Clemenza K, Levine A. Pharmacotherapy for generalized anxiety disorder in adult and pediatric patients: an evidence-based treatment review. *Expert Opin Pharmacother*. 2018;19(10):1057-1070. https://doi.org/10.1080/14656566.2018.1491966

Su VY, Chen YT, Lin WC, et al. Sleep apnea and risk of panic disorder. *Ann Fam Med*. 2015;13:325-330.

Tully PJ, Cosh SM, Baune BT. A review of the effects of worry and generalized anxiety disorder upon cardiovascular health and coronary heart disease. *Psychol Health Med*. 2013;18:627-644.

van Dis EAM, van Veen SC, Hagenaars MA, Batelaan NM, Bockting CLH, van den Heuvel RM, Cuijpers P, Engelhard IM. Long-term outcomes of cognitive behavioral therapy for anxiety-related disorders: a systematic review and meta-analysis. *JAMA Psychiatry*. 2020;77(3):265-273. https://doi.org/10.1001/jamapsychiatry.2019.3986

Wetherell JL, Petkus AJ, White KS, et al. Antidepressant medication augmented with cognitive-behavioral therapy for generalized anxiety disorder in older adults. *Am J Psychiatry*. 2013;170:782-789.

Ziffra M. Panic disorder: a review of treatment options. *Ann Clin Psychiatry.* 2021 May;33(2):124-133. doi: 10.127788/acp.0014. PMID: 33529291.

Zung WWK. A rating instrument for anxiety disorders. *Psychosomatics.* 1971;12:371-379.

Post-traumatic Stress Disorder

Ahmadpanah M, Sabzeiee P, Hosseini SM, et al. Comparing the effect of prazosin and hydroxyzine on sleep quality in patients suffering from posttraumatic stress disorder. *Neuropsychobiology.* 2014;69:235-242.

American Academy of Sleep Medicine. *International Classification of Sleep Disorders.* 3rd ed. Darien, IL: American Academy of Sleep Medicine; 2014.

American Psychiatric Association. *Practice Guideline for the Treatment of Patients with Acute Stress Disorder and Posttraumatic Stress Disorder.* Arlington, VA: American Psychiatric Association; 2017. https://psychiatryonline.org/pb/assets/raw/sitewide/practice_guidelines/guidelines/acutestressdisorderptsd-watch.pdf. Reviewed 2018.

Anderson KN, Bradley AJ. Sleep disturbance in mental health problems and neurodegenerative disease. *Nat Sci Sleep.* 2013;5:61-75.

Blevins CA, Weathers FW, Davis MT, et al. The Posttraumatic Stress Disorder Checklist for *DSM-5* (PCL-5): development and initial psychometric evaluation. *J Trauma Stress.* 2015;28:489-498.

Boland R, Verduin ML, Ruiz P. *Kaplan & Sadock's Synopsis of Psychiatry.* 12th ed. Wolters Kluwer Health; 2022.

Colvonen PJ, Straus LD, Stepnowsky C, McCarthy MJ, Goldstein LA, Norman SB. Recent advancements in treating sleep disorders in co-occurring PTSD. *Curr Psychiatry Rep.* 2018 Jun 21;20(7):48. doi: 10.1007/s11920-018-0916-9. PMID: 29931537; PMCID: PMC6645398.

Cusack K, Jonas DE, Forneris CA, Wines C, Sonis J, Middleton JC, Feltner C, Brownley KA, Olmsted KR, Greenblatt A, Weil A, Gaynes BN. Psychological treatments for adults with posttraumatic stress disorder: a systematic review and meta-analysis. *Clin Psychol Rev.* 2016 Feb;43:128-41. doi: 10.1016/j.cpr.2015.10.003. Epub 2015 Nov 2. PMID: 26574151.

Department of Veterans Affairs, Department of Defense. Clinical practice guideline for management of post-traumatic stress, version 3.0. https://www.healthquality.va.gov/guidelines/MH/ptsd/VADoDPTSDCPGFinal.pdf. Published June 2017.

Detweiler MB, Pagadala B, Candelario J, et al. Treatment of posttraumatic stress disorder nightmares at a Veterans Affairs Medical Center. *J Clin Med.* 2016;5(12):117.

De Venter M, Van Den Eede F, Pattyn T, et al. Impact of childhood trauma on course of panic disorder: Contribution of clinical and personality characteristics. *Acta Psychiatr Scand.* 2017;135:554.

Ehlers A, Grey N, Wild J, et al. Implementation of cognitive therapy for PTSD in routine clinical care: Effectiveness and moderators of outcome in a consecutive sample. *Behav Res Ther.* 2013;51(11):742-752.

Ehlers A, Hackmann A, Grey N, et al. A randomized controlled trial of 7-day intensive and standard weekly cognitive therapy for PTSD and emotion-focused supportive therapy. *Am J Psychiatry.* 2014;171(3):294-304.

Ehlers A, Wild J. Cognitive therapy for PTSD. In: Bufka LF, Wright CV, Halfond RW eds. *Casebook to the APA Clinical Practice Guideline for the treatment of PTSD.* American Psychological Association; 2020:91-121.

Gauchat A, Séguin JR, Zadra A. Prevalence and correlates of disturbed dreaming in children. *Pathol Biol (Paris).* 2014;62:311-318.

George KC, Kebejian L, Ruth LJ, et al. Meta-analysis of the efficacy and safety of prazosin versus placebo for the treatment of nightmares and sleep disturbances in adults with posttraumatic stress disorder. *J Trauma Dissociation.* 2016;17:494-510.

Gradus JL, Farkas DK, Svensson E, et al. Posttraumatic stress disorder and cancer risk: a nationwide cohort study. *Eur J Epidemiol.* 2015;30:563-568.

Greenberg MS, Tanev K, Marin MF, Pitman RK. Stress, PTSD, and dementia. *Alzheimers Dement.* 2014;10:S155-S165.

Harb GC, Phelps AJ, Forbes D, et al. A critical review of the evidence base of imagery rehearsal for posttraumatic nightmares: pointing the way for future research. *J Trauma Stress.* 2013;26:570-579.

Ho FY, Chan CS, Tang KN. Cognitive-behavioral therapy for sleep disturbances in treating posttraumatic stress disorder symptoms: a meta-analysis of randomized controlled trials. *Clin Psychol Rev.* 2016;43:90-102.

Husarewycz MN, El-Gabalawy R, Logsetty S, Sareen J. The association between number and type of traumatic life experiences and physical conditions in a nationally representative sample. *Gen Hosp Psychiatry.* 2014;36:26-32.

Jetly R, Heber A, Fraser G, Boisvert D. The efficacy of nabilone, a synthetic cannabinoid, in the treatment of PTSD-associated nightmares: a preliminary randomized, double-blind, placebo-controlled cross-over design study. *Psychoneuroendocrinology.* 2015;51:585-588.

Johannesson KB, Arinell H, Arnberg FK. Six years after the wave. Trajectories of posttraumatic stress following a natural disaster. *J Anxiety Disord.* 2015;36:15-24.

Khachatryan D, Groll D, Booij L, et al. Prazosin for treating sleep disturbances in adults with posttraumatic stress disorder: a systematic review and meta-analysis of randomized controlled trials. *Gen Hosp Psychiatry.* 2016;39:46-52.

Lehavot K, Katon JG, Chen JA, Fortney JC, Simpson TL. Posttraumatic stress disorder by gender and veteran status. *Am J Prevent Med.* 2018;54(1):e1-e9.

Levrier K, Marchand A, Belleville G, et al. Nightmare frequency, nightmare distress and the efficiency of trauma-focused cognitive behavioral therapy for post-traumatic stress disorder. *Arch Trauma Res.* 2016;5:e33051.

Littlewood DL, Gooding PA, Panagioti M, Kyle SD. Nightmares and suicide in posttraumatic stress disorder: the mediating role of defeat, entrapment, and hopelessness. *J Clin Sleep Med.* 2016;12(3):393-399.

Lohr JB, Palmer BW, Eidt CA, et al. Is post-traumatic stress disorder associated with premature senescence? A review of the literature. *Am J Geriatr Psychiatry.* 2015;23:709-725.

Mason SM, Flint AJ, Roberts AL, et al. Posttraumatic stress disorder symptoms and food addiction in women by timing and type of trauma exposure. *JAMA Psychiatry.* 2014;71:1271-1278.

Monson CM, Fredman SJ, Macdonald A, et al. Effect of cognitive-behavioral couple therapy for PTSD: a randomized controlled trial. *JAMA.* 2012;308:700-709.

Nash WP, Boasso AM, Steenkamp MM, et al. Posttraumatic stress in deployed marines: prospective trajectories of early adaptation. *J Abnorm Psychol.* 2015;124:155-171.

O'Donovan A, Cohen BE, Seal KH, et al. Elevated risk for autoimmune disorders in Iraq and Afghanistan veterans with posttraumatic stress disorder. *Biol Psychiatry.* 2015;77:365-374.

Paul F, Schredl M, Alpers GW. Nightmares affect the experience of sleep quality but not sleep architecture: an ambulatory polysomnographic study. *Borderline Personal Disord Emot Dysregul.* 2015;2:3.

Pigeon WR, Titus CE, Bishop TM. The relationship of suicidal thoughts and behaviors to sleep disturbance: a review of recent findings. *Curr Sleep Medicine Rep.* 2016;2:241-250.

Punamäki RL, Palosaari E, Diab M, et al. Trajectories of posttraumatic stress symptoms (PTSS) after major war among Palestinian children: Trauma, family- and child-related predictors. *J Affect Disord.* 2015;172:133-140.

Qiu D, Li Y, Li L, He J, Ouyang F, Xiao S. Prevalence of post-traumatic stress symptoms among people influenced by coronavirus disease 2019 outbreak: a meta-analysis. *Eur Psychiatry.* 2021 Apr 12;64(1):e30. doi: 10.1192/j.eurpsy.2021.24. PMID: 33843547; PMCID: PMC8060540.

Raskind MA, Peterson K, Williams T, et al. A trial of prazosin for combat trauma PTSD with nightmares in active-duty soldiers returned from Iraq and Afghanistan. *Am J Psychiatry.* 2013;170:1003-1010.

Roberts AL, Agnew-Blais JC, Spiegelman D, et al. Posttraumatic stress disorder and incidence of type 2 diabetes mellitus in a sample of women: a 22-year longitudinal study. *JAMA Psychiatry.* 2015;72:203-210.

Rosenberg L, Rosenberg M, Robert R, et al. Does acute stress disorder predict subsequent posttraumatic stress disorder in pediatric burn survivors? *J Clin Psychiatry.* 2015;76:1564-1568.

Schnurr PP. Focusing on trauma-focused psychotherapy for posttraumatic stress disorder. *Curr Opin Psychol.* 2017;14:56-60.

Schredl M, Reinhard I. Gender differences in nightmare frequency: a meta-analysis. *Sleep Med Rev.* 2011;15:115-121.

Seda G, Sanchez-Ortuno MM, Welsh CH, et al. Comparative meta-analysis of prazosin and imagery rehearsal therapy for nightmare frequency, sleep quality, and posttraumatic stress. *J Clin Sleep Med.* 2015;11:11-22.

Simor P, Horváth K, Gombos F, et al. Disturbed dreaming and sleep quality: altered sleep architecture in subjects with frequent nightmares. *Eur Arch Psychiatry Clin Neurosci.* 2012;262: 687-696.

Singh B, Hughes AJ, Mehta G, et al. Efficacy of prazosin in posttraumatic stress disorder: a systematic review and meta-analysis. *Prim Care Companion CNS Disord.* 2016;18(4).

Spoont MR, Williams JW Jr, Kehle-Forbes S, et al. Does this patient have posttraumatic stress disorder?: Rational clinical examination systematic review. *JAMA.* 2015;314:501-510.

Taft CT, Watkins LE, Stafford J, et al. Posttraumatic stress disorder and intimate relationship problems: a meta-analysis. *J Consult Clin Psychol.* 2011;79:22-33.

Tribl GG, Wetter TC, Schredl M. Dreaming under antidepressants: a systematic review on evidence in depressive patients and healthy volunteers. *Sleep Med Rev.* 2013;17:133-142.

U.S. Department of Veterans Affairs. PTSD: National Center for PTSD. https://www.ptsd.va.gov. Accessed November 6, 2020.

Villarreal G, Hamner MB, Cañive JM, et al. Efficacy of quetiapine monotherapy in posttraumatic stress disorder: a randomized, placebo-controlled trial. *Am J Psychiatry.* 2016;173: 1205-1212.

Waltman, SH, Shearer D, Moore BA. Management of post-traumatic nightmares: a review of pharmacologic and nonpharmacologic treatments since 2013. *Curr Psychiatry Rep.* 2018; 20(12):108.

Wichniak A, Wierzbicka A, Walęcka M, Jernajczyk W. Effects of antidepressants on sleep. *Curr Psychiatry Rep.* 2017;19(9):63.

Wilson G, Farrell D, Barron I, Hutchins J, Whybrow D, Kiernan MD. The use of eye-movement desensitization reprocessing (EMDR) therapy in treating post-traumatic stress disorder – a systematic narrative review. *Front Psychol.* 2018 Jun 6;9:923. doi: 10.3389/fpsyg.2018.00923. PMID: 29928250; PMCID: PMC5997931.

Zhang Y, Ren R, Sanford LD, Yang L, Ni Y, Zhou J, Zhang J, Wing Y, Shi J, Lu L, Tang X. The effects of prazosin on sleep disturbances in post-traumatic stress disorder: a systematic review and meta-analysis. *Sleep Med.* 2020;67:225-231.

Zhou P, Zhang Y, Wei C, et al. Acute stress disorder as a predictor of posttraumatic stress: a longitudinal study of Chinese children exposed to the Lushan earthquake. *Psych J.* 2016;5:206.

RESOURCES

Generalized Anxiety Disorder

American Academy of Child and Adolescent Psychiatry: Anxiety Disorders Resource Center
https://www.aacap.org/AACAP/Families_and_Youth/Resource_Centers/Anxiety_Disorder_Resource_Center/Home.aspx

American Counseling Association: Anxiety Resources
https://www.counseling.org/knowledge-center/mental-health-resources/anxiety

Anxiety and Depression Association of America
https://adaa.org/understanding-anxiety/generalized-anxiety-disorder-gad/resources

National Institute of Mental Health: Digital Shareables on Anxiety Disorders
https://www.nimh.nih.gov/get-involved/education-awareness/shareable-resources-on-anxiety-disorders

Post-traumatic Stress Disorder

American Academy of Child & Adolescent Psychiatry
https://www.aacap.org/App_Themes/AACAP/docs/facts_for_families/70_posttraumatic_stress_disorder_ptsd.pdf

American Psychiatric Association
https://www.psychiatry.org/patients-families/ptsd/what-is-ptsd

American Psychological Association
http://www.apa.org/topics/ptsd/

Centers for Disease Control and Prevention
https://www.cdc.gov/childrensmentalhealth/ptsd.html

Familydoctor.org: Post-Traumatic Stress Disorder (PTSD)
https://familydoctor.org/condition/post-traumatic-stress-disorder/?adfree = true

Make the Connection: PTSD
https://maketheconnection.net/conditions/ptsd/

Mayo Clinic
https://www.mayoclinic.org/diseases-conditions/post-traumatic-stress-disorder/symptoms-causes/syc-20355967

National Institute of Mental Health
https://www.nimh.nih.gov/health/topics/post-traumatic-stress-disorder-ptsd/index.shtml

Substance Abuse and Mental Health Services Administration
https://www.samhsa.gov/treatment/mental-disorders/post-traumatic-stress-disorder

Chapter 71

Obsessive-Compulsive and Related Disorders

Kim Ferguson, DNP, APRN, FNP-BC, PMHNP-BC
Karen Jennings Mathis, PhD, APRN-CNP, PMHNP-BC, FAED

OBSESSIVE-COMPULSIVE DISORDER

Obsessive-compulsive disorder (OCD) is characterized by the presence of obsessions, compulsions, or a combination of both. Only one category of symptoms is required for diagnosis. *Obsessions* are recurrent and persistent thoughts, urges, or images that are experienced as intrusive and unwanted. *Compulsions* are repetitive behaviors or mental acts that an individual feels forced to perform due to either an obsession or strict rules of conduct. Compulsions help temporarily decrease anxiety from obsessions and thus become reinforced over time.

OCD is diagnostically separate and is grouped with related disorders, including body dysmorphic disorder, hoarding disorder, trichotillomania (hair-pulling disorder), and excoriation (skin-picking) disorder. The linking feature of these ailments is repetitive behaviors, although otherwise they have differing presentations, heritability, and treatments.

Due to shame, especially resulting from aggressive or sexual thoughts, patients often delay seeking help for OCD and instead present to primary care clinicians rather than psychiatrists. OCD is the fourth most common psychiatric illness, with a lifetime prevalence of 1% to 3%, and is considered one of the leading causes of disability. As a result, it is imperative for primary care providers to recognize and screen for OCD and related disorders and to initiate treatment. Patients who do not experience an alleviation of symptoms with nonpharmacological treatment such as cognitive behavioral therapy (CBT), pharmacotherapy, or both and patients who have particularly disabling, complex, or high-risk symptoms should be referred to specialists.

EPIDEMIOLOGY AND CAUSES

OCD occurs throughout the world, spanning all cultures and races. Lifetime prevalence is estimated at 1% to 1.5%. It is a chronic disorder, with a waxing–waning course. The disorder's onset is usually in childhood, late adolescence, or early adulthood, although it can present in other age groups. The onset of OCD in childhood and adolescence can be seen both gradually and acutely. It is noted that among patients who have been diagnosed in childhood or adolescence, the condition can persist in adulthood. However, it is noted that up to 40% of these patients can have remission by early adulthood. With pediatric cases, both obsessions and compulsions can commonly be present. In children and adolescents, obsessions may be challenging to diagnose. Compulsions, however, tend to be observable and are not influenced as much by developmental factors. There is a male preponderance in earlier-onset OCD, whereas females prevail when it is diagnosed at a later age. The sex ratio is equal. In many cases, onset of OCD is acute, typically after a significant, stressful life event.

PATHOPHYIOLOGY

Although unacceptable thoughts, such as an impulse to drive one's car off the road or jump onto the tracks before an approaching train, are not uncommon in the general population, in those with OCD, these thoughts are evaluated with an exaggerated, often horrifying, sense of personal responsibility for the thoughts themselves. The obsessions are emphasized further when the individual tries to avoid thinking about them. As a result, the person becomes preoccupied with the disturbing thoughts and attempts to control them. A brutal cycle then develops in which common unacceptable thoughts develop into pathological, tormenting

Pediatric/Adolescent Considerations:
Obsessive-Compulsive Disorder

The emergence of OCD can be commonly noted in adolescence and may be associated with a sense of shame or distress. Patients with OCD will often present to primary care settings, so it is important for providers to be aware of common symptoms, proper diagnosis, and referral. Assessment of the degree of insight is also imperative to determine level of severity. Consideration of pediatric autoimmune neuropsychiatric disorders associated with streptococcus (PANDAS) as a differential diagnosis in a patient presenting with new or worsening symptoms is crucial in children and adolescents. To ensure that the patient is comfortable disclosing details about their behaviors and thoughts, a good therapeutic alliance needs to be established and maintained among the provider, patient, and family/significant others. Support and education are key from a nursing perspective.

obsessions. Compulsions follow from the obsessions. They are the patient's attempts to neutralize the irrational ideas, images, or urges for which they feel responsible. Compulsions help lessen anxiety in the short term but at the price of becoming needed tools for warding off obsessions. Accordingly, compulsions, adopting the form of behaviors or mental rituals, become ingrained and repetitive.

Individuals with OCD often have other psychopathology, requiring additional evaluation and treatment. Many have a lifetime diagnosis of an anxiety disorder (75.8%); mood disorders 63.3%), primarily major depressive disorder (MDD); impulse control disorders (56%); and/or substance-use disorders (38.6%). Up to 80% of individuals with OCD will experience a depressive episode in their lifetime, and at least one-third of patients with OCD have concurrent MDD at the time of evaluation. The commonality between OCD and depressive disorders is demonstrated by similarities in sleep electroencephalograph studies and neuroendocrine dexamethasone testing.

Genetic studies have demonstrated that both biological and environmental factors are important in the etiology of OCD. Family studies have indicated that OCD has a significant hereditable component, with relatives approximately fourfold more likely to develop OCD than the general population. Twin studies have found increased heritability estimates in pediatric (45% to 65%) compared with adult (27% to 47%) populations with OCD. Genes within the serotonin, dopamine, and glutamate pathways and those involved in white matter formation have been the focus of analyses. Although more data are needed regarding the specific cause of OCD, it is generally thought that dysregulation of serotonin is associated with the symptoms of OCD. So far, the glutamate transporter gene, *SLC1A1*, has been consistently associated with OCD.

Neurobiologically, evidence indicates that the emergence of OCD is facilitated by hyperactivity in the orbitofrontal cortex, caudate nuclei, and anterior cingulate cortex and/or by alterations to frontal cortico-striatal thalamic circuitry. Any process affecting these circuits has the potential to cause OCD. Such conditions include gross neurological insults, such as strokes, brain tumors, Huntington's disease, Sydenham's chorea, frontotemporal dementia, or brain injury to the frontal lobe or basal skull. Subtler mechanisms, involving uncommon genes or environmental factors, can also be involved.

In childhood, a unique and rare presentation consists of pediatric autoimmune neuropsychiatric disorders associated with streptococcal infection (PANDAS). It is characterized by the development of or worsening of pre-existing neuropsychiatric symptoms including symptoms of OCD and/or tics, which present/worsen abruptly and can follow a variable course. GABHS infection triggers the production of autoimmune antibodies against streptococci, which also cross-react with the basal ganglia; and this cross reaction is thought to result in neuropsychiatric symptoms, including OCD. In a 2017 study, among 1 million patients younger than 18 years, a positive strep test had an increased risk of OCD, compared with individuals without a positive test. However, a diagnosis of PANDAS remains a diagnosis of exclusion and is not universally accepted.

CLINICAL PRESENTATION

In primary care settings, patients with OCD may present with symptoms of either depression or anxiety because of distress or inability to function, rather than symptoms of OCD. These symptoms should prompt the clinician to maintain a high degree of suspicion for OCD. Patients with OCD often have good insight into their symptoms and can readily describe them, but occasionally they may have poor insight or even a delusional, fixed level of symptom intensity. Common obsessions, compulsions, and potential presentations seen in the primary care setting are in Table 71.1. The most common obsessions are fears of contamination, pathological self-doubt, intrusive thoughts, and symmetry. It is important to determine the frequency, intensity, duration, and severity of symptoms, as well as the symptoms' effects on the patient's level of functioning. One should also ask about triggers, relieving factors, and avoidance of situations or things. Individuals may begin to avoid settings that trigger their obsessions or compulsions; for example, they may stop going to restaurants or using public restrooms. The patient may believe avoidance is better than the alternative (i.e., facing one's fears). In OCD, like other anxiety disorders, avoidance worsens the illness, leading to even greater loss of functioning and decreased quality of life.

The COVID-19 pandemic may play a role in the increase in symptoms and associated dysfunctional beliefs in individuals with OCD, particularly those with an obsession of contamination and compulsions of washing. Additionally, the pandemic may affect the ability to effectively implement nonpharmacological interventions such as exposure and response prevention treatment (ERP). There is a growing amount of literature exploring the impact of COVID-19 on individuals with OCD across symptom dimensions. From a nursing perspective, it is important to assess for a change in symptoms and an increase in severity.

DIAGNOSTIC REASONING

Screening questions for OCD only take a few moments to ask. If a patient responds positively to one of the following questions, a more formal diagnostic assessment and treatment plan may be in order.

- Are you ever bothered by frequent thoughts that are senseless but that you can't get out of your head? How do you deal with them?
- Do you spend a lot of time worrying about germs? Do you wash your hands a lot?

TABLE 71.1 Common OCD Symptoms and Presentations

Type of Symptom	Examples
OBSESSIONS	
Aggressive impulses	Images of hurting a child or parent
Contamination	Becoming contaminated by shaking hands with another person
Need for order	Intense distress when objects are disordered or asymmetric
Religious	Blasphemous thoughts, concerns about unknowingly sinning
Repeated doubts	Wondering if a door was left unlocked
Sexual imagery	Recurrent pornographic images
COMPULSIONS	
Checking	Repeatedly checking locks, alarms, appliances
Cleaning	Hand washing
Hoarding	Saving trash or unnecessary items
Mental acts	Praying, counting, repeating words silently
Ordering	Reordering objects to achieve symmetry
Reassurance seeking	Asking others for reassurance
Repetitive actions	Walking in and out of a doorway multiple times

Source: Fenske JN, Schwenk TL. Obsessive-compulsive disorder: Diagnosis and management. *Am Fam Physician.* 2009;80(3):239–245. Reproduced with permission from the American Academy of Family Physicians.

- Do you find yourself counting or repeating things over and over?
- Do you repeatedly check things like locks, plugs, or burners?
- Do you arrange things in a specific order? How do you feel if someone messes them up? How much time do you spend a day doing this?
- How does it affect your day-to-day life? Have you stopped going to certain places or doing certain things?

Rating scales for OCD severity include the Yale-Brown Obsessive-Compulsive Scale (Y-BOCS), the Yale-Brown Obsessive Compulsive Scale – Second Edition, the Dimensional Yale-Brown Obsessive Compulsive Scale, and in children, the Children's Yale-Brown Obsessive Compulsive Scale (CY-BOCS). Although there are other instruments, the Y-BOCS and CY-BOCS are frequently used by clinicians.

Symptoms

The American Psychiatric Association's *Diagnostic and Statistical Manual of Mental Disorders, Fifth Edition, Text Revision* (*DSM-5-TR*) provides details for complete diagnostic criteria. Obsessions, compulsions, or both must be present. The obsessions or compulsions must be time-consuming (e.g., take up more than 1 hour a day) or cause significant distress or impairment in important areas of functioning such as social, occupational, or academic. Patients have varying degrees of insight about the accuracy of underlying beliefs about obsessive-compulsive symptoms.

Differential Diagnosis

Differential diagnoses for OCD are presented in Differential Diagnosis 71.1.

Differential Diagnosis 71.1 Obsessive-Compulsive Disorder

Disorder	Clinical Features	Distinguishing Characteristics
Body dysmorphic disorder	There is a preoccupation with perceived defects or flaws in physical appearance, leading to distress or impairment of function.	There is a preoccupation with perceived defect or overemphasis that is not significant to others. Repetitive behaviors related to the perceived physical defects are noted (checking, picking, etc.) or mental acts. Patients can have poor insight.

Continued

Differential Diagnosis 71.1 Obsessive-Compulsive Disorder—cont'd

Disorder	Clinical Features	Distinguishing Characteristics
Excoriation (skin-picking) disorder	Repeated skin picking results in skin lesions. The most common areas affected are the face, arms, and hands.	The compulsive behavior is limited to skin picking and is without the presence of obsessions
Hoarding disorder	Patients have persistent difficulty discarding or parting with objects, regardless of their actual value or importance, due to a perceived need to save them and distress associated with discarding them.	In OCD, the behaviors are unwanted and bothersome. Excessive attainment of objects is usually not present, unless there is a specific obsession for it. There is worsening over time, which is in contrast to OCD.
Trichotillomania (hairpulling) disorder	Trichotillomania entails recurrent hairpulling from any part of the body, resulting in hair loss. There are repeated attempts to stop or decrease the hairpulling.	The compulsive behavior is limited to hairpulling and is without the presence of obsessions.
Major depressive disorder	Depressed patients may have guilty or regretful ruminations, especially regarding the past. The ruminations are often mood congruent. They may not be experienced as intrusive.	Depression does not involve obsessions or compulsions. In depression, the content of the ruminations is often varied and related to an overall depressed outlook. Obsessions in OCD are also usually linked to compulsions.
Generalized anxiety disorder (GAD)	GAD involves persistent worry about real-life issues. It is also accompanied by physical symptoms of anxiety, such as muscle tension.	OCD obsessions do not constitute real-life worries and normally include content that is odd, irrational, or magical in nature. Obsessions in OCD are usually linked to compulsions.
Social anxiety disorder (social phobia)	In social anxiety disorder, the feared objects or situations are limited to social interactions. Avoidance is focused around reducing scrutiny by others.	Obsessions and corresponding compulsions are not present.
Illness anxiety disorder	There is a preoccupation with having or acquiring a serious illness, generally occurring in the absence of somatic symptoms. Patients have high anxiety about health. Patients also perform excessive health-related behaviors, such as checking their pulse.	In illness anxiety disorder, the fixations are consistent with one's sense of self and focused on having a disease. In OCD, the thoughts are intrusive, unwanted, and usually focused on fears of becoming diseased. Most patients with OCD will also have other obsessions and compulsions.
Pathological gambling/substance-use disorders/paraphilias	Gambling, substance use, and sexual behaviors can be performed repetitively by patients, not due to obsessions, but instead for pleasure. Typically, when the behaviors are given up, it is because of the consequences associated with them.	Compulsions are not pleasurable and are unwanted by the patient.
Obsessive-compulsive personality disorder (OCPD)	Despite the similarity in names, OCPD's defining feature is a pervasive pattern of preoccupation with orderliness, perfectionism, and a sense of control. OCPD begins by early adulthood and presents in a variety of contexts.	OCD requires the presence of obsessions and/or compulsions, whereas OCPD does not. OCPD is the preoccupation with orderliness, perfectionism, and control (mental, interpersonal) and limited flexibility, openness, and efficiency.
Autism spectrum disorder (ASD)	ASD patients exhibit deficits in social interactions and repetitive, restrictive ranges of interests or behaviors	OCD symptoms are common in ASD, but OCD differs from ASD behaviors because obsessions and compulsions are unwanted by patients. OCD patients do not have social impairment.
Tics	Tics are sudden, painless involuntary muscle contractions. They are preceded by localized, uncomfortable sensations, rather than thoughts, which are relieved by the tics.	Tics can be mistaken for compulsions. The behavior is considered a compulsion rather than a tic if, for example, it is performed a certain number of times, in a certain order, in response to an obsession, is intended to reduce anxiety or prevent harm, and/or is voluntary.

MANAGEMENT

In general, due to shame and embarrassment from obsessions and compulsions, a strong therapeutic alliance and building of trust with patients are crucial for ongoing care. Education should be provided regarding the chronicity of the diagnosis, treatment, and skills for self-management. Due to the increased risk, the clinician should assess for other comorbidities and risk for suicide. The patient and family/significant others should be involved and given appropriate education and resources, such as information from the International OCD Foundation (IOCDF) Web site.

Pharmacological Management

Selective serotonin reuptake inhibitors (SSRIs) are recommended as first-line pharmacological agents in the management of OCD in children and adults. Most SSRIs demonstrate efficacy; however, not all are approved by the U.S. Food and Drug Administration (FDA) for use in OCD. SSRIs have different indications for target symptoms, and therapeutic response may take longer in contrast with other disorders. SSRIs should be administered for up to 8 to 12 weeks to ensure that an appropriate time frame is instituted before augmentation or change in agent is considered. Generally, higher dosages and trials of longer duration (up to 12 weeks) of SSRIs are required to treat OCD, compared with depression or anxiety. SSRIs may be used for children and adolescents with OCD, considering the Black Box warning for SSRIs and possible increase in suicidal ideation. Although citalopram is noted as an effective treatment, cardiovascular side effects can occur at higher doses. Clomipramine, a tricyclic antidepressant, is well established as a treatment for OCD. However, the side effect profile makes use less favorable and includes risks for seizures, weight gain, and cardiovascular events. Additionally, serotonin-norepinephrine reuptake inhibitors have been used in the treatment of OCD (see Drugs Commonly Prescribed 71.1).

Drugs Commonly Prescribed 71.1: Obsessive-Complusive Disorder (OCD)

DRUG	INDICATION	ADVERSE REACTIONS AND PRESCRIBING CONSIDERATIONS
First-Line – Selective Serotonin Reuptake Inhibitors		
Fluoxetine (Prozac)	Obsessions, compulsions (ages 7 and up)	• Risk for sexual dysfunction; gastrointestinal effects (nausea, diarrhea, constipation, dry mouth, decreased appetite); CNS effects (insomnia or sedation, agitation, tremors, headache); sweating, bruising or bleeding; syndrome of inappropriate antidiuretic hormone secretion • Monitor seizures, induction of mania, serotonin syndrome, suicidal ideation. In children, monitor growth; long-term effects unknown in children • Usual dosage range: 20–60 mg/day
Fluvoxamine (Luvox, Luvox CR)	Obsessions, compulsions	• Risk for sexual dysfunction; gastrointestinal effects (nausea, diarrhea, constipation, dry mouth, decreased appetite); CNS effects (insomnia, sedation, agitation, tremors, headache, dizziness); sweating, bruising or bleeding; hyponatremia • Monitor seizures, induction of mania, serotonin syndrome, suicidal ideation. Long-term effects unknown in children • Usual dosage range: 50–200 mg/day; maximum dose: 300 mg/day
Sertraline (Zoloft)	Obsessions, compulsions	• Risk for sexual dysfunction; gastrointestinal effects (nausea, diarrhea, constipation, dry mouth, decreased appetite); CNS effects (insomnia or sedation, agitation, tremors, headache, dizziness); sweating, bruising or bleeding; hyponatremia; syndrome of inappropriate antidiuretic hormone secretion; hyponatremia or hypotension • Monitor seizures, induction of mania, serotonin syndrome, suicidal ideation. Long-term effects unknown in children • Usual dosage range: 50–200 mg/day; maximum dose: 200 mg/day
Paroxetine (Paxil, Paxil CR, Brisdelle)	Obsessions, compulsions	• Risk for sexual dysfunction; gastrointestinal effects (nausea, diarrhea, constipation, dry mouth, decreased appetite); CNS effects (insomnia or sedation, agitation, tremors, headache, dizziness); sweating, bruising or bleeding; hyponatremia; syndrome of inappropriate antidiuretic hormone secretion • Monitor weight, seizures, induction of mania, suicidal ideation, serotonin syndrome. Long-term effects unknown in children. Withdrawal effects may be noted more, compared with other SSRIs. • Usual dosage range: 20–50 mg/day

Continued

Drugs Commonly Prescribed 71.1—cont'd

DRUG	INDICATION	ADVERSE REACTIONS AND PRESCRIBING CONSIDERATIONS
Citalopram (Celexa, not FDA approved)	Obsessions, compulsions	• Risk for sexual dysfunction; gastrointestinal effects (nausea, diarrhea, constipation, dry mouth, decreased appetite); activation; CNS effects (insomnia or sedation, agitation, tremors, headache, dizziness); sweating, bruising or bleeding; hyponatremia; syndrome of inappropriate antidiuretic hormone secretion; QT prolongation • Monitor seizures, induction of mania, suicidal ideation, changes in the electrical activity of the heart, serotonin syndrome, hyponatremia (especially in older adults). Discontinue in patients with persistent QTc measurements greater than 500 ms. Long-term effects are unknown in children. • Usual dosage range: 20–40 mg/day (dependent on age); maximum dose: 40 mg/day. Doses higher than 20 mg/day should not be prescribed in patients older than 60 years.
Escitalopram (Lexapro, not FDA approved)	Obsessions, compulsions	• Risk for sexual dysfunction, gastrointestinal effects (nausea, diarrhea, constipation, dry mouth, decreased appetite); CNS effects (insomnia or sedation, agitation, tremors, headache, dizziness); sweating, bruising or bleeding; hyponatremia; syndrome of inappropriate antidiuretic hormone secretion; hyponatremia or hypotension • Monitor seizures, induction of mania, suicidal ideation, changes in the electrical activity of the heart, serotonin syndrome, hyponatremia (especially in older adults). Long-term effects are unknown in children. • Administration: 5–20 mg/day; some literature suggests a maximum dose up to 40 mg/day
Second-Line - Tricyclic Antidepressant (TCA)		
Clomipramine (Anafranil)	Obsessions, compulsions	• Risk for blurred vision, constipation, urinary retention, increased appetite, diarrhea, nausea, dry mouth, heartburn, unusual taste, weight gain (common), fatigue, weakness, dizziness, sedation, anxiety, headache, nervousness, restlessness, sexual dysfunction, sweating • Monitor seizures, paralytic ileus, hyperthermia, orthostatic hypotension, arrhythmias, tachycardia, QTc prolongation, hepatic failure, extrapyramidal symptoms, increase in intraocular pressure, induction of mania, suicidal ideation. Perform a baseline electrocardiogram in patients older than 50 years and in potentially at-risk patients. Take baseline weight, BMI, glucose, cholesterol, and monitor weight and BMI throughout treatment. Monitor serum potassium and magnesium for patients at risk for electrolyte disturbances and who are on diuretics. Death can occur with overdose. • Usual dosage: 100–200 mg/day

OCD can be refractory to treatment. Selection of adjunctive medication should take into consideration current drug treatment and comorbidities. Due to the higher doses and potential for refractory cases, it is recommended that pharmacological treatment be managed by a psychiatric mental health provider. Referral to a psychiatric mental health provider is also recommended for pediatric patients and complicated cases.

Nonpharmacological Management

CBT and ERP are regarded as first-line management, either alone or in combination with an SSRI. CBT can be delivered individually, in group sessions, or with families/significant others. CBT with ERP is one of the most effective treatments available for OCD. It is useful in both adult and pediatric populations. This technique involves repeatedly exposing patients to fear-producing stimuli in a hierarchical manner, beginning with less distressing situations and advancing to more feared encounters. During this time, patients are instructed to abstain from performing compulsive acts, thereby allowing the fear response provoked by the obsessions to reduce via habituation over time. Patients also learn that feared stimuli are not as dangerous as imagined, that anxiety is not hazardous, and that anxiety can be tolerated. In some cases, family therapy can be used to provide support to both the patient and family or significant others.

In severe cases, electroconvulsive therapy may be considered. Transcranial magnetic stimulation is another treatment recently approved by the FDA for treatment-resistant OCD (Voelker, 2018). Deep-brain stimulation (DBS) is FDA approved for OCD treatment as a last resort therapy on humanitarian grounds. The patient's OCD must be considered chronic, severe, and treatment resistant. DBS is applied to the internal capsule and/or the adjacent ventral striatal region.

FOLLOW-UP AND REFERRAL

The primary care practitioner should address medical concerns coexisting in the patient with OCD and be mindful of medication side effects or interactions. Suicide risk should be assessed at the time of diagnosis and regularly throughout the course of illness. When a medication is started, the patient should be seen weekly for the first month, and a response should be seen between 4 and 12 weeks. It may take 8 to 16 weeks to see maximum therapeutic effects. The practitioner should monitor for response, suicidality, adverse effects, and serotonin syndrome. Symptom severity can be assessed, using the aforementioned rating scales. OCD can be difficult to treat. Because each patient responds to treatment modalities quite differently and there can be variable response, it is recommended that care be provided in coordination with mental health specialists. Patients should be followed regularly, with attention paid to health maintenance issues. Referrals may be necessary for consequences of compulsive behaviors, such as referral to a dermatologist for skin excoriation or for dental care due to excessive cleaning.

Patient Education: Obsessive-Compulsive Disorder

Education of the patient, family/support people, and parents of the child with OCD is important. Web sites provide information and links to support groups. Being educated and informed about the condition helps with treatment compliance.

BODY DYSMORPHIC DISORDER

Body dysmorphic disorder (BDD) is among the obsessive-compulsive and related disorders. Its hallmark is a preoccupation with one or more perceived physical defects or flaws, often not visible or only slightly so to others. This is coupled with excessive repetitive behaviors, such as attempting to check, fix, conceal, or obtain reassurance about the perceived deformities. The course is often chronic. BDD causes significant distress and may result in decreased quality of life. It is associated with high rates of suicidality. Like OCD, it is often not recognized in clinical settings and may be misdiagnosed as OCD.

EPIDEMIOLOGY AND CAUSES

BDD is estimated to affect about 2% of the community population, and it is about as common as OCD. BDD develops mostly in adolescence and is very unlikely to appear in adults older than 40 years. Males and females are affected equally. Patients with BDD can develop suicidal ideation. Rates of suicide attempts and completed suicide appear noticeably increased, compared with the general population or individuals with OCD.

In terms of psychiatric comorbidity, about 75% have a history of MDD, which is the most common comorbid disorder. BDD usually precedes MDD in onset. Approximately 40% of patients with BDD have a history of social anxiety disorder, and almost one-third have past or current OCD. Substance-use disorders occur in 30% to 50%. Around 20% of males with muscle dysmorphia abuse anabolic steroids to increase muscle bulk.

PATHOPHYSIOLOGY

The pathophysiology of BDD is not clearly understood at this time. Results of twin studies in BDD indicate that genetic factors account for about 42% to 44% of the variance in symptoms, with the remaining difference accounted for by environmental influences. First-degree relatives of patients with BDD are thought to have a fourfold higher likelihood of developing BDD. BDD is also more common in first-degree relatives of patients with OCD. Data from visual processing studies suggest that patients with BDD actually perceive faces and objects differently than those without BDD. Patients may also have deficits with executive function (i.e., complex thinking). Neurotransmitter dysfunction, especially that of serotonin, may also play a role in BDD. Regarding the environment, a range of factors has been suggested that may influence the development of BDD, including childhood abuse, childhood neglect, and bullying.

CLINICAL PRESENTATION

Because patients feel ashamed of themselves and their bodies, they rarely report symptoms of BDD to primary care providers. Instead, patients may present with symptoms of depression or anxiety and request referrals to dermatologists, plastic surgeons, orthodontists, or maxillofacial surgeons.

Regarding symptom profiles, female patients with BDD are more likely to be concerned about their weight, breasts, hips, legs, and body hair. They may frequently check mirrors, pick their skin, or camouflage their bodies to obscure disliked areas. Many female patients have comorbid eating disorders. Male patients may be consumed by their perception of having an "undersized" body, may exhibit muscle dysmorphia, obsession over thinning hair, or disappointment with genital size. Male patients may have a comorbid substance-use disorder.

DIAGNOSTIC REASONING

Helpful screening questions include the following:

- Do you think there is something wrong with the way you look? Does everybody notice?
- Do you think you look unattractive, ugly, or even hideous?

- How long do you spend looking in the mirror or on grooming?
- Have you stopped going out? Do you feel isolated?

Screening tools that can be used for BDD include the Body Dysmorphic Disorder Questionnaire (BDDQ) and the Body Image Disturbance Questionnaire (BIDQ). The Yale-Brown Obsessive Compulsive Scale (BDD-YBOCS) is considered the standard to measure symptoms; however, it can be lengthier to use and require more training than other tools.

Symptoms

Diagnostic criteria are available in the *DSM-5-TR*. Individuals must have a preoccupation with at least one perceived defect or flaw in physical appearance that cannot be observed or is barely observable by others. Additionally, individuals must have engaged in repetitive behaviors (e.g., mirror checking, excessive grooming) or mental acts (e.g., excessive comparison to others) in response to their appearance concerns. Finally, the appearance concerns must cause significant distress or impairment in functioning. Muscle dysmorphia, or the preoccupation that one's build is too small or not muscular or lean enough, is a form of BDD that occurs almost exclusively in males. Insight varies among patients and can be good to absent. Delusional beliefs can be present in which the person is completely convinced their view of their appearance is accurate and not distorted. Thus, it is important for the clinician to rule out other disorders when establishing a diagnosis.

Differential Diagnosis

BDD deviates from normal concerns about appearance in several respects. In BDD, worries about appearance are excessive, and patients engage in time-consuming behaviors because of them. The symptoms also cause substantial distress and/or diminished functioning. Plainly visible physical defects, excluding lesions from skin picking, should not be diagnosed as BDD. The preoccupations and repetitive behaviors of BDD differ from OCD obsessions and compulsions by centering on a perceived defect in appearance. Patients with OCD are typically aware of their illness, whereas those with BDD can often lack insight. Many individuals with BDD even have delusional (false and fixed) beliefs about their appearance. This is diagnosed as BDD, not as a delusional disorder.

MANAGEMENT

Pharmacological Management

There are no FDA-approved treatments for BDD. However, high-dose SSRIs are considered the first-line pharmacological treatment for BDD. Agents prescribed have included fluoxetine, citalopram, escitalopram, fluvoxamine, and clomipramine. Dosages are typically higher than those used for depression, and the treatment is longer to prevent relapse. It is important to note that at the higher doses used for BDD, citalopram can be associated with cardiovascular side effects.

Nonpharmacological Management

BDD-focused CBT has been shown to be effective for many patients. Techniques employed include cognitive restructuring, ERP, and other specific approaches tailored to BDD, such as perceptual retraining.

FOLLOW-UP AND REFERRAL

Due to the complexity of treating BDD, referral to psychiatry and therapy is recommended. Assessment for suicide risk and appropriate follow-up are imperative for patients diagnosed with BDD. Because poor or absent insight is common in BDD, it can be difficult to engage and retain patients in treatment.

> **Patient Education: Body Dysmorphic Disorder**
>
> Educating patients and family/support people about BDD is vital to enhance diagnosis, increase support, and improve treatment compliance. The IOCDF (website: https://iocdf.org/?_ga=2.167023289.681147211.1652273905-766020909.1652273905) provides information and links to other resources, including support groups, on its Web site.

HOARDING DISORDER

In the past, hoarding was considered a subtype of OCD or a symptom of obsessive-compulsive personality disorder, but it is now recognized as a distinct diagnostic entity. Patients usually do not present complaining of hoarding but rather may be brought to clinical attention by a family member or friend who is distressed by the individual's many possessions and the state of their living environment.

EPIDEMIOLOGY AND CAUSES

Hoarding disorder (HD) is estimated to affect about 2.5% of the general population. Males and females are affected equally. Its prevalence is greater in unmarried or divorced individuals. The course can start early in life and often increases in severity as the individual becomes older. Most patients with HD have comorbid psychiatric illnesses such as post-traumatic stress disorder, generalized anxiety disorder, OCD, or MDD. In some individuals, symptoms of attention deficit-hyperactivity disorder (ADHD) are present.

PATHOPHYSIOLOGY

The pathophysiology of HD is unknown. Animal studies suggest that the dopaminergic system—as well as the subcortical limbic structures and the ventromedial prefrontal cortex—is involved in hoarding behavior. Neuroimaging studies suggest correlations between hoarding symptoms and specific brain regions (e.g., structural abnormalities in the prefrontal regions); however, results have been inconsistent, and most research has focused on hoarding as a subtype of OCD. Much more research is needed to further delineate the pathophysiology of HD.

CLINICAL PRESENTATION

The most prominent feature of HD is a cluttered home due to a patient's difficulty discarding commonplace items such as magazines, plastic bags, empty containers, newspapers, or clothes. Some individuals collect animals. Patients often lack insight into their hoarding behaviors, as well as the effects on their level of functioning and on their home environment, and they can be resistant to change. Patients can also have delusional beliefs regarding items. HD can result in hazardous living conditions. Different infections can present, related to adverse environmental conditions. Due to clutter, patients, especially older adults, are at risk for falls and possible fractures or trauma. Blocked windows and exits can make fires deadly.

DIAGNOSTIC REASONING

Symptoms

The essential features of HD are a persistent, perceived need to save items and difficulty discarding or parting with possessions, which results in accumulation of clutter and congested living areas such that they cannot be used for their intended purposes (e.g., inability to walk between rooms because piles of books and papers block most of the hallways). HD is diagnosed when the behavior results in significant impairment in functioning, including the provision of a safe environment. Diagnostic criteria for HD are available in the *DSM-5-TR.*

The saved items may have little perceived value to others. Reasons given for needing to save or having difficulty discarding or parting with possession may include the following:

- Perceived future utility of the items
- Perceived aesthetic value of the items
- A strong sentimental attachment to the possessions
- A sense of responsibility for the possessions
- A desire to avoid being wasteful
- Fearfulness of losing important information

Level of insight may vary, and some individuals do not report distress and are significantly distressed by any attempts to discard or clear the possessions. Procrastination, avoidance, indecisiveness, difficulty organizing, and perfectionism are commonplace.

Assessment scales, such as the Structured Interview for Hoarding Disorder (SIHD) and the Hoarding Rating Scale, are available to help with the diagnosis of HD. Activities of Daily Living for Hoarding (ADL-H) and the Saving Inventory—Revised are additional scales that can assist in determining the extent to which an individual is hoarding.

Differential Diagnosis

Other physical or psychiatric conditions must be excluded before a diagnosis of HD is made. HD is not diagnosed if the symptoms are a consequence of obsessions or compulsions. In OCD, the excessive acquisition of objects is usually not present, unless the individual has a specific obsession for it, and then it functions as a compulsion, as the individual does not have a genuine desire to possess the items. In OCD, the behavior is also generally undesirable and tormenting. The individual derives no pleasure from it.

MANAGEMENT

Nonpharmacological Management

CBT with ERP, as used in OCD, is generally not effective for HD. Instead, a specialized CBT approach for hoarding is employed. It involves office sessions and home visits, which are often the best way to begin the process of discarding possessions. Weekly meetings spanning 6 months or more may be needed, depending on the extent of the hoarding and the severity of the patient's resistance to discarding objects. Follow-up home visits are conducted to ensure that the individual is following through with the cleaning and discarding process.

Pharmacological Management

Pharmacological studies of SSRIs have had mixed results. There is some research indicating that venlafaxine and paroxetine may have efficacy in treating HD. An approach is to use CBT, pharmacological management, and support from family and significant others/support persons.

FOLLOW-UP AND REFERRAL

Due to the complex nature of the treatment for HD, most patients should be referred to specialists. However, primary care practitioners should address medical concerns in patients, discuss home safety, and be mindful of medication side effects or interactions, if they are prescribed. Continued follow-up visits are vital to help prevent relapse.

Patient Education: Hoarding Disorder

Patient and family/support person education about HD is critical to enhance diagnosis, increase support, improve home safety, and encourage treatment compliance. Motivational interviewing may help individuals with HD to connect their values and goals with their behaviors and identify ways to change behaviors to align with their values and goals. Support groups are beneficial in helping individuals with HD to connect to others in a shame-free environment. Skills training and CBT can be helpful with organization, problem-solving, decision making, and cognitive restructuring.

Helping someone with HD can be frustrating, and it produces feelings of hopelessness and anger, which can then lead to conflict. Educating and reminding family/support people about the importance of harm reduction and effective communication such as motivational interviewing techniques are key. The primary care provider may refer patients and family/support people to mental health professionals who specialize in HD and provide unique interventions, such as Family-as-Motivators training.

REFERENCES

General

American Psychiatric Association. Obsessive-Compulsive and Related Disorders. Diagnostic and statistical manual of mental disorders. 5th ed. Arlington, VA: American Psychiatric Association; 2013.

Sadock B, Sadock V, Ruiz P. (2014). Kaplan and Sadock's Synopsis of Psychiatry. (11th Ed.) Philadelphia PA Lippincott.

Stahl SM. (2020). Stahl's essential psychopharmacology: Prescriber's guide, 7th Ed. Cambridge: Cambridge University Press.

Body Dysmorphic Disorder

American Psychiatric Association. Obsessive-Compulsive and Related Disorders. Diagnostic and statistical manual of mental disorders. 5th ed. Arlington, VA: American Psychiatric Association; 2013.

Beilharz F, Castle DJ, Grace S, et al. A systematic review of visual processing and associated treatments in body dysmorphic disorder. Acta Psychiatr Scand. 2017 Jul;136(1):16-36. doi: 10.1111/acps.12705. Epub 2017 Feb 12. PMID: 28190269.

Buhlmann U, Teachman BA, Naumann E, et al. The meaning of beauty: Implicit and explicit self-esteem and attractiveness beliefs in body dysmorphic disorder. J Anxiety Disord. 2009;23(5): 694–702.

Corazza O, Simonato P, Demetrovics Z, et al. The emergence of Exercise Addiction, Body Dysmorphic Disorder, and other image-related psychopathological correlates in fitness settings: A cross sectional study. PLoS One. 2019 Apr 3;14(4):e0213060. doi: 10.1371/journal.pone.0213060. PMID: 30943200; PMCID: PMC6447162.

Greenberg JL, Mothi SS, Wilhelm S. Cognitive-behavioral therapy for adolescent body dysmorphic disorder: A pilot study. Behav Ther. 2016;47(2):213–224.

Hong K, Nezgovorova V, Hollander E. (2018). New perspectives in the treatment of body dysmorphic disorder. F1000Research, 7, 361. https://doi.org/10.12688/f1000research.13700.1

Hong K, Nezgovorova V, Uzunova G, et al. (2019). Pharmacological Treatment of Body Dysmorphic Disorder. Current neuropharmacology, 17(8), 697–702. https://doi.org/10.2174/1570159X16666180426153940

Kaplan RA, Rossell SL, Enticott PG, et al. Own-body perception in body dysmorphic disorder. Cogn Neuropsychiatry. 2013;18(6): 594-614. doi: 10.1080/13546805.2012.758878. Epub 2013 Feb 26. PMID: 23441837.

Krebs G, Fernández de la Cruz L, Mataix-Cols D. Recent advances in understanding and managing body dysmorphic disorder. Evid Based Mental Health. 2017;20:71–75.

Nordsletten AE, Fernández de la Cruz L, Pertusa A, et al. The Structured Interview for Hoarding Disorder (SIHD): Development, usage and further validation. J Obsessive Compuls Relat Disord. 2013;2:346–350.

Phillips KA. Body dysmorphic disorder: Clinical aspects and relationship to obsessive-compulsive disorder. Focus. 2015;13(2):162–174.

Singh AR, Veale D. (2019). Understanding and treating body dysmorphic disorder. Indian journal of psychiatry, 61(Suppl 1), S131–S135. https://doi.org/10.4103/psychiatry.IndianJPsychiatry_528_18

Veale D, Gledhill LJ, Christodoulou P, et al. Body dysmorphic disorder in different settings: A systematic review and estimated weighted prevalence. Body Image. 2016;18:168–186.

Wilhelm S, Greenberg JL, Rosenfield E, et al. The Body Dysmorphic Disorder Symptom Scale: Development and preliminary validation of a self-report scale of symptom specific dysfunction. Body Image. 2016;17:82–87.

Wilhelm S, Phillips KA, Didie E, et al. Modular cognitive-behavioral therapy for body dysmorphic disorder: A randomized controlled trial. *Behav Ther.* 2014;45(3):314–327.

Hoarding Disorder

Brakoulias V, Eslick GD, Starcevic V. A meta-analysis of the response of pathological hoarding to pharmacotherapy. Psychiatry Res. 2015;229(1–2):272–276.

Bratiotis C, Steketee G. Hoarding disorder: Models, interventions, and efficacy. Focus. 2015;13(2):175–183.

Mataix-Cols D. Hoarding Disorder. The New England Journal of Medicine 370.21 (2014): 2023–2030.

Mataix-Cols D, Pertusa A, Snowdon J. Neuropsychological and neural correlates of hoarding: a practice-friendly review. J Clin Psychol. 2011 May;67(5):467-76. doi: 10.1002/jclp.20791. Epub 2011 Feb 23. PMID: 21351104.

Mathews CA, Delucchi K, Cath DC, et al. Partitioning the etiology of hoarding and obsessive-compulsive symptoms. Psychol Med. 2014;44:2867–2876.

Nakao T, Kanba S. Pathophysiology and treatment of hoarding disorder. Psychiatry Clin Neurosci. 2019 Jul;73(7):370-375. doi: 10.1111/pcn.12853. Epub 2019 May 20. PMID: 31021515.

Nordsletten AE, Reichenberg A, Hatch SL, et al. Epidemiology of hoarding disorder. Br J Psychiatry. 2013;203:445–452.

Piacentino D, Pasquini M, Cappelletti S, et al. (2019). Pharmacotherapy for Hoarding Disorder: How did the Picture Change since its Excision from OCD? Current neuropharmacology, 17(8), 808–815. https://doi.org/10.2174/1570159X17666190124153048

Saxena S, Sumner J. Venlafaxine extended-release treatment of hoarding disorder. Int Clin Psychopharmacol. 2014;29(5):266–273.

Williams M, Viscusi JA. Hoarding disorder and a systematic review of treatment with cognitive behavioral therapy. *Cogn Behav Ther.* 2016;45(2):93–110.

Obsessive-Compulsive and Related Disorders

Alonso P, Cuadras D, Gabriëls L, et al. Deep brain stimulation for obsessive-compulsive disorder: A meta-analysis of treatment outcome and predictors of response. PLoS One. 2015;10(7):e0133591.

American Psychiatric Association. Practice guideline for obsessive compulsive disorder. http://www.guideline.gov/search/search.aspx?term=obsessive+compulsive. Published November 2007 (reaffirmed 2012).

Cocchi L, Zalesky A, Nott Z, et al. Transcranial magnetic stimulation in obsessive-compulsive disorder: A focus on network mechanisms and state dependence. Neuroimage Clin. 2018 May 23;19: 661-674. doi: 10.1016/j.nicl.2018.05.029. PMID: 30023172; PMCID: PMC6047114.

Davide P, Andrea P, Martina O, et al. (2020). The impact of the COVID-19 pandemic on patients with OCD: Effects of contamination symptoms and remission state before the quarantine in a preliminary naturalistic study. Psychiatry research, 291, 113213. https://doi.org/10.1016/j.psychres.2020.113213

Del Casale A, Kotzalidis GD, Rapinesi C, et al. (2019). Current Psychopharmacology of Obsessive-Compulsive Spectrum Disorders. Current neuropharmacology, 17(8), 668–671. https://doi.org/10.2174/1570159X17081907091448 20

Fenske JN, Petersen K. (2015). Obsessive-Compulsive Disorder: Diagnosis and Management. American Family Physician, 92(10), 896-903. Retrieved February 19, 2021, from https://www.aafp.org/afp/2015/1115/p896.html

Fineberg NA, Brown A, Reghunandanan S, et al. (2012). Evidence-based pharmacotherapy of obsessive-compulsive disorder. International Journal of Neuropsychopharmacology, 15(8), p. 1173–1191, Retrieved February 23, 2021, from https://doi.org/10.1017/S1461145711001829

Goodman WK, Grice DE, Lapidus KA, et al. Obsessive-compulsive disorder. Psychiatr Clin North Am. 2014 Sep;37(3):257-267. doi: 10.1016/j.psc.2014.06.004. Epub 2014 Jul 23. PMID: 25150561.

Grant JE. Obsessive–compulsive disorder. N. Engl J Med. 2014;371:646–653.

Guglielmi V, Vulink NC, Denys D, et al. Obsessive-compulsive disorder and female reproductive cycle events: Results from the OCD and reproduction collaborative study. Depress Anxiety. 2014;31(12):979–987.

Janardhan Reddy YC, Sundar AS, Narayanaswamy JC, et al. (2017). Clinical practice guidelines for Obsessive-Compulsive Disorder. Indian journal of psychiatry, 59(Suppl 1), S74–S90. https://doi.org/10.4103/0019-5545.196976

Jelinek L, Moritz S, Miegel F, et al. (2021). Obsessive-compulsive disorder during COVID-19: Turning a problem into an opportunity? Journal of anxiety disorders, 77, 102329. https://doi.org/10.1016/j.janxdis.2020.102329.

Khosravani V, Aardema F, Samimi Ardestani SM, et al. (2021). The impact of the coronavirus pandemic on specific symptom dimensions and severity in OCD: A comparison before and during COVID-19 in the context of stress responses. Journal of obsessive-compulsive and related disorders, 29, 100626. https://doi.org/10.1016/j.jocrd.2021.100626

Kim SW, Dysken MW, Kuskowski M. The Symptom Checklist—90: Obsessive-compulsive subscale: A reliability and validity study. Psychiatry Res. 1992;41:37–44.

Kim SW, Dysken MW, Kuskowski M. The Yale-Brown Obsessive—Compulsive Scale: A reliability and validity study. Psychiatry Res. 1990;34:99–106.

Koran LM, Simpson HB. (2013). Guideline Watch (March 2013): Practice Guideline for the Treatment of Patients with Obsessive-Compulsive Disorder. American Psychiatric Association. Downloaded from https://psychiatryonline.org/pb/assets/raw/sitewide/practice_guidelines/guidelines/ocd-watch.pdf

Krebs, G, Heyman I. (2015). Obsessive-compulsive disorder in children and adolescents. Archives of disease in childhood, 100(5), 495–499. https://doi.org/10.1136/archdischild-2014-306934

Mathes BM, Morabito DM, Schmidt NB. Epidemiological and Clinical Gender Differences in OCD. Curr Psychiatry Rep. 2019 Apr 23;21(5):36. doi: 10.1007/s11920-019-1015-2. PMID: 31016410.

Orlovska S, Vestergaard CH, Bech BH, et al. Association of streptococcal throat infection with mental disorders: Testing key aspects of the PANDAS hypothesis in a nationwide study. JAMA Psychiatry. 2017;74:740–746.

Pallanti S, Grassi G, Sarrecchia ED, et al. Obsessive-compulsive disorder comorbidity: Clinical assessment and therapeutic implications. Front Psychiatry. 2011;2:70.

Palmer E, Fuller M. Obsessive-compulsive disorder in pediatrics and adolescents: Review of treatment and future directions. Mental Health Clinician 1 June 2013; 2 (12): 406–411. doi: https://doi.org/10.9740/mhc.n155509

Rapp AM, Bergman RL, Piacentini J, et al. Evidence-Based Assessment of Obsessive-Compulsive Disorder. J Cent Nerv Syst Dis. 2016;8: 13-29. Published 2016 Aug 21. doi:10.4137/JCNSD.S38359

Shavitt RG, de Mathis MA, Oki F, et al. Phenomenology of OCD: Lessons from a large multicenter study and implications for ICD-11. J Psychiatr Res. 2014;57:141–148.

Storch EA, Sheu JC, Guzick AG, et al. (2021). Impact of the COVID-19 pandemic on exposure and response prevention outcomes in adults and youth with obsessive-compulsive disorder. Psychiatry research, 295, 113597. https://doi.org/10.1016/j.psychres.2020.113597

U.S. Food and Drug Administration. (12/15/2017). FDA Drug Safety Communication: Revised recommendations for Celexa (citalopram hydrobromide) related to a potential risk of abnormal heart rhythms with high doses. Retrieved February 26, 2021, from https://www.fda.gov/drugs/drug-safety-and-availability/fda-drug-safety-communication-revised-recommendations-celexa-citalopram-hydrobromide-related.

Veale D, Miles S, Smallcombe N, et al. Atypical antipsychotic augmentation in SSRI treatment refractory obsessive-compulsive disorder: A systematic review and meta-analysis. *BMC Psychiatry.* 2014;14:317.

Veale D, Roberts A. Obsessive-compulsive disorder. BMJ. 2014;348:g2183.

Voelker R. (2018). Brain Stimulation Approved for Obsessive-Compulsive Disorder. *JAMA*, 320(11), 1098. https://doi.org/10.1001/jama.2018.13301

RESOURCES

Body Dysmorphic Disorder

American Family Physician
https://www.aafp.org/afp/2008/0715/p217.html

Anxiety and Depression Association of America
https://adaa.org/understanding-anxiety/related-illnesses/other-related-conditions/body-dysmorphic-disorder-bdd#

Body Dysmorphic Disorder Foundation
http://bddfoundation.org/

Cleveland Clinic
https://my.clevelandclinic.org/health/diseases/9888-body-dysmorphic-disorder

John Hopkins Medicine
https://www.hopkinsmedicine.org/healthlibrary/conditions/mental_health_disorders/body_dysmorphic_disorder_134,216

Massachusetts General Hospital Research Institute
https://www.massgeneral.org/psychiatry/about/patient-education/ocd

Mayo Clinic
https://www.mayoclinic.org/diseases-conditions/body-dysmorphic-disorder/symptoms-causes/syc-20353938

Semel Institute for Neuroscience and Human Behavior
https://www.semel.ucla.edu/bdd

U.S. National Library of Medicine National Institute of Health
https://www.ncbi.nlm.nih.gov/pmc/articles/PMC3181960/

World Psychiatry
https://www.ncbi.nlm.nih.gov/pmc/articles/PMC1414653/

Hoarding Disorder

American Psychiatric Association
https://www.psychiatry.org/Patients-Families/Hoarding-Disorderhttps://www.psychiatry.org/patients-families/hoarding-disorder/patient-story

https://www.psychiatry.org/patients-families/hoarding-disorder/what-is-hoarding-disorder

International OCD Foundation
https://hoarding.iocdf.org/

Obsessive Compulsive Disorder (OCD)

American Academy of Family Physicians
https://familydoctor.org/condition/obsessive-compulsive-disorder/

Anxiety and Depression Association of America
https://adaa.org/understanding-anxiety/obsessive-compulsive-disorder-ocd

International OCD Foundation
https://iocdf.org/

Mayo Clinic
https://www.mayoclinic.org/diseases-conditions/obsessivecompulsive-disorder/symptoms-causes/syc-20354432

National Alliance on Mental Illness
https://www.nami.org/Learn-More/Mental-Health-Conditions/Obsessive-Compulsive-Disorder

National Institute of Mental Health
https://www.nimh.nih.gov/health/topics/obsessive-compulsive-disorder-ocd/index.shtml

---

Chapter 72

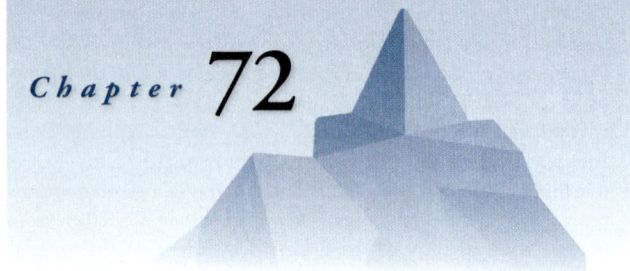

Other Psychiatric Disorders

Karen Jennings Mathis, PhD, APRN-CNP, PMHNP-BC, FAED

Meredith Kells, PhD, RN, CPNP

FEEDING AND EATING DISORDERS

OVERVIEW

Eating disorders are a group of chronic psychiatric illnesses related to food consumption and are associated with a significant impact on physical and mental health and social functioning. Eating disorders have high rates of psychiatric comorbidity as well as the highest mortality rates among psychiatric illnesses. The *Diagnostic and Statistical Manual of Mental Disorders, Fifth Edition, Text Revision* (*DSM-5-TR*) outlines the diagnostic criteria for six disorders including pica, rumination disorder, avoidant/restrictive food intake disorder (ARFID), anorexia nervosa (AN), bulimia nervosa (BN), and binge-eating disorder (BED). Additionally, the category of other specified feeding or eating disorder (OSFED) captures individuals who exhibit feeding- or eating-related impairment but fail to meet full criteria for one of the six disorders outlined earlier. For the purposes of this review to encompass most common eating disorders found in primary care, this chapter will not cover pica or rumination disorder.

AN is a restrictive illness in which individuals fail to maintain expected body weight and struggle with significant body shape or weight disturbance. AN is further categorized into either restrictive or binge-eating/purging subtypes, such that individuals with AN may engage in binge-eating and/or purging behaviors. This disease is associated with medical complications across body systems, mostly because of sustained malnutrition. BN is characterized by binge eating followed by methods to prevent associated weight gain, known as *compensatory mechanisms,* as well as body image disturbances. The key factor in classifying a binge-eating episode versus overeating is loss of control, in that individuals who experience binge eating report that they are unable to stop. BED is recurrent binge-eating episodes without the use of compensatory mechanisms; and individuals with BED describe high levels of distress related to their binge eating. ARFID is characterized by the inability to maintain adequate nutrition unrelated to body image disturbance. Most commonly occurring in childhood, those with ARFID may have sensory concerns or experienced an adverse eating-related event such as choking or vomiting. Refer to the *DSM-5-TR* for detailed diagnostic criteria.

EPIDEMIOLOGY

Among U.S. adults, lifetime prevalence of AN ranges from 0.6% to 0.8%. BN affects 0.3% to 1.3% of U.S. adults in their lifetime, and BED has a lifetime prevalence of 0.9% to 2.8%. As one of the newest additions to feeding and eating disorders in the *DSM-5-TR*, there is limited data on the prevalence of ARFID. However, among pediatric samples, prevalence of ARFID ranged from 1.5% to 23% depending on the setting (emergency department, gastroenterology clinic, eating disorder program). The combined prevalence of OSFED types (atypical AN, subthreshold BN and BED, and purging disorder) has been reported as high as 13.1%.

AN and BN affect more females and typically begin in adolescence and young adulthood (peak incidence at ages 15 to 19 years for AN and 16 to 20 years for BN). In contrast, a higher percentage of males are diagnosed with ARFID and BED, although there remains a female predominance. ARFID is more commonly diagnosed in younger children and early adolescence, and BED more often in early adulthood (mean age of onset 25.4 years). Historically, screening and assessment for eating disorders was largely focused on young, thin, cisgender, white females. However, eating disorders are prevalent across all sexual orientations, gender identifications, and racial and ethnic groups, and may vary in presentation. For example, transgender and gay youth may have higher rates of eating disorder symptoms and body dysmorphia than their cisgender or heterosexual peers. Research suggests that differences in prevalence rates of eating disorders between white and non-white populations may reflect access to care and provider bias more than differential rates. Recognition across diverse groups is imperative for screening, access to care, and culturally sensitive treatment.

Comorbid psychiatric disorders are common across the spectrum of eating disorders. In one large national survey, 56.2% of individuals with AN, 94.5% with BN, and 78.9% with BED met criteria for at least one other psychiatric disorder. Anxiety disorders, mood disorders, and substance-use disorders are the most often reported co-occurring psychiatric illnesses in AN, BN, and BED. Likewise, individuals with ARFID are more likely than the general population to be diagnosed with comorbid anxiety disorders; however, unlike other eating disorders, ARFID is less likely to be associated with mood disorders.

Eating disorders are associated with high rates of self-harm. As many as one-third of individuals with eating disorders report nonsuicidal self-injury, with higher rates among those who experience more body dissatisfaction. Up to 43% of individuals diagnosed with AN, BN, or BED endorse suicidal ideation. Nonfatal suicide attempts are seen across the diagnostic spectrum, most often in individuals diagnosed with AN binge/purge subtype and BN. Death by suicide is found in 1 in 5 individuals who die because of AN, and individuals with AN have been found to be 31 times more likely to die by suicide than age-matched peers. Death by suicide is also higher in those with BN and BED compared with the general population.

Although a comprehensive definition of recovery from eating disorders has yet to be established, recovery is thought to entail resolution of eating disorder behaviors (e.g., restriction, binge eating), normalized eating patterns, improvement in health outcomes (weight gain or halted weight loss), and improvement in psychological components such as body image disturbance. Given the differing definitions of recovery, it is difficult to establish recovery rates.

PATHOPHYSIOLOGY

The cause of eating disorders is complex and multifactorial, although evidence suggests interaction of environmental factors and genetic predisposition results in a disease state. Studies in twins and adopted individuals have confirmed the role of underlying genetic influence; however, the specific interplay between genetics and environment has yet to be fully established.

Western societal ideals interwoven into media exposure is thought to be a factor. The "thin ideal," or an overly romanticized thin body type, is a common theme portrayed in Western cultures. Greater internalization of the thin ideal and thin expectancies or thoughts of a better life because of thinness are associated with higher likelihood of eating disorder pathology. This is particularly true for individuals who identify as female in Western cultures where the thin ideal is more normative for female bodies than for their male counterparts. Greater media exposure to the thin ideal is associated with worsening of these concepts and increased pathology. Dieting in childhood or adolescence is thought to be a key predictor in development of an eating disorder later. Furthermore, environmental stressors such as acculturation, discrimination, and racism, may contribute to the onset and maintenance of eating disorder behaviors.

Several personality traits and neurocognitive processes may be implicated in eating disorder etiology. Specifically, negative emotionality and neuroticism, perfectionism, and cognitive flexibility have been suggested as risk factors for restrictive eating disorders; whereas impulsivity, negative urgency, and inhibitory control have been implicated in binge-eating and purging predominant disorders. Other environmental factors such as parenting style, parental personality, and history of childhood abuse have been identified as correlates of eating disorder etiology. Finally, biological factors such as neurotransmitter (serotonin, dopamine) disturbances and hormonal regulation may play a role in the onset of eating disorders.

CLINICAL PRESENTATION

Primary care settings are particularly equipped to screen for eating disorders with access to growth trajectory and nutritional and activity history. Early recognition and intervention are critical, as timely identification and care provision are associated with improved outcomes. Eating disorders should be suspected in any individuals who present with rapid weight loss, failure to gain weight or difficulty gaining weight, body image disturbance, obsessive food practices or thoughts about weight or shape, and growth stunting or pubertal delay in children and adolescents. Sudden changes in eating or exercise patterns are also notable for further investigation. Eating disorders occur across the weight spectrum and in individuals of diverse backgrounds; thus, they should be considered regardless of age, race, ethnicity, or weight. ARFID should be investigated in cases where individuals present with poor growth trajectory, nutritional deficiencies, use of nutritional supplements to maintain adequate nutrition, or significant sensory or aversive behaviors regarding foods.

The primary care provider should take responsibility for initial assessment and the initial coordination of care, including the determination of the need for emergency medical or psychiatric assessment (see Box 72.1). Where management is shared between providers (e.g., pediatrics, adolescent/internal medicine, psychiatry), there should be a clear agreement in writing as to who will be monitoring the patient on a regular basis. It should be shared with the patient and their support system to promote clarity on responsibilities related to care.

It is important to remember that organ systems throughout the body are affected by rapid weight loss, malnutrition, and weight loss behaviors, regardless of absolute weight or body mass index (BMI). Symptoms resulting from malnutrition or disordered eating may trigger further evaluation, and individuals or concerned parents or significant others may present to care for these symptoms primarily rather than concerns regarding eating. Examples of these symptoms include dizziness or fainting, abdominal pain, amenorrhea, and others. Alternatively, providers may note telltale signs of disordered eating or weight loss behaviors on comprehensive examination, such as abrasions on the knuckles because of self-induced vomiting (Russell's sign), lanugo, or parotid gland swelling. Vital sign changes such as bradycardia, hypotension, and orthostatic changes may indicate malnutrition. Physical signs and symptoms of eating disorders can be found in Table 72.1

A thorough history should be undertaken including past medical history, family history of eating disorders and other psychiatric illnesses, social history incorporating recent changes and or/stressors, substance use, physical or sexual abuse, changes in mood or behaviors. Review of systems with specific focus on signs and symptoms of malnutrition (e.g., dizziness, cold intolerance, menstrual irregularities) should be performed, along with complete nutritional history with 24-hour dietary recall, changes in eating habits, change in weight and duration of changes, and exercise. Box 72.2 outlines the assessment components.

Box 72.1 Criteria for Medical Hospitalization

- Less than or equal to 75% median body mass index for age and height
- Electrolyte disturbance (hypokalemia, hypophosphatemia, hyponatremia)
- Electrocardiogram (ECG) abnormalities (QT prolongation)
- Heart rate fewer than 50 beats/min at rest
- Blood pressure less than 90/45 mm Hg
- Orthostatic vital sign changes: increase in pulse by more than 20 beats/min or decrease blood pressure by 20 mm Hg after 2 minutes laying followed by 2 minutes standing
- Failure of outpatient treatment
- Acute food refusal (24 hours)
- Inability to secure appropriate psychiatric placement
- Dehydration

Source: Society for Adolescent Health and Medicine, Golden NH, Katzman DK, Sawyer SM, Ornstein RM, Rome ES, Garber AK, Kohn M, Kreipe RE. Position Paper of the Society for Adolescent Health and Medicine: medical management of restrictive eating disorders in adolescents and young adults. *J Adolesc Health.* 2015;56(1):121-125. https://doi.org/10.1016/j.jadohealth.2014.10.259

Box 72.2 Assessment Components for Suspected Eating Disorder

- Complete history—medical, family, social
- Nutrition history—changes in eating habits, duration of weight loss, 24-hour dietary recall
- Menstrual history—age at menarche, frequency and duration of menstrual periods
- Complete physical examination
- Height, weight, body mass index, and growth charts
- Vital signs including orthostatic heart rate and blood pressure (lying for 2 minutes followed by standing for 2 minutes)
- Laboratory studies—complete blood count, electrolytes, blood urea nitrogen, creatinine, liver function tests, thyroid function tests, celiac panel, serum glucose
- Urinalysis
- Electrocardiogram

Sources: Academy for Eating Disorders. *Eating Disorders: A Guide to Medical Care*, 4th ed. Reston, VA: Academy for Eating Disorders, 2021; Lock J, La Via MC, American Academy of Child and Adolescent Psychiatry. Practice parameter for the assessment and treatment of children & adolescents with eating disorders. *J Am Acad Child Adolesc Psychiatry.* 2015;54(5):412-425; American Psychiatric Association. *Diagnostic and Statistical Manual of Mental Disorders, Text Revision.* 5th ed. Arlington, VA: American Psychiatric Association, 2022.

blame, shame, and opening lines of communication to foster successful treatment. Providers should also review the serious effects of disordered eating behaviors and malnutrition to frame the importance of sufficient weight restoration and symptom resolution. Guidance on available resources, including programs, multidisciplinary care providers, and insurance considerations should be included in conversations with patients and families. See Box 72.4 for steps that the primary care provider can take to provide support to patients and families/support persons.

SLEEP–WAKE DISORDERS

Description and classification of sleep–wake disorders have been expanded in *DSM-5-TR* to reflect the important diagnostic overlay of medical conditions that affect normal sleep patterns. Of particular importance to primary care are insomnia disorder, restless legs syndrome (RLS), obstructive sleep apnea-hypopnea (OSAH) (see Chapter 29), and substance/medication-induced disorder (see Chapter 67). Insomnia disorder is presented in detail because it is an underpinning of each of these disorders. The criteria and important contributing factors for insomnia disorder and RLS are discussed.

INSOMNIA DISORDER

Insomnia disorder, or difficulty sleeping, is a common problem, yet it is one that is etiologically complex. It is defined as difficulty falling or staying asleep, waking up too early in the morning, or any combination of these. Insomnia disorder can be situational, persistent, or recurrent.

> **Box 72.4 Education and Referral for Patients With Eating Disorders**
>
> - Provide information on eating disorder programs.
> - Review nutritional information and refer to a registered dietitian.
> - Provide education on health effects of disordered behaviors and malnutrition.
> - Reinforce the long-term nature of these disorders and the need for follow-up and treatment.
> - Point out that under stress, regressive behaviors can occur.
> - Involve the family in symptoms to identify and report.
> - Encourage regular dental care for those who purge.
> - Teach strategies for managing self-destructive behaviors in ways that do not reinforce them.
> - Provide referral for individual or family therapy.
>
> Source: Vitousek KB, Orimoto L. Cognitive-behavioral models of anorexia nervosa, bulimia nervosa, and obesity. In: Kendall P, Dobson KS, eds. *Psychopathology and Cognition*. San Diego, CA: Academic Press; 1993:191.

EPIDEMIOLOGY AND CAUSES

Lifetime prevalence of sleep disorders is about one-third of the U.S. adult population. Each year, up to 40% of adults report difficulty with sleep and about 17% of adults report the problem to be serious. It is estimated that 10% to 15% of the primary care population report daytime impairment because of insomnia and that 6% to 10% meet criteria for insomnia disorder. Difficulty maintaining sleep is the most common complaint.

Females appear to be slightly more affected than males, which may be attributed to hormonal variations during the menstrual cycle and menopause that may cause disruptions to sleep. Although onset is more common in young adulthood, insomnia complaints are more common among middle-aged and older adults. The increased prevalence with older adults can partially be explained by increased likelihood of chronic health-related conditions including chronic pain and medication regimens that may cause sleep disruptions.

Acute insomnia may be precipitated by physical or emotional discomfort. Examples include pain; acute illness; and environmental disturbances such as noise, light, and temperature. Sleeping at a time that is inconsistent with daily biological (circadian) rhythms because of plane travel across time zones (jet lag) or shift work may also precipitate acute insomnia. Pain may contribute to wakefulness; indeed, often the question "Does the pain awaken you at night?" is an important piece of information in determining the severity of pain.

PATHOPHYSIOLOGY

Normal sleep is a periodic state of rest accompanied by varying degrees of unconsciousness and relative inactivity. It is normally an easily reversible, regular, recurrent state. The functions of sleep are restorative and hemostatic, critical for normal thermoregulation and energy conservation. Sleep disturbance may be an early symptom of impending mental illness.

Two physiological states compose sleep: non–rapid eye movement (NREM) and rapid eye movement (REM) sleep. In NREM sleep, most physiological functions are markedly lower than in wakefulness, although there may be episodic, involuntary body movements during NREM sleep. In contrast, REM sleep is characterized by physiological activity levels similar to those in wakefulness and a high level of brain activity and is sometimes called *paradoxical sleep*. NREM sleep is composed of stages 1 through 4, with stages 3 and 4 being deep sleep. Typically, NREM sleep is punctuated with an REM cycle every 90 to 100 minutes during the night. The first REM period tends to be the shortest, lasting less than 10 minutes; later REM periods may last 15 to 40 minutes each. Most REM periods occur in the last third of the night; most stage 4 sleep occurs in the first third of the night.

These sleep patterns change over the course of a person's life. In young adulthood, REM comprises about 25% of sleep, and NREM approximately 75%. These figures remain fairly constant in normal sleep, although there is a reduction in both slow-wave sleep and REM sleep in older persons. NREM sleep increases after exercise and starvation and is thus thought to be associated with satisfying metabolic needs.

Daily variations in a variety of physiological functions affecting the endocrine, thermoregulatory, cardiac, pulmonary, renal, gastrointestinal, and neurobehavioral systems, as well as sleep–wake cycles, are governed by the 24-hour circadian rhythm in humans. The timing and internal architecture of sleep are coupled directly to the output of the endogenous circadian pacemaker. Misalignment of the output of the endogenous circadian pacemaker with the desired sleep–wake cycle can, therefore, induce insomnia, decrease alertness, and impair performance of shift workers, and accounts for the phenomenon of jet lag. Sleep deprivation for prolonged periods can lead to hallucinations, ego disorganization, and delusions, and REM-deprived patients may exhibit irritability and lethargy.

CLINICAL PRESENTATION

Insomnia may not be the chief reason for an office visit. It may be detected, however, by incorporating sleep-related questions into the general review of systems. Direct inquiry is important because patients with chronic insomnia often have never discussed their problem or have lived with it for so long that they think nothing can be done about it. The primary consequences of acute insomnia are sleepiness, negative mood, and impairment of performance, with severity related to the amount of disrupted sleep over several nights. Patients with chronic insomnia frequently complain of fatigue, mood changes (e.g., depression, irritability), difficulty concentrating, and impaired daytime functioning.

The assessment should include questions about sleep, as well as questions about daytime functioning, where the full effects of altered sleep are manifested. The amount of sleep required for each individual to subjectively feel refreshed varies markedly. Although the ability to maintain sleep alters with age, the individual's need for sleep does not change significantly. The patient's medical history and comorbidities are other important parameters that should be documented. Many medical problems, such as gastroesophageal reflux disease, worsen at night because they may be aggravated by recumbency.

Focus on History: Insomnia Disorder

Questions to ask:

- How has the person been sleeping recently?
- How long has the person had difficulty sleeping?
- Does the person have any underlying psychiatric or medical conditions?
- Is the person's sleep environment conducive to sleep? For example, are there any problems that would make sleeping difficult, such as noise, temperature, light, or space?
- Does the person employed in shift work or odd hours?
- What does the person do in the evenings and to prepare for sleep?
- What time does the person usually go to bed? How long does it take for the person to fall asleep?
- What time does the person wake up? Get out of bed? Are these hours the same on weekdays versus weekend days?
- Does the person travel frequently?
- Does the person use caffeine, alcohol, drugs, or tobacco? If so, how much, and when was the last use?
- Does the person have difficulty staying awake or report dozing off during normal daily activities?
- Does the person report any daytime consequences of having difficulties sleeping?
- Does the person take daytime naps?
- Does the person (or their partner) report:
    - Loud snoring, gasping, or breathing stoppage at night? (sleep apnea)
    - Legs or arms jerking during sleep? (periodic limb movement)
    - Creeping, crawling, or uncomfortable feelings in the legs that are relieved by moving them? (RLS)

It may also be helpful for the patient to keep a sleep diary over 2 to 4 weeks. A sleep diary is a useful tool to track when and under what conditions the patient sleeps, and may help reveal the underlying problem. The sleep diary also helps further define the nature of the sleep problem, as patients should document what time they got into bed, what they did until they fell asleep, what time they recall falling asleep, any nighttime awakenings (including ability to fall back asleep), and what time they awoke in the morning. A diary or record of exercise and physical activity as well as dietary intake and substance use may also prove helpful. Consider screening for insomnia as part of regular patient care.

DIAGNOSTIC REASONING

Symptoms

Refer to the *DSM-5-TR* for complete diagnostic criteria for insomnia disorder. Symptoms should occur at least 3 nights per week, for at least 3 months, and must cause significant distress or impairment in areas of functioning. Difficulty sleeping cannot be an effect of a medication or drug. Common symptoms include the following:

- Poor quality or quantity of sleep (difficulty falling asleep, difficulty staying asleep, and/or early morning awakening with inability to return to sleep), despite sufficient opportunity for sleep.

- Fatigue or daytime sleepiness
- Preoccupation with sleep
- Distress because of inability to fall and/or stay asleep
- Decreased energy
- Mood disturbances

Collateral information from family or bed partners can be helpful to corroborate the diagnosis. Excessive daytime sleepiness can be assessed using the Epworth Sleepiness Scale. Polysomnography (sleep study) cannot distinguish those with insomnia from those without, and is indicated to further assess for sleep apnea, periodic limb movements, or a REM sleep behavior disorder.

Differential Diagnosis

It is necessary to rule out potential underlying causes of insomnia. Boxes 72.5 and 72.6 list medical and psychiatric causes of and contributors to insomnia. A thorough medication history must be taken, including all over-the-counter drugs such as decongestants and cough syrups that contain decongestants, which act as stimulants. In addition, a complete history of herbal remedies used, especially teas that may contain caffeine or ginseng, and a variety of other central nervous system stimulants, should be obtained. The patient also should be screened for any illicit drug and alcohol use.

MANAGEMENT

Pharmacological Management

The choice to use medication in the short term for insomnia should be based on shared decision making and the benefits, adverse effects, and financial costs should be discussed. Advantages of the sedative-hypnotics are that they hasten sleep onset, decrease the number of nighttime awakenings, increase total amount of sleep time (varies with medication duration of action), and make sleep more refreshing. Disadvantages include alterations in sleep architecture over time by decreasing slow-wave sleep and REM sleep, residual sedation, psychomotor and cognitive impairment, psychological dependence in vulnerable individuals, and rebound insomnia.

Medications indicated for insomnia disorders include benzodiazepines, benzodiazepine-receptor agonist medications, melatonin receptor agonists, and orexin receptor antagonist medication (see Drugs Commonly Prescribed 72.1). The advantages and disadvantages of a given duration of action must be assessed based on the patient's needs. All agents have some potential for abuse and dependence, thus, they are classified as Schedule IV by the Drug Enforcement Administration. Benzodiazepines should be avoided especially in older adults because of risk of falls and rebound insomnia. Clinical trials suggest that sleep can improve without medication based on patients who received a placebo reporting improvement in sleep. In sleep studies, a placebo is not "inactive" treatment because study participants must adhere to nonpharmacological regimens (such as going to bed and getting up at regular hours, not napping, avoiding caffeine and alcohol) that are recognized as effective remedies for insomnia.

Other agents often used to treat insomnia include antihistamines (diphenhydramine), antidepressants (trazodone, mirtazapine, doxepin), antipsychotics (quetiapine, olanzapine), melatonin, and the melatonin receptor agonist ramelteon. Of these, only doxepin and ramelteon are approved by the FDA for insomnia, with limited evidence for the others, despite their widespread use. Depression is the most common comorbid psychiatric diagnosis with chronic insomnia; however, antidepressants should be used most often in the setting of comorbid depression. Concurrent treatment of insomnia disorder and an underlying psychiatric comorbidity may result in greater improvements for the patient.

Nonpharmacological Management

CBT is the first-line treatment option for individuals with insomnia disorder. Insomnia can be a chronic, lifelong illness, and given the chronic nature of this problem,

---

Box 72.5 Medical Causes of and Contributors to Insomnia

- Painful conditions, such as arthritis and muscle cramps
- Fibromyalgia
- Delirium or dementia ("sundowning")
- Gastroesophageal reflux disease or duodenal ulcers
- Conditions causing shortness of breath
- Thyroid disease
- Obesity (also associated with sleep apnea)
- Substance use, intoxication, or withdrawal
- Pregnancy or postpartum
- Nocturia
- Side effect of a medication

Source: Gutierrez C, Brady P. Obstructive sleep apnea: a diagnostic and treatment guide. J Fam Pract. 2013;62(10):565-572.

Box 72.6 Psychiatric Causes of and Contributors to Insomnia

- Major depressive disorder
- Generalized anxiety disorder
- Manic episode
- Psychotic illness, such as schizophrenia
- Traumatic events precipitating acute insomnia
- Post-traumatic stress disorder leading to hyperarousal
- Poor sleep hygiene
- Other sleep–wake disorders (OSAH, RLS)

Source: Roth T. Comorbid insomnia: current directions and future challenges. Am J Manag Care. 2009;15:S6-S13.

Drugs Commonly Prescribed 72.1: Sedatives and Hypnotics

DRUG	INDICATION	ADVERSE REACTIONS AND PRESCRIBING CONSIDERATIONS
Benzodiazepines		
All Benzodiazepines		• Category IV controlled substance. • Risk of anterograde amnesia, CNS depression, paradoxical reactions, sedation, memory deficits, ataxia. • Use caution with narrow-angle glaucoma. • Association with falls and injury in older adults. • Use caution with patients who are depressed, have substance-use disorder, or have impaired hepatic or renal function. • Most contraindicated in obstructive sleep apnea. • Many drug–drug interactions (CYP pathways). • Withdrawal symptoms with abrupt discontinuation. The onset of withdrawal symptoms is usually seen on the first day without drug and lasts 5–7 days—slow taper. • Treatment longer than 4 months should be reevaluated to determine the patient's need for the drug. • Avoid valerian, St. John's wort, kava kava, gotu kola, alcohol, and other sedatives. • Potential severe allergic reactions (anaphylaxis, angioedema). • Risk of complex sleep-related behaviors, which may include driving, cooking, or eating food while asleep and making phone calls while asleep.
Estazolam (Prosom)	Insomnia, short-term	• Intermediate acting. • No active metabolites.
Flurazepam (Dalmane)	Insomnia, short-term	• Long acting. • Avoid in older adults and debilitated patients. • Active metabolites with extended half-lives may lead to delayed accumulation and adverse effects.
Temazepam (Restoril)	Insomnia, short-term	• Intermediate acting. • Administer 30 minutes before bedtime. • Lack of active metabolites—excellent option for older adults.
Triazolam (Halcion)	Insomnia, short-term	• Short acting. • In older patients, higher incidence of CNS adverse reactions; not a drug of first choice.
Quazepam (Doral)	Insomnia, short-term	• Long-acting with half-life of 39 hours. • Risk of daytime sedation and fatigue. • May prevent withdrawal symptoms when stopped.
Benzodiazepine-Receptor Agonists ("Z-drugs")		
		• Category IV controlled substance. • Risk of daytime sedation, anterograde amnesia, rebound insomnia. • Less anxiolytic properties than the benzodiazepines. • All patients should be advised of residual morning effects and of complex sleep-related behaviors (sleep-driving, having sex, cooking and eating food while asleep, making phone calls). • All patients should be advised to get at least 4 hours of sleep after taking a short-acting agent and at least 7 hours of sleep with a long-acting agent.
Eszopiclone (Lunesta)	Insomnia, long-term	• Half-life of 6 hours; good for sleep initiation and maintenance. • Advise to get 8 or more hours of sleep. • No hangover effect; may have metallic taste. • Risk of headache, dizziness, and somnolence. • Potentiates CNS depressants.

Drugs Commonly Prescribed 72.1: Sedatives and Hypnotics—cont'd

DRUG	INDICATION	ADVERSE REACTIONS AND PRESCRIBING CONSIDERATIONS
Zaleplon (Sonata)	Insomnia, short-term	• Short half-life, about 1 hour. • Good for patients that have difficulty falling asleep, not for sleep maintenance. • Advise to get at least 4 hours of sleep. • Dosage adjustment for hepatic impairment.
Zolpidem (Ambien)	Insomnia, short-term	• Half-life 1.4–2.4 hours. • Good for patients who have difficulty with falling asleep. • Risk of CNS depression, headache, dizziness, and somnolence. • Take with liquid—food can delay absorption. • No known rebound insomnia or hangover effect. • Reduced dosage in females and geriatric populations.
Zolpidem CR (Ambien CR [extended release])	Insomnia, long-term	• Half-life 1.4–2.4 hours, released over a longer duration. • Risk of headache, dizziness, and somnolence. • Sleep may be impaired after discontinuation. • Abuse potential low. • Reduced dosage in females and geriatric populations. • Complex sleep-related behaviors, which may include driving, cooking, and eating food while asleep, and making phone calls while asleep.
Melatonin Receptor Agonist		
Ramelteon (Rozerem)	Insomnia	• Indicated to promote sleep onset. • Peak concentrations within 1 hour if fasting, avoid high-fat meal. • No withdrawal or rebound insomnia. • Does not affect REM sleep. • May affect testosterone and prolactin levels. • Risk of somnolence, dizziness, fatigue, nausea, and exacerbated insomnia. • Monitor liver transaminases.
Orexin Receptor Antagonist		
Suvorexant (Belsomra)	Insomnia	• Indicated to promote sleep onset and/or sleep maintenance. • Half-life: 12 hours • Risk for drowsiness, dizziness, headaches, unusual dreams, dry mouth, cough, diarrhea, anxiety, heart palpitations and increased heart rate, psychomotor hyperactivity; more serious: temporary inability to move or speak up to a few minutes while going to sleep or waking up, temporary leg weakness during the day or night • Complex sleep-related behaviors including but not limited to driving cars, preparing and eating food, having sex, making phone calls • Works faster if taken on an empty stomach
Antihistamine		
Diphenhydramine (Benadryl)	Insomnia, short-term use less than 2 weeks	• Over the counter. • Many patients have used previously for other indications (suggests tolerance). • May have next-day sedation, dry mouth, decreased cognitive function. • Potentiates CNS depression. • Caution with asthma, other respiratory disorders; glaucoma; hyperthyroidism. • Can have a paradoxical effect in children and older adults.

Abbreviations: CNS, central nervous system; CYP, cytochrome P-450; REM, rapid eye movement.

long-term treatment is often advisable. There are various methods of providing CBT, including in-person, telephone, web-based, and self-help books, and can occur in an individual or group setting. Primary care providers should review sleep hygiene strategies with the patient and their support persons, as well as identify any barriers to implementation (see Box 72.7). Mindfulness and relaxation techniques can also be helpful in promoting sleep. Coexisting medical, psychiatric, or pain conditions should be adequately treated.

Reassurance and supportive counseling are essential; insomnia is not a complaint that should be taken lightly. For example, issues of caregiving for young children or older adults living in the home may be a part of the clinical picture. Again, lifestyle changes and situational support may be more effective than pharmacological measures for patients. Sleep parameters can be reviewed and reemphasized several times during return visits before resorting to pharmacological measures (see Table 72.2).

FOLLOW-UP AND REFERRAL

Transient insomnia may become chronic insomnia. For this reason, treatment is essential. Insomnia disorder can resolve with patience, support, and treatment. Patients should be followed until their insomnia has resolved. Referral may be needed for supportive counseling and CBT.

Box 72.7 Sleep Hygiene Strategies

- Maintain a regular sleep and wake schedule, 7 days a week.
- Eat regular meals every day.
- Develop a relaxing bedtime routine.
- Limit amount of liquid consumed in the evening.
- Limit amount of caffeine consumed later in the day.
- Avoid tobacco and alcohol late in the day.
- Avoid daytime naps.
- Exercise regularly.
- Limit exposure to bright lights in the evening; keep the bedroom as dark as possible; limit use of screens (phones, tablets, computers, TV) while in bed.
- The bed should be used for sleeping and sex only; avoid doing other activities in bed that require wakefulness (e.g., reading) so that the bed is associated with sleepiness.
- Turn any clocks to face away from the bed to avoid constant checking of the time.
- If not asleep after 20 minutes, get out of bed and engage in a quiet activity, such as reading, outside of the bedroom before reattempting to fall asleep.

Source: Sateia MJ, et al. Clinical practice guideline for the pharmacological treatment of chronic insomnia in adults: an American Academy of Sleep Medicine Clinical Practice Guideline. *J Clin Sleep Med.* 2017;13(2):307-349.

TABLE 72.2 Advanced Practice Nursing Interventions for Insomnia

Behavioral treatment	Relaxation therapy (progressive muscle relaxation therapy), autogenic training, electromyogram, biofeedback.
Sleep restriction therapy	Poor sleepers often increase their time in bed. Sleep restriction therapy curtails this time. For example, if a person reports sleeping only 5 hours per night, they should be counseled to stay in bed only 5 hours per night. As sleep improves, increase time in bed in 15- to 30-minute intervals. It works best to alter bedtime and keep rising time constant. Do not reduce sleep to less than 5 hours per night.
Stimulus control therapy	Functions on premise that insomnia is a conditioned response to temporal (bedtime) and environmental (bed/bedroom) cues. Objective is to reassociate the bed and bedroom with rapid sleep onset. Stimulus control therapy counsels: (1) Go to bed only when sleepy. (2) Use the bed only for sleep. (3) Get out of bed and go into another room when awake; go back into the bedroom only when sleepy. (4) Maintain a regular rise time, regardless of sleep deprivation during the night. (5) Avoid daytime napping.
Cognitive therapy	Identify dysfunctional ideas about sleep and replace them with more functional approaches; e.g., 8 hours of sleep is not necessary for everyone; insomnia and less sleep does not have to destroy one's life. This approach helps minimize anticipatory anxiety around sleep.
Exercise	Regular physical activity will assist with sleep. Advise the patient not to exercise too close to bedtime.
Massage	Weekly massage may assist with relaxation.
Reassurance and support	Active listening and patience; encourage expression of feelings, especially if stress is a component of the insomnia.

> **Patient Education: Insomnia Disorder**
>
> All patients and support persons should receive education about sleep hygiene and be encouraged to practice good sleep hygiene as outlined in Box 72.7. Patients and supports should be educated about using the bed for sleep and sexual activity only (no television, phones, tablets, reading). The entire environmental situation of the patient and their support persons should be assessed. Are there caregiver issues involved, and can external and additional support be provided or arranged? Is there a need for diversionary activities, or a need to increase the individual's physical activity level? If sleep apnea is suspected, a polysomnogram should be ordered.

RESTLESS LEGS SYNDROME

RLS is a neurological, sensorimotor condition that is typified by uncomfortable sensations in the lower extremities, such as burning, tingling, crawling, or itching, and an uncontrollable desire to move the legs, with associated sleep disturbance. Relief of symptoms is usually obtained once the individual moves their legs.

EPIDEMIOLOGY AND CAUSES

Prevalence rates of RLS vary from 2% to 7%, with females up to twice as likely as males to have RLS. The prevalence of RLS during pregnancy is up to three times greater than the general population and tends to peak during the third trimester and resolve after delivery. The prevalence of RLS increases with age, with onset typically occurring in the second or third decade of life. Those with familial RLS typically have an earlier age of onset and more progressive disease course. There is significant comorbidity with periodic limb movements of sleep, with up to 90% of individuals with RLS demonstrating periodic limb movements on polysomnogram.

PATHOPHYSIOLOGY

Dysfunction of dopaminergic systems is implicated in the pathophysiology of RLS, as evidenced by improvement of symptoms when dopaminergic drugs are administered. Because low iron levels can contribute to symptoms, patients should have iron levels assessed and appropriate supplementation should be implemented when necessary.

CLINICAL PRESENTATION

Symptoms occur when the patient is at rest and often worsen at night when attempting to initiate sleep. Patients often present complaining of an uncontrollable urge to move their legs that impairs their ability to initiate and maintain sleep. This leads to excessive daytime sleepiness and impaired functioning the next day. Bed partners may also notice the excessive movement during sleep. Many patients will report a family history of RLS.

DIAGNOSTIC REASONING

The diagnosis is based primarily on patient self-report, although a complete neurological examination and appropriate laboratory testing can help to rule out other possible diagnoses. In addition, patients should be referred for polysomnography.

Symptoms

Diagnosis is based on *DSM-5-TR* criteria for RLS; please refer to *DSM-5-TR* for complete diagnostic criteria. Symptoms should occur at least 3 days per week and for at least 3 months. They include:

- An urge to move the legs
- An uncomfortable sensation in the legs
- The urge or discomfort begins or worsens when at rest, at night, or attempting to sleep
- The urge or discomfort is relieved by movement

Differential Diagnosis

RLS needs to be differentiated from leg cramps or positional discomfort. Important medical differential diagnoses are arthritis, peripheral neuropathy, peripheral vascular disease/ischemia, numbness, and radiculopathy, which may be associated with pain or discomfort in the extremities, but less often with the urge to move the extremities. Psychiatric comorbidity includes depressive disorders, anxiety disorders, panic disorder, and post-traumatic stress disorder.

MANAGEMENT

The management of RLS includes reinforcing sleep hygiene strategies listed in Box 72.7. Other interventions that can help include baths, whirlpool, massage, and exercise. The American Academy of Sleep Medicine indicates that there is good evidence for use of the FDA-approved dopaminergic agents pramipexole (0.125 to 0.5 mg 2 to 3 hours before bedtime) and ropinirole (0.25 to 4.0 mg 1 to 3 hours before bedtime) in the treatment of RLS when there is moderate to severe impairment in sleep or daytime functioning.

FOLLOW-UP AND REFERRAL

All patients should be encouraged to maintain good sleep hygiene and keep a sleep diary. Patients with suspected RLS should be referred for polysomnography. Patients who have complex sleep difficulties or are nonresponsive to first-line agents should be referred to a sleep specialist. In addition, patients with additional psychiatric comorbidity should be referred to a mental health provider for further assessment and management.

Patient Education: Restless Legs Syndrome

The patient and support persons need to be reassured and counseled regarding the transient nature of RLS, including lifestyle changes that can assist with sleep. Again, appropriate sleep hygiene strategies should be emphasized. Care should be used with pharmacological therapies because of the possible adverse effects and their potential for drug dependency, especially in older patients.

REFERENCES

Eating Disorders

American Psychiatric Association. *Diagnostic and Statistical Manual of Mental Disorders.* 5th ed. Washington, DC; 2013.

Andrés-Pepiñá S, Plana MT, Flamarique I, Romero S, Borràs R, Julià L, Gárriz M, Castro-Fornieles J. Long-term outcome and psychiatric comorbidity of adolescent-onset anorexia nervosa. *Clin Child Psychol Psychiatry.* 2020;25(1):33-44. https://doi.org/10.1177/1359104519827629

Arcelus J, Mitchell AJ, Wales J, Nielsen S. Mortality rates in patients with anorexia nervosa and other eating disorders. A meta-analysis of 36 studies. *Arch Gen Psychiatry.* 2011;68(7):724-731. https://doi.org/10.1001/archgenpsychiatry.2011.74

Bardone-Cone AM, Hunt RA, Watson HJ. An overview of conceptualizations of eating disorder recovery, recent findings, and future directions. *Curr Psychiatry Rep.* 2018;20(9):79. https://doi.org/10.1007/s11920-018-0932-9

Bohrer BK, Foye U, Jewell T. Recovery as a process: exploring definitions of recovery in the context of eating-disorder-related social media forums. *Int J Eat Disord.* 2020;53(8):1219-1223. doi:10.1002/eat.23218

Brigham KS, Manzo LD, Eddy KT, Thomas JJ. Evaluation and treatment of avoidant/restrictive food intake disorder (ARFID) in adolescents. *Curr Pediatr Rep.* 2018;6(2):107-113. https://doi.org/10.1007/s40124-018-0162-y

Burke NL, Schaefer LM, Hazzard VM, Rodgers RF. Where identities converge: the importance of intersectionality in eating disorders research. *Int J Eat Disord.* 2020;53:1605-1609. https://doi.org/10.1002/eat.23371

Campbell K, Peebles R. Eating disorders in children and adolescents: state of the art review. *Pediatrics,* 2014;134(3):582-592. https://doi.org/10.1542/peds.2014-0194

Costa CB, Xandre PE, Mathis KJ. Treating individuals with eating disorders: Part 2. *J Psychosoc Nurs Ment Health Svc.* 2020 Apr;58(4): 9-15. doi: 10.3928/02793695-20200310-01.

Crow SJ. Pharmacologic treatment of eating disorders. *Psychiatric Clin North Am.* 2019;42(2):253-262. https://doi.org/10.1016/j.psc.2019.01.007

Culbert KM, Racine SE, Klump KL. Research review: What we have learned about the causes of eating disorders—a synthesis of sociocultural, psychological, and biological research. *J Child Psychol Psychiatry Allied Disc.* 2015;56(11):1141-1164. https://doi.org/10.1111/jcpp.12441

Davis H, Attia E. Pharmacotherapy of eating disorders. *Curr Opin Psychiatry.* 2017;30(6):452-457. https://doi.org/10.1097/YCO.0000000000000358

Derenne J. The role of higher levels of care for eating disorders in youth. *Child Adolesc Psychiatr Clin North Am.* 2019;28(4):573-582. doi:10.1016/j.chc.2019.05.006

Fogarty S, Smith CA, Hay P. The role of complementary and alternative medicine in the treatment of eating disorders: a systematic review. *Eat Behav.* 2016;21:179-188. https://doi.org/10.1016/j.eatbeh.2016.03.002

Forman SF, Grodin LF, Graham DA, Sylvester CJ, Rosen DS, Kapphahn CJ, Callahan ST, Sigel EJ, Bravender T, Peebles R, Romano M, Rome ES, Fisher M, Malizio JB, Mammel KA, Hergenroeder AC, Buckelew SM, Golden NH, Woods ER, National Eating Disorder QI Collaborative. An eleven site national quality improvement evaluation of adolescent medicine-based eating disorder programs: predictors of weight outcomes at one year and risk adjustment analyses. *J Adolesc Health.* 2011;49(6): 594-600. https://doi.org/10.1016/j.jadohealth.2011.04.023

Galmiche M, Déchelotte P, Lambert G, Tavolacci MP. Prevalence of eating disorders over the 2000-2018 period: a systematic literature review. *Am J Clin Nutr.* 2019;109(5):1402-1413. https://doi.org./10.1093/ajcn/nqy342

Gorrell S, Loeb KL, Le Grange D. Family-based treatment of eating disorders: a narrative review. *Psychiatr Clin North Am.* 2019;42(2):193-204. https://doi.org/10.1016/j.psc.2019.01.004

Gorrell S, Trainor C, Le Grange D. The impact of urbanization on risk for eating disorders. *Curr Opin Psychiatry.* 2019;32(3):242-247. doi:10.1097/YCO.0000000000000497

Heruc G, Hurst K, Casey A, et al. ANZAED eating disorder treatment principles and general clinical practice and training standards. *J Eat Disord* 2020;8:63. https://doi.org/10.1186/s40337-020-00341-0

Katzman DK, Norris ML, Zucker N. Avoidant restrictive food intake disorder. *Psychiatr Clin North Am.* 2019;42(1):45-57. doi:10.1016/j.psc.2018.10.003

Kornstein SG. Epidemiology and recognition of binge-eating disorder in psychiatry and primary care. *J Clin Psychiatry.* 2017;78 (Suppl 1):3-8. doi: 10.4088/JCP.sh16003su1c.01

Mandelli L, Arminio A, Atti AR, De Ronchi D. Suicide attempts in eating disorder subtypes: a meta-analysis of the literature employing DSM-IV, DSM-5, or ICD-10 diagnostic criteria. *Psychol Med.* 2019; 49(8):1237-1249. https://doi.org 10.1017/S0033291718003549

Mathis KJ, Costa CB, Xandre PE. Treating individuals with eating disorders: Part 1. *J Psychosoc Nurs Ment Health Serv.* 2020 Mar 1;58(3): 7-13. doi: 10.3928/02793695-20200217-02. PMID: 32129875.

McClain Z, Peebles R. Body image and eating disorders among lesbian, gay, bisexual, and transgender youth. *Pediatr Clin North Am.* 2016;63(6):1079-1090. doi: 10.1016/j.pcl.2016.07.008

Mikhail ME, Klump KL. A virtual issue highlighting eating disorders in people of black/African and Indigenous heritage. *Int J Eat Disord.* 2021;54:459-467. https://doi.org/10.1002/eat.23402

Norris ML, Spettigue WJ, Katzman DK. (2016). Update on eating disorders: current perspectives on avoidant/restrictive food intake disorder in children and youth. *Neuropsychiatr Dis Treat.* 2016;12:213-218. https://doi.org/10.2147/NDT.S82538

Pérez S, Marco JH, Cañabate M. Non-suicidal self-injury in patients with eating disorders: prevalence, forms, functions, and body image correlates. *Compr Psychiatr.* 2018;84:32-38. https://doi.org/10.1016/j.comppsych.2018.04.003

Qian J, Wu Y, Liu F, et al. An update on the prevalence of eating disorders in the general population: a systematic review and meta-analysis [published online ahead of print, 2021 Apr 8]. *Eat Weight Disord.* 2021;10.1007/s40519-021-01162-z. doi:10.1007/s40519-021-01162-z

Richmond TK, Woolverton GA, Mammel K, et al. How do you define recovery? A qualitative study of patients with eating disorders, their parents, and clinicians. *Int J Eat Disord.* 2020;53(8):1209-1218. doi:10.1002/eat.23294

Rodgers RF. The role of the "Healthy Weight" discourse in body image and eating concerns: an extension of sociocultural theory. *Eat Behav.* 2016;22:194-198. doi:10.1016/j.eatbeh.2016.06.004

Rodgers RF, Berry R, Franko DL. Eating disorders in ethnic minorities: an update. *Curr Psychiatry Rep.* 2018;20(10):90. Published 2018 Aug 29. doi:10.1007/s11920-018-0938-3

Sangvai D. Eating disorders in the primary care setting. *Prim Care.* 2016;43(2):301-312. https://doi.org/10.1016/j.pop.2016.01.007

Smink FR, van Hoeken D, Hoek HW. Epidemiology of eating disorders: incidence, prevalence and mortality rates. *Curr Psychiatr Rep.* 2012;14(4):406-414. https://doi.org/10.1007/s11920-012-0282-y

Smink FR, van Hoeken D, Hoek HW. Epidemiology, course, and outcome of eating disorders. *Curr Opin Psychiatr.* 2013;26(6):543-548. https://doi.org/10.1097/YCO.0b013e328365a24f

Smith AR, Zuromski KL, Dodd DR. Eating disorders and suicidality: what we know, what we don't know, and suggestions for future research. *Curr Opin Psychol.* 2018;22:63-67. https://doi.org/10.1016/j.copsyc.2017.08.023

Stice E, Marti CN, Rohde P. Prevalence, incidence, impairment, and course of proposed DSM-5 eating disorder diagnoses in an 8-year prospective community study of young women. *J Abnorm Psychol.* 2013;122(2):445-457. https://doi.org/10.1037/a0030679

Streatfeild J, Hickson J, Austin SB, et al. Social and economic cost of eating disorders in the United States: evidence to inform policy action. *Int J Eat Disord.* 2021;54:851-868. https://doi.org/10.1002/eat.23486

Treasure J, Duarte TA, Schmidt U. Eating disorders. *Lancet (London, England).* 2020;395(10227):899-911. https://doi.org/10.1016/S0140-6736(20)30059-3

Ulfvebrand S, Birgegård A, Norring C, Högdahl L, von Hausswolff-Juhlin Y. Psychiatric comorbidity in women and men with eating disorders results from a large clinical database. *Psychiatr Res.* 2015;230(2):294-299. https://doi.org/10.1016/j.psychres.2015.09.008

Westmoreland P, Krantz MJ, Mehler PS. Medical complications of anorexia nervosa and bulimia. *Am J Med.* 2016;129(1):30-37. doi:10.1016/j.amjmed.2015.06.031

Wolfe BE, Dunne JP, Kells MR. Nursing care considerations for the hospitalized patient with an eating disorder. *Nurs Clin North Am.* 2016;51(2):213-235. https://doi.org/10.1016/j.cnur.2016.01.006

Zimmerman J, Fisher M. Avoidant/restrictive food intake disorder (ARFID). *Curr Prob Pediatr Adolesc Health Care.* 2017;47(4):95-103. https://doi.org/10.1016/j.cppeds.2017.02.005

Insomnia Disorders

Allen RP, et al. Comparison of pregabalin with pramipexole for restless legs syndrome. *N Engl J Med.* 2014;370:621-631.

American Family Physician. *Treatment of Chronic Insomnia in Adults: ACP Guideline.* 2017. Retrieved from https://www.aafp.org/afp/2017/0515/p669.html

Aurora RN, et al. The treatment of restless legs syndrome and periodic limb movement disorder in adults—an update for 2012: practice parameters with an evidence-based systematic review and meta-analyses. *Sleep.* 2012;35(8):1039-1062.

Buysse DJ, et al. Clinical management of insomnia disorder. *JAMA.* 2017;318(20):1973-1974.

Edinger JD, Arnedt JT, Bertisch SM, et al. Behavioral and psychological treatments for chronic insomnia disorder in adults: an American Academy of Sleep Medicine clinical practice guideline. *J Clin Sleep Med.* 2021;17(2):255-262.

Gutierrez C, Brady P. Obstructive sleep apnea: a diagnostic and treatment guide. *J Fam Pract.* 2013;62(10):565-572.

Qaseem A, Kansagara D, Forciea MA, Cooke M, Denberg TD. Management of chronic insomnia disorder in adults: a clinical practice guideline from the American College of Physicians. *Ann Intern Med.* 016;165(2):125-133. doi:10.7326/M15-2175

Sateia MJ, et al. Clinical practice guideline for the pharmacologic treatment of chronic insomnia in adults: an American Academy of Sleep Medicine clinical practice guideline. *J Clin Sleep Med.* 2017;13(2):307-349.

Winkelman JW. Insomnia disorder. *N Engl J Med.* 2015;373:1437-1444.

RESOURCES

Eating Disorders

Academy for Eating Disorders (AED)
   http://www.aedweb.org
Andrea's Voice
   http://andreasvoice.org
Compulsive Eaters Anonymous—HOW
   http://www.ceahow.org
Eating Disorders Anonymous (EDA)
   http://www.eatingdisordersanonymous.org
Eating Disorders Coalition
   http://www.eatingdisorderscoalition.org
Eating Disorders Referral Information Center
   http://www.edreferral.com
Food Addicts Anonymous
   http://www.foodaddictsanonymous.org
Healthy Choices for Mind and Body
   http://www.healthychoicesformindandbody.org
International Association of Eating Disorders Professionals
   http://www.iaedp.com
Maudsley Parents
   http://www.maudsleyparents.org
Multi-Service Eating Disorders Association
   http://www.medainc.org
National Alliance for Eating Disorder
   http://www.allianceforeatingdisorders.com
National Association to Advance Fat Acceptance
   http://www.naafa.org
National Association of Anorexia Nervosa and Associated Disorders
   http://www.anad.org
National Eating Disorder Information Centre
   http://www.nedic.ca
National Eating Disorders Association
   http://www.nationaleatingdisorders.org
National Institute of Mental Health
   http://www.nimh.nih.gov
Overeaters Anonymous (OA)
   https://oa.org/

Restless Legs Syndrome

Restless Legs Syndrome. American Sleep Association
https://www.sleepassociation.org/patients-general-public/restless-legs-syndrome/

Restless Legs Syndrome: Brochure. National Institute of Neurological Disorders and Stroke
https://catalog.ninds.nih.gov/ninds/product/Restless-Legs-Syndrome/17-4847

Restless Leg Syndrome. American Academy and Sleep Medicine
https://sleepeducation.org/sleep-disorders/restless-legs-syndrome/

Restless Leg Syndrome Fact Sheet: Patient and Caregiver Education. National Institute of Neurological Disorders and Stroke
https://www.ninds.nih.gov/Disorders/Patient-Caregiver-Education/Fact-Sheets/Restless-Legs-Syndrome-Fact-Sheet

Understanding RLS. Restless Legs Syndrome Foundation
https://www.rls.org/understanding-rls

Sleep-Wake Disorders

Insomnia. American Academy of Family Physicians
https://familydoctor.org/condition/insomnia/?adfree=true

Insomnia. National Library of Medicine
https://medlineplus.gov/insomnia.html

Insomnia Overview, Symptoms, Causes, Risk Factors, Complications, and Prevention. Mayo Clinic
https://www.mayoclinic.org/diseases-conditions/insomnia/symptoms-causes/syc-20355167?p=1

Insomnia: What is it? National Heart, Lung, and Blood Institute
https://www.nhlbi.nih.gov/health-topics/insomnia

Narcolepsy Fact Sheet: National Institute of Neurological Disorders and Stroke
https://www.ninds.nih.gov/Disorders/Patient-Caregiver-Education/Fact-Sheets/Narcolepsy-Fact-Sheet

Narcolepsy & Hypersomnia. Stanford Medicine Center for Narcolepsy
https://med.stanford.edu/narcolepsy/symptoms.html

Narcolepsy Network
https://narcolepsynetwork.org/

Sleep Disorders. Sleep Foundation
https://www.sleepfoundation.org/sleep-disorders

Sleep Disorders. American Academy and Sleep Medicine
https://sleepeducation.org/sleep-disorders/.
https://narcolepsynetwork.org/resources/

Understanding Sleep: Brain Basics Brochure. National Institute of Neurological Disorders and Stroke
https://catalog.ninds.nih.gov/ninds/product/Understanding-Sleep-Brain-Basics-/17-NS-3440-C

Chapter 73

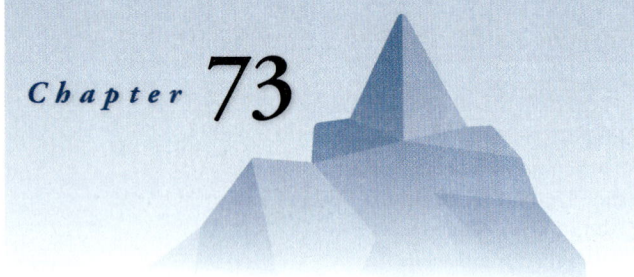

Sexual Assault

Katerina Melino, MS, PMHNP

Karen Jennings Mathis, PhD, APRN-CNP, PMHNP-BC, FAED

Sexual assault is defined by the National Institute of Justice as any unwanted sexual behavior against the person's will or lack of ability to consent due to age, disability, or being under the influence of alcohol or drugs. Sexual assault could be an actual event or threat of the following:

- Intentional touching of the victim's genitals, anus, groin, or breasts
- Voyeurism
- Exposure to exhibitionism
- Undesired exposure to pornography
- Public display of images that were taken in a private context or when the victim was unaware

Perpetrators may use emotional coercion, psychological or physical force, or manipulation to coerce a victim into nonconsensual sexual contact. Some perpetrators will use threats to force a victim to comply, such as threatening to hurt the victim or their family or other intimidation tactics.

Most perpetrators are someone known to the victim. Approximately 7 of 10 sexual assaults are committed by someone known to the victim, such as in the case of intimate partner sexual violence, acquaintance rape, or "date rape." In fact, acquaintance rape is far more common than rape by strangers. Sexual assault also includes sexual abuse of a child, sexual hate crimes, incest, sexual assault of males, sexual harassment, stalking, intimate partner rape, and sexual exploitation by trusted professionals including health-care providers, therapists, teachers, priests, and police officers.

Rape is a form of sexual assault, but not all sexual assault is rape. The term *rape* is often used as a legal definition. As of 2013, the term specifically includes a definition of sexual penetration without consent. For its Uniform Crime Reports, the Federal Bureau of Investigation (2013) defines *rape* as "penetration, no matter how slight, of the vagina or anus with any body part or object, or oral penetration by a sex organ of another person, without the consent of the victim." Attempted rape includes verbal threats of rape.

EPIDEMIOLOGY AND CAUSES

In 2019 in the United States, there were 212,230 reported victims (age 12 or older) of rape and sexual assault. Teenagers and young adults aged 12 to 34 years have the highest rates of sexual assault of any age group. It is estimated that only one in six sexual assaults is reported to law enforcement. Data collected in the United States between 2005 and 2010 indicate that women who are young, unmarried, and in a lower-income group are the most frequent victims of sexual assault. Divorced and single women experience higher rates of sexual assault than married or widowed females, and those in lower-income populations experience higher rates of assault than females in moderate or higher-income groups. In addition, in the United States, women of color report sexual assault twice as frequently as do white women, with black, Indigenous/Alaskan, and those of mixed race reporting the highest lifetime rates of rape or attempted rape. Remember that both survivors and perpetrators of sexual assault can be of any gender. Sexual assault is more likely to occur in the survivor's home (43%) or in the home of a friend (15%). Most sexual assaults (65%) occur in the evening and during the summer months. Finally, most sexual assault survivors (78%) know their perpetrators. When the sexual assault is committed by a stranger, 31% of the time, the sexual assault takes place in the home of the survivor or a friend's home. In some cases, sexual assault is part of the larger picture of intimate partner violence. Thirty-four percent of rapes involve alcohol.

The Violence Against Women Act of 2005 created the Sexual Assault Services Program, which is federally funded and dedicated to direct intervention and related assistance for survivors of sexual assault. State and local communities have responded as well to combat sexual assault. Annually, rape costs the United States more than any other crime ($127 billion), followed by assault ($93 billion), murder ($71 billion), and drunk driving ($61 billion). Indeed, health-care costs are 16% higher for adult females who were sexually abused as children, which speaks to the profound physical health effects of trauma.

PATHOPHYSIOLOGY

Sexual assault is an act of violence and humiliation that is expressed through sexual means. Power and anger are expressed through rape or sexual assault and are often part of another crime. Sexual assault can be a life-threatening event. Perpetrators may urinate or defecate on their victims, ejaculate into their faces and hair, force intercourse, insert foreign objects into the vagina and/or rectum, and cause other physical injury, including death.

Sexual assault is a highly traumatic event that can have long-term effects on the physiological and psychological well-being of the survivor. After the sexual assault, the survivor may have an acute stress reaction to the trauma. They may experience numbness, shame, confusion, humiliation, fear, and rage. Survivors may develop post-traumatic stress disorder (PTSD), depression, suicidal ideation, and/or substance-use disorders. However, not all survivors have these reactions.

Pediatric/Adolescent Considerations:
Sexual Assault

Adolescents and young adults are at highest risk for sexual assault for several reasons. Developmentally, they are exploring the world and how to form relationships with others and establishing their emotional and physical boundaries. They may also be in situations more often where they and others are using alcohol and illicit substances.

Adolescent rape victims presenting to emergency departments are more likely than adult victims to have used substances before the sexual assault and are less likely to incur nonanogenital injury during a rape. Adolescent female victims are more likely to delay seeking medical care after a sexual assault and are less likely to wish to press charges compared with adult females.

Research on adolescent sexual assault demonstrates that survivors' first disclosures are more likely to be to their peers, rather than to health-care professionals or law enforcement. Subsequently, adolescent survivors tend to disclose to parents for emotional support and/or guidance on how to enter formal systems. When sexual assaults occur in the context of other events or behaviors for which the adolescent fears they may be judged (hanging out with older peers, using substances, staying out without permission), they are less likely to disclose the sexual assault to adults and consequently less likely to receive examination or treatment. While adopting an empathic, open, nonjudgmental approach to survivor disclosure is always paramount, it appears to be even more salient to ensuring emotional and physical safety in the adolescent population. With the adolescent's consent, involving supportive parents in the interview and decision-making process can offer developmentally appropriate guidance and care.

Mental health care follow-up is also crucial for this population. Studies of adolescent survivors have found that sexual assault during childhood is associated with younger age at first voluntary intercourse; lower rates of contraception; a greater number of pregnancies and abortions; higher rates of sexually transmitted infections (STIs); and increased risks of victimization by older partners. Increases are also noted in mental health problems including higher rates of depression, suicidal ideation and suicide attempts, and other self-harm behaviors, such as self-mutilation and eating disorders, among adolescent sexual assault victims. Principles of examination, evidence collection, and treatment for sexual assault are the same for adolescents and adults.

CLINICAL PRESENTATION

Through their work with sexual assault survivors, experts have identified a set of immediate and long-term effects of sexual assault called the *sexual assault trauma syndrome*. Sexual assault trauma syndrome is considered a normal response to sexual assault. There are two identified phases of survivor responses—the initial or acute phase, characterized by a period of disorganization, and the long-term phase, characterized by a period of reorganization.

Initial or Acute Phase

During the initial or acute phase, many sexual assault survivors experience both physical symptoms and emotions such as fear, shock, and disbelief. Four major categories of physical symptoms have been identified:

- Physical trauma: symptoms include soreness and bruising from physical attack, often in the areas of the hands, throat, neck, breasts, thighs, legs, arms, back, buttocks, head, and/or face.
- Skeletal muscle tension: symptoms include tension headaches, fatigue, and sleep disturbances.
- Gastrointestinal irritability: symptoms include stomach pains, nausea, and decreased appetite.
- Genitourinary disturbance: symptoms include vaginal and/or anal bleeding, and bladder and vaginal infections.

Several researchers have observed in their study of sexual assault survivors that survivors tended to have one of two emotional response patterns—expressed or controlled. The expressed style is the expression of fear, anger, and anxiety through behaviors such as crying, sobbing, paradoxical smiling, restlessness, and tenseness. The controlled style masks the psychological distress with a calm, composed, subdued affect. Research has indicated equal numbers of both expressed and controlled response styles among sexual assault survivors. As clinicians, remember that there is no "right" way for a person to feel after being sexually assaulted. Trauma responses can take many forms.

Long-Term Phase

In the long-term phase, psychological symptoms such as depression, anxiety, and fear are prominent. This phase has three components:

- Motor activity: sexual assault survivors may exhibit an increase in activities such as changing their residence and telephone number and adopting a variety of personal safety and security measures. They may turn to family and friends for assistance with these activities. Survivors may make special trips home or to some location that symbolizes safety.
- Nightmares: nightmares after sexual assault are often upsetting, and violent dreams can occur for months after the sexual assault, as with any trauma. The nightmares may contain images that are clearly connected to the sexual assault, but nightmare content may also fail to be obviously related to the sexual assault.
- Trauma-phobia: as the term implies, *trauma-phobia* is a phobic reaction to trauma in which the phobia develops as a psychological defense against the sexual assault experience. This is also captured in the American Psychiatric Association's *Diagnostic and Statistical Manual of Mental Disorders, Fifth Edition, Text Revision (DSM-5-TR)* under the criteria for PTSD, as intrusion and avoidance symptoms. Common phobias are fear of being indoors, fear of being outdoors, fear of being alone, fear of being in crowds, fear of having people behind the individual, and sexual fears. Fear of STIs, including HIV, is also a powerful source of psychological trauma. It has been estimated that 4% to 30% of sexual assault survivors are diagnosed with an STI because of the sexual assault.
- Some survivors of sexual assault may not report the assault to anyone. Consider unreported sexual assault as an explanation for atypical anxiety; abdominal pain not otherwise specified; sexual relationship problems; significant changes in sexual behavior patterns; unexplained, sudden onset of phobias; and chronic low self-esteem.

DIAGNOSTIC REASONING

The diagnosis of sexual assault is made by patient complaint. It is important to note that particularly with adult survivors, physical examination may or may not indicate any observable evidence of sexual assault (e.g., abrasions or hematomas in the genital area). This does not mean that sexual assault has not taken place. Physical evidence of sexual assault is more likely to be observed in children and adolescents; however, these patients tend to come forward with a complaint of sexual assault after time has passed rather than in a crisis presentation. This makes physical examination less likely to reveal relevant findings.

MANAGEMENT

Initial treatment for sexual assault survivors includes crisis intervention, physical examination, pharmacological treatment, and the sexual assault interviewing and forensic evidence collection with patient approval. During the initial or acute phase, sexual assault survivors may present to emergency departments, rape crisis centers, primary care offices, or police stations. If the sexual assault has occurred within the last 5 days, forensic physical evidence may be collected, guided by the patient history. Using a trauma-informed, patient-driven approach to interviewing, assessing, and collecting evidence is crucial to establishing psychological safety for the survivor and allowing them to regain as much control over their immediate circumstance as possible.

The Sexual Assault Nurse Examiner (SANE RN)

The use of a sexual assault nurse examiner (SANE), if one is available, is highly recommended. These nurses receive special training in providing crisis intervention, offering sexual assault-related medications, and collecting forensic evidence. SANE providers offer a number of advantages over emergency department practitioners. For example, the survivor is seen by one specialist rather than by several practitioners, which decreases the time a sexual assault survivor spends in the emergency department and ensures that they receive sensitive, nonjudgmental care by a sexual assault specialist. Equally important, the nurse is skilled in the collection of forensic evidence, resulting in higher prosecution rates of sexual assault.

Crisis Intervention

Crisis intervention with sexual assault survivors includes validating feelings of fear, anger, shame, guilt, shock, or numbness that arise; identifying concerns related to the sexual assault; and creating a physical and psychological safety plan. Psychological support is necessary to address the patient's needs and should be done before the sexual assault interview. A supportive approach and focusing on restoring the patient's sense of adequacy and control over their life are the best means for supporting the survivor, provided there is no severe underlying pathology that might warrant a different treatment plan. Survivors of sexual assault fare best when they receive immediate support and can express their feelings or experiences to loved ones, supportive clinicians, and/or law enforcement officials. A longitudinal study of sexual assault survivors showed that negative social reactions and blame of the victim were associated with worsened PTSD symptoms.

Pharmacological Treatment

Medications to treat STIs and pregnancy should be offered regardless of whether the patient wishes to have forensic evidence collected. Empiric treatment with azithromycin or doxycycline and ceftriaxone for gonorrhea and chlamydia that may have been transmitted during the assault should be offered. Metronidazole should also be offered empirically for trichomoniasis. A tetanus booster is necessary if patients who experienced lacerations or abrasions have not been adequately immunized. HIV counseling, as well as testing and prophylaxis, should be offered to all survivors. Provider encouragement was shown to have an association with the patient's decision to start HIV prophylaxis treatment. Referral to an infectious disease specialist should be considered to guide antiretroviral therapy. Hepatitis B surface antibody testing with vaccination should be offered and hepatitis B immunoglobulin should be offered if there is a high risk of exposure by a known hepatitis B–positive assailant. Emergency contraception should be offered after penile-vaginal assault. Referral to an obstetrician/gynecologist and a urology specialist may be needed for treatment for specific traumatic injuries that require further care.

The Sexual Assault Interview

The formal sexual assault interview is the first step in completing a legal forensic evidence kit. Before the interview, the capacity of the patient to consent to a forensic examination should be assessed. This can be done by evaluating understanding and appropriate responses when obtaining the diagnostic history. Drugs, alcohol, developmental disability, or young age may cause a delay in obtaining the patient's consent. In the case of severe head or critical injury, law enforcement may provide a court order to proceed with forensic evidence collection. Before doing an interview and physical examination for evidence collection, it is imperative to address psychological issues related to the examination itself. Patients presenting after sexual assault have undergone an experience that denied them the right to consent. There are important psychological and legal implications with obtaining forensic evidence, and the patient's consent and opportunity for a family member, friend, or patient advocate to be present should not be undervalued.

The sexual assault interview is performed in a room away from the waiting areas and examination rooms, while the survivor is still fully clothed, often with a police officer present. It should not be rushed and, again, should be conducted using a patient-driven, trauma-informed approach. The sexual assault interview begins with general health information, including drug allergies, current medications including birth control, surgical history, tetanus, and hepatitis B immunization if relevant, major health problems, pregnancy status if known, first day of last menstrual period, gravidity, parity, history of STIs, and most recent consensual sexual contact.

Questions about the sexual assault follow the general health information questions. Although this history may be difficult for the patient to report, it is important to obtain an accurate history for collection of forensic evidence for the examiner to locate all points of physical contact and penetration, as well as documenting the survivor's activity immediately after the sexual assault.

The sexual assault survivor is asked the date, time, and place of the sexual assault. Inquire about the use of force or threats of force, including threats of future harm to the patient or others, presence of a weapon, or threats to expose a personal secret. Notation of the type of force; use of restraints; number of assailants; and type of assault, such as fondling, kissing, licking, penetration or attempted penetration of the mouth, vagina, or anus by finger, object, or penis need to be documented. "Drug-facilitated sexual abuse" may be suspected when the patient also reports lapses in consciousness. Ask whether a condom was used. Ask about activities since the assault, such as bathing, urinating, defecating, douching, gargling, eating, brushing teeth, and washing or wiping self.

Physical Examination

A complete physical examination must be offered to the patient to assess injuries related to the sexual assault, independent of pursuing evidence collection. The Violence Against Women and Department of Justice Reauthorization Act of 2005 (and reauthorized in 2013) provides that states may not require those who have experienced sexual assault to participate in the criminal justice system or cooperate with law enforcement to be provided with a forensic medical examination. Under this provision, a state must ensure access to an examination free of charge even if the survivor chooses not to report to the police or otherwise cooperate with the criminal justice system.

All physical examinations and procedures should be fully explained with ample opportunities for clarification as needed. The physical examination can be traumatic for survivors; thus, survivors should be allowed to control the examination as much as possible. This can be accomplished by letting survivors know they can refuse any part of the examination or stop the procedure at any time. Sexual assault survivors should be encouraged to have a support person, such as a friend, spouse, or family member with them during the examination. In addition, a counselor or patient advocate from the local rape crisis center may be available to support the sexual assault survivor during the examination.

Forensic Evidence Collection

Remember that collecting an evidence kit is purely for legal purposes and does not offer any health benefits to the patient. If the survivor does wish to pursue legal action, but wants to remain anonymous, a "Jane Doe Rape Kit" enables forensic evidence to be collected without revealing identifying information. Survivors are given a code number that can be used to identify themselves if they choose to report later. The practitioner needs to be aware of state guidelines for evidence collection. The sexual assault evidence collection kit, available in most states, should contain all materials needed. Become familiar with the forms before doing the sexual assault examination. Gloves should be worn throughout the physical examination to preserve evidence.

Evidence collection begins with collecting each item of clothing worn at the time of the sexual assault and placing in a separate bag. Physical forensic evidence that can be found on clothing includes hair, blood, semen, and saliva. Document the general appearance of the patient and complete a head-to-toe assessment for signs of trauma, including an oral examination, skin examination for lacerations, swelling, broken fingernails, and foreign material such as leaves, grass, fibers, dried blood, and dried secretions anywhere on the body. Forensic evidence includes samples of the individual's hair (head and pubic) and saliva; oral, vaginal, and rectal swabs; and fingernail scrapings. It is important to label specimens accurately, noting the collection time and date and the signature of each person who provided and received them.

A detailed anogenital examination is performed to assess for injury. Pelvic, vaginal, and rectal examinations are completed at the end. Colposcope and/or toluidine blue dye can be used to assess genital injury, providing permanent documentation of injuries that may heal very quickly and avoiding subjecting the patient to reexamination or potential loss of evidence. Toluidine blue dye is a nuclear stain that adheres to the areas of injury on subepithelial nucleated cells but not to intact epithelial cells; therefore, it is not useful for mucosal surfaces, such as the vagina or anus. Almost half of genital examinations done with a colposcope of female patients who have been raped will have a normal examination. Anoscopy is utilized to view the extent of rectal injuries. Genital injuries can also be detected when female patients participate in consensual intercourse. Although forensic evidence should be collected as soon as possible, examinations performed several days after the sexual assault can still produce findings.

Laboratory testing for STIs is recommended only if treatment is deferred. STI testing at this time would detect only preassault infection. Consider testing in minors because they are unable to give consent to engage in intercourse. Serological testing for HIV, hepatitis B, and syphilis is recommended because the efficacy of prophylactic treatment is not complete. Seroconversion that is attributed to the assault may be covered by the Victims of Violent Crimes Fund. Further collection of blood, buccal, and urine specimens is recommended for crime laboratory testing for DNA, pregnancy testing for all female survivors of childbearing age, and toxicology analysis if indicated. A 6-year, retrospective study of 1421 sexual assault patients who presented to the emergency department found that 12% reported drug-facilitated sexual assault. This group had a longer delay in presentation to the emergency department, less often had police involvement, and had a decreased occurrence of genital and other injury compared with others. Hospitalization may be necessary to treat unstable medical conditions or to provide surgical intervention or psychiatric stabilization.

FOLLOW-UP AND REFERRAL

Sexual assault survivors should be encouraged to use the support services available from community rape counseling centers, such as individual therapy, group therapy, and self-defense training, as well as legal follow-up. Most rape counseling centers offer 24-hour crisis hotlines. Many individuals may not feel they need this support or that their family and friends are there for them. Survivors continue to be at risk for long-term problems, however. They may have grief and mourning needs long after the immediate crisis has passed, and significant others have come to believe that the crisis is over. Rape counseling center personnel understand the long-term course of events of sexual assault. Some rape counseling centers provide advocates to support survivors as they deal with the legal and judicial systems. These services are often offered free of charge or at greatly reduced rates.

Medical follow-up after the initial visit includes reassessment of any traumatic injuries, review of laboratory results, post-HIV test counseling, and reassessment of psychological status and recovery. Retesting for pregnancy should be considered if the patient has not had the expected menstrual period. Repeat HIV, hepatitis B, and STI testing should be performed as indicated.

Patient Education: Sexual Assault

Education begins with the first patient encounter, allowing the survivor to regain control and become an active participant in their recovery, incorporating person-centered care. Include education about the diagnostic work-up, management, psychological and medical recovery, and advice about community support services, as well as discussion of the long-term effects of sexual assault. The most common long-term effect of sexual assault is the development of PTSD. Recent research has indicated that sexual assault survivors may be the largest single group of individuals with PTSD. Researchers have found that 94% of adult females who had been sexually assaulted met the criteria for acute stress disorder 12 days after the sexual assault and that 46% of these patients still met the criteria 3 months later.

In addition to having higher rates of PTSD, sexual assault survivors report higher rates of substance use, depression, attempted suicide, anxiety, obsessive-compulsive disorder (OCD), and medical care use. Female sexual assault survivors are 13.4 times more likely to have had alcohol-use disorders and 26 times more likely to have had other substance-use disorders compared with females who were not sexually assaulted. Female survivors are also three times more likely to have had a major episode of depression, four times more likely to have had thoughts about suicide, and 13 times more likely to have attempted suicide compared with other females. Finally, survivors of sexual assault report more symptoms of illness across all body systems and perceive their health less favorably than do others. Male sexual assault survivors are equally at risk for adverse outcomes, compounded further by frequent lack of available resources as well as social stereotypes about masculinity and power. Symptoms that are diagnosed at a much higher rate in sexual assault survivors include chronic pelvic pain, gastrointestinal disorders, headaches, general pain, and premenstrual symptoms. Every effort should be made to encourage the patient to initiate long-term support for dealing with the trauma of sexual assault.

REFERENCES

Abrahams N, Devries K, Watts C, et al. Worldwide prevalence of non-partner sexual violence: a systematic review. *Lancet.* 2014;383:1648-1654.

American Psychiatric Association. *Diagnostic and Statistical Manual of Mental Disorders: Diagnostic and Statistical Manual of Mental Disorders.* 5th ed. Arlington, VA: American Psychiatric Association; 2013.

Astrup BS, Ravn P, Thomsen JL, Lauritsen J. Patterned genital injury in cases of rape—a case-control study. *J Forensic Leg Med.* 2013;20:525-529.

Brawner BM, Sommers MS, Moore K, et al. Exploring genitoanal injury and HIV risk among women: menstrual phase, hormonal birth control, and injury frequency and prevalence. *J Acquir Immune Defic Syndr.* 2016;71(2):207-212.

Breiding MJ, Smith SG, Basile KC, et al. Prevalence and characteristics of sexual violence, stalking, and intimate partner violence victimization—National Intimate Partner and Sexual Violence Survey, United States, 2011. *MMWR Surveill Summ.* 2014;63:1.

Bryant RA. Acute stress disorder as a predictor of posttraumatic stress disorder: a systematic review. *J Clin Psychiatry.* 2011;72:233-239.

Bryant RA, Nickerson A, Creamer M, et al. Trajectory of posttraumatic stress following traumatic injury: 6-year follow-up. *Br J Psychiatry.* 2015;206:417-423.

Bureau of Justice Statistics. Female victims of sexual violence, 1994-2010. https://www.bjs.gov/content/pub/pdf/rsavcaf9513.pdf. Revised May 31, 2016. Accessed February 23, 2022.

Bureau of Justice Statistics. Rape and sexual assault. https://www.bjs.gov/index.cfm?ty=tp&tid=317. Published 2017. Accessed September 4, 2018.

Bureau of Justice Statistics. Violence against women: estimates from the redesigned survey. https://www.bjs.gov/content/pub/pdf/FEMVIED.PDF. Accessed February 23, 2018.

Campbell R, Bybee D, Kelley KD, Dworkin ER, Patterson D. The Impact of Sexual Assault Nurse Examiner (SANE) Program Services on Law Enforcement Investigational Practices: a mediational analysis. *Criminal Justice Behav.* 2012;39:169-184.

Carr ME, Moettus AL. Developing a policy for sexual assault examinations on incapacitated patients and patients unable to consent. *J Law Med Ethics.* 2010;38:647-653.

Chivers-Wilson KA. Sexual assault and posttraumatic stress disorder: a review of the biological, psychological and sociological factors and treatments. *McGill J Med.* 2020;9.

Cowley R, Walsh E, Horrocks J. The role of the sexual assault nurse examiner in England: nurse experiences and perspectives. *J Forensic Nurs.* 2014;10:77-83.

Crawford-Jakubiak JE, Alderman EM, Leventhal JM. Care of the adolescent after an acute sexual assault. *Pediatrics.* 2017;139.

Delgadillo DC. When there is no sexual assault nurse examiner: emergency nursing care for female adult sexual assault patients. *J Emerg Nurs.* 2017;43:308-315.

Du Mont J, Macdonald S, White M, et al. Client satisfaction with nursing-led sexual assault and domestic violence services in Ontario. *J Forensic Nurs.* 2014;10:122-134.

Dworkin ER, Menon SV, Bystrynski J, Allen NE. Sexual assault victimization and psychopathology: A review and meta-analysis. *Clin Psychol Rev.* 2017;56:65-81.

Fantasia HC, Fontenot HB. The sexual safety of adolescents. *J Obstet Gynecol Neonatal Nurs.* 2011;40:217-224.

Ford N, Irvine C, Shubber Z, et al. Adherence to HIV postexposure prophylaxis: a systematic review and meta-analysis. *AIDS.* 2014;28:2721-2727.

Gilmore AK, Ward-Ciesielski EF, Smalling A, Limowski AR, Hahn CK, Jaffe AE. Managing post-sexual assault suicide risk. *Arch Women's Ment Health.* 2020;23:673-679.

Hagemann CT, Nordbø SA, Myhre AK, et al. Sexually transmitted infections among women attending a Norwegian Sexual Assault Centre. *Sex Transm Infect.* 2014;90:283.

Kaiser J, Hanschmidt F, Kersting A. The link between masculinity ideologies and posttraumatic stress: a systematic review and meta-analysis. *Psychol Trauma.* 2020;12:599-608.

Larsen ML, Hilden M, Lidegaard Ø. Sexual assault: a descriptive study of 2500 female victims over a 10-year period. *BJOG.* 2015;122:577.

Linden JA. Clinical practice. Care of the adult patient after sexual assault. *N Engl J Med.* 2011;365:834-841.

Morgan RE, Truman, J. Criminal victimization, 2019. Bureau of Justice Statistics National Crime Victimization Survey (NCVS), 2019. Department of Justice, Office of Justice Programs. https://www.bjs.gov/content/pub/pdf/cv19.pdf. Published 2020.

Muldoon KA, Drumm A, Leach T, Heimerl M, Sampsel K. Achieving just outcomes: forensic evidence collection in emergency department sexual assault cases. *Emerg Med J.* 2018;35:746-752.

National Institute of Justice. Rape and sexual violence. https://www.nij.gov/topics/crime/rape-sexual-violence/Pages/welcome.aspx. Published 2017.

Peterson ZD, Voller EK, Polusny MA, Murdoch M. Prevalence and consequences of adult sexual assault of men: Review of empirical findings and state of the literature. *Clin Psychol Rev.* 2011;31:1-24.

Planty M, Langton L, Krebs C, Berzofsky M, Smiley-McDonald H. Female victims of sexual violence, 1994-2010. Washington, DC: US Department of Justice, Office of Justice Programs, Bureau of Justice Statistics; March 2013. Available at: https://www.bjs.gov/content/pub/pdf/fvsv9410.pdf.

Seña AC, Hsu KK, Kellogg N, et al. Sexual assault and sexually transmitted infections in adults, adolescents, and children. *Clin Infect Dis.* 2015;61(suppl 8):S856-S864.

Tiihonen Möller A, Bäckström T, Söndergaard HP, Helström L. Identifying risk factors for PTSD in women seeking medical help after rape. *PLoS One.* 2014;9:e111136.

U.S. Department of Justice. Office of Justice Programs. National best practices for sexual assault kits: a multidisciplinary approach. https://www.ncjrs.gov/pdffiles1/nij/250384.pdf. Published August 2017.

U.S. Department of Justice. Office on Violence Against Women. A national protocol for sexual abuse medical forensic examinations: pediatric. April 2016. https://www.justice.gov/ovw/file/846856/download

U.S. Department of Justice. Office on Violence Against Women. *National Protocol for Sexual Assault Medical Forensic Examinations,* 2nd ed. Updated September 2013. https://www.ojp.gov/pdffiles1/ovw/241903.pdf

Vrees RA. Evaluation and management of female victims of sexual assault. *Obstet Gynecol Surv.* 2017;72:39-53.

Walker G. The (in)significance of genital injury in rape and sexual assault. *J Forensic Leg Med.* 2015;34:173-178.

Walters ML, Chen J, Breiding MJ. The National Intimate Partner and Sexual Violence Survey (NISVS): 2010 findings on victimization by sexual orientation. Retrieved from the Centers for Disease Control and Prevention, National Center for Injury Prevention and Control. https://www.cdc.gov/violenceprevention/pdf/nisvs_sofindings.pdf. Published 2013. Accessed February 22, 2018.

Wang MJ, Khodadadi AB, Turan JM, White K. Scoping review of access to emergency contraception for sexual assault victims in emergency departments in the united states. *Trauma Violence Abuse.* 2021;22(2):413-442.

Wegner R, Davis KC. How men's sexual assault victimization experiences differ based on their sexual history. *J Interpers Violence.* 2020;2017;35:2624-2633.

WHO Guidelines Approved by the Guidelines Review Committee. *Responding to intimate partner violence and sexual violence against women: WHO clinical and policy guidelines.* Geneva, Switzerland: World Health Organization; 2013. https://apps.who.int/iris/bitstream/handle/10665/85240/9789241548595_eng.pdf

Young-Wolff KC, Sarovar V, Klebaner D, et al. Changes in psychiatric and medical conditions and health care utilization following a diagnosis of sexual assault: a retrospective cohort study. 2018;56:649-657.

RESOURCES

Centers for Disease Control and Prevention
  https://www.cdc.gov/violenceprevention/pdf/campusvsummary.pdf
  https://www.cdc.gov/violenceprevention/sexualviolence/
  https://www.cdc.gov/violenceprevention/pdf/SV-Prevention-Technical-Package.pdf

Human Rights Campaign
  https://www.hrc.org/resources/sexual-assault-and-the-lgbt-community

Mental Health America
  http://www.mentalhealthamerica.net/conditions/sexual-assault-and-mental-health

Ohio Alliance to End Sexual Violence
  https://oaesv.org/

Rape, Abuse & Incest National Network (RAINN)
  https://www.rainn.org/articles/sexual-assault-men-and-boys
  https://www.rainn.org/articles/sexual-assault
  https://www.rainn.org/statistics/victims-sexual-violence

U.S. Department of Veterans Affairs
  https://www.ptsd.va.gov/professional/treat/type/sexual_assault_female.asp

Chapter 74

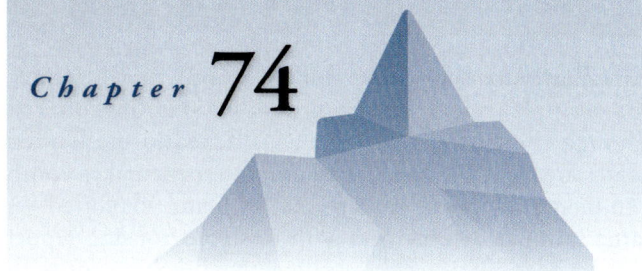

Human Trafficking

John Fraleigh, MSN, RN, CFRN

Karen Jennings Mathis, PhD, APRN-CNP, PMHNP-BC, FAED

Human trafficking, defined as the use of force, fraud, or coercion to control victims and manipulate them into performing labor, services, or a commercial sex act against their will, is considered a form of modern-day slavery and continues to operate with minimal detection globally (see Figure 74.1). Indeed, this multibillion-dollar industry thrives within the United States. Many people unknowingly interact with victims of human trafficking during their routine workday, and health care is no exception. Up to 88% of survivors report having sought health care while in the process of being trafficked, yet many went unrecognized.

There are different types of human trafficking. *Sex trafficking* is defined as the recruitment, harboring, transportation, provision, or obtaining of a person for the purposes of a commercial sex act, in which the commercial sex act is induced by force, fraud, or coercion, *or* in which the person induced to perform such an act has not attained 18 years of age. A *commercial sex act* means any sex act on account of which anything of value is given to or received by any person, and "anything of value" includes food, water, shelter, clothing, and money. *Labor trafficking* is defined as the recruitment, harboring, transportation, provision, or obtaining of a person for labor or services, using force, fraud, or coercion for the purpose of subjection to involuntary servitude, peonage, debt bondage, or slavery. For example, although someone may be smuggled into a country, it does not become labor trafficking until force, fraud, or coercion is used to make the person work in exchange for food, shelter, or debt repayment. These individuals who seek health care are less likely to report being in the country illegally for fear of deportation. They are more likely to return to inadequate living arrangements or unsafe working conditions after being discharged from the health-care setting, without reporting or understanding their victimization. However, labor trafficking can occur independently of human smuggling or importing persons into a country by deliberately evading immigration law and includes transporting or harboring persons who are in the country illegally.

A crucial step in proving a case for human trafficking is the required identification of the action, means, and purpose (AMP; see Figure 74.2). One element from each category is required to meet the U.S. federal definition of human trafficking. In cases involving minors, force, fraud, or coercion are not required to prove sex trafficking.

EPIDEMIOLOGY AND CAUSES

Why Does Human Trafficking Exist?

Although exact figures are difficult to discern, the International Labour Organization (ILO) estimates human trafficking generates over $150 billion worldwide, with $99 billion from commercial sexual exploitation alone. This minimal risk, high-profit business relies on the support of several industries, which may or may not be aware of the criminal enterprise operating within. The Polaris Project's classification system provides information about where human trafficking may occur (Table 74.1).

Elements of Force, Fraud, and Coercion

Force	Fraud	Coercion

• Physical restraint
• Physical harm
  - Sexual assault
  - Beatings
• Monitoring and confinement
	(False promises of)
	• Employment
	  - Role
	  - Wages
	  - Working conditions
	• Relationship
	  - Love or marriage
	  - Promise of a "better life"
		• Threats of serious harm
		• Psychological abuse
		  - Isolation
		• Document confiscation
		• Blackmail
		  - Photos/internet
		• Threats
		  - Reports to authorities
		    • Law enforcement
		    • Immigration

Referred to as "breaking," force is often used to stop the victim from resisting in the earlier stages.	As "unforeseen problem" will result in a change in employment status, compensation, living arrangement, debt agreement, or nature of relationship.	This is used to induce fear and shame

Figure 74.1 Examples of force, fraud, and coercion.

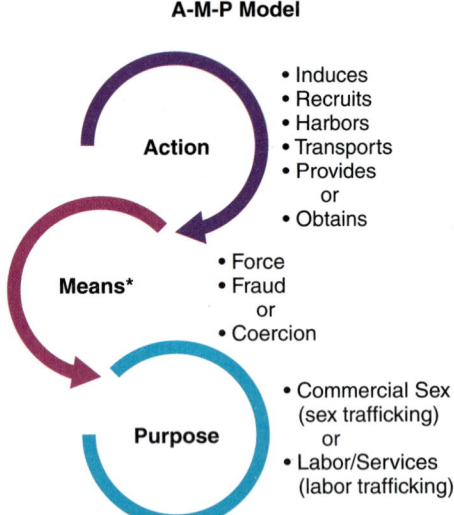

Figure 74.2 AMP Model.

Who Is at Risk?

Accurate statistics related to human trafficking are difficult to obtain; however, common themes are discernable. Although the average age for a child to be trafficked in the United States is 15 years old, some states such as Arizona report an average age of 14 years old, and some victims as young as 9 years old. Traffickers prey on younger victims to exploit vulnerabilities related to immature cognitive ability, less life experience, and poor decision-making capability. Although human trafficking occurs across the life span, sex trafficking is more prevalent among children and adolescents, whereas adults make up larger numbers of labor trafficking victims. Although U.S. statistics demonstrate larger percentages of female sex-trafficked victims, upward of 95%, it is believed that males are misrepresented. Youth who identify as LGBTQ+ are highly susceptible to victimization and less likely to report because of fear and stigma. According to the Human Trafficking Hotline, environmental factors contribute to the vulnerability of potential victims; for example, relocation from another state or country. Though the majority of people trafficked in the United States are legal U.S. residents, homelessness makes youth exponentially more susceptible to being exploited. A large number of survivors with unstable housing report having been victimized despite active involvement with the social services and histories of interaction with Child Protective Services.

Additional vulnerabilities include substance use/abuse, medical problems, or behavioral health issues. For example, traffickers may use illicit drugs to create an addiction, only to withhold drugs as a form of punishment or coercion. Another example is that needed medication such as insulin might be rationed or confiscated to discipline a victim who has diabetes. Those victims with complications related to mental health may lack the ability to fend for themselves and be deprived of needed treatment and medication.

How Does This Happen?

It is important to avoid stereotypes and understand that victims of human trafficking often know their trafficker. In some instances, the trafficker is a close relative or even a parent. Victims are rarely kidnapped and most began a relationship with their trafficker in a respectful, kind, and consensual manner. Whether a family member, partner, spouse, or a trusted friend, the relationship is exploited and the victim becomes trapped. Most children are not kidnapped off the street or caught walking in "bad neighborhoods," but contacted in their own homes. The advancing technology of Internet gaming, phone apps, and other online activity allows traffickers to connect with children, and quite often, parents remain unaware. Traffickers tend to befriend the victim, and on meeting them, the "grooming process" begins.

The "grooming process" involves gaining trust, perhaps through a shared secret, a promise not to tell, bonding over a problem/situation, or conveyance of deep understanding. Once trust is established, the trafficker seeks to

TABLE 74.1 Typology of Human Trafficking					
Typology of Human Trafficking					
Escort services	Hotels and hospitality	Restaurants and food service	Landscaping		Remote interactive sexual acts
Illicit massage	Outdoor solicitation	Peddling and begging	Illicit activities		Carnivals
Bars, strip clubs, and cantinas	Residential	Agriculture and animal husbandry	Arts and entertainment		Forestry and logging
Pornography	Domestic work	Health and beauty services	Commercial cleaning services		Health care
Personal sexual servitude	Traveling sales crews	Construction	Factories and manufacturing		Recreational facilities

Source: Polaris. (2020b, January 13). The typology of modern slavery. https://polarisproject.org/the-typology-of-modern-slavery/

fulfill a need or solve a problem, including physical items, employment, housing, transportation, or a friendship or romantic relationship. Next, the trafficker begins to isolate the victim from friends, family, and school, thus decreasing the victim's ability to seek help. Then, the trafficker will exploit the person by asking them to do something that they may not be comfortable doing. Quite often, the request is presented as a "one-time thing" to "help" the trafficker who is now in need of a favor. Once the victim fulfills the request(s), the trafficker will eventually become verbally, psychologically, and sometimes physically abusive toward the victim. At this point, the victim is controlled by the trafficker and trapped in a new world known as "the life."

CLINICAL PRESENTATION

There is no "typical" presentation for a victim of human trafficking. Like domestic violence or child abuse, a victim of human trafficking may have unexplained injuries, bruising, or scars. A majority of sex-trafficked survivors in the United States report histories of physical violence resulting in open wounds, fractures, burns, and head injuries. With concern for physical appearance in the case of sex trafficking, injuries tend to be inflicted on areas of the body that are easily concealed, such as cigarette/cigar burns to the bottom of the feet or head injuries that are hidden by hair. Patches of missing hair may result from being dragged, violently yanked, or repeatedly hit in the head.

Victims of sex trafficking might present with indications of sexual assault, including anogenital trauma from forced, unprotected, nonlubricated penetration by numerous offenders on a daily basis. Oral trauma such as a displaced jaw and broken or missing teeth are not uncommon. A torn frenulum of the lip or tongue may result from forced oral rape. Poor dentition and mouth sores are indicative of delayed or absent dental care. Bladder damage may result from untreated/recurring sexually transmitted infections (STIs) or trauma.

Females who are victims of sex trafficking may be forced to use items to stop menstruation such as make-up sponges, condoms, paper towels, napkins, or baby wipes. Multiple retained tampons without strings are a highly suspicious finding. Repeated injury to the reproductive system may cause structural damage, leading to infertility. On the other hand, multiple unplanned/unwanted pregnancies may result in damage as well.

Most survivors report having had neurological symptoms while being trafficked. Less obvious yet more prevalent complaints such as headaches, dizziness, blurred vision, and difficulty concentrating are among the most common. Symptoms associated with malnutrition might be caused by poor dietary intake, from little food availability, or an actual eating disorder. Gastrointestinal (GI) symptoms such as abdominal pain, nausea and vomiting, diarrhea, and rectal bleeding should be explored as they may result from diet, stress, or trauma.

Although victims may be hesitant to disclose injuries, performing thorough assessments and remaining watchful for subtle signs are key. A lack of preventive care or delay in seeking help for acute conditions may result in a more complicated situation than expected. Nonadherence to the medical regimen and poor hygiene are only a few examples of deficient self-care. It is crucial for the nurse to remain nonjudgmental and provide accurate information at the patient's level of understanding. Victims must be treated in a way they feel welcome to return at any time, and the provider should understand they might never see that patient again.

Using a *trauma-informed approach,* defined as collaboration with community resources to empower individuals to determine their own futures, will not only ensure the patient remains in charge of their care but also will maximize comfort and result in a better experience throughout care. Additionally, providers must be careful with language, refraining from using terms such as "noncompliance" or "unwise decision making." Finally, providers must remember that although the actions and statements by the health-care team are important to monitor, the team's nonverbal cues are magnified by a person who already feels ashamed and alone.

Some victims may be fearful and silent or may defer conversation to their companion. If the trafficker is present, the victim might look to them for permission to speak. If the victim speaks a different language, the trafficker may insist on interpreting for them. In this instance, it is important for the nurse to inform them of hospital policy and the requirement of using a medically certified interpreter. If the guest insists, document this exchange as it may be further evidence of something more serious. Protocol might require additional measures to ensure patient and staff safety.

Lack of eye contact can be commonplace. The emotional state of the victim may be centered around feelings of abandonment, loss, and neglect. Some victims will present as feeling numb or having suicidal ideation, whereas others exhibit anger or rage. For sex trafficking, there may be psychological effects from physical force and torture, as many victims are raped multiple times a day by complete strangers. Unfortunately, many victims are manipulated to being fearful of their own arrest and thus may panic at the sight of law enforcement.

One of the tactics used by traffickers to dominate a person is to control their identity. Thus, the victim may present with few or no personal possessions, no identification/passport, and no money. They might be required to check in frequently or leave their cell phone on speaker mode to allow conversations to be monitored by the trafficker. As victims are moved to various locations, they may lack knowledge of their whereabouts. Some may say, "I'm just visiting" or "I just moved here," to hide the fact they don't know what city they are in.

Although a tattoo does not automatically indicate human trafficking, tattoos with the words "property of" may be used as branding. The number "304" could represent an area code but it also spells "hOE" if the 7-segment light-emitting diode (LED) number is turned upside down. In referring to themselves as "kings," a trafficker may use branding to indicate royalty, such as a crown. Symbols like dollar signs, money, guns, and diamonds are also common. The absence of a tattoo, however, does not mean that someone is not being trafficked any more than having one indicates that someone is a victim of human trafficking. During an assessment, simple conversation such as, "What does this tattoo mean?" will allow a person to converse about their "artwork." A person upset by the conversation or unwilling to explain is not automatically a victim; however, additional assessment findings may indicate otherwise.

It's Not What You Think

Patients do not necessarily present to primary care with an unknown person. In fact, many survivors report being trafficked by people they know, including their own family members. Furthermore, human trafficking does not always involve violent crimes of force and kidnapping, as most traffickers use psychological manipulation and threats to control their victims. Some health-care workers believe that victims are being physically held against their will or locked up. Although this is true for some victims, most individuals are trapped and manipulated through physically nonviolent methods (such as withholding something or providing something that the victim cannot survive without). In many cases, the victim is afraid to leave and feels that they are in more danger if they do. However, victims tend not to identify as being under "control" of the trafficker. In fact, as health-care workers often ask, "Are you safe at home?," the victim may answer yes because they do not perceive their situation as dangerous.

Nursing Situation: Human Trafficking

A 16-year-old female lives with her 23-year-old female friend. They are both involved with substance use and host parties every weekend. During these events, the 16-year-old often engages in sexual activity with partygoers selected by the friend. After 1 month, the 16-year-old is unable to pay rent and talks to her friend. She is told, "That's OK, you're supercool and my friends love you. We can keep partying." As time goes on, the 16-year-old continues to engage in sexual activity at weekly parties. Though consensual, she sometimes feels pressured and would rather skip out on some nights. One day, the 16-year-old suspects that she may have a bladder infection and presents to the emergency department for evaluation. On completing the intake process, the triage nurse asks, "Are you safe at home?" The girl looks oddly at the nurse and says, "Yes. What kind of question is that?"

The patient believes she is "safe" because she gets along with her roommate and feels as if she has never been "forced" to do anything she doesn't want to do. Although acknowledging that her living arrangements could be better, she accepts them as "fine." The standard assessment question, "Do you feel safe at home?" was believed to reveal the truth if asked directly. In this case, the patient does not realize she is a victim. She believes she is having consensual sex in "less than ideal" situations. The better question in this case is: "If you were to stop having sex at these parties, could you still remain there, rent-free?" If the answer is "no," the sexual activity is in exchange for shelter, thus a "commercial sex act," and she is a victim of sex trafficking. The "commercial" component is what separates "sex trafficking" from the crimes of sexual assault, rape, or child molestation. Although those charges might be added to a case of sex trafficking, assault is not necessary to prove for a victim to have been trafficked. Further, force, fraud, or coercion is not required to substantiate sex trafficking when a minor is involved.

Where Do They Go for Care?

Traffickers tend to control their victims by limiting access to health care. The emergency department is the most common facility sought for treatment; however, Table 74.2 lists other health-care locations where providers may encounter victims of human trafficking. Unfortunately, often victimhood remains unnoticed when the patient interacts with health-care providers. Negative interactions such as poor treatment, victim blaming, and even harassment present other barriers to victims receiving help.

DIAGNOSTIC REASONING

It is important to note that physical examination may or may not indicate any observable evidence of human trafficking. This does not mean that human trafficking

TABLE 74.2 Common Places for Health-Care Services		
• Emergency department	• OB/GYN clinic	• Urgent care
• Dental clinics	• School nurse	• Primary care clinic
• Substance-use treatment	• Outpatient clinics	• Ambulance

Source: Polaris. On-ramps, intersections, and exit routes: a roadmap for systems and industries to prevent and disrupt human trafficking. https://polarisproject.org/wp-content/uploads/2018/08/A-Roadmap-for-Systems-and-Industries-to-Prevent-and-Disrupt-Human-Trafficking-Health-Care.pdf. Published July 2018.

has not taken place. Because a victim of human trafficking will not necessarily present with a full list of indicators, the provider may notice small findings within the physical assessment, story or intake, nonverbal cues, companion(s), and social interaction. It is not the provider's responsibility to "rescue" the victim but to acknowledge the potential of human trafficking and assess the patient's needs and concerns. In many cases, listening is the best assistance a clinician can provide, along with the promise of a safe place to return when ready. The patient's privacy is of utmost importance as it may be linked to their safety. Resources provided may need to be verbal, as the victim cannot return to the trafficker with such information. Calling 911 from the primary care setting may endanger the victim or others involved.

As mandated reporters, health-care providers must contact law enforcement and/or state agency assigned to protect children for any person under the age of 18 years suspected of being a victim of trafficking. Although visible injury makes the decision easier, the subtle signs of human trafficking might leave the provider hesitant, second-guessing their decision. The provider is simply obligated to report based on their assessment findings. There is no penalty for being wrong. Unfortunately, health-care providers tend to be cautious and fear overreacting. If there is any indication that the child is not safe, the provider should discuss the situation with their supervisor or other providers to determine next steps.

MANAGEMENT

Initial treatment for victims of human trafficking includes crisis intervention, physical examination, and psychiatric evaluation. Providers should use a trauma-informed approach by communicating their intention to keep the patient safe, such as by stating, "My first priority is your safety." Allowing multiple health-care workers to approach the patient at once may be frightening. Yet, leaving the patient alone may further isolate them, resulting in feelings of abandonment. Although the provider may have many items to document, patience is crucial. Answers may come slowly, and the primary care provider should ensure the assessment is not a harsh verbal interrogation.

As a primary care provider, it is important to be present, approachable, and nonjudgmental with every patient interaction. Although the provider may be unaware that they are speaking with a victim of human trafficking, each encounter is crucial in "planting the seed" and creating a comfortable experience to enable the patient to one day return or seek help elsewhere. There is no particular question that compels a victim to disclose their situation. Tables 74.3 and 74.4 provide questions to ask to help establish and maintain trust while eliciting information about possible human trafficking. The primary care provider should use thoughtful, nonthreatening questions throughout the interaction. If the patient is identified as a victim of human trafficking, they are not the only uncomfortable person in the room. Only about 5% of frontline health-care workers feel some degree of confidence in their ability to identify victims of human trafficking, and only 7.7% are confident in treating these patients. Unfortunately, many survivors of human trafficking report that they did not disclose their situation because "the nurse seemed busy."

Regarding documentation, primary care providers should record objectively, as stated by the patient, including sexual assault and allegations related to injuries. Documentation should use direct quotes, without including the provider's judgment.

Awareness of human trafficking is the first step. Like treating a medical or psychological condition, prevention is key and requires additional focus, methodology, and outcomes. Primary care providers can help by identifying human trafficking as a public health issue, promoting campaigns that focus on respect for others, and providing targeted education for children and adolescents about relationships (importance of healthy relationships and friendships, defining what it means to be respectful of others and respected by others).

FOLLOW-UP AND REFERRAL

The most valuable resource is the National Human Trafficking Hotline (see Resources). Available to victims, health-care workers, or anyone seeking information, they provide contact numbers for shelters, law enforcement agencies, and other resources available for a particular

TABLE 74.3 Basic Statements and Questions to Build Trust	
• "I am here to help you."	• "Where are you staying?"
• "Who is with you?"	• "What sort of work do you do?"
• "Would you like to talk in private?"	• "Do you have any ID?"
• "When was the last time you were in the hospital or saw your doctor?"	• "Do you have a cell phone?" • "Where do you usually keep it?"
• "When was your last meal?" • "What was it?"	• "Do you play any sports?"

TABLE 74.4 Higher-Level Questions

Higher-Level Questions

- "Are you scared, nervous, or anxious?"
  - "Why do you think that is?"
- "Have you ever had to do things that you did not want to do in order to stay somewhere?"
- "Did someone hurt you?"
  - "Was it on purpose?"
- "Has anyone ever taken pictures of you and put them on the Internet?"
- "Have you ever had to trade sex for money or something else you needed?"

area. Staffed 24 hours a day in all 50 states, this number is answered by a live person with training in working with victims of human trafficking. Because the hotline is not part of law enforcement, using this resource does not fulfill the need for making a mandated report.

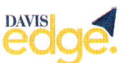 Go to Davis Edge for practice Q&A.

REFERENCES

2020 Trafficking in Persons Report. United States Department of State. https://www.state.gov/reports/2020-trafficking-in-persons-report/. Published January 15, 2021.

Chapter 78—Trafficking Victims Protection. (n.d.). Office of the Law Revision Counsel of the United States House of Representatives. Retrieved February 14, 2021. https://uscode.house.gov/view.xhtml?path=/prelim@title22/chapter78&edition=prelim

Chisolm-Straker M, Richardson LD, Cossio T. Combating slavery in the 21st century: the role of emergency medicine. *J Health Care Poor Underserved.* 2012;23(3): 980-987. doi: 10.1353/hpu.2012.0091

Department of Homeland Security. Human Trafficking 101 Information Sheet. https://www.dhs.gov/blue-campaign/materials/human-trafficking-101. Published June 30, 2020.

International Labour Organization. Economics of forced labour. International Labour Organization. Retrieved from https://www.ilo.org/global/about-the-ilo/newsroom/news/WCMS_243201/lang—en/index.htm. Published May 20, 2014.

Lederer LJ, Wetzel CA. The health consequences of sex trafficking and their implications for identifying victims in healthcare facilities. *Ann Health Law.* 2014;23(1):61-91.

National Human Trafficking Hotline. Federal Law. Retrieved from https://humantraffickinghotline.org/what-human-trafficking/federal-law. Published July 14, 2020.

National Human Trafficking Hotline. (n.d.). The Traffickers. Retrieved February 14, 2021. https://humantraffickinghotline.org/what-human-trafficking/human-trafficking/traffickers

National Human Trafficking Hotline. (2019a). Myths & facts. Retrieved from https://humantraffickinghotline.org/what-human-trafficking/myths-misconceptions.

National Human Trafficking Training and Technical Assistance Center (NHTTAC). (n.d.). Trauma-informed approach. NHTTAC. Retrieved February 14, 2021. https://nhttac.acf.hhs.gov/soar/eguide/respond/Trauma_Informed_Care

National Human Trafficking Hotline. (2019b). What is human trafficking? Retrieved from https://humantraffickinghotline.org/what-human-trafficking.

Office of Trafficking in Persons. Fact sheet: human trafficking. Administration for Children & Families Doc No: OTIP-FS-18-01; November 2017.

Office of Trafficking in Persons. What is human trafficking? https://www.acf.hhs.gov/otip/about/what-human-trafficking. Published December 24, 2020.

Polaris. On-ramps, intersections, and exit routes: a roadmap for systems and industries to prevent and disrupt human trafficking. https://polarisproject.org/wp-content/uploads/2018/08/A-Roadmap-for-Systems-and-Industries-to-Prevent-and-Disrupt-Human-Trafficking-Health-Care.pdf. Published July 2018.

Polaris. The 2019 Trafficking victims protection reauthorization act: a topical summary & analysis of four bills. Polarisproject.Org. https://polarisproject.org/wp-content/uploads/2020/01/Polaris-TVPRA-2019-Analysis.pdf. Published 2019.

Polaris. (2020a, February 18). How human trafficking happens. https://polarisproject.org/how-human-trafficking-happens/

Polaris. (2020b, January 13). The typology of modern slavery. https://polarisproject.org/the-typology-of-modern-slavery/

Polaris. (2021a). Human trafficking and the healthcare industry. https://polarisproject.org/human-trafficking-and-the-healthcare-industry/

Polaris. (2021b). Love and trafficking: how traffickers groom & control their victims. Polarisproject.Org. https://polarisproject.org/blog/2021/02/love-and-trafficking-how-traffickers-groom-control-their-victims/

Saad BL. U.S. ethics ratings rise for medical workers and teachers. Gallup.Com. https://news.gallup.com/poll/328136/ethics-ratings-rise-medical-workers-teachers.aspx. Published January 14, 2021.

TRUST Arizona. (n.d.). Human trafficking 101. TrustAZ.Org. Retrieved February 14, 2021. https://trustaz.org/human-trafficking-information/human-trafficking-101/

U.S. Immigration and Customs Enforcement. Human Trafficking and Smuggling. ICE. https://www.ice.gov/factsheets/human-trafficking. Published January 16, 2013.

RESOURCES

National Human Trafficking Hotline
  Phone: 888-373-7888
  Text: "HELP" to 233733 (BEFREE)
  https://humantraffickinghotline.org/

Trafficking of Victims Reauthorization Act of 2019
  https://www.dhs.gov/human-trafficking-laws-regulations

Section 14: URGENT CARE PROBLEMS

SECTION EDITOR
Jill E. Winland-Brown, EdD, APRN, FNP-BC, FAANP

Chapter 75

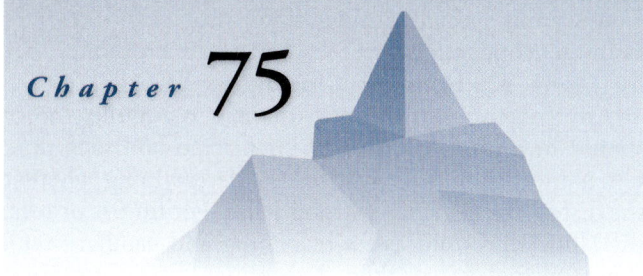

Common Injuries

Jill E. Winland-Brown, EdD, APRN, FNP-BC, FAANP
Brian Oscar Porter, MD, PhD, MPH, MBA

WOUNDS AND LACERATIONS

Wounds and lacerations result in a disruption of the continuity of skin commonly related to trauma. The mechanism and energy of the force causing the defect determine the type and severity of the wound. Wounds can range from trivial lacerations or abrasions (e.g., common childhood playground injuries) to more severe injuries such as stabbings or shootings that may require immediate surgical care. All wounds have the potential of becoming infected and should be evaluated for more serious occult injury and retained foreign bodies. Proper evaluation and care will reduce the morbidity associated with wounds.

EPIDEMIOLOGY AND CAUSES

Statistics vary in the number of patient visits to urgent care and primary care settings for wounds and lacerations. Because many clinicians do not suture in the office, most individuals seek urgent care clinics or emergency departments (EDs) where they know they can be treated. Nevertheless, most clinicians will encounter patients with wounds at some point and need to be cognizant of their care. Wounds in adults become infected about 5% of the time, whereas wounds in children become infected 1.2% of the time. Almost 75% of patients with wounds are men, with an average age in the early 20s.

It is prudent in any case for the clinician to perform a thorough assessment and maintain complete documentation of wound care. Wound management accounts for a significant percentage of malpractice claims. Although culturing the wound can identify infectious complications and subsequently guide treatment, it is essential that the clinician visually appraise the wound initially for signs of infection to determine whether more invasive action is necessary and to select the proper antibiotic.

PATHOPHYSIOLOGY

The skin is made up of several layers, which are divided into the epidermis and dermis. The skin acts as a barrier to entry into the body, regulates body temperature, aids in the elimination of waste, and helps prevent dehydration. It also contains the cutaneous nerves, is a reservoir for nutrient stores and water, and is a source of vitamin D when exposed to sunlight. The ability of bacteria and other substances to penetrate the skin is related to the depth of the wound. Wounds that do not penetrate the stratum germinativum—the basement layer of the skin—do not leave scars.

Wound healing involves many processes that occur simultaneously:

- *Injury phase.* This phase involves coagulation and platelet release. This process enhances the inflammatory response in the wound.
- *Inflammatory phase.* This phase is characterized by increased capillary permeability, which allows white blood cells (WBCs) to migrate into the wound. Neutrophils and monocytes act as scavengers and rid the wound of debris and bacteria. In addition to providing wound defenses, inflammation stimulates other monocytes to promote fibroblast replication and neovascularization.
- *Epithelialization phase.* This phase begins within hours of tissue injury and involves the migration of cells at the wound edges from one side of the incision to the other. Within 24 to 48 hours, incisional wounds are epithelialized. Lacerations may heal by primary intention when the edges of the wound are approximated with sutures and allowed to heal by secondary intention from the inside out, as granulation tissue fills in open lacerations whose edges are not approximated. Collagen synthesis in the healing wound peaks at day 7 post-trauma, and the tensile strength (which determines the ability of the wound to remain intact) increases rapidly at this stage. Typically, the wound will have only 15% to 20% of its normal tensile strength at 3 weeks and 60% by 4 months.

- *Remodeling phase.* In this final phase, the process involves wound contraction and tissue formation. This process begins on the third day after the injury and continues for up to 6 months. The appearance of the wound can change during this period; for this reason, plastic surgeons will usually wait 6 months before considering revising a scar.

CLINICAL PRESENTATION

Subjective

A thorough history of the injury must be obtained and documented. The mechanism of wounding is useful in determining the likelihood of deep structure injury, infection risk, extent of tissue damage, and likelihood of associated injuries. Questions regarding medical history should also be included. For example, a patient with diabetes or a history of vascular problems has a higher possibility of infection (see Focus on History: Wounds and Lacerations).

> **Focus on History: Wounds and Lacerations**
>
> History
> - Mechanism of injury
> - Potential for foreign body
> - Potential for injury to underlying (deep) tissues
> - Potential for infection
> - Type of injury
> - Age of wound
> - Delayed or immediate presentation
> - Tetanus immunization status
> - Allergies
> - Comorbidities (especially vascular problems)
>
> Physical Examination
> - Vital signs
> - General examination
> - Vascular injury
> - Nerve involvement
> - Location over joint
> - Tendon damage
> - Association with fracture (open or closed)
> - Range of motion
> - Wound contamination
> - Foreign body
> - Avulsion injury
> - Puncture

Objective

A description of any wound should include the length and depth (in centimeters) and the type of defect found. The depth of the wound is described as *partial thickness* if all layers of the skin have not been violated. If any subdermal tissue can be seen in the wound, it is considered a *full-thickness* defect. Wounds this deep may involve injuries to deeper structures, and further evaluation is necessary.

Different types of wounds are associated with specific types of associated injuries and special considerations. Refer to Advanced Assessment 75.1 for various types of wounds and special considerations associated with their assessment and treatment. See Therapeutic Procedure 75.1 for step-by-step instructions for abscess drainage.

Any extremity that has sustained a wound injury should be evaluated for distal circulation and sensation. Circulation should be assessed by determining whether the distal extremity has a strong pulse. For fingers or toes, the clinician should assess blanching and capillary refill time (normal is less than 2 seconds). Distal sensation should be checked to rule out nerve injury. A gross neurological screening examination comparing sensation on bilateral extremities should be done on all patients who present with wounds to the extremities.

All wounds must be explored to identify any deep structure injuries or foreign bodies and to help determine the type of closure required. After the wound is anesthetized, a bright light should be used to illuminate the wound. Wound edges should be retracted, but it is important not to cause trauma to the tissue that may impede normal healing. Blindly probing a wound can cause additional tissue destruction or nerve or vascular injury. Using Adson forceps with teeth or tissue retractors, the clinician should hook the wound edge and retract it to expose deep structures. The clinician should probe the wound with gloved fingers only.

For large wounds, it is important to examine the full length of the wound because only a small section of the wound may be deep enough to cause deep structure injury. The defect should be examined for any tendon injury. Exposed tendon will appear as a shiny white structure in the wound. The range of motion of an affected extremity or digit should be tested carefully against resistance in all planes in which the extremity can be moved. Pain during movement can indicate a partial tendon laceration.

Examination for injuries to underlying muscular fascia is required. If a large defect is found, the fascia must be closed to prevent herniation of the muscle in the future. If the wound is near a joint, violation of the joint capsule must be ruled out. The joint capsule is lined with a synovial membrane and contains synovial fluid, which lubricates the joint and also provides cushioning for the joint. If the synovial capsule is violated, the joint may become seeded (contaminated) with bacteria, in which case the possibility of developing a septic joint is likely.

The joint capsule is a shiny white structure; if it has been penetrated, bone ends are palpable and can be visualized. Again, the joint must be examined through the full range of motion to look for a defect. If a joint violation is suspected but cannot be confirmed by visualization, the clinician should order an x-ray of adhesive is very fluid and can run into the eye, essentially gluing it shut. If this happens, the clinician must apply an antibiotic eye ointment to aid in slowly dissolving the adhesive. If it cannot be removed for an eye examination, the patient should see an ophthalmologist immediately.

For 2-octylcyanoacrylate tissue adhesive application, the skin must be clean and dry. The wound is approximated with sterile fingers or tissue forceps, taking care not to injure the tissue with the forceps. Once the wound is well approximated, with the fingers at least 1 cm away, the adhesive is applied in concentric circles, allowing 15 seconds between applications. The patient should be advised not to scrub the adhesive and not to apply any antibiotic ointment to the wound, because this can dissolve the adhesive. Adhesive tape should also not be placed directly over the site.

Another application for 2-octylcyanoacrylate tissue adhesive is in the repair of skin tears. Once the skin tear has been cleansed, the torn skin should be unfurled, teasing the curled-up pieces of skin back to their previous locations. The clinician should not cut off the torn skin because it may be used as an allograft. The 2-octylcyanoacrylate adhesive can then be applied with excellent results. This tissue adhesive also serves as a barrier against common bacterial microbes.

To decrease tension in high-tension areas, subcutaneous stitches are helpful. To avoid obvious scars and poor cosmetic results, landmarks and skin layers must be meticulously aligned, with the first suture being placed in the center of the wound. Suturing techniques are illustrated in Therapeutic Procedure 75.2. Scarring will be minimized if the following adage is followed: "approximate, don't strangulate."

Wound Dressings

The wound should be kept clean, dry, and covered. For sites that are difficult to keep bandaged, a thin layer of antibiotic ointment should be applied to protect the wound. Bandages should be changed daily or if they become wet or dirty. It is helpful to apply antibiotic ointment to the wound when the dressing is changed.

Antibiotic Therapy

Antibiotic prophylaxis for most wounds is not indicated. The risk of infection of a clean, recently injured wound in a well-vascularized area is low (only 3% to 5%). Grossly contaminated wounds or wounds that involve areas of diminished vascular supply—such as the fingers, toes, and ears—may benefit from prophylactic antibiotics. Wounds that have an increased risk of infection include the following:

- Crush injuries
- Dirty wounds
- Jagged wounds
- Wounds with devitalized tissue
- Wounds that are more than 12 to 19 hours old
- Bite wounds, especially from humans (particularly if they are meat eaters), cats, and dogs
- Wounds with retained foreign bodies
- Wounds closed with subcutaneous stitches

Patients with diabetes mellitus or who have a history of vascular compromise should be started on antibiotics prophylactically. Parenteral administration of ampicillin/sulbactam or ceftriaxone is the initial treatment of choice. This should be followed by oral therapy with amoxicillin/clavulanate, cephalexin, or cefadroxil. If the patient has allergies to penicillin or cephalosporins, the clinician should consider prescribing doxycycline with or without clindamycin, or ciprofloxacin.

When treating cellulitis or established infections, the clinician should consider initial parenteral therapy with ampicillin/sulbactam, cefoxitin, or ceftriaxone. The clinician should consider wound cultures before starting antibiotics for grossly infected wounds. If the patient has allergies to penicillin and cephalosporins, the clinician should consider using doxycycline, clindamycin, or ciprofloxacin. All parenteral therapy should be followed with oral antibiotic therapy for 7 to 10 days. Appropriate choices for oral therapy include cephalexin or cefadroxil for most infections. Wounds with a high risk of infection with anaerobic bacteria (i.e., wounds contaminated by mucus or feces) need to have broader antibiotic coverage with clindamycin or amoxicillin-clavulanate. See Evidence-Based Nursing Practice 75.1 for information about prescribing antibiotics for abscesses.

Severe infections require inpatient IV therapy. Outlining the area of erythema with a tissue marker during the initial visit will allow subsequent practitioners to assess treatment response more easily. Any extremity or digit that is infected should be immobilized to reduce the inflammatory response related to mechanical movement of the affected region. Close follow-up is important for the first 8 to 24 hours after therapy has been started. If the infection appears to be responding to therapy, the patient should continue oral therapy, with additional follow-up as indicated by the extent of the injury and infection.

FOLLOW-UP AND REFERRAL

After the initiation of outpatient therapy, patients with high-risk wounds should be instructed to follow up with the clinician who treated the wound or another provider in 1 to 2 days, so that the wound can be evaluated for healing and signs of infection. Home health-care nursing is an effective mode of wound care follow-up in the outpatient setting.

Sutures must remain in place long enough to allow adequate tensile strength to develop during the healing process. The amount of time before suture removal varies with the location of the wound and the cosmetic importance of the wound site. Sutures that are not removed in

Therapeutic Procedure 75.2: Suturing Techniques/Materials

SUTURE TECHNIQUE	ADVANTAGES	DISADVANTAGES
Buried suture	Allows good approximation of wound edges	Minimal eversion occurs.
Running continuous suture	Quick, good for children; evenly distributed tension	Entire suture must be removed.
Interrupted suture	Permits precise adjustments between sutures; allows selection of sutures	Increased risk of uneven tension over the suture line; higher incidence of "railroad track" scarring.

Therapeutic Procedure 75.2: Suturing Techniques/Materials—cont'd

SUTURE TECHNIQUE	ADVANTAGES	DISADVANTAGES
Wound-closure strips	Minimal wound trauma; more resistant to wound infection	Poor wound eversion; more difficult wound edge approximation.

SUTURE MATERIALS	CLINICAL CONSIDERATIONS
Nonabsorbable	
Silk	Not recommended due to frequent tissue reaction
Nylon	Most common
Polypropylene	Best for subcuticular and continuous suturing Easiest to remove
Absorbable (metabolized after ~3 weeks—used in inner tissues)	
Synthetic polymers	For deep layers Absorbed by hydrolysis (not used for skin)
Surgical catgut	Dissolves in an unpredictable time frame Excites tissue reaction during its destruction
Tissue Adhesives	
	"Glue"-type adhesive of *n*-butyl 2-cyanoacrylate monomer is used in combination with or as an alternative to sutures for wound closure

SUTURE SIZE	USES
From smallest to largest size: 10/0—9/0—8/0—7/0—6/0—5/0—4/0—3/0—2/0—0—1—2—3—4—5—6—7—8—9—10 6/0 is thinner than a human hair; used for delicate suturing (e.g., eye surgery). Family practice clinicians primarily use 3/0 and 4/0.	
Fine sizes (5/0 to 10/0)	Plastic surgery Ophthalmic surgery Pediatric surgery Vascular surgery
Medium sizes (3/0 and 4/0)	All other kinds of surgery
Heavy sizes (2/0 and greater)	Retention Anchoring bone

a timely fashion can cause scarring, and the healing tissue can cover the sutures if left in too long; however, sutures over joints or areas of high skin tension must remain in place longer than at other sites. If staples are used, follow-up will need to be with a clinician equipped with the appropriate staple removal equipment.

The following time frames are recommended for the removal of sutures at various bodily sites:

- Face: 4 to 6 days; after suture removal, reinforce wound closure with adhesive strips (Steri-Strips)
- Scalp: 6 to 10 days

- Trunk: 7 to 10 days
- Arms: 10 to 14 days
- Legs: 10 to 14 days
- Joints: 14 days

Patient Education: Wounds and Lacerations

The patient may shower 12 to 24 hours after the initial wound repair. Wound healing processes form a protective barrier that will prevent bacterial invasion after as little as 8 hours. The wound should not be submerged in water, however, until after suture removal or scar formation. Aloe vera may provide mild pain relief, but it does not improve wound healing or reduce the risk of wound infection. Patients should be advised that taking ibuprofen (Motrin) or another NSAID will serve the same function.

Patients should monitor the wound for signs of infection, including redness surrounding the wound area (cellulitis), red streaks extending from the wound (angioedema), and any purulent discharge from the wound (infection). Other secondary signs of infection include worsening pain, fever, and chills. Patients with high-risk wounds should understand the importance of follow-up in 1 to 2 days to evaluate for appropriate healing or signs of infection. Topical vitamin E preparations should be avoided because it is a weak steroid that can delay healing and cause dehiscence of high-tension wounds. Oral intake of vitamin E during the healing process is beneficial, although a well-balanced diet will provide a sufficient amount. Box 75.1 presents discharge instructions for patients with wounds and lacerations. As smoking and malnutrition are some of the risk factors related to impaired wound healing, patients should be advised to stop smoking and follow a healthy diet.

Box 75.1 Discharge Instructions: Wounds and Lacerations

- Keep the injured extremity elevated above the level of the heart if possible.
- Cleanse the wound daily with warm, soapy water. Gently remove debris and any scab that is present.
- Lacerations over joints should be immobilized until the sutures are removed to prevent further injury from mechanical irritation.
- For lower extremities, the patient should be advised to do isometric exercises to prevent a deep vein thrombosis while wearing a splint.
- Watch for signs of infection: redness, warmth, increased pain, swelling, fever, red streaks progressing up the extremity, any purulent discharge (pus) from the wound.
- Check wound as needed for any signs of infection—up to every 24 hours for high-risk wounds.

ANIMAL AND HUMAN BITES

An animal bite is a bite wound to humans from dogs, cats, snakes, or other animals, including other humans. In most cases, bites result in puncture wounds, possible lacerations, and, in some cases, crush injuries. All bites, regardless of the source, are considered to be contaminated wounds and have a substantial risk of infection.

EPIDEMIOLOGY AND CAUSES

Two to five million animal bites occur annually in the United States. Of these bites, 80% result in only minor injury, but 1% to 2% of these wounds result in hospitalization. Bite wounds occur in all age-groups but are most common in children. Animal bites cause more than 30 deaths annually in the United States and involve mostly infants and small children.

Dogs inflict approximately 90% of all mammalian bites, with an overall infection rate of 15% to 20%. Risks of infection from dog bites are greatest for puncture wounds, crush injuries, and bites to the hand. Dog bites in general have a 5% infection rate, but dog bites to the hand carry a 40% infection rate. The most common infectious organisms isolated from dog bites are *Staphylococcus aureus*, *Pasteurella multocida*, *Corynebacterium* species, and α-hemolytic *Streptococcus* species. Most dog bite victims are children, with males between 5 and 9 years of age the most common. The majority of dog bite wounds are from a domestic pet known to the victim, with pit bulls being responsible for the most human deaths related to dog bites each year, followed by Rottweilers and Huskies.

Cats inflict approximately 10% of mammalian bites. Their needle-like teeth result in puncture wounds with a high incidence of infection—around 50%. Specifically, cat bites are more common in adult females although, in general, males receive more animal bite injuries than females. In more than 50% of cat bite wounds, *P. multocida* is isolated; this bacterium causes wound infections that develop within 24 hours of the bite, resulting in an intense inflammatory response and joint infection.

The third most common type of mammalian bites are those from other human beings. These bites account for 2% to 3% of all animal bites reported. Human bite injuries received during fistfights are common in teenagers and in alcohol-intoxicated males aged 30 to 35 years. Accidental human bites occur most commonly in children. Common infectious agents isolated from human bite wounds include *S. aureus*, *Streptococcus*, *Corynebacterium* species, *Bacteroides* species, and *Eikenella corrodens*.

Two percent of reported animal bites are from rodents. Some sick or injured wild animals—such as squirrels, skunks, and bats—will attack humans without provocation and may carry rabies caused by rhabdovirus. Clinicians should be familiar with state laws and regulations regarding bite wounds from mammals and rabies prophylaxis, especially in areas where rabies infection is endemic.

Venomous snake bites affect 7,000 to 8,000 people in the United States annually. Of the 3,000 species of snakes worldwide, 600 are venomous. In the United States, venomous snakes include rattlesnakes, copperheads, cottonmouths or water moccasins, and coral snakes. About 5% of snake bite victims die of envenomation (i.e., a venomous bite). Approximately 10% to 45% of patients with rattlesnake bites have permanent injuries, most commonly due to the loss of a finger.

PATHOPHYSIOLOGY

The risk of bite wound infection depends on the wound location, tissue damage, patient characteristics, time elapsed before treatment, and the type of animal that inflicted the bite. Wounds should be classified as low risk or high risk to facilitate decision making regarding antibiotic therapy and wound suturing. *Low-risk wounds* include lacerations involving the extremities, face, and body. Wounds at low risk for infection include bites on the face, ears, scalp, and mouth. Large, clean lacerations and bites by rodents pose a low risk for infection. *High-risk wounds* include those in the distal extremities (hand, wrist, or foot), the scalp of an infant, a wound over a joint, or a penetrating wound of the cheek. Puncture wounds and nondébridable crush injuries are high risk. Patients at high risk for infection are those older than age 50 years, (see Geriatric Considerations later in this chapter) individuals with prosthetic joints or heart valves, asplenia, diabetes mellitus, altered immune status, or peripheral vascular disease, and patients who are on chronic corticosteroid therapy. Bites from venomous snakes, domestic cats, large cats, primates, pigs, or humans (especially bites to the hand) present the highest risk of infection.

Human bites in locations other than the hand have no greater risk of infection than a dog bite, if treated promptly. Most human bites are sustained in fights, but 15% to 20% of bites reported in one study were secondary to "love nips" (related to sexual activity). A closed-fist injury ("fight bite") occurs from a laceration over the metacarpophalangeal (MCP) joint caused by striking an opponent's tooth. When this occurs, infectious organisms from the mouth are inoculated directly into the bone or joint, which can lead to septic arthritis or osteomyelitis. Also, when the fingers of the closed fist are extended, the injured extensor tendons retract proximally, sealing off the tissues. This sets the stage for a rapidly progressive infection of the tendon and adjacent tissue layers.

CLINICAL PRESENTATION

Subjective

The circumstances of the bite injury should be determined. These include the area(s) of the body injured, time elapsed since the injury, type of animal (including breed), current location of the animal, relationship of the animal to the victim, vaccination and health status of the animal, and whether the attack was provoked or unprovoked. The patient should be asked about their occupation; medical history and comorbid conditions; medication allergies; tetanus immunization status; any history of immunological compromise; and any specific musculoskeletal, neurological, or vascular complaints resulting from the bite. If the bite is on the patient's hand, the clinician should ask the patient which is the patient's dominant hand. Some additional subjective findings with snake bites may include disturbed vision and/or a metallic, minty, or rubbery taste in the mouth.

Objective

More than 70% of bite wounds are located on the extremities where the victim either handled or attempted to avoid the animal or another person. Injuries to the head and neck are the next most common locations and are seen mostly in children. The clinician should inspect the skin and soft tissues, noting the presence or absence of lacerations, punctures, scratches, abrasions, swelling, crush injuries, and/or devitalized tissue. All puncture wounds should be examined carefully for injury to structures beneath the skin. A vascular examination should be performed, noting skin temperature, capillary refill time, and relevant pulses. The range of motion of all affected areas should be assessed, evaluating the functional status of potentially involved tendons. Motor and sensory nerve function should also be evaluated. To assess sensory function of the hand, the clinician should note sensation to light touch and two-point discrimination on the volar pads of the fingertips. The patient should be able to detect stimuli less than 5 mm apart in the axis of the digit, and the response should be compared with the uninjured side. The patient should be evaluated for skeletal injury and carefully assessed for neurovascular, joint, tendon, or osseous injury.

If the patient does not present with the bite wound until several hours to several days after the injury, the clinician should perform a careful search for evidence of local or systemic infection and regional adenopathy. Infection will be evidenced by increased pain, swelling, erythema, warmth, decreased range of motion at joints, or drainage from a puncture wound site. A high index of suspicion should always be maintained for the possibility of a retained foreign body in the wound, especially when an infection develops at a puncture wound site. In addition, the patient with a venomous snake bite may have nausea, vomiting, diarrhea, labored breathing, a rapid and weak heartbeat, hypotension, increased salivation, diaphoresis, numbness or tingling around the face and extremities, and/or muscle twitching.

DIAGNOSTIC REASONING

Diagnostic Tests

A radiograph of the affected area should be obtained if a fracture is suspected; a foreign body is present (e.g., tooth fragments, which are more common in bites from older animals); a bone, joint, or tendon has been penetrated; or a puncture wound has become infected. If the patient presents with a localized wound infection several hours or days after the bite, the clinician should obtain a wound-site Gram stain and both aerobic and anaerobic cultures after superficial decontamination of the wound but before débridement of devitalized tissues. Cultures of wounds are also indicated in cases in which an immunocompromised patient is infected, where there is sepsis, or when antibiotic therapy has failed. To obtain optimal wound cultures, the clinician should perform percutaneous or deep wound aspiration. If significant blood loss has occurred, it is important to obtain a CBC to assess for anemia.

If the patient is seriously ill with a bite wound infection, diagnostic tests should include a thorough laboratory evaluation (including a CBC with platelets, serum electrolyte panel, glucose level, blood urea nitrogen [BUN] and creatinine, and PT/partial thromboplastin time), at least two blood cultures, wound-site Gram stain and culture, and appropriate x-ray studies.

Differential Diagnosis

The diagnosis of animal bites is typically straightforward to determine by history, although the etiology of some bite wounds may be unclear in infants, young children, or incapacitated adults who cannot communicate the source of the bite. To properly direct management, it is critical that the animal source and extent (e.g., depth, affected structures) of the bite wound be characterized as thoroughly as possible.

MANAGEMENT

First Aid for a Venomous Snake Bite

Medical attention must be sought as soon as possible for venomous snake bites, as antivenom (antivenin) needs to be started to prevent irreversible damage or death. If possible, a picture of the snake should be taken at a safe distance to help guide the proper treatment. There is an old adage to remember to determine whether a snake is poisonous by looking at the placement of the colors on the snake: "Red next to black, friend of Jack. Red next to yellow, kill a fellow."

Jewelry should be removed from an infected extremity. Pressure bandage immobilization is controversial. It is recommended for snake bites with venoms that cause paralysis with minimal tissue damage but not recommended for bites with venom associated with significant local tissue necrosis, as the localization of toxin may worsen tissue damage.

Analgesia

Pain management is commonly provided by analgesic agents such as NSAIDs and acetaminophen (Tylenol). If nonnarcotic oral agents are ineffective and the patient is in severe pain, ketorolac (Toradol) 30 to 60 mg may be effective.

Wound Cleansing

Bites and scratches should be cleansed with mild soap and water or 1% povidone-iodine (Betadine) solution to remove the animal's saliva from the wound, as well as any particulate matter. If the bite was caused by a potentially rabid wild animal (e.g., skunk, raccoon), the clinician, wearing protective gloves, should thoroughly irrigate the wound with 1% benzalkonium chloride, which has demonstrated effectiveness in inactivating the rabies virus.

Local Anesthesia

Using a 25-gauge or smaller needle, the clinician should infiltrate the wound edges with 1% lidocaine without epinephrine (to avoid tissue ischemia) before closure if indicated. The maximum dose of lidocaine for local infiltration is 4 mg/kg (0.4 mL/kg of a 1% solution).

Wound Irrigation

The wound should be irrigated with 500 to 2,000 mL of normal saline. For wounds considered to be at high risk for infection, the clinician can use a 1% povidone-iodine (Betadine) solution. For irrigation, a 30-mL syringe with an 18- to 20-gauge plastic catheter should be used to achieve an irrigation pressure of 5 to 8 psi. This method of irrigation has been shown to reduce wound infection.

Wound Débridement

The clinician should remove foreign material, devitalized tissue, and eschar from the wound. The margins of puncture wounds should be débrided to approximately a 1- to 2-mm rim to allow for better drainage and improved cleaning.

Wound Closure

Approximately 10% of bite wounds require suturing and follow-up care. Fresh facial bites without signs of inflammation should be closed with sutures after thorough wound cleansing and preparation. Bite wounds of the hand should not be sutured. For bites to other areas in need of closure or bites greater than 24 hours old, delayed primary closure may be considered. A layer of fine-mesh gauze can be applied to the wound, which should be packed open, dressed, and followed closely. If there is no purulence or erythema of the wound margins at a 3- to 5-day clinic follow-up, wound closure may be performed.

Tetanus Immunization

Bite wounds are tetanus-prone injuries. If the patient has received a primary immunization series but not a booster shot within the past 5 years, a tetanus booster should be administered. For patients with absent or incomplete primary immunization, 250 units of tetanus immune globulin should be given, in addition to the primary vaccination.

Antimicrobial Therapy

Patients should receive antibiotic prophylaxis for 3 to 5 days if the wound is a fresh bite wound; they were bitten by a cat; have a hand bite; have moderate to severe tissue damage; have a wound that may involve a tendon, bone, or joint; have one or more puncture wounds; or have a suppressed immune system. Patients with infected wounds should be given antibiotic therapy based on the results of aerobic and anaerobic cultures. Antimicrobial prophylaxis for cat bites, high-risk dog bites (e.g., bites to the hand or bites with considerable tissue damage), and human bites can be provided with amoxicillin/clavulanate for 3 to 5 days. An alternative that has fewer gastrointestinal (GI) side effects is cefuroxime, also for 3 to 5 days. Hospital admission and parenteral antibiotic therapy will be necessary for all significant human bites to the hand, especially closed-fist injuries and bites involving penetration of the bone or joint.

Positioning

The injured area should be elevated for several days after injury. For bites located over joints, the joint should be immobilized for 3 to 5 days in a proper position, depending on the bite location: 20 degrees wrist extension, 70 to 90 degrees flexion for metacarpophalangeal joints, and 10 degrees flexion for proximal interphalangeal and distal interphalangeal joints.

Antivenom

Antivenom (antivenin) is the primary treatment for serious snake envenomation. Although there remains a risk of an adverse reaction, antivenom may be lifesaving. There are two different types of antivenom that consist of animal immunoglobulins developed against whole snake venom molecules. Monovalent antivenom antibodies are developed against a single species of snake and are only effective for bites by that particular snake or group of snakes. Polyvalent antivenoms use venoms from multiple types of snakes, typically from a large geographical region, and can treat any snake bites from that area. Whether to administer antivenom depends on weighing the potential benefit versus the risk of adverse reactions. In the event of a severe envenomation, the use of antivenom is a necessity. The World Health Organization (WHO) maintains a list of antivenoms at https://cdn.who.int/media/docs/default-source/medicines/antivenom-assessment.pdf?sfvrsn=3bb378e7_2.

Rabies Prophylaxis

Rabies is caused by a rhabdovirus that can be found in the saliva of many mammals. The rabies virus is highly neurotoxic and can be fatal. The clinician should refer questions about postexposure prophylaxis to a local health department or infectious disease specialist familiar with the rabies risk profile of the specific geographical area. After biting a human, if a dog or cat is healthy and available for 10 days of observation and shows no signs of rabies, then no treatment of the exposed person is necessary. About 85% of all cases of animal rabies in the United States now occur in wildlife. Skunks, foxes, bats, raccoons, coyotes, bobcats, and other carnivores should be considered rabid unless proven negative by laboratory assessments. The risk of rabies in lagomorphs (e.g., rabbits, hares) and rodents (e.g., mice, rats, chipmunks, and squirrels) is small.

If postexposure rabies is strongly suspected, both rabies immune globulin (RIG) and rabies human diploid-cell vaccine (HDCV) or rabies vaccine adsorbed (RVA) should be given as soon as possible before the completion of confirmatory laboratory testing. However, the vaccine course should be discontinued if fluorescent antibody tests for rabies of the sacrificed animal's neural tissue are negative. Dosing is as follows:

- RIG: 20 IU/kg. If anatomically possible, one-half of the dose should be infiltrated around the wound and the other half given intramuscularly (IM) into the gluteal muscle.
- HDCV: 1 mL should be given IM into the deltoid region on days 0, 3, 7, 14, and 28 if the patient has not been previously vaccinated.
- RVA: 1 mL should be given IM in the deltoid region on days 0, 3, 7, 14, and 28 if the patient has not been previously vaccinated.

Individuals who have been previously vaccinated with either HDCV or RVA should not receive RIG; they should, however, receive 1-mL "booster" doses IM of either HDCV or RVA on days 0 and 3.

Hepatitis B and C Assessment

The clinician should also evaluate the potential for transmission of hepatitis B or C virus (HBV or HCV) in human bites. The type of intervention is dependent on prior receipt of the HBV vaccination series (no vaccination for HCV is currently available). If HBV prophylaxis is indicated (e.g., confirmed hepatitis B surface antigen positivity in the source of the animal bite), hepatitis B immune globulin 0.06 mL/kg IM should be administered immediately and repeated in 30 days. The primary HBV vaccine series should be completed, if not already done, and a "booster" shot should be given if a protective postvaccination titer has not been confirmed. If HCV exposure is suspected, the patient should be assessed for HCV antibodies within 48 hours and, if positive, tested further for the presence of HCV RNA, which would be indicative of preexisting disease. If negative, follow-up testing should occur after at least 3 weeks because positive results likely indicate new infection, which should then be referred for further treatment.

Postexposure HIV Prophylaxis

Although the risk of HIV transmission from a human bite is low, the clinician must also consider whether a human bite was from a known HIV-infected carrier, particularly if that individual had any bleeding in the mouth (such as from severe periodontal disease or from oral trauma during a fight). For example, health-care workers working with combative HIV-positive patients may be victims of human bite wounds, be exposed to needlestick injuries, or have mucous membrane exposure to infectious fluids from their HIV-positive patients. The section on HIV infection in Chapter 64 discusses postexposure HIV prophylaxis in detail, which is considered an emergency problem that requires immediate intervention to minimize the risk of infection.

FOLLOW-UP AND REFERRAL

The patient should be discharged to home after thorough and meticulous wound management, with follow-up assessment within 48 hours. Infection, cellulitis, abscess, osteomyelitis, septicemia, tenosynovitis, septic joint (suppurative arthritis), rabies, and the loss of an injured body part are all potential complications of animal bites. Other systemic diseases that can occur as complications of animal bites are bubonic plague, cat-scratch disease, rat-bite fever, leptospirosis, tularemia, tetanus, and sporotrichosis.

Patients with severe cellulitis; systemic manifestations of infection; failure to respond to appropriate outpatient treatment within 48 hours; or bite wound infections that involve a bone, joint, tendon, or nerve should be admitted to the hospital. The practitioner should obtain early consultation with an infectious disease specialist, if needed. Septic arthritis, osteomyelitis, and closed-fist wounds ("fight bites") require orthopedic consultation.

> **Patient Education: Animal Bites**
>
> If the bite was inflicted by a wild animal or occurred in an unprovoked attack by a domestic animal, the practitioner should ask the patient to have the animal that inflicted the bite evaluated for rabies, if possible. The patient or the family should contact the local health department and consult with an animal control officer about the patterns of rabies among animals in the local area. Individuals should be taught the importance of not petting or feeding unfamiliar or wild animals.
>
> Patients should be reminded to elevate injured extremities to prevent swelling and to return for follow-up if signs of fever, redness, or swelling occur, given the subsequent risk of infection. The clinician should instruct patients to watch for red streaks, increased warmth at the wound site, increasing pain, foul odor, or increased drainage from the bite wound—all of which should trigger the patient to seek urgent assessment in the clinic or ED.

ARTHROPOD BITES AND STINGS

Arthropods are members of Arthropoda, a large phylum of animal life characterized by an external body support structure known as an exoskeleton, which includes lobsters and crabs, as well as mites, ticks, spiders, and insects. Arthropod bites and stings involve penetration of the skin by some part of the animal, typically accompanied by the release of venom that can cause local or systemic symptoms. Some arthropods, such as ticks, can also transmit disease via infectious microorganisms. The majority of complications caused by bites and stings of arthropods are from spider bites; bee, wasp, and ant stings; caterpillar spine irritation; interactions with sucking bugs, beetles, flies, and other winged insects; bites from lice, fleas, mites, and ticks; and scorpion stings.

EPIDEMIOLOGY AND CAUSES

Millions of people in the United States are injured by venoms produced by insects and other arthropods each year, with a notable number of deaths. In one 10-year period, 65 deaths were reported to have been caused by spiders in the United States. Of these, 63 deaths were from black widow spider bites. Bee and wasp (*Hymenoptera*) stings cause more deaths annually than any other venomous animal. There are 40 to 50 fatalities each year from *Hymenoptera* stings. These insect stings result in a rapid progression of toxic effects: 80% of the deaths result from anaphylactic shock less than 1 hour after the sting. Spider bites, however, have a longer time interval between bites and time of death, with nearly 90% of deaths occurring more than 12 hours after being bitten.

Ninety-five percent of all venomous animal fatalities occur from April to October, when animals and potential victims are most active in outdoor settings, heightening the risk of exposure. The risk of insect bites further increases with lack of protective measures and in areas with heavy insect infestations. Previous exposure to venom can predispose the victim to anaphylaxis upon reexposure to venom from the same arthropod via venom-specific immunoglobulin (Ig)E-mediated mechanisms.

Wasps

The yellow jacket is the major cause of *Hymenoptera* insect-sting reactions. The yellow jacket, hornet, and other wasps feed on sugary sources and are attracted to foods commonly found in garbage cans and at picnics. When a wasp stings, it injects a venomous fluid under the skin. Yellow jackets, wasps, and hornets nest under logs, in the ground, or in walls; care should be taken to avoid disturbing these insects during gardening and landscaping.

Fire Ants

The imported fire ant is a small, light reddish brown to dark brown, wingless stinging insect that is responsible for an increasing number of acute allergic reactions. This insect attaches itself to its victim by biting with its jaws and then pivoting its body around its head, stinging in multiple sites in a circular pattern with its stinger located on the end of its abdomen. The fire ant's venom causes hemolysis, depolarization of cellular membranes, activation of the alternate complement pathway, and general tissue destruction.

Fire ants inhabit loose dirt and make nests that produce up to 200,000 ants during a 3-year period. They swarm if provoked and may attack in great numbers. The two species of imported fire ants (originally from Brazil) are found predominantly in nine southern states, particularly along the Gulf Coast. However, these colonies are gradually spreading westward and northward, accounting for increased exposure each year.

Brown Recluse Spiders

The natural habitat of the brown recluse spider (*Loxosceles reclusa*) is along the Mississippi River Valley, especially in northwestern Arkansas and southern Missouri. Because this spider can live in old boxes and furniture, it is easily transported to other states. The brown recluse spider prefers warm, dry locations, such as woodpiles, cellars, and abandoned buildings; it is generally active nocturnally. Also known as a "fiddleback" spider, the brown recluse spider has a characteristic violin-shaped marking on the dorsum of its cephalothorax (head and body section). The spider's venom contains sphingomyelinase D; it is chiefly cytotoxic, causing local tissue destruction. The resulting tissue necrosis (occurring in about 10% of spider bites) is caused by an aggregation of leukocytes and platelets that forms a hemostatic plug in venules and arterioles, effectively blocking blood flow.

Black Widow Spiders

Black widow spiders (*Latrodectus mactans*) are relatively aggressive. They are found throughout the United States, predominantly in the South. Around houses, the black widow spider is found in protected places, such as garages, storage sheds, crawl spaces under buildings, and rainspouts. Female spiders of the genus *Latrodectus* carry the characteristic orange-red hourglass-shaped marking on the ventral abdomen. The *Latrodectus* venom is a neurotoxin that acts on the myoneural junction and exerts its damage by releasing acetylcholine and norepinephrine. Black widow spiders are the most feared of all spiders because they injure their victims by injecting one of the most potent venoms secreted by any animal and subsequently account for the vast majority of spider bite–related deaths in the United States.

Scorpions

Found throughout the world, scorpions are nocturnal and spend the day under rocks, logs, and floors. The only species that is particularly dangerous, *Centruroides exilicauda* (the bark scorpion), is found mostly in the southwestern United States. This small Mexican scorpion is usually less than 2 inches long, yellow to brown, and possibly striped. The last segment of the scorpion's taillike structure contains the venom glands and stingers. Most scorpions are relatively harmless, producing only local reactions, but the venom of *Centruroides exilicauda* has effects similar to those of black widow spider venom, producing severe systemic toxicity. The venom is predominantly a neurotoxin that causes repetitive firing of axons by the activation of sodium channels.

Ticks

Some of the more common ticks in the United States are the brown dog tick and the American dog tick. Ticks are frequently encountered by hikers and people who work outdoors. When feeding, ticks make a small hole in the skin, attach themselves with a modification of one of their mouthparts (which has teeth that curve backward), and insert barbed, piercing mouthparts to remove blood. The American dog tick (*Dermacentor variabilis*) may transmit Rocky Mountain spotted fever (caused by the intracellular bacteria *Rickettsia rickettsii*), tularemia (caused by the coccobacillus *Francisella tularensis*), and other diseases from animals to people. This tick has also been reported to cause paralysis if it attaches at the base of the skull or along the spinal column, due to a paralytic toxin secreted by the feeding tick.

Lyme disease (caused by the spirochete bacterium *Borrelia burgdorferi*) is also transmitted by ticks. Most disease transmission occurs in the New England states, where the primary vector is the deer tick/black-legged tick (*Ixodes scapularis*). Species that are close relatives of the deer tick, such as the western black-legged tick (*Ixodes pacificus*), are also capable of transmitting the disease.

Fleas

Fleas are wingless, blood-sucking insects, some species of which transmit arboviruses to humans by acting as a host or vector for the organism. Certain species of fleas transmit plague, murine typhus, and tularemia. Unfortunately, if a house has been previously occupied by pets that were infested with fleas, the abandoned hungry fleas may form a welcoming party for the newly arrived "human guests."

Chiggers

Chiggers, or "red bugs," are the larvae of harvest mites. Infestations of chiggers are caused by mite larvae that feed on the host's skin cells. In other parts of the world such as India, Central and Southeast Asia, and Australia, chiggers may transmit scrub typhus (caused by the rickettsial bacteria *Orientia tsutsugamushi*). Chiggers become active in the spring, although in southern states such as Florida, they may be active all year. Chiggers attach themselves to the skin, hair follicles, or pores of human or rodent hosts by inserting their piercing mouthparts. They prefer to attach themselves to parts of the human body where clothing fits tightly or where the flesh is thin, tender, or wrinkled; in rodents, they are often found clustered on the inner skin of the ears.

During feeding, chiggers inject digestive enzymes into the skin, dissolving tissue. Chiggers feed by sucking up the liquefied tissues; they do not burrow in the skin. After 3 days, when the larva is engorged, it drops off the human host. Chiggers are most often found in low, damp areas where vegetation is heavy, although some species prefer dry areas. They are most abundant in areas covered with shrubs and small trees where rodents are numerous.

Biting Flies

Several species of blood-sucking flies can produce allergic reactions, including deerflies, blackflies, horseflies, and sandflies. Fly bites can also result in cutaneous myiasis, in which parasitism by fly larvae occurs. When a fly, such as the human botfly, deposits an egg on human skin, the egg hatches immediately, and the larva enters the skin through the bite or through another small break in the skin. The larvae grow to 15 to 20 mm under the skin, as a growing red, pruritic papule develops into a tender furuncle, with eventual emergence of the fly larvae.

Stinging Caterpillars

Stinging caterpillars include the puss caterpillar, saddleback caterpillar, and the hag moth caterpillar. These caterpillars are found primarily in the southeastern United States, especially in Texas and Florida. These caterpillars have spines that are hollow hairs containing poison sacs. When the spines break off, a toxin flows from the spines onto the victim's skin, causing a burning sensation.

Mosquitoes

Mosquitoes are blood-sucking arthropods attracted to hosts by moisture, carbon dioxide, estrogens, sweat, and/or warmth. They are vectors for many infectious diseases, and their bites also cause IgE-mediated immediate hypersensitivity reactions (i.e., erythematous urticarial lesions).

PATHOPHYSIOLOGY

The venoms produced by venomous insects and other arthropods can be classified according to their effects:

- Vesicating toxins (e.g., blister beetles, certain stinging caterpillars, and millipedes) produce blisters.
- Neurotoxins (e.g., black widow spiders, bark scorpions, certain ticks, wheel bugs, and *Hymenoptera* [honeybees, bumblebees, wasps, hornets, yellow jackets, and fire ants]) attack the central nervous system (CNS).
- Cytotoxic and hemolytic toxins (e.g., *Hymenoptera*, ground scorpions, mites, chiggers, wheel bugs, and the brown recluse spider) destroy tissue.
- Hemorrhagic toxins (e.g., lice, fleas, ticks, mites, true bugs [*Hemiptera*], and biting flies) prevent blood from clotting.

The typical reaction after an insect sting entails local erythema, pain, pruritus, and swelling. Insect stings almost always cause pain. This initial reaction should subside in 1 to 2 hours. The more significant reactions to insect bites can be categorized as large local reactions, toxic reactions, systemic or anaphylactic reactions, delayed reactions, or unusual reactions.

A *large local reaction* can spread more than 6 inches beyond the sting and is characterized by prolonged and marked edema at the site of the sting injury, peaking at 48 hours and lasting as long as 1 week. This reaction may be accompanied by nausea, vomiting, and fatigue. A large local reaction can involve one or more neighboring joints and may even produce airway obstruction due to tissue swelling if the sting occurs in the mouth or throat. The history of a large local reaction is typically not associated with the risk of anaphylaxis upon future stings.

A *toxic reaction* occurs when there is a history of multiple stings, often more than 10 in number. Toxic reactions are caused by nonantigenic properties of *Hymenoptera* venom. They resemble systemic reactions but have a greater frequency of GI disturbances. Diarrhea, nausea, vomiting, light-headedness, and syncope are common signs. The patient may also have headache, drowsiness, fever, involuntary muscle spasms, edema without urticaria, and occasionally seizures. Urticaria and bronchospasm are not present, and symptoms usually subside within 48 hours.

Systemic or *anaphylactic reactions* may range from mild to fatal. The majority of such reactions occur within the first 15 minutes, and nearly all will occur within 6 hours after the insect sting, but some may not occur until 24 to 36 hours later. The shorter the interval between the sting and the onset of symptoms, the more severe the reaction. Fatalities that occur usually result from either hypotension or airway obstruction. The patient will present initially with generalized urticaria, pruritic eyes, a dry cough, and facial flushing. These symptoms may progress rapidly to chest or throat constriction, dyspnea, wheezing, laryngeal stridor, frothy sputum, cyanosis, diarrhea, abdominal cramps, nausea, vomiting, chills and fever, vertigo, shock, loss of consciousness, and involuntary loss of bowel and bladder function.

When an individual predisposed to *Hymenoptera* allergy is initially stung, there is an increase in the production of antigen-specific IgE antibodies. The antibodies become attached to mast cells and basophils, and the individual becomes sensitized to undergo an anaphylactic reaction after a subsequent sting. Anaphylaxis is a type I immediate hypersensitivity immune response to a triggering antigen/allergen found in insect venom. In this type of reaction, once introduced into the body, the circulating venom antigen binds to antigen-specific IgE molecules that are in turn bound to mast cells and basophils. Binding of two or more cell membrane–bound IgE molecules to the same antigen (a process known as antibody cross-linking) leads to the degranulation of mast cell and basophil cytoplasmic contents and the release of preformed vasoactive mediators including histamine and tryptase. These substances are potent systemic vasodilators, accounting for the immediate flushing and life-threatening symptoms of hypotension, angioedema, and mucosal swelling with potential airway compromise in the anaphylactic patient.

Infusion of histamine into normal subjects causes the following effects and can be diminished by antagonists of specific histamine H_1 or H_2 receptors: flushing (H_1 plus H_2), hypotension (H_1 plus H_2), tachycardia (H_1), headache (H_1 plus H_2), pruritus (H_1), rhinorrhea (H_1), and bronchospasm (H_1). Honeybee venom contains histamine; wasp venom contains histamine and serotonin; hornet venom contains histamine, serotonin, and acetylcholine. The fact that histamine acts through both H_1 and H_2 receptors emphasizes the importance of administering both H_1- and H_2-blocking antihistamines during allergic reactions. However, the only reliable method of countering the life-threatening hypotension and mucosal edema associated with anaphylactic histamine release is immediate administration of epinephrine, a potent vasoconstrictor.

After this immediate response, through complex lymphocyte (e.g., T-cell) and granulocyte interactions, other inflammatory vasoactive cytokines including prostaglandins, leukotrienes, and bradykinin begin to form several hours after venom exposure. These substances contribute to a second, later phase of anaphylaxis that typically occurs 6 to 12 hours after acute exposure to the triggering antigen. Leukotrienes and prostaglandins are responsible in part for vascular permeability, vasodilation, smooth muscle contraction, and mucus secretion. Downregulation of the inflammatory response caused by these *de novo* mediators is the goal of corticosteroid treatment in anaphylaxis, which blocks the formation of these newly formed substances.

Another type of *delayed reaction* to insect venom can appear 10 to 14 days after an insect bite or sting; this reaction is also antibody mediated, but by IgG or IgM, rather than by IgE. This type of reaction presents as a serum sicknesslike illness, which is a type III antigen–antibody hypersensitivity response in which immune complexes are deposited in the various tissues of the body. The patient's signs and symptoms may include malaise, headache, fever, urticaria, lymphadenopathy, and polyarthritis.

Additional *unusual reactions* may be neurological or vascular in nature. They include nephrosis, vasculitis, serum sickness, encephalitis, and neuritis. The etiology of these reactions varies but may be due to an immunological pathogenesis.

CLINICAL PRESENTATION

Subjective

The primary care practitioner should determine the history of the sting or bite, including the exact time of injury and a precise description of the arthropod or species of insect, if possible. As the skin is inspected for signs of the insect or spider bite, the patient should first be evaluated for any anaphylactic symptoms or signs of a systemic reaction. The clinician should also determine whether the patient has had previous allergies to insect bites, a history of allergies or asthma, or any known allergies to horses or horse serum, given the composition of certain antisera. A family history of anaphylaxis to bites or stings should also be elicited, as this increases the risk of anaphylaxis in the patient as well.

With stinging insects, the patient will usually remember the insult because the sting induces immediate pain. For biting insects, there may be some delay between the actual bite and the pruritus that follows. The patient's history should be carefully pursued to identify the probable source of exposure. For indoor exposure, fleas are common offenders, although spider bites are also responsible for indoor bites. The primary care practitioner should also inquire about whether pets have recently occupied the dwelling or if the patient has been to a home with pets.

Objective

Hymenoptera (bee and wasp) stings produce immediate pain and a red papule surrounded by a pale zone of edema, with varying amounts of local swelling. Large local reactions are common, spreading more than 6 inches (15.2 cm) beyond the sting, peaking at 48 hours, and lasting as long as 1 week. A mildly hypersensitive person may experience hives, malaise, wheezing, conjunctivitis, rhinitis, fever, and nausea. A severely sensitive person is more likely to suffer diffuse urticaria, facial swelling, laryngeal edema, bronchospasm, vomiting, cyanosis, abdominal pain, cardiac arrhythmias, and hypotension. Most fatalities occur within 1 hour of the sting.

Fire ant stings produce vesicles that become sterile pustules; these pustules subsequently become necrotic within several hours and may take up to 10 days to heal. If broken, the pustules may become infected. Systemic symptoms include nausea, vomiting, syncope (fainting), headache, fever, numbness, and muscle spasms.

Brown recluse spider bites are unusual in that people bitten usually do not feel pain for 2 to 3 hours. A single necrotic lesion occurs, usually measuring 0.5 to 2 cm in size, self-limited in spread, and lacking adenopathy or sustained generalized toxicity. The typical bull's-eye lesion is created when the red blister is encircled by a pale, irregularly shaped, and ischemic halo, which in turn is surrounded by extravasated blood. The pustule may gradually grow to form a craterlike lesion over 3 to 4 days, with associated lymphadenopathy and low-grade fever. Rarely, there is a generalized systemic reaction 24 to 48 hours after the spider bite, with fever, malaise, arthralgias, rash, and hemolysis.

Black widow spider bites create an initial puncture wound that disappears rapidly, leaving a local swelling where tiny red spots appear. Symptoms of envenomation occur within 10 to 60 minutes, including severe pain in the bitten extremity and muscle spasms of the abdomen and trunk. Diffuse paresthesias, ptosis, and hyperactive deep tendon reflexes may be noted. Victims experience agonizing pain and may develop hypertension, headache, muscular rigidity and spasm, hyperreflexia, vomiting, abdominal pain, agitation, and/or psychosis. Symptoms peak at 2 to 3 hours after the bite and may last up to 24 hours.

Scorpion stings are immediately intensely painful, with little or no erythema or swelling. Generalized reactions may occur within 1 hour and progress to maximum severity in 5 hours. The reactions can be graded as follows:

- Grade I: Local pain and paresthesias at the site of envenomation
- Grade II: Pain and paresthesias remote from the sting bite, along with local findings
- Grade III: Either somatic skeletal or cranial nerve (CN) neuromuscular dysfunction, including blurred vision, wandering eye movements, hypersalivation, difficulty swallowing, upper airway obstruction, slurred speech, jerking of the upper extremities, restlessness, arching of the back, severe involuntary shaking, and jerking
- Grade IV: Both CN and somatic skeletal neuromuscular dysfunction

Hypertension, nausea, vomiting, hyperthermia, tachycardia, and respiratory distress may also occur. Children younger than 10 years of age are more likely to have severe or prolonged reactions to scorpion stings. Older children and adults usually recover within 10 to 12 hours.

Tick bites can produce lesions that vary from small pruritic nodules to extensive ulceration, induration, and erythema. The lesions may be accompanied by malaise, fever, and chills. Tick-induced paralysis occurs more frequently during the spring and summer, when ticks are feeding. Symptoms of this neurological complication occur 5 to 6 days after the adult female tick attaches to the host and include irritability, restlessness, and paresthesias in the hands and feet. Over the next 24 to 48 hours, ascending, symmetric, and flaccid paralysis occurs, along with the loss of deep tendon reflexes. Within 1 to 2 days, severe generalized weakness may develop, accompanied by respiratory paralysis.

Flea bites produce lesions that are similar to those of lice and scabies, so much so that distinguishing these different etiologies is often difficult. Flea bites produce itchy papules found in zigzag lines, especially on the legs and in the waist area. The lesions present as central hemorrhagic puncta surrounded by erythematous and urticarial patches. Pruritus is intense. Once the lesions clear, dull red spots may persist. Impetigo may develop as a complication. If the fleas remain in the environment, new lesions are likely to continue to appear.

Itching from *chigger bites* is usually noticed 4 to 8 hours after chiggers have attached or have been removed. Initially, a papule develops and ultimately enlarges over 24 to 48 hours to form a nodule. Pruritus peaks on the second day. The fluid injection of the chigger's saliva causes nodules to appear, which may last for 2 weeks. Patients who exhibit an allergic reaction to the saliva will develop severe soft tissue edema, pruritus, and fever. Chigger bites usually occur around the ankles, waistline, knees, or in the armpits. Mite infestations may be associated with an erythema multiformelike rash and fever.

Biting flies can cause pain and subsequent pruritus when they pierce the skin, and allergic reactions can occur. If flies inject their eggs under the skin, the patient can also develop myiasis. As the fly larvae hatch and grow under the skin, the initial pruritic papule becomes a furuncle with a central opening that exudes serosanguineous fluid. The tip of the fly larva may even protrude from the central opening, or bubbles produced by its respiration may be seen.

The *puss caterpillar's sting* causes intense, immediate pain, often in spasms. This is followed by local edema, pruritus, and a rash of red blotches and ridges. The lesions consist of red or white papules and vesicles, often forming perfect grid-like markings where the caterpillar made contact. Ordinarily no systemic manifestations occur, and localized symptoms typically subside within 24 hours. In some patients, the intense pain can cause nausea and vomiting, as well as headache, fever, and lymphadenopathy. The papular or urticarial rash usually subsides within a few hours to 1 to 2 days after contact, but it can persist for up to 1 week.

Immediate skin reactions to *mosquito bites* include erythema, wheal formation, and severe pruritus. A delayed reaction 12 to 24 hours later consists of more intense redness, edema, and burning pruritus. Blistering and necrosis can also occur. The immediate reaction is of short duration, whereas the delayed reaction may persist for hours, days, and even weeks. Some individuals have a history of allergy to mosquito saliva, consistent with an increasing reaction to seasonal exposures accompanied by progressively more pronounced edema and pruritus. The allergic response can be accompanied by fever, generalized malaise, nausea, vomiting, and necrosis, with resultant scarring.

DIAGNOSTIC REASONING

Diagnostic Tests

For an arthropod bite or sting that results in systemic involvement, the clinician providing emergent care should order blood typing and crossmatching studies, coagulation tests, CBC, serum electrolytes, blood urea nitrogen, creatinine, and urinalysis. Serial arterial blood gases and pulse oximetry may also be necessary. For suspected tick-borne diseases such as Rocky Mountain spotted fever and Lyme disease, further laboratory studies are in order. For example, spirochetes can be seen in a blood smear in 70% of cases of tick-borne relapsing fever. Lyme disease, Rocky Mountain spotted fever, and tularemia, which all occur from tick bites, are diagnosed by specific antibody titers. However, results from these antibody titer assays are often not available for days to weeks, with empiric treatment often initiated before this. Thus, these tests are usually sent for confirmation only when a strong suspicion already exists for the infections and should not be sent indiscriminately. Acute infection is associated with elevated disease-specific IgM titers, whereas past exposure (including from cleared infection) is characterized by elevated disease-specific IgG levels in the absence of corresponding IgM.

Differential Diagnosis

Consultation with a regional poison control center may be indicated to correctly identify, diagnose, and/or treat arthropod bites and stings. It is helpful to know the specific arthropods that are indigenous to the local area, especially those that have caused recent infestations and injuries. Bites of fleas, lice, and scabies mites produce similar lesions that can complicate differentiation. Cercariae (i.e., larval schistosomes that develop in nonhuman hosts) cause similar lesions that appear after a patient has been exposed to infected water. Scabies has a more gradual onset but should also be considered in the differential diagnosis. The diagnosis of chigger infestations can usually be made on the basis of typical skin lesions in the setting of an outdoor exposure history. Patients who present with a "bull's-eye" rash after a suspected deer tick bite should be tested for Lyme disease.

When examining an urticarial reaction to an insect bite, other causes of urticaria should be considered, but if the hive (wheal) has a central punctum, its cause is likely an insect bite. Other foreign bodies can produce pruritic papules in the skin. Dermatitis herpetiformis (commonly seen in celiac disease) should be included in the differential diagnosis, particularly when only excoriations are found. Eruptions associated with viruses or with atopic dermatitis, allergic or irritant contact dermatitis, or drug reactions must also be considered. An uncommon idiopathic disorder Mucha-Habermann disease also presents with scattered necrotic papules and vesicles, but this type of rash is usually more generalized and symmetric. Some of the other skin conditions that may be confused with local or systemic reactions to arthropod stings and bites include streptococcal necrotizing fasciitis, focal cutaneous necrosis, various infections, local thromboses, emboli to the skin, punctures, trauma, vasculitis, purpura, Arthus (type III hypersensitivity or serum sickness) reactions, and other bites that leave small puncture wounds.

Anaphylaxis from an insect sting may be confused with a vasovagal reaction, which is a disorder of central vasoregulation caused by increased parasympathetic tone mediated by the vagus nerve (CN X). A vasovagal reaction typically produces pallor, nausea, bradycardia, extreme diaphoresis, and hypotension that may result in syncope, whereas flushing, hypotension, tachycardia, and mucosal edema with severe bronchoconstriction are seen in anaphylaxis. Severe reactions to scorpion stings may present with symptoms similar to those of insecticide poisoning, with direct CNS effects.

Confirmation of stinging insect allergy is made by the detection of venom-specific IgE. This can be performed through an immediate reaction skin prick test, which measures the cutaneous histaminic response to dilute doses of allergen after scratching the skin surface with an antigen-coated needle tip, allowing for binding of allergen to IgE on tissue mast cells with subsequent degranulation and a quantifiable wheal reaction on the skin surface in allergic patients. Yellow jacket, honeybee, yellow hornet, bald-faced hornet, and wasp extracts are available for diagnosis and treatment of stinging insect allergies. A patient is considered sensitive if a skin reaction of 1+ or greater occurs at a venom concentration of 1 mg/mL or less, provided that the 1+ reaction is greater than that of a diluent control. This is the most sensitive test for detecting allergic states and is commonly used as an allergy screening tool. However, it lacks specificity and may thus overestimate allergic states. In turn, as with all skin prick test results, its utility lies mainly in its negative predictive value in ruling out allergies to specific stinging insects.

IgE antibodies reacting with venom also may be measured by a serum detection assay known as the radioallergosorbent test (RAST), although fluorescently labeled antibody tests are now recommended as the preferred methodology of serum testing for venom-specific IgE. In these tests, a patient's serum is applied to a culture plate surface coated with the specific allergen of interest, allowing for specific antibody-binding to the plate. After excess serum is rinsed away, a second fluorescently labeled antibody specific for the constant region of IgE is applied to the plate to reveal any of the patient's antigen-specific IgE that bound to the plate during the first step of the assay. Thus, the greater the amount of fluorescence, the higher the concentration of antigen-specific IgE in the patient's serum. Venom-specific serum IgE tests are not as sensitive as immediate reaction skin prick tests, although they are more specific and thus are more effective in ruling in, rather than ruling out, an allergic state, depending on the level of specific IgE detected.

MANAGEMENT

Emergency Management

Anaphylactic shock and respiratory distress are true emergencies. The clinician should focus on stabilizing the patient while arranging for immediate transport to the emergency department. It should be understood that anaphylaxis may be triggered by etiologies other than bites and stings. Anaphylactic reactions may also be caused by medications iatrogenically, environmental exposures, or certain food allergies, which are quite common. The treatment for anaphylaxis is standard and should be familiar to all practitioners who provide primary care, urgent care, or emergency care.

The clinician should place a conscious patient in a comfortable position, ensuring unimpeded ventilation. Hypotensive patients should be placed supine or in a modified Trendelenburg position if respiratory status allows. The clinician must help the patient maintain an adequate upper airway and give supplemental oxygen by mask or nebulizer with inhaled racemic epinephrine (0.5 mL of 2.25% epinephrine in 2 mL of normal saline), not to exceed three treatments in 60 minutes. However, racemic (nebulized) epinephrine should not be considered an adequate substitute for systemic (injected) epinephrine in the case of a life-threatening attack. In the case of impending upper airway compromise, inadequate oxygenation, or profound shock, the clinician must prepare for immediate administration of systemic epinephrine and endotracheal intubation if necessary to maintain an open airway. Cricothyrotomy by a trained professional would be needed if severe angioedema precludes intubation via the oral route.

Epinephrine maintains blood pressure through beta-adrenergic cardiovascular effects, causes bronchial dilation, and antagonizes the adverse actions of the mediators of anaphylaxis. It also reduces the subsequent release of anaphylactic mediators through its action on mast cells and basophils. In the case of airway edema, bronchospasm, and/or cardiovascular instability (with or without cutaneous manifestations of urticaria or angioedema), the clinician should immediately administer aqueous epinephrine 1:1,000 IM into the upper outer thigh, which provides the most rapid entry into the systemic circulation. The dose is 0.3 to 0.5 mg every 10 to 20 minutes as indicated. An injection of 0.1 to 0.2 mg of the epinephrine can go directly into the sting or bite, causing vasoconstriction and reduction of swelling. If the reaction is limited to urticaria and pruritus, there is no wheezing or facial swelling, and the victim is older than 45 years of age, epinephrine can be withheld unless the patient's condition worsens. In addition to the immediate administration of epinephrine, albuterol may be used to treat bronchospasm, administered via nebulizer every 20 minutes as needed.

Antihistamines may be included in the treatment regimen, but they are not an adequate substitute for systemic epinephrine. With H_1-blocking antihistamines, the primary care practitioner may administer diphenhydramine by mouth (PO) (in severe anaphylaxis, 100 mg may be administered IV initially) or hydroxyzine IM as needed. H_1 blockers such as cetirizine, fexofenadine, and desloratadine are less sedating, may be as effective as first generation agents, and can be used if the patient can take oral medications. For H_2-blocking antihistamines, the clinician may administer cimetidine or ranitidine. If available, cimetidine is the preferred H_2 blocker because it has greater peripheral effects than does ranitidine, which is more specific for the GI tract. Of note, in the first half of 2020, an increasing number of product recalls for ranitidine and nizatidine (another H_2-blocking antihistamine) occurred at the urging of the U.S. Food and Drug Administration (FDA), given concerns that unacceptably high levels of the contaminant N-nitrosodimethylamine (NDMA) accumulated in these products with long-term storage.

Circulatory support should be provided as needed in hypotensive patients. The clinician may infuse 0.5 to 1 L of either normal saline or lactated Ringer's solution every 20 to 30 minutes as needed to support blood pressure at a level higher than 90 mm Hg systolic. The need for further fluid resuscitation should be determined by monitoring blood pressure, cardiac rate and rhythm, and urine output. Usually, a total of 3 L can be given rapidly to an otherwise healthy adult without adverse effects. However, caution is needed in patients with heart failure or older adults (see Geriatric Considerations later in chapter), given the risk of fluid overload and pulmonary edema.

Hypotension refractory to IV colloids requires treatment with IV pressor agents (e.g., norepinephrine, phenylephrine, dopamine) in a hospital setting. Glucagon may be needed in patients who are on beta-blocking agents, given that it stimulates inotropic and chronotropic cardiac function independent of the beta blockade.

If the allergic reaction is prolonged or severe or if the patient is regularly medicated with corticosteroids, the clinician should parenterally administer hydrocortisone, methylprednisolone, or dexamethasone, followed by a 10-day oral taper. If corticosteroid therapy is initiated orally, the clinician should administer prednisone 60 to 100 mg daily. Even in the case of reactions that do not appear to be prolonged, systemic corticosteroid therapy should be administered for 24 to 48 hours after the onset of the initial reaction to minimize the chance of late-phase anaphylactic reactions, which may manifest up to 24 hours after the initial reaction and may be as severe as early-phase reactions.

General Management

Typical uncomplicated reactions to arthropod bites and stings do not require treatment other than local applications of a cold compress (ice) and oral or topical analgesics. NSAIDs such as ibuprofen PO are effective if given immediately because they block *de novo* formation of prostaglandins, which mediate these typical reactions. Secondary infections are common with pruritic bites or stings that lead to frequent scratching. A topical antimicrobial ointment such as mupirocin 2% (Bactroban) should be applied three times daily for 5 days to sites of secondary infection.

Large Local Reactions

Large local reactions to arthropod bites or stings are treated with H_1- and H_2-blocking antihistamines, such as diphenhydramine and cimetidine, respectively. Intramuscular administration of diphenhydramine is not usually done because of the pain involved and the fact that the drug is absorbed very rapidly when administered orally. A corticosteroid such as methylprednisolone tapered over 5 days will hasten resolution of a large local reaction to a bee or wasp sting. Tapering slowly prevents a rebound flare-up of symptoms. Some clinicians also administer calcium gluconate. Importantly, large local reactions are not associated with the risk of anaphylaxis on future stings by the same type of insect.

Treatment of painful cases of venomous stings or bites with large local reactions may include nerve block anesthesia with 2% lidocaine, which can be repeated up to three times at 30- to 60-minute intervals. Oral analgesics may also be useful. In moderate and severe cases, which occur mainly in children, antivenin (antivenom) serum is indicated.

Delayed Serum Sickness–Type Reactions

Delayed serum sickness–type reactions in response to multiple bee, wasp, or fire ant stings can be managed with a corticosteroid such as prednisone (Deltasone) 60 to 100 mg tapered over 2 weeks. The pruritus caused by these reactions can be controlled by a variety of oral antihistamines. Hydroxyzine is commonly prescribed because its dosage is flexible, and it produces few anticholinergic adverse effects. If patients are driving or working during the day, they should reserve the hydroxyzine for nighttime use to help with sleep. Treatment of urticaria may also require an H_2-blocking antihistamine, such as cimetidine.

For arthropod bites, when topical corticosteroids are used, class I (e.g., betamethasone dipropionate) or class II (e.g., fluocinonide) topical preparations may be applied twice daily. Lesions may take weeks to resolve. Topical antipruritics include lotions with 0.25% menthol, 1% phenol, or both (Sarna lotion), as well as topical anesthetics such as pramoxine (Pramosone). Topical antihistamines and benzocaine are not recommended because of their potential for allergic sensitization. Topical doxepin (Zonalon) is available and is effective. Infected insect bites can be treated with topical mupirocin 2% (Bactroban) or neomycin. Extensive impetigo will need treatment with oral antibiotics, such as dicloxacillin or erythromycin.

Hymenoptera Stings

When a patient is stung by a honeybee, the stinger should be removed by scraping it away from the skin with a dull object. The stinger should not be grasped and pulled because this contracts the venom sac, thus releasing more toxin into the wound. Wasps and other bees do not leave a stinger in the patient's skin and are capable of stinging many times. The site should be cleaned, and an antiseptic should be applied. Blisters from fire ant stings should not be broken open. Ice should be applied with a cold compress pack, with or without a paste of papain (unseasoned meat tenderizer), and the affected body part should be elevated.

There is no specific antivenin for *Hymenoptera* stings. If the reaction is extensive or if there is envenomation from multiple stings, systemic epinephrine may be needed as described in the section on Emergency Management, and additional aggressive therapy may be indicated in a hospital setting. This includes administering calcium gluconate IV (for muscle spasms) with an antihistamine such as diphenhydramine IV or PO (for urticarial lesions). Oral prednisone 40 mg daily for 2 to 3 days can be helpful in reducing localized swelling. Tetanus prophylaxis should be completed. In severe envenomation, an IV corticosteroid such as hydrocortisone 2 mg/kg should also be administered at the earliest opportunity to prevent late-phase reactions (see the section on anaphylactic reactions).

Brown Recluse Spider Bites

The patient should apply cold compresses intermittently over a sterile dressing for the first 4 days after the bite. A 10-day course of oral antibiotics such as dicloxacillin, cephalexin, or erythromycin can be administered. Elevation of the affected body part may be beneficial. Drug treatment is controversial; many brown recluse spider bites are minor and heal without specific treatment other than tetanus prophylaxis. One treatment for a severe wound in patients who screen negative for glucose-6-phosphate dehydrogenase (G6PD) deficiency is dapsone (Avlosulfon) 50 mg orally twice daily for 10 days. If G6PD deficiency is ultimately documented in a patient who has started dapsone empirically, the patient should discontinue dapsone immediately to avoid severe hemolysis.

Black Widow Spider Bites

The natural course of the envenomation is to resolve completely after a few days, with pain persisting for 1 week or more. Ice should be applied judiciously to the bite wound. The patient may require a narcotic analgesic, such as morphine. Opioids have a histaminic agonist effect, however, so these medications should be avoided in cases with significant histaminic responses. Muscle relaxants such as anxiolytic diazepam (Valium) may also be given for spasms. Of note, the abuse potential of opioids and anxiolytics should be considered when prescribing these.

The patient should be monitored for hypertension and administered a centrally acting or vasodilating antihypertensive if necessary. Inpatients may be given calcium gluconate via slow IV infusion to alleviate muscle spasms. Antivenin is reserved for seriously ill infants or older patients and is administered in a hospital-based critical care setting only, given the risk of anaphylaxis. Because many antivenins are derived from horse serum, horse serum sensitivity testing is needed to screen for potential anaphylactic reactions. One vial of antivenin is sufficient for most patients.

Scorpion Bites

The patient should apply ice for 30 minutes each hour to relieve local pain. Intense cooling should be avoided, and the affected body part should be immobilized but without a tourniquet. Opiate analgesics should be avoided because they potentiate the toxicity of the venom and may lead to apnea. The clinician should administer diazepam or phenobarbital to control seizures, along with an antihypertensive sympathetic antagonist agent to control hypertension. Hyperthermia from uncontrolled muscular contractions can be managed with cooling. The administration of antivenom (antivenin) is controversial, given the risk of anaphylaxis and the need for inpatient dosing. Horse serum sensitivity testing is done to rule out a potential anaphylaxis reaction to most antivenom preparations.

Tick Bites

The clinician should always remove ticks by covering with alcohol, machine oil, mineral oil, salad oil, or gasoline applied with a tissue or gauze pad. This blocks the tick's breathing pores and causes it to withdraw from the skin. It may take 30 minutes for the tick to disengage its mouthparts. Ticks should not be removed manually because squeezing the tick's body may inject more viral or bacterial pathogens into the victim. The clinician should observe for a local reaction or infection at the site of the tick bite. Most victims of tick paralysis will show improvement within hours of tick removal and return to their baseline status in several days. Patients with Rocky Mountain spotted fever or Lyme disease will require further treatment, including antibiotics and follow-up monitoring for chronic health problems.

Flea Bites

The patient should clean the bite lesions well with soap and water and apply a topical antiseptic ointment. To relieve pruritus and discomfort, calamine lotion with phenol can be applied. A systemic antihistamine such as hydroxyzine (Atarax) can be administered to control pruritus.

Chigger Bites

Chiggers are easily removed from the skin by taking a hot bath or shower and lathering with soap several times. The bath will kill attached chiggers. For moderate to severe cases, topical corticosteroid creams and oral antihistamines may provide some relief. Systemic corticosteroids will also provide relief for severe pruritus. Topical antibiotic therapy is indicated for secondary infection.

Mosquito Bites

Immediately after the person is bitten, they should apply a cold (ice) pack. A topical corticosteroid ointment can be applied to the site. Oral corticosteroids such as prednisone should be used only when the reaction is prolonged and severe, given these medications' potential adverse effects.

Fly Bites

Fly bites are treated the same as mosquito bites. In addition, if the patient presents with cutaneous myiasis, the clinician should exert pressure to extrude the fly larva. The larva may emerge if its breathing hole in the skin is occluded with heavy oil, nail polish, or bacon fat. Alternatively, the clinician can inject 2 mL of local anesthetic into the base of the lesion, thus extruding the larva by fluid pressure. Care should be taken not to rupture the larva because an inflammatory reaction may result.

Caterpillar Spine Irritation

Broken-off spines in the skin can be removed by applying adhesive tape, a commercial facial peel, or a thin layer of rubber cement over the affected area. Then an oral antihistamine and/or NSAID can be administered. If the dermatitis is persistent and severe, the clinician should prescribe oral prednisone 60 to 100 mg for adults, to be tapered over 10 days.

FOLLOW-UP AND REFERRAL

After a severe allergic reaction to an arthropod sting or bite, further delayed reactions with a severe recurrence of symptoms are possible, particularly as the effects of treating medications decrease. Thus, patients may benefit from repeated doses of antihistamines and glucocorticoids over the next several days. All patients with severe allergic reactions who are discharged home should have a follow-up visit in 24 to 48 hours, and all such patients should be referred to an allergy specialist for confirmatory testing and to establish an appropriate management plan for future stings or bites.

Individuals who have experienced a serious anaphylactic reaction should be prescribed three devices for the rapid self-administration of epinephrine by injection (EpiPen, Auvi-Q) and instructed in their use. These patients should also keep oral diphenhydramine and cimetidine readily available with injectable epinephrine in a portable kit. One kit should be kept in a bag or purse that is carried with the individual at all times, a second kit in the school or work setting, and a third kit should be kept in the home. Many individuals also keep a kit in the glove compartment of a personal vehicle; however, it is important to explain to the patient that extremes of heat and cold can affect the stability of many medicines, including lifesaving epinephrine. Thus, storing a kit in the glove compartment of a vehicle is not recommended.

Individuals with a history of an acute allergic reaction (including systemic cutaneous reactions) with positive venom skin tests or a serum sickness–type reaction after an insect sting are considered at risk for subsequent sting reactions. Venom immunotherapy to prevent IgE-mediated allergic reactions to various types of *Hymenoptera* may be recommended, and referral to an allergist is required for specialized assessment that includes allergy testing (venom skin testing and venom-specific serum IgE testing). Of note, venom immunotherapy will not prevent future type III immune complex–mediated serum sickness reactions because these do not involve the allergic IgE antibody. In addition, patients with large local reactions are not considered candidates for venom immunotherapy and do not require venom skin tests, because these reactions are not associated with the risk of anaphylaxis from future stings. Patients who have been treated for anaphylaxis and who use beta-adrenergic blocking agents should be switched to alternative medications, given the inhibitory effects of beta blockers on epinephrine.

Patient Education: Arthropod Bites and Stings

Patient education information regarding arthropod bites and stings is provided in Box 75.2.

Box 75.2 Patient Education: Arthropod Bites and Stings

- Avoid mowing lawns or working with flowering ornamental plants when bees and wasps are collecting nectar.
- Stand still if a stinging insect is near you. If it attacks, brush it off (do not slap at it) to prevent a sting.
- Do not walk in the yard in bare feet.
- Wear gloves when gardening.
- Keep garbage cans covered outdoors. Sweet items like soft drinks, ripened fruits, and watermelons attract bees and wasps and should be covered or placed in a sealed container when brought outdoors for consumption.
- Avoid perfumes, hair sprays, aftershave lotions, and colognes when outdoors, as they can attract insects.
- Pick fruit as it ripens and dispose of rotten fruit.
- If you are attacked by a swarm of bees, wasps, yellow jackets, or hornets, leave the area immediately, using your arms to protect your face.
- Control wasps by applying insecticides to the nest.
- Avoid areas where insect exposure is likely to occur and always wear shoes when outdoors.
- Avoid wearing brightly colored clothing outdoors because it may attract insects.
- If you are severely allergic to bee or wasp stings or to any medication, wear medical identification jewelry indicating the anaphylaxis-causing substance or event.
- Check bathrobes and bedsheets for spiders if you use the items after a long absence.
- When entering an attic or storeroom to open cardboard boxes, give brown recluse spiders a chance to vacate because they will avoid humans if they can.
- After experiencing a spider bite, have someone try to capture the spider for identification; immediately seek health care and contact the local poison control center.
- Treat pets for ticks by using dusts, dips, or sprays.
- When entering tick-infested areas, keep clothing buttoned, shirts tucked inside trousers, and trousers tucked inside boots.
- Wear light-colored clothing because this makes it easier to spot ticks; lighter clothing is also less attractive to biting flies.
- Do not sit on the ground or on logs in brush-filled areas.
- Keep brush cleared or pruned along frequently traveled areas. Use repellents to protect exposed skin; however, be aware that ticks will crawl over treated skin to untreated parts of the body.
- For treatment of flea infestations, treat not only the pet but also professionally fumigate the house.
- If you are going into areas suspected of being infested with chiggers, wear protective clothing and use insect repellents.
- Apply an insect repellent containing *N,N*-diethyl-3-methylbenzamide and wear permethrin-impregnated fabric.
- Apply insect repellents to legs, ankles, cuffs, waist, and sleeves, either to clothing or directly to the body as directed by the repellant's label.
- Avoid unnecessary use of lights at campsites and camp at a site that is high, dry, open, and uncluttered.

BURNS

According to the 2016 Fact Sheet of the American Burn Association, on average, 486,000 serious burn injuries warrant medical treatment each year in the United States, with 3,275 fire-related and smoke inhalation deaths (2,745 from residential fires, 310 from vehicle crash fires, and 220 from other sources). The survival rate for a burn injury is 96.8%, with the majority of burn injuries being treated in the outpatient setting. Thus, it is important for clinicians to possess the knowledge and skills to treat burns. In fact, contact burns (thermal burns from hot objects) was the theme for National Burn Awareness Week in 2020.

EPIDEMIOLOGY AND CAUSES

The risk of all types of burns is highest in adults aged 18 to 35 years. The male-to-female ratio is 2:1 for both burn injuries and death. Burns are the sixth most common cause of accidental death in the United States. Approximately 73% of burns occur in the home, 8% at work, 5% on the street or highway, 5% from recreational or sport injuries, and 9% at other locations. Of note, the use of grills results in many burn injuries, with 19,700 people seeking emergency care each year due to fires resulting from grill use and more than 10,000 home fires being caused by grill use each year.

Although the death rate from burns in patients older than 65 years is three times greater than that of the overall burn population, mortality rates from burns have significantly decreased over the past four decades. This improvement in mortality rates is the result of a better understanding of the need for early resuscitation, metabolic support after the injury, early wound excision and closure, and control of infection.

About 40% of all reported occupationally related injuries concern the skin, and about 25% of these are caused by chemical burns. Common household chemical burns are caused by lye (found in drain cleaners and paint removers), sodium hypochlorite (found in disinfectants and bleach products), sulfuric acid (found in toilet bowl cleaners), and phenols (found in deodorizers and sanitizers). The body sites most often burned by chemicals are the face, eyes, and extremities.

Burn-type injuries and other health problems can also result from overexposure to sunlight caused by ultraviolet (UV) radiation, which is commonly split into three bands: UVA, UVB, and UVC. UVB is particularly effective at damaging DNA, which contributes to melanoma and other types of skin cancer. UVC radiation is extremely dangerous but is absorbed by ozone and normal oxygen. Thus, overexposure to UV radiation not only results in painful sunburns but also causes malignant melanoma, basal cell carcinomas, squamous cell carcinomas, actinic keratoses, premature aging of the skin, cataracts, immune system suppression, sun poisoning (phototoxicity), and contact photodermatitis.

Sun poisoning (*phototoxicity*), also called *sun sensitivity*, is a systemic or allergic reaction to sun overexposure, usually occurring in conjunction with sunburn. The risk of sun poisoning is increased in people who take medications that cause photosensitivity, such as oral contraceptives, tetracyclines, amoxicillin, sulfa drugs, and thiazide diuretics. The risk of sun poisoning also increases with metabolic disorders such as diabetes mellitus or thyroid disease, as well as underlying infection. Patients who have had previous episodes of sun poisoning or who use immunosuppressive drugs are also at increased risk. Other contributing factors include medical disorders such as discoid lupus, systemic lupus erythematosus, and porphyria. Exposure to industrial light sources, such as welding arcs, also places people at greater risk for phototoxicity.

Contact photodermatitis is an acute or chronic inflammatory skin reaction resulting from the combined effects of a photosensitizing substance plus UV light, resulting in immunological delayed-type hypersensitivity. Agents that may photosensitize the skin include oral antidiabetic agents, NSAIDs, antibiotics, phenothiazines, sulfones/sulfonamides, chlorothiazides, and griseofulvin. PABA (*p*-aminobenzoic acid) in sunscreen lotion may also paradoxically cause photosensitivity dermatitis.

PATHOPHYSIOLOGY

Local Response

Cellular injury from heat results in the release of intracellular enzymes and proinflammatory vasoactive substances, such as histamine, kinins, serotonin, prostaglandins, leukotrienes, and interleukin-1. Complement is also activated. As a result, vascular permeability is altered, and significant hemodynamic, metabolic, and immunological effects occur locally and systemically. At the capillary level, there is a significant shift of protein molecules, fluid, and electrolytes from the intravascular space to the extravascular space. Lymph flow increases initially but subsequently decreases or ceases because the lymphatic vessels become blocked by serum proteins leaking through the walls of damaged capillaries.

In extensive burn injuries (involving more than 25% of the total body surface area [TBSA]), edema forms in both burned and unburned areas because of a generalized increase in capillary permeability and hypoproteinemia. A decrease in cell transmembrane potential also occurs in extensive burns, causing a shift of extracellular sodium and water into the cell that results in cellular swelling. With adequate resuscitation, cell membrane potential is restored within 24 to 36 hours. However, edema may also result from the volume and oncotic pressure effects of large fluid resuscitation volumes during initial therapy.

Maximum edema is typically seen 18 to 24 hours after a burn injury.

Systemic Response

The response of all organ systems to a burn injury occurs in a biphasic pattern of hypofunction followed by hyperfunction. For example, even sunburn can alter the distribution and function of WBCs up to 24 hours after sun exposure. The degree of physiological change is proportionate to the extent of the burn, with a maximum response reached in patients with burns over 50% TBSA.

The metabolic response is one of the most significant alterations after a burn injury. Protein wasting and weight loss occur in response to a severe burn, and the extensive healing process requires a rapid metabolic rate to support tissue anabolism, which reaches its peak 6 to 10 days after a burn injury. Hypermetabolism begins as resuscitation is completed and is probably mediated by the secretion of catecholamines. When a burn wound is closed, oxygen consumption and metabolic rate slowly return to normal.

Wound Healing

When a burn injury disrupts the integumentary system, the body automatically responds with a series of overlapping physiological changes to repair and restore epithelial continuity. The *inflammatory response* begins at the moment of injury and lasts from 3 to 4 days after injury. Localized edema, erythema, heat, and tenderness are characteristic signs of the inflammatory response. During the *fibroblastic phase*, which occurs approximately 4 to 20 days after the injury, cells needed for tissue repair and reconstruction proliferate. Fibroblasts at the wound site migrate over the new capillary network, laying down a bed of granulation tissue (collagen) to fill the wound space. During *wound contraction*, which occurs as granulation tissue forms, myofibroblasts cause the wound edges to pull toward the center.

Epithelial cells from the burn margins then migrate across the wound and eventually reproduce to form a protective barrier. This process is called *epithelialization*. Epithelial cells also migrate from the hair follicles and sweat glands, forming small islands of cells known as *epithelial buds*. Newly forming epithelial cells are easily damaged by mechanical trauma and desiccation. If allowed to dry, the wound will form *neo-eschar*, retarding the healing process. The epithelial cells must secrete enzymes to dissolve the eschar in their path. The *maturation phase* occurs when immature granulation tissue becomes highly organized and serves to restore tissue strength. This phase begins approximately 20 days after the burn injury and continues beyond 1 year. Contractures can occur if a burn wound heals with extensive scar tissue formation over a joint. A *contracture* is the fixation of a joint or area of skin into a flexed or fixed position. This is caused by atrophy and shortening of muscle fibers or by scar formation and the loss of the normal skin elasticity.

Under optimal conditions, a partial-thickness burn heals in 2 to 6 weeks. The persistence of eschar on a full-thickness burn may delay healing; if the area involved is large, this will cause the patient to remain in a hypermetabolic state. As bacteria proliferate beneath the eschar, there is a possibility of infection. Approximately 2 weeks after a burn injury, the eschar will begin to separate from the underlying tissue as a result of microbial and leukocytic action on subeschar collagen fibers. Separation generally occurs from the wound margins inward but may occur in patches. Eschar may be removed earlier by surgical excision to facilitate healing.

CLINICAL PRESENTATION

Sun poisoning may present with urticaria, an erythematous rash accompanied by edema, fever, fatigue, dizziness, GI symptoms, or malaise. Hematuria, casts, and proteinuria may also occur. Contact photodermatitis results in pruritic papules with erythema and occasional vesicles 24 hours or more after sun exposure. The skin rash will occur in the area where the triggering chemical was applied and sun exposure occurred.

In the past, burn injuries were classified as first through third degree. Currently second- and third-degree burns are classified as either partial-thickness or full-thickness. Partial-thickness injuries can be further categorized as superficial or deep. The signs and symptoms of the various depths of burn are as follows:

- *Superficial (first-degree) burns.* These burns involve the epidermal layer only. The patient presents with pain, hyperemia, and erythema. The surface is dry, with no vesicles or blisters, and blanches with pressure. The wound heals in approximately 5 days without scarring. The prototype of a first-degree burn is a mild sunburn. If this type of burn occurs over a large surface area, it can result in fever, weakness, chills, and vomiting.
- *Superficial partial-thickness (second-degree) burns.* These burns involve the epidermis along with the upper layer of dermis. Signs and symptoms include erythema, hyperemia, pain, moist skin, and hypersensitivity to touch. Vesicles and blisters appear several hours after the injury. The healing time is within 21 days with minimal scarring.
- *Deep partial-thickness (second-degree) burns.* These burns produce destruction of the epidermis, along with most of the dermis. Epidermal cells lining hair follicles and sweat glands remain intact. This level of burn may convert to a full-thickness injury. The burn wound is typically pale, mottled, pearly white, mostly dry, often insensate, and difficult to differentiate from a full-thickness burn. The burn will heal by wound contraction and reepithelialization within 3 to 6 weeks. Often, excision and grafting are done

to provide a better functional cosmetic result and to decrease the healing time.
- *Full-thickness (third-degree) burns.* These burns result in destruction of all layers of the skin, down to or past the subcutaneous fat layer, sometimes involving fascia, muscle, and bone. The nerves are also typically destroyed. Hair will pull easily out of the follicles, but in a painless manner. The clinical picture typically includes a thick, dry, leathery eschar, with a wound that is white, cherry red, or brown/black in color. The tissue is insensate, with thrombosed blood vessels. These wounds typically require skin grafting.

DIAGNOSTIC REASONING

Diagnostic Tests

Initial laboratory studies for a patient with a major burn include a CBC, serum electrolyte panel, BUN and creatinine, and serum glucose. Pulse oximetry and arterial blood gas determinations should be done, given the effects that significant burns have on the circulatory system and oxygenation. In addition, because smoke inhalation injury is associated with significant fire-related burns, a carboxyhemoglobin (COHb) level should be checked to determine the percentage of hemoglobin bound to carbon monoxide and unavailable for oxygen transport. The following COHb levels correlate with typical clinical symptoms:

- Less than 10% COHb: No symptoms
- 20% COHb: Headache, nausea, vomiting, loss of dexterity
- 30% COHb: Confusion, lethargy, ST-segment depression on electrocardiogram
- 40% to 60% COHb: Coma
- More than 60% COHb: Death

If the COHb level is less than 40%, treatment should consist of 100% oxygen administered by a high-humidity flow mask. A patient with a COHb level of 40% or higher should be considered for transfer to a hyperbaric chamber, given its life-threatening consequences.

Differential Diagnosis

Although thermal injury is the most common cause of burn wounds, several other etiologies of burns exist. For example, chemical burns occur in industrial, military, home, agricultural, school, and research laboratory settings. For clinicians affiliated with these settings, especially student health-care settings that include a chemistry laboratory, it is important to have knowledge of the initial care of chemical burn injuries. Various agents that can cause burn injuries are listed in Table 75.1.

Photodermatitis should be differentiated from contact dermatitis that may develop from one of the many substances in suntan lotions and oils. Sensitivity to the sun's rays may also be part of a more serious condition such as erythropoietic protoporphyria, systemic lupus erythematosus, pellagra, or porphyria cutanea tarda.

MANAGEMENT

If a patient with a major burn presents to an outpatient setting, it is necessary to assess and stabilize the patient so that they can be safely transported by emergency medical services (EMS) to a hospital ED or preferably a burn

TABLE 75.1 Burn Injuries	
Type of Injury	Characteristics
Chemical	• *Damage:* Destruction of tissues from coagulation or desiccation of tissue protein; damage continues until agent is removed; skin penetration by many chemicals leads to systemic toxicity • *Effects:* Injury is generally deeper than it appears; small percentage of admissions to burn units
Cold liquids/gases	• *Damage:* Frostbite (freezing of tissue) results in ice crystal formation, which draws water out of the cells and into the extracellular space; crystals expand, causing mechanical destruction of cell membranes and organelles • *Effects:* Cellular destruction; serum electrolyte imbalances
Electrical	• *Damage:* Destruction of tissues from heat generated by electric current passing through tissues; arc burn or thermal injury • *Effects:* Injury is usually more extensive than it appears; cardiac conduction system may be affected, leading to sudden death or arrhythmias; severe muscle contraction can produce long bone or vertebral fractures; severe muscle destruction leads to release of myoglobin, which can affect kidney function
Radiation	• *Damage:* Occurs primarily by gamma or x-ray particles; affects the reproductive mechanisms of tissue cells, leading to cellular death • *Effects:* Proportional to the extent of injury and depth of tissue damage
Thermal heat	• *Damage:* Destruction of tissues from flames, scalding liquids, or steam • *Effects:* Proportional to extent of injury and depth; thermal burns account for highest percentage of admissions to burn units.

center. Therefore, all practitioners should understand the fundamentals of the initial assessment and treatment of burn injuries. See Figure 75.1 to estimate the extent of a burn injury using the "Rule of Nines." When burns are scattered on the body, a rule of thumb is that the size of the patient's palm is equal to approximately 1% TBSA.

Major Burns

A patient with a major burn should be immediately transported to a burn center or ED. A *major burn* is defined as follows:

- Partial-thickness burn greater than 25% TBSA in a person 10 to 50 years of age *or* greater than 20% TBSA in a child younger than 10 years of age or an adult older than 50 years of age
- Full-thickness burn greater than 10% TBSA in any individual
- Serious burn involving the hand, face, foot, or perineum
- A burn complicated by smoke or chemical inhalation injury
- An electrical burn
- A burn in an infant, an immunocompromised patient, or an older patient

Initial management of a patient with a major burn injury should include maintaining the patient's airway, breathing, and circulation. If there is time before transportation to an ED or burn center, the patient's clothing should be removed if further damage to the skin can be avoided. Jewelry should also be removed and secured in a safe place. The patient should be placed on and covered with a clean, warm sheet and clean blankets with overhead warmers if available. No other wound care is typically required until the patient reaches the ED or burn center.

For airway management, the clinician should assess the patency of the patient's airway while maintaining the head and neck in a neutral position. If a spinal cord injury is probable, the clinician should apply a cervical collar, sandbags, and backboard as appropriate.

For respiratory management, while the clinician is maintaining the patient's breathing, they should simultaneously observe the patient's skin color, monitor oxygen saturation via pulse oximetry (SpO_2), and auscultate the lungs to ensure effective bilateral ventilation. The clinician should be alert for signs of smoke inhalation and thermal airway injury if the patient was exposed to fire in an enclosed space. Signs and symptoms include facial burns; presence of soot around the mouth and nose and in the sputum; singed nasal hairs; coughing up of carbonaceous black sputum; difficulty swallowing; signs of hypoxemia including tachycardia, dysrhythmias, anxiety, or lethargy; increased or decreased respiratory rate; use of accessory muscles for breathing; intercostal or sternal retractions; inspiratory stridor; hoarseness; and expiratory stridor.

Once an airway injury has occurred, no measures are typically effective in limiting its progress, and complete airway obstruction can occur. If signs of airway injury are present, the patient will need to be intubated. After extensive swelling has occurred, intubation will be very difficult, so the decision to insert an artificial airway should be made early in the assessment of a burn patient with airway injury. In a nonintubated patient, humidified oxygen at 5 to 10 L/min should be administered by face mask along with a bronchodilator such as albuterol via metered-dose inhaler with a spacer, every 15 to 20 minutes as needed. If the patient has signs of carbon monoxide poisoning (e.g., headache, nausea, vomiting, dizziness, loss of manual dexterity, confusion, lethargy, unconsciousness, and cherry-red skin color), 100% oxygen should be administered via a nonrebreathing mask.

For circulatory management, if the patient presents in the outpatient setting with thermal injuries that involve more than 20% TBSA, the patient will need to be transported to a hospital ED or burn center. If there is evidence of burn-related shock and the patient can still take fluids orally, they should receive oral rehydration with balanced salt solutions. The patient should be encouraged to drink enough fluid to keep the urine clear and copious. If this is not possible, a large-bore (16- or 18-gauge) IV catheter should be inserted in an upper extremity vein, preferably through unburned skin. The clinician should infuse lactated Ringer's solution at an initial rate of 500 mL/hr.

Patients with major burns should receive tetanus prophylaxis. If the patient has not received a full primary vaccination series of at least three doses of tetanus toxoid, tetanus vaccine and tetanus immune globulin 250 U should be immediately administered, with the remaining vaccinations in the series administered according to

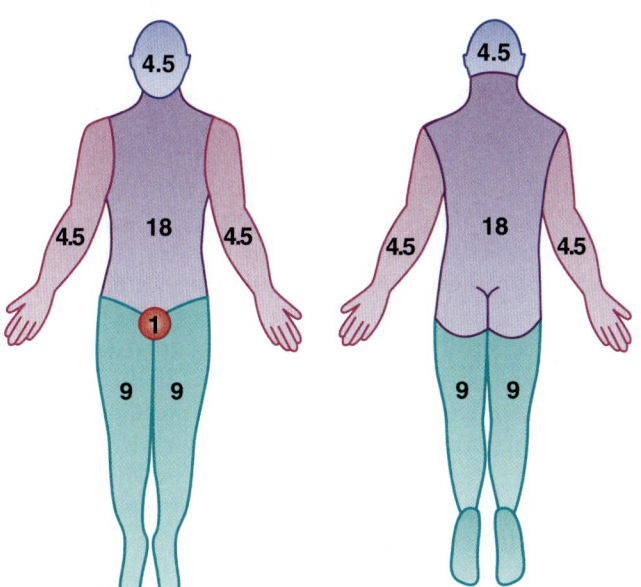

Figure 75.1 The Rule of Nines.

Minor Burns

A patient with minor burn injuries can usually be treated in an outpatient setting. Minor burn injuries include a burn of less than 15% TBSA in a patient 10 to 50 years of age or less than 10% TBSA in a child younger than 10 years of age or an adult older than 50 years of age.

Superficial (First-Degree) Burns

These burns should be cooled with wet compresses. Ice should not be placed directly on the skin. Aloe vera gel can be applied topically to the burn. Remedies (anesthetic sprays) with benzocaine or lidocaine may provide relief from pain, but these medications produce sensitivity reactions in some people. The patient can be given ibuprofen (Motrin) 800 mg every 8 hours, aspirin, or another NSAID, which work by blocking the production of prostaglandins that are mediators of pain in sunburned skin. If the sunburn is severe, the clinician should administer oral prednisone in a rapid taper: day 1, 80 mg; day 2, 60 mg; day 3, 40 mg; day 4, 20 mg; day 5, 10 mg. There are no benefits to prescribing topical corticosteroid ointments or creams.

Superficial Partial-Thickness and Deep Partial-Thickness (Second-Degree) Burns

These burns should be gently irrigated with cool water or saline solution to remove all loose dirt and skin. If the burn is chemical in nature, the caustic agent should be washed off with large amounts of water. Any necrotic skin should be peeled off or trimmed. Small, thick blisters should be left intact. Thin, fluid-filled blisters greater than 1 inch in diameter should be drained and the dead skin trimmed, using aseptic technique.

There are multiple methods for the outpatient management of superficial partial-thickness burns. One is to apply a topical antimicrobial preparation to the wound. Agents typically used are presented in Drugs Commonly Prescribed 75.1. Silver sulfadiazine (Silvadene) is the most frequently used topical agent, although it cannot be used in patients with sulfa allergies or on the face because of silver staining. Alternative topical agents for facial burns include gentamicin ophthalmic ointment, Neosporin, or bacitracin. When these ointments are applied to the face, no overlying dressing should be used. If antibiotic creams are unavailable, aloe vera gel can be applied to the burn.

Burn wounds on areas other than the face should be covered with a dressing, which should be removed twice a day at home. The burn should be washed with mild antiseptic soap and water, and then antibiotic ointment and a clean dressing should be reapplied. This regimen should continue for 7 to 10 days until the burn is healed. This particular method of treatment has some disadvantages in the outpatient setting. Some antimicrobial agents (such as Sulfamylon) encourage wound maceration and therefore cannot be used under a dressing. Also, most topical agents lose their potency in 6 to 24 hours after application, making frequent dressing changes necessary.

An alternative dressing for the superficial partial-thickness burn is to cover the affected area with a fine-mesh gauze (e.g., Xeroform gauze) without a topical antibiotic. This gauze is covered with gauze pads, and then a bulky absorbent dressing (e.g., Kerlix) is wrapped around the wound to provide protective bulk. The clinician should inspect the wound and change the dressing the next day because the maximum amount of wound seepage occurs within the first 24 hours. The same type of dressing is reapplied, and the burn wound should also be assessed for infection, which should be aggressively treated.

The burn is then reevaluated after 4 days, and the bulky dressing is removed. If a fluid collection has occurred beneath the fine-mesh gauze, the dressing will need to be removed, the wound cleansed, and new fine-mesh gauze applied. If the fine-mesh gauze is still in place without any apparent fluid collection, it should be left in place and the burn rewrapped. Another follow-up visit should be scheduled for reexamination in 5 days. At that time, the fine-mesh gauze, impregnated with the crust from the burn, should separate from the epithelium, revealing healed epithelium underneath. Once the wound is left open, it must be kept clean and protected from extremes of temperature. The wound should epithelialize in approximately 3 weeks. Epithelialization, however, may not occur for 2 to 3 months if the wound is a deep partial-thickness burn in which the only skin remnants are the hair follicles or sweat glands.

Another method for outpatient burn wound management is to place a semisynthetic occlusive dressing (e.g., Biobrane), a xenograft, a moisture vapor-permeable dressing (e.g., Opsite), or a hydrocolloid dressing (e.g., DuoDerm) over the wound. These dressings are less readily available, however, and tend to be expensive. They are most useful for the immunocompromised patient because they minimize the risk of infection. They can be used on flat-surface superficial partial-thickness burns of the extremities and trunk. The goal is for the dressing to adhere to the wound surface and for there to be no exudate or fluid between the dressing and the burn. The dressing is usually removed after 7 to 10 days because the wound is typically healed by then. If there is leaking or nonadherence at any time, the dressing must be changed. Superficial partial-thickness burn wounds heal faster, using this method, and patients usually find this method more comfortable and easier to maintain with fewer dressing changes.

Oral antibiotics should be given only if the burn becomes infected, as prophylactic antibiotic therapy is not supported in acute burns. Any partial-thickness burn

Drugs Commonly Prescribed 75.1: Burns

TOPICAL	INDICATIONS	DOSAGE AND COMMENTS
Antimicrobial Agents		
Bacitracin ointment	Antimicrobial, especially for sensitive areas (e.g., lips, eyelids)	Apply to cleansed area two to three times daily. It does not penetrate eschar
Clotrimazole cream (Lotrimin)	Fungal infections of burn wounds	Apply thin coat to wound; wait 20 minutes before applying dressing. It is not for ophthalmic use. It may cause skin irritation and blistering.
Mafenide acetate (Sulfamylon)	Active against most gram-positive and gram-negative organisms. Drug of choice for electrical and ear burns	Apply one to two times daily, using sterile gloves; do not use with dressings (may reduce effectiveness and cause skin maceration). Monitor for signs of acidosis, intake and output, and signs of allergic skin reaction. This penetrates eschar better than other agents. Pain occurs on application to partial-thickness burns and for 30 minutes thereafter. Allergic maculopapular skin rash may occur. Use with caution in patients with impaired renal or pulmonary function. Hyperchloremic metabolic acidosis may occur. Superinfection with fungi is possible.
Silver nitrate	Active against wide spectrum of bacterial pathogens and fungal infections. Used for patients with sulfa allergy or toxic epidermal necrolysis syndrome	Apply 0.5% solution via wet dressings two to three times a day; ensure dressings remain moist. Preserve solution in a light-resistant container. Protect area with plastic to prevent staining from spills or splashes, as solution stains surfaces black (including unburned skin). It has poor penetration of eschar. Electrolyte imbalances may occur. Methemoglobinemia may occur.
Silver sulfadiazine (Silvadene)	Active against wide spectrum of microbial pathogens. Most frequently used agent for partial-thickness and full-thickness thermal injuries	Apply once or twice daily, using sterile gloves; leave wounds exposed or apply gauze dressing over wound. Do not use if cream is dark in color. Transient neutropenia may occur after 2 to 3 days. It offers only moderate penetration of eschar. Bone marrow suppression may occur. Use with caution in patients with impaired hepatic or renal function.

will convert to a full-thickness burn if it becomes infected, especially with *Streptococcus*. If infection occurs, the patient may have to be admitted to a hospital for IV antibiotics. Signs of infection include pus, foul odor, cloudy blisters, increased swelling and redness in the normal skin around the burn, and fever greater than 101°F (38.3°C). Patients with infected minor burns should receive tetanus prophylaxis as described for major burns.

Chemical Burns

Consultation from clinicians at a burn center should be obtained for the treatment of chemical injuries. When a patient with a chemical burn is assessed, the clinician should don protective clothing and gloves. The first priority is to stop the burning process and arrange for rapid transportation to an ED or burn center. Any of the patient's garments that have become saturated with the chemical should be rapidly removed, and the patient should be quickly transported to a shower irrigation area. All other garments should be removed from the patient before the irrigation is complete. If the agent is a powderlike material, such as lime, the clinician should brush off as much as possible from the patient before irrigating the burned area. The hair and the areas under the nails and between the toes should be checked for collections of the chemical. The patient may be more comfortable on a chair in a running shower, but any patient who is unstable should be kept in a horizontal position during the irrigation.

A chemical burn should be irrigated with water for no less than 30 minutes and preferably for 60 minutes. Irrigation may need to be continued for hours in the case of alkali burns. Irrigation decreases the concentration of the chemical agent and physically removes it from the wound; the rate and severity of reaction between the chemical and the exposed tissue will thus be decreased. After irrigation in the outpatient setting, the clinician should place wet towels over the patient and arrange for transportation to the hospital. Although wet towels help to relieve pain and continue to dilute the chemical, caution is needed to prevent hypothermia if the burned area is extensive. If possible, the patient should bring samples of the chemical agent with a product label to the ED. Use of pH-detection litmus paper may help determine the continued presence of alkali or acid in burn wounds. After irrigation and débridement of any remaining particles and devitalized tissue, antimicrobial agents should be used and tetanus prophylaxis updated as needed, as described for major burns.

For midsized to large burns caused by hot tar or asphalt, the wound should be rapidly cooled with a large volume of water. The tar can then be removed, using a petrolatum-based product such as an antibiotic ointment (e.g., Neosporin). When a large body surface area is involved, a new (unopened) jar of mayonnaise will suffice. The wound can be dressed with a petrolatum-based dressing (e.g., Xeroform gauze). Tar can be removed from the cornea or conjunctiva with a polysorbate-containing neomycin sulfate preparation, although consultation with an ophthalmologist is recommended. Special consideration should be given to chemical or thermal burns that cause acute iritis (inflammation of the iris). Individuals will present with excess lacrimation, decreased vision, photophobia, and pain. Management should include consultation with an ophthalmologist and the use of a cycloplegic drug, as well as possibly topical corticosteroids.

Although not commonly considered a chemical burn, if a patient presents with skin that is adhered together with a fast-setting epoxy glue, the adhesive can be removed with acetone. If the glue is on the mucous membranes, the area can be swabbed with vegetable oil until the glue is removed. For glue in the eyes, the clinician should use an ophthalmic antibiotic ointment to facilitate removal. Referral to an ophthalmologist may be indicated, as care must be taken or else the drying glue can cause a corneal abrasion.

Some chemical exposures call for specialized agents as directed by an ED or burn center. If exposure to hydrofluoric acid (used in glass etching) or oxalic acid has caused a chemical burn, the affected area should be irrigated with water and then neutralized with subcutaneous injections of 10% calcium gluconate. However, this should be done only after consultation with clinicians at a burn center. If phenol (an acidic alcohol used in sanitizers and disinfectants) is the causative agent, the area should be irrigated with water if a high-density shower is available. Of note, phenol is more soluble in polyethylene glycol; therefore, a 50% solution of this agent should be used to irrigate the skin as soon as possible.

FOLLOW-UP AND REFERRAL

Although dressing changes for some types of burns may not be recommended until 5 to 7 days after the injury, all patients with a burn injury must still be reassessed in 24 hours to reevaluate the depth and extent of the burn. Infected burns must also be assessed within 1 to 2 days after starting antibiotic therapy to ensure improvement on the selected regimen.

Referral to an ED or specialized burn center is indicated for major burns, as well as minor burns that do not begin healing as expected. In addition, both thermal and chemical burns to highly sensitive parts of the body require rapid referral to appropriate specialty care (e.g., ophthalmology for eye injuries).

Patient Education: Burns

Patients should be advised to elevate the burned area, especially if it involves an extremity, and to return to the clinician's office or the ED if signs of an infection appear. Patients should also be given a prescription for analgesic medication. Given the risk of chemical burns from home-based cleaning products and other solvents, all parents should have the national Poison Control Center Help Line (1-800-222-1222) readily available in the case of chemical injury.

Patients with sunburns should be informed that sunscreens with PABA may cause photosensitivity dermatitis. Photoplex broad-spectrum sunscreen lotion not only provides protection from UVB radiation but also offers absorbent protection from UVA rays and may be beneficial for patients who experience photosensitivity activated by UVA. Other useful substitutes are sunshades that contain titanium dioxide, zinc oxide, or talc. Patients should be informed about the sun protection factor (SPF) index—a system of evaluating the effectiveness of various formulations for protecting the skin from sun exposure. Protective agents are rated one to 50 by the U.S. FDA. An SPF of 15 means that the sunscreen provides 15 times more protection from the sun, compared with unprotected skin. A patient information sheet on sun exposure safety tips should be given to all patients, especially those who have sustained a sunburn severe enough to require treatment (see Box 75.3). Given the risk of infection to sun-damaged skin, the patient should also notify the health-care provider if pain and fever persist for more than 48 hours.

HEAD TRAUMA

Types of head trauma that may be encountered in a primary care setting include cerebral contusions, concussions, skull fractures, and epidural or subdural hematomas. In contrast, subarachnoid hemorrhage typically results from the spontaneous rupture of intracranial aneurysms, rather than from a traumatic etiology. The majority of head trauma patients will need to be transported to the nearest ED for emergent evaluation and care.

Box 75.3 Patient Information: Sunburn

- Always wear sunscreen when outdoors on a sunny day. A sunscreen with a sun protection factor (SPF) of at least 15 will block most harmful ultraviolet (UV) radiation. For the average adult, the recommended dose is 1 ounce per application. Reapply every 2 hours after being in the water or after exercising and sweating.
- Use broad-spectrum sunscreens—those that contain active ingredients absorbing at least 85% of UVA and UVB rays of the sun.
- Protect sensitive areas such as the nose and rims of the ears.
- Use a lip balm containing a sunscreen. This can help keep some people from getting cold sores.
- Minimize exposure to the sun during the hours when the sun is directly overhead and exposure is most damaging, from 8 a.m. to 4 p.m. Sun (UV) exposure before 8 a.m. or after 4 p.m., when the sun is lower on the horizon, is typically only one-third that at midday. If your shadow is shorter than you are (around midday), you are being exposed to high levels of UV radiation.
- Wear sunglasses that block 99% or all UV radiation. Babies and children should also be protected with sunglasses to prevent cataracts that may develop later in life.
- Wear a hat with a wide brim to provide protection to your eyes, ears, face, and the back of your neck.
- Wear tightly woven, loose-fitting clothing during prolonged periods in the sun.
- Avoid sunlamps and tanning parlors.
- Monitor the UV Index, as reported by the U.S. Environmental Protection Agency and consistent with World Health Organization guidelines:
  - UV Index 0–2 (minimal): Precautions include wearing a hat.
  - UV Index 3–4 (low): Precautions include wearing a hat and using a sunscreen with an SPF of at least 15.
  - UV Index 5–6 (moderate): Precautions include wearing a hat, using a sunscreen with an SPF of at least 15, and staying in shady areas when outside.
  - UV Index 7–9 (high): Precautions include wearing a hat, using a sunscreen with an SPF of at least 15, staying in shady areas when outside, and staying indoors between the hours of 10 a.m. and 4 p.m.
  - UV Index 10+ (very high): Precautions include staying indoors as much as possible and taking other precautions when outdoors.
- Be aware that UV radiation increases 5% for every 1,000 feet of altitude. In North America, the sun is closest to the Earth on June 21. Snow and water can also reflect the sun's rays, making sun exposure more intense.

EPIDEMIOLOGY AND CAUSES

Head trauma is a leading cause of morbidity and mortality in the United States, resulting in about 30% of all injury deaths. Falls constitute the leading cause of head injury (disproportionately affecting the youngest and oldest age-groups, followed by being struck by or hitting an object, and motor vehicle accidents were the third leading cause [Centers for Disease Control and Prevention, 2017]). Although it is estimated that approximately 3.8 million concussions occur in the United States annually during competitive sports and recreational activities, one-half of those go unreported. In people older than 65 years of age, falls account for the majority of head injury deaths (see Geriatric Considerations for common injuries). Falls are the most common reason for an injury-related visit to an ED. Traumatic brain injury (TBI) may also be the result of drug or alcohol use, violence (fights or physical abuse), and sports-related injuries, with football, ice hockey, soccer, boxing, and rugby having the highest incidence.

PATHOPHYSIOLOGY

Mild head trauma is usually the result of a sudden deceleration injury or rotational force that causes shearing forces within the brain. These forces cause axonal and blood vessel damage. Injuries to small blood vessels can manifest as petechial hemorrhages. If the bridging veins connecting the cortex to the venous sinuses are involved, acute subdural hematomas can occur that are potentially

Geriatric Considerations: Common Injuries

Patients older than 50 years of age are at higher risk for infection from all wounds, especially if they have a chronic disease such as diabetes mellitus or hypertension or they are immunocompromised. Assess these individuals diligently.

For older adults needing circulatory support if they are hypotensive, avoid overloading them with fluids due to a propensity for heart failure.

The majority of head injury deaths occur in individuals older than 65 years. Prevention is most important to reduce falls and potential mortality. Some prevention measures include:

- Having good lighting at night
- For males with nocturia, possibly having a urinal at the bedside
- Removing throw rugs
- Having shower grab bars installed
- Reviewing medications with the clinician
- Making sure they have a recent eye examination

fatal. In contrast, subarachnoid hemorrhages, with their resultant meningeal findings including extreme headache and neck stiffness, result far more commonly from ruptured intracranial saccular (berry) aneurysms (in greater than 80% of cases), rather than from trauma.

The area of cerebral injury becomes ischemic and edematous. As edema increases, the autoregulatory control of intracranial vessels is lost. The blood–brain barrier breaks down, resulting in increased loss of fluid into the brain parenchyma, which in turn results in elevated intracranial pressure (ICP). As ICP increases, cerebral blood flow decreases, leading to tissue hypoxia, a decrease in the serum pH level, and an increase in carbon dioxide level. This process leads to cerebral vasodilation and edema, which further increases ICP (resulting in a vicious cycle). The increased ICP compromises cerebral perfusion and, if not treated and reversed, leads to increasing hypoxia and secondary brain injury. If left untreated, the brain herniates downward toward the brainstem, causing irreversible brain damage.

Cerebral Contusion

A *cerebral contusion* is a focal brain injury involving cortical bruising and, at times, vessel lacerations. This is one of the most common cerebral injuries; it is associated with hemorrhage, edema, and brain swelling. Contusions are classified as *coup* (injury directly beneath the point of impact) or *contrecoup* (injury directly opposite the point of impact). Temporal and frontal lobes are the most commonly affected sites. Contusions are graded as mild or severe and superficial or deep. Superficial contusions usually involve the cortical and subcortical tissues, whereas deep contusions penetrate the white matter.

Concussion

A *concussion* involves diffuse brain injury. It is associated with a transient loss of consciousness (LOC) that occurs immediately after nonpenetrating blunt head trauma. Most patients with only a brief LOC (less than 5 minutes) are not admitted to the hospital if their subsequent neurological examination remains within normal limits. However, close observation by a responsible adult educated in the warning signs of neurological deterioration is critical for at least the next 24 hours.

More than 90% of concussions are not accompanied by loss of consciousness. A classic concussion typically produces retrograde and post-traumatic amnesia and mild neurological impairment. The duration of amnesia can be a predictor of severity, as the longer the amnesia, the more severe the concussion. Multiple systems exist for the grading of concussions, as there are no universally agreed-upon criteria to categorize severity. Some clinicians consider a mild concussion to be one with no LOC but rather characterized by other neurological manifestations, such as confusion, disorientation, and, at times, retrograde amnesia (i.e., an inability to recall events surrounding the injury) or post-traumatic amnesia. However, other experts feel that, by definition, concussions must involve LOC. Even with mild concussions, although confusion and disorientation immediately after the injury may last only minutes, recurrent dizziness, headache, and difficulty concentrating may last for months. More severe concussions with a greater LOC usually still present with a normal computed tomography (CT) scan of the head. Nonetheless, these patients should be admitted to the hospital for close observation, given the risk of significant neurological sequelae.

Postconcussion syndrome is usually associated with mild head trauma and may follow any type of concussion. LOC does not have to occur for postconcussion syndrome to develop, and it is estimated that up to 50% of patients who suffer mild head trauma will experience this syndrome. The syndrome consists of the following signs and symptoms, which can start as early as 24 hours post-trauma and persist for up to 6 months after the injury:

- Headaches
- Dizziness
- Fatigue
- Irritability
- Insomnia
- Anxiety
- Impaired concentration
- Loss of memory

Skull Fracture

A *skull fracture* may occur with a severe blow to the head. A skull fracture increases the risk of an underlying epidural or subdural hematoma. In addition, patients with suspected or confirmed skull fractures require careful examination of the CNs, particularly those that are most likely to be injured: olfactory nerve (CN I), optic nerve (CN II), oculomotor nerve (CN III), trochlear nerve (CN IV), trigeminal nerve (CN V), abducens nerve (CN VI), facial nerve (CN VII), and acoustic nerve (CN VIII).

A basilar skull fracture (i.e., a fracture of the base of the skull) can occur as an extension of a fracture in another area of the skull. Basilar skull fractures can cause leakage of cerebrospinal fluid (CSF), an entry point for bacteria leading to meningitis, and/or pneumocephalus (air entry into the CSF-filled spaces within the head). Several clinical manifestations can be associated with basilar skull fracture, including CSF leak through the cribriform plate of the skull causing nasal CSF rhinorrhea, hemotympanum (blood behind the tympanic membrane), ecchymosis over the mastoid process ("Battle's sign"), or periorbital ecchymosis ("raccoon eyes"). Routine x-rays may not reveal a skull fracture; therefore, radiographs are usually nondiagnostic and can cost precious minutes of critical care time. Thus, the clinician should be aware that basilar skull fracture is a clinical diagnosis and proceed immediately to the ED with EMS transport, if suspected.

Epidural Hematoma

Severe head trauma can cause intracranial bleeding that can put pressure on the brain tissue. The brain is surrounded by the *meninges,* three layers of protective membranes. The layers from the cranial bone going interiorly

Ears

Removal of inanimate objects is not always straightforward. If the patient is uncooperative or if the foreign body is difficult to grasp, ear, nose, and throat (ENT) consultation is suggested. If the object becomes lodged too deeply, it will be difficult to remove, and the patient may need general anesthesia for successful removal. If the object is small, irrigation is an option. If the object is appropriately shaped and accessible, alligator or bayonet forceps may be used to grasp and remove it. Suctioning may also assist in the removal of an object. A Yankauer suction catheter has a small orifice and a firm catheter tip that may facilitate foreign body removal.

A live insect trapped in the ear canal usually causes great distress. The patient will present with agitation, nausea, and tearing. The initial therapy is to immobilize the insect. This can be done by placing 2% lidocaine in the external ear canal, which will terminate the movement of the insect. The insect can then be removed using forceps.

After successful removal of the object, the ear canal needs to be checked for infections, superficial scratches, and tympanic membrane perforation. If there is no evidence of infection, the patient may be discharged home. If an infection is present, it should be treated as an otitis with appropriate antibiotics.

Nose

If the patient is uncooperative, a restraining device or sedation may be needed. If the patient is cooperative, the following steps may be used to remove the foreign body:

- Help the patient to blow their nose to see if the foreign object will be expelled.
- If the mucosa appears swollen, soak a pledget in a liquid decongestant such as phenylephrine (Neo-Synephrine) nasal spray and insert it into the affected naris to reduce swelling; care should be taken not to push the foreign body further into the nose.
- Using a nasal speculum and alligator or bayonet forceps, visualize the foreign body and gently remove it. Other methods include using an ear curette, single skin hook, or right-angle ear hook. Another method that has been used is to pass a small urinary catheter superior to (beyond) the object, inflate the balloon, and pull the object out, although this method should only be attempted by a properly trained clinician.
- All of these methods can be successful if the patient is cooperative. Care must be taken not to push the foreign body down the back of the patient's throat, where it may be aspirated into the trachea.

After successfully removing the object, the clinician should inspect the nares for other foreign bodies. No further treatment is necessary unless local infection is apparent, in which case appropriate antibiotic therapy is indicated. If removal is unsuccessful, however, referral to an ENT specialist may be necessary.

Throat

Although most swallowed objects will pass spontaneously, up to 10% to 20% require some type of intervention. There are several physiologically narrow spaces in the esophageal-gastrointestinal tract that may restrict the movement of objects. In the pediatric population, the cricopharyngeal area is the most common site for obstruction, followed by (in order of frequency) the thoracic inlet, aortic arch, tracheal bifurcation, and hiatal narrowing. The majority of obstructions in adults occur at the distal end of the esophagus. Usually, once the object has passed through the pylorus, it will pass through the rest of the GI tract without difficulty. If the object has sharp edges, however, it can injure the intestines and/or become lodged anywhere in the gastrointestinal tract.

Ingested foreign bodies can also cause airway obstruction or perforation. If there is a possible foreign body ingestion, a chest x-ray should be ordered to see if the object is lodged in the esophagus, although foreign bodies will only be visualized if they are radiopaque. If the object is in the stomach, the patient should be monitored for passage of the object through the GI tract. The stool will need to be examined. If the object is not found, an abdominal flat-plate x-ray can be used to determine the location of the object. Objects that fail to be expelled may have to be removed by invasive procedures such as colonoscopy or surgery.

The treatment for ingestion of a sharp object is controversial. Most practitioners recommend that sharp objects be removed so that they do not cause a perforation before they pass into the intestine.

A food bolus is usually the cause of ingested foreign bodies in the adult population. Typically, inadequately chewed meat is the main culprit. If the patient is unable to swallow salivary secretions, a chest x-ray should be obtained. Glucagon, a smooth-muscle relaxant, may be administered IV to relax the esophagus: a 1-mg dose is given IV and may be repeated after 20 minutes, if the object has not passed. The patient will usually vomit, which causes the foreign body to be expelled; it is important to ensure that the patient does not aspirate the vomitus. If glucagon has not produced the desired outcome, a GI consultation should be obtained. Some references recommend a barium swallow to visualize where the obstruction is located; however, most GI specialists prefer that no barium be given because it can obstruct the view of the bolus during endoscopy.

If a coin becomes lodged in the esophagus, it should be removed by endoscopy by a trained professional. Two other methods that may be tried by properly trained clinicians include passing an indwelling urinary catheter behind the object, inflating it, and pulling the object out. Smaller objects that become lodged in the esophagus can also be safely pushed into the stomach by a small urinary catheter.

Ingestion of button batteries is a true emergency situation. The batteries can cause burns to the gastrointestinal mucosa and must be removed quickly, as mucosal perforations may prove fatal.

Vagina

Typically, the only medical treatment necessary is removal of the foreign body, as most of the discharge and foul odor will disappear after the foreign body is removed. Privacy must be maintained to avoid undue embarrassment. If the foreign body is lodged in the sidewall of the vagina, the clinician should irrigate the area with normal saline to gently remove the object from the wall. If a foreign body is suspected in a small child, referral to an ED or hospital setting for general anesthesia for exploration should be considered, if the object is not visible and cannot be removed by gently pulling on the labia.

Systemic signs of infection require an immediate referral to a more advanced clinical setting, given the risk of toxic shock syndrome from retained foreign material in the vagina. Antibiotic therapy is indicated, and a more thorough evaluation may be needed to ensure all foreign material has been successfully removed from the vagina.

Rectum

Foreign objects are usually found in the rectal ampulla and are palpable with digital examination. All patients presenting with the chief complaint of a foreign body in the rectum need x-ray examinations of the abdomen to reveal the position, shape, and number of foreign bodies in the rectum. A lateral decubitus abdominal film will also show if free air is present in the abdomen. This is indicative of a perforation of the bowel, which is the most serious potential complication and requires immediate ED referral.

Removal of a foreign body from the rectum requires that the rectal sphincter be relaxed. If a brief attempt at removing the foreign body is unsuccessful, the practitioner should refer the patient to an ED for possible conscious sedation to relax the sphincter muscle. Conscious sedation requires close monitoring and is best carried out in an inpatient or emergency care setting. If there is any possibility of perforation, an emergent GI consultation is needed.

FOLLOW-UP AND REFERRAL

Follow-up is usually not indicated once the foreign body is removed. However, the patient should be alerted to signs and symptoms of an infection should one occur after removal, given the risk of severe systemic infection associated with retained foreign material in the genitourinary tract, in particular. If a rectal perforation has occurred as a result of a foreign body insertion or during its removal, an emergency gastroenterology referral is indicated.

Patient Education: Foreign Body Obstruction

Because children are usually involved in foreign body obstruction incidents, prevention is essential. Parents should be encouraged to buy age-appropriate toys and to keep small objects out of the reach of children. A particular risk in young children is the insertion of small removable parts of larger toys, such as small plastic shoes or removable jewelry/accessories from dolls or action figures. Regardless of age, children should be taught not to put objects in the various orifices of their bodies.

It should also not be assumed that foreign body obstructions in adults always occur accidentally, and an open and frank discussion of the risks of certain sexual practices or self-care (hygiene) behaviors may be needed if it becomes apparent that the insertion of foreign bodies into the vagina or rectum was voluntary. Moreover, a domestic violence assessment with appropriate social service and police referrals should be completed on any patient presenting with a genitourinary or GI foreign body obstruction, as a nonaccidental insertion may nonetheless be involuntary for the patient.

REFERENCES

Animal and Human Bites

National Institute for Occupational Safety and Health (NIOSH). CDC Control and Prevention. Venomous snakes. https://www.cdc.gov/niosh/topics/snakes/default.html. Accessed 7/12/20.

Rivera J. Animal bite accident statistics. LegalMatch. http://www.legalmatch.com/law-library/article/animal-bite-accident-statistics.html. Published 2018. Accessed July 18, 2020.

World Health Organization. Snakebite. https://www.who.int/health-topics/snakebite#tab=tab_1. Accessed 12/5/2020.

Arthropod Bites and Stings

Haddad Junior V, Amorim PC, Haddad Junior WT, et al. Venomous and poisonous arthropods: identification, clinical manifestations of envenomation, and treatments used in human injuries. *Rev Soc Bras Med Trop*. 2015;48(6):650–657.

Burns

American Burn Association. Burn incidence fact sheet. Burn incidence and treatment in the United States: 2016. http://ameriburn.org/who-we-are/media/burn-incidence-fact-sheet/. Accessed July 17, 2020.

American Burn Association (ABA) National Burn Awareness Week 2020. https://ameriburn.org/national-burn-awareness-week-2020/. Accessed 7/18/20.

Foreign Body Obstruction

Colyar MR. *Advanced practice nursing procedures*. 2nd ed. Philadelphia, PA: FA Davis; 2015.

Head Trauma

Centers for Disease Control and Prevention, National Center for Injury Prevention and Control, Division of Unintentional Injury

Prevention. Traumatic brain injury & concussion. https://www.cdc.gov/traumaticbraininjury/get_the_facts.html. Published 2017. Accessed 7/17/20.

Csenkey A, Jozsa G, Gede N, et al. (2019). Systemic antibiotic prophylaxis does not affect infectious complications in pediatric burn injury: A meta-analysis. *PLOS ONE.* Sept. 25, 2019. https://journals.plos.org/plosone/article?id=10.1371/journal.pone.0223063. Accessed 11/22/2020.

Pneumothorax and Hemothorax

Kong VY, Sartorius B, Clarke DL. (2015). The accuracy of physical examination in identifying significant pathologies in penetrating thoracic trauma. Eur J Trauma Emerg Surg. 2015;41(6):647.

Olesen WH, Katballe N, Sindby JE, et al (2017), Cannabis increased the risk of primary spontaneous pneumothorax in tobacco smokers: a case-control study. Eur J Cardiothorac Surg. 2017;52(4):679.

Wounds and Lacerations

Daum RS, Miller LG, Immergluck L, et al. A placebo-controlled trial of antibiotics for smaller skin abscesses. *N Engl J Med.* 2017;376:2545–2555.

Ludtke H. Abscess incision and drainage. Society for Academic Emergency Medicine. https://www.saem.org/cdem/education/online-education/m3-curriculum/group-emergency-department-procedures/abscess-incision-and-drainage. Accessed 7/17/20.

Wernick B, Nahirniak P, Stawicki SP. (2020). Impaired Wound Healing. https://www.ncbi.nlm.nih.gov/books/NBK482254/. Accessed 12/5/2020.

RESOURCES

Animal and Human Bites

Venomous snakes distribution and species risk categories. World Health Organization. 2010.
https://www.cdc.gov/niosh/topics/snakes/default.html

Arthropod Bites and Stings

University of Iowa Hardin Library for the Health Sciences
http://www.lib.uiowa.edu/hardin/md/insectbites.html

Burns

American Burn Association
https://www.ameriburn.org
The Burn Survivor Resource Center
https://www.burnsurvivor.com
UV Index. United States Environmental Protection Agency
https://www.epa.gov/sunsafety/uv-index-scale-1

Head Trauma

American Association of Neurological Surgeons/Congress of Neurological Surgeons (AANS)
https://www.aans.org
CDC HEADS UP
https://www.cdc.gov/headsup/about/index.html
MedlinePlus: Traumatic Brain Injury
https://medlineplus.gov/traumaticbraininjury.html

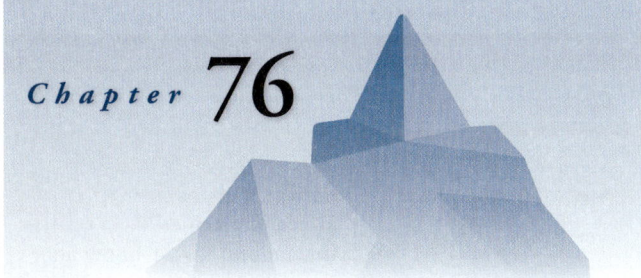

Chapter 76

Toxic and Environmental Exposures

Jill E. Winland-Brown, EdD, APRN, FNP-BC, FAANP
Brian Oscar Porter, MD, PhD, MPH, MBA

POISONING

Poisons encompass a wide variety of toxic compounds, including pesticides, overdosed drugs, carbon monoxide (CO), and other toxins such as household chemicals and venom from biting or stinging animals such as spiders, snakes, and scorpions (venom exposure is discussed in Chapter 75).

EPIDEMIOLOGY AND CAUSES

According to 2019 data compiled by the U.S. Centers for Disease Control and Prevention (CDC), poisoning is the leading cause of injury-related death in the United States, with up to 65,000 deaths reported annually. In children younger than 5 years of age, poisonings are most often due to accidental ingestion. In the adolescent population, trauma and intentional self-harm are the first and second leading causes of death, and most adolescent and adult poisonings are self-inflicted and secondary to intentional ingestion.

It has been estimated that approximately 2.2 million accidental poisonings occur each year. Nearly half of these incidents involve children, and more than 90% of all poisonings occur in the home. Toxicity events in adults due to poisonings account for 80% to 90% of all hospital admissions. Most adult poisonings involve intentional ingestions, such as recreational drug exposures or suicidal gestures/attempts by drug overdose. The American

Association of Poison Control Centers maintains a Toxic Exposure Surveillance System, which is a database of detailed toxicological information on more than 24 million poison exposures reported to U.S. poison control centers. It was estimated in 2019 that every 12 seconds someone sought information from a poison control center in the United States.

PATHOPHYSIOLOGY

The pathophysiology of poisonings varies widely, depending on the substance that the individual is exposed to and whether it is inhaled, topically applied, or ingested. The effects of most poisonings are dose dependent. The diagnosis is usually made clinically and then supported by key laboratory evaluations.

For example, inhalation of motor vehicle exhaust leads to the chemical binding of CO to hemoglobin in the blood, thereby resulting in the formation of carboxyhemoglobin (COHb), commonly known as carbon monoxide poisoning. COHb prevents oxygen from binding to hemoglobin and the subsequent transport of oxygen to bodily tissues. Although increasing COHb levels in the blood correlate to more severe clinical presentations, carbon monoxide poisoning may initially present in a clinically benign or ambiguous manner, such as with only a headache.

In contrast, a tricyclic antidepressant overdose (e.g., with amitriptyline, nortriptyline, or imipramine) can result in severe toxic cardiovascular and central nervous system (CNS) effects. These symptoms are secondary to the anticholinergic effects of the medication and alterations in cardiac cell conductivity, which lead to conduction disturbances such as QTc prolongation. Toxicology screening can confirm exposure to these medications through qualitative testing of urine or blood samples.

With a barbiturate overdose (e.g., phenobarbital), there is decreased neuronal neurotransmitter activity, depressed central sympathetic tone, and inhibition of cardiac contractility. Barbiturates act directly on inhibitory gamma-aminobutyric acid (GABA) receptors by increasing the affinity of the GABA ligand to its cognate receptor, resulting in an increase in the average opening time of chloride ion channels and a potentiation of CNS depressant activity. Benzodiazepines such as lorazepam (Ativan), alprazolam (Xanax), and diazepam (Valium) are also CNS depressants that enhance GABA receptor activity, but at a molecularly distinct portion of the receptor. Benzodiazepines increase ligand affinity and the frequency of ion channel opening, but not the duration of time that the channel remains open. Given this mechanistic difference, benzodiazepines have less potential for toxicity than barbiturates due to their saturable effects. Qualitative testing can confirm exposure to either barbiturates or benzodiazepines.

CLINICAL PRESENTATION

Given the wide range of potential poison exposures, the primary care practitioner should consider the clinical presentation of the specific type of poisoning suspected and confirm exposure with blood and urine toxicology screens when clinically warranted. Signs and symptoms of various types of poisonings are listed in Table 76.1.

TABLE 76.1 Common Poisonings

Name/Type	Signs and Symptoms	Diagnosis	Management
Drugs			

Acetaminophen (Tylenol)	Varies; may be asymptomatic to severe
	Nausea
	Vomiting
	24 to 48 hours postingestion:
	  Hepatic necrosis with jaundice
	  Hepatic encephalopathy
	  Renal failure
	  Possible death
		Acetaminophen level	Activated charcoal
			N-acetylcysteine IV (Acetadote) for 21 hours after ingestion

Barbiturates: Phenobarbital (phenobarb) Pentobarbital sodium (Nembutal)	Decreased level of consciousness Drowsiness Confusion Ataxia Vertigo Slurred speech Shallow respirations Bradycardia Headache Cyanosis Hypothermia Cardiovascular collapse	Toxicology screen (urine or blood)	Gastric lavage with activated charcoal and cathartic agent Airway maintenance Ventilatory assistance Cardiovascular support

Chapter 76 Toxic and Environmental Exposures 1377

TABLE 76.1 Common Poisonings—cont'd			
Name/Type	Signs and Symptoms	Diagnosis	Management
Benzodiazepines: Clorazepate dipotassium (Tranxene) Diazepam (Valium) Alprazolam (Xanax)	Central nervous system (CNS) depression Drowsiness Dizziness Headache Ataxia Hypotension Memory impairment	Toxicology screen (urine or blood)	Gastric lavage Symptomatic treatment Airway maintenance Ventilatory assistance Cardiovascular support
CNS stimulants: Methylphenidate (Ritalin, Concerta), amphetamine mixture (Adderall)	Vomiting Emotional lability Nervousness Fever Dizziness Hypertension Tachycardia Psychosis Dyskinesias Tourette syndrome Seizures	Toxicology screen (urine or blood)	Supportive care
Cocaine	Nervous system stimulation Restlessness Hallucinations Tachycardia Dilated pupils Chills Fever Abdominal pain Vomiting Muscle spasms Irregular respirations progressing to death	History of cocaine use Toxicology screen (urine or blood)	Diazepam (Valium) IV Emetic Gastric lavage Oxygen Symptomatic treatment
Heroin	Euphoria Flushing Pruritus Miosis Decreased level of consciousness Bradycardia Shallow, slow respirations Hypotension Hypothermia	History of heroin use Toxicology screen (urine or blood)	Maintain airway patency Oxygen Symptomatic treatment Naloxone (Narcan) 2 mg IV
Lithium (Lithobid, Lithotabs, Duralith)	Vomiting Diarrhea Slurred speech Decreased coordination Drowsiness Muscle weakness or twitching	Cerebrospinal fluid lithium level Toxicology screen (urine or blood)	Gastric lavage Osmotic and saline diuresis (if renal function is normal) Urine alkalization Hemodialysis
Salicylates (aspirin, methyl salicylate)	Nausea Vomiting Gastritis Hyperpnea Tachypnea Tinnitus Agitation Confusion Coma Seizures Cardiovascular collapse Pulmonary edema Hyperthermia Possible death	Elevated prothrombin time Toxicology screen (blood) with a level greater than 100 mg/dL Arterial blood gases reveal respiratory alkalosis (early) with underlying metabolic acidosis	Activated charcoal Gastric lavage Sodium bicarbonate IV Possible hemodialysis

Continued

TABLE 76.1 Common Poisonings—cont'd

Name/Type	Signs and Symptoms	Diagnosis	Management
Tricyclic antidepressants: Amitriptyline (Elavil), imipramine (Tofranil), nortriptyline (Pamelor) Selective serotonin reuptake inhibitors (SSRIs) are relatively safe, even in overdose	Confusion Dizziness Decreased level of consciousness Hypotension Tachycardia Hyperthermia Mydriasis Dry mucous membranes Cardiac dysrhythmias Seizures	Toxicology screen (urine or blood)	Gastric decontamination with activated charcoal and cathartic agent Symptomatic treatment
FOODS			
General food poisoning (foods consumed with toxins present)	Vomiting Abdominal cramping Afebrile	Toxins can be detected in food or stool specimens: *Staphylococcus aureus* *Bacillus cereus* *Clostridium perfringens* *Shigella* *Salmonella*	Fluids and electrolyte replacement Ciprofloxacin (use with caution, given adverse effect profile) Antimotility drugs Condition is usually self-limited
Poisonous fish	Abdominal cramps Nausea Vomiting Diarrhea Paresthesias Hypotension Respiratory paralysis	History of ingesting fish	Supportive treatment for symptoms
Scombroid fish poisoning (scombrotoxin [histamine]-producing bacteria)	30 minutes to 2 hours after ingestion: peppery sensation on the tongue Urticarial pruritic rash Headache Dizziness Periorbital edema Nausea Vomiting	History of ingesting fish	Gastric lavage Antihistamines Symptomatic treatment
OTHER SUBSTANCES			
Arsenic	Metallic taste Garlic odor to breath Burning pain throughout gastrointestinal tract Vomiting Dehydration Shock Seizures	Toxicology screen and/or attempt to discover type of material ingested by investigating all suspect containers	Gastric lavage Fluid and electrolyte management Treat shock and pulmonary edema Possible blood transfusion

TABLE 76.1 Common Poisonings—cont'd

Name/Type	Signs and Symptoms	Diagnosis	Management
Carbon monoxide (CO)	Deep respirations Pink (cherry red) tissues and skin (with COHb increased 30%) Initial bradycardia, progressing to tachycardia Pounding pulse Dizziness Paresis Tinnitus Headache Faintness Nausea Dilated pupils	COHb increase	Supplemental oxygen via nonrebreather mask 100% oxygen under hyperbaric pressure (moderate to severe CO poisoning) Symptomatic treatment
Corrosive materials: Lysol, tincture of iodine, carbolic acid (phenol)	Burned tissues along gastrointestinal tract Brownish stains on lips and tongue Stridor from laryngeal swelling Nausea Vomiting Abdominal cramps Hematemesis Watery, mucoid, or bloody stools Violet or black mucous membranes—prolonged state of shock Carbolic acid—white or gray mucous membranes Hydrochloric acid—grayish mucous membranes Nitric acid—yellowish mucous membranes Sulfuric acid-tan or dark-stained mucous membranes	Order toxicology screen and/or attempt to discover type of material ingested by investigating all suspect containers	Opiates for pain Possible tracheostomy Aggressive fluid and electrolyte resuscitation Antibiotics Corticosteroids
Iodine	Brown stains on lips and mouth Burning pain in mouth and throat Yellow emesis (blue, if starch is present)	Diagnosis based on symptoms and open or empty container found at scene	Cornstarch or flour solution: 15 g in 2 cups of water, given orally if patient is conscious or via gastric lavage if patient is comatose Morphine sulfate for pain
Lead: lead-based paints, lead-contaminated dust, hobbies (e.g., stained-glass window-making)	Colicky abdominal pain Constipation Headache Irritability Coma Convulsions Chronic poisoning—learning disorders in children Motor neuropathy (wrist drop)	Blood levels: 10 to 50 mcg/dL—mild toxicity 50 to 70 mcg/dL—moderate toxicity 70 to 100 mcg/dL—severe toxicity Microcytic anemia	*Up to moderate toxicity:* Edetate calcium disodium (EDTA) Oral chelator-succimer (dimercaptosuccinic acid [DMSA]) *Severe toxicity:* EDTA IV (continuous infusion) dimercaprol (British Anti-Lewisite or BAL) intramuscularly (IM)
Strychnine	Sense of suffocation Cyanosis Dyspnea Hypoventilation Tachycardia Muscle rigidity Contractions Seizures	Lactic acidosis Metabolic acidosis	Gastric lavage Oxygen Sedatives Supportive care

Subjective

When evaluating an individual for a potential toxic exposure, patient history is equally as important as the physical examination of the encounter. The interview process can give the clinician an opportunity to recognize possible exposures and understand the time line of events. The clinician should consider obtaining additional information from friends and family who may provide supplemental details, especially in emergent settings in which the patient's responsiveness is limited. Additionally, the clinician must remain mindful that a lack of symptoms does not preclude the possibility of an ingestion or exposure.

Objective

A toxic syndrome, or toxidrome, is a constellation of signs and symptoms associated with a distinct group of xenobiotics. Early assessment and clinical recognition can assist the provider in identifying potential ingestions and anticipate complications of toxicity. The five most common toxidromes are classified as follows: sympathomimetic, anticholinergic, cholinergic, sedative hypnotic/ethanol, and opioid. Each syndrome is characterized by vital sign and end-organ manifestations associated with several bodily systems, as summarized in Table 76.2.

Evaluation of the patient who is poisoned begins with the primary survey: airway, breathing, and circulation (ABC). Barring clinical decompensation, evaluation for signs of trauma and CNS involvement should subsequently commence. Furthermore, individuals with a reported toxic ingestion or overdose should undergo an electrocardiogram (ECG), as specific findings can suggest exposure to certain agents. Radiographic studies may identify radiopaque foreign bodies (e.g., coins, needles) or capture substantial ingestions (e.g., concretion of pills, illicit drug body packers).

DIAGNOSTIC REASONING

Diagnostic Tests

Diagnostic testing will vary depending on the potential toxin(s). Laboratory testing includes a basic metabolic panel, liver function test panel, coagulation profile (prothrombin time [PT]/international normalized ratio [INR], partial thromboplastin time [PTT]), lactic acid level, acetaminophen level, acetylsalicylic acid level, and urinalysis. A urine toxicology screen can be obtained, although the presence of a toxin does not confirm poisoning, but rather only exposure. In the setting of a known ingestion, quantitative levels of the specific substance can be obtained. However, depending on available laboratory testing equipment, specimens may need to be sent to an outside reference laboratory for certain tests.

TABLE 76.2 Common Toxidromes: Clinical Manifestations

Toxidrome	Vital Signs	Mental Status	Pupils	Gastrointestinal	Skin	Other
Sympathomimetic	↑ BP ↑ HR ↑ T	Agitated	Mydriasis	Normal/hypoactive bowel sounds	Flushed Diaphoresis	Tremors Seizures
Anticholinergic	↑ BP ↑ HR ↑ T	Delirium	Mydriasis	Hypoactive bowel sounds	Flushed Dry	Urinary retention Dry mucous membranes
Cholinergic	±BP ±HR ↓ T	Normal Confusion Weakness	Varies	Hyperactive bowel sounds	Diaphoresis	SLUDGE: Salivation Lacrimation Urination Diarrhea Gastrointestinal distress Emesis
Sedative hypnotic/ethanol	↓ BP ↓ HR ↓ RR ↓ T	Depressed Confusion Coma	Varies	Hypoactive bowel sounds	Normal	Hyporeflexia
Opioid	↓ BP ↓ HR ↓ RR ↓ T	Depressed Confusion Coma	Miosis	Hypoactive bowel sounds	Normal	Hypoventilation Hyporeflexia

Abbreviations: BP, blood pressure; HR, heart rate; RR, respiratory rate; T, temperature; ↑, increased; ↓, decreased; ±, variable.

Differential Diagnosis

A variety of clinical conditions can mimic each of the toxidromes; therefore, clinicians should maintain a broad differential diagnosis for suspected poisonings, systematically eliminating possible alternative diagnoses. The list of differential diagnoses for toxidrome presentations is extensive and can vary from psychiatric disorders and sepsis to stroke-related symptoms. In the patient presenting with altered mental status, the primary care practitioner should always consider head injury and other organic etiologies. Numerous xenobiotics produce gastrointestinal (GI), symptoms; thus, GI tract disorders should also be ruled out.

MANAGEMENT

In suspected poisonings, the priority of the clinician is to treat the immediate medical condition. Although psychiatric evaluation becomes secondary to emergent treatment, a mental health evaluation and treatment is nonetheless an important and necessary component when treating the poisoned patient, given the strong association of poisonings with intentional ingestion, self-harm, depression, and suicidality. The American Association of Poison Control Centers has 55 poison information centers in the United States to help prevent and treat poison exposures. These centers function 24 hours a day, 7 days a week. They can be reached at any time through the national U.S. Poison Help Line at 1-800-222-1222 or on the Internet at https://www.PoisonHelp.org.

Emergency Management

Utilizing the primary survey, the patient's ABCs are assessed. Emergency medical services should be immediately mobilized to transfer the poisoned patient to the nearest emergency department (ED), while concomitantly monitoring the individual's respiratory and cardiovascular status. The patient is placed on a continuous cardiac monitor and treated conservatively with IV fluids and antiemetics. The local poison control center may be contacted for additional treatment recommendations, if needed.

General Management

A xenobiotic is a pharmacologically, endocrinologically, or toxicologically active substance not endogenously produced and therefore foreign to the patient. Toxicity occurs when a substance reaches a target end organ and overwhelms natural protective mechanisms against damaging biochemical processes. By limiting the amount of a substance that reaches target tissues, these effects can be mitigated. For management principles of common poisonings, see Table 76.1.

In the setting of a toxic ingestion, the xenobiotic must first dissolve in the GI tract before it can be absorbed and enter the systemic circulation. Therefore, GI decontamination aims to restrict the amount of xenobiotic from reaching the systemic circulation. Accepted modalities include activated charcoal, gastric lavage, and whole bowel irrigation.

Historically, syrup of ipecac was used as a form of decontamination, and parents were advised to keep a bottle readily accessible for unintentional childhood ingestions of toxins or medications. Children who were given syrup of ipecac would experience induced vomiting and theoretically prevent potential toxins from gaining access to the systemic circulation. However, in 2003, the American Academy of Pediatrics released a policy statement that no longer recommended the use of ipecac for the treatment of poisoning because studies showed a discordance in efficacy between times of ingestion among individuals.

The most common form of GI decontamination is the use of activated charcoal. To treat poisonings, charcoal is processed into a slurry that is introduced into the stomach through ingestion or via an orogastric tube. The charcoal particles act as an adsorbent material, binding xenobiotic molecules of a certain size, thus hindering the absorption of potential toxins across the GI lumen. This results in the fecal elimination of unwanted substances. Nonetheless, activated charcoal has limitations. Its utility is optimized when it is administered within 1 hour of ingestion, and delayed administration reduces its efficacy. In addition, activated charcoal does not adsorb nor protect against heavy metals, alcohol, caustic agents, or cyanide.

The dose of activated charcoal for children is 1 to 2 g/kg (25 to 50 g per dose), and for adults, the dose is 1 g/kg (25 to 100 g per dose). Activated charcoal may be given with or without sorbitol as a cathartic agent to assist in charcoal elimination through the GI tract, especially with multidose regimens. Of note, sorbitol may produce dehydration that can lead to an electrolyte imbalance in young children; therefore, it should be used with caution. The local poison control center should be consulted for guidance with dosing and administration.

Gastric lavage attempts to evacuate toxins from the stomach before they can be broken down, dissolved, and absorbed through the GI tract. This modality is accomplished with the insertion of a large-bore orogastric tube and instillation of a normal saline solution into the stomach, followed by aspiration of stomach contents. Gastric lavage should only be performed in a patient with a protected airway, either in a conscious individual or someone who is intubated. The process is repeated until the aspirate is clear of particulate matter. Gastric lavage is often followed by the administration of activated charcoal to adsorb any remaining xenobiotics.

Whole bowel irrigation incorporates the use of a polyethylene glycol-electrolyte solution (PEG-ELS) to flush the contents of the GI tract before toxins can be absorbed through the GI membrane. This method produces liquid stool that is generated through a large volume of PEG-ELS (2 L/hr in adults and 0.5 L/hr in children), which is maintained until the rectal effluent matches the appearance of the solution entering the body. Many patients are unable to sustain the recommended rate of ingestion; therefore, a nasogastric tube may be needed to consistently administer the irrigation fluid.

Indications for whole bowel irrigation include the elimination of xenobiotics that may have delayed absorption or illicit drug "body stuffers" with the potential to become symptomatic (e.g., from ruptured swallowed drug packets). Body stuffers differ from body packers in relation to the vehicle that encases the swallowed illicit substance. Body packers, also known as "drug mules," carry tightly sealed packages within their GI tract for illegal transportation into a country and eventual expulsion for distribution. In contrast, body stuffers are usually averting law enforcement and ingest baggies of illicit substances urgently. These baggies can subsequently dissolve and release contents into the GI tract.

Forced diuresis and alteration of urine pH can be used to remove certain toxins that undergo renal elimination. Acidic toxins can be trapped in alkaline urine and alkaline toxins can be trapped in acidic urine. Sodium bicarbonate administration is used to alkalinize urine to a pH of greater than 7. Additionally, toxins can be eliminated through extracorporeal removal means such as dialysis, plasmapheresis, and exchange transfusion. However, elimination of toxins is limited to xenobiotics that are water soluble, unbound to protein, and have a low volume of distribution. Hyperbaric oxygen may be indicated in moderate to severe CO poisoning, and chelation therapy is used for the removal of heavy metals such as lead. Of note, chelation is also often falsely claimed by unlicensed practitioners as a method of "detoxification" of various substances, with no evidentiary basis.

Adults who present with an undifferentiated depressed mental state may require dextrose, thiamine, and naloxone to address potential hypoglycemia or opioid overdose. Hypoglycemia can masquerade as a coma or even stroke, therefore necessitating its immediate reversal with 50 to 100 mL of 50% dextrose as an IV bolus. In malnourished patients or patients with suspected alcohol abuse, Wernicke encephalopathy (ophthalmoparesis with nystagmus, ataxia, and confusion due to thiamine deficiency) should be considered and treatment initiated with 100 mg of IV thiamine. Respiratory and mental status depression due to opioid (e.g., heroin, oxycodone) toxicity can be reversed with naloxone 0.4 to 2 mg IV. Depending on the strength and chemical nature of the opioid, higher naloxone doses of 5 to 10 mg may be required, as the goal of opioid reversal is to alleviate respiratory depression as the most life-threatening manifestation.

FOLLOW-UP AND REFERRAL

Follow-up and referral will depend on the nature of the poisoning or overdose and the patient's clinical condition. If the poisoning or overdose is a suicide attempt or gesture, a psychiatric referral is indicated, which should be coordinated with the clinician. The patient with suicidal ideation or an attempt should never be discharged home without having a psychiatric evaluation clearly documented and appropriate follow-up care arranged.

In addition, for unintentional poisonings, although urgent care or emergent intervention typically occurs in the ED setting, follow-up care should be coordinated with the clinician to provide critical patient education for risk management against future toxic exposures in the home or workplace.

Patient Education: Poisons

In teaching the patient and family about poisonings, the clinician should advise friends and family to call the Poison Help Line (1-800-222-1222) of the American Association of Poison Control Centers.

General teaching points for the prevention of poisonings include the following:

- Keep all medications and hazardous products locked up and out of the reach of children.
- Keep all medications in child-resistant containers.
- Never refer to medication as "candy" when administering to children.
- Dispose carefully all unused or expired medications (wrap medication containers carefully and dispose of in the garbage, rather than flushing medications down the toilet, as the latter practice can lead to contaminated water supplies).
- Do not leave medications on countertops or tables, especially if children are present.
- Never transfer hazardous material from one container to another; keep all medications or other toxins in their original containers with appropriate labeling.
- Do not mix chemicals unless you know what the resultant reaction may be.

HEAT-RELATED ILLNESSES

Heat-related illnesses include heat rash, heat cramps, heat syncope, heat exhaustion, and heat stroke. It is important to understand that heat-related illnesses are actually a continuum of conditions, ranging from mild to severe (see Table 76.3). Heat-related deaths are usually preventable.

Heat rash, also known as prickly heat or miliaria, is a group of skin conditions caused by environmental heat and excessive perspiration. The condition occurs when sweat is trapped under the skin due to closed pores. This forms an uncomfortable and often pruritic rash ranging

TABLE 76.3 Types of Heat-Related Illnesses

Type of Illness	Signs and Symptoms	Management
Heat rash	Pruritic rash of pinpoint or small, clear-to-red vesicles, usually on face and neck	Typically self-limited May use calamine lotion or topical corticosteroids for more severe cases
Heat cramps	Cramps, especially in the large muscle groups, such as shoulders, thighs, and abdominal wall muscles, after significant exercise in hot environment and profuse diaphoresis	Stop activity and rest; move to cool environment Muscle stretching Fluid and electrolyte replacement with oral electrolyte-balanced "sports drinks" or IV normal saline Monitor for progression to heat exhaustion and heat stroke Gradual acclimatization if exercising in hot or humid environments
Heat syncope	Orthostatic syncopal episode and dizziness due to vasodilation and peripheral pooling of blood, volume deficit, or sluggish vasomotor tone	Place the patient in a supine position Oral fluid replacement Cool environment and rest
Heat exhaustion	Prolonged fluid loss (e.g., from perspiration, diarrhea, or diuretic use) results in thirst, anxiety, anorexia, muscle cramps, malaise, syncope, headache, dehydration, tachycardia, muscle weakness, orthostatic hypotension, nausea and vomiting, cutaneous flushing, and/or possible elevated temperature greater than 37.8°C	Remove the patient from hot environment into shady or cool location Elevate legs for postural hypotension Oral fluid replacement if no gastrointestinal symptoms and if alert and oriented: replace fluids and electrolytes at about 1 L/hr for several hours (recovery expected within 2 to 3 hours; otherwise, patient may need additional interventions)
Heat stroke	Medical emergency requiring rapid assessment at treatment, with core body temperature of at least 104°F (40°C), acute mental status changes, absent sweat, tachypnea, decreased urinary output, hypotension, seizures, nausea and vomiting, diarrhea, dilated and nonresponsive pupils, decerebrate posturing	Rapid cooling (e.g., ice packs in groin and axilla) Monitor rectal temperature Supplemental oxygen, with intubation if necessary IV fluids (usually 0.9% normal saline)

from pinpoint to small, clear-to-red vesicles. The rash usually occurs on the face and neck. It is more common in older adults, overweight persons, and infants.

Heat cramps are muscle spasms that usually occur in large muscle groups like the calves, abdomen, thighs, and shoulders, during or shortly after exercising in the heat. The mechanism is thought to occur from either altered neuromuscular control of contraction caused by excessive muscle fatigue or electrolyte depletion from excessive perspiration or dilutional effects from excessive water consumption.

Risk factors for heat cramps include the following:

- A personal history of heat cramps
- An impaired ability to self-regulate body temperature, especially in the young and older persons
- Alcohol use
- The use of certain medications, including anticholinergics, sympathomimetics, and diuretics

Heat syncope is a heat-related fainting episode. It may occur because of vasodilation and peripheral pooling of blood to release body heat, circulatory volume deficits, or sluggish vasomotor tone. Syncope occurs when the venous return of blood flow does not support the required cardiac output. Thus, heat syncope can result from inadequate cardiac output and postural hypotension. Typically, recovery is immediate once the patient lies flat.

Heat exhaustion occurs when the body overheats and is unable to maintain a normal core temperature. Symptoms may include thirst, heavy sweating, tachycardia, dizziness, nausea, vomiting, and weakness. Heat exhaustion or exertional heat illness (EHI) is usually caused by strenuous work in hot and/or humid environments. Therapeutic interventions include rest, moving to a cooler environment, removal of clothing that prevents evaporative cooling, and hydration. Cold, electrolyte-balanced beverages ("sports drinks") are the best source of oral hydration. IV 0.9% normal saline may also be given. Risk factors for EHI include strenuous exercise in high temperatures and humidity, poor physical condition, obesity, dehydration, acute illness, advanced age, and age younger than 5 years. The diagnosis is made by the presence of positive symptoms after heat exposure, with a body temperature up to 104°F. Heat exhaustion can be prevented by proper hydration when exposed to heat, gradual acclimatization to hot environments, utilizing proper cool-down periods after physical exertion, avoiding alcohol, and wearing clothing that allows for evaporative cooling. Patients with heat exhaustion should be monitored for more severe symptoms of heat stroke until all symptoms have resolved and core body temperature has stabilized. The clinician may choose to perform diagnostic testing in patients with heat exhaustion to confirm proper kidney function, electrolyte balance, and the absence of breakdown of muscle tissue (rhabdomyolysis).

Heat stroke or sunstroke is characterized by a core body temperature of 104°F (40°C) or higher, mental confusion, and more severe clinical manifestations that progress beyond the signs and symptoms of heat exhaustion. Heat stroke occurs when the body's internal heat production is greater than its heat loss. There may be damage to multiple organ systems and rhabdomyolysis, and mortality may be as high as 10%. The clinical presentation may include hot, dry skin; decreased level of consciousness; tachycardia; tachypnea; decreased urinary output; hypotension; seizures; nausea and vomiting; decerebrate posturing; diarrhea; and dilated, nonresponsive pupils. If a patient presenting in a primary care setting has heat stroke, emergency medical services should be initiated while the patient's respiratory and cardiovascular status are evaluated and supported as indicated. The patient must then be transported to an ED immediately.

EPIDEMIOLOGY AND CAUSES

An average of 650 persons die each year of heat-related illnesses in the United States. Heat stroke is ranked third—behind head and neck trauma and cardiac disorders—as a cause of death among high school athletes in the United States. Factors associated with an increased risk of heat-related illnesses include age (both very young children and older adults are at higher risk); a history of a chronic illness, such as cardiovascular, endocrine, neurological, or psychiatric disease; use of certain medications, such as antihistamines, beta blockers, and diuretics; fever or dehydration; a previous history of heat stroke; and heavy clothing that restricts evaporative heat loss.

Specifically, certain medications and medical conditions that impair the body's ability to self-regulate core temperature in the face of environmental heat extremes can contribute to the more severe forms of heat-related illness, such as heat exhaustion and heat stroke. Cholinergic blockade, beta-adrenergic blockade, and autonomic neuropathy are often unrecognized contributors to heat-related illnesses. Many drugs possess anticholinergic side effects that may result in an inability to perspire, and individuals on beta blockers may have a diminished ability to cope with heat. Monoamine oxidase inhibitors and sympathomimetics can cause a core temperature disturbance, leading to rapidly occurring muscle rigidity, extensive rhabdomyolysis, and electrolyte disorders that can prove fatal. Autonomic neuropathy associated with diabetes mellitus is an important risk factor for faulty heat dissipation and can also result in heat-related illnesses. Certain living conditions, such as densely populated urban environments, living alone, and a lack of air conditioning during hot weather, are additional risk factors for heat-related illnesses. Exertion-related heat exhaustion and heat stroke may also be a complication of unconditioned amateur participants involved in strenuous athletic competitions.

PATHOPHYSIOLOGY

Heat loss is dependent on radiation, convection, conduction, and evaporation. Radiation and conduction result in direct transfer of heat from the body to the environment. When environmental temperatures reach 95°F (35°C), these mechanisms for heat transfer are no longer effective. Convection is heat loss related to air circulation, which is a process that relies on wind velocity. Evaporation of sweat is the only physiological mechanism for eliminating heat in an environment hotter than 95°F.

The body's ability to sweat is affected by skin conditions (e.g., sunburn), systemic diseases that affect the ability to sweat (e.g., cystic fibrosis), and drugs that inhibit sweating (e.g., phenothiazines). Increased core temperatures stimulate peripheral vasodilation and sweating and have effects on multiple end organs. Venous return to the heart increases, resulting in increased cardiac output and heart rate. A concurrent sympathetic response decreases blood flow to the kidneys, which can damage the kidneys if this process continues, with myoglobin produced as a by-product. If this condition is not aggressively treated, it can lead to rhabdomyolysis. Respiratory function may be compromised by pulmonary edema. Hepatic function is often worsened because of the general decrease in perfusion. Clotting abnormalities with severe heat illness can range from thrombocytopenia to disseminated intravascular coagulation. As the metabolic rate rises, sweat production can increase to 1.5 L/hr, which may result in dehydration.

Acclimatization is a term that refers to the body's ability to adapt to heat stress. This adaptation primarily involves the sweating mechanism. In an unacclimatized person, each liter of sweat contains 30 to 50 mEq of sodium. This sodium level decreases to as little as 5 mEq/L in the fully acclimatized person, and the rate of sweating can be increased to 1.5 to 3 L/hr. This means that although the acclimatized person doubles sweat production, they lose only one-third to one-fifth of the total amount of sodium as the unacclimatized person.

Potassium wasting compensates for these sodium losses. Therefore, a fluid and electrolyte imbalance can develop quickly in an unacclimatized person. Cardiac output increases with acclimatization, as does aerobic muscle metabolism, which is more efficient metabolically. As the heart muscle responds to higher ambient temperatures, cutaneous circulation increases with peripheral vasodilation, thereby augmenting heat dissipation. The body develops a new, lower temperature set point at which sweating begins. Finally, increased secretion of aldosterone aids in sodium conservation by the kidneys and sweat glands in the setting of increased perspiration. This retained sodium drives increased extracellular fluid volume, which plays a part in accelerated cutaneous blood flow and heat dissipation.

CLINICAL PRESENTATION

Subjective

For any heat-related illness, a complete history of the circumstances preceding the incident should be obtained. Any past history that may assist with the differential diagnosis is crucial. Medications that the patient is currently taking should be reviewed.

Objective

A complete physical examination should be performed, including monitoring the patient's cardiac status, vital signs, and core temperature.

DIAGNOSTIC REASONING

Diagnostic Tests

Serum electrolytes should be assessed with more severe forms of heat-related illness (severe heat cramps, heat syncope, heat exhaustion, heat stroke) to assess for electrolyte imbalances or depletion, which may be corrected with IV saline infusion. With heat stroke in particular, hepatic and renal function tests should also be done to assess for end-organ dysfunction.

Differential Diagnosis

The differential diagnosis of heat stroke includes CNS infections, cerebrovascular accidents, and diabetic ketoacidosis. If the patient has recently traveled to countries in tropical or other endemic areas (e.g., certain countries in Africa and Asia), the primary care practitioner should consider malaria or typhoid fever in the differential. Additionally, with more severe presentations of heat exhaustion or heat stroke, the clinician should consider thyroid storm, meningitis, encephalitis, or brain abscess. Some toxicological issues to consider include salicylate, anticholinergic, phencyclidine (PCP), cocaine, or amphetamine toxicity.

MANAGEMENT

Treatment of heat-related illnesses is driven by the severity of presenting symptoms and the degree of electrolyte imbalance and end-organ damage. Treatment for milder forms such as heat rash is usually symptomatic because the condition is typically self-limited. Topical treatments include the use of calamine lotion applied directly to the rash and mild topical corticosteroids. Antibiotics may be prescribed if secondary infection develops. Heat rash can be prevented by minimizing exposure to heat and humidity, avoiding the use of tight-fitting clothing, and curtailing the use of creams and lotions. Heat cramps may be treated with muscle rest, but underlying causes must also be eliminated, such as dehydration and the use of contributing medications. Fluid-imbalances should also be addressed. Similarly, as patients suffering heat syncope often recover as soon as they lie flat and postural hypotension is eliminated, treatment is focused on eliminating underlying aggravating factors.

For more severe forms of heat-related illness, such as heat exhaustion and heat stroke, general management focuses on cooling the patient. The safest and most practical method is to remove all clothing and spray lukewarm water over the patient's entire body surface to facilitate evaporative cooling. Heat evaporation can be augmented with the use of fans, which should circulate air over as much of the patient's body surface as possible. If ice packs are utilized, they should be placed in the axilla and groin, with the skin protected from local injury by a barrier between the skin and ice pack (e.g., cloth or towel). Extremities should not be packed in ice, especially in older patients, because this treatment is poorly tolerated. Supplemental oxygen is also often administered.

Emergent referral to an ED is required for all patients with severe symptoms for further correction of fluid and electrolyte imbalances and directed therapy for any organ-specific damage (e.g., large-volume crystalloid infusions for rhabdomyolysis). The goal is to reduce the temperature to 102°F (38.8°C) within the first hour. To avoid hypothermia, further active cooling should cease when a core temperature of 101°F (38.3°C) is achieved. Antipyretics are ineffective in lowering the temperature in heat-related illnesses. IV fluids, such as normal saline or dextrose and half normal saline, are usually given. Chlorpromazine (Thorazine) 25 to 50 mg IV or diazepam (Valium) 5 to 10 mg IV may be given initially to control shivering and then every 4 hours. In addition, the patient's urinary output, rectal temperature, and cardiac status should be monitored.

FOLLOW-UP AND REFERRAL

As with other urgent care problems, follow-up assessments for heat-related illness depend on the severity and nature of symptoms and the risk of recurrence (e.g., due to persistent unavoidable environmental heat exposure). For example, although the immediate signs and symptoms of more severe forms of heat-related illness may be quickly corrected in the ED setting, outpatient follow-up by the primary care practitioner is critical for patient teaching and to ensure contributing risk factors and underlying causes of heat-related illness have been eliminated to avoid repeated episodes.

Similarly, referral of patients with heat-related illness to an ED is driven by the severity of symptoms and the potential for subsequent sequelae. For example, some cases of heat exhaustion and heat syncope may require further evaluation in the ED setting if these symptoms are felt to portend a more significant underlying disorder. Likewise, all cases of heat stroke require immediate ED evaluation and treatment to prevent permanent organ damage. In contrast, heat rash may be treated within the outpatient setting, and similarly, the primary care practitioner can typically assess for contributing factors to heat cramps to minimize recurrence without the need for ED referral.

Patient Education: Heat-Related Illnesses

Heat-related illnesses, with their devastating effects, can be avoided or at least reduced in severity through simple preventive measures. These include the following:

- Pacing physical activity and becoming acclimatized to hot environments
- Avoiding alcohol consumption during exposure in hot, humid environments
- Wearing protective, light-colored clothing and a hat when outdoors in hot weather
- Ingesting adequate amounts of electrolyte-balanced liquids (e.g., Gatorade, "sports drinks") to maintain fluid and electrolyte balance, avoid dehydration, and maintain homeostasis

Patients should understand that if they have experienced a heat-related illness in the past, they are more prone to heat-related illnesses in the future. Patients should be taught to gradually build up time spent in hotter conditions (acclimatization) and moderate physical activity until their bodies have adapted to the hot surroundings. It should be stressed that the higher the temperature and humidity in one's environment, the greater the risk for heat illness. In these settings, fluids must be consumed even before there is an urge to drink, and prehydration is important if exercising. The ideal fluids are plain water or a low-sugar electrolyte drink.

Education about heat-related illnesses should also be a part of health maintenance, especially with regard to younger patients and older adults. The primary care practitioner should warn parents of the risks of leaving children in cars unattended. Older adults should be cautioned about the increased risk of heat-related illnesses, especially if they have medical conditions or are taking medications that increase the risk of heat-related illnesses. Athletes should drink more fluids and try to exercise during the coolest part of the day.

COLD-RELATED ILLNESSES

HYPOTHERMIA

Hypothermia is a medical emergency that can threaten life and limb and is defined by a core temperature of less than 95°F (35°C). If not treated promptly and accurately, the diagnosis carries a high mortality rate, with patient outcomes dependent on underlying medical conditions and the duration of exposure to the elements.

EPIDEMIOLOGY AND CAUSES

The incidence and prevalence of hypothermia are difficult to quantify, because not all cases are reported. The hypothermic patient is more likely to be older (with a mean age of 45 years), to be uninsured, and to utilize more critical care than most other patients seen in the ED setting. Approximately 700 people die in the United States from accidental primary hypothermia (due to environmental temperatures) each year. The condition of hypothermia tends to affect economically disadvantaged patients due to unintentional environmental exposures to cold weather and is preventable with community engagement and social support for these patients. Problems with alcohol-use disorders, homelessness, and psychiatric disorders are common to patients presenting with hypothermia. The other category of affected individuals are adventure seekers, including hunters, skiers, mountain climbers, boaters, and swimmers. Despite in-hospital treatment, 40% of patients with moderate to severe hypothermia die.

PATHOPHYSIOLOGY

The reduction in body core temperature pathognomonic of hypothermia starts with a cascade of events. First, there is a loss of heat from the body. This can involve evaporation; convection; conduction; respiration; and, most importantly, radiation, through which 50% of body heat is lost rapidly. Common contributing factors to hypothermia include prolonged exposure to lower extremes of outdoor temperatures without protective clothing, alcohol and drug use, homelessness, and advanced age. The prognosis is highly dependent on the length of exposure to environmental cold extremes, as well as the healthcare provider's recognition of the condition and rapid therapeutic intervention. For example, progressive organ failure increases as core body temperature decreases; however, this situation is potentially reversible with adequate rewarming.

CLINICAL PRESENTATION

Subjective

The hypothermic patient may arrive with a core body temperature ranging from lower than 82.4°F to 95°F (28°C to 35°C). Depending on the core temperature, the patient may or may not be conscious enough to give a subjective history. If the patient is conscious, the primary complaint is coldness accompanied with a feeling of exhaustion.

Objective

In addition to an abnormally low body temperature, the physical signs of hypothermia depend on the degree of temperature decline.

Mild hypothermia is defined as a core temperature of 89.6°F to 95°F (32°C to 35°C):

- The cardiopulmonary response includes vasoconstriction, hypertension, tachycardia, and tachypnea.
- The renal response is cold diuresis and defective distal tubular absorption of water and sodium.
- The neurological response involves shivering, ataxia, slowed mental processes, and an apathetic affect.

Moderate hypothermia is defined as a core temperature of 82.4°F to 89.6°F (28°C to 32°C):

- The cardiopulmonary response includes hypotension, bradycardia, respiratory depression, and a J wave on ECG; atrial fibrillation and junctional bradycardia are both associated with a high mortality rate.
- The renal circulatory system clamps down (vasoconstricts) and urine output decreases.
- The neurological response leads to a diminished level of consciousness, dilated pupils, decreased reflexes (including the gag reflex), and an inability to mount a shivering reflex.

Severe hypothermia is defined as a core temperature of less than 82.4°F (28°C):

- The cardiopulmonary response may reveal profound bradycardia with ventricular dysrhythmias or asystole, accompanied by pulmonary edema and/or apnea. Severe hypothermia can cause ventricular fibrillation and other malignant cardiac rhythms. Minimizing motion and jerking movements can help prevent these.
- Renal blood flow is greatly diminished, leading to oliguria.
- Neurologically, the patient loses consciousness, and coma rapidly ensues; the pupils are nonreactive.

DIAGNOSTIC REASONING

Diagnostic Tests

Given the emergent nature of the diagnosis, a laboratory work-up is initiated in the ED setting, after rapid transfer to a higher level of care. Initial laboratory tests consist of an arterial blood gas (ABG) to assess respiratory status and acid-base balance, complete blood count, basic metabolic panel with blood urea nitrogen and creatinine levels, alcohol and drug levels, coagulation studies including PT/INR and PTT, as well as a chest x-ray and an ECG. All tests may need to be repeated frequently during rewarming to assess for physiological recovery.

Differential Diagnosis

The clinician should consider head injury, stroke, myocardial infarction, diabetic hypoglycemia or hyperglycemia, drug or alcohol intoxication, sepsis, and hypothyroidism. Typically, the patient's exposure history, as revealed by family or friends who accompany the patient, reveals the diagnosis. Unconscious hypothermic patients who present without accompanying persons to provide a reliable medical history require a comprehensive diagnostic assessment, while aggressively treating the underlying hypothermia.

MANAGEMENT

Hypothermia is a medical emergency, and patients should be transported to the nearest hospital as quickly as possible. However, prehospital management should include prevention of heat loss, initiation of rewarming, and the avoidance of dysrhythmias. Wet clothing should be removed and replaced with warm blankets while drying the skin to avoid shivering, which depletes glycogen stores. Emergent management consists of assessing and ensuring airway patency, providing respiratory support if needed, and monitoring circulation, with initiation of basic life support measures as appropriate.

General management includes gradually rewarming the body by 1°C to 2°C (1.8°F to 3.6°F) per hour via supportive care with warm IV fluids, cardiac monitoring, frequent vital signs, supplemental oxygen if needed, and repeated monitoring of serum electrolytes, ABGs, and ECGs as needed. The clinician should be aware of the pathophysiological changes in acid-base balance on initiating treatment. During rewarming, the pH remains constant until the core body temperature reaches 89.6°F (32°C). At this temperature, there is a decline in calcium (Ca^{2+}) and magnesium (Mg^{2+}), accompanied by an increase in pH. Serial ABGs and repeated serum electrolyte panels are essential to monitor acid-base balance.

FOLLOW-UP AND REFERRAL

After discharge from ED or in-hospital care, the clinician needs to consider the patient's age, psychological and medical status, and their living situation to plan appropriate follow-up care. If the patient is homeless, a wide social network must be engaged to prevent the recurrence of hypothermia, and a case manager should be consulted. The clinician may have to discern if the patient has a home or a shelter in which to stay during the winter months and whether they have adequate clothing, including a winter coat, as well as adequate food availability.

Patient Education: Hypothermia

Each patient will have different educational needs, depending on the underlying risk factors for hypothermia. Basic education includes advice on dressing appropriately for cold weather and keeping the body dry and well-covered when outdoors. The clinician should warn the patient to avoid alcohol and drug use, as well as overexertion during extremely cold temperatures.

FROSTBITE

Frostbite is freezing of an exposed area, usually the ears, cheeks, nose, fingers, or toes. If a previously frostbitten area becomes frostbitten again after it has healed, permanent tissue damage can occur, resulting in necrosis of that body part.

EPIDEMIOLOGY AND CAUSES

Because of the growing prevalence of homelessness and the increasing number of individuals participating in outdoor activities during cold weather, frostbite is a growing concern. The individuals at greatest risk for frostbite are adults aged 30 to 49 years. A cold environmental temperature is a universal risk factor for frostbite, but it is not the only factor. The duration of exposure to cold weather has a greater effect on frostbite severity and resultant tissue injury than the actual temperature itself.

In addition, ambient humidity, wind exposure, inadequate cold weather clothing, and preexisting medical conditions such as atherosclerosis, diabetes mellitus, and previous cold-related injuries predispose individuals to frostbite. In addition, alcohol consumption, tobacco smoking, poor self-care, immobility, drug use, and altered mental status all increase the risk of frostbite.

Although prolonged contact with a cold object can produce frostbite, it is cold humidity that contributes most to evaporative heat loss, as wet skin is more conducive to ice crystal formation. Wind exposure contributes to an increasing loss of heat at higher wind-chill factors. In addition to inadequate body coverage from clothing, overly constrictive clothing can also contribute to an increased incidence of frostbite, as constrictive clothing can reduce circulation to the extremities.

PATHOPHYSIOLOGY

The pathophysiology of frostbite occurs in several stages: tissue freezing, hypoxia, and the release of inflammatory mediators. As tissues cool, the circulation slows, allowing ice crystals to form, first extracellularly and then intracellularly, which damages cell membranes. Crystals that form extracellularly exert osmotic force and pull fluid from the intracellular space into the extracellular space, resulting in cellular dehydration and increasing damage to cell membranes. Intracellular crystals that subsequently form cause more harm to the cell as they expand within it.

Hypoxia results from cold-induced local vasoconstriction, which leads to acidosis and increased local blood viscosity, as well as hypoxia. Although the body has a natural defensive mechanism against the cold (called *cold-induced vasodilation* or the "hunting response," which prevents rapid freezing of the skin), prolonged exposure to the cold eventually causes this response to fail and freezing occurs. As capillary blood flow ceases, arterioles and venules thrombose, leading to the release of inflammatory mediators. The release of prostaglandins and thromboxane promotes vasoconstriction, platelet aggregation, and blood vessel thrombosis, which worsen endothelial damage. If left unchecked, this process will lead to cell death and widespread tissue necrosis.

CLINICAL PRESENTATION

Subjective

Initially, the patient complains of a tingling sensation of the affected body part, followed by pain and eventual numbness.

Objective

The anatomical regions at greatest risk for injury are the hands and feet, which account for 90% of frostbite injuries. The ears, nose, cheeks, and penis are also prone to frostbite. Classically, the clinical presentation of frostbite has been categorized according to four degrees of injury. The classification should be applied after some rewarming has been initiated because most victims of frostbite initially present similarly, with tingling and redness followed by pallor and numbness.

- **First-degree frostbite (partial skin freezing):** Erythema, edema, hyperemia, no blisters or necrosis, occasional skin desquamation (5 to 10 days later), transient stinging and burning, and possible throbbing and aching; the patient may also have hyperhidrosis (excessive sweating).
- **Second-degree frostbite (full-thickness injury):** Erythema, substantial edema, vesicles with clear fluid, blisters that desquamate and form blackened eschar, numbness, and vasomotor disturbances in severe cases.
- **Third-degree frostbite (full-thickness injury and subcutaneous freezing):** Violaceous/hemorrhagic blisters, skin necrosis, and blue-gray discoloration; initially, no sensation (tissue feels like a block of wood), but shooting pains, burning, throbbing, and aching develop later.
- **Fourth-degree frostbite (full-thickness injury and subcutaneous tissue, muscle, tendon, and bone freezing):** Initially, skin is mottled, deep red, or cyanotic; later,

skin becomes dry, black, and mummified. Minimal edema is present, with possible joint discomfort.

DIAGNOSTIC REASONING

Diagnostic Tests

There are no definitive diagnostic studies for frostbite, especially within the first week of injury. Doppler studies may be helpful to assess blood flow in the affected body part.

Differential Diagnosis

Differential diagnoses for frostbite include the following:

- Frostnip—a mild form of cold injury.
- Chilblains (erythema pernio)—tender red to red-blue itchy nodules on the extremities triggered by cold weather and thought to result from chronic vasospasm; there is no actual freezing of the tissue.
- Immersion foot—hyperhidrosis (excessive perspiration) of the feet causing thickening, maceration, and tenderness of the skin due to prolonged submersion in water or cold (also called trench foot, because it affected soldiers camped for days in trenches during times of war).
- Hypothermia—see previous section for full description.

MANAGEMENT

Frostbite is a medical emergency because of the potential for extensive tissue necrosis and loss of limb. If the patient presenting to a primary care setting has frostbite, the area should be rewarmed, and hot liquids such as coffee, tea, or broth should be administered. The basis of treatment for frostbite is to reverse the pathological effects of ice crystal formation, vasoconstriction, and the release of inflammatory mediators. Treatment should not be started if there is a possibility of refreezing. If it is suspected that the patient has second- to fourth-degree frostbite, hospitalization should be considered.

The first measure is to rewarm the affected area. Rewarming is accomplished by using warm water (104°F [40°C] to 108°F [42.2°C]). Care must be taken not to rub the affected area. If possible, the affected body part should be placed in water for 10 to 30 minutes until the tissue is pliable and red. This process can be very painful; therefore, opioids may be administered and titrated for comfort.

Blister management in patients with frostbite is somewhat controversial. Blisters containing clear or milky fluid should be débrided and covered with aloe vera every 6 hours. Aloe vera is a potent antiprostaglandin agent. Hemorrhagic blisters should be left intact and covered with aloe vera. The affected area should be wrapped with a sterile dressing, splinted, and elevated. Topical Silvadene and bacitracin ointment have proven to be effective as antibacterials; however, use of these ointments may interfere with the effects of aloe vera.

It is unclear whether prophylactic antibiotic use is warranted for frostbite. The use of penicillin G 500,000 units IV every 6 hours for the first 72 hours has proven effective. Ibuprofen 400 mg PO every 4 to 6 hours should be administered for its antiprostaglandin activity. Ibuprofen is also a potential inhibitor of thromboxane and is more potent than other NSAIDs. The patient's tetanus status should also be assessed, given the risk of infection through compromised skin. Patients who are being treated for frostbite should not be allowed to smoke, given the vasoconstrictive effects of tobacco smoke.

Patients may need daily hydrotherapy to débride devitalized tissue. In some instances, referral to a surgeon for a fasciotomy or escharotomy may be needed if there is limited range of motion in an extremity or if the possibility of compartment syndrome develops. Compartment syndrome occurs when any structure such as a nerve or tendon is constricted in a closed space, such as an extremity. The sheath or tendon becomes enlarged because of the inflammation and is no longer able to move freely in the bodily compartment. This results in a restriction of circulation—a critical condition that may result in loss of a limb. Thus, compartment syndrome is an emergent situation that requires immediate referral to an ED.

FOLLOW-UP AND REFERRAL

The majority of patients with frostbite injuries should be admitted to the hospital for 2 to 4 days. If dressings are in place, the patient should be monitored every 2 to 3 days to assess healing. If débridement or grafting is necessary, the patient should be referred to a dermatologist or a vascular surgeon.

> ### Patient Education: Frostbite
>
> Patients should be taught to watch for signs of infection, take all medications as prescribed, and use extreme care regarding further exposure to cold. The following preventive measures should also be recommended:
>
> - Do not go outdoors in cold weather for prolonged periods of time.
> - Wear a hat or earmuffs, mittens, and dress in layers.
> - Keep dry and change out of wet clothing.
> - Dress in natural materials such as cotton or wool.
> - Avoid caffeine, tobacco, and alcohol when going outdoors in the cold, because these substances leave the skin more prone to thermal injury.
> - Check the skin every 12 to 20 minutes for signs of frostbite when exposed to cold environments.

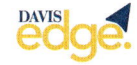 Go to Davis Edge for practice Q&A.

REFERENCES

Frostbite

Fudge JR, Bennett BL, Simanis JP, Roberts WO. Medical evaluation for exposure extremes: Cold. *Wilderness Environ Med.* 2015; 26(Suppl 4):S63-S68.

Heat-Related Illnesses

Epstein Y, Yanovich R. Heatstroke. *N Engl J Med.* 2019. June 20; 380(25):2449-2459.

Vaidyanathan A, Malilay J, Schramm P, et al. Heat-related deaths—U.S., 2004-2018. *MMWR Morb Mortal Wkly Rep.* 2020 June 19; 69(24):729-734.

Hypothermia

Danzi D. Accidental hypothermia. In: Auerback PS, Cushing TA, Harris, NS, eds. *Wilderness Medicine.* 7th ed. Elsevier, Philadelphia; 2017:135.

Poisoning

Gummin DD, Mowry JB, Spyker DA, et al. 2016 Annual Report of the American Association of Poison Control Centers' National Poison Data System (NPDS): 34th Annual Report. *Clin Toxicol.* 2017;55(10):1072-1252.

Korioth T. More health care facilities calling poison control. *AAP News & Journals Gateway.* https://www.aappublications.org/news/2019/03/18/fyipoison031819. Published 2019. Accessed November 22, 2020.

Saleh N. CDC releases top 10 causes of injury in the U.S. https://www.mdlinx.com/article/cdc-releases-top-10-causes-of-injury-in-the-us/lfc-4148. Published August 8, 2018. Accessed 8/16/20.

RESOURCES

Heat- and Cold-Related Illnesses

Medical Services: Army Public Health Program.
https://armypubs.army.mil/epubs/DR_pubs/DR_a/pdf/web/ARN16450_R40_5_FINAL.pdf. Accessed November 23, 2020.

Poisoning

American Association of Poison Control Centers
http://www.aapcc.org

National Toxic Substance Incidents Program (NTSIP) of the Agency for Toxic Substances and Disease Registry (ATSDR)
https://www.atsdr.cdc.gov/ntsip/

Unit **III**

Caring-Based Nursing
The Practice

Section 1 CARE OF VULNERABLE POPULATIONS

Chapter 77

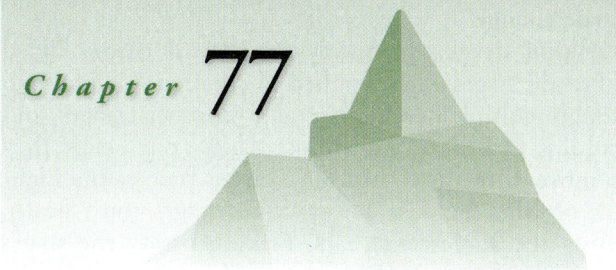

Primary Care of Adolescents

Carol Savrin, CNP, CPNP, FNP-BC, FAANP, RN
Debera J. Thomas, PhD, RN, ANP/FNP

ADOLESCENCE OVERVIEW

Adolescence is the tie between the end of childhood, generally considered to start at age 11 years, until the beginning of adulthood, generally considered to be the age of 20 or 21 years. Adolescence is the transition from the complete dependence of childhood to the independence of adulthood and can be a challenging time for both the adolescent and the parents or guardians. Each adolescent is very different depending on their temperament, their history to this time, and their experiences both within the family and the community, and each adolescent should be treated differently. The child in these formative years deserves the appropriate attention and care from the health-care provider to help them become a productive adult.

Adolescents are at risk for many preventable health problems, and many of the best ways to address these problems are through public health measures. *Healthy People 2030* lists 100 objectives, including public health objectives, research objectives, and objectives for which there are not yet good baseline data (https://health.gov/healthypeople/objectives-and-data/browse-objectives/adolescents). These comprehensive data address most of the issues and concerns that adolescents face. The health-care provider should be aware of the issues and work with the parent/guardian and the teen to provide the best positive health behaviors.

Likewise, adolescent years are a time during which the physical and developmental growth can enable some remarkable achievements. Physical capabilities are often at their peak and so many star athletes are adolescents. As the cognitive abilities expand, some extraordinary accomplishments may occur. Consider the Olympic athletes, the musical scores written, the poetry written, and the public health movements started by people in their teens.

Adolescents and their parents/guardian may be faced with situations that they are not well prepared to meet. As health-care providers, we need to assist them by providing as much information as practicable to facilitate a smooth transition to adulthood. This chapter will address many of the concerns faced by the teen and the parent or guardian. A considerable number of concerns may be addressed through anticipatory guidance, providing some resources before they are needed. Other concerns must be addressed as they occur.

Role of the Primary Care Provider

The primary care provider is in a unique position when working with the adolescent. Younger adolescents are often antiadult in general, and the provider needs to be able to communicate with the teen without being adversarial. The middle adolescent will often simply ignore adults in general, so again communication is key. Teens are very connected to and concerned about peers, so the interaction with the provider may be based on previous communications with peers. However, whether the adolescent is antiadult or simply ignoring adults, they are much more likely to communicate with an adult who is not a parent or guardian. The provider should always indicate respect for the teen, should communicate as an adult, and not attempt to be a friend or a peer. The provider should be familiar with slang that is commonly used among teens, but should not use slang terminology during the visit unless the patient does not understand standard language. The provider needs to inform the adolescent that their conversations are private unless there is a concern that they might harm themselves or others. The provider should communicate to the teen that with freedom comes personal responsibility. Communicating a sense of future and concern without sounding condescending can sometimes be a challenge for the provider; however, if respect and understanding are communicated, working with the adolescent can be very rewarding.

When the provider is caring for an adolescent, they must also communicate and work with the parent or guardian. Often, the communication with the adult can be as challenging as with the teen. Some parents or guardians have difficulty acknowledging that the teen is moving toward adulthood, and that, as mentioned earlier, they should be given freedom in tandem with the accompanying responsibilities. In addition to listening to the concerns of the caregiver, the role of the provider is to furnish information on the growth and development of the teen and share some possible ways to deal with the inevitable conflicts that arise. The adolescent may often have swings in temperament likely due to hormones; at times they may act like a young child and at other times like a mature adult. When the parent or guardian does not realize that this is normal, it can become a source of agitation. It is often the role of the provider to communicate this information.

Theorists

The ages of adolescence have been described in cognitive and developmental terms, as well as physical terms. There are a number of pediatric developmental theorists who evaluated the different ages of adolescence and discuss cognitive development and other aspects of development. Two of the most well-known theorists are Piaget and Erikson. There are many others, but these two will be discussed in this chapter (Table 77.1).

Piaget described cognitive development starting at birth. During adolescence, he talks about the child going from the concrete operational stage to the formal operational stage. In formal operations, the teen begins to understand that if A = B and B = C, then A = C. Before formal operations, the child did not understand this concept. During teen years, they begin to understand that there are multiple points of view, and they can start to see things from these perspectives. During adolescence, the teen begins to understand the abstract form of thinking and thus can grasp more complex issues in school and the community.

One of the ways that Piaget describes this transition is with the example of ethical dilemmas. The adolescent begins to understand issues surrounding something occurring "on purpose" as opposed to "by accident." However, although the adolescent can begin to see other points of view, they are still very idealistic and may be fiercely opposed to that point of view. The teen is searching for societal values that mimic their own; thus, teens are often at the forefront of new movements such as climate change.

Erikson developed his developmental theory based on Freud's stages when applied to children. Children go through multiple developmental psychosocial stages, and according to Erikson, they must achieve one before they can move to the next. Erikson calls his process the Eight Ages of Man because he describes stages until death. During the adolescent years, Erikson breaks the stages into two sections: the first is from about 11 or 12 years until about 18 years; the second stage is from age 18 years until adulthood.

During stage one, Erikson says that the primary task of the child is to determine their identity versus role confusion. The teen is trying to determine the similarities and differences between how the teen sees self and how others see them. If one is familiar with the teen's activities, one can clearly see the fluctuations that occur in this time frame. The young teen often moves from one "clique" or group of friends to another. The teen is working out who they are and to what group they belong. The older the adolescent gets, the more their individual personality and persona become clear.

The second stage, intimacy versus isolation, starts at about age 18 years and often moves later into adulthood. Erikson says that once the teen has a reasonably strong sense of their identity, they can find someone else to connect with and establish intimacy. According to Erikson, teens in this stage need to be comfortable with their sexual identity and with the roles of self and others and to establish a connection with others verbally and emotionally, as well as sexually.

These theorists give us some sense of where the adolescent and the family are coming from and what the healthcare provider needs to understand to be able to assist with healthy lifestyle and health promotion.

Physical Examination

Bright Futures (Hagan, 2017) and *Guidelines for Adolescent Preventive Services* (GAPS) (Elster and Kuznets, 1994) recommended that adolescents visit their health-care provider once a year and that a complete physical examination occur at least once in early adolescence (11 to 14 years), once in middle adolescence (15 to 17 years), and once in late adolescence (18 to 21 years). Some adolescents are seen more frequently for sports physicals (see Chapter 78) and episodic health concerns, but many adolescents are rarely seen in these formative years.

When the provider is dealing with an adolescent patient, because the teen is not yet of legal age to provide

TABLE 77.1 Theories of Erikson and Piaget

	Young Adolescent	Middle Adolescent	Late Adolescent
Erikson	Identity vs. role confusion	Identity vs. role confusion	Intimacy vs. isolation
Piaget	Tail end of concrete thinking	Formal operations	Formal operations
Puberty landmarks	Breast buds, testicular enlargement	Menarche, enlarged breasts, pubic hair, penis and testicular enlargement, body hair	Adult body with additional height in males

consent, the parent or guardian must be involved to some extent. In the early adolescent years, the parent or guardian generally brings the patient to the encounter and the majority of the history is done with the parent and teen together. However, even in the early teen years, the parent or guardian should be asked to leave the examination room and retire to the waiting area while the provider does the physical examination and asks more sensitive questions of the teen. Before the conversation related to sensitive issues, the provider needs to let the teen know that the information will be held in strict confidence unless there is information that may indicate that there could be harm to the patient or others. If there is a danger of harm to self or others, then the parent or guardian must be informed. All adolescents should be queried about sexual activity; sexual preference; and use of drugs, alcohol, and tobacco. In addition, some questions about availability of weapons, gang awareness, and interpersonal relationships should be asked. All teens should be queried about self-harm or suicidal thoughts. In the early adolescent female, the provider should ask questions about menses. All teens should be asked about their relationships in school and situations with friends. Frequently, the early adolescent will indicate that the parent or guardian can stay in the room. As the provider, it is important to indicate that for all adolescents at any age, the parent is asked to leave. That sets the tone for later encounters and begins to establish autonomy and independence for the teen.

During the middle adolescent years, the situation is generally very similar to the previously mentioned format. Often, the middle adolescent is less comfortable with the parent/guardian staying in the room during the physical examination and knows that the sensitive questions might upset that person. During the middle adolescent years, the likelihood of experimentation with risky behaviors increases. During age 15 to 17 years, many teens may begin to have sexual encounters and experiment with drugs, tobacco, or alcohol, often when at parties with other adolescents. If a teen has tried risky activities, they likely are not going to share that with the parent or guardian, but may be willing to do so with a nonjudgmental health-care provider.

The clinical encounter with the teen in the late adolescent years can be challenging. The age of consent differs from state to state, ranging from 16 years in 32 states plus the District of Columbia, 17 years in 8 states, and 18 years in 11 states. Many clinical sites have the parent or guardian sign a blanket permission once a year so if the adolescent does come to the visit alone, the permission is on file. If the older teen is unaccompanied, then clearly the entire visit is performed with the teen alone. However, the provider still needs to let the teen know that the information is confidential with the same caveat discussed earlier about harm to self or others. Often, adolescents who are 18 or 19 years old believe that they are now adults. Although in many ways their physical habitus is adult, they often are still in a developmental stage of a younger adolescent. The provider needs to be aware of the potential conflict of emotion and activity.

The provider will occasionally encounter older adolescents who, because their parent or guardian has not shared a lot of family medical history with them, may not know their risk for certain diseases. The clinical encounter with an adolescent can be challenging, but when the provider is nonjudgmental and understands the potential cognitive, developmental, and physical ambivalence, it can also be very fulfilling.

Screenings

According to Bright Futures, the adolescent should be seen each year and height, weight, body mass index (BMI), and blood pressure (BP) should be measured. Vision and hearing should also be evaluated once each in early, middle, and late adolescence. If family history indicates hypercholesterolemia, then a lipid profile should be done. If family history is indicative of diabetes mellitus (DM) or if the teen is overweight or obese, glucose should be measured as well. If there is significant concern for DM type 2 then a nonfasting in-office glucose can be done.

One of the major concerns in the adolescent years is inappropriate sexual activity. If the teen is sexually active, a urine test can be obtained for gonorrhea and chlamydia, as well as a test for human papillomavirus (HPV). Currently, unless there is a concern, according to national guidelines, a Papanicolaou (Pap) test is not recommended until adult years (ACOG, 2017; USPTF, 2018). However, if the HPV is positive, a Pap should be obtained. Much of the remainder of the visit in the adolescent years is related to health promotion, healthy lifestyle education, and risk prevention.

Puberty

Adolescents change significantly from the early stages of the 11 or 12 year old through the late stages of the 19 or 20 year old. Any parent or caregiver can tell you about the physical changes and the seemingly overnight growth in height and weight. Children move through adolescence by going through puberty, which is an exciting time as well as extremely stressful for the teen. The health-care provider needs to evaluate the stages of puberty and make sure that the teen is meeting appropriate milestones. The method of evaluation that is used is Tanner staging, which was developed by Marshall and Tanner after 20 years of observation and published in 1969 and 1970. Knowledge of Tanner staging is extremely important for the health-care provider, because adolescents often have great concerns about puberty. The stages of puberty occur in order, although the ages are not necessarily exact (Table 77.2).

Females go through the stages of puberty earlier than males. Both males and females should follow the progression shown in the Tanner staging. Often, when the female

TABLE 77.2 Physical Changes of Puberty

Female

Stage	Age Range (Years)	Breast Growth	Pubic Hair Growth	Other
I	0–8	No change from child	None	No change
II	8–14	Breast budding (thelarche); areolar hyperplasia with small amount of breast tissue	Sparse, downy pubic hair near the labia, with breast budding or shortly after	Peak growth occurs soon after stage II
III	11–12.5	Further enlargement of breast tissue and areola, with no separation of their contours	Increase in amount, curliness and pigmentation of hair	Menarche occurs in 2% of girls late in stage III
IV	11–13	Separation of contours; areola and nipple form secondary mound above breasts tissue	Adult in type but not in distribution	Menarche occurs in most girls in stage IV, 1–3 years after thelarche

TABLE 77.2 Physical Changes of Puberty—cont'd

Female

Stage		Age Range	Description	Pubic Hair	Other
V		12.5–18	Large breast with single contour	Adult in distribution	Menarche occurs in 10% of girls in stage V.

Male

Stage		Age Range (Years)	Testes Growth	Penis Growth	Pubic Hair Growth	Other
I		0–11	Child size testes (<2.5 cm)	Child size	None	
II		10–15	Enlargement of testes; pigmentation of scrotal sac	Minimal or no enlargement	Downy hair, appearing several months after testicular growth	
III		11–16.5	Further enlargement	Significant enlargement, especially in diameter	Increase in amount; curling	
IV		12–16	Further enlargement	Further enlargement	Adult in type but not in distribution	Development of axillary hair and facial hair
V		13–18	Adult in size	Adult in size	Adult in distribution	Body hair continues to grow and muscles continue to increase in size 20% of boys reach peak growth velocity during this period

begins to develop breast tissue, there is asymmetry. The provider can assure the teen and the caregiver that this is normal. Similarly, on occasion, the male will have gynecomastia, which can also be a normal manifestation of puberty and generally will disappear as hormones balance and muscles mass increases. When working with the teen and the caregiver, the provider should be careful to evaluate the Tanner stage to reassure the family. If a teen is of short stature and wants to play basketball but is still Tanner stage II, they are likely to continue to grow and basketball might be suitable. On the other hand, if the teen is Tanner stage IV, they may not grow a great deal more. This information can be very helpful for family.

For females, there should be breast development by age 13 years and menarche by age 16 years. For males, there should be testicular enlargement by age 14 years. If an adolescent has not begun to show these physical signs of pubertal development, there may be delayed puberty. Delayed puberty can be caused by diseases like hypothyroidism or conditions like anorexia nervosa. If a child begins to go through puberty earlier than predicted (age 8 years for females and age 9 years for males), they may have a hormonal imbalance or an adrenal tumor. For either of these situations, the child should be referred to a pediatric endocrinologist for further evaluation.

Immunizations

There are several immunizations that are specifically recommended for adolescents. All older children or early adolescents should have the HPV vaccine. Unfortunately, there has been some pushback against the HPV vaccine primarily by parents or guardians who think that it may create a permissive atmosphere in which their children may feel that it is acceptable to have sexual intercourse if they are immunized. The parent may then decide not to have the child immunized, assuming that if the teen is not immunized, they will decide not to have sexual intercourse. The parent often does not realize that lack of the HPV vaccine will not affect the thought process of the adolescent in the same way as it does an adult. The vaccines that are recommended by the Centers for Disease and Prevention (CDC 2021) start in early adolescence with the HPV and the meningococcal vaccine. All teens need two doses of the HPV 6 to 12 months apart. If the second dose is 5 months or less after the first, the series needs to be restarted. There are two forms of meningitis vaccine. Meningococcal conjugate (MenACWY) vaccine protects against four types (serogroups A, C, W, and Y) of *Neisseria meningitidis* bacteria. Serogroup B meningococcal (MenB) vaccine protects against one type (serogroup B) of *N. meningitidis*. It is recommended that the MenACWY be given at age 11 years with a booster recommended at age 16 years. The MenB is recommended for late adolescents before they go off to college or military, for instance. The MenB is also a two-shot vaccine 1 month apart. The MenB is only a recommendation, but it is possible that some colleges and universities may require it.

In addition to the vaccines that are new for the adolescent, they should be getting the flu vaccine each year, and they will be due for a booster of their Tdap. All of these immunizations are important to keep the adolescent healthy. As the COVID vaccine is tested on children and adolescents, this may also become a recommended vaccine for this age group. Information on immunizations can be found on the CDC website, which can be suggested to parents and adolescents.

Healthy Lifestyle

Unhealthy lifestyle choices often begin in adolescence, and there are many behaviors that need to be discussed and healthy lifestyle choices encouraged. Each yearly visit should include conversations about lifestyle choices such as nutrition, exercise, sleep, and mental health. During adolescence, teens often make unhealthy choices that can affect long-term health; for example, substance use experimentation can have an impact on cardiac health and poor dietary choices can cause obesity, which affects overall adult health. The health-care provider should ask about many lifestyle behavioral choices and provide guidance about positive changes when necessary. Motivational interviewing techniques may be used to change behaviors as needed.

Nutrition

Adolescence is a period of immense physical growth and requires increased nutritional intake. The National Health and Nutrition Examination Survey (NHANES) collects data every fiscal year on varying age groups. Longitudinal NHANES data show that obesity rates for children and adolescents has tripled since the 1970s and severe obesity (greater than the 95th percentile for weight by age) has more than quintupled during this same time period. A BMI above the 85th percentile for adolescents increases the likelihood that they will be obese by age 35 years. Obesity in adolescence increases the risk of chronic diseases throughout adulthood including hypertension, dyslipidemia, endothelial dysfunction, metabolic syndrome, insulin resistance hyperglycemia, and fatty liver disease. Dietary guidelines from the U.S. Department of Agriculture (USDA) are updated every 5 years based on the NHANES data and give a good baseline for everyone to follow. These guidelines recommend a diet that is high in vegetables of all types—red, green, and orange. They also recommend whole fruits and whole grains. Diets for adolescents should include low-fat milk, yogurt, and cheese, as well as proteins like poultry, lean meat, fish, lentils, and nuts. Oils should be included in limited amounts. The latest guidelines recommend limiting processed sugar and salt for everyone.

Unfortunately, any provider who has worked with adolescents is aware that many adolescents' diets consist largely of fast food, pizza, snack foods, and sugary drinks. They tend to have diets that are high in fat, sugar, and salt, and low in fruits, vegetables, and whole grains. That is not true of all adolescents; however, many do not pay much attention to their nutrition and eat what is fast and what their friends are eating. In addition, adolescents tend to skip breakfast and then many are hungry and eat late in the day. A recent survey done by the USDA (2019) found that almost 30% of teens eat and drink high-calorie foods late in the day. Those who did so had higher overall calorie intake for the day. The health-care provider needs to determine not only what the teen is eating, but when. All teens should be encouraged to eat breakfast even if it is on the go, such as a banana or protein bar, and limit late-evening snacking. Obesity has doubled among teens in the last 10 years and late-evening snacking can lead to that problem. The provider should make recommendations regarding nutritious foods (tailored to individual preference and culture), the time of eating, and potential weight loss if needed. Motivational interviewing may be useful. Chapter 60 discusses obesity in more detail.

Not all adolescents tend to overeat or eat inappropriate foods; some teens do not eat adequate calories to maintain their weight. Because of the idealism and focus on their pubertal changes, some teens are at risk for anorexia nervosa and bulimia. This is a high-risk time for these diseases and the provider must be careful to screen for these problems as well. Adolescents should be weighed in a gown, and all adolescents should be plotted on a growth chart from the CDC (https://www.cdc.gov/growthcharts/data/set1clinical/cj41c021.pdf) at each visit through age 20 years. If a teen is found to have fallen two or more percentile lines on the growth chart, this is an indication of either a major health issue or anorexia nervosa. This weight loss should be carefully followed up (see Chapter 71).

Sleep

Sleep can be a major problem in the adolescent years. Often, teens have a large number of activities in addition to school, and generally have many hours of homework. Because many teens are heavily involved with sports, music, dance, theater, and other extracurricular activities, they may not even start to tackle homework until late in the evening. For many teens, that means that they may not complete the homework until midnight. They then are often caught up in social media and spend time on their phones or other screens even longer. Once they do get to sleep they get up early in the morning to get ready for school, which may begin as early as 7:30 or 8:00 a.m., meaning that they may not have more than 5 or 6 hours of sleep; as noted later, they should have 8 to 10 hours of sleep. One study by Mireku et al. (2019) showed that teens in the late adolescent years averaged much less than 7 hours of sleep a night, which has been determined to be an inadequate amount of sleep for anyone but especially during puberty and growth spurts. In fact, teens actually need more sleep than adults (Table 77.3). It is recommended that adolescents get at least 8 hours of sleep each night. This lack of sleep has been correlated with psychological problems, as well as an increase in injury and risk. When measured with electroencephalograms (EEGs) it was determined that in late adolescence when there are so many activities and a decrease in sleep that females slept better, went to sleep faster, and in general did better than males. This is likely because puberty in females is usually accomplished by late adolescence, whereas many males are still going through pubertal changes. One of the primary goals of the adolescent years is to successfully complete high school, and in many cases transition to college. Unfortunately, lack of sleep has a detrimental effect on learning and cognitive abilities. Lack of sleep and general sleepiness hampers learning in teens and adults. Because of all of the negative effects of inadequate sleep, it is important for the provider to evaluate sleep and recommend adequate sleep behaviors.

One of the ways that adolescents and adults lose sleep is through the use of blue screen electronics before or in bed. Studies have showed that nighttime mobile phone and television use was associated with higher risk of insufficient sleep duration on weekdays. It has been shown that the use of screens either right before bed or in bed interrupts that circadian rhythm by suppressing melatonin and interrupting the circadian cycle. This causes the adolescent to have difficulty falling asleep and consequent sleepiness in the morning. Inadequate sleep is negatively associated with academic performance, physical health, unintentional injury risk, and the ability to complete tasks of daily living in general. As teens begin to drive, this lack of sleep may result in car accidents and injuries. The health-care provider should work with the parent or guardian and the teen to devise a plan to limit screen time before and in bed.

TABLE 77.3 National Sleep Foundation Recommendations

	Age Range	Recommended Hours of Sleep
Newborn	0–3 months old	14–17 hours
Infant	4–11 months old	12–15 hours
Toddler	1–2 years old	11–14 hours
Preschool	3–5 years old	10–13 hours
School-age	6–13 years old	9–11 hours
Teen	14–17 years old	8–10 hours
Young Adult	18–25 years old	7–9 hours
Adult	26–64 years old	7–9 hours
Older Adult	65 or more years old	7–8 hours

Source: Hirshkowitz M, Whiton K, Albert SM, et al. National Sleep Foundation's sleep time duration recommendations: methodology and results summary. *Sleep Health*. 2015;1(1):40–43.

Physical Activity

Adolescents tend to fall into one of two lifestyle categories regarding physical activity. There are many teens who are extremely active in sports and participate in some organized sport every season and frequently are active in off seasons. There are other adolescents who are not active in any organized sports, they spend inordinate amounts of time in front of a screen, and do not do any physical activity. There are few teens who fall in between these two categories with respect to physical activity. *Healthy People 2030* has goals of increasing physical activity, muscle strengthening, and in general, moving more while reducing screen time. The recommendations for middle and late adolescents are actually similar to adult physical education recommendations. Currently, 20% of students in grades 9 through 12 were physically active for at least 60 minutes on all 7 days of the past week and participated in muscle-strengthening activity on 3 or more days of the past week. In terms of simply measuring physical activity, the percentages are higher; 26% engage in physical activity. Approximately 53% of teens are engaged in organized sports, so approximately half of adolescents are getting reasonable physical activity and half are not. In general, the health-care provider needs to determine into which category the teen falls and help identify activities that they enjoy and will agree to engage in.

Anticipatory Guidance

When health-care providers work with children and adolescents, one of the primary activities is to provide anticipatory guidance to the adolescent and the parent or guardian. It is important to address not only current issues and concerns but to let the family know what changes are coming and what they might expect to encounter in the future. This is extremely important for the adolescent who will encounter multiple challenges as they move through the transition from early adolescent through to early adulthood. The health-care provider needs to take a role in guiding the parent/guardian and child in negotiating the tasks that will arise. These various topics will be discussed separately.

Early Adolescence

During early adolescence, the thinking is often closer to that of later childhood. The teen is thinking more concretely, but physical changes are either beginning or coming very soon. The anticipatory guidance should focus on these developments, preparing both the teen and the parent/guardian for the changes. During this time, the adolescent is beginning to focus more on peers, so discussion of the types of peers that might best suit the teen would be beneficial. It is important to discuss with the adolescent the concept of sexual intercourse, how to deal with pressure for sex, and pregnancy and sexually transmitted infection prevention before the situation arises. These issues should be discussed with the parent/guardian as well, and this is the time to begin separating the adolescent from the parent/guardian as standard office behavior.

Middle Adolescence

Often, this is a time of conflict between the teen and the parent/guardian as there is increased independence, with the ability to drive often coming at this stage. Teens often are able to get a job so they have money of their own and desire to spend it in ways of which the parent or guardian may not approve. These increased responsibilities and freedoms need to be discussed with both teens and parents/guardians. Abstract thinking increases during this time, so discussion with the adolescent can take place on a more theoretical level. There should be continued discussion about sexual intercourse and interpersonal relationships.

Late Adolescence

During these years, the adolescent is getting ready to launch from the family. This can be very stressful for both the family and the teen. Preparation for this separation is paramount in the late adolescent years. Discussion of the future should occur with both the adolescent and the parent/guardian. Discussion of responsibilities—which are increasing at this age, such as voting rights, and those that are not yet legal, such as purchasing alcohol—is of great importance. In some situations, transition to a new health-care provider needs to be addressed as well.

When the provider is working with adolescents, there is a variety of acronym tools that can be helpful when doing the history and guidance of the teen and the parent/guardian. These tools assist in asking important questions of the teen and working with the parent/guardian to develop plans with the teen. These acronyms include GAPS, CRAFFT, and HEADSS, among others (Table 77.4). These tools help the health-care provider remember the important topics to discuss with the teen and parent/guardian. They are particularly useful to the provider when discussion revolves around one topic when another topic also needs to be covered. GAPS is the Guideline for Adolescent Preventive Services, and there are three separate forms for early, middle, and late adolescents with an additional form that can be used for parents or guardians. CRAFFT is an evaluation of drugs and alcohol, and HEADSS is an acronym to guide the history in any adolescent.

Mental Health

The primary goal of the adolescent years is to build positive self-esteem of the adolescent patient. Adolescents are facing many challenges, and throughout these years, they need to know that they are still developing appropriately and that they will become a productive adult. An adolescent who has a goal is likely an adolescent who will come

TABLE 77.4 Anticipatory Guidance Tools—CRAFFT and HEADSS

Car	Have you either driven or been in **Car** driven by someone who was on drugs?
Relax	Do you ever use drugs or alcohol to **Relax**?
Alone	Do you ever use drugs or alcohol when you are **Alone**?
Forget	Do you ever **Forget** things when using drugs or alcohol?
Family or Friends	Do your **Friends** or **Family** ever tell you that you need to cut down on your drugs or alcohol use?
Trouble	Have you ever gotten into **Trouble** when you were using drugs or alcohol?

Source: American Academy of Pediatrics. Bright Futures: Prevention and Health Promotion for Infants, Children, and their Families. Published in 2022. https://brightfutures.aap.org/

Home	Where do you call home? Who lives with you? Do you feel safe at home?
Education Employment	Where do you go to school? What do you like best/least about school? How are you doing in school? Do you have a job? Where? How often do you work?
Activities	Do you have activities during/after school? Do you have a best friend at these? Do you drive? If so, do you wear a seat belt? Do you text and drive?
Drugs	Do your friends do drugs/smoke? Have you tried drugs/smoking? How often?
Sex	Sexual orientation? Do you have a boyfriend/girlfriend? Have you had sex? Oral? Anal? How many partners? Condoms?
Suicide	Have you ever thought of taking your life? Have you ever made a plan?

Sources: Cohen E, MacKenzie RG, Yates GL. HEADSS, a psychosocial risk assessment instrument: Implications for designing effective intervention programs for runaway youth. *J Adolesc Health*. 1991;12 (7): 539–544; Moreno, MA. Adolescent health and medical ethics. *AMA J Ethics*. 2005;7(3):203–264. https://journalofethics.ama-assn.org/issue/ethics-adolescent-medicine

through these challenging years in good mental health and do well. Sometimes, the goal may not be realistic—such as a 5-foot 6-inch adolescent becoming an Olympic basketball player; however, just the fact that they have a goal and are working toward that goal is a positive for building self-esteem.

On the other hand, there are many adolescents who have mental health concerns. Depression and anxiety are very prevalent in adolescence. Because of all of the changes in body habitus and development of identity and formal operations, the teen has a significant number of challenges to face. Puberty alone puts major stress on the hormonal balances in the body. At the same time, they are trying to identify who they are according to Erikson and facing increasingly difficult academic challenges at school. When a parent tells the provider that one minute the teen acts like a 10-year-old and the next acts more like a 20-year-old, it is not surprising. All of the challenges occur within an environment with many other adolescents all going through similar changes and challenges. Given all of this, one may wonder that any adolescent turns out well. Most do develop well, but some have mental health concerns along the way.

Any adolescent who indicates during the health-care provider's evaluation that they are extremely sad, have thought about suicide, or have major anxiety problems should be referred for counseling. It can be extremely helpful to have the adolescent complete the Pediatric Symptom checklist before seeing the provider. The provider can then ask about some of the concerns that might have been checked on this questionnaire. Unfortunately, most locations have a paucity of health-care providers who can do counseling for the child or adolescent. Because that is true in many places, the primary-care provider may be called on to do some counseling, as well as provide medication on occasion. All providers need to be aware that selective serotonin reuptake inhibitors (SSRIs) all have U.S. Food and Drug Administration (FDA) black box warnings related to provisions to adolescents. However, the FDA has approved fluoxetine (Prozac) for use in adolescents with depression. When necessary, SSRIs can be prescribed, but the provider needs to be vigilant about follow-up and must get the family involved in watching for signs of further depression or suicidal ideation. On occasion, the school system can provide counseling and that may be helpful. For further discussion, see Chapters 68 and 69.

Another aspect of adolescence that can cause major concerns for the teen is the development of sexual identity. During adolescence, the teen may realize that they are attracted to persons of the same sex. Depending on the family background and the community in which the adolescent resides, this can be a particular problem. In general, the majority of students in any given high school identify as heterosexual so if one adolescent perceives that they are different, that may be a cause of depression or anxiety. In addition, there are some communities and some context in which the preference for same sex is strongly prohibited, and that can clearly create great anxiety for the teen. A teen who identifies as LGBTQ+ in an area that has a large concentration of those who by religious faith believe that to be a sin may have a great deal of anxiety and depression. The mental health of these adolescents should be assessed carefully.

The other concern with the adolescent who identifies as LGBTQ+ is that, as indicated in the section on Erikson, this is a time when teens are trying to determine exactly what their identity is. An adolescent may believe that they are pulled toward the LGBTQ+ lifestyle for a while and then may later decide that that lifestyle really did not fit them after all. That can cause great distress for the teen, their friends, and family. It is important for the health-care provider to discuss with the teen and the parent or guardian the concept of developing identity and to allow the teen to change their preference if they find that a previous preference no longer works for them. It also is incumbent on the provider to help the parent understand that the preference may change over time and suggest that the parent recognize this possibility.

Sex

Part of the developmental tasks for the middle and late adolescent is to establish intimacy. Many people find that establishing intimacy includes experience with sexual intimacy and sexual intercourse. This is an area that can cause great concern for the parent or guardian, as well as on occasion for the teen. The provider needs to be nonjudgmental when interviewing the teen about sexual encounters. Many clinics and offices have questionnaires, such as the GAPS, that the teen completes before the encounter. The questionnaires can assist the provider when discussing sensitive issues with the teen. The questionnaires have questions for the teen to complete on sexuality, drug and alcohol use, tobacco use, and so on. It is then easy for the provider to say, "I see that you are sexually active. Can you tell me more about that?" If one of the surveys is not completed, then the provider needs to ask about it. In addition to sexual intercourse, questions about oral and anal sexual encounters are important as well.

There are multiple potential concerns with sexual encounters. The teen needs to be advised about sexually transmitted infections and the need for the use of condoms in all situations. The teen likely will need to be taught how to put on and take off a condom. In addition to sexually transmitted infections, there is always the concern about potential pregnancy. That means that the adolescent female should be educated about contraception. Currently, the contraception that is being recommended for adolescents is the long-acting reversible contraception (LARC; ACOG 2017). LARC forms include intrauterine devices (IUD), implantable progestin-only rods that are implanted in the upper arm (Implanon), and Depo-Provera injections. Depo-Provera is only recommended for maximum of 2 years, whereas the IUD is effective for up to 6 years and up to 3 years for the Implanon.

If the LARC is not considered an option for contraception, the adolescent can use oral contraceptive pills or the contraceptive patch. The guidelines recommend the LARC so that the teen does not have to remember to take a pill or change a patch. In addition, many teens find that the anonymity of the LARC to be preferable for their lifestyle. For all contraception, the provider has to be aware of side effects of the progestin-only forms, as well as the combined hormonal formats of contraception. The side effects of progestin-only are different from those of combined hormonal contraception (Chapter 47). Follow-up at each visit is mandatory.

Not all adolescents are going to follow the appropriate guidelines, and on occasion mistakes are going to occur. Emergency contraception routinely should be included in discussions about contraception, including access issues. This should be discussed before the need arising so that the teen can decide what they want to do if a slip or a mistake does occur. The adolescent needs to know how to access emergency contraception. The health-care provider does, however, need to make the teen aware that emergency contraception is NOT an alternative to long-term use of a regular form of contraception.

Another area regarding adolescent sexual encounters that needs to be addressed is the age of the participants. If a teen is 15 and having sexual intercourse with another teen who is 16, the consequences of intercourse need to be addressed and all of the conversations about contraception and use of condoms needs to occur. However, if the teen is 15 and having sexual intercourse with someone who is 27, in most states that is considered statutory rape and needs to be reported to the child protective agency. The adolescent may think this behavior is perfectly fine, and it may take persuasion on the part of the provider to let them know that it is not acceptable.

When discussing sexual behavior, the sexual preference of the teen needs to be addressed. Often, adolescents are not sure what their preference really happens to be, or the preference changes over time. The provider should listen in a nonjudgmental way and allow the teen to talk about their thoughts. Often, just listening is helpful. If the adolescent is in the late phase of development, it is beneficial to have local resources that are adept at dealing with LGBTQ+ adolescents that you can share with the teen. Chapter 79 addresses the primary care for patients who are transgender.

Other Adolescent Concerns

The greatest cause of death in adolescents is unintentional injury. Automobile accidents account for 20% of all unintentional deaths in adolescents. Auto accidents may occur if the driver has been drinking alcohol or using drugs. Teens often use drugs and alcohol in groups and then may challenge one another to participate in risky behaviors, resulting in injury and death. In many states, marijuana is legal, although not for anyone under age 21 years, but like alcohol, teens may obtain and use marijuana and may have health-related problems. One of the side effects of cannabis use may be severe abdominal pain and hyperemesis. On occasion, the cannabis can also cause diarrhea when taken in high doses. When adolescents present with these symptoms, unless the provider has gotten information about marijuana usage, a multitude of imaging studies and bloodwork may ensue. Adolescents may also illegally use prescription medications, both those prescribed to them and taken from others. Opioids and attention-deficit/hyperactivity disorder (ADHD) medications taken from someone else may result in problems for the adolescent. Careful attention to drug and alcohol use and abuse must be part of the adolescent interview.

Another significant cause of unintentional injury is the use or misuse of firearms. There may be guns in the home that the teen has access to, or there may be intentional use of guns for hunting. If an adolescent is planning to use a gun to hunt, they should have education on the safety and use of the gun before going out for the first time. However, if the adolescent simply has access to guns in the home, safety is paramount. The health-care provider needs to discuss gun safety with both the parent/guardian and the teen. If the parent/guardian has a gun, it should be kept locked and the ammunition kept separate from the gun. This is true for all children and adolescents. If an adolescent is going to use a gun, they should not be left unattended with a firearm.

Adolescents may try tobacco or vaping. Again, a good way to approach the topic would be to ask if the teen's friends have tried tobacco or vaping. Both tobacco and vaping are on the increase in adolescents, particularly in the middle and late adolescent population. Many e-cigarettes have more nicotine than traditional cigarettes and vaping has been known to cause potentially lung-damaging pneumonia, especially in adolescents. The long-term health concerns with traditional cigarettes is well known, but there may be similar problems and even other long-term health problems with e-cigarettes. It has been shown that vaping can actually lead to other tobacco use. There are several reasons that teens become involved with vaping; the first is that e-cigarettes are small and easily hidden, another is that e-cigarettes come in many flavors that appeal to the adolescent. It can be quite challenging to get the teen to consider stopping. All health-care providers can assist with adolescent e-cigarette use by advocating for public policy to reduce the availability of e-cigarettes to teens. Appealing to the teen regarding the long-term health consequences is rarely effective. Teens are rarely interested in discussing what might occur in 20 years; they are more concerned with the time between today and next week. Generally, smoking cessation tools such as gums and patches are not used in adolescents as they may cause as many problems as the tobacco or vaping (see Chapter 33).

Another area of concern for adolescents today is social media. Unfortunately, although there may be positive aspects to social media, there are also many problems that arise for adolescents. Social media is a big part of many teens' lives. A 2018 Pew Research Center survey of nearly 750 13- to 17-year-olds found that 45% are online almost constantly, and 97% use a social media platform, such as YouTube, Facebook, Instagram, or Snapchat. Research has shown that teens who use social media are more susceptible to mental health issues. In addition, many of the same concerns that face adolescents such as bullying and sexuality are magnified on social media. Cyberbullying and sexting have become major problems for the adolescent and are clearly more of an issue the more the teen engages with social media. Adolescents can benefit from use of social media through connecting with friends and promoting positive social activities, but they can also have major psychosocial issues if they are the victim of cyberbullying or if they participate in cyberbullying. Some teen cyberbullying victims have become so distraught that they died by suicide. Sexting, sending sexual texts or images over digital media, can also be a problem. On occasion, the images have gotten adolescents into trouble either at the time or later in life when they are applying for a job or for college. The adolescent does not think of the future when posting this sort of content.

Bullying has been described as aggressive intentional behavior within a situation of an imbalance of power against victims who cannot easily defend themselves. Cyberbullying is this activity performed through electronic media such as chat rooms, phone texts, and e-mail. This negative behavior can have a major impact on a teen's mental health. Between 20% and 50% of adolescents have been the victim of cyberbullying at some point. In general, male teens are more often the bullies and female teens are more often the victims. It is important that the health-care provider ask about cyberbullying and then have a conversation with the parent/guardian and the teen about ways to cope. It may be helpful for the teen to be able to talk about cyberbullying with a trusted person, and the issue may be reported to the school if it persists. If the teen tries to ignore it or internalizes the thoughts, this can lead to depression and anxiety. Actively talking about it and changing the thought focus may help.

Another issue for adolescents is tattoos. In 45 states, adolescents are not old enough to consent to a tattoo until they are 18 years old. Many adolescents want "to get inked" before that, and therefore would need parental or legal guardian consent. Often, parents do not agree. The major concern arises when the teen finds a non–state-approved tattoo artist and gets the tattoo without parental knowledge or consent. The non–state-approved locations may not follow appropriate hygiene or health rules and the needles can transmit diseases such as hepatitis. The ink can cause a serious allergic reaction (rarely), and serious infections at the site have been reported. If an adolescent wants a tattoo, they should go to a state-approved tattoo establishment. The artist should wear gloves when working, and needles should be changed for each patient. Ideally, the ink should be changed for each patient as well. If the parent/guardian is involved, they can make sure these rules are followed and that the teen is properly immunized against hepatitis and tetanus. Generally, a parent/guardian or health-care provider might suggest that the tattoo be in a location that is easily covered. Often, the teen does not think about what they might be doing in the future. For example, if the teen gets a tattoo on the neck and then decides that they want to go into the military, they can be barred. The other concern with tattoos is that they may be "addictive" and the teen may want to continue to get them. Any addictive behavior is problematic.

Tanning beds can also be an issue in the adolescent population. Melanoma is the second most frequently diagnosed cancer overall among individuals aged 15 to 29 years and is the most frequent cancer diagnosed among those aged 25 to 29 years at 18% of all cancers in this age group. Tanning beds and all sources of artificial ultraviolet (UV) light are a major modifiable factor in adolescent and young adult skin cancer. Between 15% and 18% of adolescents use tanning beds and that number increases as the adolescent gets into young adulthood. Educating adolescents about the use of sunscreen should be a discussion at every visit. Currently, tanning beds do not have an age restriction, so providing guidance and recommending use of sunscreen is the most that the provider can do.

CONCLUSION

Adolescence can be a stressful time for the parent or guardian as well as the teen. Although there are potentially many concerns that may arise during adolescence, and there are significant changes that occur both physically and mentally, the joys of dealing with an adolescent can be just as great. Adolescents, with their idealism, have made great changes in society over the years. As a health-care provider, if one is nonjudgmental and listens to the teen and to the parent/guardian, one can learn a great deal and can often help the family significantly in dealing with their challenges. When the provider prepares the parent/guardian and child for the changes that will occur and makes recommendations about things like alcohol, tattoos, and other challenges, the process of having an open discussion can go a long way in avoiding conflict.

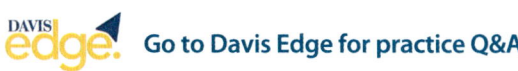 Go to Davis Edge for practice Q&A.

REFERENCES

Alderman EM, Breuner CC, Committee on Adolescence. Unique needs of the adolescent. *Pediatrics*. December 2019;144(6):e20193150. https://doi.org/10.1542/peds.2019-3150

American Academy of Pediatrics. Mental health screening and assessment tools for primary care. https://www.aap.org/en-us/advocacy-and-policy/aap-health-initiatives/mental-health/documents/mh_screeningchart.pdf. Accessed December 2020.

American College of Obstetricians and Gynecologists. Health care for lesbians and bisexual women. Care for transgender adolescents. (2017) Committee Opinion No. 685. *Obstet Gynecol*. 2017;129:e11-6N.

American Medical Association. *Implementing the Guidelines for Adolescent Preventive Services (GAPS)*. https://www.aafp.org/afp/1998/0501/p2181.html

Anderson N, Jiang J. (2018). Teens, social media, & technology 2018. *Pew Research Center*. http://publicservicesalliance.org/wp-content/uploads/2018/06/Teens-Social-Media-Technology-2018-PEW.pdf

Bleyer A, Viny A, Barr R. Cancer in 15- to 29-year-olds by primary site. *Oncologist*. 2006;11(6):590-601.

Centers for Disease Control and Prevention. Adolescents and school health. Module 5: health services. http://www.cdc.gov/healthyyouth/. Accessed June 24, 2022.

Cohen E, MacKenzie RG, Yates GL. HEADSS, a psychosocial risk assessment instrument: Implications for designing effective intervention programs for runaway youth. *J Adolesc Health*. 1991;12(7):539-544.

Cunningham RM, Walton MA, Carter PM. (2018) The major causes of death in children and adolescents in the United States. *N Engl J Med*. 2018;379(25):2468-2475.

Elster A, Kuznets N. *AMA Guidelines for Adolescent Preventive Services (GAPS)*. Baltimore, Maryland: Williams & Wilkins;1994. https://www.ncbi.nlm.nih.gov/books/NBK138588/

Fobian AD, Avis K, Schwebel DC. Impact of media use on adolescent sleep efficiency. *J Dev Pediatr*. 2017;37(1):9-14.

Gandini S, Autier P, Boniol M. Reviews on sun exposure and artificial light and melanoma. *Prog Biophys Mol Biol*. 2011;107(3):362-366.

Hagan JF, Shaw JS, Duncan PM, eds. *Bright Futures: Guidelines for Health Supervision of Infants, Children, and Adolescents*. 4th ed. Elk Grove Village, IL: American Academy of Pediatrics;2017. https://brightfutures.aap.org/materials-and-tools/guidelines-and-pocket-guide/Pages/default.aspx. Accessed 6/16/21.

Henry TS, Kligerman SJ, Raptis CA, Mann H. Imaging findings of vaping-associated lung injury. *Am J Roentgenol*. 2020;214:498-505.

Jones K, Saltzan GA. The vaping epidemic in adolescents. *Missouri Med*. 2020;117(1):56-58.

Kim S, Colwell SR, Kata A, et al. Cyberbullying victimization and adolescent mental health: evidence of differential effects by sex and mental health problem type. *J Youth Adolesc*. 2018;47:661-672. https://doi.org/10.1007/s10964-017-0678-4

Kirby KC, Versek B, Kerwin ME, Meyers K, Benishek L, Bresani E. Developing community reinforcement and family training (CRAFT) for parents of treatment-resistant adolescents. *J Child Adolesc Subst Abuse*. 2015;24(3):155-165.

Knight JR, Sherritt L, Shrier LA, Harris SK, Chang G. Validity of the CRAFFT substance abuse screening test among adolescent clinic patients. *Arch Pediatr Adolesc Med*. 2002;156:607-614.

Knishkowy B, Palti H. (1997). GAPS (AMA guidelines for adolescent preventive services). where are the gaps? *Arch Pediatr Adolesc Med*. 151(2):123-128

Lenzer, J. FDA panel urges "black box" warning for antidepressants. *BMJ* 2004;329(7468):702.

Marshall WA, Tanner JM Variations in pattern of pubertal changes in girls. *Arch Dis Child*. June 1969;44 (235):291-303. Accessed January 18, 2021.

Marshall WA, Tanner JM. Variations in the pattern of pubertal changes in boys. *Arch Dis Child* 1970;45(239):13-23. Accessed January 18, 2021. doi: 10.1136/adc.45.239.13

Mireku MO, Barker MM, Mutz J, Thomas MSC, Roosli M, Elliott P, Toledano MB. Night-time screen-based media device use and adolescents' sleep and health-related quality of life. *Environ Int.* 2019;124:66-78.

Richardson LP, Rockhill C, Russo JE. Evaluation of the PHQ-2 as a brief screen for detecting major depression among adolescents. *Pediatrics.* 2010;125:e1097-e1103.

Sebastian RS, Wilkinson C, Goldman JD, Moshfegh AJ. Late evening food and beverage consumption by adolescents in the U.S. what we eat in America. Published 2016. https://www.ars.usda.gov/ARSUserFiles/80400530/pdf/DBrief/25_Late_Evening_Food_and_Beverage_Consumption_by_Adolescents_in_the_U.S._1316.pdf

Tarokh L, Saletin JM, Carskadori MA. (2016) Sleep in adolescence: physiology, cognition and mental health. *Neurosci Biobehav Rev.* 2016 Nov;70:182-188. doi: 10.1016/j.neubiorev.2016.08.008. Accessed January 29, 2021.

USDA, Dietary Guidelines for Americans 2020-2025. https://www.dietaryguidelines.gov/sites/default/files/2020-12/DGA_2020-2025_ExecutiveSummary_English.pdf. Published 2019.

U.S. Department of Health and Human Services. Healthy People 2030: adolescents. https://health.gov/healthypeople/objectives-and-data/browse-objectives/adolescents

U.S. Preventive Services Task Force. (2018). Cervical cancer: screening. https://www.uspreventiveservicestaskforce.org/uspstf/recommendation/cervical-cancer-screening.

Vollink T, Bolman CAW, Dehue F, Jacobs NCL. Coping with cyberbullying: differences between victims, bully-victims and children not involved in bullying. *J Commun Appl Soc Psychol.* 2013;23:7-24.

White MC, Shoemaker ML, Park S, Neff LJ, Carlson SA, Brown DR, Kanny D. Prevalence of modifiable cancer risk factors among U.S. adults aged 18–44 years. *Am J Prevent Med.* 2017;53(3S1): S14-S20.

Zuckerbrot RA, Cheung A, Jensen PS, Stein REK, Laraque D, GLAD-PC Steering Group. Guidelines for adolescent depression in primary care (GLAD-PC): part 1. Practice preparation, identification, assessment, and initial management. *Pediatrics.* 2018;141(3):e20174081. doi: https://doi.org/10.1542/peds.2017-4081

RESOURCES

American Academy of Pediatrics: Adolescent Sexual Health
   https://www.aap.org/en-us/advocacy-and-policy/aap-health-initiatives/adolescent-sexual-health/Pages/Caring-for-the-Adolescent-Patient.aspx

Centers for Disease Control and Prevention
   https://health.gov/healthypeople/objectives-and-data/browse-objectives/adolescents
   https://www.cdc.gov/healthyyouth/healthservices/index.htm

Chapter 78

Sports Physicals

Michael E. Zychowicz, DNP, ANP, ONP, FAAN, FAANP

INTRODUCTION

In the United States, millions of children participate in organized sports annually. Athletic participation has a benefit of enhancing mental and physical well-being. One way clinicians can enhance safe athletic participation is to perform a preparticipation physical evaluation (PPE), or sports physical, for young athletes. Although the main goal for performing the PPE is to promote safe sports participation, it is not meant as a means to exclude athletes from participation. Less than 2% of athletes who have a PPE are disqualified from sport due to examination findings.

By performing a PPE the clinician can identify risks for injury or illness, as well as high risk for potentially life-threatening conditions based on history and physical findings. The clinician may identify some prior injuries or conditions that have not fully resolved and require management or rehabilitation before safe sport participation. The monograph, *Preparticipation Physical Evaluation, 5th ed.*, published by the American Academy of Pediatrics (AAP), is a foundational resource for clinicians performing presports physicals including a standardized history and physical form.

Unfortunately, for some children, the PPE may be their only interaction with a health-care provider. This may be due to a variety of reasons, including insurance policy restrictions. The clinician should keep this in mind as they engage the patient. The PPE visit can be utilized to assess the overall health and general fitness level of the child. The clinician can also use this time to engage the patient in health education, health-risk assessment, or nutritional counseling.

Although laws vary from state to state, most states require a PPE to be performed by a clinician before participating in school or organized sports. Aside from state law, these may also be a requirement of the sponsoring organization's insurance. Objectives of the PPE are listed in Box 78.1.

Sports are divided into degrees of contact and intensity that the provider must consider when assessing an athlete for sports participation. A list of sports by level of contact and intensity is shown on Table 78.1.

Box 78.1 Objectives of the Sports Physical

Objectives

- Promote healthy and safe athletic participation
- Assess an athlete's general level of physical health
- Assess an athlete's general level of mental health
- Detect conditions that may be life-threatening or disabling
- Detect conditions that may predispose the athlete to injury or illness
- Create an opportunity to engage and educate the athlete about health, wellness, and lifestyle
- Provide an opportunity to engage with a health-care provider for those athletes who do not routinely have access to preventive health care

Source: Bernhardt DT, Roberts WO. *Preparticipation Physical Evaluation*. 5th ed. McGraw-Hill; 2019.

TABLE 78.1 Examples of Sports by Level of Contact and Intensity

Contact/Collision	Limited Contact	Noncontact
Basketball	Baseball/softball	Archery
Boxing	Bicycle	Crew
Field hockey	Cheerleading	Golf
Football	Fencing	Riflery
Ice hockey	Gymnastics	Running
Lacrosse	Ice skating	Scuba
Martial arts	Skiing/	Swimming
Rodeo	snowboarding	Tennis
Rugby	Volleyball	Track
Soccer		Weightlifting
Wrestling		

Low Dynamic/ Low Static	Low Dynamic/ High Static	High Dynamic/ Low Static	High Dynamic/ High Static
Bowling	Archery	Basketball	Boxing
Golf	Gymnastics	Lacrosse	Downhill skiing
Riflery	Rodeo	Racquetball	Football
	Waterskiing	Soccer	Water polo
	Weightlifting	Volleyball	Wrestling

Source: Miller SM, Peterson AR. The sports preparticipation evaluation. *Pediatr Rev.* 2019;40(3):108–128.

EXAMINATION TIMING

For some, the PPE is an annual formal requirement before participation in school or other organized sports. Others may be required to have an examination before each sports season over a few seasons per year. Individual state law may dictate how often a child will be required to have a PPE before sports participation.

Recommendations from the AAP state a young child or adolescent should have a comprehensive PPE at least every 2 to 3 years. An evaluation of an updated health history should be conducted annually with a problem-focused physical examination as needed. For college athletes, a comprehensive history and physical examination should minimally be conducted during the first year of participation. Additionally, an annual assessment of an updated health history along with a problem-focused physical examination should be performed as needed.

Ideally, the PPE is not performed at the last minute before participating in athletics. The PPE should be performed at least 6 to 8 weeks before the first sport practice. This gives adequate lead time if additional testing or specialist evaluation needs to be conducted. Between 3.1% and 13.9% of students who undergo a PPE will need further evaluation of some type before being cleared for sport. Additionally, performing the PPE early gives some time for the athlete to engage in rehabilitation, should that be needed, before the beginning of sport.

EXAMINATION FORMATS

Three formats or settings for conducting the PPE are commonly utilized. These examinations are office based, assembly line or mass examination, and station based. There is limited data to demonstrate a significant difference in the rate of clearing athletes for sport among the PPE formats.

1. Office-based examination—A single provider examines one athlete in the office setting. This may be in a retail health setting, an urgent care, a primary care practice, or a school health office. Office-based examinations allow for privacy in counseling at important stages of life, establishes the importance of preventive care, provides privacy for open communication, and provides continuity of care. A greater continuity of care, understanding of the patient's medical and family history, and full access to the patient's health records can occur when the patient's primary care provider performs the PPE.
2. Assembly line or mass examination—A single provider examines several athletes, one athlete after the other. This format frequently involves several athletes examined en masse in a gym. Although this approach might be cheaper and quicker, it lacks individual attention, causes possible communication problems, increases the risk that insufficient medical history is taken, and lacks continuity. This eliminates privacy for the athletes, which may limit athletes' disclosure of history or complaints. Additionally, these mass examinations can be distracting or noisy, decreasing the examiner's ability to hear findings with the stethoscope.
3. Station-based examination—Multiple examiners do different parts of the examination. For example, a station-based examination may include an orthopedist, neurologist, ophthalmologist, primary care provider, and cardiologist all conducting different parts of the examination. This type of examination allows for specialists to examine specific body systems. Although this may seem more thorough, there are limited data to demonstrate benefit of this type of examination over other models to assess athletes for sport. This format may be impersonal, lack privacy, and may feel rushed to the athlete. In addition, there may be a tendency toward disorganization, as well as potential for inadequate integration of all findings. Utilizing a sports medicine or a primary care provider to collate the data from specialists and clear the athlete for participation may aid in synthesizing physical assessment data.

COMPONENTS OF SPORTS PHYSICAL: HISTORY, PHYSICAL EXAMINATION, AND CLEARANCE

No matter what format is chosen, the sports physical can be divided into three main components: history, physical examination, and determination of clearance.

History

The athlete's history gives the provider most of the information needed to make an informed decision about clearing or disqualifying an athlete. The athlete and parent/guardian should complete the history together before the examination to ensure that the most accurate and complete information is available for the clinician to review. Specific items to screen for in the medical history, specific sports history, and family history are listed in Box 78.2.

Some states or athletic organizations may have their own unique history and physical forms to be completed. The clinician may need to explore positive findings on the health history or additional areas of the athlete's health history that may not be on a standard form. The clinician should also understand what sport(s) the athlete is planning to engage in because certain history or physical examination findings may preclude the athlete from participating in specific sports. For example, patients with a history of seizure disorder can participate in a wide variety of sports; however, the athlete would be disqualified from scuba diving. A clinician should also inquire if an athlete has ever been medically disqualified from participating in sport in the past or if their participation has been restricted. If they have been disqualified or restricted, explore why this occurred. If this was due to a medical condition or injury, explore if that condition has resolved, been effectively managed, or rehabilitated and no longer poses a risk to safe athletic participation.

The recommended baseline history includes the following areas:

- Any current health concerns
- Medical conditions and diseases

> **Box 78.2 History Components of Sports Physical**
>
> **Past Medical History**
>
> Allergies
> Asthma or exercise-induced bronchospasm
> Burning/stinging pain, numbness, or tingling caused by a contact injury
> Congenital disorder
> Infectious diseases
> - Chickenpox
> - Hepatitis
> - Measles
> - Mononucleosis
> - Pneumonia
> - Rheumatic fever
> - Skin infections/rashes
> - Tuberculosis
>
> Diabetes
> Disqualification from sports previously
> Eating disorders
> Glasses/contacts use and visual disturbance
> Heart murmur
> Heart conditions (i.e., arrhythmia or palpitations)
> Heat injury/illness
> Hernia
> Hypertension/hypotension
> Immunization status
> Kidney disease
> Medications (prescription, over the counter, supplements)
> Menstrual history
> Mental health disorders (i.e., anxiety, depression, suicidality)
> Paired organ injury or loss
> Sickle cell disease/trait
> Seizures
> Surgeries
>
> **Sports-Specific History**
>
> Chest pain with exercise
> Concussions
> Dental trauma
> Excessive shortness of breath
> Excessive fatigue with exercise
> Feeling faint or passing out with exercise
> Orthopedic injuries
> - Sprains/strains
> - Traumatic or stress fractures
> - Dislocations
> - Back or neck injuries
>
> **Family History**
>
> Diabetes
> Heart disease
> Hypertension
> Unexpected death before age 50
>
> Source: Bernhardt DT, Roberts WO. *Preparticipation Physical Evaluation*. 5th ed. McGraw-Hill; 2019.

- Surgeries
- Heat or musculoskeletal injuries
- Orthotics or bracing used
- Hospitalizations
- Medications (prescription, over the counter, supplements)
- Allergies (medications, insects, environmental)
- Immunization status
- Cardiac history
- Menstrual history
- Psychosocial history (depression, anxiety, disordered eating, substance-use disorder)

Additional information that should be elicited include the following:

- **Asthma**—Exercise-induced asthma is a common cause of exertional chest pain in young athletes and can be a sign of left ventricular outflow tract obstruction or coronary artery anomalies. If this is a new condition, the athlete should be referred to a pulmonologist. Asthma is not a condition that would disqualify an athlete from participation. It is important for the clinician to reinforce the need to have an asthma action plan and for the athlete to have a metered-dose inhaler readily available while engaged in sport.
- **Cognitive or physical disability**—The principles of safe athletic participation need to guide the clinician's approach to the athlete with cognitive or physical disability. The clinician needs to keep in mind associated physical conditions that exist with specific disabilities that can affect clearance for specific sport or activity. For example, athletes who have Down's syndrome have a greater incidence of ligamentous laxity and atlantoaxial instability, placing them at greater risk for joint and cervical spinal cord injury.
- **Concussion**—For athletes with a concussion history, the provider should determine the number of concussions the athlete has had, their duration, frequency, recovery time, and risk factors. Athletes should have further neurocognitive assessment if they report having experienced multiple prior concussions. A clinician should give consideration to holding clearance, and obtain further evaluation, for athletes who have experienced concussion due to lesser force or impact, with increasing frequency, increasing severity of symptoms, increasing time to recover, or incomplete recovery of symptoms. Athletes with signs and symptoms of concussion (brief loss of consciousness after an injury, memory problems, confusion, drowsiness or feeling

sluggish, dizziness, double or blurred vision, headache) or postconcussion syndrome (headaches, dizziness, fatigue, irritability, anxiety, insomnia, loss of concentration and memory, and noise and light sensitivity) should not be cleared for participation until all symptoms have resolved. Formal balance testing, such as the Balance Error Scoring System [BESS] (Table 78.2) and neuropsychological testing, can be done before sports participation and when head injury occurs to determine when the athlete can return to play. Although some clinicians utilize this baseline testing, the AAP does not generally recommend it.

- **Diabetes**—Athletes with a medical history of diabetes should have a good understanding of caloric intake/expenditure and glycemic control before, during, and after exercise. These athletes need to pay close attention to blood glucose, hydration, insulin, and diet. The athlete should be encouraged to wear a diabetic alert bracelet and to ensure the coach or athletic trainer understands how to deliver emergency medications. Although athletes with diabetes can participate in most sports, certain activities are considered high risk because of the consequences if the athlete experiences hypoglycemia. These sports include rock climbing, scuba diving, and skydiving.

- **Dyspnea on exertion**—Dyspnea on exertion and becoming easily fatigued may simply represent poor conditioning. However, primary pulmonary hypertension, profound anemia, exercise-induced asthma, or an underlying cardiovascular disorder should be suspected. The athlete should be referred for a work-up before participation.

- **Family history of premature sudden cardiac death (SCD)**—A family history of premature (younger than 50 years) SCD is particularly relevant in identifying athletes who have an increased risk of experiencing SCD themselves. SCD is estimated to occur in young athletes at a rate of between 1:40,000 and 1:80,000 athletes. This incidence is greater in males and African American athletes. Hypertrophic cardiomyopathy is a major risk factor, believed to account for up to 35% of SCDs. Long QT syndrome, arrhythmogenic right ventricular cardiomyopathy, Marfan syndrome (detailed later), and congenital coronary artery anomalies are other identified common causes. The American Heart Association (AHA) has developed a 14-element cardiovascular screening checklist for congenital and genetic heart disease, which can be used by clinicians to screen athletes for cardiovascular risk. Electrocardiography (ECG) is generally not recommended as a screening tool for all athletes. For athletes who have positive history findings and increased risk for SCD, further evaluation should be performed, including an ECG, echocardiography, exercise stress testing, and lipid panels to evaluate for occult cardiovascular disease. In addition, a cardiology referral should be considered.

- **Hematological disorders**—Athletes with bleeding disorders such as hemophilia and von Willebrand

TABLE 78.2 Balance Error Scoring System Testing for Concussion

Test	Component	Timing
DOUBLE LEG STANCE		
• Stand with feet pelvic width apart • Hands on hips • Eyes closed	On firm surface	20 seconds
SINGLE LEG STANCE		
• Stand on the nondominant leg with contralateral limb in approximately 20° of hip flexion, 45° of knee flexion • Hands on hips • Eyes closed	On firm surface	20 seconds
TANDEM STANCE		
• Dominant foot in front of the nondominant foot • Heel of the anterior foot touching the toe of the posterior foot • Hands on hips • Eyes closed	On firm surface	20 seconds
DOUBLE LEG STANCE		
• Stand with feet pelvis width apart • Hands on hips • Eyes closed	On foam surface	20 seconds
SINGLE LEG STANCE		
• Stand on the nondominant leg with contralateral limb in approximately 20° of hip flexion, 45° of knee flexion • Hands on hips • Eyes closed	On foam surface	20 seconds
TANDEM STANCE		
• Dominant foot in front of the nondominant foot • Heel of the anterior foot touching the toe of the posterior foot • Hands on hips • Eyes closed	On foam surface	20 seconds

Note: No shoes should be worn.
Scoring: Count balance errors—opening the eyes; hands coming off hips; a step, stumble, or fall; moving the hips more than 30°; lifting the forefoot or heel; or remaining out of testing position for more than 5 seconds. Compare with presports participation score.
Source: Mucha A, Trbovich A. Considerations for diagnosis and management of concussion. *J Orthop Sports Phys Ther*. 2019;49(11):787–798.

disease should be encouraged to engage in athletics. A hematologist should provide guidance, counseling, bleeding prophylaxis, and surveillance. Children with hemophilia who exercise regularly have a lower rate of spontaneous bleeding than children who do not exercise regularly. Guidelines from the CDC, National Hemophilia Foundation, and the World Federation of Hemophilia give recommendations for sports to engage in for athletes with hemophilia. In general, these athletes should avoid contact activities and sports that have a high risk for injury such as basketball, wrestling, bodybuilding, and waterskiing. Those with sickle cell trait may participate in most activities, but athletes with sickle cell disease should have decisions about clearance made on a case-by-case basis. They are frequently recommended to participate in low-intensity activities, including swimming, golf, and running. Exercise at high altitude, especially in humid or hot environments and without acclimatization, dehydration, and illness, poses risks for exertional sickness. Vaso-occlusion and ischemia occur due to the exertional sickling, which in turn can lead to acute rhabdomyolysis. In athletes, acute exertional rhabdomyolysis is a leading atraumatic cause of death.

- **Infectious mononucleosis**—Athletes who have had a recent mononucleosis infection should be evaluated for pharyngitis, lymphadenopathy, fever, and splenomegaly during physical examination. Due to associated splenomegaly, these athletes are at risk for splenic injury. Because the majority of splenic injuries occur within 3 weeks of illness, it is recommended that the athlete rest for at least 3 weeks. If at 3 weeks the athlete's symptoms have resolved, the athlete can begin light activity at week 4. A clinician can consider clearance for sport at week 5 on a case-by-case basis and based on patient assessment.
- **Mental health**—A mental health screening of athletes can easily be included in the PPE. The Patient Health Questionnaire (PHQ)-9 and PHQ-4 are easy tools to use to screen for depression and anxiety during the PPE. Athletes who experience anxiety or depression without suicidal ideation should not be prevented from sport participation. Athletes in weight-sensitive sports (boxing, wrestling) and aesthetic sports (diving, figure skating, dance, cheerleading) are at risk for eating disorders such as anorexia and bulimia. An athlete who consistently does not consume enough calories relative to their level of activity can develop a syndrome called *relative energy deficiency in sports* (RED-S). Although this can affect both males and females, in females this is commonly known as *female athlete triad* (disordered eating, amenorrhea/oligomenorrhea, low bone mineral density). Other common symptoms include stress fractures, fatigue, hair loss, low body mass index, and anemia. This has the potential for long-term multisystem adverse effects. During the PPE, the clinician should evaluate athletes for potential substance-use disorder. This could include alcohol, opiate, stimulant, tobacco, or anabolic steroid use.
- **Musculoskeletal**—The most common reasons for an athlete being disqualified for sport are musculoskeletal conditions. The clinician should ask about any current complaints and prior injuries that caused the athlete to not be able to participate in sport. Inquire about any treatment or rehabilitation. The athlete should be asked about any bracing, taping, or orthotics used during sport participation.
- **Paired organs**—For athletes who have an absence or injury of one of a paired organ (eye, ovary, testicle, or kidney), they need to ensure protective equipment is worn during sport to protect the remaining solitary organ. An athletic cup should be worn to protect a solitary testicle and a protective kidney guard can be worn to protect a solitary kidney. Sports such as skiing, cycling, and horseback riding have an increased risk for renal injury. Wrestling, baseball, soccer, and lacrosse have an increased risk of testicular injury for athletes. An athlete with one functional eye must wear protective eyewear, preferably athletic goggles with polycarbonate lenses and secured to the athlete with a head strap. Standard eyewear or contact lenses provide little to no eye protection for the athlete. Athletes with a single functional eye are recommended against participating in boxing or full-contact martial arts. The risk for injury to the remaining solitary organ in relation to the athletic activity should be assessed. The athlete and parent/guardian should fully understand the risk of injury to the remaining organ and the consequences if an injury should occur.
- **Palpitations**—Palpitations may signify supraventricular tachycardia, sinus tachycardia, right ventricular cardiomyopathy, or long QT syndrome. Abruptness of onset, heart rate, and frequency of episodes should be evaluated. A sudden onset of a fast heart rate suggests supraventricular tachycardia, especially if it can be resolved with vagal maneuvers. A gradual onset and relief of palpitations on exertion suggests sinus tachycardia. The athlete should be asked about use of tobacco, caffeine, alcohol, over-the-counter medications, supplements, and illicit drugs. Sports participation should be restricted, and the athlete should be referred for a basic work-up (i.e., electrolyte testing, thyroid function testing, and careful ECG evaluation) with consideration for a cardiology evaluation. If the etiology of palpitations is not clear, then further evaluation for malignant arrhythmia with Holter monitoring should be done.
- **Seizures**—Athletes with well-controlled seizures can participate in most sports, including contact sports. The exceptions are those sports that could be fatal, such as skydiving, hang-gliding, and scuba diving, if the athlete experienced a seizure during participation. For those with poorly controlled or uncontrolled seizure disorder, evaluation and clearance needs to be performed on a case-by-case basis.

- **Syncope and presyncope**—Athletes with exercise-related syncope or presyncope may have left ventricular outflow tract obstruction, arrhythmia, or congenital coronary anomalies and require further evaluation to rule out structural cardiovascular disease. They should not participate in sports until cleared by a cardiologist. The patient will likely have further evaluation with an ECG and echocardiogram. A congenital coronary anomaly, most often a coronary artery that arises from the opposite aortic sinus, should also be suspected when an athlete presents with chest pain or syncope.
- **Transgender athletes**—Although controversy may exist around certain aspects of transgender athlete participation in organized sport, such as competition categories or hormone levels, clearance for sport for the transgender athlete is generally the same as for other athletes.

Physical Examination

The physical examination is a screening tool that emphasizes the areas of greatest concern in sports participation. Table 78.3 lists areas to focus on in each system.

Vital Signs

The usual pulse, respirations, blood pressure, and temperature should be assessed in the athlete. Approximately 6% of athletes will be found to have hypertension on PPE. Athletes who are febrile should have clearance held until they are no longer febrile. Fever can increase an athlete's risk for heat stroke or exhaustion, dehydration, decreased cardiac output, and hypotension. Height and weight can be utilized to evaluate growth and development of the young athlete. This can also be an indicator of obesity or anorexia. Obesity and anorexia are not contraindications to athletic participation; however, they do increase the risk for other conditions such as heat injury, slipped capital femoral epiphysis, and stress fractures.

Head, Ears, Eyes, Nose, and Throat

Visual acuity is the focus of the eye examination. If the athlete's vision is greater than 20/40 in one or both eyes, they should be referred for an eye examination. Monocular vision and detached retina disqualify the athlete from contact sports. People who are legally blind are not disqualified from participating in athletics. The United States Association of Blind Athletes details several sports

TABLE 78.3 Physical Examination Focus Points and Considerations

Area	Focus Points and Considerations
General appearance	Appearance of characteristic signs of Marfan syndrome
Height/weight	Anorexia, bulimia, obesity, any evidence of disordered eating or relative energy deficiency in sports (RED-S) or female athlete triad
Head	Concussion, unexplained hair loss
Eyes/ear/nose/throat	Visual acuity, monocular vision, detached retina, high narrow palate, oral/dental health, cerumen, gross hearing assessment, equality of pupils, nasal polyps, deviated septum
Pulses	Irregular rhythm, rate, symmetry or quality, aortic coarctation
Blood pressure	Hypertension/hypotension
Heart	Murmurs or abnormal heart sounds, valve prolapse or regurgitation, exertional syncope, dizziness, chest pain with activity, palpitations
Lungs	Wheezing or abnormal lung sounds, frequent cough, pectus carinatum or excavatum, active tuberculosis, uncontrolled asthma, pulmonary insufficiency, and history of spontaneous pneumothorax
Abdomen	Hepatomegaly, splenomegaly, abdominal rigidity, pain, masses
Genitourinary	Costovertebral angle tenderness, kidney disorder, single kidney, discomfort with urination
Genitalia (boys)	Femoral or inguinal hernia, singular testicle, undescended testicle, testicular masses
Skin	Contagious skin lesions (tinea, boils, impetigo, herpes simplex), stretch marks from Marfan or weight loss
Musculoskeletal	Range of motion, strength, joint stability, symmetry or deformity, pain, joint locking, giving way or crepitus, scoliosis. Pes planus, hammer toes, joint laxity, long fingers and toes from Marfan
Neurological	Sensory loss, numbness, tingling, reflexes

Source: Bernhardt DT, Roberts WO. *Preparticipation Physical Evaluation.* 5th ed. McGraw-Hill; 2019.

their members compete in. These include limited or no-contact sports such as running, powerlifting, swimming, soccer, and goalball. An otoscope examination of the ears, nose, and throat should be done, but abnormalities rarely indicate disqualification from sports participation. Any cerumen impaction should be cleared before participating in sport. Nasal polyps or a deviated nasal septum do not disqualify an athlete from participation.

Cardiovascular System

All peripheral pulses should be assessed and all four valves of the heart auscultated. A diminished femoral pulse compared with radial pulses is a sign of aortic coarctation. The clinician should assess heart sounds with the patient in at least two positions (e.g., standing and supine). For any identified irregular heart sounds or murmur that have not been detected previously, the athlete should be referred for an echocardiogram. The most common cause of SCD in athletes is hypertrophic cardiomyopathy. A systolic murmur heard along the right upper sternal border that increases with a Valsalva maneuver (decreasing cardiac preload) and standing, but decreases with handgrip and squat maneuvers, is a classic sign. Symptoms usually occur during peak physical exertion or in volume-depleted states. Any irregularity of heart rate should be checked by ECG, as a prolonged QT interval can be a cause of sudden death. Serious arrhythmias are usually detectable when the athlete holds their breath.

Normal blood pressure for children is less than the 90% percentile (less than 120/80 mm Hg). Hypertension must be controlled before sports participation. The AAP Clinical Practice Guideline for Screening and Management of High Blood Pressure in Children and Adolescents can serve as guidance for clinicians. Clinicians need to remember that a diagnosis of hypertension in a child is based on three or more findings of elevated blood pressure greater than the 95% percentile for height, weight, and age. These should be measured on separate occasions, not a singular blood pressure measurement identified on a single office visit. The clinician should explore the use of tobacco, caffeine, or other stimulants as a component for the athlete's elevated blood pressure.

AAP recommends no limitations on athletic eligibility for those athletes with elevated blood pressure (previously called *prehypertension*) greater than or equal to the 90th percentile to less than the 95th percentile or 120/<80 mm_Hg to 129/<80. Children with stage 1 hypertension (greater than or equal to the 95th percentile to less than the 95th percentile + 12 mm Hg, or 130/80 to 139/89 mm Hg), without end-organ damage, are eligible for sport participation. Lifestyle modifications, follow-up repeat blood pressure measurement, and referral for those with confirmed stage 1 hypertension is appropriate. For children with stage 2 hypertension (greater than or equal to the 95th percentile + 12 mm_Hg, or greater than or equal to 140/90 mm Hg) without end-organ damage, sports such as weightlifting and cycling with a high static component should be restricted. Appropriate referral should be made for blood pressure management.

A consensus statement by the American College of Cardiology and the AHA includes guidelines for eligibility for athletes who have previously been diagnosed with cardiac conditions based on the intensity of the sport. The guidelines allow athletes with known hypertrophic cardiomyopathy to participate in low-intensity activities, but recommend exclusion from most strenuous activities.

Respiratory System

The respiratory rate should be measured and all lung fields auscultated, both anteriorly and posteriorly. Assess for the presence of any wheezing on examination. The clinician should inquire about any wheezing that the athlete perceives during sport, which may be consistent with exercise-induced bronchospasm and may not be found on a resting examination. Uncontrolled asthma and exercise-induced deoxygenation are reasons to restrict contact sports participation.

Neuromuscular

A key component of the neuromuscular examination is symmetry. This includes symmetry in range of motion, muscle strength, sensation, and reflexes. Range of motion should be full, symmetrical, and pain-free in all directions assessed. Asymmetry should be further examined. Asymmetry in reflexes, with hyperreflexia, may be indicative of a central nervous system (CNS) lesion. Asymmetry in strength or range of motion may be a sign of a prior or unresolved injury. Athletes who have had a recent injury for which they have been receiving treatment may seek input from the treating provider regarding clearance for sport. Athletes with pain, weakness, atrophy, joint instability, or joint locking should have further evaluation.

Although the typical neuromuscular examination on PPE consists of a brief screening, some additional assessments can be predictive of injury risk. For example, the box drop test can be moderately predictive of risk for anterior cruciate ligament injury.

Range of motion of the neck should be evaluated. The athlete should be able to flex the cervical spine forward, extend backward, laterally bend to the right and left, and should be able to rotate the head from right to left. Motion should be full in all directions, symmetrical, and pain free. If the athlete reports burning pain, weakness, numbness, or tingling in the upper extremities, cervical nerve impingement should be suspected. Other possible conditions are stenosis, congenital fusions, and disc herniation. Athletes with Down's syndrome have a greater risk for atlantoaxial instability.

Inspect for symmetry of the shoulder girdle. Asymmetry of muscle bulk may be a sign of suprascapular nerve impingement. Asymmetry of shoulder height may be an indication of scoliosis. Assessment includes trapezius muscle strength, deltoid muscle strength, and glenohumeral range of motion. The athlete should shrug and abduct their shoulders against resistance. External and internal rotation of the shoulders should be observed. This can easily be performed by asking the athlete to put their hands behind their back and then place their hands behind their neck. Strength and motion assessment should be pain free, full, and symmetrical.

Range of motion of the elbows should be assessed. The athlete should be able to extend and flex the elbows, and then pronate and supinate the forearm fully, symmetrically, and without pain.

Range of motion of the wrists with plantar flexion, dorsiflexion, and internal and external rotation should be assessed. For the hands and fingers, the athlete should be instructed to make a fist and then spread the fingers. Bilateral grip should be tested to evaluate upper extremity strength. Strength and motion should be symmetrical, full, and pain free.

The spine should be assessed for scoliosis and range of motion, as well as hamstring flexibility. The athlete should be instructed to stand up straight, flex forward at the waist, extend back, bend laterally, and then rotate to both sides. Range of motion should be symmetrical and without pain. Discomfort into the lower extremities with range of motion of the back may be a sign of tight hamstring muscles or could be a sign of a lumbar spine nerve impingement. Back pain with lumbar extension may be a sign of spondylolysis, a defect or stress fracture of the vertebral arch, which could be the result of an acute or repetitive sport injury.

An athlete with scoliosis can have asymmetry in height of the shoulder girdles, asymmetry of the pelvic girdle, and a unilateral elevation of the thoracic cage ("rib hump") with an Adams' forward bending test. To perform the Adams' test, the examiner stands behind the athlete to visualize the thorax, then the athlete bends forward at the waist. The examiner visualizes any asymmetry of the thoracic cage. Athletes with scoliosis should be able to participate in sport; however, they should be further evaluated with assessment for further progression of the spinal curve.

Strength, balance, and range of motion of hips, knees, and ankles are tested by instructing the athlete to squat down and duck-walk four steps. Calf strength, symmetry, and balance are assessed by instructing the athlete to walk on tiptoe and walk on heels. Although the box drop test mentioned earlier is frequently not part of the standard PPE, the test is simple to perform and can be moderately predictive of risk for anterior cruciate ligament (ACL) injury. The athlete jumps down to the floor from a step then immediately springs up, jumping to a maximal height. Athletes unable to perform this, who have imbalance, or whose knee(s) deviate medially (valgus) should have further assessment.

Gastrointestinal System

The abdomen should be palpated to check for pain or masses, and the liver and spleen size should be assessed because of the risk of rupture in contact sports. Any costovertebral angle tenderness may indicate kidney problems. Clearance should be held until further work-up for athletes with masses, tenderness, hepatosplenomegaly, or abdominal rigidity.

Hernias

An inguinal hernia check should be done on all male athletes, and they should be taught how to do a testicular self-examination and what to look for. Athletes with a symptomatic inguinal hernia should be referred for surgical consultation. The need for a genital examination is an area of controversy among sports medicine physicians.

Skin

The athlete should be asked to show any skin lesions to the examiner. Contagious skin lesions such as tinea corporis, boils, impetigo, scabies, and herpes lesions will disqualify the athlete until corrected.

Assessment for Marfan Syndrome

Marfan syndrome is an inherited autosomal-dominant disorder that affects connective tissue and commonly the heart, eyes, blood vessels, and skeleton. Signs an athlete has Marfan syndrome include long arms, legs, and fingers; tall, thin body type; kyphoscoliosis; pectus carinatum or excavatum; hyperflexible joints; pes planus; and hammer toes. Oral examination may show crowded teeth and a high, narrow palate. Stretch marks on the skin may be noted that are not related to weight gain or loss. Because aortic root dilation is common with Marfan syndrome and can cause aortic dissection and sudden death, the AHA recommends including examination for the physical signs of Marfan syndrome, auscultation of all four heart valves for heart murmurs, palpation of peripheral pulses, and brachial artery blood pressure taken in the sitting position. On auscultation of the heart, listen for evidence of aortic stenosis, mitral valve prolapse, or aortic murmur. Marfan syndrome can affect the eyes, leading to retinal detachment, glaucoma, or myopia.

Evaluation including ECG, slit-lamp eye examination, and echocardiography to assess the aortic root is also recommended for males taller than 6 feet (1.83 m) and females taller than 5 feet 10 in (1.78 m) who have two or more physical manifestations of Marfan syndrome.

Clearance

Ultimately, clearance for sport is done on a case-by-case basis and based on the history and physical examination findings during the PPE, keeping in mind the basic principle of promoting safe athletic participation. Although less than 2% of athletes are disqualified from sport, up to 13% will require some type of additional work-up or evaluation after the PPE. If any problems were identified, the clinician should consider if the athlete or the athlete's competitors are at increased risk for injury or illness if this athlete participates in their selected sport.

If there are problems identified on examination, consider if the athlete can fully participate with protective gear, with medication management, and/or while engaged in rehabilitation for the problem. If the athlete is not safe to engage in full participation, consider engaging the athlete in limited participation or an alternate sport.

Clearance can be divided into five categories:

1. **Unrestricted clearance**—Athletes have full, unrestricted clearance to engage in any and all sports and all levels of participation appropriate for their age.
2. **Cleared for sport, no restrictions, but with recommendations for further evaluation and treatment**—The athlete is cleared to participate in sports activity, but it is determined that he or she should have further evaluation and treatment for an identified condition. This is for a condition that would not affect the athlete's ability to participate safely in athletics. For example, an athlete who is experiencing mild depression may be referred for therapy or counseling, but should be able to participate in athletics without restriction.
3. **Not cleared for sport until after completion of further evaluation or rehabilitation**—If the athlete has a health issue that needs evaluation or treatment or has suspicious signs or symptoms, further work-up or treatment may be needed before sports participation is safe. Clearance after completion of further evaluation or rehabilitation should be chosen.
4. **Disqualification or no clearance for certain types of sports**—Disqualification is the appropriate category when a known condition prohibits an athlete's safe participation in the given sport. Disqualification from one sport typically does not preclude the athlete from participating in another sport. Examples of conditions that can limit participation for types of sport activities are shown in Table 78.4.
5. **Disqualification for any and all sports**—This category conveys that it is completely unsafe for the person to participate in any sporting activity, no matter what the category or intensity. Less than 1% of PPE will result in this type of disqualification.

TABLE 78.4 Sports Participation and Qualification			
Problem	**Contact/Collision**	**Limited Contact**	**Noncontact**
Acute infections: respiratory, genitourinary, mononucleosis, hepatitis, rheumatic fever, tuberculosis	X	X	X
Hemorrhagic disease—hemophilia and von Willebrand disease	X	J	J
Diabetes—inadequately controlled	X	X	X
Diabetes—controlled	O	O	O
Eyes—single eye or detached retina	X	O (w/protective eyewear)	O (w/protective eyewear)
Corrected visual acuity <20/200	X	J	J
Glaucoma	X	X	O
Exercise-induced bronchospasm with/without asthma (controlled)	O	O	O
Respiratory—*severe pulmonary insufficiency	X	X	X
Resolved spontaneous pneumothorax	J	J	J
Cardiovascular—*mitral/aortic valve stenosis/prolapse, aortic insufficiency, coarctation of aorta, cyanotic heart disease, recent carditis	X	X	X
Hypertension—*uncontrolled	X	X	X
Hypertension—controlled	O	O	O
Previous heart surgery	J	J	J
Hepatomegaly (acute)	X	X	X
Hepatomegaly (chronic)	J	J	J
Splenomegaly	X	X	X

> **Box 79.1 Collecting Medical and Social Histories**
>
> **Medical History**
>
> - Gender-related surgical interventions: what specific procedures have been performed and to what extent; what are the plans for continued surgeries; medication/hormone therapies. (Note: it is also important to ask about family history as it relates to the patient's use or potential use of hormone therapies.)
> - Reproductive history: specific to transgender men; pregnancies, births, complications, hysterectomy (partial or full), PCOS.
>
> **Social History**
>
> - Sexual history: approach this topic gradually and sensitively. Assess sexual behaviors including vaginal or anal intercourse, oral sex, and other sexual activities; number and gender of partners (do not assume); sexual function; comfort during sex; high-risk sexual activity; sexual orientation.
> - Psychiatric history: assess for mood disorders and anxiety disorders; past trauma; gender dysphoria. Also assess self-care activities.
> - Family, socioeconomic, and social supports: elicit information regarding social rejection, isolation, discrimination, workplace struggles, family relationships.
> - Spiritual/religious history: assess for type of religion or lack thereof; effect of religion or spiritual beliefs on transgender status/transition; shame or guilt based on spirituality.
> - Unwanted gender-conforming behaviors:
>   - Assess for "tucking" in transgender women, the hiding of the penis and scrotum, which includes tucking the testicles into the inguinal canal; can be very harmful. Continual tucking may result in significant discomfort and the development of inguinal defects and hernias.
>   - Assess for chest binding in transgender men, minimizing the appearance of the breasts by tightly wrapping or taping them down to have a flat appearance; continual binding can cause significant discomfort to the chest, shoulders, back, and abdomen; may cause skin irritation or result in respiratory problems (shortness of breath).

Commonly, transgender patients may present to primary care with some type of mental health complaint. The most common mental health complaints are gender dysphoria, anxiety, and depression. Screening for all of these conditions should take place in the primary care setting. Specifically, the use of screening tools, including the Patient Health Questionnaire-9 and the Generalized Anxiety Disorder-7 scales, can be easily implemented in primary care settings to screen for depression and anxiety, respectively. If any these symptoms or diagnoses are present at the time of the examination, the provider should fully assess these complaints and provide the appropriate intervention.

Laboratory Assessment

Currently, there are no recommendations specific to transgender patients related to normal laboratory values. Therefore, the normal laboratory reference ranges should be used. Providers should keep in mind the current use of hormonal therapies and their effect on laboratory values. In trans women, the creatinine levels may be slightly elevated compared with the normal reference range due to preserved muscle mass, and hematocrit may be slightly low due to reduced testosterone. Conversely, trans men may have an elevated hematocrit because of their use of testosterone supplementation.

COMMON GENDER-AFFIRMING TREATMENTS – TRANS MEN

Often, the priorities for trans men (female-to-male or FTM) seeking gender-affirming treatment include the induction of physical changes to match their gender identity. This may consist of hormonal therapy or surgery, including gender-reassignment surgeries. It is important to note that not all trans men choose to undergo gender-affirming treatments (hormonal or surgical), so the provider should identify treatment goals early in the encounter.

Hormonal Therapy

In trans men, the most important medication used for hormone therapy is testosterone. The goal of testosterone use is to cease menses and induce virilization (deepening of voice, growing sexual and facial hair, and increasing muscle mass).

Surgery

Some of the surgeries trans men may undergo include:

- Oophorectomy—the removal of ovaries
- Hysterectomy—the removal of the uterus (partial hysterectomy) and cervix (total hysterectomy)
- Vaginectomy—the removal of the vagina
- Chest reconstruction—the rebuilding of the chest wall
- Mastectomy—the removal of breast tissue
- Metoidioplasty—the construction of a neopenis involving changing the clitoris into a penis. The urethra is lengthened and positioned through the neopenis using the skin of the labia minora to allow the trans man to urinate while standing.
- Phalloplasty—the creation of a neopenis by using skin from the arm, thigh, back, or abdomen. After this procedure, the trans man may choose to have a penile implant to be able to achieve an erection. Compared with a metoidioplasty, this procedure results in a larger neopenis.

- Scrotoplasty—the creation of a scrotum by hollowing out and repositioning the labia majora and inserting testicular implants.

COMMON GENDER-AFFIRMING TREATMENTS – TRANS WOMEN

Trans women (male-to-female or MTF) have specific goals related to their gender-affirming treatments. Usually of priority is the reduction and elimination of facial hair growth, reduction of muscle, and the induction of breast formation. Trans women may also choose to undergo gender-reassignment surgery, at which time a referral to a surgical specialist is indicated. Again, it is important to note that not all individuals choose to undergo gender-affirming treatments (hormonal or surgical); therefore, discussing treatment goals with the patient is important.

Hormonal/Medication Therapy

There are multiple types of medications trans women use as part of gender-affirming treatment, including:

- Androgen blockers
- Estrogens
- Gonadotropin-releasing hormones
- Finasteride

Surgery

Some of the surgeries trans women may undergo include:

- Orchiectomy—to remove both testicles and the source of endogenous testosterone
- Penectomy—the removal of the penis
- Vaginoplasty—the creation of a vagina, including a vaginal canal and external genitalia, often created by using the skin of the scrotum and penis
- Breast augmentation—the creation of or increase in size of breasts

PHARMACOLOGICAL CONSIDERATIONS

There are important pharmacological considerations in transgender patients related to the common medications used for gender affirmation. The medications commonly used in the transgender population are listed in Drugs Commonly Prescribed 79.1.

Drugs Commonly Prescribed 79.1: Medications Used for Gender Affirmation

DRUG	GOALS OF TREATMENT	DOSING	MONITORING	ADVERSE EFFECTS
Transgender Men				
Testosterone: Available in multiple formulations: gel, patch, buccal tablets, intramuscular injection	Masculinizing effects 1) Deepen voice. 2) Promote hair growth on upper lip, chin, cheeks. 3) Increase muscle mass and contour as a male; decrease fat. 4) Clitoral enlargement. 5) Increase sexual desire. Cease menstruation 1) Menses usually stop within a few months of starting testosterone therapy. If bleeding persists, the addition of an oral progestin may be warranted (medroxyprogesterone).	Transdermal: 1%–1.6%, 2.5–10 g/day IM: 50–100 mg weekly Available in gel, patch, intramuscular, and buccal tablet formulations.	1) Goal for serum levels to be at the same levels as their cisgender counterparts (400–700 ng/dL) 2) Recommended serum testosterone monitoring every 3 months for the first 12 months, then once or twice annually 3) Estradiol less than 50 pg/mL 4) Serum hematocrit—may be elevated 5) Weight 6) Blood pressure 7) Bone mineral density—testosterone increases bone demineralization	Adverse effects 1) Heart disease 2) Erythrocytosis 3) Persistent bleeding

Drugs Commonly Prescribed 79.1: Medications Used for Gender Affirmation—cont'd

DRUG	GOALS OF TREATMENT	DOSING	MONITORING	ADVERSE EFFECTS
Transgender Women				
Androgen blockers	1) Decrease hair growth. 2) Reduce testosterone secretion.	Spironolactone: 100–300 mg/day Cyproterone acetate: 25–50 mg/day	1) Blood pressure 2) Electrolytes	Hypotension
Estrogens	1) Suppress androgen secretion.	Oral: 2–10 mg/day (varies by formulation). Transdermal: 50–100 μg/day Note: If testes remain intact, a higher dose may be needed for androgen suppression.	1) Serum testosterone levels every 3 months for the first 12 months, then once or twice annually. 2) Bone mineral density	1) Venous thromboembolism (VTE) 2) Increased incidence of breast cancer. Contraindications 1) VTE 2) Cardiovascular disease 3) Cerebrovascular accident 4) Liver dysfunction 5) Breast cancer
Gonadotropin-releasing hormones	1) Suppress testicular testosterone production. 2) Stop undesired pubertal changes in adolescents.	Available as injection, implant and infusion. Dose varies significantly by drug.	1) Cardiovascular disease 2) Cerebrovascular disease 3) Seizures 4) Bone density loss	
Finasteride	1) Inhibits conversion of testosterone to dihydrotestosterone, which is more potent than testosterone. 2) Treats benign prostatic hypertrophy in transgender women with prostate still intact. 3) Helps prevent hair loss.	1–5 mg orally	None required. Prostate-specific antigen optional.	1) Angioedema 2) Prostate cancer 3) Breast cancer 4) Male infertility

GENDER-APPROPRIATE CARE

Throughout this chapter, there has been emphasis on the importance of referring to the patient using the correct gender terminology, although it is essential to remember their biological sex when considering pathology. Transgender individuals remain susceptible to the same ailments as their cisgender counterparts. It is important for the provider to assess early in the encounter what state of transition (gender reassignment surgery, hormone therapy, etc.) the patient is in to be able to identify the appropriate assessment needs.

Both trans men and trans women are susceptible to osteoporosis, cardiovascular disease, and mental health ailments. Estrogen and testosterone are both important for bone mineral density, so when these levels are altered, there is increased risk for demineralization and the development of osteoporosis. This may be further influenced by the introduction of hormone-replacement therapy in transgender individuals undergoing sex reassignment. Screening for osteoporosis is recommended for trans women older than age 65 and for trans women aged 50 to 65 who have been off estrogen for more than 5 years (Feldman, 2016). Trans men do not require routine screening for osteoporosis unless they have not maintained physiological male levels of testosterone, or if they are high risk because of other factors shown in their history and physical examination.

Cardiovascular disease should also be considered in the assessment and health promotion of transgender individuals. The effects of cross-sex hormones in this population increase the risk of cardiovascular complications. Oral estrogen has been noted to induce prothrombotic coagulation factors, and testosterone use in trans men has resulted in increased total cholesterol and triglycerides, and reductions in high-density lipoproteins. In addition, smoking is more prevalent in the transgender population than in the general population, further increasing cardiovascular risk. Therefore, smoking cessation, cholesterol management, exercise, and weight management are all important health promotion recommendations for these patients.

As with any patient, it is important to assess the mental health of transgender patients. Of particular importance in this population is identification and treatment of gender dysphoria. Gender dysphoria is commonly the cause for other mental health diagnoses including depression, mood disorders, anxiety disorders, and suicidality in transgender individuals, and the rates are much higher in this population compared with their cisgender counterparts. Transgender patients, however, experience less gender dysphoria when provided access to gender-affirming hormone therapy earlier, emphasizing the importance of early access to comprehensive care.

Trans Men

Trans men have many of the same considerations in primary care as their cisgender (female) counterparts, and therefore need the appropriate screening. Among trans men who have not had a chest surgery, they remain at increased risk for breast cancer. Therefore, ordering mammograms annually for trans men aged 45 to 54, and every other year after the age of 55 is essential in identifying breast cancers early. For trans men who have not had a hysterectomy, they remain at risk for ovarian, cervical, and endometrial cancers. Therefore, pelvic examination with Papanicolaou test is recommended every 3 years for ages 21 to 29, and every 5 years for human papillomavirus screening for ages 30 to 65 years. Trans men who have not had a hysterectomy are also at risk for pregnancy if they are engaging in sexual intercourse with biological males, and therefore eliciting information about menstrual cycle and performing urine pregnancy testing is necessary.

Trans Women

Just as trans men have the same considerations as their cisgender counterparts, so do trans women. Of particular importance is the screening for prostate cancer in all trans women. Prostatectomy is not a procedure performed during sex reassignment surgery, which leaves the organ susceptible to cancer. Therefore, the provider and patient should determine whether digital rectal examinations and prostate-specific antigen screenings should be considered as part of routine screening.

Unfortunately, transgender individuals often experience obstacles or blockades to appropriate treatment. Due to stigmatization, access to care for transgender individuals may be reduced compared with their cisgender counterparts. For example, trans men may not be welcomed in a gynecological office where many of the previously mentioned examinations may be performed because of their gender identity. As a result, the primary care provider may become responsible for completing these examinations or the patient may not receive the care they need. Conversely, providers may not consider the need for prostate examinations if they are not comfortable with the aspects of caring for a trans woman.

CONCLUSION

Care for transgender patients is an important component of the role of primary care providers. Caring for this population is not complex and does not require specialized training, but it does necessitate an understanding of and sensitivity to the needs of transgender individuals. The provider needs to strive to build trust with the patient by expressing compassion and empathy, and by using correct gender-related terminology. Identifying the patient's treatment goals is essential to developing a comprehensive and appropriate plan of care of the transgender person. Once these goals are known, the primary care provider will be able to meet the needs of the patient and collaborate with specialists in the care of transgender individuals. Primary care providers can also go above and beyond the direct care of the patient and promote the creation of community, regional, and national priorities to improve health care for transgender individuals.

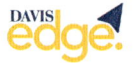 Go to Davis Edge for practice Q&A.

REFERENCES

American Psychiatric Association Publishing. Diagnostic and Statistical Manual of Mental Disorders: DSM-5-TR 5th edition, text revision; 2022.

Aitken S. The primary health care of transgender adults. *Sex Health*. 2018;14(5):477-483.

Beckwith N, McDowell MJ, Reisner SL, Zaslow S, Weiss RD, Mayer KH, Keuroghlian AS. Psychiatric epidemiology of transgender and nonbinary adult patients at an urban health center. *LGBT Health*. 2019;6(2):51-61.

Bonvicini KA. LGBT healthcare disparities: What progress have we made? *Patient Educ Couns*. 2017;100(12):2357-2361.

Casey LS, Reisner SL, Findling MG, Blendon RJ, Benson JM, Sayde JM, Miller C. Discrimination in the United States: experiences of lesbian, gay, bisexual, transgender, and queer Americans. *Health Serv Res*. 2019;54:1454-1466.

Center of Excellence for Transgender Health. *Primary Care Protocol for Transgender Patient Care*. 2nd ed. Deutsch MB, ed. University of California, San Francisco; 2016.

Cicero EC, Reisner SL, Silva SG, Merwin EI, Humphreys JC. Healthcare experiences of transgender adults: an integrated mixed research literature review. *ANS.* 2019;42(2):123-138.

Dilaveri C, Klassen C, Fazzio R, Ghosh K. Breast cancer screening for women at average risk. *J Clin Immunol.* 2019;11:123-128.

Elamin MB, Garcia MZ, Murad MH, Erwin PJ, Montori VM. Effect of sex steroid use on cardiovascular risk in transsexual individuals: a systematic review and meta-analysis. *Clin Endocrinol.* 2010; 72:1-10.

Feldman J. Preventive care of the transgender patient: an evidence based approach. In: Ettner R, Monstrey S, Coleman E, eds. *Principals of Transgender Medicine and Surgery.* 2nd ed. New York: Routledge; 2016:100-120.

Flores AR, Herman JL, Gates GJ, et al. How many adults identify as transgender in the United States? Los Angeles: The Williams Institute; 2016. https://williamsinstitute.law.ucla.edu/publications/trans-adults-united-states/. Accessed February 3, 2021.

Grant J, Mottet L, Tanis J, Herman JL, Harrison J, Keisling M. National transgender discrimination survey report on health and health care. Published 2010. Retrieved from https://scholar.google.com/scholar?q=the+National+Transgender+Discrimination+Survey:+Report+on+Health+and+Health+Care&hl=en&as_sdt=0&as_vis=1&oi=scholart. Accessed February 3, 2021.

Hembree W, Cohen-Kettenis P, Gooren L. Endocrine Treatment of Gender-Dysphoric/Gender-Incongruent Persons: An Endocrine Society Clinical Practice Guideline. *J Clin Endocrinol Metab.* 2017;102(11):3869-3903.

Johnson AH, Hill I, Beach-Ferrara J, Rogers BA, Bradford A. Common barriers to healthcare for transgender people in the U.S. Southeast. *Int J Transgend Health.* 2020;21(1):70-78.

King WM, Hughto J, Operario D. Transgender stigma: a critical scoping review of definitions, domains, and measures used in empirical research. *Soc Sci Med.* 2020;250:112867.

Lakkis NA, Mahmassani DM. Screening instruments for depression in primary care: a concise review for clinicians. *Postgrad Med.* 2015;127(1):99-106.

Oeffinger KC, et al. American Cancer Society. Breast cancer screening for women at average risk: 2015 guideline update from the American Cancer Society. *JAMA.* 2015;314(15):1599-1614.

Roberts TK, Kraft CS, French D, et al. Interpreting laboratory results in transgender patients on hormone therapy. *Am J Med.* 2014;127(2):159-162.

Roselli CE. Neurobiology of gender identity and sexual orientation. *J Neuroendocrinol.* 2018;30(7):e12562.

Safer JD, Coleman E, Feldman J, et al. Barriers to healthcare for transgender individuals. *Curr Opin Endocrinol Diabetes Obes.* 2016;23(2):168-171.

Safer JD, Tangpricha V. Care of the transgender persons. *New Engl J Med.* 2019;381:2451-2460.

Sapra A, Bhandari P, Sharma S, Chanpura T, Lopp L. Using Generalized Anxiety Disorder-2 (GAD-2) and GAD-7 in a primary care setting. *Cureus.* 2020;12(5):e8224.

Sawaya GF, Kulasingam S, Denberg TD, Qaseem A. Cervical cancer screening in average-risk women: best practice advice from the Clinical Guidelines Committee of the American College of Physicians. *Ann Int Med.* 2015;162(12):851-859.

Sevelius JM. Gender affirmation: a framework for conceptualizing risk behavior among transgender women of color. *Sex Roles.* 2013;68:675-689.

Stanczyk FZ, Archer DF, Bhavnani BR. Ethinyl estradiol and 17betaestradiol in combined oral contraceptives: pharmacokinetics, pharmacodynamics and risk assessment. *Contraception.* 2013;87:706-727.

Whitlock BL, et al. Primary care in transgender persons. *Endocrinol Metab Clin. North Am.* 2019;48(2):377-390.

Wierckx K, Mueller S, Weyers S, Van Caenegem E, Roef G, Heylens G, T'Sjoen G. Long-term evaluation of cross-sex hormone treatment in transsexual persons. *J Sex Med.* 2012;9:2641-2651.

Williams Institute. Race and ethnicity of adults who identify as transgender in the United States. 2016. https://williamsinstitute.law.ucla.edu/wp-content/uploads/Race-Ethnicity-Trans-Adults-US-Oct-2016.pdf. Accessed February 3, 2021.

RESOURCES

Resources for Health Care Providers

Eight Best Practices for HIV Prevention Among Trans People
   https://prevention.ucsf.edu/

Glossary of Terms for Health Care Teams (Fenway)
   https://www.lgbtqiahealtheducation.org/publication/lgbtqia-glossary-of-terms-for-health-care-teams/

Health Equity for Diverse Populations
   https://www.hrsa.gov/about/organization/bureaus/ohe/populations/diverse-populations.html#lgbt

Healthy People 2030: LGBT
   https://health.gov/healthypeople/objectives-and-data/browse-objectives/lgbt

Meeting the Needs of Transgender Individuals
   https://www.lgbtqiahealtheducation.org/wp-content/uploads/Sari-slides_final1.pdf

Transgender Health Resources
   https://www.amsa.org/advocacy/action-committees/gender-sexuality/transgender-health/

Resources for Transgender and Gender-Diverse Individuals

CDC HIV Reduction Tool
   https://hivrisk.cdc.gov/

Know Your Rights in Healthcare
   https://transequality.org/know-your-rights/healthcare

Ten Things Transgender Persons Should Discuss with their Healthcare Provider (GLMA)
   http://www.glma.org/index.cfm?fuseaction=Page.viewPage&pageID=692

The Trevor Project (Crisis Resource)
   866-488-7386

Trans Lifeline (Crisis Resource)
   877-565-8860

Transgender Organizations

Gender Diversity
   http://www.genderdiversity.org/

National Center for Transgender Equality
   https://transequality.org/

Transgender Americans Veterans Association (TAVA)
   http://transveteran.org/

Trans Latina Coalition
   https://www.translatinacoalition.org/

Trans People of Color Coalition
   https://www.glaad.org/tags/trans-people-color-coalition

Chapter 80

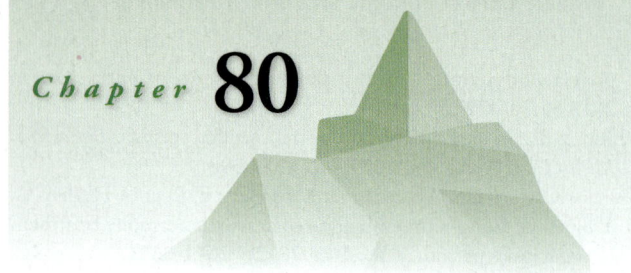

Primary Care of Veterans

Michael E. Zychowicz, DNP, ANP, ONP, FAAN, FAANP
Sherley Belizaire, DNP, PMHNP-BC, FNP-BC
Janet G. Campbell, DNP, ANP-BC, ACNS, COHN-S
Angela Richard-Eaglin, DNP, MSN, FNP-BC, CNE, FAANP
Michelle Gibson, MSN, PMHNP-BC, CARN-AP
Michael Anthony Moore, MSN, NP-C, RN, HIV-PCP
Susan Wilkinson, MSN, PMHNP-BC

INTRODUCTION

In the United States, there are more than 20 million veterans who have served our country during times of peace or wartime, accounting for nearly 10% of the U.S. population. This includes veterans who have served in World War II, the Korean War, the Vietnam War, and the wars in Iraq and Afghanistan. Veterans are at greater risk for and have a greater incidence of many health conditions, including musculoskeletal (MSK) problems, mental health conditions, and exposure to hazards and toxins. To say the least, veterans' health care is complex. Veterans who have been deployed and endured combat or transitioning and reintegrating to civilian life are at greater risk for suicide, depression, substance-use disorder (SUD), traumatic brain injury (TBI), and post-traumatic stress disorder (PTSD).

More than 9 million veterans receive care in the Veterans Health Administration (VHA) system. The VHA has 1,255 health-care facilities under the administration of the Under Secretary for Health. This includes 1,074 outpatient clinics and 170 medical centers. The VA health-care facilities distributed across the United States and its territories are grouped into 18 regional Veterans Integrated Service Networks (VISNs). The regional grouping of facilities allows the health-care systems within the VISN to work together, enhancing access to care and meeting local or regional health-care needs. Within areas of each VISN, regional medical centers and clinics may come together as a health-care system to offer veterans services in a more efficient, convenient, and coordinated fashion. As a component of regional health-care systems, community-based outpatient clinics (CBOCs) can be convenient options for veterans to obtain primary care or various outpatient specialty services. These clinics allow the VHA to expand veterans' access to care away from the medical centers. Lastly, community living centers (CLCs), or skilled nursing facilities, within the VHA system can provide long-term care, rehabilitation, or hospice care to veterans.

With more than 300,000 full-time health-care providers, the VHA is the largest integrated health-care system in the United States, providing a wide range of services. These include surgery, emergency and critical care, mental health, orthopedics, pharmacy, radiology, and physical therapy. Most VHA medical centers will offer specialty or advanced services such as audiology and speech pathology, dermatology, dental, geriatrics, neurology, oncology, organ transplant, podiatry, plastic surgery, prosthetics, urology, and vision care.

The mission of the VHA is to "Honor America's veterans by providing exceptional health care that improves their health and well-being." In a systematic review by O'Hanlon et al. (2017), VA health-care facilities were found to be comparable or favorable to non-VA health-care facilities regarding safety, which includes measures of morbidity, mortality, and complications. Effectiveness of VA care, which includes quality of preventive care, recommended care, end-of-life care, nonambulatory care, and medication management were seen to be similar or superior in comparison to non-VA health-care systems.

Although less than 50% of veterans receive care at the VHA, a majority obtain care in the community from providers who are not VA health-care providers. These veterans may live too far away from a VHA facility or in a rural and underserved area. A veteran may also be ineligible for VA benefits due to a dishonorable discharge or another reason. More than half of veterans receive health care from community providers who may know little of the unique health-care needs of veterans. One VHA program, the Veterans' Choice Program, facilitates veterans' ability to receive care for service-connected conditions outside the VA system in cases of a demonstrated excessive travel burden or wait time to obtain an appointment with a VA provider. With this, it is essential for community non-VA health-care providers to understand the unique health-care needs of veterans.

NON-VA HEALTH-CARE PROVIDERS

Non-VA health-care providers who deliver care to veterans need to have some understanding of the special needs of their veteran patient population. Veteran patients have unique needs and experiences that stem from military service in addition to the same health-care needs as anyone in the general population. Deployments, engaging in combat, and specific military occupations add to the complexity of veterans' needs. Providers who have greater competence in veteran-centric care and needs may help enhance veterans' health-care outcomes.

A study by Vest et al. (2018) demonstrated non-VA health-care providers have limited awareness of how military service could potentially require modification of the health-care delivered. Additionally, they found many non-VA health-care providers have little or uneven understanding of military culture, the scope of services the VA provides, or the stressors of military life and deployment. The study also states that non-VA health-care providers have diminished self-efficacy in evaluating and managing veteran-specific health-care needs. Additionally, some non-VA providers assume that the VA will be the only provider for all military service-related care to veterans.

Although it is important to ask about military service, less than 20% of non-VA primary care providers will seek this information. Knowing veteran status and perhaps adding it to electronic health records can potentially prompt for veteran-centric screening tools to identify common health-care conditions such as PTSD or TBI.

The VA provides some general guidance for those non-VA providers about questions to ask veterans. Asking veterans questions about their service can help the clinician understand service-related medical or mental health problems and patient concerns. A clinician may want to start by asking for permission to ask about the patient's military experience. Some patients may not want to share painful experiences or even feel ashamed of things they have done during combat. The clinician should ask questions in a safe and private space. Use good eye contact and supportive tone of voice. If the veteran discloses painful, stressful, personal, or traumatic experiences, thank them for sharing those feelings and experiences with you.

Ask the veteran what branch of service they were in and what their occupation was, as this can potentially reveal specific occupation-related exposures or hazards. Knowing when the veteran served also helps guide the clinician to consider the health risks and exposures related to different military service eras. Ask if they were ever deployed, how many times, and if they were ever in combat. Ask about any illnesses or injuries and any residual effects or disability that occurred while in the military. Depending on the patient's answers, the clinician may want the patient to elaborate or to ask some follow-up questions. See Table 80.1 for sample questions a provider can ask about a patient's military health history.

MILITARY SEPARATION

Roughly 200,000 service members separate from military service each year. This transition from active-duty service back to civilian life is a significant stressor for those separating from military service. This time of military separation is a critical time that can significantly affect veterans and their families going into the future.

Nearly half of veterans report personal difficulty during this period of transition back to civilian life. Some new veterans have difficulty moving to civilian life with significantly less structure, supervision, and camaraderie, as well as loss of close friendships. Some veterans contend with homelessness and socioeconomic problems.

Veterans receive screening and referral for mental health and SUD on separation from service; however, this screening and referral to services may not be adequate. Roughly half of veterans experience anger, strained family relationships, and frequent outbursts after separation. Separation adjustment, among other mental health conditions including SUD, PTSD, and depression, is another concern after transition. Among active-duty service members, more than a quarter report moderate to heavy alcohol use, which frequently continues after military separation.

MILITARY AND VETERAN FAMILIES

Military service poses unique challenges to the families of service members while on active duty. The stress that accompanies separation from service, discussed previously, is yet another stressor on the veteran and the family. The mental and physical health conditions that veterans may experience certainly can impact and affect the entire family.

TABLE 80.1 Military Health History Questions	
General questions	**Would it be OK if I talked with you about your military experience?**
	When and where did you/do you serve and in what branch?
	What type of work did you/do you do while in the service?
	Did you have any illnesses or injuries while in the service?
	Did you ever become ill while you were in the service?
	Were you or a buddy wounded, injured, or hospitalized?
	Did you have a head injury with loss of consciousness, loss of memory, "seeing stars," or being temporarily disoriented?

Continued

TABLE 80.1 Military Health History Questions—cont'd	
General questions	**Would it be OK if I talked with you about your military experience?**
	Did you see combat, enemy fire, or casualties?
	Were you a prisoner of war?
Compensation and benefits	Do you have a service-connected condition?
	Would you like assistance in filing for compensation for injuries or illnesses related to your service?
Living situation	Would it be OK to talk about your living situation?
	Where do you live and whom do you live with?
	Is your housing safe?
	Are you in any danger of losing your housing?
	Do you need assistance in caring for yourself and/or dependents?
Unwanted sexual experiences in the military	May I ask you about stressful experiences that men and women can have during military service?
	Did you have any unwanted sexual experiences in the military? For example, threatening or repeated sexual attention, comments, or touching?
	Did you have any sexual contact against your will or when unable to say no, such as being forced, or when asleep or intoxicated? **If Yes**: I am sorry; thank you for sharing that. VA refers to this as "military sexual trauma" or "MST" and offers free MST-related care. **If No**: Okay, thank you. I ask all veterans because VA offers free care related to these experiences.
Exposure concerns	Would it be OK if I asked about some things you may have been exposed to during your service?
	What _____ were you exposed to? (chemicals, biologics, psychological trauma or abuse, physical injury or exposure)
	What precautions were taken? (avoidance, PPE, treatment)
	How long was the exposure?
	How concerned are you about the exposure?
	Where were you exposed?
	When were you exposed?
	Who else may have been affected? Unit name, etc.
Behavior	Would it be OK if we talked about emotional responses during your service?
	Have you been concerned that you might suffer from post-traumatic stress disorder? Symptoms can include reexperiencing symptoms such as nightmares or unwanted thoughts, hyperarousal/being "on guard," avoiding situations that remind you of the trauma, and/or numbing of emotions.
	Have you been experiencing sadness, feelings of hopelessness/helplessness, lack of energy, difficulty with concentrating, and/or poor sleep?
	Have you had thoughts of harming yourself or others?
Blood-borne viruses (hepatitis and HIV)	Do you have tattoos?
	Have you ever injected or snorted drugs, such as heroin, cocaine, or methamphetamine?
	Have you ever been tested for hepatitis C or HIV? If not, would you like to be tested for these?

Source: Adapted from U.S. Department of Veterans Affairs, Veterans Health Administration. Military Health History Pocket Card for Health Professionals Trainees & Clinicians. https://www.va.gov/OAA/archive/Military-Health-History-Card-for-print.pdf

Regular separation of the service member from their family for prolonged training or deployment puts a significant strain on the family members. This includes growing apart from one's spouse, shifting of marital or parenting roles, and changing home responsibilities. Stressors can contribute to possible spousal depression, anxiety, and adjustment disorder. Longer deployment is associated with greater risk for divorce.

Another stressful component of military life for families is frequent geographical relocation, which can disrupt social networks and support systems, affect spousal employment, and potentially negatively affect financial and family well-being. Families of service members or veterans who are grappling with effects of PTSD or combat stress have a greater risk for domestic or intimate partner violence as well as child maltreatment.

Although military families and families of veterans can experience many stressors, there are also some characteristic adaptive strengths. Military families develop resilience, adaptability, and flexibility in their family roles and responsibilities due to service member deployments or assignment for training. Military families can be described as confident, independent, patriotic, and proud.

EXPOSURE TO RISKS FOR ILLNESS AND INJURY

Throughout history, service members have been subject to a variety of physical, environmental, and psychological stressors and exposures associated with military service. Some exposures can result in acute episodic illness or injury, whereas other exposures can result in lifelong illness. Veterans may face certain unique health challenges depending on when and where they served. Although there may be some overlap in the types of health issues, each service era also has some issues that are unique. These war eras include World War II, the Korean War, the Vietnam War, the Cold War era, the Persian Gulf War (Operations Desert Shield and Desert Storm), the Iraq war (Operations Iraqi Freedom [OIF] and Operation New Dawn), and the Afghanistan war (Operation Enduring Freedom [OEF]). Health-care providers should be aware of the risks and prevalence of diseases and conditions during each of these eras (see Table 80.2) to enhance the probability of veterans achieving optimal health outcomes.

Environmental Exposures

Veterans, particularly those having served in combat, have the potential to be exposed to environmental toxins or irritants. Service during OEF and OIF potentiated environmental exposure to air pollution from burn pits, depleted uranium (DU), contaminated food/water, petrochemicals, chemical weapons, biological or radiological warfare agents, vaccines including the anthrax vaccine, prophylactic medicines, insect bites, insect repellants, and herbicides. Airborne hazards from burning trash or oil fires have been associated with reports of chronic respiratory conditions and decreased lung function.

Gulf War–era veterans were also exposed to asbestos and chemical-biological agents. They have a higher

TABLE 80.2 Health Issues, Risks, and Exposures Related to Military Service Era

	World War II (September 1, 1939 to September 2, 1945)	Korean War (June 25, 1950 to July 27, 1953)	Vietnam War (November 1, 1965 to April 30, 1975)	Cold War Era (Between 1945 and 1991)	Gulf War (After August 2, 1990)	Iraq War (March 19, 2003 to December 15, 2011)	Afghanistan War (After October 7, 2001)
Noise injury/hearing loss	X	X	X	X	X	X	X
Radiation exposure	X			X	X (depleted uranium)	X (depleted uranium)	X (depleted uranium)
Extreme cold	X	X					X
Extreme heat					X	X	X
Chemical or biological weapons	X (mustard gas)				X (mustard gas)	X	X
Pesticides and herbicides			X (Agent Orange)	X (Agent Orange)	X		

Continued

TABLE 80.2 Health Issues, Risks, and Exposures Related to Military Service Era—cont'd							
	World War II (September 1, 1939 to September 2, 1945)	Korean War (June 25, 1950 to July 27, 1953)	Vietnam War (November 1, 1965 to April 30, 1975)	Cold War Era (Between 1945 and 1991)	Gulf War (After August 2, 1990)	Iraq War (March 19, 2003 to December 15, 2011)	Afghanistan War (After October 7, 2001)
Infectious disease			X (hepatitis C)		X	X	X
Sand, dust, and particulate exposure					X	X	X
Smoke					X (oil well fires)	X (burn pits)	X (burn pits)
Toxic embedded fragments (shrapnel)					X	X	X
Traumatic brain injury						X	X
Rabies						X	X
Occupational hazards from chemicals, paints, radiation, etc.	X	X	X	X	X	X	X
Chemical Agent Resistant Coating (CARC) paint					X		
Side effects of antimalarial Mefloquine						X	X

Source: Adapted from U.S. Department of Veterans Affairs. (n.d.) Veterans health issues related to service history. https://www.va.gov/health-care/health-needs-conditions/health-issues-related-to-service-era/

incidence of chronic fatigue, joint pain, and cognitive deficits, also referred to as *Gulf War illness* (GWI), compared with nondeployed veterans. DU is both a chemo-toxic and a radio-toxic element. Possible harmful effects from exposure to DU are related to damage of mitochondrial DNA and may be one of the causes of GWI.

Many veterans who served during the Vietnam War have developed chronic disease resulting from exposure to Agent Orange (see Table 80.3), an herbicide used to clear foliage to enhance visualization of enemy forces. The VA has identified several illnesses associated with Agent Orange exposure including B-cell leukemia, Hodgkin disease, lung and prostate cancers, ischemic heart disease, and type 2 diabetes mellitus. Advanced practice nurses should obtain the veteran patient's health history including military service dates to help the clinician gather knowledge of potential environmental exposures.

Infectious Diseases and Blood-borne Pathogens

Traumatic injuries commonly lead to infections, including skin and soft tissue infection, osteomyelitis, and urinary tract infection. Infectious diseases related to military service, particularly in Southwest Asia, include malaria, brucellosis, *Campylobacter jejuni*, *Coxiella burnetii* (Q fever), *Mycobacterium tuberculosis*, nontyphoid salmonella, shigella, leishmaniasis, and West Nile virus (Table 80.4).

These diseases can have a delayed presentation, emphasizing the need to ask veterans about overseas military service. For returning veterans who present with relapsing-remitting fevers, fatigue, muscle or joint aches,

TABLE 80.3 Conditions Resulting From Agent Orange Exposure	
Cancers	**Other Health Conditions**
• AL amyloidosis • Chronic B-cell leukemias • Chloracne • Type 2 diabetes • Hodgkin's disease • Ischemic heart disease • Multiple myeloma • Non-Hodgkin's lymphoma	• Parkinson's disease • Early onset peripheral neuropathy • Porphyria cutanea tarda • Prostate cancer • Respiratory cancers • Soft tissue sarcomas

Source: U.S. Department of Veterans Affairs. (n.d.) Veterans' Diseases Associated with Agent Orange. https://www.publichealth.va.gov/exposures/agentorange/conditions/index.asp

TABLE 80.4 Infectious Diseases Related to Military Service in Southeast Asia and Afghanistan

Malaria	An infectious disease caused by a parasite transmitted by mosquitoes. Symptoms include chills, fever, and sweats.
Brucellosis	A bacterial disease with symptoms such as profuse sweating and joint and muscle pain. The illness may be chronic and persist for years.
Campylobacter jejuni	A bacterial disease with symptoms such as abdominal pain, diarrhea, and fever.
Coxiella burnetii (Q fever)	A bacterial disease with symptoms such as fever, severe headache, and gastrointestinal problems such as nausea and diarrhea. In chronic cases, the illness may cause inflammation of the heart.
Mycobacterium tuberculosis	A bacterial illness that primarily affects the lungs and causes symptoms such as chest pain, persistent cough (sometimes bloody), weight loss, and fever.
Nontyphoid salmonella	A condition characterized by symptoms such as nausea, vomiting, and diarrhea.
Shigella	A bacterial illness characterized by symptoms such as fever, nausea, vomiting, and diarrhea.
Visceral leishmaniasis	A parasitic disease characterized by symptoms such as fever, weight loss, enlargement of the spleen and liver, and anemia.
West Nile virus	A viral disease spread by mosquitoes characterized by symptoms such as fever, headache, muscle pain or weakness, nausea, and vomiting. Symptoms may range from mild to severe.

persistent cough, and/or nonhealing skin ulcers, consideration should be given to the diagnoses presented earlier.

Hepatitis C and HIV

Chronic hepatitis C virus (HCV) is the most prevalent blood-borne pathogen in the United States. Veterans have been disproportionately affected by this condition. HCV seropositivity predictors include demographic factors, Vietnam War–era military service, health-care utilization, and lifestyle factors. More than one-third have reported at least a traditional risk factor of transfusion or intravenous drug use.

In 2013, 174,302 HCV-infected veterans were seeking care for HCV at VA facilities, making the VA the world's largest provider of care for HCV. Most veterans living with a diagnosis of HCV were born between 1945 and 1965 and were subsequently infected with HCV between 1970 and 1990. HCV-related complications such as cirrhosis, hepatocellular carcinoma (HCC), and mortality are the sequelae and primary aims of the VA's aggressive viral eradication efforts.

The VHA continues to provide unrestricted access to HCV treatments, including prescribing direct-acting antiviral (DAA) therapy. This has shown success in achieving cure in a majority of the VA's overall caseload. DAAs became available in January 2014, leading to greater than 92,000 HCV-infected veterans achieving a cure rate exceeding 90%. The overall incidence of HCV-related HCC among VHA patients decreased after the viral eradication efforts between 2014 and 2016. The VA continues to make testing, treating, and curing HCV infection a priority and has treated more than 123,000 veterans and cured more than 105,000 with HCV. All veterans enrolled in VA health care are eligible to receive serology testing for HCV. Advanced practice nurses should ask veterans about their periods of military service and whether they have been screened for HCV. Although there are many veterans who receive primary health care at the VA, a considerable portion of veterans may receive care in the private sector, making screening a vital step toward identification of HCV infection and subsequent referral for appropriate treatment.

The VA currently cares for more than 30,000 veterans with HIV across the country and is the single largest provider of HIV care. Greater than 43% of all veterans enrolled in VA for care are tested for HIV, which is representative of the commitment to ensuring all veterans continue to have access to testing and high-quality HIV care at diagnosis.

Prevention of HIV remains an essential aim with recommendation for testing at least once, and for those with higher risk to be tested at least annually. Veterans who test positive should be linked to care immediately. There are great tools to help prevent HIV, including pre-exposure prophylaxis (PrEP). PrEP is a daily pill that is highly effective at preventing HIV. Education is another primary strategy in preventing HIV. This should include discussion about practicing safe sex and avoiding needle-sharing. Veterans can ask their VA providers about condoms, PrEP, or local syringe service programs. Advanced practice nurses should ask veterans if they have been screened for HIV. Community and federal partners play a critical role in extending care to veterans for the prevention, early detection, and treatment of HIV.

Noise-Induced Hearing Loss

Hazardous noise exposure causes injury to the hearing mechanisms in the inner ear. The symptoms of acoustic trauma are hearing loss, tinnitus, aural fullness, ear pain with loud noise, difficulty localizing sounds, difficulty hearing in a noisy background, and vertigo. Hearing loss, tinnitus, and acoustic trauma are commonly related to veteran combat and weapons training experiences. Disability resulting from acoustic trauma affects 13% to 18% of the veteran population. Permanent hearing loss resulting from hazardous noise exposure may stem from an acute injury or cumulative exposure from high-caliber weapons and explosives. Hearing loss secondary to acoustic trauma is significant due to the highly sensitive structure of the tympanic membrane, which can easily perforate and is vulnerable to the effects of blast injury described later.

Hearing loss can have a profound effect on personal safety, impaired communication, and balance secondary to vestibular deficits, which may present as vertigo. Tinnitus is linked to significant cognitive and psychological comorbidities, sharing many characteristics with PTSD.

Patients should be referred for specialty otolaryngology and audiology evaluation and testing based on symptom presentation. This would include findings such as debris in the external ear canal that does not clear with topical ear drops, inability to visualize the tympanic membrane, persistent dizziness, and noticeable communication problems or tinnitus that interferes with the patient's daily activities.

Blast Injuries and Traumatic Brain Injury

Blast injuries are complex and are a direct result of either a direct impact, rapid acceleration/deceleration, or blast injury sustained from traditional ordnance or improvised explosive devices (IEDs). The most frequent blast injury sustained by U.S. service members deployed to Iraq or Afghanistan is mild TBI (mTBI), or concussion, most often caused by blast waves from an IED or other explosive ordnance. A TBI is one of the most significantly debilitating conditions identified in combat veterans. The direct effect of blast waves and extent of injury is determined by the proximity to the source of the blast subjecting the brain to concussive injury. Advanced practice nurses should ask veterans about a history of TBI and treat related conditions accordingly.

VETERAN MENTAL HEALTH NEEDS

Post-Traumatic Stress Disorder

People can develop PTSD after exposure to a traumatic event, serious injury, violence, and/or death. This may include directly experiencing or witnessing a traumatic event. This can also include learning about a traumatic event that occurred to a close friend or family member. For veterans who may have experienced these types of traumatic exposures while in service, it is not difficult to understand that they have a greater risk for the development of PTSD. Service-related traumatic exposures may accompany combat experiences such as firefights, personal injury, or injury and death of fellow service members. PTSD may also follow noncombat trauma such as military sexual trauma (MST).

An overwhelming majority of veterans and military service members will be exposed to some type of potentially PTSD-causing traumatic event at some time in their life. The prevalence of PTSD among Vietnam, Persian Gulf, OEF, and OIF veterans is between 10% and 13%. National Guard and Reserve members of the military, who were called to active duty and deployed, have a greater risk for developing PTSD than full-time active-duty service members. This is significant in that U.S. combat operations after the 9/11 attacks relied heavily on deploying National Guard and Reserve service members. There is a greater risk for PTSD in veterans who were enlisted service members, have a history of depression, have decreased social support, experienced sexual or physical assault, or experienced a disabling combat-related injury or illness.

PTSD is characterized by several symptoms, including recurrent, involuntary, and intrusive thoughts or distressing dreams. People with PTSD can experience dissociative states, commonly known as *flashbacks*. A trigger event may lead to a significant physiological reaction or psychological distress, which can be prolonged and intense. People may also attempt to avoid things that are connected with the traumatic event. This includes people, places, memories, feelings, discussion, activities, or objects. Cognition, mood, reactivity (i.e., exaggerated startle), and arousal (i.e., sleep disturbance) may be altered as well with PTSD. The PTSD checklist for *Diagnostic and Statistical Manual of Mental Disorders, Fifth Edition, Text Revision* (DSM-5-TR; PCL-5) is commonly used as a screening tool to evaluate for PTSD in patients. To diagnose a patient with PTSD, symptoms must be present for more than a month, other potential causes for the symptoms (i.e., medication or alcohol) should be excluded, and the symptoms have led to clinically significant distress or impaired social or occupational relationships.

PTSD not only affects the mental health of veterans, but their physical health as well. Veterans who experience PTSD have a higher incidence of health problems and greater health-care utilization. Evidence exists demonstrating greater mortality rate for veterans with PTSD in comparison to those without PTSD. Death due to homicide, suicide, and accident are greater for veterans with PTSD compared with those without PTSD. Veterans with PTSD have a greater risk for obesity; tobacco use; dyslipidemia; hypertension; cardiovascular disease; and inflammatory, autoimmune, and MSK disorders. Evaluation and management strategies for PTSD are detailed in Chapter 70.

Suicide

Suicide is a significant public health problem in the United States. The pain that families, loved ones, and communities experience after a person dies by suicide is immeasurable. Suicide among military veterans has historically been lower than the general population but has always been a public health concern. The rate of suicide among military service members and veterans has increased since the beginning of OIF. In 2008, the rate of suicide among military members was greater than the general population. The VA health-care system has placed a high priority on preventing and reducing veteran suicide through increasing attention and availability of mental health services.

Veterans currently have a 21% greater rate of suicide compared with the general population. More than 20 veterans per day will die by suicide. There is a significantly greater risk of suicide among veterans who do not utilize VA services in comparison to those who engage with VA health care. In comparing male and female veterans who do not use VA services, females have a significantly greater rate of suicide than males. Generally, there is a greater rate of veteran suicide in western states and a greater number of suicides in highly populated areas of the United States. A majority of veteran suicides are the result of firearm injuries. Although there is a larger number of veteran suicides among middle-aged and older veterans, the younger veteran population (18 to 29 years) has a greater rate of suicide per capita.

Assessing veterans for suicide risk factors is a significant role of the primary care or mental health clinician. The Patient Health Questionnaire 9 (PHQ-9) is a good tool that is widely used for screening for suicide risk. Another commonly used tool is the Columbia Suicide Severity Rating Scale (C-SSRS). Unfortunately, suicide screening tools are believed to have a low degree of accuracy and high rate of false positives.

Treatment of those with self-injurious thoughts and behaviors is complex. Management may include hospitalization or psychotherapy. Cognitive behavioral therapy can reduce suicidal ideation, suicide behaviors, and feelings of hopelessness. Lethal means counseling among patients, their family/significant others, and providers is aimed at identifying potential lethal means (e.g., firearms, opioids, or poisons) and developing a plan for reducing or eliminating lethal means for suicide. Evaluation and management of suicidal thoughts and behaviors are described in greater detail in Chapter 69.

Traumatic Brain Injury

TBI can result in permanent or temporary cerebral dysfunction. This can be the result of blast injury, direct impact, or acceleration/deceleration injury. TBI is thought to be one of the signature injuries of the OEF/OIF military engagements. As a result of the increase in IEDs used in the OEF/OIF conflicts, service members wear body armor to provide protection. A combination of body armor use and advances in combat casualty care have led to a greater survival rate after a blast injury. With this, more service members are living with TBI after blast injuries that would have killed them just a few decades ago.

Veterans with an mTBI (loss of consciousness of less than 30 minutes) will have a significantly greater rate of head, neck, and back pain. A common comorbidity that accompanies TBI is chronic pain. Chronic pain is reported at a five to seven times greater rate in veterans with TBI compared with those who have not experienced a TBI. Veterans who experience a TBI because of a blast injury also have an increased risk for developing PTSD, among other mental health conditions. PTSD is a greater risk for those who experienced a loss of consciousness after TBI compared with those who did not lose consciousness. Additionally, suicidal ideation and behavior may be greater for those who have experienced a TBI.

The proximity to detonated blast munitions may affect memory. Veterans exposed to close-range blasts are more likely to demonstrate clinically meaningful memory deficits that should be considered during assessment. mTBI also gives rise to neuroendocrine effects that include chronic pituitary gland dysfunction. Associated symptoms include cognitive deficits, mood disorders, sleep disturbance, significant changes in metabolism and body composition, and increased cardiovascular disease risk.

Treatment for patients with TBI includes therapies such as speech pathology, occupational therapy, physical therapy, rehabilitation, and cognitive behavioral therapy. Sleep disturbance affects many patients after a TBI. A comorbid underlying condition, such as obstructive sleep apnea, needs to be ruled out. Sleep disturbance can exacerbate comorbid mental health conditions, such as PTSD, and can also lead to cognitive impairment. Sleep hygiene, relaxation techniques, physical activity, and environmental and dietary modifications can be used as part of the management plan. Patients may receive acetaminophen or NSAIDs to manage headaches. Medications such as gabapentin and baclofen may be used to manage neuropathic pain or muscle spasm and tension headaches. Tricyclic antidepressants (TCAs) or serotonin and norepinephrine reuptake inhibitors (SNRIs) may augment the management of a patient with a TBI. Evaluation and management of head trauma and TBI are described in greater detail in Chapter 75.

Substance-Use Disorder

SUD is relatively common among military service members and veterans. As with civilians, SUD can significantly negatively affect and disrupt a veteran's life. Substance use among the veteran population increases the risk for homelessness. Veterans' mental health and medical conditions can be negatively affected and complicated with substance use.

While on active duty, military service members experience life stressors that increase their risk for using substances and developing SUD. These stressors include deployments, engagement in combat action, and the stress of military separation and reintegration into civilian life. Common substance use among active military service members includes tobacco (31%), heavy alcohol use (20%), illicit drug use (12%), and misuse of prescription medication (11%). More than half of service members report binge drinking after returning from a combat deployment. Veterans are at increased risk for mortality, decreased overall health, and interpersonal violence if they use or abuse alcohol.

Among combat veterans, substance misuse/abuse and dependence occur at a higher rate than the civilian population. More than 10% of veterans meet the criteria for a diagnosis of SUD when they present to the VA health system for the first time. Tobacco and alcohol SUD among veterans is the most prevalent.

Tobacco dependence is 15% greater in the veteran population compared with the civilian population. For veterans with cardiovascular disease, there is a greater likelihood that they smoke than nonveterans. Smoking also contributes to cancer deaths among veterans. Nearly half of veteran cancer deaths affect current smokers, whereas former smokers account for a quarter of veteran cancer deaths.

Female veterans with a diagnosis of PTSD have a greater risk of developing SUD. A history of MST, childhood sexual abuse, and domestic violence can contribute to an increased risk for a female developing SUD. Female veterans with an SUD, compared with female veterans without SUD, have a greater risk for abuse, trauma, or violence at some point in their life. Some people may have made the decision to join the military so they can escape an adverse or abusive home environment. This history can contribute to a service member or veteran's risk for developing SUD.

Although development of an SUD can be due to stressors of military life, it can also accompany a mental health problem such as depression or PTSD. Veterans with mental health conditions have a greater risk for opiate-use disorder, as well as adverse events related to opiate use. This can include injury, violence, or overdose. Veterans with mental health disorders may have a greater likelihood of being prescribed opioid medication. For patients with PTSD, there is an increased likelihood they may be prescribed a higher dose of an opioid than a veteran without PTSD. Evaluation and management of SUDs are described in greater detail in Chapter 67.

Military Sexual Trauma

MST refers to sexual assault or repeated, threatening sexual harassment experienced during military service. Service members of different races, sexual orientations, and every service era (e.g., Vietnam) report having experienced MST. MST can involve threats, offensive remarks about a person's body or sexual activities, unwelcome sexual advances, touching or grabbing, or unwanted oral/anal/vaginal penetration with an object and/or sexual intercourse. A veteran may be physically forced into participation, unable to consent, or pressured into sexual activities. MST can occur on or off base and while a veteran is on or off duty (Table 80.5).

Most MST survivors remain silent or wait many years before disclosing this trauma. Many are hesitant because they do not think they would be believed or that anything would happen as a result of speaking up. Other reported factors include fear of retaliation and feelings of shame, guilt, or disbelief.

The VA national screening program data revealed that approximately 1 in 3 females and 1 in 50 males responded "yes" to experiencing MST, when screened by their VA provider (U.S. Department of Veterans Affairs, 2020). The rates are higher among females because there are many more males in the military. This incidence of MST is believed to be underreported, however. In males, this is most likely due to stigma, shame, rape myths, lack of empathic response, and one's masculinity and sexuality. Furthermore, approximately 70% of female veterans are not enrolled in VA health care. This is likely a choice due to the VA system reminding female veterans of the military as a male-dominated environment.

There are many contributing factors to a veteran's response to MST, including the type, severity, duration, prior history of trauma, and type of responses from others at the time of the MST. Race, ethnicity, religion, sexual orientation, and cultural variables also affect a veteran's response to the trauma. Veterans may have strong emotions; feelings of numbness; trouble sleeping; or difficulties with attention, concentration, and memory. Those who have experienced MST reported problems with substances, their relationships, or anything that reminds them of trauma. MST survivors may experience headaches, gastrointestinal

TABLE 80.5	Service Member Risk Factors for MST Episode
Sociodemographics	Age between 17 and 24 Earlier in military career Racial minorities Sexual minorities Unmarried Adverse childhood experiences (ACEs)
Aspects of military services	Marines and Navy—Highest Air Force—Lowest Enlisted members—Higher rates
Other contributing factors	High alcohol use, particularly binge drinking Previous trauma Combat exposure

difficulties, chronic pain, fatigue, sexual dysfunction, and eating disorders as a result of their trauma.

It should be noted that not every veteran exposed to MST develops related conditions that affect their functionality. Common symptoms and problems that a veteran may experience because of MST are listed in Box 80.1.

MST is not a diagnosis nor a mental condition. However, it can result in a cluster of symptoms experienced by veterans who have PTSD or other trauma-related disorders. Diagnostic work-up begins with sensitively screening for MST. When screening for MST, remember your ABCs; **A**sk, **B**e authentic, and **C**onnect to care. Good screening practices include a safe environment that ensures privacy and confidentiality. Make eye contact with the veteran, speak in a calm and unrushed tone. Use clear, simple questions with examples and provide empathy and validation. The National Center for Posttraumatic Stress Disorder suggests two screening questions for MST:

1. While you were in the military, did you experience any unwanted sexual attention, such as verbal remarks, touching, or pressure for sexual favors?
2. Did anyone ever use force or threat of force to have sex with you against your will?

If either of these questions are answered affirmatively, it is recommended to use the Primary Care PTSD Screen for DSM-5-TR (PC-PTSD-5) for further screening. Additional screening tools used by mental health providers recommended by the VA/Department of Defense (DoD) include Clinician Administered PTSD Scale (CAPS-5) PTSD Checklist (PCL-5) Life Events Checklist (LEC-5) Post-traumatic Diagnostic Scale (PDS) PTSD Symptom Scale Interview (PSS-I-5).

MST and related sequalae are extremely difficult life experiences. Evidence-based treatments have been shown to mitigate the effects of this life experience. It should be noted that not all veterans who have experienced MST receive their care in the VA. Therefore, it is important for non-VA primary care providers to provide primary screening for MST with their veteran patients. With appropriate and timely treatment, evidence has shown that symptom abatement and sustained recovery are possible. The key is timely treatment and continued support.

The most studied and evidence-based treatment is psychotherapy. Trauma-informed or trauma-focused modalities include cognitive processing therapy (CPT), eye movement desensitization and processing (EMDR), prolonged exposure (PE), narrative exposure therapy (NET), specific cognitive behavioral therapies for PTSD, brief eclectic psychotherapy (BEP), and written narrative exposure. Comprehensive MST management includes assessing for PTSD, major depression, and SUD.

When a veteran has a positive screen for MST, validation and empathy are first-line treatment. Provide MST education, assess the patient's health status, and ask them about their support systems. Due to elevated risk for hyperarousal symptoms, pharmacological treatment may not be effective nor indicated. Of note, pharmacological treatment is not first-line treatment for MST.

There are not many pharmacological treatments approved by the U.S. Food and Drug Administration (FDA) for MST-related PTSD or PTSD in general. Sertraline, paroxetine, fluoxetine, and venlafaxine have a moderate quality of evidence for the management of PTSD and are recommended by the VA/DoD Clinical Practice Guideline for the Management of PTSD and Acute Stress Disorder (2020). Selective serotonin reuptake inhibitors (SSRIs) are some of the most prescribed first-line treatment for symptoms related to depression and anxiety. Prazosin, an alpha-1 blocker medication used to treat hypertension, is often prescribed for PTSD-related nightmares.

The follow-up and referral for MST is similar to PTSD and sexual assault. MST may have a stronger correlation with PTSD than sexual assault in civilians (Bell, 2013). Encourage MST survivors to seek treatment and support services at their local VA facilities. Every VA provides MST-related mental health outpatient services including psychological assessment and evaluation, psycho-pharmacotherapy, and individual/group psychotherapy. In addition to VA facilities, MST outpatient counseling can occur at the Veteran Centers. Veteran Centers are VA community-based counseling centers that provide social and psychological treatments to service members and

---

Box 80.1   Common Symptoms and Problems of MST

- Extremes of emotion or emotional lability
- Emotional disengagement or flatness
- Difficulties with attention, concentration, and memory
- Reexperiencing and strong emotional reactions to reminders of MST
- Hypervigilance
- Trouble sleeping, nightmares
- Suicidal thoughts or behaviors
- Self-harm
- Disordered eating
- Alcohol or substance use
- Difficulties with hierarchical environments
- Sexual dysfunction
- Difficulties in core areas of functioning and well-being
  - Interpersonal difficulties or avoidance of relationships
  - Getting and maintaining employment
  - With school
  - With parenting
  - Identity and sense of self
  - Spirituality issues/crisis of faith
- Homelessness
- Problems related to crime or interaction with the legal system

veterans. Intensive treatment and support are available for MST-related mental health care at inpatient and residential programs at the VA. Gender-specific MST-related treatment programs are available at various sites.

Veterans with a history of MST are entitled to receive MST-related care even if they are not eligible for other VA services. They can receive care for any MST-related physical and/or mental health illnesses without any cost to them. There are MST coordinators at all VA facilities to assist the veteran with issues related to MST. MST coordinators are advocates who can assist the veteran in accessing VA programs and services, federal and state benefits, and community resources. The veteran may also contact Disabled American Veterans (DAV) to speak with the benefits experts, who are veterans as well, to file a claim with the VA. The veteran needs no documentation of MST experiences nor VA disability compensation to receive treatment. The veteran should be encouraged to call the VA's general benefit information hotline at 1-800-827-1000. Sexual assault is discussed further in Chapter 73.

Musculoskeletal Disorders

MSK conditions are a pervasive problem globally. The global burden of MSK disease is substantial and is the second greatest cause of disability. The burden of MSK disease within the military and veteran community occurs at a significantly greater rate than in the civilian population. Veterans will experience a chronic physical health condition at a two to three times greater rate than those in the general population. These conditions can be a result of either combat injury or nonbattle injuries. A majority of the MSK injuries sustained are nonbattle injuries.

In the military population, there is a five times greater occurrence of anterior cruciate ligament (ACL) injury and shoulder dislocation compared with the civilian population. Military veterans have a three times greater incidence of neck and back conditions as nonveterans. Veterans are also more likely than nonveterans to experience some type of activity-limiting condition at a younger age. Due to the physical demands and repetitive stress injury that accompanies military duty, veterans have nearly twice the incidence of osteoarthritis than nonveterans. Although osteoarthritis can be due to overuse and joint strain, it can also be secondary to a traumatic limb injury (post-traumatic osteoarthritis).

The nature and demands of the training and work military members engage in places them at greater risk for nonbattle injury. Nonbattle injuries have a three times greater occurrence than battle injuries. Sprains, strains, fractures, overuse injuries, and other acute injuries are among the common nonbattle injuries. Working and training with weapons, heavy machinery and vehicles, and other occupational hazards increases the risk for injury. Engaging in strenuous activity while carrying heavy loads over challenging terrain can set the stage for acute, overuse, or chronic nonbattle injuries. Wearing body armor and heavy packs contributes to stress and strain of the neck, back, and upper extremities. Activities such as long marches, parachuting, and running contribute to the nonbattle injuries of the lower extremities. For both active-duty military and veterans, back pain is the most common MSK condition they experience. Among active-duty service members, 22% will experience neck and back pain and 28% will have some type of nontraumatic joint disorder.

The nature of combat-related injuries has evolved. Surgical and emergency care of the battlefield-injured service member has advanced. The survival rate for a battlefield-injured person is greater than 90%. In addition, the emergency first-aid and lifesaving training service members receive, as well as the use of body armor, have contributed to increased survival of battlefield-injured veterans.

Given that more service members will live after injuries that would have killed them just a few decades ago, many will live with chronic MSK conditions and disability. Approximately 80% of combat-injured veterans serving in Iraq and Afghanistan experienced blast-type injuries. This is greater than prior conflicts the United States has engaged in (Vietnam War, 65%; Korean War, 69%; WWII, 73%; WWI, 35%; Civil War, 9%). Although the use of body armor during the U.S. wars in Iraq and Afghanistan has helped to protect service members from lethal torso injuries, it does not provide protection for the limbs. Limb amputations account for approximately 5% to 10% of battlefield injuries.

Differences exist between the MSK injury patterns among male and female service members and veterans. Female service members are generally at greater risk for experiencing an MSK injury either while deployed or during training. Female service members have a 1.3 times greater number of military medical visits for noncombat MSK injuries. Females who are new to active duty (in basic training) have a 1.6% to 2.4% greater risk for MSK injury compared with females on active duty who have completed their initial training. Osteoarthritis rate is 20% greater in female compared with male veterans.

Some factors that contribute to a greater prevalence of MSK injury for females include lower bone mineral density, smaller body mass, and a comparatively lower level of fitness when entering the service. A predictor for females developing an MSK injury during military service includes greater body fat. Although females are less likely than males to experience spine, knee, and upper extremity injuries, they are more likely to experience foot, ankle, and hip conditions.

One of the greatest causes for medical discharge from the military is an MSK condition. The leading cause of disability discharge from military service is noncombat MSK injury. When considering those with severe MSK combat injury, between 82% and 92% will not return to military duty. These MSK disabilities put a significant strain on the DoD medical system, as well as the VA and nongovernmental health systems after discharge from the military.

Veterans who experience chronic MSK conditions have a greater risk for decreased quality of life, increased health-care utilization, and greater long-term disability. Chronic MSK conditions and disability are often accompanied by chronic pain. A greater number of veterans, compared with nonveterans, experience chronic pain mainly due to the larger number of veterans with chronic MSK conditions. Of those post 9/11 veterans, more than 50% are affected by chronic pain and an MSK condition.

Veterans with chronic pain and an MSK injury are at greater risk for anxiety, mood disorders, PTSD, and SUD. Due to disability, there is a greater risk for obesity as well as cardiovascular morbidity and mortality. Additionally, there may be a negative financial impact if an injured veteran is unable to work due to a disability and chronic pain.

Burden of veteran MSK disease and disability on the VA and nonfederal health-care systems is significant. Approximately 60% of health care delivered in the VA system is related to an MSK condition. A large portion of veterans have some type of service-connected disability. For those veterans with a normal, nonmedical military separation, nearly half had some type of MSK condition that was considered service-connected and therefore eligible for VA care, benefits, and compensation. In 2013, approximately 3.5 million veterans were receiving disability compensation for service-connected injuries, totaling $54 billion annually. As of 2019, more than 1 million veterans had a service-connected neck or back condition.

The long-term follow-up and care for veterans with chronic MSK injuries, complications from injury, and disability hold a significant cost. As an example, the lifetime cost for disability and treatment for a veteran who is diagnosed with post-traumatic arthritis at age 24 is approximately $1 million. In fact, for the care of veterans with an MSK injury, the VA pays more than $43 billion annually.

Veterans with the highest percentage of service-connected MSK disability are male, white, not married, and have a high school education. Although males comprise the largest percent of disability because of the greater proportion of males in service, females have a greater likelihood to have a service-related disability compared with males. Interestingly, noncombat veterans are more likely than combat veterans to experience service-connected MSK disability. Army veterans have a greater percentage (53%) of service-connected MSK disability while Navy, Marine, and Air Force veterans comprise less than 20% of total service-connected MSK disability. Coast Guard veterans account for less than 1%.

Female Veterans

Females, as a subset of the veteran population, have needs that are different from their male counterparts. Females continue to play an expanding role in military service. Historically, females in the military were predominantly thought of as serving in roles such as nurse; however, females currently have more combat-forward roles. Over the past several decades, the roles of female service members have been evolving, with an increasing number on active duty. By 2030, females are projected to make up nearly 14% of the U.S. veteran population, up from 9%. Although female veterans are at greater risk for mental health conditions, endocrine disorders, MSK conditions, or physical injury and disability that are service-related, less than 25% will receive all or part of their health care at the VA.

LGBTQI Veterans' Issues

Lesbian, gay, bisexual, transgender, queer, and intersex (LGBTQI) veterans carry disproportionate health disparities due to the stigma of being a sexual orientation and/or gender minority in addition to the disparities already carried by veterans. It is difficult to assign population health statistics for the LGBTQI community. Data on LGBTQI veteran's health trends are limited as the VHA has not effectively collected data on veterans' sexual orientation or sexual identity (U.S. Government Accountability Office [GAO], 2020).

Many veterans have served in a military that did not want to know about the service member's gender identity or sexual orientation. Between 1993 and 2011, the U.S. military enforced a policy of "Don't Ask, Don't Tell," which actively prohibited people from serving openly as LGBTQI in the armed services. This had an effect on the health of military members because both they and their health-care providers were hesitant to discuss sexuality and gender. It is estimated that about 78,000 LGBTQI active members and about 900,000 veterans were affected with the repeal of the Don't Ask, Don't Tell policy in 2011. With the Supreme Court decision on *Obergefell v. Hodges* in 2015, the VHA is now required to recognize same-sex marriages in order to honor spousal VA benefits.

LGBTQI veterans have experienced discrimination and prejudice by many in society, including health-care providers. The fear of discrimination or prejudice may lead a veteran to not disclose their sexual or gender identity to their health-care provider. In turn, the clinician may not provide appropriate health screenings or education. Even if a veteran discloses their sexual or gender identity, many clinicians can be underprepared to provide appropriate LGBTQI-competent health care.

Two areas that may underappreciated and inadequately assessed by the clinician for the LGBTQI veteran is the risk of MST and death by suicide. Suicide is the fifth leading cause of death for LGBTQI veterans. Although the rate of suicide among veterans is higher than the rate in the U.S. civilian population, the rate of suicide among LGBTQI veterans is higher than that of the veteran population broadly. MST is also disproportionately experienced by LGBTQI military members, including higher rates of harassment, stalking, and assault than non-LGBTQI peers.

With clinicians often unaware of LGBTQI concerns, they may fail to assess for risk of suicide or MST, or the converse may also occur where the LGBTQI veteran does not feel comfortable disclosing these issues to their clinician.

Transgender and gender-affirming care for veterans at the VHA can be difficult to navigate. Under the 2011 VHA Directive 1341, transgender veterans cannot receive gender-affirmation surgery through the VA health-care system. However, Directive 1341 does provide for other medically necessary care such as hormone replacement therapy (HRT), pre- and postoperative care, and other types of care. As mentioned earlier, transgender veterans may not feel comfortable disclosing their gender identity to their clinicians therefore removing the opportunity for the veteran to receive such care at the VHA.

CONCLUSION

Veterans' health-care needs are complex and varied. Although the VA can provide world-class care and be a leader in several areas, the health-care system does have some areas for improvement. Despite being the largest integrated health-care system in the United States delivering outstanding care, a majority of veterans seek to obtain their care outside of the VA. This may be due to ineligibility for VA health-care benefits, living too far away from a VA health-care facility, or simply choosing not to seek care there for a variety of reasons. Knowing that a majority of veterans will seek care outside of the VA health-care system in the community, it is essential for non-VA health-care providers to understand the unique and varied physical and mental health-care needs of the veterans they care for in their practices.

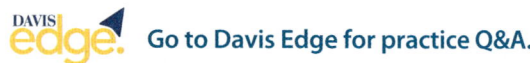 Go to Davis Edge for practice Q&A.

REFERENCES

General

Cogan A, Cervelli L, Dillahunt-Aspillaga T, Rossiter AG. Treating military service members and veterans in the private sector: Information and resources for clinicians. *Arch Phys Med Rehab*. 2018;99(12): 2659-2661. https://doi.org/10.1016/j.apmr.2018.06.006

Derefinko KJ, Hallsell TA, Isaacs MB, Colvin LW, Salgado Garcia FI, Bursac Z. Perceived needs of veterans transitioning from the military to civilian life. *J Behav Health Serv Res*. 2019;46(3): 384-398. https://doi.org/10.1007/s11414-018-9633-8

Meffert BN, Morabito DM, Sawicki DA, Hausman C, Southwick SM, Pietrzak RH, Heinz AJ. US veterans who do and do not utilize veterans affairs health care services: demographic, military, medical, and psychosocial characteristics. *Prim Care Companion CNS Disord*. 2019;21(1):18m02350. https://doi.org/10.4088/PCC.18m02350

Muirhead L, Hall P, Jones-Taylor C, Clifford GD, Felton-Williams T, Williams K. Critical questions: advancing the health of female veterans. *J Am Assoc Nurse Pract*. 2017;29(10):571-580. https://doi.org/10.1002/2327-6924.12490

O'Hanlon C, Huang C, Sloss E, Anhang Price R, Hussey P, Farmer C, Gidengil C. Comparing VA and non-VA quality of care: A systematic review. *J Gen Int Med*. 2017;32(1):105-121. https://doi.org/10.1007/s11606-016-3775-2

Vest BM, Kulak J, Hall VM, Homish GG. Addressing patients' veteran status: primary care providers' knowledge, comfort, and educational needs. *Fam Med*. 2018;50(6):455-459. https://doi.org/10.22454/FamMed.2018.795504

Vest BM, Kulak JA, Homish GG. Caring for veterans in US civilian primary care: qualitative interviews with primary care providers. *Fam Pract*. 2019;36(3):343-350. https://doi.org/10.1093/fampra/cmy078

Yedlinsky NT, Neff LA, Jordan KM. Care of the military veteran: selected health issues. *Am Fam Physician*. 2019;100(9):544-551.

Exposures

Belperio PS, Chartier M, Ross DB, Alaigh P, Shulkin D. Curing hepatitis C virus infection: best practices from the U.S. Department of Veterans Affairs. *Ann Int Med*. 2017;167(7):499-504. https://doi.org/10.7326/M17-1073

Beste LA, Green P, Berry K, Belperio P, Ioannou GN. Hepatitis C-related hepatocellular carcinoma incidence in the Veterans Health Administration after introduction of direct-acting antivirals. *JAMA*. 2020;324(10):1003-1005. https://doi.org/10.1001/jama.2020.10121

Beste LA, Ioannou GN. Prevalence and treatment of chronic hepatitis C virus infection in the US Department of Veterans Affairs. *Epidemiol Rev*. 2015;37:131-143. https://doi.org/10.1093/epirev/mxu002

Bjørklund G, Pivina L, Dadar M, Semenova Y, Rahman MM, Chirumbolo S, Aaseth J. Depleted uranium and Gulf War Illness: updates and comments on possible mechanisms behind the syndrome. *Environ. Res*. 2020;181:108927. https://doi.org/10.1016/j.envres.2019.108927

Clifford RE, Baker D, Risbrough VB, Huang M, Yurgil KA. Impact of TBI, PTSD, and hearing loss on tinnitus progression in a US Marine cohort. *Mil Med*. 2019;184(11-12):839-846. https://doi.org/10.1093/milmed/usz016

Esquivel CR, Parker M, Curtis K, Merkley A, Littlefield P, Conley G, Wise S, Feldt B, Henselman L, Stockinger Z. Aural blast injury/acoustic trauma and hearing loss. *Mil Med*. 2018;183(suppl 2): 78-82. https://doi.org/10.1093/milmed/usy167

Grande LJ, Robinson ME, Radigan LJ, Levin LK, Fortier CB, Milberg WP, McGlinchey RE. Verbal memory deficits in OEF/OIF/OND veterans exposed to blasts at close range. *JINS*. 2018;24(5): 466-475. https://doi.org/10.1017/S1355617717001242

McAndrew LM, Teichman RF, Osinubi OY, Jasien JV, Quigley KS. Environmental exposure and health of Operation Enduring Freedom/Operation Iraqi Freedom veterans. *J Occup Environ Med*. 2012;54(6):665-669. https://doi.org/10.1097/JOM.0b013e318255ba1b

Moring JC, Peterson AL, Kanzler KE. Tinnitus, traumatic brain injury, and posttraumatic stress disorder in the military. *Int J Behav Med*. 2018;25(3):312-321. https://doi.org/10.1007/s12529-017-9702-z

Schram B, Orr R, Rigby T, Pope R. An analysis of reported dangerous incidents, exposures, and near misses amongst Army soldiers.

Int J Environ Res Publ Health. 2018;15(8):1605. https://doi.org/10.3390/ijerph15081605

Self-reported illness and health status among Gulf War veterans. a population-based study. The Iowa Persian Gulf Study Group. (1997). *JAMA.* 277(3):238-245.

Undurti A, Colasurdo EA, Sikkema CL, Schultz JS, Peskind ER, Pagulayan KF, Wilkinson CW. Chronic hypopituitarism associated with increased post-concussive symptoms is prevalent after blast-induced mild traumatic brain injury. *Front Neurol.* 2018;9:72. https://doi.org/10.3389/fneur.2018.00072

U.S. Department of Veterans Affairs. *Agent Orange.* Retrieved February 28, 2021. https://www.publichealth.va.gov/exposures/agentorange/index.asp. Published October 13, 2020.

U.S. Department of Veterans Affairs. Annual Benefits Report Fiscal Year 2019. https://www.benefits.va.gov/REPORTS/abr/. Published 2019.

U.S. Department of Veterans Affairs. *Infectious diseases and Gulf War veterans.* Retrieved February 28, 2021. https://www.publichealth.va.gov/exposures/gulfwar/infectious_diseases.asp. Published May 5, 2016.

Conditions by Service Era

U.S. Department of Veterans Affairs. *Airborne hazards and burn pit exposures.* Published January 27, 2021. https://www.publichealth.va.gov/exposures/burnpits/index.asp. Retrieved February 27, 2021.

U.S. Department of Veterans Affairs. *Cold War veterans health issues.* Published April 30, 2020. https://www.va.gov/health-care/health-needs-conditions/health-issues-related-to-service-era/cold-war/. Retrieved February 27, 2021.

U.S. Department of Veterans Affairs. *Gulf War veterans health issues.* Published April 30, 2020. https://www.va.gov/health-care/health-needs-conditions/health-issues-related-to-service-era/gulf-war/. Retrieved February 27, 2021.

U.S. Department of Veterans Affairs. *Military sexual trauma: treatment.* Published 2020.

U.S. Department of Veterans Affairs. *Sand, dust and particulates.* Published July 12, 2018. https://www.publichealth.va.gov/exposures/sand-dust-particulates/index.asp. Retrieved February 27, 2021.

U.S. Department of Veterans Affairs. *Vietnam War exposures.* Published March 27, 2020. https://www.publichealth.va.gov/exposures/wars-operations/vietnam-war.asp. Retrieved February 28, 2021.

U.S. Department of Veterans Affairs. *World War II veterans health issues.* Published April 30, 2020. https://www.va.gov/health-care/health-needs-conditions/health-issues-related-to-service-era/world-war-ii/. Retrieved February 28, 2021.

Mental Health

Barth SK, Kimerling RE, Pavao J, McCutcheon SJ, Batten SV, Dursa E, Peterson MR, Schneiderman AI. Military sexual trauma among recent veterans: correlates of sexual assault and sexual harassment. *Am J Prevent Med.* 2016;50(1):77-86. https://doi.org/10.1016/j.amepre.2015.06.012

Bell M. *Military sexual trauma: what civilian providers need to know* [PowerPoint Slides]. Published November 14, 2013. Association of American Medical Colleges' Joining Forces Wellness Week. Retrieved on March 25, 2021. https://mentalhealth.va.gov/docs/mst/MST-Overview-for-Civilian-Providers.pdf

Calhoun PS, Schry AR, Dennis PA, Wagner HR, Kimbrel NA, Bastian LA, Beckham JC, Kudler H, Straits-Tröster K. The association between military sexual trauma and use of VA and non-VA health care services among female veterans with military service in Iraq or Afghanistan. *J Interpers Violence.* 2018;33(15):2439-2464. https://doi.org/10.1177/0886260515625909

Gibson CJ, Maguen S, Xia F, Barnes DE, Peltz CB, Yaffe K. Military sexual trauma in older women veterans: prevalence and comorbidities. *J Gen Int Med.* 2020;35(1):207-213. https://doi.org/10.1007/s11606-019-05342-7

Johnson JM, Capehart BP. Psychiatric care of the post-September 11 combat veteran: a review. *Psychosomatics.* 2019;60(2):121-128. https://doi.org/10.1016/j.psym.2018.11.008

Lofgreen A, Carroll K, Dugan S, Karnik N. An overview of sexual trauma in the U.S. military. *Psychiatry Online.* 2017;15(4):411-419. doi: 10.1176/appi.focus.20170024

Monteith LL, Bahraini NH, Matarazzo BB, Gerber HR, Soberay KA, Forster JE. The influence of gender on suicidal ideation following military sexual trauma among veterans in the Veterans Health Administration. *Psychiatry Res.* 2016;244:257-265. https://doi.org/10.1016/j.psychres.2016.07.036

Pulverman CS, Christy AY, Kelly UA. Military sexual trauma and sexual health in women veterans: a systematic review. *Sex Med Rev.* 2019;7(3):393-407. https://doi.org/10.1016/j.sxmr.2019.03.002

Sall J, Brenner L, Millikan Bell AM, Colston MJ. Assessment and management of patients at risk for suicide: synopsis of the 2019 U.S. Department of Veterans Affairs and U.S. Department of Defense Clinical Practice Guidelines. *Ann Int Med.* 2019;171(5):343-353. https://doi.org/10.7326/M19-0687

Teeters JB, Lancaster CL, Brown DG, Back SE. Substance use disorders in military veterans: prevalence and treatment challenges. *Subst Abuse Rehab.* 2017;8:69-77. https://doi.org/10.2147/SAR.S116720

U.S. Department of Veterans Affairs. *Military sexual trauma: treatment.* Published 2020. https://www.mentalhealth.va.gov/msthome/treatment.asp

U.S. Department of Veterans Affairs & Department of Defense. *VA/DOD Clinical Practice Guideline for the Management of Posttraumatic Stress Disorder and Acute Stress Disorder.* Published 2020. https://www.healthquality.va.gov/guidelines/MH/ptsd/VADoDPTSDCPGFinal012418.pdf

MSK Conditions

Cogan A, Cervelli L, Dillahunt-Aspillaga T, Rossiter AG. Treating military service members and veterans in the private sector: information and resources for clinicians. *Arch Phys Med Rehab.* 2018;99(12):2659-2661. https://doi.org/10.1016/j.apmr.2018.06.006

Derefinko KJ, Hallsell TA, Isaacs MB, Colvin LW, Salgado Garcia FI, Bursac Z. Perceived needs of veterans transitioning from the military to civilian life. *J Behav Health Serv Res.* 2019;46(3):384-398. https://doi.org/10.1007/s11414-018-9633-8

Grimm PD, Mauntel TC, Potter BK. Combat and noncombat musculoskeletal injuries in the U.S. military. *Sports Med Arthrosc Rev.* 2019;27(3):84-91. https://doi.org/10.1097/JSA.0000000000000246

Gundlapalli AV, Redd AM, Suo Y, Pettey W, Brignone E, Chin DL, Walker LE, Poltavskiy EA, Janak JC, Howard JT, Sosnov JA, Stewart IJ. Predicting and planning for musculoskeletal service-connected disabilities in VA using disability for active duty OEF/OIF military service members. *Mil Med.* 2020;185(Suppl 1):413-419. https://doi.org/10.1093/milmed/usz223

Haskell SG, Brandt C, Bastian L, Driscoll M, Bathulapalli H, Dziura J. Incident musculoskeletal conditions among men and women

Veterans returning from deployment. *Med Care*. 2020;58(12):1082-1090. https://doi.org/10.1097/MLR.0000000000001403

Martino S, Lazar C, Sellinger J, Gilstad-Hayden K, Fenton B, Barnett PG, Brummett BR, Higgins DM, Holtzheimer P, Mattocks K, Ngo T, Reznik TE, Semiatin AM, Stapley T, Rosen MI. Screening, brief intervention, and referral to treatment for pain management for Veterans seeking service-connection payments for musculoskeletal disorders: SBIRT-PM study protocol. *Pain Med (Malden, Mass.)*. 2020;21(12 Suppl 2):S110-S117. https://doi.org/10.1093/pm/pnaa334

Meffert BN, Morabito DM, Sawicki DA, Hausman C, Southwick SM, Pietrzak RH, Heinz AJ. US veterans who do and do not utilize Veterans Affairs health care services: demographic, military, medical, and psychosocial characteristics. *Prim Care Companion CNS Disord*. 2019;21(1):18m02350. https://doi.org/10.4088/PCC.18m02350

Muirhead L, Hall P, Jones-Taylor C, Clifford GD, Felton-Williams T, Williams K. Critical questions: advancing the health of female veterans. *J Am Assoc Nurse Pract*. 2017;29(10):571-580. https://doi.org/10.1002/2327-6924.12490

O'Hanlon C, Huang C, Sloss E, Anhang Price R, Hussey P, Farmer C, Gidengil C. Comparing VA and non-VA quality of care: a systematic review. *J Gen Int Med*. 2017;32(1):105-121. https://doi.org/10.1007/s11606-016-3775-2

Reyes J, Shaw LE, Lund H, Heber A, VanTil L. Chronic musculoskeletal pain among active and retired military personnel: a prevalence systematic review protocol. *JBI Evid Synth*. 2020;19(2):426-436. https://doi.org/10.11124/JBISRIR-D-19-00392

Vest BM, Kulak JA, Hall VM, Homish GG. Addressing patients' Veteran status: primary care providers' knowledge, comfort, and educational needs. *Fam Med*. 2018;50(6):455-459. https://doi.org/10.22454/FamMed.2018.795504

Vest BM, Kulak JA, Homish GG. Caring for veterans in US civilian primary care: qualitative interviews with primary care providers. *Fam Pract*. 2019;36(3):343-350. https://doi.org/10.1093/fampra/cmy078

LGBTQI Vet Issues

Agron RT, Gale S, Neavins TM, Stassinos MG, Tarro-Zylema RE, Volpp BD, ... Swislocki AL. (2020). Evaluation of healthcare for transgender veterans. *Endocr Metab Sci*. 2021;2(100072).

Lynch KE, Gatsby E, Viernes B, Schliep KC, Whitcomb BW, Alba PR, ... Blosnich JR. Evaluation of suicide mortality among sexual minority US Veterans from 2000 to 2017. *JAMA Netw Open*. 2020;3(12):e2031357-e2031357.

National Resource Center on LGBT Aging, & SAGE Services & Advocacy for Gay, Lesbian, Bisexual & Transgender Elders. Fact sheet: LGBT veterans [Pamphlet] Published 2021. https://www.lgbtagingcenter.org/resources/pdfs/SAGE_Veterans_Fact_Sheet_final_update_2015_2016.pdf

Ruben MA, Livingston NA, Berke DS, Matza AR, Shiperd JC. Lesbian, gay, bisexual, and transgender veterans' experiences of discrimination in health care and their relation to health outcomes: a pilot study examining the moderating role of provider communication. *Health Equity*, 2019;3(1):480-488.

Shrader A, Casero K, Casper B, Kelley M, Lewis L, Calohan J. Military lesbian, gay, bisexual, and transgender (LGBT) awareness training for health care providers within the military health system. *J Am Psychiatr Nurses Assoc*. 2017;23(6):385-392.

U.S. Government Accountability Office. (2020, October 19). VA health care: better data needed to assess the health outcomes of lesbian, gay, bisexual, and transgender veterans (GAO-21-69). Published October 19, 2020. https://www.gao.gov/products/gao-21-69

Chapter 81

Primary Care of the Patient With Cancer

Anna L. Schwartz, PhD, FNP-BC, FAAN

INTRODUCTION

Currently, there are more than 16.9 million cancer survivors in the United States. In 2040, the population of adult cancer survivors is expected to reach 26.1 million. This number includes childhood and adult cancer survivors who, with effective treatments, are living longer and experiencing age-related comorbidities. As the number of cancer survivors grows, there is a looming shortage of oncology services to care for them and no clear path to integrate their needs into primary care. Despite practice-level resources, there is little systematic primary care provided to cancer survivors. Primary care providers have divergent views on their roles and responsibilities in caring for cancer survivors.

People living with and beyond cancer face a life journey that begins at diagnosis and may continue to affect their health for the remainder of their lives. Although treatments for cancer have become more effective and cancer survivors are being cured or are living for extended periods of time with their disease, practitioners are seeing new long-term and late side effects of treatments. The most common cancers are breast, lung, prostate, and colorectal cancers (https://www.cancer.gov/types/common-cancers). New cancer treatments, although highly efficacious for certain types of cancer, cause lingering side effects. For example, the new immunotherapies and other targeted treatments can impair multiple organs.

In 2020, the American Cancer Society reported that among cancer survivors, approximately two-thirds are older than 60 years. Only 6% of cancer survivors are younger than 40 years. As people living with and beyond cancer transition out of active treatment, care must focus on monitoring for disease recurrence, health promotion, and disease prevention. This chapter will focus on primary care during the acute and long-term phases and on late effects of treatment faced by cancer survivors, and it will provide essential knowledge needed to care for these patients.

Cancer survivorship generally begins at diagnosis and continues through end of life. The acute phase is the time from diagnosis through the completion of active treatment. This phase is focused on getting the individual through treatment and controlling side effects to improve treatment tolerance. At this point, the oncology team manages the majority of treatment-related side effects. The long-term effects phase begins after the completion of treatment through the first 1 to 2 years of recovery. During this time, many of the acute side effects of treatment resolve. Late effects may extend throughout the remainder of the patient's life. Distinct and unique late effects of treatment pose health challenges that necessitate action by the primary care provider. Once treatment is completed, preventive screening is recommended.

Developing a plan of care for survivors in all phases of treatment and recovery requires an understanding of not only the individual's type and stage of cancer and their treatment regimen(s) but also other comorbid conditions that may affect the patient's ability to function and engage in health-promoting activities such as exercise. Comorbid conditions that may also result from the treatment itself include hypothyroidism, hypertension, cardiac arrhythmias, chronic obstructive pulmonary disease, asthma, diabetes, osteoporosis, and diseases of aging such as cognitive decline, cerebrovascular attack, essential tremors, or Parkinson's disease. Although a detailed discussion of these individual disorders is beyond the scope of this chapter, an understanding of how the different impairments and limitations resulting from various comorbid conditions may compound the long-term and late effects of cancer is paramount in developing safe and effective treatment and health-promotion regimens.

Acute Phase

The acute effects phase is the period of active treatment, when patients see their oncology team regularly for treatment, blood work, and side-effect and symptom management. The primary care provider's role is focused on health maintenance and management of basic symptoms that may arise. Common side effects of cancer treatments include nausea, vomiting, diarrhea, rash, fatigue, impaired physical function, depression, anxiety, and other declines in quality of life. Table 81.1 details common acute, long-term, and late effects of treatment.

Cancer-related fatigue is the most common and persistent side effect during the acute phase. It is an effect of treatment (surgery, chemotherapy, immunotherapy, radiation therapy) and may compound or be compounded by inactivity, depression, anxiety, and disrupted sleep. The most effective intervention for fatigue is exercise. Although this is counterintuitive, it reduces the decline in functional ability that is caused by increased sedentary behavior. Exercise during treatment is safe, and people with cancer need to exercise regularly. The evidence base is overwhelmingly strong to support exercise to reduce many of the side effects of cancer (e.g., fatigue, weakness, depression, declines in quality of life), and steps are in

TABLE 81.1 Examples of Acute, Long-term, and Late Effects of Cancer

	Acute	Long Term	Late	Causative Agent
Nausea/vomiting	X			Chemotherapy, radiation therapy
Fatigue	X	x	x	Chemotherapy, immunotherapy, surgery, radiation therapy
Decreased functional ability	X	x	x	Chemotherapy, immunotherapy, surgery, radiation therapy
Weakness	X	x	x	Chemotherapy, immunotherapy, surgery, radiation therapy
Alopecia	X			Chemotherapy, radiation
Pain	X	x	x	Chemotherapy, immunotherapy, surgery, radiation therapy
Peripheral neuropathy	X	x	x	Paclitaxel, oxaliplatin
Lymphedema	X	x	x	Surgery
Infertility	X	x	x	
Premature menopause	X	x		Chemotherapies, surgery, radiation therapy
Congestive heart failure, coronary artery disease, arrhythmia	X	x	x	Trastuzumab, doxorubicin, daunorubicin, epirubicin, cyclophosphamide, osimertinib
Hypertension	X	x	x	Bevacizumab, sorafenib, sunitinib
Decreased lung function, fibrosis		x	x	Bleomycin, carmustine, methotrexate
Hypothyroid	X	x	x	
Osteoporosis, bone and soft tissue problems		x	x	Chemotherapy, steroids, hormonal therapy, immunotherapy
Hearing loss	X	x	x	Cisplatin, brain radiation
Stroke		x	x	Brainstem radiation
Cognitive problems	X	x	x	Chemotherapy, immunotherapy, high-dose radiation
Dental problems (gum disease, dry mouth, loss of tooth enamel)		x	x	Chemotherapy, head and neck radiation
Cataracts		x	x	Steroids, radiation
Emotional problems (e.g., fear recurrence, depression, anxiety, anger)	X	x	x	Cancer experience
Secondary cancers (breast cancer, acute leukemia, myelodysplasia)			x	Chemotherapy, immunotherapy, radiation
Recurrence	X	x	x	

process by the American College of Sports Medicine to make exercise rehabilitation the standard of care for all people diagnosed with and living beyond cancer.

When young adults are treated for cancer, fertility preservation is a concern. Patients should be informed of the risk for infertility and given the opportunity to bank sperm or eggs before chemotherapy or radiation therapy is started. This is a discussion that should begin at diagnosis, and the primary care provider is a trusted person who can initiate this discussion. Unfortunately, in the rush to treatment, fertility preservation is often overlooked.

Another important role of the primary care provider is to assess functional ability at every visit. Ask the patient if they feel ready to exercise on their own or need some supervision and assistance and then refer the patient to either a physical therapist or rehabilitation specialist, an exercise trainer with specialization in exercise oncology, or a home-based program that can be self-directed. Guiding a patient to maintain or even improve their functional ability allows them to continue working and pursuing meaningful activities.

Long-term Effects Phase

The long-term effects phase extends beyond treatment for 1 to 2 years. This is the recovery period when most side effects resolve, but some may linger. In this phase, nausea, vomiting, mouth sores, and alopecia resolve, but fatigue, peripheral neuropathy, depression, anxiety, and fear of recurrence may linger. This is also a time when the patient doesn't see their oncology team as often. The usual follow-up schedule is once every 3 months, so management of lingering symptoms may be assumed by either the oncology or primary care team.

A side effect that may begin to resolve in the long-term phase is chemotherapy-induced peripheral neuropathy (CIPN). Peripheral neuropathy is a feeling of tingling, numbness, or shooting pains, and CIPN may be induced by drugs (oxaliplatin, carboplatin, cisplatin) that are commonly used to treat colorectal cancer, breast cancer, and many other cancers. It can become so severe that buttoning a shirt is difficult and balance is compromised. Currently, there are no treatments to minimize or resolve CIPN, and this side effect becomes a lifelong challenge.

The nerve pain of CIPN can be managed, to some degree, with drugs such as gabapentin or pregabalin.

The primary care provider needs to be aware of management of acute symptoms that now become long-term side effects of treatment and be aware of the potential for development of new health problems that are secondary to treatment. This is a time to monitor for recurrence and begin to assess for development of secondary cancers. Table 81.2 details common tumor markers and laboratory measures to monitor for new disease. In the long-term

TABLE 81.2 Tumor Markers for Monitoring for Recurrence		
Tumor Marker	**Associated Cancer**	**Sample**
Alpha Fetoprotein (AFP)	Liver, ovarian, testicular	Blood
B-cell immunoglobulin gene rearrangement	B-cell lymphoma	Bone marrow, tissue, body fluid, blood
Beta-2 microglobulin	Multiple myeloma, some leukemias and lymphomas	Blood, urine, cerebrospinal fluid (CSF)
BCR-ABL	Chronic myeloid leukemia (CML) and acute lymphocytic leukemia (ALL)	Blood, bone marrow
CA15-3	Breast, lung, ovarian	Blood
CA19-9	Pancreatic, bile duct, gallbladder, stomach, colon	Blood
CA27.29	Breast	Blood
CA125	Ovarian, endometrial, peritoneal, fallopian tube cancers	Blood
Calcitonin	Medullary thyroid carcinoma, C-cell hyperplasia, lung and leukemias	Blood
Carcinoembryonic antigen (CEA)	Colon, pancreatic, lung, breast, ovarian, medullary thyroid	Blood
Chromogranin A (CgA)	Carcinoid	Blood
Chromosomes 3, 7, 9p21	Bladder	Urine
Cytokeratin fragment 21-1	Lung	Blood
Des-gamma-carboxy prothrombin (DCP)	Hepatocellular carcinoma	Blood
Fibrin/Fibrinogen	Bladder	Blood, urine
Gastrin	G-cell hyperplasia, gastrinoma	Blood
HE4	Ovarian	Blood
5-HIAA	Carcinoid	Urine
Lactate dehydrogenase (LDH)	Testicular, germ cell tumors, lymphoma, leukemia, melanoma, neuroblastoma	Blood
Monoclonal immunoglobulins	Multiple myeloma	Blood, urine
PML/RARA fusion gene	Acute promyelocytic leukemia	Blood, bone marrow
Prostate specific antigen (PSA)	Prostate	Blood
Soluble mesothelin-related peptides (SMRP)	Mesothelioma	Blood
T-cell receptor gene rearrangement	T-cell lymphoma	Blood, bone marrow, body fluid
Thyroglobulin	Thyroid	Blood, tissue

National Cancer Institute. *Tumor Markers in Common Use.* https://www.cancer.gov/about-cancer/diagnosis-staging/diagnosis/tumor-markers-list

effects phase, new health problems may also develop as a result of treatment. The most common of these is thyroid dysfunction. Many chemotherapy and immunotherapy regimens can impair thyroid function, and any radiation to that area may completely suppress thyroid function. It is important to routinely screen for hypothyroid disease, which can potentiate cancer-related fatigue.

Monitoring for Long-term and Late Effects

Long-term and late effects of cancer can include dental problems; hearing loss; infertility; early menopause; impaired heart, lung, immune, and endocrine function; and secondary malignancies (Table 81.3). The physical changes often occur insidiously over time. Primary care providers need to be vigilant about signs and symptoms of recurrence, second cancers, and development of long-term and late effects of treatment and to offer prompt evaluation, treatment, and, if needed, referral to a specialist.

Second Cancers and Screening for Recurrence

Chemotherapy and radiation therapy can increase the risk for secondary cancers. Chemotherapy-induced leukemias may occur 2 to 5 years after treatment. The risk for secondary cancers begins declining 10 years after treatment. Alkylating agents increase the risk for solid tumor development in the lung, gastrointestinal tract, bladder, and breast and sarcomas of the bone or connective tissue. Radiation-induced secondary malignancies are influenced by the dose, field of radiation, and age at treatment. These malignancies typically have a latency period of at least 5 to 10 years. The most frequent childhood cancers

TABLE 81.3 Examples of Long-term and Late Effects of Cancer Treatment

Organ System	Chemotherapy Effect	Radiation Therapy Effect
Bone and soft tissue	Avascular necrosis, osteoporosis, loss of muscle mass	Fibrosis, osteonecrosis, atrophy, short stature (children)
Cardiovascular	Cardiomyopathy, arrythmias, reduced ejection fraction, coronary artery disease	Pericardial effusion, pericarditis, coronary artery and peripheral vascular disease
Pulmonary	Fibrosis, interstitial pneumonitis, abnormal pulmonary functions	Pulmonary fibrosis, reduced lung volume
Neurological	Leukoencephalopathy, peripheral neuropathy, hearing loss, vision loss	Neurocognitive impairment, radiation necrosis, brachial plexopathy, lumbosacral plexopathy
Hematological	Myelodysplastic syndromes and secondary leukemias	Myelodysplastic syndromes
Renal	Decreased creatinine clearance, hypertension, kidney failure	Decreased creatinine clearance, hypertension
Genitourinary	Bladder fibrosis, hemorrhagic cystitis, bladder cancer	Bladder fibrosis, contractures
Gastrointestinal	Abnormal liver function tests, hepatic fibrosis, cirrhosis, diabetes	Malabsorption, strictures, radiation proctitis, second cancers
Endocrine	Adrenal-pituitary axis dysfunction, hypothyroidism, diabetes	Deficient growth hormone and pituitary, metabolic syndrome, obesity, diabetes, hyper- or hypothyroidism, nodules, thyroid cancer
Reproductive	Males: Sterility Females: Sterility, premature menopause	Males: Sterility Females: Ovarian failure, premature menopause
Ophthalmic	Cataracts, dry eye	Cataracts
Dental	Caries, xerostomia	Xerostomia, caries
Skin	Dyspigmentation, contractures, nail and hair changes	Second cancers
Immunological	Hypogammaglobulinemia, common variable immune deficiency	
Psychological	Fatigue, depression, anxiety, fear of recurrence, sleep problems, sexual dysfunction, pain, opioid dependence, financial concerns	Fatigue, depression, anxiety, fear of recurrence, sleep problems, sexual dysfunction, pain, opioid dependence, financial concerns

are acute lymphoblastic leukemia, Hodgkin's lymphoma, and astrocytoma, with 6.9% of survivors developing secondary malignancies over a 22.5-year follow-up period that include breast and thyroid cancers.

Screening of pediatric and adult cancer survivors for recurrent disease and new cancer should follow the guidelines of the Children's Oncology Group, American Cancer Society, and the U.S. Public Health Service. Special screening guidelines for breast, colorectal, lung, and other cancers should be followed for survivors treated with radiation therapy to the abdomen, pelvis, chest, axilla, and/or spine or with total body irradiation (TBI). Similar to the general population, age-appropriate screening is recommended for other cancers such as prostate and cervical, with special attention to the skin, thyroid, and other organs that are prone to radiation effects.

Body Composition and Bone Health

Many cancer treatments negatively affect body composition. It is not uncommon for patients to gain weight during treatment. Whether patients gain weight or not, most demonstrate an increased fat mass and loss of muscle mass and bone density because of inactivity. The declines in bone density can be further compounded by the bone-wasting effects of many drugs for cancer treatment (e.g., adriamycin, dexamethasone, estrogen, and testosterone ablation in breast and prostate cancer), leading to osteopenia and osteoporosis. Early screening for osteopenia and osteoporosis is important and should begin at younger ages, depending on the age an individual was treated for cancer. The importance of a healthy diet and regular weight-bearing exercise must be stressed to the patient.

Cardiovascular Function

Cancer survivors have an average of two to six times higher cardiovascular mortality risk than the general population. In a study of more than 3 million U.S. cancer survivors from 1973 to 2012, 38% died from cancer and 11.3% died from cardiovascular disease (CVD). Younger cancer survivors had a higher risk for heart disease, and those diagnosed before age 55 years had a 10-fold higher risk for CVD mortality than the general population. Most deaths occurred within the first year after diagnosis, which may be due in part to the interaction of preexisting CVD, cardiovascular toxicities of treatment, and cardiovascular risk associated with tumor burden. A proactive approach to managing cardiovascular health is critically important for survivors.

Cardiomyopathies can be induced by chemotherapy and may lead to changes in blood pressure, arrhythmias, myocarditis, pericarditis, myocardial infarction, left ventricular failure, and congestive heart failure. Cardiomyopathies may present as reduced heart function or be asymptomatic, presenting only with a murmur or fatigue. Commonly used drugs that can cause cardiomyopathies are doxorubicin and trastuzumab. Doxorubicin, an anthracycline, causes cellular death and permanent cardiac damage. In contrast, trastuzumab causes cellular dysfunction that can be reversible. The degree of damage is dose dependent, but late effects of anthracycline cardiotoxicity can occur decades after chemotherapy has ended.

Although cardiovascular disease is increased in cancer survivors, it is often undertreated. For unknown reasons, cardioprotective therapies are prescribed less frequently in cancer survivors. Cardioprotective therapies include the use of statins and P2Y12 blockers after myocardial infarction. Compared with patients without cancer, cancer survivors are less likely to receive statins (61.2% vs. 63.8%), antiplatelet therapy (58% vs. 75.3%), angiotensin-converting enzyme inhibitors or angiotensin-receptor blockers (55.1% vs. 61.4%), and beta blockers (62.3% vs. 70.1%). Unfortunately, although cancer treatments are getting better, there is poor management of cardiovascular risk.

Pulmonary Function

Pulmonary dysfunction may emerge as a late effect of treatment. Impairments to pulmonary function may be caused by bleomycin and mediastinal radiation. Pulmonary dysfunction may manifest as pulmonary fibrosis, bronchiectasis, chronic pleural effusions, and/or recurrent pneumonia. Reduced lung function can contribute to fatigue and lead to declines in functional ability. There may be a correlation between declines in physical function, fatigue, and cardiac and pulmonary dysfunction.

Endocrine Function

Among the late effects of cancer treatment, endocrine dysfunctions are the most common. The hypothalamus and pituitary gland can be damaged by cranial radiation. Immune checkpoint inhibitors can cause a variety of endocrine dysfunctions including hypophysitis. The thyroid can be damaged from radiation, chemotherapy agents, and checkpoint inhibitors.

Growth hormone deficiency manifests as increased body fat, decreased lean body mass and bone mineral density, abnormal lipid profile, increased cardiovascular morbidity, and reduced quality of life. Early detection and treatment are important to prevent its effects. Growth hormone deficiency can occur at any age.

Infertility from treatment as a child or young adult is likely when treated with alkylating chemotherapy agents or radiation to the gonads. In males, treatment impairs germ cell function and sperm production. Males should be monitored for hypoandrogenism. Females receiving the same therapies will have a reduced production of estrogen and progesterone and impaired ovulation. Both prepubescent males and females may fail to enter puberty. Sperm banking and oocyte cryopreservation may be important options for these patients. Radiation to the hypothalamic/pituitary area also may cause gonadotropin deficiencies.

Cardiometabolic effects of cancer include obesity, hypertension, dyslipidemias, and impaired glucose metabolism. Metabolic syndrome, the occurrence of insulin resistance, obesity, atherogenic dyslipidemia, and hypertension, occur in almost 66% of pediatric cancer survivors. These late effects are associated with TBI or abdominal radiation, both of which may impair the hypothalamus, which controls metabolism, weight, and body composition. The cardiometabolic effects increase the risk for cardiovascular disease.

Neurological Issues

Chemotherapy causes many neurotoxicities. CIPN increases fall risk and is a prevalent side effect of many cancer treatments. CIPN is noted in 50% to 60% of patients who are treated with taxanes, especially paclitaxel. CIPN symptoms include dysesthesias and paresthesias, diminished deep tendon reflexes, pain, and diminished strength. CIPN is a chronic condition that has a significant impact on quality of life, poorer physical function, and higher prevalence of disability and falls.

Ototoxic cancer therapy is associated with hearing loss and risk of neurocognitive deficits in long-term childhood cancer survivors 20 years after diagnosis. Severe hearing loss occurs in 84.9% of patients after platinum-based therapy and 38.3% after cranial radiation. Neurotoxicity also occurs in adults who received platinum-based therapy or cranial radiation. These treatments may cause negative sequelae on daily function, ability to work, and quality of life.

Pain

Chronic pain occurs in cancer survivors 1 to 3 years after cancer treatment. For one-half of these patients, pain is severe enough to limit their lives and ability to work. Even 16 years after diagnosis, the prevalence of chronic pain is almost 35%, which is comparable to the prevalence of pain noted within a year of diagnosis (Jiang et al., 2019). There are socioeconomic disparities in cancer pain management. Cancer pain is more prevalent and poorly managed in patients on Medicaid, in part because they often cannot afford their medications. Primary care providers need to assess and manage pain in people living with and beyond cancer. When patients can't work because of pain, there is a burden to the individual and society. It is the responsibility of the primary care provider to learn how to manage chronic cancer pain or know where to refer patients for appropriate resources.

Reproductive Health

The primary care provider should initiate a discussion of sexual health with the cancer survivor. Sexual function, or dysfunction, may become apparent in this phase of recovery. Young females often experience premature menopause and must cope with the physical and emotional side effects and consequences of infertility. Common problems for females of all ages include vaginal dryness, atrophy, painful intercourse, and infertility. Males may also experience infertility. Erectile dysfunction may require the use of agents devised to promote erection. Phosphodiesterase type 5 (PDE5) inhibitors can help males with erectile dysfunction, but the medications may take a long time to take effect. Surgical interventions may be offered to patients who do not respond to medical therapy. These problems can be managed by primary care providers with referral, as needed, to an appropriate specialist.

Immune Function

Immune function can be impaired from aggressive and often prolonged treatment after B-cell lymphoma or blood and marrow transplant. Immunotherapy (i.e., rituximab) and radiation therapy are associated with immune dysfunction. The impairment can range from transient hypogammaglobulinemia to loss of B-cell function and development of common variable immune deficiency. When B-cell function is impaired, there are a loss of vaccine response and increased risk for severe bacterial, fungal, and viral infection.

Cancer-related Fatigue

Cancer-related fatigue is often persistent after treatment and may become a chronic problem for long-term survivors. The side effect is complicated as it can be compounded by other late effects of cancer, such as hypothyroidism, cardiac or pulmonary dysfunction, or depression. Fatigue can be related to aging and other comorbid conditions, but as a persistent late effect of treatment, it is primarily related to declines in cardiopulmonary function and loss of muscle strength. Many interventions have been studied to reduce fatigue, and moderate exercise has a strong and clear benefit in reducing fatigue.

Emotional Health and Well-being

Anxiety, depression, and fear of cancer recurrence are commonly reported by survivors. Although anxiety and depression can be medically treated, fear of cancer recurrence cannot. Fear of cancer recurrence can affect a survivor throughout their life. Every cough or pain may be interpreted as a possible recurrence. As many as 70% of breast cancer survivors report clinically significant fear of cancer recurrence. Acceptance and commitment therapy (ACT) has been found to reduce the fear of cancer recurrence. ACT is a skills-based intervention that helps cancer survivors learn to focus on the present moment through mindfulness meditation.

Economic Well-being

Job lock, the inability to change jobs due to health insurance being provided by an employer, is common among cancer survivors. Job lock can negatively affect career trajectory and potential for increased income and quality of life. Almost 20% of cancer survivors report job lock, with a higher prevalence among females than males (36%

vs. 28%). Most survivors affected earn incomes between 138% and 400% of the federal poverty level, which makes them ineligible for Medicaid.

Caregiver Considerations

The burden of cancer not only affects the person living with and beyond cancer but also their caregivers and loved ones. Caregivers are often untrained in caregiving, yet the patient may be physically and emotionally dependent on that person. The impact of caregiving is significant. It is an unpaid role that can be overwhelming and cause significant stress. The caregiver often has to learn to negotiate the health-care system and insurance regulations and to communicate with the health-care team and the patient's other support person(s). The caregiver not only tries to support the patient but also face the uncertainty of the patient's serious, often life-threatening, disease. They need to understand that it is normal to feel sad and grieve the change in life circumstance. The caregiver needs to be aware that there is supportive care available to help them through the experience.

HEALTH PROMOTION

The primary care provider should be the leader in health promotion and prevention for cancer survivors. In addition to seeing that the patient gets regular cancer screenings, the provider needs to ensure that the patient is getting appropriate follow-up for the type of cancer the patient had. The primary care provider is the care coordinator for cancer survivors and must have a good understanding of the specific health-promotion needs of cancer survivors. Four key areas of preventive health recommendations focus on a healthy lifestyle: exercise, nutrition and weight control, smoking cessation, and immunization. The American Cancer Society's recommendations for a healthy lifestyle include preserving lean body mass, maintaining or achieving a healthy weight, preventing nutritional deficiencies, and maximizing quality of life. Paramount to optimal health after cancer treatment are assuring proper immunization or reimmunization after blood or marrow transplant, following a healthy diet for weight maintenance, avoiding smoking and excess alcohol, and getting regular exercise.

Exercise

Regular exercise decreases not only the risk for recurrence and development of second cancers, but it also reduces the risk for seven other cancers (colon, breast, kidney, endometrial, bladder, and stomach cancer and esophageal adenocarcinoma). Exercise is regarded as a safe and helpful way for cancer survivors to lessen the impact of cancer treatment on their physical and mental health, both during and after treatment. It is an intervention that reduces fatigue, depression, and anxiety and helps to regulate sleep.

The updated American College of Sports Medicine cancer exercise guidelines create specific "exercise prescriptions" to address different health outcomes relative to cancer survivors. The recommended minimum exercise prescription for cancer survivors is to exercise three times a week by engaging in both aerobic and resistance exercise for approximately 30 minutes per session. As the person living with and beyond cancer gets stronger, the exercise goal should be to increase the total time of exercise to 300 minutes of aerobic exercise per week and at least 2 days a week of resistance exercise. Exercise may need to be tailored to an individual's ability and potential physical limitations from cancer, such as CIPN, lymphedema, bone metastasis, osteoporosis, venous access lines, or ostomies. An exercise program needs to begin slowly and gradually increase in duration and intensity to progressively improve aerobic function and muscle strength.

Ideally, the primary care provider would assess, advise, and refer the patient to the appropriate exercise program, such as a medically supervised rehabilitation with physiatrist, physical therapist, or occupational therapist; community-based supervised exercise with a cancer exercise trainer or a group such as Livestrong at the YMCA; or a home-based exercise program. Each of these exercise programs is progressive in that as the person living with or beyond cancer gets stronger, they should progress from a medically supervised exercise program to a community-based supervised program with a trainer and then to a home-based program. Although primary care providers do not need to know how to adapt an exercise program, they should know what resources are available in their community for appropriate referral.

The number of people living with and beyond cancer continues to grow. Caring for these patients presents unique challenges and requires special knowledge and expertise. Primary care providers must work collaboratively with the oncology team and other specialists (e.g., rehabilitation specialists, cardiologist, endocrinologist, immunologist, etc.) who may provide expertise and care directed toward the unique health concerns patients experience during and after cancer treatment.

Diet and Alcohol

The World Cancer Research Fund (WCRF), the American Institute for Cancer Research (AICR), and the American Cancer Society (ACS) all recommend cancer survivors eat a plant-based diet and limit the consumption of red and processed meat. They also recommend limiting the consumption of alcohol. Cancer survivors should strive to achieve a healthy weight and limit the consumption of calorie-dense foods and beverages and focus on a diet that is high in vegetables, fruits, and whole grains.

Smoking Cessation

Smoking cessation reduces the chance of dying from cancer and improves overall health and quality of life. Discussing different ways to quit smoking is the first step in developing an individualized approach to quitting that may include a combination of behavioral therapy and medications. Medications to aid smoking cessation include nicotine replacement therapies that are available over the counter as patches, gum, and lozenges. Two prescription drugs, varenicline and bupropion, are generally well tolerated; however, they may be contraindicated for a patient with a history of seizures or psychiatric illness.

Dental Care

Most cancer survivors are not at risk for dental complications from cancer treatment. However, cancer survivors may experience long-lasting toxicities, and they are at risk for dental complications if they received bone-modifying or antiangiogenic agents, radiation therapy for head or neck cancer, chemotherapy for childhood cancer, or are patients who received high-dose chemotherapy and stem cell transplant. The loss of normal salivation can increase the risk for dental caries and periodontal disease. Regular long-term oral health screenings coordinated by the dental and oncology teams are important for patients at high risk for late complications.

Infection Precautions

Once cancer treatment is complete and hematological recovery has occurred, the patient is no longer at increased risk of infection. Immune function generally recovers within 6 to 12 months after chemotherapy. The exception concerns patients who were treated with immunotherapeutics (e.g., rituximab) or radiation therapy because they may develop profound immune deficiency. Immune deficiency is often diagnosed in patients who have persistent infections, particularly sinus infections or severe pneumonia. For cancer survivors with immune deficiency, this becomes a lifelong complication of treatment.

Vaccinations

Vaccinations are important for all adults, including cancer survivors. The U.S. Centers for Disease Control and Prevention (CDC) recommends immunization schedules for cancer survivors and urges maintenance of vaccinations for people with weakened immune systems and cancer survivors. Vaccines with a live virus should be avoided by patients who are currently receiving cancer treatment or who have recently completed treatment. These vaccines include the nasal spray version of the influenza; varicella; measles, mumps, and rubella; and zoster virus vaccines.

REFERENCES

American Cancer Society. Cancer Treatment & Survivorship Facts & Figures 2019-2021. American Cancer Society, Atlanta, 2019. https://www.cancer.org/content/dam/cancer-org/research/cancer-facts-and-statistics/cancer-treatment-and-survivorship-facts-and-figures/cancer-treatment-and-survivorship-facts-and-figures-2019-2021.pdf (Accessed on October 20, 2020).

Bluethmann SM, Mariotto AB, Rowland JH. Anticipating the "silver tsunami": prevalence trajectories and comorbidity burden among older cancer survivors in the United States. Cancer Epidemiol Bio-markers Prev. 2016; 25(7): 1029-1036.

Chao C, Bhatia S, Xu L, et al. Incidence, risk factors, and mortality associated with second malignant neoplasms among survivors of adolescent and young adult cancer. JAMA: Network Open, 2019:2(6):1-15.

Crabtree BF, Miller WL, Howard J, et al. Cancer survivorship care roles for primary care physicians. Annals of Family Medicine, 2020:18(3):202-209.

Jiang C, Wang H, Wang Q, et al. Prevalence of chronic pain and high-impact chronic pain in cancer survivors in the United States. JAMA Oncology, 2019:5(8):1224-1226.

Johns SA, Stutz PV, Talib TL, et al. Acceptance and commitment therapy for breast cancer survivors with fear of cancer recurrence: a 3-arm randomized controlled trial. Cancer, 2020:126(1): 211-218.

Kelley GA, Kelley KS. Exercise and cancer-related fatigue in adults: a systematic review of previous systematic reviews with meta-analyses. BMC Cancer, 2017:17:article 693.

Kok JL, Teepen JC, van der Pal HJ, et al. Incidence of and risk factors for histologically confirmed solid benign tumors among long-term survivors of childhood cancer. JAMA Oncology, 2019:5(5): 671-680.

Nekhlyudov L, O'malley DM, Hudson SV. Integrating primary care providers in the care of cancer survivors: gaps in evidence and future opportunities. Lancet Oncology, 2017:18(1):e30-e38.

Patel AV, Friedenreich CM, Moore SC, et al. American College of Sports Medicine Roundtable Report on Physical Activity, Sedentary Behavior, and Cancer Prevention and Control. Medicine and Science in Sports & Exercise, 2019:51(11):2391-2402. https://www.regenhealthsolutions.info/wp-content/uploads/2019/10/American_College_of_Sports_Medicine_Roundtable.24.pdf

Rubinstein EB, Miller WL, Hudson SV, et al. JAMA Internal Medicine, 2017:177(12):1726-1732.

Schmitz KH, Campbell AM, Stuiver MM, et al. Exercise is medicine in oncology: Engaging clinicians to help patients move through cancer. CA: A Journal for Clinicians, 2019:69(6):468-484.

Sklar CA, Antal Z, Chemaitilly W, et al. Hypothalamic-pituitary and growth disorders in survivors of childhood cancer: an endocrine society clinical practice guideline. Journal of Clinical Endocrinology and Metabolism, 2018:103(8):2761-2784.

Tsui J, Hudson SV, Rubinstein EB, et al. A mixed-methods analysis of the capacity of the patient-centered medical home to implement care coordination services for cancer survivors. Translational Behavioral Medicine, 2018:8(3):319-327.

Turcotte LM, Liu Q, Yasui Y, et al. Chemotherapy and risk of subsequent malignant neoplasms in the childhood cancer survivor study cohort. Journal of Clinical Oncology, 2019:37(34):3310-3319.

Untaru R, Chen D, Kelly C, et al. Suboptimal use of cardioprotective medications in patients with a history of cancer. JACC Oncology, 2020:2(2):312-315.

Veiga LH, Curtis RE, Morton LM, et al. Association of breast cancer risk after childhood cancer with radiation dose to the breast and anthracycline use: a report from the Childhood Cancer Survivor Study. JAMA Pediatrics. 2019:173(12):1171-1179.

Winters-Stone KM, Horak F, Jacobs PG, et al. Falls, functioning and disability among women with persistent symptoms of chemotherapy-induced peripheral neuropathy. Journal of Clinical Oncology, 2017:35(23):2604-2612.

RESOURCES

American Cancer Society, Guidelines for Cancer Survivors
https://www.cancer.org/health-care-professionals/american-cancer-society-survivorship-guidelines.html

American College of Sports Medicine, Moving Through Cancer
https://www.exerciseismedicine.org/support_page.php/moving-through-cancer/

American Society of Clinical Oncology, Guidelines on Survivorship Care
https://www.asco.org/practice-policy/cancer-care-initiatives/prevention-survivorship/survivorship-compendium-0

Children's Oncology Group, Long-Term Follow-Up Guidelines
https://www.childrensoncologygroup.org/long-term-follow-up-care-226

Livestrong at the YMCA
https://www.livestrong.org/what-we-do/program/livestrong-at-the-ymca

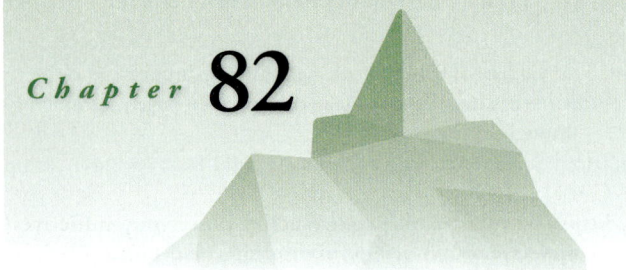

Chapter 82

Primary Care of Older Adults

Deirdre Carolan, PhD, ANP-BC, GNP-BC, FAANP
Lynne M. Dunphy, PhD, APRN, FNP-BC, FAAN, FAANP

INTRODUCTION

Over the course of a lifetime, an older adult develops a unique physiology, specific to the changes of aging, their living environment and lifestyle, their genetic makeup, and their health care. This distinctive aging process and subsequent care ramifications remained unrecognized and unaddressed until the 1980s. Dr. Donald Berwick, a pediatrician, president emeritus and senior fellow of the Institute for Healthcare Improvement (IHI) stated, "…as a student of performance and improvement of healthcare, I am embarrassed that it took so long for the needs and circumstances of people of older age to receive this needed specialized recognition." This, he noted, had been recognized for decades in the youngest population, the specialty of pediatrics. The primary care practitioner's awareness and familiarity with the needs and uniqueness of the older adult population are mandated by the ethics of delivering appropriate and evidence-based care. All primary care providers need to be familiar with the special needs of this unique, valuable, and often vulnerable population.

The organic process of aging is called *senescence,* the medical study of the aging process is called *gerontology,* and the study of diseases that affect older adults is called *geriatrics.* Aging presents unique challenges for older adults, their loved ones and families, their surrounding communities, and their health-care providers. The human life cycle—or "life expectancy"—varies from country to country. Old age is not a definite biological stage, as the chronological age denoted as "old age" varies culturally and historically. For purposes of this chapter, an older adult is one who is aged 65 or older because life expectancy in the United States exceeds that of many—but certainly not all—other countries.

Hirth (2011) describes geriatrics as the field of medicine that strives to provide patient care in the most comprehensive way; some geriatricians have even noted that geriatrics is essentially good "nursing care."

It considers not just diagnosis and treatment but also the patient's preferences for care; the cultural and ethnic background that affect how the patient receives, interprets, and conceptualizes their illness; and consequently how this affects the patients' decision making and interaction with health-care professionals. It fits within the Circle of Caring. It weighs the risks and benefits of treatment in the balance of the patient's physical functioning, living situation, and health-care priorities as well as the strength or weakness of the evidence for a particular intervention.

DEMOGRAPHICS AND THE CHANGING FACE OF AGING

The older adult population growth is increasing exponentially, according to the U.S. Census Bureau (U.S. Census Bureau, 2020), and despite the preponderance of chronic diseases and morbidity, the older population is *overall* a healthier, more functional group. Older adults are generally categorized as *young-old* at 65 to 75 years; *old,* which is 76 to 85 years; and *old-old,* which are those patients 85 years and older. The group most rapidly increasing in size consists of those individuals older than 85 years. Those 85 and older are projected to more than double from 6.6 million in 2019 to 14.4 million in 2040, a 118% increase. The United States has the highest absolute number of centenarians in the world, with 97,000 living in the country. Japan comes second with 79,000 people who are 100 years or older (2016 and 2020) (Projected Age Groups and Sex Composition of the Population: Main Projections Series for the United States, 2017–2060, 2018).

The U.S. population of those 65 years and older has multiplied rapidly from 2009 to 2019 and continues to increase, growing by more than a third (36%) in the past 10 years. The 2020 Profile of Older Americans (ACL, May 2021) reports that in 2019, there were more than 54.1 million adults aged 65 years and older living in the United States; this represents 16% of the population, about one in every seven Americans. This group consisted of 30 million women and 24.1 million men age 65 and older, which is 125 women for every 100 men at age 85. Between 2020 and 2030 alone—when the last of the Baby Boom cohorts reaches age 65—the number of older adults is projected to increase by almost 18 million, and 2040 projections see those older than 65 years numbering 80.8 million, more than twice as many as in 2000.

The increase in the number of older adults correlates with increasing diversity. Minority populations in the United States are expected to outnumber the majority of white, non-Hispanic people by 2044. In 2019, nearly one in four older adults (24%), representing 12.9 million people, was a person of color (ACL, 2021). The percentages of people aged 65 years or older within each racial and ethnic group were as follows:

- African Americans (not Hispanic): 12%
- Asian Americans (not Hispanic): 13%
- Native Hawaiians and other Pacific Islanders (not Hispanic): 10 %
- American Indians and Alaskan Natives (not Hispanic): 12%
- Hispanics: 8%
- People identifying as two or more groups: 6%

For decades, U.S. life expectancy, defined as the average number of years a baby born in a given year might expect to live, continued to increase. Life expectancy is an important snapshot of the overall health of a nation. This positive trend in increasing life expectancy, however, turned around, beginning in 2015, and life expectancy continued to decline from 2016 to 2018. This was attributed, in part, to opioid overdoses, termed by some as "deaths of despair." There were increases in deaths by suicide in different age groups and injuries from gun violence. By 2019, overall life expectancy had leveled off at age 78 and 10 months. However, CDC reported in July 2021, based on nearly final 2020 data, that life expectancy in 2020 had decreased to 77 years and 4 months, the lowest since 2003. Male life expectancy (74.6) was the lowest recorded since 2003; and female life expectancy (80.2) was the lowest since 2005. Concerningly, life expectancy for black Americans dropped nearly 2.9 years, to 71 years 10 months; Hispanic Americans had the largest decline of 3 years in 2020, from 81.8 years life expectancy to 78.8; and the white population lost 1.2 years. These statistics again confirm the disparities in health care of people of color. Much of this was related to COVID-19 (74% of the overall life expectancy decline). More than 3.3 million Americans died in 2020, more than any other year in U.S. history. More than 80% of 2020's COVID deaths were people aged 65 years and older, according to CDC.

More promisingly, levels of independent function and higher education among older adults continue to increase. In 2020, 89% of the population older than age 65 years had completed high school, and approximately one-third had a bachelor's degree or higher. Educational levels alone for older adults have risen 5% since 2017, impacting household incomes. Additionally, many older adults are choosing to work longer, and people in this age-group currently comprise 6.6% of the U.S. labor force, with 9.8 million (18%) older Americans working or actively seeking work, down slightly from 2019 when 10.7 million (20.2%) were employed. From 2018 to 2019, older adults had an increase of 6.5% in household income. Households of families headed by people 65 years and older reported a median income of $70,254 in 2019. About 5% of families headed by people aged 65 and older had incomes of less than $15,000, and 81% had incomes of $35,000 or more. This equates to nearly one in 10 older adults (8.9% or 4.8 million) living below the poverty level. Older Hispanic females who lived alone (32.1%) and older African American females living alone (31.7%) experienced the highest poverty rate, again confirming long standing economic disparities. In 2019, about 1.1 million people aged 60 years and older were responsible for the basic needs of at least one grandchild.

The majority (95%) of older adults live in the community independently, and many own their own homes. In 2019, 45% of older householders spent one-third *or more* of their incomes on housing costs: 36% for homeowners and 76% for renters. Three percent of the older adult population resides in nursing homes; however, 2.8% are temporary residents receiving rehabilitation services. Two percent of older adults live in group homes or assisted living facilities. More males than females over the age of 65 years live with their spouses, predominantly due to differences in longevity between males and females. Nine percent of older adults continue to live in poverty, with an imbalance of females (10.6%) to males (7.6%). Fragile older adults older than 90 years are more likely to have increased care needs and a higher risk of living in an institution (Harper, Lyons, Potter, 2019).

This population's continued independence, functional level, and health care depend on many factors—genetics, environment, and lifestyle choices. Older adults may also be affected by the caregiver's familiarity with the physiology of aging, the impact of normal changes of aging, characteristics of this population, socioeconomic factors, health and health behaviors, health status, risks, and available resources. Those clinicians privileged to care for older adults need specialized knowledge to provide the most current, evidence-based standards of care.

PROCESSES OF AGING

Theories of Aging

Aging theories fall into two categories, evolutionary theories and physiological theories. Evolutionary theories address why aging exists and its evolution. Physiological theories of aging include cellular and structural changes that affect the organism's function (Table 82.1). Aging affects all aspects of the organism, from cellular organelles to cells to tissues to organs to the individual person. This aging process occurs differently in each human person.

Heterogeneity of Older Adults

Each older adult for whom we care presents differently. There exists far more heterogeneity in this population than any other age-group. Health-care decisions and judgments should never be based strictly on chronological age. Care or procedures should not be discounted as options due to age alone.

The normal aging process is accompanied by numerous physiological changes within different body systems.

TABLE 82.1 Theories of Aging

Category	Theory	Description
EVOLUTIONARY		
	Mutation Accumulation	Aging is a nonadaptive trait. No selective pressure is brought on older postreproductive organisms expressing a mutation with minimal effect on fitness.
	Antagonistic Pleiotropy	Considers aging an adaptive trait. Pleiotropic genes have beneficial effects on early fitness but harmful effects on late fitness.
PHYSIOLOGICAL		
	Target Theory of Genetic Damage	Aging is heavily influenced by genes. DNA is subject to damage by ionizing radiation, toxins, and alkylating agents that harm DNA structure.
	Mitochondrial DNA Damage Theory	The inner mitochondrial membrane houses the mitochondrial DNA (mDNA). In this area, damage occurs 20 times faster than in nuclear DNA. This is more harmful as 100% of mDNA is shared with the cells as opposed to 50% of nuclear DNA.
	Free Radical Theory	Free radicals are generated in metabolism. The higher the metabolic rate, the larger and more rapid the production of free radicals. This overwhelms the enzymes, inactivating them.
	Telomere Theory	The DNA replication process cannot make a copy of the end of a chromosome (telomere). There is progressive shortening of the telomere with each replication. This hypothesis offers that telomere shortening causes aging.
	Accumulation Theories	Aging is associated with an accumulation of cellular and extracellular components with altered structure that impair cellular function.

Source: Harper G, Lyons W, Potter J. (ed) (2019). Geriatrics Review Syllabus: A Core Curriculum in Geriatric Medicine. 10th Edition. New York: American Geriatrics Society 2019.

Visible manifestations of this aging process include male pattern baldness, graying of hair, thinning and wrinkling of skin, and other changes that reflect normal aging. The aging process results in the loss of physiological reserve and impaired homeostasis. Pathologies occur at higher rates in older adults, and the nurse practitioner (NP) must be able to differentiate normal from pathology.

Even in the absence of disease, these physiological changes increase older adults' vulnerability to morbidity and mortality. Many of these alterations involve decline in functional reserves with a reduced physiological response to stressors. For example, when older adults experience a physical stressor such as infection, their immune response is slower and less effective than that of a younger person. Normal age-related changes can adversely affect health and functionality and require corrective strategies to adapt to the changes. Too often, the older adult or their family members incorrectly accept the individual's decline in functionality as inevitable. Many of the physiological changes associated with aging are listed in Table 82.2, and changes in the laboratory values for older adults are listed in Table 82.3.

Normal changes of aging can cause altered or atypical presentations of common conditions, responses to treatments, and outcomes. For example, when a younger adult experiences a myocardial infarction, it is usually accompanied by crushing chest pain and diaphoresis. In the older adult, myocardial infarction often causes less obvious signs, such as nausea, confusion, and generalized weakness.

Genetic differences affect aging; however, except in rare genetic mutations, they only account for 15% of the aging process. Environmental stressors, socioeconomic status, and nutrition together more strongly affect the aging process. Habits of smoking, alcohol use, and lack of exercise affect the rate at which we age. This process results in substantial loss of physiological reserve (Nguyen et al, 2020).

Older adults often have more limited regenerative abilities and are more susceptible to acute illnesses and complications that typically are more complex than in younger populations. Additionally, older adults have a higher prevalence of chronic diseases that occur as the overall strength and resilience of the body declines. The older population also faces social issues around retirement, such as poverty, loneliness, and ageism.

A FOCUS ON HEALTHY AGING

Populations around the world are rapidly aging, with some of the fastest changes occurring in low- and middle-income countries. Promoting healthy aging, emphasizing health promotion and disease prevention, and building systems to meet the needs of older adults are sound

TABLE 82.2 Physiological Influences of the Aging Process

Age-Related Change	Appearance or Functional Change	Implication
INTEGUMENTARY SYSTEM		
Loss of dermal and epidermal thickness	Loss of subcutaneous tissue and thin epidermis	Prone to skin breakdown and injury
Decreased vascularity	• Atrophy of sweat glands resulting in decreased sweat production • Decreased body odor • Decreased heat loss • Dryness	• Alteration in thermoregulatory response • Fluid requirements that may change seasonally • Loss of skin water • Increased risk of heat stroke
RESPIRATORY SYSTEM		
Decreased lung tissue elasticity	Decreased vital capacity	Reduced overall efficiency of ventilatory exchange
Cilia atrophy	Change in mucociliary transport	Increased susceptibility to infection
Decreased respiratory muscle strength	Reduced ability to handle secretions and reduced effectiveness against noxious foreign particles Partial inflation of lungs at rest	Increased risk of atelectasis
CARDIOVASCULAR SYSTEM		
Heart valves thicken and become fibrotic.	Reduced stroke volume, cardiac output; may be altered	Decreased responsiveness to stress
Fibroelastic thickening of the sinoatrial node; decreased number of pacemaker cells	Slower heart rate	Increased prevalence of arrhythmias
Decreased baroreceptor sensitivity (stretch receptors)	Decreased sensitivity to changes in blood pressure	Prone to loss of balance, which increases the risk for falls
GASTROINTESTINAL SYSTEM		
Liver becomes smaller.	Decreased storage capacity	
Decreased muscle tone	Altered motility	Increased risk of constipation, functional bowel syndrome, esophageal spasm, diverticular disease
Decreased basal metabolic rate (rate at which fuel is converted into energy)		May need fewer calories

investments in a future where older people have the freedom to be who they are and do what they value.

With more Americans living longer and overall healthier lives, there is an increasing need to focus on health promotion in older adult populations and their specialized health-related needs. Health promotion and disease prevention in the older adult population require close collaboration among health, social welfare, and community services. Health-care providers and policymakers must rethink fundamental values related to the health care of older adults to include emotional, social, educational, and financial issues, as well as medical diagnoses and treatments. This is congruent with the Circle of Caring approach of this text, and it reemphasizes the need for nursing-based approaches in this population including person-centered care and teamwork.

The U.S. Department of Health and Human Services' *Healthy People 2030* addresses population health and supports plans to improve both individual and population health status. The overarching goal for older adults is to "improve health and wellbeing for older adults," by focusing on reducing health problems and improving quality of life. It is projected that nearly 25% of the U.S. population will be 65 and older by the year 2060. Currently, this population of older adults has high rates of comorbid conditions, such as diabetes, cardiovascular issues, osteoporosis, and dementia. Older adults fall more frequently than younger individuals. Falling is a major event and results in injury in those 65 years and older, and as many as one-third of older adults fall each year. Spending time exercising each week is a preventive intervention for chronic disease, falls, and injuries from

TABLE 82.3 Changes in Laboratory Values for Older Adults

Laboratory Test	Normal Values	Changes With Age	Comments
URINALYSIS			
Protein	0–5 mg/100 mL	Rises slightly	May be due to kidney changes with age, urinary tract infection, renal pathology
Specific gravity	1.005–1.020	Lower maximum in older persons 1.016–1.022	Decline in nephrons impairs ability to concentrate urine.
HEMATOLOGY			
Erythrocyte sedimentation rate	Males: 0–20 Females: 0–30	Significant increase	Neither sensitive nor specific in aged
Iron binding	50–160 mcg/dL 230–410 mcg/dL	Slight decrease	
Hemoglobin	Males: 13–18 g/100 mL Females: 12–16 g/100 mL	Males: 10–17 g/mL Females: none noted	Anemia common in older adults
Hematocrit	Males: 45%–52% Females: 37%–48%	Slight decrease speculated	Decline in hematopoiesis
Leukocytes	4,300–10,800/mm^3	Drop to 3,100–9,000/mm^3	Decrease may be due to drugs or sepsis and should not be attributed immediately to age.
Lymphocytes	500–2,400 T cells/mm^3 50–200 B cells/mm^3	T-cell and B-cell levels fall.	Infection risk higher; immunization encouraged
Platelets	150,000–350,000/mm^3	No change in number	
BLOOD CHEMISTRY			
Albumin	3.5–5/100 mL	Decline	Related to decrease in liver size and enzymes; protein-energy malnutrition common
Globulin	2.3–3.5 g/100 mL	Slight increase	
Total serum protein	6–8.4 g/100 mL	No change	Decreases may indicate malnutrition, infection, liver disease.
Blood urea nitrogen	Males: 10–25 mg/100 mL Females: 8–20 mg/100 mL	Increases significantly up to 69 mg/100 mL	Decline in glomerular filtration rate; decreased cardiac output
Creatinine	0.6–1.5 mg/100 mL	Increases to 1.9 mg/100 mL seen	Related to lean body mass decrease
Creatinine clearance	104–124 mL/min	Decreases 10% per decade after age 40 years	Used for prescribing medications for drugs excreted by kidney
Glucose tolerance	62–110 mg/dL after fasting; less than 120 mg/dL after 2 hours postprandial	Slight increase of 10 mg/dL/decade after 30 years of age	Diabetes increasingly prevalent; drugs may cause glucose intolerance
Alkaline phosphatase	13–39 IU/L	Increase by 8–10 IU/L	Elevations greater than 20% usually due to disease; elevations may be found with bone abnormalities, drugs (e.g., narcotics), and eating a fatty meal

falls. The older adult experiences more infections and is hospitalized for these infectious diseases at a higher rate. Preventive care and vaccines have protective effects in preserving function and quality of life.

The general objectives for this population of older adults include physical activity in a larger percentage of those suffering from physical or cognitive health problems, reduced rate of pressure injury–related hospital admissions, and reduction of hospital admissions for diabetic issues. Additionally, *Healthy People 2030, Older Adults* addresses goals related to dementia that include improved detection and earlier treatment, decreasing preventable hospitalizations, and increasing discussion of symptoms with a provider; promoting safe practices such as hand washing and using separate cutting boards and the like to help decrease foodborne illnesses; regular oral hygiene and dental care for prevention of oral conditions, such as tooth loss, and treating periodontitis; screening for osteoporosis and increasing physical activity including strength training to help prevent progression of the disease; supporting immune system function with a healthy diet to prevent respiratory infections; and screening for hearing loss and vision loss to decrease sensory or communication disorders that also lead to falls (see https://health.gov/healthypeople/objectives-and-data/browse-objectives/older-adults for greater detail).

To promote healthy aging, the World Health Organization named 2021 to 2030 the *Decade of Healthy Ageing*. This new initiative emphasizes health prevention and the need to build systems to meet the needs of older adults, with the goal of realizing a future where older people have the freedom to be who they are, free of ageism, and to do what they value. The strategy has two goals:

- Five years of evidence-based action to maximize functional ability that reaches every person
- Establish evidence and partnerships necessary to support a Decade of Healthy Ageing from 2021 to 2030

The strategy has five objectives:

1. Commitment to action on healthy aging in every country
2. Developing age-friendly environments
3. Aligning health systems to the needs of older populations
4. Developing sustainable and equitable systems for providing long-term care (home, communities, institutions)
5. Improving measurement, monitoring, and research on healthy aging

This initiative presents an "opportunity to bring together government, civil society, international agencies, professionals, academia, the media and the private sector for ten years of concerted, catalytic and collaborative action to improve the lives of older people, their families and the communities in which they live." (What Is the Decade of Healthy Ageing? WHO, 2020).

Health-Care System Change

Not only do the numbers of older adults continue to increase, but the cost of providing care to them also escalates yearly (Coe, Skira, & Larson, 2018). Providers and payers will need to find ways to provide needed care while holding costs to a sustainable level. *Healthy People 2030* lists the following emerging issues in the health care of older adults:

- Person-centered care planning that includes caregivers and families
- Quality measures of care and monitoring of health conditions
- Fair pay and compensation standards for formal and informal caregivers
- Minimum levels of geriatric training for all health professionals
- Enhanced data on certain subpopulations of older adults, including the aging LGBTQ+ populations

Sixty-eight percent of older adults have two or more chronic diseases (National Council on Aging, 2020) that require a potentially complex plan of care centered around the wishes of the patient and family. Creating an effective care plan that functions across a continuum of settings, providers, and living conditions can improve the overall quality of life for older adults.

Health systems have traditionally been designed to respond to episodic health needs than the more complex and chronic health needs that tend to arise with increasing age. There is an urgent need to develop and implement comprehensive and coordinated primary health-care approaches that can prevent, slow, or reverse declines in intrinsic capacity and where these declines are unavoidable, to help older people compensate in ways that maximize their functional ability. Integrated-care approaches should be community based, designed around the needs of the older person rather than the provider, and coordinated effectively with long-term care systems.

Services should be oriented around the needs of older people rather than the needs of the services themselves. Services should respond to a diversity of older people that ranges from those with high and stable levels of intrinsic capacity through those with declining capacity to people whose capacity has deteriorated to the point of needing the care and support of others. According to the WHO Guidelines on Integrated Care for Older People (ICOPE, 2016), important elements of integrated care at the community level are as follows:

- A comprehensive assessment and care plan shared with all providers
- Common care and treatment goals across different providers
- Community outreach and home-based interventions
- Support for self-management
- Comprehensive referral and monitoring processes
- Community engagement and caregiver support (WHO, 2016)

Delivering ICOPE can support a transformation in the way health systems are designed and operate. One of the most successful methods to help older adults improve their quality of life while meeting all their health-care needs is to use a team approach to care throughout care management. Geriatric care management helps older adults and their families find resources and manage stress. The care manager can be a medical office–based provider or a consultant available to older adults for a fee or through insurance coverage (Box 82.1). In primary-care settings with many older adult patients, a list of local care

Box 82.1 Services Provided by a Care Manager

- Assessment to determine what is needed to maximize patient's quality of life
- Complete evaluations and referral recommendations for where to turn and what to do for specific types of care
- Design, implement, and manage a comprehensive plan of care to relieve uncertainty, educate patient about available services, and help older adults and their families understand the language and programs involved in eldercare
- Family meetings to provide a safe space and a neutral party to listen to family concerns and help work toward resolving disagreements
- Coordination of services, appointments, and follow-up, based on individual needs and decisions
- Assistance with living arrangement transitions
- Advocacy for older patients at doctor visits and hospital stays and review of their care
- Assistance with screening, arranging, and monitoring services

Source: Aging Life Care Association. (2020). https://www.aginglifecare.org/ALCA/About_Aging_Life_Care/What_you_need_to_know/ALCA/About_Aging_Life_Care/What_you_need_to_know.aspx

managers might be useful to patients and families, especially when older adults do not live in the same vicinity as their family members. Names and locations of geriatric care managers are available using their professional organization, found at https://www.aginglifecare.org.

Images of older adults and old age are changing. Single-focused interventions for health promotion often do not "fit" with the interrelatedness of older adult health-promotion challenges, and thus, clear age-specific preventive health guidelines for the older population are only recently becoming available. Many disorders in older adults encompass multiple risk factors that involve several systems and interventions to achieve outcomes; this presents a challenge when measuring and synthesizing evidence and reporting outcomes (Harper, Lyons, Potter, 2019). Medicare will only pay for A- and B-level recommendations that meet the U.S. Preventive Services Task Force (USPSTF) stringent evidence guidelines, leaving other beneficial interventions without coverage (see Table 82.4). Another confounding factor is the way that outcomes for screening are measured in terms of years of life saved; for older adults, quality of life or functional life is a more realistic goal (van Leeuwen, van Loon, van Nes, et al, 2019).

TABLE 82.4 Screening Guidelines for Older Adults

Clinical Recommendation	Evidence Rating	Reference
The USPSTF concludes that the current evidence is insufficient to assess the balance of benefits and harms of screening for hearing loss in asymptomatic adults aged 50 years or older.	I	USPSTF, 3/9/2021
The USPSTF recommends annual screening for lung cancer with low-dose computed tomography in adults aged 50–80 years who have a 20 pack-year smoking history and currently smoke or have quit within the past 15 years.	B	USPSTF, 3/9/2021
The USPSTF recommends against screening for asymptomatic carotid artery stenosis in asymptomatic adults.	D	USPSTF, 2/2/2021
The USPSTF recommends clinicians ask about tobacco use, advise cessation, and provide behavioral interventions and US FDA-approved pharmacotherapy for cessation for adults who use tobacco.	A	USPSTF, 1/19/2021
The USPSTF recommends screening for hepatitis B virus in (adolescents and) adults at increased risk of infection.	B	USPSTF, 12/15/2020
The USPSTF recommends offering or referring adults with cardiovascular disease risk factors to behavioral counseling interventions to promote a healthy diet and physical activity.	B	USPSTF, 11/24/2020
The USPSTF recommends behavioral counseling for all sexually active (adolescents and) adults who are at increased risk for sexually transmitted infections.	B	USPSTF, 8/18/2020
The USPSTF recommends screening by asking questions about unhealthy drug use in adults aged 18 years and older. Screening should be implemented when services for accurate diagnosis, effective treatment, and appropriate care can be offered or referred.	B	USPSTF, 6/9/2020
The USPSTF recommends screening for hepatitis C virus infection in adults aged 18–79 years.	B	USPSTF, 3/2/2020
The USPSTF concludes that the current evidence is insufficient to assess the balance of benefits and harms of screening for cognitive impairment in older adults.	I	USPSTF, 2/25/2020
The USPSTF recommends one-time screening for abdominal aortic aneurysm with ultrasonography in males aged 65–75 who have ever smoked.	B	USPSTF, 12/10/2019

TABLE 82.4 Screening Guidelines for Older Adults—cont'd		
Clinical Recommendation	**Evidence Rating**	**Reference**
The USPSTF recommends that clinicians offer to prescribe risk-reducing medications, such as tamoxifen, raloxifene, or aromatase inhibitors, to females who are at increased risk for breast cancer and at low risk for adverse medication effects.	B	USPSTF, 9/3/2019
The USPSTF recommends that primary care clinicians assess females with a personal or family history of breast, ovarian, tubal, or peritoneal cancer or who have an ancestry associated with breast cancer susceptibility 1 and 2 gene mutations with an appropriate brief familial risk assessment tool. Females with a positive screen should receive genetic counseling, and if indicated, genetic testing.	B	USPSTF, 8/20/2019
The USPSTF recommends screening for unhealthy alcohol use in primary care settings in adults 18 years and older and providing people engaged in hazardous drinking with brief behavioral counseling interventions to reduce unhealthy alcohol use.	B	USPSTF, 11/13/2018
The USPSTF recommends that clinicians offer or refer older adults with a body mass index of 30 or higher to intensive, multicomponent behavioral interventions.	B	USPSTF, 9/18/2018
The USPSTF recommends against screening for cervical cancer in females older than 65 years who have an adequate prior screening and are not otherwise at high risk for cervical cancer.	D	USPSTF, 8/21/2018
The USPSTF recommends screening for osteoporosis with bone measurement testing to prevent osteoporotic fractures in females 65 years and older.	B	USPSTF, 6/26/2018
The USPSTF recommends against PSA screening for prostate cancer in males 70 years and older. The American Cancer Society offers that males who choose to be tested who have a PSA less than 2.5 ng/mL may be retested every 2 years. Screening should be done annually for those with a PSA of 2.5 ng/mL or higher.	D	USPSTF, 5/8/18 Smith, Andrews, Brooks, et al, 2018
The USPSTF recommends against daily supplementation with 400 IU or less of vitamin D and 1,000 mg or less of calcium for the primary prevention of fractures in community-dwelling postmenopausal females.	D	USPSTF, 4/17/2018
The USPSTF recommends exercise interventions to prevent falls in community-dwelling adults 65 years or older who are at increased risk of falls.	B	USPSTF, 4/17/2018
The USPSTF recommends that clinicians selectively offer multifactorial interventions to prevent falls to community-dwelling adults 65 years or older who are at increased risk of falls. Furthermore, clinicians should consider the balance of benefits and harms, based on the circumstances of prior falls, presence of comorbid medical conditions, and the patient's values and preferences.	C	USPSTF, 4/17/2018
The USPSTF recommends against screening for ovarian cancer in asymptomatic females without a known high risk hereditary cancer syndrome.	D	USPSTF, 2/13/2018

Abbreviations: CVD, cardiovascular disease; USPSTF, U.S. Preventive Services Task Force.
Evidence ratings: A, consistent, good-quality, patient-oriented evidence; B, inconsistent or limited-quality, patient-oriented evidence; C, consensus, disease-oriented evidence, offer or provide this service for selected patients depending on individual circumstances; D, discourage service; I, insufficient evidence.
Sources: USPSTF (n.d.); Smith RA, Andrews KS, Brooks D, et al. Cancer screening in the United States, 2019: A review of current American Cancer Society guidelines and current issues in cancer screening. CA Cancer J Clin. 2019 May;69(3):184–210.

HEALTH SCREENING FOR OLDER ADULTS

Care must respect patient preferences with regard to particular preventive measures and possible treatment. Screening for conditions for which the patient would refuse treatment is inappropriate for that patient. The benefits and harm conferred on each individual patient must be assessed before the screening. Consideration of the patient's life expectancy and their wishes is paramount. The patient's ability to comply with the recommended treatments or interventions as a result of screening is affected by cognitive, psychological, and functional status in addition to a functioning support system and environment (Bolenius et al, 2019).

"Welcome to Medicare" Visit/Annual Wellness Visit

This benefit, begun in 2005, allows all new beneficiaries to receive a preventive examination without a copayment within 1 year of beginning Medicare coverage. Components of this visit include a review of medical and family history and measurement and recording of blood pressure and body mass index. Screening for cognitive impairment, depression, functional ability, and level of safety takes place. A written schedule for recommended screening and preventive services is designed in collaboration with the patient. Education, counseling, and referrals for other personalized preventive services are implemented. Discussion of care planning, patient wishes, and goals of care support the development of an end-of-life plan.

A new Medicare benefit, the annual wellness visit (AWV), became available in 2011 with the implementation of the Patient Protection and Affordable Care Act. The Alzheimer's Association developed and published guidelines on incorporation of cognitive assessment into the AWV. The initial AWV includes height, weight, vital signs, medical and family history review, cognitive assessment, depression screening, functional assessment and review of current providers, medications, and plans for further preventive assessments. The Centers for Medicare & Medicaid Services (CMS) included cognitive function assessment as a component of the AWV secondary to organizations' and experts' input and recommendations made during the public comment period (2020 Alzheimer's Disease Facts and Figures, 2020).

The American Geriatrics Society (AGS) recommends incorporating a rapid screen containing basic components of a geriatric assessment into the AWV. These components have the potential to be related to cognition but could also identify age-related issues affecting function (Resnick, 2019). The AGS rapid screen includes a brief assessment in the domains of functional status, mobility, nutrition, vision, hearing, cognition, and depression (Table 82.5). Function is assessed by asking if the patient requires assistance with the five tasks of bathing, walking, meal preparation, medication management, and household finances. The Timed Up and Go (TUG) test assesses a person's mobility and their skill for static and dynamic balance. The clinician times the patient as they rise from sitting, walk 3 meters, turn around, walk back to the chair, and sit down (Resnick, 2019). Normal mobility is performing the test in 10 seconds or less, but taking 11 to 20 seconds indicates some disability or frailty. The risk of patient falls correlates with increased test time. The TUG test has excellent reliability (Resnick, 2019).

Unintentional weight loss of 5% or more over 6 months or low body weight is part of the third domain and an indicator of nutritional issues (Resnick, 2019). Vision is assessed, using a Snellen chart, and hearing assessment is assessed, using the whisper test. Administration of the Mini-Cog screens for cognitive impairment. The patient is given three words to remember and repeat back to the examiner; next, the patient draws a clock, placing the numbers correctly and adding hands indicating a time of 11:10. The examiner then elicits the earlier three words. Mood is assessed, using two questions about feeling down, depressed, or hopeless in the past month and having little interest or pleasure in doing things in the past month (Resnick, 2019).

TABLE 82.5 Strategy for Rapid Screening

Domain	Rapid Screen
Functional status	Answers "yes" to one or more of the following: Because of a health or physical problem, do you need help to: a) Take a bath or shower b) Walk across the room c) Prepare meals d) Manage medications e) Manage household finances
Mobility	"Timed Up and Go" test: Unable to complete in less than 15 seconds Usual gait speed: Unable to walk 50 feet in less than 20 seconds
Nutrition	Unintentional weight loss equal to or greater than 5% in prior 6 months
Vision	If unable to read a newspaper headline and sentence while wearing corrective lenses, test each eye with Snellen chart: Unable to read greater than 20/40
Hearing	Acknowledges hearing loss when questioned or unable to perceive a letter/number combination whispered at 2 feet
Cognitive function	Three-item recall: Unable to remember all three items after 1 minute Mini Cog: Recall = 0 or recall is less than 3 and abnormal clock
Depression	Answers "yes" to either of the following: In the past month, have you often been bothered by: a) Feeling down, depressed, or hopeless b) Having little interest or pleasure in doing things

Source: Harper G, Lyons W, Potter J. (2019). Assessment. Geriatrics Review Syllabus (10th Edition). American Geriatrics Society, New York.

This rapid screen assesses the older adult for indicators of cognitive decline, allowing for earlier identification, evaluation, and possible treatment in the primary care setting. The AGS and the Alzheimer's Association have identified key criteria for cognitive assessment, which include valid and reliable instruments. These can be administered in 5 minutes or less; are easily administered by ancillary staff; have good to excellent psychometric properties; are free from educational, language, and cultural bias; and are available for clinicians in the public domain (Resnick, 2019).

Approach to the Older Adult

Each encounter with the older adult presents an opportunity to observe their present function, gait, and stability. The experienced clinician will escort the patient from the waiting area and accompany them to the examination room, offering the ability to observe the patient arising from a chair, gathering their belongings, and walking (if able) to the examination room. The optimal environment is well lit, without backlighting. Avoid or minimize noise and interruptions. Face the patient directly, preferably sitting at eye level. Speak slowly, validate the ability to hear, and compensate as needed. Questions may be printed in large print, if needed. Ensure sufficient time for the patient to answer questions and provide information. Utilize patient education materials that are appropriate for the patient's level of health literacy (Harper, Lyons, Potter, 2019).

Age-related changes in vision and/or pathology potentially impair the older adult's ability to report signs or symptoms of disease or cognitive impairment, present at higher rates with advancing age. A detailed physical examination must include blood pressure, vital signs, and BMI at a minimum. Additional assessments should be added, based on symptoms, underlying medical conditions, effects of disease progression, and adverse effects of treatment, in addition to gait and sensory impairment (Resnick, 2019).

It is always important to remember, given the increasing heterogeneity associated with aging, the atypical presentation of illness in older adults in every setting where older adults are seen—acute and primary care and long-term care settings. The older adult may present vague (nonspecific) symptoms and history; certain serious and treatable conditions may be missed because they are considered by the person or family to be a normal part of aging; or they may be reluctant to report certain issues as they do not want further tests or hospitalization. Communication deficits and provider bias may also lead to underreporting. Additionally, and commonly, older adults frequently present with altered (atypical) presentation, meaning "no signs and symptoms, unrelated to or even the opposite of what is usually expected" (Resnick, 2022).

Health-promotion activities should be incorporated into every patient encounter, as opposed to being addressed selectively, and they should be individualized to the patient. Recent efforts focus on partnering population-based, community-centered programs with personal health initiatives in older adults to make interventions more available and more economical and to increase socialization opportunities and harness the power of group support.

Healthy Lifestyle Counseling and Health Promotion

Throughout the life span, healthy lifestyle and health promotion remain essential components of medical care. When collaborating with the older adult patient regarding screening and routine health maintenance examinations, the benefits should be weighed against the patient's goals of care, life expectancy, and the feasibility of testing in regard to functional status. The challenge facing most health promotion efforts comes from the goal of maximizing longevity and avoiding death, when the correct goal focuses on maintaining function and reducing dependency.

The Welcome to Medicare visit provides an ideal opportunity for healthy lifestyle counseling, along with a thorough history and assessment of home safety and depression. Healthy lifestyle counseling should be addressed at each visit, using brief motivational interviewing (Harper, Lyons, Potter, 2019).

Physical Activity

Older adults are the least active age-group, although recent trends show an increase in physical activity in older adults. The American College of Sports Medicine and the American Heart Association issued updated recommendations for physical activity in all adults, with additional recommendations tailored to adults older than 65 years and adults aged 50 to 64 years with chronic conditions that are clinically significant or result in functional limitations. Counseling on physical activity should include any type of activity that the patient is able and willing to do. The health benefits of regular physical activity are well-documented and include flexibility, increased muscle mass, maintenance of desirable weight, decreased insulin resistance, decreased peripheral vascular resistance, lower blood pressure, and a sense of well-being. Whenever possible, the components of aerobic activity (low to moderate), flexibility, balance, and strengthening (weight training) should be included, and the physical activity prescription should be individualized to the patient.

Active hobbies, such as gardening, golfing, tennis, dancing, bowling, hiking, and swimming, are beneficial. Tai chi and yoga are helpful for stretching and balance. Frail older adults or those with impaired mobility can benefit from armchair exercises and modified ambulation; a recent study showed a decrease in risk of death in older adults with multiple morbidities who engaged in regular physical activity (Harper, Lyons, Potter, 2019).

Patients need to be reassured that expensive equipment or fitness memberships are not necessary to increase physical activity; motivation is the key. There are also many community exercise programs targeted to older adults, as well as Web sites that can be shared if the patient has access to the Internet. These include Exercise is Medicine, the American Association of Retired Persons, the National Council on Aging, and the National Institute on Aging. Many programs are now targeting exercise and brain health to prevent cognitive decline. Several government and community group programs have handouts for patients. Before embarking on an exercise program, all patients should have an evaluation of health history, including medications, present physical activity and functional level, potential barriers to exercise, and a physical examination. Older adults with known or suspected cardiac risk factors should have a stress test before engaging in vigorous exercise. All participants should be reminded of the need for adequate hydration and the use of caution during extreme weather conditions.

Nutrition

The heterogeneity of older adults is evident in the wide range of nutritional issues affecting them. Before initiating counseling on diet, obtain baseline information on current dietary intake and activity pattern and combine this with height and weight data and other health status information. For patients in the long-term care setting, this information is obtained easily from chart documentation. For community-dwelling older adults, a brief nutrition screening tool such as the Mini Nutritional Assessment (MNA) can be helpful. The abbreviated MNA consists of six questions, and there is a patient questionnaire that can be downloaded or mailed in advance of the visit. The MNA Web site contains a section on tools for clinicians, including a user guide and streaming video. It is available in multiple languages as well.

The importance of a healthy, balanced diet to the overall health of older adults cannot be overemphasized. Chronic illness and disability can interfere with the activities of daily living such as shopping or preparing meals. Financial hardship can limit food choices. Prescribed medications can affect absorption of nutrients, sense of taste, or appetite. Depression or social isolation can contribute to poor nutrition. Another problem commonly seen in community-dwelling older adults is obesity. Close to one-half of U.S. older adults are overweight or obese (Jun et al, 2020). A recent systematic review of interventions targeting obesity in older adults found that programs combining physical activity and diet had better outcomes, although the findings were of low to moderate quality (Jun et al, 2020). There is a need for further research to guide clinical interventions to decrease obesity. Overweight and obesity are associated with heart disease, certain types of cancer, type 2 diabetes, breathing difficulties, stroke, arthritis, and psychological problems. Although there is a decline in the prevalence of overweight and obesity after age 60 years, it remains a problem for many older adults. It is a major risk factor for decreased mobility and functional impairment, as well as a cardiovascular risk. General guidelines for dietary counseling include:

- Limit fat and cholesterol.
- Maintain a balanced caloric intake.
- Emphasize the daily inclusion of grains, fruits, and vegetables.
- Ensure an adequate dietary calcium intake, especially for females.
- Limit alcohol, if used, to one drink daily for females and two drinks daily for males: one drink = 12 oz beer, 5 oz wine, or 1.5 oz of 80-proof distilled spirits.

Safety

Prevention of injury in the older adult is of paramount importance to continuing functionality and quality of life. Part of this counseling involves reinforcement of extant recommendations, including wearing lap and shoulder seat belts in a motor vehicle, avoiding drinking and driving, having working smoke detectors in the residence, and keeping hot water set below 120°F. For older adults who drive a motor vehicle, periodic assessment of their ongoing ability to drive safely is vital to the older adult and the public at large. Most motor vehicle accidents involve young drivers and/or older drivers.

Additionally, screening for firearms may need to be considered to ensure the safety of the older adult. The first step involves the safe storage and removal of firearms. Possession of a firearm combined with depression, caregiver stress, irreversible illness, or decline in functional abilities can invite self-inflicted injury, suicide pacts, or other acts of violence. Counsel patients to avoid having firearms in the home and to use alternative means for self-protection, such as alarm systems and pepper or mace spray.

Another recommendation involves the prevention of falls, the leading cause of nonfatal injuries and unintentional death from injury in older people. See the section on falls later in this chapter for more detail.

Aging in Place

Aging in place as a concept refers "to the ability to live in one's own home and community safely, independently and comfortably, regardless of age, income or ability level" (Bosch-Farré et al, 2020). Most older adults wish to remain in their own homes as they age. Today, older adults have multiple options supporting this desire, including support in their homes, gated retirement communities, continuing care communities, and naturally occurring retirement communities (NORCs). Housing design elements increase accessibility for the older adult and those with disabilities, increasing the likelihood that the older adult has the option to remain in their current setting (Wick, 2017).

Aging in place as an option is affected by a number of factors. Key factors contributing to the ability to age in place are safe environment, sufficient income to meet care needs, and support from family and friends in conjunction with access to supportive and effective primary care (Bosch-Farré et al, 2020). Models supporting this concept include programs of support within communities and optional community living. Two successful programs exist in NORCs and the village model. These models may be seen scattered throughout the United States and in Europe.

Eighty-nine percent of older adults voiced a preference for remaining in their homes (Wick, 2017). Cost of long-term care in a facility or nursing home ranges from

$82,000 to $100,000 per year, dependent on the location. Assisted living facilities average $44,000 per year. Older adults aging in place can expect to pay an average of $25,000 per year (Wick, 2017). Quality of life for older adults correlates directly with the ability to remain in their homes. Autonomy—the ability to take care of oneself or direct needed care at home—enhances the quality of life of the older adult (see The Patient's Voice 82.1). This option is increased by the expanded use of universal design and technological advances (Bosch-Farré et al, 2020).

Available technologies can assist patients with activities of daily living (ADLs) while simultaneously providing information to remote caregivers. Personal emergency response systems, in wide use, can alert systems when help is needed. Technology can support medication administration and tracking, vital sign monitoring, and virtual connections to caregivers and telemedicine services (Resnick, 2019). In the past few years, technology such as smart homes and sensors have been introduced to facilitate aging in place. Most of these technologies are still in their infancy but offer hope in delaying institutionalization and promoting healthy functioning at home. Other programs, primarily in European countries, are targeting at-risk "oldest old" and have designed comprehensive interventions to maintain them at home (Dahlin-Ivanoff et al, 2016). Japan, for example, has fully integrated the use of care-providing robots into the care of older adults at home and on their own. These trends continue to accelerate, and they were also fueled by the move to online service delivery during COVID.

Older adults aging in the community—whether in their own home, a continuing care community, or some assisted living facilities—benefit from interprofessional team care, typically including nurses, rehabilitation professionals, social workers, caregivers, and the primary care provider. The interprofessional team in the community setting is directed by the primary care provider, and the patient usually receives their care at a variety of outpatient settings coordinated by their primary care provider. It is incumbent on the provider to coordinate referrals and then to follow up on findings and recommendations. A documented face-to-face encounter is needed to certify the patient's eligibility for home health services or outpatient services, which may be covered by Medicare (Resnick, 2019).

Home-bound patients have functional impairments and benefit from a comprehensive geriatric assessment. This assessment supports patient evaluation of individual functional abilities and baseline, cognitive baseline, and monitoring the course of chronic illness. Home visits facilitate assessment of the patient's home environment for safety related to the individual's needs. Some providers and their associates will make house calls to facilitate the care of home-bound older adults. In-home assessment differs from office-based assessment as performance-based functional assessment focuses on ADL performance by direct observation. Safety issues in the patient environment are identified quicker. Caregiver needs for support, education, and counseling are addressed more efficiently. Environmental barriers are easily identified by the provider, but usually a Medicare home safety assessment is utilized to recommend modifications and compensatory strategies. There are community-based services that provide wide ranges of social and support services to the patient while they continue to live in their home. Options include adult day care, day hospitals, the Program of All-inclusive Care for the Elderly (PACE), and long-term care programs (Resnick, 2019).

Assisted living facilities are as diverse as individual patients. They continue to grow as the population ages. Many individuals prefer to receive care in a social model as opposed to the medical model of long-term care settings. Assisted living may be covered by long-term care insurance. Medicare and usually Medicaid do not cover assisted living settings. Family involvement continues in this alternate setting. Assisted living settings vary in whether they have a provider who comes to the setting or the patient continues to see their own provider in the office (Resnick, 2019).

Sexuality

Assumptions regarding lack of sexual expression in the healthy older adult are unfounded. With the possibility of pregnancy eliminated, many mature adults feel less restraint. As a result of divorce or widowhood, they may

---

The Patient's Voice 82.1

MY CHILDREN ARE COMING TODAY

My children are coming today. They mean well. But they worry.
  They think I should have a railing in the hall. A telephone in the kitchen.
  They want someone to come in when I take a bath.
  They really don't like my living alone.
  Help me be grateful for their concern. And help them to understand that I have to do what
  I can as long as I can.
  They're right when they say there are risks. I might fall. I might leave the stove on.
  But there is no challenge, no possibility of triumph, no real aliveness without risk.
  When they were young and climbed trees and rode bicycles and went away to camp, I was terrified. But I let them go.
  Because to hold them would have hurt them.
  Now our roles are reversed. Help them see.
  Keep me from being grim and stubborn about it. But don't let them smother me.

Source: Maclay E. (1977). Green Winters: Celebrations of Old Age. NY: Reader's Digest Press distributed by Thomas Y. Crowell Co.

seek satisfaction with new partners yet lack the knowledge to protect themselves from sexually transmitted diseases, especially HIV. More than 42% of those living with HIV in the United States in 2013 were in people older than 50 years (Centers for Disease Control and Prevention [CDC], 2017), and 39% of deaths from HIV in 2014 were in adults older than 55 years (CDC, 2017). Older adults need to be taught methods for safe sex with use of a barrier to avoid sexually transmitted diseases, including HIV and hepatitis B. Using the patient's sexual history, explore patient needs, preferences, and medical or psychological obstacles to sexual expression. This exploration facilitates counseling and interventions to promote healthy sexual behavior.

Dental Health

Counseling regarding dental health in the older adult includes the need for regular visits to the dental-care provider, daily flossing, and brushing with fluoride toothpaste. Many older adults have dentures or dental implants and assume that dental checkups are no longer necessary. Oral screening for cancer is still indicated, as is periodic assessment of denture fit and functionality. Another concern is for the condition of the remaining teeth of some older adults. Periodontal disease, erosion of dentin, or other problems may render the teeth nonfunctional for chewing and a potential source for infection. Dependence on others for transportation or lack of available dental resources for patients in long-term care settings further complicates the problem. Caregivers simply may overlook this aspect of preventive health, or financial considerations may preclude treatment. Patient and family education regarding dental health is essential.

Substance Use

Counseling about substance use (tobacco, alcohol, and drugs) and injury prevention can be combined naturally within the issue of safety. Smoking is the leading preventable cause of death in the United States. Smoking cessation yields many benefits to former smokers in terms of reduction of risk for several chronic illnesses and stabilization of pulmonary status. Clear and specific guidelines are available to help health-care providers advise tobacco users to quit and to provide them with follow-up encouragement and relapse prevention management. Quitting smoking may not be a choice for the institutionalized older adult but rather dictated by the policy of the institution. Health-care providers can offer support and encouragement, emphasizing the positive health changes that will result.

Counseling regarding alcohol or other drug use can be preventive or interventional, depending on the initial assessment. The Michigan Alcohol Screening Test (MAST), the CAGE questionnaire, or the Alcohol Use Disorders Identification Test (AUDIT) can be used to assess risk. The dangers of drinking and driving and the increased risk of falling while under the influence of alcohol or any drug that acts on the central nervous system should be emphasized. Patients should be informed about the coincidental interactions between alcohol and many prescription drugs, over-the-counter preparations such as acetaminophen, and herbal remedies. The contribution of alcohol use to problems, such as insomnia, depression, aggressive behaviors, and deteriorating social relationships, should be addressed. Likewise, the problem of dependence on prescription drugs, such as analgesics, hypnotics, tranquilizers, and anxiolytics, should be assessed and addressed. Counseling in the form of individual follow-up sessions, group support, or outpatient or inpatient rehabilitation may be indicated. In a group-living situation, the governing body (i.e., resident council) may become involved if the patient's behavior threatens the safety or well-being of the other group members.

IMMUNIZATIONS

The influenza vaccine is now recommended annually for all adults older than 50 years, unless contraindicated. Residents of long-term care facilities that house people with chronic medical conditions are at especially high risk for developing the disease. Health-care workers also should receive the vaccine. Patients with a severe egg allergy or severe reaction to the influenza vaccine in the past and patients with a prior history of Guillain-Barré syndrome should talk with their health-care provider before getting the vaccine.

The tetanus-diphtheria toxoids with acellular pertussis vaccine (Tdap) is administered as a once-in-a-lifetime booster to every adult. After this, a tetanus-diphtheria (Td) booster is recommended every 10 years.

Pneumococcal vaccine should be administered as a one-time dose to PCV13-naïve adults at age 65 years, followed by a dose of PPSV23 12 months later.

Hepatitis B vaccine is recommended for high-risk people such as IV drug users, persons who are sexually active with multiple partners, those living with someone with chronic hepatitis B, patients younger than 60 years with diabetes, and all desiring protection from hepatitis B. The initial dose is given, followed 1 month later by the second dose, and then the third dose is given 4 to 6 months after the second dose.

Zostavax is recommended for all people older than 60 years as a single dose. People who have had a prior episode of zoster should be vaccinated (Advisory Committee on Immunization Practices, 2018).

GERIATRIC SYNDROMES

Geriatric syndromes are not related to one specific disease, such as bladder control problems, sleep problems, delirium, dementia, falls, gait and balance, depression, visual acuity, or weight loss. Some of these conditions result from a combination of several diseases and may require detailed assessment, diagnosis, and treatment. A tool called "SPICES," developed in 2003, lists markers of early geriatric syndromes (Shannon, Bellantoni, Weiner, 2020; Wallace & Fulmer, 2003) (Box 82.2).

Geriatric syndromes are not inevitable among older adults, and early implementation of preventive therapies and safety measures is important. Prevention is best provided using an interdisciplinary team approach with health-care providers who are geriatric centered in their education and approach. The failure of health-care providers to identify, diagnose, and treat the underlying causes of geriatric syndromes can adversely affect the health of older adults. Early detection and correction of problems such as sensory deficits, confusion, and gait and balance issues can increase independence and longevity among this group. The focus of all health-care providers should be on maintaining function, dignity, and individual control to promote health and quality of life.

Geriatric syndromes are associated with substantial morbidity and poor outcomes (Lundy et al, 2020). Geriatric syndromes are multifactorial, and although each is distinct, they share several risk factors. For example, older age, cognitive impairment, functional impairment, and mobility impairment are risk factors for falls, functional decline, delirium, and pressure injuries. Therefore, identification of these risk factors must prompt an evaluation for multiple conditions. The following discussion focuses on geriatric syndromes and emphasizes their overlapping risk factors as well as overlapping symptoms.

Cognition

Mental status change in older adults is not uncommon and often caused by three problems: depression, delirium, and dementia (see Chapters 6 and 8).

Delirium describes a state of mental confusion that develops suddenly and can fluctuate over time. Symptoms of delirium include hallucinations, delusions, and a dreamlike state of incoherence and mental confusion. One in 10 hospitalized older patients has episodes of delirium, and these patients often have poor outcomes. Common causes of delirium in older adults include infection (often urinary tract infection), anticholinergic medications, sedatives, antidepressant drugs, steroids, dehydration and electrolyte imbalance, metabolic encephalopathy, vitamin deficiencies, diabetes, and thyroid disease. An easy way to remember the causes of delirium in the older adult is the mnemonic DELIRIUM:

- D: Drugs
- E: Electrolyte imbalance
- L: Lack of drugs (withdrawal, uncontrolled pain)
- I: Infection
- R: Reduced sensory input (vision or hearing loss)
- I: Intracranial (e.g., cerebral vascular accident or subdural hematoma)
- U: Urinary retention or fecal impaction
- M: Myocardial/pulmonary

Prevention of delirium is best accomplished by treating or avoiding possible underlying causes. Unlike dementia, delirium has an underlying cause that, if corrected, can reduce or eradicate the delirium. Therefore, treatment of delirium begins with recognizing and treating the underlying cause, maintaining a quiet environment, and using simple communication methods and reassurance. In severe cases, antipsychotic drugs can reduce anxiety, hallucinations, aggressive behaviors, and delusion. However, use of drugs should not replace identification and treatment of the underlying cause of the delirium.

Dementia is another cause of confusion in older adults, and it differs significantly from delirium. Dementia has a gradual onset over months or even years. Over time, these symptoms become severe enough to impair the patient's ability to complete activities of daily living. See Chapter 8 for more specific information about dementia.

Team-based care with a social worker and access to a geriatric care manager is essential. Local and regional resources that offer education about the disease, emotional support, and financial and legal advice are important for families who care for someone with dementia (see Resources at the end of this chapter). Learning to manage challenging behaviors, feelings of grief and loss, a need for respite care (a break from caregiving duties), safety, medical care, stress relief, and planning for the future are all important issues that should be addressed with dementia caregivers. In the end-stages of dementia, placement in a care facility and hospice services are often required for these patients.

Falls

As early as 2000, falls were identified as the leading cause of older adult injury-related visits to emergency departments in the United States (Fuller, 2000). Each year 2.8 million older adults are treated in the emergency department because of a fall; that is one person every 11 seconds (National Council on Aging, 2020). However, less than one-half of those who fall tell their health-care providers.

Box 82.2   SPICES Geriatric Syndrome Markers

- Sleep Disturbances
- Problems with eating or feeding
- Incontinence
- Confusion
- Evidence of falls
- Skin breakdown

Source: Fulmer T. (2019). Fulmer SPICES: An Overall Assessment Tool for Older Adults. Hartford Institute for Gerontologic Nursing. New York. Retrieved from https://hign.org/consultgeri/try-this-series/fulmer-spices-overall-assessment-tool-older-adults

Risk factors for falls include previous falls, increasing age, medications, and cognitive deficits (CDC, 2020). Falls among older adults constitute the most common cause of traumatic injury, and adjusted for inflation, they result in direct medical costs of $31 billion annually. Each year, 800,000 older adults, one in five, are hospitalized because of a fall, most often because of a hip or head fracture. Older adults who have fallen or who feel they might fall should be evaluated for fall risk. Fall risk assessment can reduce the risks of falls, decrease the morbidity and mortality associated with falls in older adults, and improve the quality of life for both the patient and loved ones.

The CDC has created Stopping Elderly Accidents, Deaths and Injuries (STEADI), a free fall-risk assessment and prevention program for health-care professionals (CDC, 2016). This program includes physical assessment tools to assess for fall risk; instructions about how to identify patients at low, moderate, and high risk for falls; and forms to track falls among older adults. Provider guidelines for fall prevention are summarized, using the memory device RITUAL:

- Review self-assessment from older adults.
- Identify risk factors (e.g., scatter rugs in the home, lack of grab bars in bathrooms, stairs, and poor home lighting or poor vision).
- Test gait and balance (recommendation of programs such as yoga, tai chi, Zumba, and other programs for older adults to improve strength, gait, and balance).
- Undertake multifactorial assessment.
- Apply interventions (e.g., order appropriate fall prevention devices such as canes, walkers, and bathroom grab bars).
- Later follow-up.

Three questions are used to identify older adults who are at risk for falls:

1. Have you fallen in the past year?
2. Do you feel unsteady when standing or walking?
3. Do you worry about falling?

These questions are easily asked in the health-care provider's office. If the answer to any of these questions is yes, the STEADI program provides step-by-step instruction for further assessment, intervention, and treatments. Once fall risk is identified, the health-care provider is prompted to identify modifiable risk factors and offer effective interventions to prevent falls.

Fall risk is best reduced when a team effort is applied to the problem, including pharmacy, physical therapy, nursing, and medicine. Key interventions to reduce falls include patient education, enhancing strength and balance, modification of medications, management of hypotension, vitamin D and calcium supplementation, addressing foot and footwear issues, assessment of vision, and implementing home safety precautions.

MEDICATIONS IN THE OLDER ADULT

Normal changes of aging result in altered pharmacodynamics and pharmacokinetics in the older adult. These changes greatly increase the risk of adverse drug reactions (ADRs) in the older adult. This population makes up 13% of the population but has 50% of the ADRs reported. Polypharmacy can cause great harm in older adults and unfortunately is common because older adults often have multiple chronic diseases that require multiple medications (Guharoy, 2017; Jirón et al, 2016). *Polypharmacy* is defined as the practice of administering many different medications concurrently for a single disease or to treat coexisting conditions, a practice that increases the risk of ADRs (Rambhade et al, 2012). Many older adults see numerous health-care providers; each provider may prescribe medications for the condition that they are treating. Many studies in ambulatory care define polypharmacy as a medication count of five or more medications. However, current medical practice guidelines often require multiple medications to treat each chronic disease state for optimal clinical benefit. Therefore, an older patient with at least two disease states, such as heart failure and chronic obstructive pulmonary disease, will usually exceed this arbitrary threshold of more than five medications (Boyd et al, 2005). The concurrent use of multiple medications by a patient to treat frequently coexisting conditions may result in ADRs.

Health-care providers are not always aware of other medications taken by the older adult, whether prescribed by another provider or in the form of over-the-counter products that the patient chooses to use. Additionally, the older adult population is at greater risk of ADRs from medications due to age-related changes in the absorption, distribution, metabolism, and elimination of medications (Breton et al, 2011; Garg et al, 2004).

Risks of Polypharmacy

Management of both prescribed and over-the-counter medications, including herbal substances, presents a special and significant challenge for older adults. Older patients may become confused about how to correctly take medications, especially when multiple medications are prescribed to be taken several times daily. Additionally, changes in how medications look—changes in shape and color of the pill itself related to various compounding processes among different pharmaceutical suppliers—have been demonstrated to also interfere with correct medication adherence and to be confusing to the consumer in general. The costs of medications, as well as side effects, may also lead to noncompliance. Enhanced drug coverage for older adults has been shown to be a powerful incentive to improve the use of beneficial therapies (Saeed & Mehta, 2020).

Unfortunately, polypharmacy has been linked to an increase in adverse events, including falls, confusion, extrapyramidal symptoms, and syncope (Fernando et al, 2017; George & Verghese, 2017). The risk of falling, for example, is directly correlated with the number of health conditions an older person has (Fernando et al, 2017; George & Verghese, 2017). Furthermore, not to be underestimated is underutilization of prescribed drugs, not just overutilization (Fick et al, 2021). Some sources say that in general, less than 50% of people take medications as ordered and that this increases with age (Fick et al, 2021).

Factors leading to unintended underutilization include clinicians not recognizing medication benefit in the older population, affordability, and dose availability (Fick et al, 2021).

Management of Polypharmacy

One strategy that may reduce the risks of polypharmacy is medication reconciliation. Medication reconciliation is the process of obtaining a list of all medications that a person is taking including dose and frequency and comparing that list to what has been ordered. This can provide valuable information on duplicate or overlapping drug regimens (Aronson, 2017). Asking older patients to bring all their medications in the original containers to each office visit can facilitate accurate medication reconciliation. The need for adoption of this strategy has grown, as older adults often see numerous healthcare providers and are treated in different settings including hospitals, clinics, and physician offices (Fick et al, 2021; Sirois et al, 2017). Patients' medications can change rapidly, which may result in confusion or inappropriate medication administration, and periodic assessment of the benefits of individual medications in comparison to their risks is essential (Fick et al, 2021; Sirois et al, 2017).

Another strategy to reduce polypharmacy risks is to be aware of which drugs frequently cause problems in this age group. The AGS Beers Criteria (Fick et al, 2021) is a valuable resource for providers when prescribing medications. The criteria identify medications for which the risks may be greater than the benefits for individuals aged 65 years and older. It includes the following classifications:

- Medications that are potentially inappropriate for use in older adults
- Medications that are potentially inappropriate for use in older adults due to drug–disease interactions or drug–syndrome interactions
- Medications that should be used with caution in older adults

Health-care providers should use the Beers Criteria as a guide for prescribing in all settings except for palliative care and hospice care (Fick et al, 2021; Sirois et al, 2017; Nicoteri, 2019).

SPECIAL TOPICS IN AGING

LGBTQ+

A specific aging minority, LGBTQ+ older adults, is an extremely underserved population. This population suffers large care disparity. They are five times less likely to receive usual care, and receive less care specific to their unique needs. Currently, there are 1 to 2 million older LGBTQ+ adults living in the United States. This population is expected to increase considerably by 2030. Their numbers are underrepresented due to stigmatization preventing self-identification. Females identifying as lesbian and bisexual have higher rates of cardiovascular disease and obesity and lower rates of screening mammography, compared with heterosexual older females. Gay and bisexual older males have higher rates of poor physical health and are more likely to live alone than heterosexual older males. Transgender older adults are challenged with health concerns and disparities related to their gender identity, fear of discrimination, victimization, internalized stigma, and financial barriers, related to fear of accessing health services. Older LGBTQ+ adults have higher rates of disability, poor mental health, smoking, and excessive drinking, compared with older heterosexual adults. When asking about sexual orientation, create an environment that respects the patient and allows the patient to disclose information. Ask questions sensitively by asking general questions regarding living situation, relationships, and support system. The older LGBTQ+ patient may not disclose their sexual orientation or identity and are less likely to identify than younger LGBTQ+ patients. This population has increased risk from cardiovascular disease, anal cancer, prostate cancer, breast cancer, cervical cancer, HIV/AIDS, anxiety, and substance abuse. Transgender older adults encounter health issues corresponding to their sex at birth. Significant distress may result in coping with a disease associated with their prior gender and the associated examinations.

LGBTQ+ adults are up to twice as likely to report mood and anxiety disorders. Managing social stressors such as prejudice, stigma, and homophobia over an extended time results in higher risks of depression, suicide, and substance abuse. LGBTQ+ older adults may have strained relationships with family or children related to their sexuality or efforts to conceal sexual preferences. Clinicians must recognize the patient's family of choice and be alert to isolation and loneliness.

Loneliness

Loneliness, experienced more frequently by the older adult than in younger individuals, is described as "a depressed feeling related to perceived social isolation and a lack of meaningful companionship" (Lee & Cagle, 2017). Loneliness may be experienced in all life stages. It is a complex phenomenon and does not relate to a lack of belonging or absence of companionship. In early work, Victor, Scambler, and Bond (2012) discuss it as the difference between desired social connection and the person's perception of their actual relationships. "Lonely people are at risk for reduced health and well-being, including poor life satisfaction, depression, low self-esteem and reduced hope, negative affect and impaired function in activities of daily living" (O'Rourke, Collings, & Sidani, 2018). There are multiple scales available; however, they are all measured against the UCLA Loneliness Scale. The instrument includes 20 items; 11 items are negatives (i.e., expressing loss or missing elements) while nine are positives (i.e., I feel connected) (Ausín et al, 2019).

Interventions to counter loneliness range from regular chores and activities, even if solitary activities, to counseling to support reframing a person's outlook on life or their relationships. Researchers found that one of the strongest interventions was social support. However, they further examined this factor and found that the "giving of social support was more positive than receiving. Helping others made people feel needed" (O'Rourke, Collings, & Sidani, 2018).

These researchers also categorized the interventions found to be effective into categories: personal contact, activity/discussion groups, animal contact, skills courses, multifaceted programs, models of care, reminiscence, support group, and public broadcast (O'Rourke, Collings, & Sidani, 2018). The researchers recommended that each action be systematically tested for effectiveness of the distinct type of intervention.

COVID-19 and the Older Adult

The older adult has the highest risk for hospitalization and death secondary to COVID-19. The CDC reports the greatest risk for severe illness related to COVID is among those 85 years and older (COVID-19 [2021]. Your Health: Older Adults. Centers for Disease Control and Prevention). Eighty percent of COVID-19 U.S. deaths reported occurred in adults 65 years and older. The population of people 65 years and older suffered twice the risk of becoming ill, 95 times the risk of hospitalization, and 8,700 times the risk of death compared with other populations (COVID-19 [2021]. Your Health: Older Adults. Centers for Disease Control and Prevention). Older adults constitute approximately 15% of the population but have accounted for over 25% of patient deaths from COVID.

Long-term care facilities, especially nursing homes, felt the effects of COVID disproportionately, sustaining a death rate of 10% as of March 2021 (Curiskis et al. What We Know—and What We Don't Know—About the Impact of the Pandemic on Our Most Vulnerable Community. The COVID Tracking Project. The Atlantic. March 31, 2021). Those older adults in congregate living sustained this higher risk due to the communal setting facilitating the spread among residents. Consequently, residents experienced hardship imposed by the facility lockdowns, eliminating all visitors from the building. They have suffered social isolation, limited mobility, and fewer activities and services at a time when families could not intervene or may not have even been aware. This is heightened in the older adult with cognitive impairment unable to understand their loved ones' absences and why they have not visited. A pervasive sense of abandonment is the new norm.

Older adults living independently in congregate settings have declined functionally due to apartment or living quarter restrictions. Older adults regularly walking 1 to 2 miles a day around their residential campus now have their ability to walk limited to the length of their apartment. Functional loss has been the disastrous result. Social distancing and remaining home have placed some older adults at greater risk for the unintended consequence of social isolation. Social isolation and loneliness are linked to higher risks for a variety of health problems. These potential health problems include hypertension, anxiety, depression, cognitive decline, functional decline, and even death (O'Sullivan et al, 2021). This population experienced increased risks of debility and death from numerous other treatable comorbid conditions due to delayed or avoided care or emergency visits due to fear of contracting COVID.

Due to the disproportionate impact of COVID on older adult population, the American Geriatrics Society convened an expert panel. This panel discussed the impact of COVID-19 on older adults, based on principles of justice of resource allocation, legal considerations. This AGS panel adopted seven position statements (Box 82.3).

The older adult population commonly experiences vague symptomatology in their presentation of many

---

Box 82.3 American Geriatrics Society Position Statement on the Impact of COVID-19

1. Age should not be used as a means for excluding anyone from care.
2. Assessment should include comorbidities and consideration of the disparate impact of social determinants of health.
3. Encourage decision makers to focus primarily on potential short-term (not long-term) outcomes.
4. Ancillary criteria such as "life years saved" and "long-term predicted life expectancy" should be avoided due to its impact to disadvantage older adults.
5. Creation of staffing triage committees tasked with allocation of scarce resources.
6. Develop transparent institutional resources allocation strategies.
7. Appropriate advanced care planning should be facilitated.

Source: Farrell T, Ferrante L, Brown T, et al. (2020). AGS Position Statement: Resource Allocation Strategies and Age- Related Consideration in the COVID-19 Era and Beyond. Journal of the American Geriatrics Society. 68: 1136–1142.

pathologies. COVID presented in the senior care settings with vague nonspecific symptomatology. Subsequently, COVID-19 in older adults went unrecognized in the early days of the pandemic. Presentations of lethargy, anorexia, and increased falls went unrecognized. Currently, most congregate living settings have high rates of vaccination of both staff and residents, reporting vaccination rates between 85% and 98%. Increased awareness has resulted in frequent preventive isolation, even in those vaccinated individuals returning from acute care to a rehab setting. Frequent testing is occurring with each transition of care and even between areas of a continuing care community (Curiskis et al, 2021).

These interventions have been effective. The CDC COVID data reported weekly since early 2020 demonstrated massive improvements. The peak impact of COVID in the nursing home setting occurred the week ending December 20, 2020. The reported rate of cases was 30.45 and reported rate of deaths was 5.57 in the nursing home setting. The most recent CDC data from the week ending May 9, 2021, shows a decrease in the case rate to 0.85 and in the death rate to 0.37 (CDC [2021a]). The population 65 years and older in the United States has a vaccine completion rate of 73% (CDC [2021c]).

END-OF-LIFE DECISION MAKING

Older adults should be asked about their end-of-life (EOL) preparations at annual office visits, when entering the hospital, or when undergoing an outpatient procedure. For this reason, older people, even those who are healthy, should be encouraged to document their wishes for EOL care and discuss these instructions with their physicians. See Chapter 84 for more specific information about end-of-life care.

CONCLUSION

The number of older adults in the U.S. population and around the world continues to grow, and older adults represent a larger segment of society. Caring for the health of older adults and acting as a primary care provider for this group present unique challenges and require special knowledge and expertise. Although people are living longer, they often struggle with multiple chronic diseases and geriatric syndromes that diminish quality of life for both themselves and their families. Creating care plans specific to older adults enables the primary care provider to improve the quality of life and longevity of older adults and aids families caring for their older loved ones.

REFERENCES

Ahn M, Kang J, Kwon HJ. The Concept of Aging in Place as Intention. Gerontologist. 2020 Jan 24;60(1):50-59. doi: 10.1093/geront/gny167. PMID: 30605499

Alldred DP, Kennedy MC, Hughes C, et al. Interventions to optimise prescribing for older people in care homes. *Cochrane Database Syst Rev.* 2016;2:CD009095.

Alzheimer's Disease Facts and Figures. (2020). Alzheimer's Association Report. Alzheimers & Dementia 16(3). 385-580.

Arias E, Tejada-Vera B, Ahmad F. (2021). Provisional Life Expectancy Estimates for January through June, 2020. NVSS Vital Statistics Rapid Release. Report No. 010. Hyattsville, MD.

Ausín B, Muñoz M, Martín T, et al. (2019). Confirmatory factor analysis of the Revised UCLS Loneliness Scale (UCLA LS-R) in individuals over 65, Aging and Mental Health. 23(3).

Bell HT, Steinsbekk A, Granas AG. Elderly users of fall-risk-increasing drug perceptions of fall risk and the relation to their drug use—a qualitative study. *Scand J Prim Health Care.* 2017;35(3):247–255.

Bleijenberg N, Imhof L, Mahrer-Imhof R, et al. Patient characteristics associated with a successful response to nurse-led care programs targeting the oldest-old: A comparison of two RCTs. *Worldviews Evid Based Nurs.* 2017;14(3):210–222.

Bölenius K, Lämås K, Sandman PO, et al. (2019). Perceptions of self-determination and quality of life among Swedish home care recipients—a cross-sectional study. *BMC Geriatr* 19, 142.

Bosch-Farré C, Malagón-Aguilera MC, Ballester-Ferrando D, et al. (2020). Healthy Ageing in Place: Enablers and Barriers from the Perspective of the Elderly. A Qualitative Study. *International journal of environmental research and public health, 17*(18), 6451.

Boulos C, Salameh P, Barberger-Gateau P. Social isolation and risk for malnutrition among older people. *Geriatr Gerontol Int.* 2016;17:286–294.

Brown-O'Hara P. (2014). Geriatric Syndromes and Their Implications for Nursing. Journal of Legal Nurse Consulting, 25(2):8–11.

Brown JD, Hutchison LC, Li C, et al. Predictive validity of the Beers and Screening Tool of Older Persons' Potentially Inappropriate Prescriptions (STOPP) criteria to detect adverse drug events, hospitalizations, and emergency department visits in the United States. *J Am Geriatr Soc.* 2016;64(1):22–30.

Burnes D, Sheppard C, Henderson CR Jr, et al. (2019). Interventions to Reduce Ageism Against Older Adults: A Systematic Review and Meta-Analysis. *American journal of public health, 109*(8), e1–e9. https://doi.org/10.2105/AJPH.2019.305123

Centers for Disease Control. (2021a). Confirmed COVID-19 Cases and Deaths among Residents and Rate per 1,000 Resident-Weeks in Nursing Homes, by Week—United States. Retrieved from https://covid.cdc.gov/covid-data-tracker/#nursing-home-residents

Centers for Disease Control and Prevention. (2021b). COVID-19: Your Health: Older Adults.

Centers for Disease Control and Prevention. (2021c). Federal Pharmacy Partnership for Long Term Care Program. COVID Data Tracker. Retrieved from https://covid.cdc.gov/covid-data-tracker/#vaccinations-ltc

Centers for Disease Control and Prevention. Healthy aging & the built environment. http://www.cdc.gov/healthyplaces/healthtopics/healthyaging.htm. Published 2015.

Centers for Disease Control and Prevention. STEADI—older adult fall prevention. https://www.cdc.gov/steadi/. Published 2016.

Coe N, Skira M, Larson E. (2018). A Comprehensive Measure of the Costs of Caring for a Parent: Differences According to Functional Status. Journal of the American Geriatrics Society. 66(10).

Courtin E, Knapp M. (2017). Social isolation, loneliness and health in old age: a scoping review. Home and Social Care in the Community, 25 (3): 799-812.

Curiskis A, Kelly C, Kissane E, et al. (2021). What We Know—and What We Don't Know—About the Impact of the Pandemic on Our Most Vulnerable Community. The COVID Tracking Project. The Atlantic. March 31, 2021

Dahlin-Ivanoff S, Eklund K, Wilhelmson K, et al. For whom is a health-promoting intervention effective? Predictive factors for performing activities of daily living independently. *BMC Geriatr.* 2016;6:271.

Davidoff AJ, Miller GE, Sarpong EM, et al. Prevalence of potentially inappropriate medication use in older adults using the 2012 Beers criteria. *J Am Geriatr Soc.* 2015;63:486.

Family Caregiver Alliance. Alzheimer's disease and caregiving. https://www.caregiver.org/alzheimers-disease-caregiving. Published 2021.

Farrell T, Ferrante L, Brown T, et al. (2020). AGS Position Statement: Resource Allocation Strategies and Age- Related Consideration in the COVID-19 Era and Beyond. Journal of the American Geriatrics Society. 68: 1136-1142.

Fernando E, Fraser M, Hendriksen J, et al. Risk factors associated with falls in older adults with dementia: A systematic review. *Physiother Can.* 2017;69(2):161–173.

Fick D, Cooper J, Wade W, et al. (2021). Updating the BEERS Criteria for Potentially Inappropriate Medication Use in Older Adults. Archives of Internal Medicine 163: 2716-2724.

George C, Verghese J. Polypharmacy and gait performance in community-dwelling older adults. *J Am Geriatr Soc.* 2017;65(9):2082–2087.

Harper G, Lyons W, Potter J. (ed) (2019). Geriatrics Review Syllabus: A Core Curriculum in Geriatric Medicine. 10th Edition. New York: American Geriatrics Society 2019.

Hazzard WR, Blass JP, Halter JB, et al. *Principles of geriatric medicine and gerontology.* 6th ed. New York, NY: McGraw-Hill; 2016.

Hirth V, Wieland D, Dever-Bumba M. (2011). Why Geriatrics and Gerontology? Case-Based Geriatrics: A Global Approach. McGraw Hill Publishing. Sykesville, Maryland.

Hofman, MR, van den Hanenberg F, Sierevelt IN, et al (2017). Elderly patients with an atypical presentation of illness in the emergency department. Netherland Journal of Medicine, 75 (6):241-46.

Hong SH, Park H. A meta-analysis of the risk factors related to falls among elderly patients with dementia. *Kor J Adult Nurs.* 2017;29(1):51-62. doi:10.7475/kjan.2017.29.1.51

Hung L, Liu C, Woldum E, et al. (2019). The benefits of and barriers to using a social robot PARO in care settings: a scoping review. *BMC geriatrics*, 19(1), 232. https://doi.org/10.1186/s12877-019-1244-6

Jun S, Cowan AE, Bhadra A, et al. (2020). Older adults with obesity have higher risks of some micronutrient inadequacies and lower overall dietary quality compared to peers with a healthy weight, National Health and Nutrition Examination Surveys (NHANES), 2011-2014. *Public health nutrition*, 23(13), 2268–2279.

Kennedy-Malone L, Martin-Plank L, Duffy E. (2018), *Advanced practice nursing in the care of older adults.* 2nd Edition. Philadelphia, PA: FA Davis.

Kovačević SV, Miljković B, Ćulafić M, et al. Evaluation of drug-related problems in older polypharmacy primary care patients. *J Eval Clin Pract.* 2017;23(4):860–865.

Kuhn-Thiel AM, Weiß C, Wehling M, et al. Consensus validation of the FORTA (Fit fOR The Aged) List: a clinical tool for increasing the appropriateness of pharmacotherapy in the elderly. *Drugs Aging.* 2014;31:131.

Lee J, Cagle J. (2017). Validating the 11-Item Revised University of California Los Angeles Scale to Assess Loneliness Among Older Adults. American Journal of Geriatric Psychiatry 25(11).

Lee WW, Choi KC, Yum RW, et al. Effectiveness of motivational interviewing on lifestyle modification and health outcomes of clients at risk or diagnosed with cardiovascular diseases: A systematic review. *Int J Nurs Stud.* 2016;53:331–341.

Lomas-Vega R, Obrero-Gaitán E, Molina-Ortega FJ, et al. Tai chi for risk of falls. A meta-analysis. *J Am Geriatr Soc.* 2017;65(9):2037–2043.

Lundy J, Hayden D, Pyland S, et al. (2020). An Age Friendly Health System. Journal of the American Geriatrics Society. 69(3).

Martinez-Gomez D, Guallar-Castillon P, Garcia-Esquinas E, et al. Physical activity and the effect of multimorbidity on all-cause mortality in older adults. *Mayo Clin Proc.* 2017;92(3):376–382.

Medina L, Sabo S, Vespa J. (2020). Life Expectancy in the United States: Population Estimates and Projections. United States Census Bureau, February 2020

National Council on Aging. Chronic disease management. https://www.ncoa.org/article/evidence-based-chronic-disease-self-management-education-programs. Published 2020.

National Council on Aging. (2021). Get the Facts on Chronic Disease Self-Management. Center for Healthy Aging. National Council on Aging. Washington, D. C. retrieved 4/6/21 from https://www.ncoa.org/article/get-the-facts-on-chronic-disease-self-management

Nguyen Q, Moodie E, Forget M, et al. (2020). Health Heterogeneity in Older Adults: Exploration in the Canadian Longitudinal Study on Aging. Journal of the American Geriatrics Society 69(3):678-687.

Nicoteri, JAL. (2021). Practical Use of the American Geriatric Society Beers Criteria® 2019 Update. The Journal for Nurse Practitioners 17 (2012): 789-794. (https://doi.org/10.1016/j.nurpra.2021.04.014 accessed Aug. 1, 2021).

O'Connor MN, O'Sullivan D, Gallagher PF, et al. Prevention of hospital-acquired adverse drug reactions in older people using screening tool of older persons' prescriptions and screening tool to alert to right treatment criteria: A cluster randomized controlled trial. *J Am Geriatr Soc.* 2016;64:1558.

Office of Disease Prevention and Health Promotion. *Healthy People 2020.* https://www.healthypeople.gov/2020/topics-objectives. Published 2014.

O'Rourke H, Collins L, Sidani S. (2018). Interventions to address social connectedness and loneliness for older adults: A scoping review. British Medical Journal – Geriatrics. 18: 214.

Ortman J, Velkoff V. Hogan H. An aging nation: The older population in the United States population estimates and projections. U.S. Census Bureau. https://www.census.gov/. Published 2014.

Osborn R, Moulds D, Squires D, et al. International survey of older adults finds shortcomings in access, coordination, and patient centered care. *Health Affairs.* 2014;33(12):2247–2255.

O'Sullivan R, Lawlor B, Burns A, et al. (2021). Will the Pandemic Reframe Loneliness and Social Isolation? The Lancet. 2(2).

Paliwal Y, Slattum PW, Ratliff SM. Chronic health conditions as a risk factor for falls among the community-dwelling US older adults: A zero-inflated regression modeling approach. *Biomed Res Int.* 2017;2017: 5146378.

Pilotto A, Cella A, Pilotto A, et al. Three decades of comprehensive geriatric assessment: Evidence coming from different healthcare settings and specific clinical conditions. *J Am Med Directors Assoc.* 2016;18(2):192e1–192e11.

Resnick B. (Ed.). Chapter 5: Assessment. In: *Geriatric Nursing Review Syllabus: A Core Curriculum in Advanced Practice Geriatric Nursing.* 6th ed. New York, New York: American Geriatrics Society; 2019.

Resnick, B. (ed) (2022). *Geriatrics Nursing Review Syllabus: A Core Curriculum in Advanced Practice Geriatric Nursing.* 7th Edition, Page 12. New York. American Geriatrics Society.

Saeed A, Mehta L.(2020). Statin Therapy in Older Adults for Primary Prevention of Atherosclerotic Cardiovascular Disease: The Balancing Act. American College of Cardiology. October 1, 2020. Washington, DC. Retrieved from: https://www.acc.org/latest-in-cardiology/articles/2020/10/01/11/39/statin-therapy-in-older-adults-for-primary-prevention-of-atherosclerotic-cv-disease

Saraf AA, Petersen AW, Simmons SF, et al. Medications associated with geriatric syndromes and their prevalence in older hospitalized adults discharged to skilled nursing facilities. *J Hosp Med.* 2016;11:694.

Sirois C, Laroche ML, Guénette L, et al. (2017). Polypharmacy in Multimorbid Older Adults: Protocol for a Systematic Review. Systematic Reviews. 104.

Siu HY-H, White J, Sergeant M, et al. Development of a periodic health examination form for the frail elderly in long-term care. *Can Fam Physician.* 2016;62(2):147–155.

Smith RA, Andrews KS, Brooks D, et al. Cancer screening in the United States, 2019: A review of current American Cancer Society guidelines and current issues in cancer screening. CA Cancer J Clin. 2019 May;69(3):184-210. doi: 10.3322/caac.21557. Epub 2019 Mar 15. PMID: 30875085.

Terrery CL, Nicoteri JL. The 2015 American Geriatric Society Beers Criteria: Implications for nurse practitioners. *J Nurse Pract.* 2016;12(3):192–200.

Tommelein E, Mehuys E, Van Tongelen I, et al. Community pharmacists' evaluation of potentially inappropriate prescribing in older community-dwelling patients with polypharmacy: observational research based on the GheOP^{3}S tool. *J Pub Health.* 2017;39(3):583–592.

Tanioka T, Yokotani T, Tanioka R, et al. (2021) Development Issues of Healthcare Robots: Compassionate Communication for Older Adults with Dementia. *International Journal of Environmental Research and Public Health* 18:9, 4538.

U.S. Census Bureau. Selected characteristics of families by total money income. https://www.census.gov/data/tables/time-series/demo/income-poverty/cps-finc/finc-01.html. Published 2016.

U.S. Census Bureau. (2018). Projected Age Groups and Sex Composition of the Population: Main Projections Series for the United States, 2017-2060. U.S. Census Bureau Population Division: Washington, DC.

U.S. Census Bureau. (2020). 2019 Population Estimates by Demographic Characteristics. United States Census Bureau, Washington DC.

U.S. Department of Health and Human Services. Administration for Community Living (ACL) Administration on Aging (AOA) (May 2021). 2020 Profile of Older Americans: 1-21.

U.S. Department of Health and Human Services, Office of Disease Prevention and Health Promotion. (2021). Healthy People 2030. Older Adults. Retrieved 3/1/21 from https://health.gov/healthypeople/objectives-and-data/browse-objectives/older-adults

van Leeuwen KM, van Loon MS, van Nes FA, et al. (2019). What does quality of life mean to older adults? A thematic synthesis. *PloS one,* 14(3).

Veronese N, Stubbs B, Noale M, et al. Polypharmacy is associated with higher frailty risk in older people: An 8-year longitudinal cohort study. *J Am Med Directors Assoc.* 2017;18(7):624–628.

Victor C, Scambler S, Bond J. (2009). The Social World of Older People: Understanding Loneliness and Social Isolation in Later Life. McGraw Hill Education. New York.

Vonnes C, El-Rady R. (2020). When You Hear Hoof Beats, Look for Zebras: Atypical Presentation of Illness in the Older adults. The Journal for Nurse Practitioners 17: 458-461. https://doi.org/10.1016/j.nurpra.2020.10.017 (accessed Aug. 1, 2021).

Wallace M, Fulmer T. Fulmer SPICES: An overall assessment tool of older adults. *Ala Nurse.* 2020;30(3):26.

Wick JY. Aging in Place: Our House Is a Very, Very, Very Fine House. Consult Pharm. 2017 Oct 1;32(10):566-574.

Wimmer BC, Cross AJ, Jokanovic N, et al. Clinical outcomes associated with medication regimen complexity in older people: A systematic review. *J Am Geriatr Soc.* 2017;65:747.

World Health Organization. The global strategy and action plan on ageing and health, 2016–2000. Retrieved from http://www.who.int/publications/i/item/9789241513500. Published 2016.

World Health Organization. (2020). What is the Decade of Healthy Ageing? Decade of Healthy Ageing. Retrieved 2/1/21 from https://www.who.int/initiatives/decade-of-healthy-ageing.

World Health Organization. WHO guidelines on Integrated Care for Older People (ICOPE). https://www.who.int/publications/i/item/WHO-FWC-ALC-19.1. Published 2017.

Wu S, Bellantoni M, Weiner J. (2020). Geriatric Syndrome Risk Factors Among Hospitalized Postacute Medicare Patients. American Journal of Managed Care. 26(10).

Wyman MF, Shiovitz-Ezra S, Bengel J. (2019). Ageism in the health care system: Providers, patients, and systems, Contemporary perspectives on Aging, Cham Switzerland: Springer International Publishing; 193-2012.

Zia A, Kamaruzzaman SB, Tan MP. The consumption of two or more fall risk-increasing drugs rather than polypharmacy is associated with falls. *Geriatr Gerontol Int.* 2017;17(3):463–470.

RESOURCES

Ageing. World Health Organization
http://www.who.int/ageing/en/

Ageing: Trends in Population Ageing, Demographic Drivers of Population Ageing, Key Conferences on Ageing. United Nations
https://www.un.org/en/global-issues/ageing

Alzheimer's Foundation of America
https://alzfdn.org/

American Geriatrics Society (AGS)
http://www.americangeriatrics.org/

American Geriatrics Society 2019 Updated AGS Beers Criteria® for Potentially Inappropriate Medication Use in Older Adults. J Am Geriatr Soc, 67: 674-694.
https://doi.org/10.1111/jgs.15767

Centers for Medicare and Medicaid Services
https://www.cms.gov/Medicare/Medicare.html

End-of-Life Issues and Care. American Psychological Association
http://www.apa.org/topics/death/end-of-life.aspx

Fact Sheet: Aging in the United States. Population Reference Bureau
https://www.prb.org/resources/fact-sheet-aging-in-the-united-states/

Gerontological Advanced Practice Nurses Association (GAPNA)
https://www.gapna.org/

Gerontological Society of America
https://www.geron.org/

Health for Older Adults. National Council on Aging (NCOA)
https://www.ncoa.org/older-adults/health/

Long-Term-Care Systems. World Health Organization
https://www.who.int/ageing/health-systems/icope/icope-consultation/ICOPE-Global-Consultation-Background-Paper-3.pdf?ua=1

Making End-of-Life Decisions: What Are Your Important Papers? Family Caregiver Alliance: National Center on Caregiving
https://www.caregiver.org/making-end-life-decisions-what-are-your-important-papers

Medicines and You: A Guide for Older Adults. U.S. Department of Health and Human Services: U.S. Food & Drug administration
https://www.fda.gov/Drugs/ResourcesForYou/ucm163959.htm

Nestlé Nutritional Institute. Mini Nutritional Assessment Tool.
https://www.mna-elderly.com/sites/default/files/2021-10/mna-mini-english.pdf

Older Adult Falls. Centers for Disease Control and Prevention: Home and Recreation Safety
http://medbox.iiab.me/modules/en-cdc/www.cdc.gov/homeandrecreationalsafety/falls/index.html

Older Adults: Behavioral Health Identification and Treatment, Screening and Assessment Tools, Evidence-Based Practices, Workforce, Financing, Resources for Individual and Families, and Federal and National Entities for Older Adults' Health. SAMHSA-HRSA Center for Integrated Health Solutions
https://www.samhsa.gov/resources-serving-older-adults

Promoting Health for Older Adults. Centers for Disease Control and Prevention: Healthy Aging
https://www.cdc.gov/chronicdisease/resources/publications/factsheets/promoting-health-for-older-adults.htm.

The Demographics of Aging. Transgenerational Design Matters
http://transgenerational.org/aging/demographics.htm

The Growth of the U.S. Aging Population. SeniorCare.com
https://www.seniorcare.com/featured/aging-america/

World Health Organization. (2015). Measuring the age-friendliness of cities: a guide to using core indicators. World Health Organization.
https://apps.who.int/iris/handle/10665/203830

Chapter 83

Pain Management

Didier Demesmin, MD, MBA
Lynne M. Dunphy, PhD, APRN, FNP-BC, FAAN, FAANP
Brian Oscar Porter, MD, PhD, MPH, MBA

The ongoing opioid crisis lies at the intersection of substantial public health challenges—reducing the burden of suffering from pain and containing the toll of the harms that can result from the use of opioid medications.

—Pain Management and the Opioid Epidemic:
Balancing Societal and Individual Benefits
and Risks of Prescription Opioid Use;
National Academies of Sciences,
Engineering, and Medicine, 2017

INTRODUCTION

The above statement, cited in a *Pain Management Best Practices Inter-Agency Task Force Report* (2019), remains even truer today. The ravages of the COVID-19 epidemic have only accelerated and heightened the ongoing opioid epidemic, even though the root causes are better understood. Pain continues to be a multifaceted complex public health concern globally and nationally. It is estimated that 100 million Americans suffer from chronic, noncancer pain, and according to *Healthy People 2030,* one in 12 Americans live with high-impact chronic pain. Many Americans experience acute pain for a variety of reasons, such as trauma, burns, injuries, and surgeries, many of which are short-term and self-limiting. However, improperly managed acute pain can lead to high-impact chronic pain. The economic burden of chronic pain accounts for more than $600 billion annually in direct medical costs and lost productivity. In fact, general pain—both acute and chronic—is one of the most common reasons that patients seek help from a primary care provider, accounting for as many as 50% of physician visits per year in the United States.

There are many definitions of pain. The International Association for the Study of Pain (IASP) defines *pain* as "an aversive sensory and emotional experience typically caused by, or resembling that caused by, actual or potential tissue injury" (IASP Pain Task Force, 2021). This new definition of pain emphasizes that a person's experience of pain is not always supported by evidence of tissue damage, and as such, the experience of pain cannot be reduced to the activity of sensory neurons. It also reinforces that nonverbal pain indicators should be considered and a patient's report of pain should be accepted (see Fig. 83.1). Many patients may experience pain in the absence of noxious stimuli, and this definition supports a view of pain as a complex biopsychosocial phenomenon that involves an interplay of sensory-physiological, cognitive-affective, and behavioral processes. Pain can also be thought of as a motivational state that engenders goal-directed action.

PAIN MECHANISMS: PATHOPHYSIOLOGY

An important concept central to a thorough understanding of pain mechanisms, pathophysiology, and treatments is the concept of *somatosensation*. Somatosensation is the activation of physical stimuli by neural substrate, resulting in the perception of touch, pressure, and pain. Nociceptors are sensory receptors that respond to noxious stimuli; they are specialized neurons that detect a noxious stimulus and then conduct it to the central nervous system (CNS). Nociceptors transduce mechanical, chemical, and thermal stimuli into electrical activity to the CNS where it is processed and interpreted as pain. Nociceptors have been identified in all tissues and organs throughout the body except the nervous system. Noxious stimuli are transmitted from the injured tissue such as skin, muscle, or viscera to the cerebral cortex. This information is projected to higher cortical levels to the thalamus and to the somatosensory cortex of the cerebral cortex where pain perception occurs.

A basic understanding of the anatomy and physiology of pain transmission is essential in evaluating different pain states and associated pharmacological and interventional treatments. The nervous system can transmit and modulate various nociceptive stimuli. Pain stimuli are transmitted via nociceptors, which are peripheral afferent nerve fibers that detect noxious stimuli—thermal, mechanical, or chemical. These stimuli are conducted from these first-order neurons peripherally to the spinal cord via spinal roots at each cervical, thoracic, lumbar, and sacral level. These first-order neurons may ascend two to four spinal cord segments in Lissauer's tract before synapsing with second-order neurons in the gray matter of the ipsilateral dorsal horn. These second-order neurons then cross to the contralateral side of the spinal cord and ascend via the spinothalamic tract to the thalamus, where third-order neurons project to the cerebral cortex.

Peripheral nociceptors have their cell bodies residing in the dorsal root ganglion, which lies within the intervertebral foramina at each spinal level. Nociceptors are pseudounipolar, and they travel in a bidirectional fashion

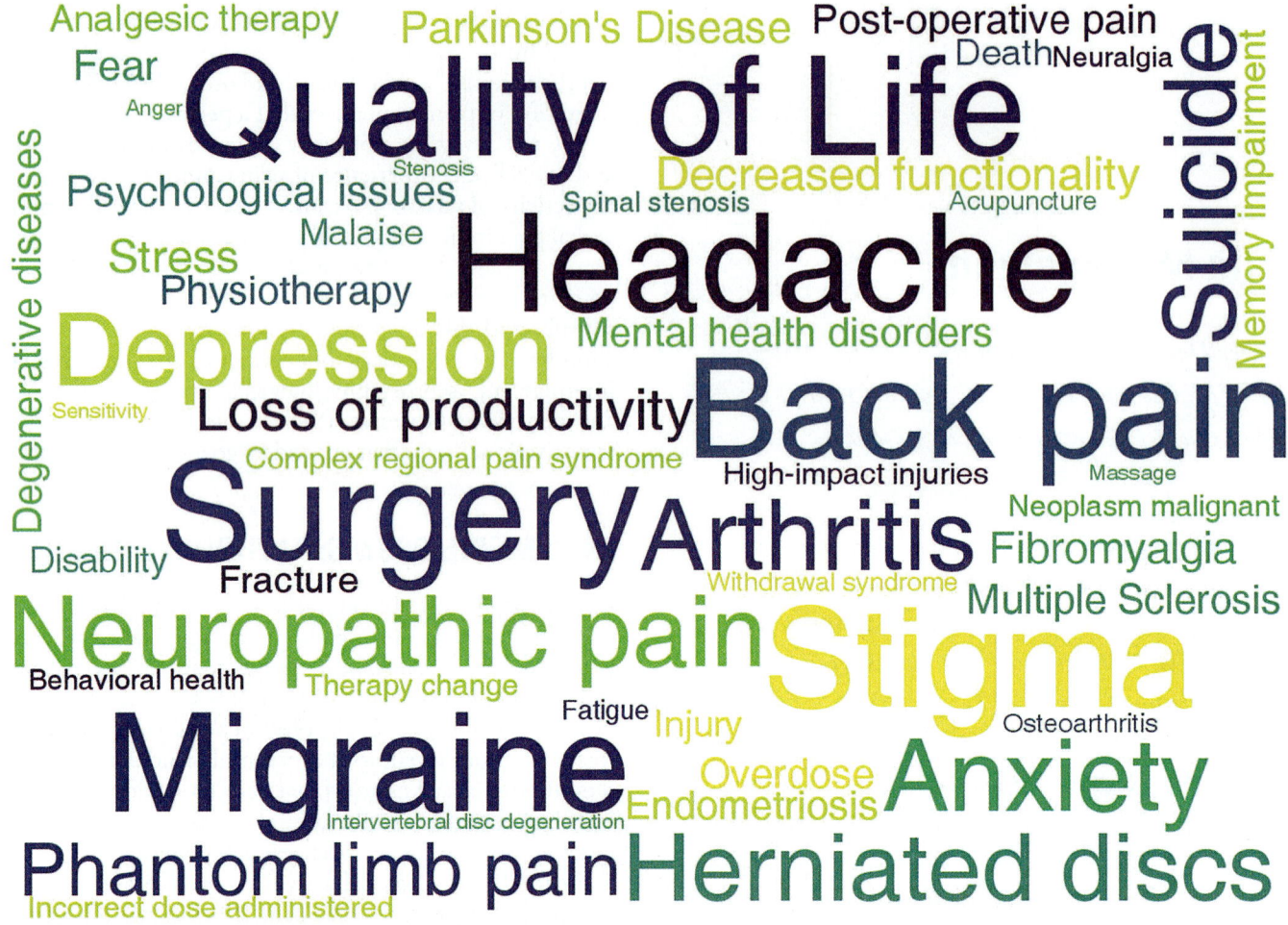

Figure 83.1 Pain cloud. *Source: U.S. Department of Health and Human Services (2019, May). Pain Management Best Practices Inter-Agency Task Force Report: Updates, Gaps, Inconsistencies, and Recommendations.*

from the periphery to the spinal cord and from the spinal cord to the peripheral organs and tissues. Thus, their axons travel both centrally to the spinal cord and higher brain centers and transmit impulses peripherally to the skin and other organs. There are two major classes of pain-transmitting fibers: A delta fibers, which are of medium diameter and thinly myelinated, and C fibers, which are of small diameter and unmyelinated. The A delta and C fibers can detect thermal, mechanical, or chemical stimuli. The A delta and C fiber nociceptors encode and transmit information to the CNS concerning the intensity, location, and duration of noxious stimuli. A delta fibers mediate acute and precisely localized pain, whereas C fibers mediate poorly localized and delayed pain.

Somatosensory perception of pain involves four processes: transduction, transmission, modulation, and perception (see Fig. 83.2). Transduction is the basis of creating a chemical event that progresses to an electrical event. Transduction occurs in the peripheral terminals of primary afferent neurons. These primary afferent first-order neurons respond to mechanical, chemical, and thermal stimuli. The axonal membrane of these primary afferent neurons has transduction channels that once an action potential is sufficient to depolarize the axon will generate potentials that are then transmitted through the nervous system. Noxious substances that facilitate pain production include bradykinin, tumor necrosis factor (TNF), histamine, prostaglandins, hydrogen ions, and potassium ions. Transmission is the process by which, as this stimulus progresses, the action potential depolarizes the neuron, allowing for the release of chemicals that facilitate the pain stimulus of the afferent primary neuron to the dorsal horn of the spinal cord. Modulation of pain from the higher CNS occurs via the descending inhibitory tracts and can occur at the nociceptor peripherally, in the dorsal horn of the spinal cord and in supraspinal structures. Modulation of pain stimulus therefore can be facilitated or inhibited to stop the progression up the CNS. This process involves the release of neurotransmitters, which can either reduce activity of pain transmission or can enhance the pain signal. In order words, modulation of pain transmission can either increase or decrease the pain stimulus. Perception occurs in the cerebral cortex and involves the process by which neural activity in the pain transmission pathway results in the subjective sensation of pain.

Chapter 83 Pain Management

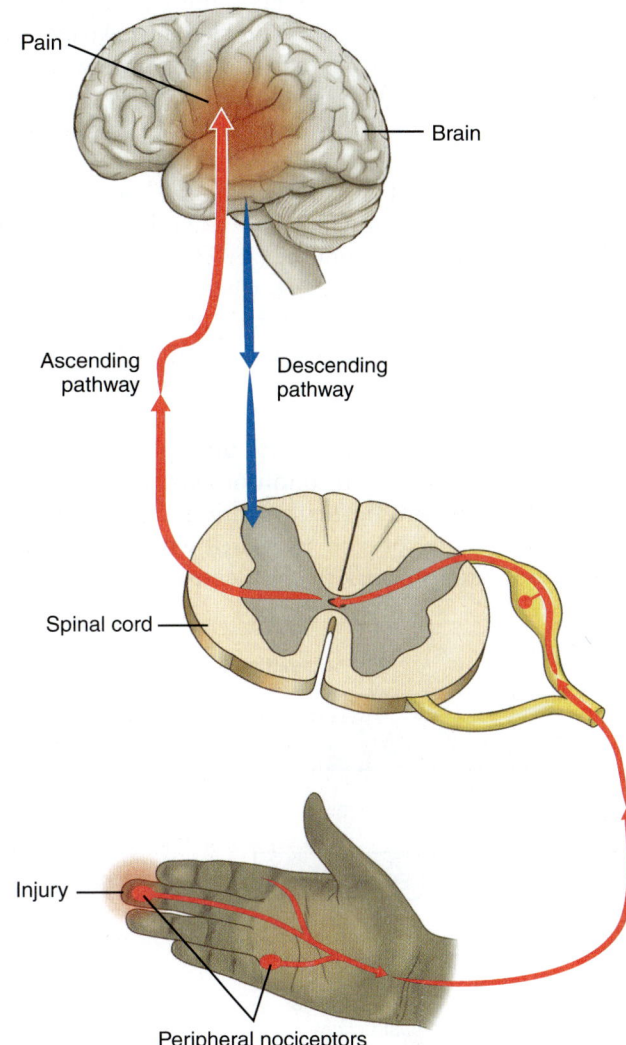

Figure 83.2 Physiology of pain perception.

Afferent nociceptive fibers release several neuropeptides and excitatory amino acids to the spinal cord to mediate pain. Some of these neurotransmitters include substance P, glutamate, and calcitonin gene-related peptide (CGRP). Substance P, once released by the primary afferent neuron where it is synthesized, facilitates the transmission of pain and causes various biochemical cascades including mast cell degranulation, vasodilation, and chemoattraction for leukocytes. Conversely, several neuropeptides are involved in the inhibition of nociceptive input via descending neural activity from supraspinal centers. Glycine, gamma-aminobutyric acid (GABA), serotonin, and norepinephrine are inhibitory neurotransmitters that inhibit nociceptive transmission. Glycine and GABA inhibit segmental pain transmission in the spinal cord, whereas serotonin and norepinephrine inhibit nociceptive transmission supraspinally both pre- and postsynaptically. Hence, the clinical effect of monoamine oxidase inhibitors (MAOIs) and tricyclic antidepressants (TCAs) for pain works by blocking the reuptake of serotonin and norepinephrine, thereby inhibiting pain transmission. Endogenous opioids such as beta-endorphins act presynaptically, whereas synthetic opioids such as morphine produce analgesia by inhibiting the release of substance P postsynaptically in the substantia gelatinosa of the dorsal horn.

Pain is also a uniquely individual and subjective experience. Each patient will experience a distinct level of pain tolerance or emotional and affective response to pain. The pain threshold is the lowest tolerable level in each individual, in which a stimulus can cause and be perceived as pain.

CLASSIFICATIONS OF PAIN

Pain is basically classified into nociceptive or neuropathic pain, which helps in categorizing different pain conditions to organize treatment modalities and pharmacological therapies. Nociceptive pain is initiated by tissue injury. It can be secondary to trauma, an incision, inflammation, or a disease process. The degree of pain is usually somewhat proportional to the degree of the injury. There are two types of nociceptive pain, somatic and visceral pain. Nociceptive pain represents a normal response to tissue injury. This type of pain is divided into two categories: (1) somatic pain, which is pain arising from muscles, joints, and cutaneous tissues, to name a few; and (2) visceral pain, which is pain arising from organs and smooth muscle. Somatic pain is sharper, discrete, and intense, and it has a more localized sensation within the body, whereas visceral pain is more diffuse, cramplike, and characterized as a poorly localized discomfort (see Fig. 83.3). Somatic pain is carried by sensory fibers, whereas visceral pain is carried along autonomic sympathetic fibers.

Neuropathic pain is caused by lesions to the peripheral nervous system as in diabetic neuropathy, postherpetic neuralgia, lumbar radiculopathy, or a lesion of the CNS such as poststroke pain, multiple sclerosis, or what could be acquired in conditions such as HIV neuropathy (see Fig. 83.3). Neuropathic pain is nonnociceptive. The degree of pain associated with neuropathic pain is not proportional to the degree of injury. It is often caused by an abnormal sensory processing of the nervous system.

From a neurobiological perspective, pain can be classified in three distinct ways. First, pain can be regarded as an early warning sign of impending tissue injury. In this instance, pain can be regarded as an adaptive and protective mechanism to warn individuals to withdraw from a noxious stimulus to avoid tissue injury. Pain can also warn an individual to seek medical help as it is often the first warning sign of a physiological disturbance. This type of pain is often referred to as *nociceptive pain*.

A second type of pain may also arise, inflammatory pain, as a response to an injury. This is a "mixed" pain type (see Fig. 83.4). This type of pain also has adaptive and protective functions. It occurs in response to tissue damage, for instance, after a surgical procedure. Inflammatory pain will create an environment where the patient will avoid physical contact and manipulation of the painful site. This type of pain is caused by activation of an inflammatory cascade that is often seen because of tissue injury, infection, or trauma.

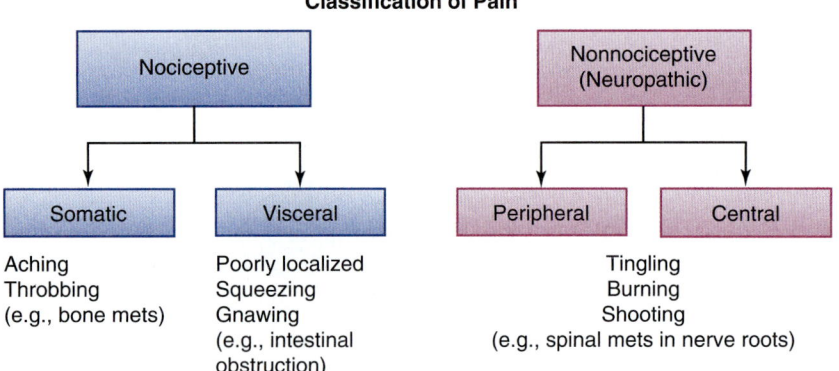

Figure 83.3 Classification of pain.

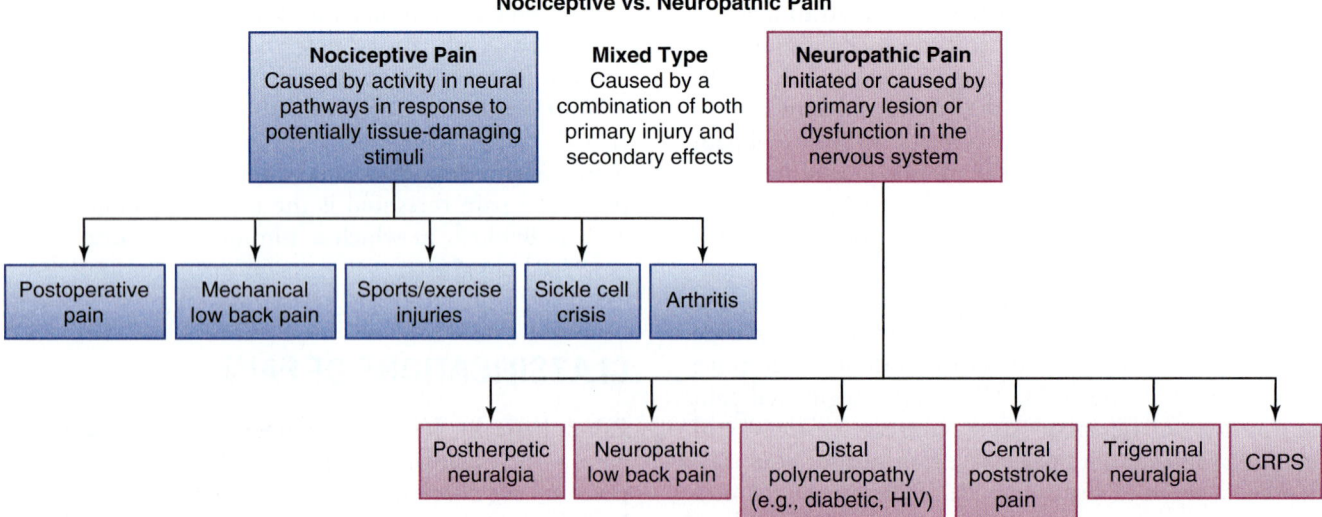

Figure 83.4 Nociceptive vs. neuropathic pain. *Data from Portenoy RK, Kanner RM. (1996). Pain Management Theory and Practice. Philadelphia, PA: F.A. Davis Company, 4; Galer BS, Dworkin RH. (2000). A Clinical Guide to Neuropathic Pain. Minneapolis, MN: The McGraw-Hill Companies Inc., 8–9*

The third type of pain does not have a protective function and is considered rather maladaptive. This type of pain is called *neuropathic pain* and results from an insult to the nervous system. Although pain serves as a vital protective function, pain can become a disease as it transforms from an acute physiological response to tissue injury to a chronic maladaptive condition in the absence of tissue damage.

Differentiating between nociceptive and neuropathic pain is important because these two types of pain conditions influence selection of pharmacological or interventional modalities. Neuropathic pain responds poorly to both opioid analgesics and NSAID agents but often responds well to antiepileptic drugs, antidepressants, and local anesthetics (see Fig. 83.5).

Additionally, pain is classified as either acute or chronic. Acute pain is a normal, predictable, physiological response to pain that has a sudden onset and a short duration. It often has an identifiable cause such as trauma, injury, or surgery. It is usually nociceptive in nature and results from nociceptor activation. This type of pain is not as difficult to manage as chronic pain because it has a short and often an identifiable cause. Once the injury heals, the pain usually goes away; however, acute pain that is inadequately managed may lead to chronic pain. The continuum from acute to chronic pain is influenced by the initial pain experience and various biophysiological and psychosocial factors. Moderate to severe acute pain has many physiological multiorgan consequences (Table 83.1). These effects obviate the need for proper assessment and diligent treatment of acute pain.

Chronic pain persists beyond the course of a reasonable time from injury to healing. Typically, pain is considered chronic if it persists 3 to 6 months or longer. Chronic pain can be nociceptive, neuropathic, or mixed. In addition to physical and physiological problems, chronic pain is often accompanied by a psychological and emotional component where the patient can present with fear, anger, depression, anxiety, or a reduced ability to interact with other people or engage in any social activities. Therefore, the practitioner must always assess for depression and other associated psychological stress when customizing a treatment plan for a patient with chronic pain, as well as alcohol and drug use in an attempt to control pain. Chronic pain is often encountered in patients with musculoskeletal disorders such as chronic low back pain and joint abnormalities, cancer, neuropathic conditions, and chronic visceral disorders, to name a few.

A thorough physical examination and history will help the primary care practitioner assess if this is a person who should be referred or treated within the practice.

ASSESSMENT OF ACUTE AND CHRONIC PAIN

When assessing a patient with pain, the assessment should be approached in an orderly and logical fashion. The difficulty when assessing a patient with pain is the reliance on the patient's report of the symptoms, as pain lacks physiological markers or any objective test that can accurately measure the patient's pain levels.

As with any patient evaluation, the practitioner should begin with the history part of the evaluation. The chief complaint should be in the patient's own words as the content of the patient's complaint is usually subjective.

History of Present Illness

Documentation of the date of onset of the pain will help determine an acute versus a chronic condition, traumatic versus atraumatic process, acute versus insidious. Characteristic of the pain should also be elicited to distinguish between a nociceptive versus neuropathic process. A nociceptive process will be described as sharp, achy, or throbbing; often it will have an identifiable cause; and the patient will be able to localize the pain. A neuropathic process would be described as piercing, stabbing, burning, shooting, tingling, or radiating, and the pain may be more difficult to assess and localize. The location and intensity of the pain are important, as well any associated factors such as weakness, numbness, bladder disturbance, or any other neurological disturbance. The practitioner should explore

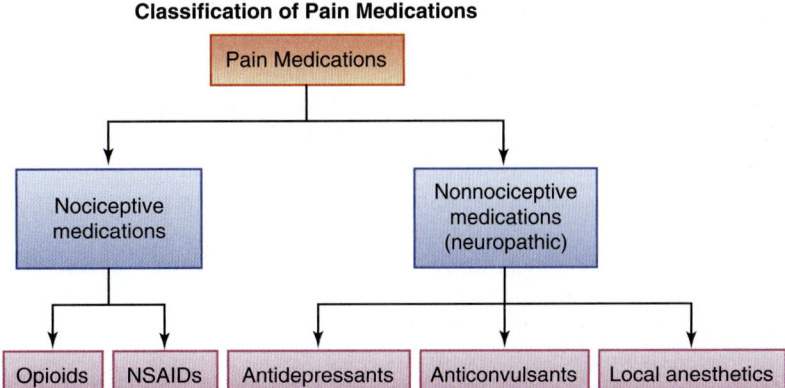

Figure 83.5 Classification of pain medications.

TABLE 83.1 Effects of Chronic Pain on Body Systems	
Body System	Effect
Cardiovascular	Tachycardia, hypertension, myocardial strain, increased myocardial oxygen demand; can lead to myocardial ischemia; triggered by the accompanied sympathetic discharge and neuroendocrine stress response
Pulmonary	Increased total body oxygen consumption, which can increase the work of breathing
Gastrointestinal	Hypersecretion of gastric acid, which can lead to ulceration, nausea, and vomiting
Genitourinary	Urinary retention
Hematological	Increased platelet adhesiveness, hypercoagulability
Immune	Leukocytosis, predisposition to infection
Endocrine	Increased catecholamine release, decreased insulin and testosterone

all exacerbating and alleviating factors, and the temporal onset of the pain will determine an acute or chronic process.

Pain-related anxiety and pain "catastrophizing" are considered transdiagnostic factors among people with chronic pain, as well as anxiety sensitivity as a contributory factor to greater pain impairment/persistence. *Distress intolerance,* defined as the perceived inability to tolerate negative emotional and/or other aversive states, has been shown in some studies to correlate with substance addiction.

Medical and Surgical History

Assessment of the patient's medical history can be useful in determining the etiology of pain, especially in the case of known medical conditions that can lead to pain such as diabetes, cancer, and surgical interventions and outcomes.

Medication History

A thorough review of the patient's medication list should include prescribed medications, over-the-counter medications, and home remedies including herbal supplements. Additionally, review all alcohol and drug usage in pursuit of pain relief. A patient's prior response or lack of response to any particular analgesics including indication, dosage, duration, and side effects should also be explored.

Diagnostic studies including x-rays, magnetic resonance imaging (MRI), computed tomography (CT), electromyograms (EMGs), nerve conduction velocity (NCV) tests, and various laboratory studies are useful for therapeutic and diagnostic purposes.

A thorough review of systems and constitutional symptoms may reveal problems that were not previously noted during the patient's history. All systems including neurological, rheumatological, genitourinary, musculoskeletal, psychiatric, endocrine, cardiovascular, and pulmonary should be explored.

Because of the subjective nature of pain, making the pain visible to the practitioner is necessary to determine therapeutic interventions and evaluate efficacy of treatment. Pain diagrams and other assessment tools are being used in clinical practice. Some frequently used pain and functional scales include the numerical rating scale, the visual analog scale (VAS), and the McGill Pain Questionnaire. The Wong-Baker Faces Pain Rating Scale is used for children 3 years of age and older.

The physical examination should include a mental status, and joint, motor and sensory, and neurological examinations.

Individualized patient care consists of a diagnostic evaluation that results in an integrative treatment plan that includes all necessary treatment options.

PAIN MANAGEMENT

The biopsychosocial model of pain management (Fig. 83.6) has become widely accepted and is analogous to the Circle of Caring model. This model includes

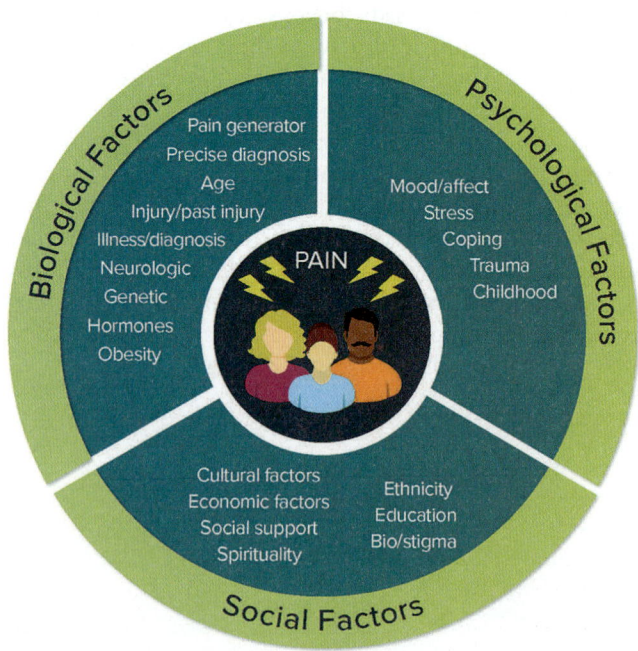

Figure 83.6 The Biopsychosocial Model of Pain Management. *Source: U.S. Department of Health and Human Services (2019, May). Pain Management Best Practices Inter-Agency Task Force Report: Updates, Gaps, Inconsistencies, and Recommendations.*

biological, psychological, and social factors that include culture, economic, social support, spirituality, ethnicity, education, and access to care/stigma. All aspects of the person's life, including their social circumstances, must be considered when assessing and creating a treatment plan in concert with the patient and family/significant others as appropriate. A therapeutic alliance must be formed between the person in pain and the practitioner. This begins with taking the history, performing a physical examination, and developing an individualized integrative treatment plan. Special considerations for different ages and populations are addressed later in this chapter. The application of this model implies an individualized approach affecting many aspects of a person's life. The Inter-Agency Task Force Report on *Pain Management: Best Practices* (2019) specifies an individualized, multimodal, multidisciplinary approach to acute and chronic pain management. Although medication remains a cornerstone and the chapter discusses pharmacological management first, the chapter also outlines a range of therapies, including:

- Restorative therapies
- Interventional procedures
- Behavioral health approaches
- Complementary and integrative health

Some of these approaches, such as interventional procedures, are clearly beyond the scope of primary care practice and require referrals. Likewise, some of these approaches—such as physical therapies—also require referral and a team-based, multimodal, multidisciplinary approach requiring coordination by the primary care provider.

Pharmacological Management of Pain

The pharmacotherapy of chronic pain requires knowledge of various classes of drugs, including the mechanisms of action and side-effect profiles. The prescriber must also understand drug, synergistic, and antagonistic interactions and must consider the underlying medical conditions of the patient. Pharmacological interventions to treat chronic pain include acetaminophen, NSAIDs, neuropathic agents, anticonvulsants, antidepressants, opioids, and medical marijuana. There is no one-size-fits-all approach to treat acute and chronic pain, because the causes vary and the practitioner must consider the patient's comorbid conditions. Given the multiple pain complaints that a practitioner will encounter during a patient visit, choosing a medication that fits the patient's overall need for pain control is crucial. It is very important for the practitioner to explain to the patient the reasoning for the prescribed medications and the side-effect profiles of the medications and to provide a mechanism to alert the practitioner about any side effects or ineffective medications. Often, a patient will stop a medication without an adequate trial and without telling the provider. Common reasons for this include side effects such as confusion, lightheadedness, nausea, and constipation, or the patient may stop because they perceive the medication to be ineffective. Determining the type of pain is also very important when considering the medication to treat it. Having a good understanding of nociceptive pain and neuropathic pain, as well as somatic and visceral pain, is also critical in using the appropriate medication therapy.

Acetaminophen

Acetaminophen (Paracetamol) is an oral analgesic and antipyretic agent. It inhibits central prostaglandin synthesis with minimal inhibition of peripheral prostaglandin synthesis. It lacks significant anti-inflammatory activity. Acetaminophen has a good side-effect profile; however, it can be hepatotoxic at high doses. It does not have any adverse effects on platelet function or the gastric mucosa. A small portion of acetaminophen is bound to plasma proteins, and elimination from the body is primarily by the formation of glucuronide and sulfate conjugates in a dose-dependent manner. The maximum daily dose of acetaminophen is 3,000 mg per day, reduced from a previously recommended limit of 4,000 mg per day. An IV formulation of acetaminophen is now available for the treatment of mild to moderate pain.

NSAIDs

NSAIDs have showed great effectiveness for treating nociceptive pain. NSAIDs have analgesic, antipyretic, and anti-inflammatory activity. Prostaglandins are synthesized from arachidonic acid via the cyclooxygenase-2 pathway (COX 2). They play an important role in the inflammatory response, thrombocyte aggregation, sensitizing pain receptors, and in the induction of fever. The mechanism of action of NSAIDs is by blocking the synthesis of prostaglandins from arachidonic acids by reversibly or irreversibly inhibiting cyclooxygenase (COX). COX is present in two isoforms: COX-1 and COX-2. COX-1 is constitutive throughout the body in most cell types and is responsible for renal blood flow regulation, protection of the gastric mucosa, and platelet aggregation and activation. COX-1 inhibition is responsible for the side effects of nonselective COX-1 inhibitors, namely renal dysfunction, gastrointestinal side effects, and cardiovascular side effects (see Drugs Commonly Prescribed 83.1).

Renal Effects. Prostaglandins are necessary for maintenance of renal blood flow. Inhibition of prostaglandins from NSAIDs results in reduction of renal blood flow with subsequent risk of developing renal insufficiency. This risk is higher in patients with existing congestive heart failure; existing renal disease; concomitant drug therapy with diuretics, beta blockers, or angiotensin-converting enzyme inhibitors (ACEIs); and advanced age.

Cardiovascular Effects. All NSAIDs have been shown to increase cardiovascular thrombotic events

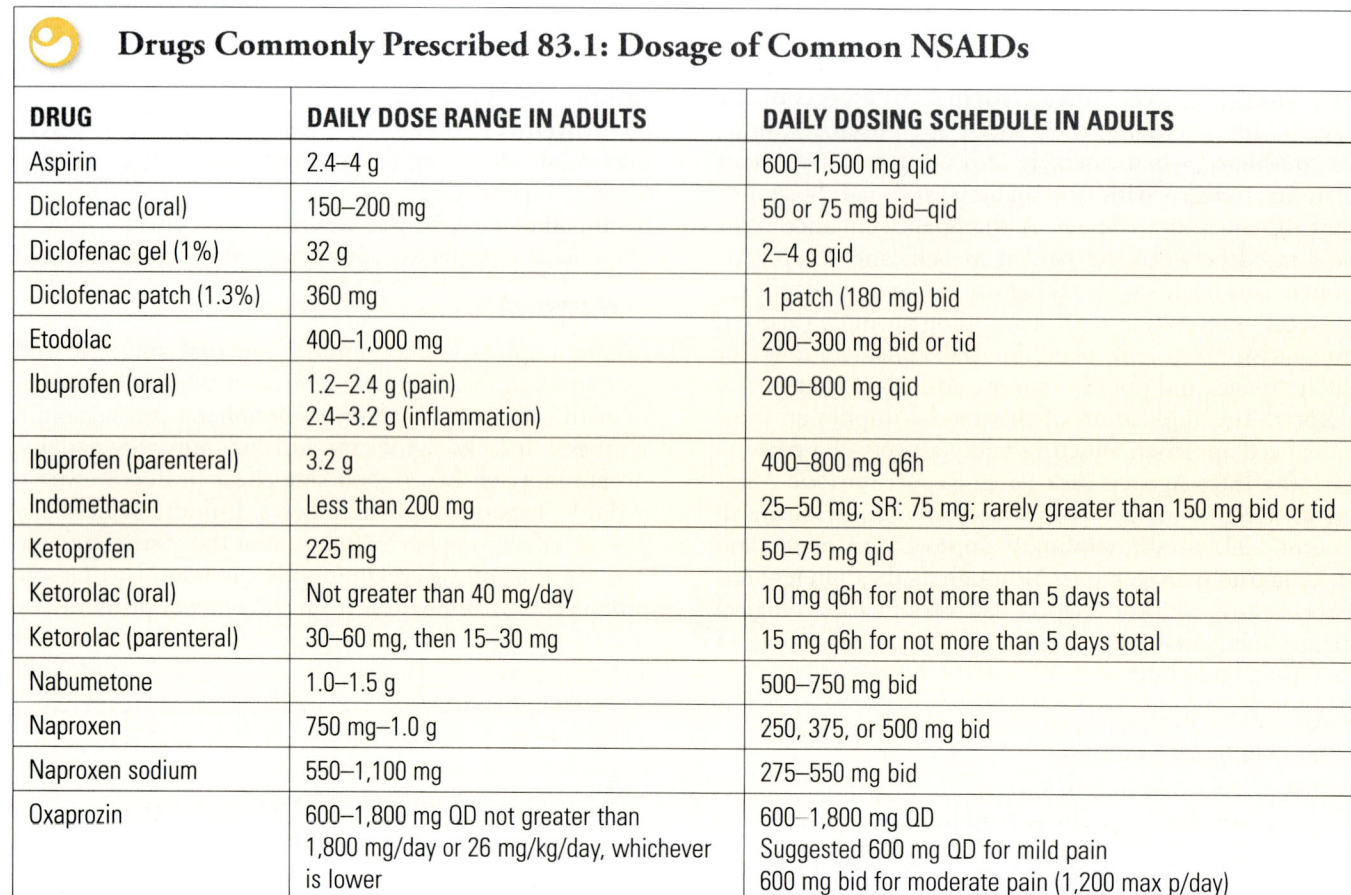

Drugs Commonly Prescribed 83.1: Dosage of Common NSAIDs

DRUG	DAILY DOSE RANGE IN ADULTS	DAILY DOSING SCHEDULE IN ADULTS
Aspirin	2.4–4 g	600–1,500 mg qid
Diclofenac (oral)	150–200 mg	50 or 75 mg bid–qid
Diclofenac gel (1%)	32 g	2–4 g qid
Diclofenac patch (1.3%)	360 mg	1 patch (180 mg) bid
Etodolac	400–1,000 mg	200–300 mg bid or tid
Ibuprofen (oral)	1.2–2.4 g (pain) 2.4–3.2 g (inflammation)	200–800 mg qid
Ibuprofen (parenteral)	3.2 g	400–800 mg q6h
Indomethacin	Less than 200 mg	25–50 mg; SR: 75 mg; rarely greater than 150 mg bid or tid
Ketoprofen	225 mg	50–75 mg qid
Ketorolac (oral)	Not greater than 40 mg/day	10 mg q6h for not more than 5 days total
Ketorolac (parenteral)	30–60 mg, then 15–30 mg	15 mg q6h for not more than 5 days total
Nabumetone	1.0–1.5 g	500–750 mg bid
Naproxen	750 mg–1.0 g	250, 375, or 500 mg bid
Naproxen sodium	550–1,100 mg	275–550 mg bid
Oxaprozin	600–1,800 mg QD not greater than 1,800 mg/day or 26 mg/kg/day, whichever is lower	600–1,800 mg QD Suggested 600 mg QD for mild pain 600 mg bid for moderate pain (1,200 max p/day) And max dose 1,800 mg in divided doses for severe pain

from the imbalance that occurs between COX-1 and COX-2. The nonselective inhibition of COX reduces the synthesis of thromboxane (TX) and prostacyclin. Thromboxane is a vasoconstrictor and increases platelet aggregation. Thus, inhibition of TX can prevent the formation of a hemostatic plug by inhibiting platelet activation, which is one of the reasons aspirin therapy is recommended to reduce the risk of thrombotic events. Aspirin irreversibly inhibits platelet-dependent COX-1 for the life of the platelet. Selective COX-2 inhibitors were developed because of their better gastroprotective effect.

Gastrointestinal Effects. GI bleeding is one of the most common complications reported from NSAID use. Endoscopic studies have shown that more than 30% of patients develop gastric erosions within a week of starting an NSAID regimen (Sostres et al, 2013). More than 100,000 hospitalizations and at least 2,600 deaths each year in the United States are attributed to NSAID-associated gastropathy. One of the most important factors predicting the incidence of GI bleeding is the duration of use of NSAID therapy. Celecoxib (Celebrex) has been associated with significantly fewer mucosal erosions, bleeding, and perforation compared with other NSAIDs. Using an NSAID with a proton pump inhibitor (PPI) for high-risk patients is recommended when using Celebrex or any other NSAID.

Neuropathic Pain Medications

Neuropathic pain is defined by the IASP as pain caused by lesion(s) or disease of the somatosensory nervous system. Neuropathic pain is described when there is insult to the peripheral nervous system or the CNS with or without associated autonomic changes or CNS dysfunction. The neuropathic pain category includes several disorders of the nervous system including painful diabetic neuropathy, postherpetic neuralgia, central neuropathic pain, complex regional pain syndrome, HIV-associated polyneuropathy, trigeminal neuralgia, and multiple sclerosis, among others. Neuropathic pain is often described as burning, piercing, stabbing, or tingling. After tissue injury and inflammation, the thresholds needed to activate A delta and C fibers decrease. In addition, sodium and calcium channels help proliferate hyperexcitability in central and peripheral neurons. Mechanistically, neuropathic pain presents with an abnormal firing of nerves and abnormal amplification or propagation of nerve signals. There is also altered descending inhibitory signaling of the pain pathway. It has been shown that after nerve injury, the number of ion channels accumulate, leading to spontaneous firing of sensory nerves in the dorsal root ganglion of the injured primary afferent neuron.

Understanding the neurotransmitters and neuropeptides activities on specific receptors in the pain pathway is important in determining which medication for neuropathic pain will be used to help propagate or attenuate pain signals. Hence, neuropathic pain medication helps either enhance or suppress neurotransmitters and neuropeptides.

Various groups of medications have been used in the treatment of neuropathic pain including anticonvulsant drugs, which block voltage-gated sodium and calcium channels. Neuropathic pain may require treatment with more than one medication at once, and each individual medication should have a different mechanism of action to follow what is described as rational polypharmacy for the treatment of neuropathic pain.

Anticonvulsant Medications. Anticonvulsant medications have been used for the treatment of neuropathic pain (see Drugs Commonly Prescribed 83.2). These medications block voltage-gated calcium or sodium channels and have been shown to suppress spontaneous neural discharge postulated to play a role in neuropathic pain disorders. Gabapentin is FDA approved for the treatment of seizures, restless leg syndrome, and postherpetic neuralgia. Pregabalin is FDA approved for partial-onset seizures, fibromyalgia, and diabetic polyneuropathy. Gabapentin and pregabalin are structural analogs of GABA; however, they do not bind to the GABA receptors. These medications bind the alpha 2 subunit of the N-type calcium channels, which results in the release of GABA, an inhibitory neurotransmitter. The most common side effects of these medications include nausea, somnolence, dizziness, ataxia, swollen legs, and abdominal discomfort.

Antidepressant Medications. Antidepressants have also been used in the treatment of neuropathic pain. Usually, analgesia from antidepressants to treat neuropathic pain occurs at a much lower dose than that needed for antidepressant activity (see Drugs Commonly Prescribed 83.3).

Drugs Commonly Prescribed 83.3: Antidepressants

DRUG	STARTING DOSE	DAILY DOSING SCHEDULE (MAXIMUM DAILY DOSE)
Selective Serotonin Reuptake Inhibitors		
Citalopram (Celexa)	10 mg qd	20–40 mg qd (60 mg)
Fluoxetine (Prozac)	10 mg qd	20–40 mg qd (80 mg)
Fluvoxamine (Luvox)	25 mg qd	50–100 mg bid (300 mg)
Paroxetine (Paxil)	5–10 mg qd	20–40 mg qd (60 mg)
Sertraline (Zoloft)	25 mg qd	50–150 mg qd (200 mg)
Tricyclic Antidepressants		
Amitriptyline (Elavil)	10–25 mg qd	75–150 mg qd (300 mg)
Amoxapine (Asendin)	25 mg bid	75–200 mg bid (600 mg)
Clomipramine (Anafranil)	25 mg qd	150–250 mg qd (250 mg)
Desipramine (Norpramin)	10–25 mg qd	75–150 mg qd (300 mg)
Doxepin (Sinequan)	10–25 mg qd	75–150 mg qd (300 mg)
Nortriptyline (Pamelor)	10–25 mg qd	75–150 mg qd (200 mg)
Protriptyline (Vivactil)	5 mg qd	10 mg tid (60 mg)

Antidepressants' mechanism of action includes presynaptic reuptake of serotonin, norepinephrine, or both. Tricyclic antidepressants (TCAs) such as amitriptyline, nortriptyline, desipramine, and imipramine work by inhibiting reuptake of serotonin and norepinephrine in the synaptic cleft of the neurons. The side-effect profiles of TCAs should be carefully considered when selecting this class of medication for the treatment of pain. Tertiary TCAs, such as imipramine, amitriptyline, and doxepin, have equal reuptake inhibition of both serotonin and norepinephrine. They are considered more effective analgesics, compared with the secondary amines, which exhibit more selective norepinephrine reuptake inhibition. Examples of secondary TCAs include desipramine, nortriptyline, and maprotiline. Common side effects seen in TCAs include constipation, dry mouth, blurry

Drugs Commonly Prescribed 83.2: Anticonvulsant Drugs

DRUG	STARTING DOSE	MAXIMUM DAILY DOSE
Gabapentin (Neurontin)	300–900 mg tid	3,600 mg
Levetiracetam (Keppra)	500 mg bid	3,000 mg
Pregabalin (Lyrica)	150 mg/day	600 mg
Topiramate (Topamax)	50–200 mg/day	400 mg

vision, glaucoma, urinary retention, visual problems, lower seizure thresholds, and prolongation of the QTC interval.

Opioids

Opioids are potentially the most effective analgesics available. Opioids are indicated in patients with moderate to severe pain that is acute and/or chronic, cancer pain, and any patients not showing improvement with nonopioid therapy. In theory, opioids have no ceiling effect and are only limited by the various adverse effects that often accompany opioid therapy, including addiction.

Opioids are derived from opium obtained from the juice of opium poppy, *Papaver somniferum*. Opioids are classified as naturally occurring, semisynthetic, or synthetic (Fig. 83.7). Morphine, codeine, papaverine, and thebaine are naturally occurring (Fig. 83.8). Semisynthetic opioids are derived from morphine, codeine, and thebaine. They have the morphine ring structure, but they do not occur naturally (Fig. 83.9). The semisynthetic opioids are oxycodone, hydromorphone, hydrocodone, heroin, and buprenorphine. The synthetic opioids are methadone, propoxyphene, meperidine, fentanyl, sufentanil, and alfentanil. The synthetic and semisynthetic opioids are produced by reducing the five-ring structure of morphine to a four-ring structure of the semisynthetic compound and further reduced to the three-ring synthetic product.

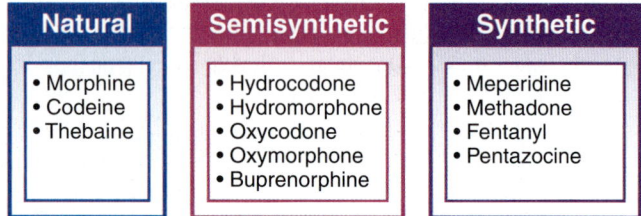

Figure 83.7 Opioid classification: origin. *Data from Charles P. O'Brien. Hardman JG, Limbird LE, Gilman AG, editors. (2001). Goodman & Gilman's The Pharmacological Basis of Therapeutics, 10th edition. New York: McGraw-Hill; Cherny NI. Drugs. 1996; 51: 714–737.*

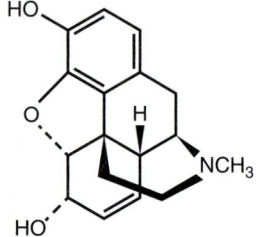

Figure 83.8 Chemical structure of morphine.

The mechanism of action of opioids occurs by binding to the opioid receptors found in the CNS, gastrointestinal tract, and to a lesser extent, the peripheral tissues. There are four main types of opioid receptors: mu, kappa, delta, and sigma. Each receptor plays a different role in pain inhibition and the analgesic effects and adverse-effect profile of opioids. Opioids exert their activity over wide dose ranges and can be administered via many routes such as oral, parenteral, transdermal, intraspinal, rectal, sublingual, and buccal.

The clinical actions of all opioids are similar in part. They all produce varying degrees of analgesia for pain control and have varying degrees of adverse effects such as sedation, constipation, cardiovascular depression, cognitive impairment, respiratory depression, euphoria, and dysphoria in a dose-dependent fashion.

Morphine. Morphine is the standard by which all other opioids are compared. It is considered a strong opioid. Morphine is metabolized in the liver, and the major metabolites are morphine-3-glucuronide (M3G) and morphine-6-glucuronide (M6G). M3G is inactive, whereas M6G is active and considered 100 times more potent than morphine itself and has a longer half-life. Morphine is renally cleared and should be used with caution in patients with renal failure, as morphine has been shown to produce a prolonged effect and sedation in this population. It is believed that the active metabolite, M6G, is largely responsible for the side effects observed in patients with renal disorders. The half-life of morphine is 2 to 4 hours in adults, 6 to 8 hours in neonates, and 10 hours in premature infants.

Codeine. Codeine is considered a weak opioid and is not effective for severe pain. It has good antitussive activity. It is believed that the analgesia produced by codeine is from its biotransformation to morphine. The half-life of codeine is about 2 to 4 hours. Codeine is available in combination with acetaminophen and aspirin.

Oxycodone. Oxycodone is considered a strong opioid. It has a potency like morphine. It is available as an immediate-release in the form of Oxy IR or plain oxycodone and often in combination with acetaminophen (Percocet) or with aspirin (Percodan). The sustained-release preparation OxyContin is used in chronic pain and in patients with cancer. The half-life of oxycodone is 3.5 to 4 hours, and the sustained-release oxycodone lasts about 12 hours.

Fentanyl. Fentanyl is commonly used in transdermal preparations for severe chronic cancer pain. Fentanyl can also be given orally as well. It is lipid soluble, compared with the other opioids, which are primarily water-soluble. Fentanyl is used for severe pain and may be effective for neuropathic pain. Its mechanism of action involves binding to the N-methyl-D-aspartate (NMDA) receptor and muscarinic receptor and releases serotonin and norepinephrine. It is effective in relieving headaches and

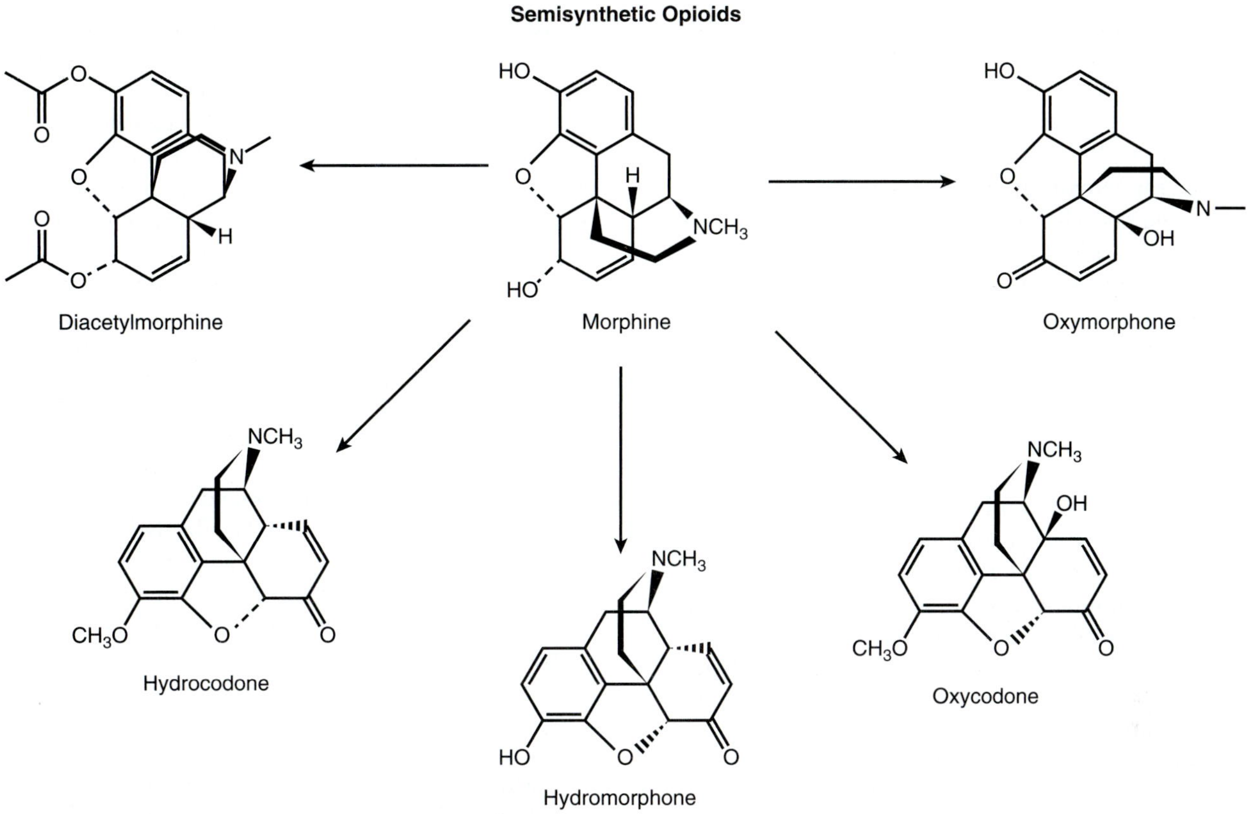

Figure 83.9 Chemical structures of semisynthetic opioids.

cancer-related pain. Fentanyl has a slow onset and long duration of action and half-life.

Tramadol. Tramadol is essentially a synthetic analog of codeine. Its mechanism of action is binding to the mu receptors and inhibiting serotonin and norepinephrine reuptake. Tramadol has been found to be effective in treating neuropathic pain associated with polyneuropathy, given its dual mechanism of action. The most common adverse events associated with tramadol administration include dizziness, nausea, constipation, somnolence, and orthostatic hypotension. Tramadol has been shown to reduce the seizure threshold; therefore, it is important to screen for previous history of seizure or increased risk of developing seizures before initiating therapy with tramadol. Careful monitoring is necessary with concomitant use of tramadol and a selective serotonin reuptake inhibitor (SSRI) or TCA, given the risk of developing serotonin syndrome.

Hydromorphone. Hydromorphone (Dilaudid) is structurally similar to morphine; however, it is up to eight times more potent than morphine. It is more lipid soluble than morphine and therefore has a faster penetration of the blood-brain barrier. The IV half-life of hydromorphone is about 2 to 3 hours. After onset of IV administration, levels of hydromorphone rise rapidly, which makes it a good option for severe acute pain relief in a hospital or emergency department setting. Hydromorphone is also available as an oral preparation in 2-, 4-, and 8-mg tablets.

Meperidine. Meperidine (Demerol) is highly protein bound. The oral and parenteral doses are similar. Meperidine is given at about 50 to 100 mg initially and can be titrated to effect. Meperidine's analgesic onset usually peaks 15 minutes after an oral dose and about 10 minutes after a parenteral dose. Clinical duration of meperidine's analgesic effect is 2 to 4 hours. Meperidine has anticholinergic effects causing urinary retention and is the only opioid that may produce tachycardia. Meperidine is metabolized to normeperidine, which is not reversible by naloxone. Normeperidine can accumulate in patients with reduced renal and hepatic activity, and its half-life can be in between 15 to 20 hours. Normeperidine can cause tremors, convulsions, and muscle twitching in large doses. Meperidine blocks the reuptake of serotonin and norepinephrine and should not be combined with a serotonin reuptake inhibitor such as fluoxetine. Meperidine should also be avoided in patients taking a monoamine oxidase inhibitor (MAOI) as the combination can trigger hyperpyrexia, convulsions, severe respiratory depression, and delusions. Meperidine is available as an injectable preparation in doses of 25, 50, 75, and 100 mg/mL. An oral tablet form is available in 50- and 100-mg dosages.

Methadone. Methadone is a synthetic opioid that is a mu-1 receptor agonist, an NMDA antagonist, and also a reuptake inhibitor of both serotonin and norepinephrine. These properties can reduce the risk of opioid tolerance and therefore can be used in opioid rotation. Given its unique mechanism of action, methadone has also been effective in treating neuropathic and central pain such as poststroke and spinal cord–injury pain. Its analgesic duration is 4 to 6 hours, and its elimination half-life is between 15 and 60 hours. Because of this long half-life, methadone can be used for detoxification and a maintenance program for opioid addicts. Methadone prolongs QTc interval and can enhance the risk of developing torsades de pointes.

Tolerance, dependence, and addiction occur with long-term exposure to all opioids, and the risk for abuse and aberrant drug behavior must be monitored. *Tolerance* refers to decreased effectiveness of an opioid with repeated exposure to the drug. To achieve the same analgesic effectiveness, escalating doses of the opioid may be required.

Cross-tolerance refers to tolerance to a class of drugs with the same structure and mechanism of action within that class. Incomplete cross-tolerance occurs when selective tolerance at different types of opioid receptor subunit occurs, producing a variable response to different opioids. For example, if a patient has intolerable opioid side effects such as severe sedation without the benefit of the analgesic effect, transitioning to a different opioid within the same class may confer better analgesia without the negative side effects.

Opioid rotation refers to switching one opioid to another to achieve better analgesia and/or reduce side effects. By rotating the opioid, improved benefit from the new opioid may result from varying activities at the mu receptor, such as improved analgesia and reduction of adverse events.

Special Considerations in Opioid Prescribing. A study (Tong, Hochheimer, Brooks, et al, 2019) documented that 45% of all opioid prescriptions in the United States are written by primary care clinicians. Diversion and abuse of prescription opioid medications have been growing over the last three decades. Nearly 841,000 people have died since 1999 from drug overdoses. More than 70% of drug overdose deaths in 2019 involved a synthetic opioid, and the number of deaths attributed to opioid overdose has increased in parallel with the number of opioid prescriptions written. Not only is this a sad statistic, but it is also detrimental to all of society through increased crime rates, increased medical costs, and lost productivity. As new drugs and drug combinations are created (such as mixing fentanyl with heroin), it is evident that law enforcement alone is inadequate in combating this epidemic. Efforts to control the pace of the epidemic focus on three areas: (1) monitoring patient need, (2) shortening the amount of time medication is prescribed, and (3) reducing the overall number of opioid prescriptions in medical practice. Another important effort is subsidized access to evidence-based, medication-assisted treatment for opioid use disorder (OUD).

Health-care providers are often faced with balancing the risk of OUD with treatment of chronic pain syndromes. There are documented cognitive-affective transdiagnostic factors associated with vulnerability to alcohol and opioid use in the context of pain. Most health-care providers have not been educated to treat substance use disorders in routine clinical practice, and there is a shortage of health-care providers who have expertise in this area. There are also conflicting societal pressures on health-care providers working with patients who have an OUD. For example, providing an opioid user with naloxone to prevent overdose and death is seen by some as supporting the opioid use rather than working with the patient. More research is needed to provide evidence-based recommendations about how to diagnose and treat OUDs in the health-care setting.

Binswanger and Gordon (2016) suggest the following to help health-care professionals understand the opioid epidemic and assist patients dealing with substance use disorders:

- Labeling those who require opioids for pain management as weak or lazy is unlikely to be effective in resolving this complex problem. Creating a public dialogue about the complex issues in pain management and providing a venue for honest discourse founded on compassion and understanding could improve outcomes of pain management and avoid opioid overuse.
- The use of criminal sanctions against patients who use opioids and their providers is not helpful to stem the tide of the epidemic. OUD is a complex condition with medical, socioeconomic, and legal implications. Often, the criminalization of opioid use alienates, disempowers, and abandons the patient at the time of need. The stigma of OUD is strengthened by pejorative language and attitudes that actually increase the risks and problems associated with the disorder.
- Opioid overuse occurs in people of all backgrounds—young, old, homeless, wealthy, isolated, and living with loving families. This diversity makes assessment, diagnosis, and treatment difficult.
- Effective pharmacological treatment of opioid disorder requires assistive medications and medication management that may not be supported by families and partners. Evidence-based recommendations for the treatment of OUDs are lacking. Although health-care providers are anxious to avoid more deaths and create an effective treatment plan for people with OUD, observational data alone are not sufficient to overcome this epidemic.

How should health-care providers approach opioid prescribing and identifying patients who may be at risk for OUD? One example of an evidence-based program for OUD comes from the Johns Hopkins Bloomberg School of Public Health (Johns Hopkins, 2015). This program is designed to inform action with evidence and intervene comprehensively to promote appropriate and safe use of prescription opioids. This program was presented at a conference hosted by the Bloomberg School of Public Health and the Clinton Health Matters Initiative. Steps in this program include the following:

- Increase education for providers and strengthen prescribing guidelines for opioid prescriptions.

- Mandate prescriber prescription drug monitoring programs and allow third-party payers to use these data.
- Increase education related to overdose and naloxone use.
- Provide education and information on treatment for substance use disorders including expanded access to buprenorphine (Suboxone) and methadone.
- Develop patient-centered treatments for opioid overuse and study the outcomes and effectiveness of these programs.

Medical Marijuana

Cannabinoids exert their mechanism of action by binding to cannabinoid receptors and endogenous ligands. Suppression of calcium conductance and reduction of neuronal activities have been associated with reduction of inflammation. Cannabinoids have been found to be effective in the setting of visceral and neuropathic pain but has limited effectiveness in nociceptive somatic pain. It has also demonstrated effectiveness in the setting of fibromyalgia, multiple sclerosis–related pain, nausea in people with cancer, and HIV-related neuropathy. The side-effect profile of cannabinoids includes sedation, dizziness, and impaired balance. Hallucinations and psychotic behaviors also have been reported. Controversies surround its use in pain management as it is perceived as a possible gateway drug to abuse of other illicit drugs.

Nonpharmacological Management of Pain

Treating the whole person frequently necessitates a team-based, integrative treatment plan that may include pharmacological agents and/or various other modalities.

Restorative therapies may include treatment by physical therapists (PTs) and/or occupational therapists (OTs) but also may involve therapeutic exercise, physiotherapy, and other movement modalities, such as tai chi, Pilates, and yoga. Such therapy can occur in a variety of settings; it focuses on positive outcomes such as improvements in function. Inconsistent reimbursement policies may complicate the use of these adjuvant therapies. Transcutaneous electrical nerve stimulation (TENS) is considered a safe self-administered option, but evidence as to effectiveness is unclear. Massage therapy is considered a restorative therapy, and deep-tissue massage often provides subjective relief from trigger-point pain. Traction for low-back pain and/or neck pain is a PT technique whose efficacy is not well-documented. Cold and heat are ancient remedies for relief of pain; the synonym RICE (rest, ice, compression, elevation) is a standard cold treatment for acute, usually minor, injuries. The efficacy of heat wraps has been scientifically established for acute low back pain. Short-term bracing (immobilization) may be effective. Long-term bracing is known to contribute to deconditioning and muscle atrophy.

Interventional pain management would more likely necessitate referral to a pain specialist. Interventional procedures vary by invasiveness and degree of complexity. Trigger-point injections, joint injections, and peripheral nerve injection may be done in the primary care setting. Epidural steroid injections (ESIs), which deliver anti-inflammatory medication directly into the epidural space, have been shown to be effective, potentially reducing health-care costs. They can provide significant pain relief and decrease the need for surgical intervention.

Behavioral health approaches also play a large part in pain management. There is a well-documented relationship between pain and psychological health. There are a broad variety of approaches in this field, and finding the best fit between the practitioner and the person seeking treatment is critical. Some practitioners take an eclectic approach; others adhere more to one school of thought than others, such as mindfulness-based stress reduction (MBSR) or the currently popular dialectical behavioral therapy (DBT). Cognitive behavioral therapy (CBT) can improve functioning and decrease maladaptive behaviors. Primary care medical homes are more likely to have a behavioral counselor or an acupuncturist available for team-based approaches. It takes a "village," consistent with the Circle of Caring model.

Acupuncture is a restorative therapeutic approach that also includes massage and manipulative therapies, MBSR, yoga, and tai chi, as well as Reiki. Spirituality also falls under this rubric. As can be seen from Farshaad's story (see the Patient's Voice 83.1), frequent combinations—a multimodal, flexible approach and a

---

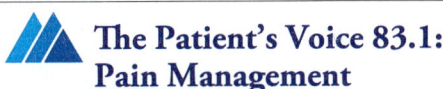

The Patient's Voice 83.1: Pain Management

FARSHAAD'S STORY

I was diagnosed with ulcerative colitis and eventually complex pain. Additionally, I have an allergy to medication that made it worse. I had a surgical removal of my colon, and it was replaced with a J-pouch. Two years after, I had surgery again, which resulted in severe pain. At that time, we left Canada and moved to the U.S.

Ultimately, I was referred to a pain management clinic and offered trigger-point injections, which turned out to be extremely effective. Physical therapy was coordinated with these injections and also helped me a lot. I regained my life. I also have severe pain from migraines. Botox injections on my neck and forehead were a huge breakthrough, too. I am pain-free for 4 months, then I need another injection. Reiki, or touch healing, also helps me. It doesn't cure anything, but it gives me power to face problems and calms me. I also very rarely take an opioid pain pill, Tylenol #3, for severe acute flares of my pain. Not everybody who takes that kind of pill should be considered an addict, however.

Adapted from: U.S. Department of Health and Human Services (2019, May). Pain Management Best Practices Inter-Agency Task Force Report: Updates, Gaps, Inconsistencies, and Recommendations.

willingness to try new things—of therapeutic options, individualized through an open therapeutic alliance, may yield the best results.

VULNERABLE AND SPECIAL POPULATIONS

Health Disparities in Pain Management

In 2003, the Institute of Medicine published a report titled, *Unequal Treatment: Confronting Racial and Ethnic Disparities in Health Care*. After reviewing more than 100 studies, the report concluded that "bias, prejudice, and stereotyping" contributed to widespread differences in health care by race and ethnicity (Smedley et al, 2003). In 2015, the *New England Journal of Medicine* published an article titled, "#BlackLivesMatter—A Challenge to the Medical and Public Health Communities" (Bassett, 2015). The author, New York City's health commissioner Mary T. Bassett, was once again bringing the attention of the entire medical community to the recalcitrant issue of black and white life expectancy and ongoing inequities and health disparities and urging action by the biomedical community writ large. In 2021, the *New England Journal of Medicine* published an article titled, "How Structural Racism Works—Racist Policies as a Root Cause of U.S. Racial Health Inequities" (Bailey et al). These authors make the case that understanding susceptibility to disease is racialized, which also has implications for our current understanding of pain and pain relief. This article makes the case that modern American medicine has "historical roots in scientific racism and the eugenics movement" (p 770), noting that: "Scientific racism reified the concept of race as an innate biological, and later genetic, attribute using culturally influenced scientific theory and inquiry" (Jackson et al., 2005).

As late as 2016, a study to assess racial attitudes discovered that half of white medical students and residents held unfounded beliefs about intrinsic biological differences between white and black people. Black patients' pain was still assessed as being less severe than that of white patients, leading to inadequate treatment of pain.

As noted earlier, the biopsychosocial model of pain management (Fig. 83.6) is composed of biological, psychological, and social factors and is an instructive lens for viewing health disparities in pain management. Biological factors such race and sex are inherited. Race distinguishes groups of people according to physical characteristics such as hair and eye color, physical build, and skin color, all of which are genetically determined, as is one's sex determined by X or Y chromosomes. These have important implications for disease prevalence, manifestations, and responses to treatment. Genetics, epigenetics, and hormones of biological sex and race influence physiology and pathology, including manifestations such as pain, and yield useful but incomplete data for overall pain management.

Additionally, emerging research on the cumulative effects of chronic stress and life events and trauma has led to the development of the concept of allostatic load (McEwen & Stellar, 1993). Different biological and physiological responses to stress interact and are triggered at varying degrees of activity, such as rises in cortisol and glucose. When external challenges such as the environment exceed the individual's ability to cope, allostatic load occurs (Guidi et al, 2021). This allopathic load can be measured through the use of biomarkers and clinical criteria, and higher levels of allostatic load have been associated with poorer health outcomes. Allostatic overload affects both physical and mental health across a variety of settings. This physiological "storm" invariably affects pain perceptions and outcomes.

Social constructs of gender and ethnicity also play a large role in pain manifestations and assessment, as do various other social and psychological factors, as outlined in the biopsychosocial model of pain management. Broadly, social constructs of gender and ethnicity also affect the overall community, as well as the behavior of clinicians and access to quality care. Consideration of race, sex, ethnicity, culture, and gender by the primary care provider yields a more complete approach to diagnosis, prevention, and treatment of disease, including pain management, and is an important, fundamental step toward precision medicine, which will benefit all populations.

Race and Ethnicity

Health disparities exist when treatment protocols differ solely based on racial or ethnic differences without taking the underlying health conditions or treatment preferences of the patient into consideration. Disparities in pain management have been well-documented. Disparities are observed not only in populations of color, but also include gender, sexual orientation, age, disability, religion, socioeconomic status, and geographical location.

The experience of pain activates stress-related physiological responses across differing ethnic groups, and different groups use different coping strategies. Overall, African Americans suffer a greater burden of pain and pain-related suffering. As an example, children with sickle cell anemia who presented to hospital emergency departments with pain were less likely to have their pain assessed than were children with long bone fractures. Other studies have shown that physicians tend to prescribe fewer analgesic medications for black Americans than white Americans. It was also found that blacks were less likely than their white counterparts to obtain prescription medication for adequate pain relief based on reported pain severity and the dose of analgesic provided, as well as access to pharmacies that carried prescription pain relievers. These pain management disparities may be secondary to racial bias and the fact that some clinicians may still hold false beliefs about biological differences between racial and ethnic groups.

Sex and Gender

Historically, females have been documented to consistently report a higher prevalence of chronic pain than males. Females have also been found to report more pain from certain diseases, compared with males. Some studies found that females with cancer report greater pain, as well as a higher rate of depression, compared with males (Green et al, 2011). Some chronic pain syndromes occur predominantly in females, including chronic fatigue syndrome, fibromyalgia, interstitial cystitis, and temporomandibular disorders. Females have reported both lower pain thresholds and tolerance, linked in part to hormonal levels (Fillingim et al, 2009). The role of sex hormones in nociception as well as coping strategies and psychological factors has been theorized to explain these differences. Other disparities found in females have been an increase in adverse drug effects and complications. Hormonal factors, physiology, and psychological and sociocultural factors have been implicated in differences in response to analgesics between females and males (Fillingim et al, 2009). Additionally, females have been found to have greater risk of pain misdiagnosis, delays in correct diagnosis, and improper and unproven treatments stemming from these biases (Campaign to End Chronic Pain in Women, 2010).

However, more current research that emphasizes longstanding gender stereotyping, as well as structural factors discussed earlier—delays in correct diagnosis, access to care, and the like—forces an ongoing examination of sex and gender. There is well-established current evidence that "…robust sex and gender influences… exist across leading causes of death and morbidity globally" (Mauvais-Jarvis et al, 2020). These authors provide recommendations across biomedical research, education, and practice focused on providing education and training of all clinicians to provide culturally and clinically appropriate care for the LGBTQ+ community (Fig. 83.10).

Pain Management in Children and Adolescents

Disparities have also been found as the cause of suboptimal pain management in children and adolescents. Undertreatment of pain in the acute setting such as patients with sickle cell crises, fractures, or burns has been found to be more pronounced in racial and ethnic minorities (Goyal et al, 2015). Some causes cited by providers for this undertreatment involve concerns about the risks of adverse effects and addiction with opioids.

Education, training, and research are critically necessary to provide better pain management and improve the quality of care among groups that are affected by these health disparities.

Pain Management in the Geriatric Population

Chronic pain in the geriatric population affects physical functioning and quality of life. This population undergoes age-related physiological and physical changes, which increase their susceptibility to chronic pain.

Pain Management During the COVID-19 Pandemic

The COVID-19 pandemic has affected the lives and health of many people around the world. The virus had left

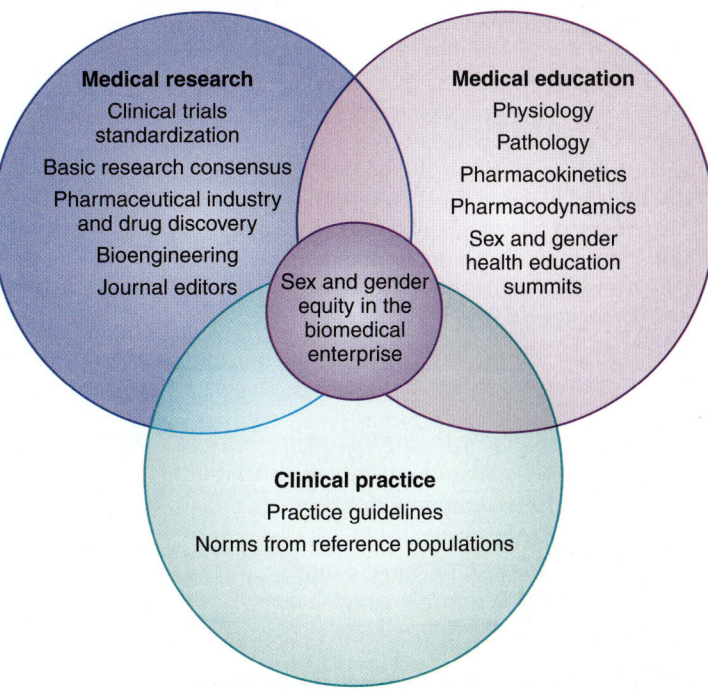

Figure 83.10 Summary of recommendations to promote sex and gender equity in the biomedical enterprise. *Source: Mauvais-Jarvis F, Bairey Merz N, Barnes PJ, et al. (2020). Sex and gender: modifiers of health, disease, and medicine. Lancet, 396(10250), 565–582.*

Pediatric/Adolescent Considerations: Pain Management

Effective pain management in the pediatric population requires a good line of communication between the child/patient, the patient's family, and the medical professional. Often a multidisciplinary and comprehensive approach is the cornerstone in the assessment and treatment of pain in the pediatric population. Setting realistic goals should be aimed at improving the function and quality of life of the pediatric patient. Abdominal pain and headaches are the most common chronic pain complaints in the pediatric population. Sickle cell disease is the most common type of acute pain complaint in the pediatric population other than traumas/accidents. Pain in sickle cell crises occurs during vaso-oclusive periods. Medical management of these pain crises include NSAIDs, hypertransfusions, and treatment of any medical and physiological stressors. Behavior modification techniques such as biofeedback, self-hypnosis, and relaxation techniques can be helpful.

Opioids at times are underused because of fear of addiction, which often leads to inadequate analgesia in this population. The painful crisis often does not respond to nonnarcotic interventions, and adolescent patients are sometimes labeled as drug seekers due to this inadequate analgesia. Several investigations have found that up to 50% of adolescents who present to primary care for headaches or sports injuries received an opioid medication (DeVries et al, 2014; Veliz et al, 2014). Another study found that 20% of adolescents with currently prescribed opioid medications reported using them intentionally to get high or increase the effects of alcohol or other drugs (McCabe et al, 2013). Misuse of opioid medications before high school graduation is associated with a 33% increase in the risk of later opioid misuse. Opioid misuse in adolescents is strongly associated with later-onset heroin use (Miech et al, 2015).

Geriatric Considerations: Pain Management

The geriatric patient with pain is more prone to develop depression and anxiety and may lack the proper support system to help them cope with these issues. Practitioners should be vigilant to the fact that geriatric patients tend to underreport pain because of their belief that pain is a normal part of the aging process.

From a physiological perspective, chronic pain management in the geriatric population needs to be carefully assessed when it comes to pharmacological therapies. From a pharmacokinetic and pharmacodynamic point of view, the geriatric population requires careful medication dose titration. Practitioners must carefully evaluate all the medications that geriatric patients are taking, as the potential for adverse events increases due to polypharmacy. The geriatric patient's comorbid conditions such as decreased renal function and hepatic metabolism, cardiac disease, and higher ratio of fat to lean muscle greatly puts the patient at increased risk from various pain medications. The prescriber must constantly evaluate geriatric patients for concerns about disorientation, confusion, and unintentional overdose.

many patients living with chronic pain, overburdened by not just psychological and emotional issues but also with reduced or delayed ongoing treatment for their chronic pain symptoms as routine clinics have been less accessible or closed. Limited interpersonal contacts, fear of contracting the virus, and economic strain have everyone around the world under stress. These stressors may exacerbate pain even in the absence of the viral illness. The COVID-19 virus itself has manifested as myalgia, fatigue, headaches, arthralgias, abdominal pain, poor sleep, and multiorgan–specific symptoms. These factors may also contribute to an increase in chronic pain symptoms, especially in older patients and those with other comorbid conditions.

Moderate to severe cases of COVID-19 have required intensive care unit (ICU) admission and management. Those afflicted by the virus have presented not only with respiratory impairment but also with multiorgan failure including cardiac, renal, hematological, and neurological systems (Kemp et al, 2020). Patients who have survived critical illnesses have been shown to have increased risk of developing chronic pain (Fig. 83.11). Factors that increase this risk in this population include sustained periods of immobilization, critical illness myopathy, critical illness polyneuropathy, muscle atrophy, and multiorgan dysfunction. Post-ICU patients will present with weakness, deconditioning, orthopedic-related pain such as arthropathies, and motor and sensory dysfunction (Kemp 2020). There has been growing evidence of COVID-19–related neurological sequelae in both the peripheral nervous system and the CNS in the form of headache, neuropathy, dizziness, and confusion. These neurological effects are secondary to neural tissue injuries associated with axonopathic polyneuropathy observed in both cerebrospinal fluid (CSF) and brain tissue (Ding et al, 2004). Other causes of neuropathic pain in COVID-19 patients include Guillain-Barré syndrome and therapeutic agents used to treat the virus such as ritonavir and hydroxychloroquine.

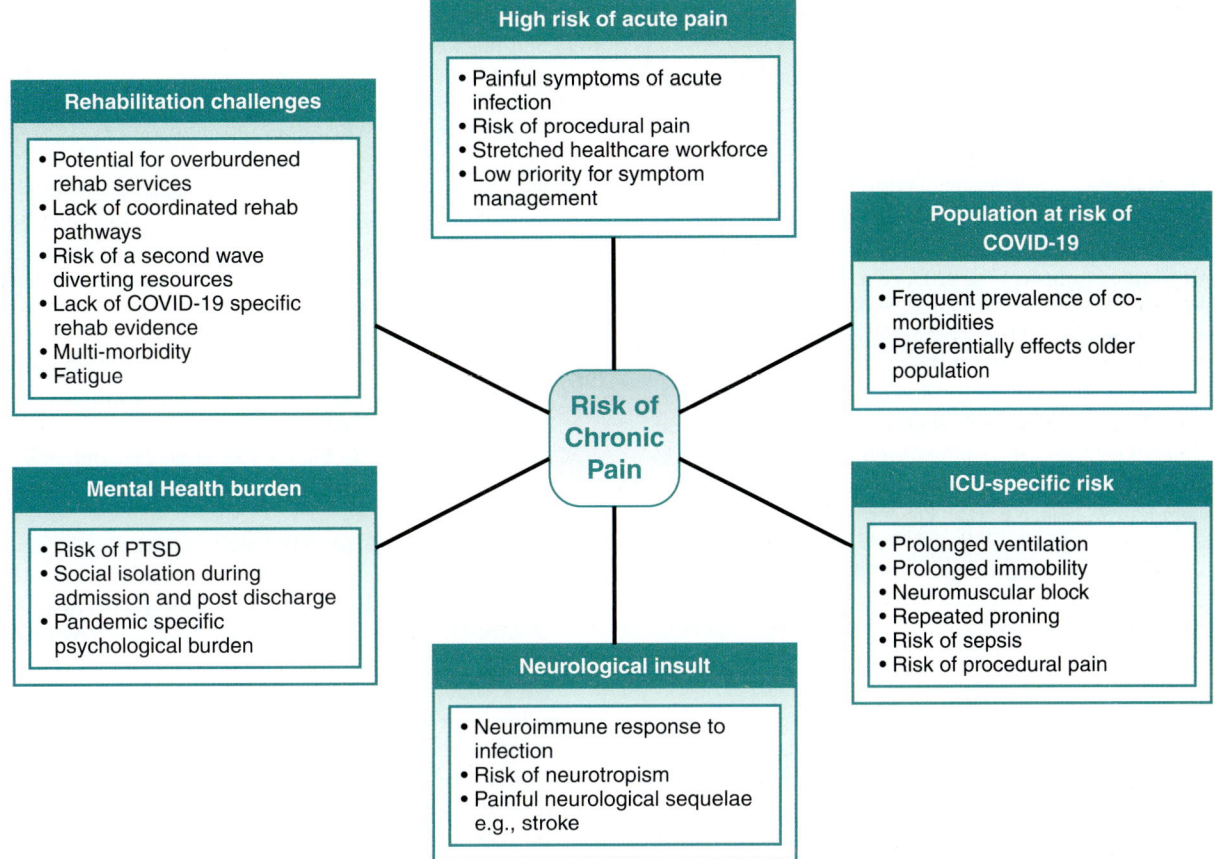

Figure 83.11 Potential risk factors for chronic pain development after COVID-19. *Source: Kemp HI, Corner E, Colvin LA. Chronic pain after COVID-19: implications for rehabilitation. Br J Anaesth. 2020 Oct; 125(4): 436–440.*

Multidisciplinary programs should be implemented to rehabilitate these patients from a physical and psychological perspective. A multimodal pain strategy involving psychologists, PTs, and pain-management physicians must be implemented in treating acute and chronic pain in this population.

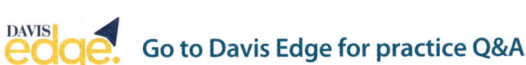 Go to Davis Edge for practice Q&A.

REFERENCES

Bailey ZD, Feldman JM, Bassett MT. (2021). How structural racism works – Racist policies as a root cause of US racial health inequities. NEJM, 384:8: 768-772.

Bally M, Dendukuri N, Rich B, et al. Risk of acute myocardial infarction with NSAIDS in real world use: Bayesian meta-analysis of individual patient data. *BMJ.* 2017:367:j 1909.

Bassett MT (2015). #BlackLivesMatter — A challenge to the medical and public health community. NEJM, 372: 1085-87. Feb 2021. DOI: 10.1056/NEJMp1500529

Campaign to end chronic pain in women. (2010). *The TMJ Association, Ltd.* https://tmj.org/news/campaign-to-end-chronic-pain-in-women/

Campbell CM, Edwards RR. (2012). Ethnic differences in pain and pain management. Pain management, 2(3), 219–230. https://doi.org/10.2217/pmt.12.7

Cintron A, Morrison RS. Pain and ethnicity in the United States: a systematic review. Journal of Palliative Medicine. Dec 2006. 1454-1473. http://doi.org/10.1089/jpm.2006.9.1454

Clauw DJ, Häuser W, Cohen SP, et al. Considering the potential for an increase in chronic pain after the COVID-19 pandemic, PAIN: August 2020 - Volume 161 - Issue 8 - p 1694-1697.

Dahlhamer J, Lucas J, Zelaya C, et al. (2018). Prevalence of Chronic Pain and High-Impact Chronic Pain Among Adults — United States, 2016. *Morbidity and Mortality Weekly Report, 67*(36), 1001–1006.

De Mesa C, Sheth S, Keenan C, et al. Primary Care Pain Management. Wolters Kluwer, 2019.

DeVries A, Koch T, Wall E, et al. A. Opioid use among adolescent patients treated for headache. *J Adolesc Health.* 2014;55:128–133.

Dowell D, Haegerich TM, Chou R. CDC Guideline for prescribing opioids for chronic pain—United States, 2016. *MMWR Recomm Rep.* 2016;65(No. RR-1):1–49. https://www.cdc.gov/mmwr/volumes/65/rr/rr6501e1.htm.

El-Tallawy SN, Nalamasu R, Pergolizzi JV, et al. Pain Management During the COVID-19 Pandemic. *Pain Ther* 9, 453–466 (2020). https://doi.org/10.1007/s40122-020-00190-4

Fillingim RB, King CD, Ribeiro-Dasilva MC, et al. (2009). Sex, gender, and pain: a review of recent clinical and experimental findings. *J Pain.* 10(5):447-85. doi: 10.1016/j.jpain.2008.12.001.

Gaskin DJ, Richard P. The economic costs of pain in the United States. *J Pain* 2012;13(8):715-724.

Green CR, Anderson KO, Baker TA, et al. (2003). The Unequal Burden of Pain: Confronting Racial and Ethnic Disparities in Pain, *Pain Medicine*, Volume 4, Issue 3, September 2003, Pages 277–294. https://doi.org/10.1046/j.1526-4637.2003.03034.x

Green CR, Hart-Johnson T, Loeffler DR. (2011). Cancer-related chronic pain: examining quality of life in diverse cancer survivors. *Cancer*. 117(9):1994-2003. doi: 10.1002/cncr.25761.

Goyal MK, Kuppermann N, Cleary SD, et al. (2015). Racial disparities in pain management of children with appendicitis in emergency departments. *JAMA Pediatr*. 169(11):996-1002. doi: 10.1001/jamapediatrics.2015.1915.

Guidi J, Lucente M, Sonino N, et al. Allostatic Load and Its Impact on Health: A Systematic Review. Psychotherapy and Psychosomatics. 2021;90(1):11-27. doi: 10.1159/000510696. Epub 2020 Aug 14. PMID: 32799204.

Han B, Compton W, Blanco C, et al. Prescription opioid use, misuse, and use disorders in U.S. adults: 2015 National Survey on Drug Use and Health. *Ann Int Med*. 2017;167(5):293–301. doi: 10.7326/M17-0865.

Hill KP. Medical Marijuana for Treatment of Chronic Pain and Other Medical and Psychiatric Problems: A Clinical Review. *JAMA*. 2015;313(24):2474–2483. doi:10.1001/jama.2015.6199

Hoffman KM, Trawalter S, Axt JR, et al. Racial bias in pain assessment and treatment recommendations, and false beliefs about biological differences between blacks and whites. Proc Natl Acad Sci U S A 2016; 113: 4296-301.

IASP. (2021). *Pain Reports*. https://www.iasp-pain.org/publications/pain-reports/

Jackson J, Weidman NM, Rubin G (2005). The origins of scientific racism. Journal of Blacks Higher Education, 50: 66-79.

Jones RC 3rd, Lawson E. Backonja M. Managing neuropathic pain. *Med Clin North Am* 2016;100(1):151-167.

Kemp HI, Corner E, Colvin LA (2020). Chronic Pain after COVID-19: Implications for Rehabilitation. British Journal of Anaesthesia Vol 124 Number 4 October 2020: 436-449 Doi: 10.1016/j.bja.2020.05.021

Lazaridou A, Elbaridi N, Edwards RR, et al. (2019). Chapter 5 - Pain Assessment, Eds: Benzon H, Raja S, Liu S, et al. Essentials of Pain Medicine, 4th ed. Elsevier: 39-46.e1, ISBN 9780323401968.

Lee P, Le Saux M, Siegel R, et al. Racial and ethnic disparities in the management of acute pain in US emergency departments: Meta-analysis and systematic review. *The American Journal of Emergency Medicine (37)*9, 2019. https://doi.org/10.1016/j.ajem.2019.06.014

Lozada MJ, Raji MA, Goodwin JS, et al. Opioid Prescribing by Primary Care Providers: a Cross-Sectional Analysis of Nurse Practitioner, Physician Assistant, and Physician Prescribing Patterns. J Gen Intern Med. 2020 Sep;35(9):2584-2592. doi: 10.1007/s11606-020-05823-0. Epub 2020 Apr 24. PMID: 32333312; PMCID: PMC7459076.

Mao J. Gold MS, Backonja MM. Combination drug therapy for chronic pain: a call for more clinical studies. *J Pain*. 2011;12(2): 157-166.

Martin WR, History and development of mixed opioid agonists, partial agonists and antagonists, *Br J Clin Pharmacol*. 1979;7(Suppl3): 273S-279S.

Mauvais-Jarvis F, Bairey Merz N, Barnes PJ, et al. (2020). Sex and gender: modifiers of health, disease, and medicine. Lancet (London, England), 396(10250), 565–582. https://doi.org/10.1016/S0140-6736(20)31561-0

Maxwell JC. The pain reliever and heroin epidemic in the United States: Shifting winds in a perfect storm. *J Addict Dis*. 2015;34(2–3): 127–140.

McCabe SE, West BT, Boyd CJ. Medical use, medical misuse and nonmedical use of prescription opioids: Results from a longitudinal study. *Pain*. 2013;154 (5):708–713.

McEwen BS, Stellar E. Stress and the individual. Mechanisms leading to disease. Arch Intern Med. 1993 Sep; 153(18): 2093–101.

Meints S, Wang V, Edwards RR. (2018). Sex and race differences in pain sensitization among patients with chronic low back pain. The Journal of Pain Volume: 19 Issue 12 (2018) ISSN: 1526-5900 Online ISSN: 1528-8447.

Merskey H, Bogduk N. Classification of pain. IASP Pain Terminol. 1994. **https://www.iasp-pain.org/PublicationsNews/Content.aspx?ItemNumber=1673**

Miech R, Johnston L, O'Malley PM, et al. Prescription opioids in adolescence and future opioid misuse. *Pediatrics*. 2015;136: e1169–1177.

Mossey JM. Defining racial and ethnic disparities in pain management. In: *Clinical orthopedics and Related Research*, 2011:1859-1870.

Muench U, Spetz J, Jura M, et al. Opioid-prescribing Outcomes of Medicare Beneficiaries Managed by Nurse Practitioners and Physicians. Med Care. 2019 Jun;57(6):482-489. doi: 10.1097/MLR.0000000000001126. PMID: 31008896.

Pizzo PA, Clark NM, Carter-Pokras O, et al. Relieving Pain in America: *A Blueprint for Transforming Prevention, Care, Education, and Research*. Institute of Medicine: 2011.

Rogers AH, Kauffman BY, Bakhshaie J, et al. Anxiety sensitivity and opioid misuse among opioid-using adults with chronic pain. *Am J Drug Alcohol Abuse*. 2019;45(5):470-478. https://doi.org/10.1080/00952990.2019.1569670

Simons JS, Gaher RM. The Distress Tolerance Scale: Development and validation of a self-report measure. *Motiv Emot*. 2005;29(2): 83-102. https://doi.org/10.1007/s11031-005-7955-3

Smedley BD, Stith AY, Nelson AR (2003) Unequal treatment: Confronting racial and ethnic disparities in health care. Washington, D.C.: The National Academies Press. 764 p.

Sostres C, Lanas Á. Appropriate prescription, adherence and safety of non-steroidal anti-inflammatory drugs. *Medicina Clínica* (English Edition), Volume 146, Issue 6, 2016. **https://doi.org/10.1016/j.medcle.2016.05.006**

Stefanick ML, Schiebinger L. (2020). Analysing how sex and gender interact. *Lancet, (398)* Nov. 14, 2020.

Stewart SH, Asmundson GJ. Anxiety sensitivity and its impact on pain experiences and conditions: A state of the art. *Cogn Behav Ther*. 2006;35(4):185-188. https://doi.org/10.1080/16506070601090457

Tong ST, Hochheimer CJ, Brooks EM, et al. (2019). Chronic Opioid Prescribing in Primary Care: Factors and Perspectives. *Annals of family medicine*, *17*(3), 200–206. https://doi.org/10.1370/afm.2357

Trawalter S, Hoffman KM, Waytz A (2012) Racial Bias in Perceptions of Others' Pain. PLoS ONE 7(11): e48546. doi:10.1371/journal.pone.0048546

U.S. Department of Health and Human Services (2007) National healthcare disparities report. Agency for Healthcare Research and Quality website. **http://archive.ahrq.gov/qual/nhdr07/nhdr07.pdf**. Accessed 7-25-21.

U.S. Department of Health and Human Services (2019, May). Pain Management Best Practices Inter-Agency Task Force Report: Updates, Gaps, Inconsistencies, and Recommendations. Retrieved from U. S. Department of Health and Human Services website: **https://www.hhs.gov/opioids/prevention/pain-management-options/index.html**

Veliz P, Epstein-Ngo QM, Meier E, et al. Painfully obvious: A longitudinal examination of medical use and misuse of opioid medication among adolescent sports participants. *J Adolesc Health.* 2014;54:333–340.

Vlaeyen JWS, Crombez G. Behavioral conceptualization and treatment of chronic pain. *Annu Rev Clin Psychol.* 2020;16(1):187-212. https://doi.org/10.1146/annurev-clinpsy-050718-095744.

Watson CP: The treatment of neuropathic pain: antidepressants and opioids. *Clin J Pain* 16:S49-S55, 2000.

Zale EL, Powers JM, Ditre JW. (15 July 2021). Cognitive-Affective Transdiagnostic Factors Associated With Vulnerability to Alcohol and Prescription Opioid Use in the Context of Pain. Alcohol Research: Current Reviews, Volume 41 Issue 1 (https://experts.syr.edu/en/publications/cognitive-affective-transdiagnostic-factors-associated-with-vulne Accessed 7/19/2021).

Zis P, Daskalaki A, Bountouni I, et al. Depression and chronic pain in the elderly: links and management challenges. *Clin Interv aging* 2017;12:709-720.

Zvolensky MJ, Rogers AH, Garey L, et al. The role of anxiety sensitivity in the relation between pain intensity with substance use and anxiety and depressive symptoms among smokers with chronic pain. *Int J Behav Med.* 2020;27(6):668-676. https://doi.org/10.1007/s12529-020-09914-4

Cannabis/cannabinoids, 1211, 1216
   adolescents and, 1403
   for pain, 1481
Capnocytophaga canimorsus, 199
Carbonic anhydrase inhibitors, 294
Carbon monoxide (CO) poisoning, 421, 1379t
Carboxyhemoglobin (COHb) levels, 1358
Carbuncles. *See* Furuncles and carbuncles
Cardiac and associated risk disorders
   acute coronary syndrome (ACS), 553–565, 553t, 554t, 556f, 556t, 557f, 558f, 561f, 562f
   coronary heart disease (CHD), 547–552
   dyslipidemia, 543–547, 543t, 545t
   heart failure (HF), 565–573, 566t
   hypertension (HTN), 529–542, 530b, 531t, 533t, 535b
   premature sudden cardiac death (SCD), 1410
Cardiovascular complaints
   after cancer, 1443
   with aging, 1451t
   chest pain, 521–523, 522f
   dyspnea, 419–421, 524–526
   eating disorders and, 1307t
   leg aches, 526
   palpitations, 523–524, 525f
   peripheral edema, 526–528, 527f
   syncope, 524
Cardiovascular examination in sports physicals, 1411–1412
Caregivers of cancer patients, 1445
Caring in advanced practice nursing, 19–21
   advocacy in, 20–21
   authentic presence in, 20
   commitment in, 21
   courage in, 20
   knowing in, 21
   patience in, 21
   processes in, 22–23
   self-care and, e1558–e1559
   spirited, 22–23
Cariprazine, 1233
Carpal tunnel syndrome (CTS)
   clinical presentation of, 941–942
   diagnosis of, 942
   epidemiology and causes of, 941
   follow-up and referral for, 942–943
   management of, 942
   pathophysiology of, 941
   patient education on, 943
Carpopedal spasm, 979
Cash/private pay patients, e1535–e1536
Cataracts, 286t
   clinical presentation of, 289
   diagnosis of, 289–290
   epidemiology and causes of, 288
   follow-up and referral for, 290
   management of, 290
   pathophysiology of, 288–289
   patient education on, 290
Cauda equina syndrome (CES)
   clinical presentation of, 929–930
   diagnosis of, 930
   epidemiology and causes of, 928–929, 929t
   follow-up and referral for, 930
   management of, 930
   pathophysiology of, 929
   patient education on, 930
Causalgia, 892
Celiac disease
   clinical presentation of, 658
   diagnosis of, 658
   epidemiology and causes of, 657
   follow-up and referral for, 658
   management of, 658
   pathophysiology of, 657–658
   patient education on, 658

Cellulitis, 199–200, 1336
   clinical presentation of, 201–202
   diagnosis of, 202
   epidemiology and causes of, 200–201
   follow-up and referral for, 204
   management of, 202–203, 203t
   pathophysiology of, 201
   patient education on, 204
Centers for Disease Control and Prevention (CDC)
   on smoking cessation, 514
   Stopping Elderly Accidents, Deaths and Injuries (STEADI), 1462
Centers for Medicare and Medicaid Services (CMS), e1526–e1527. *See also* Medicare
Center to Advance Palliative Care, 1189
Central apnea. *See* Sleep apnea
Central hypothyroidism, 994
Central nervous system (CNS)
   dizziness and vertigo due to disorders of, 77
   paresthesia and paresis due to disorders of, 90
   seizure disorders and, 95, 96
Central retina artery occlusion, 287
Cephalosporins for lower urinary tract infections (UTIs), 718
Cerebral contusion, 1364
Cerebral hemorrhage, 118
Cerebral ischemia, 117–118
Cerebral perfusion, 118
Cerebrospinal fluid (CSF), 126
Cerebrovascular accident (CVA)
   clinical presentation of, 119–120, 121t
   diagnostic reasoning for, 120–122
   epidemiology and causes of, 117
   follow-up and referral for, 123
   headache and, 81
   iceberg of stroke, 124f
   management of, 122–123
   paresthesia and paresis with, 90
   pathophysiology of, 117–118
   types of, 116–117
Cerumen, 303
Cervical cancer, 750–751
   clinical presentation of, 821
   diagnosis of, 821–823, 822t, 824b
   epidemiology and causes of, 819–820
   follow-up and referral for, 824
   management of, 823–824
   pathophysiology of, 820–821
   patient education on, 824
Cervical cap, 769
Cervical muscle strain
   clinical presentation of, 911–912
   diagnosis of, 912
   epidemiology and causes of, 910–911
   follow-up and referral for, 913
   management of, 912–913
   pathophysiology of, 911
   patient education on, 913
Cervical spondylosis
   clinical presentation of, 914
   diagnosis of, 914–915
   epidemiology and causes of, 913–914
   follow-up and referral for, 915
   management of, 915
   pathophysiology of, 914
   patient education on, 915
Cessation, smoking, 514–516, 515f, 519–521. *See also* Smoking addiction
CFTR modulators, 437, 438
CGRP antagonists, 88
Chaemolyticum, 393
Chalazion. *See* Hordeolum and chalazion
Chamomile, 222
Champus/Tricare, e1535
CHAMPVA, e1535

Chancroid, 867t
Chemical burns, 1361–1362
Chemotherapy
   breast cancer, 806
   colorectal cancer, 676
   leukemia, 1100–1101
   lung cancer, 505–506
   malignant melanoma, 260
   ovarian cancer, 829–830
   pancreatic cancer, 689
   testicular cancer, 862, 864
Chemotherapy-induced peripheral neuropathy (CIPN), 1441
Chest pain
   diagnosis of, 521–523, 522f
   evidence-based nursing for, 521
Chest reconstruction, 1419
Chest wall syndrome (CWS), 523
Chiggers, 1348, 1350, 1354
Children
   pain management in, 1483
   sports physicals for, 1406–1417
Children's Yale-Brown Obsessive Compulsive Scale (CY-BOCS), 1295
Chlamydia pneumoniae, 442
   acute otitis media (AOM) and, 342–343
   pharyngitis and tonsillitis and, 393
Chlamydia trachomatis, 867t
   acute otitis media (AOM) and, 343
   epididymitis and, 854
   pharyngitis and tonsillitis and, 393
   prostatitis and, 840
   red eye/conjunctivitis and, 282
   as sexually transmitted infection (STI), 866, 870t, 872
Chloasma, 152
Chlorpromazine, 1231
Cholecystitis, 678–679
   clinical presentation of, 680
   diagnosis of, 680
   epidemiology and causes of, 679
   follow-up and referral for, 681
   management of, 680–681
   pathophysiology of, 679–680
   patient education on, 681
Cholesteatoma, 337
Cholesterol levels. *See* Dyslipidemia
Cholinergics
   glaucoma and, 294
   nausea and vomiting and, 617
Cholinesterase inhibitors for Alzheimer's disease (AD), 109
Chronic bronchitis. *See* Chronic obstructive pulmonary disease (COPD)
Chronic diarrhea with acquired immunodeficiency syndrome (AIDS), 1168
Chronic fatigue syndrome (CFS), 1124
   clinical presentation of, 1126
   diagnosis of, 1126–1127, 1126t
   epidemiology and causes of, 1125
   follow-up and referral for, 1128
   management of, 1127
   pathophysiology of, 1125–1126
   patient education on, 1128
Chronic glaucoma, 286t
Chronic hepatitis, 630
Chronic kidney disease (CKD)
   clinical presentation of, 737–738
   diagnosis of, 738–739, 738b
   epidemiology and causes of, 736
   follow-up and referral for, 742
   management of, 739–741, 740t
   pathophysiology of, 736–737
   patient education on, 742
Chronic lymphocytic leukemia (CLL). *See* Leukemia

Chronic myelogenous leukemia (CML). *See* Leukemia
Chronic obstructive pulmonary disease (COPD)
   clinical presentation of, 477–479, 478t
   diagnosis of, 479–480
   epidemiology and causes of, 475–476
   evidence-based nursing for, 486
   follow-up and referral for, 484
   management of, 480–484
   pathophysiology of, 476–477
   patient education on, 484–485
   pneumothorax and hemothorax, 1369–1371, 1371b
Chronic otitis externa (COE), 334, 337
Chronic otitis media (COM), 343
Chronic pancreatitis
   clinical presentation of, 686
   diagnosis of, 686–687
   epidemiology and causes of, 685–686
   follow-up and referral for, 687–688
   management of, 687
   pathophysiology of, 686
   patient education on, 688
Chronic pelvic pain syndrome
   in females, 753–754
   in males, 754–755
Chronic/subacute meningitis, 126t
Chronic tension-type headache, 82
Chronic venous insufficiency, 596–597
   clinical presentation of, 598–599
   diagnosis of, 599
   epidemiology and causes of, 597
   follow-up and referral for, 600
   management of, 599–600
   pathophysiology of, 597–598
   patient education on, 600
Churg-Strauss syndrome, 488b
Chvostek's sign, 979
Cigarette smoking. *See* Smoking addiction
CINAHL, 65
Circle of Caring practice model, 3, 13–15, 14f, 15–16, 19, 22, 542
   clinical judgment and, 38–39
   community-based, 27, 27f
   contextualized approach in, 13
   creative approach to therapeutics and interventions in, 14–15
   EBP clinical decision making and, 68–69, 68f
   grief and, 1181
   nature of patient responses in, 13–14
   self-care in, e1558
Cirrhosis and liver failure
   clinical presentation of, 692–693
   diagnosis of, 693–695
   epidemiology and causes of, 690–691, 690b
   follow-up and referral for, 698
   management of, 695–698, 696–697b
   pathophysiology of, 691–692
   patient education on, 698
Citalopram, 1298
Civil Health and Medical Program of the Uniformed Services (Champus), e1535
Civilian Health and Medical Program of the Department of Veterans Affairs (CHAMPVA), e1535
Cleansing, wound, 1338
   after animal and human bites, 1344
Clinical alignment, 40
Clinical decision making, EBP, 68–69, 68f
Clinical judgment
   Circle of Caring and, 38–39
   communication and, 40
   ethics and, 54–55
   purpose and goal of diagnosis of, 39

Clinical practice. *See* Primary care practice
Clinical practice guidelines. *See* Evidence-based practice (EBP)
Clinical process
   critical thinking in, 40–41
   developing expertise in, 41, 41t
   human memory limitations in, 40
   intuition in, 41
Clomipramine, 1298
Closed-angle glaucoma. *See* Glaucoma
Clostridium spp.
   diarrhea and, 607, 609
   gastroenteritis and, 619, 620–621t
Closure, wound, 1338–1339, 1340–1341
   after animal and human bites, 1344–1345
Clozapine, 1232
Cluster headache, 79t, 80, 83
   clinical presentation of, 84f, 85
Clustering history, 42
Cocaine poisoning, 1377t
Codeine, 1478
Cognition in older adults, 1460–1462
Cognitive behavioral skills building (CBSB), e1551, e1552–e1553
Cognitive behavioral therapy (CBT), e1552–e1554, e1554f
   anxiety disorders and, 1275
   bipolar and related disorders (BD) and, 1262
   eating disorders and, 1310
   generalized anxiety disorder (GAD) and, 1280, 1280b
   hoarding disorder (HD) and, 1301
   improving assertiveness and problem-solving skills, e1554
   increasing pleasurable activation, e1553–e1554
   insomnia disorder and, 1316t
   irritable bowel syndrome (IBS) and, 656
   major depressive disorder (MDD) and, 1244
   obsessive-compulsive disorder (OCD) and, 1298
   pain management and, 1481
   panic disorder and, 1283
   post-traumatic stress disorder (PTSD) and, 1289
   reducing negative thoughts, e1553, e1554f
   schizophrenia spectrum disorders and, 1235
Cognitive impairment, 102
   sports physicals and, 1409
   treatment guidelines for community-acquired pneumonia from, 449
Cognitive processing therapy (CPT), 1288
Cognitive restructuring, e1553, e1554f
Cohort studies, 61–62
Colchicine, 1059
Cold-related illnesses
   frostbite, 1388–1389
   hypothermia, 1386–1388
Collaboration, e1525–e1526
Collagen vascular diseases, 487b
Colonoscopy, 667–668
Colorectal cancer, 672–673
   clinical presentation of, 674–675
   diagnosis of, 675
   epidemiology and causes of, 673
   follow-up and referral for, 676–677
   management of, 675–676
   pathophysiology of, 673–674, 674t
   patient education on, 677
Columbia-Suicide Severity Rating Scale (C-SSRS), 1266
Combination analgesics, 88
Comedones, 240
Commercial sex act, 1327
Commitment, 21
Common cold, 433
Communication and clinical judgment, 40
Community-acquired pneumonia (CAP). *See* Pneumonia

Community-based Circle of Caring, 27, 27f
Community influences on health promotion, 33–34
Compassion fatigue, e1560–e1561
Compensatory mechanisms, 1304
Complementary and alternative therapies
   atopic dermatitis, 222
   benign prostatic hyperplasia (BPH), 838
   coronary heart disease (CHD), 550, 551–552
   eating disorders, 1310
   endometriosis, 816, 817
   osteoarthritis (OA), 961, 962
   for pain in palliative care, e1506–e1513
   premenstrual syndrome (PMS) and premenstrual dysphoric disorder (PMDD), 782, 783
   psoriasis, 237
Compliance planning, e1546–e1547
Comprehensive Addiction and Recovery Act (CARA), e1527
Comprehensive End of Life Care (CELC) Initiative, e1489
COMT (Catechol-O-Methyl Transferase) inhibitors, 113
Concussion, 1364
   sports physicals, 1409–1410, 1409t
Condoms
   female, 768
   male, 768
Conductive hearing loss (CHL), 310, 312t, 316
Confidentiality, e1516b, e1517–e1518
Confusion
   defined, 73
   delirium, 73
   dementia, 73, 75–76t
   diagnostic reasoning algorithm, 74f
   differential diagnosis, 73
   infectious process, 76
   metabolic disturbances, 73, 76
   neoplasm, 76
   tissue hypoxia and ischemia, 76
Conjunctivitis. *See* Red eye/conjunctivitis
Constipation, 604, 606, 606b
   diagnosis of, 606–607, 608f
   management of, 607, 609, e1503t
   palliative care and, e1502, e1503t
Contact dermatitis
   clinical presentation of, 224
   diagnosis of, 224–225
   epidemiology and causes of, 223
   follow-up and referral for, 225
   management of, 225
   pathophysiology of, 223–224
   patient education on, 226
Contact photodermatitis, 1356
Continuous glucose monitoring (CGM), 1023
Continuous positive airway pressure (CPAP), e1499
Contraception and family planning, 760–761, 762f
   abortion, 770–771
   adolescents and, 1402
   barrier methods, 768–769
   contraceptive patch, 766–767
   contraceptive vaginal ring, 767
   etonogestrel implant, 763
   fertility awareness methods, 769–770
   intrauterine device (IUD), 761–762
   medroxyprogesterone acetate (DMPA) injections, 768
   oral contraceptive pills (OCPs), 750, 751, 763–766
   patient education on, 771
   postcoital controls, 770
   sterilization, 770
Contraceptive foam, cream, film, jelly, and suppository, 769
Contraceptive patch, 766–767
Contraceptive vaginal ring, 767

Control studies, 61–62
Contusions, cerebral, 1364
Coronary heart disease (CHD)
  clinical presentation of, 548
  complementary therapies for, 550, 551–552
  diagnosis of, 548–550
  epidemiology and causes of, 547
  follow-up and referral for, 550
  management of, 550
  pathophysiology of, 547–548
  patient education on, 550
Cor pulmonale, 567
Corrosive materials, exposure to, 1379t
Corticosteroids
  allergic reactions and, 1110, 1111–1112
  arthropod bites and stings and, 1353
  carpal tunnel syndrome (CTS) and, 942
  gout and, 1059–1060
  inflammatory bowel disease (IBD) and, 670
  intra-articular injections for osteoarthritis (OA), 964
  rheumatoid arthritis (RA) and, 1121–1122
  rhinitis and, 359–361
  rhinosinusitis and, 373
  tendinitis/tenosynovitis and, 940
Cortisone acetate, 1010
Corynebacterium diphtheriae
  acute otitis media (AOM) and, 343
  pharyngitis and tonsillitis and, 392, 393
  upper respiratory infections (URIs) and, 433
Costochondritis, 888
Cough
  conditions and diseases associated with, 417
  diagnosis of, 417–419
  management of, 419, e1500
  palliative care and, e1500
  patient education on, 419
Courage, 20
COVID-19, 3, 7, 36, 440
  bipolar and related disorders (BD) and, 1262
  clinical presentation of, 443–444, 443b
  depression and, 1241
  follow-up and referral for, 451–452
  grief and, 1179, 1180
  Home Health Care Planning Improvement Act and, e1527–e1528
  impact on reimbursement, e1534
  intimate partner violence (IPV) and, 1183
  life expectancy reduced by, 6
  management of pneumonia and, 448–451
  maskne and, 240
  obsessive-compulsive disorder (OCD) and, 1294
  older adults and, 1464–1465, 1464b
  pain management and, 1483–1484, 1485f
  patient education on, 452
  psychosocial complaints and, 1173–1174
  self-care and, e1558, e1559–e1560
  speed of vaccine development for, 13
  stress and, e1551
  substance use disorders (SUDs) and, 1209, 1210, 1212b
  telehealth use and, 53
  treatment of, 450–451
  vaccine for, 1398
  value-based health care and, e1526
  verification of vaccine against, 44
CPR (cardiopulmonary resuscitation), e1495
CRAFFT screening tool, 1400, 1401t
Cramps, muscle, 893
Creative thinking, 41
Crisis intervention
  sexual assault, 1323
  suicide prevention, 1268
Critical thinking, 40–41
Crohn's disease (CD). *See* Inflammatory bowel disease (IBD)

Cross-tolerance, 1480
Cruciate ligament injury, 951
Crusted scabies, 163, 165
Cryosurgery
  actinic keratosis, 255
  seborrheic keratoses, 253
Cryptococcosis with acquired immunodeficiency syndrome (AIDS), 1169
Cryptococcus linguae-pilosasae, 384
Cryptosporidiosis with acquired immunodeficiency syndrome (AIDS), 1169
Cryptosporidium, 625t
Current procedural terminology (CPT) coding, e1540–e1544
  evaluation and management documentation, e1541–e1543, e1542b
  "incident to," 1543
  level II codes, e1543
  modifiers and add-on codes, e1542, e1542b
  new requests, e1542
  unlisted codes, e1542
Cushing response/reflex, 1367
Cushing's syndrome, 1089
  clinical presentation of, 1007–1008
  diagnosis of, 1008–1009
  epidemiology and causes of, 1006
  follow-up and referral for, 1009–1010
  management of, 1009
  pathophysiology of, 1006–1007
  patient education on, 1010–1011
Cyclothymic disorder, 1252t, 1255–1256
Cystic fibrosis (CF), 439
  clinical presentation of, 436–437
  diagnosis of, 437
  epidemiology and causes of, 436
  follow-up and referral for, 437–438
  management of, 437
  pathophysiology of, 436
  patient education on, 438
Cytomegalic inclusion virus (CMV), 443
Cytomegalovirus (CMV)
  AIDS and, 1168–1169
  HIV and, 1066
  infectious mononucleosis and (*See* Infectious mononucleosis)

D

Daily Enhancement of Meaningful Activity (DEMA) intervention, 110
Data collection, 41–42
D-dimer assay, 599
Deafness. *See* Hearing loss
Death
  leading causes of, 34, 34f, 1402–1403
  life expectancy and, e1491–e1492
  sites of, e1492
Débridement, wound, 1338
  after animal and human bites, 1344
Decongestants
  for rhinitis, 358–361
  for rhinosinusitis, 372
Deep-brain stimulation (DBS), 1298
Deep folliculitis, 195
Deep partial-thickness burns, 1357–1358, 1360–1361
Deep vein thrombosis (DVT), 596–597
  clinical presentation of, 598–599
  diagnosis of, 599
  epidemiology and causes of, 597
  follow-up and referral for, 600
  management of, 599–600
  pathophysiology of, 597–598
  patient education on, 600
Degenerative disorders
  Alzheimer's disease (AD), 104–109, 108f
  amyotrophic lateral sclerosis (ALS), 114–115

cervical spondylosis, 896, 913–915
  dementia, 102–104, 102t
  osteoarthritis (OA), 956–967, 959b, 960t, 963f
  osteoporosis, 967–975, 970t, 972f, 973t
  Parkinson's disease, 109–114, 110f
Degenerative joint disease (DJD), 956
Delayed serum sickness-type reactions, 1353
Delayed-type cellular hypersensitivity response, 1106
Delirium
  defined, 73
  versus dementia, 75–76t
  in older adults, 1461
  palliative care and, e1503–e1505, e1504b
Delusional disorder, 1226t
Dementia
  clinical presentation of, 103
  defined, 73, 102
  versus delirium, 75–76t
  diagnostic reasoning for, 103
  epidemiology and causes of, 102, 102t
  follow-up and referral for, 104
  management of, 103–104
  in older adults, 1461
  pathophysiology of, 103
Demodex, 249
Dental health
  in cancer survivors, 1446
  in older adults, 1460
Deontology, e1515
Deprescribing medications, e1505
Depression, 1178–1179, 1178t, 1201b, 1209
  cancer and, 1444
  diagnosis of, 1178–1179
  evidence-based practice for, 1239
  major depressive disorder (MDD), 1178, 1188b, 1226t, 1239–1250, 1296
  screening tools for, 1175t
  types of, 1179
De Quervain's tenosynovitis
  clinical presentation of, 943
  diagnosis of, 944
  epidemiology and causes of, 943
  follow-up and referral for, 944
  management of, 944
  pathophysiology of, 943
  patient education on, 944
De Quervain thyroiditis, 995
Dermatitis
  atopic, 215–223, 221b
  contact, 223–226
  psoriasis, 228–238
  seborrheic, 226–228
Dermatology Life Quality Index, 230
Dermatophytoses
  clinical presentation of, 181–183
  diagnosis of, 183
  epidemiology and causes of, 180–181
  follow-up and referral for, 185–186
  management of, 183–185
  pathophysiology of, 181
  patient education on, 186
Descriptive research, 62
Desensitizing immunotherapy, 363
Dexamethasone, 1010
Diabetes and sports physicals, 1410
Diabetes distress, 1026–1027
Diabetes mellitus (DM) type 1. *See also* Hypoglycemia
  clinical presentation of, 1017–1018
  diagnosis of, 1018–1019
  epidemiology and causes of, 1014–1016, 1015f

follow-up and referral for, 1025–1027
management of, 1019–1025, 1019t, 1020t, 1023t
pathophysiology of, 1016–1017
patient education on, 1027
Diabetes mellitus (DM) type 2
clinical presentation of, 1029, 1030t
diagnosis of, 1030–1031
epidemiology and causes of, 1027–1028
follow-up and referral for, 1037–1039
management of, 1031–1037, 1032t
pathophysiology of, 1028–1029
patient education on, 1039
Diabetes mellitus (DM) type 3C
clinical presentation of, 1039–1040
diagnosis of, 1040
epidemiology and causes of, 1039
follow-up and referral for, 1041
management of, 1040–1041
pathophysiology of, 1039
patient education on, 1041
Diabetic ketoacidosis (DKA), 1020, 1020t
Diabetic kidney disease, 1038
Diabetic nephropathy, 736–737
Diabetic retinopathy, 286t
clinical presentation of, 295–296
diagnosis of, 296
epidemiology and causes of, 295
follow-up and referral for, 296
management of, 296
pathophysiology of, 295
patient education on, 296
Diagnosis
clinical judgment and Circle of Caring in, 38–39
clinical process in, 40–41
current trends in, 49–50
developing a management plan after, 48–49
diagnostic tests and, 46–47, 46t
differential, 47–48
documentation of, 50–52
evidence-based practice (EBP) and, 49
functional health patterns in, 44–46
genetic influences and, 47
history in, 42, 43–44, 43b, 44f
of interrelated problems, 42
outcome considerations and, 50
physical examination in, 46
process elements, 42–49
process example, 49
process overview, 41–42
purpose and goal of diagnostic reasoning in, 39
review of systems in, 44
shared decision making and, 49–50
uncertainty in, 39
unique aspects of primary care and, 39
working, 42
Diagnostic and Statistical Manual of Mental Disorders, fifth edition (DSM-5), 1174, 1187
on acute stress disorder, 1286
on agoraphobia, 1283
on anxiety disorders, 1176, 1274
on body dysmorphic disorder (BDD), 1300
on delirium, e1503
on dementia, 102
on eating disorders, 304
on gender dysphoria, 1417
on generalized anxiety disorder (GAD), 1277
on insomnia disorder, 1312
on intellectual disability (ID), 1199–1200
on major depression, 1242
on obsessive-compulsive disorder (OCD), 1295
on panic disorder, 1283
on post-traumatic stress disorder (PTSD), 1287–1288, 1322
on psychiatric diagnoses, e1551
on schizophrenia spectrum disorders, 1228
on substance use disorders (SUDs), 1209

Diagnostic reasoning, 39
critical thinking in, 40–41
Diagnostic tests, 46–47, 46t
Alzheimer's disease (AD), 107
cerebrovascular accident (CVA), 120–122
dementia, 103
headache, 85–86
Parkinson's disease, 112
Dialectical behavioral therapy (DBT)
eating disorders and, 1310
pain management and, 1481
Diaphragm, 769
Diarrhea, 607, 609–610, 610–611f
chronic, with acquired immunodeficiency syndrome (AIDS), 1168
Diet modifications. *See* Lifestyle and diet
Differential diagnosis, 47–48
Digitalis, arrhythmias associated with, 577
Dimensional Yale-Brown Obsessive Compulsive Scale, 1295
Dipeptidyl peptidase-4 inhibitors, 1035
Direct inguinal hernias, 651
Disease
definition of, 7
prevalence and incidence rates of, 35, 35t
Disease-modifying antirheumatic drugs (DMARDs), 1122–1123
Dissociative disorders, 1177
Diuretics
for chronic obstructive pulmonary disease (COPD), 483
for hypertension (HTN), 538
Diverticular disease, 661–662
clinical presentation of, 662–663
diagnosis of, 663
epidemiology and causes of, 662
follow-up and referral for, 664
management of, 663–664
pathophysiology of, 662
patient education on, 664
Dix-Hallpike maneuver, 77, 323
Dizziness and vertigo, 76–77, 78f
vestibular disorders, 320–321, 321f
DNR (Do Not Attempt Resuscitation order), e1495
Dock, Lavinia, 9
Documentation, 50–52
electronic medical record (EMR) systems for, 52, 53b
SOAP (subjective, objective, assessment, and plan) format for, 50–52
Domains, AACN, 9
Dopamine agonists, 113
Dopamine/norepinephrine reuptake inhibitor, 1192
Dopaminergic medications, 113
Double-blinding studies, 61
Down syndrome. *See* Intellectual disability (ID)
Dressings, wound, 1339
Drug-induced hyperpigmentation, 152
Drug-induced pulmonary disease, 488b
Dry eye syndrome (DES), 267–268
clinical presentation of, 275–276
diagnosis of, 276
epidemiology and causes of, 274
follow-up and referral for, 277
management of, 276–277
pathophysiology of, 274–275
patient education on, 277, 277b
Dupuytren's contracture, 945
Dyslipidemia
chronic kidney disease (CKD) and, 741
clinical presentation of, 544
diagnosis of, 544–545, 545t
epidemiology and causes of, 543, 543t
follow-up and referral for, 546

management of, 545–546
pathophysiology of, 543–544
patient education on, 547
Dysmenorrhea
clinical presentation of, 812–813
diagnosis of, 813
epidemiology and causes of, 812
follow-up and referral for, 814
management of, 813
pathophysiology of, 812
patient education on, 814
Dyspareunia, 751–752
Dyspepsia and heartburn, 611–612, 613f
Dysphagia, 615, 617–618
Dysphonia, 415
clinical presentation of, 412–413, 413b
diagnosis of, 305, 413–414
epidemiology and causes of, 412
follow-up and referral for, 415
management of, 414
pathophysiology of, 412
patient education on, 415
Dyspnea, 419–420, 524–526
assessment of, e1499–e1500
diagnosis of, 420–421
management of, 421, e1500, e1501b, e1501t
palliative care and, e1499–e1500, e1500b, e1501b, e1501t
sports physicals and, 1410
Dystonia, 1234t
Dysuria, 701

E

Ear, inflammatory and infectious disorders of
otitis externa (swimmer's ear), 334–341
otitis media (OM), 341–349, 348t
Ear, nose, and throat complaints
dysphonia, 305, 412–415, 413b
ear pain (otalgia), 303
epistaxis, 306
foreign body obstruction, 1372–1374
hearing loss (*See* Hearing loss)
mouth sores, 304–305
neck masses, 307
sinus complaints, 307
sore throat, 305–306
tinnitus (*See* Tinnitus)
Ear examination in sports physicals, 1411
Ear pain, 303
Eating Attitudes Test-26 (EAT-26), 1307, 1307b
Eating Disorder Examination Questionnaire (EDE-Q), 1307, 1307b
Eating Disorder Inventory (EDI-2), 1307
Eating disorders, 1304–1311
in adolescents, 1399
assessment components for suspected, 1306b
clinical presentation of, 1306–1307, 1306b, 1307b, 1307t
criteria for medical hospitalization for, 1306b
diagnosis of, 1307–1309
epidemiology of, 1305
excessive eating, 983–984, 983f
follow-up and referral for, 1310
management of, 1309–1310
overview of, 304–305
pathophysiology of, 1305–1306
patient education on, 1310–1311, 1311b
Eating Disorder Screen for Primary Care (EDS-PC), 1307, 1307b
Eating Disorders Inventory, Second Edition (EDI-2), 1307b
Eating Disorders in Youth Questionnaire (EDY-Q), 1307, 1307b
E-cigarettes, 510. *See also* Smoking addiction
Economic well-being and cancer, 1444–1445
Ecthyma, 191, 192t

Eczema. *See* Atopic dermatitis
Eczematous rash. *See* Atopic dermatitis
Edema, peripheral, 526–528, 527f
Edinburgh Postnatal Depression (EPSD) scale, 1242
Effectiveness and Efficiency: Random Reflections on Health Services, 58
Effect size, 59
Eikenella corrodens, 199
Elbow pain, 899–900
Electrocardiogram (ECG)
   acute coronary syndrome (ACS), 556–559, 556f, 556t, 557f, 558f
   heart failure (HF), 569–570
Electronic cigarettes, 510. *See also* Smoking addiction
Electronic health records (EHR), e1559
   evaluation and management documentation, e1541–e1543, e1542b
Electronic medical record (EMR) programs, 52–53, 53b
Embolism, 117
Emergent conditions
   acute musculoskeletal injury (*See* Acute musculoskeletal injury)
   cauda equina syndrome (CES), 928–930, 929t
   malignant hypertension (HTN), 532
   seizures, 101b
Emphysema. *See* Chronic obstructive pulmonary disease (COPD)
Encephalitis
   clinical presentation of, 130
   diagnosis of, 130–131
   epidemiology and causes of, 129, 130t
   follow-up and referral for, 131
   management of, 131
   pathophysiology of, 129–130
   patient education on, 131
Endemic events, 35, 36t
Endocrine and metabolic complaints. *See also* Glandular disorders
   after cancer, 1443–1444
   eating disorders and, 1307t
   gynecomastia (GM), 980–981
   hirsutism, 981–982
   hypocalcemia, 979–980
   increased neck size, 982–983
   polydipsia, polyphagia, and polyuria, 983–984, 983f
End-of-life care. *See* Palliative care
End-of-life decision making for older adults, 1465
Endometrial cancer
   clinical presentation of, 825–826
   diagnosis of, 826
   epidemiology and causes of, 824–825
   follow-up and referral for, 827
   management of, 826–827
   pathophysiology of, 825
   patient education on, 827
Endometriosis
   clinical presentation of, 815, 818
   diagnosis of, 815
   epidemiology and causes of, 814
   follow-up and referral for, 816
   management of, 815–816, 817
   pathophysiology of, 814–815
   patient education on, 817
Endophthalmitis, 287
End-stage renal disease (ESRD). *See* Chronic kidney disease (CKD)
Energy field therapies, e1562
Entamoeba histolytica, 625t
Enterobacter, 840
Enterococcus
   lower urinary tract infections (UTIs) and, 715
   mastitis and, 795
   pyelonephritis and, 721

Environmental exposures. *See* Toxic and environmental exposures
Enzyme-linked immunosorbent assay test (ELISA), 218
Eosinophilic folliculitis (EF), 194
Epidemics, 35, 36t
Epidemiology, practical, 34–36, 35t, 36t
Epidermolysis bullosa, 384
Epidermophyton. See Dermatophytoses
Epididymitis
   clinical presentation of, 855
   diagnosis of, 855
   epidemiology and causes of, 854
   follow-up and referral for, 856
   management of, 855–856
   pathophysiology of, 854–855
   patient education on, 856
Epidural hematomas, 118, 1364–1365, 1365f
Epidural steroid injections (ESIs), 1481
Epigastric hernias, 651
Epilepsy. *See* Seizure disorders
Epinephrine for arthropod bites and stings, 1352, 1354
Epiphora. *See* Excessive tearing (epiphora)
Epistaxis, 306
   clinical presentation of, 403–404, 404b
   diagnosis of, 404
   epidemiology and causes of, 401–402, 401b
   follow-up and referral for, 405–406
   management of, 404–405
   pathophysiology of, 402–403, 403f
   patient education on, 406
Epithelialization phase of wounds, 1333, 1357
Epley maneuver, 325
Epstein-Barr virus (EBV), 392, 1139. *See also* Infectious mononucleosis
   acquired immunodeficiency syndrome (AIDS) and, 1170
Epworth Sleepiness Scale (ESS), 427
Equianalgesics, e1507b
Erectile dysfunction (ED)
   clinical presentation of, 850
   diagnosis of, 850–851
   epidemiology and causes of, 847–849, 848f, 849b
   follow-up and referral for, 854
   management of, 851–853
   pathophysiology of, 849–850
   patient education on, 854
Ergot derivatives, 87
Erikson, Erik, 1394, 1394t
Erysipelas, 200b
Erythroplakia, 391
Escherichia coli
   acute otitis media (AOM) and, 343
   epididymitis and, 854
   folliculitis and, 194
   gastroenteritis and, 621–622t
   lower urinary tract infections (UTIs) and, 715
   mastitis and, 795
   prostatitis and, 840
   pyelonephritis and, 721
   rhinitis and, 351
Escitalopram, 1298
Escort services, 1328t
Essential hypertension, 529–531
Estrogen therapy for osteoporosis, 972
Ethics, 54–55, e1513–e1529
   autonomy, e1516–e1517, e1516b
   beneficence, e1516b, e1517
   confidentiality, e1516b, e1517–e1518
   defined, e1513
   ethical dilemmas and, e1514, e1518–e1519
   fidelity, e1516b, e1518
   Golden Rules in, e1513, e1513t

   Institutional Ethics Committees (IECs) and, e1520–e1521
   issues for health-care providers, e1514–e1515
   justice, e1516b, e1518
   nonmaleficence, e1516b, e1517
   principles in, e1515–e1518, e1516b
   professional codes of, e1514
   relationship between law and, e1521
   resolution guidelines, e1519–e1520, e1520f
   skill of ethical action and, e1513–e1514
   theoretical approaches to, e1515
   veracity, e1516b, e1517
Etonogestrel implant, 763
Eubacterium, 619
Evaluation and management documentation, e1541–e1543, e1542b
Evening primrose, 222
Evidence-based practice (EBP), 49
   aims of nursing research for clinical application in, 56–58, 57f
   application of, 63–64
   atopic dermatitis, 219
   breast cancer, 808
   brief history of, 58
   chest pain, 521
   chronic obstructive pulmonary disease (COPD), 486
   clinical decision making in, 68–69, 68f
   Daily Enhancement of Meaningful Activity (DEMA) intervention, 110
   defined, 56
   depression, 1239
   developing point-of-care strategy in, 65–68, 67–68b
   development of, 59, 60–61t
   development of best practice guidelines and, 58–62, 60–61t
   environmental and sociocultural influences on, 69
   evaluation of, 63–64
   examples of, 64
   grading the evidence for, 59
   heart failure (HF), 570
   human immunodeficiency virus (HIV), 1162
   integrated with nursing research-based practice, 65, 66–67b
   interprofessional education, e1526
   key steps in implementing, 56, 56b
   level I evidence—systematic review or meta-analysis of RCTs, 59
   level II evidence—single well-designed RCTs, 59, 61
   level III evidence—well-designed controlled trials without randomization, 61
   level IV evidence—well-designed case-control or cohort studies, 61–62
   level V evidence—systematic reviews of descriptive and qualitative studies, 62
   level VI evidence—single descriptive or qualitative studies, 62
   level VII evidence—opinion of authorities and/or reports of expert committees, 62–63
   literature searches and, 64–65, 65b
   malpractice, e1525
   moral distress, e1521
   multiple sclerosis (MS) and, 144
   practice standards in, 58–59
   Sjögren's syndrome (SS), 1129
   smoking addiction, 519
   sources of, 63, 63b
   wounds and lacerations, 1337
Excessive tearing (epiphora), 268
   clinical presentation of, 278
   diagnosis of, 278
   epidemiology and causes of, 277
   follow-up and referral for, 280

management of, 278–279
pathophysiology of, 277–278
patient education on, 280
Exclusive provider organizations (EPOs), e1533
Excoriation, 1296
Exercise. *See* Physical activity
Expectorants for chronic obstructive pulmonary disease (COPD), 483
Expertise and experience, 41, 41t
Exposure and response prevention (ERP)
   hoarding disorder (HD) and, 1301
   obsessive-compulsive disorder (OCD) and, 1298
Exposure therapy for phobias, 1285
Extrapyramidal symptoms, 1233, 1234t
Eye complaints. *See also* Visual disturbances and impaired vision
   blepharitis, 270–272, 272b
   dry eye syndrome (DES), 267–268, 274–277, 277t
   excessive tearing (epiphora), 268, 277–280
   hordeolum and chalazion, 272–273, 274b
   overview of, 267
   pain, 268, 268t
   red eye/conjunctivitis, 268–269, 280–284, 283t
Eye examination in sports physicals, 1411
Eye movement desensitization and reprocessing (EMDR), 1288

F

Falls, 1461–1462, e1505, e1505t
Family-based therapy (FBT) for eating disorders, 1310
Family history, 44, 44f
   of premature sudden cardiac death (SCD), 1410
Fatigue, 1064
   cancer-related, 1444
Fear Survey Schedule for Children, 1275
Feeding disorders. *See* Eating disorders
Felitti, Vincent, e1551–e1552
Female athlete triad, 1410
Females
   chronic pelvic pain in, 753–754
   contraception and family planning (*See* Contraception and family planning)
   dyspareunia in, 751–752
   fertility problems (*See* Fertility problems)
   hirsutism in, 981–982
   pain management disparities in, 1483
   puberty in, 1395–1398, 1396–1397t
   transgender, 1417–1423
   vaginal, uterine, and ovarian disorders (*See* Vaginal, uterine, and ovarian disorders)
   veterans, 1435
   as victims of human trafficking, 1329
   vulvovaginitis in, 756–759
Femoral hernias, 651
Fentanyl, 1478–1479
Fertility awareness methods, 769–770
Fertility problems
   clinical presentation of, 773–774
   diagnosis of, 774–776, 775t
   epidemiology and causes of, 771–772
   follow-up and referral for, 778
   management of, 776–778, 777b
   pathophysiology of, 772–773
   patient education on, 778
Fetal alcohol syndrome. *See* Intellectual disability (ID)
Fever, 1064–1065
Fibrocystic disease, 749
Fibromyalgia syndrome (FMS), 1124
   clinical presentation of, 1126
   diagnosis of, 1126–1127, 1126t
   epidemiology and causes of, 1125
   follow-up and referral for, 1128

management of, 1127
pathophysiology of, 1125–1126
patient education on, 1128
Fidelity, e1516b, e1518
Finasteride, 149–150
Fine-needle aspiration (FNA), head and neck, 381
Finkelstein's test, 901
Fire ants, 1347, 1350
Firearms, 1403
First-degree burns, 1357, 1360
First generation sulfonylureas, 1034
First-line TB drugs, 459
Fish poisoning, 1378t
5-aminosalicylic acid agents, 670
Flashing lights (vision), 269
Flat warts. *See* Warts
Fleas, 1348, 1350, 1354
Floaters (vision), 269
Fludrocortisone, 1010
Fluid and electrolytes
   eating disorders and, 1307t
   management in chronic kidney disease (CKD), 740–741
Fluoride for osteoporosis, 974
Fluoxetine, 1297, 1310
Fluphenazine, 1231
Fluvoxamine, 1297
Focal onset seizures, 94–95
Folic acid antagonists, 1122
Folic acid deficiency, 1080–1081
Follicular thyroid cancer. *See* Thyroid cancer
Folliculitis
   clinical presentation of, 195
   diagnosis of, 195–196
   epidemiology and causes of, 194
   follow-up and referral for, 197
   management of, 196–197
   pathophysiology of, 194–195
   patient education on, 197
Food poisoning, 1378t
Foot disorders
   interdigital neuroma, 953–954
   plantar fasciitis, 953
Foot pain, 906–907
Forefoot problems, 906–907
Foreign body obstruction, 1371–1374
   clinical presentation of, 1371–1372
   diagnosis of, 1372
   epidemiology and causes of, 1371
   follow-up and referral for, 1374
   management of, 1372–1374
   pathophysiology of, 1371
   patient education on, 1374
Forensic evidence collection after sexual assault, 1324
Forward failure, 566
Fosphenytoin, 100
Fractures, 889–893
   ankle, 891
   hip, 890–891
   osteoporosis (*See* Osteoporosis)
   skull, 1364
   vertebral, 931–933
Fragile X syndrome. *See* Intellectual disability (ID)
Francisella tularensis, 392
Frostbite, 1388–1389
   clinical presentation of, 1388–1389
   diagnosis of, 1389
   epidemiology and causes of, 1388
   follow-up and referral for, 1389
   management of, 1389
   pathophysiology of, 1388
   patient education on, 1389
Frozen shoulder, 945–946
Full-thickness burns, 1358
Full-thickness defect, 1334

Functional Activities Questionnaire (FAQ), 106
Functional Assessment Staging Test (FAST), e1497–e1498, e1499f
Functional health patterns, 44–46
Functional incontinence, 708t, 713
Fungal culture, 188
Fungal skin infections
   candidiasis, 172–180
   dermatophytoses, 180–186
   onychomycosis, 187–189
Furuncles and carbuncles
   clinical presentation of, 198
   diagnosis of, 198
   epidemiology and causes of, 197
   follow-up and referral for, 199
   management of, 198–199
   pathophysiology of, 197–198
   patient education on, 199
Fusobacterium, 619
Future of Nursing 2020-2030: Charting a Path to Achieve Health Equity, 3, 4b, e1526, e1559
Future of Nursing: Leading Change, Advancing Health, The, 3

G

Gallbladder and jpancreatic disorders
   acute pancreatitis, 681–685, 682b, 684b, 684t
   cholecystitis, 678–681
   chronic pancreatitis, 685–688
   pancreatic cancer, 688–689
Gallstones. *See* Cholecystitis
Gambling disorder, 1296
Gamekeeper's thumb, 901
Gamma-aminobutyric acid (GABA), 96
   generalized anxiety disorder (GAD) and, 1276
Ganglion cyst, 944
Gastric and intestinal disorders
   abdominal hernias, 650–653, 652f
   bowel obstruction, 659–661
   celiac disease, 657–658
   colorectal cancer, 672–677, 674t
   diverticular disease, 661–664
   gastroesophageal reflux disease (GERD), 640–645, 641f, 642b
   hemorrhoids, 648–650, 649t
   inflammatory bowel disease (IBD), 664–672, 665t
   irritable bowel syndrome (IBS), 653–657
   peptic ulcer disease (PUD), 645–648
Gastroenteritis, 614–615, 615b
   clinical presentation of, 625–626
   diagnosis of, 626–627
   epidemiology and causes of, 618–619, 620–625t
   follow-up and referral for, 627
   management of, 627
   pathophysiology of, 619
   patient education on, 628
Gastroesophageal reflux disease (GERD)
   clinical presentation of, 642
   diagnosis of, 643
   epidemiology and causes of, 640–642, 641f, 642b
   follow-up and referral for, 644–645
   management of, 643–644
   pathophysiology of, 642
   patient education on, 645
Gastrointestinal complaints
   with aging, 1451t
   with eating disorders, 1307t
Gastrointestinal disorders, infectious
   appendicitis, 635–639
   gastroenteritis, 618–628, 620–625t
   hepatitis, 628–635, 628t, 631t, 632t, 633t
Gastrointestinal examination in sports physicals, 1413

Gender-affirming treatments
 trans men, 1419
 trans women, 1419
Gender and pain management disparities, 1483, 1483f
Gender dysphoria, 1417
Gender identity, 1417–1417, 1417t
Generalized anxiety disorder (GAD), 1188b, 1256t, 1275–1281, 1296
 clinical presentation of, 1276–1277
 diagnosis of, 1277, 1277b
 epidemiology and causes of, 1275–1276
 follow-up and referral for, 1280
 management of, 1277–1280, 1280b
 pathophysiology of, 1276
 patient education on, 1281
Generalized Anxiety Disorder-7 (GAD-7) Scale, 1275
Generalized onset seizures, 95
Genetic influences and diagnosis, 47
Genital herpes simplex virus (HSV), 868t
Geographic tongue, 386–387
Geriatric considerations. *See also* Older adults
 Alzheimer's disease (AD), 106
 anti-allergy medications, 1107
 antipsychotic medications, 1233
 arrhythmias, 576
 benign prostatic hyperplasia (BPH), 837
 common abdominal complaints, 617
 common injuries, 1363
 common neurological complaints, 93
 community-acquired pneumonia, 439
 dry eye syndrome (DES), 275
 dysphonia, 412
 epistaxis, 402
 eye conditions, 286
 fracture, 890
 generalized anxiety disorder (GAD), 1280
 hearing loss, 310
 hematuria, 703
 herpes zoster, 133
 hypertension (HTN), 536
 influenza, 432
 major depressive disorder (MDD), 1249
 musculoskeletal injury, 886
 pain management, 1483
 posterior vitreous detachment (PVD), 269
 prostate cancer, 842
 rotator cuff tear, 948
 seborrheic keratosis, 251
 sexual health in menopause, 788
 sexually transmitted infections (STIs), 872
 substance use disorders (SUDs), 1212
 urinary incontinence (UI), 706
 urinary tract infection (UTI), 714
Geriatric Depression Scale (GDS), 1242
Geriatric syndromes, 1460–1462, 1461b
Giant cell arteritis (GCA), 81, 85
Giardia lamblia, 624t
Glandular disorders. *See also* Endocrine and metabolic complaints
 adrenal insufficiency, 1011–1013
 Cushing's syndrome, 1006–1011, 1089
 hyperthyroidism, 984–993, 985t, 987t, 989t
 hypothyroidism, 993–1002, 994t, 997t, 1001b
 thyroid cancer, 378, 985, 985t, 1003–1005
Glasgow Coma Scale, 1366
Glaucoma
 acute, 286t
 chronic, 286t
 clinical presentation of, 292
 diagnosis of, 292–293
 epidemiology and causes of, 291
 follow-up and referral for, 294
 management of, 293–294
 pathophysiology of, 291–292
 patient education on, 294–295

Gleason score, 845
Glomerular filtration rate (GFR), 738–739, 738b
Glomerulonephritis (GN), 737
Glossitis. *See* Stomatitis and glossitis
Glucagon-like peptide-1 analogues, 1035, 1036
Glutamate, 96
 generalized anxiety disorder (GAD) and, 1276
Glycemic control, 1040–1041
Golden rules, e1513, e1513t
Goldenseal, 222
Gonorrhea. *See Neisseria gonorrhoeae*
Gout
 clinical presentation of, 1057
 diagnosis of, 1057–1059
 epidemiology and causes of, 1055
 follow-up and referral for, 1061
 management of, 1059–1061, 1059t
 pathophysiology of, 1055–1057, 1056t
 patient education on, 1061–1062
Government health initiatives, 29–32
 Healthy People 2030, 29–32, 30b, 31b, 33
 National Prevention Strategy, 29
 U.S. Preventive Services Task Force, 31–32
Graves' disease, 985, 985t, 986, 990–992
Greater trochanteric pain syndrome (GTPS), 903, 949
Grief, 1179–1180
 diagnosis of, 1180–1181
Grooming process in human trafficking, 1328–1329
Gufoni maneuver, 325–326
Guided imagery, e1508–e1513
Guidelines for Adolescent Preventive Services (GAPS), 1394
Guillain-Barré syndrome (GBS)
 diagnosis of, 137
 epidemiology and causes of, 137
 management of, 138
Gulf War illness (GWI), 1428
Gum, nicotine, 517
Guns, 1403
Gynecomastia (GM), 980–981

H

H2-receptor antagonists for peptic ulcer disease (PUD), 647
Haemophilus ducreyi, 866, 867t
Haemophlus influenzae
 acute otitis media (AOM) and, 342
 cellulitis and, 199
 laryngitis and, 433
 pharyngitis and tonsillitis and, 393
 pneumonia and, 441
 rhinosinusitis and, 366, 371
Hair loss. *See* Alopecia
Hair tongue, 386
Hairy black tongue, 386
Hallucinogens, 1216
Haloperidol, 1231
Hamilton Anxiety Rating Scale, 1275
Hand and wrist disorders
 carpal tunnel syndrome (CTS), 941–943
 de Quervain's tenosynovitis, 943–944
 Dupuytren's contracture, 945
 ganglion cyst, 944
 pain, 900–901, 902
 tendon injuries of the hand, 945, 945f
 trigger finger, 944–945
Hastings Center Report on Prevention, 9
HDL cholesterol. *See* Dyslipidemia
Headache, 77, 79
 clinical presentation of, 83–85, 84f
 cluster, 79t, 80, 83
 complementary therapies for, 89
 diagnostic reasoning for, 85–86
 drugs prescribed for, 87–88

epidemiology and causes of, 79–81, 80b
 follow-up and referral for, 87, 89–90
 management of, 86–89
 migraine, 79t, 80, 80b, 82–85, 84f, 89–90
 pathophysiology of, 81–83, 82f
 tension-type, 79–80, 79t, 82
 types of, 79, 79t
Head examination in sports physicals, 1411
Head impulse test (HIT), 331
Head Impulse test, Nystagmus, and Test of Skew (HINTS) examination, 77
HEADSS screening tool, 1400, 1401t
Head thrust, 331
Head trauma/traumatic brain injury (TBI), 1362–1369
 cerebral contusion, 1364
 clinical presentation of, 1365–1368
 concussion, 1364
 diagnosis of, 1368
 epidemiology and causes of, 1363
 epidural hematoma, 118, 1364–1365, 1365f
 follow-up and referral for, 1368
 management of, 1368
 pathophysiology of, 1363–1365, 1365f
 patient education on, 1369
 skull fracture, 1364
 subdural hematoma, 81, 85, 118, 1365
 in veterans, 1431
Health
 components of, 25, 25f
 definition of, e1490
 pain management disparities, 1482
Healthcare Common Procedure Coding System (HCPCS), e1538
Health-care power of attorney (HCPOA), e1494
Health coaching, e1552–e1554, e1554f
Health insurance plans, e1530
Health Insurance Portability and Accountability Act (HIPAA), e1518, e1527
 value-based health care and, e1546
Health literacy, 29
Health maintenance organizations (HMOs), e1533
Health promotion
 cancer prevention, 1445–1446
 Circle of Caring in, 27, 27f
 community as partner in, 27, 27f
 community influences on, 33–34
 defined, 25–26
 government initiatives and, 29–32, 30b, 31b
 health literacy and, 29
 immunization practices and, 32
 individual influences on, 32–33
 influences on, 33–34
 information on leading causes of death and, 34, 34f
 for older adults, 1457
 practical epidemiology and, 34–36, 35t, 36t
 prevention as, 8–9, 26–27
 primary, secondary, and tertiary, 28, 28t
 risk factors in, 28–29, 29b
 screening tests and, 26, 26b
Healthy People 2030, 4, 16, 29–32, 30b, 31b, 33, 36, 69, 1451, 1452, 1469, e1514, e1514b, e1518
Hearing and balance disorders
 benign paroxysmal positional vertigo (BPPV), 321–327, 322t, 323b, 324t, 325t, 326t
 hearing loss, 303–304, 309–316, 311f, 312b, 312t, 314–315t
 Ménière's disease, 326t, 327–330
 tinnitus, 304, 316–320, 318b, 319b
 vestibular disorders, 320–321, 321f
 vestibular neuritis (VN) and labyrinthitis, 330–332
Hearing loss
 clinical presentation of, 311–313, 312b, 312t
 diagnosis of, 313–315, 314–315t

epidemiology and causes of, 303–304, 309–310
follow-up and referral for, 316
management of, 315–316
pathophysiology of, 310–311, 311f, 312t
patient education on, 316
in veterans, 1429–1430
Heart blocks, 576–577
clinical presentation of, 582–583
epidemiology and causes of, 577, 579f
management of, 585
pathophysiology of, 581
Heartburn, 611–612, 613f
Heart failure (HF)
clinical presentation of, 568–569
diagnosis of, 569–570
epidemiology and causes of, 565, 566t
evidence-based nursing for, 570
follow-up and referral for, 572
management of, 570–572
pathophysiology of, 565–568
patient education on, 572–573
Heart murmurs. See Valvular disorders and murmurs
Heat cramps, 1383, 1383t
Heat exhaustion, 1383–1384, 1383t
Heat rash, 1382–1383, 1383t
Heat-related illnesses, 1382–1386
clinical presentation of, 1385
diagnosis of, 1385
epidemiology and causes of, 1384
follow-up and referral for, 1385–1386
management of, 1385
pathophysiology of, 1384–1385
patient education on, 1386
Heat stroke, 1383t, 1384
Heat syncope, 1383, 1383t
Helicobacter pylori
dyspepsia and, 612
peptic ulcer disease (PUD) and, 645, 646
rosacea and, 249
Hematological and immunological complaints
bruising, 1063–1064
eating disorders and, 1307t
fatigue, 1064
fever, 1064–1065
lymphadenopathy, 1065–1066
Hematological disorders
anemia, 1066–1067
leukemia, 1092–1102, 1093–1094t, 1099b
macrocytic anemia, 1079–1083
microcytic anemia, 1067–1074, 1070–1071t
normocytic anemia, 1074–1079
polycythemia, 1088–1092
sickle cell anemia, 1083–1088
sports physicals and, 1410
Hematomas
epidural, 118, 1364–1365, 1365f
subdural, 81, 85, 118, 1365
Hematuria, 701–702
diagnosis of, 703–704
Hemic murmur, 588
Hemochromatosis, 697–698
Hemoglobin formation, 1067–1068
Hemophilia, 1410
Hemoptysis
diagnosis of, 421–422
management of, 422
patient education on, 422
Hemorrhoids, 648–649
clinical presentation of, 649
diagnosis of, 649
epidemiology and causes of, 649
follow-up and referral for, 650
management of, 650
pathophysiology of, 649, 649t
patient education on, 650

Hemothorax. See Pneumothorax and hemothorax
Henderson, Virginia, 9–10
Hepatitis
A, 628, 631t, 633
B, 629, 631t, 633, 633t, 1345–1346
C, 629, 631t, 633, 636, 1345–1346, 1429
causes of acute, 628, 628t
chronic, 630
clinical presentation of, 632, 632t
D, 629–630, 631t, 633
diagnosis of, 632–634, 633t
E, 630, 631t, 633–634
epidemiology and causes of, 628–630, 631t
follow-up and referral for, 635
management of, 634–635, 636
pathophysiology of, 630–631
patient education on, 635
in veterans, 1429
Herbal therapy. See Aroma and herbal therapy
Hernias, abdominal
clinical presentation of, 651–652, 652f
diagnosis of, 652
epidemiology and causes of, 650–651
follow-up and referral for, 653
management of, 653
pathophysiology of, 651
patient education on, 653
sports physicals and, 1413
Herniated lumbar disc (herniated nucleus pulposus)
clinical presentation of, 923–924
diagnosis of, 924–925
epidemiology and causes of, 922–923
follow-up and referral for, 926
management of, 925–926
pathophysiology of, 923
patient education on, 926
Heroin poisoning, 1377t
Herpes simplex infections
acquired immunodeficiency syndrome (AIDS) and, 1169
clinical presentation of, 211–212
diagnosis of, 212
epidemiology and causes of, 210
follow-up and referral for, 214
genital, 868t
management of, 212–214, 214b
pathophysiology of, 210–211
patient education on, 214
stomatitis and glossitis, 383, 385, 386
types of, 210, 210t
Herpes zoster, 90
acquired immunodeficiency syndrome (AIDS) and, 1169
clinical presentation of, 132
diagnosis of, 132
epidemiology and causes of, 131
follow-up and referral for, 133
management of, 132–133
pathophysiology of, 131–132
patient education on, 133–134
High-dose amiodarone, 985, 985t
Hindfoot problems, 907
Hip disorders
avascular necrosis (AVN), 949–950
bone tumors, 950–951
greater trochanteric pain syndrome (GTPS), 949
meralgia paresthetica, 949
Hip fracture, 890–891
Hip pain, 901, 903
Hippocratic Oath, e1517
Hirsutism, 981–982
Histoplasmosis with acquired immunodeficiency syndrome (AIDS), 1169

Historical perspectives on advanced practice nursing, 9–10, 9f
changing models of medical practice, 12–13
History, 42
autism spectrum disorder (ASD), 1195
as component of sports physicals, 1408–1411, 1408b, 1409t
diarrhea, 609–610
eye complaints, 267
family, 44, 44f
herpes simplex virus infections, 211–212
insomnia disorder, 1312
low back pain, 918
musculoskeletal problems, 878
pain, 1473–1474
past medical (PMH), 43–44
of present illness (HPI), 43, 43b
pruritus, 154
rash, 157
risk of HIV infection, 1150–1151
scabies, 164
signs and symptoms of prostatitis, 841
social, 44
taking an occupational and environmental, 490
transgender persons, 1418, 1418b
wounds and lacerations, 1334
HIV. See Human immunodeficiency virus (HIV)
HMG-CoA reductase inhibitors, 546
Hoarding disorder (HD), 1296
clinical presentation of, 1301
diagnosis of, 1301
epidemiology and causes of, 1300–1301
follow-up and referral for, 1301–1302
management of, 1301
pathophysiology of, 1301
patient education on, 1302
Hoarseness. See Dysphonia
Hodgkin's lymphoma, 156
Holistic approaches, 12, 15
Home Health Care Planning Improvement Act, e1527–e1528
Home oxygen for chronic obstructive pulmonary disease (COPD), 483
Hordeolum and chalazion
clinical presentation of, 273
diagnosis of, 273
epidemiology and causes of, 272
follow-up and referral for, 273
management of, 273, 274b
pathophysiology of, 273
patient education on, 273
Hormonal therapy
acne vulgaris, 244–245, 246–247
breast cancer, 806–807
erectile dysfunction (ED), 851–852, 853
gender-affirming treatment for trans men, 1419, 1420
gender-affirming treatment for trans women, 1419, 1420–1421
menopause, 788–790
Hospice. See also Palliative care
advance directives and, e1494–e1495
differences between palliative and, e1490–e1491
DNR (Do Not Attempt Resuscitation order) and, e1495
history of, e1489
relieving suffering in, e1493–e1494
utilization of, e1491
Hot tub folliculitis, 195, 242
Human bites. See Animal and human bites
Human Genome Project, 54
Human herpesvirus-8, 1169
Human immunodeficiency virus (HIV). See also Acquired immunodeficiency syndrome (AIDS)
ARVs for initial HIV-1 infection, 1160–1161

Index I-17

shoulder pain, 898–899
sports physicals and, 1410
in veterans, 1434–1435
wrist and hand pain, 900–901, 902
Music therapy, e1508
Myasthenia gravis (MG)
   diagnosis of, 138
   epidemiology and causes of, 138
   management of, 138
Mycobacterium avium complex (MAC) and AIDS, 1169–1170
Mycobacterium tuberculosis. See also Tuberculosis (TB)
   acute otitis media (AOM) and, 343
   AIDS and, 1170
   bursitis and, 936
   mastitis and, 795
   pneumonia and, 440
Mycoplasma genitalium, 866, 870t
Mycoplasma hominis, 722
Mycoplasma pneumoniae, 442
   acute otitis media (AOM) and, 342
   pharyngitis and tonsillitis and, 393
My Five Wishes, e1494
Myocardial infarction (MI). See Acute coronary syndrome (ACS)
Myocardial ischemia. See Acute coronary syndrome (ACS)
Myoclonic jerks, 95
Myofascial pain, 894–895
Myopia, 285, 286, 286t
Myxedema, 996, 1001b

N

Narrative exposure therapy (NET), 1289
Nasal spray, nicotine, 517, 518
Nasolacrimal duct system (NLDO), 277
National Center for Health Statistics, 34
National Childhood Vaccine Injury Act of 1986, 32
National Comprehensive Cancer Network (NCCN), e1493
National Health and Nutrition Examination Survey (NHANES), 1398
National Hospice and Palliative Care Organization (NHPCO), e1491
National Hospice Organization (NHO), e1489
National Practitioner Data Bank (NPDB), e1525
National Prevention Strategy: America's Plan for Better Health and Wellness, 29
National Provider Identifier (NPI) numbers, e1524
National Strategy for Suicide Prevention, 1267
National Suicide Prevention Lifeline, 1250
Nature of Nursing, The, 9–10
Nausea and vomiting, 614–615, 615b, 616f, 617
   palliative care and, e1501–e1502
Neck masses, 307
   clinical presentation of, 379–381, 380b, 380f
   diagnosis of, 381–382
   epidemiology and causes of, 377–379, 378f
   follow-up and referral for, 382
   management of, 381
   pathophysiology of, 379, 379f
   patient education on, 382
Neck pain, 895–896
Neck size, increased, 982–983
Necrotizing fasciitis, 200b
Necrotizing otitis externa, 335, 337
Necrotizing ulcerative gingivitis, 387
Neisseria gonorrhoeae
   epididymitis and, 854
   laryngitis and, 433
   pharyngitis and tonsillitis and, 393
   prostatitis and, 840
   red eye/conjunctivitis and, 282
   as sexually transmitted infection (STI), 866, 870t

Neoplasm, confusion due to, 76
Nephrolithiasis
   clinical presentation of, 725
   diagnosis of, 725–726, 726t
   epidemiology and causes of, 724
   follow-up and referral for, 727
   management of, 726–727, 727t
   pathophysiology of, 724–725, 725t
   patient education on, 727–728
Nephropathy, 1025–1026
Nerve entrapment syndrome, 90
Neurodevelopmental disorders, 1187
   attention deficit-hyperactivity disorder (ADHD), 1188–1194, 1188b, 1190b
   autism spectrum disorder (ASD), 1194–1197, 1195b, 1196b
   intellectual disability (ID), 1197–1201, 1199b, 1200t, 1201b
   tic disorders, 1201–1204, 1202b, 1202t
Neurological complaints
   after cancer, 1444
   confusion, 73–76, 74f, 75–76t
   dizziness and vertigo, 76–77, 78f
   eating disorders and, 1307t
   headache, 77, 79–90, 79t, 80b, 82f, 84f
   paresthesia and paresis, 90, 91f
   tremors, 90, 92–93, 92f
Neurological disorders, infectious and inflammatory
   Bell's palsy, 136–138
   encephalitis, 129–131, 130t
   Guillain-Barré syndrome (GBS), 137–138
   herpes zoster, 131–134
   meningitis, 126–129, 126t
   multiple sclerosis (MS), 138–144, 140b
   myasthenia gravis (MG), 138
   trigeminal neuralgia, 134–135
Neuromuscular examination in sports physicals, 1413
Neuropathic pain, 1472, 1472f, 1473
   medications for, 1476–1478
Neuropathy, 90
   diabetes mellitus (DM) type 1 and, 1026
   diabetes mellitus (DM) type 2 and, 1038–1039
   palliative care and, e1507b
Neurotransmitters and depression, 1241
Nevus, 252t
Newest Vital Scale (NVS), 29
Nicotine. See Smoking addiction
Nicotine replacement therapies, 516–518
Nightingale, Florence, 8, 9
   research utilization (RU) model, 58
N-methyl-D-aspartate receptor antagonist, 109
Nocardia lingualis, 384
Nociceptive pain, 1471–1472, 1472f
Nocturia in males, 752, 837
Nocturnal myoclonus, 428
Nodular scabies, 163, 165
Noise-induced hearing loss in veterans, 1429–1430
Nonalcoholic fatty liver disease (NAFLD), 690–691, 690b, 695
Nonallergic rhinitis. See Rhinitis
Nonbullous impetigo, 191, 192t
Nonmaleficence, e1516b, e1517
Nonmelanomatous skin cancers, 261–264, 264t
Nonoxynol-9, 768
Nonpharmacological management
   acne vulgaris, 248
   atopic dermatitis, 219–220
   attention deficit-hyperactivity disorder (ADHD), 1192
   autism spectrum disorder (ASD), 1197
   bipolar and related disorders (BD), 1262
   body dysmorphic disorder (BDD), 1300
   constipation, e1502
   dyspnea, e1501t

   eating disorders, 1310
   generalized anxiety disorder (GAD), 1280, 1280b
   hoarding disorder (HD), 1301
   impetigo, 192
   insomnia disorder, 1313
   intellectual disability (ID), 1201
   low back pain (LBP), 920–921
   major depressive disorder (MDD), 1244
   obsessive-compulsive disorder (OCD), 1298
   osteoarthritis (OA), 961
   of pain, 1481–1482
   panic disorder, 1283
   phobias, 1285
   post-traumatic stress disorder (PTSD), 1288–1289
   schizophrenia spectrum disorders, 1230, 1235
   tic disorders, 1204
Nonpsychotic mental disorders, 1177
Non-rapid eye movement (NREM) sleep, 1311–1312
Nonscarring alopecia, 147, 148–149
Non-small-cell lung cancer (NSCLCs). See Lung cancer
Non-ST-elevation MI. See Acute coronary syndrome (ACS)
Nonsteroidal anti-inflammatory drugs (NSAIDs), 1475–1476
   adhesive capsulitis and, 946
   animal and human bites and, 1344
   carpal tunnel syndrome (CTS) and, 942
   cervical muscle strain and, 912–913
   conjunctivitis and, 279
   De Quervain's tenosynovitis and, 944
   dysmenorrhea and, 813
   elbow pain and, 900
   epididymitis and, 855
   gout and, 1059
   headache and, 86–87, 88
   herniated lumbar disc (herniated nucleus pulposus) and, 925
   impingement syndrome and, 947
   low back pain (LBP) and, 921
   lumbar spinal stenosis and, 928
   osteoarthritis (OA) and, 962–964, 963f, 965
   premenstrual syndrome (PMS) and premenstrual dysphoric disorder (PMDD) and, 782
   rheumatoid arthritis (RA) and, 1121
   rhinitis and, 359
   rhinosinusitis and, 372
   rotator cuff tear and, 948
   sprains and strains and, 889
   systemic lupus erythematosus (SLE) and, 1136
   tendinitis/tenosynovitis and, 940
   trigger finger and, 945
Norepinephrine-dopamine reuptake inhibitors (NDRIs), 1243–1244, 1247
Normocytic anemia
   clinical presentation of, 1076
   diagnosis of, 1076–1077
   epidemiology and causes of, 1074
   follow-up and referral for, 1079
   management of, 1077–1079
   pathophysiology of, 1074–1076
   patient education on, 1079
Norwalk virus, 624t
Nose, sinuses, mouth, and throat, inflammatory and infectious disorders of
   neck masses, 307, 377–382, 378f, 379f, 380b, 380f
   oral cancer, 389–392
   pharyngitis and tonsillitis, 392–398, 396b
   rhinitis, 350–365, 350b, 363–364f
   rhinosinusitis, 365–377, 366f
   stomatitis and glossitis, 382–389, 388b

Nosebleed. *See* Epistaxis
Nose examination in sports physicals, 1411
Nosocomial pneumonia. *See* Pneumonia
Notes on Nursing, 9
NS3/4A protease inhibitors, 636
NS5A inhibitors, 636
NS5B nonnucleos(t)ide polymerase inhibitor, 636
NS5B nucleos(t)ide polymerase inhibitor, 636
Nucleic acid VEGF inhibitor, 299
Nurse Coaching, 11
Nurse practitioners (NPs), 3, 6. *See also* Advanced practice nursing
   licensure and certification of, e1522–e1523
   medical model and, 40
   -patient dialogue, 11
   practical knowledge and healing role of, 10–11
   reimbursement, e1524
   role in value-based health care, e1539–e1540
   self-care for, e1558–e1559
   unique aspects of primary care and, 39
Nursing research, 56–58, 57f
   integration of evidence-based practice and, 65, 66–67b
Nutrition. *See* Lifestyle and diet

O

Obesity, 1047
   in adolescents, 1398
   clinical presentation of, 1050–1051
   diagnosis of, 1051
   epidemiology and causes of, 1048, 1048t
   follow-up and referral for, 1053–1054, 1054b
   management of, 1051–1053
   pathophysiology of, 1049–1050, 1049b
   patient education on, 1054
Obsessive-compulsive disorder (OCD), 1293–1299
   clinical presentation of, 1294, 1295t
   diagnosis of, 1295–1296
   epidemiology and causes of, 1188b, 1293
   follow-up and referral for, 1299
   management of, 1297–1298
   pathophysiology of, 1293–1294
   patient education on, 1299
   symptoms of, 1295
Obsessive-compulsive disorders
   body dysmorphic disorder (BDD), 1177, 1299–1300
   hoarding disorder (HD), 1296, 1300–1302
   obsessive-compulsive disorder (OCD), 1188b, 1293–1299, 1295t
Obsessive-compulsive personality disorder (OCPD), 1296
Obstructive lung diseases. *See* Chronic obstructive pulmonary disease (COPD)
Obstructive sleep apnea (OSA). *See* Sleep apnea
Occupational therapy for osteoarthritis (OA), 961
Olanzapine, 1232
OLD CART mnemonic, 43, 43b
Older adults, 1448–1465. *See also* Geriatric considerations
   aging in place, 1458–1459
   approach to, 1456–1457
   categories of, 1448
   changes in laboratory values for, 1452t
   cognition in, 1461
   COVID-19 and, 1464–1465, 1464b
   demographics and changing face of aging and, 1448–1449
   dental health in, 1460
   end-of-life decision making for, 1465
   falls by, 1461–1462
   geriatric syndromes in, 1460–1462, 1461b
   headache in, 80–81
   health-care system change for, 1453–1454, 1454b
   health screening for, 1454–1455t, 1455–1460
   healthy aging for, 1450–1454, 1454b
   healthy lifestyle counseling and health promotion for, 1457
   heterogeneity of, 1449–1450
   immunizations for, 1460
   loneliness in, 1463–1464
   medications in, 1462–1463
   nutrition in, 1458
   pain management in, 1483
   physical activity in, 1457–1458
   processes of aging and, 1449–1450, 1450t
   psychosocial complaints of, 1174
   safety for, 1458
   sexuality in, 1459–1460
   substance use by, 1460
   suicide in, 1265–1266
On Death and Dying, e1489
Onychomycosis
   clinical presentation of, 187–188
   diagnosis of, 188
   epidemiology and causes of, 187
   follow-up and referral for, 189
   management of, 188–189
   pathophysiology of, 187
   patient education on, 189
Oophorectomy, 1419
Open-angle glaucoma. *See* Glaucoma
Open-ended questions, e1497
Opioids, 88
   chemical structure of, 1478, 1479f
   classification of, 1478, 1478f
   codeine, 1478
   constipation and, e1502
   cross-tolerance of, 1480
   for dyspnea, e1500
   fentanyl, 1478–1479
   hydromorphone, 1479
   mechanism of action of, 1478
   meperidine, 1479
   methadone, 1479–1480
   morphine, 1478
   oxycodone, 1478
   for pain management in palliative care, e1506, e1508b
   rotation of, 1480
   special considerations in prescribing, 1480
   tramadol, 1479
Opioid use disorder (OUD), 1211, 1217, 1480–1481
   in adolescents, 1403
Oppositional defiant disorder/conduct disorder, 1188b
Opsonization, 1106
Oral appliances for sleep apnea, 429
Oral cancer
   clinical manifestations of, 390
   diagnosis of, 390–391
   epidemiology and causes of, 389–390
   follow-up and referral for, 391
   management of, 391
   pathophysiology of, 390
   patient education on, 391–392
Oral candidiasis, 173
Oral contraceptive pills (OCPs), 750, 751
   adverse effects of, 765–766
   discontinuing use of, 766
   eligibility criteria for combined, 763
   instructions for use of, 764
   missed doses of, 764
   noncontraceptive benefits of, 765
   progestin-only pill, 763–764
   special considerations with, 764–765
Oral H_2-receptor antagonists, 1110
Oral hairy leukoplakia, 1170
Oral lesions, 304–305
Oral mucolytics, 373
Oral potentially malignant disorders (OPMD), 389
Oral secretions, e1500–e1501
Oral sympathomimetics, 1110
Orbital cellulitis, 287
Orchiectomy, 1419
Orthopnea, 526
Osmotic diarrhea, 607
Osteoarthritis (OA)
   clinical presentation of, 958, 959b
   diagnosis of, 958–960, 960b
   epidemiology and causes of, 956–957
   follow-up and referral for, 966
   management of, 961–966, 963f
   pathophysiology of, 957
   patient education on, 966–967
Osteonecrosis, 949–950
Osteophytes, 896
Osteoporosis
   clinical presentation of, 969–970
   diagnosis of, 970–971, 970t
   epidemiology and causes of, 967–968
   follow-up and referral for, 974
   management of, 971–974, 972f, 973t
   pathophysiology of, 968–969
   patient education on, 974–975
   postmenopausal, 790–791, 967
Otalgia, 303
Other specified feeding or eating disorder (OSFED), 304
   diagnosis of, 1309
Otitis externa (swimmer's ear)
   clinical presentation of, 335–336
   diagnosis of, 336–338
   epidemiology and causes of, 334
   follow-up and referral for, 341
   management of, 338–341
   pathophysiology of, 334–335
   patient education on, 341
Otitis media (OM), 336, 337
   acute, 342–343
   clinical presentation of, 343
   diagnosis of, 344
   with effusion (OME), 343
   epidemiology and causes of, 342
   follow-up and referral for, 348
   management of, 344–348, 348t
   patient education on, 348–349
   types of, 341–342
Otitis media with effusion (OME), 343
Ottawa Ankle and Foot Rules, 889
Outcome considerations, 50
Ovarian cancer
   clinical presentation of, 828–829
   diagnosis of, 829
   epidemiology and causes of, 827–828
   follow-up and referral for, 830
   management of, 829–830
   pathophysiology of, 828
   patient education on, 830
Overactive bladder, 712
Overflow incontinence, 708t, 712–713
Overuse syndrome. *See* Tendinitis/tenosynovitis
Oxycodone, 1478
Oxygen, home, for chronic obstructive pulmonary disease (COPD), 483

P

P. acnes, 240
Paget's disease, 157–158
Pain, 1469–1487
   abdominal, 603–604, 604–606f
   acute versus chronic, 1473–1474
   animal and human bites, 1344
   ankle, 905
   arthropod bites and stings, 1350

assessment of, 1473–1474
back, 896–898
biopsychosocial model of management of, 1474–1475, 1474f
bursitis, 936–937
cancer, 1444
cervical muscle strain, 911–912
chest, 521–523, 522f
chronic pelvic pain syndrome in females, 753–754
chronic pelvic pain syndrome in males, 754–755
classifications of, 1471–1473, 1472f
COVID-19 and, 1483–1484, 1485f
defined, 1469
dysmenorrhea, 812–814
dyspareunia, 751–752
dysuria, 701
ear, 303
effects of chronic, 1474t
elbow, 899–900
endometriosis, 814–817
eye, 268, 268t
foot, 906–907
health disparities in management of, 1482, 1483f
hip, 901, 903
knee, 903–905
leg, lumbar spinal stenosis and, 927
leg aches, 526
low back, 915–922, 917t, 920f
mechanisms of, 1469–1471
myofascial, 894–895
neck, 895–896
nephrolithiasis, 726
nonpharmacological management of, 1481–1482
osteoarthritis (OA), 958, 959b
otitis externa (swimmer's ear), 339
palliative care and, e1505–e1513, e1506–e1508b, e1507b, e1507t
perception of, 1469–1471, 1471f
pharmacological management of, 1475–1481
pharyngitis and tonsillitis, 396, 396b
shoulder, 898–899
sore throat, 305–306
stomatitis and glossitis, 388b
strains and sprains, 889
suffering and, e1493–e1494
tendinitis/tenosynovitis, 938–939
testicular, 755–756
testicular torsion, 856–857
types of medications for, 1473f
varicocele, 859
vertebral fracture, 931–932
vulvodynia, 830–832
wrist and hand, 900–901, 902
Pain Management Best Practices Inter-Agency Task Force Report, 1475
Paired organs in sports physicals, 1411
Paliperidone, 1232
Palliative care, e1489–e1516
advance directives and, e1494–e1495
anorexia and cachexia in, e1502–e1503
constipation in, e1502, e1503t
cough in, e1500
delirium in, e1503–e1505, e1504b
deprescribing medications in, e1505
differences between hospice and, e1490–e1491
DNR (Do Not Attempt Resuscitation order) and, e1495
dyspnea in, e1499–e1500, e1500b
falls in, e1505, e1505t
goals of, e1490
history of, e1489–e1490
LGBTQ+ persons in, e1496

nausea and vomiting in, e1501–e1502
oral secretions in, e1500–e1501
pain in, e1505–e1513, e1506–e1508b, e1507t
pediatric, e1495–e1496
professional education efforts to improve practice of, e1492–e1493
racial disparities in, e1496–e1497
relieving suffering in, e1493–e1494
role of primary care provider in, e1497, e1513–e1514
symptom management in, e1498–e1513
utilization of, e1492
Palliative Performance Score (PPS), e1497–e1498, e1498f
Palmar fibromatosis, 945
Palpitations, 523–524, 525f
sports physicals and, 1411
Pancreatitis, acute, 681–682
clinical presentation of, 682–683
diagnosis of, 683–684, 684b, 684t
epidemiology and causes of, 682, 682b
follow-up and referral for, 685
management of, 684–685
pathophysiology of, 682
patient education on, 685
Pancreatitis, chronic
clinical presentation of, 686
diagnosis of, 686–687
epidemiology and causes of, 685–686
follow-up and referral for, 687–688
management of, 687
pathophysiology of, 686
patient education on, 688
Pandemics, 35–36, 36t
Panic disorder, 1177–1178, 1184, 1281–1284
clinical presentation of, 1282
diagnosis of, 1282–1283
epidemiology and causes of, 1281–1282
follow-up and referral for, 1284, 1284b
management of, 1283
pathophysiology of, 1282
patient education on, 1284, 1284b
Panic Disorder Severity Scale, 1275, 1283
Papillary thyroid cancer. *See* Thyroid cancer
Papilloma, 391
Pap test, 822–823, 822t
Paradoxical sleep, 1311
Paraneoplastic syndromes, lung cancer, 500, 500t
Paraphilias, 1296
Parasitic skin infestations
pediculosis, 167–171
scabies, 163–167
Parathyroid hormone (PTH), 974, 979–980
Parentalism, e1516
Paresis, 90, 91f
Paresthesias, 90, 91f, 894
Parietal pain, 603
Parkinson's disease
clinical presentation of, 111–112
defined, 109–110
diagnostic reasoning for, 112–113
drugs prescribed for, 113–114
epidemiology of, 110–111
follow-up and referral for, 114
management of, 113–114
pathophysiology and causes of, 111
Paroxetine, 1297
Partial hospitalization (PHP) for eating disorders, 1309
Partial thickness wound, 1334
Pasteurella multocida, 199
Past medical history (PMH), 43–44
Patience, 21
Patient-centered medical homes (PCMHs), 9, 11, 15, 1174

Patient education
abdominal hernias, 653
acne vulgaris, 248, 249b
acquired immunodeficiency syndrome (AIDS), 1171
actinic keratosis, 256
acute coronary syndrome (ACS), 564–565
acute kidney injury (AKI), 735
acute pancreatitis, 685
adrenal insufficiency, 1013
allergic reactions, 1113
Alzheimer's disease (AD), 109
animal bites, 1346
appendicitis, 639
arrhythmias, 585, 586t
arthropod bites and stings, 1355, 1355b
asthma, 474
atopic dermatitis, 222
attention deficit-hyperactivity disorder (ADHD), 1193–1194, 1194b
autism spectrum disorder (ASD), 1197
Bell's palsy, 137
benign paroxysmal positional vertigo (BPPV), 326–327
benign prostatic hyperplasia (BPH), 839
bipolar and related disorders (BD), 1263–1264
bladder tumors, 747
blepharitis, 272
body dysmorphic disorder (BDD), 1300
bowel obstruction, 661
breast cancer, 807–808
burns, 1362, 1363b
bursitis, 937
candidiasis, 180
carpal tunnel syndrome (CTS), 943
cataracts, 290
cauda equina syndrome (CES), 930
celiac disease, 658
cellulitis, 204
cerebrovascular accident (CVA), 123–125
cervical cancer, 824
cervical muscle strain, 913
cervical spondylosis, 915
cholecystitis, 681
chronic fatigue syndrome (CFS) and fibromyalgia syndrome (FMS), 1128
chronic kidney disease (CKD), 742
chronic obstructive pulmonary disease (COPD), 484–485
chronic pancreatitis, 688
cirrhosis, 698
colorectal cancer, 677
contact dermatitis, 226
contraception and family planning, 771
coronary heart disease (CHD), 550
cough, 419
Cushing's syndrome, 1010–1011
cystic fibrosis (CF), 438
deep vein thrombosis (DVT)/chronic venous insufficiency, 600
de Quervain's tenosynovitis, 944
dermatophytoses, 186
diabetes mellitus (DM) type 1, 1027
diabetes mellitus (DM) type 2, 1039
diabetes mellitus (DM) type 3C, 1041
diabetic retinopathy, 296
diverticular disease, 664
dry eye syndrome (DES), 277, 277b
dyslipidemia, 547
dysmenorrhea, 814
dysphonia, 415
eating disorders, 1310–1311, 1311b
encephalitis, 131
endometrial cancer, 827
endometriosis, 817
epididymitis, 856

epistaxis, 406
erectile dysfunction (ED), 854
excessive tearing (epiphora), 280
fertility problems, 778
folliculitis, 197
foreign body obstruction, 1374
frostbite, 1389
furuncles and carbuncles, 199
gastroenteritis, 628
gastroesophageal reflux disease (GERD), 645
generalized anxiety disorder (GAD), 1277, 1281
glaucoma, 294–295
gout, 1061–1062
head trauma, 1369
hearing loss, 316
heart failure (HF), 572–573
heat-related illnesses, 1386
hemoptysis, 422
hemorrhoids, 650
hepatitis, 635
herniated lumbar disc (herniated nucleus pulposus), 926
herpes simplex infections, 214
herpes zoster, 133–134
hoarding disorder (HD), 1302
hordeolum and chalazion, 273
human immunodeficiency virus (HIV), 1163
hydrocele, 859
hypertension (HTN), 542
hyperthyroidism, 993
hypoglycemia, 1046
hypothermia, 1388
hypothyroidism, 1001–1002
impetigo, 193–194
infectious mononucleosis, 1142
inflammatory bowel disease (IBD), 672
insomnia disorder, 1317
intellectual disability (ID), 1201
interstitial lung disease (ILD), 493, 493b
irritable bowel syndrome (IBS), 657
leiomyomas (uterine fibroids), 819
leukemia, 1102
low back pain (LBP), 922
lower urinary tract infections (UTIs), 721
lumbar spinal stenosis, 928
lung cancer, 506–507
Lyme disease, 1147
macrocytic anemia, 1083
macular degeneration, 300
major depressive disorder (MDD), 1250
malignant melanoma, 260
mastitis, 798
Ménière's disease, 330
meningitis, 129
menopause, 791–792
microcytic anemia, 1074
migraine headache, 89–90
multiple sclerosis (MS), 143
musculoskeletal trauma, 893
neck masses, 382
nephrolithiasis, 727–728
nonmelanomatous skin cancers, 264, 264t
normocytic anemia, 1079
obesity, 1054
obsessive-compulsive disorder (OCD), 1299
onychomycosis, 189
oral cancer, 391–392
osteoarthritis (OA), 966–967
osteoporosis, 974–975
otitis externa (swimmer's ear), 341
otitis media (OM), 348–349
ovarian cancer, 830
panic disorder, 1284, 1284b
Parkinson's disease, 114
pediculosis, 170–171
peptic ulcer disease (PUD), 648
peripheral artery disease (PAD), 596
pharyngitis and tonsillitis, 398
phobias, 1285
pneumonia, 452
pneumothorax and hemothorax, 1371
poisoning, 1382
polycythemia, 1091
post-traumatic stress disorder (PTSD), 1289
premenstrual syndrome (PMS) and premenstrual dysphoric disorder (PMDD), 782
prostate cancer, 846
prostatitis, 842
psoriasis, 237–238
pyelonephritis, 723
red eye/conjunctivitis, 284
refractive errors, 288
renal tumors, 744
restless legs syndrome (RLS), 1318
rheumatoid arthritis (RA), 1124
rhinitis, 364–365
rhinosinusitis, 377
rosacea, 251
scabies, 167
schizophrenia spectrum disorders, 1235–1236
seborrheic dermatitis, 228
seborrheic keratosis, 253
seizure disorders, 101
sexual assault, 1325
sexually transmitted infections (STIs), 874–875
sickle cell anemia, 1088
Sjögren's syndrome (SS), 1132
sleep apnea, 430–431
smoking addiction, 518–520
sports physicals, 1415
stomatitis and glossitis, 389
substance use disorders (SUDs), 1221–1222
suicide, 1269
systemic lupus erythematosus (SLE), 1138
temporomandibular disorders (TMDs), 411
tendinitis/tenosynovitis, 940
testicular cancer, 865
testicular torsion, 857
thyroid cancer, 1005
tic disorders, 1204
tinnitus, 320
trigeminal neuralgia, 135
tuberculosis (TB), 463–464
upper respiratory infections (URIs), 435–436
urinary incontinence (UI), 714
valvular disorders and murmurs, 592–593
varicocele, 860
vertebral fracture, 933
vestibular neuritis (VN) and labyrinthitis, 332
vulvodynia, 832
warts, 209, 209b
wounds and lacerations, 1342, 1342b
Patient Health Questionnaire-9 (PHQ-9), 1242, 1249, 1275, 1307
sports physicals and, 1410
Patient Health Questionnaire-Somatic, Anxiety, and Depressive Symptoms Screener (PHQ-SADS), 1275
Patient Protection and Affordable Care Act of 2010. *See* Affordable Care Act of 2010
Patient Self-Determination Act (PSDA), e1489
Peak expiratory flow rate (PEFR), 421
Pediatric/adolescent considerations
acne vulgaris, 242
amenorrhea, 811
bone health, 968
congenital hypothyroidism, 994
COVID-19, 447–448
cruciate ligament injury, 952
epistaxis, 403
gynecomastia (GM), 980
hypertension (HTN), 531
infectious mononucleosis, 1140
major depressive disorder (MDD), 1249
meningitis, 127
mental disorders, e1553
musculoskeletal injury, 884
obesity, 1048
obsessive-compulsive disorder (OCD), 1293
palliative care, e1495–e1496
panic disorder, 1282
red eye/conjunctivitis, 281
reproductive issues, 760
schizophrenia spectrum disorders, 1227
seizure disorder, 102
sexual assault, 1321
sexually transmitted infections (STIs), 866
smoking addiction, 510
substance use disorders (SUDs), 1210
Wilson's disease, 110
Pediatric Anxiety Rating Scale (PARS), 1275
Pediculosis
clinical presentation of, 167–168
diagnosis of, 168
epidemiology and causes of, 167
follow-up and referral for, 169–171
management of, 168–169
pathophysiology of, 167
patient education on, 170–171
Pediculus humanus capitis. *See* Pediculosis
Pediculus humanus corporis. *See* Pediculosis
Pelvic pain, 753–754
Pelvic steal syndrome, 851
Pender, Nola, 33
Penectomy, 1419
Penile and testicular disorders
epididymitis, 854–856
erectile dysfunction (ED), 847–854, 848f, 849b
hydrocele, 857–859
testicular cancer, 860–865, 863–864t
testicular torsion, 856–857
varicocele, 859–860
Penile prostheses, 853
Penile revascularization, 853
Peptic ulcer disease (PUD)
clinical presentation of, 646
diagnosis of, 646
epidemiology and causes of, 645
follow-up and referral for, 647
management of, 646–647, 648
pathophysiology of, 645
patient education, 648
Peptostreptococcus
otitis externa (swimmer's ear) and, 335
rhinosinusitis and, 366, 371
Performance improvements, e1546–e1547
Periodic limb movements (PLMs), 428
Periorbital cellulitis, 200b
Peripartum depression (PPD), 1240
Peripheral artery disease (PAD)
clinical presentation of, 595
diagnosis of, 595
epidemiology and causes of, 594
follow-up and referral for, 596
lumbar spinal stenosis and, 927
management of, 595–596
pathophysiology of, 594–595
patient education on, 596
Peripheral edema, 526–528, 527f
Peripheral vascular disease (PVD), 526
Peripheral vestibular disease, 77
Perphenazine, 1231
Personalized medicine, 1276b
Personal sexual servitude, 1328t
Phalen's test, 901
Phalloplasty, 1419

Pharyngitis and tonsillitis, 305–306
   clinical presentation of, 393–394
   diagnosis of, 394–396
   epidemiology and causes of, 392
   follow-up and referral for, 397–398
   management of, 396–397, 396b
   pathophysiology of, 392–393
   patient education on, 398
Phenobarbital, 100
Phenytoin, 100
Phobias, 1284–1285
Phosphodiesterase$_4$ (PDE$_4$) inhibitors, 482
Photopsia, 269
Phototoxicity, 1356
Physical activity
   adolescents and, 1400
   cancer prevention and, 1445
   diabetes mellitus (DM) type 1 and, 1024–1025
   diabetes mellitus (DM) type 2 and, 1032
   headache and, 89
   insomnia disorder and, 1316t
   low back pain (LBP) and, 922
   lumbar spinal stenosis and, 928
   obesity and, 1052
   by older adults, 1457–1458
   sports physicals and, 1406–1417
Physical disability and sports physicals, 1409
Physical examination
   of adolescents, 1394–1395
   in diagnostic process, 46
   in palliative care, e1497–e1498, e1498f
   for sexual assault, 1324
   sports physicals, 1411–1414, 1412t
   of transgender persons, 1418–1419
Physical therapy for osteoarthritis (OA), 961
Physicians, collaboration with, e1525–e1526
Piaget, Jean, 1394, 1394t
Pica, 304
Pigmentation changes, 150
   Addison's disease, 152
   differential diagnosis, 151–153
   drug-induced hyperpigmentation, 152
   melasma and chloasma, 152
   normal variations of pigmentation and, 150–151
   vitiligo, 151–152
Pinhole test, 287
Pituitary adenoma, 985, 985t
Plantar fasciitis, 953
Plantar warts. *See* Warts
Platelet-rich plasma (PRP) injections for osteoarthritis (OA), 965
Pleurisy, 440
Pleuritis, 440
Plummer's disease, 985, 985t
Pneumocystis jiroveci, 439, 442–443
   AIDS and, 1170
Pneumonia
   COVID-19-associated (*See* COVID-19)
   diagnosis of, 444–448
   epidemiology and causes of, 438–440, 439b
   pathophysiology of, 440–443, 441f
Pneumothorax and hemothorax, 1369–1371
   clinical presentation of, 1370
   diagnosis of, 1370
   epidemiology and causes of, 1369
   follow-up and referral for, 1370–1371
   management of, 1370, 1371b
   pathophysiology of, 1369–1370
   patient education on, 1371
Point-of-care strategy, 65–68, 67–68b
Point-of-service plans (POS), e1533
Poisoning
   clinical presentation of, 1376–1379t, 1376–1380, 1380t
   common toxidromes, 1380, 1380t
   diagnosis of, 1380–1381

   epidemiology and causes of, 1375–1376
   follow-up and referral for, 1382
   management of, 1381–1382
   pathophysiology of, 1376
   patient education on, 1382
Polycythemia
   clinical presentation of, 1090
   diagnosis of, 1090–1091
   epidemiology and causes of, 1088
   follow-up and referral for, 1092
   management of, 1091–1092
   pathophysiology of, 1088–1089
   patient education on, 1091
Polydipsia, 983–984, 983f
Polyglandular autoimmune disease type 2, 1016
Polymorphonuclear leukocytes (PMNs), 194
Polymyositis-dermatomyositis, 487b
Polyphagia, 983–984, 983f
Polypharmacy, 1462–1463
Polyuria, 983–984, 983f
Pornography, 1328t
Positioning after animal and human bites, 1345
Positive intentionality, e1561
Positive shopping cart sign, 927
Postcoital controls, 770
Posterior cruciate ligament (PCL) injuries, 951
Posterior vitreous detachment (PVD), 269
Postexposure HIV prophylaxis, 1346
Postherpetic neuralgia (PHN), 132, 133
Postphlebitic syndrome, 598
Postrenal azotemia, 731
Post-traumatic stress disorder (PTSD), 1173, 1177, 1183b, 1184, 1188, 1256t, 1285–1289
   clinical presentation of, 1287
   diagnosis of, 1287–1288
   epidemiology and causes of, 1286–1287
   management of, 1288–1289
   pathophysiology of, 1287
   patient education on, 1289
   sexual assault and, 1322
   in veterans, 1430
Postvention, 1269
Poultices for headache, 89
Practice standards, 58–59
Precision health care, 54, 1276b
Prednisolone, 1010
Prednisone, 1010
Preferred provider organizations (PPOs), e1533
Pregnancy
   diabetes mellitus (DM) type 1 in, 1026
   diabetes mellitus (DM) type 2 in, 1039
   hyperthyroidism in, 985t
   hypothyroidism in, 997, 1000
   and trophoblastic tumors, 985, 985t
Premalignant lesions
   actinic keratosis, 254–256
   cervical, 819–824, 822t, 824b
Premature atrial contractions (PACs), 575, 582, 584
Premature ventricular contractions (PVCs), 582, 585
Premenstrual syndrome (PMS) and premenstrual dysphoric disorder (PMDD)
   clinical presentation of, 779–780
   diagnosis of, 780–781
   epidemiology and causes of, 779
   follow-up and referral for, 782
   management of, 781–782
   patient education on, 782
   symptoms of, 778, 779
Preparticipation physical evaluation (PPE). *See* Sports physicals
Prerenal azotemia, 730
Presbyopia, 286, 286t
Prescriptive authority, e1523–e1524
Presence, authentic, 20

Present-centered therapy (PCT), 1289
Presyncope and sports physicals, 1411
Prevention as health promotion, 8–9
   primary, secondary, and tertiary, 28, 28t
PRICE therapy, 889, 939
Primary adrenal insufficiency. *See* Addison's disease
Primary biliary cirrhosis (PBC), 690b, 691, 695
Primary Care: America's Health in a New Era, 5
Primary care practice. *See also* Advanced practice nursing; Value-based health care
   with adolescents, 1393–1394
   challenges in access to quality, 5–6
   clinical judgment in, 38–40
   gender-appropriate, 1421–1422
   nursing perspectives needed for, 6–7
   with older adults, 1448–1465
   palliative care, e1497, e1513–e1514
   PCMH model for, 9, 11, 15
   prevention as health promotion in, 8–9
   reports on future of nursing and, 3–5, 4b, 5b, 5t
   as tip of the iceberg, 7–8, 7f
   uncertainty in, 39
   unique aspects of, 39
   with veterans (*See* Veterans)
Primary Care PTSD Screen for *DSM-5* (PC-PTSD-5), 1287
Primary prevention, 28, 28t
Primary sclerosing cholangitis (PSC), 690b, 691
Problem-solving skills, e1554
Professional Quality of Life (ProQOL) scale, e1561
Progestin-only pill, 763–764
Prognostication, e1493–e1494
Progressive multifocal leukoencephalopathy (PML), 1171
Progressive systemic sclerosis (scleroderma), 487b
Prolonged exposure (PE), 1288
Propylthiouracil (PTU), 991
Prostaglandin analogs, 294
Prostate cancer
   clinical presentation of, 843
   diagnosis of, 843–845
   epidemiology and causes of, 842–843
   follow-up and referral for, 846
   management of, 845–846
   pathophysiology of, 843
   patient education on, 846
Prostate disorders
   benign prostatic hyperplasia (BPH), 752, 833–839, 835t
   prostate cancer, 842–846
   prostatitis, 840–842
Prostate specific antigen (PSA) test, 843–844
Prostatitis
   clinical presentation of, 840–841
   diagnosis of, 841
   epidemiology and causes of, 840
   follow-up and referral for, 842
   management of, 841–842
   pathophysiology of, 840
   patient education on, 842
Prostheses, penile, 853
Proteinuria, 704–705, 705t
Proteus spp.
   lower urinary tract infections (UTIs) and, 715
   mastitis and, 795
   prostatitis and, 840
   pyelonephritis and, 721
   rhinitis and, 351
Proton pump inhibitor (PPI) therapy
   gastroesophageal reflux disease (GERD) and, 643–644
   peptic ulcer disease (PUD) and, 647
Providencia, 715
Provider comparison web sites, e1547
Provider Enrollment Chain and Ownership System (PECOS), e1527

Proximal femoral (hip) fracture, 890–891
Pruritic urticarial papules and plaques of pregnancy (PUPPP), 159
Pruritus
  differential diagnosis of, 153–155
  management of, 155–156
Pseudomonas aeruginosa
  diabetes mellitus (DM) type 1 and, 1017
  epididymitis and, 854
  folliculitis and, 194, 195
  lower urinary tract infections (UTIs) and, 715
  mastitis and, 795
  otitis externa (swimmer's ear) and, 334, 335
  pneumonia and, 441
  prostatitis and, 840
  pyelonephritis and, 721
  rhinosinusitis and, 366
Pseudoparkinsonism, 1234t
Psoriasis
  clinical presentation of, 230–231
  diagnosis of, 231–234
  epidemiology and causes of, 228–229
  follow-up and referral for, 237
  management of, 234–237
  pathophysiology of, 229–230
  patient education on, 237–238
Psoriasis Area and Severity Index, 230
Psychogenic nonepileptic seizures (PNES), 95
Psychosocial complaints
  anxiety disorders, 1175t, 1176–1178
  depressed mood, 1178–1179, 1178t, 1226t
  diabetes mellitus (DM) type 2, 1033
  grief, 1179–1181
  intimate partner violence (IPV), 1182–1184, 1183b, 1184b
  overview of, 1173–1176, 1175t
  screening tools for, 1175t
  substance use disorder, 1175t, 1181–1182
Psychotic disorder, 1256t
Pthirus pubis. See Pediculosis
Puberty, 1395–1398, 1396–1397t
PubMed, 65
Punch biopsy, 231
Purulent OM. See Otitis media (OM)
Puss caterpillar, 1351
Pyelonephritis
  clinical presentation of, 722
  diagnosis of, 722–723
  epidemiology and causes of, 721
  follow-up and referral for, 723
  management of, 723
  pathophysiology of, 721–722
  patient education on, 723
Pyrimidine synthesis inhibitors, 1122

Q

Qualitative studies, 62
Quasi-experimental research designs, 61
Quetiapine, 1232
Quick Inventory of Depressive Symptomatology (QIDS-SR), 1242

R

Rabies prophylaxis, 1345
Race and ethnicity
  health disparities and, 6
  life expectancy and, 5–6
  older adults and, 1449
  pain management disparities and, 1482
  palliative care and, e1496–e1497
Radiation therapy
  breast cancer, 804–806
  colorectal cancer, 676
  endometrial cancer, 827
  lung cancer, 506
  malignant melanoma, 260
  ovarian cancer, 829–830
  testicular cancer, 862
Radioactive iodine, 991–992
Radioallergosorbent test (RAST), 217–218
Ramsay-Hunt syndrome, 132, 136
Randomized clinical trials (RCTs), 59–62
Range of motion (ROM) testing, 880–881, 896, 903
  in sports physicals, 1413
Ranson's criteria for acute pancreatitis, 683–684, 684t
Rape. See Sexual assault
Rapid Estimate of Adult Literacy in Medicine-Short Form, 29
Rapid eye movement (REM) sleep, 1311–1312
Rash, 156–157
  differential diagnosis of, 157–158
  eczematous (See Atopic dermatitis)
  Paget's disease, 157–158
  toxic shock syndrome (TSS), 158
Rebound rhinitis, 363
Rectum, foreign body obstruction in, 1372, 1374
Red eye/conjunctivitis, 268–269
  clinical presentation of, 281–282
  diagnosis of, 282–284, 283t
  epidemiology and causes of, 280–281
  follow-up and referral for, 284
  management of, 284
  pathophysiology of, 281
  patient education on, 284
Reflexology for headache, 89
Refractive errors
  clinical presentation of, 287
  diagnosis of, 287
  epidemiology and causes of, 285–286
  follow-up and referral for, 288
  management of, 287
  pathophysiology of, 287
  patient education on, 288
Regular insulin, 1022
Reiki, e1562
  for pain in palliative care, e1513
Reimbursement, e1524. See also Value-based health care
  Affordable Care Act of 2010, 3, 34, e1526–e1527, e1531–e1535, e1536t
  auto liability, workers' compensation, Champus/Tricare, and CHAMPVA, e1535
  billing and coding rules, e1540–e1544, e1542b
  cash/private pay patients, e1535–e1536
  impact of COVID-19 on, e1534
  indemnity and managed care organizations, e1533
  Medicaid, 5, e1527
  Medicare Access and CHIP Reauthorization Act (MACRA), 52, e1538–e1539
  Medicare for All proposal, e1539
  Medicare parts, e1527
  Medicare physician and nonphysician practitioner fee schedule (PFS), e1543–e1544
  performance-based care and value-based, e1541t, e1544–e1547
  third-party payer rules, e1526–e1529
Relative energy deficiency in sports (RED-S), 1410
Relative polycythemia, 1088, 1091, 1092
Relaxation therapy
  for generalized anxiety disorder (GAD), 1281
  for headache, 89
Religious distress, e1493
Remodeling phase of wounds, 1334
Renal calculi. See Nephrolithiasis
Renal tumors
  clinical presentation of, 743
  diagnosis of, 743–744, 743f
  epidemiology and causes of, 742
  follow-up and referral for, 744
  management of, 744
  pathophysiology of, 742–743
  patient education on, 744
Reproductive issues. See also Vaginal, uterine, and ovarian disorders
  cancer and, 1444
  contraception and family planning, 760–771, 762f
  fertility problems, 771–778, 775t, 777b
  menopause, 782–792
  premenstrual syndrome (PMS) and premenstrual dysphoric disorder (PMDD), 778–782, 779b
  prostate disorders (See Prostate disorders)
  vaginal, uterine, and ovarian disorders (See Vaginal, uterine, and ovarian disorders)
Reproductive system complaints
  abnormal uterine bleeding (AUB), 750–751
  breast mass, 749–750
  chronic pelvic pain syndrome in females, 753–754
  chronic pelvic pain syndrome in males, 754–755
  dyspareunia, 751–752
  nocturia in males, 752
  testicular pain, 755–756
  testosterone deficiency, 756
  vulvovaginitis, 756–759
Research, nursing, 56–58, 57f
  integration of evidence-based practice and, 65, 66–67b
Research utilization (RU) model, 58
Residential care for eating disorders, 1309
Resilience, e1561
Resolution guidelines for ethical issues, e1519–e1520, e1520f
Respiratory disorders, infectious
  COVID-19 (See COVID-19)
  cystic fibrosis (CF), 436–438, 439
  pneumonia, 438–443, 439b, 441f
  tuberculosis (TB), 452–464, 455t, 456b, 456t, 460b, 462–463t
  upper respiratory infections (URIs), 431–436, 432b
Respiratory disorders, inflammatory
  asthma, 465–475, 467b, 468t, 470–471f, 474b, 475b
  chronic obstructive pulmonary disease (COPD), 475–486, 478t, 485f
  interstitial lung disease (ILD), 486–493, 487–488b, 493b
Respiratory Distress Observation Scale (RODS), e1500
Respiratory disturbance index (RDI), 423
Respiratory examination in sports physicals, 1412–1413
Respiratory problems
  after cancer, 1443
  with aging, 1451t
  cough, 417–419
  dyspnea, 419–421
  eating disorders and, 1307t
  hemoptysis, 421–422
Restless legs syndrome (RLS), 1317–1318
Rest tremor, 111–112
Retention hyperkeratosis, 240
Retinal detachment, 287
Retinopathy, 1025, 1038
Revascularization, penile, 853
Review of systems, 44
Rheumatoid arthritis (RA), 487b
  clinical presentation of, 1115–1116
  diagnosis of, 1116–1117
  epidemiology and causes of, 1113–1114
  follow-up and referral for, 1124

management of, 1117–1124, 1118–1120t
pathophysiology of, 1114–1115
patient education on, 1124
Rheumatoid disease, 936
Rhinitis
clinical presentation of, 351–355
diagnosis of, 355–356
epidemiology and causes of, 350–351
follow-up and referral for, 364
forms of, 350, 350b
pathophysiology of, 351
patient education on, 364–365
Rhinosinusitis, 350, 366f
clinical presentation of, 367
diagnosis of, 367–368
epidemiology and causes of, 365–366
follow-up and referral for, 376
management of, 368–376
pathophysiology of, 366–367
patient education on, 377
Rings, removing, 902
Rinne test, 313
Risk factors in health promotion, 28–29, 29b
Risk management, e1546–e1547
Risperidone, 1232
Rogers, Martha, 10
Rosacea, 242
clinical presentation of, 249–250
diagnosis of, 250
epidemiology and causes of, 248–249
follow-up and referral for, 251
management of, 250
pathophysiology of, 249
patient education on, 251
Rotator cuff syndrome, 899
Rotator cuff tear, 947–948
Rotavirus, 624t
Rule of Nines, 1359, 1359f
Rumination disorder, 304
Running continuous suture, 1340

S

Safety
medical error reduction and, 52
for older adults, 1458
Salicylates poisoning, 1377t
Salicylate sulfonamides, 1122
Saline-load test, 1337
Salmonella, 623t
SAMHSA Suicide Assessment Five-Step Evaluation and Triage (SAFE-T), 1266
Sarcoidosis, 488b
SARS-CoV-2. *See* COVID-19
Saunders, Cicely, e1489
Scabies
clinical presentation of, 163–164
diagnosis of, 164–165
epidemiology and causes of, 163
follow-up and referral for, 165–167
management of, 165
pathophysiology of, 163
patient education on, 167
Scarring alopecia, 147, 148, 149
Schizoaffective disorder, 1226t
Schizophrenia spectrum disorders, 1209, 1226–1227, 1226t
clinical presentation of, 1228
diagnosis of, 1228–1230, 1229b
epidemiology and causes of, 1227
follow-up and referral for, 1235
management of, 1230–1235, 1231t, 1234t
pathophysiology of, 1227–1228
patient education on, 1235–1236
weight loss with, 1309
Schizophreniform, 1226t
Schwabach test, 313

SCOFF Questionnaire, 1307, 1307b
Scombroid fish poisoning, 1378t
Scorpions, 1347, 1350, 1354
Screen for Child Anxiety-Related Emotional Disorders (SCARED), 1275
Screening tests, 26, 26b, 47
for adolescents, 1395, 1400, 1401t
eating disorders, 1307, 1307b
for older adults, 1454–1455t, 1455–1460
Scrotoplasty, 1419
Seborrheic dermatitis
clinical presentation of, 226
diagnosis of, 226–227
epidemiology and causes of, 226
follow-up and referral for, 228
management of, 227–228
pathophysiology of, 226
patient education on, 228
Seborrheic keratosis
clinical presentation of, 251
diagnosis of, 252, 252t
epidemiology and causes of, 251
follow-up and referral for, 253
management of, 252–253
pathophysiology of, 251
patient education on, 253
Secondary hypertension, 531
Secondary hypothyroidism, 994
Secondary prevention, 28, 28t
Second-degree burns, 1357–1358, 1360–1361
Second generation antipsychotics (SGAs), 1198
Second generation sulfonylureas, 1034, 1036
Second-line TB drugs, 459
Secretions, oral, e1500–e1501
Secretory diarrhea, 607
Sedative-hypnotics and anxiolytics, 1217
Seizure disorders
absence seizures, 95
clinical presentation of, 96–97
defined, 94
drugs prescribed for, 99–100
emergent care for, 101b
epidemiology and causes of, 95
focal onset seizures, 94–95
follow-up and referral for, 100–101
generalized onset seizures, 95
management of, 97–100
pathophysiology of, 96
psychogenic nonepileptic seizures (PNES), 95
sports physicals and, 1411
tonic-clonic seizures, 95
types of, 94, 94f
Selective serotonin reuptake inhibitors (SSRIs)
anxiety disorders and, 1275
attention deficit-hyperactivity disorder (ADHD) and, 1191
body dysmorphic disorder (BDD) and, 1300
eating disorders and, 1310
generalized anxiety disorder (GAD) and, 1278
hoarding disorder (HD) and, 1301
major depressive disorder (MDD) and, 1243–1244, 1245–1246
obsessive-compulsive disorder (OCD) and, 1297–1298
panic disorder and, 1283
Self-actualization, 8–9
Self-assessment, e1561
Self-care, e1558–e1564
caring and, e1558–e1559
challenges to, e1559–e1560
for compassion fatigue and burnout, e1560–e1561
defined, e1558–e1559
goal setting for, e1561
implementing strategies in, e1562
importance of, e1563b
osteoarthritis (OA), 961

principles of, e1561
process of, e1561–e1562
self-assessment in, e1561
Self-monitoring, blood glucose levels, 1022–1023, 1023t, 1033
Semont liberatory maneuver, 325
Senile keratosis. *See* Actinic keratosis
Sensorineural hearing loss (SNHL), 310, 312t, 316
Serotonin modulators, 1247
Serotonin norepinephrine reuptake inhibitors (SNRIs)
attention deficit-hyperactivity disorder (ADHD) and, 1191, 1192
eating disorders and, 1310
generalized anxiety disorder (GAD) and, 1278
major depressive disorder (MDD) and, 1243–1244, 1246
panic disorder and, 1283
Serotonin receptor antagonists for nausea and vomiting, 617
Serotonin transporter gene (5-HTT), 1241
Serratia, 715
Sertraline, 1297
Sex and pain management disparities, 1483, 1483f
Sex trafficking, 1327
Sexual assault, 1320–1326
clinical presentation of, 1322
diagnosis of, 1322
epidemiology and causes of, 1321
follow-up and referral for, 1324–1325
management of, 1322–1324
military sexual trauma (MST) and, 1432–1434, 1432t, 1433b
pathophysiology of, 1321
patient education on, 1325
Sexual assault interview, 1323–1324
Sexual assault nurse examiner (SANE RN), 1323
Sexual assault trauma syndrome, 1322
Sexuality
in adolescents, 1402
in older adults, 1459–1460
Sexually transmitted infections (STIs)
clinical presentation of, 872–873
common, 866, 867–871t
diagnosis of, 873–874
epidemiology and causes of, 866, 872
follow-up and referral for, 874
management of, 874
pathophysiology of, 872
patient education on, 874–875
SHARE approach, 40
Shared decision making, 49–50
Shigella, 623t
Shingles. *See* Herpes zoster
Short-acting beta-agonists (SABAs)
asthma and, 471–472
chronic obstructive pulmonary disease (COPD) and, 481
Short Post-Traumatic Stress Disorder Rating Interview, 1287
Shoulder disorders
adhesive capsulitis, 945–946
calcific tendinitis, 947
impingement syndrome, 946–947
rotator cuff tear, 947–948
Shoulder fracture, 890
Shoulder pain, 898–899
Shoulder sprains, 886
Shuler Nurse Practitioner Practice Model, 11
Shur-Clens, 1338
Sickle cell anemia
clinical presentation of, 1085–1086
diagnosis of, 1086–1087
epidemiology and causes of, 1083–1084

follow-up and referral for, 1088
management of, 1087
pathophysiology of, 1084–1085
patient education on, 1088
Sideroblastic anemia, 1069, 1072, 1073, 1074
Sinus complaints, 307
Sjögren's syndrome (SS)
clinical presentation of, 1130
diagnosis of, 1130–1131
epidemiology and causes of, 1128–1129
evidence-based nursing for, 1129
follow-up and referral for, 1132
management of, 1131–1132
pathophysiology of, 1129–1130
patient education on, 1132
Skier's thumb, 901
Skin cancer, 152–153, 378
clinical presentation of, 262–263
diagnosis of, 263
epidemiology and causes of, 261
follow-up and referral for, 263–264
management of, 263
nonmelanomatous, 261–264, 264t
pathophysiology of, 261–262
patient education on, 264, 264t
tanning beds and, 1404
urticaria, 158–161, 160f
Skin infections, bacterial
cellulitis, 199–204, 200b, 203t
folliculitis, 194–197
furuncles and carbuncles, 197–199
impetigo, 190–194, 192t
Skin infections, fungal
candidiasis, 172–180
dermatophytoses, 180–186
onychomycosis, 187–189
Skin infections, viral
herpes simplex infections, 210–214, 210t, 214b
warts, 205–209, 208t, 209b
Skin infestations, parasitic
pediculosis, 167–171
scabies, 163–167
Skin lesions
acne vulgaris, 239–248, 241f, 245b
actinic keratosis, 254–256
malignant melanoma, 256–260, 259b
nonmelanomatous skin cancers, 261–264, 264t
rosacea, 248–251
seborrheic keratosis, 251–253
Skin-picking disorder, 1296
Skin problems
with aging, 1451t
alopecia, 147–150
animal and human bites, 1342–1346
arthropod bites and stings, 1346–1355
burns, 1356–1362
dermatitis (*See* Dermatitis)
eating disorders and, 1307t
pigmentation changes, 150–153
pruritus, 153–156
rash, 156–158
sports physicals and, 1414
wounds and lacerations, 1333–1342
Skin tags, 252t
Skull fracture, 1364
Sleep apnea
clinical presentation of, 425–427, 426b, 426f
diagnosis of, 427–428
epidemiology and causes of, 424
follow-up and referral for, 430
management of, 428–430
pathophysiology of, 424–425
patient education on, 430–431
possible consequences of, 423–424, 423b
types of, 423

Sleep recommendations for adolescents, 1399, 1399t
Sleep restriction therapy, 1316t
Sleep-wake disorders
insomnia disorder, 1311–1317, 1313b, 1316b, 1316t
restless legs syndrome (RLS), 1317–1318
Small-cell lung cancer (SCLC). *See* Lung cancer
Smoking addiction
acute effects of nicotine use, 511–512, 511b
in adolescents, 1403
cancer and, 1446
chronic effects of nicotine use, 512
chronic obstructive pulmonary disease (COPD) and, 476–477
clinical presentation of, 512–513
consequences of, 508, 509t
diagnosis of, 513
epidemiology and causes of, 508–511
follow-up and referral for, 518
lung cancer and, 495
management of, 513–518, 515f
osteoporosis and, 968
pathophysiology of, 511–512, 511b
patient education on, 518–520
pharyngitis and tonsillitis and, 393
stomatitis and glossitis and, 383
Smoking cessation programs, 514
Snake bites, 1343, 1344, 1345
Snellen eye chart, 287
SOAP (subjective, objective, assessment, and plan) documentation format, 50–52
Social anxiety disorder, 1188b, 1296
Social determinants of health (SDOH), 5t, 6, 7
Social history, 44
Social media, 1403
Social phobia, 1188b, 1296
Sodium-glucose transport-2 inhibitors, 1035
Soft tissue disorders
adhesive capsulitis, 945–946
avascular necrosis (AVN), 949–950
bone tumors, 950–951
bursitis, 935–937
calcific tendinitis, 947
carpal tunnel syndrome (CTS), 941–943
cruciate ligament injury, 951
de Quervain's tenosynovitis, 943–944
Dupuytren's contracture, 945
ganglion cyst, 944
greater trochanteric pain syndrome (GTPS), 949
impingement syndrome, 946–947
interdigital neuroma, 953–954
medial collateral ligament (MCL) injury, 951–952
meniscus tear, 952
meralgia paresthetica, 949
plantar fasciitis, 953
rotator cuff tear, 947–948
tendinitis/tenosynovitis, 937–940, 937t
tendon injuries of the hand, 945, 945f
trigger finger, 944–945
Solar keratosis. *See* Actinic keratosis
Somatic symptom and related disorders, 1177
Sore throat, 305–306
Specific phobia disorders, 1177
Spinal disorders
cauda equina syndrome (CES), 928–930, 929t
cervical muscle strain, 910–913
cervical spondylosis, 913–915
herniated lumbar disc (herniated nucleus pulposus), 922–926
low back pain (LBP), 915–922, 917t, 920f
lumbar spinal stenosis, 926–928
vertebral fracture, 931–933
Spinal stenosis. *See* Lumbar spinal stenosis
Spirited caring, 22–23

Spirit-focused nursing model, 11
Spirituality, e1493
transgender persons and, 1417
Spondyloarthritis, 1118–1120t
Spondylolisthesis, 917
Spondylosis, 896
cervical, 913–915
Sporadic outbreaks, 35–36, 36t
Sports physicals, 1406–1417
clearance, 1414, 1414–1415t
examination formats for, 1407–1408
examination timing for, 1406–1407
history component of, 1408–1411, 1408b, 1409t
introduction to, 1406
by level of contact and intensity, 1407t
objectives of, 1406, 1407b
patient education on, 1415
physical examination component of, 1411–1414, 1412t
Spurling's maneuver, 895
Squamous cell carcinoma (SCC), 254
clinical presentation of, 262–263
diagnosis of, 263
epidemiology and causes of, 261
follow-up and referral for, 263–264
lung cancer, 496
management of, 263
oral, 391
pathophysiology of, 261–262
patient education on, 264, 264t
Stable angina. *See* Acute coronary syndrome (ACS)
Standard bismuth quadruple therapy, 648
Standard nonbismuth quadruple therapy, 648
Stanford Sleepiness Score (SSS), 427
Staphyloccus aureus
acute otitis media (AOM) and, 342
atopic dermatitis and, 216
bursitis and, 936
cellulitis and, 199
epididymitis and, 854
folliculitis and, 194, 197
gastroenteritis and, 623t
hordeolum and chalazion and, 273
impetigo and, 190–191
lower urinary tract infections (UTIs) and, 715
mastitis and, 794, 795
otitis externa (swimmer's ear) and, 334, 335
pharyngitis and tonsillitis and, 393
pneumonia and, 442
prostatitis and, 840
pyelonephritis and, 721
red eye/conjunctivitis and, 281
rhinitis and, 351
rhinosinusitis and, 366, 371
as sexually transmitted infection (STI), 866
valvular disorders and murmurs and, 588
Staphylococcal scalded skin syndrome (SSSS), 191, 192t
Staphylococcus saprophyticus, 715
Statins, 546
ST-elevation MI. *See* Acute coronary syndrome (ACS)
Stellate or flap laceration, 1335
Stem cell injections for osteoarthritis (OA), 965–966
Stenosing tenosynovitis of the flexor tendons, 944–945
Stereotypic movement disorder, 1201b
Sterilization, 770
Steroids, 88
Stetler Model, 58
Stills murmu, 588
Stimulants, 1217–1218
poisoning, 1377t

Stimulus control therapy, 1316t
Stinging caterpillars, 1348, 1351, 1354
Stings. See Arthropod bites and stings
Stomatitis and glossitis, 382–383
    diagnosis of, 385–387
    epidemiology and causes of, 383
    follow-up and referral for, 389
    management of, 387–389, 388b
    pathophysiology of, 383–384
    patient education on, 389
Stopping Elderly Accidents, Deaths and Injuries (STEADI), 1462
Straight-leg-raise test, 897
Strains and sprains, 884–889, 888t
    ankle, 886–887, 888t, 953
    cervical muscle strain, 910–913
Streptococcus pneumoniae, 441
Streptococcus pyogenes, group A
    laryngitis and, 433
    otitis externa (swimmer's ear) and, 335
    pharyngitis and tonsillitis and, 397
Streptococcus spp.
    acute otitis media (AOM) and, 342
    bursitis and, 936
    cellulitis and, 199
    impetigo and, 190–191
    mastitis and, 795
    pharyngitis and, 305
    pharyngitis and tonsillitis and, 393
    pneumonia and, 440, 441
    prostatitis and, 840
    rhinitis and, 351
    rhinosinusitis and, 366, 371
Streptococcus viridans, 588
Stress
    adverse childhood experiences (ACEs) and, e1551–e1552
    brain changes in response to counseling and, e1552
    COVID-19 and, e1551
    toxic, e1552
Stress fractures, 891
Stress incontinence, 708t, 710
Stress inoculation therapy (SIT), 1289
Stroke. See Cerebrovascular accident (CVA)
Structured Clinical Interview for DSM Disorders, DSM-5 (SCID-5-SV), 1254t
Struma ovarii, 985, 985t
Strychnine poisoning, 1379t
Stye. See Hordeolum and chalazion
Subacute thyroiditis, 985, 985t, 986
Subarachnoid hemorrhage (SAH), 118
Subclinical hyperthyroidism. See Hyperthyroidism
Subclinical hypothyroidism. See Hypothyroidism
Subdural hematomas, 81, 85, 118, 1365
Substance Abuse and Mental Health Services Administration (SAMHSA), 1250
Substance use disorders (SUDs), 1181–1182, 1188b, 1256t, 1296
    in adolescents, 1402–1403
    clinical presentation of, 1213–1218, 1215t
    diagnosis of, 1182, 1218
    epidemiology and causes of, 1210–1211, 1212b
    follow-up and referral for, 1220–1221
    management of, 1218–1220, 1219b
    in older adults, 1460
    pathophysiology of, 1212–1213
    patient education on, 1221–1222
    screening tools for, 1175t
    types of, 1209–1210, 1210b
    in veterans, 1431–1432
Subungual candida, 173, 174
Sudden cardiac death (SCD) and sports physicals, 1410
Sudeck atrophy, 892
Suffering, e1493–e1494

Suicide, 1175t, 1264–1269
    assessment for, 1250
    bipolar and related disorders (BD) and, 1254
    clinical presentation of risk of, 1266
    diagnosis of risk factors for, 1266–1267
    epidemiology and causes of, 1265–1266
    follow-up and referral for, 1268–1269
    management for preventing, 1267–1268, 1268t
    pathophysiology of, 1266
    patient education on, 1269
    by veterans, 1265, 1431
Sulfonamides for lower urinary tract infections (UTIs), 717
Sunburns, 1363b
Sun poisoning, 1356
Superficial burns, 1357, 1360
Superficial folliculitis, 195
Superficial partial-thickness burns, 1357, 1360–1361
Suppurative OM. See Otitis media (OM)
Supraventricular tachycardia (SVT), 575–576, 582, 584–585
Surgical treatments
    acne vulgaris, 248
    actinic keratosis, 255–256
    benign prostatic hyperplasia (BPH), 838–839
    bowel obstruction, 661
    breast cancer, 804
    cataracts, 290
    cauda equina syndrome (CES), 930
    cervical cancer, 824
    for chronic obstructive pulmonary disease (COPD), 483–484
    chronic pancreatitis, 687
    colorectal cancer, 675–676
    diverticular disease, 664
    endometrial cancer, 827
    epididymitis, 855–856
    gender-affirming, 1419
    glaucoma, 293–294
    herniated lumbar disc (herniated nucleus pulposus), 925–926
    hydrocele, 858–859
    hyperthyroidism, 992
    laser-assisted *in situ* keratomileusis (LASIK), 287
    lung cancer, 504–505
    malignant melanoma, 260
    myomectomy, 819
    nephrolithiasis, 726–727, 727t
    nonmelanomatous skin cancers, 263
    obesity, 1053
    osteoarthritis (OA), 966
    ovarian cancer, 829–830
    pancreatic cancer, 689
    pancreatic or extrapancreatic tumors, 1045
    penile revascularization, 853
    for pharyngitis and tonsillitis, 397
    prostate cancer, 846
    pyelonephritis, 723
    rosacea, 250
    seborrheic keratosis, 253
    septoplasty, 363
    for sleep apnea, 429–430
    testicular cancer, 862
    testicular torsion, 857
    thyroidectomy, 1005
    varicocele, 860
    warts, 207–208
Suturing, 1340–1342, 1344–1345
Swimmer's ear. See Otitis externa (swimmer's ear)
Syncope, 524
    sports physicals and, 1411
Synthetic L-thyroxine, 1000
Syphilis. See *Treponema pallidum*
Systemic disorders, dizziness and vertigo due to disorders of, 77

Systemic granulomatous vasculitis, 487–488b
Systemic lupus erythematosus (SLE), 487b
    clinical presentation of, 1134–1135
    diagnosis of, 1135–1136, 1136f
    epidemiology and causes of, 1132–1133
    follow-up and referral for, 1138
    management of, 1136–1138
    pathophysiology of, 1133–1134
    patient education on, 1138
Systemic therapy
    acne vulgaris, 244, 246–247
    for asthma, 473
    breast cancer, 806
    candida and tinea infections, 174–175
    glaucoma, 294
    impetigo, 193
    onychomycosis, 189
    pediculosis, 169, 170
    psoriasis, 236–237
    rosacea, 250
    scabies, 165, 166
Systolic dysfunction, 566

T

Tanning beds, 1404
Tardive dyskinesia, 1234t
Tattoos
    adolescents and, 1403–1404
    human trafficking and, 1330
Technology
    artificial intelligence (AI), 53–54
    electronic medical record (EMR), 52–53, 53b
    precision health care and, 54
    telehealth, 53
Telehealth, 52–53
Teleology, e1515
Temporal arteritis, 81
Temporomandibular disorders (TMDs)
    clinical presentation of, 407–408
    diagnosis of, 408
    epidemiology and causes of, 407
    follow-up and referral for, 411
    management of, 408–410, 410f
    pathophysiology of, 407, 407f
    patient education on, 411
Temporomandibular joint (TMJ) disease, 407
Tendinitis/tenosynovitis
    clinical presentation of, 938–939
    diagnosis of, 939
    epidemiology and causes of, 937–938, 937t
    follow-up and referral for, 940
    management of, 939–940
    pathophysiology of, 938
    patient education on, 940
Tendon injuries, 1336
    of the hand, 945, 945f
Tension pneumothorax, 1370, 1371b
Tension-type headache, 79–80, 79t
    chronic, 82
    clinical presentation of, 83–85, 84f
Tertiary prevention, 28, 28t
Testicular cancer
    clinical presentation of, 861
    diagnosis of, 861–862
    epidemiology and causes of, 860–861
    follow-up and referral for, 864–865
    management of, 862–864, 863–864t
    pathophysiology of, 861
    patient education on, 865
Testicular pain, 755–756
Testicular torsion
    clinical presentation of, 856–857
    diagnosis of, 857
    epidemiology and causes of, 856

follow-up and referral for, 857
management of, 857
pathophysiology of, 856
patient education on, 857
Test of Functional Health Literacy in Adults, 29
Testosterone deficiency, 756
Tests
diagnostic, 46–47, 46t
screening, 26, 26b, 47
Tetanus immunization after animal and human bites, 1345
Thalamus, 82
Thalassemia, 1068–1069, 1071–1072, 1073, 1074
Therapeutic touch (TT), e1562
Thiazolidinediones, 1035, 1036
Third-degree burns, 1358
Third-party payer rules, e1531–e1536
Thirst, excessive, 983–984, 983f
Thoracic outlet syndrome, 894
Three-pillow orthopnea, 526
Thrombosis, 117
Thrush, 173
Thunderclap headache, 81
Thyroid cancer, 378, 985, 985t
clinical presentation of, 1004
diagnosis of, 1004–1005
epidemiology and causes of, 1003
follow-up and referral for, 1005
management of, 1005
pathophysiology of, 1003–1004
patient education on, 1005
Thyroid gland
cancer of, 378, 985, 985t, 1003–1005
hyperthyroidism, 984–993, 985t, 987t, 989t
hypothyroidism, 993–1002, 994t, 997t, 1001b
increased neck size and, 982–983
weight loss and, 1309
Thyrotoxicosis, 984, 985, 985t
Tic disorders, 1296
clinical presentation of, 1201–1202, 1202b
diagnosis of, 1202–1203, 1202b
epidemiology and causes of, 1201
follow-up and referral for, 1204
management of, 1203–1204
pathophysiology of, 1201, 1202t
patient education on, 1204
Tic douloureux. *See* Trigeminal neuralgia
Tick bites, 1347–1348, 1350, 1354
Tilt-table testing, 583
Tinea capitis, 181, 182, 184–185
Tinea corporis, 181, 182, 185
Tinea cruris, 181, 182, 185
Tinea manuum, 185
Tinea pedis, 182–183, 185
Tinea unguium. *See* Onychomycosis
Tinea versicolor, 182, 183, 185
Tinel's sign, 901
Tinnitus, 304, 316–317
clinical presentation of, 317–318, 318b
diagnosis of, 318–319
epidemiology and causes of, 317
follow-up and referral for, 320
management of, 319–320, 319b
pathophysiology of, 317
patient education on, 320
Tissue hypoxia, confusion due to, 76
TMJ myofascial pain syndrome. *See* Temporomandibular disorders (TMDs)
TNM system, 259, 259b
Tobacco use. *See* Smoking addiction
Tonic-clonic seizures, 95
Tonic seizures, 95
Tonsillitis. *See* Pharyngitis and tonsillitis
Topical therapy
acne vulgaris, 243–244, 245–246, 245b
actinic keratosis, 255

candida and tinea infections, 176–177
nonmelanomatous skin cancers, 263
onychomycosis, 188–189
pediculosis, 169, 170
psoriasis, 234–236
rosacea, 250
scabies, 165, 166
Topiramate, 100
Torus planus, 386
Toxic and environmental exposures
frostbite, 1388–1389
heat-related illnesses, 1382–1386, 1383t
hypothermia, 1386–1388
poisoning, 1375–1382
veterans and, 1427–1428, 1427–1428t
Toxic multinodular goiter, 985, 985t, 986
Toxic reactions to arthropod bites and stings, 1348–1349
Toxic shock syndrome (TSS), 158
Toxic stress, e1552
Toxoplasma gondii, 1141
acquired immunodeficiency syndrome (AIDS) and, 1166, 1168, 1171
bipolar and related disorders (BD) and, 1251
Tramadol, 1479
Transcranial direct current stimulation (tDCS), 1280
Transcranial magnetic stimulation (TMS), 1280
Transcutaneous electrical nerve stimulation (TENS), 1481
Transdermal contraceptive patch, 766–767
Transdermal nicotine patch, 517, 518
Transesophageal echocardiography (TEE), 583
Transgender persons, 1417–1423. *See also* LGBTQ+ population
assessment of, 1417–1419, 1418b
gender-affirming treatments, 1419
gender-appropriate care for, 1421–1422
introduction to, 1417–1417, 1417t
prevalence and demographics of, 1417
sports physicals for, 1411
Transient ischemic attack (TIA), 116–117. *See also* Cerebrovascular accident (CVA)
clinical presentation of, 119–120
headache and, 81
paresthesia and paresis with, 90
Trauma, head. *See* Head trauma/traumatic brain injury (TBI)
Trauma- and stressor-related disorders, 1177. *See also* Post-traumatic stress disorder (PTSD)
Trauma-focused psychotherapy, 1288
Trauma-informed approach to human trafficking victims, 1329
Trauma Screening Questionnaire (TSQ), 1287
Traumatic brain injury. *See* Head trauma/traumatic brain injury (TBI)
Traumatic ulcer, oral, 387
Treatment
documentation of, 50–52
reduction of medical errors in, 52
Tremors, 90, 92–93, 92f
Treponema pallidum
Ménière's disease and, 328
pharyngitis and tonsillitis and, 393
as sexually transmitted infection (STI), 866, 869t
stomatitis and glossitis and, 385–386
Trichomonas vaginalis, 840, 866, 869t
Trichophyton. See Dermatophytoses
Trichotillomania disorder, 1296
Tricyclic antidepressants (TCAs)
attention deficit-hyperactivity disorder (ADHD) and, 1192
eating disorders and, 1310
major depressive disorder (MDD) and, 1243–1244, 1247–1248

for neuropathic pain, 1477
obsessive-compulsive disorder (OCD) and, 1298
panic disorder and, 1283
poisoning, 1378t
temporomandibular disorders (TMDs) and, 409
urinary incontinence (UI) and, 711
Trigeminal nerve, 81, 82f
Trigeminal neuralgia
clinical presentation of, 134–135
diagnosis of, 135
epidemiology and causes of, 134
follow-up and referral for, 135
management of, 135
pathophysiology of, 134
patient education on, 135
Trigger finger, 944–945
Triptans, 87
Trousseau's sign, 979
Tuberculosis (TB)
clinical presentation of, 454, 455t
diagnosis of, 455–458, 456b, 456t
epidemiology and causes of, 452–453
follow-up and referral for, 461–463, 462–463t
management of, 458–461, 460b
pathophysiology of, 453–454
patient education on, 463–464
Tumor necrosis factor (TNF)-alpha blockers, 1122
Tumor-node-metastasis (TNM) stage grouping
bladder tumors, 746, 746t
breast cancer, 803t
colorectal cancer, 673–674, 674t
lung cancer, 500, 501–502t
prostate cancer, 845
testicular cancer, 862–864, 863–864t
Tumors
bladder, 744–747, 746t
bone, 950–951
renal, 742–744, 743f
Turmeric, 222
2-octylcyanoacrylate, 1338–1339
Type I (Mobitz I) block, 579f
Type II (Mobitz II) block, 579f

U

Ulcerative colitis (UC). *See* Inflammatory bowel disease (IBD)
Umbilical hernias, 651
Unequal Treatment: Confronting Racial and Ethnic Disparities in Health Care, 1482
Unipolar episodes, 1257b
Unstable angina. *See* Acute coronary syndrome (ACS)
Upper respiratory infections (URIs), 431–432
clinical presentation of, 433–434
diagnosis of, 434
epidemiology and causes of, 432, 432b
follow-up and referral for, 435
management of, 434–435
pathophysiology of, 433
patient education on, 435–436
Upper urinary tract infection (UTI). *See* Pyelonephritis
Ureaplasma
lower urinary tract infections (UTIs) and, 715
prostatitis and, 840
pyelonephritis and, 721–722
Urge incontinence, 708t, 710
Urinary complaints
dysuria, 701
hematuria, 701–704
lower urinary tract infections (UTIs), 714–721
nephrolithiasis, 724–728, 725t, 726t, 727t
polyuria, 983–984, 983f
proteinuria, 704–705, 705t
pyelonephritis, 721–723

Urinary incontinence (UI)
  clinical presentation of, 708–709
  diagnosis of, 709–710
  epidemiology and causes of, 706, 708t
  follow-up and referral for, 713–714
  management of, 710–713, 713b
  pathophysiology of, 706–707, 707f
  patient education on, 714
Urinary tract infections (UTIs), lower
  clincal presentation of, 715–716
  diagnosis of, 716
  epidemiology and causes of, 714
  follow-up and referral for, 720–721
  management of, 716–720
  pathophysiology of, 715
  patient education on, 721
Urinary tract infections (UTIs), upper
  clinical presentation of, 722
  diagnosis of, 722–723
  epidemiology and causes of, 721
  follow-up and referral for, 723
  management of, 723
  pathophysiology of, 721–722
  patient education on, 723
Urine ketone testing, 1025
Urticaria
  differential diagnosis of, 158–159
  management of, 159–161, 160f
Urticarial plaques, 1104
U.S. Department of Veterans Affairs (VA) Final Rule, e1527
U.S. Preventive Services Task Force (USPSTF), 31–32, 36, 59
  guidelines on screening tests, 47
Uterine cancer, 750–751
Uterine fibroids. See Leiomyomas (uterine fibroids)

V

Vaccine Adverse Event Reporting System, 32
Vaccines. See Immunizations
Vacuum constriction devices, 853
Vaginal, uterine, and ovarian disorders. See also Reproductive issues
  amenorrhea, 809–811
  dysmenorrhea, 812–814
  endometrial cancer, 824–827
  endometriosis, 814–817
  foreign body obstruction, 1372, 1374
  leiomyomas (uterine fibroids), 817–819
  ovarian cancer, 827–830
  precancerous lesions and cancer of the cervix, 819–824, 822t, 824b
  vulvodynia, 830–832
Vaginal candidiasis, 173
Vaginal contraceptive sponge, 769
Vaginectomy, 1419
Vaginoplasty, 1419
Valproic acid, 100
Value-based health care, e1530–e1550
  Affordable Care Act and, e1536–e1540, e1536t
  billing and coding rules and, e1540–e1544, e1542b
  COVID-19 impact on reimbursement for third-party payers and, e1534
  development of, e1539–e1540
  Health Insurance Portability and Accountability Act (HIPAA) and, e1546
  introduction to, e1530–e1531
  Medicare Access and CHIP Reauthorization Act (MACRA) and, 52, e1538–e1539
  Medicare for All proposal, e1539
  nurse practitioners' role in, e1539–e1540
  provider comparison web sites, e1547
  quality metrics-inpatient services, e1545
  quality metrics-physician services, e1541t, e1545–e1546, e1546t
  risk management, compliance planning, and performance improvements in, e1546–e1547
  third-party payer rules and, e1531–e1536
Valvular disorders and murmurs
  clinical presentation of, 588–589
  diagnosis of, 589–591
  epidemiology and causes of, 588
  follow-up and referral for, 592
  management of, 591–592
  pathophysiology of, 588
  patient education on, 592–593
  types of, 586–588, 587t
Vaping, 510. See also Smoking addiction
Variant angina. See Acute coronary syndrome (ACS)
Varicocele
  clinical presentation of, 859
  diagnosis of, 859–860
  epidemiology and causes of, 859
  follow-up and referral for, 860
  management of, 860
  pathophysiology of, 859
  patient education on, 860
Vascular endothelial growth factor (VEGF)-receptor fusion protein, 299
Vascular system disorders
  deep vein thrombosis (DVT)/chronic venous insufficiency, 596–600
  peripheral artery disease (PAD), 594–596
Vasoactive therapy for erectile dysfunction (ED), 852, 853
Vasodilators, 540
Ventricular arrhythmias, 576
  epidemiology and causes of, 577, 578f
  pathophysiology of, 581
Ventricular tachycardia (VT), 582
Veracity, e1516b, e1517
Verruca vulgaris. See Warts
Vertebral fracture
  clinical presentation of, 931–932
  diagnosis of, 932
  epidemiology and causes of, 931
  follow-up and referral for, 933
  management of, 932–933
  pathophysiology of, 931
  patient education on, 933
Vertigo, 76–77, 78f
Vestibular disorders, 320–321, 321f
Vestibular neuritis (VN) and labyrinthitis
  clinical presentation of, 330–331
  diagnosis of, 331
  epidemiology and causes of, 330
  follow-up and referral for, 332
  management of, 331
  pathophysiology of, 330
  patient education on, 332
Vestibulo-ocular reflex (VOR), 331
Veterans, 1424–1436, e1535
  blast injuries and traumatic brain injury in, 1430
  exposure to risks for illness and injury in, 1427–1428t, 1427–1430
  families of, 1425, 1427
  female, 1435
  hepatitis C and HIV in, 1429
  infectious diseases and blood-borne pathogens in, 1428–1429, 1429t
  introduction to, 1424
  LGBTQI, 1435–1436
  mental health needs of, 1430–1436, 1432t, 1433b
  military separation and, 1425
  military sexual trauma (MST) in, 1432–1434, 1432t, 1433b
  musculoskeletal disorders in, 1434–1435
  noise-induced hearing loss in, 1429–1430
  non-VA health-care providers and, 1424–1425, 1424–1425t
  post-traumatic stress disorder (PTSD) in, 1430
  substance-use disorder in, 1431–1432
  suicide by, 1265, 1431 (See also Post-traumatic stress disorder (PTSD))
  traumatic brain injury (TBI) in, 1431
Veterans Health Administration (VHA) system, 1424
Vibrio spp., 199
  gastroenteritis and, 622t
Viral meningitis, 126–127, 126t
Viral pneumonia, 442
Viral skin infections
  hepatitis B and C from animal and human bites, 1345–1346
  herpes simplex infections, 210–214, 210t, 214b
  warts, 205–209, 208t, 209b
Virchow's triad, 596–598
Visceral pain, 603
Viscosupplementation, 964–965
Visual analog scale (VAS), 1474
Visual disturbances and impaired vision, 269
  cataracts, 286t, 288–290
  diabetic retinopathy, 286t, 295–296
  glaucoma, 286t, 291–295
  macular degeneration, 286t, 296–300
  refractive errors, 285–288, 286t
Vital signs in sports physicals, 1411
Vitamins
  for headache, 89
  vitamin B_{12} deficiency and macrocytic anemia, 1080
  vitamin D and osteoporosis, 971–972
Vitiligo, 151–152
Vocal cords. See Dysphonia
Vomiting. See Nausea and vomiting
Von Willebrand disease, 1410
Vulvodynia
  clinical presentation of, 831
  diagnosis of, 831
  epidemiology and causes of, 830–831
  follow-up and referral for, 831–832
  pathophysiology of, 831
  patient education on, 832
Vulvovaginitis, 756–759

W

Wald, Lillian, 9
Warfarin, 586t
Warts
  clinical presentation of, 206
  diagnosis of, 206
  epidemiology and causes of, 205
  follow-up and referral for, 208–209
  management of, 206–208, 208t
  pathophysiology of, 205
  patient education on, 209, 209b
Wasps and bees, 1347, 1350, 1353
Wear and tear arthritis. See Osteoarthritis (OA)
Weber test, 313
Wegener's granulomatosis, 487b
Whiplash, 896
White blood cells (WBCs), 126, 127
  in inflammatory phase of wounds, 1333
"White coat" hypertension, 531–532
Wilson's disease, 110, 690b, 691, 697–698
Wolff-Chaikoff effect, 986
Wolff-Parkinson-White (WPW) syndrome, 580, 580f
Wong-Baker Faces Pain Rating Scale, 1474
Wood's lamp examination, 278
Workers' compensation, e1535

World Health Organization (WHO)
  on anemia, 1066
  on antivenoms, 1345
  on cataracts, 288
  Decade of Health Ageing, 1453
  definition of health, 25
  on depression, 1241
  designation of 2020 as "Year of the Nurse and Midwife," 1513
  Guidelines on Integrated Care for Older People, 1454
  on hearing loss, 309
  on herpes simplex virus infections, 210
  on HIV, 1147
  on influenza, 433
  in interprofessional collaborative practice (IPCP), 19
  on intimate partner violence, 1182–1183
  on nonoxynol-9 use with condoms, 768
  on obesity, 1047, 1048
  on osteoporosis, 970
  on pancreatogenic diabetes, 1039
  on scabies, 163
  on schizophrenia, 1226
  on self-care, e1558
  on sexual health in menopause, 788
  on sexually transmitted infections, 872
  on sunburn prevention, 1363
  on tobacco use, 508
Wound-closure strips, 1341
Wounds and lacerations, 1333–1342
  burn, 1357
  clinical presentation of, 1334–1337
  diagnosis of, 1337–1339
  epidemiology and causes of, 1333
  evidence-based nursing practice, 1337
  follow-up and referral for, 1339, 1341–1342
  management of, 1338–1341
  pathophysiology of, 1333–1334
  patient education on, 1342, 1342b
Wrist. *See* Hand and wrist disorders
Written narrative exposure, 1289

X
Xerosis, 154
X-rays
  animal and human bites, 1344
  of wounds and lacerations, 1338

Y
Yale-Brown Obsessive Compulsive Scale (BDD-YBOCS), 1300
Yale-Brown Obsessive-Compulsive Scale (Y-BOCS), 1295
Yale-Brown Obsessive Compulsive Scale – Second Edition, 1295
Yersinia enterocolitica, 623t
Young Mania Rating Scale (YMRS), 1254t
Youth Anxiety Measure for *DSM-5* (YAM-5), 1275

Z
Ziprasidone, 1232
Zonisamide, 100
Zung Self Rating Anxiety Scale, 1275